Jeanne Duus Johansen · Peter J. Frosch
Jean-Pierre Lepoittevin
Editors

Contact Dermatitis

Fifth Edition

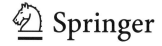 Springer

Prof. Jeanne Duus Johansen
Copenhagen University Hospital Gentofte
National Allergy Research Centre
Department of Dermato-allergology
Niels Andersens Vej 65
2900 Hellerup
Denmark
jedu@geh.regionh.dk

Prof. Dr. Peter J. Frosch
Hautklinik
Klinikum Dortmund gGmbH
Beurhausstr. 40
44137 Dortmund
Germany
peter.frosch@klinikumdo.de

Prof. Jean-Pierre Lepoittevin
Institut le Bel, Labo. Dermatochimie
4, rue Blaise Pascal
67070 Strasbourg cedex
France
jplepoit@unistra.fr

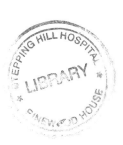

ISBN: 978-3-642-03826-6   e-ISBN: 978-3-642-03827-3

DOI: 10.1007/978-3-642-03827-3

Springer Heidelberg Dordrecht London New York

Library of Congress Control Number: 2010923774

Cover design: eStudio Calamar, Figueres/Berlin

Printed on acid-free paper

Springer is part of Springer Science+Business Media (www.springer.com)

Contact Dermatitis

Fifth Edition

To Kelly for her continuous support of my scientific activities.

Peter J. Frosch

Preface to the Fifth Edition

This is the fifth edition of the book since 1992. A lot of changes have been made over the years, but the biggest transformation came with the fourth edition in 2005: many new chapters, easy overview, and core messages providing all the clinical photos and diagrams. All these advantages have been retained for the fifth edition, where an extensive update of chapters has been made including new versions and authors for several topics.

Contact dermatitis is one of the major problems in occupational skin diseases. This is reflected in the book, where new chapters on occupational contact dermatitis have been written: a general chapter, which gives an overview of the subject, provides clear definitions and gives valuable guidance for the investigation of patients suspected of occupational contact dermatitis; followed by specific chapters on three high-risk professions.

The popular dictionary of contact allergens and lists of patch test concentrations have been expanded and provide the tool for evidence-based investigation and information of patients with contact dermatitis.

Contact dermatitis is a frequent, disabling and expensive disease. This brings both primary and secondary prevention in focus of research. A solid basis has already been established for intervention on a personal, organizational and regulatory level. The significant level of knowledge in these areas is summarised in three new chapters, which also cover therapy, a previous somewhat neglected subject in the book. Other chapters on different aspects of prevention have gone through a significant updation and revision. Basic understanding of pathophysiology within the fields of genes, skin barrier and chemistry has taken a leap forward and these new developments are reflected in new and former chapters of the book.

With this edition, Torkil Menné has resigned from the editorial group. Torkil Menné was one of the initiators of this textbook and has been part of the editorial board since then. The editors would like to express their sincere thanks to Torkil Menné for his invaluable contributions to the book and to the field of contact dermatitis over many years.

The fourth edition was a great success, and even though it seemed an impossible task to surpass it, we think we have done so with the fifth edition. This has, of course, only been possible with the help of the many great contributors and the editors are very grateful to each and every one of them.

Last but not the least, we would like to thank Springer-Verlag for their excellent support to this project.

Hellerup, Denmark   Jeanne Duus Johansen
Dortmund, Germany   Peter J. Frosch
Strasbourg, France   Jean-Pierre Lepoittevin

Contents

Contents

J.-M. Lachapelle
Department of Dermatology, Catholic University of Louvain, 30, Clos Chapelle-aux-Champs, UCL 3033, 1200 Brussels, Belgium
e-mail: lachapelle@uclouvain.be

1.1 Introduction

Contact dermatitis, an inflammatory skin reaction to direct contact with noxious agents in the environment, was most probably recognized as an entity even in ancient times, since it must have accompanied mankind throughout history. Early recorded reports include Pliny the Younger who, in the first century A.D., noticed that some individuals experienced severe itching when cutting pine trees. A review of the ancient literature could provide dozens of similar, mostly anecdotal, examples, and some are cited in modern textbooks, monographs, and papers.

It is interesting to note that the presence of idiosyncrasy was suspected in some cases of contact dermatitis reported in the nineteenth century, many decades before the discovery of allergy by von Pirquet. For instance, in 1829, Dakin, describing *Rhus* dermatitis, observed that some people suffered from the disease, whereas others did not. He therefore posed the question: "Can it be possible that some peculiar structure of the cuticule or rete mucosum constitutes the idiosyncrasy?"

The history of contact dermatitis in the twentieth century is indistinguishable from the history of patch testing, which is considered the main tool for unmasking the causative chemical culprits. Nevertheless, starting in the early 1980s, additional tests (within the scope of patch testing) have been introduced, such as the open test, the semi-open test, the repeated open application test (ROAT) and its variants, referred to as "use tests." Moreover, prick testing, which has been underestimated for decades in dermato-allergology, has gained popularity, as an investigatory tool for immediate contact hypersensitivity.

J.D. Johansen et al. (eds.), *Contact Dermatitis*,
DOI: 10.1007/978-3-642-03827-3_1, © Springer-Verlag Berlin Heidelberg 2011

1

Core Message

> Historical aspects of contact dermatitis are indistinguishable from those of patch testing and prick testing.

1.2 Historical Aspects of Patch Testing

Historical aspects of patch testing are reviewed by Foussereau [1] and Lachapelle [2]. A selection of important forward steps has been made for this short survey.

1.2.1 The Pre-Jadassohn Period

During the seventeenth, eighteenth, and nineteenth centuries [1], some researchers occasionally reproduced contact dermatitis by applying the responsible agent (chemical, plant, etc.) to intact skin. Most of the observations are anecdotal, but some deserve special attention.

In 1847, Städeler [3] described a method devised to reproduce the lesions provoked by *Anacardium occidentale* (Städeler's blotting paper strip technique) on human skin, which can be summarized as follows: "Balsam is applied to the lower part of the thorax on an area measuring about 1 cm². Then, a piece of blotting paper previously dipped in the balsam is applied to the same site. Fifteen minutes later, the subject experiences a burning sensation, which increases very rapidly and culminates after about half an hour. The skin under the blotting paper turns whitish and is surrounded by a red halo. As the burning sensation decreases, the blotting paper is kept in place for 3 h." This observation is important because it was the first time that any test was actually designed and described in full detail [1].

In 1884, Neisser [4] reviewed a series of eight cases of iodoform dermatitis triggered by a specific influence. Neisser wrote that it was a matter of idiosyncrasy, dermatitis being elicited in these cases by iodoform application. The symptoms were similar to those subsequent to the application of mercurial derivatives, and a spread of the lesions that was much wider

than the application site was a common feature to both instances.

In retrospect, this presentation can be considered an important link between casuistical writings of older times and a more scientifically orientated approach of skin reactions provoked by contactants. It was a half-hidden event that heralded a new era, which blossomed at the end of the nineteenth century.

Core Message

> The first experimental – clinically orientated – attempts to relate contact dermatitis to a causative agent were made during the nineteenth century, both anecdotal and unscheduled.

1.2.2 Josef Jadassohn, the Father of Patch Testing in Dermatology

Josef Jadassohn (Fig. 1.1) is universally acknowledged as the father of patch testing ("*Funktionelle Hautprüfung*"), a new diagnostic tool offered to dermatologists [5]. At the time of his discovery, Jadassohn was a young Professor of Dermatology at Breslau University (Germany); he most probably applied and expanded – in a practical way

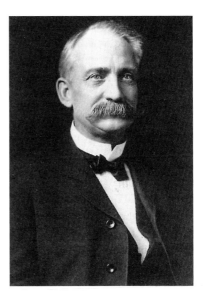

Fig. 1.1 Josef Jadassohn (1863–1936) (used with kind permission from the Institut für Geschichte der Medizin der Universität Wien)

– the observations and interpretations previously made by his teacher Neisser [4]. Summing up the different sources of information available, we can reasonably assume that: (1) the birthday and birthplace of the patch test is Monday, 23 September 1895 at the Fünfter Congress der Deutschen Dermatologischen Gesellschaft held in Graz (Austria), where Jadassohn made his oral presentation "*Zur Kenntnis der medicamentösen Dermatosen*"; (2); the birth certificate is dated 1896, when the proceedings of the meeting were published [6].

As recorded by Sulzberger in 1940 in his classic textbook [7], the key message of Jadassohn's paper was the fact that he recognized the process of delayed hypersensitivity to simple chemicals:

1. In his original publication, Jadassohn describes the following two occurrences: A syphilitic patient received an injection of a mercurial preparation and developed a mercurial dermatitis which involved all parts of the skin except a small, sharply demarcated area. It was found that the spared area was the site previously occupied by a mercury plaster which had been applied in the treatment of a boil.
2. In a second observation, a patient who had received an injection of a mercurial preparation developed an acute eczematous dermatitis which was confined to the exact sites to which gray ointment (Hg) had been previously applied in the treatment of pediculosis pubis. In this patient, the subsequent application of a patch test (Funktionelle Hautprüfung) with gray ointment to unaffected skin sites produced an eczematous reaction consisting of a severe erythematous and bullous dermatitis.

When put together, those two observations reflect a double-winged discovery: the local elicitation of a mercury reaction and the local elicitation of refractoriness to reaction.

Concerning the technical aspects of the "*Funktionelle Hautprüfung*," the methodology was quite simple: gray mercury ointment was applied on the skin of the upper extensor part of the left arm and covered by a 5-cm^2 piece of tape for 24 h. Many comments can be made at this point: (1) from the beginning, the patch test appears as a "closed" or occlusive testing technique, (2) the size of the patch test material is large

(2.3–2.3 cm) compared to the current available materials, (3) the amount of ointment applied is not mentioned (the technique is therefore considered as qualitative), and (4) the duration of the application is limited in the present case to 24 h.

It should be remembered that soon after developing the patch test, Jadassohn was appointed as the Professor of Dermatology (1896) at the University of Bern (Switzerland) where he stayed for several years, before coming back (in 1917) to his native Silesia, in Breslau again. One of his major accomplishments there was the observation of a specific anergy in patients suffering from sarcoidosis or Hodgkin's disease, for example.

> **Core Message**
>
> › A careful analysis of the historical literature clearly indicates that Josef Jadassohn is the initiator of aimed patch testing in dermatology.

1.2.3 Jean-Henri Fabre's Experiments

Another description of a patch test technique was given by the French entomologist Jean-Henri Fabre (1823–1915), who lived in Sérignan-du-Comtat, a village in Provence (Fig. 1.2). This work was

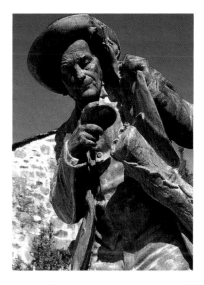

Fig. 1.2 Jean-Henri Fabre, French entomologist (1823–1915)

contemporaneous with Jadassohn's experiments, but it is described here because it was not designed primarily for dermatological diagnosis [8]. Fabre reported in 1897 (in the sixth volume of the impressive encyclopedia *Souvenirs entomologiques*, translated into more than 20 languages) that he had studied the effect of processionary caterpillars on his own skin. A square of blotting paper, a novel kind of plaster, was covered by a rubber sheet and held in place with a bandage. The paper used was a piece of blotting paper folded 4 times, so as to form a square with 1-in. sides, which had previously been dipped into an extract of caterpillar hair. The impregnated paper was applied to the volar aspect of the forearm. The next day, 24 h later, the plaster was removed. A red mark, slightly swollen and very clearly outlined, occupied the area that had been covered by the "poisoned" paper.

In these and further experiments, he dissected various anatomical parts of the caterpillars in order to isolate noxious ones (barbed hairs) that provoked burning or itching. Rostenberg and Solomon [9] have emphasized the importance of Fabre's methodology to dermatology, so often used in the past decades by dermato-allergologists. For instance, many similar attempts were made during the twentieth century to isolate noxious agents (contact allergens and irritants), not only from different parts of plants, woods, and animals, but also from various other naturally occurring substances and industrial products encountered in our modern environment.

In my view, Fabre's experiments are gratifying for an additional reason: they reproduce another common skin reaction of exogenous origin, contact urticaria [10]. It is well known today that a protein, thaumetopoietin (molecular weight 28 kDa), is responsible for the urticarial reaction. In an attempt to reproduce Fabre's experiments, I applied caterpillars' barbed hairs to my skin, using a plastic square chamber designed by Van der Bend as patch test material, which was kept in place for 2 h. After the removal of the patch, two types of reactions were recorded consecutively: (1) at 20 min, an urticarial reaction (considered to be nonimmunological), which faded slowly during the next 2 h, and (2) at day 2, an eczematous reaction, spreading all around the application site and interpreted as an experimentally induced immunological protein contact dermatitis.

Core Message

> Surprisingly, the first steps of patch testing were introduced – at the same time as Jadassohn's experiments – by an entomologist, Fabre, when he was working on processionary caterpillars.

1.2.4 A General Overview of Patch Testing During the Period 1895–1965

It is difficult, in retrospect, to assess the importance of the patch test technique for the diagnosis of contact dermatitis between 1895 and the 1960s. Some points are nevertheless clear: (1) the technique was used extensively in some European clinics, and ignored in others, (2) no consensus existed concerning the material, the concentration of each allergen, the time of reading, the reading score, etc., and (3) differential diagnosis between irritant and allergic contact dermatitis was very often unclear.

It is no exaggeration to say that patch testers were acting like skilled craftsmen [11], though – step by step – they provided new information on contact dermatitis.

When covering this transitional period, we should recall the names of some outstanding dermatologists who directly contributed to our present knowledge and to the dissemination of the patch test technique throughout the world.

1.2.5 Bruno Bloch's Pioneering Work in Basel and in Zurich

Bruno Bloch is considered by the international community as one of the more prominent pioneers in the field of patch testing, continuing and expanding Jadassohn's clinical and experimental work. In many textbooks or papers, patch testing is often quoted as the Jadassohn–Bloch technique.

The major contributions made by Bloch to patch testing are the following:

1. When he was in Basel, in 1911, he described [12] in detail the technique of patch testing. The allergen should be applied to a linen strip

which is put on the back, covered with a slightly larger piece of gutta-percha and fixed in place with zinc oxide adhesive plaster; the test should then be left for 24 h. The size of the patch was chosen to be 1 cm². For the first time in the history of patch testing, he graded the stages of the skin reaction from simple erythema to necrosis and ulceration, and stressed that a normal and a sensitized subject differ fundamentally in that only the latter reacts.

2. In collaboration with the chemist Paul Karrer, who first synthesized vitamin C and received the Nobel Prize in 1937, Bloch discovered and successfully synthesized primin, the specific chemical in *Primula obconica* that is responsible for allergic contact dermatitis in persons contacting the common plant [13].

3. He also conceived the concept of cross-sensitization in contact dermatitis by studying the reactivity patterns of iodoform, a commonly used topical medication at that time.

4. He described the first cases of systemic contact dermatitis, illustrated forever by moulages of the Zurich collection (moulageur: Lotte Volger).

5. The idea of developing a standard series of allergens was also developed extensively by Bruno Bloch in Zurich [14]. The substances with which standard tests were made were the following: formaldehyde (1–5%), mercury (1% sublimate or ointment of white precipitate of mercury), turpentine, naphthalene (1%), tincture of arnica, *P. obconica* (piece of the leaf), adhesive plaster, iodoform (powder), and quinine hydrochloride (1%).

As far as we can understand by consulting various sources of information, Bruno Bloch acted as a group leader for promoting and disseminating the idea of applying a limited standard series in each patient. This was made in close connection with Jadassohn in Breslau (his former teacher when he was in Bern), Blumenthal and Jaffé in Berlin, and – later on – Sulzberger in New York. In Bloch's clinic, Hans Stauffer and Werner Jadassohn worked on determining the adequate concentration and vehicle for each allergen.

> **Core Message**
>
> › Bruno Bloch's devotion to patch testing methodology at Zurich University led to its expansion and initial standardization (including standard series) throughout the world.

1.2.6 The Influence of Poul Bonnevie in Scandinavian Countries

Poul Bonnevie, a former assistant of Bruno Bloch at Zurich University, was a professor of Occupational Medicine in Copenhagen. He expanded Bloch's limited standard series of tests and published it in his famous textbook of environmental dermatology [15].

This list (Table 1.1) can be considered as the prototype of the standard series of patch tests. It was built

Table 1.1 The standard series of patch tests proposed by Poul Bonnevie [20]

Allergen	Concentration (%)	Vehicle
Turpentine	50	Olive oil
Colophony	10	Olive oil
Balsam of Peru	25	Lanolin
Salicylic acid	5	Lanolin
Formaldehyde	4	Water
Mercuric chloride	0.1	Water
Potassium dichromate	0.5	Water
Silver nitrate	2	Water
Nickel sulfate	5	Water
Resorcinol	5	Water
Primula obconica	As is	
Sodium perborate	10	Water
Brown soap	As is	
Coal tar	Pure	
Wood tars	Pure	
Quinine chlorhydrate	1	Water
Iodine	0.5	Ethanol
Pyrogallol	5	Petrolatum
p-Phenylenediamine	2	Petrolatum
Aminophenol	2	Petrolatum
Adhesive plaster	As is	

on the experience gained at the Finsen Institute in Copenhagen regarding the occurrence of positive reactions to various chemicals among patch-tested patients. It is remarkable that the list was used in Copenhagen without any change from 1938 to 1955, which allowed Marcussen to publish, in 1962 [16], a most impressive epidemiological survey concerning time fluctuations in the relative occurrence of contact allergies. Of the 21 allergens listed by Bonnevie, seven are still present in the standard series of patch tests used currently.

> **Core Message**
>
> › Poul Bonnevie is the author of the first modern textbook on occupational dermatology. The key role played by a standard series of patch tests for investigating contact dermatitis is obvious in his personal approach.

1.2.7 A Controversial Period: The Pros and Cons of a Standard Series

In the 1940s and 1950s, the standard series did not blossom throughout Europe. Some authors refused to adhere to the systematic use of a standard series in all patients and championed the concept of "selected epicutaneous tests." Two former assistants of Bruno Bloch, Hans Stauffer and Werner Jadassohn, were particularly keen on this concept of selection.

Werner Jadassohn (son of Josef), Professor of Dermatology at Geneva University, had a strong influence on many colleagues in this respect. The principle of "choice" or "selection" was based upon a careful recording of anamnestic data, especially in the field of occupational dermatology [17].

A similar view was defended in France by Foussereau; [18] this was a source of intense debates at meetings. This discussion is obsolete nowadays due to a general agreement as regards the practical interest of using standard and additional patch test series in daily practice.

1.2.8 Marion Sulzberger, the Initiator of Patch Testing in North America and Alexander Fisher, a World Leader in the Field of Contact Dermatitis

Sulzberger was one of the most brilliant assistants of Bruno Bloch in Zurich, and later of Josef Jadassohn in Breslau. In both the places, he was considered as the beloved American fellow worker. When Sulzberger came back to New York and became one of the Professors of Dermatology there, he modified considerably the spirit of the discipline, which was at that time very static in the New World.

But it is acknowledged that the "master" in the field of contact dermatitis and patch testing in the United States is Alexander Fisher, through more than 50 years of pioneering work in New York City. He has become more closely identified with this subject than any other physician in the world. He has published countless papers, describing his methodology in the search of new contact allergens, and also suggesting hypoallergenic substitutes. This proved to be a very useful and stimulating approach; when lecturing, he often recalled attention on "doing so patients are not doomed to repeated attacks." His famous book: "Contact Dermatitis," now in its sixth edition, actualized by Rietschel and Fowler [19], is an undisputed source of insight for all clinicians.

> **Core Message**
>
> › Marion Sulzberger was the initiator of patch testing in the United States. Alexander Fisher was the propagator of the technique throughout the New World. He published countless papers in the field, and, when describing new contact allergens, he suggested hypoallergenic substitutes.

1.2.9 The Founding of Groups

A Scandinavian Committee for Standardization of Routine Patch Testing was formed in 1962. In 1967, this committee was enlarged, resulting in the formation of the International Contact Dermatitis Research Group (ICDRG). The founder members of the ICDRG were Bandmann, Calnan, Cronin, Fregert, Hjorth, Magnusson, Maibach, Malten, Meneghini, Pirilä, and Wilkinson. The major task for its members was to standardize at an international level the patch testing procedure, for example, the vehicles used for allergens, the concentration of each allergen, and so on.

Niels Hjorth (1919–1990) in Copenhagen was the vigorous chairman of the ICDRG for more than 20-years. He organized the first international symposium on contact dermatitis at Gentofte, Denmark, in October 1974; this symposium was followed by many others, which led to an increasing interest in contact dermatitis throughout the world, and, consequently, to the establishment of numerous national and/or international contact dermatitis groups. Hjorth's contribution to promoting our knowledge of contact dermatitis was enormous; it is true to say that he ushered in a new era in environmental dermatology. All the contributors to this textbook are greatly indebted to him; he showed us the way forward.

Etain Cronin wrote in 1980 an extensive book entitled "Contact Dermatitis" [20], which can be compared in its spirit to Alexander Fisher's textbook.

In the meantime, in the United States, the North American Contact Dermatitis Group (NACDG) was founded, working towards similar aims. Howard Maibach acted as a constant link between both the groups.

Core Message

> The founding of groups played a great part in the development and standardization of patch testing throughout the world.

1.2.10 The Founding of the European Environmental and Contact Dermatitis Research Group (EECDRG) and the European Society of Contact Dermatitis (ESCD)

During the 1980s, an increasing interest for all facets of contact dermatitis was evident in many European countries. This led some dermatologists and basic scientists to join their efforts to improve knowledge in the field. The EECDRG was born and the first meeting initiated

by John Wilkinson, took place at Amersham, England (28 June to 1 July, 1985). Later, two meetings were organized each year. At that time, the members of the group were: Andersen, Benezra, Brandao, Bruynzeel, Burrows, Camarasa, Ducombs, Frosch, Goossens, Hannuksela, Lachapelle, Lahti, Menné, Rycroft, Scheper, Wahlberg, White, and Wilkinson. The main goal was to perform joint studies to clarify the allergenicity (and/or irritant potential) of different chemicals. Studies were planned following the principles of "newborn" evidence-based dermatology. The adventure was fruitful and many joint papers were published.

From the early days of its founding, the group felt the need to disseminate the acquired expertise to other experienced colleagues. Peter Frosch was the leader of this new policy, by organizing a Symposium in Heidelberg, Germany in May 1988, that – obviously – was a great success. This event was the starting point of the ESCD. The new society was involved in the organization of congresses, on a 2-year schedule. The first congress took place in Brussels, Belgium in 1992, under the chair of Jean-Marie Lachapelle and has been followed by nine others, so far!

Additional aims of the Society were: the publication of the *Textbook of Contact Dermatitis* (first edition in 1992) and the creation of subgroups of specialists, devoted to the study of specific research projects. The *Journal Contact Dermatitis* is the official publication of the ESCD.

1.2.11 Dermatochemistry and Contact Dermatitis

The introduction of dermatochemistry in the scope of contact dermatitis proved to be of uppermost interest. The leader in the field was Claude Benezra in Strasbourg (France). After his premature accidental death, new developments were achieved by his successor, Jean-Pierre Lepoittevin.

1.2.12 Recent Advances in the Management of Patch Testing

Recent history has forwarded some new insights to reach a better significance of patch test results, either positive or negative. First of all, in case of doubt,

1

additional tests are available, among which the ROAT, standardized by Hannuksela and Salo [21] and completed by other variants of use tests, provides a more accurate answer in some difficult cases.

In addition, efforts have been made to determine more precisely the relevance (or non relevance) of positive patch test results [22], which is the ultimate goal in dermato-allergology.

Much attention has been paid to the dose–response relationships in the elicitation of contact dermatitis, a concept that modifies our views in the matter.

A new ready-to-use patch test system, the TRUE test, was introduced in 1985 by Fischer and Maibach [23]. It represents a more sophisticated approach in the technology of patch testing, taking into account the parameter of optimal penetration and delivery of allergens through the skin. The allergens are incorporated in hydrophilic gels. The gel is adapted to each individual allergen. For protection against light and air, the strips are contained in airtight and opaque aluminum poaches.

TRUE test represents an alternative way of patch testing [24], which intends to avoid variations of the allergens applied on the skin.

1.3 Historical Aspects of Prick Testing

The historical aspects of prick testing are rather difficult to circumscribe.

Blackley [25] was probably the first to suggest that allergens could be introduced into the skin to detect sensitization. Schloss [26] used a scratch technique in the studies of food allergy between 1910 and 1920. The "codified" methodology of prick testing was described as early as 1924 by Lewis and Grant, but became widely used only after its modification by Pepys [27], almost exclusively by allergologists and pneumologists.

In dermato-allergology, it was introduced routinely in the late 1980s, in relation to expanding knowledge on contact urticaria, immediate allergy to latex proteins, and also protein contact dermatitis considered a well-defined entity.

Nowadays, it is an undisputed tool of investigation in the field of contact dermatitis.

> **Core Message**
>
> > Historically, prick testing was developed independently from patch testing; today, it is considered an important tool of investigation in contact urticaria and/or protein contact dermatitis.

References

1. Foussereau J (1984) History of epicutaneous testing: the blotting–paper and other methods. Contact Dermat 11: 219–223
2. Lachapelle JM (1996) A century of patch testing. First Jadassohn Lecture (ESCD) Jadassohn's Centenary Congress, London, 9–12 Oct 1996
3. Städeler J (1847) Über die eigenthümlichen Bestandtheile der Anacardium Früchte. Ann Chemie Pharmacie 63: 117–165
4. Neisser A (1884) Über Jodoform-Exantheme. Dtsch Med Wochenschr 10:467–468
5. Adams RM (1993) Profiles of greats in contact dermatitis. I: Josef Jadassohn (1863–1936). Am J Contact Dermat 4: 58–59
6. Jadassohn J (1896) Zur Kenntnis der medicamentösen Dermatosen. Verhandlungen der Deutschen Dermatologischen Gesellschaft, V Congress, Vienna (1895). Braumüller, Vienna, pp 103–129
7. Sulzberger MD (1940) Dermatologic allergy. Thomas, Springfield, Illinois, p 88
8. Fabre JH (1897) Souvenirs entomologiques, vol 6. Delagrave, Paris, pp 378–401
9. Rostenberg A, Solomon LM (1968) Jean Henri Fabre and the patch-test. Arch Dermatol 98:188–190
10. Lachapelle JM, Frimat P, Tennstedt D, Ducombs G (1992) Précis de Dermatologie Professionnelle et de l'Environnement. Masson, Paris
11. Sézary A (1936) Méthodes d'exploration biologique de la peau. Les tests cutanés en dermatologie. Encyclopédie médico-chirurgicale, Paris, 12010, pp 1–8
12. Bloch B (1911) Experimentelle Studien über das Wesen der Jodoformidiosynkrasie. Z Exp Pathol Ther 9:509–538
13. Bloch B, Karrer P (1927) Chemische und biologische Untersuchungen über die Primelidiosynkrasie. Beibl Vierteljahrsschr Naturforsch Gesell Zürich 72:1–25
14. Bloch B (1929) The role of idiosyncrasy and allergy in dermatology. Arch Dermatol Syphilis 19:175–197
15. Bonnevie P (1939) Aetiologie und Pathogenese der Ekzemkrankheiten. Klinische Studien über die Ursachen der Ekzeme unter besonderer Berücksichtigung des Diagnostischen Wertes der Ekzemproben. Busch, Copenhagen/Barth, Leipzig
16. Marcussen PV (1962) Variations in the incidence of contact hypersensitivities. Trans St Johns Hosp Dermatol Soc 48: 40–49
17. Jadassohn W (1951) A propos des tests épicutanés "dirigés" dans l'eczéma professionnel. Praxis 40:1–4
18. Foussereau J, Benezra C (1970) Les eczémas allergiques professionnels. Masson, Paris

19. Rietschel RL, Fowler JF Jr (2008) Fisher's contact dermatitis, 6th edn. BC Decker, Hamilton, Ontario
20. Cronin E (1980) Contact dermatitis. Churchill Livingstone, Edinburgh
21. Hannuksela M, Salo H (1986) The repeated open application test (ROAT). Contact Dermat 14:221–227
22. Lachapelle JM, Maibach HI (2009) Clinical relevance of patch test reactions, Chapter 8. In: Lachapelle JM, Maibach HI (eds) Patch testing and prick testing. A practical guide. Springer, Berlin, pp 113–120
23. Fischer T, Maibach HI (1985) The thin layer rapid use epicutaneous test (TRUE Test), a new patch test method with high accuracy. Br J Dermatol 112:63–68
24. Fischer T, Kreilgard B, Maibach HI (2001) The true value of the TRUE test for allergic contact dermatitis. Curr Allergy Asthma Reports 1:316–322
25. Blackley CH (1873) Experimental research on the causes and nature of catarrhus aestivus. Baillere, Tindall and Cox, London
26. Schloss OM (1920) Allergy in infants and children. Am J Dis Child 19:433–436
27. Pepys J (1975) Skin testing. Br J Hosp Med 14:412

Part I

Basic Features

Genetics and Individual Predispositions in Contact Dermatitis

2

Axel Schnuch and Berit Christina Carlsen

Contents

Abbreviations

AFMU	5-acetylamino-6-formylamino-3-methyluracil
ACD	Allergic contact dermatitis
ACE	Angiotensin-converting enzyme
AD	Atopic dermatitis
Ala	Alanin
Au	Gold
CA	Contact allergy
CD	Cluster of differentiation
CI	Confidence interval
Cr	Chromate
CYP	Cytochrome P
D	Deletion
DC	Dendritic cell
DNCB	2,4 dinitrochlorobenzene
DTH	Delayed-type hypersensitivity
DZ	Dizygote
FLG	Filaggrin
GST	Glutathione S-transferase
GWAS	Genome wide association studies
Hg	Mercury
HLA	Human leukocyte antigen
I	Insertion
ICD	Irritant contact dermatitis
I/D	Insertion/deletion
IFN	Interferon
IL	Interleukin
LT	Lymphotoxin
MDBGN	Methyldibromo glutaronitrile
MHC	Major histocompatibility complex
MMP	Matrix metalloproteinase
MnSOD	Manganese superoxide dismutase
MZ	Monozygote
MX	Methylxantin

A. Schnuch (✉)
IVDK-Zentrale, Institut an der Universität Göttingen,
von-Sieboldstraße 3, 37075 Göttingen, Germany
e-mail: aschnuch@med.uni-goettingen.de

B.C. Carlsen
Department of Dermato-Allergology, Copenhagen University
Hospital Gentofte, Niels Andersens Vej 65, 2900 Hellerup,
Denmark

J.D. Johansen et al. (eds.), *Contact Dermatitis*,
DOI: 10.1007/978-3-642-03827-3_2, © Springer-Verlag Berlin Heidelberg 2011

2

NAT   *N*-acetyltransferase
NDMA   *p*-nitroso-dimethylanilin
Ni   Nickel
OR   Odds ratio
PPD   *p*-phenylenediamine
ROS   Reactive oxygen species
SNP   ("snip") Single nucleotide polymorphism
TAP   Transporter associated with antigen presentation
TEWL   Transepidermal water loss
TNF   Tumor necrosis factor
Val   Valine

2.1 General Introduction

Contact dermatitis cannot develop without exposure to substances in the environment. Conversely, only a part of individuals exposed to the same exogenous stimulus develop contact dermatitis, allergic or irritant. In addition, several cofactors are involved. Hence, the notion of a complex disease, with probably many genes and many environmental factors contributing to the observed phenotypes. There are essentially two reasons to study genetic factors: (a) to get further insights into the pathogenesis, and (b) to get information about how and where to target preventive measures. However, there has been a lack of conclusive results in the study of the genetics of allergic and irritant contact dermatitis, and even more, a complete ignorance of the interplay between endogenous factors of individual susceptibility and exposure to noxious agents. In some instances, the environmental factor may override any genetic predisposition. In others, the genetic factor may prevail, with the consequence that the disease is confined to a specific subpopulation, the "noxious agent" doing no harm to the vast majority of people. The problem becomes more complex, even insurmountable, if a quantitative approach is taken [1]. One should have in mind the critical remark of HARDY and SINGELTON: "To state that most complex diseases are caused by an interaction between genome and environment is a cliché. Such interactions, while likely, have for the most part not been demonstrated, and we should be cautious about universally subscribing to this belief without evidence" [2]. This is the challenge for those few dealing with the genetics of contact dermatitis and a reminder for those (many)

being involved in research, treatment, and prevention of contact dermatitis.

2.2 Genetic Factors in Allergic Contact Dermatitis[1]

People probably differ in susceptibility to allergen exposure [3, 1]. However, it would be premature to attribute susceptibility to genetic traits only. Susceptibility to sensitization may be acquired as in patients with leg dermatitis [1], and susceptibility to elicitation may be increased through a high induction dose of the allergen [4] or through interfering coexisting factors like irritation of the skin [1]. The "internal milieu" may temporarily be influenced by endocrinological or pharmacological factors, going along with an increased or decreased susceptibility to contact allergy (CA) (Table 2.1). One should have in mind or even exclude these confounding causes of different susceptibilities when studying the genetics of CA.

Table 2.1 Acquired or inherent factors probably influencing susceptibility to CA, notwithstanding possible genetic variations of these factors themselves (e.g., venous insufficiency/leg dermatitis [165] or irritability of the skin [166, 57])

High induction dose of the allergen [4]
Irritant contact dermatitis [59]
"Status eczematicus" [1]
Leg dermatitis [167]
Drugs [168, 133, 169]
Climatic conditions [170]
Psychological stress [171, 172]
Gender [173, 174]
Age [167, 175]
Ethnicity [176, 177, 178]

[1]This article is partly based on A. Schnuch, G. Westphal, R. Mössner, K. Reich: Genetic factors in contact allergy–Review and future goals Contact Dermatitis (submitted)

2.2.1 Early Studies in the Genetics of Contact Allergy

In the past, different approaches were taken to study the question of inheritance in CA in humans and animals (Table 2.2). Studies up to 1985 were comprehensively reviewed by Menné and Holm [5], and recent studies on nickel allergy by Shram and Warshaw [6].

2.2.1.1 Experimental Sensitization

After Sulzberger and Rostenberg had noticed interindividual differences in experimental sensitization to *p*-nitroso-dimethylanilin (NDMA) and 2,4 dinitrochlorobenzene (DNCB), Landsteiner et al. reanalyzed these data and concluded that the susceptibility to sensitization is not general (equally expressed regardless of the nature of the chemical), but most probably chemical-specific

Table 2.2 Summary of studies in the genetics of ACD

Authors	Study	Results	References
Experimental sensitization			
Sulzberger and Rostenberg (1939)	Sensitization to *p*-nitroso-dimethylanilin (NDMA) and 2,4 dinitrochlorobenzene (DNCB) in humans	Interindividual differences in susceptibility to sensitization; impact of preexisting eczema	[7]
Landsteiner, Rostenberg and Sulzberger (1939)	Reanalysis of the above study	Susceptibility to sensitization is chemical-specific. Individuals sensitized to one allergen are more easily sensitized to others	[3]
Chase (1941)	Sensitization of guinea pigs with DNCB and poison ivy; identification of high and low responders. Controlled breeding of the two colonies	The offspring of the high reactors reacted also intensely; the other group reacted poorly, although induction was even higher. Sensitivities (to organic compounds) not substance specific	[179]
Polak, Barnes and Turk (1968)	Sensitization of different inbred strains of guinea pigs with metal compounds	One strain could be sensitized to potassium dichromate, but not to mercury chloride; reverse sensitivity of the other strain. Sensitivities (to metal compounds) substance specific	[180]
Family studies			
Walker, Smith and Maibach (1967)	Experimental sensitization of parents and their children of 99 families with DNCB and NDMA	Sensitization of children more frequent if parents were sensitized (only NDMA, not DNCB)	[8]
Forsbeck, Skog and Ytterborn (1971)	Relatives (*n*=404) of patients with ACD (*n*=94) were patch tested with 23 standard allergens	Pos. reactions in female relatives more frequent than in controls (30/18%)	[10]
Fleming, Burden and Forsyth (1999)	Relatives (*n*=209) of patients with Ni – ACD (*n*=39) were questioned about intolerance to nickel	The risk ratio for first degree relatives of Ni positive patients was 2.83 (CI 2.45–3.27). Remark: confounders were not controlled for!	[11]
Twin studies			
Menné and Holm (1983)	Based on a questionnaire on a possibly nickel allergy mailed to 1.546 female twins from the Danish Twin register, 115 pairs were investigated (patch test in *n*=75)	Difference between concordance rate for Ni allergy among MZ and DZ pairs. The heritability for nickel allergy was ~60%. For a medium potent sensitizer (Ni), genetic factors may play a role (see Table 2.3)	[9]
Forsbeck, Skog, and Ytterborn (1968)	101 twin pairs from the Swedish twin register	Insignificant concordance among the MZ pairs	[12]
	Patch tested with 23 standard allergens Sensitization with DNCB (see comment in Table 2.3)	No difference in sensitization between MZ and DZ pairs Conclusion: no evidence for genetic background	

(continued)

2

Table 2.2 (continued)

Authors	Study	Results	References
Bryld et al. (2004)	A sample of female twins with hand eczema from the Danish twin register was patch tested with nickel (n=630)	Patch test positive to nickel: $n=146$. Only a small tendency for larger odds ratio in MZ (OR: 1.28, 95% CI 0.33–5.00). Ni allergy mainly caused by environmental factors. Cave: selection criterion!	[13]
Studies of immunogenetic markers			
Ishii et al. (1990-1998)	Genetic control of metal sensitization in mice	Various polymorphism in the I-A region	[18, 20, 21, 19]
Asherson et al. (1990)	sensitization and IFNγ release in CBA (H-2k) and BALB/c (H-2d) mice	The H-2d haplotype determines contact sensitivity and poor IFNγ response to several antigens	[181]
Okuda, Ishii et al. (1980)	Genetic control of DNFB sensitization in mice	Controlled by I-A region of H-2, and non-H-2 loci	[22]
In humans	*Significant findings only*	For further results see	[5, 24, 6]
Walton et al. (1986)	Associations of nickel allergy with MHC loci	HLA-B35	[25]
Önder et al. (1995)	Dito	DQA1*061; DR15 decreased	[26]
Silvennoinen-Kassinen et al. (1997)	Association with TAP genes, encoding the ABC (ATP-binding cassette) transporter associated with antigen processing (TAP)	RR for the alleles TAP2B increased, for TAP2C decreased (both significantly)	[27]

[3, 7]. Nevertheless, it was shown that individuals sensitized to one allergen are more easily sensitized to others. However, the question of the cause of different susceptibilities remained unsettled.

2.2.1.2 Family Studies

A genetic influence became more evident through the study done by Walker et al. [8], probably one of the most convincing human studies. The authors studied experimental sensitization with NDMA and DNCB in 99 families with a total of 301 individuals. Interestingly, children were sensitized to (the strong allergen) DNCB independent of successful sensitization to their parents, but in case of the weaker allergen NDMA, children were sensitized significantly more often, when their parents were sensitized (Table 2.3). One may conclude that a very potent allergen can be considered to overpower genetic influences [8]. In contrast, in sensitization to weaker allergens (like NDMA or nickel), genetic factors may play a role [8, 9]. With regard to other types of family studies [10, 11], Menné and Holm raise several shortcomings of such studies, e.g.,

Table 2.3 Difference in sensitization rates in children of sensitized and nonsensitized parents

Status of parents	Percentage of children sensitized	
	DNCB (%)	NDMA (%)
Sensitized	65	51
Not sensitized	52	29
	$p<0.10$	$p<0.01$

"The potent allergen DNCB is probably overpowering genetic influences" (Walker, Smith, Maibach [8])

difference in exposure time for parents and offspring, or changing exposure patterns over time [5].

2.2.1.3 Twin Studies

Clustering of diseases in families may either be the result of shared genetic influences or shared family environment. With regard to nickel CA, the results of twin studies are controversial [9, 12, 13] (Table 2.2). In a more recent study, Bryld et al. recruited a sample of female twins with hand eczema from the Danish twin register [13]. In the final analysis, 630 females were included, of which 146 had a positive patch test to nickel. There was a trend toward an increased risk for nickel allergy among MZ (OR: 1.28, 95% CI 0.33–5.00). The authors concluded that allergic contact dermatitis (ACD) to nickel is mainly caused by environmental and, only to a lesser degree, genetic factors [13]. The limitations of this study (admitted by the authors) included the use of the heterogeneous phenotype "hand eczema" as a selection criterion and a relatively small sample size per age group [14]. Furthermore, MZ and DZ twins might share a different degree of allergen exposure leading to a systematic error in twin studies [15].

2.2.1.4 Studies of Immunogenetic Markers

Early studies have used the proteins (HLA-"antigens") of the MHC class I (HLA-A/-B/-C) and MHC class II (HLA-DP/-DQ/-DR) as serological immunogenetic markers. Meanwhile, they were complemented by the typing of genomic (g) DNA, relating the phenotype (serotype) to genotypes. Up to now, >1,200 class I and >336 class II alleles were identified [16]. MHC-variations (HLA-phenotype and/or genotype) were found to be associated with disease susceptibility, mainly in autoimmune and infectious diseases [17]. Studies of immunogenetic markers in CA were performed in animals and humans. It is generally believed that the genetic control of delayed-type hypersensitivity (DTH) reactions in mice relies on the I-A subregion of H-2, the murine MHC, and is antigen-specific, at least in some instances, as was shown for nickel (Ni) [18], Mercury (Hg) [19], Chromium (Cr) [20], Gold (Au) [21], and organic haptens [22, 23].

Numerous studies on MHC I and MHC II in humans with contact sensitization were performed during the last three decades (reviews: [5, 24, 6]). Class I and class II MHC molecules differ greatly among individuals. Most of the associations of HLA loci with CA were not significant, with the exception of HLA-B35 [25] and DQA1*061 [26], which were increased, and DR15, which was decreased in nickel allergic patients [26]. In addition, polymorphisms of genes encoding the TAP transporter proteins located in the HLA class II region and of genes encoding complement factor B (component of the C3 convertase enzyme activating the alternative pathway), particularly the subtype BF*FB, located in the MHC class III region, were found to be associated with nickel allergy [27, 28]. But

even if MHC-disease associations exist, they would not necessarily be causal, since they might be caused by genetic linkage. In almost all studies only nickel allergy was considered, which may be a further reason for the lack of significant findings, as nickel may bind to nearly every HLA-molecule and may even act in an HLA independent manner [29, 30]. Rarely, HLA polymorphisms were studied in individuals sensitized to organic compounds, again with inconclusive results [31, 32, 33, 34].

Core Message

> It is believed that ACD is a complex disease, in which the cause is considered to be a combination of genetic effects and environmental influences. Particularly studies performed in humans and in animals suggest that genetic factors may play a role in ACD (Table 2.2), in addition to environmental factors, namely the various conditions of allergen exposure.

2.2.2 In Search of the Phenotype of Contact Allergy: Polysensitization

The phenotype, the observable characteristics of an individual, results from the interaction of genotype and environment. In CA, the phenotype corresponds hypothetically to unknown genotypes. For many reasons, the genes involved in CA have not yet been found. One of them may be the variety of chosen (operationalized) "phenotypes." Most often, only sensitization to nickel (or to other metals) was considered (assuming that nickel allergy could be considered a valid paradigm for CA in general). In other experiments, organic haptens were used, but they differed in sensitization potency, blurring the view on possible genetic influences. The problem became more complicated through the notion that CA is not an all-or- none, but a graded phenomenon [35]. Different doses (1), different potencies (2) of the allergen, and different susceptibilities of the individual (3) result together in different grades of sensitization (Review: [1]). As in principle, every human being is equipped with the immunological tools to mount a

2

DTH reaction, such reaction cannot reasonably be understood as a "disease" (or its "phenotype"). On the other hand, a carefully well-defined phenotype is of utmost importance in genetic studies of a disease [2]. Therefore, the focus of research should be "*increased susceptibility* to CA," which could serve as the phenotype to be studied. But what can we understand of "increased susceptibility" [1]?

It was the seminal work of a group from the UK done 20 years ago that contributed essentially to the notion of susceptibility [36]. With a set of intriguing experiments using DNCB sensitization they found (in a rather small study group) that patients with multiple sensitization (to three and more unrelated contact allergens) were more easily (with lower doses) sensitized and exhibited stronger reactions upon rechallenge. Consequently, a study was done to determine whether there was an association between multiple sensitization and HLA molecules [32]. No statistically significant association was found. More recently, however, the concept of polysensitization has experienced a new turn (review: [1]):

1. The risk to be sensitized to an index allergen gradually increased with the number of cosensitization. This was shown for a group of quite heterogeneous allergens (neomycin, the fragrance mix, paraphenylendiamine (PPD), bufexamac, nickel, cobalt chromate).
2. The risk to react in patch testing to an index allergen (the fragrance mix) with stronger (++/+++) reactions increased with the number of cosensitization.
3. The risk to be sensitized to the weak allergen paraben-mix (compared to sensitization to the stronger allergen MDBGN) increased with the number of cosensitization.
4. The prevalence of polysensitization remained stable over a 20-year periode [37], despite generally decreasing sensitization rates in the background population [38].

One will easily agree that all three elements (induction and elicitation increased, sensitization even to weak allergens) are suitable to make up the meaning of "increased susceptibility." There is sufficient evidence that this increased susceptibility is unequivocally indicated by polysensitization.

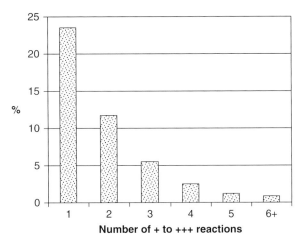

Fig. 2.1 Distribution of the number of positive reactions (+, ++, or +++) to allergens of the standard series. 6+: 6 or more than 6 reactions. Total number of patients $n=58{,}268$. Number of patients with no positive reaction to standard series allergens: $n=31{,}865$ (54.7%) [1]

Interestingly, the distribution of graded susceptibility (as expressed by increasing polysensitization) follows the general distribution of quantitative traits of multifactorial disorders (i.e., complex diseases like blood pressure) (Fig. 2.1) [39] (p. 248).

Core Message

❯ Studies on the genetics of CA should focus on increased susceptibility, and therefore, studied in patients with polysensitization.

2.2.3 Polymorphisms in Allergic Contact Dermatitis

In many diseases, susceptibility loci on defined chromosomes or polymorphisms (variation present at greater than 1% in the population) located in specific DNA sequences were detected and found to be associated with the disease (e.g., psoriasis [40]), thereby substantiating more and more the notion of disease genes. However, genes at the root of ACD have not yet been identified. Linkage or association studies have been done until now without convincing success, and thus, almost no putative susceptibility loci were identified (with the exception of a few HLA loci). Therefore, a group of investigators from the University of Göttingen/Germany opted for the "candidate gene" approach [41, 42, 43, 44, 45]. Candidate genes are those whose characteristics (e.g., protein product) suggest that they may be responsible for a genetic disease. The existing knowledge on the biologic relevant steps in CA may point the way [46, 47].

Contact allergens are low-molecular weight chemicals, their permeation into the skin being a function of the molecular structure of the allergen and of the skin barrier (which is elsewhere discussed [48]). Some molecules may require metabolic activation in the skin to become an active prohapten. Others may be deactivated by early metabolic conversion (detoxication). Sensitization to the allergen may then depend on the capabilities of the organism to metabolize a chemical to a protein-reactive metabolite [47]. Individuals differ with regard to these metabolizing capabilities. This is caused by various genetic polymorphisms of xenobiotic metabolizing enzymes, such as N-acetyltransferases (NAT) and glutathione S-transferases (GST) [49, 50].

Sensitization itself – the immunological step – is a complex process leading up finally to the activation of allergen-specific T-cells (mainly CD8+) [46]. One of the pivotal steps is the activation, maturation, and migration of antigen-presenting dendritic cells (DCs), namely dermal DCs and (epidermal) Langerhans cells [51]. The whole process is orchestrated by several important changes in the skin, involving *cytokines and chemokines, adhesion molecules,* and *matrix metalloproteinases* (e.g., MMP-9) [46]. Interleukin 1-beta (IL-1-beta) and tumor necrosis factor (TNF) can be regarded as the key cytokines during this process, although many other factors were shown to be indispensable for sensitization to take place [51]. However, getting this gearing going is by no means allergy specific [52]. Unspecific stimuli (e.g., irritants), not to forget microbes via activation of the innate immune system [53], are able to start the machinery as well [52, 54, 55]. Even more, allergens need these nonspecifically activated stimuli by virtue of their own (most contact allergens dispose of irritating properties) [56] or by interference of external factors (preexisting or induced inflammation) [57, 58]. This interplay resulted in the concept of the "danger model," introducing, as indispensable elements, inflammatory processes into the pathogenesis of ACD [59].

As important elements within the pathogenetic relevant steps of ACD, metabolically active enzymes and various cytokines were studied [41, 42, 43, 44, 45].

2.2.3.1 Tumor Necrosis Factor (TNF)

Following a change in nomenclature in 1998, TNFα and TNFβ were renamed TNF and LTα (lymphotoxin α). TNF is a proinflammatory cytokine, mainly produced by macrophages, playing an essential role in host defense against infections [60]. Its role is, however, far more complex: This cytokine is involved in the *physiological* regulation of a wide spectrum of biological processes (e.g., cell proliferation, differentiation, apoptosis, skin barrier homeostasis) and implicated in a diverse range of *pathological* conditions, particularly inflammatory (rheumatoid arthritis, psoriasis) and infectious (sepsis) [60, 61, 62].

The gene encoding TNF is located on chromosome 6p21.33, within the MHC Class III complex (Fig. 2.2). Several gDNA variants or single nucleotide polymorphisms ("SNPs") have been identified, e.g., TNF – 238 G→A, TNF – 308 G→A, TNF – 857 C→T, TNF – 1031 T→C. More than 90 case-control studies for the TNF-308 promoter SNP and disease were accumulated [63, 61].

Studies of TNF Polymorphisms in ACD
(See Table 2.4)

1. The first study investigating the relationship between polymorphisms of the TNF gene and ACD found that the distribution of TNF – 308 genotypes, but not TNF-238, was significantly different in cases with ACD and healthy controls, with carriers of the A allele being more frequent among polysensitized patients [44].
2. Individuals from Germany and the Netherlands sensitized to PPD ($n = 181$) and controls without history of ACD ($n = 161$), age- and gender-matched to cases, were selected for genotyping for the TNF-308 gene polymorphism [64]. The frequency of the rare A allele was significantly higher in cases than in controls (22.1 vs. 12.4%). A logistic regression analysis, using

Fig. 2.2 Scheme depicting the MHC on chromosome 6p21.33, TNF and flanking genes in the TNF region (LTBA/LTBB: lymphotoxin α/β), and the promoter polymorphisms. Numbering is descending from the +1 of the transcription start site ([63], modified)

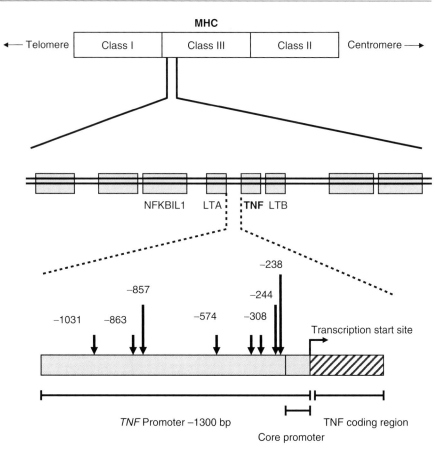

Table 2.4 Studies of probably functional relevant polymorphisms in contact allergic patients from the Göttingen/IVDK group[a] (row I;1–5) from more recent studies (row I;6–9) and replication studies (row IV)

Polymorphisms	Results	Reference	Replicated
Genotype and phenotype of N-acetyltransferase (NAT) 2	Genotype and phenotype of "rapid acetylators" (rap. Acet.) increased	[41]	[105, 104]
NAT 1 and 2 in patients allergic to "para compounds"	NAT2*4 allele (rap. Acet) increased	[42]	[105, 104]
	NAT2*5b/2*6a (slow Acet) decreased		
	Genetic linkage of NAT1*10 with NAT2*4		
Glutathione S-transferases (GST) M1 and T1	Combined deletion (GSTT1-/GSTM-1) in patients allergic to organic mercury compounds compared to controls and to para group allergics	[43]	[65][b]
Cytokines: ILB-511, ILB + 3953, ILRN, IL-6-174, TNFA-238, TNFA-308	TNFA-308 (G→A): increased (in polysensitized)	[44]	[65][b] [64][c]
Cytokine: IL-16	IL-16–295 (T→C) increased (in polysensitized)	[45]	
Cytokine IL-4	No difference between Cr allergics and controls with regard to IL-4–590 polymorphism	[65][b]	
Angiotensin- I-converting-enzyme (insertion/deletion polymorphism)	Insertion (I) or deletion (D) of a 287-base pair in intron 16/I-polymorphism (~low ACE activity) increased	[135][c]	

Table 2.4 (continued)

Polymorphisms	Results	Reference	Replicated
Manganese superoxide dismutase (MnSOD)	Valine (Val) to alanine (Ala) at amino acid – 9 (Ala-9Val) polymorphism No difference between allergics[c] and controls	[130][c]	
Filaggrin null mutations (combined genotypes for R501× and 2282del4)	*Results inconclusive*		
	Not associated with ACD[d]	[149][d]	
	when compared to other controls: risk increased	[150][d]	
	Not associated with ACD[d]	[148][d]	
	Associated with relevant sensitization to nickel only	[152]	

[a]University of Göttingen (department of occupational medicine, department of dermatology) and department of dermatology joining the IVDK

[b]allergic to chromate

[c]allergic to PPD

[d]sensitization not specified

sex, age, and TNF (A/A + A/G) vs. GG as explanatory variables, confirmed the risk associated with the combined TNF (A/G + A/A) genotypes.

3. In a cohort study in cement workers ($n = 153$) conducted in Taiwan [65], those sensitized to chromate (cases, n = 19; 12.4%) were compared to nonsensitized with regard to TNF – 308 G/A and IL-4–590 (C/T) gene polymorphisms. The TNF – 308 G/A genotype was found to be a significant risk factor for ACD to chromate (RR: 3.9; CI: 1.14–13.2), whereas the distribution of genotypes of the IL-4 polymorphism (C/T) did not differ between cases and controls. Assuming an identical exposure, the different outcomes are most likely due to different susceptibilities for which the genetic variation found (TNF and GST (see below)) may partly account for.

These consistent findings support the concept that the promoter polymorphism at position – 308 of the TNF gene might be a risk factor for acquiring ACD. In particular, in one study, the rare *TNFA* – 308A polymorphism was more frequent among polysensitized patients supporting the notion that polysensitization is in fact the relevant phenotype. Although DTH reactions differ in some aspects from ACD, the finding of an increased granulomatous (DTH) response to lepromin in carriers of the TNF – 308 A allele supports the above results [66]. As TNF is also involved in irritant contact dermatitis (ICD), and as the TNF-308 A polymorphism was shown to be associated with an increased risk of ICD [67, 68], it is conceivable that this polymorphism might have an impact on ACD via unspecific trigger factors as suggested by the "danger model" [59].

Despite quite a number of studies showing a functional relevance, albeit highly context specific (increase of transcriptional activity or production of TNF), Bayley et al., summarized the results of functional in vivo and in vitro studies and concluded that the – 308 G/A polymorphism is probably not functional [63]. The definite functional role of this polymorphisms remains to be elucidated [69, 70, 71].

The starting point of most studies was the hypothesis that genetic variants of the TNF locus *are likely to* be involved in the disease *because* TNF is clearly involved in pathogenesis. However, this locus may be linked to other candidate SNPs within or outside the TNF gene (e.g., *LTA*, encoding lymphotoxin α) or unknown susceptibility markers, which may extend over a large region of the MHC including many genes [72]. Thus, it may be an extended haplotype (e.g., HLA A1, B8, DR3), and not the single SNP, that impact disease susceptibility [73], indicating the need to study frequencies of rather long-range haplotypes containing TNF*-308 together with other susceptibility marker (Fig. 2.2).

2

2.2.3.2 Interleukin-16

IL-16, originally described as a lymphocyte chemoat-tractant factor, exerts a variety of proinflammatory functions (review: [74, 75]). The active peptide (121 amino acids) is cleaved from a precursor protein by caspase three, and then self aggregates to an active homotetramer. IL-16 has been identified at sites of inflammation associated with several different disease states [74]. Its role could be to mediate directed locomotion of T-cells toward DC after these have captured antigen and attract other DC to sites of antigenic challenge, resulting in a tenfold higher accumulation of CD4+ T-cells [76]. Based on several studies, an important role for IL-16 during DTH reactions can be assumed [77, 78, 79].

The gene encoding IL-16 *(IL-16)* is located on chromosome 15q26.3. One polymorphism in the promoter region, a T/C SNP at position – 295, was dissected in Crohn's disease, atopic dermatitis (AD), asthma, and periodontitis, with, however, conflicting results [80, 81, 82, 83, 84]. Due to different effects of IL-16 in different types of disease, this polymorphism may exert an enhancing (in Th1 driven-) or protective effect (in Th2 driven- diseases) [82].

Studies of IL-16 Polymorphisms in ACD

Up to now, only one study investigated the IL-16–295 polymorphism in ACD. It was found that the IL-16–295 genotypes were differently distributed among patients with ACD and healthy controls [45]. In particular, the IL-16–295*C/C genotype was overrepresented among polysensitized individuals (7.0 vs. 1.0% in the control group; odds ratio (OR) 7.68; 95% CI 1.59–48.12). Association was found neither in monosensitized patients (sensitized to para-arylic compounds) with ACD nor in patients with AD [45].

The fact that the homozygous combination of the rare allele IL-16–295*C appeared to be more common among polysensitized patients with ACD adds, from the part of genetics, further support the concept of polysensitization as a phenotype of increased risk. The observed association both in ACD and Crohn's disease [80] thought to be driven by Th1 cytokines, as well as the lack of association in AD [81], dominated by Th2 cytokines, at least in acute lesions, is compatible with the Th1/Th2 paradigm. Despite these findings suggestive of being plausible, the study needs to be replicated.

2.2.3.3 *N*-Acetyltransferase 1 and 2 (NAT1/NAT2)

Acetylation is a major route of biontransformation for several therapeutic arylamine and hydrazine drugs (review: [85]. It plays an important role in the bioactivation as well as bioincativation of numerous potential carcinogens. *N*-acetylation is in general regarded as a detoxifying reaction, while *N*-*O*-acetylation (the acetylation of the corresponding hydroxylamine) leads to highly reactive, toxic intermediates (review: [85, 50, 86]. In humans these acetylation reactions are catalyzed by two closely related cytosolic enzymes, *N*-acetyltransferase-1 (NAT1; EC 2.3.1.5) and *N*-acetyltransferase-2 (NAT2; EC 2.3.1.5). In dermatology, the xenobiotic most studied with regard to *N*-acetlylation is the contact allergen para-phenylenediamine (PPD). It was shown that PPD is metabolized to its mono- and dicacetylated derivatives and to oxidation products such as Brandowskis Base (BB, an end-product of oxidation) [87, 88, 89, 90]. However, it can be expected that only a part of PPD is acetylated [91, 92]. The remnant, PPD and its oxidation products, could still act as sensitizer [93, 94].

The human *NAT1* and *NAT2* genes are located in close proximity on chromosome 8p22 and share 87%

nucleotide sequence identity within their protein coding regions. Until now (updated 16 Nov 2007 and 27 May 2008), 26 alleles of *NAT1* and 53 of *NAT2* have been identified (http://louisville.edu/medschool/pharmacology/NAT.html; accessed 23 March 2009). Both genes are polymorphic with regard to the "slow" and "rapid" acetylator phenotype. Epidemiological studies have provided some clues concerning the importance of variations in both NAT1 and NAT2 in altering risk for a variety of disorders, most notably cancers [50, 86], but also nonmalignant diseases [95] and, in particular, atopic diseases [96, 97, 98, 99, 100].

Studies of NAT: Polymorphisms in ACD

1. Early studies investigated the NAT *phenotype* in ACD. A "slow acetylator" NAT1 phenotype was reported to be associated with ACD [101, 102, 103]. As the studies (a) comprised patients with CA as controls, (b) used a NAT2-substrate (caffeine), and (c) their sample size was *very* small, no convincing conclusion can be drawn from the results with regard to the NAT1-phenotype in ACD patients [102, 103].

2. Actually the first *molecular-epidemiologic* study in CA determined the *NAT2* genotype and phenotype [41]. Patients allergic to para-substituted aryl compounds (but other sensitization not excluded) ($n=55$) and healthy controls ($n=85$) were compared with regard to their capacity to metabolize caffeine (phenotype) and with regard to the *NAT2* genotype. Carriage of at least one *NAT2*4 or *NAT2*12A*

allele encodes a rapid phenotype. In addition, NAT2 phenotypes (rapid and slow) were determined by the use of the ratio of the caffeine metabolites AFMU/1-MX (Fig. 2.3) in urine. Concordance between genotypes and phenotypes was >90%. Concerning the NAT2 phenotype, 48% of contact allergic patients were classified as rapid acetylators, compared to 24% in the control group (Fisher's exact test $p<0.001$) (Fig. 2.4). Genotypically, 51% of contact allergic patients were rapid acetylators, whereas in the control group only 31% "rapid" genotypes were found.

3. In a second study on NAT in a similarly characterized but extended group of patients ($n=88$) and healthy controls ($n=123$), we investigated polymorphism in the *NAT1* and the *NAT2* gene [42]. NAT2 rapid acetylators (carriers of at least one NAT2*4, or *NAT2*12A* allele) were more common in the disease group (45%) than in the control group (30%) ($p=0.029$). The carriage rate of the *NAT1*10* allele (encoding probably the NAT1 rapid acetylator phenotype) was slightly but not significantly increased in patients (43 vs. 36%; OR: 1.5; CI: 0.88–2.68). The haplotype *NAT2*4/NAT1*10* (rapid acetylators) was increased in patients (27 vs. 15%; OR: 2.1; CI:1.04–4.04). This may be due a genetic linkage between *NAT2*4* and *NAT1*10* ($p=0.0025$).

4. These findings, namely an increased risk of ACD for the "rapid" NAT2 polymorphism, were corroborated in a study from Turkey [104] and Iraq [105], although the results of the latter study are compromised by a low sample size and an unconventional, not standardized patch test technique.

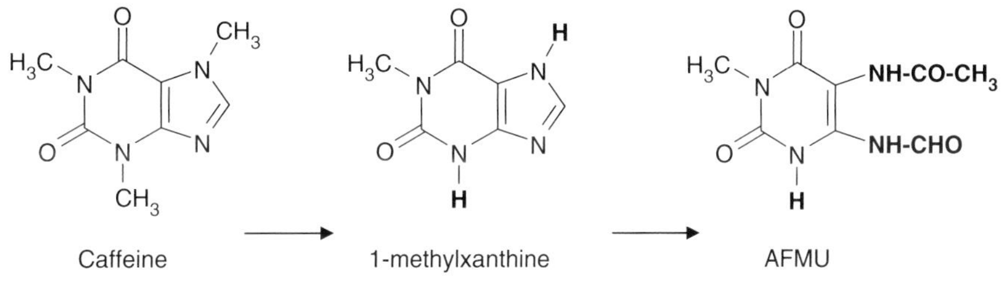

Fig. 2.3 Stepwise metabolism of caffeine catalyzed by NAT2. A ratio >1 of AFMU to methylxanthine indicates a phenotype of NAT2 "rapid acetylator" (AFMU: 5-acetylamino-6-formylamino-3-metyhuracil)

Caffeine → 1-methylxanthine → AFMU

2

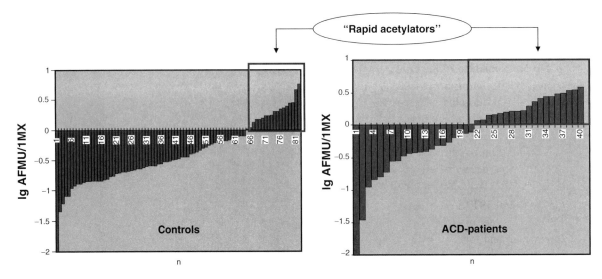

Fig. 2.4 Ratio of the caffeine metabolites AFMU and 1 MX (Fig. 2.3) in patients with ACD ($n=52$) and healthy controls ($n=85$). The values were logarithmically transformed and the cut-off point set at 0, separating slow (ratio <0) and rapid (ratio >0) acetylators ($p<0.001$) [41]

At first sight, the concept of reduced detoxifying competence (slow acetylators) associated with an increased risk of CA seems intriguing [103, 87]. However, N-acetylation may be involved in the development of CA through activation (e.g., N-O-acetylation of the corresponding hydroxylamines), leading to higher levels of reactive metabolites. NAT enzymes may also play a role beyond xenobiotic metabolism and may address endogenous substrates (like folic acid and derivatives or other unknown substrates), or internal signaling pathways [106, 107, 108]. Grant et al. pointed at the paradox that acetylated xenobiotics are less water soluble than their parent compounds, which would make it unlikely that these enzymes evolved specifically in order to accelerate elimination of foreign chemicals [85].

Core Message

> The NAT2 rapid acetylator phenotype and genotype is probably a risk factor of increased susceptibility to ACD.

2.2.3.4 Glutathione Transferases M1 and T1 (GSTM1 and GSTT1)

Cytosolic/soluble glutathione transferases (GST) are a superfamily of phase II enzymes. GST conjugate electrophilic substrates with the nucleophilic tripeptide glutathione (GSH). As a general rule, this leads to decreasing reactivity of toxicants. The cytosolic GSTs are subdivided into seven main classes, including the most studied families GST μ (mu, M) and θ (theta, T). Although some substrates are metabolized by several GST, others are specific for particular isozymes (reviews: [50, 109]). The observed substrate specificities (e.g., genotoxic aromatic epoxides, mono and dihaloalkanes, aminophenols) were found in the context of specific toxicological research (on canceroge-nicity) [109], and will probably not reflect the total of the activities of these enzymes. GSH conjugation may result in toxification as well as detoxification. And, similar to NATs, GSTs may act beyond xenobiotic metabolism, and may be involved in modulating internal signaling pathways [110].

The genes encoding for the proteins GSTM1 and GSTT1 are organized on chromosome 1p13.3 and chromosome 22q11, respectively. Although there are numbers of SNPs of GSTs of class μ and θ, many of these variations have no or little effect on enzyme activity. Exceptions are the deletion polymorphisms *GSTM1*0* and *GSTT1*0*, leading to complete loss of enzyme activity. Variations (null deletions; phenotype: "nonconjugators") in both GSTM1 and GSTT1 were found to alter the risk for a variety of disorders, most notably cancers of different sites but also other diseases, such as chronic cardio vascular disease, rheumatoid arthritis, drug eruptions, and atopic asthma [109,

110, 111, 112, 113]. Although the variation itself being probably of moderate strength, these gene variations lead to synergistic effects if they are combined with other polymorphisms such as the highly active CYP1A1 gene variant [114].

Studies of GSTM1 and GSTT1 Polymorphisms in ACD

1. GSTM1 and GSTT1 may be involved in inactivation of the organic mercury compound thiomersal and of its degradation products (e.g., ethylmercury), as several organic mercury compounds were detoxified by GSH [115], these compounds may interact with GSTs [116], and GSH was shown to inhibit elicitation in patients allergic to thiomersal [117]. Therefore, the GSTM1 and GSTT1 polymorphisms were studied in patients sensitized to mercury compounds (thiomersal, phenylmercury acetate, and ammonium mercury chloride, $n = 100$) [43]. Healthy individuals ($n = 169$) and patients with CA to "para-substituted aryl compounds" ($n = 114$) served as control. GSTM1 deficiency was significantly more frequent in thiomersal allergics, and GSTT1 deficiency more frequent in patients allergic to mercury compounds other than thiomersal. More importantly, the combined deletion (GSTM 1*0 and GSTT1*0) was significantly more frequent in the thiomersal group than in healthy controls (16/91 vs. 11/169; $p = 0.0093$) and the para-compound group (16/91 vs. 7/114, $p = 0.014$). This finding suggests a "synergistic" effect of these enzyme deficiencies (synthetic genetic interaction of two genes; deletion of only one of them with no effect on the phenotype).

2. A cohort study on cement workers [65] (see above) investigated the *GSTM1* and *GSTT1* polymorphisms. While the GSTM1 deletion was equally distributed among cases (cement workers sensitized to chromate (Cr)) and controls (cement workers without sensitization to Cr), there was a higher frequency of the GSTT1 deficiency in Cr positives (3.2 vs. 18.9%, RR 5.5; CI 1.40–36.2).

Both studies point at a substrate-specific influence of GST polymorphisms. Although probably not restricted to mercury (Hg) and Cr, a general influence on pathogenetic steps in CA is less probable. However, there are allergenic metal compounds like Cr, Hg, or Ni, (but some organic compounds as well, like PPD), which generate reactive oxygen species (ROS), e.g., hydroxyl radicals, singlet oxygen, hydrogen peroxides [118, 119, 120], playing a role in the pathobiology of ACD [121, 122, 123, 124]. GSTM1 and GSTT1 exhibit GSH peroxidase activity, and thus, may protect against toxic effects of endogenous and exogenous reactive oxygens [125, 126].

> **Core Message**
>
> › The *GSTT1*0*, and in particular the combined deletion polymorphism *GSTM1*0* and *GSTT1*0*, is associated with an increased risk of enhanced susceptibility to ACD caused by Hg compounds and Cr (and probably other metals?).

2.2.3.5 Manganese Superoxide Dismutase

Manganese superoxide dismutase (MnSOD, EC 1.15.1.1) is a mitochondrial protein that scavenges potentially toxic superoxide radicals by dismuting superoxide (O_2^-) to O_2 plus H_2O_2. The gene (*SOD2*) was mapped to chromosome 6q25.3. A peptide polymorphism in the target sequence of MnSOD enzyme, Ala(16)Val, is known to disrupt proper targeting of the enzyme from cytosol to mitochondrial matrix. Several diseases were suspected to be associated with this polymorphism, but with conflicting results (e.g., cancer [127], rheumatic diseases [128], or asthma [129]).

Studies of the MnSOD Polymorphisms in ACD

In view of the pathogenetic role of ROS in ACD (see above), this polymorphism was studied in 157 patients with sensitization to PPD and compared to healthy controls ($n = 201$) [130]. No significant difference in the distribution of allelic frequencies and genotypes between cases and controls was observed, although for subgroups defined by gender and age, there was a trend

2

toward a overrepresentation of the CC carriers (Ala/Ala) (OR: 1.3; CI: 0.8–2.1) [130]. The authors concluded that the *SOD2* polymorphism studied has no strong impact on the individual susceptibility to develop sensitization to PPD.

> **Core Message**
>
> > The Ala(16)Val peptide polymorphism of the MnSOD enzyme is probably not associated with an increased risk of ACD.

2.2.3.6 Angiotensin-Converting Enzyme

Angiotensin-converting enzyme (ACE, kininase II, EC 3.4.15.1) catalyzes the conversion of angiotensin I into angiotensin II, a potent vasoconstrictor, and is involved in the inactivation of bradykinin, a potent vasodilator. Beyond these well-known substrates, ACE cleaves substance P, beta-endorphins, and other peptides [131], which may modulate Langerhans cells and T-lymphocyte functions [132]. In particular, it was shown in animal experiments that ACE modulated the inflammatory response to allergens, but not to irritants, by degrading bradykinin and substance P [133]. The gene, *ACE*, is located on chromosome 17q.23.3. The presence or absence of a 287 bp *Alu* repeat element in this gene (a repeated DNA sequence that can be cut by the *Alu* restriction enzyme), i.e., an "insertion/deletion" (I/D) polymorphism), was found to be associated with the levels of circulating enzyme, namely, that ACE levels were low for I/I homozygotes and high for D/D homozygotes [134].

Studies of the ACE Polymorphisms in ACD

Based on this functional role of the polymorphism, it was hypothesized that individuals with the I/I genotype would be at greater and those with the D/D genotype at lower risk for developing ACD. In 90 patients with ACD (patch test positive to PPD) and 160 controls, the I/D polymorphism was studied [135]. Carriers of the I allele (OR: 1.6; CI: 1.1–2.4), as well as the I/I genotype (OR 2.0; CI: 1.1–3.7), were found significantly more often in the ACD group, and carriers of the "protective" D allele were found less often in this study group (OR: 0.6 (CI 0.4–0.9).

These interesting results broaden our view on ACD beyond the chemical, immunological, and inflammatory aspects to a neuro-endocrinological network, rarely considered in the pathogenesis of ACD [136, 137]. Furthermore, they underline the importance of structural variants beyond SNPs in the study of complex traits [138].

> **Core Message**
>
> > An "insertion/deletion" (I/D) polymorphism of the *ACE* gene was found to be associated with an increased risk of ACD. This finding must be replicated.

2.2.3.7 Filaggrin

Filaggrin (FLG) (filament-aggregating protein) is a key component of the stratum corneum (review: 139, 140]). Multiple FLG peptides are cleaved from profilaggrin, which is encoded by the *FLG* gene on chromosome 1q21. FLG aggregates keratins and filaments, is a major component of the cornified envelope, and contributes – after degradation – with a mixture of hygroscopic amino acids to the pool of amino acids, metabolites, and various ions, known as "natural moisterizing factor" [141, 142]. In addition, the *N*-terminal portion cleaved from profilaggrin is a calcium binding domain, which enters the nucleus of keratinocytes and is thought to be involved in regulating the terminal differentiation of the epidermis [143]. More than 20 loss-of-function mutations within the *FLG* gene have been reported [139]. These *FLG* mutations are nonsense or frameshift mutations, each resulting in truncation of the profilaggrin molecule. Association of the *FLG* null genotype (in particular R501× and 2282del4) with AD has now been replicated in numerous studies [144, 145, 146].

Studies of FLG Mutations in ACD

FLG deficiency may lead to skin barrier defects, as was shown in AD patients with and without *FLG* mutations [141, 147]. An increase of susceptibility to chronic ICD was recently shown to be associated with

FLG null mutations (OR: 1.91; 1.02–3.59) [148]. This may also be true for ACD because a compromised skin barrier will facilitate permeation of allergens and contribute by itself to an inflammatory milieu, both favoring an allergic response [48]. A study based on a population (*n* = 183) from the Danish twin register included a small subpopulation with ACD (*n* = 45) [149]. It was reported that "FLG null alleles are not associated with....CA" [149]. A critical comment referred to the inadequate choice of controls and lack of statistical power, altogether denying a sound basis to draw such conclusions [150]. Even more, on using data from a population-based study as controls (*n* = 249) [151], a recalculated odds ratio (OR 2.87; 1.10–7.51) indicated an increased risk for CA to be associated with the combined *FLG* null genotype. In 60% of patients with ICD (out of *n* = 296), one or more type IV sensitization (not specified) was diagnosed [148]. No association to FLG deficiency was found. In a larger population-based study in Germany (KORA C), the *FLG* null mutations mentioned above had been genotyped in 1,502 adults [152]. Neither sensitization to specific allergens (nickel, the fragrance mix) nor sensitization to at least one (39.3%) or two allergens (13.2%) were significantly associated with the combined null genotype. In contrast, nickel patch test positivity together with a history of intolerance to fashion jewellery was significantly associated with the combined null genotype (OR 4.04; 1.35–12.06) [152].

These results seem to point against a major role of the FLG mutations as a risk factor for ACD. However, the results of patch testing (in terms of frequency and pattern of sensitization) differ considerably with regard to other population-based [153, 154, 155] and clinical studies [156, 157]. In particular, sensitization frequency to at least one allergen was higher by a factor >2, compared to other epidemiological studies, and surprisingly almost as high as found in selected clinical patch test populations. The frequency of sensitization to the fragrance mix exceeded that which was found in probably all larger clinical studies [158]. One explanation could be a high proportion of falsely positive cases, which cannot be excluded totally in less professional patch testing in epidemiological studies. When the diagnosis of nickel patch test positivity was strengthened by a positive history, and the patch test result thus probably not falsely positive, a significant association between ACD (to nickel) and FLG mutations was observed.

> **Core Message**
>
> ❯ The studies published so far do not answer the question; "are FLG mutations associated with CA?" instead: "we do not know" (Brown and Cordell [150]).

2.2.3.8 General Remarks on the Study of "Candidate Gene" Polymorphisms in ACD

In this review we have presented studies supporting the view that manifestation of ACD may be influenced by distinct polymorphisms. The reason to investigate these polymorphism was guided by a pathogenetic hypothesis. If a polymorphism is shown to be associated with a disease, its functional relevance should be demonstrated. In this regard, the functional role has not been proven experimentally, but the results could be regarded as plausible, at least.

Nevertheless, a number of limitations regarding the validity and the interpretation of the studies are to be addressed:

- Many studies were done in individuals sensitized to PPD only. One may argue that greater phenotype homogeneity is achieved, albeit at the expense of generalization. On the other hand, as explained above, a study group defined by the mere presence of a sensitization would be too heterogeneous with regard to susceptibility. Hence, the suggestion to investigate genetic variation in a high-risk group [1], where genetic influences can probably be more readily identified [159, 2]
- With the exception of Wang's et al. study [65], there was no control for allergen exposure. Individuals with high susceptibility but without allergen exposure (and no sensitization) may be found in the control group.
- As cytokines (e.g., TNF/IL-1β [160] or TNF/IFNγ [161]) and enzymes (cytochrome p450/GST [49]) interact in vivo, polymorphisms may act synergistically, e.g., the combination

2

of *CYP1A1* with *GSTM1*0* may increase the risk of lung cancer [109], or the combination of NAT2 and TNF polymorphisms the susceptibility for psoriasis [162]. Although a synergism between NAT1 and NAT2 and between GSTM1 and GSTT1 polymorphisms was demonstrated (see above), no further analysis, in particular between cytokine and enzyme-polymorphisms, has been done.

- Often it is unresolved as to whether a disease-associated polymorphism is itself functionally important or acting only as a marker for a coinherited, perhaps as yet, unidentified polymorphism. Thus, for instance, the association with the TNF locus may be secondary and likely to be caused by genetic linkage. Furthermore, susceptibility markers may, as in the case of TNF, extend over a large region of the MHC including many genes [72], and it may be the extended haplotype (and not the single SNP) that impact disease susceptibility. However, the structure of the extended haplotype is still not fully understood. It was suggested that the – 308 G/A polymorphism together with the MHC 8.1 ancestral haplotype (HLA A1, B8, DR3) may play a role in the altered TNF gene expression.

- In view of the poor reproducibility of the majority of studies – only six out of 600 associations were found to be consistently replicated – BAYLEY at al refer to some basic requirements of the editors of Nature Genetics: Large sample size, small *p*-values, associations that make biological sense, and alleles that have a relevant physiological function. An initial study should be accompanied by an independent replication [63, 163].

The studies of polymorphisms in ACD reviewed that all suffer essentially from a small sample size, and *p*-values are rather poor. All studies are essentially underpowered, or false positive results cannot be excluded. Nevertheless, all studies offered tentatively a plausible functional role for the polymorphisms, notwithstanding the limitations outlined above. It is noteworthy that three polymorphisms first identified by the Göttingen group to be associated with an increased risk of ACD, namely TNF, NAT, and GST, were

replicated at least once, albeit with slightly different study designs.

Taken together, the impact of the results presented here may support the view that ACD as a complex disease is influenced by genetic factors, in addition to many well-known environmental factors. However, some diseases are not simply present or absent, but can be viewed as quantitative traits expressed on a measured continuum. Only if a normal trait variation exceeds a defined threshold, it is considered as "disease" (e.g., hypertension). Alike, a variety of anthropometric and laboratory traits were also studied in GWAS (Genome Wide Association Studies), such as serum lipid levels, body mass index, and height [164]. CA was considered here as a quantitative trait, and it was suggested to study the genetics in individuals where this trait is expressed at the extreme tail of the distribution of sensitization (Fig. 2.1), namely as polysensitization [1].

> **Core Message**
>
> › ACD should be understood as a quantitative trait (like arterial hypertension). Genetic studies should focus on individuals with a phenotypically increased risk (i.e., polysensitization). Although all studies on polymorphisms in ACD are compromised by several limitations, particularly small sample size, they support the notion that ACD is influenced by genetic factors.

2.3 Irritant Contact Dermatitis

Irritant contact dermatitis (ICD) has a multifactorial pathogenesis. Exposure to irritants, e.g., water, alkalis, acids, oils, and organic solvents, is a necessity and generally considered the most important causal component. Several exogenous factors influence the irritant reaction, (see Table 2.5). Certain phenotypes have an increased risk of irritant contact dermatitis under controlled experimental settings and are considered especially susceptible. These phenotypes are discussed below and an overview is given in Table 2.5.

The irritant response shows great interindividual variability in healthy individuals [182–184]. The

Table 2.5 Causal components in irritant contact dermatitis

Causal components in irritant contact dermatitis		
Exogenous factors	Allergen	Concentration [190]
		Irritant potency [190]
	Exposure	Duration of exposure [190]
		Meteorological conditions [257, 258]
		Combined exposure to irritants [259]
		Application site [197, 226, 240]
		Friction [260]
Endogenous factors		Atopic dermatitis [201, 205–207]
		Concomitant skin disease other than atopic dermatitis [199, 237, 239]
		Age [197, 226, 227]
		Sex [207, 221, 224, 225]
		Ethnicity [230]
		Minimal erythema dosage [242]

underlying mechanism of this interindividual variability and of the different phenotypes is poorly understood. It is possibly genetically determined [185]. Genetic factors examined in relation to ICD and details of the interindividual variation are also presented below.

2.3.1 Individual Variability in Irritant Responses in Healthy Individuals

Under well-defined test conditions and in relatively homogenous populations, interindividual variability in irritant responses has repeatedly been documented both after acute irritant assaults and chronic irritant exposure [182–184]. This means that some individuals develop irritant reactions at lower doses than others and/or react more intensely on irritant exposure. They can be considered more susceptible. The variation in reaction mimics a normal distribution [184]. The interindividual variations are not only apparent by visual scoring of reactions, but also when assessing the skin changes by noninvasive objective methods [186–188].

The great interindividual variation in irritant responsiveness is not explained by intraindividual variability. Intraindividual variability is in all instances less than the interindividual variation [188,189]. Increased susceptibility toward one irritant is not always indicative of an increased susceptibility to other irritants [190].

The clinical implication of increased susceptibility to irritant reactions has been assessed in a few studies. Development of clinical hand dermatitis, type IV allergies, and enhanced allergic reactivity on elicitation is linked to an increased irritant susceptibility [191–193]. The association between type IV allergies and increased irritant susceptibility is consistent with the danger model, where an antigenic signal in itself is not enough to produce sensitization [194]. A nonantigen-specific irritant signal – danger signal – is a pivotal component for sensitization to occur. This is supported by the observations that otherwise subclinical doses of allergen produce a clinical response only in combination with irritants [195] and irritants lower the threshold for sensitization [196]. The effect on elicitation occurs both when the irritant is applied simultaneous with the allergen and when applied 24 h after allergen exposure [195]. A danger signal may more easily be produced in individuals with an inherent increased irritant susceptibility, and thus, associate with CA.

The irritant response depends on the skin barrier integrity and the inflammatory response. Variations in the skin barrier construct, skin recovery ability, and the components in the inflammatory reaction may give rise to the interindividual variations seen. Skin penetration of irritants and transepidermal water loss (TEWL) are measures of skin barrier integrity. Both measures have been found to be predictive of the acute irritant response [187, 197–200], but not of the chronic irritant response [186, 201]. Total consensus is not apparent since skin reactivity to acute irritant assault is not always related to the baseline skin barrier function [202]. Skin thickness correlates with the irritant penetration rate which indicates that skin thickness plays a role in the permeability of the skin and possibly in the response to irritant exposure [187]. Epidermal lipids are also important to the skin barrier integrity. The level of ceramides in the stratum corneum at baseline in healthy volunteers was inversely correlated to the intensity of reaction to acute irritant exposure in one study [203].

Several cytokines are involved in the inflammatory response and considerable interindividual differences in cytokines baseline levels are also observed [186, 204].

2

Baseline stratum corneum levels of two cytokines, interleukin-1 receptor antagonist and interleukin-8, respectively, have been shown to be predictive of the acute response to skin irritation [186]. The proinflammatory cytokine interleukin-1α, which is generally considered an important contributor to the early response of ICD, was not predictive of the acute irritant response under experimental settings [186]. The predictive value of the baseline level of TNF-α, another important proinflammatory cytokine in ICD, has not been assessed. A permeable skin barrier, perhaps caused by changes in epidermal lipids and skin thickness, and variations in the basal inflammatory cytokine levels seem associated with the degree of susceptibility to irritant exposure. But skin barrier and the inflammatory response are highly complex fields with innumerable components and further investigation into the underlying biological mechanisms of individually increased irritant susceptibility is warranted.

> **Core Message**
>
> ❯ Great *inter* individual variation in the irritant response exists in healthy individuals and is not explained by intraindividual variability. An altered skin barrier and variations in basal inflammatory cytokine levels might contribute to the explanation of the interindividual variability, but further investigation into the underlying mechanism is warranted.

2.3.2 Predisposition Related to Specific Phenotypes

Small variations in irritant responses might be ascribed to ethnicity, age, sex, AD, and other skin diseases. Generally, studies on the endogenous factors sex, ethnicity, and age are marked by divergent results, whereas studies on AD are more consistent. Many of the studies on predisposing factors related to specific phenotypes are small in size, and therefore, seem to lack power to determine if any difference exists. It can explain the divergent results reported. The great inter-individual variability may also mask any small impact of a certain phenotype making it difficult in small studies to determine if any difference exists. When larger studies are carried out, small differences seem to appear, e.g., when examining sex as predisposing factor for ICD. This indicates that variations in irritant responses related to phenotypes do exist, but the impact of these phenotypes is relatively small. The predisposing ability of the endogenous factors such as AD, sex, age, ethnicity, body mass index, and other skin diseases to ICD is discussed below.

2.3.2.1 Atopic Dermatitis

It is firmly established that patients with AD represent a phenotype with increased reactivity when experimentally exposed to irritants [201, 205–207]. Such increased hyperreactivity is both present in clinically normal and dry skin of patients with AD with the dry skin showing the greatest susceptibility to irritants [201, 205]. Patients with a history of AD but no active lesions do not show an increased reactivity compared with patients with active AD [208, 209]. The hyperreactivity observed in AD patients may also be positively correlated with severity of disease [210].

The higher susceptibility toward irritant reactions in AD might partly be explained by higher permeability of the skin barrier and by a greater inflammatory response. The baseline barrier function in atopic individuals has been reported not to differ from nonatopics [186, 209], but most studies report a higher baseline level of TEWL than in controls [201, 206, 211], indicating an altered skin barrier. Measures were performed in macroscopically unaffected skin. Patients with AD also have a higher penetration rate of SLS in uninvolved skin compared with nonatopics [187, 211], especially those with active AD lesions. Patients with inactive dermatitis showed intermediate values in skin diffusibility [211]. The baseline level of TEWL does not seem to be correlated with skin thickness in patients with AD, which indicate that other factors than skin thickness play a role in permeability of the skin in AD [211]. The lipid composition in stratum corneum in skin of AD is disturbed, and changes in the epidermal proliferation and differentiation in both nonlesional and lesional skin of AD have also been reported, reviewed in [212]. The indications of a compromised skin barrier may also be related to the recently found FLG mutations and association with AD [213]. Baseline cytokine levels in the stratum corneum do not differ between atopics and nonatopics in in vivo studies [186, 209], but spontaneous release of proinflammatory cytokines from keratinocytes is greater in atopics in one cultured cell study [214]. Furthermore, the cytokine response upon stimulation, including the important proinflammatory cytokines TNF-α and IL-1, seems greater in atopic patients than in controls [214]. Patients with AD also possess a higher number of TNF-α positive mast cells in the dermis [215]. Additional reading in reference [216].

The genetic basis of AD has been reviewed in [217] and [218] and common susceptibility genes between AD and ICD may be an obvious explanatory possibility of the increased irritant sensitivity in AD patients. Thirty-three SNPs in different genes and null mutations in the profilaggrin gene have so far been associated with AD, but only associations between AD and five of the SNPs and the FLG mutations have been replicated [217, 218]. Besides FLG mutations, none of the other genetic markers for AD – which have been replicated – have been examined in relation to ICD.

> ### Core Message
>
> > AD is a risk factor for increased susceptibility to ICD, which might be ascribed to an altered skin barrier and greater cytokine release.

2.3.2.2 Sex

Conflicting data exist on the role of the sex as predisposing factor for ICD. Epidemiological studies consistently show a higher rate of women among patients with irritant hand eczema, but most experimental studies cannot confirm any differences between the sexes in acute or cumulative irritant reactivity [183, 198]. Also no differences in baseline TEWL or barrier recovery rate has been observed between sexes [183, 219, 220]. This stands in contrast to the generally perception of women having more sensitive skin. Total consensus does not exist since a few studies have reported an increased irritant susceptibility in women compared with men [207, 221]. Cyclic variation in baseline TEWL and acute irritant response has also been reported for women in accordance with menstrual cycle [222, 223].

In more recent studies, men reacted to a greater degree on irritant exposure than did women [224, 225].

One of these studies compiled data from previous studies and represents one of the largest studies regarding sex as predisposing factor. A large number of test subjects may reveal an endogenous factor with a relatively small impact on the irritant response, which is not revealed by a smaller number of test subjects. The finding has been confirmed in one recent study, where male sex was a risk factor for irritant reaction, but the effect of the male sex was relatively weak [225]. Overall, no consensus on the role of the sex as predisposing factor of ICD is yet reached.

2.3.2.3 Age

Few studies have been conducted on age and irritant reactivity and the results are not uniform. Most studies point at a decreased reactivity in the elderly both after acute and chronic irritant assaults [197, 226, 227]. In one study, this age difference was most apparent for strong irritants [224]. Cultured cell studies show a decreased inflammatory cytokine production after irritant exposure in intrinsic aged skin supporting a reduced response in the elderly compared with younger age [228]. The basal barrier function measured as TEWL in the elderly is not altered [220], but other histological abnormalities of the skin barrier are apparent and the recovery of elderly skin is slower than in younger skin, reviewed in [229]. In contrast, age above 40 years was a risk factor for irritant responses in one study; however, a rather weak risk factor [225]. Larger studies are needed for further elucidation.

2.3.2.4 Ethnicity

Interethnic variations in irritant reactions have been assessed between Asians and Caucasians, Blacks and Caucasians, and Hispanics and Caucasians. Divergent reports on interethnic variations in irritant reactions have been given and no consensus on the topic exists. The topic is reviewed in [230].

When different irritants with differing potencies were compared, no consistent differences in the level of response was observed between Caucasians and Asians [190]. Both increased responsiveness in Japanese vs. Caucasian skin and decreased responsiveness in Chinese vs. Caucasian skin have been reported [231, 232]. Increasing the number of test subjects by compiling earlier studies revealed that the number of responders and intensity of reactions were greater among Asians than Caucasians for all irritants examined [224]. This reflects that a small impact of ethnicity, nevertheless, exists. Baseline levels of TEWL and barrier recovery rate do not seem to vary between Asians and Caucasians [219]. Within the Asian population, differences have also been reported between Chinese and Malaysian subjects, but not between Indian and Chinese or Indian and Malaysian subjects [221]. This contributes to the complexity of ethnicity as predisposing factor in ICD.

Several studies have undertaken the mission to investigate the difference in irritant reactivity between Black and Caucasian skin. Studies based on visual scoring of irritant responses have reported a decreased reactivity in Black skin [233], whereas studies based on objective parameters have resulted in increased reactivity, similar reactivity, or decreased reactivity, but for the most part decreased reactivity in Black skin compared with Caucasian skin [230, 234, 235]. The decreased reactivity in blacks was eliminated after removing the stratum corneum with tape stripping and repeating the irritant assault [233]. This indicates that the stratum corneum plays a main role in the interethnic differences observed. Structural differences in the stratum corneum might exist between Black skin and Caucasian skin [236]. The amount of cell layers and intercellular cohesion of the stratum corneum have been reported to be greater in Black skin, but the thickness of stratum corneum is the same [236]. The intercellular lipid content also seems to be greater in Black skin [236].

No differences in response to an irritant assault was observed between Hispanics and Caucasians, but has only been assessed in one study [200].

2.3.2.5 Other Skin Diseases

Hand eczema is accompanied by increased reactivity and increased skin barrier impairment to acute irritant assaults and hand eczema patients also seem to heal slower after irritant exposure compared with controls [199]. Acute rather than chronic or healed eczema show such increased irritant susceptibility [199]. The basal barrier function did not, however, differentiate between eczema patients and controls [199]. In contrast, patients with irritant contact dermatitis taken together as a whole did not show an increased response to acute irritant assault compared with healthy controls, whereas patients with seborrhoiec dermatitis did

[237]. Patients with seborrhoiec dermatitis have higher levels of the important proinflammatory cytokine IL-α in the skin [238]. Cancer lowers the reaction to irritants [239].

2.3.2.6 Regional Differences

Variations in the response to irritant exposure are also seen between different anatomical skin sites. The thigh has the highest reactivity and the palms the lowest reactivity [226]. The skin on the volar forearm shows a graded susceptibility from the wrist to the cubital fossa, with the cubital fossa being most susceptible and the wrist the least suspectible [240]. The face is more susceptible to irritant exposure than the forearm [197].

2.3.2.7 Skin Type

Human skin can be subdivided into six groups based on their pigmentation status and tanning ability in response to sunlight. No difference in acute irritant threshold response has been noted between individuals according to their skin type [198, 241], but measures of minimal erythema dosage seem to inversely correlate with the degree of reaction to irritant exposure [242], making persons with low minimal erythema dosages more susceptible. Baseline skin integrity seems to be the same in skin type II/III vs. skin type V/VI, but the recovery rate after tape stripping was markedly greater in skin types V/VI [219]. Responses to chronic irritant exposure might vary on this account, but has not been assessed.

2.3.2.8 Body Mass Index

High body mass index does not influence skin susceptibility to irritant, but seem to influence the basal biophysical parameters of the skin [243].

> **Core Message**
>
> › Studies on the predisposing ability of endogenous factors for ICD are marked by divergent results, small study sizes, and for some phenotypes, few studies. AD is a certain predisposing factor for increased skin reactivity upon irritant exposure.

2.3.3 Genetic Predisposing Factors

Monozygotic twins show a greater concordance of irritant reactions than do dizygotic twins and healthy controls pairs. This points at a genetic parameter as the underlying mechanism in sensitivity to irritants [185]. Identification of genetic factors that can explain any increased sensitivity to irritants has received limited attention. Only genetic polymorphisms in a small number of cytokines and mutations in the gene of one epidermal structural protein have been assessed in relation to ICD. An overview is given in Table 2.6.

A SNP (G/A substitution) in the TNF-α gene at position – 308 in the promoter region is associated with ICD [244, 245]. TNF-α is a proinflammatory cytokine, is released in response to irritants, and is considered an important contributor to the ICD pathogenesis [246]. Occurrence of the SNP leads to an increased production of TNF-α [247] because of increased transcription activity [248] and may, therefore, contribute to an increased irritant response and to the interindividual variations observed in irritant responses. This is supported by the finding that an irritant response is elicited at lower concentrations in healthy volunteers with SNP at position – 308 in the TNF-α gene compared to healthy volunteers without this SNP [245]. In patients with ICD, the observed association between the TNF-α – 308 A variant and ICD is only representative in patients

with low exposure to wet work and irritants. High exposure to irritants seemed to mask any effect of this variant genotype [244]. The polymorphism is not unique for ICD. It is related to ACD, AD, and other inflammatory diseases [244, 249, 250]. The higher frequency of the TNF-α – 308 A variant in AD also contributes to the explanation of the enhanced irritant reactivity in AD. A SNP at position – 238 in the promoter region of the TNF-α gene does not seem to increase the risk of ICD [244].

A SNP (C/T substitution) in the interleukin-1α (IL-1α) gene at position – 889 in the promoter region is not associated with ICD, but seems to be protective of hand dermatitis in apprentices in training for high-risk occupations for ICD [244]. The effect of the SNP has not been examined in relation to experimentally induced irritant responses. Interleukin-1α is also an important proinflammatory cytokine and is produced in the skin after an acute irritant insult [246] but tends to decrease after repeated irritant exposure [186]. Occurrence of the SNP leads to an increased transcriptional activity as well as increased mRNA and protein levels of IL-1-α in cytoplasma in peripheral blood mononuclear cells [251]. On the contrary, protein levels of IL-1-α are decreased in the stratum corneum of individuals with the variant genotype [252], which relates to the protective function observed. IL-1α – 889 SNP is also in linkage disequilibrium with the SNP IL-1α +4,845 and may not be functionally important in itself. Further investigation into the biological influence of the IL-1-α – 889 SNP is warranted to reach consensus on the influence of this SNP and on the significance of this SNP on ICD and hand dermatitis. IL-1α – 889 SNP is also associated with other inflammatory diseases [249].

SNPs in the genes of other inflammatory cytokines have also been assessed, but only in one study. They were not linked to ICD. The SNPs in questions are IL-1β position – 31 and position – 511, in IL-8 position – 251, and in IL-10 position – 1,082 and position – 592 [244]. The lack of association needs to be confirmed.

An important constituent in the skin barrier is the protein FLG. Lack of FLG in the skin as a consequence of mutations in the profilaggrin gene is associated with an increased TEWL, reduced stratum corneum hydration, and increased stratum corneum thickness [253, 254]. Some of these factors have been shown to be predictive of the acute irritant response. One study has linked FLG mutations to ICD [255]. The frequency of mutations was 12.5% in ICD patients, contrary to 6.9%

Table 2.6 Genetic factors examined for their predisposing capacity in relation to irritant contact dermatitis (ICD)

	Genetic markers	Association with ICD
Cytokines	IL-1-α −889	− [244]
	IL-1-α +4,845	− [244]
	IL-1-β −31	− [244]
	IL-1-β −511	− [244]
	IL-8−251	− [244]
	IL-10 −592	− [244]
	IL-10 −1082	− [244]
	TNFα −238	− [244]
	TNFα −308	+ [244, 245]
Epidermal structural proteins	Filaggrin (R501×/2282del4)	+ [255]

− No association

+ Significant association

2

in controls. FLG mutations are important predisposing factors to AD, and AD is a risk factor for ICD. Further clarification of the relationship between FLG mutations and ICD corrected for AD is, therefore, warranted before any conclusions can be drawn. Mutations in the profilaggrin gene are also associated with other diseases [256].

Only a small fraction of the important constituents in the inflammatory response to irritant exposure and in the skin barrier has been examined and the findings are based on very few studies. Further, these factors act in concert and may affect each other, contributing to the complexity of examination of genetic predisposing factors. Examination of additional genetic variants and confirmatory studies is warranted before any conclusions can be drawn on genetic predisposing factors. It is still a rather unexplored area. The balance between genetic predisposing factors and environmental exposure also needs to be considered. The genetic basis of individual predisposition to ICD might in some circumstances be outbalanced by environmental causal factors as was seen for TNF-α.

Core Message

> Only a limited part of the genetic basis of important constituents in the irritant response has been examined. The TNF – 308 G/A polymorphism is probably a risk factor for ICD. The IL-1α – 889 C/T polymorphism might be protective of hand dermatitis and FLG null mutations might be a risk factor for ICD. However, confirmatory studies are warranted before any conclusions can be drawn on genetic predisposing factors for ICD.

References

Allergic Contact Dermatitis

1. Schnuch A, Brasch J, Uter W (2008) Polysensitization and increased susceptibility in contact allergy: a review. Allergy 63:156–167
2. Hardy J, Singleton A (2009) Genomwide association studies and human disease. N Engl J Med 360:1759–1768
3. Landsteiner K, Rostenberg A, Sulzberger MB (1939) Individual differences in susceptibility to eczematous sensitization with simple chemical substances. J Invest Dermatol 2:25–29
4. Hostynek JJ, Maibach HI (2004) Thresholds of elicitation depend on induction conditions. Could low level exposure induce sub-clinical allergic states that are only elicited under the severe conditions of clinical diagnosis? Food Chem Toxicol 42:1859–1865
5. Menne T, Holm NV (1986) Genetic susceptibility in human allergic contact sensitization. Semin Dermatol 5:301–306
6. Shram SE, Warshaw EM (2007) Genetics of nickel allergic contact dermatitis. Dermatitis 18:125–133
7. Sulzberger MB, Rostenberg A (1939) Acquired specific supersensitivity (allergy) to simple chemicals. IV. A method of experiemntal sensitization; and demonstration of increased susceptibility in individuals with eczematous dermatitis of contact type. J Immunol 36:17–27
8. Walker FB, Smith PD, Maibach HI (1967) Genetic factors in human allergic contact dermatitis. Int Arch Allergy Appl Immunol 32:453–462
9. Menne T, Holm NV (1983) Nickel allergy in a female twin population. Int J Dermatol 22:22–28
10. Forsbeck M, Skog E, Ytterborn KH (1971) Allergig diseases among relatives of patients with allergic contact dermatitis. Acta Derm Venereol (Stockh) 51:123–128
11. Fleming CJ, Burden AD, Forsyth A (1999) The genetics of allergic contact hypersensitivity to nickel. Contact Dermat 41:251–253
12. Forsbeck M, Skog E, Ytterborn KH (1968) Delayed type of allergy and atopic disease among twins. Acta Derm Venereol (Stockh) 48:192–197
13. Bryld LE, Hindsberger C, Kyvik KO, Agner T, Menne T (2004) Genetic factors in nickel allergy evaluated in a population- based female twin sample. J Invest Dermatol 123: 1025–1029
14. Bataille V (2004) Genetic factors in nickel allergy. J Invest Dermatol 123:xxiv–xxv
15. Bataille V (1999) The role of twin studies in the genetics of skin diseases. Clin Exp Dermatol 24:286–290
16. Holdsworth R, Hurley CK, Marsh SGE, Lau M, Noreen HJ, Kempenich JH, Setterholm M, Maiers M (2009) The HLA dictionary 2008: a summary of HLA-A,-B,-C, DRB1/3/4/5, and DQB1 alleles and their association with serologically defined HLA-A, -B, -C, -DR, and -DQ antigens. Tissue Antigens 73:95–170
17. Fernando MM, Stevens CR, Walsh EC, DeJager PL, Goyette P, Plenge RM, Vyse TJ, Rioux JD (2008) Defining the role of the MHC in autoimmunity: a review and pooled analysis. PLoS Genet 4(4):e100024.doi:10.1371/journal.pgen.000024
18. Ishii N, Ishii H, Ono H, Horiuchi Y, Nkajima H, Aoki I (1990) Genetic control of nickel sulfate delayed-type hypersensitivity. J Invest Dermatol 94:673–676
19. Ishii N, Ishii H, Nakajima H, Aoki I, Shimoda N (1991) Contact sensitivity to mercuric chloride is associated with I-A region in mice. J Dermatol Sci 2:268–273
20. Ishii N, Takahashi K, Kawaguchi H, Nakajima H, Tanaka S, Aoki I (1993) Genetic control of delayed-type hypersensitivity to chromium chloride. Int Arch Allergy Immunol 100:333–337
21. Ishii N, Takahashi K, Ishiwa M, Sugita Y, Nakajima H (1998) Genetic control of delayed-type hypersensitivity to gold antigens in mice. J Dermatol Sci 16:104–110
22. Okuda K, Ishii N, Ikezawa Z, Tani K, Ishigatsubo Y (1980) Genetic control of contact hypersensitivity. I. I-A subregion

as well as non-H-2 loci codes for the gene of 2, 4-dinitro-1-fluorobenzene antigen. Eur J Immunol 10:969–971

23. Kato H, Hayashi M, Fukumori Y, Kaneko H (2002) MHC restriction in contact hypersensitivity to dicyclohexylcarbodiimide. Food Chem Toxicol 40:1713–1718

24. Emtestam L, Zetterquist H, Olerup O (1993) HLA-DR, -DQ and -DP alleles in nickel, chromium, and/or cobalt-sensitive individuals: genomic analysis based on restriction fragment length polymorphisms. J Invest Dermatol 100:271–274

25. Walton S, Keczkes K, Learoyd PA, Rajah SM (1986) HLA-A, -B and DR antigens in nickel sensitive females. Clin Exp Dermatol 11:636–640

26. Önder M, Aksakal B, Gulekon A, Makki S, Gurer MA, Barut A (1995) HLA DR, DQA, DQB and DP antigens in patients allergic to nickel. Contact Dermat 33:434–435

27. Silvennoinen-Kassinen S, Ikäheimo I, Tiilikainen A (1997) TAP1 and TAP2 genes in nickel allergy. Int Arch Allergy Immunol 114:94–96

28. Orecchia G, Perfetti L, Finco O, Dondi E, Cuccia M (1992) Polymorphisms of HLA class III genes in allergic contact dermatitis. Dermatology 184:254–259

29. Moulon C, Wild D, Dormoy A, Weltzien HU (1998) MHC-dependent and -independent activation of human nickel-specific CD8+ cytotoxic T cells from allergic donors. J Invest Dermatol 111:360–366

30. Gamerdinger K, Moulon C, Karp DR, VanBergen J, Koning F, Wild D, Pflugfelder U, Weltzien HU (2003) A new type of metal recognition by human T cells: contact residues for peptide- independent bridging of T cell receptor and major histocompatibility complex by nickel. J Exp Med 197:1345–1353

31. Valsecchi R, Bontempelli M, Vicari O, Scudeller G, Cainelli T (1981) HLA antigens and contact sensitivity to para group. Ital Gen Rev Dermatol 18:99–103

32. White SI, Friedmann PS, Stratton A (1986) HLA antigens and Langerhans cell density in contact dermatitis. Br J Dermatol 115:447–452

33. Hegyi E, Busova B, Niks M (1990) HLA-A and -B antigens in IPPD- sensitive persons. Contact Dermat 22:228–229

34. Wilkinson SM, Morrey K, Hollowood K, Heagerty AH, English JS (1993) HLA-A, -B and -DR antigens in hydro-cortisone contact hypersensitivity. Contact Dermat 28: 295–297

35. Friedmann PS (1991) Graded continuity, or all or none-studies of the human immune response. Clin Exp Dermatol 16:79–84

36. Moss C, Friedmann PS, Shuster S, Simpson JM (1985) Susceptibility and amplification of sensitivity in contact dermatitis. Clin Exp Immunol 61:232–241

37. Carlsen BC, Menné T, Johansen JD (2007) 20 years of standard patch testing in an eczema population with focus on patients with multiple contact allergies. Contact Dermat 57:76–83

38. Thyssen JP, Linneberg A, Menné T, Nielsen NH, Johansen JD (2009) Contact allergy to allergens of the TRUE test (panels 1 and 2) has decreased modestly in the general population. Br J Dermatol 161:1124–1129

39. Jorde LB, Carey JC, Bamshad MJ, White RL (2006) Medical genetics, 3rd edn. Aufl, Mosby, St. Louis

40. Reich K, Huffmeier U, Konig IR, Lascorz J, Lohmann J, Wendler J, Traupe H, Mossner R, Reis A, Burkhardt H (2007) TNF polymorphisms in psoriasis: association of

psoriatic arthritis with the promoter polymorphism TNF*-857 independent of the PSORS1 risk allele. Arthritis Rheum 56:2056–2064

41. Schnuch A, Westphal GA, Müller MM, Schulz TG, Geier J, Brasch J, Merk HF, Kawakubo Y, Richter G, Koch P, Fuchs Th, Gutgesell C, Reich K, Gebhardt M, Becker D, Grabbe J, Szliska C, Lischka G, Aberer W, Hallier E (1998) Genotype and phenotype of N-acetyltransferase 2 (NAT2) polymorphism in patients with contact allergy. Contact Dermat 38:209–211

42. Westphal GA, Reich K, Schulz TG, Neumann C, Hallier E, Schnuch A (2000) N-Acetyltransferases 1 and 2 polymor-phisms in para-substituted arylamine-induced contact allergy. Br J Dermatol 142:1121–1127

43. Westphal G-A, Schnuch A, Schulz T-G, Reich K, Aberer W, Brasch J, Koch P, Wessbecher R, Szliska C, Bauer A, Hallier E (2000) Homozygous gene deletions of the glutathione S-transferases M1 and T1 are associated with thimerosal sensitization. Int Arch Occup Environ Health 73:384–388

44. Westphal G-A, Schnuch A, Moessner R, Koenig IR, Kränke B, Hallier E, Ziegler A, Reich K (2003) Cytokine gene poly-morphisms in allergic contact dermatitis. Contact Dermat 48:93–98

45. Reich K, Westphal G, König IR, Mössner R, Krüger U, Ziegler A, Neumann C, Schnuch A (2003) Association of allergic contact dermatitis with a promoter polymorphism in the IL16 gene. J All Clin Immunol 112:1191–1194

46. Rustemeyer T, van-Hoogstraten IMW, von-Blomberg BME, Scheper RJ (2006) Mechanisms in allergic contact dermati-tis. In: Frosch PJ, Menné T, Lepoittevin J-P (eds) Contact dermatitis, 4th edn. Aufl, Springer, Berlin, pp S11–S43

47. Smith CK, Hotchkiss SAM (2001) Allergic contact dermati-tis. Chemical and metabolic mechanisms. Taylor & Francis, London

48. Schnuch A, Uter W, Reich K (2005) Allergic contact derma-titis and atopic eczema. In: Ring J, Przybilla B, Ruzicka T (Hrsg) Handbook of atopic eczema, Kapit. 17, 2nd Aufl. Springer, Berlin, pp S176–S199

49. Wormhoudt LW, Commandeur JNM, Vermeulen NPE (1999) Genetic polymorphisms of human N-acetyltrans-ferase, cytochrome p450, glutathione-S-transferase, and epoxide hydrolase enzymes. relevance to xenobiotic metab-olism and toxicity. Crit Rev Toxicol 29:59–124

50. Thier R, Bruning T, Roos PH, Rihs HP, Golka K, Ko Y, Bolt HM (2003) Markers of genetic susceptibility in human envi-ronmental hygiene and toxicology: the role of selected CYP, NAT and GST genes. Int J Hyg Environ Health 206:149–171

51. Toebak MJ, Gibbs S, Bruynzeel DP, Scheper RJ, Rustemeyer T (2009) Dendritic cells: biology of the skin. Contact Dermat 60:2–20

52. Jacobs JJ, Lehe CL, Hasegawa H, Elliott GR, Das PK (2006) Skin irritants and contact sensitizers induce Langerhans cell migration and maturation at irritant concentration. Exp Dermatol 15:432–440

53. Martin SF, Dudda JC, Bachtanian E, Lembo A, Liller S, Durr C, Heimesaat MM, Bereswill S, Fejer G, Vassileva R, Jakob T, Freudenberg N, Termeer CC, Johner C, Galanos C, Freudenberg MA (2008) Toll-like receptor and IL-12 signal-ing control susceptibility to contact hypersensitivity. J Exp Med 205:2151–2162

54. Zepter K, Häffner A, Soohoo LF, De-Luca D, Tang HP, Fisher P, Chavinson J, Elmets CA (1997) Induction of biologically active IL-1-beta-converting enzyme and mature IL-1 beta in human keratinocytes by inflammatory and immunologic stimuli. J Immunol 159:6203–6208

55. Yazdi AS, Ghoreschi K, Rocken M (2007) Inflammasome activation in delayed-type hypersensitivity reactions. J Invest Dermatol 127:1853–1855

56. Grabbe S, Steinert M, Mahnke K, Schwartz A, Luger TA, Schwarz T (1996) Dissection of antigenic and irritative effects of epicutaneously applied haptens in mice. Evidence that not the antigenic component but nonspecific proinflammatory effects of haptens determine the concentration-dependent elicitation of allergic contact dermatitis. J Clin Invest 98:1158–1164

57. Bonneville M, Chavagnac C, Vocanson M, Rozieres A, Benetiere J, Pernet I, Denis A, Nicolas JF, Hennino A (2007) Skin contact irritation conditions the development and severity of allergic contact dermatitis. J Invest Dermatol 127:1430–1435

58. Pedersen LK, Johansen JD, Held E, Agner T (2004) Augmentation of skin response by exposure to a combination of allergens and irritants – a review. Contact Dermat 50:265–273

59. Smith HR, Basketter DA, McFadden JP (2002) Irritant dermatitis, irritancy and its role in allergic contact dermatitis. Clin Exp Dermatol 27:138–146

60. Clark IA (2007) How TNF was recognized as a key mechanism of disease. Cytokine Growth Factor Rev 18:335–343

61. Bradley JR (2008) TNF-mediated inflammatory disease. J Pathol 214:149–160

62. Tracey D, Klareskog L, Sasso EH, Salfeld JG, Tak PP (2008) Tumor necrosis factor antagonist mechanisms of action: a comprehensive review. Pharmacol Ther 117:244–279

63. Bayley JP, Ottenhoff TH, Verweij CL (2004) Is there a future for TNF promoter polymorphisms? Genes Immun 5:315–329

64. Blömeke B, Brans R, Dickel H, Bruckner T, Erdmann S, Heesen M, Merk HF, Coenraads PJ (2009) Association between TNFA-308 G/A polymorphism and sensitization to paraphenylenediamine: a case-control study. Allergy 64:279–283

65. Wang BJ, Shiao JS, Chen CJ, Lee YC, Guo YL (2007) Tumour necrotizing factor-alpha promoter and GST-T1 genotype predict skin allergy to chromate in cement workers in Taiwan. Contact Dermat 57:309–315

66. Moraes MO, Duppre NC, Suffys PN, Santos AR, Almeida AS, Nery JAC, Sampaio EP, Sarno EN (2001) Tumor necrosis factor-alpha promoter polymorphism TNF2 is associated with a stronger delayed-type hypersensitivity reaction in the skin of borderline tuberculoid leprosy patients. Immunogenetics 53:45–47

67. Allen MH, Wakelin SH, Holloway D, Lisby S, Baadsgaard O, Barker JNWN, McFadden JP (2000) Association of TNFA gene polymorphism at position -308 with susceptibility to irritant contact dermatitis. Immunogenetics 51:201–205

68. deJongh CM, John SM, Bruynzeel DP, Calkoen F, vanDijk FJ, Khrenova L, Rustemeyer T, Verberk MM, Kezic S (2008) Cytokine gene polymorphisms and susceptibility to chronic irritant contact dermatitis. Contact Dermat 58:269–277

69. Taudorf S, Krabbe KS, Berg RM, Moller K, Pedersen BK, Bruunsgaard H (2008) Common studied polymorphisms do not affect plasma cytokine levels upon endotoxin exposure in humans. Clin Exp Immunol 152:147–152

70. Kroeger KM, Steer JH, Joyce DA, Abraham LJ (2000) Effects of stimulus and cell type on the expression of the -308 tumour necrosis factor promoter polymorphism. Cytokine 12:110–119

71. Heesen M, Kunz D, Bachmann-Mennenga B, Merk HF, Bloemeke B (2003) Linkage disequilibrium between tumor necrosis factor (TNF)-alpha-308 G/A promoter and TNF-beta NcoI polymorphisms: association with TNF-alpha response of granulocytes to endotoxin stimulation. Crit Care Med 31:211–214

72. Stenzel A, Lu T, Koch WA, Hampe J, Guenther SM, DeLaVega FM, Krawczak M, Schreiber S (2004) Patterns of linkage disequilibrium in the MHC region on human chromosome 6p. Hum Genet 114:377–385

73. Lio D, Candore G, Romano GC, D'Anna C, Gervasi F, DiLorenzo G, Modica MA, Potestio M, Caruso C (1997) Modification of cytokine patterns in subjects bearing the HLA-B8, DR3 phenotype: implications for autoimmunity. Cytokines Cell Mol Ther 3:217–224

74. Glass WG, Sarisky RT, Vecchio AM (2006) Not-so-sweet sixteen: the role of IL-16 in infectious and immune-mediated inflammatory diseases. J Interferon Cytokine Res 26:511–520

75. Cruikshank WW, Kornfeld H, Center DM (2000) Interleukin-16. J Leukoc Biol 67:757–766

76. Laberge S, Ghaffar O, Boguniewicz M, Center DM, Leung DY, Hamid Q (1998) Association of increased CD4+ T-cell infiltration with increased IL-16 gene expression in atopic dermatitis. J Allergy Clin Immunol 102:645–650

77. Yoshimoto T, Wang CR, Yoneto T, Matsuzawa A, Cruikshank WW, Nariuchi H (2000) Role of IL-16 in delayed-type hypersensitivity reaction. Blood 95:2869–2874

78. Masuda K, Katoh N, Soga F, Kishimoto S (2005) The role of interleukin-16 in murine contact hypersensitivity. Clin Exp Immunol 140:213–219

79. Stoitzner P, Ratzinger G, Koch F, Janke K, Schöller T, Kaser A, Tilg H, Cruikshank WW, Fritsch P, Romani N (2001) Interleukin-16 supports the migration of Langerhans cells, partly in a CD4-independent way. J Invest Dermatol 116:641–649

80. Glas J, Torok HP, Unterhuber H, Radlmayr M, Folwaczny C (2003) The -295T-to-C promoter polymorphism of the IL-16 gene is associated with Crohn's disease. Clin Immunol 106:197–200

81. Reich K, Westphal G, Konig IR, Mossner R, Schupp P, Gutgesell C, Hallier E, Ziegler A, Neumann C (2003) Cytokine gene polymorphisms in atopic dermatitis. Br J Dermatol 148:1237–1241

82. Burkart KM, Barton SJ, Holloway JW, Yang IA, Cakebread JA, Cruikshank W, Little F, Jin X, Farrer LA, Clough JB, Keith TP, Holgate S, Center DM, O'Connor GT (2006) Association of asthma with a functional promoter polymorphism in the IL16 gene. J Allergy Clin Immunol 117:86–91

83. Akesson LS, Duffy DL, Phelps SC, Thompson PJ, Kedda MA (2005) A polymorphism in the promoter region of the human interleukin- 16 gene is not associated with asthma or atopy in an Australian population. Clin Exp Allergy 35:327–331

84. Folwaczny M, Glas J, Torok HP, Tonenchi L, Paschos E, Malachova O, Bauer B, Folwaczny C (2005) Prevalence of the

-295 T-to-C promoter polymorphism of the interleukin (IL)-16 gene in periodontitis. Clin Exp Immunol 142:188–192

85. Grant DM, Goodfellow GH, Sugamori KS, Durette K (2000) Pharmacogenetics of the human arylamine *N*-acetyltransferases. Pharmacology 61:204–211

86. Agundez JA (2008) Polymorphisms of human *N*-acetyltransferases and cancer risk. Curr Drug Metab 9:520–531

87. Kawakubo Y, Merk HF, Masaoudi TA, Sieben S, Blomeke B (2000) *N*-Acetylation of paraphenylenediamine in human skin and keratinocytes. J Pharmacol Exp Ther 292:150–155

88. Krasteva M, Nicolas J-F, Chabeau G, Garrigue J-L, Bour H, Thivolet J, Schmitt D (1993) Dissociation of allergenic and immunogenic functions in contact sensitivity to paraphenylenediamine. Int Arch Allergy Immunol 102:200–204

89. Lisi P, Hansel K (1998) Is benzoquinone the prohapten in cross – sensitivity among aminobenzene compounds? Contact Dermat 39:304–306

90. White JM, Kullavanijaya P, Duangdeeden I, Zazzeroni R, Gilmour NJ, Basketter DA, McFadden JP (2006) p-Phenylenediamine allergy: the role of Bandrowski's base. Clin Exp Allergy 36:1289–1293

91. Goebel C, Hewitt NJ, Kunze G, Wenker M, Hein DW, Beck H, Skare J (2009) Skin metabolism of aminophenols: Human keratinocytes as a suitable in vitro model to qualitatively predict the dermal transformation of 4-amino-2-hydroxytoluene in vivo. Toxicol Appl Pharmacol 235: 114–123

92. Aeby P, Sieber T, Beck H, Gerberick GF, Goebel C (2009) Skin sensitization to p-phenylenediamine: the diverging roles of oxidation and *N*-acetylation for dendritic cell activation and the immune response. J Invest Dermatol 129:99–109

93. Sieben S, Kawakubo Y, Al Masaoudi T, Merk HF, Blomeke B (2002) Delayed-type hypersensitivity reaction to paraphenylenediamine is mediated by 2 different pathways of antigen recognition by specific alphabeta human T-cell clones. J Allergy Clin Immunol 109:1005–1011

94. Coulter EM, Jenkinson C, Wu Y, Farrell J, Foster B, Smith A, McGuire C, Pease C, Basketter D, King C, Friedmann PS, Pirmohamed M, Park BK, Naisbitt DJ (2008) Activation of T-cells from allergic patients and volunteers by p-phenylenediamine and Bandrowski's base. J Invest Dermatol 128:897–905

95. Ladero JM (2008) Influence of polymorphic *N*-acetyltransferases on non-malignant spontaneous disorders and on response to drugs. Curr Drug Metab 9:532–537

96. Orzechowska-Juzwenko K, Milejski P, Patkowski J, Nittner-Marszalska M, Malolepszy J (1990) Acetylator phenotype in patients with allergic diseases and its clinical significance. Int J Clin Pharmacol Therap Toxicol 28:420–425

97. Kosmadakis G, Bulovskaya L, Rudinski K, Lintsov A (1996) Acetylator phenotype in patients with bronchial asthma. Eur J All Clin Immunol 51(30 Suppl):70

98. Zielinska E, Niewiarowski W, Bodalski J, Stanczyk A, Bolanowski W, Rebowski G (1997) Arylamine *N*-acetyltransferase (NAT2) gene mutations in children with allergic diseases. Clin Pharmacol Ther 62:635–642

99. Gawronska-Szklarz B, Luszawska-Kutrzeba T, Czaja-Bulsa G, Kurzawski G (1999) Relationship between acetylation polymorphism and risk of atopic diseases. Clin Pharmacol Ther 65:562–569

100. Brocvielle H, Muret P, Goydadin A-C, Boone P, Broly F, Kantelip J-P, Humbert P (2003) *N*-Acetyltransferase 2 acetylation polymorphism: prevalence of slow acetylators does not differ between atopic dermatitis patients and healthy subjects. Skin Pharmacol Appl Skin Physiol 16:386–392

101. Olszewska Z, Jablkowska-Gajdzinska J, Majewska E (1984) Acetylation phenotype in patients with eczema. Prezeg Dermatol LXXI:213–214

102. Kawakubo Y, Nakamori M, Schoepf E, Ohkido M (1995) Acetylator phenotyping in patients with p-phenylenediamine (PPD) allergy. Skin Pharmacol 8(11):273

103. Kawakubo Y, Nakamori M, Schöpf E, Ohkido M (1997) Acetylator phenotype in patients with p-phenylenediamine allergy. Dermatology 195:43–45

104. Nacak M, Erbagci Z, Aynacioglu AS (2006) Human arylamine *N*-acetyltransferase 2 polymorphism and susceptibility to allergic contact dermatitis. Int J Dermatol 45: 323–326

105. Najim RA, Al-waizt M, Al-Razzuqi RA (2005) Acetylator phenotype in Iraqi patients with allergic contact dermatitis. Ann Saudi Med 25:473–476

106. Butcher NJ, Ilett KF, Minchin RF (2000) Inactivation of human arylamine *N*-acetyltransferase 1 by the hydroxylamine of p- aminobenzoic acid. Biochem Pharmacol 60:1829–1836

107. Butcher NJ, Ilett KF, Minchin RF (2000) Substrate-dependent regulation of human arylamine *N*-acetyltransferase-1 in cultured cells. Mol Pharmacol 57:468–473

108. Gillam EMJ (2001) The dark side of a 'detoxification' mechanism. Trends Pharmacol Sci 22:11

109. Bolt HM, Thier R (2006) Relevance of the deletion polymorphisms of the glutathione *S*-transferases GSTT1 and GSTM1 in pharmacology and toxicology. Curr Drug Metab 7:613–628

110. Hayes JD, Flanagan JU, Jowsey IR (2005) Glutathione transferases. Annu Rev Pharmacol Toxicol 45:51–88

111. Ates NA, Tursen U, Tamer L, Kanik A, Derici E, Ercan B, Atik U (2004) Glutathione *S*-transferase polymorphisms in patients with drug eruption. Arch Dermatol Res 295:429–433

112. Brasch-Andersen C, Christiansen L, Tan Q, Haagerup A, Vestbo J, Kruse TA (2004) Possible gene dosage effect of glutathione- *S*-transferases on atopic asthma: using real-time PCR for quantification of GSTM1 and GSTT1 gene copy numbers. Hum Mutat 24:208–214

113. Holla LI, Stejskalova A, Vasku A (2006) Polymorphisms of the GSTM1 and GSTT1 genes in patients with allergic diseases in the Czech population. Allergy 61:265–267

114. Lira MG, Provezza L, Malerba G, Naldi L, Remuzzi G, Boschiero L, Forni A, Rugiu C, Piaserico S, Alaibac M, Turco A, Girolomoni G, Tessari G (2006) Glutathione *S*-transferase and CYP1A1 gene polymorphisms and non-melanoma skin cancer risk in Italian transplanted patients. Exp Dermatol 15:958–965

115. Bohets HH, Van Thielen MN, VanderBiest I, Van Landeghem GF, D'Haese PC, Nouwen EJ, DeBroe ME, Dierickx PJ (1995) Cytotoxicity of mercury compounds in LLC-PK1, MDCK and human proximal tubular cells. Kidney Int 47:395–403

116. Almar MM, Dierickx PJ (1990) In vitro interaction of mercury, copper (II) and cadmium with human glutathione transferase pi. Res Commun Chem Pathol Pharmacol 69:99–102

117. Santucci B, Cannistraci C, Cristaudo A, Camera E, Picardo M (1998) Thimerosal positivities: the role of SH groups and divalent ions. Contact Dermat 39:123–126
118. Picardo M, Zompetta C, Marchese C, de Luca C, Faggioni A, Schmidt RJ, Santucci B (1992) Paraphenylenediamine, a contact allergen, induces oxidative stress and ICAM-1 expression in human keratinocytes. Br J Dermatol 126: 450–455
119. Valko M, Morris H, Cronin MT (2005) Metals, toxicity and oxidative stress. Curr Med Chem 12:1161–1208
120. Kaur S, Zilmer M, Eisen M, Rehema A, Kullisaar T, Vihalemm T, Zilmer K (2004) Nickel sulphate and epoxy resin: differences in iron status and glutathione redox ratio at the time of patch testing. Arch Dermatol Res 295:517–520
121. Rutault K, Alderman C, Chain BM, Katz DR (1999) Reactive oxygen species activate human peripheral blood dendritic cells. Free Radic Biol Med 26:232–238
122. Young CN, Koepke JI, Terlecky LJ, Borkin MS, Boyd SL, Terlecky SR (2008) Reactive oxygen species in tumor necrosis factor-alpha-activated primary human keratinocytes: implications for psoriasis and inflammatory skin disease. J Invest Dermatol 128:2606–2614
123. Mizuashi M, Ohtani T, Nakagawa S, Aiba S (2005) Redox imbalance induced by contact sensitizers triggers the maturation of dendritic cells. J Invest Dermatol 124: 579–586
124. Bruchhausen S, Zahn S, Valk E, Knop J, Becker D (2003) Thiol antioxidants block the activation of antigen-presenting cells by contact sensitizers. J Invest Dermatol 121: 1039–1044
125. Kalergis AM, Lopez CB, Becker MI, Diaz MI, Sein J, Garbarino JA, De Ioannes AE (1997) Modulation of fatty acid oxidation alters contact hypersensitivity to urushiols: role of aliphatic chain beta-oxidation in processing and activation of urushiols. J Invest Dermatol 108:57–61
126. Christensson JB, Matura M, Backtorp C, Borje A, Nilsson JL, Karlberg AT (2006) Hydroperoxides form specific antigens in contact allergy. Contact Dermat 55:230–237
127. Bag A, Bag N (2008) Target sequence polymorphism of human manganese superoxide dismutase gene and its association with cancer risk: a review. Cancer Epidemiol Biomark Prev 17:3298–3305
128. Yen JH, Chen CJ, Tsai WC, Lin CH, Ou TT, Hu CJ, Liu HW (2003) Manganese superoxide dismutase and cytochrome P450 1A1 genes polymorphisms in rheumatoid arthritis in Taiwan. Hum Immunol 64:366–373
129. Mak JC, Leung HC, Ho SP, Ko FW, Cheung AH, Ip MS, Chan-Yeung MM (2006) Polymorphisms in manganese superoxide dismutase and catalase genes: functional study in Hong Kong Chinese asthma patients. Clin Exp Allergy 36:440–447
130. Brans R, Dickel H, Bruckner T, Coenraads PJ, Heesen M, Merk HF, Blomeke B (2005) MnSOD polymorphisms in sensitized patients with delayed-type hypersensitivity reactions to the chemical allergen para-phenylene diamine: a case-control study. Toxicology 212:148–154
131. Scholzen TE, König S, Fastrich M, Bohm M, Luger TA (2007) Terminating the stress: peripheral peptidolysis of proopiomelanocortin-derived regulatory hormones by the dermal microvascular endothelial cell extracellular

peptidases neprilysin and angiotensin-converting enzyme. Endocrinology 148:2793–2805
132. Scholzen T, Armstrong CA, Bunnett NW, Luger TA, Olerud JE, Ansel JC (1998) Neuropeptides in the skin: interactions between the neuroendocrine and the skin immune systems. Exp Dermatol 7:81–96
133. Scholzen TE, Stander S, Riemann H, Brzoska T, Luger TA (2003) Modulation of cutaneous inflammation by angiotensin-converting enzyme. J Immunol 170:3866–3873
134. Rigat B, Hubert C, Alhenc-Gelas F, Cambien F, Corvol P, Soubrier F (1990) An insertion/deletion polymorphism in the angiotensin I-converting enzyme gene accounting for half the variance of serum enzyme levels. J Clin Invest 86:1343–1346
135. Nacak M, Erbagci Z, Buyukafsar K, Yurtsever AS, Tiftik RN (2007) Association of angiotensin-converting enzyme gene insertion/deletion polymorphism with allergic contact dermatitis. Basic Clin Pharmacol Toxicol 101:101–103
136. Masek K, Slansky J, Petrovicky P, Hadden JW (2003) Neuroendocrine immune interactions in health and disease. Int Immunopharmacol 3:1235–1246
137. Hendrix S (2008) Neuroimmune communication in skin: far from peripheral. J Invest Dermatol 128:260–261
138. Frazer KA, Murray SS, Schork NJ, Topol EJ (2009) Human genetic variation and its contribution to complex traits. Nat Rev Genet 10:241–251
139. Brown SJ, McLean WHI (2009) Eczema genetics: current state of knowledge and future goals. J Invest Dermatol 129:543–552
140. Sandilands A, Smith FJ, Irvine AD, McLean WH (2007) Filaggrin's fuller figure: a glimpse into the genetic architecture of atopic dermatitis. J Invest Dermatol 127:1282–1284
141. Kezic S, Kemperman PM, Koster ES, deJongh CM, Thio HB, Campbell LE, Irvine AD, McLean WHI, Puppels GJ, Caspers PJ (2008) Loss-of-function muations in the filaggrin gene lead to reduced level of natural moisterizing factor in the stratum corneum. J Invest Dermatol 128:2117–2119
142. Irvine AD, McLean WH (2006) Breaking the (un)sound barrier: filaggrin is a major gene for atopic dermatitis. J Invest Dermatol 126:1200–1202
143. O'Regan GM, Sandilands A, McLean WH, Irvine AD (2008) Filaggrin in atopic dermatitis. J Allergy Clin Immunol 122:689–693
144. Brown SJ, Relton CL, Liao H, Zhao Y, Sandilands A, Wilson IJ, Burn J, ReynoldsNJ, McLean WH, Cordell HJ (2008) Filaggrin null mutations and childhood atopic eczema: a population-based case-control study. J Allergy Clin Immunol 121:940–946.e3
145. Weidinger S, O'Sullivan M, Illig T, Baurecht H, Depner M, Rodriguez E, Ruether A, Klopp N, Vogelberg C, Weiland SK, McLean WH, von Mutius E, Irvine AD, Kabesch M (2008) Filaggrin mutations, atopic eczema, hay fever, and asthma in children. J Allergy Clin Immunol 121: 1203–1209.e1
146. Baurecht H, Irvine AD, Novak N, Illig T, Buhler B, Ring J, Wagenpfeil S, Weidinger S (2007) Toward a major risk factor for atopic eczema: meta-analysis of filaggrin polymorphism data. J Allergy Clin Immunol 120:1406–1412
147. Nemoto-Hasebe I, Akiyama M, Nomura T, Sandilands A, McLean WH, Shimizu H (2009) Clinical severity correlates

with impaired barrier in filaggrin-related eczema. J Invest Dermatol 129:632–639

148. de Jongh CM, Khrenova L, Verberk MM, Calkoen F, van Dijk FJ, Voss H, John SM, Kezic S (2008) Loss-of-function polymorphisms in the filaggrin gene are associated with an increased susceptibility to chronic irritant contact dermatitis: a case- control study. Br J Dermatol 159:621–627

149. Lerbaek A, Bisgaard H, Agner T, Ohm-Kyvik K, Palmer CN, Menne T (2007) Filaggrin null alleles are not associated with hand eczema or contact allergy. Br J Dermatol 157:1199–1204

150. Brown SJ, Cordell HJ (2008) Are filaggrin mutations associated with hand eczema or contact allergy?–we do not know. Br J Dermatol 158:1383–1384

151. Weidinger S, Rodriguez E, Stahl C, Wagenpfeil S, Klopp N, Illig T, Novak N (2007) Filaggrin mutations strongly predispose to early-onset and extrinsic atopic dermatitis. J Invest Dermatol 127:724–726

152. Novak N, Baurecht H, Schäfer T, Rodriguez E, Wagenpfeil S, Klopp N, Heinrich J, Behrendt H, Ring J, Wichmann E, Illig T, Weidinger S (2008) Loss-of-function mutations in the filaggrin gene and allergic contact sensitization to nickel. J Invest Dermatol 128:1430–1435

153. Nielsen NH, Menne T (1992) Allergic contact sensitization in an unselected danish population – the Glostrup allergy study, Denmark. Acta Derm Venereol (Stockh) 72: 456–460

154. Nielsen NH, Linneberg A, Menne T, Maden F, Frolund L, Dirksen A, Jorgensen T (2001) Allergic contact sensitization in an adult Danish population: two cross-sectional surveys eight years apart (The Copenhagen Allergy Study). Acta Derm Venereol 81:31–34

155. Schnuch A, Uter W, Geier J, Gefeller O (2002) Epidemiology of contact allergy: an estimation of morbidity employing the clinical epidemiology and drug utilisation research (CE-DUR) approach. Contact Dermat 47:32–39

156. Uter W, Ludwig A, Balda B-R, Schnuch A, Pfahlberg A, Schäfer T, Wichmann H-E, Ring J (2004) The prevalence of contact allergy differed between population-based and clinic-based data. J Clin Epidemiol 57:627–632

157. Schnuch A, Geier J, Uter W, Frosch PJ, Lehmacher W, Aberer W, Agathos M, Arnold R, Fuchs T, Laubstein B, Lischka G, Pietrzyk PM, Rakoski J, Richter G, Rueff F (1997) National rates and regional differences in sensitization to allergens of the standard series. Population adjusted frequencies of sensitization (PAFS) in 40.000 patients from a multicenter study (IVDK). Contact Dermat 37:200–209

158. Schnuch A, Lessmann H, Geier J, Frosch PJ, Uter W (2004) Contact allergy to fragrances: frequencies of sensitization from 1996 to 2002. Results of the IVDK. Contact Dermat 50:65–76

159. Hayes JD, Strange RC (2000) Glutathione S-transferase polymorphisms and their biological consequences. Pharmacology 61:154–166

160. Cumberbatch M, Dearman RJ, Kimber I (1997) Langerhans cells require signals from both tumour necrosis factor-alpha and interleukin-1 beta for migration. Immunology 92: 388–395

161. Bartee E, Mohamed MR, McFadden G (2008) Tumor necrosis factor and interferon: cytokines in harmony. Curr Opin Microbiol 11:378–383

162. Reich K, Westphal G, Schulz T, Müller M, Zipprich S, Fuchs T, Hallier E, Neumann C (1999) Evidence for a synergistic effect of polymorphisms of N-actetyltransferase 2 and TNF- alpha promoter as susceptibility factors for psoriasis in males. J Invest Dermatol 113:214–220

163. Balding DJ (2006) A tutorial on statistical methods for population association studies. Nat Rev Genet 7:781–791

164. Manolio TA, Brooks LD, Collins FS (2008) A HapMap harvest of insights into the genetics of common disease. J Clin Invest 118:1590–1605

165. Wallace HJ, Vandongen YK, Stacey MC (2006) Tumor necrosis factor-alpha gene polymorphism associated with increased susceptibility to venous leg ulceration. J Invest Dermatol 126:921–925

166. Willis CM (2002) Variability in responsiveness to irritants: thoughts on possible underlying mechanisms. Contact Dermat 47:267–271

167. Uter W, Geier J, Pfahlberg A, Effendy I (2002) The spectrum of contact allergy in elderly patients with and without lower leg dermatitis. Dermatology 204:266–272

168. Descotes J (1988) Immunotoxicology of drugs and chemicals. Elsevier, Amsterdam, New York, Oxford

169. Elliott JC, Picker MJ, Nelson CJ, Carrigan KA, Lysle DT (2003) Sex differences in opioid-induced enhancement of contact hypersensitivity. J Invest Dermatol 121:1053–1059

170. Uter W, Hegewald J, Kranke B, Schnuch A, Gefeller O, Pfahlberg A (2008) The impact of meteorological conditions on patch test results with 12 standard series allergens (fragrances, biocides, topical ingredients). Br J Dermatol 158:734–739

171. Saint-Mezard P, Chavagnac C, Bosset S, Ionescu M, Peyron E, Kaiserlian D, Nicolas JF, Berard F (2003) Psychological stress exerts an adjuvant effect on skin dendritic cell functions in vivo. J Immunol 171:4073–4080

172. Choi EH, Brown BE, Crumrine D, Chang S, Man MQ, Elias PM, Feingold KR (2005) Mechanisms by which psychologic stress alters cutaneous permeability barrier homeostasis and stratum corneum integrity. J Invest Dermatol 124:587–595

173. Lübbe D, Fiedler H (1991) Experimentelle DNCB-Kontaktallergie, eine 10-Jahresstudie bei 137 Probanden. Z Hautkr 66:954–956

174. Rees JL, Friedmann PS, Matthews JNS (1989) Sex differences in susceptibility to development of contact hypersensitivity to dinitrochlorobenzene (DNCB). Br J Dermatol 120:371–374

175. Kwangsukstith C, Maibach HI (1995) Effect of age and sex on the induction and elicitation of allergic contact dermatitis. Contact Dermat 33:289–298

176. Kligman AM (1966) The identification of contact allergens by human assay: II. Factors influencing the induction and measurement of allergic contact dermatitis. J Invest Dermatol 47:375–391

177. DeLeo VA, Taylor S, Belsito DV, Fowler JF Jr, Fransway AF, Maibach HI, Marks JG Jr, Mathias T, Nethercott J, Pratt MD, Rietschel RL, Sherertz EF, Storrs FJ, Taylor J (2000) North American Contact Dermatitis Group patch test results: ethnic differences. Am J Contact Derm 11:197

178. Dickel H, Taylor JS, Evey P, Merk HF (2001) Comparison of patch test results with a standard series among white and black racial groups. Am J Contact Derm 12:77–82

179. Chase MW (1941) Inheritance in Guinea pigs of the susceptibility to skin sensitization with simple chemical compounds. J Exp Med 73:711–726
180. Polak L, Barnes M, Turk JL (1968) The genetic control of contact densitization to inorganic metal compounds in guinea pigs. Immunology 14:707–711
181. Asherson GL, Dieli F, Gautam Y, Siew LK, Zembala M (1990) Major histocompatibility complex regulation of the class of the immune response: the H-2d haplotype determines poor interferon-gamma response to several antigens. Eur J Immunol 20:1305–1310

Irritant Contact Dermatitis

182. Basketter DA, Griffiths HA, Wang XM, Wilhelm KP, McFadden J (1996) Individual, ethnic and seasonal variability in irritant susceptibility of skin: the implications for a predictive human patch test. Contact Dermat 35:208–213
183. Lammintausta K, Maibach HI, Wilson D (1987) Irritant reactivity in males and females. Contact Dermat 17:276–280
184. Judge MR, Griffiths HA, Basketter DA, White IR, Rycroft RJ, McFadden JP (1996) Variation in response of human skin to irritant challenge. Contact Dermat 34:115–117
185. Holst R, Moller H (1975) One hundred twin pairs patch tested with primary irritants. Br J Dermatol 93:145–149
186. de Jongh CM, Verberk MM, Withagen CE, Jacobs JJ, Rustemeyer T, Kezic S (2006) Stratum corneum cytokines and skin irritation response to sodium lauryl sulfate. Contact Dermat 54:325–333
187. de Jongh CM, Jakasa I, Verberk MM, Kezic S (2006) Variation in barrier impairment and inflammation of human skin as determined by sodium lauryl sulphate penetration rate. Br J Dermatol 154:651–657
188. Agner T, Serup J (1990) Individual and instrumental variations in irritant patch-test reactions–clinical evaluation and quantification by bioengineering methods. Clin Exp Dermatol 15:29–33
189. Pinnagoda J, Tupker RA, Smit JA, Coenraads PJ, Nater JP (1989) The intra- and inter-individual variability and reliability of transepidermal water loss measurements. Contact Dermat 21:255–259
190. Robinson MK, Perkins MA, Basketter DA (1998) Application of a 4-h human patch test method for comparative and investigative assessment of skin irritation. Contact Dermat 38:194–202
191. Smith HR, Holloway D, Armstrong DK, Basketter DA, McFadden JP (2000) Irritant thresholds in subjects with colophony allergy. Contact Dermat 42:95–97
192. Smith HR, Armstrong DK, Holloway D, Whittam L, Basketter DA, McFadden JP (2002) Skin irritation thresholds in hairdressers: implications for the development of hand dermatitis. Br J Dermatol 146:849–852
193. Smith HR, Kelly DA, Young AR, Basketter DB, McFadden JP (2002) Relationship between 2, 4-dinitrochlorobenzene elicitation responses and individual irritant threshold. Contact Dermat 46:97–100
194. McFadden JP, Basketter DA (2000) Contact allergy, irritancy and 'danger'. Contact Dermat 42:123–127
195. McLelland J, Shuster S, Matthews JN (1991) 'Irritants' increase the response to an allergen in allergic contact dermatitis. Arch Dermatol 127:1016–1019
196. Kligman AM (1966) The identification of contact allergens by human assay. II. Factors influencing the induction and measurement of allergic contact dermatitis. J Invest Dermatol 47:375–392
197. Marrakchi S, Maibach HI (2006) Sodium lauryl sulfate-induced irritation in the human face: regional and age-related differences. Skin Pharmacol Physiol 19:177–180
198. Tupker RA, Coenraads PJ, Pinnagoda J, Nater JP (1989) Baseline transepidermal water loss (TEWL) as a prediction of susceptibility to sodium lauryl sulphate. Contact Dermat 20:265–269
199. Agner T (1991) Skin susceptibility in uninvolved skin of hand eczema patients and healthy controls. Br J Dermatol 125:140–146
200. Berardesca E, Maibach HI (1988) Sodium-lauryl-sulphate-induced cutaneous irritation. Comparison of white and Hispanic subjects. Contact Dermat 19:136–140
201. Tupker RA, Pinnagoda J, Coenraads PJ, Nater JP (1990) Susceptibility to irritants: role of barrier function, skin dryness and history of atopic dermatitis. Br J Dermatol 123:199–205
202. Wilhelm KP, Maibach HI (1990) Susceptibility to irritant dermatitis induced by sodium lauryl sulfate. J Am Acad Dermatol 23:122–124
203. Di Nardo A, Sugino K, Wertz P, Ademola J, Maibach HI (1996) Sodium lauryl sulfate (SLS) induced irritant contact dermatitis: a correlation study between ceramides and in vivo parameters of irritation. Contact Dermat 35:86–91
204. de Jongh CM, Lutter R, Verberk MM, Kezic S (2007) Differential cytokine expression in skin after single and repeated irritation by sodium lauryl sulphate. Exp Dermatol 16:1032–1040
205. Werner Y, Lindberg M (1985) Transepidermal water loss in dry and clinically normal skin in patients with atopic dermatitis. Acta Derm Venereol 65:102–105
206. Agner T (1991) Susceptibility of atopic dermatitis patients to irritant dermatitis caused by sodium lauryl sulphate. Acta Derm Venereol 71:296–300
207. Cowley NC, Farr PM (1992) A dose-response study of irritant reactions to sodium lauryl sulphate in patients with seborrhoeic dermatitis and atopic eczema. Acta Derm Venereol 72:432–435
208. Loffler H, Effendy I (1999) Skin susceptibility of atopic individuals. Contact Dermat 40:239–242
209. Basketter DA, Miettinen J, Lahti A (1998) Acute irritant reactivity to sodium lauryl sulfate in atopics and non-atopics. Contact Dermat 38:253–257
210. Tupker RA, Coenraads PJ, Fidler V, De Jong MC, Van der Meer JB, De Monchy JG (1995) Irritant susceptibility and weal and flare reactions to bioactive agents in atopic dermatitis. I. Influence of disease severity. Br J Dermatol 133:358–364
211. Jakasa I, de Jongh CM, Verberk MM, Bos JD, Kezic S (2006) Percutaneous penetration of sodium lauryl sulphate is increased in uninvolved skin of patients with atopic dermatitis compared with control subjects. Br J Dermatol 155:104–109
212. Proksch E, Folster-Holst R, Jensen JM (2006) Skin barrier function, epidermal proliferation and differentiation in eczema. J Dermatol Sci 43:159–169

213. Palmer CN, Irvine AD, Terron-Kwiatkowski A, Zhao Y, Liao H, Lee SP, Goudie DR, Sandilands A, Campbell LE, Smith FJ, O'regan GM, Watson RM, Cecil JE, Bale SJ, Compton JG, Digiovanna JJ, Fleckman P, Lewis-Jones S, Arseculeratne G, Sergeant A, Munro CS, El HB, McElreavey K, Halkjaer LB, Bisgaard H, Mukhopadhyay S, McLean WH (2006) Common loss-of-function variants of the epidermal barrier protein filaggrin are a major predisposing factor for atopic dermatitis. Nat Genet 38:441–446
214. Pastore S, Corinti S, La PM, Didona B, Girolomoni G (1998) Interferon-gamma promotes exaggerated cytokine production in keratinocytes cultured from patients with atopic dermatitis. J Allergy Clin Immunol 101:538–544
215. de Vries I, Langeveld-Wildschut EG, van Reijsen FC, Dubois GR, van den Hoek JA, Bihari IC, van WD, de Weger RA, Knol EF, Thepen T, Bruijnzeel-Koomen CA (1998) Adhesion molecule expression on skin endothelia in atopic dermatitis: effects of TNF-alpha and IL-4. J Allergy Clin Immunol 102:461–468
216. Schnuch A, Uter W, Reich K (2005) Allergic contact dermatitis and atopic eczema. In: Ring J, Przybilla B, Ruzicka T (eds) Handbook of atopic eczema. Springer, Berlin, Heidelberg, New York, pp 176–199
217. Kiyohara C, Tanaka K, Miyake Y (2008) Genetic susceptibility to atopic dermatitis. Allergol Int 57:39–56
218. Brown SJ, McLean WH (2009) Eczema genetics: current state of knowledge and future goals. J Invest Dermatol 129: 543–552
219. Reed JT, Ghadially R, Elias PM (1995) Skin type, but neither race nor gender, influence epidermal permeability barrier function. Arch Dermatol 131:1134–1138
220. Wilhelm KP, Cua AB, Maibach HI (1991) Skin aging. Effect on transepidermal water loss, stratum corneum hydration, skin surface pH, and casual sebum content. Arch Dermatol 127:1806–1809
221. Goh CL, Chia SE (1988) Skin irritability to sodium lauryl sulphate–as measured by skin water vapour loss-by sex and race. Clin Exp Dermatol 13:16–19
222. Harvell J, Hussona-Saeed I, Maibach HI (1992) Changes in transepidermal water loss and cutaneous blood flow during the menstrual cycle. Contact Dermat 27:294–301
223. Agner T, Damm P, Skouby SO (1991) Menstrual cycle and skin reactivity. J Am Acad Dermatol 24:566–570
224. Robinson MK (2002) Population differences in acute skin irritation responses. Race, sex, age, sensitive skin and repeat subject comparisons. Contact Dermat 46:86–93
225. Uter W, Geier J, Becker D, Brasch J, Loffler H (2004) The MOAHLFA index of irritant sodium lauryl sulfate reactions: first results of a multicentre study on routine sodium lauryl sulfate patch testing. Contact Dermat 51:259–262
226. Cua AB, Wilhelm KP, Maibach HI (1990) Cutaneous sodium lauryl sulphate irritation potential: age and regional variability. Br J Dermatol 123:607–613
227. Schwindt DA, Wilhelm KP, Miller DL, Maibach HI (1998) Cumulative irritation in older and younger skin: a comparison. Acta Derm Venereol 78:279–283
228. Suh DH, Youn JI, Eun HC (2001) Effects of 12-O-tetradecanoyl-phorbol-13-acetate [corrected] and sodium lauryl sulfate on the production and expression of cytokines and proto-oncogenes in photoaged and intrinsically aged human keratinocytes. J Invest Dermatol 117:1225–1233

229. Ghadially R, Brown BE, Sequeira-Martin SM, Feingold KR, Elias PM (1995) The aged epidermal permeability barrier. Structural, functional, and lipid biochemical abnormalities in humans and a senescent murine model. J Clin Invest 95:2281–2290
230. Modjtahedi SP, Maibach HI (2002) Ethnicity as a possible endogenous factor in irritant contact dermatitis: comparing the irritant response among Caucasians, blacks, and Asians. Contact Dermat 47:272–278
231. Robinson MK (2000) Racial differences in acute and cumulative skin irritation responses between Caucasian and Asian populations. Contact Dermat 42:134–143
232. Foy V, Weinkauf R, Whittle E, Basketter DA (2001) Ethnic variation in the skin irritation response. Contact Dermat 45:346–349
233. Weigand DA, Gaylor JR (1974) Irritant reaction in Negro and Caucasian skin. South Med J 67:548–551
234. Astner S, Burnett N, Rius-Diaz F, Doukas AG, Gonzalez S, Gonzalez E (2006) Irritant contact dermatitis induced by a common household irritant: a noninvasive evaluation of ethnic variability in skin response. J Am Acad Dermatol 54:458–465
235. Hicks SP, Swindells KJ, Middelkamp-Hup MA, Sifakis MA, Gonzalez E, Gonzalez S (2003) Confocal histopathology of irritant contact dermatitis in vivo and the impact of skin color (black vs white). J Am Acad Dermatol 48:727–734
236. Berardesca E, Maibach H (2003) Ethnic skin: overview of structure and function. J Am Acad Dermatol 48: S139–S142
237. Van der V, Nater JP, Bleumink E (1985) Vulnerability of the skin to surfactants in different groups of eczema patients and controls as measured by water vapour loss. Clin Exp Dermatol 10:98–103
238. Faergemann J, Bergbrant IM, Dohse M, Scott A, Westgate G (2001) Seborrhoeic dermatitis and Pityrosporum (Malassezia) folliculitis: characterization of inflammatory cells and mediators in the skin by immunohistochemistry. Br J Dermatol 144:549–556
239. Johnson MW, Maibach HI, Salmon SE (1971) Skin reactivity in patients with cancer. Impaired delayed hypersensitivity or faulty inflammatory response? N Engl J Med 284: 1255–1257
240. Van der Valk, Maibach HI (1989) Potential for irritation increases from the wrist to the cubital fossa. Br J Dermatol 121:709–712
241. McFadden JP, Wakelin SH, Basketter DA (1998) Acute irritation thresholds in subjects with type I–type VI skin. Contact Dermat 38:147–149
242. Frosch PJ, Wissing C (1982) Cutaneous sensitivity to ultra-violet light and chemical irritants. Arch Dermatol Res 272:269–278
243. Loffler H, Aramaki JU, Effendy I (2002) The influence of body mass index on skin susceptibility to sodium lauryl sulphate. Skin Res Technol 8:19–22
244. de Jongh CM, John SM, Bruynzeel DP, Calkoen F, van Dijk FJ, Khrenova L, Rustemeyer T, Verberk MM, Kezic S (2008) Cytokine gene polymorphisms and susceptibility to chronic irritant contact dermatitis. Contact Dermat 58: 269–277
245. Allen MH, Wakelin SH, Holloway D, Lisby S, Baadsgaard O, Barker JN, McFadden JP (2000) Association of TNFA gene polymorphism at position -308 with susceptibility to irritant contact dermatitis. Immunogenetics 51:201–205

2

246. Corsini E, Galli CL (2000) Epidermal cytokines in experimental contact dermatitis. Toxicology 142:203–211

247. Louis E, Franchimont D, Piron A, Gevaert Y, Schaaf-Lafontaine N, Roland S, Mahieu P, Malaise M, De GD, Louis R, Belaiche J (1998) Tumour necrosis factor (TNF) gene polymorphism influences TNF-alpha production in lipopolysaccharide (LPS)-stimulated whole blood cell culture in healthy humans. Clin Exp Immunol 113:401–406

248. Wilson AG, Symons JA, McDowell TL, McDevitt HO, Duff GW (1997) Effects of a polymorphism in the human tumor necrosis factor alpha promoter on transcriptional activation. Proc Natl Acad Sci USA 94:3195–3199

249. Hollegaard MV, Bidwell JL (2006) Cytokine gene polymorphism in human disease: on-line databases, Supplement 3. Genes Immun 7:269–276

250. Castro J, Telleria JJ, Linares P, Blanco-Quiros A (2000) Increased TNFA*2, but not TNFB*1, allele frequency in Spanish atopic patients. J Investig Allergol Clin Immunol 10:149–154

251. Dominici R, Cattaneo M, Malferrari G, Archi D, Mariani C, Grimaldi LM, Biunno I (2002) Cloning and functional analysis of the allelic polymorphism in the transcription regulatory region of interleukin-1 alpha. Immunogenetics 54:82–86

252. de Jongh CM, Khrenova L, Kezic S, Rustemeyer T, Verberk MM, John SM (2008) Polymorphisms in the interleukin-1 gene influence the stratum corneum interleukin-1 alpha concentration in uninvolved skin of patients with chronic irritant contact dermatitis. Contact Dermat 58:263–268

253. Nemoto-Hasebe I, Akiyama M, Nomura T, Sandilands A, McLean WI, Shimizu H (2009) Clinical severity correlates with impaired barrier in filaggrin-related eczema. J Invest Dermatol 129:682–689

254. Kezic S, Kemperman PM, Koster ES, de Jongh CM, Thio HB, Campbell LE, Irvine AD, McLean IW, Puppels GJ, Caspers PJ (2008) Loss-of-function mutations in the filaggrin gene lead to reduced level of natural moisturizing factor in the stratum corneum. J Invest Dermatol 128:2117–2119

255. de Jongh CM, Khrenova L, Verberk MM, Calkoen F, van Dijk FJ, Voss H, John SM, Kezic S (2008) Loss-of-function polymorphisms in the filaggrin gene are associated with an increased susceptibility to chronic irritant contact dermatitis: a case-control study. Br J Dermatol 159:621–627

256. Rodriguez E, Illig T, Weidinger S (2008) Filaggrin loss-of-function mutations and association with allergic diseases. Pharmacogenomics 9:399–413

257. Uter W, Hegewald J, Pfahlberg A, Pirker C, Frosch PJ, Gefeller O (2003) The association between ambient air conditions (temperature and absolute humidity), irritant sodium lauryl sulfate patch test reactions and patch test reactivity to standard allergens. Contact Dermat 49:97–102

258. Loffler H, Happle R (2003) Influence of climatic conditions on the irritant patch test with sodium lauryl sulphate. Acta Derm Venereol 83:338–341

259. Pedersen LK, Johansen JD, Held E, Agner T (2004) Augmentation of skin response by exposure to a combination of allergens and irritants – a review. Contact Dermat 50:265–273

260. McMullen E, Gawkrodger DJ (2006) Physical friction is under-recognized as an irritant that can cause or contribute to contact dermatitis. Br J Dermatol 154:154–156

Mechanisms of Irritant and Allergic Contact Dermatitis

3

Thomas Rustemeyer, Ingrid M.W. van Hoogstraten,
B. Mary E. von Blomberg, Sue Gibbs, and Rik J. Scheper

Contents

T. Rustemeyer (✉) and S. Gibbs
Department of Dermatology, VU University Medical Center
Amsterdam, De Boelelaan 1117, 1081 HV Amsterdam,
Netherlands
e-mail: t.rustemeyer@vumc.nl

I.M. Hoogstraten, B.M.E. Blomberg
and R.J. Scheper
Department of Pathology, VU University Medical Center
Amsterdam, De Boelelaan 1117, 1081 HV Amsterdam,
Netherlands

3.1 Introduction

Contact dermatitis describes the skin reaction resulting from exposure to irritants (irritant contact dermatitis) or allergens (allergic contact dermatitis). In most patients, irritant and allergic contact dermatitis (ACD) are clinically indistinguishable. Also histopathologically, no distinguishing markers have been identified. This is in line with the fact that in irritant and ACD, principal inflammatory pathways are essentially similar. The pivotal different factor in ACD is the involvement of "allergen-specific" T cells as initiators of the inflammatory skin reaction. In irritant contact dermatitis (ICD), the inflammatory reaction mainly depends on either or both chemical and physical irritation. The most frequent chemical irritative factors are long-lasting and repetitive contacts to water, detergents, solvents, or a combination of these factors, often aggravated by too high or too low humidity. Inflammatory reactions to irritants are not triggered by one specific substance or cause, and do not show rapid amplification of severity by repeated insults and are thus called "unspecific."

In the following chapter the immunopathological mechanisms of ICD and ACD reactions will be discussed further in detail.

3.2 Irritant Contact Dermatitis

3.2.1 Skin Barrier Perturbation Can Lead to Irritant Contact Dermatitis

The skin functions as a barrier protecting an individual from dehydration, mechanical trauma, irradiation, microbial insults, and direct exposure to harmful sensitizing or

J.D. Johansen et al. (eds.), *Contact Dermatitis*,
DOI: 978-3-642-03827-3_3, © Springer-Verlag Berlin Heidelberg 2011

43

irritant chemicals [1, 2]. Perturbation of the skin barrier can result in ICD. The barrier function is provided by the uppermost layer of the epidermis, the stratum corneum. The epidermis consists of more than 90% keratinocytes. Proliferating basal keratinocytes undergo a commitment to terminally differentiate and, in doing so, form a compact multilayered cellular compartment consisting of, depending on the skin region, approximately eight living cell layers (approximately 50–100 µm thick). As the keratinocytes become more differentiated, they approach the outermost layers and ultimately form the stratum corneum (10–20 µm thick). The stratum corneum consists of dead, terminally differentiated keratinocytes (corneocytes) embedded in extracellular lipid. The corneocytes and the lipid component of the stratum corneum can be considered as bricks and mortar and form the barrier to the environment and potentially harmful substances [3–5]. In order for a potential irritant to cause an irritant reaction, it must first penetrate or damage the stratum corneum to exert its effect on the viable epidermal and dermal layers below.

A chemical can penetrate the skin via three routes: the intercellular lipid route, the transcellular route across cornified cells and lipid bilayers, and via diffusion along hair follicles and sweat glands [4, 6–9]. Chemicals can also penetrate at sites of skin trauma (wounds) and where the barrier function is impaired by other diseases. Hydrophobic substances have the potential to penetrate via the lipid layers, whereas hydrophilic substances preferentially penetrate via the hair follicles and sweat lands. The lipid bilayer is the primary target for common skin damaging factors such as solvents and soaps since these substances degrade the lipid bilayer directly and expose the underlying viable epidermal layers to the irritant. Once an irritant has penetrated the stratum corneum, it may exert cytotoxic effects on the keratinocytes and trigger keratinocytes to release alarm signals in the form of cytokines and chemokines. In this way, the innate immune system is triggered and the ICD reaction is initiated.

3.2.2 Pathogenesis of Acute Irritant Contact Dermatitis

Thus, ICD reflects an innate inflammatory response of the skin to direct injury. Frequency and intensity of skin contacts with harmful agents determine the outcome. For acute ICD, the reaction is often caused by a single exposure to the irritant and the skin manifestations usually disappear within days to weeks. The source of the irritant is most often a chemical or abrasion to the skin. One of the major initial events before skin damage is observed is the release of proinflammatory cytokines. This in turn amplifies the inflammatory reaction by releasing chemokines, resulting in vasodilation and infiltration of cells (e.g., lymphocytes, eosinophils, macrophages, neutrophils, T cells) into the epidermis and dermis. The resulting physiological signs of irritation are damage to the epidermis as observed by spongiosis and microvesicle formation, erythema, induration, and edema leading to localized painful areas of skin [10–13] (Fig. 3.1).

However, the clinical appearance is often very variable and, moreover, difficult to distinguish from ACD [14, 15]. ACD shows all the features of ICD, but in an accelerated and/or augmented fashion due to the involvement of allergen-reactive T cells. Proinflammatory cytokines locally released by the latter, such as IFN-γ, IL-4, and IL-17, as will be discussed below, serve to amplify the overall inflammatory reactivity and protect the body against potentially harmful agents. Indeed, clinical observations show a clear role for irritancy in ACD: virtually all allergens have irritant properties, whereas irritated skin is easier to sensitize than nonirritated skin. During both an ACD and an ICD reaction, alarm signals provided by skin barrier disruption, epidermal cellular changes and cytokine/chemokine release, stimulate the initial trafficking of immune cells to the site under attack.

Core Message

> In acute ICD, similar immunological mechanisms are involved as in acute ACD. However, the crucial difference is the involvement of specific T cells in ACD. Major events in acute contact dermatitis include damage of the epidermal skin barrier by contact irritants and subsequent activation of unspecific innate immune responses.

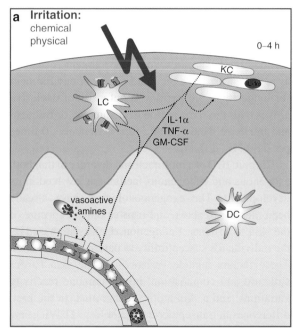

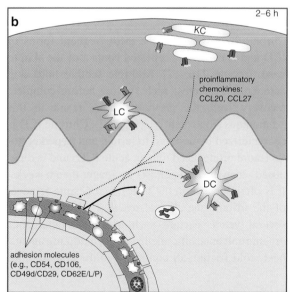

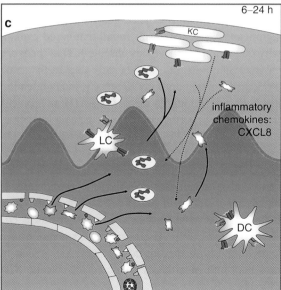

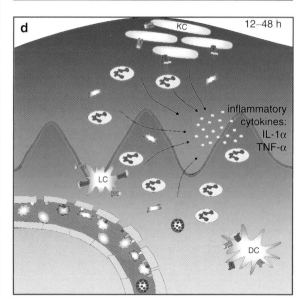

Fig. 3.1 (**a–d**) Immunological events in irritant contact dermatitis (ICD). (**a**) Physical and/or chemical irritation triggers the fast release of prestored cytokines and other inflammatory mediators, termed "danger signals." (**b**) In response to the release of these danger signals proinflammatory chemokines from resident epidermal and dermal cells. (**c**) Subsequently, inflammatory chemokines are secreted from resident cells and already infiltrated inflammatory cells. A major cytokine is this process is CXCL8 (formerly known as IL-8). (**d**) As a consequence, from the producion of inflammatory chemokines, more and more inflammatory cells, including neutrophils (☜), are attracted and, under the influence of inflammatory triggers, secrete inflammatory mediators. This results in the clinically visible acute ICD

3.2.3 Development of Chronic Irritant Contact Dermatitis

Chronic ICD is one of the most frequent forms of ICD and is caused by repeated contact of the skin to weak irritants [16, 17]. Multiple subthreshold skin damaging exposures, each starting before complete recovery from the previous insult, result in this eczematous skin condition (Fig. 3.2). Chronic ICD is characterized by dryness, fissuring, and hyperkeratosis (more pronounced than in acute ICD) and is diagnosed when the ICD persists for longer than 6 weeks. It is often located on the hands, and despite removal of the irritant, the clinical reaction may remain for several years. Factors such as water, detergents, organic solvents, oils, alkalis, acids, oxidizing agents, heat, cold friction all contribute to the elicitation of

chronic ICD [16, 17]. Such factors are frequently associated with a wet working environment, and therefore, chronic ICD is a frequent work-related dermatitis [18, 19]. A wet work environment is defined as regular work with the hands in a wet environment for longer than 2 h per day, regular use of occlusive gloves over the same period of time, and / or frequent and intensive hand washing (approximately 20 times per day) [18, 20].

Chronic ICD is a multifactorial disorder in that both exogenous and endogenous factors are involved in its development. The exogenous factors have already been mentioned above and involve direct exposure of the skin to irritants. Endogenous factors are based on the individual's susceptibility to develop chronic ICD. These factors include variations in the skin barrier structure and composition, innate immune reactivity variations, and a skin atopic background. In the past, differences in transepidermal water loss (TEWL), erythema, irritation thresholds, and gender-related differences have been investigated [21–27]. However, no significant differences were found that could explain why one individual develops chronic ICD at the work environment, whereas another individual in the same work environment does not. Recently, much attention has been paid to atopic dermatitis (AD) as a potentially important predisposing factor since a history of AD more than quadruples the risk of hand eczema in cases of skin exposure in a wet work environment [28]. It was shown that penetration of the irritant SLS and subsequent increase in TEWL and erythema was higher in subjects with AD than in healthy individuals indicating that more permeable skin is more susceptible to irritants [29]. Also, genetic risk factors have been linked with the development of AD, which in turn may influence the development of chronic ICD [30–34].

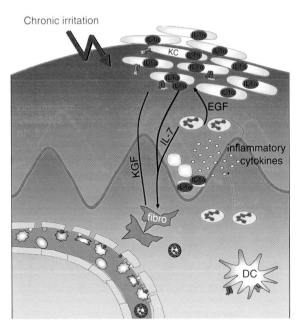

Fig. 3.2 Chronic ICD results from the continuing presence of various inflammatory triggers. Keratinocytes at skin sites of former inflammatory skin reactions contain higher levels of stored IL-1α. Upon exposure to unspecific inflammatory triggers, IL-1α is easily secreted and stimulates the activation of the inflammatory cascade. As a consequence of continuing exposure to inflammatory triggers, epidermal, dermal, and infiltrated inflammatory cells produce different growth factors, including epidermal growth factor (EGF) and keratinocyte growth factor (KGF). These growth factors stimulate proliferation of fibroblasts and keratinocytes, which results in the hyperkeratotic and desquamating clinical phenotype of chronic ICD

Core Message

> In chronic ICD, repetitive skin contacts to different contact irritants cause substantial and prolonged skin barrier damage. A skin atopic background is a strong risk factor for developing chronic ICD.

3.2.4 Genetic Risk Factors in Irritant Contact Dermatitis and Atopic Dermatitis

AD is a hereditary disease and, as already mentioned, is an important predisposing factor for chronic ICD. It is associated with hyperreactivity of the skin to irritants, aero-allergens, microbes, and scratching. Next to overexpression of the epithelial cell and fibroblast-produced cytokine TSLP [35], recently two loss-of-function polymorphisms in the gene encoding for filaggrin have been described as strong predisposing factors for AD [33]. Depending on the disease phenotype, 16–56% of patients with AD carry one or more filaggrin null mutations compared to only 5–10% of the general European population [33, 34, 36–39]. Filaggrin is involved in the formation of corneocytes, and therefore, in the formation of the stratum corneum [37]. Once cornification is complete, filaggrin is degraded into free amino acids. These free amino acids contribute to the natural moisturizing factor component of the stratum corneum by retaining water. Therefore, it is possible that filaggrin null alleles may be responsible in part for the dry skin characteristic of AD. De Jong et al. showed that FLG null alleles are associated with increased susceptibility to chronic ICD; however, whether or not the filaggrin null allele is an independent risk factor needs further study [32].

Until now, no genetic factors have been identified that contribute to hand eczema in the absence of AD. However, it is possible that unidentified polymorphisms in cytokines and chemokines may be involved in chronic ICD. Indeed, such polymorphisms have already been reported in several other inflammatory diseases e.g., rheumatoid arthritis and multiple sclerosis [40]. A case–control study in 197 patients with chronic ICD vs. 217 healthy individuals showed that polymorphisms in several cytokine genes (IL-1α, IL-1β, IL-8, IL-10 and TNF-α) and the two loss-of-function polymorphisms in the filaggrin gene did not provide a substantial risk factor for development of chronic ICD [30]. However, the study did show that (1) both the variant TNFA-308A allele and the filaggrin null alleles predispose to flexural eczema, (2) the variant TNFA-308A allele can increase susceptibility to chronic ICD, and (3) the IL1A-889T allele might protect against hand dermatitis. Here, the ratio of IL-1 receptor antagonist (IL-RA)/IL-1α increased 2–3-fold, corresponding to a reduced level of agonistic IL-1a in the stratum corneum in subjects expressing the variant genotype as compared to the wild type genotype. In conclusion, genetic polymorphisms of TNFA-308 and IL1A-889 may influence the susceptibility of chronic ICD.

3.2.5 Cellular Immunological Changes in Irritant Contact Dermatitis

Next to its barrier function, the skin is recognized as an immunologically active organ. Barrier perturbation results in the generation of the first alarm signal. Skin epidermal cells, notably keratinocytes, melanocytes and Langerhans cells (LC), respond to nonspecific irritant stimuli by producing cytokines, adhesion molecules, and chemotactic factors [41–43]. Keratinocyes are the major source of skin derived cytokines. Epidermal cytokines diffuse into the dermis and trigger dermal cells (e.g., fibroblasts and endothelial cells) to also secrete chemokines [44, 45]. In this way the proinflammatory response is amplified and a chemotactic gradient is introduced directing infiltrating cells into the site of tissue damage. The initial proinflammatory response can result in Langerhans' cell migration out of the epidermis, potentially contributing to allergenicity, and infiltration of monocytes, neutrophils, macrophages, and lymphocytes into the skin. This skin innate immune response is rapid, provides the initial line of defense against damage caused by irritants, is antigen-nonspecific, and lacks immunological memory [13, 46, 47].

As stated, ACD and ICD reactions share alarm signal(s) [14, 48, 49]. This is supported by several in vivo and in vitro studies in which both allergen and irritant exposures result in increased cytokine levels in keratinocytes and fibroblasts [41, 45]. So, which is the initiating cytokine, and is it prestored or does de novo synthesis occur? Of all the cytokines produced by keratinocytes, only IL-1α, IL-1β, and TNF-α activate a sufficient number of effector mechanisms to independently trigger cutaneous inflammation [47]. Furthermore, large stores of preformed and biologically active IL-1α have also been detected as a depot in the stratum corneum and within the epidermis [50, 51]. In contrast, other cytokines such as TNF-α and IL-8 are detectable only at low amounts deep within the stratum corneum

[50, 52]. These results strongly suggest that the release of prestored IL-1α upon barrier perturbation is the initiating cytokine signal, which triggers the induction of other inflammatory mediators. Upon release, IL-1α stimulates further release of IL-1α and the production and release of other cytokines. While resting keratinocytes produce some cytokines constitutively, exposure to irritants induces production of (pro-) inflammatory cytokines (IL-1α, TNF-α), chemotactic cytokines (IL-6, IL-8, CCL20, CCL27), growth-promoting cytokines (GM-CSF, TGF-β), and cytokines regulating specific immune responses (IL-10, IL-12, IL-18) [11, 43]. Thus, via cytokine cascades, an inflammatory response can be rapidly generated. In this way, keratinocytes act as proinflammatory signal transducers, responding to nonspecific external stimuli with the production of inflammatory cytokines, adhesion molecules, and chemotactic factors, stimulating the dermal stroma to amplify the response.

In this context, it should be mentioned that in the skin, TNF-α is stored in dermal mast cells, and following stimulation, it is produced by keratinocytes and LC. Antibodies to TNF-α abolish many inflammatory skin reactions, including allergic and ICD [53]. An in vitro study using a full thickness human skin equivalent model showed that antibodies directed against either TNF-α or IL-1α were able to completely inhibit inflammatory chemokine secretion by dermal fibroblasts [45]. Therefore, taken together, these findings suggest that both TNF-α and IL-1α are pivotal cytokines in mediating irritant induced skin inflammation. In conclusion, several cell types and downstream mechanisms act in concert in inducing different types of skin irritant responses. Determining the cell source, kinetics of production, and the regulation of inflammatory mediators in the skin will be the key to predicting and treating irritant responses arising from different environmental agents (Table 3.1).

Table 3.1 Cytokines, chemokines, and growth factors expressed by epidermal cells and dermal fibroblasts

Cell type	Cytokine/chemokine/growth factors
Epidermal cells Keratinocyte	Cytokines: IL-1α, IL-1β, IL-1RA, IL-3 (mouse), IL-6, IL-7, IL-8 (human), IL-10, IL-12, IL-15, IL-18, IL-20, IL-23, IL-24, IL-33, TNF-α, TGF-α, TGF-β Chemokines: CCL2, CCL5, CCL20, CCL27, CXCL1, CXCL10, CXCL14 (mouse) Growth factors: G-CSF, GM-CSF, M-CSF
Langerhans' cell	Cytokines: IL-1α, IL-1β, IL-6, IL-15, IL-18, IL-23, TNF-α, TGF-β Chemokines: CCL3, CXCL1, CXCL14
Melanocyte	Cytokines: IL-1α, IL-1β, IL-6, IL-7, IL-8, IL-10, IL-12, IL-24, TNF-α, TGF-α, TGF-β Chemokines: CCL2, CCL5, CXCL1, CXCL14 (mouse) Growth factors: G-CSF, GM-CSF, M-CSF
Dermal fibroblast	Cytokines: TNF-α, IL-8, IL-6 Chemokines: CCL2, CCL5, CCL20, CXCL1, CXCL12

Cytokines may be constitutively expressed or induced upon irritant stimuli [11, 41, 43–47]

3.3 Introduction Allergic Contact Dermatitis

During the past few decades, our understanding of why, where, and when ACD might develop has rapidly increased. Critical discoveries include the identification of T cells as mediators of cell-mediated immunity, their thymic origin and recirculation patterns, and the molecular basis of their specificity to just one or few allergens out of the thousands of allergens known. Progress has also resulted from the identification of genes that determine T-cell function and the development of monoclonal antibodies that recognize their products. Moreover, the production of large amounts of recombinant products, e.g., cytokines and chemokines, and the breeding of mice with disruptions in distinct genes (knock-out mice) or provided with additional genes of interest (transgenic mice) have allowed in-depth analysis of skin-inflammatory processes, such as those taking place in ACD.

Although humoral antibody-mediated reactions can be a factor, ACD depends primarily on the activation of allergen-specific T cells [54], and is regarded as a

> **Core Message**
>
> › Unspecific innate immune reactions cause the development of ICD reactions. Some genetic risk factors including polymorphisms in TNF-α genes have been detected. Further research is needed to unravel the inflammatory innate immune cascades involved in ICD.

prototype of delayed hypersensitivity, as classified by Turk [55] and Gell and Coombs (type IV hypersensitivity) [56]. Evolutionarily, cell-mediated immunity has developed in vertebrates to facilitate eradication of microorganisms and toxins. Elicitation of ACD by usually nontoxic doses of small molecular-weight allergens indicates that the T-cell repertoire is often slightly broader than one might wish. Thus, ACD can be considered to reflect an untoward side effect of a well-functioning immune system.

Subtle differences can be noted in macroscopic appearance, time course, and histopathology of allergic contact reactions in various vertebrates, including rodents and man [57]. Nevertheless, essentially all basic features are shared. Since both mouse and guinea pig models, next to clinical studies, have greatly contributed to our present knowledge of ACD, both data sets provide the basis for this chapter.

In ACD, a distinction should be made between induction (also known as sensitization or primary) and effector (also known as elicitation or secondary) phases [58] (Fig. 3.3). The induction phase includes the events following a first contact with the allergen and is complete when the individual is sensitized and capable of giving a positive ACD reaction. The effector phase begins upon elicitation (challenge) and results in clinical manifestation of ACD. The entire process of the induction phase requires at least 4 days to several weeks, whereas the effector phase reaction is fully developed within 1–4 days. Main episodes in the induction phase (steps 1–5) and effector phase (step 6) are:

1. *Binding of allergen to skin components.* The allergen penetrating the skin readily associates with all kinds of skin components, including major histocompatibility complex (MHC) proteins. These molecules, in humans encoded for by histocompatibility antigen (HLA) genes, are abundantly present on epidermal antigen presenting cells, called LC.

2. *Hapten-induced activation of allergen-presenting cells.* Allergen-carrying LC become activated, mature, and travel via the afferent lymphatics to the regional lymph nodes, where they settle as so-called interdigitating cells (IDC) in the paracortical T-cell areas.

3. *Recognition of allergen-modified LC by specific T cells.* In nonsensitized individuals the frequency of T cells with certain specificities is usually far below one per million. Within the paracortical areas, conditions are optimal for allergen-carrying IDC to encounter naïve T cells that specifically recognize the allergen–MHC molecule complexes. The dendritic morphology of these allergen-presenting cells strongly facilitates multiple cell contacts, leading to binding and activation of allergen-specific T cells.

4. *Proliferation of specific T cells in draining lymph nodes.* Supported by interleukin (IL)-1, released by the allergen-presenting cells, activated T cells start producing several growth factors, including IL-2. A partly autocrine cascade follows since at the same time receptors for IL-2 are upregulated in these cells, resulting in vigorous blast formation and proliferation within a few days.

5. *Systemic propagation of the specific T-cell progeny.* The expanded progeny is subsequently released via the efferent lymphatics into the blood flow and begins to recirculate. Thus, the frequency of specific effector memory T cells in the blood may rise to as high as one in a thousand, whereas most of these cells display receptor molecules facilitating their migration into peripheral tissues. In the absence of further allergen contacts, their frequency gradually decreases in subsequent weeks or months, but does not return to the low levels found in naive individuals.

6. *Effector phase.* By renewed allergen contact, the effector phase is initiated, which depends not only on the increased frequency of specific T cells, and their altered migratory capacities, but also on their low activation threshold. Thus, within the skin, allergen-presenting cells and specific T cells can meet, and lead to plentiful local cytokine and chemokine release. The release of these mediators, many of which have a proinflammatory action, causes the arrival of more inflammatory cells, thus further amplifying local mediator release. This leads to a gradually developing eczematous reaction that reaches its maximum after 18–72 h and then declines.

In the following sections, we will discuss these six main episodes of the ACD reaction in more detail. Furthermore, we will discuss local hyperreactivity, such as flare-up and retest reactivity, and hyporeactivity, i.e., upon desensitization or tolerance induction.

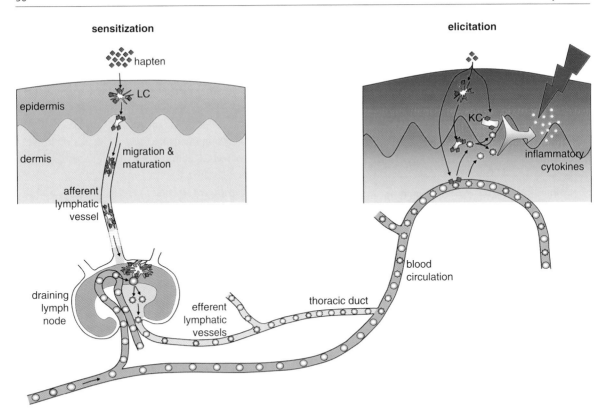

Fig. 3.3 Immunological events in allergic contact dermatitis (ACD). During the induction phase (*left*), skin contact with a hapten triggers migration of epidermal Langerhans cells (*LC*) via the afferent lymphatic vessels to the skin-draining lymph nodes. Haptenized LC home into the T cell-rich paracortical areas. Here, conditions are optimal for encountering naïve T cells that specifically recognize allergen–MHC molecule complexes. Hapten-specific T cells now expand abundantly and generate effector and memory cells, which are released via the efferent lymphatics into the circulation. With their newly acquired homing receptors, these cells can easily extravasate peripheral tissues. Renewed allergen contact sparks off the effector phase (*right*). Due to their lowered activation threshold, hapten-specific effector T cells are triggered by various haptenized cells, including *LC* and keratinocytes (*KC*), to produce proinflammatory cytokines and chemokines. Thereby, more inflammatory cells are recruited further amplifying local inflammatory mediator release. This leads to a gradually developing eczematous reaction, reaching a maximum within 18–48 h, after which reactivity successively declines

3.3.1 Binding of Contact Allergens to Skin Components

3.3.1.1 Chemical Nature of Contact Allergens

Most contact allergens are small, chemically reactive molecules with a molecular weight less than 500 Da [59] (Fig. 3.4). Since these molecules are too small to be antigenic themselves, contact sensitizers are generally referred to as haptens.

Upon penetration through the epidermal horny layer, haptens readily conjugate to endogenous epidermal and dermal molecules. Sensitizing organic compounds may covalently bind to protein nucleophilic groups, such as thiol, amino, and hydroxyl groups, as is the case with poison oak/ivy allergens (reviewed in [60, 61]). Examples of contact allergens containing electrophilic components include aldehydes, ketones, amides, or polarized bonds. Metal ions, e.g., nickel cations, instead form stable metal–protein chelate complexes by coordination bonds [62]. The most reactive nucleophilic side chains are those found in the amino acids lysine, cysteine and histidine [63]. Of note, their degree of ionization and hence nucleophilicity is dependent on the pH of the microenvironment, which is influenced by surrounding amino acids as well as protein location within the epithelium [64]. Predicting the chemicals that can function as haptens in ACD as well as identifying cutaneous proteins

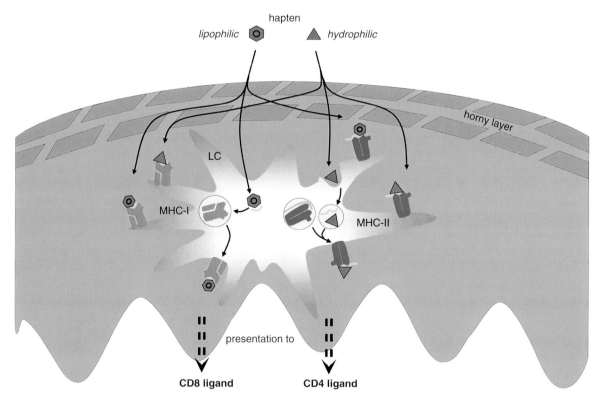

Fig. 3.4 Hapten presentation by epidermal Langerhans cells. Allergen penetrating into the epidermis readily associates with all kinds of skin components, including major histocompatibility complex (*MHC*) proteins, abundantly present on epidermal Langerhans cells (*LC*). Both MHC class I and class II molecules may be altered directly or via intracellular hapten processing and, subsequently, be recognized by allergen-specific CD8+ and CD4+ T cells

involved in hapten–protein complexes is the subject of current intense investigations [65, 66] and discussed in more detail elsewhere in this textbook.

3.3.1.2 Hapten Presentation by Langerhans Cells (LC)

Sensitization is critically dependent on direct association of haptens with epidermal LC-bound MHC molecules, or peptides present in the groove of these molecules. Both MHC class I and class II molecules may be altered this way, and thus give rise to allergen-specific CD8+ and CD4+ T cells, respectively. Distinct differences between allergens can, however, arise from differences in chemical reactivity and lipophilicity (Fig. 3.4), since association with MHC molecules may also result from internalization of the haptens, followed by their intracellular processing as free hapten

molecules or hapten–carrier complexes. Lipophilic haptens can directly penetrate into LC, conjugate with cytoplasmic proteins, and be processed along the "endogenous" processing route, thereby favoring association with MHC class I molecules [67]. In contrast, hydrophilic allergens such as nickel ions may, after conjugation with skin proteins, be processed along the "exogenous" route of antigen processing and thus favor the generation of altered MHC class II molecules. Thus, the chemical nature of the haptens can determine to what extent allergen-specific CD8+ and/ or CD4+ T cells will be activated [68–70].

3.3.1.3 Pre and Prohaptens

Whereas most contact allergens can form hapten–carrier complexes spontaneously, some need activation first. Contact allergens requiring activation outside the body, e.g., by UV-light or oxygen, are called prehaptens [71, 72]. The typical photoallergen tetrachlorosalicylanilide is a prototype of this. Tetrachlorosalicylanilide, which undergoes photochemical dechlorination with UV irradiation, ultimately provides photoadducts with skin proteins [73]. Contact allergens dependent on activation inside the body, e.g., by enzyme-induced metabolic conversion, are referred to as prohaptens. A classical prohapten is *p*-phenylenediamine, which needs to be oxidized by *N*-acetyltransferases to a reactive metabolite that can form a trimer, known as Bandrowski's base [74, 75]. Reduced enzyme activity in certain individuals, related to genetic enzyme polymorphisms, explains the reduced risk of sensitization to prohaptens that need enzymatic activation [76, 77]. Subsequent chapters of this book will present in extensive detail the numerous groups of molecules that have earned disrepute for causing ACD.

Core Message

> Allergenicity depends on several factors determined by the very physicochemical nature of the molecules themselves, i.e., their capacity to penetrate the horny layer, lipophilicity, and chemical reactivity. The sensitizing property of the majority of contact allergens could be predicted from these characteristics [63, 78]. Two other factors, however, further contribute to the allergenicity of chemicals, viz their proinflammatory activity and capacity to induce maturation of LC. These issues will be dealt with in more detail in the following sections.

3.3.2 Hapten-Induced Activation of Allergen-Presenting Cells

3.3.2.1 Physiology of Langerhans Cells

Although originally thought to be neurons based on their staining properties and cellular morphology [79], LC were subsequently surmised to function as "professional" antigen-presenting-cells [80]. They form a contiguous network within the epidermis and represent 2–5% of the total epidermal cell population [81]. Their principal functions are internalization, processing,

transport, and presentation of skin-encountered antigens [82, 83]. As such, LC play a pivotal role in the induction of cutaneous immune responses to infectious agents as well as to contact sensitizers [84–86]. Recent studies of LC indicate that this cell type has direct epidermal innervations and can respond to a number of neurotransmitters (among them are calcitonin gene-related peptide, α-melanocyte stimulating hormone, and substance P). Most of the experimental evidence to date indicates a suppressive effect of the neurohormones and neuropeptides on Langerhans cell function and cutaneous inflammation, but it has become evident lately that the timing of exposure to a stimulus is critical to the outcome of the immune response. Thus, administration of a stress hormone or exposure to a stressor before the LC encounters an allergen may diminish the immune response toward that substance, while a stressor may enhance immune function when acting on a maturing LC or before reexposure to the allergen [87]. LC originate from CD34+ bone marrow progenitors, entering the epidermis via the blood stream [88]. Their continuous presence in the epidermis is also assured by local proliferation [89, 90]. They reside as relatively immature DC, characterized by a high capacity to gather antigens by macropinocytosis, whereas their capacity to stimulate naïve T cells is still underdeveloped at this stage [91]. Their prominent dendritic morphology and the presence of distinctive Birbeck granules were observed long ago [79, 92, 93]. In the last decade, their pivotal function in the induction of skin immune responses was explained by high expression of molecules mediating antigen-presentation (e.g., MHC class I and II, CD1), as well as of cellular adhesion and costimulatory molecules (e.g., CD54, CD80, CD86, and cutaneous lymphocyte antigen [CLA]) [94–96].

3.3.2.2 Hapten-Induced LC Activation

Upon topical exposure to contact sensitizers, or other appropriate stimuli (e.g., trauma, irradiation), up to 40% of the local LC become activated [97, 98], leave the epidermis, and migrate, via afferent lymphatic vessels, to the draining lymph nodes [99] (Fig. 3.5). This process of LC migration results from several factors, including contact allergen-induced production of cytokines favoring LC survival [100–102] and loosening from surrounding keratinocytes [103–105]. Thus,

Fig. 3.5 (**a–d**) Hapten-induced migration of Langerhans cells. (**a**) In a resting state, epidermal Langerhans cells (*LC*) reside in suprabasal cell layers, tightly bound to surrounding keratinocytes (*KC*), e.g., by E-cadherin. (**b**) Early after epidermal hapten exposure, LC produce IL-1β and IL-18, which induce the release of IL-1α, TNF-α, and GM-CSF from keratinocytes. Together, these three cytokines facilitate migration of LC from the epidermis toward the lymph nodes. (**c**) Emigration of LC starts with cytokine-induced disentanglement from surrounding keratinocytes (e.g., by downregulation of E-cadherin) and production of factors facilitating penetration of the basal membrane (e.g., matrix metalloproteinases) and interactions with extracellular matrix and dermal cells (e.g., integrins and integrin ligands). (**d**) Once in the dermis, LC migration is directed toward the draining afferent lymphatic vessels, guided by local production of chemokines (e.g., CCL19 and CCL21) acting on newly expressed chemokine receptors, such as CCR7, on activated LC. Along their journey, haptenized LC further matures as characterized by their increased dendritic morphology and expression of costimulatory and antigen-presentation molecules

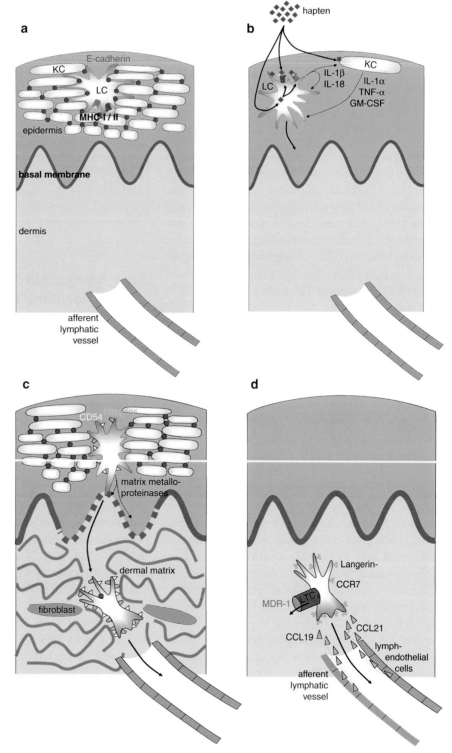

within 15 min after exposure to a contact sensitizer, production of IL-1β mRNA is induced [106, 107]. Along with this, caspase-1, formerly known as interleukin-1-converting enzyme, is activated and cleaves the active IL1β cytokine from the translated precursor-IL1β protein. Caspase-1 activates also IL-18 from its precursor form. These inflammatory processes are now viewed at as making up the "inflammasome" [108]. IL-1β in concert with IL-18 stimulates release of tumor necrosis factor (TNF)-α and granulocyte–macrophage colony-stimulating factor (GM-CSF) from keratinocytes [108]. Together these three cytokines facilitate migration of LC from the epidermis toward the lymph nodes [109]. IL-1β and TNF-α downregulate membrane-bound E-cadherin expression and thus cause disentanglement of LC from surrounding keratinocytes (Fig. 3.5) [104, 105, 110]. Simultaneously, adhesion molecules are upregulated promoting LC migration by mediating interactions with the extracellular matrix and dermal cells, such as CD54, α_6 integrin, and CD44 variants [111–115]. Also, production of the epidermal basement membrane degrading enzyme metalloproteinase-9 is upregulated in activated LC [116].

Next, LC migration is directed by hapten-induced alterations in chemokine receptor levels [117]. Upon maturation, LC downregulate expression of receptors for inflammatory chemokines (e.g., CCR1, 2, 5, and 6), whereas others (including CCR4, 7, and CXCR4) are upregulated (Fig. 2.3) (reviewed by [118] and [119–121]). Notably, CCR7 may guide maturing LC into the draining lymphatics and the lymph node paracortical areas, since two of its ligands (CCL19 and 21) are produced by both lymphatic and high endothelial cells [122, 123]. Importantly, the same receptor-ligand interactions cause naive T cells, which also express CCR7, to accumulate within the paracortical areas [124]. Migratory responsiveness of both cell types to CCR7 ligands is promoted by leukotriene C4, released from these cells via the transmembrane transporter molecule Abcc1 (previously called MRP1) [117, 125–127]. Interestingly, Abcc1 belongs to the same superfamily as the transporter associated with antigen-processing TAP, known to mediate intracellular peptide transport in the "endogenous route" which favors peptide association with MHC Class I molecules. Final positioning of the LC within the paracortical T-cell areas may be due to another CCR7 ligand, EBI1-ligand chemokine (ELC, CCL19), produced by resident mature DC [128].

Core Message

> Along with their migration and settling within the draining lymph nodes, haptenized LC further mature, as characterized by their increased expression of costimulatory and antigen-presentation molecules [129, 130]. In addition, they adopt a strongly veiled, interdigitating appearance, thereby maximizing the chances of productive encounters with naive T lymphocytes and recognition of altered self [131–133].

3.3.3 Recognition of Allergen-Modified Langerhans' Cells by Specific T Cells

3.3.3.1 Homing of Naive T Cells Into Lymph Nodes

More than 90% of naive lymphocytes present within the paracortical T-cell areas have entered the lymph nodes by high endothelial venules (HEV) [134]. These cells are characterized not only by CCR7 but also by the presence of a high molecular-weight isoform of CD45 (CD45RA) [134, 135]. Entering the lymph nodes via HEV is established by the lymphocyte adhesion molecule L-selectin (CD62L), which allows rolling interaction along the vessel walls by binding to peripheral node addressins (PNAd), such as GlyCAM-1 or CD34 [136–138]. Next, firm adhesion is mediated by the interaction of CD11a/CD18 with endothelial CD54, resulting in subsequent endothelial transmigration. Extravasation and migration of naïve T cells to the paracortical T-cell areas are supported by chemokines such as CCL18, 19, and 21 produced locally by HEV and by hapten-loaded and resident DC [125, 139–141]. In nonsensitized individuals, frequencies of contact allergen-specific T cells are very low, and estimates vary from 1 per 109 to maximally 1 per 106 [134, 142]. Nevertheless, the preferential homing of naive T cells into the lymph node paracortical areas and the large surface area of IDC make allergen-specific T-cell activation likely with only few dendritic cells exposing adequate densities of haptenized-MHC molecules [143, 144].

3.3.3.2 Activation of Hapten-Specific T Cells

As outlined in "Binding of Contact Allergens to Skin Components," the chemical nature of the hapten determines its eventual cytoplasmic routing in antigen-presenting cells (APC), and thus whether presentation will be predominantly in context of MHC class I or II molecules (Fig. 3.4). T cells, expressing CD8 or CD4 molecules, can recognize hapten-MHC class I or II complexes showing stabilized MHC membrane expression [145, 146]. Chances of productive interactions with T cells are high since each MHC-allergen complex can trigger a high number of T-cell receptor (TCR) molecules ("serial triggering") [147]. Moreover, after

contacting specific CD4[+] T cells, hapten-presenting DC may reach a stable superactivated state, allowing for efficient activation of subsequently encountered specific CD8[+] T cells [148]. The actual T-cell activation is executed by TCRξ-chain mediated signal transduction, followed by an intracellular cascade of biochemical events, including protein phosphorylation, inositol phospholipid hydrolysis, increase in cytosolic Ca^{2+} [149, 150], and activation of transcription factors, ultimately leading to gene activation (Fig. 3.6) [151].

For activation and proliferation, TCR triggering ("signal 1") is insufficient, but hapten-presenting APC also provide the required costimulation ("signal 2"; Fig. 3.7) [152, 153]. The costimulatory signals may

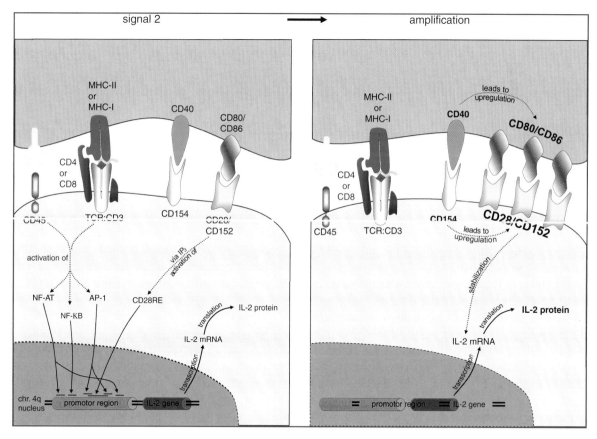

Fig. 3.6 Activation of hapten-specific T cells. T-cell receptor (TCR) triggering by hapten-major histocompatibility complex (*MHC*) complexes ("signal 1") is insufficient for T-cell activation. But "professional" antigen-presenting cells (*APC*), such as Langerhans cells, can provide the required costimulation ("signal 2") involving secreted molecules, such as cytokines, or sets of cellular adhesion molecules present on the outer cellular membranes of APC and T cells. T cells, stimulated in this way, activate nuclear responder elements (e.g., CD28RE). Together with nuclear transcription factors (*NF*) produced upon TCR trig-

gering, these nuclear responder elements enable transcription of T-cell growth factors, e.g., IL-2. APC–T cell interaction gives rise to mutual activation ("amplification"): on APC, ligation of CD40 with CD154 molecules on T cells induces overexpression of several costimulatory molecules, including CD80 and CD86. In turn, these molecules bind to and increase expression of CD28 on T cells. This interaction stabilizes CD154 expression, causing amplified CD154–CD40 signaling, and preserves strong IL-2 production, finally resulting in abundant T-cell expansion

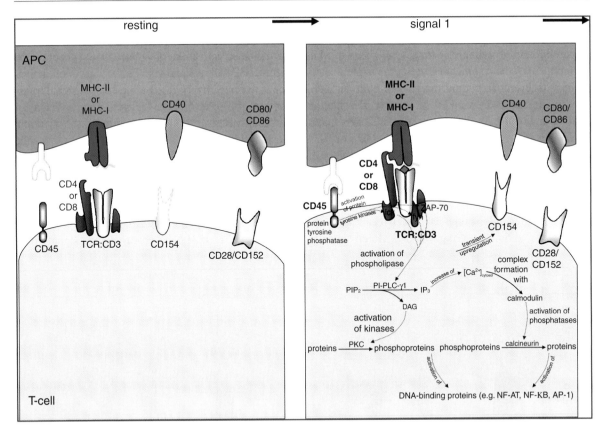

Fig. 3.6 (continued)

involve secreted molecules, such as cytokines (IL-1), or sets of cellular adhesion molecules (CAMs) and their counter-structures present on the outer cellular membranes of APC and T cells. Expression levels of most of these CAMs vary with their activational status, and thus can provide positive stimulatory feedback-loops. For example, as mentioned above, after specific TCR binding and ligation of CD40L (CD154) on T cells with CD40 molecules, APC reach a superactivated state, characterized by overexpression of several CAMs, including CD80 and CD86 (Fig. 3.6) [154, 155]. In turn, these molecules bind to and increase expression of CD28 on T cells. This interaction stabilizes CD154 expression, causing amplified CD154–CD40 signaling [155, 156].

The activational cascade is, as illustrated above, characterized by mutual activation of both hapten-presenting APC and hapten-reactive T cells. While this activation protects the APC from apoptotic death and prolongs their life to increase the chance of activating their cognate T cells, only the latter capitalize on these interactions by giving rise to progeny. As discussed below, to promote T-cell growth, cellular adhesion stimuli need

to be complimented by a broth of cytokines, many of which are released by the same APC. Together, elevated expression levels of (co-)stimulatory molecules on APC and local abundance of cytokines overcome the relatively high activation threshold of naive T cells [157].

> **Core Message**
>
> › The intricate structure of lymph node para-cortical areas, the differential expression of chemokines and their receptors, the characteristic membrane ruffling of IDC, and the predominant circulation of naïve T lymphocytes through these lymph node areas provide optimal conditions for T-cell receptor binding, i.e., the first signal for induction of T-cell activation [158]. Intimate DC–T cell contacts are further strengthened by secondary signals, provided by sets of CAMs, and growth-promoting cytokines (reviewed in [159, 160]).

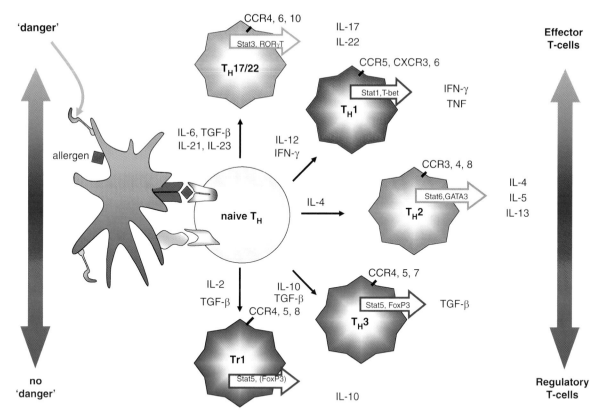

Fig. 3.7 Spectrum of allergen driven CD4$^+$ T cell differentiation: current schematic view. Depending on the immunological microenvironment (amount of allergen, danger signals, and other soluble mediators), activated naïve T cells are skewed into distinct phenotypes. The presence of allergen and sufficient danger signals leads to the development of effector T cell phenotypes of ACD. Presence of IL-6, TGF-β, IL-21, and IL-23 stimulates the generation of TH17/Th23 cells. Development of TH1 cells is stimulated by the presence of IL-12 and IFN-γ, and the development of TH2 is favored by IL-4. The absence of sufficient danger signals stimulates the development of tolerogenic phenotypes, including TH3 and Tr1 [165–167, 175, 201, 239, 241]

3.3.4 Proliferation and Differentiation of Specific T Cells

3.3.4.1 T-Cell Proliferation

Upon their activation, naive allergen-specific T cells start producing several cytokines, including IL-2, the classical T-cell growth factor [161, 162]. In particular, ligation of T cell-bound CD28 receptors unleashes full-scale IL-2 production in T cells by increasing IL-2 transcription and mRNA stabilization [163]. T-cell IL-2 production peaks within 24 h, and declines subsequently (Villarino 2007). Concomitant upregulation of the IL-2 receptor α-chain facilitates the assembly of high affinity IL-2 receptor complexes that augment autocrine T-cell responsiveness, thus providing a positive feedback loop leading to T-cell clonal expansions up to 1,000-fold [164]. The process of proliferation can be visible as an impressive, sometimes painful lymph node swelling.

3.3.4.2 T-Cell Differentiation

Whereas allergen-specificity remains strictly conserved along with their proliferation, within few days T cells show distinct expression of transcription factors associated with varying cytokine production profiles and [165–168]. Thus, the recent offspring of allergen-specific CD4$^+$ T cells can show at least five distinct cytokine profiles, generally associated with helper/effector or regulatory/suppressive functions (Fig. 3.7). Type 1 Th cells are characterized by a predominant release of IFN-γ, IL-2, and TNF-β, all known as proto-typical proinflammatory and cytotoxic cytokines. Type 2 Th cells secrete IL-4, IL-5, and IL-13, which have distinct proinflammatory activities, but are most prominent in promoting humoral antibody production, e.g., along mucosal surfaces where IgA contributes to exclusion of microbial entry [169, 170]. Next, the Th3 subset is distinguished by its release of transforming growth factor (TGF)-β, which displays anti-inflammatory activities [170]. Recently, Th-17 cells have been recognized as a separate lineage of proinflammatory T cells, characterized by the production of IL-17A and IL-17E, as well as IL-22, all of which play pivotal roles in auto-immune diseases, e.g., by recruiting neutrophils and macrophages [171, 172]. Finally, still another subset of CD4+ T cells is recognized for its strong regulatory role in controlling inflammatory reactivities, i.e., the Tr1 cells or "inducible Tregs," characterized by the secretion of IL-10 [166, 167]. This CD4+ T cell population is phenotypically remarkably heterogeneous, with part of the cells expressing high amounts of the high affinity IL-2 receptor ("CD25high"), either or not accompanied by expression of the transcription factor FoxP3 [173–175] (Fig. 3.7). Tr1 cells have essential roles in the maintenance of immune homeostasis, regulating effector T-cell responses and preventing their potentially pathogenic effects by various indirect ways, e.g., by suppressing macrophage functions [176, 177]. Each of these five cytokine profiles is under control of distinct sets of transcription factors that are shown in Fig. 3.7, but are discussed further elsewhere (e.g., [165, 166, 178–180].

To some extent, the same distinct cytokine profiles may develop in CD8+ T cells, where at least type 1 and 2 cytokine releasing CD8+ cells are known to contribute to ACD [68, 181].

Several factors are thought to contribute to the above described polarized cytokine production profiles in allergen-specific T cells, including (1) the site and cytokine environment of first allergenic contact, (2) the molecular nature and concentrations of the allergen, and (3) the neuroendocrine factors.

3.3.4.3 Cytokine Environment

In the skin-draining lymph nodes, allergen-activated LC and dermal dendritic cells rapidly produce large amounts of IL-12, switching off IL-4 cytokine production, thereby promoting the differentiation of Th1 cells [182–184]. Of note, since Th1 cells retain, next to IL12R, high IL-4R expression, they remain sensitive to IL-4 as a growth factor [185]. Thus, they also retain the capacity to shift cytokine production toward the type 2 profile. In contrast, type-2 T cells, e.g., developing in mucosa-draining lymph nodes, rapidly lose the genes encoding the IL-12-R β2 chain and thus type-2 differentiation is irreversible [186, 187].

Early differentiation of type-1 T cells is promoted by microbial danger-signal-induced IL-12 and IL-18, leading to IFN-γ release by nonspecific "bystander" cells, e.g., DC and NK cells, within the lymph nodes [188, 189]. IFN-γ interferes with skewing toward other cytokine profiles. Since Th1 cells rapidly lose functional IFN-γR expression, these cells, in contrast to Th2, Th3, and Th17 cells, become refractory to the growth-inhibitory effects of IFN-γ [190–192]. Interestingly, T-cell skewing may also be facilitated by primary contact-mediated signals, e.g., Th1 skewing by CD154 ligation through APC-bound CD40 [193] or Th2 skewing by ligation of CD134 (OX40) through APC-bound CD252 [194, 195].

In the process of T-cell skewing toward the other major cytokine profiles, TGF-β plays a central role. TGF-β can be produced by various cell types, including Th3 cells themselves, but is most prominently produced by mucosal epithelial cells [166, 192, 196]. Apparently, in conjunction with IL-10 production, e.g., produced by mucosal B cells, allergen-stimulated T cells rapidly initiate endogenous TGF-β production thus revealing the Th3 phenotype [197]. These cells may stimulate IgA production along the mucosae, but elsewhere immunosuppressive activities prevail. Interestingly, in conjunction with abundant local IL-2 production, such as induced by strong antigenic stimulation involving most effective CD28 triggering, TGF-β favors skewing toward IL-10 production, thereby providing an effective immunoregulatory feedback loop [198, 199]. Still, in the presence of strong and persistant microbial molecule-induced danger/growth signals, e.g., IL-6, IL-21, and IL-23, TGF-β induces the development of Th17 and/or Th22 cells, which both have been postulated to contribute to various allergic and autoimmune disorders [168, 172, 192, 200, 201] (Fig. 3.7).

Thus, ACD may be caused by any combination of at least three distinct types of effector T cells, releasing type-1, -2, and –17/22 cytokines, respectively. Considering that contact allergens will mainly enter via the skin, type-1 proinflammatory T cells are thought to represent the primary effector cells in ACD [202, 203]. Nevertheless, in sensitized individuals, type-2 T cells also play a role, as shown by both IL-4 production and allergen-specific type-2 T cells in the blood and at ACD reaction sites (see Sect. 3.3.6) [204–206]. Their role may increase along with the longevity of sensitization, since several factors contribute to shifting type-1 to type-2 responses, including reversibility of the former and not of the latter T cells, as mentioned above [207, 208]. Still, other sets of cytokines, including IL-17 and/or IL-22, are important in immune defense mechanisms, and thus Th17 and or Th22 cells have also been found to mediate allergic and autoimmune disorders [209]. Given rapid local release of both IL-4 and TGF-β within mucosal tissues, mucosal allergen contacts, if accompanied by strong danger signals, may lead in particular to Th2 and Th17 effector cells. Without these signals, rather immunoregulatory subsets (Th3, Tr1) would develop, as is observed in the induction of "oral tolerance" (see below) [210].

3.3.4.4 Nature of the Allergen

A second factor in determining T-cell cytokine production profiles, although still poorly understood, is the molecular character of the contact allergen itself, and the resulting extent of TCR triggering [211, 212]. For both protein and peptide antigens, high doses of antigen might favor type-2 responses, whereas intermediate/low doses would induce type-1 T-cell responses [211, 213]. Strong antigenic stimulation was also shown to upregulate CD40L expression on T cells and, in combination with microbial-induced IL-6, to promote Th17 differentiation. To what extent this translates to contact allergens is still unclear. Certainly, endogenous capacities of contact allergens to provide danger signals and activate the "inflammasome," in combination with their capacity to induce differentiation-skewing cytokines (in particular IL-4, IL-6, IL-12, and IL-23), will affect the outcome [214, 215]. In this respect, some contact allergens are notorious for inducing type-2 responses, even if their primary contact is by the skin route, e.g., trimellitic acid, which is also known as a respiratory sensitizer [216].

3.3.4.5 Neuroendocrine Factors

Diverse neuroendocrine factors codetermine T-cell differentiation [217–219]. An important link has been established between nutritional deprivation and decreased T cell-mediated allergic contact reactions [220]. Apparently, adipocyte-derived leptin, a hormone released by adequately nourished and functioning fat cells, is required for type-1 T-cell differentiation. Administration of leptin to mice restored ACD reactivity in mice during starvation [220]. Also, androgen hormones and adrenal cortex-derived steroid hormones, e.g., dehydroepiandrosterone (DHEA), promote type-1 T-cell and ACD reactivity. DHEA, like testosterone, may favor differentiation of type-1 T cells by promoting IFN-γ and suppressing IL-4 release [221, 222]. In contrast, the female sex hormone progesterone furthers the development of type-2 CD4$^+$ T cells and even induces, at least transient, IL-4 production and CD30 expression in established type-1 T cells [223, 224]. Type-2 T-cell polarization is also facilitated by adrenocorticotrophic hormone (ACTH) and glucocorticosteroids [225], and by prostaglandin (PG)E$_2$ [226]. PGE$_2$, released from mononuclear phagocytes, augments intracellular cAMP levels, resulting in inhibition of proinflammatory cytokine, like IFN-γ and TNF-α, production [227–230] and thus can influence the development of effector T cells in ACD.

> **Core Message**
>
> › In healthy individuals, primary skin contacts with contact allergens lead to differentiation and expansion of allergen-specific effector T cells displaying Th1, Th2, and/or Th17 cytokine profiles. The same allergens, if encountered along mucosal surfaces, favor the development of allergen-specific Th2 and Th17 effector cells, and/or Th3 and Tr1 allergen-specific regulatory T cells. While the first two subsets may assist or replace Th1 cells in proinflammatory effector functions, the latter two subsets are mainly known for downregulating immune responsiveness. For most, if not all allergens, along with prolonged allergenic contacts, the role of Th2 cells as effector cells gradually increases given reduced longevity of Th1 responses.

> The respective contributions of similar subsets o f allergen-specific CD8+ T cells are still unknown, but distinct effector roles of allergen-specific Tc1 and Tc2 have been postulated.

3.3.5 Systemic Propagation of the Specific T-Cell Progeny

3.3.5.1 T-Cell Recirculation

Upon sensitization via the skin, the progeny of primed T cells is released via the efferent lymphatic vessels

of the skin-draining lymph nodes and the thoracic duct into the blood (Fig. 3.8). If the first encounter with allergen occurs via the intestinal route, (e.g., along with induction of oral tolerance), priming will take place in the Peyer's patches and mesenteric lymph nodes, and primed T cells will be released from there to the circulation. The subsequent recirculation and homing pattern of primed T cells is guided by adhesion molecules and chemokine receptors, which they express on the cell membrane (Table 3.2). As outlined below, expression of these molecules is determined by the site of priming, as well as by the activational state of the T cells. In addition, there is a distinct relationship between the sets of chemokine

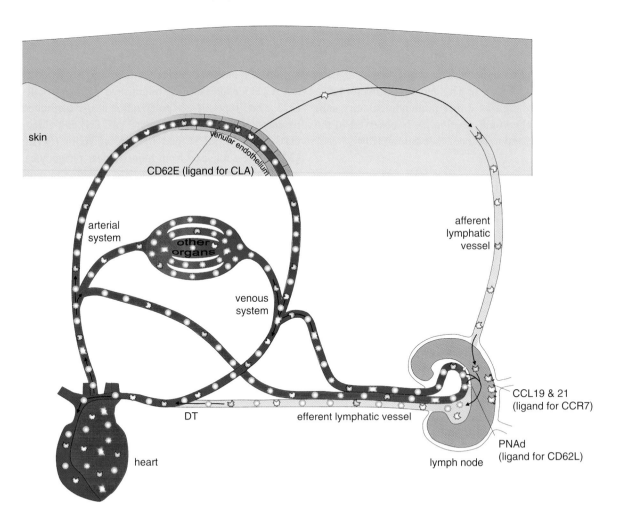

Fig. 3.8 Systemic propagation of hapten-specific T cells. From the skin-draining lymphoid tissue, the progeny of primed T cells is released via the efferent lymphatic vessels and the thoracic duct (*DT*) into the blood and becomes part of the circulation. Like their naïve precursors, these CCR7+ effector/memory T cells can still enter lymphoid tissues and settle in paracorticale areas by binding to its ligands CCL19 and CCL21. But increased expression of skin-homing molecules, e.g., cutaneous lymphocyte antigen (*CLA*), facilitates their spontaneous migration in the skin

Table 3.2 Molecules involved in the migration of hapten-specific T lymphocytes

Receptor/ligand	T-cell	Ligand/receptor	Cell	Tissue	References
CD62L (L-selectin)		CD34, GlyCAM-1 (PNAd)	HEV		Janeway [436], Sallusto [212]
CCR7		CCL19, CCL21	Stromal cells, DC	lymph node	Sallusto [212]
CD11a/CD18 (αL:β2-integrin, LFA-1)	increased upon activation	CD54, CD102 (ICAM-1, ICAM-2)	Endothelial cells		Janeway [436]
CD49d (α4:β1-integrin, VLA-4)	increased upon activation	CD106, fibronectin (VCAM-1)	Endothelial cells		Janeway [436]
CD162 (P-selectin ligand, PSGL-1)	increased upon activation	CD62P (P-selectin)	Endothelial cells		Woodland [461]
CLA	skin homing	CD62E (E-selectin)	Cutaneous endothelial cells		Woodland [461]
CCR4	Th2	CCL17 (TARC)	Keratinocytes	Skin	Woodland [461]
CCR5	Th1	CCL2 (MCP-1)? CCL3 (MIP-1α)	Keratinocytes (a.o.)		Meller [479], Gaga [490]
CCR6	Th17	CCL20 (MIP-3α / LARC)	Langerhans cells Endothelial cells		Larsen [455] Meller [479]
CCR10	Th22, CLA+	CCL27 (CTACK)	Keratinocytes Langerhans cells		Duhe [462], Homey [491], Kagami [492], Woodland [461]
CXCR3	Th1	CXCL9 and CXCL10 (Mig and IP-10)	Keratinocytes		Moed [285], Meller [479]
α4:β7-integrin	gut homing	MAdCAM-1	Endothelial cells		Janeway [436]
CCR9	T-cells	CCL25 (TECK)	Epithelial cells	gut	Grimm [493]; Miles [460]

and homing receptors expressed by T cells and their type of differentiation.

First, primed T cells have different homing receptors depending on the site of priming, a process called "imprinting" [231, 232]. During priming of allergen-specific T cells in the skin-draining lymph nodes, both CD4+ and CD8+ T cells are stimulated to express CLA [233] and the chemokine receptors CCR4 and CCR10, a phenotype that predisposes for eventual migration to the skin. In the mesenteric lymph nodes, on the other hand, T cells are stimulated to express the integrin α4:β7 and the chemokine receptor CCR9, a phenotype which predisposes for gut homing. An instructive role

of the peripheral tissues in this imprinting process was demonstrated in a mouse model on T cell priming by dendritic cells, where either dermal or intestinal cells were added to the cultures, resulting in T cells expressing mouse "CLA" or α4:β7 integrin, respectively [231]. For the imprint of gut homing, retinoic acid was identified as a crucial factor, while for the imprint of skin homing, the active metabolite of vitamin D3 was shown to be essential, because it induces CCR10 expression in T cells [234]. Still, for induction of CLA and thus for establishing the full skin-homing profile, cell–cell contact and/or other mediators, like IL-12, seem to be required [231].

After priming and imprinting, circulating gut homing memory T lymphocytes, bearing the $\alpha4{:}\beta7$ integrin, can attach to intestinal endothelial cells by binding to the mucosal vascular addressin MAdCAM-1. Further infiltration in the mucosa is guided by chemokines, such as CCL25, produced by small intestinal epithelial cells [235]. Thus, along the gut, T lymphocyte progeny is attracted that has been generated in other mucosal tissues. Likewise, in the skin, CLA-positive cells that have been generated in skin-draining lymph nodes are attracted. CLA binds to E-selectin (CD62E) on dermal endothelial cells, while CCR4 and CCR10 expression allow the lymphocytes to migrate in the skin toward CCL17 and CCL27 produced by keratinocytes in the epidermis.

At least as important for the recirculation and homing characteristics of T cells is the activational state of the cells. In this respect, primed T cells can be divided into two main subsets: the central memory T cells (T_{CM}) and the effector memory T cells (T_{EM}). Like their naive precursors, T_{CM} can still enter the peripheral lymphoid tissues due to the fact that they continue to express CD62L and CCR7, allowing for binding to HEV in the lymph nodes and migration into the paracortical areas. T_{EM}, on the other hand, have lost these molecules and migrate, due to simultaneous upregulation of several other adhesion molecules, preferentially to peripheral inflamed tissues. T_{EM} are characterized by rapid effector function upon antigenic stimulation, but, in the absence of antigenic stimuli, T_{EM} eventually convert to T_{CM} by reacquiring CCR7 and CD62L. In turn, T_{CM} may convert to T_{EM} upon antigenic restimulation [167, 232, 236, 237].

Peripheral endothelial binding and extravasation of T cells to inflamed tissues require the expression of both selectins and integrins on the T cell membrane, such as LFA-1, VLA-4, and PSGL-1. The vascular expression of their respective ligands (Table 3.2) is strongly increased by cytokines released at inflammatory sites. The density of adhesion molecules on the T cell membrane is generally upregulated upon activation, in particular in T_{EM}. Since their expression is highest only for short periods after activation, only recently activated T cells show a unique propensity to enter skin sites and exert effector functions.

Third, the differentiation of T cells (Th1, Th2 etc.) is clearly associated with distinct homing characteristics. T cells biased toward a proinflammatory phenotype show a higher propensity to enter skin sites, as compared to mucosal tissues [233, 238]. [201, 239] In mice, the early influx of type-1 T cells into delayed-type hypersensitivity (DTH) reactions was found to be more efficient than that of type-2 T cells, although both cell types expressed CLA. Here, CD162, highly expressed by type-1 T cells, was found to be important for this preferential homing [240]. Also, the pattern of chemokine receptors differs between the Th subsets (Table 3.2). Some receptors, such as CXCR3, are preferentially expressed on Th1 cells, whereas others, such as CCR4 and CCR8, are in particular expressed by Th2 cells [167, 175, 241, 242]. The latter chemokine receptors are not only overexpressed on type-2 cytokine-producing T cells, but also on basophils and eosinophils. Together these cells strongly contribute to local immediate allergic hyperresponsiveness. The more recently described Th17 and Th22 lymphocyte subsets expressing CCR4, CCR6, and CCR10 [239, 241] are attracted to the skin by epidermal CCL17, CCL20, and CCL27, respectively (Table 3.2). Overall, results obtained thus far favor the view that the proinflammatory subsets (Th1 and Th17/22) will be the first to enter skin sites upon local inflammatory stimuli, their primary function being an early control of antigenic pressure, e.g., through amplification of macrophage effector functions. The ACD reaction is, however, a dynamic process, in which the first influx of cells influences the local chemokine environment and determines the type of subsequent infiltrating cells. Thus, upon repeated exposure to contact allergens, gradually Th2 cells and regulatory cells may dominate [243]. Interestingly, also at the T cell level modulation of the cytokine and chemokine receptor profiles may occur, thereby maintaining plasticity of the immune response [167, 180]. The actual composition of the T cell infiltrate in ACD skin lesions does not only depend on the influx of lymphocytes, but should rather be regarded as the resultant of infiltration, apoptosis and retention of lymphocytes, next to their emigration to the lymphatics.

Finally, the antigen specificity of T cells contributes to their migration pattern. Allergens penetrated via the epidermis and displayed at the dermal endothelial surface may be recognized by allergen-specific T cells, thereby resulting in activation, immobilization, and transendothelial migration of these cells at sites of allergen exposure [241].

Core Message

> Priming via the skin results in CLA-positive T cells, which upon inflammatory stimuli preferentially enter the skin; on the other hand, gut homing T cells have been primed and generated along mucosal surfaces. Upon priming, T cells loose much of their capacity to recirculate via the lymph nodes, but gain the capacity to enter the tissues. In particular, recently activated T cells will enter skin-inflammatory sites. ACD reactions are primarily infiltrated by CD4 and/or CD8 proinflammatory cells, later reactions may be dominated by Th2 cells and regulatory T cells. Skin infiltration by T cells is fine tuned by sets of adhesion molecules and chemokine receptors, whose expression is not rigid, but can be modulated by microenvironmental factors.

3.3.5.2 Allergen-Specific T-Cell Recirculation: Options for In Vitro Testing

The dissemination and recirculation of primed, allergen-specific T cells in the body suggests that peropheral blood offers a most useful and accessible source for T-cell based in vitro assays for ACD. A major advantage of in vitro testing would be the noninterference with the patient's immune system, thereby eliminating any potential risk of primary sensitization and boosting by in vivo skin testing. Although such tests have found several applications in fundamental research, e.g., on recognition of restriction elements, cross-reactivities, and cytokine profile analyses, their use for routine diagnostic purposes is still limited. Even in highly sensitized individuals, frequencies of contact allergen-specific memory/effector cells may still be below 1 per 10^4 [244–246]. Given the relatively small samples of blood obtainable by venepuncture (at only one or a few time points), numbers of specific T cells in any culture well used for subsequent in vitro testing would typically be below 100 cells/well. For comparison, in vivo skin test reactions recruit at least 1,000 times more specific T cells from circulating lymphocytes passing by for the period of testing, i.e., at least 24 h [247].

Therefore, the sensitivity of in vitro assays, e.g., allergen-induced proliferation or cytokine production, may not always be sufficient to pick up weak sensitization. Intermediate or strong sensitization is, however, readily detected in vitro by both proliferation and cytokine production assays [245, 248–250]. With respect to the latter, both the "Elispot" assay, where allergen-induced cytokine production is evaluated at the single cell level, and the cytokine evaluation in allergen-stimulated culture supernatants provide adequate information [249, 251, 252]. Notably with respect to cytokine production, type-2 cytokines appear to provide most specific parameters for contact sensitization in these assays, [251, 253] although generally both Th1 and Th2 cytokines are being produced in vitro by allergic individuals, upon allergen exposure [250, 254].

Importantly, most of the above mentioned successful in vitro studies evaluated hydrophilic allergens, such as nickel, chromium, and palladium salts. Reports on successful in vitro assays with other hydrophobic and more toxic allergens are scarce [250, 255, 256]. Appropriate allergen presentation is a major hurdle in in vitro studies because of the broad range of requirements for different allergens with unique solubilities, toxicities, and reactivity profiles. Moreover, in the absence of LC, monocytes are the major source of APC, and their numbers in peripheral blood vary substantially within and between donors. Of note, optimal APC function is particularly critical for in vitro activation of resting memory T cells, since in the absence of repeated allergenic contacts, activated effector memory T cells (T_{EM}) may finally revert to a more naïve phenotype, with a higher threshold for triggering [236, 257]. Supplementing in vitro test cultures with appropriate mixtures of cytokines may, however, compensate for suboptimal APC function [250, 251, 258].

Core Message

> After antigenic activation the progeny of primed T cells is released via the efferent lymphatics into the bloodstream. Circulating allergen-specific cells can be challenged in vitro to provide diagnostic parameters for contact hypersensitivity. At least for water-soluble

allergens, such as metal salts, the degree of allergen-specific proliferation and cytokine production, in particular type-2 cytokines, correlates with clinical allergy. For routine application of a broad spectrum of allergens, culture conditions still need to be improved. For mechanistic in vitro studies in ACD, however, with selected sets of relatively nontoxic allergens, peripheral blood provides an excellent source of lymphocytes and APC.

3.3.6 The Effector Phase of Allergic Contact Dermatitis

3.3.6.1 Elicitation of ACD

Once sensitized, individuals can develop ACD upon reexposure to the contact allergen. Positive patch test reactions mimic this process of allergen-specific skin hyperreactivity. Thus, skin contacts induce an inflammatory reaction that, in general, is maximal within 2–3 days and, without further allergen supply, declines thereafter (Fig. 2.8). Looked at superficially, the mechanism of this type of skin hyperreactivity is straightforward: allergen elicitation or challenge leads to the (epi)dermal accumulation of contact allergen-specific memory/effector T lymphocytes, which, upon encountering allergen-presenting cells, are reactivated to release proinflammatory cytokines. These, in turn, spark the inflammatory process, resulting in macroscopically detectable erythema and induration. As compared to immediate allergic reactions, developing within a few minutes after mast-cell degranulation, ACD reactions show a delayed time course, since both the migration of allergen-specific T cells from the dermal vessels and local cytokine production need several hours to become fully effective. Still, the picture of the rise and fall of ACD reactions is far from clear. Some persistent issues are discussed below, notably: (1) irritant properties of allergens, (2) role of early phase reactivity, (3) T-cell patrol and specificity, (4) effector T-cell phenotypes, and (5) downregulatory processes.

3.3.6.2 Irritant Properties of Allergens

Within a few hours after allergenic skin contact, immunohistopathological changes can be observed, including vasodilatation, upregulation of endothelial adhesion molecules [259, 260], mast-cell degranulation [261, 262], keratinocyte cytokine and chemokine production, [45, 263] influx of leucocytes [264, 265], and LC migration toward the dermis [112, 266–268]. These proinflammatory phenomena, which are also observed in nonsensitized individuals [269] and in T cell-deficient nude mice [270], strongly contribute to allergenicity [58]. Clearly most, if not all, of these effects can also be caused by irritants and, therefore, do not unambiguously discriminate between irritants and contact allergens [45, 271–273]. Apparently, true differences between these types of compounds depend on whether or not allergen-specific T cells become involved. Thus, only after specific T-cell triggering, distinctive features might be observed, e.g., local release of certain chemokines such as the Th1 associated chemokines CXCL9, CXCL10 (IP-10), and CXCL11 (I-TAC/IP-9) [263, 274] or the Th2 related chemokines CCL11, CCL17, and CCL22 [263, 274]. Certainly, proinflammatory effects of contact allergens increase, in many ways, the chance of allergen-specific T cells meeting their targets. The first cells affected by skin contact, i.e., keratinocytes and LC, are thought to represent major sources of pivotal mediators such as IL-1β and TNF-α [106, 275]. First, as described in "Hapten-Induced Activation of Allergen-Presenting Cells," these cytokines cause hapten-bearing LC to mature and migrate toward the dermis [94, 131, 268]. But these cytokines also cause (over)expression of adhesion molecules on dermal postcapillary endothelial cells, and loosen intercellular junctions. In that way, extravasation of leucocytes, including allergen-specific T cells, is strongly promoted [241, 275–278]. Moreover, haptens can stimulate nitric oxide (NO) production of the inducible NO-synthase (iNOS) of LC and keratinocytes, which contributes to local edema, vasodilatation, and cell extravasation [279, 280].

Histopathological analyses support the view that the major causative events take place in the papillary dermis, close to the site of entry of allergen-specific T cells, for instance at hair follicles, where haptens easily penetrate and blood capillaries are nearby [281]. Here, perivascular mononuclear cell infiltrates develop, giving the highest chance of encounters between

allergen-presenting cells and specific T cells. Once triggered, extravasated T cells will readily enter the lower epidermal layers, in which haptenized keratinocytes produce lymphocyte-attracting chemokines, such as CXCL9/10, CCL17, CCL20, and CCL27 ([201, 232, 263, 274]; Table 3.2). Subsequently, since effector memory T cells can also be triggered by "nonprofessional" APC, including KC, fibroblasts, and infiltrating mononuclear cells, ACD reactivity is amplified in the epidermis [157, 159, 269]. Together, these events result in the characteristic epidermal damage seen in ACD, such as spongiosis and hyperplasia. Notably, in ongoing ACD reactions, the production of chemokines attracting lymphocytes and monocytes/macrophages, in addition to the production of cytokines, adds to the nonspecific recruitment and activation of leucocytes [119, 282, 283]. Thus, like the very early events in the effector phase reaction, the final response to a contact allergen is antigen-nonspecific. It is, therefore, not surprising that allergic and irritant reactions are histologically alike.

3.3.6.3 Early Phase Reactivity

In the elicitation phase allergen-specific T cells are triggered by MHC-bound allergen, just like in the afferent phase. The role of LC in allergen presentation upon elicitation is, however, less prominent, and also other cells such as mast cells, macrophages, and keratinocytes may now contribute, since effector T cells are easily triggered and do not require professional antigen presentation. The role of keratinocytes in the onset of the ACD reaction is important because of the cytokines and chemokines they produce upon hapten application [237, 263], thereby facilitating the influx of effector T cells. In addition, a variety of other cells and mediators may contribute to the initiation of the ACD reaction, as summarized below.

The role of neutrophils in the onset of ACD reactions has not been well-established, though recent studies in mice demonstrate that skin reactivity to haptens largely depends on CXCL1, released from endothelial cells when the first hapten-specific CD8 T cells encounter the allergen and produce IL-17. CXCL1 may then attract neutrophils to the elicitation site, thus facilitating further influx of allergen-specific T cells [284]. In the human system, neutrophil infiltration was also observed in skin biopsies from nickel patch tests,

presumably as a result of IL-17/IL-22 mediated inflammation [201]. Moreover, it has been shown that IL-8/CXCL8, a potent neutrophil chemoattractant, is readily produced by human antigen-presenting cells upon hapten exposure [285]; this could also contribute to an early influx of neutrophils in ACD reactions.

The role of an antibody-mediated early-phase reaction in the development of ACD is still unclear in man, although Askenase and his colleagues have generated robust data to support this view in murine models [286]: Hapten-specific IgM, produced upon sensitization by distant hapten-activated B-1 cells, can bind antigen early after challenge and activate complement. The resulting C5a causes the release of serotonin and TNF-α from local mast cells and platelets, leading to vascular dilatation and permeabilization, detectable as an early ear swelling peaking at 2 h [287]. Furthermore, C5a and TNF-α induce the upregulation of adhesion molecules on local endothelial cells [288, 289], thereby contributing to the recruitment of T cells in hapten challenge sites [289, 290]. In addition, human T cells were found to express the C5a receptor and are chemoattracted to endothelium-bound C5a [291]. However, against most contact allergens, including nickel, no antibodies have been detected in man, arguing against humoral mechanisms playing more than a minor role in clinical ACD [292, 293]. Interestingly in mice, immunoglobulin light chains, which have long been considered as the meaningless remnants of a spillover in the regular immunoglobulin production of B cells, were discovered to mediate very early hypersensitivity reactions by mast cell activation [294].

In addition to an auxiliary role of B cells and antibodies, natural killer (NK) cells have been reported to play a role in the onset of ACD reactions. Mice lacking both T and B cells (RAG2−/−) could still be sensitized to contact allergens, and Thy1+ NK cells were identified here as effector cells with a prominent role for the activating NK receptor NKG2D [295]. Interestingly, another NK-like cell, the invariant NKT cell, that recognizes CD1d bound glycolipids resulting in rapid IL-4 and IFN-γ release, was also found to play a role in the elicitation of contact sensitivity in mice: blocking of CD1d prevented both sensitization and elicitation by contact allergens [296]. Notably, in human ACD reactions relatively high frequencies of invariant NKT cells have been observed, ranging from 1.7 to 33% of total infiltrating T cells, which is 10–100-fold higher than the frequency found in the circulation [297]. Also, other

T cells with relatively restricted TCR repertoire, such as Tγδ cells, have been reported to contribute in a nonantigen-specific, probably non-MHC-restricted manner, to (early) elicitation responses [298].

To conclude, using various mouse models, different types of early allergen-specific reactivity have been claimed to play initiating roles in ACD, but clinical evidence for such mechanisms is still lacking.

3.3.6.4 T-Cell Patrol and Specificity of T-Cell Infiltrates

Whereas early nonspecific skin reactivity to contact allergens is pivotal for both sensitization and elicitation, full-scale development of ACD, of course, depends on allergen-specific T cells within the (epi) dermal infiltrates. In healthy skin there is a constant flow of memory T cells ending up in the draining lymph nodes: about 200 T cells/h/cm^2 skin [115]. Since one single antigen-specific T cell can already trigger visible skin inflammation [299, 300], randomly skin-patrolling memory/effector T cells might account for the initiation of the allergen-specific effector phase. However, since frequencies of hapten-specific T cells in sensitized individuals may still remain below 1 in 10,000, this does not seem to be a realistic scenario. Thus, augmented random and/or specific T-cell infiltration accompanies the development of ACD. Apparently, local chemokine release upon allergen contact is pivotal in this respect (see *T-Cell recirculation*; 482). Chemokine gene expression evaluated 48 h after NiSO4 application was increased for both Th1 related cytokines (CXCL9, CXCL10, and CXCL11) and Th2 related cytokines (CCL11, CCL17, and CCL22). On the other hand, CCL27 that attracts preferentially CCR10 bearing Th17/22 cells is constitutively produced in resting skin, but is rapidly released upon allergen contact to accumulate in the draining lymph nodes.

The question concerning the specificity of ACD T-cell infiltrates has so far received little attention. In a guinea pig model, preferential entry of dinitrochlorobenzene (DNCB)-specific T cells was observed within 18 h after elicitation of skin tests with DNCB, as compared to nonrelated compounds [301]. Probably, extravasation of hapten-specific T cells benefits from T-cell receptor-mediated interactions with endothelial MHC molecules, presenting hapten penetrated from

the skin [241]. Within minutes after epicutaneous application, hapten can indeed be found in dermal tissues and on endothelial cells [259, 302, 303]. Indeed, the frequency of allergen-specific cells in positive patch tests to urushiol was found to be 10–100-fold higher than in the blood [246]. Interestingly, whereas preferential entry may already contribute to relatively high frequencies of allergen-specific T cells (within 48 h up to 10%) [205, 299], at later stages, when the ACD reaction fades away, the local frequency of allergen-specific T cells may increase even further, due to allergen-induced proliferation and rescue from apoptosis. Thus, at former skin reaction sites, these cells can generate "local skin memory" (see Sect. 3.3.7).

3.3.6.5 Effector T-Cell Phenotypes

The debate on phenotypes of effector T cells in ACD is still ongoing and the number of T cell subsets potentially involved is growing every year (Fig. 3.7). Consensus exists, however, on the phenotype of the skin-homing T cell, i.e., CLA positive. This molecule enables binding to cutaneous endothelial cells via E-selectin (CD62E) and thus migration into the dermis.

Since cutaneous infiltrates show a clear preponderance of CD4$^+$ T cells, it is not surprising that these cells have most often been held responsible for mediating ACD. In nickel allergic individuals, indeed, allergen responding cells were found to be CD4$^+$CLA$^+$ memory T cells [304]. Other studies, however, revealed CD8$^+$CLA$^+$ nickel reactive T cells as most discriminating for allergic individuals, since CD4$^+$ nickel reactive T cells were also found in healthy controls [244]. While the effector mechanism of CD4$^+$T cells is mainly based on cytokine production, CD8+ T cells may mediate skin inflammation also through killing of hapten-bearing target cells. In mice, generally CD8$^+$ T cells are found to cause contact sensitivity reactions, certainly to strong allergens, like DNFB [284, 297]. In mice CD4$^+$ T cells are rather found to be regulatory, as shown by the fact that contact sensitization to weak allergens succeeded only after depletion of the CD4$^+$ T cells [305]. Of note, most model allergens studied in mice are hydrophobic molecules such as DNFB and oxazolone, whereas in human studies, very often, water-soluble metal salts, such as NiSO4, are used as model allergen. This could, at least partly, explain the different T cell subsets involved (Fig MHCI/II presentation). So, taken together, it has become clear that both CD4+ and CD8+ T cells can act as effector cells in DTH and ACD reactions. Likewise, neither of these subsets can be regarded simply as regulatory or suppressor cells, although both of these subsets may, depending on the allergen models and read-out assays, play such roles [68, 306].

An essentially similar conclusion holds true for T-cell subsets (whether CD4+ or CD8+), releasing type-1, type-2, or type-17 cytokines or combinations thereof. While type-1 cytokines, in particular IFN-γ, display well-established proinflammatory effects by fi increasing MHC and ICAM-1 expression [284, 307], thereby contributing to improved allergen presentation and infiltration, IL-4, a hallmark type-2 cytokine, can cause erythema and induration, when released in the skin [308, 309]. Indeed, blockage of IL-4 can interfere with ACD [309]. IL-17 plays a role in recruitment and activation of neutrophils. It was shown to be produced both by CD8+ T cells (in mouse models with DNFB; 483) and by CD4+ T cells (in human nickel patch tests; 456). The latter study shows, interestingly, that within a few hours after challenge, CCL20 expression is upregulated in the skin, attracting CCR6 positive cells. Since all Th17 cells do express this receptor, an early preferential influx of Th17 and, as a consequence, IL-17 and IL-22 production could be an essential early event in the development of the ACD reaction.

Thus, a picture emerges in which ACD reactions can be caused both by allergen-specific type-1, type-2, and type-17 T cells [168, 201, 244, 251, 297, 304]. In retrospect, the downregulatory effects of IL-4 on ACD reactions observed earlier in some mouse models [310] might be ascribed to accelerated allergen-clearance, rather than to blunt suppression. Still, both with time and repeated allergen-pressure, type-2 responsiveness may rapidly take over [243, 311]. Allergen-specific T cells isolated from skin test sites of sensitized individuals, as compared to blood, showed a strong bias toward type-2 cytokine profiles [204]. Additional local IFN-γ release seems, however, indispensable, since for a broad panel of contact allergens, clinical ACD reactions were characterized by increased expression of mRNA encoding IFN-γ-inducible chemokines [274]. In addition, transgenic mice expressing IFN-γ in the epidermis showed strongly increased ACD reactivity [312].

3.3.6.6 Downregulatory Processes

Resolution of ACD reactions and risk factors for the development of chronicity are not yet fully understood. Of course, if the allergen source is limited, as with skin testing, local concentrations of allergen usually rapidly decrease, thus taking away the critical trigger of the ACD reaction cascade. Since even ACD reactions due to chronic exposure to allergen seldomly result in permanent tissue destruction and scarification, immunoregulatory factors most likely contribute to prevention of excessive cytotoxicity and fatal destruction of the basal membrane. Both IL-1 and heparinase, secreted from activated keratinocytes and T cells, protect keratinocytes from TNF-α-induced apoptosis [313, 314]. Moreover, activated effector T cells can undergo activation-induced cell death (AICD) during the resolution phase [315]. Notably, proinflammatory type-1 T cells, expressing high levels of Fas-ligand (CD95L) and low amounts of apoptosis-protecting FAP-1 protein, are more susceptible to AICD than type-2 cells [316]. This may partly explain the shift toward type-2 reactivity that is observed upon prolonged allergen exposure [311]. Moreover, during the late phase of ACD, keratinocytes, infiltrated macrophages, and T cells start producing IL-10 [317–319], which has many anti-inflammatory activities, including suppression of antigen-presenting cell and macrophage functions [320, 321]. In addition, the release of factors, such as PGE$_2$ and TGF-β, derived from activated keratinocytes and infiltrated leucocytes, e.g., type-3 T cells, contribute to dampening of the immune response [322, 323]. Release of PGE$_2$, on the one hand, inhibits production of proinflammatory cytokines [230, 324] and, on the other hand, activates basophils [325]. These may constitute up to 5–15% of infiltrating cells in late phase ACD reactions [326] and are also believed to contribute to downregulation of the inflammatory response [327, 328]. TGF-β silences activated T cells and inhibits further infiltration by downregulating the expression of adhesion molecules on both endothelial and skin cells [236]. Regulatory cells producing these suppressive mediators might even predominate in skin sites, frequently exposed to the same allergen, and known to show local (allergen-specific) hyporesponsiveness [329]. It is of interest in this context that CD4+ memory T cells expanded from late DTH reactions could be educated to become CD4+CD25++ regulatory T cells expressing Foxp3.

Core Message

> ACD reactions can be mediated by classical effector cells, i.e., allergen-specific CD4$^+$ type-1 T cells, which, upon triggering by allergen-presenting cells, produce IFN-γ to activate non-specific inflammatory cells such as macrophages. However, CD8$^+$ T cells and other cytokines, including IL-4, IL-17, and IL-22, can also play major roles in ACD. The conspicuous difference with DTH reactions induced by intradermal administration of protein antigens, i.e., the epidermal infiltrate, can largely be attributed to hapten-induced chemokine release by keratinocytes.

3.3.7 Flare-Up and Retest Reactivity

3.3.7.1 Local Allergen Retention

Flare-up reactivity of former ACD and patch test reaction sites is sometimes observed [330–332]. From the basic mechanisms of ACD, it can be inferred that allergen-specific flare-up reactions depend either on local allergen or T-cell retention at these skin sites. Upon short-lasting, low-dose contacts, e.g., by skin testing, local allergen retention usually does not exceed a 2-week period, which is actually long enough to exceed the time required for active sensitization. In experimental guinea pig studies, we observed that skin tests with DNCB, chromium, or penicillin could become positive even if primary sensitization was postponed to 1 week after skin testing. Apparently effector T cells released into the circulation at that late time still detected sufficient residual allergen at the former skin test sites to cause flare-up reactivity (Scheper et al., unpublished results). Maximum allergen-persistence for around 14 days was also reported by Saint-Mezard et al., [58] using the hapten fluorescein-isothiocyanate in a mouse model for flare-up reactivity. Also in humans flare-up reactions due to locally persisting allergen can be observed, when from about 4–6 days after primary sensitization, peripheral effector T cell frequency increases [333]. Clinically, this phenomenon can explain anomalous results from patch testing with multiple contact allergens. When a patient suspected for penicillin allergy was patch tested with cross-reactive penicillin derivatives, a regular 24–72 h reaction was only observed to one of the penicillins, but all others also became positive from about 8–9 days after skin testing. The first penicillin derivative turned out to release formaldehyde to which the patient was found to be allergic. Positive reactivity to formaldehyde apparently had potentiated primary sensitization to penicillin, causing the other previously negative reaction sites to flare-up (Neering, personal communication). Thus, skin test sites may occasionally flare-up if the testing dose itself led to the release or activation of sufficiently high numbers of effector T cells in the circulation.

3.3.7.2 Local T-Cell Retention

In contrast, allergen-specific T cells may persist for at least several months in the skin causing "local skin memory" (Figs. 3.9 and 3.10) [334, 335]. Thus, locally increased allergen-specific hyperreactivity, detectable through either accelerated "retest" reactivity (after repeated allergenic contact at the same skin site) or flare-up reactivity (after allergen entry from the circulation, e.g., derived from food ingestion), may be observed for long periods of time at former skin reaction sites [336–338]. Typically, the erythematous reactions peak between 2 and 6 h after contact with the allergen. Histological examination of such previously positive skin reaction sites shows that the majority of remaining T cells is CD4$^+$ CCR10$^+$ [335]. The remarkable flare-up reactivity at such sites can be understood by considering that just one specific effector T cell can be sufficient to generate macroscopic reactivity [300]. Moreover, a very high frequency of the residual T cells may be specific for the allergen, as discussed above in Sect. 3.3.6. Apparently, local specific T cell retention is highly advantageous in combating microbial infections, since memory T cells localized in peripheral tissues contribute to robust protection, e.g., to viral infections [232]. Only in highly sensitized individuals unrelated skin test sites may also show flare-up reactions [334] and even generalized erythematous macular eruptions can be observed with higher allergen doses [339]. The latter reactivities probably relate to the fact that recently activated T cells show strong expression of adhesion and homing molecules, e.g., CLA and chemokine receptors such as CCR5, facilitating random migration into peripheral tissues and thus allergen-specific T cell patrol in the skin [232, 340]. Upon subsequent allergen entry from the circulation, these allergen-specific T cells could mediate generalized erythematous reactions [331].

Interestingly, local allergen-specific T cell retention/ "local skin memory" can be clinically exploited to discriminate between simultaneous sensitization to different sensitizers ("concomitant sensitization") and cross-reactivity between different sensitizers [341–343]. Using several different combinations of contact allergens in a guinea pig model, we retested guinea pigs previously sensitized to DNCB and methyl

methacrylate (MMA), with the same allergens and some other methacrylate congeners. Accelerated retest reactivities were observed with the latter congeners on the former MMA, but not DNCB, patch test sites [341]. Thus, with preferential local retention of MMA-specific T cells at the MMA skin test site, no accelerated retest reactivity could be elicited with DNCB, but to varying degrees with all four MMA-related compounds. In clinical practice using this approach, Matura [342] confirmed positive cross-retest reactions for cloprednol and tixocortol pivalate, both belonging to group A, and budesonide, amcinonide, and triamcinolone, all belonging to group B corticosteroids (see also [344]).

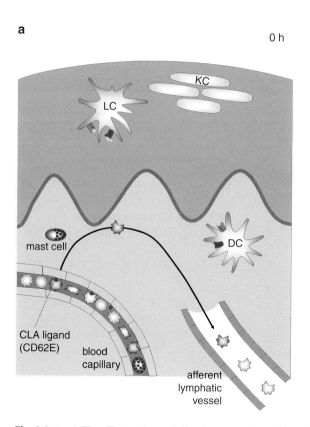

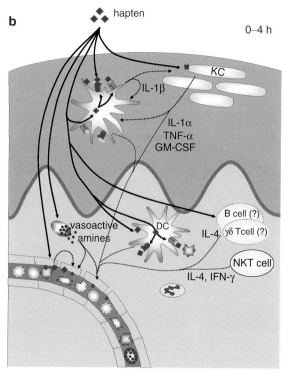

Fig. 3.9 (**a–c**) The effector phase of allergic contact dermatitis. (**a**) *0 h:* In resting skin relatively few randomly patrolling, skin-homing CLA⁺ T cells are present. (**b**) *0–4 h:* Reexposure of the contact allergen, binding to (epi)dermal molecules and cells, induces release of proinflammatory cytokines. (**c**) *2–6 h:* Influenced by inflammatory mediators, activated epidermal Langerhans cells (*LC*) start migrating toward the basal membrane and endothelial cells express increased numbers of adhesion molecules. Endothelial cell-bound hapten causes preferential extravasation of hapten-specific T cells, which are further guided

by inflammatory chemokines. (**d**) *4–8 h:* Hapten-activated T cells release increasing amounts of inflammatory mediators, amplifying further cellular infiltration. (**e**) *12–48 h:* The inflammatory reaction reaching its maximum, characterized by (epi) dermal infiltrates, edema, and spongiosis. (**f**) *48–120 h:* Gradually, downregulatory mechanisms take over, leading to decreased inflammation and disappearance of the cellular infiltrate. Finally, primordial conditions are reconstituted except for a few residual hapten-specific T cells causing the local skin memory. *KC* keratinocyte; *DC* dendritic cell

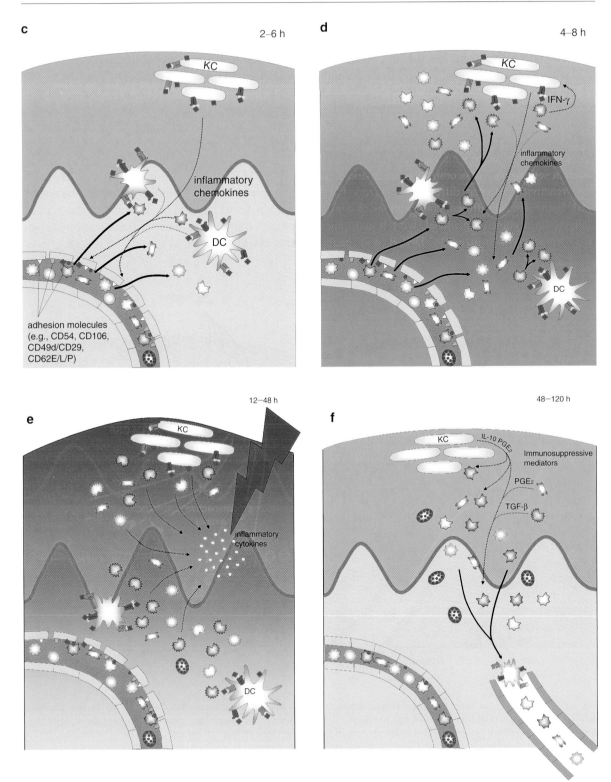

Fig. 3.9 (continued)

weeks/months after ACD reaction   retest reaction

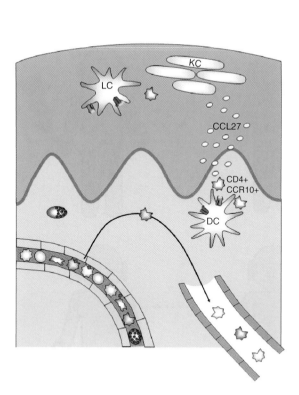
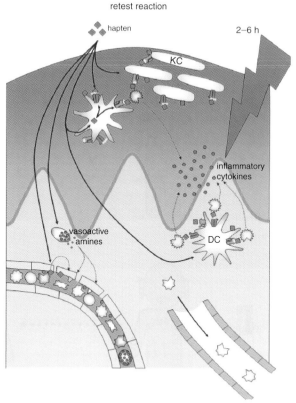

Fig. 3.10 Local skin memory. In former allergic contact dermatitis sites, a few hapten-specific T cells can remain, mainly close to dermal dendritic cells (*DC*). Retest reaction: renewed hapten contact can induce a rapid onset of an erythematous reaction, sparked off by the residual hapten-specific T cells. *KC* keratinocyte; *LC* Langerhans cell

3.3.8 Hyporeactivity: Tolerance and Desensitization

Of course, uncontrolled development and expression of T cell-mediated immune function would be detrimental to the host. During evolution, several mechanisms developed to curtail lymph node hyperplasia or prevent excessive skin damage upon persisting antigen exposure.

3.3.8.1 Regulation of Immune Responses

First, allergen contacts, e.g., by oral or intravenous administration, may lead to large-scale presentation of allergen by cells other than skin DC (Fig. 3.11). In the absence of appropriate costimulatory signals (as described above in Sect. 3.3.3), allergen presented by, e.g., immature Langerhans' cells may anergize naive T cells, i.e., cause receptor-downregulation associated with an unresponsive state, eventually leading to their death by apoptosis (Fig. 3.12) [345–347]. With increasing densities of MHC-antigen complexes on the surface of professional APC, at least three different levels of T-cell tolerance may be induced, characterized by active suppression, anergy, or deletion [348, 349]. Unresponsiveness of T cells, induced by allergenic contacts at skin sites where LC/DC functions have been damaged, e.g., by UV irradiation, or are naturally absent, e.g., in the tail skin of mice, may be ascribed to T-cell anergy, frequently associated with TCR/CD4 or CD8 downregulation, and apoptosis/deletion [350, 351]. Whereas anergy and deletion reflect "passive" unresponsiveness, tolerance by active suppression may also be induced under similar circumstances [352].

antigen ingestion   skin contact(s)   48 h after
                                                                                     reexposure

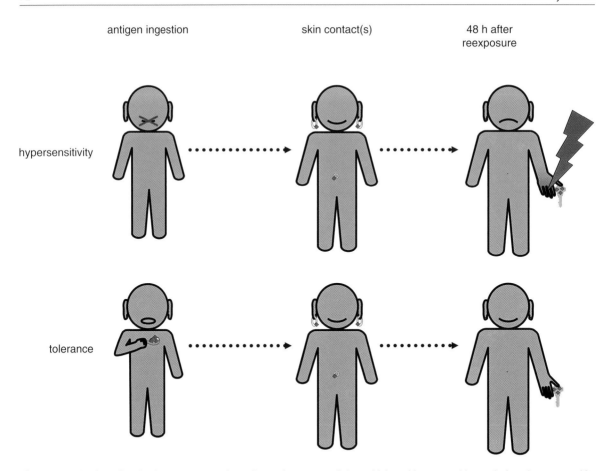

hypersensitivity

tolerance

Fig. 3.11 Induction of oral tolerance. Hapten ingestion, prior to potential sensitizing skin contact(s), can induce hapten-specific tolerance

Actually, with increasing dose and exposure times, even regular epicutaneous allergenic contacts induce not only T effector cells but also lymphocytes controlling T-cell proliferation (afferently acting regulatory cells) and/or causing decreased skin reactivity (regulatory cells of effector phase). Thus, allergic contact hypersensitivity is the resultant of a delicate balance between effector and regulatory mechanisms [329, 353].

3.3.8.2 Cellular Basis of Active Tolerance

Upon preferential stimulation of regulatory cells, e.g., by feeding nonprimed, naïve individuals with contact allergens, strong, and stable allergen-specific, active tolerance may develop [354–356]. The concept of active regulatory ("suppressor") cells controlling ACD is based on the fact that in experimental animal models, such allergen-specific tolerance can be transferred

by lymphoid cells from tolerant to naive animals [298, 357]. Active suppression, as revealed by these adoptive cell transfers, is a critical event in regulating T-cell responses to contact sensitizers and to all possible peptide/ protein antigens, including bacterial, autoimmune, and graft rejection antigens [358–360].

Like effector T cells in ACD, regulatory cells are not a single subpopulation of cells. As outlined above, depending on, e.g., the nature of the allergen and route of exposure, ACD can be mediated by both CD4+ and CD8+ T cells, either or both releasing Th1, Th2, Th3, Th17/22 cytokines. With distinct effector phenotypes for particular allergens, each of the other phenotypes can act as regulatory cells ([361, 362]: CD8+ Treg). Notwithstanding, type-2 cytokine-producing cells are prominent in regulating ACD, with allergic contact hypersensitivity enhanced and tolerance reversed by interfering with type-2 T cell functions [363–366]. Also, interferons and IL-12, both impairing Th2 and Th17/22 cells, were shown to inhibit regulatory cells

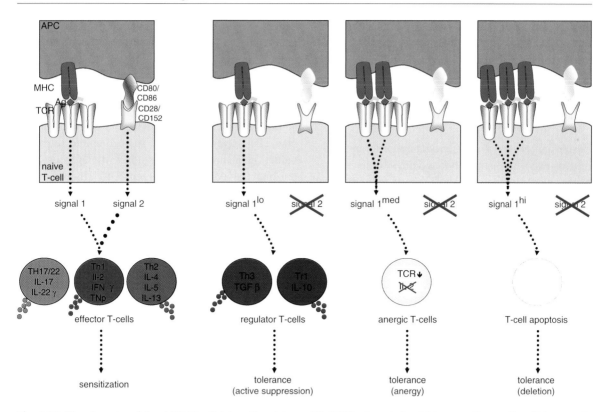

Fig. 3.12 The character of the APC–T cell interaction determines the immunological outcome. Sensitization: Naïve T cells, activated by antigen-presenting cells (*APC*) providing both hapten-specific ("signal 1") and appropriate costimulatory ("signal 2") signals, develop into effector T cells, characterized by Th-17/22, -1, and -2 cytokine secretion profiles. Tolerance: In the absence of appropriate costimulatory signals, immunological tolerance may develop. With increasing density of MHC–hapten complexes on the surface of APC, activating "signal 1" T-cell pathways, multiple levels of T-cell tolerance might be induced

and stimulate effector cell functions in mouse models [367–369]. In particular, after mucosal allergen contact stimulation, T cells producing IL-10 and/or TGF-β (type-3 cytokine profile), many of which coexpressing CD4, CD25, and the transcription factor Foxp3 (Treg), may act as regulatory cells [174, 370, 371]. These T cells promote anti-inflammatory immunity, e.g., by switching antibody production to IgA, which mediates secretory immunity and thus contributes to antigen exclusion in the lumen, e.g., of the gastro-intestinal tract [372]. Of note, TGF-β strongly suppresses development of both type-1 and -2 effector T cells, and can silence T cells in a seminaïve state [236].

3.3.8.3 Regulatory Mechanisms of the Effector Phase

A critical feature of the regulatory principles involving mutual regulation of T-cell subpopulations by Th1, Th2,

Th3, and Th17/22 cytokines is that regulatory functions are most effective during initiation of immune responses (Fig. 3.7). Thus, once established, effector T cell and cytokine profiles show remarkable stability and refractoriness to regulatory forces. Downregulation of allergic skin reactions may, therefore, take considerable time. Of course, the preliminary factor facilitating decreased allergic skin reactivity is the removal of hapten by exudate and innate immune cells of the inflammatory infiltrate. But, at chronically exposed sites, specific regulatory mechanisms can also be involved, such as CD8[+] T cells, acting either as regulator/ suppressor (CD28[−]CD11b[+]) or cytotoxic (CD28[+]CD11b[−]) T cells [373, 374], which may downregulate skin reactivity by targeting allergen-presenting DC [374]. Multiplicity and redundancy of regulatory mechanisms have thus far hampered development of robust clinical treatments exploiting regulatory T cell functions to provide for allergen-specific downregulation of the effector phase of ACD. The development of potential therapeutic applications of regulatory cells in various disorders, such as ACD and autoimmune diseases, therefore, needs much more time than envisioned earlier [375].

3.3.8.4 Redundancy of Tolerance Mechanisms

Besides regulatory T cells, producing different cytokines or exerting distinct cytotoxicities, other mechanisms may also contribute to immune regulation and tolerance. Clearly, the risk of excessive immune reactivity should be very low. These mechanisms involve allergen-specific T cells shedding truncated TCRs, acting as antagonists and blocking allergen presentation [376], and high-dose allergen-induced anergic T cells [349]. Possibly, the latter cells, by actively suppressing DC functions, can function as "active" suppressor cells [377, 378]. Interestingly, DC, becoming suppressive by this mechanism [378] or by suppressive cytokines like IL-10 and PGE_2 [230, 379, 380], can, in turn, act themselves as suppressor cells by conferring antigen-specific anergy to subsequently encountered T cells [377, 378, 381]. Although, at present, consensus has been reached about a critical role of regulatory/ suppressor cells in the development and expression of ACD, the relative contributions of each of the various mechanisms are still far from clear.

3.3.8.5 Induction of Lasting Tolerance Only in Naive Individuals

Both clinical and experimental findings indicate that full and persistent tolerance can only be induced prior to any sensitizing allergen contacts [356, 382, 383]. Upon primary allergenic contacts, naive T cells differentiate to produce polarized cytokine profiles (Figs. 3.7 and 3.11). Once polarized, however, T-cell profiles are irreversible, due to loss of cytokine (receptor) genes, or at least very stable, due to the mutually suppressive activities of T-cell cytokines. An important corollary of the latter concept of active suppression is the bystander effect, in which the response to any antigen can be downregulated by immunosuppressive cytokines acting in a local tolerogenic microenvironment [384]. The latter was observed for both protein antigens [385] and methacrylate contact allergens [357]. Stable polarization/ skewing may also

explain why even low, nonsensitizing doses of nickel applied to the skin prevented subsequent tolerance induction by feeding the metal allergen [386]. Apparently, the progeny of naïve allergen-specific cells, once "on the stage," has been triggered to a "sub-clinical" degree toward effector cell differentiation and becomes refractory to regulatory cell action. This may also have contributed to incomplete tolerance induction in earlier clinical studies when feeding with poison ivy-/oak-derived allergens [387]. Indeed, to our knowledge, permanent reversal of existing ACD in healthy individuals has, as yet, never been achieved. Nevertheless, as described above, effector cells still seem susceptible, though transiently, to the downregulation of allergen reactivity, as was observed in desensitization procedures [386, 388].

3.3.8.6 Transient Desensitization in Primed Individuals

For dermatologists, methods by which patients might be desensitized for existing ACD would be a welcome addition to the currently prevailing symptomatic therapies, and investigators have made a wide variety of attempts to achieve this goal. Unfortunately, as mentioned above, therapeutic protocols involving ingestion of poison ivy allergen, penicillin, or nickel sulfate were of only transient benefit to the patients [387–391]. Similarly, in animal models, only a limited and transient degree of hyposensitization was obtained by Chase [392] when feeding DNCB-contact-sensitized guinea pigs with the allergen, whereas for achieving persistent chromium-unresponsiveness in presensitized animals, Polak and Turk [393] needed a rigorous protocol involving up to lethal doses of the allergen. As outlined above, mechanisms underlying specific desensitization in ACD probably depend on direct interference of allergen with effector T-cell function by blocking or downregulating TCRs, leading to anergy and apoptosis [394]. As the onset of desensitization is immediate, no suppressor mechanisms may initially be involved. Apparently in the absence of LC, MHC class II-positive keratinocytes can serve as APC and are very effective in rendering allergen-specific effector cells anergic [395]. Moreover, at later stages active suppression may come into play resulting from secondary inactivation of DC function by anergized T cells [350]. Nevertheless, major problems with in vivo desensitization procedures relate to the refractoriness of effector T cells to regulatory cell functions, and the rapid replacement of anergized effector cells by naïve T cells from relatively protected peripheral lymphoid tissues provides a source of new effector cells upon sensitizing allergen contacts. The same conclusions can be drawn from attempts to achieve local desensitization. It was found that local desensitization by repeatedly applying allergen at the same skin site did not result from local skin hardening or LC inactivation, as local reactivity to an unrelated allergen at the site was unimpaired [329]. Persistence of cellular infiltrates, in the absence of erythematous reactivity, at a desensitized skin site could reflect local anergy, but also locally active regulatory cells. Upon discontinuation of allergen exposure, however, local unresponsiveness was rapidly (within 1 week) lost. Collectively, this data illustrate the problems encountered in attempting to eradicate established effector T-cell function, not only in ACD but also in autoimmune diseases [356, 360].

3.4 Summary and Conclusions

Extensive research has led to a better understanding of the mechanisms of ICD and ACD. The primary role of innate immune cells in coping with exogenous potential harmful threats is rapidly being uncovered. Also, the basic immunology of ACD is now well-defined, including T-cell migratory patterns, recognition of distinct allergens, interactions with other inflammatory cells to generate inflammation, and cytokine profiles. But new complexities have emerged. For instance, in contrast to earlier belief, many of the currently known T-cell subpopulations can act either or both as effector and regulatory cells, depending on the nature of the allergen, the route of entry, frequency of exposure, and many other still ill-defined factors. In particular, the poor understanding of regulatory mechanisms in ACD still hampers further therapeutic progress. So far, no methods of permanent desensitization have been devised.

Nevertheless, next to the established anti-inflammatory drugs, recently defined cellular interaction molecules and mediators provide promising targets for new generations of anti-inflammatory drugs, some of which have already entered clinical trials. Clearly, drugs found to be effective in preventing severe T-cell-mediated conditions, e.g., rejection of a vital organ graft, should be very safe before their use in ACD

would seem appropriate. To date, prudence favors alternative measures to prevent ICD and ACD, be it through legal action to outlaw the use of certain materials or through avoiding personal contact with these materials. In the meantime, for difficult-to-avoid allergens, further studies on the potential value of tolerogenic treatments prior to possible sensitization seem warranted.

References

1. Elias PM (2005) Stratum corneum defensive functions: an integrated view. J Invest Dermatol 125:183–200
2. Elias PM (2007) The skin barrier as an innate immune element. Semin Immunopathol 29:3–14
3. Bouwstra JA, Ponec M (2006) The skin barrier in healthy and diseased state. Biochim Biophys Acta 1758:2080–2095
4. Elias PM (1983) Epidermal lipids, barrier function, and desquamation. J Invest Dermatol (80 suppl):44s–49s
5. Elias PM (2004) The epidermal permeability barrier: from the early days at Harvard to emerging concepts. J Invest Dermatol 122(2):xxxvi–xxxix
6. Hadgraft J, Lane ME (2005) Skin permeation: the years of enlightenment. Int J Pharm 305:2–12
7. Herkenne C, Alberti I, Naik A, Kalia YN, Mathy FX, Preat V, Guy RH (2008) In vivo methods for the assessment of topical drug bioavailability. Pharm Res 25:87–103
8. Moser K, Kriwet K, Naik A, Kalia YN, Guy RH (2001) Passive skin penetration enhancement and its quantification in vitro. Eur J Pharm Biopharm 52:103–112
9. Schaefer H, Lademann J (2001) The role of follicular penetration. A differential view. Skin Pharmacol Appl Skin Physiol (14 suppl 1):23–27
10. Basketter DA, Gerbrick F, Kimber I, Willis C (1999) Contact irritation mechanism. In: Toxicology of contact dermatitis. Wiley, Chichester
11. Enk AH, Katz SI (1992) Early events in the induction phase of contact sensitivity. J Invest Dermatol 99:39S–41S
12. Le TK, Schalkwijk J, van de Kerkhof PC, van HU, van der V (1998) A histological and immunohistochemical study on chronic irritant contact dermatitis. Am J Contact Dermatitis 9:23–28
13. Welss T, Basketter DA, Schroder KR (2004) In vitro skin irritation: facts and future. State of the art review of mechanisms and models. Toxicol In Vitro 18:231–243
14. Levin CY, Maibach HI (2002) Irritant contact dermatitis: is there an immunologic component? Int Immunopharmacol 2:183–189
15. Smith HR, Basketter DA, McFadden JP (2002) Irritant dermatitis, irritancy and its role in allergic contact dermatitis. Clin Exp Dermatol 27:138–146
16. Chew AL, Maibach HI (2003) Occupational issues of irritant contact dermatitis. Int Arch Occup Environ Health 76:339–346
17. English JS (2004) Current concepts of irritant contact dermatitis. Occup Environ Med 61(8):722–726, 674

18. Dickel H, Kuss O, Schmidt A, Kretz J, Diepgen TL (2002) Importance of irritant contact dermatitis in occupational skin disease. Am J Clin Dermatol 3:283–289

19. McDonald JC, Beck MH, Chen Y, Cherry NM (2006) Incidence by occupation and industry of work-related skin diseases in the United Kingdom, 1996-2001. Occup Med (Lond) 56:398–405

20. Diepgen TL, Coenraads PJ (1999) The epidemiology of occupational contact dermatitis. Int Arch Occup Environ Health 72:496–506

21. Bauer A, Bartsch R, Stadeler M, Schneider W, Grieshaber R, Wollina U, Gebhardt M (1998) Development of occupational skin diseases during vocational training in baker and confectioner apprentices: a follow-up study. Contact Dermatitis 39:307–311

22. Berndt U, Hinnen U, Iliev D, Elsner P (1999) Is occupational irritant contact dermatitis predictable by cutaneous bioengineering methods? Results of the Swiss Metalworker' Eczema Study (PROMETES). Dermatology 198:351–354

23. John SM, Uter W, Schwanitz HJ (2000) Relevance of multiparametric skin bioengineering in a prospectively-followed cohort of junior hairdressers. Contact Dermatitis 43:161–168

24. Koopman DG, Kezic S, Verberk MM (2004) Skin reaction and recovery: a repeated sodium lauryl sulphate patch test vs. a 24-h patch test and tape stripping. Br J Dermatol 150:493–499

25. Schmid K, Broding HC, Uter W, Drexler H (2005) Transepidermal water loss and incidence of hand dermatitis in a prospectively followed cohort of apprentice nurses. Contact Dermatitis 52:247–253

26. Smith HR, Armstrong DK, Holloway D, Whittam L, Basketter DA, McFadden JP (2002) Skin irritation thresholds in hairdressers: implications for the development of hand dermatitis. Br J Dermatol 146:849–852

27. Smith HR, Rowson M, Basketter DA, McFadden JP (2004) Intra-individual variation of irritant threshold and relationship to transepidermal water loss measurement of skin irritation. Contact Dermatitis 51:26–29

28. Coenraads PJ, Diepgen TL (1998) Risk for hand eczema in employees with past or present atopic dermatitis. Int Arch Occup Environ Health 71:7–13

29. Jakasa I, De Jongh CM, Verberk MM, Bos JD, Kezic S (2006) Percutaneous penetration of sodium lauryl sulphate is increased in uninvolved skin of patients with atopic dermatitis compared with control subjects. Br J Dermatol 155:104–109

30. De Jongh CM, John SM, Bruynzeel DP, Calkoen F, van Dijk FJ, Khrenova L, Rustemeyer T, Verberk MM, Kezic S (2008) Cytokine gene polymorphisms and susceptibility to chronic irritant contact dermatitis. Contact Dermatitis 58:269–277

31. De Jongh CM, Khrenova L, Kezic S, Rustemeyer T, Verberk MM, John SM (2008) Polymorphisms in the interleukin-1 gene influence the stratum corneum interleukin-1 alpha concentration in uninvolved skin of patients with chronic irritant contact dermatitis. Contact Dermatitis 58:263–268

32. De Jongh CM, Khrenova L, Verberk MM, Calkoen F, van Dijk FJ, Voss H, John SM, Kezic S (2008) Loss-of-function polymorphisms in the filaggrin gene are associated with an increased susceptibility to chronic irritant contact dermatitis: a case-control study. Br J Dermatol 159:621–627

33. Palmer CN, Irvine AD, Terron-Kwiatkowski A, Zhao Y, Liao H, Lee SP, Goudie DR, Sandilands A, Campbell LE, Smith FJ, O'Regan GM, Watson RM, Cecil JE, Bale SJ, Compton JG, DiGiovanna JJ, Fleckman P, Lewis-Jones S, Arseculeratne G, Sergeant A, Munro CS, El HB, McElreavey K, Halkjaer LB, Bisgaard H, Mukhopadhyay S, McLean WH (2006) Common loss-of-function variants of the epidermal barrier protein filaggrin are a major predisposing factor for atopic dermatitis. Nat Genet 38:441–446

34. Sandilands A, Terron-Kwiatkowski A, Hull PR, O'Regan GM, Clayton TH, Watson RM, Carrick T, Evans AT, Liao H, Zhao Y, Campbell LE, Schmuth M, Gruber R, Janecke AR, Elias PM, van Steensel MA, Nagtzaam I, van GM, Steijlen PM, Munro CS, Bradley DG, Palmer CN, Smith FJ, McLean WH, Irvine AD (2007) Comprehensive analysis of the gene encoding filaggrin uncovers prevalent and rare mutations in ichthyosis vulgaris and atopic eczema. Nat Genet 39:650–654

35. Demehri S, Morimoto M, Holtzman MJ, Kopan R (2009) Skin-derived TSLP triggers progression from epidermal-barrier defects to asthma. PLoS Biol 7(5)

36. Marenholz I, Nickel R, Ruschendorf F, Schulz F, Esparza-Gordillo J, Kerscher T, Gruber C, Lau S, Worm M, Keil T, Kurek M, Zaluga E, Wahn U, Lee YA (2006) Filaggrin loss-of-function mutations predispose to phenotypes involved in the atopic march. J Allergy Clin Immunol 118:866–871

37. Sandilands A, Sutherland C, Irvine AD, McLean WH (2009) Filaggrin in the frontline: role in skin barrier function and disease. J Cell Sci 122:1285–1294

38. Smith FJ, Irvine AD, Terron-Kwiatkowski A, Sandilands A, Campbell LE, Zhao Y, Liao H, Evans AT, Goudie DR, Lewis-Jones S, Arseculeratne G, Munro CS, Sergeant A, O'Regan G, Bale SJ, Compton JG, DiGiovanna JJ, Presland RB, Fleckman P, McLean WH (2006) Loss-of-function mutations in the gene encoding filaggrin cause ichthyosis vulgaris. Nat Genet 38:337–342

39. Stemmler S, Parwez Q, Petrasch-Parwez E, Epplen JT, Hoffjan S (2007) Two common loss-of-function mutations within the filaggrin gene predispose for early onset of atopic dermatitis. J Invest Dermatol 127:722–724

40. Hollegaard MV, Bidwell JL (2006) Cytokine gene polymorphism in human disease: on-line databases, Supplement 3. Genes Immun 7:269–276

41. Corsini E, Galli CL (2000) Epidermal cytokines in experimental contact dermatitis. Toxicology 142:203–211

42. Jacobs JJ, Lehe CL, Hasegawa H, Elliott GR, Das PK (2006) Skin irritants and contact sensitizers induce Langerhans cell migration and maturation at irritant concentration. Exp Dermatol 15:432–440

43. Williams IR, Kupper TS (1996) Immunity at the surface: homeostatic mechanisms of the skin immune system. Life Sci 58:1485–1507

44. Ouwehand K, Santegoets SJ, Bruynzeel DP, Scheper RJ, de Gruijl TD, Gibbs S (2008) CXCL12 is essential for migration of activated Langerhans cells from epidermis to dermis. Eur J Immunol 38:3050–3059

45. Spiekstra SW, Toebak MJ, Sampat-Sardjoepersad S, van Beek PJ, Boorsma DM, Stoof TJ, von Blomberg BM, Scheper RJ, Bruynzeel DP, Rustemeyer T, Gibbs S (2005) Induction of cytokine (interleukin-1alpha and tumor necrosis factor-alpha) and chemokine (CCL20, CCL27, and CXCL8) alarm signals after allergen and irritant exposure. Exp Dermatol 14:109–116

46. Effendy I, Löffler H, Maibach HI (2000) Epidermal cytokines in murine cutaneous irritant responses. J Appl Toxicol 20:335–341

47. Kupper TS (1990) Immune and inflammatory processes in cutaneous tissues. Mechanisms and speculations. J Clin Invest 86:1783–1789

48. McFadden JP, Basketter DA (2000) Contact allergy, irritancy and 'danger'. Contact Dermatitis 42:123–127

49. Slodownik D, Lee A, Nixon R (2008) Irritant contact dermatitis: a review. Australas J Dermatol 49:1–9

50. De Jongh CM, Verberk MM, Spiekstra SW, Gibbs S, Kezic S (2007) Cytokines at different stratum corneum levels in normal and sodium lauryl sulphate-irritated skin. Skin Res Technol 13:390–398

51. Wood LC, Elias PM, Calhoun C, Tsai JC, Grunfeld C, Feingold KR (1996) Barrier disruption stimulates interleukin-1 alpha expression and release from a pre-formed pool in murine epidermis. J Invest Dermatol 106: 397–403

52. De Jongh CM, Verberk MM, Withagen CE, Jacobs JJ, Rustemeyer T, Kezic S (2006) Stratum corneum cytokines and skin irritation response to sodium lauryl sulfate. Contact Dermatitis 54:325–333

53. Piguet PF, Grau GE, Hauser C, Vassalli P (1991) Tumor necrosis factor is a critical mediator in hapten induced irritant and contact hypersensitivity reactions. J Exp Med 173:673–679

54. Bergstresser PR (1989) Sensitization and elicitation of inflammation in contact dermatitis. In: Norris DA (ed) Immune mechanisms in cutaneous disease. Dekker, New York, pp 219–246

55. Turk JL (1975) Delayed hypersensitivity, 2nd edn. North-Holland, Amsterdam

56. Gell PDH, Coombs RRA, Lachman R (1975) Clinical aspects of immunology, 3rd edn. Blackwell, London

57. Mestas J, Hughes CC (2004) Of mice and not men: differences between mouse and human immunology. J Immunol 172:2731–2738

58. Saint-Mezard P, Krasteva M, Chavagnac C, Bosset S, Akiba H, Kehren J, Kanitakis J, Kaiserlian D, Nicolas JF, Berard F (2003) Afferent and efferent phases of allergic contact dermatitis (ACD) can be induced after a single skin contact with haptens: evidence using a mouse model of primary ACD. J Invest Dermatol 120:641–647

59. Bos JD, Meinardi MMHM (2000) The 500 Dalton rule for the skin penetration of chemical compounds and drugs. Exp Dermatol 9:165–169

60. Roberts DW, Lepoittevin J-P (1998) Allergic Contact Dermatitis. In: Lepoittevin J-P, Basketter DA, Goossens A, Karlberg A-T (eds). Springer, Berlin Heidelberg New York, pp 81–1118

61. Eliasson E, Kenna JG (1996) Cytochrome P450 2E1 is a cell surface autoantigen in halothane hepatitis. Mol Pharmacol 50:573–582

62. Budinger L, Hertl M (2000) Immunologic mechanisms in hypersensitivity reactions to metal ions: an overview. Allergy 55:108–115

63. Gerberick F, Aleksic M, Basketter D, Casati S, Karlberg AT, Kern P, Kimber I, Lepoittevin JP, Natsch A, Ovigne JM, Rovida C, Sakaguchi H, Schultz T (2008) Chemical reactivity measurement and the predicitve identification of skin sensitisers. The report and recommendations of ECVAM Workshop 64. Altern Lab Anim 36(2):215–242

64. Divkovic M, Pease CK, Gerberick GF, Basketter DA (2005) Hapten-protein binding: from theory to practical application in the in vitro prediction of skin sensitization. Contact Dermatitis 53(4):189–200

65. Mutschler J, Giménez-Arnau E, Foertsch L, Gerberick GF, Lepoittevin JP (2009) Mechanistic assessment of peptide reactivity assay to predict skin allergens with Kathon CG isothiazolinones. Toxicol In Vitro 23(3):439–446

66. Gerberick F, Aleksic M, Basketter D, Casati S, Karlberg AT, Kern P, Kimber I, Lepoittevin JP, Natsch A, Ovigne JM, Rovida C, Sakaguchi H, Schultz T (2008) Chemical reactivity measurement and the predicitve identification of skin sensitisers. The report and recommendations of ECVAM Workshop 64. Altern Lab Anim 36(2):215–242

67. Blauvelt A, Hwang ST, Udey MC (2003) Allergic and immunologic diseases of the skin. J Allergy Clin Immunol 111:S560–S570

68. Kimber I, Dearman RJ (2002) Allergic contact dermatitis: the cellular effectors. Contact Dermatitis 46:1–5

69. Liberato DJ, Byers VS, Ennick RG, Castagnoli N (1981) Region specific attack of nitrogen and sulfur nucleophiles on quinones from poison oak/ivy catechols (urushiols) and analogues as models for urushiol-protein conjugate formation. J Med Chem 24:28–33

70. Kalish RS, Wood JA, LaPorte A (1994) Processing of urushiol (poison ivy) hapten by both endogenous and exogenous pathways for presentation to T cells in vitro. J Clin Invest 93:2039–2047

71. Naisbitt DJ (2004) Drug hypersensitivity reactions in skin: understanding mechanisms and the development of diagnostic and predictive tests. Toxicology 194:179–196

72. Lepoittevin JP (2006) Metabolism versus chemical transformation or pro- versus prehaptens? Contact Dermatitis 54(2):73–74

73. Epling GA, Wells JL, Yoon UC (1988) Photochemical transformations in salicylanilide photoallergy. Photochem Photobiol 47:167–171

74. Krasteva M, Nicolas JF, Chabeau G, Garrigue JL, Bour H, Thivolet J, Schmitt D (1993) Dissociation of allergenic and immunogenic functions in contact sensitivity to paraphenylenediamine. Int Arch Allergy Immunol 102: 200–204

75. Merk HF, Abel J, Baron JM, Krutmann J (2004) Molecular pathways in dermatotoxicology. Toxicol Appl Pharmacol 195:267–277

76. Schnuch A, Westphal GA, Muller MM, Schulz TG, Geier J, Brasch J, Merk HF, Kawakubo Y, Richter G, Koch P, Fuchs T, Gutgesell T, Reich K, Gebhardt M, Becker D, Grabbe J, Szliska C, Aberer W, Hallier E (1998) Genotype and phenotype of N-acetyltransferase 2 (NAT2) polymorphism in patients with contact allergy. Contact Dermatitis 38:209–211

77. Karlberg AT, Bergström MA, Börje A, Luthman K, Nilsson JL (2008) Allergic contact dermatitis–formation, structural requirements, and reactivity of skin sensitizers. Chem Res Toxicol 21(1):53–69

78. Patlewicz GY, Basketter DA, Pease CK, Wilson K, Wright ZM, Roberts DW, Bernard G, Arnau EG, Lepoittevin JP (2004) Further evaluation of quantitative structure–activity relationship models for the prediction of the skin sensitization potency of selected fragrance allergens. Contact Dermatitis 50:91–97

79. Langerhans P (1868) Über die Nerven der menschlichen Haut. Virchows Arch Pathol Anat 44:325–337

80. Wilson NS, Villadangos JA (2004) Lymphoid organ dendritic cells: beyond the Langerhans cells paradigm. Immunol Cell Biol 82:91–98

81. Hoath SB, Leahy DG (2003) The organization of human epidermis: functional epidermal units and phi proportionality. J Invest Dermatol 121:1440–1446

82. Breathnach SM (1988) The Langerhans cell. Centenary review. Br J Dermatol 119:463–469

83. Romani N, Holzmann S, Tripp CH, Koch F, Stoitzner P (2003) Langerhans cells – dendritic cells of the epidermis. APMIS 111:725–740

84. Kimber I, Dearman RJ (2003) What makes a chemical an allergen? Ann Allergy Asthma Immunol 90:28–31

85. Inaba K, Schuler G, Witmer MD, Valinsky J, Atassi B, Steinman RM (1986) Immunologic properties of purified epidermal Langerhans cells. Distinct requirements for stimulation of unprimed and sensitized T lymphocytes. J Exp Med 164:605–613

86. Kimber I, Cumberbatch M (1992) Dendritic cells and cutaneous immune responses to chemical allergens. Toxicol Appl Pharmacol 117:137–146

87. Seiffert K, Granstein RD (2006) Neuroendocrine regulation of skin dendritic cells. Ann N Y Acad Sci 1088(1):195–206

88. Dieu M-C, Vanbervliet B, Vicari A, Bridon J-M, Oldham E, Ait-Yahia S, Brière F, Zlotnik A, Lebecque S, Caux C (1998) Selective recruitment of immature and mature dendritic cells by distinct chemokines expressed in different anatomic sites. J Exp Med 188:373–386

89. Stingl G, Katz SI, Clement L, Green I, Shevach EM (1978) Immunological functions of Ia-bearing epidermal Langerhans cells. J Immunol 121:2005–2013

90. Czernielewski SM, Demarchez M (1987) Further evidence for the self-reproducing capacity of Langerhans cells in human skin. J Invest Dermatol 88:17–20

91. Streilein JW, Grammer SF (1989) In vitro evidence that Langerhans cells can adopt two functionally distinct forms capable of antigen presentation to T lymphocytes. J Immunol 143:3925–3933

92. Birbeck M (1961) An electron microscope study of basal melanocytes and high level clear cells (Langerhans cells) in vitiligo. J Invest Dermatol 37:51–56

93. Braathen LR (1980) Studies on human epidermal Langerhans cells. III. Induction of T lymphocyte response to nickel sulphate in sensitized individuals. Br J Dermatol 103:517–526

94. Kimber I, Dearman RJ, Cumberbatch M, Huby RJ (1998) Langerhans cells and chemical allergy. Curr Opinion Immunol 10:614–619

95. Kimber I, Basketter DA, Gerberick GF, Dearman RJ (2002) Allergic contact dermatitis. Int Immunopharmacol 2:201–211

96. Park SH, Chiu YH, Jayawardena J, Roark J, Kavita U, Bendelac A (1998) Innate and adaptive functions of the CD1 pathway of antigen presentation. Semin Immunol 10:391–398

97. Weinlich G, Heine M, Stössel H, Zanella M, Stoitzner P, Ortner U, Smolle J, Koch F, Sepp NT, Schuler G, Romani N (1998) Entry into afferent lymphatics and maturation in situ of migrating murine cutaneous dendritic cells. J Invest Dermatol 110:441–448

98. Richters CD, Hoekstra MJ, van Baare J, Du Pont JS, Hoefsmit EC, Kamperdijk EW (1994) Isolation and characterization of migratory human skin dendritic cells. Clin Exp Immunol 98:330–336

99. Jakob T, Ring J, Udey MC (2001) Multistep navigation of Langerhans/dendritic cells in and out of the skin. J Allergy Clin Immunol 108:688–696

100. Ozawa H, Nakagawa S, Tagami H, Aiba S (1996) Interleukin-1b and granulocyte-macrophage colony stimulating factor mediate Langerhans cell maturation differently. J Invest Dermatol 106:441–445

101. Wong BR, Josien R, Lee SY, Sauter B, Li HL, Steinman RM, Choi YW (1997) TRANCE (Tumor necrosis factor [TNF]-related activation-induced cytokine), a new TNF family member predominantly expressed in T cells, is a dendritic cell-specific survival factor. J Exp Med 186:2075–2080

102. Aiba S, Tagami H (1999) Dendritic cell activation induced by various stimuli, eg exposure to microorganisms, their products, cytokines, and simple chemicals as well as adhesion to extracellular matrix. J Dermatol Sci 20:1–13

103. Inaba K, Schuler G, Steinman RM (1993) GM-CSF – a granulocyte/macrophage/dendritic cell stimulating factor. In: Van Furth R (ed) Hemopoietic growth factors and mononuclear phagocytes. Karger, Basel, pp 187–196

104. Jakob T, Udey MC (1998) Regulation of E-Cadherin mediated adhesion in Langerhans cell-like dendritic cells by inflammatory mediators that mobilize Langerhans cells in vivo. J Immunol 160:4067–4073

105. Schwarzenberger K, Udey MC (1996) Contact allergens and epidermal proinflammatory cytokines modulate Langerhans cell E-cadherin expression in situ. J Invest Dermatol 106:553–558

106. Enk AH, Katz SI (1992) Early molecular events in the induction phase of contact sensitivity. Proc Natl Acad Sci U S A 89:1398–1402

107. Enk AH, Angeloni VL, Udey MC, Katz SI (1993) An essential role for Langerhans cell-derived IL-1b in the initiation of primary immune responses in skin. J Immunol 150:3698–3704

108. Iversen L, Johansen C (2008) Inflammasomes and inflammatory caspases in skin inflammation. Expert Rev Mol Diagn 8(6):697–705

109. Wang B, Esche C, Mamelak A, Freed I, Watanabe H, Sauder DN (2003) Cytokine knockouts in contact hypersensitivity research. Cytokine Growth Factor Rev 14:381–389

110. Tang A, Amagai M, Granger LG, Stanley JR, Udey MC (1993) Adhesion of epidermal Langerhans cells to keratinocytes mediated by E-cadherin. Nature 361:82–85

111. Ma J, Wing J-H, Guo Y-J, Sy M-S, Bigby M (1994) In vivo treatment with anti-ICAM-1 and antiLFA-1 antibodies inhibits contact sensitization-induced migration of epidermal Langerhans cells to regional lymph nodes. Cell Immunol 158:389–399

112. Rambukhana A, Bos JD, Irik D, Menko WJ, Kapsenberg ML, Das PK (1995) In situ behaviour of human Langerhans cells in skin organ culture. Lab Invest 73:521–531

113. Price AA, Cumberbatch M, Kimber I (1997) α6 integrins are required for Langerhans cell migration from the epidermis. J Exp Med 186:1725–1735

114. Weiss JM, Sleeman J, Renkl AC, Dittmar H, Termeer CC, Taxis S, Howells N, Hofmann M, Kohler G, Schöpf E, Ponta H, Herrlich P, Simon JC (1997) An essential role for CD44 variant isoforms in epidermal Langerhans cell and blood dendritic cell function. J Cell Biol 137:1137–1147

115. Brand CU, Hunger RE, Yawalkar N, Gerber HA, Schaffner T, Braathen LR (1999) Characterization of human skin-derived CD1a-positive lymph cells. Arch Dermatol Res 291:65–72

116. Kobayashi Y (1997) Langerhans cells produce type IV collagenase (MMP-9) following epicutaneous stimulation with haptens. Immunology 90:496–501

117. Randolph GJ (2001) Dendritic cell migration to lymph nodes: cytokines, chemokines, and lipid mediators. Semin Immunol 13:267–274

118. Sallusto F, Lanzavecchia A, Mackay CR (1998) Chemokines and chemokine receptors in T-cell priming and Th1/Th2-mediated responses. Immunol Today 19:568–574

119. Zlotnik A, Morales J, Hedrick JA (1999) Recent advances in chemokines and chemokine receptors. Crit Rev Immunol 19:1–47

120. Caux C, Ait-Yahia S, Chemin K, de Bouteiller O, Dieu-Nosjean MC, Homey B, Massacrier C, Vanbervliet B, Zlotnik A, Vicari A (2000) Dendritic cell biology and regulation of dendritic cell trafficking by chemokines. Springer Semin Immunopathol 22:345–369

121. Sallusto F, Palermo B, Lenig D, Miettinen M, Matikainen S, Julkunen I, Forster R, Burgstahler R, Lipp M, Lanzavecchia A (1999) Distinct patterns and kinetics of chemokine production regulate dendritic cell function. Eur J Immunol 29:1617–1625

122. Saeki H, Moore AM, Brown MJ, Hwan ST (1999) Secondary lymphoid-tissue chemokine (SLC) and CC chemokine receptor 7 (CCR7) participate in the emigration pathway of mature dendritic cells from the skin to regional lymph nodes. J Immunol 162:2472–2475

123. Gunn MD, Tangemann K, Tam C, Cyster JG, Rosen SD, Williams LT (1998) A chemokine expressed in lymphoid high endothelial venules promotes the adhesion and chemotaxis of naïve T lymphocytes. Proc Natl Acad Sci U S A 95:258–263

124. Kim CH, Broxmeyer HE (1999) Chemokines: signal lamps for trafficking of T and B cells for development and effector function. J Leuk Biol 65:6–15

125. Robbiani DF, Finch RA, Jager D, Muller WA, Sartorelli AC, Randolph GJ (2000) The leukotriene C(4) transporter MRP1 regulates CCL19 (MIP-3beta, ELC)-dependent mobilization of dendritic cells to lymph nodes. Cell 103:757–768

126. Honig SM, Fu S, Mao X, Yopp A, Gunn MD, Randolph GJ, Bromberg JS (2003) FTY720 stimulates multidrug transporter- and cysteinyl leukotriene-dependent T cell chemotaxis to lymph nodes. J Clin Invest 111:627–637

127. van de Ven R, Scheffer GL, Scheper RJ, de Gruijl TD (2009) The ABC of dendritic cell development and function. Trends Immunol 30(9):421–429

128. Sallusto F, Schaerli P, Loetscher P, Schaniel C, Lenig D, Mackay CR, Qin S, Lanzavecchia A (1998) Rapid and coordinated switch in chemokine receptor expression during dendritic cell maturation. Eur J Immunol 28: 2760–2769

129. Cumberbatch M, Dearman RJ, Kimber I (1997) Interleukin 1-beta and the stimulation of Langerhans cell migration – comparisons with tumour necrosis factor alpha. Arch Dermatol Res 289:277–284

130. Heufler C, Koch F, Schuler G (1988) Granulocyte/macrophage colony-stimulating factor and interleukin 1 mediate the maturation of epidermal Langerhans cells into potent immunostimulatory dendritic cells. J Exp Med 167:700–705

131. Steinman RM, Hoffman L, Pope M (1995) Maturation and migration of cutaneous dendritic cells. J Invest Dermatol 105:2S–7S

132. Furue M, Chang CH, Tamaki K (1996) Interleukin-1 but not tumor necrosis factor a synergistically upregulates the granulocyte-macrophage colony-stimulating factor-induced B7–1 expression of murine Langerhans cells. Br J Dermatol 135:194–198

133. Schuler G, Steinman RM (1985) Murine epidermal Langerhans cells mature into potent immune-stimulatory dendritic cells in vitro. J Exp Med 161:526–546

134. Haig DM, Hopkins J, Miller HRP (1999) Local immune responses in afferent and efferent lymph. Immunology 96:155–163

135. Altin JG, Sloan EK (1997) The role of CD45 and CD45-associated molecules in T cell activation. Immunol Cell Biol 75:430–445

136. Schon MP, Zollner TM, Boehncke WH (2003) The molecular basis of lymphocyte recruitment to the skin: clues for pathogenesis and selective therapies of inflammatory disorders. J Invest Dermatol 121:951–962

137. Von Andrian UH, Mrini C (1998) In situ analysis of lymphocyte migration to lymph nodes. Cell Adh Comm 6:85–96

138. Vestweber D, Blanks JE (1999) Mechanisms that regulate the function of the selectins and their ligands. Physiol Rev 79:181–213

139. Adema GJ, Hartgers F, Verstraten R, de Vries E, Marland G, Menon S, Foster J, Xu Y, Nooyen P, McClanahan T, Bacon KB, Figdor CG (1997) A dendritic-cell-derived C-C chemokine that preferentially attracts naïve T cells. Nature 387:713–717

140. Ngo VN, Tang LH, Cyster JG (1998) Epstein-Barr virus-induced molecule 1 ligand chemokine is expressed by dendritic cells in lymphoid tissues and strongly attracts naïve T cells and activated B cells. J Exp Med 188:181–191

141. Nagira M, Imai T, Hieshima K, Kusuda J, Ridanpaa M, Takagi S, Nishimura M, Kakizaki M, Nomiyama H, Yoshie

O (1997) Molecular cloning of a novel human CC chemokine secondary lymphoid-tissue chemokine that is a potent chemoattractant for lymphocytes and mapped to chromosome 9p13. J Biol Chem 272:19518–19524

142. Rustemeyer T, von Blomberg BME, de Ligter S, Frosch PJ, Scheper RJ (1999) Human T lymphocyte priming in vitro by dendritic cells. Clin Exp Immunol 117:209–216

143. Crivellato E, Vacca A, Ribatti D (2004) Setting the stage: an anatomist's view of the immune system. Trends Immunol 25:210–217

144. Itano AA, Jenkins MK (2003) Antigen presentation to naive CD4 T cells in the lymph node. Nat Immunol 4:733–739

145. Griem P, Wulferink M, Sachs B, Gonzales JB, Gleichmann E (1998) Allergic and autoimmune reactions to xenobiotics: how do they arise? Immunol Today 19:133–141

146. Moulon C, Vollmer J, Weltzien H-U (1995) Characterization of processing requirements and metal crossreactivities in T cell clones from patients with allergic contact dermatitis to nickel. Eur J Immunol 25:3308–3315

147. Li QJ, Dinner AR, Qi S, Irvine DJ, Huppa JB, Davis MM, Chakraborty AK (2004) CD4 enhances T cell sensitivity to antigen by coordinating Lck accumulation at the immunological synapse. Nat Immunol 5:791–799

148. Schoenberger SP, Toes REM, Vandervoort EIH, Offringa R, Melief CJM (1998) T-cell help for cytotoxic T lymphocytes is mediated by CD40-CD40L interactions. Nature 393:480–483

149. Gascoigne NR, Zal T (2004) Molecular interactions at the T cell-antigen-presenting cell interface. Curr Opin Immunol 16:114–119

150. Cantrell D (1996) T cell receptor signal transduction pathways. Annu Rev Immunol 14:259–274

151. Kuo CT, Leiden JM (1999) Transcriptional regulation of T lymphocyte development and function. Annu Rev Immunol 17:149–187

152. Davis SJ, van der Merwe PA (2003) TCR triggering: co-receptor-dependent or -independent? Trends Immunol 24:624–626

153. Trautmann A, Randriamampita C (2003) Initiation of TCR signalling revisited. Trends Immunol 24:425–428

154. Acuto O, Michel F (2003) CD28-mediated co-stimulation: a quantitative support for TCR signalling. Nat Rev Immunol 3:939–951

155. Quezada SA, Jarvinen LZ, Lind EF, Noelle RJ (2004) CD40/CD154 interactions at the interface of tolerance and immunity. Annu Rev Immunol 22:307–328

156. Dong C, Nurieva RI, Prasad DV (2003) Immune regulation by novel costimulatory molecules. Immunol Res 28:39–48

157. Viola A, Lanzavecchia A (1996) T cell activation determined by T cell receptor number and tunable thresholds. Science 273:104–106

158. Banchereau J, Steinman RM (1998) Dendritic cells and the control of immunity. Nature 392:245–252

159. Hommel M (2004) On the dynamics of T-cell activation in lymph nodes. Immunol Cell Biol 82:62–66

160. Cella M, Sallusto F, Lanzavecchia A (1997) Origin, maturation and antigen presenting function of dendritic cells. Curr Opin Immunol 9:10–16

161. Crispín JC, Tsokos GC (2009) Human TCR-alpha beta+ CD4- CD8- T cells can derive from CD8+ T cells and dis-

play an inflammatory effector phenotype. J Immunol 183(7):4675–4678

162. Malek TR, Yu A, Zhu L, Matsutani T, Adeegbe D, Bayer AL (2008) IL-2 family of cytokines in T regulatory cell development and homeostasis. J Clin Immunol 28(6):635–639

163. Pei Z, Lin D, Song X, Li H, Yao H (2008) TLR4 signaling promotes the expression of VEGF and TGFbeta1 in human prostate epithelial PC3 cells induced by lipopolysaccharide. Cell Immunol 254(1):20–27

164. Lan RY, Selmi C, Gershwin ME (2008) The regulatory, inflammatory, and T cell programming roles of interleukin-2 (IL-2). J Autoimmun 31(1):7–12

165. Dong C (2008) TH17 cells in development: an updated view of their molecular identity and genetic programming. Nat Rev Immunol 8(5):337–348

166. Zhu J, Paul WE (2008) CD4 T cells: fates, functions, and faults. Blood 112(5):1557–1569

167. Sallusto F, Lanzavecchia A (2009) Human Th17 cells in infection and autoimmunity. Microbes Infect 11(5):620–624

168. Oboki K, Ohno T, Saito H, Nakae S (2008) Th17 and allergy. Allergol Int 57(2):121–134

169. Dabbagh K, Lewis DB (2003) Toll-like receptors and T-helper-1/T-helper-2 responses. Curr Opin Infect Dis 16:199–204

170. Faria AM, Weiner HL (2006) Oral tolerance and TGF-beta-producing cells. Inflamm Allergy Drug Targets 5(3):179–190

171. Korn T, Bettelli E, Oukka M, Kuchroo VK (2009) IL-17 and Th17 cells. Annu Rev Immunol 27:485–517. Review. PubMed PMID: 19132915

172. Louten J, Boniface K, de Waal Malefyt R (2009) Development and function of TH17 cells in health and disease. J Allergy Clin Immunol 123(5):1004–1011

173. Romagnani S (2006) Regulation of the T cell response. Clin Exp Allergy 36(11):1357–1366

174. Feuerer M, Hill JA, Mathis D, Benoist C (2009) Foxp3+ regulatory T cells: differentiation, specification, subphenotypes. Nat Immunol 10(7):689–695

175. Cavani A (2008) Immune regulatory mechanisms in allergic contact dermatitis and contact sensitization. Chem Immunol Allergy 94:93–100

176. Wu K, Bi Y, Sun K, Wang C (2007) IL-10-producing type 1 regulatory T cells and allergy. Cell Mol Immunol 4(4):269–275

177. Shevach EM (2009) Mechanisms of foxp3+ T regulatory cell-mediated suppression. Immunity 30(5):636–645

178. Basso AS, Cheroutre H, Mucida D (2009) More stories on Th17 cells. Cell Res 19(4):399–411

179. Zhou L, Littman DR (2009) Transcriptional regulatory networks in Th17 cell differentiation. Curr Opin Immunol 21(2):146–152. Review

180. Wilson CB, Rowell E, Sekimata M (2009) Epigenetic control of T-helper-cell differentiation. Nat Rev Immunol 9(2):91–105

181. Coulter EM, Jenkinson C, Farrell J, Lavergne SN, Pease C, White A, Aleksic M, Basketter D, Williams DP, King C, Pirmohamed M, Park BK, Naisbitt DJ (2010) Measurement of CD4+ and CD8+ T-lymphocyte cytokine secretion and gene expression changes in p-phenylenediamine allergic patients and tolerant individuals. J Invest Dermatol 130(1):161–174

182. Nakamura T, Lee RK, Nam SY, Podack ER, Bottomly K, Flavell RA (1997) Roles of IL-4 and IFN-g in stabilizing

the T helper cell type-1 and 2 phenotype. J Immunol 158:2648–2653

183. Kang KF, Kubin M, Cooper KD, Lessin SR, Trinchieri G, Rook AH (1996) IL-12 synthesis by human Langerhans cells. J Immunol 156:1402–1407

184. Pulendran B (2004) Modulating TH1/TH2 responses with microbes, dendritic cells, and pathogen recognition receptors. Immunol Res 29:187–196

185. Kubo M, Ransom J, Webb D, Hashimoto Y, Tada T, Nakayama T (1997) T-cell subset-specific expression of the IL-4 gene is regulated by a silencer element and STAT6. EMBO J 16(13):4007–4020

186. Rogge L, Barberis-Maino L, Biffi M, Passini N, Presky DH, Gubler U, Sinigaglia F (1997) Selective expression of an interleukin-12 receptor component by human T helper 1 cells. J Exp Med 185:825–831

187. Zhou L, Chong MM, Littman DR (2009) Plasticity of CD4+ T cell lineage differentiation. Immunity 30(5):646–655. Review. PubMed PMID: 19464987

188. Nakamura T, Kamogawa Y, Bottomly K, Flavell RA (1997) Polarization of IL-4- and IFN-gamma-producing CD4($^{+}$) T cells following activation of naive CD4($^{+}$) T cells. J Immunol 158:1085–1094

189. Orange JS, Biron CA (1996) An absolute and restricted requirement for IL-12 in natural killer cell IFN-g production and antiviral defense. J Immunol 156:1138–1142

190. Groux H, Sornasse T, Cottrez F, de Vries JE, Coffman RL, Roncarolo MG, Yssel H (1997) Induction of human T helper cell type-1 differentiation results in loss of IFN-g receptor b-chain expression. J Immunol 158:5627–5631

191. Gajewski TF, Fitch FW (1988) Antiproliferative effect of IFN-gamma in immune regulation. I. IFN-gamma inhibits the proliferation of Th2 but not Th1 murine helper T lymphocyte clones. J Immunol 140:4245–4252

192. Takatori H, Kanno Y, Chen Z, O'Shea JJ (2008) New complexities in helper T cell fate determination and the implications for autoimmune diseases. Mod Rheumatol 18(6):533–541

193. Cella M, Scheidegger D, Palmer-Lehmann K, Lane P, Lanzavecchia A, Alber G (1996) Ligation of CD40 on dendritic cells triggers production of high levels of interleukin 12 and enhances T cell stimulatory capacity. J Exp Med 184:747–752

194. Ohshima Y, Tanaka Y, Tozawa H, Takahashi Y, Maliszewski C, Delespesse C (1997) Expression and function of OX40 ligand on human dendritic cells. J Immunol 159:3838–3848

195. Croft M (2009) The role of TNF superfamily members in T-cell function and diseases. Nat Rev Immunol 9(4):271–278

196. Iliev ID, Mileti E, Matteoli G, Chieppa M, Rescigno M (2009) Intestinal epithelial cells promote colitis-protective regulatory T-cell differentiation through dendritic cell conditioning. Mucosal Immunol 2(4):340–350

197. Izcue A, Coombes JL, Powrie F (2009) Regulatory lymphocytes and intestinal inflammation. Annu Rev Immunol 27:313–338

198. Hoyer KK, Dooms H, Barron L, Abbas AK (2008) Interleukin-2 in the development and control of inflammatory disease. Immunol Rev 226:19–28

199. Létourneau S, Krieg C, Pantaleo G, Boyman O (2009) IL-2- and CD25-dependent immunoregulatory mechanisms in the homeostasis of T-cell subsets. J Allergy Clin Immunol 123(4):758–762

200. Oukka M (2008) Th17 cells in immunity and autoimmunity. Ann Rheum Dis 67(suppl 3):iii26–iii29

201. Larsen JM, Bonefeld CM, Poulsen SS, Geisler C, Skov L (2009) IL-23 and T(H)17-mediated inflammation in human allergic contact dermatitis. J Allergy Clin Immunol 123(2):486–492

202. Edele F, Esser PR, Lass C, Laszczyk MN, Oswald E, Strüh CM, Rensing-Ehl A, Martin SF (2007) Innate and adaptive immune responses in allergic contact dermatitis and autoimmune skin diseases. Inflamm Allergy Drug Targets 6(4):236–244

203. Fyhrquist-Vanni N, Alenius H, Lauerma A (2007) Contact dermatitis. Dermatol Clin 25(4):613–623

204. Werfel T, Hentschel M, Kapp A, Renz H (1997) Dichotomy of blood- and skin-derived IL-4-producing allergen-specific T cells and restricted V beta repertoire in nickel-mediated contact dermatitis. J Immunol 158:2500–2505

205. Probst P, Küntzlin D, Fleischer B (1995) T$_{H}$2-type infiltrating T cells in nickel-induced contact dermatitis. Cell Immunol 165:134–140

206. Grewe M, Bruijnzeel-Koomen CA, Schöpf E, Thepen T, Langeveld-Wildschut AG, Ruzicka T, Krutmann J (1998) A role for Th1 and Th2 cells in the immunopathogenesis of atopic dermatitis. Immunol Today 19(8):359–361

207. Perez VL, Lederer JA, Lichtman AH, Abbas AK (1995) Stability of Th1 and Th2 populations. Int Immunol 7:869–875

208. Ulrich P, Grenet O, Bluemel J, Vohr HW, Wiemann C, Grundler O, Suter W (2001) Cytokine expression profiles during murine contact allergy: T helper 2 cytokines are expressed irrespective of the type of contact allergen. Arch Toxicol 75(8):470–479

209. van Beelen AJ, Teunissen MB, Kapsenberg ML, de Jong EC (2007) Interleukin-17 in inflammatory skin disorders. Curr Opin Allergy Clin Immunol 7(5):374–381

210. Mucida D, Salek-Ardakani S (2009) Regulation of TH17 cells in the mucosal surfaces. J Allergy Clin Immunol 123(5):997–1003

211. Constant SL, Bottomly K (1997) Induction of Th1 and Th2 CD4+ T cell responses: the alternate approaches. Annu Rev Immunol 15:297–322

212. Constant SL, Pfeiffer C, Woodard A, Pasqualini T, Bottomly K (1995) Extent of T cell receptor ligation can determine the functional differentiation of naïve CD4+ T cells. J Exp Med 5:1591–1596

213. Bretscher PA, Ogunremi O, Menon JN (1997) Distinct immunological states in murine cutaneous leishmaniasis by immunizing with different amounts of antigen: the generation of beneficial, potentially harmful, harmful and potentially extremely harmful states. Behring Inst Mitt 98: 153–159

214. Toebak MJ, Moed H, von Blomberg MB, Bruynzeel DP, Gibbs S, Scheper RJ, Rustemeyer T (2006) Intrinsic characteristics of contact and respiratory allergens influence production of polarizing cytokines by dendritic cells. Contact Dermatitis 55(4):238–245

215. Watanabe H, Gehrke S, Contassot E, Roques S, Tschopp J, Friedmann PS, French LE, Gaide O (2008) Danger signaling through the inflammasome acts as a master switch

between tolerance and sensitization. J Immunol 180(9):5826–5832

216. Kanerva L, Hyry H, Jolanki R, Hytonen M, Estlander T (1997) Delayed and immediate allergy caused by methyl-hexahydrophthalic anhydride. Contact Dermatitis 36:34–38

217. Geenen V, Brilot F (2003) Role of the thymus in the development of tolerance and autoimmunity towards the neuroendocrine system. Ann N Y Acad Sci 992:186–195

218. Luger TA, Lotti T (1998) Neuropeptides: role in inflammatory skin diseases. J Eur Acad Derm Venereol 10:207–211

219. Luger TA (2002) Neuromediators – a crucial component of the skin immune system. J Dermatol Sci 30(2):87–93

220. Lord GM, Matarese G, Howard LK, Baker RJ, Bloom SR, Lechler RI (1998) Leptin modulates the T-cell immune response and reverses starvation-induced immunosuppression. Nature 394:897–901

221. Morfin R, Lafaye P, Cotillon AC, Nato F, Chmielewski V, Pompon D (2000) 7 alpha-hydroxy-dehydroepiandrosterone and immune response. Ann N Y Acad Sci 917: 971–982

222. Cutolo M, Seriolo B, Villaggio B, Pizzorni C, Craviotto C, Sulli A (2002) Androgens and estrogens modulate the immune and inflammatory responses in rheumatoid arthritis. Ann N Y Acad Sci 966:131–142

223. Kidd P (2003) Th1/Th2 balance: the hypothesis, its limitations, and implications for health and disease. Altern Med Rev 8:223–246

224. Piccinni MP, Giudizi MG, Biagiotti R, Beloni L, Giannarini L, Sampognaro S, Parronchi P, Manetti R, Annuziato F, Livi C, Romagnani S, Maggi E (1995) Progesterone favors the development of human T helper cells producing Th2-type cytokines and promotes both IL-4 production and membrane CD30 expression in established Th1 cell clones. J Immunol 155:128–133

225. Vieira PL, Kalinski P, Wierenga EA, Kapsenberg ML, Dejong EC (1998) Glucocorticoids inhibit bioactive IL-12P70 production by in vitro-generated human dendritic cells without affecting their T cell stimulatory potential. J Immunol 161:5245–5251

226. Calder PC, Bevan SJ, Newsholme EA (1992) The inhibition of T-lymphocyte proliferation by fatty acids is via an eicosanoid-independent mechanism. Immunology 75: 108–115

227. Uotila P (1996) The role of cyclic AMP and oxygen intermediates in the inhibition of cellular immunity in cancer. Cancer Immunol Immunother 43:1–9

228. Demeure CE, Yang LP, Desjardins C, Raynauld P, Delespesse G (1997) Prostaglandin E-2 primes naïve T cells for the production of anti-inflammatory cytokines. Eur J Immunol 27:3526–3531

229. Abe N, Katamura K, Shintaku N, Fukui T, Kiyomasu T, Lio J, Ueno H, Tai G, Mayumi M, Furusho K (1997) Prostaglandin E2 and IL-4 provide naïve CD4+ T cells with distinct inhibitory signals for the priming of IFN-gamma production. Cell Immunol 181:86–92

230. Kalinski P, Hilkens CMU, Snijders A, Snijdewint FGM, Kapsenberg ML (1997) IL-12 deficient dendritic cells, generated in the presence of prostaglandin E₂, promote type-2 cytokine production in maturing human naïve T helper cells. J Immunol 159:28–35

231. Edele F, Molenaar R, Gütle D, Dudda JC, Jakob T, Homey B, Mebius R, Hornef M, Martin SF (2008) Cutting edge: instructive role of peripheral tissue cells in the imprinting of T cell homing receptor patterns. J Immunol 181(6):3745–3749

232. Woodland DL, Kohlmeier JE (2009) Migration, maintenance and recall of memory T cells in peripheral tissues. Nat Rev Immunol 9(3):153–156

233. Fuhlbrigge RC, Kieffer JD, Armerding D, Kupper TS (1997) Cutaneous lymphocyte antigen is a specialized form of PSGL-1 expressed on skin-homing T cells. Nature 389:978–981

234. Sigmundsdottir H, Butcher EC (2008) Environmental cues, dendritic cells and the programming of tissue-selective lymphocyte trafficking. Nat Immunol 9(9):981–987

235. Miles A, Liaskou E, Eksteen B, Lalor PF, Adams DH (2008) CCL25 and CCL28 promote alpha4 beta7-integrin-dependent adhesion of lymphocytes to MAdCAM-1 under shear flow. Am J Physiol Gastrointest Liver Physiol 294(5):G1257–G1267

236. Sallusto F, Geginat J, Lanzavecchia A (2004) Central memory and effector memory T cell subsets: function, generation, and maintenance. Annu Rev Immunol 22:745–763

237. Sallusto F, Lenig D, Förster R, Lipp M, Lanzavecchia A (1999) Two subsets of memory T lymphocytes with distinct homing potentials and effector functions. Nature 401(6754):708–712

238. Austrup F, Vestweber D, Borges E, Lohning M, Brauer R, Herz U, Renz H, Hallmann R, Scheffold A, Radbruch A, Hamann A (1997) P- and E selectin mediate recruitment of T-helper-1 but not T-helper-2 cells into inflamed tissues. Nature 385:81–83

239. Duhen T, Geiger R, Jarrossay D, Lanzavecchia A, Sallusto F (2009) Production of interleukin 22 but not interleukin 17 by a subset of human skin-homing memory T cells. Nat Immunol 10(8):857–863

240. Borges E, Tietz W, Steegmaier M, Moll T, Hallmann R, Hamann A, Vestweber D (1997) P-selectin glycoprotein ligand-1 (PSGL-1) on T helper 1 but not on T helper 2 cells binds to P-selectin and supports migration into inflamed skin. J Exp Med 185:573–578

241. Ward SG, Marelli-Berg FM (2009) Mechanisms of chemokine and antigen-dependent T-lymphocyte navigation. Biochem J 418(1):13–27

242. Hudak S, Hagen M, Liu Y, Catron D, Oldham E, McEvoy LM, Bowman EP (2002) Immune surveillance and effector functions of CCR10(+) skin homing T cells. J Immunol 169(3):1189–1196

243. Kitagaki H, Ono N, Hayakawa K, Kitazawa T, Watanabe K, Shiohara T (1997) Repeated elicitation of contact hypersensitivity induces a shift in cutaneous cytokine milieu from a T helper cell type 1 to a T helper cell type 2 profile. J Immunol 159(5):2484–2491

244. Cavani A, Mei D, Guerra E, Corinti S, Giani M, Pirrotta L, Puddu P, Girolomoni G (1998) Patients with allergic contact dermatitis to nickel and nonallergic individuals display different nickel-specific T cell responses. Evidence for the presence of effector CD8+ and regulatory CD4+ T cells. J Invest Dermatol 111:621–628

245. Lindemann M, Rietschel F, Zabel M, Grosse-Wilde H (2008) Detection of chromium allergy by cellular in vitro methods. Clin Exp Allergy 38(9):1468–1475

246. Kalish RS (1990) The use of human T-lymphocyte clones to study T-cell function in allergic contact dermatitis to urushiol. J Invest Dermatol 94(6 suppl):108S–111S

247. von Blomberg BME, Bruynzeel DP, Scheper RJ (1991) Advances in mechanisms ofallergic contact dermatitis: in vitro and in vivo research. In: Marzulli FN, Maibach HI (eds) Dermatotoxicology, 4th edn. Hemisphere Publishing Corporation, New York, pp 255–362

248. Bordignon V, Palamara F, Cordiali-Fei P, Vento A, Aiello A, Picardo M, Ensoli F, Cristaudo A (2008) Nickel, palladium and rhodium induced IFN-gamma and IL-10 production as assessed by in vitro ELISpot-analysis in contact dermatitis patients. BMC Immunol 9:19

249. Minang JT, Troye-Blomberg M, Lundeberg L, Ahlborg N (2005) Nickel elicits concomitant and correlated in vitro production of Th1-, Th2-type and regulatory cytokines in subjects with contact allergy to nickel. Scand J Immunol 62(3):289–296

250. Moed H, von Blomberg BM, Bruynzeel DP, Scheper RJ, Gibbs S, Rustemeyer T (2005) Regulation of nickel-induced T-cell responsiveness by CD4+CD25+ cells in contact allergic patients and healthy individuals. Contact Dermatitis 53(2):71–74

251. Rustemeyer T, von Blomberg BME, van Hoogstraten IMW, Bruynzeel DP, Scheper RJ (2004) Analysis of effector and regulatory immune-reactivity to nickel. Clin Exp Allergy 34(9):1458–1466

252. Spiewak R, Moed H, von Blomberg BM, Bruynzeel DP, Scheper RJ, Gibbs S, Rustemeyer T (2007) Allergic contact dermatitis to nickel: modified in vitro test protocols for better detection of allergen-specific response. Contact Dermatitis 56(2):63–69

253. Minang JT, Areström I, Ahlborg N (2008) ELISpot displays a better detection over ELISA of T helper (Th) 2-type cytokine-production by ex vivo-stimulated antigen-specific T cells from human peripheral blood. Immunol Invest 37(4):279–291

254. Minang JT, Areström I, Troye-Blomberg M, Lundeberg L, Ahlborg N (2006) Nickel, cobalt, chromium, palladium and gold induce a mixed Th1- and Th2-type cytokine response in vitro in subjects with contact allergy to the respective metals. Clin Exp Immunol 146(3):417–426

255. Wahlkvist H, Masjedi K, Gruvberger B, Zuber B, Karlberg AT, Bruze M, Ahlborg N (2008) The lipophilic hapten parthenolide induces interferon-gamma and interleukin-13 production by peripheral blood-derived CD8+ T cells from contact allergic subjects in vitro. Br J Dermatol 158(1):70–77

256. Skazik C, Grannemann S, Wilbers L, Merk HF, Coenraads PJ, Breuer S, Blömeke B (2008) Reactivity of in vitro activated human T lymphocytes to p-phenylenediamine and related substances. Contact Dermatitis 59(4):203–211

257. Boyman O, Létourneau S, Krieg C, Sprent J (2009) Homeostatic proliferation and survival of naïve and memory T cells. Eur J Immunol 39(8):2088–2094

258. Rustemeyer T, von Blomberg BME, de Ligter S, Frosch PJ, Scheper RJ (1999) Human T lymphocyte priming in vitro by haptenated autologous dendritic cells. Clin Exp Immunol 117:209–216

259. Goebeler M, Meinardus-Hager G, Roth J, Goerdt S, Sorg C (1993) Nickel chloride and cobalt chloride, two common contact sensitizers, directly induce expression of intercellular adhesion molecule-1 (ICAM-1), vascular cell adhesion molecule-1 (VCAM-1), and endothelial leukocyte adhesion molecule (ELAM-1) by endothelial cells. J Invest Dermatol 100:759–765

260. Goebeler M, Roth J, Brocker EB, Sorg C, Schulze-Osthoff K (1995) Activation of nuclear factor-kappa B and gene expression in human endothelial cells by the common haptens nickel and cobalt. J Immunol 155:2459–2467

261. Walsh LJ, Lavker RM, Murphy GF (1990) Determinants of immune cell trafficking in the skin. Lab Invest 63: 592–600

262. Waldorf HA, Walsh LJ, Schechter NM, Murphy GF (1991) Early molecular events in evolving cutaneous delayed hypersensitivity in humans. Am J Pathol 138:477–486

263. Meller S, Lauerma AI, Kopp FM, Winterberg F, Anthoni M, Müller A, Gombert M, Haahtela A, Alenius H, Rieker J, Dieu-Nosjean MC, Kubitza RC, Gleichmann E, Ruzicka T, Zlotnik A, Homey B (2007) Chemokine responses distinguish chemical-induced allergic from irritant skin inflammation: memory T cells make the difference. J Allergy Clin Immunol 119(6):1470–1480

264. Bangert C, Friedl J, Stary G, Stingl G, Kopp T (2003) Immunopathologic features of allergic contact dermatitis in humans: participation of plasmacytoid dendritic cells in the pathogenesis of the disease? J Invest Dermatol 121: 1409–1418

265. Houck G, Saeed S, Stevens GL, Morgan MB (2004) Eczema and the spongiotic dermatoses: a histologic and pathogenic update. Semin Cutan Med Surg 23:39–45

266. Silberberg-Sinakin I, Thorbecke GJ, Baer RL, Rosenthal SA, Berezowsky V (1976) Antigen-bearing Langerhans cells in skin, dermal lymphatics, and in lymph nodes. Cell Immunol 25:137–151

267. Hill S, Edwards AJ, Kimber I, Knight SC (1990) Systemic migration of dendritic cells during contact sensitization. Immunology 71:277–281

268. Toebak MJ, Gibbs S, Bruynzeel DP, Scheper RJ, Rustemeyer T (2009) Dendritic cells: biology of the skin. Contact Dermatitis 60(1):2–20

269. Sterry W, Künne N, Weber-Matthiesen K, Brasch J, Mielke V (1991) Cell trafficking in positive and negative patch test reactions: demonstration of a stereotypic migration pathway. J Invest Dermatol 96:459–462

270. Herzog WR, Meade R, Pettinicchi A, Ptak W, Askenase PW (1989) Nude mice produce a T cell-derived antigen-binding factor that mediates the early component of delayed-type hypersensitivity. J Immunol 142:1803–1812

271. Willis CM, Young E, Brandon DR, Wilkinson JD (1986) Immunopathological and ultrastructural findings in human allergic and irritant contact dermatitis. Br J Dermatol 115:305–316

272. Brasch J, Burgard J, Sterry W (1992) Common pathways in allergic and irritant contact dermatitis. J Invest Dermatol 98:166–170

273. Hoefakker S, Caubo M, van 't Herve EHM, Roggeveen MJ, Boersma WJA, van Joost TH, Notten WRF, Claassen E (1995) In vivo cytokine profiles in allergic and irritant contact dermatitis. Contact Dermatitis 33:258–266

274. Flier J, Boorsma DM, Bruynzeel DP, van Beek PJ, Stoof TJ, Scheper RJ, Willemze R, Tensen CP (1999) The

CXCR3 activating chemokines IP-10, MIG and IP-9 are expressed in allergic but not in irritant patch test reactions. J Invest Dermatol 113:574–578

275. Kondo S, Sauder DN (1995) Epidermal cytokines in allergic contact dermatitis. J Am Acad Dermatol 33:786–800

276. Wardorf HA, Walsh LJ, Schechter NM (1991) Early cellular events in evolving cutaneous delayed hypersensitivity in humans. Am J Pathol 138:477–486

277. Pober JS, Bevilacqua MP, Mendrick DL, Lapierre LA, Fiers W, Gimbrone MA Jr (1986) Two distinct monokines, interleukin 1 and tumor necrosis factor, each independently induce biosynthesis and transient expression of the same antigen on the surface of cultured human vascular endothelial cells. J Immunol 136:1680–1687

278. Shimizu Y, Newman W, Gopal TV, Horgan KJ, Graber N, Beall LD, van Seventer GA, Shaw S (1991) Four molecular pathways of T cell adhesion to endothelial cells: roles of LFA-1, VCAM-1, and ELAM-1 and changes in pathway hierarchy under different activation conditions. J Cell Biol 113:1203–1212

279. Ross R, Gilitzer C, Kleinz R, Schwing J, Kleinert H, Forstermann U, Reske-Kunz AB (1998) Involvement of NO in contact hypersensitivity. Int Immunol 10:61–69

280. Rowe A, Farrell AM, Bunker CB (1997) Constitutive endothelial and inducible nitric oxide synthase in inflammatory dermatoses. Br J Dermatol 136:18–23

281. Szepietowski JC, McKenzie RC, Keohane SG, Walker C, Aldridge RD, Hunter JA (1997) Leukaemia inhibitory factor: induction in the early phase of allergic contact dermatitis. Contact Dermatitis 36:21–25

282. Yu X, Barnhill RL, Graves DT (1994) Expression of monocyte chemoattractant protein-1 in delayed type hypersensitivity reactions in the skin. Lab Invest 71:226–235

283. Buchanan KL, Murphy JW (1997) Kinetics of cellular infiltration and cytokine production during the efferent phase of a delayed-type hypersensitivity reaction. Immunology 90:189–197

284. Kish DD, Li X, Fairchild RL (2009) CD8 T cells producing IL-17 and IFN-gamma initiate the innate immune response required for responses to antigen skin challenge. J Immunol 182(10):5949–5959

285. Toebak MJ, Pohlmann PR, Sampat-Sardjoepersad SC, von Blomberg BM, Bruynzeel DP, Scheper RJ, Rustemeyer T, Gibbs S (2006) CXCL8 secretion by dendritic cells predicts contact allergens from irritants. Toxicol In Vitro 20(1):117–124

286. Askenase PW, Kawikova I, Paliwal V, Akahira-Azuma M, Gerard C, Hugli T, Tsuji R (1999) A new paradigm of T cell allergy: requirement for the B-1 cell subset. Int Arch Allergy Immunol 118(2–4):145–149

287. Van Loweren H, Meade R, Askenase PW (1983) An early component of delayed type hypersensitivity mediated by T cells and mast cells. J Exp Med 157:1604–1617

288. Foreman KE, Vaporciyan AA, Bonish BK, Jones ML, Johnson KJ, Glovsky MM, Eddy SM, Ward PA (1994) C5a-induced expression of P-selectin in endothelial cells. J Clin Invest 94:1147–1155

289. Groves RW, Allen MH, Ross EL, Barker JN, MacDonald DM (1995) Tumor necrosis factor alpha is pro-inflammatory in normal human skin and modulates cutaneous adhesion molecule expression. Br J Dermatol 132:345–352

290. Tsuji RF, Geba GP, Wang Y, Kawamoto K, Matis LA, Askenase PW (1997) Required early complement activation in contact sensitivity with generation of local C5-dependent chemotactic activity, and late T cell interferon g: a possible initiating role of B cells. J Exp Med 186:1015–1026

291. Nataf S, Davoust N, Ames RS, Barnum SR (1999) Human T cells express the C5a receptor and are chemoattracted to C5a. J Immunol 162:4018–4023

292. Wilkinson SM, Mattey DL, Beck MH (1994) IgG antibodies and early intradermal reactions to hydrocortisone in patients with cutaneous delayed-type hypersensitivity to hydrocortisone. Br J Dermatol 131:495–498

293. Shirakawa T, Kusaka Y, Morimoto K (1992) Specific IgE antibodies to nickel in workers with known reactivity to cobalt. Clin Exp Allergy 22:213–218

294. Redegeld FA, Nijkamp FP (2003) Immunoglobulin free light chains and mast cells: pivotal role in T-cell-mediated immune reactions? Trends Immunol 24:181–185

295. O'Leary JG, Goodarzi M, Drayton DL, von Andrian UH (2006) T cell- and B cell-independent adaptive immunity mediated by natural killer cells. Nat Immunol 7(5):507–516

296. Nieuwenhuis P, Ford WL (1976) Comparative migration of B- and T-Lymphocytes in the rat spleen and lymph nodes. Cell Immunol 23(2):254–267

297. Gober MD, Fishelevich R, Zhao Y, Unutmaz D, Gaspari AA (2008) Human natural killer T cells infiltrate into the skin at elicitation sites of allergic contact dermatitis. J Invest Dermatol 128(6):1460–1469

298. Dieli F, Ptak W, Sireci G, Romano GC, Potestio M, Salerno A, Asherson GL (1998) Cross-talk between V-beta-8(+) and gamma-delta(+) T lymphocytes in contact sensitivity. Immunology 93:469–477

299. Milon G, Marchal G, Seman M, Truffa-Bachi P (1981) A delayed-type hypersensitivity reaction initiated by a single T lymphocyte. Agents Actions 11:612–614

300. Marchal G, Seman M, Milon G, Truffa-Bachi P, Zilberfarb V (1982) Local adoptive transfer of skin delayed-type hypersensitivity initiated by a single T lymphocyte. J Immunol 129:954–958

301. Scheper RJ, van Dinther-Janssen AC, Polak L (1985) Specific accumulation of hapten-reactive T cells in contact sensitivity reaction sites. J Immunol 134:1333–1336

302. Macatonia SE, Knight SC, Edwards AJ, Griffiths S, Fryer P (1987) Localization of antigen on lymph node dendritic cells after exposure to the contact sensitizer fluorescein isothiocyanate. Functional and morphological studies. J Exp Med 166:1654–1667

303. Lappin MB, Kimber I, Norval M (1996) The role of dendritic cells in cutaneous immunity. Arch Dermatol Res 288:109–121

304. Moed H, Boorsma DM, Stoof TJ, von Blomberg BM, Bruynzeel DP, Scheper RJ, Gibbs S, Rustemeyer T (2004) Nickel-responding T cells are CD4+ CLA+ CD45RO+ and express chemokine receptors CXCR3, CCR4 and CCR10. Br J Dermatol 151:32–41

305. Vocanson M, Hennino A, Cluzel-Tailhardat M, Saint-Mezard P, Benetiere J, Chavagnac C, Berard F, Kaiserlian D, Nicolas JF (2006) CD8+ T cells are effector cells of contact dermatitis to common skin allergens in mice. J Invest Dermatol 126(4):815–820

306. Abe M, Kondo T, Xu H, Fairchild RL (1996) Interferon-gamma inducible protein (IP-10) expression is mediated by CD8+ T cells and is regulated by CD4+ T cells during the elicitation of contact hypersensitivity. J Invest Dermatol 107:360–366

307. Saulnier M, Huang S, Aguet M, Ryffel B (1995) Role of interferon-gamma in contact hypersensitivity assessed in interferon-gamma receptor-deficient mice. Toxicology 102(3):301–312

308. Rowe A, Bunker CB (1998) Interleukin-4 and the interleukin-4 receptor in allergic contact dermatitis. Contact Dermatitis 38:36–39

309. Asherson GL, Dieli F, Sireci G, Salerno A (1996) Role of IL-4 in delayed type hypersensitivity. Clin Exp Immunol 103:1–4

310. Asada H, Linton J, Katz SI (1997) Cytokine gene expression during the elicitation phase of contact sensitivity – regulation by endogenous IL-4. J Invest Dermatol 108:406–411

311. Kitagaki H, Fujisawa S, Watanabe K, Hayakawa K, Shiohara T (1995) Immediate-type hypersensitivity response followed by late reaction is induced by repeated epicutaneous application of contact sensitizing agents in mice. J Invest Dermatol 105:749–755

312. Carroll JM, Crompton T, Seery JP, Watt FM (1997) Transgenic mice expressing IFN-gamma in the epidermis have eczema, hair hypopigmentation, and hair loss. J Invest Dermatol 108:412–422

313. Lider O, Cahalon L, Gilat D, Hershkoviz R, Siegel D, Margalit R, Shoseyov O, Cohen IR (1995) A disaccharide that inhibits tumor necrosis factor alpha is formed from the extracellular matrix by the enzyme heparinase. Proc Natl Acad Sci U S A 92:5037–5041

314. Kothny-Wilkes G, Kulms D, Poppelmann B, Luger TA, Kubin M, Schwarz T (1998) Interleukin-1 protects transformed keratinocytes from tumor necrosis factor-related apoptosis-inducing ligand. J Biol Chem 273:29247–29253

315. Orteu CH, Poulter LW, Rustin MHA, Sabin CA, Salmon M, Akbar AN (1998) The role of apoptosis in the resolution of T cell-mediated cutaneous inflammation. J Immunol 161:1619–1629

316. Zhang X, Brunner T, Carter L, Dutton RW, Rogers P, Bradley L, Sato T, Reed JC, Green D, Swain SL (1997) Unequal death in T helper cell (Th)1 and Th2 effectors: Th1, but not Th2, effectors undergo rapid Fas/FasL-mediated apoptosis. J Exp Med 185:1837–1849

317. Enk AH, Katz SI (1992) Identification and induction of keratinocyte-derived IL-10. J Immunol 149:92–95

318. Schwarz A, Grabbe S, Riemann H, Aragane Y, Simon M, Manon S, Andrade S, Luger TA, Zlotnik A, Schwarz T (1994) In vivo effects of interleukin-10 on contact hypersensitivity and delayed-type hypersensitivity reactions. J Invest Dermatol 103:211–216

319. Berg DJ, Leach MW, Kuhn R, Rajewsky K, Muller W, Davidson NJ, Rennick D (1995) Interleukin 10 but not interleukin 4 is a natural suppressant of cutaneous inflammatory responses. J Exp Med 182:99–108

320. Morel PA, Oriss TB (1998) Crossregulation between Th1 and Th2 cells. Crit Rev Immunol 18:275–303

321. Lalani I, Bhol K, Ahmed AR (1997) Interleukin-10 biology, role in inflammation and autoimmunity. Ann Allergy Asthma Immunol 79:469–484

322. Epstein SP, Baer RL, Thorbecke GJ, Belsito DV (1991) Immunosuppressive effects of transforming growth factor beta: inhibition of the induction of Ia antigen on Langerhans cells by cytokines and of the contact hypersensitivity response. J Invest Dermatol 96:832–837

323. Lawrence JN, Dickson FM, Benford DJ (1997) Skin irritant-induced cytotoxicity and prostaglandin E-2 release in human skin keratinocyte cultures. Toxicol Vitro 11:627–631

324. Walker C, Kristensen F, Bettens F, deWeck AL (1983) Lymphokine regulation of activated (G1) lymphocytes. I. Prostaglandin E_2-induced inhibition of interleukin 2 production. J Immunol 130:1770–1773

325. Weston MC, Peachell PT (1998) Regulation of human mast cell and basophil function by cAMP. Gen Pharmacol 31:715–719

326. Dvorak HF, Mihm MC Jr, Dvorak AM (1976) Morphology of delayed-type hypersensitivity reactions in man. J Invest Dermatol 64:391–401

327. Marone G, Spadaro G, Patella V, Genovese A (1994) The clinical relevance of basophil releasability. J Aller Clin Immunol 94:1293–1303

328. Lundeberg L, Mutt V, Nordlind K (1999) Inhibitory effect of vasoactive intestinal peptide on the challenge phase of allergic contact dermatitis in humans. Acta Derm Venereol 79:178–182

329. Boerrigter GH, Scheper RJ (1987) Local and systemic desensitization induced by repeated epicutaneous hapten application. J Invest Dermatol 88:3–7

330. Jensen CS, Menne T, Lisby S, Kristiansen J, Veien NK (2003) Experimental systemic contact dermatitis from nickel: a dose-response study. Contact Dermatitis 49:124–132

331. Hindsen M, Bruze M, Christensen OB (2001) Flare-up reactions after oral challenge with nickel in relation to challenge dose and intensity and time of previous patch test reactions. J Am Acad Dermatol 44:616–623

332. Larsson A, Moller H, Björkner B, Bruze M (1997) Morphology of endogenous flare-up reactions in contact allergy to gold. Acta Derm Venereol 77:474–479

333. Skog E (1976) Spontaneous flare-up reactions induced by different amounts of 1, 3-dinitro-4-chlorobenzene. Acta Derm Venereol 46:386–395

334. Scheper RJ, von Blomberg BME, Boerrigter GH, Bruynzeel D, van Dinther A, Vos A (1983) Induction of local memory in the skin. Role of local T cell retention. Clin Exp Immunol 51:141–148

335. Moed H, Boorsma DM, Tensen CP, Flier J, Jonker MJ, Stoof TJ, Von Blomberg BM, Bruynzeel DP, Scheper RJ, Rustemeyer T, Gibbs S (2004) Increased CCL27-CCR10 expression in allergic contact dermatitis: implications for local skin memory. J Pathol 204:39–46

336. Christensen OB, Beckstead JH, Daniels TE, Maibach HI (1985) Pathogenesis of orally induced flare-up reactions at old patch sites in nickel allergy. Acta Derm Venereol 65:298–304

337. Hindsen M, Christensen OB (1992) Delayed hypersensitivity reactions following allergic and irritant inflammation. Acta Derm Venereol 72:220–221

338. Gawkrodger DJ, McVittie E, Hunter JA (1987) Immunophenotyping of the eczematous flare-up reaction in a nickel-sensitive subject. Dermatology 175:171–177

339. Polak L, Turk JL (1968) Studies on the effect of systemic administration of sensitizers in guinea-pigs with contact sensitivity to inorganic metal compounds.II. The flare-up of previous test sites of contact sensitivity and the development of a generalized rash. Clin Exp Immunol 3:253–262

340. Moser B, Loetscher M, Piali L, Loetscher P (1998) Lymphocyte responses to chemokines. Int Rev Immunol 16:323–3244

341. Rustemeyer T, de Groot J, von Blomberg BME, Frosch PJ, Scheper RJ (2002) Assessment of contact allergen cross-reactivity by retesting. Exp Dermatol 11:257–265

342. Matura M (1998) Contact allergy to locally applied corticosteroids. Thesis, Leuven, Belgium

343. Inerot A, Moller H (2000) Symptoms and signs reported during patch testing. Am J Contact Dermatol 11:49–52

344. Isaksson M, Bruze M (2003) Late patch-test reactions to budesonide need not be a sign of sensitization induced by the test procedure. Am J Contact Dermatol 14:154–156

345. Zinkernagel RM (2004) On "reactivity" versus "tolerance". Immunol Cell Biol 82:343–352

346. Piccirillo CA, Thornton AM (2004) Cornerstone of peripheral tolerance: naturally occurring CD4+CD25+ regulatory T cells. Trends Immunol 25:374–380

347. Benson JM, Whitacre CC (1997) The role of clonal deletion and anergy in oral tolerance. Res Immunol 148:533–541

348. Ferber I, Schönrich G, Schenkel J, Mellor AL, Hämmerling GJ, Arnold B (1994) Levels of peripheral T cell tolerance induced by different doses of tolerogen. Science 263:674–676

349. Morgan DJ, Kreuwel HTC, Sherman LA (1999) Antigen concentration and precursor frequency determine the rate of CD8($^+$) T cell tolerance to peripherally expressed antigens. J Immunol 163:723–727

350. Shreedhar V, Giese T, Sung VW, Ullrich SE (1998) A cytokine cascade including prostaglandin E2, IL-4, and IL-10 is responsible for UV-induced systemic immune suppression. J Immunol 160:3783–3789

351. Semma M, Sagami S (1981) Induction of suppressor T cells to DNFB contact sensitivity by application of sensitizer through Langerhans cell-deficient skin. Arch Dermatol Res 271:361–364

352. Taams LS, van Eden W, Wauben MHM (1999) Dose-dependent induction of distinct anergic phenotypes: multiple levels of T cell anergy. J Immunol 162:1974–1981

353. Girolomoni G, Gisondi P, Ottaviani C, Cavani A (2004) Immunoregulation of allergic contact dermatitis. J Dermatol 31:264–270

354. Mayer L, Sperber K, Chan L, Child J, Toy L (2001) Oral tolerance to protein antigens. Allergy 56:12–15

355. Weiner HL, Gonnella PA, Slavin A, Maron R (1997) Oral tolerance: cytokine milieu in the gut and modulation of tolerance by cytokines. Res Immunol 148:528–533

356. Wang YH, Liu YJ (2008) The IL-17 cytokine family and their role in allergic inflammation. Curr Opin Immunol 20(6):697–702

357. Rustemeyer T, de Groot J, von Blomberg BME, Frosch PJ, Scheper RJ (2001) Induction of tolerance and cross-tolerance to methacrylate contact sensitizers. Toxicol Appl Pharmacol 176:195–202

358. Miller SD, Sy M-S, Claman HN (1977) The induction of hapten-specific T cell tolerance using hapten-modified lymphoid membranes. II. Relative roles of suppressor T cells and clone inhibition in the tolerant state. Eur J Immunol 7:165–170

359. Polak L (1980) Immunological aspects of contact sensitivity. An experimental study. Monogr Allergy 15:4–60

360. Weiner HL (1997) Oral tolerance: immune mechanisms and treatment of autoimmune diseases. Immunol Today 18:335–343

361. Weigle WO, Romball CG (1997) CD4+ T-cell subsets and cytokines involved in peripheral tolerance. Immunol Today 18:533–538

362. Arnaboldi PM, Roth-Walter F, Mayer L (2009) Suppression of Th1 and Th17, but not Th2, responses in a CD8(+) T cell-mediated model of oral tolerance. Mucosal Immunol 2(5):427–438

363. Zembala M, Ashershon GL (1973) Depression of T cell phenomenon of contact sensitivity by T cells from unresponsive mice. Nature 244:227–228

364. Boerrigter GH, Scheper RJ (1984) Local administration of the cytostatic drug 4-hydroperoxy-cyclophosphamde (4-HPCY) facilitates cell mediated immune reactions. Clin Exp Immunol 58:161–166

365. Boerrigter GH, de Groot J, Scheper RJ (1986) Intradermal administration of 4-hydoperoxy-cyclophosphamde during contact sensitization potentiates effector T cell responsiveness in draining lymph nodes. Immunopharmacology 1:13–20

366. Mokyr MB, Kalinichenko T, Gorelik L, Bluestone JA (1998) Realization of the therapeutic potential of CTLA-4 blockade in low-dose chemotherapy-treated tumor-bearing mice. Cancer Res 58:5301–5304

367. Knop J, Stremmer R, Neumann C, Dc Maeyer D, Macher E (1982) Interferon inhibits the suppressor T cell response of delayed-type hypersensitivity. Nature 296:775–776

368. Zhang ZY, Michael JG (1990) Orally inducible immune unresponsiveness is abrogated by IFN-gamma treatment. J Immunol 144:4163–4165

369. Claessen AME, von Blomberg BME, de Groot J, Wolvers DAE, Kraal G, Scheper RJ (1996) Reversal of mucosal tolerance by subcutaneous administration of interleukin-12 at the site of attempted sensitization. Immunology 88:363–367

370. Bridoux F, Badou A, Saoudi A, Bernard L, Druet E, Pasquier R, Druet P, Pelletier L (1997) Transforming growth factor beta (TGF-beta)-dependent inhibition of T helper cell 2 (Th2)-induced autoimmunity by self-major histocompatibility complex (MHC) class II-specific, regulatory CD4+ T cell lines. J Exp Med 185: 1769–1775

371. Cavani A, Nasorri F, Ottaviani C, Sebastiani S, De Pita O, Girolomoni G (2003) Human CD25+ regulatory T cells maintain immune tolerance to nickel in healthy, nonallergic individuals. J Immunol 171:5760–5768

372. Hafler DA, Kent SC, Pietrusewicz MJ, Khoury SJ, Weiner HL, Fukaura H (1997) Oral administration of myelin induces antigen-specific TGF-beta 1 secreting T cells in patients with multiple sclerosis. Ann N Y Acad Sci 835:120–131

373. Lonati A, Licenziati S, Marcelli M, Canaris D, Pasolini G, Caruso A, de Panfilis G (1998) Quantitative analysis "at the

single cell level" of the novel CD28⁻CD11b⁻ subpopulation of CD8⁺ T lymphocytes. ESDR meeting at Cologne

374. De Panfilis G (1998) CD8⁺ cytolytic T lymphocytes and the skin. Exp Dermatol 7:121–131

375. Ilan Y (2009) Oral tolerance: can we make it work? Hum Immunol 70(10):768–776

376. Kuchroo VK, Byrne MC, Atsumi Y, Greenfeld E, Connol JH, Whitters MJ, O'Hara RM, Collins M, Dorf ME (1991) T cell receptor alpha chain plays a critical role in antigen-specific suppressor cell function. Proc Natl Acad Sci U S A 88:8700–8704

377. Taams LS, Boot EPJ, van Eden W, Wauben MHM (2000) "Anergic" T cells modulate the T-cell activating capacity of antigen-presenting cells. J Autoimmun 14:335–341

378. Taams LS, van Rensen AJML, Poelen MC, van Els CACM, Besseling AC, Wagenaar JPA, van Eden W, Wauben MHM (1998) Anergic T cells actively suppress T cell responses via the antigen presenting cell. Eur J Immunol 28:2902–2912

379. Kalinski P, Schuitemaker JH, Hilkens CM, Kapsenberg ML (1998) Prostaglandin E₂ induces the final maturation of IL-12 deficient CD1a⁺CD83⁺ dendritic cells. J Immunol 161:2804–2809

380. Steinbrink K, Wolf M, Jonuleit H, Knop J, Enk AH (1997) Induction of tolerance by IL-10-treated dendritic cells. J Immunol 159:4772–4780

381. Steinbrink K, Jonuleit H, Muller G, Schuler G, Knop J, Enk AH (1999) Interleukin-10-treated human dendritic cells induce a melanoma-antigen-specific anergy in CD8(⁺) T cells resulting in a failure to lyse tumor cells. Blood 93:1634–1642

382. Van Hoogstraten IMW, Andersen JE, von Blomberg BME, Boden D, Bruynzeel DP, Burrows D, Camarasa JMG, Dooms-Goossens A, Lahti A, Menné T, Rycroft R, Todd D, Vreeburg KJJ, Wilkinson JD, Scheper RJ (1989) Preliminary results of a multicenter study on the incidence of nickel allergy in relationship to previous oral and cutaneous contacts. In: Frosch PJ, Dooms-Goossens A, Lachapelle JM, Rycroft RJG, Scheper RJ (eds) Current topics in contact dermatitis. Springer, Berlin, pp 178–184

383. Strobel S, Mowat AM (1998) Immune responses to dietary antigens: oral tolerance. Immunol Today 19:173–181

384. von Herrath MG (1997) Bystander suppression induced by oral tolerance. Res Immunol 148:541–554

385. Fowler E, Weiner HL (1997) Oral tolerance: elucidation of mechanisms and application to treatment of autoimmune diseases. Biopolymers 43:323–335

386. Van Hoogstraten IMW, von Blomberg BME, Boden D, Kraal G, Scheper RJ (1994) Non-sensitizing epicutaneous skin tests prevent subsequent induction of immune tolerance. J Invest Dermatol 102:80–83

387. Epstein WL (1987) The poison ivy picker of Pennypack Park: the continuing saga of poison ivy. J Invest Dermatol 88:7–9

388. Morris DL (1998) Intradermal testing and sublingual in desensitization for nickel. Cutis 61:129–132

389. Wendel GD, Stark BJ, Jamison RB, Molina RD, Sullivan TJ (1985) Penicillin allergy and desensitization in serious infections during pregnancy. N Engl J Med 312: 1229–1232

390. Panzani RC, Schiavino D, Nucera E, Pellegrino S, Fais G, Schinco G, Patriarca G (1995) Oral hyposensitization to nickel allergy: preliminary clinical results. Int Arch Allergy Immunol 107:251–254

391. Troost RJ, Kozel MM, van Helden-Meeuwsen CG, van Joost T, Mulder PG, Benner R, Prens EP (1995) Hyposensitization in nickel allergic contact dermatitis: clinical and immunologic monitoring. J Am Acad Dermatol 32:576–583

392. Chase MW (1946) Inhibition of experimental drug allergy by prior feeding of the sensitizing agent. Proc Soc Exp Biol Med 61:257–259

393. Polak L, Turk SL (1968) Studies on the effect of systemic administration of sensitizers in guinea pigs with contact sensitivity to inorganic metal compounds. I. The induction of immunological unresponsiveness in already sensitized animals. Clin Exp Immunol 3:245–251

394. Polak L, Rinck C (1978) Mechanism of desensitization in DNCH-contact sensitive guinea pigs. J Invest Dermatol 70:98–104

395. Gaspari AA, Jenkins MK, Katz SI (1988) Class II MCH-bearing keratinocytes induce antigen-specific unresponsiveness in hapten-specific TH1 clones. J Immunol 141:2216–2220

396. Murphy K, Travers P, Walport M (eds) (2008) Janeway's immunobiology, 7th edn. Garland Science, Taylor & Francis Group, US, UK

397. Gaga M, Ong YE, Benyahia F, Aizen M, Barkans J (2008) Kay AB.Skin reactivity and local cell recruitment in human atopic and nonatopic subjects by CCL2/MCP-1 and CCL3/MIP-1alpha. Allergy 63(6):703–711

398. Homey B, Alenius H, Müller A, Soto H, Bowman EP, Yuan W, McEvoy L, Lauerma AI, Assmann T, Bünemann E, Lehto M, Wolff H, Yen D, Marxhausen H, To W, Sedgwick J, Ruzicka T, Lehmann P, Zlotnik A (2002) CCL27-CCR10 interactions regulate T cell-mediated skin inflammation. Nat Med 8(2):157–165

399. Kagami S, Saeki H, Tsunemi Y, Nakamura K, Kuwano Y, Komine M, Nakayama T, Yoshie O, Tamaki K (2008) CCL27-transgenic mice show enhanced contact hypersensitivity to Th2, but not Th1 stimuli. Eur J Immunol 38(3):647–657

400. Grimm MC, Ng WS (2008) Road most traveled: gut-specific migration signals and leucocyte entry to the intestine. J Gastroenterol Hepatol 23(12):1775

401. Gomez J, Gonzalez A, Martinez-A C, Rebollo A (1998) IL-2-induced cellular events. Crit Rev Immunol 18:185–220

402. Berridge MJ (1997) Lymphocyte activation in health and disease. Crit Rev Immunol 17:155–178

403. Theze J, Alzari PM, Bertoglio J (1996) Interleukin 2 and its receptors: recent advances and new immunological functions. Immunol Today 17:481–486

404. Lacour M, Arrighi J-F, Müller KM, Carlberg C, Saurat J-H, Hauser C (1994) cAMP up-regulates IL-4 and IL-5 production from activated CD4⁺ T cells while decreasing IL-2 release and NF-AT induction. Int Immunol 6:1333–1343

405. Linsley PS, Ledbetter JA (1993) The role of the CD28 receptor during T cell responses to antigen. Annu Rev Immunol 11:191–212

406. Mazzoni A, Segal DM (2004) Controlling the Toll road to dendritic cell polarization. J Leukoc Biol 75:721–730

407. O'Garra A (1998) Cytokines induce the development of functionally heterogeneous T helper cell subsets. Immunity 8:275–283

408. Santana MA, Rosenstein Y (2003) What it takes to become an effector T cell: the process, the cells involved, and the mechanisms. J Cell Physiol 195:392–401

409. Burkett PR, Koka R, Chien M, Boone DL, Ma A (2004) Generation, maintenance, and function of memory T cells. Adv Immunol 83:191–231

410. Spahn TW, Kucharzik T (2004) Modulating the intestinal immune system: the role of lymphotoxin and GALT organs. Gut 53:456–465

411. Bour H, Peyron E, Gaucherand M, Garrigue JL, Desvignes C, Kaiserlian D, Revillard JP, Nicolas JF (1995) Major histocompatibility complex class I-restricted CD8+ T cells and class II-restricted CD4+ T cells, respectively, mediate and regulate contact sensitivity to dinitrofluorobenzene. Eur J Immunol 25:3006–3010

412. Paul WE, Ohara J (1987) B-cell stimulatory factor-1/interleukin 4. Annu Rev Immunol 5:429–459

413. Mackey MF, Barth RJ, Noelle RJ (1998) The role of CD40/CD154 interactions in the priming, differentiation, and effector function of helper and cytotoxic T cell. J Leuk Biol 63:418–428

414. Kuchroo V, Prabhu Das M, Brown JA, Ranger A, Zamvill MSS, Sobel RA, Weiner HL, Nabavi N, Glimcher LH (1995) B7-1 and B7-2 costimulatory molecules activate differentially the Th1/Th2 developmental pathways. Application to autoimmune disease therapy. Cell 80: 707–718

415. Ranger AM, Prabhu Das M, Kuchroo VK, Glimcher LH (1996) B7-2 (CD86) is essential for the development of IL-4 producing cells. Int Immunol 153:1549–1560

416. Schweitzer AN, Borriello F, Wong RCK, Abbas AK, Sharpe AH (1997) Role of costimulators in T cell differentiation – studies using antigen-presenting cells lacking expression of CD80 or CD86. J Immunol 158:2713–2722

417. Rulifson IC, Sperling AI, Fields PE, Fitch FW, Bluestone JA (1997) CD28 costimulation promotes the production of Th2 cytokines. J Immunol 158:658–665

418. Pernis A, Gupta S, Gollob KJ, Garfein E, Coffman RL, Schindler C, Rothman P (1995) Lack of interferon gamma receptor beta chain and the prevention of interferon signaling in Th1 cells. Science 269:245–247

419. Yoshimoto T, Takeda K, Tanaka T, Ohkusu K, Kashiwamura S, Okamura H, Akira S, Nakanishi K (1998) IL-12 up-regulates IL-18 receptor expression on T cells, TH1 cells, and B cells – synergism with IL-18 for IFN-gamma production. J Immunol 161:3400–3407

420. Zanni MP, Mauri-Hellweg D, Brander C, Wendland T, Schnyder B, Frei E, von Greyerz S, Bircher A, Pichler WJ (1997) Characterization of lidocaine-specific T cells. J Immunol 158:1139–1148

421. Rincon M, Anguita J, Nakamura T, Fikrig E, Flavell RA (1997) Interleukin (IL)-6 directs the differentiation of IL-4 producing CD4+ T cells. J Exp Med 182:1591–1596

422. Yoshimoto T, Bendelac A, Watson C, Hu-Li J, Paul WE (1995) Role of NK1.1+ T cells in a TH2 response and in immunoglobulin E production. Science 270:1845–1847

423. Hiroi T, Iwatani K, Iijima H, Kodama S, Yanagita M, Kiyono H (1998) Nasal immune system – distinctive Th0

and Th1/Th2 type environments in murine nasal-associated lymphoid tissues and nasal passage, respectively. Eur J Immunol 28:3346–3353

424. Banchereau J (1995) Converging and diverging properties of human interleukin-4 and interleukin-10. Behr Inst Mitteil 96:58–77

425. Itoh K, Hirohata S (1995) The role of IL-10 in human B cell activation, proliferation, and differentiation. J Immunol 154:4341–4350

426. Napolitano LM, Buzdon MM, Shi HJ, Bass BL (1997) Intestinal epithelial cell regulation cell regulation of macrophage and lymphocyte interleukin 10 expression. Arch Surg 132:1271–1276

427. Xu H, Banerjee A, Diulio NA, Fairchild RL (1996) T cell populations primed by hapten sensitization in contact sensitivity are distinguished by polarized patterns of cytokine production: interferon gamma-producing (Tc1) effector CD8+ T cells and interleukin (IL)-4/IL-10-producing (Th2) negative regulatory CD4+ T cells. J Exp Med 183: 1001–1012

428. Letterio JL, Roberts AB (1998) Regulation of immune responses by TGF-beta. Annu Rev Immunol 16:137–161

429. Hosken NA, Shibuya K, Heath AW, Murphy KM, O'Garra A (1995) The effect of antigen dose on CD4+ T helper cell phenotype development in a T cell receptor phenotype development in a T cell receptor alpha/beta-transgenic model. J Exp Med 182:1579–1584

430. Scholzen T, Armstrong CA, Bunnett NW, Luger TA, Olerud JE, Ansel JC (1998) Neuropeptides in the skin: interactions between the neuroendocrine and the skin immune systems. Exp Dermatol 7:81–96

431. Westerman J, Geismar U, Sponholz A, Bode U, Sparshott BEB (1997) CD4+ T cells of both the naive and the memory phenotype enter rat lymph nodes and Peyer's patches via high endothelial venules: within the tissue their migratory behaviour differs. Eur J Immunol 27:3174–3181

432. Marshall D, Haskard DO (2002) Clinical overview of leukocyte adhesion and migration: where are we now? Semin Immunol 14:133–140

433. Hall JG, Morris B (1965) The origin of cells in the efferent lymph from a single lymph node. J Exp Med 121:901–910

434. Hwang ST (2001) Mechanisms of T-cell homing to skin. Adv Dermatol 17:211–241

435. Pober JS, Kluger MS, Schechner JS (2001) Human endothelial cell presentation of antigen and the homing of memory/effector T cells to skin. Ann N Y Acad Sci 941:12–25

436. Mackay CR (1993) Homing of naïve, memory and effector lymphocytes. Curr Opin Immunol 5:423–427

437. Tietz W, Allemand Y, Borges E, Vonlaer D, Hallmann R, Vestweber D, Hamann A (1998) CD4(+) T cells migrate into inflamed skin only if they express ligands for E- and P-selectin. J Immunol 16:963–970

438. Rosen Homey B (2004) Chemokines and chemokine receptors as targets in the therapy of psoriasis. Curr Drug Targets Inflamm Allergy 3:169–174

439. Homey B, Bunemann E (2004) Chemokines and inflammatory skin diseases. Ernst Schering Res Found Workshop 4:69–83

440. Tanchot C, Rocha B (1998) The organization of mature T-cell pools. Immunol Today 19:575–579

441. Williams IR (2004) Chemokine receptors and leukocyte trafficking in the mucosal immune system. Immunol Res 29:283–292

442. Telemo E, Korotkova M, Hanson LA (2003) Antigen presentation and processing in the intestinal mucosa and lymphocyte homing. Ann Allergy Asthma Immunol 90:28–33

443. Picker LJ, Treer JR, Ferguson-Darnell B, Collins PA, Bergstresser PR, Terstappen LWMM (1993) Control of lymphocyte recirculation in man: II. Differential regulation of the cutaneous lymphocyte associated antigen, a tissue-selective homing receptor for skin homing T cells. J Immunol 150:1122–1136

444. Sunderkötter C, Steinbrink K, Henseleit U, Bosse R, Schwarz A, Vestweber D, Sorg C (1996) Activated T cells induce expression of E-selectin in vitro and in an antigen-dependent manner in vivo. Eur J Immunol 26:1571–1579

445. Tensen CP, Flier J, Rampersad SS, Sampat-Sardjoerpersad A, Scheper RJ, Boorsma DM, Willemze R (1999) Genomic organization, sequence and transcriptional regulation of the human CXCL 11 gene. Biochim Biophys Acta 1446:167–172

446. Sallusto F, Kremmer E, Palermo B, Hoy A, Ponath P, Qin SX, Forster R, Lipp M, Lanzavecchia A (1999) Switch in chemokine receptor expression upon TCR stimulation reveals novel homing potential for recently activated T cells. Eur J Immunol 29:2037–2045

447. Baggiolini M (1998) Chemokines and leukocyte traffic. Nature 392:565–568

448. Bell EB, Sparshott SM, Bunce C (1998) CD4⁺ T-cell memory, CD45R subsets and the persistence of antigen – a unifying concept. Immunol Today 19:60–64

449. Bell EB, Sparshott SM, Ager A (1995) Migration pathways of CD4 T cell subsets in vivo: the CD45RC- subset enters the thymus via alpha 4 integrin- VCAM-1 interaction. Int Immunol 11:1861–1871

450. Stoof TJ, Boorsma DM, Nickoloff BJ (1994) Keratinocytes and immunological cytokines. In: Leigh I, Lane B, Watt F (eds) The keratinocyte handbook. Cambridge University Press, Cambridge, pp 365–399

451. Tensen CP, Flier J, van der Raaij-Helmer EM, Sampat-Sardjoerpersad S, van den Schors RC, Leurs R, Scheper RJ, Boorsma DM, Willemze R (1999) Human IP-9: a keratinocyte derived high affinity CXC-chemokine ligand for the IP-10/Mig receptor (CXCR3). J Invest Dermatol 112:716–722

452. Virag L, Szabo E, Bakondi E, Bai P, Gergely P, Hunyadi J, Szabo C (2002) Nitric oxide-peroxynitrite-poly(ADP-ribose) polymerase pathway in the skin. Exp Dermatol 11:189–202

453. Ptak W, Askenase PW, Rosenstein RW, Gershon RK (1982) Transfer of an antigen-specific immediate hypersensitivity-like reaction with an antigen-binding factor produced by T cells. Proc Natl Acad Sci U S A 79:1969–1973

454. Van Loveren H, Ratzlaff RE, Kato K, Meade R, Ferguson TA, Iverson GM, Janeway CA, Askenase PW (1986) Immune serum from mice contact-sensitized with picryl chloride contains an antigen-specific T cell factor that transfers immediate cutaneous reactivity. Eur J Immunol 16:1203–1208

455. Ptak W, Herzog WR, Askenase PW (1991) Delayed-type hypersensitivity initiation by early-acting cells that are antigen mismatched or MHC incompatible with late-acting, delayed-type hypersensitivity effector T cells. J Immunol 146:469–475

456. Askenase PW, Kawikova I, Paliwal V, Akahira-Azuma M, Gerard C, Hugli T, Tsuji R (1999) A new paradigm of T cell allergy: requirement for the B-1 B cell subset. Int Arch All Appl Immunol 118:145–149

457. Hardy RR, Hayakawa K (1994) CD5⁺ B cells, a fetal B cell lineage. Adv Immunol 55:297–339

458. Feinstein A, Richardson N, Taussig MJ (1986) Immunoglobulin flexibility in complement activation. Immunol Today 7:169–173

459. Geba GP, Ptak W, Anderson GA, Ratzlaff RE, Levin J, Askenase PW (1996) Delayed-type hypersensitivity in mast cell deficient mice: dependence on platelets for expression on contact sensitivity. J Immunol 157:557–565

460. Salerno A, Dieli F (1998) Role of gamma delta T lymphocytes in immune response in humans and mice. Crit Rev Immunol 18:327–357

461. Szczepanik M, Lewis J, Geba GP, Ptak W, Askenase PW (1998) Positive regulatory gamma-delta T cells in contact sensitivity – augmented responses by in vivo treatment with anti-gamma-delta monoclonal antibody, or anti-V-gamma-5 or V-delta-4. Immunol Invest 27:1–15

462. Tang HL, Cyster JG (1999) Chemokine up-regulation and activated T cell attraction by maturing dendritic cells. Science 284:819–822

463. Vana G, Meingassner JG (2000) Morphologic and immunohistochemical features of experimentally induced allergic contact dermatitis in Gottingen minipigs. Vet Pathol 37:565–580

464. Teraki Y, Picker LJ (1997) Independent regulation of cutaneous lymphocyte-associated antigen expression and cytokine synthesis phenotype during human CD4⁺ memory T cell differentiation. J Immunol 159:6018–6029

465. Butcher EC, Picker LJ (1996) Lymphocyte homing and homeostasis. Science 272:60–66

466. Strunk D, Egger C, Leitner G, Hanau D, Stingl G (1997) A skin homing molecule defines the Langerhans cell progenitor in human peripheral blood. J Exp Med 185:1131–1136

467. Wroblewski M, Hamann A (1997) CD45-mediated signals can trigger shedding of lymphocyte L-selectin. Int Immunol 9:555–562

468. Burastero SE, Rossi GA, Crimi E (1998) Selective differences in the expression of the homing receptors of helper lymphocyte subsets. Clin Immunol Immunopathol 89:110–116

469. Wahbi A, Marcusson JA, Sundqvist KG (1996) Expression of adhesion molecules and their ligands in contact allergy. Exp Dermatol 5:12–19

470. Dailey MO (1998) Expression of T lymphocyte adhesion molecules: regulation during antigen-induced T cell activation and differentiation. Crit Rev Immunol 18:153–184

471. Oppenheimer-Marks N, Lipsky PE (1997) Migration of naïve and memory T cells. Immunol Today 18:456–457

472. Romanic AM, Graesser D, Baron JL, Visintin I, Janeway CA Jr, Madri JA (1997) T cell adhesion to endothelial cells and extracellular matrix is modulated upon transendothelial cell migration. Lab Invest 76:11–23

473. Zanni MP, von Greyerz S, Schnyder B, Brander KA, Frutig K, Hari Y, Valitutti S, Pichler WJ (1998) HLA-restricted, processing- and metabolism-independent pathway of drug recognition by human alpha beta T lymphocytes. J Clin Invest 102:1591–1598

474. Akdis CA, Akdis M, Simon HU, Blaser K (1999) Regulation of allergic inflammation by skin-homing T cells in allergic eczema. Int Arch Allergy Immunol 118:140–144

475. Okazaki F, Kanzaki H, Fujii K, Arata J, Akiba H, Tsujii K, Iwatsuki K (2002) Initial recruitment of interferon-gamma-producing CD8+ effector cells, followed by infiltration of CD4+ cells in 2, 4, 6-trinitro-1-chlorobenzene (TNCB)-induced murine contact hypersensitivity reactions. J Dermatol 29:699–708

476. Pichler WJ, Schnyder B, Zanni MP, Hari Y, von Greyerz S (1998) Role of T cells in drug allergies. Allergy 53:225–232

477. Kehren J, Desvignes C, Krasteva M, Ducluzeau MT, Assossou O, Horand F, Hahne M, Kagi D, Kaiserlian D, Nicolas JF (1999) Cytotoxicity is mandatory for CD8+ T cell mediated contact hypersensitivity. J Exp Med 189:779–786

478. Mauri-Hellweg D, Bettens F, Mauri D, Brander C, Hunziker T, Pichler WJ (1995) Activation of drug-specific CD4+ and CD8+ T cells in individuals allergic to sulfonamides, phenytoin, and carbamazepine. J Immunol 155:462–472

479. Stark GR, Kerr IM, Williams BRG, Silverman RH, Schreiber RD (1998) How cells respond to interferons. Annu Rev Biochem 67:227–264

480. Yamada H, Matsukura M, Yudate T, Chihara J, Stingl G, Tezuka T (1997) Enhanced production of RANTES, an eosinophil chemoattractant factor, by cytokine-stimulated epidermal keratinocytes. Int Arch Aller Immunol 114:28–32

481. Siveke JT, Hamann A (1998) T helper 1 and T helper 2 Cells respond differentially to chemokines. J Immunol 160:550–554

482. Qin S, Rottman JB, Myers P, Kassam N, Weinblatt M, Loetscher M, Koch AE, Moser B, Mackay CR (1998) The chemokine receptors CXCR3 and CCR5 mark subsets of T cells associated with certain inflammatory reactions. J Clin Invest 101:746–754

483. Rocha B, von Boehmer H (1991) Peripheral selection of the T cell repertoire. Science 251:1225–1228

484. Arnold B, Schönrich G, Hämmerling GJ (1993) Multiple levels of peripheral tolerance. Immunol Today 14:12–14

485. Pozzilli P, Gisella Cavallo M (2000) Oral insulin and the induction of tolerance in man: reality or fantasy? Diabetes Metab Res Rev 16:306–307

486. Röcken M, Shevach EM (1996) Immune deviation – the third dimension of nondeletional T cell tolerance. Immunol Rev 149:175–194

487. Kumar V, Sercarz E (1998) Induction or protection from experimental autoimmune encephalomyelitis depends on the cytokine secretion profile of TCR peptide-specific regulatory CD4 T cells. J Immunol 161:6585–6591

488. Strober W, Kelsall B, Marth T (1998) Oral tolerance. J Clin Immunol 18:1–30

489. Inobe J, Slavin AJ, Komagata Y, Chen Y, Liu L, Weiner HL (1998) IL-4 is a differentiation factor for transforming growth factor-beta secreting Th3 cells and oral administration of IL-4 enhances oral tolerance in experimental allergic encephalomyelitis. Eur J Immunol 28:2780–2790

490. Allan SE, Broady R, Gregori S, Himmel ME, Locke N, Roncarolo MG, Bacchetta R, Levings MK (2008) CD4+ T-regulatory cells: toward therapy for human diseases. Immunol Rev 223:391–421

491. Croft M, So T, Duan W, Soroosh P (2009) The significance of OX40 and OX40L to T-cell biology and immune disease. Immunol Rev 229(1):173–191

Molecular Aspects in Allergic and Irritant Contact Dermatitis

4

Jean-Pierre Lepoittevin

Contents

J.-P. Lepoittevin
Institut le Bel, Labo. Dermatochimie,
4, rue Blaise Pascal, 67070 Strasbourg Cedex, France
e-mail: jplepoit@unistra.fr

4.1 Introduction

Skin exposure to chemicals, natural or synthetic, may result in toxic reactions ranging from mild irritation to cutaneous allergy. These inflammatory reactions, subsequent to chemical exposure, derive from very different biological mechanisms. Very often and for classification purposes, a difference is made between nonimmunological inflammatory reactions or so-called irritant reactions and immunological inflammatory reactions or cutaneous allergies. Of course, skin toxic reactions induced by exposure to chemicals are a consequence and very often a superimposition of both the mechanisms.

Interactions between chemicals and biological systems always involve chemical interactions!

4.2 Chemical Interactions

Chemicals in contact with the skin will interact with biological systems through chemical interactions. These chemical interactions result from electronic interactions between atoms or groups of atoms and are characterized by the energy involved that reflects their stability. This energy must be provided to break the chemical interaction between the atoms. In general, a distinction is made between *weak interactions,* involving energy levels from a few joules to approximately 50 kJ/mol of complex, and *strong interactions*, covalent or coordination bonds, with energies ranging from 200 to 420 kJ/mol. Indeed, there is a continuum ranging from weak to strong interactions (Fig. 4.1).

J.D. Johansen et al. (eds.), *Contact Dermatitis*,
DOI: 10.1007/978-3-642-03827-3_4, © Springer-Verlag Berlin Heidelberg 2011

4

Fig. 4.1 Energy level of chemical bonds

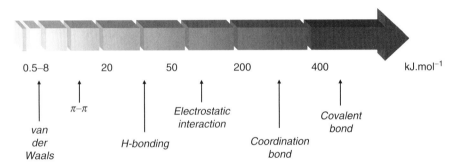

4.2.1 Weak Interactions

Weak interactions are normally grouped into three main categories: hydrophobic, dipolar, and ionic bonds. Although these weak interactions involve modest energy levels and produce complexes of low stability, they are nonetheless of great biological importance, as they control virtually all the phenomena of recognition between receptors and substrates.

Hydrophobic interactions result from the ability of organic molecules to arrange themselves in such a way as to minimize the area of contact with the aqueous medium. This is, for example, how hydrophobic molecules insert themselves into the phospholipid bilayers of cell membranes and into hydrophobic regions of proteins or membrane receptors. These hydrophobic bonds involve very low energies of about 40–90 J/Å^2/mol (1 Å = 0.1 nm), but they probably play an important role in irritant reactions to hydrophobic molecules such as organic solvents in dissolving lipids and perturbing membrane fluidity. They may also be important in allergic reactions to very lipophilic haptens, such as the allergens of poison ivy (*Rhus radicans* L.) or poison oak (*Rhus diversiloba* T.). This could also be of importance for the interaction of haptens with the lipophilic domains of antigen presenting cells.

Dipolar interactions are weak electrostatic interactions between pre-existing or induced dipoles. Electron clouds do not always have a uniform density of charge, and zones of high and low electron density can interact. In addition, dipoles can form when molecules approach one another, the electron clouds deforming at the approach of another cloud, due to repulsion and attraction of charges, and electrons moving to the interior of the cloud, thus creating a dipole. Such interactions (induced dipoles) are also known as van der Waals forces, the amount of energy involved being 0.2–2 kJ/mol. Hydrogen bonds are examples of strong dipolar interactions. They occur between a hydrogen atom, linked to an electron-withdrawing atom, and an electron-rich atom with at least one electron doublet. The energy involved can then be up to 25 kJ/mol and such hydrogen bonds can form between two different molecules in an intermolecular way or within a molecule in an intramolecular way.

Finaly, *ionic bonds* are electrostatic interactions between pre-existing and generally localized charges on organic molecules or minerals. Such interactions occur, for example, between the charged amino acids in proteins and are therefore important in phenomena of recognition.

Core Message

> Hydrophobic, dipolar, and ionic bonds are weak interactions between atoms. They lead to reversible interactions but may play an important role in biological mechanisms and irritant contact dermatitis.

4.2.2 Strong Interactions

Strong interactions, mainly *covalent bonds*, are formed between two atoms by the sharing of a pair of electrons. These bonds are classically represented in chemical formulae by dashes. When an atom is not able to stabilize itself by a loss or gain of one or two electrons, it can do so by sharing electrons with other atoms, the shared electrons stabilizing both the partners. Carbon, for example, will form four covalent bonds with four other atoms by sharing its valence electrons in order to be surrounded by eight electrons (complete electron shell). This can be seen in the case of methane, one of the simplest carbon compounds with the composition CH_4, in which the carbon atom forms four covalent bonds with four hydrogen atoms. Covalent bonds involve energies of the order of 200–420 kJ/mol and are therefore very stable compared with the weak interactions.

$$Nu^{\ominus} + E^{\oplus} \longrightarrow Nu-E$$

Fig. 4.2 Principle of nucleophilic–electrophilic reaction

shared with another atom poor in electrons; in this case, it is referred to as a reaction between a nucleophile (from *nucleus* and *philos*, abreviated Nu) which is rich in electrons, and an electrophile (from *elektron* and *philos*, abbreviated E) which is poor in electrons (Fig. 4.2). These two terms, nucleophile and electrophile, represent the ability of a molecule, or rather an atom of this molecule, to donate or accept electrons to form a covalent bond. Nucleophilic centers are rich in electrons and therefore negatively charged or partially negatively charged, while electrophilic centers, deficient in electrons, are positively charged or partially positively charged. Nucleophilic atoms can react with electrophilic centers according to several mechanisms (Fig. 4.3).

Core Message

> ❯ Covalent bonds are strong interactions between atoms. They lead to nonreversible interactions and are therefore considered as the major form of protein modification by haptens.

4.2.3 Heterolytic or Nucleophilic–Electrophilic Reactions

The two electrons required for bond formation can be contributed by both the partners, in which case it is called a radical reaction, or can be provided by one of the atoms, which is especially rich in electrons, and

---

Core Message

> ❯ Nucleophiles (electron-rich atoms) can react with electrophiles (electron poor atoms) to form a stable covalent bond.

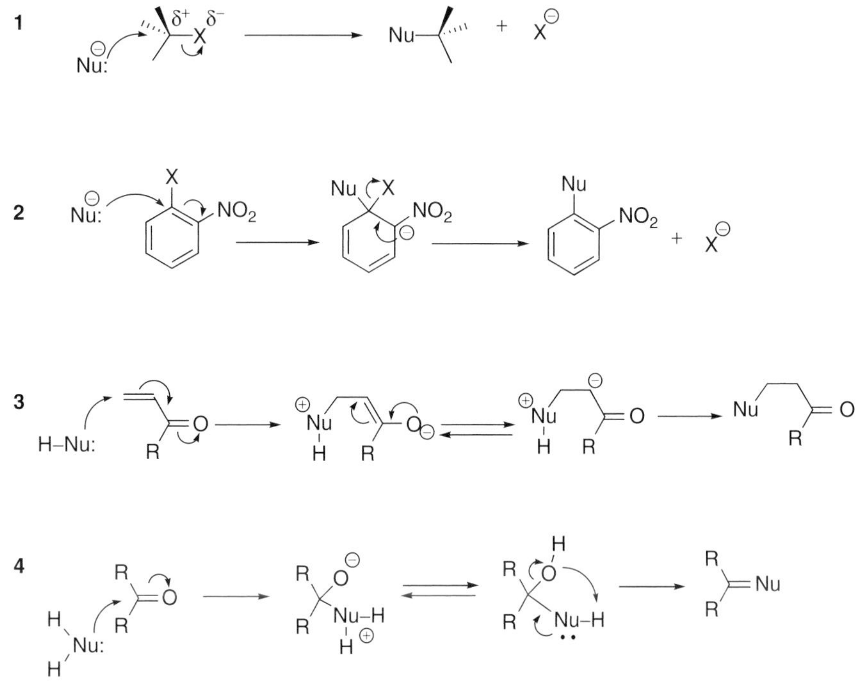

Fig. 4.3 Main nucleophilic reactions involved in allergic contact dermatitis. *1*: Nucleophilic substitution on a saturated center. *2*: Nucleophilic substitution on an unsaturated center. *3*: Michael type Nucleophilic addition. *4*: Nucleophilic addition on a carbonyl function

4

4.2.4 Homolytic or Radical Reactions

Homolytic or radical reactions arise from the homolytic cleavage of a covalent bond (Fig. 4.4). The symmetrical sharing of the common electron doublet in the covalence results in each of the two atoms retaining an electron. This leads to the formation of free radicals, which are uncharged atoms, or groups of atoms, containing an uneven number of electrons. Radical reactions are mainly the reactions of molecules with weakly polar or nonpolar bonds (hydrocarbons), and they require a radical inducer, such as ultraviolet radiation (hv) or atmospheric oxygen. The stability of radicals is relative, as they are unstable species and therefore highly reactive. For this reason, radical reactions often occur as chain reactions. Again, radicals can react through different mechanisms to form covalent bonds (Fig. 4.5).

Core Message

> Radicals can combine to form stable covalent bonds.

4.2.5 Coordination Bonds

Another type of relatively strong bond, comparable to covalent bonds, is formed between metals or metal salts and electron-rich atoms (mainly hetero-atoms, such as

$$A^{\bullet} + B^{\bullet} \longrightarrow A{-}B$$

Fig. 4.4 Principle of radical reaction

nitrogen, oxygen, sulfur, and phosphorus). These interactions, known as *coordination bonds*, permit these electron-rich groups or "ligands" to transfer part of their electron density to the positively charged metal in order to increase its stability. Coordination bonds are characterized by the number of ligands and the geometry of the complex thus formed, which is specific both for the metal and its oxidation state. The most common geometries for coordination bonds are tetrahedal and square planar when four ligands are involved, trigonal bipyramidal for five ligands, and octahedral for six ligands surrounding the metal. It is not unusual for a metal at the same oxidation level or a metal at two different oxidation levels to form complexes of different geometries. For example, cobalt II (Co^{++}) is characterized by a tetrahedral arrangement while nickel II (Ni^{++}) mainly forms square planar tetra-coordinated arrangements (Fig. 4.6). The number of ligands and the geometry of these coordination complexes determine whether the metals are allergenic and controls cross-reactions.

Core Message

> Coordination bonds are strong interactions between metals and ligands. Coordination bonds are characterized by the number of ligands and the geometry of the complex thus formed, which are specific both for the metal and its oxidation state.

4.3 Chemical Aspects of Allergic Contact Dermatitis

The skin sensitization reaction to a chemical is a multistep process with two principal stages:

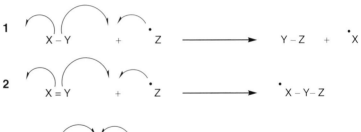

Fig. 4.5 Main radical reaction mechanisms. *1*: Substitution mechanism. *2*: Addition mechanism. *3*: Termination mechanism

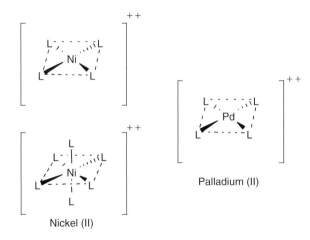

Fig. 4.6 Example of coordination bonds to metal salts

1. A state of sensitization to a chemical is induced. This may be on first exposure to the chemical or only after many exposures.
2. A sensitization response is elicited. This happens when a subject sensitive to a given chemical is exposed to, or challenged with, the same or a related chemical.

Chemical reactions and/or interactions are involved throughout these biological processes which will result in the patient developing delayed hypersensitivity, whether it be during the crossing of the cutaneous barrier (mainly controlled by the physicochemical properties of the allergen), during the formation of the hapten–protein complex (in which chemical bonds are involved) or during the phenomenon of recognition between the antigen and the T-cell receptors (TcR).

For the present purpose, a relatively simple description of the biological mechanism of skin sensitization is sufficient.

At induction, the chemical penetrates or is introduced into the epidermis, beneath the *stratum corneum*. There it binds to the protein, thus modifying the protein's structure. The modified protein is processed and presented, in a form that can be recognized as antigenic, to uncommitted T-cells. Those T-cells whose receptors match the modified protein are stimulated to multiply, producing expanded clones of circulating T-cells capable of recognizing the modified protein. The subject is now sensitized.

At elicitation or challenge, on subsequent exposure to the same chemical, or a cross-reactive chemical, the same, or a similar, protein modification is produced,

and the modified protein is recognized by the circulating T-cells which resulted from the induction stage. As a result, a chain of biochemical events is initiated, leading to the symptoms of allergic contact dermatitis.

In general, the induction of sensitization is partly, but not completely, specific to the compound applied at induction. For example, in a classic study carried out in the 1960s on alkyl catechols with a variety of R chain lengths, Baer et al. [1] found that the magnitude of cross-challenge responses decreased as the difference in R chain length between the two compounds increased. Cross-reactivity is highly relevant to human sensitization – for example, North Americans who have been sensitized by poison ivy, which grows only on the East coast, react strongly to poison oak which grows only on the West coast [2] and contains similar haptens. Typically, humans can become sensitive to industrial chemicals in the workplace, naturally occurring chemicals in the garden and in the countryside, and to chemical components of domestic products.

It follows from the above description of the biological mechanism that, for a chemical to be a sensitizer, it must have the ability to bind to protein so that a nonself antigen can be produced. The evidence indicates that normally this binding occurs by covalent bond formation, and one of the earliest structure-activity studies in skin sensitization was reported by Landsteiner and Jacobs in the 1930s [3]. Although the biological mechanism of sensitization was not at that time understood in any detail, they had already come to the view that sensitization to chemicals involved covalent binding [4] to proteins.

> **Core Message**
>
> › For a chemical to be a sensitizer, it must have the ability to first penetrate the skin and second to bind to epidermal proteins.

4.3.1 Reactive Amino Acids

In proteins, the side-chain of several amino acids contains electron-rich or nucleophilic groups capable of reacting with haptens (Fig. 4.7). Lysine and cysteine are those that are most often cited, but other amino

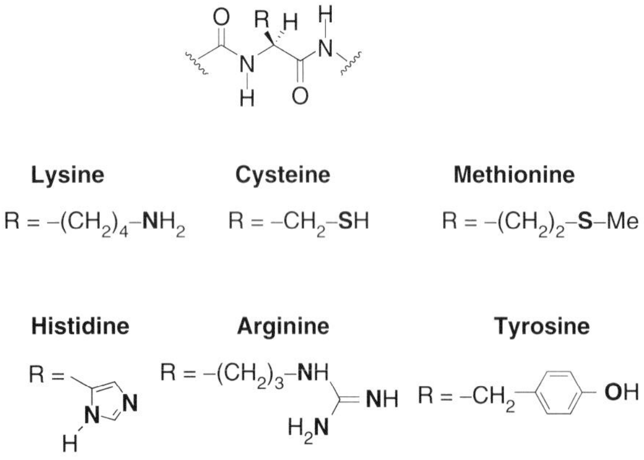

Fig. 4.7 Main nucleophilic residues on amino acids – reactive atoms are in *bold*

acids containing nucleophilic hetero-atoms, for example, histidine, methionine, tyrosine, and arginine, have been shown to react with electrophiles. Studies performed in the last few years on the mechanisms involved in the modification of proteins by small xenobiotic molecules have made it possible to demonstrate the involvement of a wide variety of mechanisms, depending on the structure of the hapten.

Core Message

> › Several amino acids lateral chains contain nucleophilic groups that are able to react with haptens.

4.3.2 Reactivity of Haptens

One direct consequence of this diversity is the existence of selectivity in the modification of amino acids (Table 4.1). Thus, it has been shown that methyl alkanesulfonates, lipophilic methylating agents, and strong allergens, modify almost exclusively histidine and methionine residues in proteins [5], while the α-methylene-γ-butyrolactones, the main allergens in plants of the Asteraceae (Compositae) family, mainly modify lysine residues [6]. Similarly, alk-2-ene-γ-sultones have been shown, in several animal models, to be particularly strong skin sensitizers [7, 8], exhibiting sensitization potential down to the

levels of approximately 1 ppm. Attention was focused on these chemicals in the mid-1970s, when the cause of a 1968 outbreak of contact dermatitis in Scandinavia was traced to 2-chloro-γ-sultones and α,β-unsaturated-γ-sultones, formed as contaminants in a batch of ether sulfate used to formulate dishwashing liquids [9]. Recent studies have shown that these molecules are highly oxophilic and are reactive mainly with tyrosine at physiological pH [10]. However, the sensitizing potential appeared to be associated with the ability to modify some lysine residues [11]. The suspected role of lysine residues was further confirmed with reactivity studies carried out on MCI and MI, the main components of Kathon CG, a well-known preservative. While both the molecules were very reactive toward cysteins [12], the strong sensitizer MCI was also shown to react with lysine and histidine residues in proteins [13, 14].

Such studies have also been applied to coordination bonds and it has been shown by nuclear magnetic resonance (NMR) that nickel sulfate interacted with histidine residues of peptides bound to MHC molecule [15].

In recent years, the radical mechanism has gained increasing interest in the discussion of the mechanism of hapten–protein binding [16]. This mechanism, which has never been firmly established, has been postulated to explain, for example, the allergenic potential of eugenol vs. isoeugenol [17]. More recently, studies indicating that radical reactions were important for haptens containing allylic hydroperoxide groups (Fig. 4.8) have been published [18–20].

Core Message

> › Each haptens has its own chemical reactivity pattern toward nucleophilic amino acids. This reactivity pattern depends on the electron density at the reactive site.

4.3.3 Mechanisms of Reactions

The selectivity of haptens for some amino acids is directly related to the electron density at the reaction site (determined by the structure of the molecule) and

Table 4.1 Examples of main adducts formed between some haptens and human serum albumin

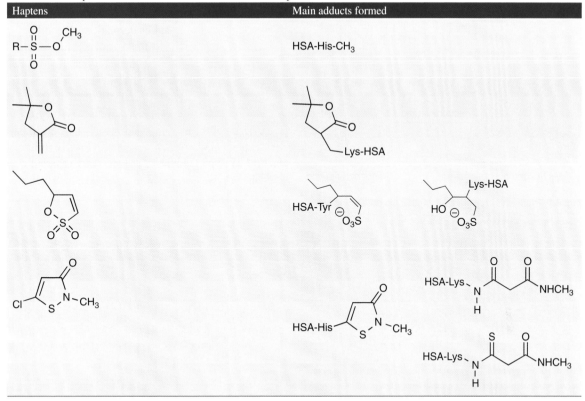

Haptens	Main adducts formed

the type of chemical reaction that takes place. The chemical reactions can be divided into several groups on the basis of their characteristics and the mechanisms involved in the breaking and forming of bonds. Thus, molecules with very similar structures can give rise to the formation of different intermediates, for example,

Fig. 4.8 Example of radical formation from allylic hydroperoxides. *Arrows* indicate major reactive sites

during metabolization, which lead to different reaction mechanisms. The case of eugenol and isoeugenol is very relevant in this respect.

These two molecules, present in many natural extracts, have very similar structures, but their sensitizing potentials are very different, eugenol being a weak, and isoeugenol a relatively strong, sensitizer. Studies in the mouse seem to indicate that these two very similar molecules are metabolized in different ways and so have different reaction mechanisms [21], which could explain the observed differences in sensitization potential. Eugenol (Fig. 4.9) could be metabolized to an electrophilic orthoquinone after a demethylation step, whereas isoeugenol (Fig. 4.10) could be directly oxidized to a quinonemethide.

Core Message

> Even similar haptens can react with proteins through different chemical mechanisms and with different amino acids.

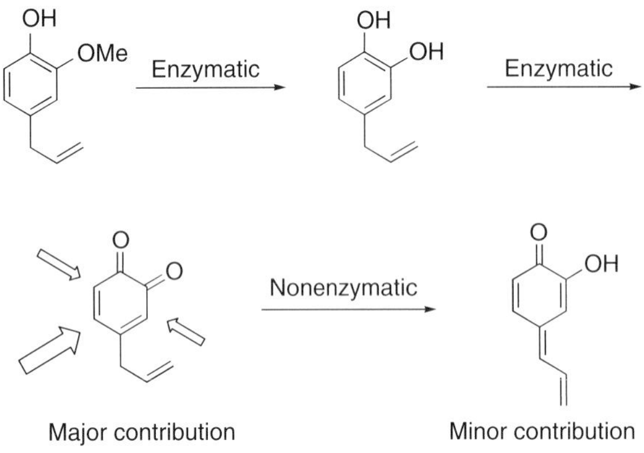

Fig. 4.9 Proposed mechanism to explain the sensitizing potential of eugenol in mice. *Arrows* indicate major reactive sites

Major contribution   Minor contribution

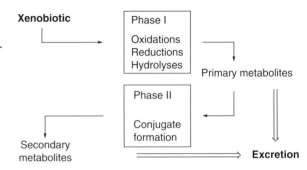

Fig. 4.11 Principles of primary and secondary metabolization of xenobiotics

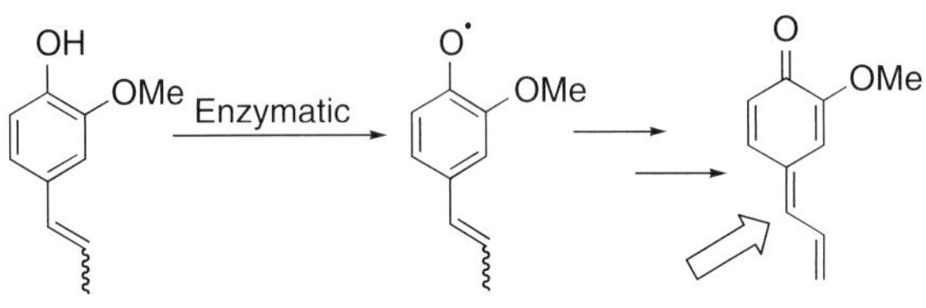

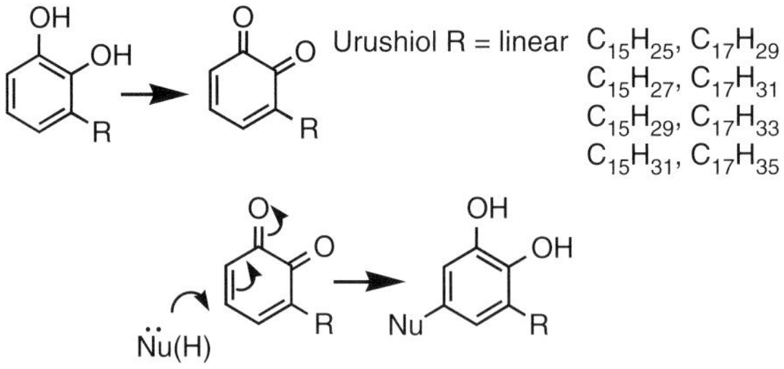

Fig. 4.10 Proposed mechanism to explain the sensitizing potential of isoeugenol in mice. *Arrows* indicate major reactive sites

Urushiol R = linear $C_{15}H_{25}$, $C_{17}H_{29}$
$C_{15}H_{27}$, $C_{17}H_{31}$
$C_{15}H_{29}$, $C_{17}H_{33}$
$C_{15}H_{31}$, $C_{17}H_{35}$

Fig. 4.12 Nucleophilic addition on the orthoquinones derived from urushiol

4.4 Modifications of Molecules

4.4.1 Enzymatic Processes: Prohaptens

Far from being an inert tissue, the skin is the site of many metabolic processes, which can result in structural modification of xenobiotics which penetrate into it (Fig. 4.11). These metabolic processes, primarily intended for the elimination of foreign molecules during detoxification, can, in certain cases, convert harmless molecules into derivatives with electrophilic, and therefore allergenic, properties. The metabolic processes are mainly based on oxido-reduction reactions via extremely powerful enzymatic hydroxylation systems, such as the cytochrome P450 enzymes [22] or flavine monooxygenase, but monoamine oxidases, which convert amines to aldehydes, and peroxidases seem to play an important role in the metabolism of haptens. When activated by the production of hydrogen peroxide during the oxidative stress following the introduction of a xenobiotic into

the skin, peroxidases convert electron-rich aromatic derivatives (aminated or hydroxylated) into quinones, which are powerful electrophiles. In this way, long-chain catechols, responsible for the severe allergies to poison ivy (*Rhus radicans* L.) and poison oak (*Rhus diversiloba* T.), are oxidized *in vivo* to highly-reactive orthoquinones (Fig. 4.12) [23], though we cannot exclude a radical participation. The same applies to para-phenylenediamine or hydroquinone derivatives, for example, the allergens from *Phacelia crenulata* Torr [24], which are converted into electrophilic paraquinones (Fig. 4.13). Metabolic reactions involving enzymatic hydrolyses can also occur in the skin. Thus tuliposides A and B, found in the bulb of the tulip (*Tulipa gesneriana* L.), are hydrolysed, releasing the actual allergens, tulipalins A and B [25].

All these molecules, which do not by themselves have electrophilic properties and therefore cannot be haptens but can be metabolized to haptens, are referred to as *prohaptens* [26, 27], and they play an important role in contact allergy because of their number and highly-reactive nature. The fact that the structure of the

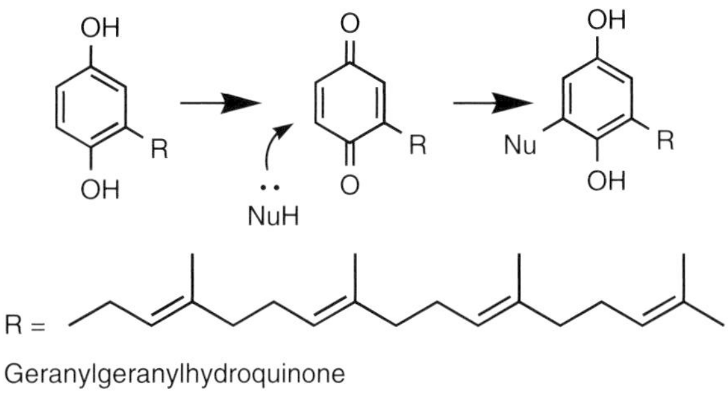

R = [structure]

Geranylgeranylhydroquinone

Fig. 4.13 Nucleophilic addition on the para-quinone derived from geranylgeranylhydroquinone

metabolized molecule can be far removed from the structure of the initial molecule can make allergologic investigations even more difficult.

Core Message

> During metabolism and detoxification steps some nonsensitizing molecules can be transformed into reactive haptens. We will refer to these molecules as prohaptens.

Δ^3-carene
Pinus palustris Mill.

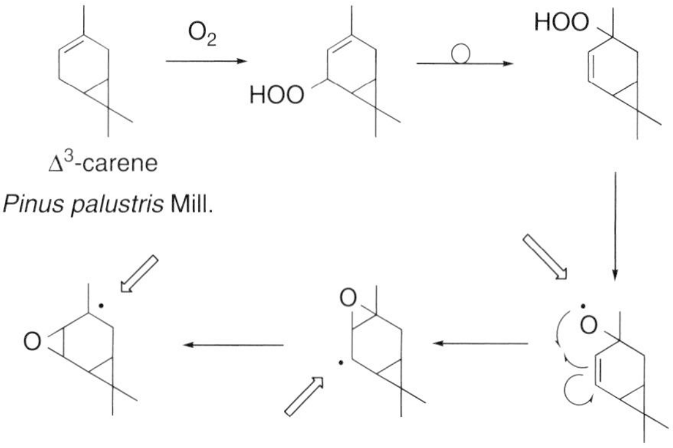

Fig. 4.14 Autoxidation of Δ^3-carene to form hydroperoxides and subsequent formation of potentially reactive radicals

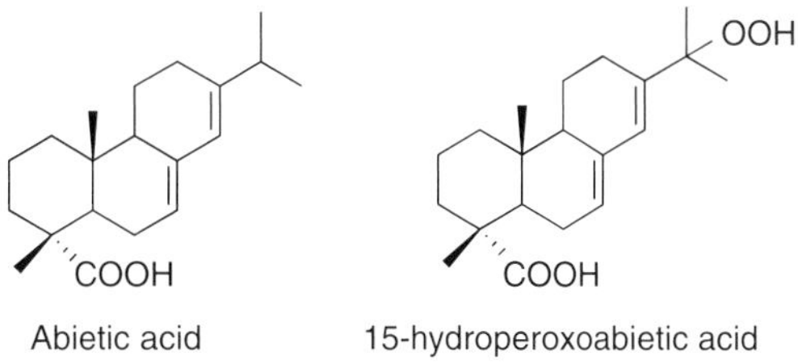

Abietic acid   15-hydroperoxoabietic acid

Fig. 4.15 Structure of abietic acid and of 15-hydroperoxoabietic acid

4.4.2 Nonenzymatic Processes: Prehaptens

Nonenzymatic processes, such as reaction with atmospheric oxygen or ultraviolet irradiation, can also induce changes in the chemical structure of molecules. Many terpenes autoxidize at air exposure, producing sensitizing derivatives. In the 50s, it was found that the allergenic activity of turpentine was mainly due to hydroperoxides of one of the monoterpene, Δ^3-carene (Fig. 4.14) [28]. This is also the case for abietic acid, the main constituent of colophony, which is converted into highly-reactive hydroperoxide (Fig. 4.15) [29] by contact with air. Such an autoxidation mechanism has also been demonstrated for another monoterpene, *d*-limonene, found in citrus fruits. *d*-Limonene itself is not allergenic, but on air exposure, hydroperoxides, epoxides, and ketones are formed which are strong allergens [30].

Core Message

> Haptens, as any molecule, are sensitive to heat, light, and oxygen. Some nonsensitizing molecules can be transformed into sensitizers by chemical modification during storage and handling. By extension, these molecules are often considered as prohaptens, but should rather be considered as prehaptens as no enzymatic process is involved.

4.5 Haptens and Cross-Allergies

The factors which control molecular recognition during the elicitation stage are primarily the nature of the chemical group and the compatibility of the spatial geometry. Although the identity of the chemical group

4

is very important and serves to define what are commonly called group allergies, it cannot account for all structure-activity relationships. Receptor molecules are highly sensitive to volume and shape, and molecules must have a similar size and spatial geometry to be recognized by the same receptor. Thus, even though the molecules tulipalin A or B and alantolactone (the allergen of *Inula helenium* L.) bear the same chemical group, α-methylene-γ-butyrolactone, they cannot give rise to cross-allergic reactions, as their spatial volumes are too different. In contrast, isoalantolactone and alantolactone produce a cross-allergic reaction [31], since they share both a *homologous chemical group and spatial volume* (Fig. 4.16). The term cross-allergy is often misused and should be restricted to the well-defined cases that can be called true cross-allergies [32, 33].

True cross-allergy between a sensitizer A and a triggering agent B can be interpreted in various ways:

- A and B are chemically and structurally similar.
- A is metabolized to a compound that is similar to B.
- B is metabolized to a compound that is similar to A.
- A and B are both metabolized to similar compounds.

The identification of cross-allergic responses can be especially difficult, particularly in man, in whom the possibility of co- or polysensitization should never be ruled out. In addition, the metabolism of

molecules can be very complex and two molecules with *a priori* little in common can be converted to derivatives that have a similar structure. Thus, the derivatives of hydroquinones and para-phenylenediamines can be converted into benzoquinone derivatives. It is therefore dangerous to draw conclusions from tests without knowing how the substances used are liable to be metabolized. Many reactions described as demonstrating cross-allergy are, without doubt, due to cosensitization. Experimental studies in animals are often the only means of being really certain of what happens during recognition. The concept of the prohapten is very important in the interpretation of results in allergy. As the structure of the metabolized molecule can sometimes be very different from that of the initial molecule, it can be difficult to establish similarities between chemical groups and structures.

> **Core Message**
>
> › Two molecules of different structure but similar in chemical reactivity and molecular shape can activate the same T-cell receptors. This is the base of the so-called cross-reaction phenomenon. A "group sensitization" refers to a series of similar molecules often giving cross-reactions in patients. It is not always easy to distinguish cross-reactions from concomitant sensitization.

4.6 Some Applications of the Chemical Knowledge

4.6.1 Understanding Cross-Reactions Among Corticosteroids

In the last few years, molecular modeling has been shown to be a powerful tool in the studies of conformational-dependent drug–receptor interactions and structure-activity relationship analysis [34]. Despite the great potential of this technique, few attempts to analyze crossreaction patterns in the field of allergic contact dermatitis have yet been reported. One reason

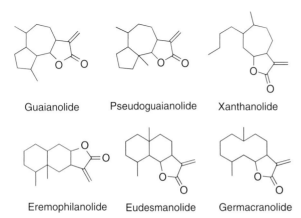

Guaianolide   Pseudoguaianolide   Xanthanolide

Eremophilanolide   Eudesmanolide   Germacranolide

Fig. 4.16 Main structures of sesquiterpene lactones

may be the heterogeneous population of patients with heterogeneous clinical histories, in which it is somewhat difficult to distinguish between actual cross-reaction and concomitant sensitization. A second reason is that, to be effective, structure-activity relationship studies need data for a wide range of molecules. The clinical investigation of contact dermatitis from corticosteroids, in which a large number of related substances are tested on a large number of patients, represents a good opportunity to carry out

such a structure-activity study. From the statistical analysis of the clinical data, it is now possible to advance an experimentally-supported hypothesis for cross-reaction patterns. Coopman et al. [35] hypothesized that cross-reactions occur primarily within certain groups of corticosteroids. They distinguished four groups, group A (Fig. 4.17) consisting of hydrocortisone, tixocortol pivalate, and related compounds, group B consisting of triamcinolone acetonide, amcinonide, and related compounds, group C (Fig. 4.18)

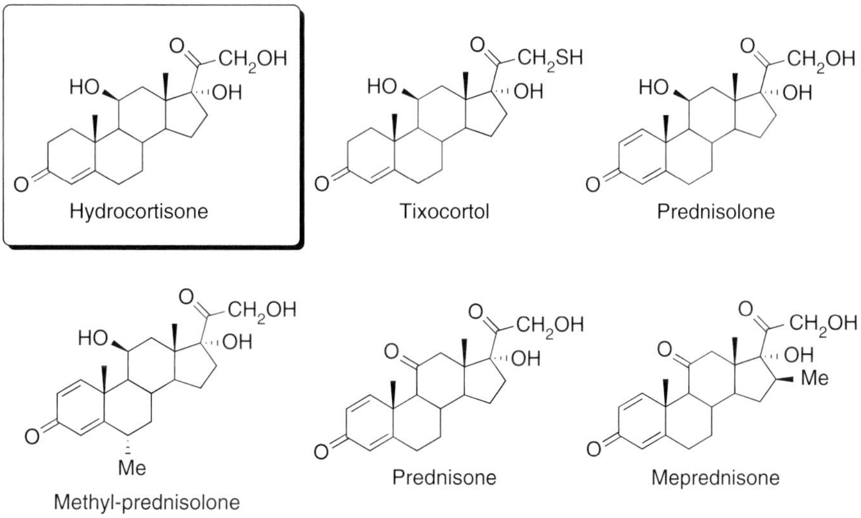

Fig. 4.17 Chemical structure of main group A corticosteroids

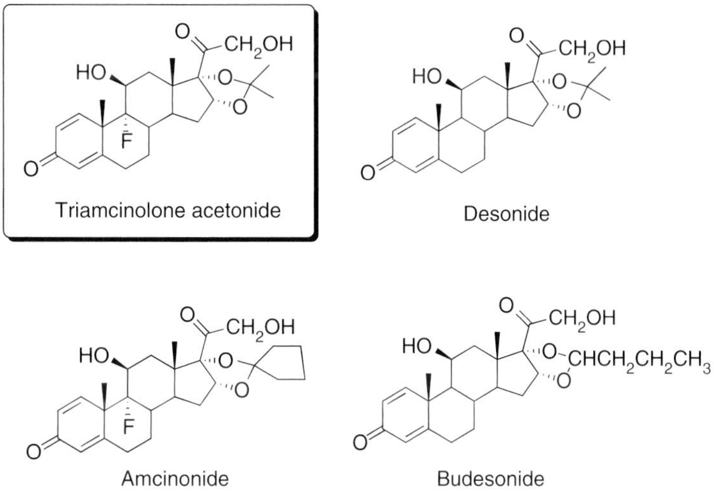

Fig. 4.18 Chemical structure of main group B corticosteroids

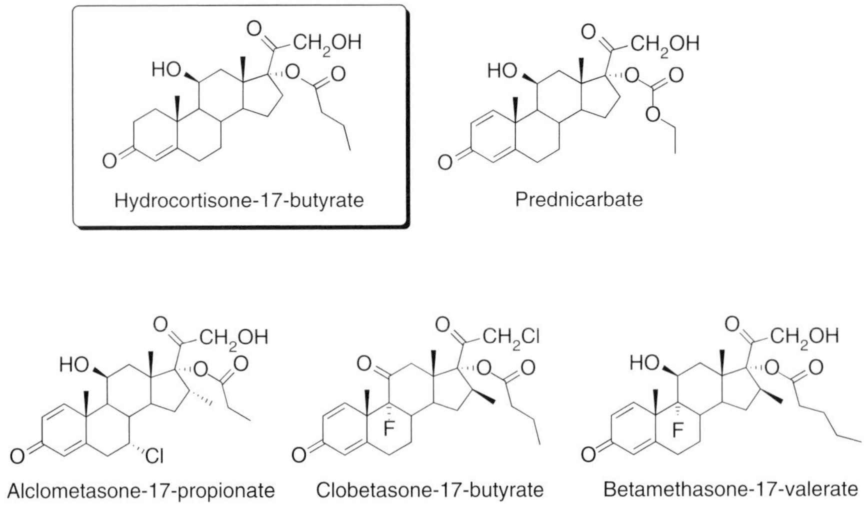

Fig. 4.19 Chemical structure of main group D corticosteroids

Hydrocortisone-17-butyrate

Prednicarbate

Alclometasone-17-propionate   Clobetasone-17-butyrate   Betamethasone-17-valerate

consisting of betamethasone, dexamethasone, and related compounds and group D (Fig. 4.19) consisting of esters such as hydrocortisone-17-butyrate and clobetasone-17-butyrate. It is now possible to correlate this with conformational characteristics and to establish a molecular basis for cross-reaction patterns in patients sensitized to corticosteroids. This could be invaluable in the prediction of potential cross-reactions to new molecules.

The conformation of corticosteroids from groups A, B, C, and D were analyzed [36]. This study was based on two hypotheses. The first was that all corticosteroids should interact with proteins in a very similar way. All corticosteroid molecules were designed to interact with the same type of receptors, and thus should be more or less metabolized in similar ways. The second hypothesis, based on chemical observations, was that esters at position 21 are readily hydrolyzed to give the free alcohol, while esters at position 17 are more resistant to hydrolysis, due to strong steric hindrance. Thus, for example, tixocortol pivalate was considered as tixocortol with a free thiol group at position 21, and alclometasone-17, 21-dipropionate was considered as alclometasone-17-propionate.

All molecules were drawn from energy-minimized building blocks and were then submitted to a multiconformational analysis in order to achieve the most energetically stable conformation. These conformations were then compared for analogies or differences in the van der Waals volumes that define the electronic shape of the molecule. As expected from the hypothesis, significant group-specific characteristics of volume and shape were found for molecules of group A, B, and D, but not for molecules of group C.

Molecular characteristics: the existence of groups A, B, and D, as defined by the analysis of cross-reaction patterns in patients sensitized to corticosteroids, is fully supported by the conformational analysis of these molecules. Molecules of the same group have very similar spatial structures, explaining the cross-reactions observed. In addition, molecules from one group are sufficiently different from molecules of another group to explain the lack of cross-reactions observed between groups A, B, and D.

The volume occupied by specific groups on the α face of ring D seems to be critical for the molecular recognition of corticosteroids by receptors of immunocompetent cells, while modifications of other parts of the molecule seem to have little effect on the recognition patterns. Each group represents a well-defined, characteristic shape (Fig. 4.20) that can be very useful for the prediction of potential cross-reactions of new corticosteroid molecules.

Fig. 4.20 General electronic shape of hydrocortisone (group A), triamcinolone acetonide (group B), and hydrocotisone-17-butyrate (group D)

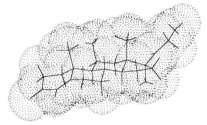

Hydrocortisone

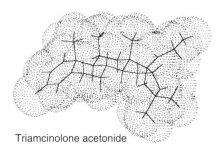

Triamcinolone acetonide

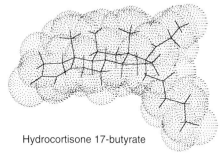

Hydrocortisone 17-butyrate

Core Message

> Four main structural groups have been identified for the cross-reactivity pattern of corticosteroids. These groups correspond to the presence of specific chemical functions on the α face of the D ring and can explain the lack of cross reactivity between molecules of the different groups.

4.6.2 Development of Quantitative Structure-Activity Relationships (QSARs)

4.6.2.1 Introduction

The main objective of the QSAR approach is to define "quantifiers" for a given biological reaction, then combine these to give a quantitative estimate of the biological activity; it therefore no longer simply answers the question whether the molecule is potentially sensitizing, but also gives a quite accurate indication of the expected intensity of the biological response. Several approaches have been reported in the literature mainly based on reactivity and lipophilicity parameters. Thus, Roberts and Williams [37] established QSARs using the relative alkylation index mathematical model.

This quantifier gives an estimate of the level of protein modifications by a potentially sensitizing molecule and assumes that the intensity of the biological response is directly related to the level of modification. This is a simple hypothesis taking into account three parameters, the dose of the product applied to the skin, its lipophilicity, and its chemical reactivity. These parameters were chosen because it has been known experimentally for a long time that the sensitizing response increases with an increase in each of these parameters.

It is thus possible to express the relative level of protein modification by the equation:

$$RAI = a\log k + b\log P + c\log D,$$

where a, b, and c represent the relative weight of each parameter. Presently, these constants are determined experimentally and are valid only for a series of molecules with the same reaction mechanism and it is for this reason that the RAI is defined as a relative index of alkylation.

This model has been used to evaluate data of various sets of skin sensitizing chemicals [38–41].

A complementary approach is to search for empirical quantitative SARs by application of statistical methods to sets of biological data and structural descriptors.

The development of the local lymph node assay (LLNA) has facilitated the use of QSARs to predict the skin sensitization potential of chemicals because it provides well-defined end points. The LLNA is described in detail in the literature [42, 43] and a given chemical is tested over a range of concentrations such that a dose–response relationship can be determined, from which the sensitizing potential is defined in terms of the concentration required to give a specified stimulation index value. Currently, the preference is to estimate the concentration of a chemical required to generate an SI of 3, the EC3 value [43].

4.6.2.2 Example of Fragrance Aldehydes

As part as an EU funded project on fragrance allergy, QSARs have been developed for sensitizing aldehydes. Aldehydes are molecules widely used by the fragrance industry because of their floral odor, but it has been known for many years that these molecules could be associated with skin sensitizations. From a chemical point, aldehydes can be classified into two main categories with respect to their reaction mechanisms toward amino groups on proteins. So-called saturated aldehydes are suspected to react with lysine residues through the formation of a Schiff's base, while unsaturated aldehydes, with a carbonyl function conjugated with one or more double bonds, are suspected to react with lysine through a Michael addition. From 71 aldehydes, a cluster analysis was used to select subsets of 10 materials from the 2 classes of Schiff base (aliphatic) and Michael addition (α,β-unsaturated) aldehydes. LLNA tests were conducted using a 4:1 acetone:olive oil vehicle to generate dose–response data for the aldehydes in order to determine EC_3 values. The negative logarithm of this molar EC_3, $\log (1/EC_3)$, was used as a quantitative measure of sensitizing potential and it was investigated how the sensitization potential varied with the chemical reactivity and lipophilicity. Chemical reactivity was modeled using Taft σ^* values. The Taft σ^* constant for a substituent R is a measure of the inductive effect of R. The σ^* values used were taken from the extensive compilation by Perrin

et al. [44]. Lipophilicity was modeled by LogP values, computed using CLogP.

A QSAR was developed for each of the Michael addition aldehydes and Schiff base aldehydes [45].

- Michael addition aldehydes:

$$\log (1/EC_3) = 0.54 + 0.17\text{LogP} + 0.49\text{R } \sigma^* + 1.31\text{R'}\sigma^*$$

$$N = 9 \; R^2 = 0.741 \; s = 0.184 \; \text{F Ratio} = 4.77$$

- Schiff's base aldehydes:

$$\log(1/EC_3) = 0.25 + 0.28\text{LogP} + 0.86 \text{ R } \sigma^*$$

$$N = 12 \; R^2 = 0.825 \; s = 0.172 \; \text{F Ratio} = 21.2592$$

These QSAR's illustrate (Fig. 4.21) that only molecules reacting through a similar mechanism, that is, Schiff's base formation or Michael addition can be correlated. Despite this restriction, a good correlation was found, and these QSARs were further validated with a new set of molecules for which a good quantitative prediction was found.

Core Message

> Quantitative Structure Activity Relationships (QSARs) based on reactivity factors and lipophilicity allow the prediction of the sensitizing potential of aldehydes.

4.6.2.3 Predictive Tests Based on Hapten Reactivity

Introduction

One of the major objectives at the end of this century is the development of "alternative" tests for the evaluation of the pharmacological and/or toxicological activity of newly developed molecules. Contact allergy is no exception to the rule and many research programs have been started to develop in vitro techniques for the detection of allergizing compounds [46]. To date, despite the considerable effort expended in the last few years, the complex character of the biological mechanism of allergy has prevented the development of a reliable test. Various promising routes are currently

Fig. 4.21 QSARs for two series of aldehydes (saturated and unsaturated)

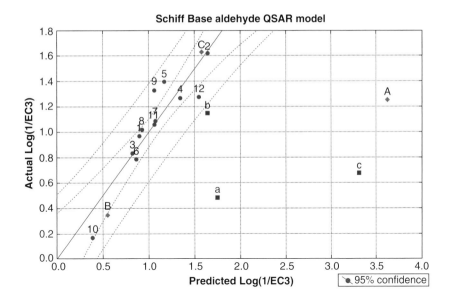

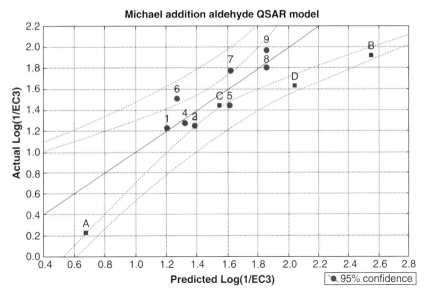

being explored, but are not expected to yield a result for several years.

In parallel with these biological studies, another approach could be based on the quantification of the chemical reactivity of haptens toward nucleophiles such as amino acids, peptides, or proteins. This approach is based on the observation already reported by Landsteiner in the 30s that a correlation exists between the chemical reactivity of a molecule and its sensitizing potential.

The Direct Peptide Reactivity Assay (DPRA)

Since reactivity is a key step in the induction of skin sensitization, it was hypothesized that reactivity could be used to screen the sensitization potential of chemicals. Therefore, a chemical-based peptide assay was developed and chemicals representing allergens of different potencies (weak to extreme) along with nonsensitizers were evaluated to determine if reactivity could be used as a potential skin sensitization screening tool [47].

4

All materials used have been evaluated in the LLNA and each assigned a skin sensitization potency category: extreme, strong, moderate, and weak. These molecules were reacted with glutathion (GSH) and two synthetic peptides containing a cystein or a lysine, respectively, as reactive function. The depletion in peptides was measured after 24 h and used as a quantifier to assess the reactivity of the molecules. These data demonstrates that a significant correlation exists between a chemical's skin sensitization potency and its ability to react with peptides containing nucleophilic amino acids such as cysteine and lysine (Fig. 4.22). Based on these results, a classification tree that allows to classify test molecules according to their chemical reactivity toward the cysteine peptide and the lysine peptide has been developed [48]. The DPRA is currently at the validation stage.

Core Message

> ❭ A significant correlation exists between a chemical's skin sensitization potency and its ability to react with peptides containing nucleophilic amino acids such as cysteine and lysine.

4.7 Molecular Aspects in Irritant Contact Dermatitis

4.7.1 Introduction

As already mentioned, a difference is very often made between immunological and nonimmunological skin reactions. In fact, this should mainly refer to the selection and activation of specific T-cells and not to the participation of actors of the immune system. Indeed, chemicals leading to irritant contact dermatitis will interact and activate the cells of the immune system leading to the release of cytokines. Molecular mechanisms associated with irritant contact dermatitis are more difficult to investigate and demonstrate as they are very often based on reversible interactions with biological systems. However, one can mention acido-basic, surfactant, and alkylating properties.

4.7.2 Acido-Basic Properties

Alkaline or acid compounds can induce irritant contact dermatitis. These reactions can be very severe in case of highly alkaline or acid properties and be associated with chemical burns. These reactions can develop very rapidly and are associated with cell and tissue necrosis. Most of the biological systems are based on molecules sensitive to pH, and intense variation of this parameter can lead to protein and DNA hydrolysis reactions and then a loss of functionality.

4.7.3 Surfactants

Cell membranes are mainly constituted of phospholipids associated by non covalent low energy interactions. This is also the case with the *stratum corneum* that contains a high proportion of organized lipids. As already mentioned, these low energy chemical interactions can be easily disturbed by molecules that either increase or decrease membrane fluidity. These properties are very well known for detergents used in biochemistry for membrane disruption. Surfactants are based on a lipophilic part associated with a hydrophilic end. Historically, soaps were obtained by alkaline hydrolysis of animal fat to form a carboxylate hydrophilic head associated with lipophilic chains. Since then, many surfactants with cationic or anionic hydrophilic heads have been developed. More recently, nonionic surfactants, supposed to be less irritating, have been marketed. These surfactants are based on hydrophilic heads (aminoacids, glycosides, etc.) associated with a lipophilic tail. Perturbation of the *stratum corneum* by surfactants can be, for example, monitored by the measure of transepidermal water loss (TEWL) [49].

4.7.4 Alkylating Agents

Electrophilic molecules or haptens, able to react with nucleophilic residues on biomolecules, will have toxic effects. As already mentioned, one of these toxic effects is cutaneous allergy resulting in modifications of epidermal proteins. However, proteins are not the only targets

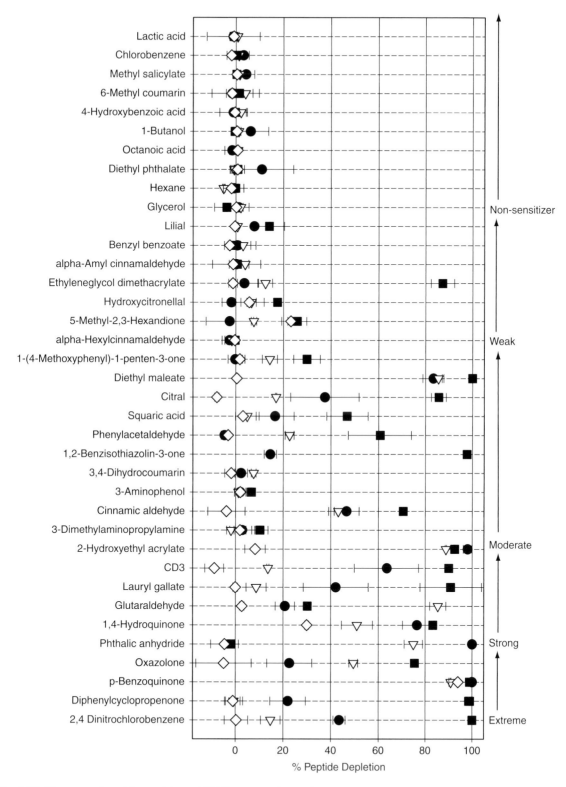

Fig. 4.22 Histogram of peptide reactivity and LLNA potency (from ref. [47])

and many other systems can be modified. Recently, mechanisms by which cells can perceive danger associated with a chemical reactivity have attracted much attention. It is now well accepted that chemical insults exert their biological effects by perturbation of cellular redox homeostasis, a condition defined as oxidative stress. The capacity of the cells to maintain homeostasis during oxidative stress resides in activation or induction of protective enzymes. Nuclear-factor-E2-related factor (Nrf-2) as a member of basic leucine zipper (bZIP) transcription factors is expressed in a variety of tissues. Transcriptional activation of antioxidant genes through an antioxidant response element (ARE) is largely dependent upon Nrf2. The genes that contain a functional ARE include those encoding heme oxygenase *(hmox)*, glutathione-*S*-transferase (*GST*), and NAD(P)H:quinone reductase *(nqo-1)* that play a role in the defense against oxidative stress [50]. Nrf-2-dependent antioxidant response can thus be considered as a cell survival signal conferring cellular protection against various insults. When dendritic cells (DC) are exposed to chemical sensitizers, a number of redox-sensitive pathways including several mitogen-activated protein kinases (MAPK) cascades are activated and are mandatory for DC maturation to occur suggesting that protection systems failed. Chemical sensitizers were also able to induce the accumulation of the Nrf-2 proteins in treated cells suggesting a specific activation of this pathway by chemical sensitizers in DCs and myeloid cell lines. Natsch et al. have also shown recently, using a large number of chemicals and a luciferase reporter system, that contact sensitizers activated the Nrf-2 pathway [51].

Core Message

> Any chemical is irritating to some extent. This can be due to a direct interaction with biological structures (DNA/protein hydrolysis, cell membrane disruption, etc.) or by the activation of dendritic cells (danger signal).

4.8 Conclusion

Although many questions are still unanswered or partly answered, the present state of understanding has proven useful in a variety of situations, for example,

in deciding whether a positive sensitization result is due to the allergenic properties of the compound under consideration or more likely due to an allergic impurity.

Current knowledge, in our experience, has led to successful predictions much more often than not. Occasionally, predictions have turned out to be incorrect: most of these cases have led to refinements in our understanding.

Ongoing research into structure-skin sensitization relationships is aimed at clarifying some of the major areas where our understanding is still insufficient to be useful for predictive purposes, in particular proelectrophile and radical mechanisms.

References

1. Baer H, Watkins RC, Kurtz AP, Byck JS, Dawson CR (1967) Delayed contact sensitivity to catechols. J Immunol 99: 307–375
2. Corbett MD, Billets S (1975) Characterization of poison oak urushiol. J Pharm Sci 64:1715
3. Landsteiner K, Jacobs J (1936) Studies on the sensitization of animals with simple chemical compounds. J Exp Med 64:625–639
4. Lepoittevin JP, Berl V (1997) Chemical basis. In: Lepoittevin JP, Basketter DA, Goossens A, Karlberg AT (eds) Allergic contact dermatitis: the molecular basis. Springer, Berlin, pp 19–42
5. Lepoittevin J-P, Benezra C (1992) ^{13}C-Enriched methylalkanesulfonates: new lipophilic methylating agents for the identification of nucleophilic amino acids of protein by NMR. Tetrahedron Lett 33:3875–3878
6. Franot C, Benezra C, Lepoittevin J-P (1993) Synthesis and interaction studies of ^{13}C labeled lactone derivatives with a model protein using ^{13}C NMR. Biorg Med Chem 1: 389–397
7. Ritz HL, Connor DS, Sauter ED (1975) Contact sensitization of guinea-pigs with unsaturated and halogenated sultones. Contact Derm 1:349–358
8. Goodwin BFJ, Roberts DW, Williams DL, Johnson AW (1983) Relationships between skin sensitization potential of saturated and unsaturated sultones. In: Gibson GG, Hubbard R, Parke DV (eds) Immunotoxicology. Academic Press, London, pp 443–448
9. Magnusson B, Gilje O (1973) Allergic contact dermatitis from dishwashing liquid containing lauryl ether sulfate. Acta Derm Venereol (Stockholm) 53:136–140
10. Meschkat E, Barratt M, Lepoittevin JP (2001) Studies of chemical selectivity of hapten, reactivity and skin sensitization potency. Synthesis and studies on the reactivity towards model nucleophiles of the ^{13}C-labeled skin sensitizers, hex-1-ene- and hexane-1,3 sultones. Chem Res Toxicol 14: 110–117

11. Meschkat E, Barratt M, Lepoittevin JP (2001) Studies of chemical selectivity of hapten, reactivity and skin sensitization potency. NMR studies of the covalent binding of the ^{13}C-labeled skin sensitizers, 2-[^{13}C] and 3-[^{13}C]-hex-1-ene- and 3-[^{13}C]-hexane-1,3-sultones to human serum albumin. Chem Res Toxicol 14:118–126

12. Alvarez-Sanchez R, Basketter D, Pease C, Lepoittevin JP (2003) Studies of chemical selectivity of hapten, reactivity and skin sensitization potency. 3. Synthesis and studies on the reactivity towards model nucleophiles of the ^{13}C-labeled skin sensitizers, 5-chloro-2-methylisothiazol-3-one (MCI) and 2-methylisothiazol-3-one (MI). Chem Res Toxicol 16:627–636

13. Alvarez-Sanchez R, Basketter DA, Pease C, Lepoittevin JP (2004) Covalent binding of the 13C-labeled skin sensitizers 5-chloro-2-methylisothiazol-3-one (MCI) and 2-methylisothiazol-3-one (MI) to a model peptide and glutathione. Bioorg Med Chem Letters 14:365–368

14. Alvarez-Sanchez R, Divkovic M, Basketter D, Pease C, Panico M, Dell A, Morris H, Lepoittevin JP (2004) Effect of glutathione on the covalent binding of the ^{13}C-labeled skin sensitizer 5-chloro-2-methylisothiazol-3-one (MCI) to human serum albumin: identification of adducts by NMR, MALDI-MS and nano-ES MS/MS. Chem Res Toxicol 17(9):1280–1288

15. Romagnoli P, Labahrdt AM, Sinigaglia F (1991) Selective interaction of nickel with an MHC bound peptide. EMBO J 10:1303–1306

16. Schmidt R, Kahn L, Chung LY (1990) Are free radicals and quinones the haptenic species derived from urushiols and other contact allergenic mono- and dihydric alkylbenzenes? The significance of NADH, glutathione and redox cuycling in the skin. Arch Dermatol Res 282:56–64

17. Barratt MD, Basketter DA (1992) Possible origin of the skin sensitization potential of eugenol and related compounds. Contact Derm 27:98–104

18. Gäfvert E, Shao LP, Karlberg A-T, Nilsson U, Nilsson JLG (1994) Contact allergy to resin acid hydroperoxides. Hapten binding via free readicals and epoxides. Chem Res Toxicol 7:260–266

19. Mutterer V, Gimenez-Arnau E, Karlberg AT, Lepoittevin JP (2000) Synthesis and allergenic potential of a 15-hydroperoxyabietic acid-like model: trapping of radical intermediates. Chem Res Toxicol 13:1028–1036

20. Giménez-Arnau E, Haberkorn L, Grossi L, Lepoittevin JP (2002) Identification of alkyl radicals derived from an allergenic cyclic tertiary allylic hydroperoxide by combined use of radical trapping and ESR studies. Tetrahedron 58: 5535–5545

21. Bertrand F, Basketter DA, Roberts DW, Lepoittevin J-P (1997) Skin sensitization to eugenol and isoeugenol in mice: possible metabolic pathways involving ortho-quinone and quinone methide intermediates. Chem Res Toxicol 10: 335–343

22. Merk HF (1997) Skin metabolism. In: Lepoittevin JP, Basketter DA, Goossens A, Karlberg AT (eds) Allergic contact dermatitis: the molecular basis. Springer, Berlin, pp 68–80

23. Dupuis G (1979) Studies of poison ivy. In vitro lymphocytes transformation by urushiol protein conjugates Brit J Dermatol 101:617–624

24. Reynolds G, Rodriguez E (1981) Prenylated hydroquinones: contact allergens from trichomes of *Phacelia minor* and *P. parryi*. Phytochemistry 20:1365–1366

25. Bergmann HH, Beijersbergen JCH, Overeem JC, Sijpesteijn AK (1967) Isolation and identification of α-methylene-γ-butyrolactone: a fungitoxic substance from tulips. Recueil des Travaux Chimiques des Pays-Bas 86:709–713

26. Landsteiner K, Jacobs JL (1936) Studies on the sensitization of animals with simple chemicals. J Exp Med 64:625–639

27. Dupuis G, Benezra C (1982) Allergic contact dermatitis to simple chemicals. Marcel Dekker, New York

28. Hellerström S, Thyresson N, Blohm SG, Widmark G (1955) On the nature of eczematogenic component of oxidized Δ3-carene. J Invest Dermatol 24:217–224

29. Karlberg AT (1988) Contact allergy to colophony. Chemical identification of allergens. Sensitization experiments and clinical experiments. Acta Dermato-Venereol 68(suppl 139):1–43

30. Karlberg AT, Shao LP, Nilsson U, Gäfvert E, Nilsson JLG (1994) Hydroperoxides in oxidized d-limonene identified as potent contact allergens. Arch Dermatol Res 286:97–103

31. Stampf JL, Benezra C, Klecak G, Geleick H, Schulz KH, Hausen B (1982) The sensitization capacity of helenin and two of its main constituents, the sesquiterpene lactones, alantolactones and isoalantolactone. Contact Derm 8:16–24

32. Baer RL (1954) Cross-sensitization phenomena. In: Mackenna (ed). Modern trends in dermatology. Butterworth, London, pp 232–258

33. Benezra C, Maibach H (1984) True cross-sensitization, false cross-sensitization and otherwise. Contact Derm 11:65–69

34. Cohen NC, Blaney JM, Humblet C, Gund P, Barry DC (1990) Molecular modeling software and methods for medicinal chemistry. J Med Chem 33:883–984

35. Coopman S, Degreef H, Dooms-Goossens A (1989) Identification of cross-reaction patterns in allergic contact dermatitis from topical corticosteroids. Brit J Dermatol 121:27–34

36. Lepoittevin JP, Drieghe J, Dooms-Goossens A (1995) Studies in patients with corticosteroid contact allergy: understanding cross-reactivity among different steroids. Arch Dermatol 131:31–37

37. Roberts DW, Williams DL (1982) The derivation of quantitative correlations between skin sensitisation and physico-chemical parameters for alkylating agents and their application to experimental data for sultones. J Theor Biol 99:807–825

38. Fraginals R, Roberts DW, Lepoittevin J-P, Benezra C (1991) Refinement of the relative alkylation index (RAI) model for skin sensitization and application to mouse and guinea-pig test data for alkylsulfonates. Arch Dermatol Res 283: 387–394

39. Franot C, Roberts DW, Basketter DA, Benezra C, Lepoittevin J-P (1994) Structure-activity relationships for contact allergenic potential of γ, γ-dimethyl-γ-butyrolactone derivatives Part II. Chem Res Toxicol 7:307–312

40. Roberts DW, Basketter DA (1997) Further evaluation of the quantitative structure-activity relationship for skin-sensitizing alkyl transfer agents. Contact Derm 37:107–112

41. Roberts DW, Basketter DA (2000) Quantitative structure-activity relationships: sulfonate esters in the local lymph node assay. Contact Derm 42:154–161

42. Basketter DA, Gerberick GF, Kimber I, Loveless SE (1996) The local lymph node assay: a viable alternative to currently accepted skin sensitization tests. Food Chem Toxicol 34: 985–997

43. Basketter DA, Lea LJ, Dickens A et al (1999) A comparison of statistical approaches to the derivation of EC3 values from local lymph node assay dose-response. J Appl Toxicol 19:261–266

44. Perrin DD, Dempsey B, Serjeant EP (1981) pKa prediction for organic acids and bases. Chapman and Hall, London, pp 109–126

45. Patlewicz GY, Wright ZM, Basketter DA, Pease CK, Lepoittevin JP, Gimenez-Arnau E (2002) Structure-activity relationships for selected fragrance allergens. Contact Derm 47:219–226

46. Barbier A, Rizova E, Stampf J-L, Lacheretz F, Pistor FHM, Bos JD, Kapsenberg ML, Becker D, Mohamadzadeh M, Knop J, Mabic S, Lepoittevin J-P (1994) Development of a predictive in vitro test for detection of sensitizing compounds (European BRIDGE project). In: Rougier A, Goldberg AM, Maibach HI (eds) In vitro skin toxicology (irritation, phototoxicity, sensitization). Liebert, New York, pp 341–350

47. Gerberick F, Vassallo J, Bailey R, Morrall S, Lepoittevin J-P (2004) Development of peptide reactivity assay for screening allergens. Toxicol Sci 81:332–343

48. Gerberick F, Vassallo J, Foertsch L, Price B, Chaney J, Lepoittevin J-P (2007) Quantification of chemical peptide reactivity for screening contact allergens. Toxicol Sci 97: 417–427

49. Levin CY, Maibach HI (2008) Animal, human, and in vitro test methods for predicting skin irritation. In: Zhai H, Maibach HI (eds) Dermatotoxicology, 7th edn. CRC press, Boca Raton, pp 383–389

50. Kang KW, Lee SJ, Kim SG (2005) Molecular mechanism of nrf2 activation by oxidative stress. Antioxid Redox Signal 7(11–12):1664–1673

51. Natsch A, Emter R (2008) Skin sensitizers induce antioxidant response element dependent genes: Application to the *In Vitro* testing of the sensitization potential of chemicals. Toxicol Sci 102:110–119

Classical References

Lepoittevin JP, Basketter DA, Goossens A, Karlberg AT (eds) (1997) Allergic contact dermatitis: the molecular basis. Springer, Berlin

Dupuis G, Benezra C (1982) Allergic contact dermatitis to simple chemicals. Marcel Dekker, New York

Smith CK, Hotchkiss SAM (2001) Allergic contact dermatitis: chemical and metabolic mechanisms. Taylor & Francis, London, New York

Bio-Guided Fractionation and Identification of Allergens in Complex Mixtures and Products

5

Elena Giménez-Arnau

Contents

E. Giménez-Arnau
Laboratoire de Dermatochimie,
Institut de Chimie de Strasbourg – ILB,
4, Rue Blaise Pascal, 67070, Strasbourg, France
e-mail: egimenez@chimie.u-strasbg.fr

5.1 Introduction

At the present time, preventive measures are claimed to play a key role in the global management of allergic contact dermatitis disease. Prevention of skin allergy to a chemical can be discussed in terms of primary prevention for nonsensitized individuals and secondary prevention for those who are already sensitized [1]. In the development of any primary prevention strategy, there is a need to identify fully the nature of chemicals responsible for causing contact allergy in the consumer, to create initiatives that regulate the exposure to those chemicals so that induction of allergic contact sensitization does not take place, and to improve risk assessment procedures. Critical factors for skin sensitization to a chemical, and for the following elicitation of allergic contact dermatitis by renewed contact, are indeed the inherent sensitizing potential of the chemical and the skin exposure concentration, given as a dose–response relationship between specific environmental exposures and health outcomes [2–4]. Hazard identification is, therefore, the first step in the safety assessment of a chemical. In the context of primary prevention, this corroborates the necessity to have suitable, sensitive, and reliable methods for the prospective identification of those novel chemicals that possess the potential to cause the sensitization of the skin.

Detecting and identifying contact allergens among the myriad of chemicals used in commercial products can be an extremely arduous task. In the case of fragrance allergy, for example, approximately 3,000 fragrance ingredients, of synthetic origin or natural products, are available to the perfumer for compounding a fragrance formula, which may consist of 10–300 or more different ingredients in a cosmetic product [5, 6]. From the standpoint of hazard identification, the present chapter describes the combined use of bioassay-guided

J.D. Johansen et al. (eds.), *Contact Dermatitis*,
DOI: 10.1007/978-3-642-03827-3_5, © Springer-Verlag Berlin Heidelberg 2011

5

chemical fractionation, chemical analysis, and structure-activity relationships studies (SARs) as a convenient tool for the identification of sensitizing molecules present in fragrance complex mixtures. Practical applications such as the cases of eaux de toilette and the allergenic natural extract oak moss are shown.

5.2 The Principle of Bioassay-Guided Fractionation

Bioassay-guided fractionation is one of the most commonly used strategies for the identification of bioactive lead compounds and new drugs [7, 8]. The principle of bioassay-guided chemical fractionation is based on the isolation of a pure chemical agent of natural origin, implying a step-by-step separation of extracted components based on the differences in their physicochemical properties, and assessing the biological activity, followed by a next round of separation and assaying. Usually, the process is initiated after a given crude, normally prepared by solvent extraction of the natural material, is considered to be "active" in a specific in vitro assay. The end-goal is the identification of the compounds that are responsible for the observed in vitro activity. The way to that end is quite simple. After fractionating the crude extract, usually by chromatographic techniques such as column chromatography and high-performance liquid chromatography, the fractions generated are tested in the in vitro assay. These steps are then repeated with active fractions until pure, active compounds are obtained for which the structure can be determined by using spectroscopic methods such as nuclear magnetic resonance (NMR) and mass spectrometry (MS).

The same kind of methodology can be applied to allergenic perfume mixtures in order to find the compound(s) responsible for the skin sensitivity declared by the patient(s) to that mixture. Ideally, the perfume mixture is chemically fractionated and the fractions obtained are tested on the patient(s) by patch testing and/or by repeated open application test (ROAT). Fractions giving a positive reaction are refractionated, and the new fractions obtained are tested on the patient(s). These steps are repeated until a positive fraction that contains one or two single compounds easily identifiable by spectroscopic techniques is obtained (Fig. 5.1a).

An example of bioassay-guided fractionation in the case of fragrance allergy can be given by a study in

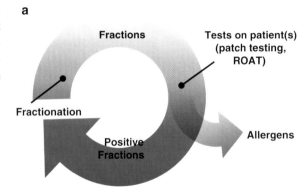

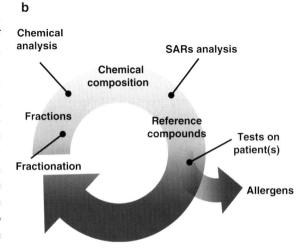

Fig. 5.1 Identification of allergens in complex mixtures. (**a**) Bioassay-guided fractionation. The mixture is chemically fractionated and the fractions obtained are tested on the patient(s) by patch testing and/or repeated open application test. Fractions giving a positive reaction are refractionated, and the new fractions obtained are tested on the patient(s). These steps are repeated until a positive fraction that contains the allergen(s) is obtained. (**b**) Bioassay-guided fractionation combined to structure-activity relationship analysis (SARs). The mixture is chemically fractionated and the chemical composition of the fractions obtained is analyzed. Potential allergenic compounds among the myriad of compounds composing the fractions are selected by SARs analysis as reference compounds and are tested on the patient(s) in order to determine the allergen(s)

which the offending allergen in a patient sensitive to her own eau de toilette but negative to the fragrance mix I (FMI) was identified [9]. At the time of the study, the fragrance mix (eugenol, isoeugenol, geraniol, hydroxycitronellal, α-amylcinnamic aldehyde, cinnamic aldehyde, cinnamic alcohol, and oak moss) was the sole existing screening tool for perfume contact allergy, and still identifies 70–80% of fragrance allergy cases [10]. However, its eight components neither represent the thousands of chemical structures found in fragrances, norall possible sensitizing molecules. A 44-year-old woman without previous skin problems developed an axillary rash using a perfumed deodorant. At the same time, she started to use the eau de toilette of the same brand and developed a rash on the neck and the trunk. The patient was patch tested positive to the deodorant and the eau de toilette, but was negative to FMI. The eau de toilette perfume concentrate was chemically fractionated by column chromatography on silica gel giving three fractions (F1–F3) that were tested on the patient in a ROAT using ethanol as the vehicle. The test material concentration was calculated so that it corresponded to the amount of the fraction present in the final formulation. Only fraction F2 gave a positive reaction and was further chemically fractionated to afford four subfractions (F2.1–F2.4) that were tested on the patient. Fraction F2.4 confirmed a positive reaction. This fraction was analyzed and found to contain simply coumarin and ethyl vanillin. The patient was negative on use testing to 1% ethyl vanillin in ethanol, but was positive to 1% coumarin in ethanol after 2 days of application. Ten control eczema patients were negative after 3 days of applying 1% coumarin to one elbow flexure. The patient was also positive at patch testing to 5% coumarin in ethanol, but negative to ethanol. This simple case of bioassay-guided fractionation on a fragrance mixture confirmed coumarin as the offending allergen. Today, coumarin, a widely used fragrance compound, is included in the FMII. The FMII was introduced this decade as an additional screening tool to FMI. It contains six other allergenic compounds (hydroxyisohexyl-3-cyclohexene carboxaldehyde or Lyral®, α-hexyl-cinnamic aldehyde, farnesol, citronellol, citral, and coumarin), frequently used in fragrance formulations and identifies additional relevant cases of contact allergy to fragrances not detected by FMI [11, 12].

> ### Core Message
>
> > Bioassay-guided fractionation can be used for the isolation of allergens in complex mixtures. It implies a step-by-step separation of components into fractions and assessment of their allergenic activity, followed by a next round of separation and analysis until pure allergenic compounds are obtained.

5.3   The Principle Behind Structure-Activity Relationships in Allergic Contact Dermatitis

The principle behind SARs is that the properties of a chemical, with respect to its mode of interaction with a defined system (i.e., a specified organism, a biological structure, a macromolecule such as a protein), are inherent in its molecular structure. SARs are developed by looking for links between structure and biological activity, based on mechanistic or empirical grounds. In other words, the biological activity of a compound is seen as a function of the structural and physicochemical properties of the chemical.

Progress in the understanding of the molecular basis of allergic contact dermatitis has helped the development of SAR analysis for sensitizing chemicals. In contact allergy, as it is the chemical that drives the immune system, it is essential to examine the extent to which it is possible to relate its chemical structure with the propensity to behave as a skin sensitizer. Already in the 30s, it was recognized that a correlation exists between the skin sensitization potential of a chemical and its reactivity toward nucleophiles [13]. Since then, a well-established connection between the ability of chemicals to react with proteins to form covalently linked conjugates and their skin sensitization potential has been identified. Indeed, the first step in the induction and the elicitation of a contact allergy is the formation of a covalent, irreversible, bond between the sensitizer and skin proteins to form an antigenic complex. It is now accepted that this occurs principally through a nucleophile–electrophile mechanism, as the majority of allergens contain in their chemical structure an electrophilic functional group which is able to react with nucleophilic amino acids in proteins [14]. It is therefore reasonable to conclude that if a chemical is capable of reacting with a protein, either directly or after a metabolism (prohaptens) or oxidation step (prehaptens), then it has the potential to be a contact allergen.

In contact allergy, the modern concept of SARs was introduced by Dupuis and Benezra, and today there is a considerable knowledge on the chemical functions present in haptens that are related to a sensitizing potential [15]. Further, relationships between chemical structures and their ability to form covalent conjugates with proteins have been established. This knowledge, relating chemical structures to skin sensitization, has been decomposed in a series of chemical rules, also called

5

"structural alerts." A "structural alert" consists of a total or partial chemical structure known to present allergizing risks. Mainly, "structural alerts" are defined by the analysis of the literature and contact allergy databases. The presence of a "structural alert" in a structure is an indication of the capacity to modify skin proteins and thus behave as a skin sensitizer. It allows the detection of a "risk." Accordingly, these structural properties can be used to predict the allergizing potential of a new molecule, for example, in "expert" computerized systems.

Expert systems are decision-aiding programs, based on the use of large databases that employ the structural, physicochemical, and electronic data of a new compound, and compare them with the data stored in memory to give an opinion on its allergizing status. One expert computerized system based on the structural alerts approach is DEREK (deductive estimation of risk from existing knowledge). It is a program that analyzes the structure of the molecules and compares it with a database consisting of "rules" in the form of molecular substructures known to be associated with an allergizing activity [16]. Examples of "rules" are shown in Table 5.1.

Modern analytical methods such as gas chromatography combined to mass spectrometry (GC–MS) and liquid chromatography–mass spectrometry (LC–MS) can give a detailed access to the composition of complex chemical mixtures. SARs studies based on the existence of "structural alerts" have, for example, been used for the evaluation of the sensitizing potential of the ingredients present in marketed deodorants and identified by GC–MS [17]. Among the 226 molecules that were identified by analyzing 71 deodorants, 84 were found to contain at least one "structural alert," and 70 to belong to, or be susceptible to being metabolized into, the chemical group of aldehydes (alkyl or aryl), ketones (alkyl or aryl) and α,β-unsaturated aldehydes, ketones, or esters. The combination of analytical methods and SARs analysis can thus be helpful for the selection of substances for supplementary investigations regarding sensitizing properties.

Core Message

> The combination of analytical methods giving the chemical composition of complex mixtures and SARs analysis on identified molecules is helpful for the selection of potentially sensitizing substances.

Table 5.1 Examples of rules and chemical structures used by DEREK to predict the sensitizing potential

Chemical function	Substituents	Structure
Aldehydes	R = alkyl, aryl	
Ketones	R, R^1 = alkyl, aryl	
Aldehydes, amides, esters, and α,β-unsaturated ketones	R = H, C, N, O (not OH) R^1 = not heteroatoms, esters, ketones R^2 = not aryl except when R = H	
Phenyl esters	R = alkyl, aryl R^1 = any	
Hydroquinones and their O-alkyl precursors	R = H, alkyl R^1 = any	
Catechols and their O-alkyl precursors	R = H, alkyl R^1 = any	
Anhydrides	R = any	
Aromatic primary and secondary amines	R = alkyl, aryl R^1 = any	
Alkyl halides	R = alkyl X = Cl, Br, I	

5.4 Combined Use of Bioassay-Guided Fractionation and SARs to Identify Allergens in Fragrance Complex Mixtures

In the course of a large number of investigations on fragrance chemical allergy, a new approach for the identification of fragrance sensitizers present in complex chemical mixtures has been developed. In this research area, a complex mixture can be, for instance, a commercial perfume such an eau de toilette, or a natural extract used in perfumery. The method is based on the combination of bioassay-guided chemical fractionation, chemical analysis, and SARs studies. The need to develop this methodology, complementing simple bioassay-guided fractionation, became apparent due to the difficulty to obtain more and more refined fractions in the case of complex fragrance mixtures.

5.4.1 General Methodology

As a general procedure, the complex fragrance mixture is first of all fractionated chemically, and the fractions obtained are tested on the patient(s) who are allergic to the mixture by patch testing and/or ROAT. Positive fractions are subjected to an extensive chemical analysis in order to identify the chemical composition and molecule structures. From the structures, a SARs analysis permits to select molecules with a suspected sensitizing potential as defined by the presence of structural alerts. These molecules (reference compounds) are then directly tested on the patient(s) for the identification of the actual sensitizer(s) (Fig. 5.1b). The major advantage of this approach is to avoid iterative fractionation/patient testing sessions that are time consuming, require considerable effort by the patients and the scientists involved, and very often are of low benefit. Two practical examples are given in the following sections.

> **Core Message**
>
> › To accelerate the process of allergen identification in complex mixtures, it is possible to combine bioassay-guided fractionation, chemical analysis, and SARs studies.

5.4.2 The Case of an Eau de Toilette

In the first study, bioassay-guided chemical fractionation, chemical analysis, and SARs studies were applied for the identification, in an eau de toilette, of fragrance allergens not included in the fragrance mix [18]. The basis for the investigation was a 45-year-old woman allergic to her own eau de toilette with infiltrated itchy erythematous papular reactions. She had a negative patch test to the fragrance mix, but a positive patch test and ROAT results to the commercial product.

The first fractionation of the perfume concentrate by column chromatography on silica gel gave six fractions (F1–F6) that were dissolved in ethanol and used for patch testing the patient. Fractions F2 and F6 elicited a clear positive reaction that was further confirmed by ROAT. Subsequently, fractions F2 and F6 were again fractionated chemically and six (F2.1–F2.6) and two (F6.1–F6.2) new fractions were obtained, respectively. Further fractionation was not considered suitable, because of the complexity to obtain more and more refined fractions by column chromatography. The GC–MS analysis of F2.1–F2.6 and F6.1–F6.2 allowed the identification of 24 compounds. Among them, nine were found to contain at least one structural alert. The nine compounds were chosen as references and were patch tested on the patient. Lilial®, which contains an aldehyde chemical function in its molecular structure, was the sole compound eliciting a positive patch test reaction, and clinical relevance was again identified by ROAT. Lilial® (p-t-butyl-α-methylhydrocinnamic aldehyde) is a synthetic fragrance, not reported to occur in nature, and is a known contact allergen [10, 19, 20]. It is actually included in the list of the 26 allergenic fragrance ingredients fixed, by the Seventh Amendment to the European Cosmetics Directive, to be labeled on commercial products [21]. This case illustrates, therefore, that the combination of fractionation, testing, analytical and SARs methods is a valuable tool for the management of contact allergy to fragrance materials.

It is important to note the necessity to perform the bioassay-guided chemical fractionation on the perfume concentrate obtained from the commercial product after removal, by evaporation, of alcohol and aqua, and not only on the perfume concentrate that the manufacturer usually supplies for the studies. This has been stressed in a second study in which another eau de toilette giving allergic reactions in a patient also negative to the fragrance mix was analyzed using the same procedure described above. This time, ingredients supplied by the manufacturer were also included in the study [22]. Benzophenone-2, Lyral®, α-hexyl-cinnamic aldehyde, and α-damascone were found to be responsible for the patient's contact allergy to the commercial product. From the first contact with the manufacturer, they informed that the eau de toilette contained the photoscreen agent benzophenone-2 and they furnished it separately of the fragrance concentrate. From the first patch test consultations, the patient showed a strong reaction to the manufacturer's benzophenone-2 and fragrance concentrate. If only the industry concentrate had been analyzed, benzophenone-2 allergizing effect would have been missed, as the compound was not present in the fragrance concentrate supplied by the manufacturer. However, analysis of the concentrate from the commercial product allowed the identification of benzophenone-2 as an allergenic compound for that patient. The concentrate obtained from the evaporation of the eau de toilette contained indeed all the formula ingredients, including fragrance components, photo-screen agents, and colorants.

5.4.3 The Case of Oak Moss

In addition to pure synthetic fragrance materials, many natural extracts are also used in the perfume industry. Like commercial eaux de toilette and perfumes, natural extracts are complex mixtures that contain several hundred different chemicals that are responsible for the complexity of the odor. Among them is the oak moss absolute, prepared from the lichen *Evernia prunastri* (L.) Arch. Because of its woody aroma and fixative properties, oak moss absolute is extensively used in perfumery as a natural fragrance, particularly for masculine products. Oak moss is considered as a major contact sensitizer and is therefore included in the FMI used for diagnosing perfume allergy. Testing with the individual constituents of the fragrance mix has shown that oak moss absolute is the most frequently documented cause of fragrance contact allergy [23, 24].

Oak moss absolute is traditionally prepared by extracting the harvested lichen with hydrocarbon solvents, and subsequently treating-of the so-called oak moss concrete with a mixture of alcohols. In the 70s and 80s, the chemical composition of oak moss absolute was extensively studied and the allergenic potential of the major components was evaluated [25, 26]. At that time, sensitivity to oak moss was associated not only with the presence of phenylbenzoates such as atranorin and evernic acid but also with usnic acid although not a phenylbenzoate [27–29]. For many years, benzene was used to prepare the oak moss concrete. However, it is no longer used and it was replaced by more polar hydrocarbons. As a consequence, the composition of oak moss absolute did change, and, even though several potential sensitizers had been identified from former benzene extracts, the constituents of oak moss absolute obtained from the new extraction procedures and their allergenic status were not clear.

The methodology previously described for the identification of fragrance allergens present in complex mixtures such as eaux de toilette was applied to oak moss absolute [30]. Patients with a previous known sensitivity to oak moss were recruited for the study. After a first round of fractionation of the natural extract by column chromatography and patch testing, attention was focused on the strongest elicitant fraction in the patients. Chemical analysis of this fraction, by gas chromatography combined to MS, identified eight chemicals derived from a resorcinol structure. A SAR analysis indicated that they all should be considered as potential sensitizers. In order to avoid too many patch tests, the most representative molecules covering the different molecular structures were selected and tested on the patients. Atranol and chloroatranol were this way identified as the major elicitant chemicals, and methyl-β-orcinol carboxylate as a minor one (Figs. 5.2 and 5.3). Freshly harvested oak

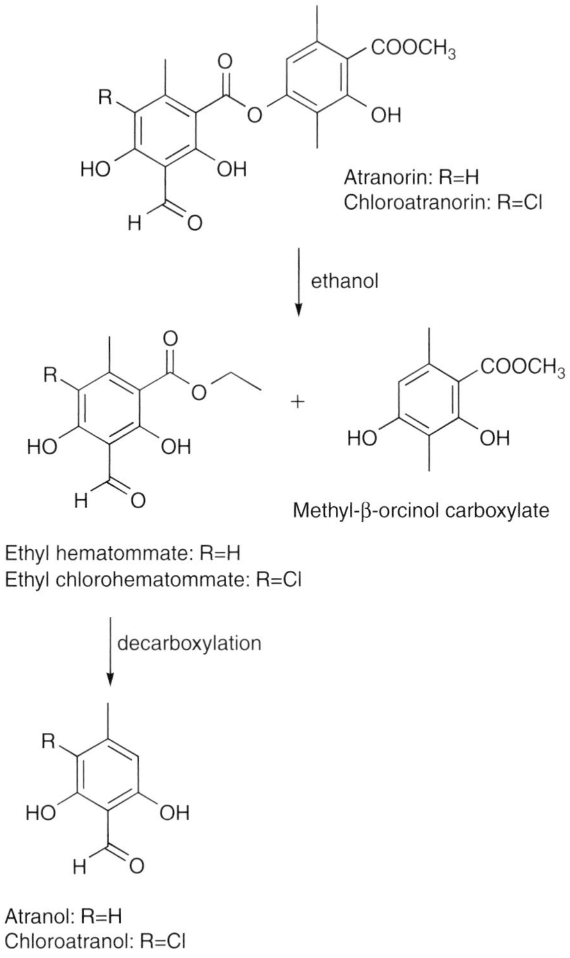

Fig. 5.2 Formation of atranol and chloroatranol from atranorin and chloroatranorin during oak moss processing

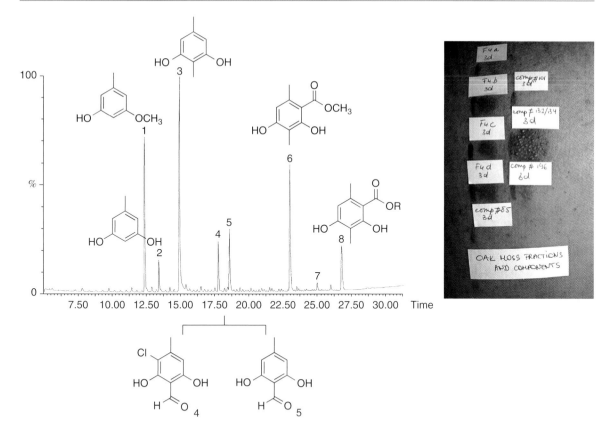

Fig. 5.3 Gas chromatogram of the strongest elicitant fraction of oak moss (F4), together with the chemical structures identified and patch test results of representative molecules and subfractions (picture by courtesy of Pr An Goossens). In the patch tests, compounds 132/134 correspond to a mixture of chloroatranol 4 and atranol 5, and compound 196 to methyl-β-orcinol carboxy-late 6. Subfractions F4c and F4d contained essentially atranol and chloroatranol, whereas subfraction F4b contained essentially methyl-β-orcinol carboxylate. The subfractions patch test results were thus in agreement with the patch test results of the selected molecules

moss has substantially no scent. The moss contains various types of depsides, which are nonvolatile, odorless, polyfunctional diaryl derivatives. Among these depsides are lecanoric acid, evernic acid, barbatic acid, atranorin and chloroatranorin. The characteristic oak moss fragrance is developed only after the cleavage of the depsides during the treatment of oak moss concrete with alcohols to give volatile, scented, monoaryl derivatives. Atranol and chloroatranol are, in fact, degradation products formed during oak moss processing, after transesterification and decarboxylation of atranorin and chloroatranorin during the ethanolic treatment (Fig. 5.2). Methyl-β-orcinol carboxylate, also obtained during this processing, is essentially responsible for the characteristic earthy-moss-like odor of oak moss products.

The results of this bioassay-guided fractionation procedure, combining testing of individuals sensitized to oak moss absolute with fractions of the fragrance material, with GC–MS analysis of positive fractions, and with chemical structure-activity relationship analysis of identified molecules, allowed the identification of atranol and chloroatranol as offending chemicals in oak moss absolute. It has been shown that both atranol and chloroatranol elicit reactions at very low levels of exposure [31]. Differences in the elicitation capacity between the two substances are counterbalanced by exposure being greater to atranol than to chloroatranol, as it has been found that oak moss absolute contains approximately 2.1% (w/w) of atranol and 0.9% (w/w) of chloroatranol [30]. Of both the compounds, chloroatranol, a hitherto unknown fragrance allergen, was identified as the main allergen in oak moss absolute. Further exposure assessment together with dose–response elicitation studies showed that chloroatranol elicited reactions by repeated open exposure at the ppm level (0.0005%), and at the ppb level on patch testing (50% of patients elicited at 0.000015%) [32, 33]. These results were described as unprecedented, chloroatranol being the most powerful allergen present in consumer products today.

5.5 Conclusion

The opening step for any prevention strategy for skin sensitization is the identification of new allergens, ideally before they are put into the market, though already present in consumer products. In this chapter, a methodology based on the combination of bioassay-guided chemical fractionation, patch test and/or use testing of individuals with fractions, detailed chemical composition analysis of positive fractions, and chemical SAR analysis of identified molecules, is presented as a valuable tool for the identification of allergens in fragrance complex mixtures. The cases of commercial eaux de toilette and a natural extract such as oak moss absolute are detailed to illustrate the methodology. Following the identification of new allergens, it is critical to conduct a complete skin sensitization risk assessment based on ingredient exposure, allergenic potency, and dose–response studies. The importance of exposure, dose–response correlation, and potency estimation has been underlined for the newly found oak moss offending allergens, atranol and chloroatranol.

References

1. Lachapelle JM (2001) Principles of prevention and protection in contact dermatitis (with special reference to occupational dermatology). In: Rycroft RJG, Menné T, Frosch PJ, Lepoittevin JP (eds) Textbook of contact dermatitis. Springer, Berlin, pp 979–993
2. Lepoittevin JP (1999) Development of structure–activity relationships (SARs) in allergic contact dermatitis. Cell Biol Toxicol 15:47–55
3. Kimber I, Basketter DA, Butler M, Gamer A, Garrigue JL, Gerberick GF, Newsome C, Steiling W, Vohr HW (2003) Classification of contact allergens according to potency: proposals. Food Chem Toxicol 41:1799–1809
4. Robinson MK, Gerberick GF, Ryan CA, McNamee P, White IR, Basketter DA (2000) The importance of exposure estimation in the assessment of skin sensitization risk. Contact Dermatitis 42:251–259
5. Bauer K, Garbe D, Surburg H (1997) Common fragrance and flavor materials. Preparation, properties and uses, 3rd edn. Wiley-VCH, Weinheim
6. Rastogi SC (1998) Contents of sensitizing fragrance materials in natural ingredient based cosmetics. In: Frosch PJ, Johansen JD, White IR (eds) Fragrances: beneficial and adverse effects. Springer, Berlin, pp 113–120
7. Pieters L, Vlietinck AJ (2005) Bioguided isolation of pharmacologically active plant components, still a valuable strategy for the finding of new lead compounds? J Ethnopharmacol 100:57–60
8. Houghton PJ, Raman A (1998) Laboratory handbook for the fractionation of natural extracts, 2nd edn. Springer, Berlin
9. Mutterer V, Giménez-Arnau E, Lepoittevin JP, Johansen JD, Frosch PJ, Menné T, Andersen KE, Bruze M, Rastogi SC, White IR (1999) Identification of coumarin as the sensitizer in a patient sensitive to her own perfume but negative to the fragrance mix. Contact Dermatitis 40:196–199
10. Larsen W, Nakayama H, Lindberg M, Fischer T, Elsner P, Burrows D, Jordan W, Shaw S, Wilkinson J, Marks J, Sugawara M, Nethercott J (1996) Fragrance contact dermatitis. A world-wide multicentre investigation (part I). Am J Contact Dermatitis 7:77–83
11. Frosch PJ, Pirker C, Rastogi SC, Andersen KE, Bruze M, Svedman C, Goossens A, White IR, Uter W, Giménez-Arnau E, Lepoittevin JP, Menné T, Johansen JD (2005) Patch testing with a new fragrance mix detects additional patients sensitive to perfumes and missed by the current fragrance mix. Contact Dermatitis 52:207–215
12. Frosch PJ, Rastogi SC, Pirker C, Brinkmeier T, Andersen KE, Bruze M, Svedman C, Goossens A, White IR, Uter W, Giménez-Arnau E, Lepoittevin JP, Johansen JD, Menné T (2005) Patch testing with a new fragrance mix – reactivity to the individual constituents and chemical detection in relevant cosmetic products. Contact Dermatitis 52:216–225
13. Landsteiner K, Jacobs J (1936) Studies on the sensitization of animals with simple chemical compounds. J Exp Med 64:625–639
14. Lepoittevin JP (2001) Molecular aspects of allergic contact dermatitis. In: Rycroft RJG, Menné T, Frosch PJ, Lepoittevin JP (eds) Textbook of contact dermatitis. Springer, Berlin, pp 59–89
15. Dupuis G, Benezra C (1982) Allergic contact dermatitis to simple chemicals. A molecular approach. Marcel Dekker, New York
16. Barratt MD, Basketter DA, Chamberlain M, Admans GD, Langowski JJ (1994) An expert system rulebase for identifying contact allergens. Toxicol In Vitro 8:1053–1060
17. Rastogi SC, Lepoittevin JP, Johansen JD, Frosch PJ, Menné T, Bruze M, Dreier B, Andersen KE, White IR (1998) Fragrances and other materials in deodorants: search for potentially sensitizing molecules using combined GC-MS and structure activity relationship (SAR) analysis. Contact Dermatitis 39:293–303
18. Giménez-Arnau E, Andersen KE, Bruze M, Frosch PJ, Johansen JD, Menné T, Rastogi SC, White IR, Lepoittevin JP (2000) Identification of Lilial® as a fragrance sensitizer in a perfume by bioassay-guided chemical fractionation and structure-activity relationships. Contact Dermatitis 43:351–358
19. Larsen WG (1983) Allergic contact dermatitis to the fragrance material lilial. Contact Dermatitis 9:158–159
20. Sugai T (1994) Group study IV-farnesol and lily aldehyde. Environ Dermatol 1:213–214

21. European Commission (2003) Directive 2003/15/EC of the European Parliament and of the Council of 27 February 2003 amending Council Directive 76/768/EEC on the approximation of the laws of the Member States relating to cosmetic products (7th Amendment to the European Cosmetics Directive). Off J Eur Union L-66:26–35

22. Giménez-Arnau A, Giménez-Arnau E, Serra-Baldrich E, Lepoittevin JP, Camarasa JG (2002) Principles and methodology for identification of fragrance allergens in consumer products. Contact Dermatitis 47:345–352

23. Buckley DA, Wakelin SH, Seed PT, Holloway D, Rycroft RJG, White IR, McFadden JP (2000) The frequency of fragrance allergy in a patch test population over a 17-year period. Br J Dermatol 142:279–283

24. Schnuch A, Lessmann H, Geier J, Frosch PJ, Uter W (2004) Contact allergy to fragrances: frequencies of sensitization from 1996 to 2002. Results of the IVDK. Contact Dermatitis 50:65–76

25. Gavin J, Tabacchi R (1975) Isolement et identification de composés phénoliques et monoterpéniques de la mousse de chêne (*Evernia prunastri* (L.) Arch.). Helv Chim Acta 58:190–194

26. Schulz H, Albroscheit G (1989) Characterization of oak moss products used in perfumery by high-performance liquid chromatography. J Chromatogr 466:301–306

27. Dahlquist I, Fregert S (1980) Contact allergy to atranorin in lichens and perfumes. Contact Dermatitis 6:111–119

28. Thune P, Solberg Y, McFadden N, Staerfelt F, Sandberg M (1982) Perfume allergy due to oak moss and other lichens. Contact Dermatitis 8:396–400

29. Gonçalo S, Cabral F, Gonçalo M (1988) Contact sensitivity to oak moss. Contact Dermatitis 19:355–357

30. Bernard G, Giménez-Arnau E, Rastogi SC, Heydorn S, Johansen JD, Menné T, Goossens A, Andersen KE, Lepoittevin JP (2003) Contact allergy to oak moss: search for sensitizing molecules using combined bioassay-guided chemical fractionation, GC-MS, and structure-activity relationship analysis. Arch Dermatol Res 295:229–235

31. Johansen JD, Bernard G, Giménez-Arnau E, Lepoittevin JP, Bruze M, Andersen KE (2006) Comparison of elicitation potential of chloroatranol and atranol–2 allergens in oak moss absolute. Contact Dermatitis 54:192–195

32. Johansen JD, Andersen KE, Svedman C, Bruze M, Bernard G, Giménez-Arnau E, Rastogi SC, Lepoittevin JP, Menné T (2003) Chloroatranol, an extremely potent allergen hidden in perfumes: a dose-response elicitation study. Contact Dermatitis 49:180–184

33. Rastogi SC, Bossi R, Johansen JD, Menné T, Bernard G, Giménez-Arnau E, Lepoittevin JP (2004) Content of oak moss allergens atranol and chloroatranol in perfumes and similar products. Contact Dermatitis 50:367–370

Role of the Permeability Barrier in Contact Dermatitis

6

Ehrhardt Proksch and Jochen Brasch

Contents

E. Proksch (✉)
Department of Dermatology, University Hospitals of Kiel,
Schittenhelmstraße 7, 24105 Kiel, Germany
e-mail: eproksch@dermatology.uni-kiel.de

J. Brasch
Department of Dermatology, University of Kiel,
24105 Kiel, Germany

6.1 Introduction

The most important function of the skin is to form an effective barrier between the "inside" and the "outside" of the organism [1]. The "inside–outside" barrier regulates transepidermal water loss (TEWL) and prevents desiccation. The "outside–inside" barrier protects against mechanical, chemical, and microbial assaults from the external environment (Fig. 6.1). Many studies have shown that a disturbance of the skin barrier is a decisive initial step in the development of occupational dermatitis that is often followed by manifest irritant and/or allergic occupational contact dermatitis [2–6]. A detailed understanding of the barrier with its physiology and functions is therefore indispensable for the comprehension, prevention, diagnosis, and treatment of occupational dermatoses.

6.2 Barrier Physiology

To perform its protective function, the skin contains different types of barriers: a physical, a chemical/biochemical (innate immunity), and an immune barrier (adaptive immune system). The physical barrier consists mainly of the stratum corneum. In addition, the nucleated epidermis, in particular the tight junctions, provides another important barrier component. The chemical/biochemical (antimicrobial) barrier consists of lipids, acids, lysozymes, and antimicrobial peptides. The immune barrier (humoral and cellular immune system) provides a barrier to infectious disease, but immune hyperactivity may lead to allergy (reviewed in: [1]).

The epidermis, the skin's outer layer, consisting primarily of keratinocytes is most important for

J.D. Johansen et al. (eds.), *Contact Dermatitis*,
DOI: 10.1007/978-3-642-03827-3_6, © Springer-Verlag Berlin Heidelberg 2011

Intact Barrier

Impaired Barrier in Eczema

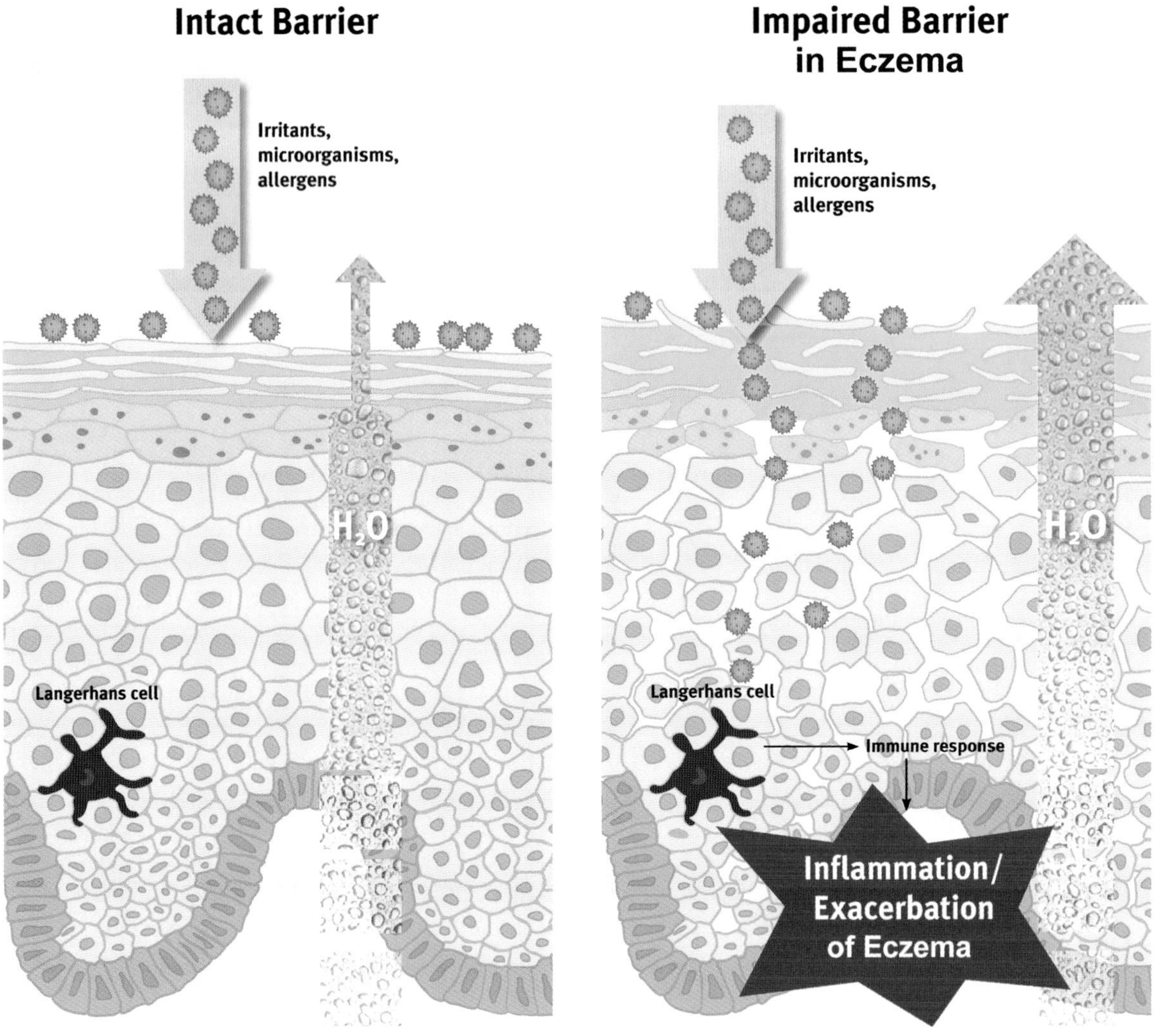

Fig. 6.1 An intact permeability barrier prevents the entry of harmful substances into the skin. In barrier-disrupted skin, irritants, allergens, and microbes may penetrate into the skin and induce immunological reactions and inflammation

skin protection and for the prevention of occupational diseases. The epidermis undergoes keratinization, a process in which the epidermal cells progressively mature from basal cells with proliferative potential to the lifeless, flattened squames of the stratum corneum. The stratum corneum serves as the principal physical barrier against the percutaneous penetration of chemical substances and microbial assaults and is capable of withstanding mechanical forces [7–9].

The 10–20 μm thick stratum corneum forms a continuous sheet of protein-enriched cells, embedded in an

intercellular matrix, enriched in nonpolar lipids, and organized as lamellar lipid layers. Keratinocytes synthesize and express numerous structural proteins and lipids during their maturation. The final steps in keratinocyte differentiation are associated with profound changes in their structure, resulting in their transformation into flat and anucleated squamous cells of the stratum corneum. The corneocytes contain abundant keratin filament proteins to withstand mechanical forces, and the cell membrane is surrounded by a cell envelope composed of cross-linked proteins (cornified envelope proteins) as well as a covalently-bound lipid envelope. Extracellular

Fig. 6.2 The skin's permeability barrier is formed during epidermal proliferation and differentiation. Structural proteins, keratins, involucrin, loricrin, and filaggrin as well as skin lipids are important for skin barrier function

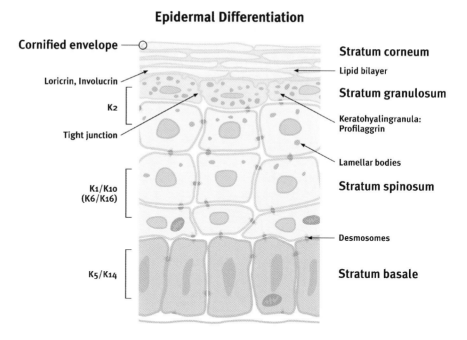

Epidermal Differentiation

nonpolar lipids surround the corneocytes to form a hydrophobic matrix. The cornified envelope proteins as well as the covalently bound lipid envelope are thought to be important for the chemical resistance of the corneocytes. Desmosomes, which interconnect adjacent keratinocytes, are important for stratum corneum cohesion and are shed during the desquamation process [10].

In the upper spinous and granular layers, characteristic lamellar vesicles appear, which are called epidermal lamellar bodies. These are enriched in polar lipids, glycosphingolipids, free sterols, phospholipids, and catabolic enzymes which deliver the lipids required for the SC's extracellular layers. The lipids derived from the lamellar bodies are subsequently modified and rearranged into intercellular lamellae positioned approximately parallel to the cell surface. The covalently-bound lipid envelope acts as a scaffold for this process. After the extrusion of the lamellar bodies into the stratum granulosum–stratum corneum interface, the polar lipids are enzymatically converted into nonpolar products. Hydrolysis of glycosphingolipids generates ceramides while phospholipids are converted into free fatty acids. These changes in lipid composition and cell structure result in the formation of a very

dense structure packed into the interstices of the stratum corneum [11] (Fig. 6.2).

6.3 Skin Lipids

Confocal laser scanning microscopy and X-ray microanalysis studies have shown that the major route of penetration results in the tortuous halfway between the corneocytes, confirming that the intercellular lipids play an irreplaceable role in regulating skin barrier function [9]. Also, creams and ointments that are most important to treat and prevent contact eczema are mainly composed of lipids or lipid-like chemical. The major physiological lipid classes in the stratum corneum are cholesterol, free fatty acids, and ceramides [12–14]. Cholesterol is probably the most abundant lipid in the entire body and part of the plasma membrane and also part of the intercellular lipid lamellae in the stratum corneum. Although the basal cells are capable of resorbing cholesterol from circulation, most cholesterol in the epidermis is synthesized in situ from acetate [15]. The epidermal keratinocyte, the main cell type in the

6

epidermis, is highly active in the synthesis of several lipids, including cholesterol and free fatty acids.

The skin contains free fatty acids as well as fatty acids bound in triglycerides, phospholipids, glycosylceramides, and ceramides. Saturated and monounsaturated fatty acids are synthesized in the epidermis, in contrast to di- and polyunsaturated acids. The nonessential monounsaturated fatty acid, the oleic acid, is a ω-9-fatty acid. The most important double unsaturated fatty acid, linoleic acid, is a ω-6 fatty acid. ω-6 fatty acids are essential fatty acids. An essential fatty acid deficient diet (EFAD) in mice leads to redness, rough and scaly skin characterized by a disturbed skin barrier function and epidermal thickening due to epidermal hyperproliferation [16]. The clinical, histological, and biochemical features of EFAD mice resemble eczema. No skin changes due to an ω-3-fatty acid deficiency are currently known; however, it has been proposed that these fatty acids are important for the resolution of inflammation. ω-3-fatty acids are obtained from fish, whereas ω-6-fatty acids are obtained from plant oils [17, 18]. Linoleic acid is part of phospholipids, glucosylceramides, ceramide 1, ceramide 4, and ceramide 9 [19]. It has been proposed that the linoleic acid metabolite γ-linoleic acid is of special importance for atopic eczema.

Ceramide (sphingolipid) is an amide-linked fatty acid containing a long-chain amino alcohol called sphingoid base. Ceramide is a major lipid component in the stratum corneum, accounting for 30–40% of lipids by weight. The stratum corneum contains at least nine different ceramides. In addition, there are two protein-bound ceramides, ceramide A and ceramide B. These ceramides are covalently bound to cornified envelope proteins, most importantly to involucrin [15, 19–21] (Fig. 6.3).

The regulation of the lipid metabolism is also important, and drugs interfering with the lipid metabolism are used to treat eczema. ABCA1 is a membrane transporter responsible for cholesterol efflux and plays a pivotal role in regulating cellular cholesterol levels. It was demonstrated that ABCA1 is expressed in cultured human keratinocytes and murine epidermis. Liver X receptor (LXR) activation and activation of peroxisome proliferator-activated receptor (PPAR)-α, PPAR-ss/δ and retinoid X receptor (RXR) increased ABCA1 expression in keratinocyte cultures. Thus the cholesterol levels for permeability barrier function are regulated by ABCA1, LXR, and PPARs. Unsaturated fatty acids used in creams and ointment for years may regulate PPARs [20]. The cellular fatty acid transport and metabolism is regulated by fatty acid-binding proteins (FABPs) [22].

6.4 Epidermal Proliferation and Differentiation

To provide this physical barrier of the stratum corneum, not only intercellular lipids, but also the corneocytes are of crucial importance [8, 23]. Keratinocytes arise from stem cells in the basal layers and transient amplification cells and move to a series of differentiation events until they are finally brought to desquamation [24]. Thus, in the normal epidermis, there is a balance between the processes of proliferation and desquamation.

Keratins are major structural proteins synthesized in keratinocytes. During the final stages of normal differentiation, keratins are aligned into highly ordered and condensed arrays through interactions with filaggrin, a matrix protein. This promotes the collapse of the cell into a flattened shape, which is characteristic of corneocytes in the cornified layer [8, 23].

The structural proteins involucrin, loricrin, trichohyalin, and the class of small proline-rich proteins are synthesized and subsequently cross-linked by transglutaminases to reinforce the cornified envelope just beneath the plasma membrane. The proteins of the cornified envelope constitute about 7–10% of the mass of the epidermis. These corneocytes provide the bulwark of mechanical and chemical protection, and together with their intercellular lipid surroundings, confer water-impermeability. The cornified cell envelope is a tough protein/lipid polymer structure formed just below the cytoplasmic membrane and subsequently resides on the exterior of the corneocytes. It consists of two parts: a protein envelope and a lipid envelope. The protein envelope contributes to the biomechanical properties of the corneocytes as a result of the cross-linking of specialized cornified envelope structural proteins by both disulfide bonds and N(epsilon)-(gamma-glutamyl)lysine isopeptide bonds formed by transglutaminases [9, 23]. The isopeptide bonds are resistant to most common proteolytic enzymes. The corneocyte-bound lipid envelope is a plasma membrane-like structure, which replaces the plasma membrane on the external aspect of the mammalian corneocytes. Involucrin, envoplakin, periplakin serve as substrates for the covalent attachment of ω-hydroxyceramides with very long chain N-acyl fatty acids by ester linkage [20, 21] (Fig. 6.2).

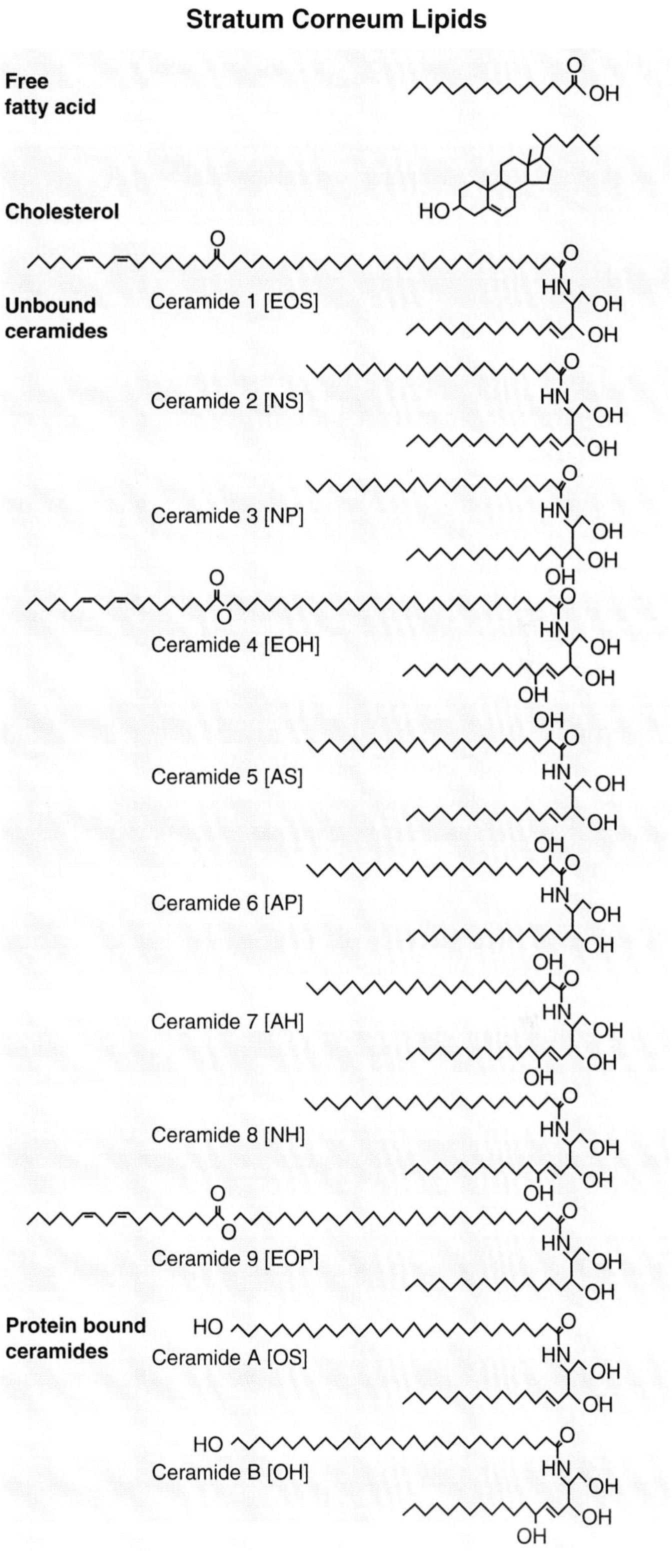

Fig. 6.3 The stratum corneum contains three classes of lipids: free fatty acids, cholesterol, and ceramides. Ceramides are unbound or protein bound, mainly to involucrin

Stratum Corneum Lipids

Free fatty acid

Cholesterol

Unbound ceramides

Ceramide 1 [EOS]

Ceramide 2 [NS]

Ceramide 3 [NP]

Ceramide 4 [EOH]

Ceramide 5 [AS]

Ceramide 6 [AP]

Ceramide 7 [AH]

Ceramide 8 [NH]

Ceramide 9 [EOP]

Protein bound ceramides

Ceramide A [OS]

Ceramide B [OH]

6

> **Core Message**
>
> › The main permeability barrier of the skin is located in the stratum corneum and consists of corneocytes and intercellular lipid bilayers. The barrier is formed during epidermal differentiation.

6.5 Tight Junctions and Desmosomal Proteins: A Second-Line Epidermal Barrier

Tight junctions are cell-junctions sealing neighboring cells and controlling the paracellular parts of molecules. The most important tight junction proteins in the human epidermis are occludin, claudins, and zonal occluding proteins (ZOs). In various diseases with perturbed SC barrier function, e.g., psoriasis vulgaris, lichen planus, acute and chronic eczema, and ichthyosis vulgaris, tight junction proteins that were formerly restricted to the stratum granulosum and upper stratum spinosum were also found in the deeper layers of the epidermis [25].

Desmogleins are desmosomal cadherins that play a major role in stabilizing cell–cell adhesion in the living layers of the epidermis. Autoantibodies against these transmembrane glycoproteins cause blisters in pemphigus vulgaris due to the loss of keratinocyte adhesion. In acute eczema, which shows disturbed skin barrier function, a reduction in keratinocyte membrane E-cadherin in areas of spongiosis has been found [26–28]. In transgenic mice in which the distribution of desmoglein 3 in epidermis was similar to that in the mucous membrane, a highly increased TEWL resulted in lethality during the first week of life due to dehydration [29, 30].

6.6 Cytokine Signaling: Regulation of Epidermal Homeostasis and Repair

Cytokines are very important for the regulation of skin barrier repair. Besides the immune cells, keratinocytes are able to produce a large variety and amount of cytokines.

Of special importance are the so-called primary cytokines TNF, IL-1, and IL-6, which are potent mitogens and stimulators of lipid synthesis. The acute increase in TNF, IL-1, and IL-6 after barrier disruption is crucial for skin barrier repair. However, if barrier disruption is prolonged and a chronic increase in cytokine production occurs as in chronic contact dermatitis, it could have a harmful effect leading to inflammation and epidermal proliferation (reviewed in: [10]).

6.7 Experimental Barrier Disruption, Lipids and Protein Modification in Epidermal Differentiation

Experimental acute or chronic barrier disruption leads to changes in skin lipids, epidermal keratin, and cornified envelope protein expression. Increase in epidermal lipids and changes in lipid processing enzymes have been described in numerous studies [31, 32]. Also, in diseases accompanied by a disturbed skin barrier function, psoriasis and different forms of eczema changes in lipid content and composition have been noted (reviewed in [10]).

Experimental skin barrier disruption also influences structural proteins of the skin. Increased expression of the basal keratins K5 and K14 and a reduction of the differentiation-related keratins K1 and K10 were noted. In addition, there was expression of the proliferation-associated keratins K6 and K16 as well as the inflammation-associated keratin K17. Experimental permeability barrier disruption leads to a premature expression of involucrin, but not loricrin (reviewed in [1]). Overexpression of filaggrin in mice in the suprabasal epidermis resulted in a delayed barrier repair [33].

Changes in epidermal proliferation and differentiation are also seen in inflammatory skin diseases with a disturbed skin barrier function. Increased proliferation is one of the main characteristics of psoriasis, but also in atopic dermatitis lesional skin there is a considerable increase in epidermal proliferation [24]. Also, changes in keratins and cornified envelope proteins occur in inflammatory skin diseases [34]. Overall, this shows that epidermal lipids, proliferation, and differentiation regulate skin barrier function.

Core Message

> ❯ Acute skin barrier disruption by mechanical forces or chemicals leads to a repair response which involves an increase in epidermal lipid synthesis, increase in proliferation, and changes in differentiation.

6.8 Barrier Disturbance in Contact Dermatitis

As was mentioned in the introduction, contact dermatitis usually starts with a disturbance of the skin barrier that in the course of disease continues to play an important role [2–6]. The most common agents that induce barrier damages under occupational conditions are water, detergents, solvents, dryness, and a diversity of chemicals. Many experimental models were applied to investigate the pathophysiology of the evolving barrier impairment under defined conditions, mostly by use of repeated applications of irritants like sodium laury sulfate (SLS, also named sodium dodecyl sulfate, SDS) to the skin or a single application of SLS in a patch test chamber for 24 h. In addition, many analytic and interventional studies were done with employees in specific working environments (metal workers, hairdressers, health care workers, etc.). In the following, the most important findings from such investigations as well as from other skin disorders with disturbed barrier function will be discussed.

Core Message

> ❯ Skin barrier disruption is the first step in the pathophysiology of irritant and allergic contact dermatitis.

6.9 Pathological Skin Barriers: Skin Barrier Function in Dermatoses

Most inflammatory skin lesions are covered with dry scales or scale-crusts due to the disturbed epidermal differentiation and a stratum corneum with poor water-holding capacity. Inflammatory skin diseases can be produced by either exogenous or endogenous causes. In contact dermatitis, disruption of the barrier by irritants and allergens is the primary event, followed by sensitization, inflammation, increased epidermal proliferation, and changes in differentiation. Dermatophytosis is accompanied by functional and anatomical alterations of the barrier [35]. Interestingly, new findings indicate that the permeability and antimicrobial barriers are coordinately regulated [36, 37]. In T-cell lymphoma (mycosis fungoides), an endogenous cause for barrier disruption, changes in epidermal proliferation, and differentiation, by expansion of clonal malignant CD4+ T-cells is obvious [25]. In atopic dermatitis and in psoriasis, it is debatable whether permeability barrier disruption is followed by inflammation or whether inflammation leads to epidermal changes including barrier dysfunction. The vast majority of reports on the pathogenesis of atopic dermatitis and even more on psoriasis focused on the primary role of abnormalities in the immune system [92]. However, others have proposed an "outside–inside" pathogenesis for atopic dermatitis and other inflammatory dermatoses with barrier abnormalities [13, 38], as an alternative to the current "inside–outside" paradigm.

6.10 Atopic Dermatitis as a Model for the Consequence of a Chronically Disturbed Barrier

It is well known from many observations that individuals suffering from atopic dermatitis have a higher risk to acquire occupational contact dermatitis under appropriate working conditions than individuals without atopic dermatitis. Also, hand eczema continuing after stopping work in which pollutions with chemicals occurs, is often caused by atopic genetic predisposition, and called atopic hand eczema. Since the existence of a defective permeability barrier function in atopic dermatitis is now widely accepted, this disorder appears to be a suitable model to study the principles and effects of barrier impairment.

A genetically impaired skin barrier function is already present in nonlesional and more pronounced in lesional skin in atopic dermatitis. Increased epidermal proliferation and disturbed differentiation, including changes in keratins and cornified envelope proteins involucrin, loricrin, and filaggrin, and in lipid composition, cause impaired barrier function in atopic dermatitis [39]. Recently, mutations in the filaggrin gene in atopic dermatitis have been described [40–42]. Two loss-of-function genetic variants in the gene encoding filaggrin are strong predisposing factors for atopic dermatitis in atopic kindreds of European origin [43, 44]. Later on, different mutations have also been found in the Japanese and in the Chinese population. Filaggrin mutations are detectable in about 20% of the patients with atopic dermatitis and in about 50% of the patients with severe disease. The mutations were also significantly associated with asthma, independent of atopic dermatitis, which means that genetic factors that compromise the epidermal barrier could also underlie mucosal atopic diseases (filaggrin is a protein that is unique to keratinizing epithelia). The atopic syndrome represents a genetically impaired skin barrier function as well as impaired nasal, bronchial, and intestinal mucous membranes leading to atopic dermatitis, allergic rhinitis, bronchial asthma, or aggravation of atopic dermatitis [45]. Defective permeability barrier function enables penetration of environmental allergens, in particular allergens from house dust mites, cat dander, and grass pollen, into the skin and initiates immunological reactions and inflammation. Recently, it was shown that a high prevalence of delayed sensitization to indoor and outdoor aeroallergens in infants with atopic dermatitis is related to a high TEWL, indicating a major role of constitutive epidermal barrier impairment in determining early atopen sensitization in infants with atopic dermatitis [46].

Filaggrin mutation is the first strong genetic factor identified in this complex disease. Filaggrin hydrolysis generates amino acids in their deiminated products such as pyrrolidon carboxylic acid and transurocanic acid, which serve as endogenous humectants [4]. This may explain the dry skin well-known in atopic dermatitis.

Whether filaggrin mutations are important for hand eczema is debatable. In one study, it was found that filaggrin null alleles are not associated with hand eczema or contact allergy [17, 47]. Others found a correlation; one study point toward an association between the filaggrin null alleles and the subgroup of patients having both hand eczema and atopic dermatitis [48–50].

The impaired skin barrier function in atopic dermatitis is also caused by reduced lipid content or impaired lipid composition in atopic dermatitis. In particular, a decreased content of the total amount and of certain types of ceramides has been described [39]. A decrease in covalently-bound ceramides [26] and a reduced sphingomyelinase activity has been found in atopic dermatitis. Also, decreased lamellar body secretion, which is predominantly composed of lipids, with subsequent entombment of lamellar bodies within corneocytes, has been reported [51].

> **Core Message**
>
> › Filaggrin mutations resulting in a disturbed skin barrier function and dry skin are found in about 20% of the patients with atopic dermatitis and may have a role in contact dermatitis.

6.11 Influence of the Permeability Barrier on the Immune System and Contact Dermatitis

The most important protection mechanism against contact dermatitis is the intact permeability barrier. Only after the impairment of the physical barrier, allergens may penetrate into the skin, come into contact with immune cells and cause immunological reactions. An injury to the skin, e.g., a wound, erosion, a scratch, burns, or irritant contact dermatitis precedes an allergic contact dermatitis. Also, occlusion by a patch test chamber leads to a disruption of the barrier by hyperhydration and this allows the allergens to penetrate into the skin [52, 53].

A pronounced disturbance of the skin barrier is present after the loss of the entire epidermis in erosions and wounds. Also in any form of inflammatory skin disease, visible as reddening of the skin, there is a disturbed skin barrier function. In burns of first and second degree there is a barrier disruption though the epidermis seems to be intact. In all kinds of eczema (dermatitis), irritant and allergic contact dermatitis, seborrheic dermatitis, and atopic dermatitis the barrier is significantly disturbed. In all of these diseases, an additional sensitization may develop after contact with allergens. Very often an allergic contact dermatitis develops after an irritant contact dermatitis. The irritant compounds may be different from the allergens; however, the compound itself may have a dual function. Many strong allergens, like poison ivy, DNCB (dinitro chloro benzene), diphenylcyclopropenone, or squaric acid dibutylester (both are used to treat alopecia areata by inducing a strong inflammation by a strong allergic reaction which may stimulate the hair follicle for hair growth) are strong irritants and may lead to an allergic contact dermatitis after the first contact. These chemicals first destroy the permeability barrier; thereafter, penetrate into the skin and cause an irritant contact dermatitis (which may not always be visible with a single contact). Subsequently, the contact of the allergens with the immune system leads to sensitization and an allergic contact dermatitis. With weak allergens like nickel, an injury of the skin must occur first like a pinprick for ear lops or repeated contact with water and detergents. Also in psoriasis, ichthyosis, and mycosis fungoides, there is inflammation and a disturbed barrier function. However, in these diseases an allergic contact dermatitis occurs very seldom. This may be due to changes in the immune surveillance. Particularly, T-cells are changed in mycosis fungoides [54].

The disturbed permeability barrier leads to different reactions of keratinocytes and immune cells, with the goal to repair the permeability barrier and to remove invaded substances from the skin. An important mechanism is the stimulation of epidermal proliferation. The proliferation rate is increased after experimental skin barrier disruption, in fungal infection and in atopic dermatitis [31, 35, 55]. A physiological increase of proliferation is known after injury to the skin and in bacterial and mycotic infections. Invaded substances will be eliminated fast if the proliferation rate is high. It is well-known that a fungal infection in young people may heal quickly because of the high proliferation rate which removes fungal hyphae, whereas a fungal infection may persist and even spread in aged people.

After penetration into the skin, Langerhans cells take up and process foreign substances and initiate an α,β-T-cell dependent immune response. Langerhans cell density is increased in chronic dermatitis [1]. It has been postulated that epidermal exposure to any penetrating substance should activate the local Langerhans cell system, including antigen processing and presentation. Furthermore, epidermal exposure to any substance should lead to the migration of immune competent cells into the dermis, to ensure antigen recognition or pathogen elimination. The extent of cellular traffic is less pronounced in positive patch test reactions, in which antigen recognition and activation of sensitized T-cells may trigger amplification mechanisms [56].

In mice, it was shown that elicitation of allergic reactions through barrier-disrupted skin decreased the expression of mRNA for IL-2 and IFN-gamma, but not for IL-4. These findings suggest that the percutaneous entry of environmental allergens through barrier-disrupted skin is strongly associated with the induction of Th2-dominant immunological responses, as is seen in atopic dermatitis [57].

We examined the interrelationship between skin barrier function and the immune system. An experimental disruption of the skin barrier was achieved by the treatment of human skin with acetone, sodium dodecylsulphate (SDS), or tape stripping. Serial biopsies were performed 6–168 h after treatment, and Langerhans cells were complexed with anti-CD1a (Leu6) or S-100 antibodies. Acetone treatment, tape stripping, or sodium laury sulfate (SDS) treatment resulted in a significant increase in epidermal Langerhans cell density [58]. There was a linear correlation between the degree of barrier disruption and the increase in epidermal Langerhans cell density. The time curves of the increase in Langerhans cell density and the increase in epidermal proliferation were similar, suggesting that there was a coordinate regulation. In contrast to the previous studies of reactions to patch tests after 24 h to allergens or irritants, disruption of barrier function neither resulted in an increased dermal Langerhans cell density, nor influenced T lymphocyte, macrophages, ICAM-1 or ELAM-1 expression in the skin. In addition, barrier disruption did not result in an increase of inflammatory cells in the dermis [59]. Occlusion by a latex wrap, which partially restored the barrier, reduced the increase in Langerhans cell density. Others showed that a subpopulation of Langerhans cells in acetone-rubbed or tape-stripped mouse skin which expressed major histocompatibility complex class II CD54 and CD86 was increased [60].

> **Core Message**
>
> › A disturbed skin barrier function influences the immune surveillance.

6

6.12 Barrier and Patch Testing

We examined the impact of the interrelation of the skin barrier and the immune system by patch test studies. Barrier disruption was induced by acetone on the upper arms in volunteers with known sensitization to nickel, fragrance mix, or p-phenylenediamine. Twenty-four hours after this treatment the relevant allergen was applied without occlusion or with Finn chambers. Twenty-four hours after the application of the allergen, clinical grading and TEWL measurements were performed and biopsies were taken. Immunohistochemical stainings for Langerhans cells and epidermal proliferation were performed. Open applications of the allergens after acetone pretreatment resulted in strong allergic test reactions. TEWL, which showed a 70% recovery 24 h after acetone treatment, was increased again fourfold by the allergic test reactions. Langerhans cell density, which was increased by 80% 24 h after acetone-induced barrier disruption, was further enhanced 2.4-fold in total. Epidermal proliferation showed a sixfold increase after open application of the allergens. Under patch test conditions after acetone pretreatment very strong bullous reactions were observed. These findings indicate that the increase in epidermal LC density induced by epidermal permeability barrier disruption is accompanied by an enhanced response in allergic contact dermatitis [59] (Table 6.1).

More than 50 years ago, a modified patch test method was described that takes advantage of a skin barrier impairment via reduction of the stratum corneum by stripping with adhesive tape prior to the application of test allergens [19]. This procedure has in fact successfully been used in occupational dermatology for patch testing with materials that were considered possible work-related allergens [61, 62]. In recent years, efforts were taken to further develop this technique and especially to establish a basis for its standardization [63–66]. The main advantages of this "strip" patch test are that due to the reduction of the stratum corneum it can be used for substances with a poor epicutaneous penetration, and due to an induction of an enhanced epidermal inflammatory background as described above, it may in fact create conditions more appropriate for the development of an unambiguous patch test reaction than a conventional patch test. Interestingly, an artificial mechanical disruption of the skin barrier prior to irritant patch testing was not found to improve the test design [67]. Due to the barrier disruption with its consequences for

Table 6.1 Langerhans cell density and epidermal proliferation after allergen application ± barrier disruption by pretreatment with acetone (acute irritant contact) (modified after [59])

	Langerhans cell density (cells/mm)	Proliferation (Ki-67+ cells/mm)
Untreated	2.08	7.1
Barrier disruption by acetone treatment[a]	3.89	11.95
Barrier disruption + allergen[b]	5.09	42.6
Barrier disruption + allergen + patch test chamber[c]	3.97	29.2
Allergen + patch test chamber (without acetone treatment)[d]	3.31	8.3

[a]Acute irritant contact by acetone disrupts the permeability barrier and leads to an increase of epidermal Langerhans cell density

[b]Allergen application enhances the effects

[c]The occlusive patch test chamber reduces the effects

[b–d]Acetone pretreatment + allergen application shows a more pronounced effect compared to the usual patch test application of the allergen alone

allergen penetration and immunological surveillance, a well-designed "strip" patch test may thus be a more sensitive test method to verify contact allergy in certain occupational dermatoses than a conventional patch test.

Core Message

> Patch testing leads to disruption of the skin barrier which allows for penetration of chemicals into the skin, followed by immune reaction.

6.13 Treatment Implications and Approaches: Restoring the Skin's Protective Function

Although it is undisputed that therapeutic interventions in occupational contact dermatitis should aim for a rapid and lasting restoration of the epidermal barrier it is far from clear as to how this can be achieved [22].

Treatment strategies in inflammatory diseases often address immunogenic abnormalities and barrier function. Treatment with corticosteroids, cyclosporin, tacrolimus, pimecrolimus, and UV light has been shown to reduce cell inflammation as well as improve barrier function to a certain degree, thus helping to normalize proliferation and differentiation. However, because of certain side effects, these treatments should be used for a limited time only.

In this context, we examined whether corticosteroids or the calcineurin inhibitors have an influence on the disrupted skin barrier in atopic dermatitis. To prevent sensitization by environmental allergens, it is essential that drugs applied in atopic dermatitis restore the impaired epidermal barrier. Stratum corneum hydration and transepidermal water loss (TEWL), a marker of the inside–outside barrier, improved under treatment with corticosteroids and the calcineurin inhibitor pimecrolimus. Dye penetration, a marker of the outside–inside barrier, was also reduced by both the drugs. Electron microscopic evaluation of the barrier structure displayed ordered stratum corneum lipid layers and regular lamellar body extrusion in pimecrolimus-treated skin, but inconsistent extracellular lipid bilayers and only partially filled lamellar bodies after betamethasone treatment. Both the drugs normalized epidermal differentiation and reduced epidermal hyperproliferation. Betamethasone was superior in reducing clinical symptoms and epidermal proliferation, however, led to epidermal thinning. It follows that both betamethasone and pimecrolimus improve clinical and biophysical parameters, and epidermal differentiation. As pimecrolimus improved the epidermal barrier and did not cause atrophy, it may be more suitable for long-term treatment of atopic dermatitis and also hand eczema [68].

The chronic use of corticosteroids should also be avoided in contact eczema because a barrier repair does not occur during that treatment. In contrast, application of bland creams and ointments containing lipids and lipid-like substances, hydrocarbons, fatty acids, cholesterol esters, and triglycerides can be used without side-effects for long-term treatment of mild to moderate inflammatory diseases. Creams and ointments partially correct or stimulate barrier repair and increase stratum corneum hydration [34, 69–71], thus influencing epidermal proliferation and differentiation [72, 73]. It has been proposed that a lipid mixture containing the three key lipid groups (ceramides, cholesterol, and free fatty acids) is able to improve skin barrier function and stratum corneum hydration in atopic dermatitis [74]. Also, the efficacy of ceramide 3 in a nanoparticle cream in atopic dermatitis has been described [75]. However, because several research groups and companies report that creams containing ceramides and a mixture of the three key lipids are not superior to "classical" cream or ointment preparations, such preparations have not yet been widely used. More research is necessary to determine the significance of ceramides and the composition of creams and ointments with the most therapeutic benefit.

Retinoids have been in use to treat hyperkeratotic skin diseases like psoriasis, ichthyosis, or the chronic form of hand eczema with fissures since many years. Recently, a new orally given drug, the retinoid alitretinoin (Toctino[R]) has been introduced to treat hand eczema. Alitretinoin is an endogenous retinoid and acts as a pan-agonist at retinoid receptors, binding with high affinity to both retinoic acid receptors and RXR [76]. Oral alitretinoin once daily is approved for use in patients with severe chronic hand eczema unresponsive to treatment with potent topical corticosteroids. Retinoids influence epidermal proliferation and differentiation and that in turn influences skin barrier function [77]. Treatment with the classical retinoids 13-*cis*-retinoic acid or the aromatic retinoids (NeoTigason) does not result in a complete barrier repair of the skin barrier in diseased skin. The influence of the more selective retinoid alitretinoin on the skin barrier has not been examined to our knowledge.

It is well accepted that bland creams and ointments help repair a disturbed skin barrier function in atopic dermatitis or contact dermatitis. However, detailed electron microscopy studies showing barrier repair or penetration studies are lacking. Numerous studies using TEWL after the use of emollients exist. However, measurements of the TEWL are only an indirect marker for the skin barrier and only for the "inside–outside" barrier which does not correlate always with the "outside–inside" barrier. TEWL depends on skin temperature and skin hydration [68, 78]. After corticosteroid treatment, the known vasoconstrictive effect of the drug shows a decrease in TEWL which mimics skin barrier repair. Measurements of the TEWL immediately after the application of an emulsion show an increased TEWL simply by the evaporation of excessive water.

6

The use of so called barrier creams is debatable. Barrier creams may improve the "outside–inside" barrier against certain chemicals. The choice of the right barrier cream for the respective chemical is crucial [79–82]. Nevertheless, the effect of barrier creams is often small [82]. Under certain circumstances, barrier creams may even enhance penetration [83, 84]. Protection against corrosive chemicals or chronic contact with irritants and allergens is much better achieved by gloves as compared to barrier creams. However, corrosive chemicals may even penetrate gloves.

Appropriate gloves can definitely protect the skin from harmful irritants, but on the other hand, their occlusive effect resulting in hyperhydration can disturb the epidermal barrier [52, 53, 85]. Hyperhydration is pronounced during exhausting labor which results in sweating. Gloves that allow for a certain degree of water binding and evaporation should be preferred.

For the follow-up of patients recovering from a barrier disturbance due to occupational dermatoses, it is of particular importance to consider that a complete barrier restoration is a long-lasting process that is not finished when the skin has regained its normal phenotype [86–91]. Therefore, care must be taken that the skin of such patients remains protected from all barrier injuries for several weeks beyond the apparent clinical healing.

In summary, an intact skin barrier is of crucial importance for the prevention of occupational skin disease. Treatment strategies must include barrier repair to prevent relapse of the disease.

Core Message

> Repair of the disturbed skin barrier is an important goal in the treatment of contact dermatitis. Corticosteroids delay skin barrier repair. In contrast, treatment with bland creams and ointments supports barrier repair and should be used after initial anti-inflammatory therapy. TEWL is not always a reliable marker of skin barrier. Patients with contact dermatitis should restart working only after complete restoration of the skin barrier.

References

1. Rosén K, Jontell M, Mobacken H, Rosdahl I (1989) Epidermal Langerhans' cells in chronic eczematous dermatitis of the palms treated with PUVA and UVB. Acta Derm Venereol 69:200–205
2. Del Rosso J (2001) Protecting the hand-skin barrier in the workplace. Occup Health Saf 70:116–120
3. Antezana M, Parker F (2003) Occupational contact dermatitis. Immunol Allergy Clin North Am 23:269–290
4. Slodownik D, Nixon R (2007) Occupational factors in skin diseases. Curr Probl Dermatol 35:173–189
5. Fluhr JW, Darlenski R, Angelova-Fischer I, Tsankov N, Basketter D (2008) Skin irritation and sensitization: mechanisms and new approaches for risk assessment. 1. Skin irritation. Skin Pharmacol Physiol 21:124–135
6. Nielsen JB, Nielsen F, Sørensen JA (2007) Defense against dermal exposures is only skin deep: significantly increased penetration through slightly damaged skin. Arch Dermatol Res 299:423–431
7. Madison KC (2003) Barrier function of the skin: "la raison d'etre" of the epidermis. J Invest Dermatol 121:231–241
8. Roop D (1995) Defects in the barrier. Science 267:474
9. Candi E, Schmidt R, Melino G (2005) The cornified envelope: a model of cell death in the skin. Nat Rev Mol Cell Biol 6:328–340
10. Proksch E, Brandner JM, Jensen JM (2008) The skin: an indispensable barrier. Exp Dermatol 17:1063–1072
11. Bouwstra JA, Pilgrim K, Ponec M (2006) Structure of the skin barrier. In: Elias PM, Feingold KR (eds) Skin barrier. Taylor & Francis, New York, pp 65
12. Elias PM (1983) Epidermal lipids, barrier function, and desquamation. J Invest Dermatol 80:44s
13. Gray GM, Yardley HJ (1975) Different populations of pig epidermal cells: isolation and lipid composition. J Lipid Res 16:441–447
14. Downing DT, Stewart ME, Wertz PW, Colton SW, Abraham W, Strauss J (1987) Skin lipids: an update. J Invest Dermatol 88:2s–6s
15. Wertz PW (2006) Biochemistry of human stratum corneum lipids. In: Elias PM, Feingold KR (eds) Skin barrier. Taylor & Francis, New York, pp 33
16. Proksch E, Feingold KR, Elias PM (1992) Epidermal HMG CoA reductase activity in essential fatty acid deficiency: barrier requirements rather than eicosanoid generation regulate cholesterol synthesis. J Invest Dermatol 99:216–220
17. Brown SJ, Cordell HJ (2008) Are filaggrin mutations associated with hand eczema or contact allergy?–we do not know. Br J Dermatol 158:1383–1384
18. Elias PM, Feingold KR (2001) Does the tail wag the dog? Role of the barrier in the pathogenesis of inflammatory dermatoses and therapeutic implications. Arch Dermatol 137:1079–1081
19. Uchida Y, Hamanaka S (2006) Stratum corneum ceramides: function, origins, and therapeutic implications. In: Elias PM, Feingold KR (eds) Skin barrier. Taylor & Francis, New York, pp 43
20. Marekov LN, Steinert PM (1998) Ceramides are bound to structural proteins of the human foreskin epidermal cornified cell envelope. J Biol Chem 273:17763–17770

21. Swartzendruber DC, Wertz PW, Madison KC, Downing DT (1987) Evidence that the corneocyte has a chemically bound lipid envelope. J Invest Dermatol 88:709
22. Schurer NY (2002) Implementation of fatty acid carriers to skin irritation and the epidermal barrier. Contact Derm 47:199–205
23. Nemes Z, Steinert PM (1999) Bricks and mortar of the epidermal barrier. Exp Mol Med 31:5–19
24. Webb A, Li A, Kaur P (2004) Location and phenotype of human adult keratinocyte stem cells of the skin. Differentiation 72:387–395
25. Brandner JM, Proksch E (2006) Epidermal barrier function: role of tight junctions. In: Elias PM, Feingold KR (eds) Skin barrier. Taylor & Francis, New York, pp 191
26. Maretzky T, Reiss K, Ludwig A, Buchholz J, Scholz F, Proksch E, de Strooper B, Hartmann D, Saftig P (2005) ADAM10 mediates E-cadherin shedding and regulates epithelial cell-cell adhesion, migration, and beta-catenin translocation. Proc Natl Acad Sci USA 102:9182–9187
27. Maretzky T, Scholz F, Köten B, Proksch E, Saftig P, Reiss K (2008) ADAM10-mediated E-cadherin release is regulated by proinflammatory cytokines and modulates keratinocyte cohesion in eczematous dermatitis. J Invest Dermatol 128:1737–1746
28. Trautmann A, Altznauer F, Akdis M, Simon HU, Disch R, Brocker EB, Blaser K, Akdis CA (2001) The differential fate of cadherins during T-cell-induced keratinocyte apoptosis leads to spongiosis in eczematous dermatitis. J Invest Dermatol 117:927–934
29. Elias PM, Matsuyoshi N, Wu H, Lin C, Wang ZH, Brown BE, Stanley JR (2001) Desmoglein isoform distribution affects stratum corneum structure and function. J Cell Biol 153:243–249
30. Tunggal JA, Helfrich I, Schmitz A, Schwarz H, Gunzel D, Fromm M, Kemler R, H Krieg T, Nissen CM (2005) E-cadherin is essential for in vivo epidermal barrier function by regulating tight junctions. EMBO J 24:1146–1156
31. Jensen JM, Fölster-Holst R, Baranowsky A, Schunck M, Winoto-Morbach S, Neumann C, Schütze S, Proksch E (2004) Impaired sphingomyelinase activity and epidermal differentiation in atopic dermatitis. J Invest Dermatol 122:1423–1431
32. Proksch E, Elias PM, Feingold KR (1990) Regulation of 3-hydroxy-3-methylglutaryl-coenzyme A reductase activity in murine epidermis modulation of enzyme content and activation state by barrier requirements. J Clin Invest 85:874
33. Ishida-Yamamoto A, Iizuka H (1998) Structural organization of cornified cell envelopes and alterations in inherited skin disorders. Exp Dermatol 7:1–10
34. Jensen JM, Proksch E, Elias PM (2006) The stratum corneum of the epidermis in atopic dermatitis. In: Elias PM, Feingold KR (eds) Skin barrier. Taylor & Francis, New York, pp 569
35. Brasch J (2009) Current knowledge of host response in human tinea Mycoses 52:304–312
36. Aberg KM, Man MQ, Gallo RL, Ganz T, Crumrine D, Brown BE, Choi EH, Kim DK, Schröder JM, Feingold KR, Elias PM (2008) Co-regulation and interdependence of the mammalian epidermal permeability and antimicrobial barriers. J Invest Dermatol 128:917–925
37. Gläser R, Meyer-Hoffert U, Harder J, Cordes J, Wittersheim M, Kobliakova J, Fölster-Holst R, Proksch E, Schröder JM, Schwarz T (2009) The antimicrobial protein psoriasin (S100A7) is upregulated in atopic dermatitis and after experimental skin barrier disruption. J Invest Dermatol 129: 641–649
38. Proksch E, Jensen JM, Elias PM (2003) Skin lipids and epidermal differentiation in atopic dermatitis. Clin Dermatol 21:134
39. Proksch E, Foelster-Holst R, Jensen JM (2006) Skin barrier function, epidermal proliferation and differentiation in eczema. J Dermatol Sci 43:159–169
40. Palmer CN, Irvine AD, Terron-Kwiatkowski A, Zhao Y, Liao H, Lee SP, Goudie DR, Sandilands A, Campbell LE, Smith FJ, O'Regan GM, Watson RM, Cecil JE, Bale SJ, Compton JG, DiGiovanna JJ, Fleckman P, Lewis-Jones S, Arseculeratne G, Sergeant A, Munro CS, El Houate B, McElreavey K, Halkjaer LB, Bisgaard H, Mukhopadhyay S, McLean WH (2006) Common loss-of-function variants of the epidermal barrier protein filaggrin are a major predisposing factor for atopic dermatitis. Nat Genet 38: 441–446
41. Ruether A, Stoll M, Schwarz T, Schreiber S, Fölster-Holst R (2006) Filaggrin loss-of-function variant contributes to atopic dermatitis risk in the population of Northern Germany. Br J Dermatol 155:1093–1094
42. Weidinger S, Illig T, Baurecht H, Irvine AD, Rodriguez E, Diaz-Lacava A, Klopp N, Wagenpfeil S, Zhao Y, Liao H, Lee SP, Palmer CN, Jenneck C, Maintz L, Hagemann T, Behrendt H, Ring J, Nothen MM, McLean WH, Novak N (2006) Loss-of-function variations within the filaggrin gene predispose for atopic dermatitis with allergic sensitizations. J Allergy Clin Immunol 118:214–219
43. Irvine AD, McLean WH (2006) Breaking the (un)sound barrier: filaggrin is a major gene for atopic dermatitis. J Invest Dermatol 126:1200–1202
44. Compton JG, DiGiovanna JJ, Fleckman P, Lewis-Jones S, Arseculeratne G, Sergeant A, Munro CS, El Houate B, McElreavey K, Halkjaer LB, Bisgaard H, Mukhopadhyay S, McLean WH (2006) Common loss-of-function variants of the epidermal barrier protein filaggrin are a major predisposing factor for atopic dermatitis. Nat Genet 38:441–446
45. Hanifin JM (2009) Evolving concepts of pathogenesis in atopic dermatitis and other czemas. J Invest Dermatol 129: 320–322
46. Boralevi F, Hubiche T, Léauté-Labrèze C, Saubusse E, Fayon M, Roul S, Maurice-Tison S, Taïeb A (2008) Epicutaneous aeroallergen sensitization in atopic dermatitis infants – determining the role of epidermal barrier impairment. Allergy 63:205–210
47. Lerbaek A, Bisgaard H, Agner T, Ohm Kyvik K, Palmer CN, Menné T (2007) Filaggrin null alleles are not associated with hand eczema or contact allergy. Br J Dermatol 157: 1199–1204
48. Giwercman C, Lerbaek A, Bisgaard H, Menné T (2008) Classification of atopic hand eczema and the filaggrin mutations. Contact Derm 59:257–260
49. Molin S, Vollmer S, Weiss EH, Ruzicka T, Prinz JC (2009) Filaggrin mutations may confer susceptibility to chronic hand eczema characterized by combined allergic and irritant contact dermatitis. Br J Dermatol 161(4):801–807
50. Novak N, Baurecht H, Schäfer T, Rodriguez E, Wagenpfeil S, Klopp N, Heinrich BH, Ring J, Wichmann E, Illig T, Weidinger S (2008) Loss-of-function mutations in the

filaggrin gene and allergic contact sensitization to nickel. J Invest Dermatol 128:1430–1435

51. Fartasch M, Bassukas ID, Diepgen TL (1992) Disturbed extruding mechanism of lamellar bodies in dry non-eczematous skin of atopics. Br J Dermatol 127:221–227

52. Friebe K, Effendy I, Löffler H (2003) Effects of skin occlusion in patch testing with sodium lauryl sulphate. Br J Dermatol 148:65–69

53. Warner RR, Stone KJ, Boissy YL (2003) Hydration disrupts human stratum corneum ultrastructure. J Invest Dermatol 120:275–284

54. Berger CL, Edelson R (2004) The life cycle of cutaneous T cell lymphoma reveals opportunities for targeted drug therapy. Curr Cancer Drug Targets 4:609–619

55. Jensen JM, Pfeiffer S, Akaki T, Schröder JM, Kleine M, Neumann C, Proksch E, Brasch J (2007) Barrier function, epidermal differentiation, and human beta-defensin 2 expression in tinea corporis. J Invest Dermatol 127:1720–1727

56. Sterry W, Künne N, Weber-Matthiesen K, Brasch J, Mielke V (1991) Cell trafficking in positive and negative patch-test reactions: demonstration of a stereotypicmigration pathway. J Invest Dermatol 96:459–462

57. Kondo H, Ichikawa Y, Imokawa G (1998) Percutaneous sensitization with allergens through barrier-disrupted skin elicits a Th2-dominant cytokine response. Eur J Immunol 28: 769–779

58. Proksch E, Brasch J, Sterry W (1996) Integrity of the permeability barrier regulates epidermal Langerhans cell density. Br J Dermatol 134:630–638

59. Proksch E, Brasch J (1997) Influence of epidermal permeability barrier disruption and Langerhans' cell density on allergic contact dermatitis. Acta Derm Venereol 77: 102–104

60. Nishijima T, Tokura Y, Imokawa G, Seo N, Furukawa F, Takigawa M (1997) Altered permeability and disordered cutaneous immunoregulatory function in mice with acute barrier disruption. J Invest Dermatol 109:175–182

61. Jung EG (1963) Nachweis der beginnenden Bichromat-Sensibilisierung von Zementekzematikern mittels des Abrisstests. Berufsdermatosen 11:93–103

62. Kühl M, Klaschka F (1990). Berufsdermatosen. Urban & Schwarzenberg München, pp 204

63. Dickel H, Bruckner TM, Erdmann SM, Fluhr JW, Frosch PJ, Grabbe J, Löffler H, Merk HF, Pirker C, Schwanitz HJ, Weisshaar E, Brasch J (2004) The strip-patch test: results of a multicentre study towards a standardization. Arch Dermatol Res 296:212–219

64. Dickel H, Geier J, Kuss O, Altmeyer P (2008) Strip patch test vs. conventional patch test to detect type IV sensitization in patients with allergic contact dermatitis. J Eur Acad Dermatol Venereol 22:1516–1517

65. Dickel H, Kamphowe J, Geier J, Altmeyer P, Kuss O (2009) Strip patch test vs. conventional patch test: investigation of dose-dependent test sensitivities in nickel- and chromium-sensitive subjects. J Eur Acad Dermatol Venereol 23(9): 1018–1025

66. Fernandez MFM, de Mello JF, Pires MC, Vizeu MC (2007) Comparative study of patch test using traditional method vs. prior skin abrading. J Eur Acad Dermatol Venereol 21: 1351–1359

67. Gebhard KL, Effendy I, Löffler HL (2004) Artificial disruption of skin barrier prior to irritant patch testing does not improve test design. Br J Dermatol 150:82–89

68. Jensen JM, Pfeiffer S, Witt M, Bräutigam M, Neumann C, Weichenthal M, Schwarz T, Fölster-Holst R, Proksch E (2009) Different effects of pimecrolimus and betamethasone on the skin barrier in patients with atopic dermatitis. J Allergy Clin Immunol 123:1124–1133

69. Ghadially R, Halkier-Sörensen L, Elias PM (1992) Effects of petrolatum on stratum corneum structure and function. J Am Acad Dermatol 26:387–396

70. Loden M, Andersson AC, Lindberg M (1999) Improvement in skin barrier function in patients with atopic dermatitis after treatment with a moisturizing cream (Canoderm). Br J Dermatol 140:264–267

71. Tabata N, O'Goshi K, Zhen YX, Kligman AM, Tagami H (2000) Biophysical assessment of persistent effects of moisturizers after their daily applications: evaluation of corneotherapy. Dermatology 200:308

72. Proksch E, Feingold KR, Man MQ, Elias PM (1991) Barrier function regulates epidermal DNA synthesis. J Clin Invest 87:1668–1673

73. Proksch E, Holleran WM, Menon GK, Elias PM, Feingold KR (1993) Barrier function regulates epidermal lipid and DNA synthesis. Br J Dermatol 128:473–482

74. Chamlin SL, Frieden IJ, Fowler A, Williams M, Kao J, Sheu M, Elias PM (2001) Ceramide-dominant, barrier repair lipids improve childhood atopic dermatitis. Arch Dermatol 137: 1110–1112

75. Berardesca E, Barbareschi M, Veraldi S, Pimpinelli N (2001) Evaluation of efficacy of a skin lipid mixture in patients with irritant contact dermatitis, allergic contact dermatitis or atopic dermatitis: a multicenter study. Contact Derm 45: 280–285

76. Garnock-Jones KP, Perry CM (2009) Alitretinoin: in severe chronic hand eczema. Drugs 69:1625–1634

77. Elias PM, Fritsch PO, Lampe M, Williams ML, Brown BE, Nemanic M, Grayson S (1981) Retinoid effects on epidermal structure, differentiation, and permeability. Lab Invest 44(6):531–540

78. Endo K, Suzuki N, Yoshida O, Sato H, Fujikura Y (2007) The barrier component and the driving force component of transepidermal water loss and their application to skin irritant tests. Skin Res Technol 13:425–435

79. Kütting B, Drexler H (2003) Effectiveness of skin protection creams as a preventive measure in occupational dermatitis: a critical update according to criteria of evidence-based medicine. Int Arch Occup Environ Health 76:253–259

80. Zhai H, Maibach HI (2007) Protection from irritants. Curr Probl Dermatol 34:47–57

81. Saary J, Qureshi R, Palda V, DeKoven J, Pratt M, Skotnicki-Grant S, Holness L (2005) A systematic review of contact dermatitis treatment and prevention. J Am Acad Dermatol 53:845

82. Winker R, Salameh B, Stolkovich S, Nikl M, Barth A, Ponocny E, Drexler H, Tappeiner G (2009) Effectiveness of skin protection creams in the prevention of occupational dermatitis: results of a randomized, controlled trial. Int Arch Occup Environ Health 82:653–662

83. Alvarez MS, Brown LH, Brancaccio RR (2001) Are barrier creams actually effective? Curr Allergy Asthma Rep 1: 337–341

84. Korinth G, Lüersen L, Schaller KH, Angerer J, Drexler H (2008) Enhancement of percutaneous penetration of aniline and o-toluidine in vitro using skin barrier creams. Toxicol In Vitro 22:812–818

85. Wetzky U, Bock M, Wulfhorst B, John SM (2009) Short- and long-term effects of single and repetitive glove occlusion on the epidermal barrier. Arch Dermatol Res 301: 595–602

86. Lee JY, Effendy I, Maibach HI (1997) Acute irritant contact dermatitis: recovery time in man. Contact Derm 36: 285–290

87. Wilhelm KP, Freitag G, Wolff HH (1994) Surfactant-induced skin irritation and skin repair: evaluation of a cumulative human irritation model by noninvasive techniques. J Am Acad Dermatol 31:981–987

88. Schürer NY, Schwanitz HJ (2004) Prevention and regeneration of barrier disturbances in occupational dermatology. J Dtsch Dermatol Ges 2:895–904

89. Scott IR, Harding CR (1986) Filaggrin breakdown to water binding compounds during development of the rat stratum corneum is controlled by the water activity of the environment. Dev Biol 115:84–92

90. Spier HW, Sixt I (1955) Untersuchungen über die Abhängigkeit des Ausfalles der Ekzem-Läppchenprobe von der Hornschichtdicke. Quantiativer Abriß-Epikutantest. Hautarzt 6:152–159

91. Macheleidt O, Kaiser HW, Sandhoff K (2002) Deficiency of epidermal protein-bound omega-hydroxyceramides in atopic dermatitis. J Invest Dermatol 119:166–173

92. Ong PY, Leung DY (2006) Immune dysregulation in atopic dermatitis. Curr Allergy Asthma Rep 6:384–389

Immediate Contact Reactions

David Basketter and Arto Lahti

Contents

D. Basketter (✉)
DABMEB Consultancy Ltd, Sharnbrook MK44 1PR, UK
e-mail: david.basketter@ukonline.co.uk

A. Lahti
Medical Center Mehiläinen Oulu, Kauppurienkatu 27–29,
0100 Oulu, Finland

7.1 Introduction

Nonimmunologic contact urticaria (NICU) and other nonimmunologic immediate contact reactions (NIICRs) of the skin comprise a group of inflammatory reactions that appear within minutes to an hour after contact with the eliciting substance and usually disappear within a few hours [1]. These reactions could also be regarded as a form of immediate-type irritancy. They form a subset of a wider panel of urticarias, which are not generally discussed here [2]. NIICRs can be caused by chemicals, or occasionally by proteins, and occur without previous immunologic sensitization in most exposed individuals. They are the most common type of immediate contact reaction [3]. In contrast to NICU, immunologic contact urticaria requires the previous induction of IgE antibody-mediated sensitization to the offending agent, not necessarily through exposure via the dermal route. Subsequent contact with the material, which is usually a protein, can then elicit the clinical symptoms, which are essentially indistinguishable from their nonimmunologic counterpart. However, in practice, from both a clinical and a mechanistic perspective, it can sometimes be difficult to be convinced (and particularly for chemicals) whether one is dealing with an immunologic or a nonimmunologic (or a combination of both) type of urticaria, although to do so can be an important guide to the most effective form of treatment. In this context, it has been noted that the onset of immunologically mediated responses tends to be faster than the nonimmune variant, but in our view, this is by no means a hard and fast rule [4, 5].

The epidemiology of immediate contact reactions of all types is not well documented. Anecdotal clinical experience suggests that they may be quite common [4]. Such a perspective is consistent with the older

7

Finnish occupational survey which indicated that almost 30% of the cases diagnosed as allergic contact dermatoses were primarily urticarial in nature [6]. Added to this, it is true that the great majority of individuals can react at least via nonimmune mechanisms if the exposure is sufficient, but in reality there is little evidence to indicate the frequency with which these problems occur in either the consumer or occupationally exposed populations. Taken together, immune and nonimmune urticarias may present a relatively common skin disorder.

7.2 Definitions, Concepts, and Symptoms

The symptoms of NIICRs are heterogeneous, and the intensity of the reaction typically varies, depending on the concentration, the vehicle, the skin area exposed, the mode of exposure, and the substance itself [7]. A further important variable is the susceptibility of the exposed individual, which can vary widely [8]. Itching, tingling, and burning accompanied by erythema are the weakest types of reactions. Sometimes, only local sensations without any visible change in the skin are reported. The redness is usually follicular at first and then spreads to cover the whole application site. A local weal and flare suggest a contact urticarial reaction. Generalized urticaria after contact with NICU agents is a rare phenomenon but has been reported more often after contact with agents eliciting immunologic IgE-mediated contact urticaria. Repeated applications of NICU agents may cause eczematous reactions. Rapidly appearing microvesicles are frequently seen after contact with food products in protein contact dermatitis, which can be caused by nonimmunologic (irritant) or immunologic (allergic) mechanisms [9, 10]. In NICU reactions, the symptoms usually appear and remain in the contact area. In addition to local skin symptoms, other organs are occasionally involved, giving rise to conjunctivitis, rhinitis, an asthmatic attack, or anaphylactic shock [11]. This is called the contact urticaria syndrome and it mostly involves IgE-mediated immunologic mechanisms [12, 13]. In some cases, NICU reactions appear only on slightly compromised skin and can be part of the mechanism responsible for the maintenance of chronic eczemas.

The precise usage of the terms "immediate contact reaction," "contact urticaria," "immediate-type irritancy," "contact urticaria syndrome," "protein contact dermatitis,"

Table 7.1 Definitions and terms

Immediate contact reactions
Immunologic (allergic) or nonreaction
Immunologic (irritant), urticarial or nonurticarial reactions.
Does not define the appearance of the reaction

Contact urticaria
Allergic and nonallergic urticarial reactions

Immediate-type irritancy
Nonallergic urticarial or nonirritancy urticarial reactions

Protein contact dermatitis
Allergic or nonallergic eczema-dermatitis immediate reactions caused by proteins or proteinaceous material

Contact urticaria syndrome
Local reactions in the skin and syndrome
Systemic symptoms in other organs, usually allergic

and "atopic contact dermatitis" varies considerably in the literature and is understandable given the obvious mechanistic overlapping between them. Immediate contact reaction is the broadest concept, which covers both immunologic (allergic) and nonimmunologic (irritant) reactions, but does not say anything about the appearance of the reaction. Contact urticaria can be either allergic or irritant. Protein contact dermatitis is caused by proteins or proteinaceous materials, and it represents either allergic (both immediate and delayed) or irritant dermatitis, which has characteristic features of acute or chronic eczema [3]. Atopic contact dermatitis is a historical term and means an immediate-type (IgE-mediated) allergic contact reaction in an atopic person [14]. It is included in the concept of allergic protein contact dermatitis (Table 7.1). Occupational contact urticaria has been reviewed alongside occupational protein contact dermatitis relatively recently [15].

7.3 Mechanisms and Clinical Aspects of Nonimmunologic Immediate Contact Reactions

7.3.1 Histamine

The mechanisms of NIICRs, as with most other irritant skin reactions, are not well understood. It was previously assumed that substances eliciting NIICRs result in nonspecific histamine release from mast cells. However, it has been shown that H_1-antihistamines hydroxyzine, and terfenadine do not inhibit reactions to benzoic acid, cinnamic acid, cinnamic aldehyde (cinnamal), methyl nicotinate, or dimethylsulfoxide, although they inhibit reactions to histamine in prick tests [7, 16]. These results suggest that histamine is not the main mediator in NIICRs to these well-known contact urticants.

7.3.2 Skin Nerves

The role of skin nerves in NIICRs has been studied using capsaicin (trans-8-methyl-*N*-vanillyl-6-nonenamide), which is known to induce the release of bioactive peptides, such as substance P, from the axons of unmyelinated C-fibers of sensory nerves. Pretreatment of the skin with capsaicin inhibits erythema reactions in histamine prick tests [17], but does not inhibit either erythema or edema elicited by benzoic acid or methyl nicotinate [18]. This suggests that NIICRs to these model substances are not a type of neurogenic inflammation of the skin. Topical anesthesia inhibits erythema reactions to histamine, benzoic acid, and methyl nicotinate, but it is not known whether the inhibitory effect is due to the influence on the sensory nerves only, or whether the anesthetic also affects other cell types or regulatory mechanisms of immediate-type skin inflammation [18].

7.3.3 Ultraviolet Light

NIICRs to benzoic acid and methyl nicotinate can be inhibited by exposure to ultraviolet B and A light. The inhibition lasts for at least 2 weeks [19]. The reactions on nonirradiated skin sites also decrease, suggesting the possibility that UV irradiation may have "systemic effects" [20]. The mechanism of UV inhibition is not known, but it does not seem to be due to the thickening of the stratum corneum, as has been speculated [21]. The inhibition of mast cell functions is one possible mechanism [22, 23].

7.3.4 Prostanoids

The NIICRs to benzoic acid, cinnamic acid, cinnamic aldehyde, methyl nicotinate, and diethyl fumarate can be inhibited by peroral acetylsalicylic acid and indometacin

[24, 25] and by topical application of diclofenac or naproxen gels [26]. The duration of inhibition from a single dose of acetylsalicylic acid can be as long as 4 days [27]. The mechanism by which nonsteroidal anti-inflammatory drugs inhibit NIICRs in human skin has not been defined, but it is probably ascribable to the inhibition of prostaglandin (PG) metabolism.

New data provide evidence that PGD_2 is the primary mediator of contact urticarial reactions to benzoic acid, sorbic acid, and nicotinic acid esters [28]. PGD_2 is dose-dependently released in human skin after the application of these agents [28–30]. It is also known that intradermal injection of PGD_2 elicits erythema and weal formation in human skin. An interesting, but still unanswered, question in human skin is that which type of cells are activated by these substances to release PGD_2. According to animal studies, good candidates are dermal macrophages and epidermal Langerhans cells [31, 32]. In rabbit skin, PGD_2 has been shown to be an intermediate in agonist-stimulated nitric oxide release, and the cutaneous vasodilatation can be inhibited by a nitric oxide synthase inhibitor [33, 34]. This suggests that vasodilatation caused by PGD_2 is mediated by nitric oxide. Whether the mechanism is similar in human skin remains to be studied.

7.3.5 Molecular Structure

Molecular structure is important for the irritant properties of an NIICR agent. Pyridine carboxaldehyde (PCA) has three isomers: 2-, 3- and 4-PCA, depending on the position of the aldehyde group on the pyridine ring (Fig. 7.1). 3-PCA is a strong, and 2-PCA a weak, irritant in both human and animal skin (guinea pig ear swelling test). A slight change in the molecular structure of a chemical may substantially alter its capacity to produce NIICRs [35].

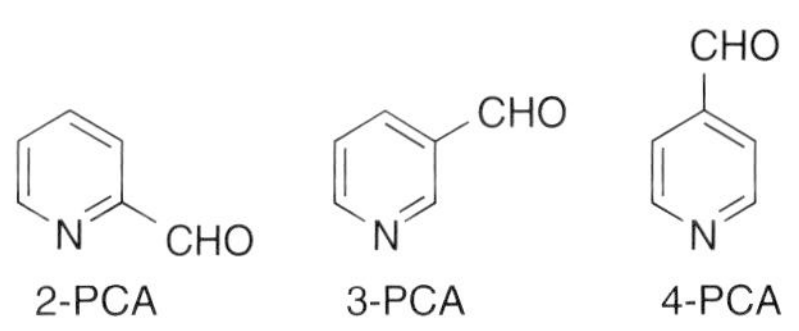

Fig. 7.1 Three isomers of pyridine carboxaldehyde (*PCA*)

7

7.3.6 Agents Producing Nonimmunologic Immediate Contact Reactions

The best-studied substances producing NIICRs are benzoic acid, sorbic acid, cinnamic acid and aldehyde and nicotinic acid esters. Under optimal conditions, most individuals react to these substances with local erythema and/or edema within 45 min after application, albeit with widely varying intensities of skin reaction [36]. Cinnamic aldehyde at a concentration of 0.01% may elicit erythema with a burning or stinging feeling in the skin. Some mouthwashes and chewing gums contain cinnamic aldehyde (cinnamal) at concentrations high enough to produce a pleasant tingling in the mouth and enhance the sale of the product. Higher concentrations may produce lip swelling. Some agents causing immediate irritant skin reactions are listed in Table 7.2.

Table 7.2 Agents producing immediate nonimmunologic contact reactions including contact urticaria

Animals
Arthropods
Caterpillars
Corals
Jellyfish
Moths
Sea anemones

Foods
Cayenne pepper
Fish
Mustard
Thyme

Fragrances and flavorings
Balsam of Peru (*Myroxylon pereirae*)
Benzaldehyde
Cassis (cinnamon oil)
Cinnamic acid
Cinnamic aldehyde (cinnamal)

Medicaments
Alcohols
Benzocaine
Camphor
Cantharides
Capsaicin
Chloroform
Dimethylsulfoxide
Friar's balsam
Iodine
Methyl salicylate
Methylene green

Myrrh
Nicotinic acid esters
Resorcinol
Tar extracts
Tincture of benzoin
Witch hazel

Metals
Cobalt

Plants
Chrysanthemum
Nettles
Seaweed

Preservatives and disinfectants
Benzoic acid
Chlorocresol
Formaldehyde
Sodium benzoate
Sorbic acid

Miscellaneous
Butyric acid
Diethyl fumarate
Histamine
Pine oil
Pyridine carboxaldehyde
Sulfur
Turpentine

7.3.7 Tests in Animal Skin

Animals models of contact urticaria have been the subject of recent review, but remain rather a "Cinderalla" topic [37]. An animal test method for determining NIICRs is available to screen for putative agents and to clarify the mechanisms. At the moment, the guinea pig ear swelling test is the best animal test available for studying NIICRs [38, 39]. A positive reaction in the guinea pig ear lobe comprises erythema and edema. Quantification of the edema by measuring the change in ear thickness is an accurate, quick, and reproducible method. Similar to human skin, the swelling response in the guinea pig ear lobe depends on the concentration of the eliciting substance. The maximal response is a roughly 100% increase in ear thickness and it appears 40–50 min after the application, depending on the vehicle.

A decrease in reactivity to NIICR agents is noticed after reapplication on the following day [40]. This tachyphylaxis phenomenon is not specific to the substance that produces it, and reactivity to other agents also decreases. The length of the refractory period is 4 days for methyl nicotinate, 8 days for diethyl fumarate and cinnamic aldehyde, and 16 days for benzoic acid, cinnamic acid, and dimethylsulfoxide.

The guinea pig ear lobe resembles human skin in many respects, including the morphology of the reaction, the timing of the maximal response, the concentrations of the eliciting substances needed to produce the reaction, the tachyphylaxis phenomenon, and the lack of an inhibitory effect of antihistamines on the NIICRs.

It must be noted that this in vivo model has not been formally validated and could not be used in the evaluation of cosmetic ingredients or products in Europe.

7.3.8 Tests in Human Skin

Special tests for NIICRs are needed, because these reactions are not seen in ordinary tests for irritancy and contact allergy. The most frequently used tests are the open test, the chamber test, and the skin prick test. Such tests may try to involve sensitive individuals, but this may present some difficulties since a particularly high reactivity to one urticant is not predictive of reactivity to other urticants [8, 36]. Full details of the test methods have been summarized in a recent overview of diagnostic testing in contact urticaria [5].

7.3.8.1 Open Test

In the open test, 0.1 mL of the test substance is spread on a 3×3-cm area of the skin on the upper back, the extensor aspect of the upper arm, or the forearm. There are marked differences between skin sites in reactivity to NIICR substances. The face (especially the cheek), the antecubital space, the upper back, the upper arm, the volar forearm, the lower back, and the leg constitute a rough order of decreasing reactivity [3, 21, 41]. A 10-μL dose to a 1×1-cm area is often used if a greater number of substances are to be tested at the same time. Petrolatum and water are the most often used vehicles [3], but it has been shown that the use of alcohol vehicles and the addition of propylene glycol to the vehicle enhance the sensitivity of the test to detect marginal immediate irritant reactions [42, 43]. The test is usually read at 20, 40, and 60 min in order to see the maximal response. In visual grading, scores for the erythema and edema components of the reaction (+ weak, ++ moderate, +++ strong) have

been used [5, 43], but objective measurement of erythema has been recommended [25, 44]. The test is usually performed on normal-looking skin, but it is sometimes useful to test suspected irritants on slightly or previously affected skin areas or on skin sites suggested by the patient's history. For example, if an immediate irritant reaction to a cosmetic cream has appeared on the face, one may see nothing if the test is performed on the back, but the reaction can be elicited by reapplication to the previously affected skin of the face. Repeated open tests on the same test site may be needed to detect weak immediate irritant reactions [45]. In a use test, the suspected product or substance is used in the same way as it was when the symptoms appeared. In recent usage, it has been suggested that there is merit in performing a second application to the skin site to enhance the sensitivity of the procedure [46].

7.3.8.2 Chamber Test

The chamber test is a routine method of patch testing for contact allergy, but it can also be used to study NIICRs. The test substances are applied in small aluminum chambers (Finn chamber, Epitest, Hyrylä, Finland) and fixed to the skin with porous acrylic tape. The occlusion time is 15 min and the test is read at 20, 40, and 60 min. Occlusion enhances percutaneous penetration and may increase the sensitivity of the test. The advantage of the chamber test is that a smaller skin area is needed than in the open test [5, 7, 8, 47].

7.3.8.3 Factors to be Considered in Skin Tests

The concentration of a NIICR agent needed in a skin test may be difficult to define, as it is in tests with classic, delayed-type irritants. Therefore, dilution series are recommended. They make it possible to determine the threshold irritant concentration for that particular patient and skin area. Examples of the concentrations often used in dilution series in alcohol vehicles are 250, 125, 62, and 31 mM for benzoic acid and 50, 10, 2, and 0.5 mM for methyl nicotinate [16, 48]. However, it is critical that a suitable panel of control subjects is tested as well so that the specificity of the diagnostic test for that material can be properly assessed.

7

It is known that oral and topical nonsteroidal anti-inflammatory drugs efficiently suppress NIICRs and may therefore cause false-negative results in testing [25, 26]. The minimum refractory period is 3 days [27]. Tanned skin has decreased reactivity to NIICR agents [49] and both UVB and UVA irradiation suppress these reactions for 2–3 weeks [19, 20]. Skin sites that are washed repeatedly may have a lowered threshold for immediate irritancy to NIICR agents [48]. The importance of the selection of the test site and the testing method has already been mentioned. These sources of false results should be kept in mind when tests for immediate irritancy are performed and the results of such tests are interpreted.

7.4 Mechanisms and Clinical Aspects of Immunologic Immediate Contact Reactions

The basic mechanisms involved are summarized in Fig. 7.2.

7.4.1 Induction

Immunologic contact urticaria is a type of immediate (type I) hypersensitivity reaction. In this manifestation of

hypersensitivity, exposure to the offending agent, most commonly a protein but in some cases a chemical hapten, stimulates the production of IgE-class antibodies. These are manufactured by B lymphocytes and typically are highly specific to the protein or the hapten–protein complex, although cross-reactions do occur. Sensitization most commonly occurs via the respiratory or gastrointestinal tracts, but can also occur through the skin, as in the case of latex and some foods. The IgE antibodies produced bind to high-affinity Fc_ receptors (Fc_ R1) on the surface of mast cells and basophils, thereby sensitizing them [50].

The ability to mount an IgE response is dependent upon a subtype of helper T lymphocytes designated Th2 and the production of specific cytokines, notably interleukin-4 (IL-4) [51]. It is likely that those individuals whose physiology is biased toward this Th2 phenotype are more likely to develop an IgE response [52]. From this group, the factors determining those who will display a contact urticarial reaction upon exposure are poorly understood, but will include the ease with which the agent penetrates the skin, the fragility of their mast cells, and their tissue sensitivity to the inflammatory mediators released.

It is interesting to note in this respect that recent observations indicate that the processes associated with the induction of IgE sensitization can occur via skin contact [53, 54] and that Th2 responses may even be favored when there is stratum corneum damage [55]. This may of course have been an important factor

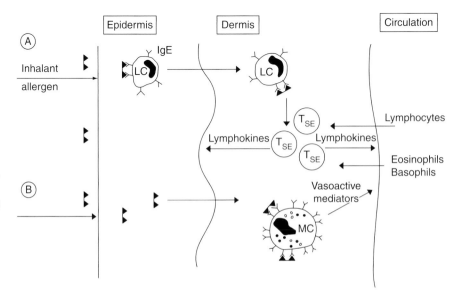

Fig. 7.2 Mechanisms by which protein allergens (pollen, mite, food, etc.) may produce delayed-type eczematous reactions (*A*) and immediate-type contact reactions (*B*) in patients with atopic dermatitis. (*LC* Langerhans cell; *MC* mononuclear cell; T_{SE} sensitized T lymphocyte)

in the epidemic of latex allergy – see the suggested reading and Sect. 7.4.3 below. It is certainly regarded as an important factor in the development of protein contact dermatitis in food handlers [10].

7.4.2 Elicitation

The typical symptoms of NIICRs have been described above. Following the induction of sensitization (a process for which the parameters are not well described), the clinical symptoms of immunologic contact urticaria are induced by direct skin contact with the antigen. Alternatively, inhalation of airborne protein or ingestion of food allergens may also lead to a more systemic expression of urticaria. This secondary exposure to the relevant urticant leads to the binding of antigen to the IgE molecules on the surface of tissue mast cells and basophils. The consequent cross-linking of IgE causes an increase in the intracellular calcium that triggers the release of both preformed and newly synthesized mediators. The most important of these mediators is the vasoactive amine histamine, the response to which can be blocked by the preinjection of compound 48/80 [56]. However, it is also likely that various leukotrienes, prostaglandins (PGD_2, PGE_2, PGI_2), platelet activating factor (PAF), and numerous other chemotactic and regulatory factors play a role [57, 58]. Furthermore, there is evidence, based on the use of the competitive inhibitor spantide, to suggest that the neuropeptide substance P, which is localized in peripheral sensory nerve endings, may be involved [59]. The importance of the role of nonhistamine mediators is reinforced by the relatively poor response of chronic idiopathic urticaria (caused by histamine-releasing autoantibodies to Fc_R1) to antihistamine treatment [60].

Of significance from a clinical perspective is the fact that, in addition to the cutaneous manifestations of immunologic contact urticaria, which arise mainly from increased vascular permeability leading to erythematous and/or edematous swelling reactions in the dermis, other symptoms, such as rhinitis, conjunctivitis, asthma, and even anaphylaxis, may also be elicited in individuals who are highly sensitized or in whom a high degree of exposure occurs [50].

In addition to the clear role of histamine-releasing tissue mast cells in immunologic contact urticaria, a number of other cell types also possess functional IgE receptors and so, at least in some cases, may also participate in the responses observed. Langerhans cells have high-affinity (Fc_R1) IgE receptors, at least in subjects with atopic dermatitis (reviewed in [61, 62]). However, Langerhans cells may express surface IgE receptors in response to the local inflammatory environment, [63] and so it may be speculated that they might play a role in skin disorders other than atopic dermatitis. In addition to Langerhans cells, eosinophils [64], circulating lymphocytes (T and B) [65], platelets [66], and monocytes [67] also have Fc receptors for IgE, although not necessarily of high affinity. However, as with Langerhans cells, the role of these receptors in immunologic contact urticaria is largely unknown.

> **Core Message**
>
> > Immunologic and nonimmunologic contact reactions are morphologically indistinguishable.

7.4.3 Agents Producing Immunologic Immediate Contact Reactions

The commonest causes of immunologic contact urticaria are food proteins (via topical contact and oral ingestion), animal proteins, and natural rubber latex. However, the catalog of chemicals and proteins reported to have been implicated in immunologic contact urticaria is extensive (Table 7.3). In principle, it might be expected that any protein capable of generating the formation of an IgE antibody response will also be capable of causing immunologic contact urticaria. Since, given appropriate exposure conditions, the majority of proteins can generate to some degree an IgE response (at least in a susceptible individual), the list in Table 7.3 is neither particularly useful in identifying those proteins that are clinically most culpable nor is it of much value in terms of clinical guidance or in risk assessment/management. Nevertheless, as mentioned above, certain materials either more commonly cause immunologic urticaria or, at least, are well recognized as such. These include foodstuffs (especially vegetables and shellfish), natural rubber latex, and proteins in the amniotic fluid of cows [68]. The relationship between food allergen ingestion and cutaneous symptoms, including urticaria, has been reviewed recently [69]. It is reported that acute

7

Table 7.3 Agents producing immediate immunologic contact reactions including contact urticaria

Animals and animal products
Amnion fluid
Blood
Brucella abortus
Bull terrier's seminal fluid
Cercariae
Cheyletus malaccensis
Chironomidae, *Chironomus thummi thummi*
Cockroach, *Blaberus giganteus*
Dander
Dermestes maculatus
Gelatin
Gut
Hair
Listrophorus gippus
Liver
Locust
Mealworm, *Tenebrio molitor*
Nereis diversicolor, worm
Oyster
Pine processionary caterpillar, Thaumetopoea pityocampa
Placenta
Saliva
Serum
Silk
Spider mite, *Tetranychus urticae*
Wool
Food
Dairy
Cheese
Milk
Fruits
Apple
Apricot
Banana
Kiwi
Litchi fruit, *Litchi chinensis*
Mango
Orange
Peach
Plum
Grains
Buckwheat
Maize
Malt
Rice
Wheat
Wheat bran
Nuts, seeds
Peanut
Sesame seed
Sunflower seed
Meats
Beef
Chicken
Lamb
Liver
Pork
Roe deer, *Capreolus capreolus*
Turkey
Seafood
Codfish
Prawns
Shrimp
Vegetables
Asparagus, *Asparagus officinalis*
Beans
Cabbage
Carrot
Celery
Chives
Cucumber
Endive
Globe artichoke, *Cynara scolymus*
Lettuce, *Lactuca sativa*

Table 7.3 (continued)

Onion

Paprika, *Capsicum annuum*

Parsley

Parsnip

Potato

Rutabaga (swede)

Soybean

Tomato

Watermelon

Fragrances and flavorings

Balsam of Peru (*Myroxylon pereirae*)

Cinnamic aldehyde

Menthol

Vanillin

Medicaments

Acetylsalicylic acid

Albendazole

Antibiotics

Amoxicillin

Ampicillin

Bacitracin

Cephalosporins

Cefotiam dihydrochloride

Cephalothin

Chloramphenicol

Cloxacillin

Gentamicin

Iodochlorhydroxyquin

Mezlocillin

Neomycin

Nifuroxime

Penicillin

Rifamycin

Streptomycin

Virginiamycin

Benzocaine

Benzoyl peroxide

Chlorothalonil

Cisplatin

Clobetasol-17-propionate

Dinitrochlorobenzene

Etofenamate

Fumaric acid derivatives

Ketoprofen

Mechlorethamine

Mexiletine

Pentamidine

Phenothiazines

Chlorpromazine

Levomepromazine

Promethazine

Pyrazolones

Aminophenazone

Methimazole

Propyl phenazone

Sodium fluoride

Tocopherol

Metals

Aluminum

Cobalt

Copper

Gold

Iridium

Mercury

Nickel

Palladium

Platinum

Rhodium

Ruthenium

Tin

Zinc

Plants and plant products

Abietic acid

Aescin, *Aesculus hippocastanum*

(*continued*)

Table 7.3 (continued)

Algae

Aster novi-belgii

Beer

Birch

Bougainvillea

Chamomile

Campanula

Castor bean

Christmas cactus, *Schlumbergera*

Chrysanthemum

Cinchona

Cnidoscolus angustidens

Colophony

Corn starch

Cotoneaster

Creeping fig, *Ficus pumila*

Devils ivy, pothos, *Epipremnum aureum*

Dianthus caryophyllus

Dill

Emetin

Eucalyptus

Fennel

Gardenia, *Gardenia jasminoides*

Garlic

Gerbera

Grevillea juniperina

Gypsophila paniculata

Hakea suaveolens

Hawthorn, *Crataegus monogyna*

Henna

Hibiscus rosa-sinensis

Hops, *Humulus lupulus*

Latex rubber

Lichens

Lily, *Lilium longiflorum*

Lime

Limonium tataricum

Loligo japonica

Lupin

Madagascar jasmine, *Stephanotis floribunda*

Mahogany

Monstera deliciosa

Mukali wood, *Aningeria robusta*

Mulberry, *Morus alba*

Mustard

Obeche wood

Papain

Poppy flower, *Papaver rhoeas*

Pelargonium

Perfumes

Phoenix canariensis

Pickles

Poinsettia, *Euphorbia pulcherrima*

Pomegranate, *Punica granatum*

Rice

Rose

Rouge

Runner bean, *Phaseolus multiflorus*

Semecarpus anacardium

Shiitake mushroom

Spathe, *Spathiphyllum*

Spices

Strawberry

Teak

Tobacco

Tradescantia

Tulip

Verbena

Weeping fig, *Ficus benjamina*

Winged bean

Preservatives and disinfectants

Benzoic acid

Benzyl alcohol

Butylated hydroxytoluene

Chlorhexidine

Table 7.3 (continued)

Chloramine

Chlorocresol

1,3-Diiodo-2-hydroxypropane

Formaldehyde

Gentian violet

Hexanetriol

p-Hydroxybenzoic acid

Parabens

2-Phenoxyethanol

Phenylmercuric propionate

o-Phenylphenate

Polysorbates

Polyvinylpyrrolidone

Sodium hypochlorite

Sorbitan monolaurate

Tropicamide

Enzymes

alpha-amylase

Cellulases

Protease (detergent)

Xylanases

Miscellaneous

Acetyl acetone

Acrylic monomer

Alcohols (amyl-, butyl-, ethyl-, isopropyl)

Aliphatic polyamide

Ammonia

Ammonium persulfate

Aminothiazole

Aziridine

Basic Blue 99

Benzonitrile

Benzophenone

Carboxymethylcellulose

Chlorothalonil

Cu(II)-acetyl acetonate

Cresylglycidyl ether

Denatonium benzoate

Di(2-ethylhexyl) phthalate (DOP)

Diethyltoluamide

Diphenylmethane-4,4'-diisocyanate

Epoxy resin

Ethylenediamine dihydrochloride

Formaldehyde resin

Glyseryl thioglycolate

2-hydroxyethyl methacrylate

HATU

HBTU

Hexahydrophthalic anhydride

Lanolin alcohols

Lindane

Methyl ethyl ketone

Methylhexahydrophthalic anhydride

Monoamylamine

Naphtha

Naphthylacetic acid

Nylon

Oleylamide

Panthenol

Para-aminophenol

Para-methylaminophenol

Paraphenylenediamine

Patent Blue dye

Perlon

Petrolatum

Phenyl glycidyl ether

Phosphorus sesquisulfide

Phthalic anhydrides

Plastic

Polypropylene

Polyethylene gloves

Polyethylene glycol

Potassium ferricyanide

Potassium persulfate

(continued)

7

Table 7.3 (continued)

Protein hydrolysates

Seminal fluid [84]

Sodium silicate

Sodium sulfide

Sorbitan sesquioleate

Sulfur dioxide

Terpinyl acetate

Textile finish

Vinyl pyridine

Xylene

Zinc diethyldithiocarbamate

urticaria is the most common food-induced adverse cutaneous reaction, occurring in approximately half of all patients with an IgE-mediated food allergy.

Immediate allergic reactions to natural rubber latex (NRL) proteins have been recognized for over 20 years as an important medical and occupational health problem [70–73]. An expert group set up in 1999 by the European Commission wrote an opinion paper on NRL allergy (http://europa.eu.int/comm/ food/fs/sc/scmp/ out31en.pdf; European Commission – Opinion on natural rubber latex allergy; adopted by the Scientific Committee on Medical Products and Medical Devices on June 2000). Thirteen different NRL allergens (www. allergen.org) have been characterized at the molecular level, as reviewed recently [74]. Prevalence studies, based on skin prick testing, indicate that 2–17% of exposed health care workers are sensitized to NRL, whereas the sensitization rate in the general population is less than 1% [75]. For the correct diagnosis of NRL allergy, the skin prick test and the measurement of NRL-specific IgE confirm the sensitization, but allergy diagnosis requires symptoms to be studied by a challenge or use test with NRL material. At the moment, there is no standardized, sufficiently allergenic material available for the latex challenge test. Delayed-type reactions to NRL proteins have recently been studied and 1% (27/2738) was found to be patch-test positive to NRL, of which 19 (70%) were considered to be clinically relevant for eczematous skin conditions [76].

Results of animal studies indicate that cutaneous sensitization to NRL proteins eluting from latex gloves can, in addition to the production of high levels of NRL-specific IgE antibodies, also contribute the development of hand eczema (Fig. 7.3) [77, 78].

In the health care sector, change of all gloves from high-protein/powdered to low-protein/nonpowdered has had a beneficial effect, but measuring the total protein cannot be deemed as a satisfactory regulatory measure to control allergen content in the future. A commercial test for measuring individual NRL allergens is available (FITkit; FIT Biotech, Tampere, Finland) and measurement of four main allergens in gloves and other rubber products is possible [79].

Allergen cross-reactions related to certain fruits and plant foods are known to be common in patients with NRL allergy [80–84]. The molecular basis for a major part of these reactions seems to be in the structural similarity between the hevein domains in NRL and the ubiquitously occurring hevein-like class I endochitinases in various plants [85]. Although accumulating evidence suggests that the peak of the NRL allergy epidemic may have already passed in the health care sector, latex allergy remains an important disease entity with many unanswered questions.

In contrast to the above, some causes of immunologic urticarial reactions are remarkably rare, for example, that to proteins in human semen [86].

The capacity of chemical haptens to provoke immunologic contact urticaria is not well studied, although a substantial number of chemicals have been implicated. However, it must be noted that the quality of the evidence

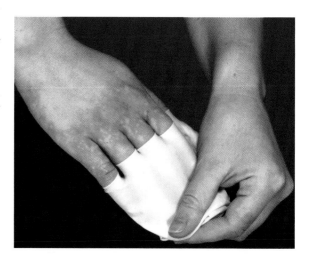

Fig. 7.3 Immunologic contact urticaria to natural rubber latex glove. (Courtesy by Arto Lahti, Department of Dermatology, University of Oulu, Oulu, Finland)

to substantiate the argument that these chemical urticants have operated via an immune mechanism has not always been of the highest order. Reasons for this are discussed below.

7.4.4 Tests in Animals

Predictive models for the specific identification of materials capable of causing immunologic contact urticaria are not well developed. Animal models have been used (e.g., [87]), but the focus has been on mechanistic aspects rather than prediction. The guinea pig can be sensitized to foreign protein, as well as to a variety of chemicals that have been reported as immunologic contact urticants, e.g., cinnamic aldehyde (cinnamal). The process for the induction of sensitization may vary from the techniques designed to examine the relative ability of proteins to behave as potential respiratory allergens (e.g., [88, 89]) to methods for the investigation of chemical respiratory sensitization (e.g., [90]) or even the evaluation of chemicals in skin sensitization tests, such as the guinea pig maximization test. In all of these procedures, once animals have been sensitized, intradermal challenge can be used to examine whether it is possible to elicit an immediate hypersensitivity response in the skin. This can readily be visualized if the animals have been given Evans blue dye (usually intracardially) prior to challenge. The reaction can be assessed some 20 min after the intradermal injection by the measurement of the diameter and intensity of blueness. However, it might not be straightforward to relate this type of reaction to immunologic contact urticaria in humans; there are no data on the sensitivity/specificity of the predictions from such models, nor are there any data on the ability to elicit immediate skin reactions following epicutaneous rather than intradermal application. In addition to the guinea pig, the rabbit has also been shown to be capable of mounting immediate hypersensitivity reactions in skin, but the use of this phenomenon as a model of immunologic contact urticaria is untried [91]. Whatever model is proposed, since it will be relatively easy to raise IgE antibodies, the key will be to find a way to determine the relevance of the predictions made.

The mouse has been proposed as a possible model of chemically induced immunologic contact urticaria. On the basis of the work with trimellitic anhydride (a chemical capable of causing both immediate and delayed types of hypersensitivity) [92], an approach has been suggested that involves topical application of the test chemical to BALB/c strain mice, followed about 1 week later by epicutaneous challenge on the ear. The urticarial reaction is measured as ear swelling over a time course of 2 h [93, 94]. The only substance examined to date has been trimellitic anhydride, so clearly a large amount of work must still be done in order to demonstrate both the validity and the relevance of this potential model. Nevertheless, it can be argued that the approach is mechanistically based, fairly straightforward to conduct, and could perhaps prove of value in the future. It is interesting to speculate as to whether the model might work with proteins shown to produce immunologic contact urticaria, such as the hevein of latex (reviewed in [95]). The most likely problem of the approach would be poor specificity, with very many proteins demonstrating an ability to produce IgE responses.

> **Core Message**
>
> › Reliable nonhuman predictive tests for either immunologic or nonimmunologic agents do not exist.

7.4.5 Tests in Humans

In contrast to animal studies, the only real purpose of human testing is to permit the diagnosis of disease. Full details of the test methods have been summarized in a recent overview of diagnostic testing in contact urticaria [5]. The typical clinical presentation of immunologic contact urticaria is essentially very similar to that of its nonimmunologic counterpart, although it is much more probable than for NICU that there may be some accompanying systemic organ involvement. However, there are a number of diagnostic test procedures that can be employed to identify the existence of an immunological mechanism. The main methods involve skin testing with the suspect substance and serological assays for specific IgE. In either situation, where a chemical hapten is the suspect material, it is normally necessary to conjugate it to a protein prior to testing. Commonly, the protein selected is human serum albumin (HSA).

7

However, the process of making a suitable hapten–protein complex should not be undertaken lightly; it may not be an easy process and insufficient attention to detail can easily result in false-negative data being obtained when the patient is assessed. Detailed guidance on the preparation of suitable hapten–protein conjugates has been published [96].

In theory, there is no reason why the tests for NIICR outlined above cannot also be applied to the investigation of immunologic contact urticaria. Simple open application of the suspect allergen may be sufficient [1]. However, the prick test approach developed many years ago for the identification of sensitization to protein respiratory allergens [97] has been adopted as a means to detect the presence of immunologic contact urticaria when the epicutaneous tests are negative. It is used as a routine method by some dermatologists, being regarded as more reliable in terms of avoiding the risk of false-negative results. It should be noted that skin testing may carry a small risk of precipitating systemic reactions and thus low concentrations of putative allergen are employed. As with diagnostic patch testing for delayed allergic reactions, it is vital to ensure that the test conditions/concentrations do not lead to nonspecific reactions. If necessary, suitable testing of a control panel may be necessary.

As an adjunct to skin testing, or as an alternative where it is contraindicated (e.g., if the patient has experienced anaphylactic-type reactions in conjunction with the urticaria), serological assessment may be carried out. In this case, the serum sample is assayed for the presence of specific IgE antibodies directed against the suspect substances. Traditionally, IgE testing has been conducted using the radioallergosorbent test (RAST), although this has recently been replaced commercially by the UNICAP system. RAST methodology was originally described over 30 years ago [98] and has proven to be of value in the identification of many immunologic urticants, including NRL [99], and is useful for the assessment of potential cross-reactivity between allergens (e.g., [100]).

In recent years, the commercial RAST system (such as that available from Pharmacia) has been replaced by a number of alternatives, but all, in essence, follow the same principle, that of measuring antigen-specific IgE.

As mentioned above, perhaps the most challenging area in the diagnosis of immunologically mediated urticarias is where the causation is by a chemical hapten. A recent publication investigating occupational contact urticaria caused by cyclic acid anhydrides provides an excellent working example of how to approach the problem [46] in which a structured mix of the above methods are deployed to identify the causative chemicals.

Core Message

> ❯ Agents causing immune-mediated urticaria can be identified by careful human testing.

References

1. Amin S, Maibach HI (1997) Immunologic contact urticaria definition. In: Amin S, Lahti A, Maibach HI (eds) Contact urticaria syndrome. CRC Press, Boca Raton, FL, pp 11–26
2. Zuberbier T (2003) Urticaria. Allergy 58:1224–1234
3. Lahti A (1995) Immediate contact reactions. In: Rycroft RJG, Menné T, Frosch PJ (eds) Textbook of contact dermatitis. Springer, Berlin Heidelberg New York, pp 62–74
4. Amin S, Lahti A, Maibach HI (2008) Contact urticaria and contact urticaria syndrome (immediate contact reactions). In: Zhai H, Wilhelm K-P, Maibach HI (eds) Dermatotoxicology, 7th edn. CRC Press, Boca Raton, pp 525–536
5. Amin S, Lauerma A, Maibach HI (2008) Diagnostic tests in dermatology: patch and photopatch testing and contact urticaria. In: Zhai H, Wilhelm K-P, Maibach HI (eds). Dermatotoxicology, 7th edn. CRC Press, Boca Raton, pp 581–586
6. Kanerva L, Toikkanen J, Jolanki R, Estlander T (1996) Statistical data on occupational contact urticaria. Contact Derm 35:229–233
7. Lahti A (1980) Non-immunologic contact urticaria. Acta Derm Venereol 60:1–49
8. Basketter DA, Wilhelm K-P (1996) Studies on non-immune immediate contact reactions in an unselected population. Contact Derm 35:237–240
9. Hannuksela M (1986) Contact urticaria from foods. In: Roe DA (ed) Nutrition and the skin, vol 10. Liss, New York, pp 153–162
10. Hjorth N, Roed-Petersen J (1976) Occupational protein contact dermatitis in food handlers. Contact Derm 2:28–42
11. Harvell J, Bason M, Maibach H (1994) Contact urticaria and its mechanisms. Food Chem Toxicol 32:103–112
12. Amin S, Lahti A, Maibach HI (1997) Contact urticaria syndrome. CRC Press, Boca Raton
13. Maibach HI, Johnson HL (1975) Contact urticaria syndrome. Contact urticaria to diethyltoluamide (immediate-type hypersensitivity). Arch Dermatol 111:726–730
14. Hannuksela M (1980) Atopic contact dermatitis. Contact Derm 6:30

15. Doutre MS (2005) Occupational contact urticaria and protein contact dermatitis. Eur J Dermatol 15:419–424

16. Lahti A (1987) Terfenadine (H1-antagonist) does not inhibit non-immunologic contact urticaria. Contact Derm 16: 220–223

17. Bernstein DI, Swift RM, Keyoumars S, Lorincz AL (1981) Inhibition of axon reflex vasodilatation by topically applied capsaicin. J Invest Dermatol 76:394–395

18. Larmi E, Lahti A, Hannuksela M (1989) Effects of capsaicin and topical anesthesia on nonimmunologic immediate contact reactions to benzoic acid and methyl nicotinate. In: Frosch PJ, Dooms-Goossens A, Lachapelle J-M, Rycroft RJG, Scheper RJ (eds) Current topics in contact dermatitis. Springer, Berlin, pp 441–447

19. Larmi E, Lahti A, Hannuksela M (1988) Ultraviolet light inhibits nonimmunologic immediate contact reactions to benzoic acid. Arch Dermatol Res 280:420–423

20. Larmi E (1989) Systemic effect of ultraviolet irradiation on nonimmunologic immediate contact reactions to benzoic acid and methyl nicotinate. Acta Derm Venereol 69: 296–301

21. Gollhausen R, Kligman AM (1985) Human assay for identifying substances which induce non-allergic contact urticaria: the NICU-test. Contact Derm 13:98–106

22. Czarnetzki BM, Rosenbach T, Kolde G, Frosch PJ (1985) Phototherapy of urticaria pigmentosa: clinical response and changes of cutaneous reactivity, histamine and chemotactic leukotrienes. Arch Dermatol Res 277:105–113

23. Kolde G, Frosch PJ, Czarnetzki BM (1984) Response of cutaneous mast cells to PUVA in patients with urticaria pigmentosa: histomorphometric, ultrastructural, and biochemical investigations. J Invest Dermatol 83:175–178

24. Lahti A, Oikarinen A, Viinikka L, Ylikorkala O, Hannuksela M (1983) Prostaglandins in contact urticaria induced by benzoic acid. Acta Derm Venereol 63:425–427

25. Lahti A, Väänänen A, Kokkonen E-L, Hannuksela M (1987) Acetylsalicylic acid inhibits non-immunologic contact urticaria. Contact Derm 16:133–135

26. Johansson J, Lahti A (1988) Topical non-steroidal anti-inflammatory drugs inhibit non-immunologic immediate contact reactions. Contact Derm 19:161–165

27. Kujala T, Lahti A (1989) Duration of inhibition of non-immunologic immediate contact reactions by acetylsalicylic acid. Contact Derm 21:60–61

28. Downard CD, Roberts LJ II, Morrow JD (1995) Topical benzoic acid induces the increased synthesis of prostaglandin D_2 in human skin in vivo. Clin Pharmacol Ther 57:441

29. Morrow JD, Awad JA, Oates JA, Roberts LJ Jr (1992) Identification of skin as a major site of prostaglandin D_2 release following oral administration of niacin in humans. J Invest Dermatol 98:812

30. Morrow JD, Minton TA, Awad JA, Roberts LJ Jr (1994) Release of markedly increased quantities of prostaglandin D_2 from the skin in vivo in humans following the application of sorbic acid. Arch Dermatol 130:1408

31. Ruzicka T, Aubock J (1987) Arachinodic acid metabolism in guinea pig Langerhans cells: studies of cyclooxygenase and lipooxygenase pathways. J Immunol 138:539

32. Urade Y, Ujihara M, Hariguchi Y, Ikai K, Hayaishi O (1989) The major source of endogenous prostaglandin D_2 production is likely antigen-presenting cells: localization of glutathione-requiring PGD synthetase in histiocytes, dendritic and Kupffer cells in various rat tissues. J Immunol 143:2982

33. Wallengren J (1991) Substance P antagonist inhibits immediate and delayed type cutaneous hypersensitivity reactions. Br J Dermatol 124:324–328

34. Warren JB, Loi KR, Wilson AJ (1994) PGD_2 is an intermediate in agonist-induced nitric oxide release in rabbit skin microcirculation. Am J Physiol 226:1846

35. Hannuksela A, Lahti A, Hannuksela M (1989) Nonimmunologic immediate contact reactions to three isomers of pyridine carboxaldehyde. In: Frosch PJ, Dooms-Goossens A, Lachapelle J-M, Rycroft RJG, Scheper RJ (eds) Current topics in contact dermatitis. Springer, Berlin, pp 448–452

36. Coverly J, Peters L, Whittle E, Basketter DA (1998) Susceptibility to skin stinging, non-immunologic contact urticaria and skin irritation - is there a relationship? Contact Derm 38:90–95

37. Lauerma A, Maibach HI (2008) Animal models of contact urticaria. In: Zhai H, Wilhelm K-P, Maibach HI (eds). Dermatotoxicology, 7th edn. CRC Press, Boca Raton, pp 577–579

38. Lahti A, Maibach HI (1984) An animal model for nonimmunologic contact urticaria. Toxicol Appl Pharmacol 76: 219–224

39. Lahti A, Maibach HI (1985a) Species specificity of nonimmunologic contact urticaria: guinea pig, rat and mouse.J Am Acad Dermatol 13:66

40. Lahti A, Maibach HI (1985) Long refractory period after one application of nonimmunologic contact urticaria agents to the guinea pig ear. J Am Acad Dermatol 13:585–589

41. Larmi E, Lahti A, Hannuksela M (1989b) Immediate contact reactions to benzoic acid and the sodium salt of pyrrolidone carboxylic acid. Comparison of various skin sites. Contact Dermatitis 20:38–40

42. Lahti A, Kopola H, Harila A, Myllylä R, Hannuksela M (1993) Assessment of skin erythema by eye, laser Doppler flowmeter, spectroradiometer, two-channel erythema meter and Minolta chroma meter. Arch Dermatol Res 285: 278–282

43. Ylipieti S, Lahti A (1989) Effect of the vehicle on non-immunologic immediate contact reactions. Contact Derm 21:105–106

44. Lahti A, Poutiainen A-M, Hannuksela M (1993) Alcohol vehicles in tests for non-immunological immediate contact reactions. Contact Derm 29:22–25

45. Hannuksela A, Niinimäki A, Hannuksela M (1993) Size of the test area does not affect the result of the repeated open application test. Contact Derm 28:299–300

46. Helaskoski E, Kuuliala O, Aalto-Korte K (2009) Occupational contact urticaria caused by cyclic adic anhydrides. Contact Derm 60:214–221

47. Hannuksela M (1995) Skin tests for immediate hypersensitivity. In: Rycroft RJG, Menné T, Frosch PJ (eds) Textbook of contact dermatitis. Springer, Berlin Heidelberg New York, pp 287–292

48. Lahti A, Pylvänen V, Hannuksela M (1995) Immediate irritant reactions to benzoic acid are enhanced in washed skin areas. Contact Derm 33:177–182

49. Feczko PJ, Simms SM, Bakirci N (1989) Fatal hypersensitivity reaction during a barium enema. Am J Roentgenol 153:275–276

7

50. Garssen J, Vandebriel RJ, Kimber I, van Loveren H (1996) Hypersensitivity reactions: definitions, basic mechanisms and localizations. In: Vos JG, Younes M, Smith E (eds) Allergic hypersensitivities induced by chemicals, recommendations for prevention. CRC Press, Boca Raton, pp 19–58

51. Finkelman FD, Katona IM, Urban JF Jr, Holmes J, Ohara T, Tung AS, Sample JG, Paul WE (1988) IL-4 is required to generate and sustain in vivo IgE responses. J Immunol 141: 2335–2341

52. Ricci M, Matucci A, Rossi O (1994) T cells, cytokines, IgE and allergic airways inflammation. J Invest Allergol Clin Immunol 4:214–220

53. Hsieh KY, Tsai CC, Wu CHH, Lin RH (2003) Epicutaneous exposure to protein antigen and food allergy. Clin Exp Allergy 33 : 1067–1075

54. Li XM, Kleiner G, Huang CK, Lee S, Schofield B, Soter N, Sampson H (2001) Murine model of atopic dermatitis associated with food hepersensitivity. J Allerg Clin Immunol 107:693–702

55. Strid J, Hourihane J, Kimber I, Callard R, Strobel S (2004) Disruption of the stratum corneum allows potent epicutaneous immunization with protein antigens resulting in a dominant systemic Th2 response. Eur J Immunol 34: 2100–2109

56. Larko O, Lindstedt G, Lundberg PA, Mobacken H (1983) Biochemical and clinical studies in a case of contact urticaria to potato. Contact Derm 9:108–114

57. Lewis RA, Austen KF (1981) Mediation of local homeostasis and inflammation by leukotrienes and other mast cell-dependent compounds. Nature 293:103

58. Schwartz LB, Austin KF (1984) Structure and function of the chemical mediators of mast cells. Prog Allergy 34:272

59. Wallengren J, Ekman R, Moller H (1986) Substance P and vasoactive intestinal peptide in bullous and inflammatory skin disease. Acta Derm Venereol 66:23–28

60. Sabroe RA, Greaves MW (1997) The pathogenesis of chronic idiopathic urticaria. Arch Dermatol 133: 1003–1008

61. Bieber T (1996) Fc epsilon R1 on antigen presenting cells. Curr Opin Immunol 8:773–777

62. Stingl G, Maurer D (1997) IgE mediated allergen presentation via Fc epsilon R1 on antigen presenting cells. Int Arch Allergy Immunol 113:24–29

63. Kraft S, Wessendorf JH, Hanau D, Bieber T (1998) Regulation of the high affinity receptor for IgE on human epidermal Langerhans cells. J Immunol 161:1000–1006

64. Capron M, Capron A, Dessaint J, Johansson S, Prin L (1981) Fc receptors for IgE on human and rat eosinophils. J Immunol 126:2087–2091

65. Yodoi J, Iskizaka K (1979) Lymphocytes bearing Fc receptors for IgE. Presence of human and rat lymphocytes with Fc receptors. J Immunol 122 : 2577–2583

66. Joseph M, Auriault C, Capron A, Vorng H, Viens P (1983) A new function for platelets: IgE dependent killing of schistosomes. Nature 303:810–812

67. Melewicz F, Spiegelberg H (1980) Fc receptors for IgE on a subpopulation human peripheral blood monocytes. J Immunol 125:1026–1031

68. Kalveram K-J, Kästner H, Frock G (1986) Detection of specific IgE antibodies in veterinarians suffering from contact urticaria. Z Hautkr 61:75–81

69. Wuthrich B (1998) Food induced cutaneous adverse reactions. Allergy 53:131–13

70. Nutter AF (1979) Contact urticaria to rubber. Br J Dermatol 101:597–598

71. Turjanmaa K, Alenius H, Mäkinen-Kiljunen S et al (1996) Natural rubber latex allergy. Review. Allergy 51:593–602

72. Turjanmaa K, Alenius H, Reunala T, Palosuo T (2002) Recent developments in latex allergy. Curr Opin Clin Immunol 2:407–412

73. Turjanmaa K (1997) Contact urticaria from latex gloves. In: Amin S, Lahti A, Maibach HI (eds) Contact urticaria syndrome. CRC Press, Boca Raton, pp 173–188

74. Yeang HY (2004) Natural rubber allergens: new developments. Curr Opin Clin Immunol 4:99–10

75. Liss GM, Sussman GL (1999) Latex sensitization: occupational versus general population prevalence rates. Am J Ind Med 35:196–200

76. Sommer S, Wilkinson SM, Beck MH et al (2002) Type IV hypersensitivity reactions to natural rubber latex: results of a multicenter study. Br J Dermatol 146:114–117

77. Laouini D, Alenius H, Bryce P et al (2003) IL-10 is critical for Th2 responses in a murine model of allergic dermatitis. J Clin Invest 112:1058–1066

78. Lehto M, Koivuluhta M, Wang G et al (2003) Epicutaneous natural rubber latex sensitization induces T helper 2-type dermatitis and strong prohevein-specific IgE response. J Invest Dermatol 120:633–640

79. Palosuo T, Alenius H, Turjanmaa K (2002) Quantitation of latex allergens. Methods 27:52–58

80. Garcia Ortiz JC, Moyano JC, Alvarez M, Bellido J (1998) Latex allergy in fruit-allergic patients. Allergy 53:532–536

81. Hannuksela M, Lahti A (1977) Immediate reaction to fruits and vegetables. Contact Derm 3:79–84

82. Köpman A, Hannuksela M (1983) Kumin aiheuttama koskeтusurtikaria. Duodecim 99:221–224

83. Mikkola JH, Alenius H, Kalkkinen N, Turjanmaa K, Palosuo T, Reunala T (1998) Hevein-like protein domains as a possible cause for allergen cross-reactivity between latex and banana. Allergy Clin Immunol 102:1005–1012

84. Pastorello EA, Ortolani C, Farioli L, Pravettoni V, Ispano M, Borga A, Bengtsson A, Incorvaia C, Berti C, Zanussi C (1994) Allergenic cross-reactivity among peach, apricot, plum, and cherry in patients with oral allergy syndrome: an in vivo and in vitro study. J Allergy Clin Immunol 94:699–707

85. Dias-Perales A, Sanchez-Monge R, Blanco C et al (2002) What is the role of the hevein-like domain of fruit class I chitinases in their allergenic capacity? Clin Exp Allergy 32:448–454

86. Shah A, Panjabi C (2004) Human seminal plasma allergy: a review of a rare phenomenon. Clin Exp Allergy 34(6): 827–838

87. Moore KG, Dannenberg AM (1993) Immediate and delayed (late phase) dermal contact sensitivity reactions in guinea pigs. Int Arch Allergy Immunol 101:72–81

88. Blaikie L, Basketter DA, Morrow T (1995) Experience with a guinea pig model for the assessment of respiratory allergens. Hum Exp Toxicol 14:743

89. Sarlo K, Fletcher ER, Gaines WG, Ritz HL (1997) Respiratory allergenicity of detergent enzymes in the guinea pig intratracheal test: association with sensitisaiton of occupationally exposed individuals. Fund Appl Toxicol 39: 44–52

90. Dearman RJ, Basketter DA, Kimber I (1996) Characterisation of chemical allergens as a function of divergent cytokine secretion profiles induced in mice. Toxicol Appl Pharmacol 138:308–316

91. Reijula KE, Kelly KJ, Kurup VP, Choi H, Bongard RD, Dawson CA, Fink JN (1994) Latex-included dermal and pulmonary hypersensitivity in rabbits. J Allergy Clin Immunol 94:891–902

92. Dearman RJ, Mitchell JA, Basketter DA, Kimber I (1992) Differential ability of occupational chemical contact and respiratory allergens to cause immediate and delayed dermal hypersensitivity reactions in mice. Int Arch Allergy Toxicol 97:315–321

93. Lauerma A, Maibach HI (1997) Model for immunologic contact urticaria. In: Amin S, Lahti A, Maibach HI (eds) Contact urticaria syndrome. CRC Press, Boca Raton, pp 27–32

94. Lauerma AI, Fenn B, Maibach HI (1997) Trimellitic anhydride sensitive mouse as an animal model for contact urticaria. J Appl Toxicol 17:357–360

95. Palosuo T (1997) Latex allergens. Rev Fr Allerg Immunol Clin 37:1184–1187

96. Bernstein JE, Zeiss CR (1989) Guidelines for preparation and characterization of chemical-protein conjugate antigens. Report of the subcommittee on preparation and characterization of low molecular weight antigens. J Allergy Clin Immunol 84 : 820–822

97. Pepys J (1972) Laboratory methods in clinical allergy – skin tests for immediate, type I, allergic reactions. Proc R Soc Med 65:271–272

98. Wide L, Bennich H, Johansson SGO (1967) Diagnosis of allergy by an in vitro test for allergen antibodies. Lancet 2:1105–1108

99. Turjanmaa K, Reunala T, Räsänen L (1988) Comparison of diagnostic methods in latex surgical glove contact urticaria. Contact Derm 20:360–364

100. Halmepuro L, Lovestein H (1985) Immunological investigation of possible structural similarities between pollen antigens and antigens in apple, carrot and celery tuber. Allergy 40:264–272

Suggested Reading

Turjanmaa K, Alenius H, Mäkinen-Kiljunen S, Reunala T, Palosuo T (1996) Natural rubber latex allergy. Review. Allergy 51:593–602

Reunala T, Alenius H, Turjanmaa K, Palosuo T (2004) Latex allergy and skin. Curr Opin Allergy Clin Immunol 4: 397–401

Mechanisms of Phototoxic and Photoallergic Reactions

8

Renz Mang, Helger Stege, and Jean Krutmann

Contents

R. Mang (✉)
Gemeinschaftspraxis für Dermatologie,
Venerologie, Allergologie, Proktologie,
Hauptstraße 36, 42349 Wuppertal, Germany
e-mail: mang@hautarzt-cronenberg.de

H. Stege
Depatement of Dermatology, Klinikum Lippe,
Röntgenstrasse 18, D-32756 Detmold, Germany

J. Krutmann
Institut für umweltmedizinische Forschung,
an der Heinrich-Heine-Universität Düsseldorf gGmbH,
Auf'm Hennekamp 50, 40225 Düsseldorf, Germany

8.1 Introduction

Solar radiation represents the most important environmental stress to which human beings are exposed. Within the spectrum of solar radiation reaching the Earth's surface, the ultraviolet (UV) and visible portions of the electromagnetic radiation are of particular importance to human skin. According to different photochemical and photobiological reactions, the UV portion of the electromagnetic spectrum is divided into different regions: UVC (wavelength 200–290 nm), UVB (290–320 nm), UVA (320–400 nm), and visible light (400–800 nm) [1–3]. UV radiation is able to penetrate the skin and blood. Its photon energy is sufficient to cause unimolecular and bimolecular chemical reactions within the skin.

The biological reactions resulting from the interaction of UV or visible radiation with human skin include physiological responses such as enhanced melanogenesis or thickening of the epidermal layers, and pathological reactions include photocarcinogenesis, photoaging, and the triggering of skin diseases characterized by an increased photosensitivity. In general, increased photosensitization is an abnormal reactivity of a biological substrate to, in principle, ineffective doses of UVA, UVB, and visible radiations. This can manifest as photodermatoses such as polymorphic light eruption or solar urticaria, as well as photoallergic and phototoxic reactions [4, 5].

For photosensitivity responses to occur, the relevant radiation must penetrate the tissue, be absorbed by biomolecules, and initiate chemical reactions in the tissue. The light-absorbing molecules are called *chromophores* or *photosensitizers*. In skin cells, the major UV-radiation-absorbing chromophores are nucleic acids, lipids, and proteins. Additionally, other molecules such as

J.D. Johansen et al. (eds.), *Contact Dermatitis*,
DOI: 10.1007/978-3-642-03827-3_8, © Springer-Verlag Berlin Heidelberg 2011

porphyrins, vitamins, or drugs are also able to absorb UV and visible radiation. In general, photosensitivity reactions result from the interaction of solar radiation with chromophores that are present constitutively in human skin or that have been topically or systemically applied [6]. Examples of endogenous molecules causing a photosensitivity reaction are porphyrins, whereas phytophotodermatitis is a prime example of an exogenous photosensitivity reaction. The combination of drugs and UV can produce both desired and undesired effects. Thus, PUVA therapy (psoralen plus UVA radiation) has long been employed for the treatment of psoriasis, and porphyrins can be used therapeutically, i.e., in photodynamic therapy [7–9].

The present chapter focuses on the mechanisms underlying phototoxic and photoallergic reactions caused by exogenous chromophores, especially drugs.

8.2 Clinical Aspects of Photoallergic and Phototoxic Reactions

Phototoxicity is the result of direct cellular damage caused by an inflammatory nonimmunological mechanism, which is initiated by a phototoxic agent and subsequent irradiation. In contrast, photoallergic reactions represent delayed or cell-mediated or type IV hypersensitivity responses, which require the specific sensitization of a given human individual to a photoactivated drug. Differentiation of phototoxic from photoallergic reactions is often difficult. This is due to the fact that most drugs are capable of causing both photoallergic and phototoxic reactions, and that the two types of photosensitivity reactions are very similar in their clinical and histological features. The following criteria can be used to differentiate between these two types of photosensitivity (Table 8.1).

Phototoxic reactions develop in most individuals if they are exposed to sufficient amounts of light and the drug. They represent an unwanted pharmacological effect. Typically, reactions appear as an exaggerated sunburn response (Figs. 8.1a, b and 8.2). Photoallergic reactions develop in only a minority of individuals exposed to the compound and light; its incidence is less than that of phototoxic skin reactions. The amount of drug required to elicit photoallergic reactions is considerably smaller than that required for phototoxic reactions. Moreover, photoallergic reactions are a delayed-type hypersensitivity; their onset is often delayed for as long as 24–72 h after exposure to the drug and light. Although the clinical appearances of phototoxic and photoallergic reactions are similar, they result from photobiologic mechanisms that can be clearly differentiated [2–4, 10].

Table 8.1 Clinical and histological features that help differentiate between the types of photosensitivity (modified after [6])

	Phototoxicity	Photoallergy
Incidence	High	Low
Pathophysiology	Tissue injury	Delayed hypersensitivity response
Required dose of agent	Large	Low
Required dose of light	Large	Small
Onset after light exposure	Minutes to hours	24 h or more
Clinical appearance	Sunburn reaction	Eczematous
Reaction after a single contact	Yes	No
Localization	Only exposed area	Exposed area; may be spread
Pigmentation changes	Frequent	Unusual
Histology	Epidermal cell degeneration; dermal edema and vasodilatation; sparse dermal mononuclear infiltrate	Epidermal spongiosis and exocytosis of mononuclear cells, dermal mononuclear cell infiltrate

Fig. 8.1 (**a**) Acute phototoxic dermatitis after contact to Cow parsnip (*Heracleum sphondylium*). (**b**) Hyperpigmentation 4 weeks later

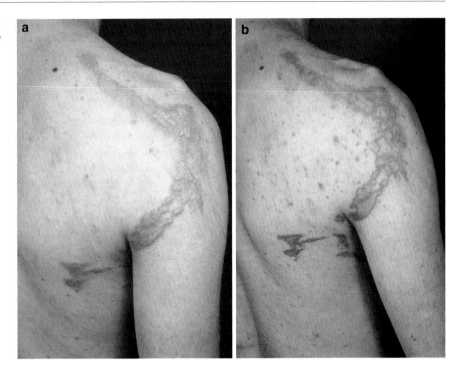

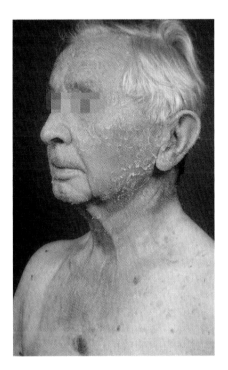

Fig. 8.2 Photoallergic dermatitis due to quinidine sulfate

Core Message

> Phototoxicity is the result of direct cellular damage caused by a nonimmunological inflammatory mechanism that results from the chemical or pharmacological structure of the used substances. In contrast, photoallergic reactions represent a cell-mediated hypersensitivity response, which requires the specific sensitization to a photoactivated drug.

8.3 Phototoxicity: General Mechanisms

In order for phototoxic reactions to occur, they require photons to be absorbed by a molecule that is the chromophore or photosensitizer. The structural requirement of this molecule to induce photosensitization is its ability to absorb radiation. Typically, these are wavelengths that penetrate the skin deeply (above 310 nm).

This characteristic absorption spectrum is determined by the chemical structure of the molecule, in particular, by the presence of single or double bonds or halogenated aromatic rings.

The absorbed photon promotes electrons within the molecule from a stable ground to an excited state, the so-called singlet or triplet state of the photosensitizer. Singlet and triplet states are higher-energy states that are defined by the spin state of the two electrons with the highest energies. When these two electrons have opposite spins, the electronic state is a singlet state; when they have the same spin, it is a triplet state. This excited singlet or triplet state is an unstable state and exists for only a very short time after photophysical formation. Typically, excited singlet states are stable for less than 10^{-10} s. Triplet states exist for a longer period, and in tissues, their lifetime is limited due to deactivation by oxygen (less than 10^{-6} s).

The excited states return to the ground state and the absorbed energy discharges by the emission of radiation (fluorescence), heat, or a chemical reaction producing a photoproduct. Complex processes are initiated by this photoproduct, which may then result in phototoxic reactions. It is important to keep in mind that not all drugs with the chemical features of a chromophore produce a photochemical reaction, because this also depends on variables such as drug absorption, metabolism, stability, and solubility. In general, phototoxicity can be produced in all individuals given a high enough dose of a photosensitizer and light irradiation. The most common skin manifestation of a phototoxic reaction is an exaggerated sunburn reaction with or without edema, blisters, and subsequent hyperpigmentation and desquamation in the exposed area. In other words, phototoxicity represents an inflammatory reaction, which results from direct cellular damage produced by the photochemical reaction between a photosensitizer and the appropriate wavelength of radiation in the UV or visible range. In contrast to photoallergic reactions, phototoxic reactions can occur during the first exposure of a given individual to this chemical in combination with irradiation and do not require a previous sensitization phase [4, 10, 11] (Fig. 8.3).

From a photochemical point of view, four pathways may be involved to exert phototoxic effects on a biological substrate. In general, these reactions can be further subdivided into oxygen-dependent photodynamic reactions and oxygen-independent nonphotodynamic reactions.

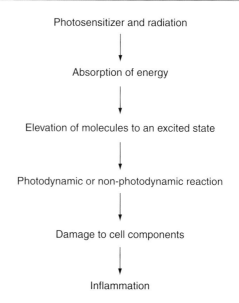

Fig. 8.3 Pathomechanism of phototoxic reactions (modified after [6])

Photosensitizer + photon photosensitizer*

1. An energy transfer from the excited photosensitizer to the oxygen produces excited singlet oxygen, which can participate in lipid and/or protein oxidation or induce DNA damage.

   *Photosensitizer** + O_2 → Photosensitizer + $^1O_2$ → $^1O_2$ + target

2. An electron or hydrogen transfer can lead to the formation of free radicals that directly attack biomolecules. In another pathway, interaction of these free radicals with ground state oxygen can result in the generation of reactive oxygen species. These include superoxide anion, singlet oxygen, hydroxyl radicals, and hydrogen peroxide.

   *(I)   Photosensitizer** → Photosensitizer˙ → Photosensitizer˙ + target*

   (II) Photosensitizer˙ + O_2 → Photosensitizer O_2 • → Photosensitizer O_2 • + target

   (II) Photosensitizer˙ + O_2 → Photosensitizer⁺ + $O_2^{-˙}$ → H_2O_2 → OH• → OH• + target

Reactive oxygen intermediates generated through this process are then capable of damaging subcellular organelles, which in turn can lead to tissue injury and inflammation. Many photosensitization reactions may be explained on the basis of these reactions.

3. In contrast, the nonphotodynamic reaction is a direct reaction and leads to the generation of stable photoproducts independent of oxygen. A prime example of a nonphotodynamic type III reaction is a photosensitivity reaction induced by psoralens [11] (Fig. 8.3).

Photosensitizer* + target →|
Photosensitizer – target

4. Finally, the photosensitizer can undergo decomposition so that the resulting photoproduct can act as either a toxin or a new photosensitizer (adapted by [12]).

Photosensitizer* → Photosensitizer· →
Photoproduct → Photoproduct + target
↓ + hv
Photoproduct* → Photoproduct* + target

Core Message

> There are direct and indirect photochemical mechanisms involved in phototoxicity.

The precise cellular target of phototoxic reactions depends on the physiochemical characteristics of the phototoxic agent. Topically applied agents are more likely to damage keratinocytes due to their higher concentration in the epidermis. Systemically applied drugs cause the greatest phototoxicity to the components of the dermis, specifically mast cells and endothelial cells. At the cellular level several organelles may be damaged by the phototoxic reaction. A hydrophilic photosensitizer mainly damages the cell membranes, whereas lipophilic substances diffuse into the cell and have been shown to destroy the components within the cell including lysosomes, mitochondria, and the nucleus [13, 14]. It should be noted that although the effects on one organelle may predominate, most photosensitizers affect more than one structure. Damage to the cells results in the release of soluble mediators that cause the inflammatory response. Among these mediators, eicosanoids, histamine, and complement have all been implicated in the generation of inflammatory responses induced by photosensitizers. Cytokines such as interleukin-1, interleukin-6, and tumor necrosis factor-α (TNF-alpha) which have been detected in UVB-induced erythema responses (sunburn reaction), may be involved in phototoxicity caused by drugs and chemicals; however, experimental evidence supporting this concept is lacking for most agents [15].

The specific wavelengths of light absorbed by a given phototoxic chemical depend on the physicochemical characteristics of the phototoxic agent. As a general rule, in most instances, the wavelengths are within the UVA range. It is important to keep in mind, however, that a few agents such as sulfonamides, vinblastine, and fibric acid derivatives absorb in the UVB range, whereas porphyrins absorb energy from the long-wave UV and visible spectrum.

In general, phototoxic drugs pertain to different therapeutic classes, i.e., antibiotics, antidiabetic drugs, antihistamines, cardiovascular drugs, diuretics, nonsteroidal anti-inflammatory drugs (NSAIDs), psychiatric drugs, and others. These drugs appear in the literature as phototoxic either in vivo or in vitro. It is problematic that it is not possible to predict phototoxic potency [16, 17].

8.4 Some Examples of Specific Agents Capable of Causing Phototoxic Reactions

The following examples are given to illustrate the different mechanisms and factors that cause and influence phototoxic reactions.

8.4.1 Psoralens

Psoralens are heterocyclic, aromatic compounds derived from the condensation of a furan ring with a coumarin ring. Phototoxic reactions induced by psoralens constitute the major therapeutic principle of PUVA (psoralen plus UVA-radiation) therapy. For PUVA therapy, linear psoralens such as 8-methoxypsoralen, 5-methoxypsoralen, and trimethylpsoralen are mostly used in combination with UVA radiation (Fig. 8.4). PUVA therapy is a mainstay in the treatment of patients with psoriasis

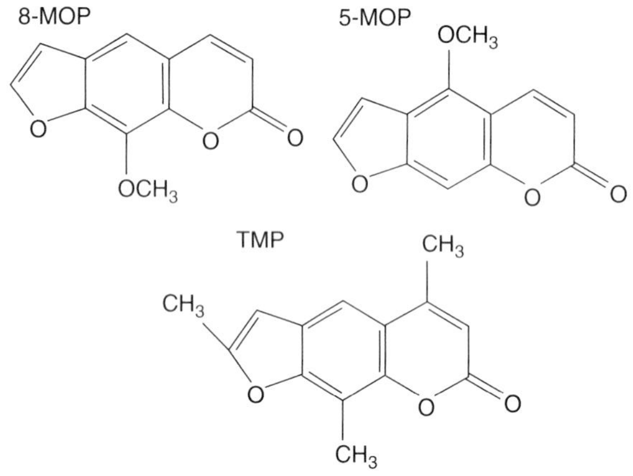

Fig. 8.4 Structure of 8-methoxypsoralen (*8-MOP*), 5-methoxy-psoralen (*5-MOP*) and 4,5,8-trimethylpsoralen (*TMP*)

vulgaris, cutaneous T-cell lymphoma, and several other inflammatory skin diseases. Psoralens are able to produce photomodifications of various biomolecules. Unlike most other photosensitizing compounds, psoralens mediate their phototoxic effect for the most part through a nonoxygen-dependent photoreaction, although photodynamic reactions may additionally contribute. As opposed to other phototoxic agents, psoralens primarily target DNA. The interaction between psoralens and DNA occurs in two separate steps. In the first step, the nonirradiated ground state of psoralen intercalates inside the nucleic acid duplex. In combination with UVA radiation, the excited psoralen molecules then form monofunctional and bifunctional psoralen–DNA photoadducts (cross-links) with pyrimidine bases – mainly thymine, but also cytosine and uracil. This mechanism may explain the antiproliferative effects of psoralens. Psoralen-induced DNA damage is responsible for adverse effects such as increased mutagenicity and skin cancer [18].

Other important targets of psoralens are specific receptors, in particular the epidermal growth factor (EGF) receptor and this interaction could provide another basis to explain the antiproliferative effect of PUVA therapy in psoriasis [19]. However, there are, also effects on other cell membrane components [20]. For example, it has been shown that psoralen–fatty acid adducts can activate a signaling transduction cascade leading to melanosynthesis in melanocytes. This effect may explain the beneficial effects of PUVA therapy in vitiligo patients [21] or the strong tanning following the treatment. More recently, it has been noticed

that PUVA therapy can induce programmed cell death (apoptosis) in skin-infiltrating T-helper lymphocytes. The resulting depletion of skin-infiltrating T-cells from psoriatic skin is thought to be one of the major mechanisms by which PUVA therapy clears psoriasis. The precise mechanism by which PUVA induces T-helper-cell apoptosis remains to be elucidated [22].

In addition to PUVA therapy, psoralen-induced photosensitivity reactions may also cause unwanted reactions, as they are observed in phytophotodermatitis and berloque dermatitis such as hyperpigmentation of a bizarre configuration, blister formation, and erythema [23, 24].

8.4.2 Porphyrins

The phototoxicity of porphyrins and their derivatives is important for the pathogenesis of cutaneous symptoms of porphyrias and the therapeutic use of porphyrins in photodynamic therapy. The photoactivation of porphyrins results in the formation of singlet oxygen and thus represents a prime example of a type II reaction. The formation of singlet oxygen and other free radicals then results in the production of peroxides, which can cause cell damage and cell death. It should be noted that the action spectrum of porphyrins does not lie within the UV range, but rather in the range of visible light (405 nm Soret band) [7, 8].

8.4.3 Fluoroquinolones

Quinolone antibiotics bearing fluorine substituent are commonly called fluoroquinolones (FQ). Chemically the parent compound is nalidixic acid. Some derivatives maintain the naphthyridinecarboxylic nucleus (enoxacin, trovafloxacin), but in others, it is replaced by the quinolinecarboxylic acid (norfloxacin, lomefloxacin, sparfloxacin, clinafloxacin, ciprofloxacin). In both the cases, the nucleus is substituted with halogens in one or two positions. Phototoxicity induced by FQ appears to be related to structural features. 8-Halogenated FQ (i.e., lomefloxacin, clinafloxacin) provokes severe reactions in the skin in comparison with the low phototoxicity exhibited by 8-methoxy derivatives. Moreover, fluorine substituent on the 8-position of the quinoline ring of FQ also induces photoallergic responses. In general, the presence of an electron-donating substituent has been suggested to confer photostability to the halogenated substituent at the 8-position, reducing the phototoxicity. Although the exact mechanism of FQ photosensitization remains unclear, basically the following processes have been indicated to justify the FQ photoreactivity:

- An oxygen singlet is produced by the zwitterionic form resulting from the dissociation of carboxylic acid and the simultaneous protonation of the piperazinyl group.
- The formation of reactive oxygen species including singlet oxygen, superoxide radical, hydroxyl radical, and hydrogen peroxide, although a mechanism based on these toxic agents does not appear to be correlated with the FQ photoreactivity.
- The photochemically induced dehalogenation generates a highly reactive carbene C-8, which reacts with some cell component.
- A combined process wherein the hemolytic defluorination leads to the formation of aryl radical which triggers the attack of the cellular substrate, whereas the oxygen reactive species could operate in a secondary or a parallel process [12, 13, 25–28].

8.4.4 Nonsteroidal Anti-Inflammatory Drugs

NSAIDs frequently cause phototoxic reactions. The capacity of NSAIDs to cause an inflammatory skin reaction contrasts with their pharmacological capacity to inhibit inflammatory responses. NSAIDs are a chemically heterogeneous group of drugs. Basically, three subclasses may be considered: the carboxylic acids (salicylates, arylalkanoic acids, and fenamates), pyrazoles, and oxicams. In any of these subclasses phototoxic and nonphototoxic molecules can be found.

It has been pointed out that their common use in clinical practice has led to multiple reports of photo-induced effects. The result is the existence of a number of mechanistic studies on this subject. There are numerous reports of phototoxic reactions resulting from the use of carprofen, ketoprofen, suprofen, tiaprofenic acid, and naproxen.

Benoxaprofen was removed from the European market in 1982 because of a high frequency of phototoxic reactions. Photochemical studies have shown that NSAID phototoxicity is mainly mediated by reactive oxygen species and free radicals. This has been worked out mainly for naproxen. For example, Diclofenac is lesser phototoxic than naproxen. Nevertheless, this drug has received attention because of its wide use. The major photoproducts of diclofenac are carbazole derivates (compounds: 8ClCb and cb). In vitro assays performed with diclofenac and its photoproducts have shown phototoxicity only for 8ClCb, which has structural similarities to the phototoxic drug carprofen [1, 12, 29–31].

8.4.5 Amiodarone

Amiodarone – an antiarrhythmic drug – often induces phototoxicity. As a clinical consequence a gray hyperpigmentation develops in the UV-exposed areas. Amiodarone and its metabolite desethylamiodarone are highly phototoxic and cause cell damage by injuring the cell membrane in an oxygen-dependent process. Because of the long half-time of amiodarone, this phototoxic reaction may persist for several months. The action spectrum of amiodarone-induced phototoxicity lies within the UVA range. This is surprising because in vitro studies have shown that the UVB range mediates the phototoxicity induced by amiodarone more efficiently than the UVA range. A possible explanation might be that the highest concentration of amiodarone in vivo was found in the dermis, which is reached preferentially by UVA, whereas the UVB portion of solar radiation is almost completely absorbed within the epidermis [32].

8.5 Photoallergic Reactions: General Mechanisms

Both phototoxic and photoallergic reactions require the presence of a chemical and radiation in the UV or visible range. Nevertheless, the mechanisms of action are completely different in both the reactions. Photoallergic reactions are classic T-cell-mediated immune mechanisms (Gell and Coombs type IV reactions) and, as a consequence, patients do not have clinical manifestations upon

8

first exposure, because sensitization to the photoallergic agent is an indispensable prerequisite. The photoallergic reaction can be produced by substances that are applied topically or systemically and, in contrast to phototoxic reactions, it does not depend on the concentration of the photosensitizer. The clinical features of photoallergic reactions closely resemble those of an eczematous reaction, as they are observed in contact dermatitis and usually occur 24–72 h after irradiation.

Agents that can cause photoallergic reactions include topical antimicrobials, fragrances, sunscreen ingredients, NSAIDs, psychiatric medications, and others. It is important to know that some of these substances might also have the potency to induce a common allergic contact dermatitis [6, 10, 32–35].

The steps involved in this photochemical reaction, which results in the formation of a complete antigen, are only poorly understood. From the mechanistic point of view, photoallergy involves covalent drug – protein photobinding (haptenization) leading to the formation of a complete photoantigen. This photoantigen may trigger a hypersensitivity reaction due to a cell-mediated immune response. In addition, the photosensitized modifications of proteins may also produce extensive structural changes associated with the loss of biological function [6, 10].

For quinidine sulfate photoallergic reactions, the presence of serum components has been implicated in the pathogenesis of the photosensitivity reaction. Accordingly, an eczematous reaction could be provoked after an intradermal injection of the drug together with patient serum into the previously UVA-irradiated skin, whereas injection of the drug alone in the absence of serum did not induce eczema. It has therefore been proposed that binding of the hapten quinidine sulfate to a potential carrier protein that is present in the serum may be of crucial importance in the pathogenesis of this particular type of photoallergic reaction [36].

In the past, most photoallergic reactions resulted from the topical use of soaps and deodorants containing halogenated salicylanilides and related compounds, whereas recently, sunscreen ingredients have been found to be among the most frequent photoallergens. Systemic photoallergens include phenothiazines, chlorpromazine as well as NSAIDs. It should been noted that the same agents can also cause phototoxic reactions. For the majority of photoallergens the action spectrum lies within the UVA range. Exceptions are sulfonamides, benzodiazepines, diphenhydramine, isotretinoin, and thiazide diuretics, which produce photoallergic reactions upon exposure to UVB radiation [34] (Fig. 8.5).

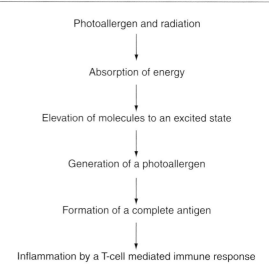

Fig. 8.5 Mechanism of a photoallergic reaction (modified after [6])

References

1. Ferguson J (1999) Drug and chemical photosensitivity. In: Hawk JLM (ed) Photodermatology. Arnold, London, pp 155–169
2. Krutmann J, Hönigsmann H, Elmets CA, Bergstresser PR (eds) (2000) Dermatological phototherapy and photodiagnostic methods. Springer, Berlin
3. Epstein JH (1989) Photomedicine. In: Smith KC (ed) The science of photobiology, 2nd edn. Plenum, New York, pp 155–192
4. Epstein JH (1983) Phototoxicity and photoallergy in man. J Am Acad Dermatol 8:141–147
5. Hölzle E, Plewig G, Lehmann P (1987) Photodermatoses – diagnostic procedures and their interpretation. Photodermatology 4:109–114
6. Gould JW, Mercurio MG, Elmets CA (1995) Cutaneous photosensitivity diseases induced by exogenous agents. J Am Acad Dermatol 33:551–573
7. Fritsch C, Goerz G, Ruzicka T (1998) Photodynamic therapy in dermatology. Arch Dermatol 134:207–214
8. Lim HW (1989) Mechanisms of phototoxicity in porphyria cutanea tarda and erythropoietic protoporphyria. Immunol Ser 46:671–685
9. Strauss GH, Bridges BA, Greaves M, Vella-Briffa D, Hall-Smith P, Price M (1980) Methoxypsoralen photochemotherapy. Lancet 122:1134–1135
10. Gonzalez E, Gonzalez S (1996) Drug photosensitivity, idiopathic photodermatoses, and sunscreens. J Am Acad Dermatol 35:871–885
11. Ljunggren B, Bjellerup M (1986) Systemic drug photosensitivity. Photodermatology 3:26–35
12. Quintero B, Miranda MA (2000) Mechanisms of photosensitization induced by drugs: a general survey. Ars Pharmadeutica 1:27–46

13. Quedraogo G, Morliere P, Santus R, Miranda CJV (2000) Damage to mitochondria of cultured human skin fibroblasts photosensitized by fluoroquinolones. J Photochem Photobiol 58:20–25

14. Kochevar KE (1991) Phototoxicity mechanisms: chlorpromazine photosensitized damage to DNA and cell membranes. J Invest Dermatol 77:59–64

15. Terencio MC, Guillen I, Gomez-Lechon MJ, Miranda MA, Castell JV (1998) Release of inflammatory mediators (PGE2, IL-6) by fenofibric acid-photosensitized human keratinocytes and fibroblasts. Photochem Photobiol 68:331–336

16. Diffey BL, Farr PM, Adams SJ (1988) The action spectrum in quinine photosensitivity. Br J Dermatol 118:679–685

17. Diffey BL, Farr PM (1988) The action spectrum in drug induced photosensitivity. Photochem Photobiol 47:49–53

18. Dall'Acqua F, Vedaldi D, Bordin F, Rodighiero G (1979) New studies on the interaction between 8-methoxypsoralen and DNA in vitro. J Invest Dermatol 73:191–197

19. Laskin JD, Lee E, Laskin DL, Gallo MA (1986) Psoralens potentiate ultraviolet light-induced inhibition of epidermal growth factor binding. Proc Natl Acad Sci USA 83:8211–8215

20. Zarebska Z (1994) Cell membrane, a target for PUVA therapy. J Photochem Photobiol B 23:101–109

21. Anthony FA, Laboda HM, Costlow ME (1997) Psoralen-fatty acid adducts activate melanocyte protein kinase C: a proposed mechanism for melanogenesis induced by 8-methoxypsoralen and ultraviolet A light. Photodermatol Photoimmunol Photomed 13:9–16

22. Coven TR, Walters IB, Cardinale I, Krueger JG (1999) PUVA-induced lymphocyte apoptosis: mechanism of action in psoriasis. Photodermatol Photoimmunol Photomed 15:22–27

23. Pathak MA, Daniels F, Fitzpatrick TB (1962) The presently known distribution of furocomarins (psoralens) in plants. J Invest Dermatol 32:225–239

24. Kavli G, Volden G (1984) Phytophotodermatitis. Photodermatology 1:65–75

25. Dawe RS, Ibbotson SH, Sanderson JB, Thomson EM, Ferguson J (2003) A randomized controlled trial (volunteer study) of sitafloxacin, enoxacin, levofloxacin and sparfloxacin phototoxicity. Br J Dermatol 149:1232–1241

26. Kawada A, Hatanaka K, Gomi H, Matsuo I (1999) In vitro phototoxicity of new quinolones: production of active oxygen species and photosensitized lipid peroxidation. Photodermatol Photoimmunol Photomed 15:226–230

27. Neumann NJ, Holzle E, Lehmann P, Rosenbruch M, Klaucic A, Plewig G (1997) Photo hen's egg test: a model for phototoxicity. Br J Dermatol 136:326–330

28. Ferguson J, Johnson BE (1993) Clinical and laboratory studies of the photosensitizing potential of norfloxacin, a 4-quinolone broad-spectrum antibiotic. Br J Dermatol 128:285–295

29. Diffey BL, Daymond TJ, Fairgreaves H (1983) Phototoxic reactions to piroxicam, naproxen and tiaprofenic acid. Br J Rheumatol 22:239–242

30. Ljunggren B (1985) Propionic acid-derived nonsteroidal anti-inflammatory drugs and phototoxicity in vitro. Photodermatology 2:3–9

31. Stern RS (1983) Phototoxic-reactions to piroxicam and other non-steroidal anti-inflammatory agents. N Engl J Med 309:186–187

32. Ferguson J, Addo HA, Jones S, Johnson BE, Frain-Bell W (1985) A study of cutaneous photosensitivity induced by amiodarone. Br J Dermatol 113:537–549

33. Elmets CA (1986) Drug-induced photoallergy. Dermatol Clin 4:231–241

34. Emmett EA (1978) Drug photoallergy. Int J Dermatol 17:370–379

35. Horio T (1984) Photoallergic reaction. Classification and pathogenesis. Int J Dermatol 23:376–382

36. Schurer NY, Holzle E, Plewig G, Lehmann P (1992) Photosensitivity induced by quinidine sulfate: experimental reproduction of skin lesions. Photodermatol Photoimmunol Photomed 9:78–82

Part II

Pathology

Histopathological and Immunohistopathological Features of Irritant and Allergic Contact Dermatitis

9

Jean-Marie Lachapelle and Liliane Marot

Contents

9.1 Introduction: General Considerations

Histopathological features of allergic and/or irritant contact dermatitis are not described in full detail in most textbooks of dermatology [1–3]. This is because they are not usually involved in the diagnostic procedures of both conditions. In most cases, contact dermatitis is suspected from anamnestic data and clinical signs [4]. Diagnosis is confirmed by patch testing and/or other tests, with additional information about the responsible agent(s). Nevertheless, in daily practice, contact dermatitis may be superimposed onto an underlying skin disease, the diagnosis of which is sometimes difficult.

In those circumstances, skin biopsy is recommended and considered a useful tool of differential diagnosis.

Among such examples, the following can be quoted:

- Nummular dermatitis (eczema) vs. parapsoriasis en plaques (benign type), psoriasis or *tinea incognito*
- Seborrhœic dermatitis vs. lupus erythematosus or rosacea
- Pompholyx vs. pustular psoriasis, palmoplantar pustulosis, bullous pemphigoid, or linear IgA disease

When an eczematous reaction is involved, the histopathological clue in diagnosis is the presence of a spongiotic (spongiform) dermatitis, notwithstanding its origin: irritant, allergic, or endogenous.

In each individual case, the histopathological picture is dependent on various parameters that can play a confounding role, such as: (1) unknown duration of the disease; (2) lesions related to scratching; (3) infections; and (4) lichenification. Clinicians are sometimes advised to perform two biopsies instead of one, in order to focus on different stages of the disease.

J.-M. Lachapelle (✉) and L. Marot
Department of Dermatology, Catholic University of Louvain,
30, Clos Chapelle-aux-Champs, UCL 3033, 1200 Brussels,
Belgium
e-mail: lachapelle@uclouvain.be
e-mail: LMarot@uclouvain.be

J.D. Johansen et al. (eds.), *Contact Dermatitis*,
DOI: 10.1007/978-3-642-03827-3_9, © Springer-Verlag Berlin Heidelberg 2011

9

A full description of the histopathological signs of allergic and/or irritant contact dermatitis is better achieved by a careful study of positive allergic and/or irritant patch test reactions.

This approach has two advantages: (1) the histopathological signs reflect a practical situation, encountered daily at the patch test clinic; (2) a positive patch test reaction is a clear-cut, unmodified reaction – the direct consequence of the application of a substance on previously intact skin.

The only possible drawback to using patch test reactions is the role played by occlusion. This might be especially true for allergic reactions, and it is the reason for this description also being based upon open (unoccluded) reactions, the use of which is becoming commoner in many clinics.

This description will be a "freeze-frame photograph" of the situation at 48, 72, or 96 h; it does not take into account the chronology of events, starting at time 0 (with the application of the substance) and continuing for instance every 6 h – until 48 or 72 h. This dynamic view has been achieved in previous research studies [5].

It has to be emphasized that this description is useful when expressed in scientific (more than practical) terms, to improve our knowledge at the microscopic level. In this respect, patch testing has been used recently as a tool for evaluating the efficacy of topical drugs, such as pimecrolimus [6] or tacrolimus, [7] vs. corticosteroids as well as regarding the outcome of allergic positive patch test reactions to nickel sulfate in volunteers. The evaluation of results has been based on visual scoring and biometrical measurements using noninvasive technology, but not on the evaluation of histopathological parameters. Indeed, biopsy is considered an invasive procedure, rejected nowadays by most ethical committees.

A lot of information delivered in the next paragraphs comes from our own material, used in former studies, at a time when legal procedures were not as strictly codified as they are today.

Core Messages

> In clinical practice, when the clinical diagnosis of allergic and/or irritant contact dermatitis is not clear-cut, skin biopsy is considered a useful tool of differential diagnosis.

> In contrast, biopsies of positive patch tests are not recommended, except for scientific purposes.

9.2 Histopathological Features of Positive Allergic Patch Test Reactions

The histopathological picture of a positive allergic patch test reaction (read at 48 h) is a typical example of a spongiotic dermatitis [3]. Features are very similar in all cases.

9.2.1 Epidermal Changes

In the epidermis, spongiosis is an almost constant sign, resulting from the accumulation of fluid around individual keratinocytes (exoserosis) and the consequent stretching of intercellular desmosome complexes (or "prickles").

Spongiosis is focally or evenly distributed along the length of the epidermis; it is either limited to the lower layers or extends from the basal to the granular layer. In some but not all cases, it spares the cells of the sweat duct unit. Hair follicles are usually involved by the spongiotic process.

A more plentiful accumulation of fluid results in the rupture of the desmosomes and the formation of vesicles. Thus, in allergic contact dermatitis, spongiotic vesiculation can be defined as an intraepidermal cavity with ragged walls and surrounding spongiosis. There is migration of inflammatory cells into the epidermis (exocytosis). These cells, mainly lymphocytes and occasionally polymorphonuclear neutrophils and eosinophils, accumulate in the spongiotic vesicles.

Some vesicles are rounded and tense; they are located in the stratum spinosum, whereas others are flat and located in the stratum corneum. They finally rupture at the surface of the epidermis and vertical channels of fluid discharge are occasionally seen on serial sections. These channels are sometimes colorfully described as "Devergie's eczematous wells." Intracellular edema of keratinocytes does occur, with accumulation of glycogen (Fig. 9.1).

At the electron microscopic level, dissolution of interdesmosomal areas, or "microacantholysis," can be demonstrated; remaining desmosomes show tension and alignment of tonofilament bundles.

In photoallergic contact dermatitis, a biopsy of the photopatch test site, when positive, clearly shows transforming keratinocytes in sunburn cells (apoptotic cells).

Fig. 9.1 Allergic positive patch test reaction to balsam of Peru (*Myroxylon pereirae*) at 2 days: spongiotic vesiculation in epidermis with exocytosis of mononuclear cells and dermal edema. Hematoxylin–eosin–saffron stain (×150)

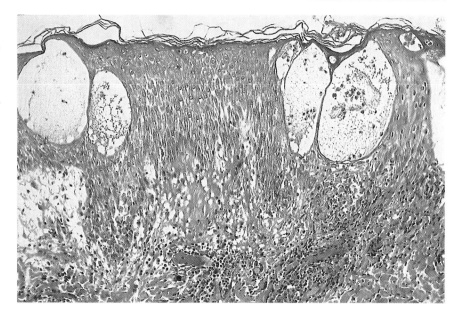

9.2.2 Dermal Changes

Papillary blood capillaries are often congested and dilated; dilatation of lymphatic vessels is very conspicuous in some but not all cases. Dermal edema is prominent with deposits of acid mucopolysaccharides. A dense mononuclear cell infiltrate is usually present around blood vessels of the lower dermis, and even (but rarely) in the subcutaneous tissue. The cells of the infiltrate migrate from the perivascular spaces to the epidermis and are found throughout the dermal tissue, either isolated or grouped in small clumps.

It is not uncommon to see a dermal infiltration of inflammatory cells around and within hair sheaths and sebaceous ducts, which show some degree of spongiosis and cellular degeneration. This picture could be partly due to direct penetration of the allergens through the pilosebaceous unit.

The infiltrate is of the lymphohistiocytic type, composed almost exclusively of mononuclear cells, varying in form and size. The occurrence of an intimate contact between the cell surfaces of lymphocytes and the cell processes of macrophages was demonstrated many years ago at the ultrastructural level. It was emphasized that, in delayed hypersensitivity, macrophages were thought to play an important role, together with lymphocytes. This view was later confirmed and broadened by the discovery of the role played by Langerhans cells (Fig. 9.2).

Polymorphonuclear neutrophils are usually absent. Some eosinophils can be found in the edematous tissue of the upper dermis, migrating toward the epidermis, but this is not a common finding.

The histopathological picture is very similar when the biopsy is taken 72 or 96 h after the application of the allergen. The dermal infiltrate around blood vessels is usually more pronounced. At this later stage, a few eosinophils can be observed very occasionally.

The role of the mast cell in allergic contact hypersensitivity remains controversial. Some studies showing histological evidence of mast cell degranulation suggest that early mast cell activation does occur [8].

In recent years, Hannuksela's repeated open application test (see Chap. 24.) has become popular for confirming the clinical relevance of positive allergic patch test reactions [9]. We have taken biopsies from positive allergic open test reactions on the volar aspect of the forearm, or the cubital fossa, 48, 72, or 96 h after the application of the allergen. In all cases, the histopathological picture was quite similar to that observed in positive allergic patch test reactions. Spongiosis in hair follicles was often prominent, explaining the clinically follicular pattern of the reactions, observed very often when practicing ROAT tests.

9

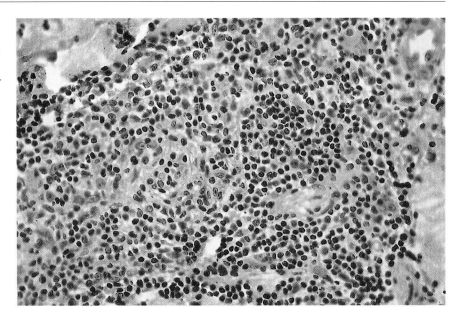

Fig. 9.2 Allergic positive patch test reaction to wool wax alcohols (lanolin alcohol) at 2 days: dense perivascular infiltrate of mononuclear cells. Hematoxylin–eosin–saffron stain (×250)

Two additional features can be observed occasionally:

- In some positive allergic patch test reactions, particularly to azo dyes, purpuric lesions are clinically present [10]. In those cases, there is an important extravasation of erythrocytes, mainly located around blood capillaries, but extending also to interstitial dermal tissue and invading epidermis (exocytosis). In reality, a mild extravasation of erythrocytes with epidermal exocytosis is noticed in almost all positive patch test reactions. This common observation is not detected at the clinical level, but is clearly identified histologically on formaldehyde-fixed skin specimens.

- In some other positive allergic patch test reactions, e.g., to gold (more often at 96 h than 48 h), the infiltrate may be lymphomatoid and mimics pseudolymphoma [11]. It is dense, with a few mitotic figures, and subtle nuclear atypia. Rarely, the lymphoid cells may be very bizarre.

Core Message

> Histopathological features of positive allergic patch test reactions are typical of a spongiotic dermatitis, similar to that observed in different eczematous (exogenous or endogenous) reactions. This includes typical epidermal lesions, and the presence of a dense lymphocytic infiltrate in upper dermis, with epidermal exocytosis of the lymphocytes.

9.3 Histopathological Features of Positive Irritant Patch Test Reactions

The histopathological picture of positive allergic patch test reactions has been shown to be very similar ("monotonous and uniform") in most cases (see above). When irritants are applied – under occlusion – on the skin, a wide range of different lesions can be seen. This kaleidoscope of lesions concerns mainly epidermal alterations.

Various factors play a role in the formation of lesions: (1) the nature of the irritant agent, and consequently its mode of deleterious action on the cells, (2) the concentration of the irritant applied on the skin, (3) the ways of penetration of the skin, and (4) the individual reactivity of the skin to a well-defined irritant.

It is therefore possible that the same irritant chemical can produce different types of lesions in different patients, even when it is applied for the same duration

Fig. 9.3 Irritant positive patch test reaction to croton oil at 2 days: spongiotic vesiculation in epidermis with exocytosis of mononuclear cells. This picture is indistinguishable from an allergic reaction. Masson's trichrome *blue* stain (×150)

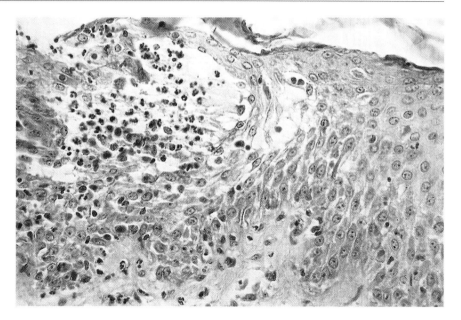

and under the same conditions. There is no general rule in this respect (Fig. 9.3).

9.3.1 Epidermal Changes

Various alterations of epidermal cells can be observed. In some cases, these alterations are limited to the superficial layers of the epidermis, the granular layer and the upper part of the spinous layer; in others, they extend to the dermo-epidermal junction, invading all layers of the epidermis. At first, cells become karyopyknotic and lose their cytoplasmic staining properties on hematoxylin and eosin sections. These changes are known as "Bandmann's achromasia" [12]. When the irritation process becomes more severe, complete necrosis (or cytolysis) of epidermal cells occurs, leading to the formation of intra- or subepidermal vesicles and bullae. "Chemical acantholysis" of epidermal cells can be seen (Fig. 9.4), mainly, but not exclusively, with certain irritants, such as cantharidin and

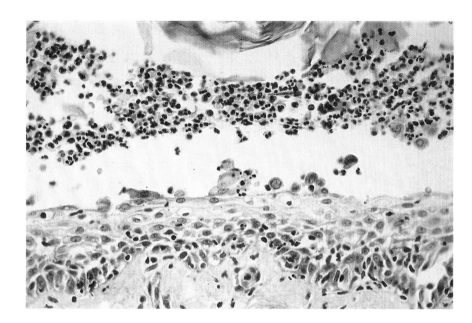

Fig. 9.4 Irritant positive patch test reaction to trichloroethylene at 2 days: epidermal necrosis with acantholytic keratinocytes, exocytosis of inflammatory cells. Masson's trichrome blue stain (×150)

9

trichloroethylene [13]. Polymorphonuclear neutrophils accumulate in the damaged epidermis, leading to the formation of subcorneal or intraepidermal pustules.

In some cases, the formation of pustules is preferentially limited to the hair follicles (Fig. 9.5). Follicular pustules are preferentially provoked by some irritants, such as croton oil ("croton oil effect"), or metal salts such as chromates, and those of mercury and nickel. Pustules due to metals are observed mainly, but not exclusively, in atopics. As already noted many years ago, some irritant reactions do not show any of the aforementioned histopathological signs; they are exclusively spongiotic (with or without vesicles).

Such observations can be made: (1) with weak irritants, (2) with strong irritants, applied on the skin at a low concentration, and (3) in the "excited" (or irritable) skin syndrome.

Table 9.1 Epidermal lesions observed in relation to certain common irritants

Irritants	Epidermal lesions
Nonchlorinated organic solvents (i.e., alkanes, such as n-hexane; toluene; xylene; white spirit; turpentine, etc.)	Achromasia; superficial necrosis; karyopyknosis; very occasional acantholysis; subepidermal vesicles and/or bullae
Chlorinated organic solvents (i.e., trichloro-ethane; trichloroethylene; carbon tetrachloride; etc.)	Acantholysis ++; karyopyknosis; complete necrosis of epidermal cells; intraepidermal vesicles and/or bullae
Acids, alkalis, surfactants, detergents, aldehydes	Achromasia; superficial or complete necrosis of epidermal cells; subepidermal vesicles and/or bullae; no acantholysis

Examples of epidermal lesions classically observed with certain categories of irritants are given in Table 9.1.

Many years ago, ultrastructural studies threw some light on the mode of action of certain irritants, including croton oil, sodium hydroxide, and hydrochloric acid. More recently, Willis et al. [14, 15] completed an extensive study comparing the action of several categories of irritants, using semi-thin section technology. They noted in particular that various kinds of detergents damaged epidermal cells in different ways when applied at a low concentration. For instance, the major response to the anionic detergent sodium lauryl sulfate was parakeratosis, indicating increased epidermal cell turnover, whilst benzalkonium chloride, a cationic detergent, caused a different type of reaction – spongiosis and exocytosis with focal necrotic damage [16].

Phototoxic reactions are characterized by the presence of eosinophilic necrotic keratinocytes ("sunburn cells").

9.3.2 Dermal Changes

Dermal changes are also related to the mechanisms involved in the mode of action of each individual irritant. Dermal edema is absent or slight. Blood capillaries and lymphatics are discretely dilated, but usually to a lesser extent than in positive allergic patch test reactions.

In some cases, there is an important inflammatory response distributed around the blood vessels of the upper and mid-dermis. It is either homogeneously

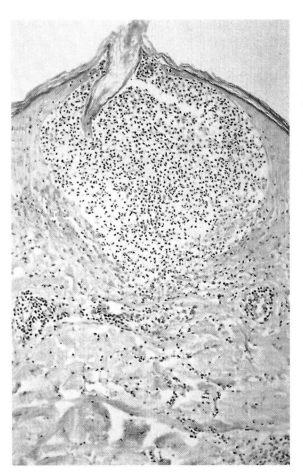

Fig. 9.5 Irritant positive patch test reaction to croton oil at 2 days: a follicular pustule is filled with neutrophils and lymphoid cells. There is a perivascular infiltrate of mononuclear cells. Masson's trichrome *blue* stain (×75)

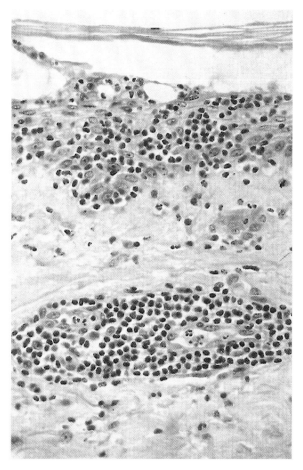

Fig. 9.6 Irritant positive patch test reaction to sodium lauryl sulfate at 2 days: the epidermis is partly necrotic with infiltration of mononuclear cells. There is a dermal perivascular infiltrate of mononuclear cells. Hematoxylin–eosin stain (×150)

mononuclear or mixed (polymorphonuclear neutrophils and lymphocytes/macrophages). Eosinophils are absent. In cases of severe irritation, it is usual to find pyknotic remnants of neutrophils in the upper part of the dermis (Fig. 9.6).

Core Message

> › Histopathological features of positive irritant patch test reactions are varied, depending on the nature and/or concentration of irritant chemicals and the individual reactivity of the skin. This "kaleidoscope" of lesions concerns mainly epidermal and/or adnexal alterations.

9.4 Histopathological Criteria for Distinguishing Between Allergic and Irritant Patch Test Reactions in Humans

In the preceding paragraphs, the various histopathological signs encountered in allergic and irritant patch test reactions have been reviewed in detail [12, 17–20]. We must remember that this description refers to "typical" cases: irritant (without allergic component) or allergic (without irritant component). Comparative signs are presented in Table 9.2. These distinctive criteria are of limited value in practice for many reasons: (1) most criteria are present in irritant as well as in allergic positive patch test reactions; (2) other criteria are predominant either in irritant or in allergic reactions, but they lack specificity; (3) most allergens also have irritant properties. Even when the allergens are patch tested at a concentration below the level of clinical irritancy to avoid "mixed" pictures, it is just possible that subclinically, at the microscopic level, they might show a mixed picture of irritation and allergy.

In practice, when a positive patch test reaction is clinically doubtful (irritant vs. allergic), the help from a biopsy is minimal, due to the differential bias explained above. As an example, the recent epidemics of allergic contact dermatitis to dimethylfumarate, a preservative agent, inserted in small bags in the lining of Chinese sofas, boots, and/or shoes led to extensive clinical investigations throughout Europe. Positive patch test reactions to dimethylfumarate, 0.1% in petrolatum, were biopsied at 48 h. The histopathological picture was a mixture of irritant (necrosis of the upper layers of epidermis) and allergic (spongiosis and vesiculation) contact dermatitis. This emphasizes that dimethylfumarate has both irritant and allergenic properties, a common feature encountered with preservatives and/or antiseptic agents.

Interestingly enough, biopsies of positive patch test reactions to dimethylfumarate, 0.01% in petrolatum, showed only spongiosis and vesiculation, without any sign of necrosis (unpublished data).

Avnstorp et al. [21] conducted a semiquantitative histopathological study of individual morphological parameters in allergic and irritant patch test reactions. Their conclusions were as follows: statistical analysis by correlation of 17 selected variables gives a diagnostic specificity of 87% and a

Table 9.2 Distinctive histopathological criteria between allergic and irritant patch test reactions in humans (modified from [8])

	Allergic reactions	Irritant reactions
Epidermis		
Spongiosis	+ to +++	+ or −
Exocytosis	+ to +++	+++
Vesicles	+ (spongiotic)	+ (rarely spongiotic)
Formation of bullae	Facultative (spongiotic)	Facultative (rarely spongiotic)
Pustules	−	+ or −
Necrosis of epidermal cells	−	+ to +++
Acantholysis of epidermal cells	−	+ or −
Distribution of the infiltrate in epidermis	Focal [21]	Diffuse [21]
Dermis		
Perivascular infiltrate	Mononuclear	Mononuclear or mixed (mononuclear + neutrophils)
Eosinophilic leucocytes	+ or −	−
Dilatation of lymphatic vessels	+ or −	−
Dilatation of blood capillaries	+ or −	+ or −
Edema	+ or −	Very unusual

sensitivity of 81% for allergic reactions. For irritant reactions, the specificity is 100% and the sensitivity 46%. By multiple regressive analysis, an index was calculated for the differentiation of allergic and irritant reactions. If this index were to be used in cases of allergic patch test reactions, all would also be reported as allergic reactions while half of the irritant reactions would be reported as allergic. Although this study has shed some light on the problem of the histopathological differentiation between allergic and irritant contact dermatitis, many difficulties remain in making such a differentiation [21].

When considering all these potential criteria of differential diagnosis, it is worth saying that spongiosis is in bulk a more consistent feature in allergic than in irritant reactions. Vestergaard et al. [22] have recently conducted a human study comparing allergic and irritant reactions. Biopsy samples were taken at a very early stage (6–8 h) after applying (1) an irritant (benzalkonium chloride) and (2) an allergen (that is colophony or quaternium-15) to

individuals with known allergy to one of these allergens, selected because they rarely give rise to unspecific or irritant reactions. The significant finding was that focal spongiosis was present only in allergic reactions.

It is likely that the aggregation of monocytes/macrophages and proliferating T-cells, along with their chemical mediators, is responsible for the epidermal spongiosis in allergic contact dermatitis [23].

In conclusion, though conventional histopathology of positive patch test reactions can provide some useful information, it is of little help in separating allergic from irritant or mixed reactions. Drawing such a conclusion at the end of this section might appear to be negative, since a different view has prevailed for decades in so many European contact dermatitis clinics. Nevertheless, it is based on a careful review of the literature and a reappraisal of our own material. It coincides with the views of the basic scientists and must be considered by practicing dermatologists as reflecting reality.

Core Message

› Histopathological differential diagnosis between allergic and irritant patch test reactions is clearly explained in Table 9.2.

9.5   Comparative Immunohistochemical and Immunocytochemical Characteristics of Allergic and Irritant Patch Test Reactions in Humans

An explosion of knowledge concerning the mechanisms involved in contact dermatitis has been taking place over the past 10 years; the discovery of the key role played by the Langerhans cells and the ability to identify subpopulations of lymphocytes by the use of monoclonal antibodies must be considered as major advances. This has raised the question as to whether the use of new immunocytopathological techniques might help in distinguishing between irritant and allergic patch test reactions.

9.5.1   Epidermal Langerhans Cells in Irritant and Allergic Positive Patch Test Reactions

Semiquantitative studies related to the number of Langerhans cells (LC; CD1, or T_6 dendritic cells) in the epidermis in positive irritant and allergic patch test reactions have been conducted. These studies have revealed a statistically significant decrease in LC 48 or 72 h after the application of various types of irritants: sodium lauryl sulfate, mercuric chloride, benzalkonium chloride, croton oil, or dithranol. There was also a significant reduction in dendritic length. These changes in density were unrelated to the intensity of the inflammatory response [24].

Similar studies in positive allergic patch test reactions show an early transitory increase in LC in the first few hours [25] following the application of allergens, though a similar response occurs at the sites of

petrolatum application [25]. This phenomenon may therefore lack specificity. Later on, at 24, 48, or 72 h after the application of the allergen, the number of LC is unchanged or decreases when compared with normal skin. It may also be reduced at the site of negative patch test reactions [26]. Current studies indicate that allergic and irritant patch test reactions cannot be differentiated reliably by counting LC, in spite of the small differences observed [27]. Moreover, lymphocyte/LC apposition is observed in both types of reactions [28, 29]. The presence of human leukocyte antigen (HLA) DR antigens on keratinocytes in allergic reactions may reflect an immunological response [30].

9.5.2   Cells of the Infiltrate in Irritant and Allergic Positive Patch Test Reactions: Immunophenotypic Studies

Early human studies showed little evidence of differential cytokine release between allergic and irritant contact dermatitis.

This strongly suggests that, although initiating events vary considerably, the cascade mechanisms responsible for the induction and release of regulating mediators are similar [31, 32]. Clearly, most, if not all, proinflammatory phenomena can be caused both by irritants and allergens. Therefore, they do not unambiguously discriminate between irritants and contact allergens [33].

In the various studies conducted so far, the composition of the infiltrates is similar in allergic and irritant reactions, and consists of T lymphocytes of helper/inducer types in association with T-cell accessory cells, that is, LC and HLA-DR-positive macrophages.

Probably, true differences between these types of compounds depend on whether or not allergen-specific T-cells become involved [33]. Thus, only after specific T-cell triggering distinctive features might be observed, e.g., local release of certain chemokines, such as CXCL10 (IP-10) and CXCL11 (I-TAC/IP9) [34].

The latter chemokines are produced by interferon-γ-activated keratinocytes and T lymphocytes [35].

9

Core Messages

> New immunocytopathological techniques are of no real help in distinguishing between irritant and allergic patch test reactions, since there is little evidence of differential cytokine release.

> Clearly, most, if not all, of proinflammatory phenomena can be caused by both irritants and allergens. Therefore, they do not discriminate between irritants and contact allergens.

9.6 Conclusions

In spite of certain differences in the histopathological lesions observed in allergic and irritant patch test reactions, there is as yet no reliable diagnostic tool (either morphological or immunophenotypic) to "label" specifically each type of reaction.

References

1. Wilkinson SM, Beck MH (2004) Contact dermatitis: irritant. In: Burns DA, Breathnach SM, Cox N, Griffiths CE (eds) Rook's textbook of dermatology, 7th edn, Chap. 19. Blackwell Science, Oxford
2. Beck MH, Wilkinson SM (2004) Contact dermatitis: allergic. In: Burns DA, Breathnach SM, Cox N, Griffiths CE (eds) Rook's textbook of dermatology, 7th edn, Chap. 20. Blackwell Science, Oxford
3. Rietschel RL, Fowler JF Jr (2008) Fisher's contact dermatitis, 6th edn. BC Decker, Hamilton
4. Rietschel RL, Conde-Salazar L, Goossens A, Veien NK (1999) Atlas of contact dermatitis. Dunitz, London
5. Kerl H, Burg G, Braun-Falco O (1974) Quantitative and qualitative dynamics of the epidermal and cellular inflammatory reaction in primary toxic and allergic dinitrochlorobenzene contact dermatitis in guinea pigs. Arch Dermatol Forsch 249:207–226
6. Queille-Roussel C, Graeber M, Thurston M, Lachapelle JM, Decroix J, de Cuyper C, Ortonne JP (2000) SDZ ASM 981 is the first non-steroid that suppresses established nickel contact dermatitis elicited by allergen challenge. Contact Dermat 42:349–350
7. Alomar A, Puig L, Gallardo CM, Valenzuela N (2003) Topical tacrolimus 0.1% ointment (Protopic®) reverses nickel contact dermatitis elicited by allergen challenge to a similar degree to mometasone furoate 0.1% with greater suppression of late erythema. Contact Dermat 49:185–188
8. Angelini G, Vena GA, Filotico R, Tursi A (1990) Mast cell participation in allergic contact sensitivity. Contact Dermat 23:239
9. Hannuksela M, Salo H (1986) The repeated open application test (ROAT). Contact Dermat 14:221–227
10. Lazarov A, Cordoba M (2000) Purpuric contact dermatitis in patients with allergic reaction to textile dyes and resins. J Eur Acad Dermatol Venereol 14:101–105
11. Fleming C, Burden D, Fallowfield M et al (1997) Lymphomatoid contact reaction to gold earrings. Contact Dermat 37:298–299
12. Lachapelle JM (1973) Comparative histopathology of allergic and irritant patch test reactions in man. Current concepts and new prospects. Arch Belg Dermatol 28:83–92
13. Mahmoud G, Lachapelle JM (1985) Evaluation expérimentale de l'efficacité de crèmes barrière et de gels antisolvants dans la prévention de l'irritation cutanée provoquée par des solvants organiques. Cah Med Trav 22:163–168
14. Willis CM, Stephens CJM, Wilkinson JD (1989) Epidermal damage induced by irritants in man: a light and electron microscopic study. J Invest Dermatol 93:695–699
15. Willis CM, Stephens CJM, Wilkinson JD (1989) Preliminary findings on the patterns of epidermal damage induced by irritants in man. In: Frosch PJ, Dooms-Goossens A, Lachapelle JM, Rycroft RJ, Scheper RJ (eds) Current topics in contact dermatitis. Springer, Berlin, pp 42–45
16. Willis CM, Stephens CJM, Wilkinson JD (1993) Differential patterns of epidermal leukocyte infiltration in patch test reactions to structurally unrelated chemical irritants. J Invest Dermatol 101:364–370
17. Medenica M, Rostenberg A (1971) A comparative light and electron microscopic study of primary irritant contact dermatitis and allergic contact dermatitis. J Invest Dermatol 56:259–271
18. Lachapelle JM (1972) Comparative study of 3H-thymidine labelling of the dermal infiltrate of skin allergic and irritant patch test reactions in man. Br J Dermatol 87:460–465
19. Grosshans E, Lachapelle JM (1982) Comparative histo- and cytopathology of allergic and irritant patch test reactions in Man. In: Foussereau J, Benezra C, Maibach H (eds) Occupational contact dermatitis. Clinical and chemical aspects. Munksgaard, Copenhagen, pp 63–69
20. Nater JP, Hoedemaeker PHJ (1976) Histopathological differences between irritant and allergic patch test reactions in man. Contact Dermat 2:247–253
21. Avnstorp C, Balslev E, Thomsen HK (1989) The occurrence of different morphological parameters in allergic and irritant patch test reactions. In: Frosch PJ, Dooms-Goossens A, Lachapelle JM, Rycroft RJ, Scheper RJ (eds) Current topics in contact dermatitis. Springer, Berlin, pp 38–41
22. Vestergaard L, Clemmensen OJ, Sorensen FB, Andersen KE (1999) Histological distinction between early allergic and irritant patch test reactions: follicular spongiosis may be characteristic of early allergic contact dermatitis. Contact Dermat 41:207–210
23. Belsito DV (1999) The molecular basis of allergic contact dermatitis. In: Dyall-Smith D, Marks R (eds) Dermatology at the millennium. The Proceedings of the 19th World Congress of Dermatology. Parthenon, New York, pp 217–223

24. Ferguson J, Gibbs JH, Beck JS (1985) Lymphocyte subsets and Langerhans cells in allergic and irritant patch test reactions: histometric studies. Contact Dermat 13:166–174
25. Christensen OB, Daniels TE, Maibach HI (1986) Expression of OKT6 antigen by Langerhans cells in patch test reactions. Contact Dermat 14:26–31
26. Brasch J, Mielke V, Kÿnne N, Weber-Matthiesen V, Bruhn S, Sterry W (1990) Immigration of cells and composition of cell infiltrates in patch test reactions. Contact Dermat 23:238
27. Kanerva L, Ranki A, Lauharanta J (1984) Lymphocytes and Langerhans cells in patch tests. An immuno-histochemical and electron microscopic study. Contact Dermat 11:150–155
28. Willis CM, Young E, Brandon DR, Wilkinson JD (1986) Immunopathological and ultrastructural findings in human allergic and irritant contact dermatitis. Br J Dermatol 115:305–316
29. Illis CM, Wilkinson JD (1990) Changes in the morphology and density of epidermal Langerhans cells (CD1 + cells) in irritant contact dermatitis. Contact Dermat 23:239
30. Scheynius A, Fischer T (1986) Phenotypic difference between allergic and irritant patch test reactions in man. Contact Dermat 14:297–302
31. Hoeffaker S, Caubo M, Van't Erve EH (1995) In vivo cytokine profiles in allergic and irritant contact dermatitis. Contact Dermat 33:258–266
32. Ulfgren AK, Klareskog L, Lindberg M (2000) An immunohistochemical analysis of cytokine expression in allergic and irritant contact dermatitis. Acta Derm Venereol (Stockh) 80:167–170
33. Rustemeyer T (2004) Immunological aspects of environmental and occupational contact allergies. Thela Thesis, Amsterdam
34. Flier J, Boorsma DM, Bruynzeel DP, van Beek PJ, Stoof TJ, Scheper RJ, Willemze R, Tensen CP (1999) The CXCR3 activating chemokines IP-10, MIG and IP-9 are expressed in allergic but not in irritant patch test reactions. J Invest Dermatol 113:574–578
35. Tensen CP, Flier J, van der Raaij-Helmer EM, Sampat-Sardjoepersad S, van den Schors RC, Leurs R, Scheper RJ, Boorsma DM, Willemze R (1999) Human IP-9: a keratinocyte derived high affinity CXC-chemokine ligand for the IP-10/Mig receptor (CXCR3). J Invest Dermatol 112:716–722

Ultrastructure of Irritant and Allergic Contact Dermatitis

10

Carolyn M. Willis

Contents

C.M. Willis
Department of Dermatology, Amersham Hospital, Amersham,
Buckinghamshire HP7 0JD, UK
e-mail: carolyn.willis@buckshosp.nhs.uk

10.1 Introduction

Electron microscopy (EM) provides a unique opportunity to scrutinize biopsies of contact dermatitis lesions at ultra-high resolution. Using conventional electron-dense stains, membranes and organelles can be observed in exquisite detail, with developments such as postfixation in ruthenium tetroxide for the visualization of intercellular lipids, further enhancing our ability to study the ultrastructure of skin subjected to irritants and allergens. However, EM undoubtedly has its limitations. Only tiny fragments of tissue can be investigated in depth, which is particularly problematic for experimental irritancy studies, where the cellular damage induced is rarely uniform across the application site. This can be mitigated to an extent by the parallel study of semi-thin plastic sections at the light microscope level, but, nevertheless, studies employing small sample sizes, with limited scrutiny of biopsies, should be viewed with caution. Linking ultrastructure to physiological function has also proven difficult, and there is a need to apply more elaborate staining and imaging tools, such as EM in-situ hybridization and Raman spectroscopy, to enhance our interpretation of the morphological changes that take place. EM also gives us only a snapshot in time of what is a highly dynamic organ system, as indeed does histology, and therefore the recently developed noninvasive, real-time technique of reflectance confocal microscopy has enormous potential as a complementary imaging technique for contact dermatitis.

J.D. Johansen et al. (eds.), *Contact Dermatitis*,
DOI: 10.1007/978-3-642-03827-3_10, © Springer-Verlag Berlin Heidelberg 2011

10

10.2 Ultrastructural Changes in the Epidermis

Being composed of keratinocytes of varying states of differentiation, interspersed with melanocytes and bone marrow-derived cells, such as Langerhans cells (LCs) and T lymphocytes, the epidermis presents a wide variety of biochemical and immunological targets for topically applied irritants and allergens. As a consequence, differing patterns of ultrastructural change are seen across the epidermis, depending upon the chemical characteristics of the agent, the nature and severity of the resulting inflammatory response, and the time of biopsy post-exposure.

10.2.1 Stratum Corneum

The outermost diffusion barrier of the skin, the stratum corneum, is a 20–30 cell-thick layer of flat, hexagonal, protein-rich corneocytes surrounded by intercellular lipids. Generally speaking, chemical irritants produce more pronounced changes to its structure and behavior, as evidenced, biophysically, by increased transepidermal water loss, than do allergens. Ultrastructural studies utilizing ruthenium tetroxide as a postfixative have greatly increased our understanding of the manner in which some chemicals interact with this region of the epidermis and contribute to the development of irritant contact dermatitis (ICD). The application of low concentrations of the anionic surfactant, sodium lauryl sulfate (SLS), to normal human skin was found by Fartasch to result not so much in an alteration to the existing lipid structure, but rather to an alteration in the synthesis of new lipids [1]. Hence, disturbance of lamellar body lipid extrusion and the transformation into the lipid bilayers occurred, in the absence of any disruption to the intercellular lipid layers of the upper stratum corneum. In contrast, acetone produced a different pattern of change. Epidermal lipid lamellae displayed disruption and loss of cohesion throughout the stratum corneum, the transformed, more unpolar, lamellar lipids showing greater disruption than the more polar lamellar body sheets [1]. A similar disruption of stratum corneum intercellular bilayers was also seen in human skin patch tested with water alone [2], which would have the effect, as pointed out by the investigators, of enhancing skin permeability and susceptibility to irritants.

10.2.2 Viable Keratinocytes

The greatest diversity of ultrastructural effects on viable keratinocytes within the epidermis is undoubtedly exerted by irritants, rather than by allergens. While both induce varying degrees of spongiosis, clearly visible by both light and EM, chemical irritants also give rise to a heterogeneity of forms of intracellular damage which are time-, dose-, and, in some cases, irritant-dependent.

10.2.2.1 Irritant Contact Dermatitis

Two early studies provided some of the first evidence that irritants can damage the skin by different mechanisms. A comparison between the effects of an acid and an alkali on human epidermis found that sodium hydroxide dissolved the contents of horny cells and disrupted tonofilament-desmosome complexes, while hydrochloric acid did not [3]. Similarly, in a comparative study of two lipid solvents, the response to acetone, which was characterized by intracellular edema of keratinized cells and vacuolation of spinous cells, was conspicuously different from that to kerosene, in which the formation of large lacunae and cytolysis of spinous cells were seen [4]. In our own study, designed to systematically compare the morphological effects of six structurally-unrelated irritants on normal human skin, EM also revealed significant differences in the nature of the cellular damage induced by different chemicals after 48 h exposure [5]. Patch test reactions to SLS were characterized by parakeratotic cells in the upper epidermis, containing dense osmiophilic cytoplasm with numerous lipid droplets and vesicles, and an absence of keratohyalin granules (Fig. 10.1). Lipid droplets were also numerous in keratinocytes within the stratum spinosum (Fig. 10.2), whilst basal keratinocytes undergoing mitosis were occasionally observed (Fig. 10.3), reflecting the increased rate of proliferation known to occur with this irritant [6]. In contrast, the cationic detergent, benzalkonium chloride, produced intracytoplasmic vacuolation within the keratinocytes of mild reactions (Fig. 10.4) through to distinct areas of necrosis in severe responses (Fig. 10.5). Application of the 12-C long chain fatty acid, nonanoic acid, resulted in the formation of tongues of dyskeratotic cells, largely composed of dense, wavy aggregates of osmiophilic keratin filaments associated with prominent

Fig. 10.1 Low power transmission electron micrograph of a 48-h patch test reaction to SLS (5%) showing a zone of parakeratotic cells with dense osmiophilic cytoplasm containing lipid droplets and membrane bound vesicles, but devoid of keratohyalin granules (original magn. ×1,400)

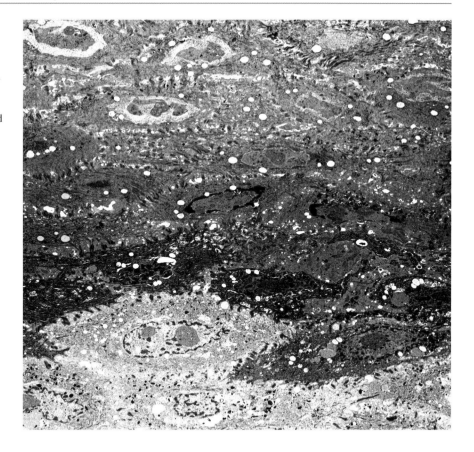

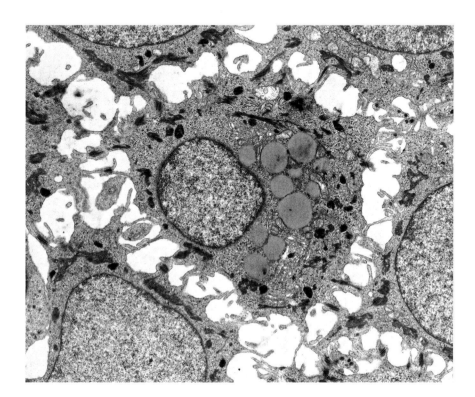

Fig. 10.2 Keratinocytes in the stratum spinosum of a 48-h SLS (5%) patch test reaction, illustrating lipid droplet accumulation (original magn. ×4,000)

10

Fig. 10.3 A mitotic
keratinocyte in the basal
epidermis of a 48-h patch
test reaction to SLS (5%)
(original magn. ×2,000)

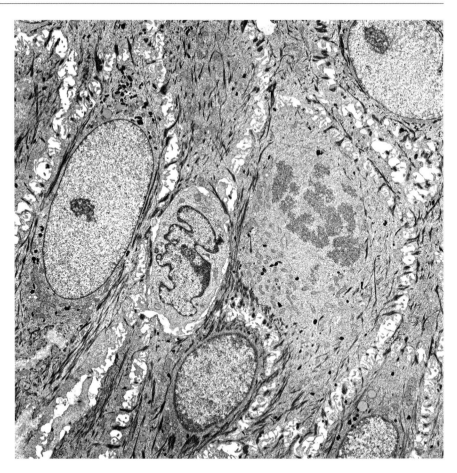

intercellular desmosomes, and containing shrunken
nuclei with condensed, marginated heterochromatin
(Fig. 10.6). Exposure to dithranol produced markedly
enlarged upper epidermal keratinocytes, containing
finely dispersed filaments and ribosomes, and, in keeping with previous findings [7, 8], disrupted mitochondria clustered around the nucleus (Fig. 10.7). Croton
oil induced reactions which were very similar to allergic contact dermatitis (ACD), the major features being
pronounced spongiosis and exocytosis, and an exocy-
totic infiltrate largely composed of mononuclear cells
(Fig. 10.8) except in severe reactions where significant
numbers of polymorphonuclear leucocytes were
present.

The concept of ultrastructural changes being irritant-
dependent was further supported by a recent study of
the effects of a wide variety of irritant chemicals on the
skin of hairless guinea pigs [9]. Although the skin

changes described were not identical to those seen in
human skin, partly perhaps as a result of concentration
differences, it was clear, for example, that, again, the
nature of the epidermal damage elicited by SLS differed markedly from that of benzalkonium chloride.

The ultrastructural changes to the viable cells in the
epidermis which have been variously described by investigators during the last three decades [3–11] (Table 10.1)
are, in the main, indicative of autolysis or cytolysis,
which would eventually lead to the disintegration of the
cell. In some cases, however, certain alterations, such as
condensation of chromatin and cytosol, clumping of
tonofilaments and budding of membrane-bound cell
fragments, may be suggestive of another form of cell
death, that of apoptosis. Often ultrastructurally indistinguishable from dyskeratotic cells in the early stages,
apoptotic keratinocytes have been described in reactions
to a number of well-studied irritants [12–14].

Fig. 10.4 Intracytoplasmic vacuolation within keratinocytes of the stratum spinosum in a mild 48 h reaction to benzalkonium chloride (0.5%) (original magn. ×2,000)

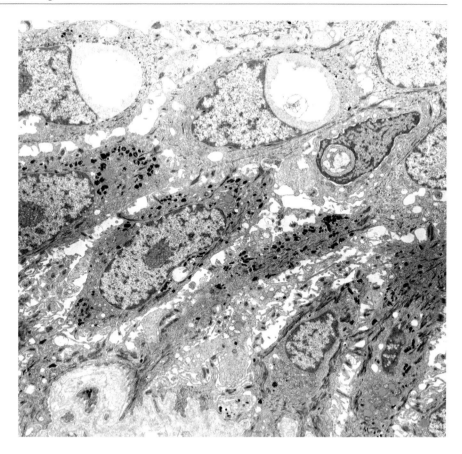

10.2.2.2 Allergic Contact Dermatitis

Intercellular edema or spongiosis, characterized by dilated intercellular spaces, stretched or absent tonofilament-desmosome complexes, and the aggregation of tonofilaments into short bundles, is a consistent feature of the viable epidermal layers in ACD (Fig. 10.9), and one which is detectable in sensitized individuals by EM as early as 3 h after exposure to hapten [15]. Vesiculation frequently occurs as the reaction progresses, with exocytosis of predominantly mononuclear cells (Fig. 10.10). Intracellular changes to keratinocytes, such as vacuolation and endoplasmic reticulum dilatation, are also seen, but since the majority of allergens are also intrinsically irritant in nature, ascribing such changes with any degree of certainty to the process of sensitization itself is very difficult. Indeed, in a study of chromium reactions in man and guinea pig, the authors concluded that keratinocyte intracellular reaction patterns were nonspecific and could not be distinguished from those of vehicle or occlusion alone [16].

10.2.3 Langerhans Cells

Much of the ultrastructural data relating to LC behavior in contact dermatitis focus on ACD rather than ICD. Contradictory EM findings exist, stimulating debate as to whether overt cellular damage to LC is an inherent feature of allergic contact reactions, and the extent to which the changes seen are specific to ACD. Nevertheless, there is no doubt that this antigen-presenting cell plays a pivotal role in ACD [17]. As to whether LCs have a functional role in ICD remains a matter of speculation, although there is certainly evidence of migration into the dermis in common with ACD [17] and a considerable degree of morphological change apparent within epidermal LC.

10.2.3.1 Allergic Contact Dermatitis

As early as 1973, ultrastructural observations led to speculation that LCs might play a role in allergic contact reactions [18]. Close apposition to mononuclear cells was

10

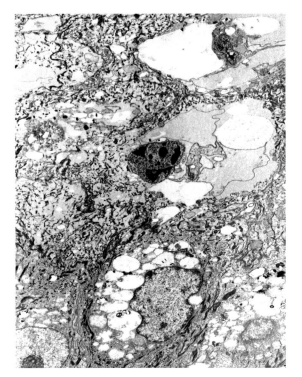

Fig. 10.5 An area of necrosis induced in the mid epidermis by 48-h patch testing with benzalkonium chloride (0.5%). Keratinocytes show extensive vacuolation, pyknotic nuclei and disrupted organelles and membranes (original magn. ×2,700)

described as being an exclusive feature of ACD, and a variety of cellular changes suggestive of targeted physiological activity were seen. In the intervening years, numerous ultrastructural studies designed to elucidate the behavior of LC have been conducted, some of which are summarized in Table 10.2. From these, it would appear that there is early metabolic activation, as indicated by prominent rough endoplasmic reticulum and Golgi apparatus, during the early stages of induction and elicitation, followed later by degenerative changes, such as membrane disruption and condensation of nuclear chromatin. In a rare ultrastructural study linking LC function and morphology, Rizova et al. described an alteration in the pattern of endocytosis of major histocompatibility complex class II (HLA-DR) molecules specific to allergens. Sensitiser-treated LCs internalized HLA-DR preferentially in lysosomes collected near the nucleus, whereas irritant-treated and nontreated LCs internalized the molecules in prelysosomes located near the cell membrane [19].

10.2.3.2 Irritant Contact Dermatitis

Current immunological evidence does not support the concept of any specific functional activities for LC

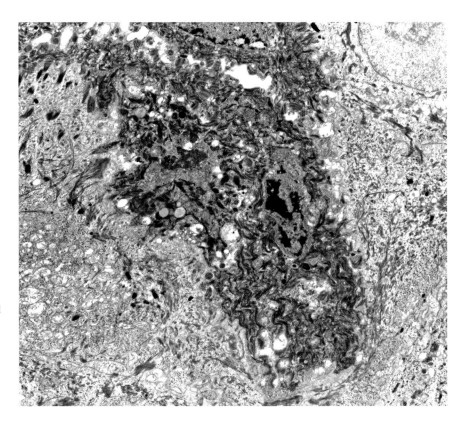

Fig. 10.6 A tongue of dyskeratotic upper epidermal cells, containing dense, wavy aggregates of osmiophilic keratin filaments, produced by 48 h patch testing with nonanoic acid (80%) (original magn. ×4,000)

Fig. 10.7 Enlarged upper epidermal keratinocyte, with cytoplasm containing finely dispersed filaments and ribosomes and perinuclearly clustered mitochondria, in a 48-h patch test reaction to dithranol (0.2%) (original magn. ×2,000)

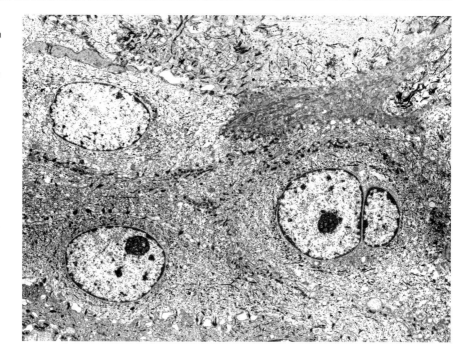

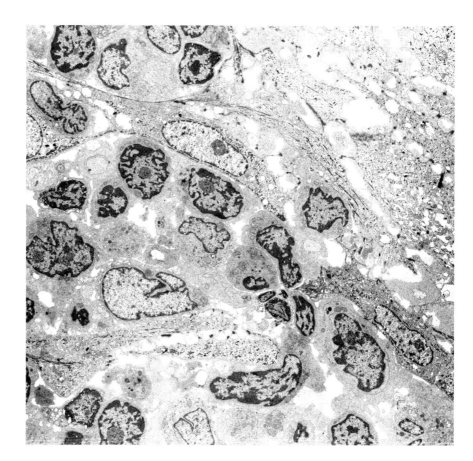

Fig. 10.8 Low power micrograph of the upper epidermis of a 48-h patch test reaction to croton oil (0.8%) showing spongiosis and exocytosis of predominantly mononuclear cells (original magn. ×1,400)

10

Table 10.1 Ultrastructural changes induced in the viable epidermis by acute exposure to selected irritants

Irritant	Ultrastructural changes
Sodium lauryl sulfate	Spongiosis, vesiculation, nuclear/intracytoplasmic/mitochondrial vacuolation, lipid droplet accumulation, hydropic swelling, decreased desmosomes with aggregation of tonofilaments
Benzalkonium chloride	Nuclear/intracytoplasmic vacuolation, nuclear pyknosis, mitochondrial swelling, organelle disruption, hydropic swelling, spongiosis
Dithranol	Hydropic swelling, mitochondrial membrane disruption, spongiosis, intracytoplasmic vacuolation, dyskeratosis, apoptosis, colloid bodies
Croton oil	Marked spongiosis, intracytoplasmic vacuolation, pyknotic/enlarged nuclei
Nonanoic acid	Dyskeratosis, nuclear/intracytoplasmic vacuolation, vesiculation, lipid droplet accumulation, pyknotic nuclei
Acetone	Acantholysis, spongiosis, nuclear/intracytoplasmic oedema and vacuolation
Sodium hydroxide	Disrupted tonofilament-desmosome complexes

Changes are irritant, concentration and time-dependent

Combined human and animal data [3–13]

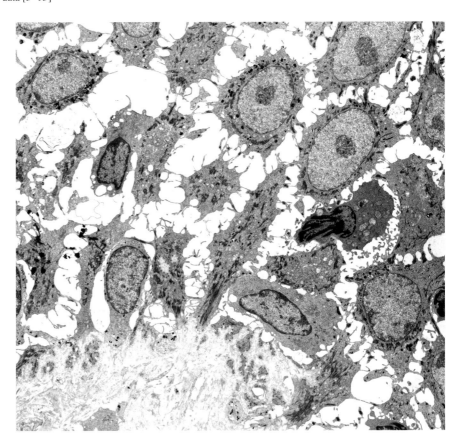

Fig. 10.9 Marked basal spongiosis in a 48-h patch test reaction to nickel sulfate (5%) (original magn. 1,400)

during the evolution of ICD, other than perhaps as a contributor to the milieu of inflammatory mediators, through their production and release of cytokines such as IL-1 [20]. Morphological evidence, however, certainly points to their participation in ICD, which, within the epidermis, shows variability with respect to time, severity of insult and the chemical nature of the irritant applied [21]. Table 10.3 provides a summary of some of the ultrastructural studies in this area, which provide evidence for LC being both activated and in a

Fig. 10.10 Vesiculation and exocytosis of mononuclear cells in a 48-h patch test reaction to balsam of Peru (original magn. ×1,400)

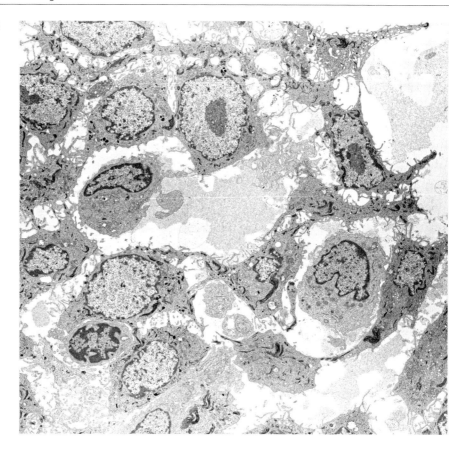

Table 10.2 A summary of the major ultrastructural changes induced in Langerhans cells by selected chemical allergens

Allergen(s)	Langerhans cell changes	References
Various (man, 4–72 h)	Apposition to mononuclear cells. Prominent rough endoplasmic reticulum and Golgi complexes, glycogen accumulation, presence of polyribosomes, lysosome-like projections, ruffled cell membranes. Disruption to membranes	[18]
DNCB (guinea pig, 2–48 h)	Early cellular vacuolar and granular changes, with apposition to mononuclear cells. Later migration to/loss from, the horny layer	[29]
Nickel, thiuram mix, epoxy resin, neomycin (man, 72 h)	Apposition to other cells, marked endocytosis with greatly increased cytoplasmic content of vesicles, the latter having trilaminar membranes and specific granules. Dark cytoplasmic vesicles (nickel). No evidence of cell damage	[30]
DNCB (guinea pig, 2 h to 14 days)	Early activation (6 h), with prominent rough endoplasmic reticulum and Golgi, and numerous lysosomes and vacuoles. After 12 h, cell damage, evidenced by disruption of cell membranes etc	[31]
Various (man, 3–168 h)	Increased metabolic activity in some cells, with distended endoplasmic reticulum, pronounced microtubules and increased numbers of Birbeck granules. Also occasional necrotic cells, with condensed chromatin and shrunken cytoplasm	[32]

(continued)

10

Table 10.2 (continued)

Allergen(s)	Langerhans cell changes	References
Various (man, 3–72 h)	No morphological changes indicative of damage	[33]
Picryl chloride, DNFB (mouse, 1–96 h)	1–24 h, activation with enlargement of cell and nucleus and increase in mitochondria, Golgi and endoplasmic reticulum. After 48 h, degenerative changes	[34]
DNFB (induction) (guinea pig, 15 min to 24 h)	Activation from 15 min, with LC showing intense endocytotic activity – numerous coated vesicles and Birbeck granules	[35]
Various (man, 72 h)	Increased numbers of LC, increased synthesis and cell surface expression of HLA class II molecules	[36]
DNFB (mouse, 1–96 h)	During induction phase, cellular and endocytotic activation. Degenerative changes, including membrane rupture, cytoplasmic oedema and irregular condensation of nuclear chromatin, in the late elicitation phase	[37]

DNCB dinitrochlorobenzene; *DNFB* dinitrofluorobenzene

Table 10.3 A summary of the predominant ultrastructural changes induced in Langerhans cells by acute exposure to selected chemical irritants

Irritant(s)	Langerhans cell changes	References
Mercuric chloride, soap, SLS (man, 24–48 h)	No apposition to mononuclear cells. Glycogen accumulation	[18]
Dithranol, nonanoic acid (man, 6–72 h)	Apposition to mononuclear cells. Ultrastructural evidence of both stimulation and degeneration	[22]
Dithranol (man, 24–48 h)	Fine structural changes in the mitochondria	[23]
BC (man, 3–168 h)	Evidence of both increased metabolic activity (distended endoplasmic reticulum and increased numbers of mitochondria and Birbeck granules) and necrosis (condensed chromatin and shrunken cytoplasm)	[32]
CO, BC, SLS (mice, 1–96 h)	Degenerative changes, with mitochondrial swelling and irregular cytoplasmic vacuolization, followed by membrane disruption and disorganization of the cellular components. With low concentration of CO, prior activation of LC, with increased numbers of mitochondria and enlargement of nuclei	[34]
Six irritants of varying chemical structure (man, 48 h)	Varying numbers of damaged cells displaying vesiculation, loss of integrity of organelles and membranes, condensed nuclear heterochromatin and lipid accumulation. Frequent activated LC, with numerous Birbeck granules in reactions to benzalkonium chloride	[21]

These are irritant, dose, time and species-dependent
SLS sodium lauryl sulfate; *BC* benzalkonium chloride; *CO* croton oil

state of degeneration during the evolution of ICD. Earlier beliefs that apposition of LC to mononuclear cells within the epidermis was unique to ACD [17] have now been set aside, following numerous reports of its occurrence also in ICD [22, 23].

Figure 10.11a–f give examples of some of the common features of LC seen in patch test reactions to allergens and irritants.

10.3 Ultrastructural Changes in the Dermis

Commonly seen changes within the dermis of both ACD and ICD lesions include edema and capillary dilatation (Fig. 10.12), with disruption and degeneration of collagen being an additional feature of some irritant reactions [24]. In their recent light and electron

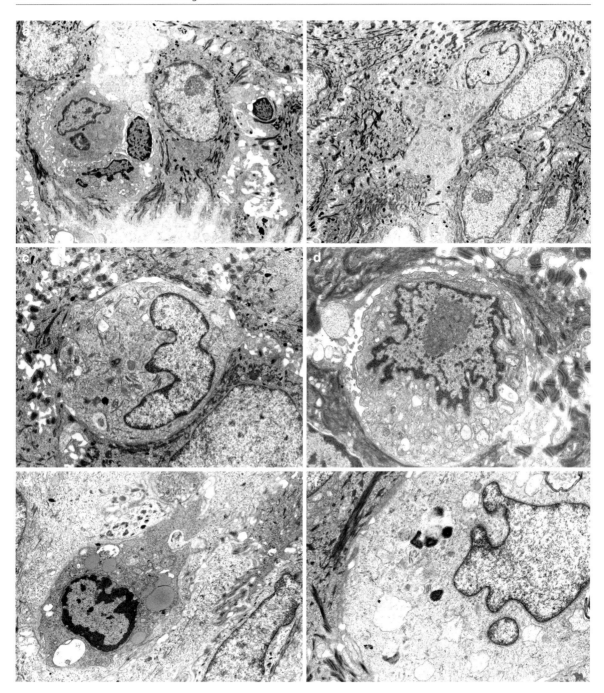

Fig. 10.11 A collection of micrographs showing the variation in Langerhans cell (LC) morphology within ACD and ICD patch test reactions. Apposition of LC to lymphocytes is a common feature in allergic reactions, but is also frequently seen in irritant reactions, particularly those induced by dithranol where clustering of lymphocytes around LC occurs (**a**; 48 h reaction to dithranol [0.02%]; original magn. ×2,700). Activated LC containing widened rough endoplasmic reticulum and numerous mitochondria and Birbeck granules are seen in patch test reactions to both allergens (**b**; 48 h nickel sulfate [5%] patch test; original magn. ×2,700) and irritants (**c**; 48 h benzalkonium chloride [0.5%] reaction; original magn. ×5,000). Degenerative changes to LC, including vacuolation, disrupted organelles and membranes, lipid accumulation and condensation of nuclear chromatin, are also observed in 48 h biopsies of ACD and ICD patch test reactions (**d**, balsam of Peru, original magn. ×8,000; **e**, nonanoic acid [80%], original magn. ×5,000; **f**, benzalkonium chloride [0.5%], original magn. ×6,700)

10

Fig. 10.12 A dilated blood vessel in the dermis of a severe 48 h patch test reaction to benzalkonium chloride (0.5%). Polymorphonuclear leucocytes in addition to lymphocytes have been attracted to the site. An extravasating red blood cell can be seen on the *left* (original magn. ×2,000)

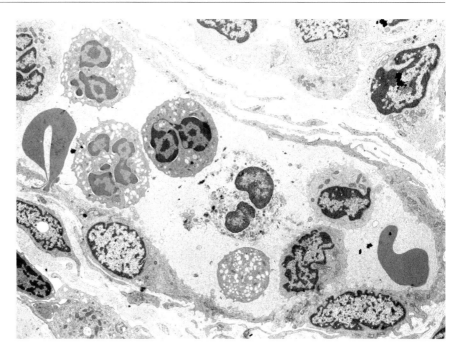

microscopical investigation of the effects of a range of chemical irritants on the skin of hairless guinea pigs, Sueki and Kligman [9] observed variations in the dermis which were, to a degree, irritant-dependent. Exposure to SLS and to organic solvents affected the dermis relatively little. In contrast, benzalkonium chloride and various urticariogens and comedogenic agents induced marked dilation of lymphatic vessels, as well as capillaries. Increased numbers of granules within dermal mast cells were also described for the latter irritants, although this was not quantified in any way.

An earlier light and EM study conducted in hairless mice revealed that many irritant chemicals cause, in addition to the above changes, enlargement or hyperplasia of sebaceous glands, with basal cells displaying morphological signs of enhanced metabolic activity, such as increases in rough endoplasmic reticulum and sebum droplets [25]. Ultrastructural evidence has also led to the belief that platelets lining the dermal venular endothelium during irritant reactions contribute significantly to the pathogenesis of the overall response, at least in mice, being closely linked to the formation of edema [26].

10.4 Ultrastructural Changes in Chronic Contact Dermatitis

Little information is available regarding the ultrastructural changes associated with chronic contact dermatitis. This is largely because of the difficulty in accurately characterizing the disorder. Most clinical cases of chronic contact dermatitis are attributable to a complex admix of endogenously and exogenously-derived provocation factors. Atopy often plays a role and even where sensitization to a relevant hapten is proven, the influence of concomitant irritant exposure is difficult to disentangle. However, recently, Shah and Palmer [27] have attempted to document the variations in the ultrastructural appearance of chronic occupational hand dermatitis linked to chromate allergy. Examination of a broad spectrum of clinical disease, in terms of intensity and duration, revealed cellular features within the epidermis common to other inflammatory dermatoses. These included marked spongiosis and intracellular vacuolation, particularly within the basal layers. However, the authors also described, for the first time in chromate dermatitis, the presence of spindle-shaped granular cells, possibly mast cells, in the upper dermis, closely opposed to the dermo-epidermal junction.

10.5 Summary

The past two or three decades have seen the publication of a wealth of information on the ultrastructural morphology of acute allergic and ICD. However, we still know relatively little about the cellular features of the chronic forms of contact dermatitis. The introduction of modified tissue preparative techniques, such as postfixation in ruthenium tetroxide, has greatly improved visualization of the stratum corneum and increased our understanding of the damage caused by topical exposure to chemicals. Similarly, complementary imaging by semi-thin section light microscopy, reflectance confocal microscopy [28] and flourescence confocal laser scanning microscopy [38] should all assist in the interpretation of ultrastructural observations. However, the challenge remains to fully utilize correlative functional and morphological techniques so that we can more meaningfully translate electron microscopic findings into pathophysiological events.

References

1. Fartasch M (1997) Ultrastructure of the epidermal barrier after irritation. Microsc Res Tech 37:193–199
2. Warner RR, Boissy YL, Lilly NA, Spears MJ, McKillop K, Marshall JL, Stone KJ (1999) Water disrupts stratum corneum lipid lamellae: damage is similar to surfactants. J Invest Dematol 113:960–966
3. Nagao S, Stroud JD, Hamada T, Pinkus H, Birmingham DJ (1972) The effect of sodium hydroxide and hydrochloric acid on human epidermis. Acta Dermatovenereol (Stockh) 52:11–23
4. Lupulescu AP, Birmingham DJ, Pinkus H (1973) An electron microscopic study of human epidermis after acetone and kerosene administration. J Invest Dermatol 60:33–45
5. Willis CM, Stephens CJM, Wilkinson JD (1989) Epidermal damage induced by irritants in man. A light and electron microscopy study. J Invest Dermatol 93:695–700
6. Willis CM, Stephens CJM, Wilkinson JD (1992) Differential effects of structurally unrelated chemical irritants on the density of proliferating keratinocytes in 48h patch test reactions. J Invest Dermatol 99:449–453
7. Swanbeck G, Lundquist PG (1972) Ultrastructural changes of mitochondria in dithranol treated psoriatic epidermis. Acta Dermatovenereol (Stockh) 52:94–98
8. Molière P, Dubertret L, Sa E, Melo MT, Salet C, Fosse M, Santus R (1985) The effect of anthralin (dithranol) on mitochondria. Br J Dermatol 112:509–515
9. Sueki H, Kligman AM (2003) Cutaneous toxicity of chemical irritants on hairless guinea pigs. J Dermatol 30:859–870
10. Metz J (1972) Elecktronenmikroskopische Untersuchungen an allergischen und toxischen Epicutantestreaktionen des Menschen. Arch Derm Forsch 245:125–146
11. Tovell PWA, Weaver AC, Hope J, Sprott WE (1974) The action of sodium lauryl sulphate on rat skin – an ultrastructural study. Br J Dermatol 90:501–506
12. Lindberg M, Forslind B, Wahlberg JE (1982) Reactions of epidermal keratinocytes in sensitized and non-sensitized guinea pigs after dichromate exposure: an electron microscopic study. Acta Dermatovener (Stockh) 62:389–396
13. Kanerva L (1990) Electron microscopic observations of dyskeratosis, apoptosis, colloid bodies and fibrillar degeneration after skin irritation with dithranol. J Cutan Pathol 17:37–44
14. Forsey RJ, Shahidullah H, Sands C, McVittie E, Aldridge RD, Hunter JA, Howie SE (1998) Epidermal Langerhans cell apoptosis is induced in vivo by nonanoic acid but not by sodium lauryl sulphate. Br J Dermatol 139:453–461
15. Komura J, Ofuji S (1980) Ultrastructural studies of allergic contact dermatitis in man. Arch Dermatol Res 267:275–282
16. Forslind B, Wahlberg JE (1978) The morphology of chromium allergic skin reactions at electron microscopic resolution: studies in man and guinea pig. Acta Dermatovener (Stockh) Suppl 79:43–51
17. Toebak MJ, Gibbs S, Bruynzeel DP, Scheper RJ, Rustemeyer T (2009) Dendritic cells: biology of the skin. Contact Dermat 60:2–20
18. Silberberg I (1973) Apposition of mononuclear cells to Langerhans cells in contact allergic reactions. An ultrastructural study. Acta Dermatovener (Stockh) 53:1–12
19. Rizova H, Carayon P, Barbier A, Lacheretz F, Dubertret L, Michel L (1999) Contact allergens, but not irritants, alter receptor-mediated endocytosis by human epidermal Langerhans cells. Br J Dermatol 140:200–209
20. Kimber I (1999) Contact sensitisation mechanisms. In: Basketter DA (ed) Toxicology of contact dermatitis; allergy, irritancy and urticaria, Chap 5. Wiley, Chichester
21. Willis CM, Stephens CJM, Wilkinson JD (1990) Differential effects of structurally-unrelated chemical irritants on the density and morphology of epidermal CD1a+ cells. J Invest Dermatol 95:711–716
22. Kanerva L, Ranki A, Mustakallio K, Lauharanta J (1983) Langerhans cell-mononuclear cell contacts are not specific for allergy in patch tests. Br J Dermatol 109(Suppl 25):64–67
23. Kanerva L, Ranki A, Lauharanta J (1984) Lymphocytes and Langerhans cells in patch tests. Contact Dermat 11:150–155

24. Willis CM (1995) The histopathology of irritant contact dermatitis. In: van der Valk PGM, Maibach HI (eds) The Irritant contact dermatitis syndrome. CRC, Boca Raton, pp 297–298

25. Lesnik RH, Kligman LH, Kligman AM (1992) Agents that cause enlargement of sebaceous glands in hairless mice. I. Topical substances. Arch Dermatol 284:100–105

26. Senaldi G, Piguet P-F (1997) Platelets play a role in the pathogenesis of the irritant reaction in mice. J Invest Dermatol 108:248–252

27. Shuh M, Palmer IR (2002) An ultrastructural study of chronic chromate hand dermatitis. Acta Derm Venereol 82:254–259

28. Astner S, González E, Cheung AC, Rius-Díaz F, Doukas AG, William F, González S (2005) Non-invasive evaluation of the kinetics of allergic and irritant contact dermatitis. J Invest Dermatol 124(2):351–359

29. Hunziker N, Winkelman RK (1978) Langerhans cells in contact dermatitis of the guinea pig. Arch Dermatol 114:1309–1313

30. Falck B, Andersson A, Elofsson R, Sjöborg S (1981) New views on epidermis and its Langerhans cells in the normal state and in contact dermatitis. Acta Dermatovener (Stockh) Suppl 99:3–27

31. Bian Z, Bing-He W (1985) Cytochemical and ultrastructural studies of the Langerhans cells. Int J Dermatol 24:653–659

32. Willis CM, Young E, Brandon DR, Wilkinson JD (1986) Immunopathological and ultrastructural findings in human allergic and irritant contact dermatitis. Br J Dermatol 115:305–316

33. Giannotti B, De Panfilis G, Manara GC (1986) Langerhans cells are not damaged in contact allergic reactions in humans. Am J Dermatopathol 8:220–226

34. Kolde G, Knop J (1987) Different cellular reaction patterns of epidermal Langerhans cells after application of contact sensitizing, toxic, and tolerogenic compounds. A comparative ultrastructural and morphometric time-course analysis. J Invest Dermatol 89:19–23

35. Hanau D, Fabre M, Schmitt DA (1989) ATPase and morphologic changes in Langerhans cells induced by epicutaneous application of a sensitizing dose of DNFB. J Invest Dermatol 92(5):689–694

36. Mommaas AM, Wijsman MC, Mulder AA, van Praag MC, Vermeer BJ, Koning F (1992) HLA class II expression on human epidermal Langerhans cells in situ: upregulation during elicitation of allergic contact dermatitis. Hum Immun 34:99–106

37. Kolde G (1996) Turnover and kinetics of epidermal Langerhans cells and their dendritic precursor cells in experimental contact dermatitis. Arch Dermatol Res 288:197–202

38. Suihko C, Serup J (2008) Fluorescence confocal laser scanning microscopy for in vivo imaging of epidermal reactions to two experimental irritants. Skin Res Technol 14:498–503

Epidemiology

11

Pieter-Jan Coenraads, Wolfgang Uter, and Thomas Diepgen

Contents

P.-J. Coenraads (✉)
Dermatology Department, University Medical Centre
Groningen, Hanzeplein 1, 9713 GZ Groningen,
The Netherlands
e-mail: p.j.coenraads@med.umcg.nl

W. Uter
Department of Medical Informatics, Biometry and
Epidemiology, Univ. Erlangen/Nürnberg, Waldstraße 6,
91054 Erlangen, Germany

T. Diepgen
Department Clinical Social Medicine, University of
Heidelberg, Thibautstraße 3, 69115 Heidelberg,
Germany

11.1 Introduction

Contact dermatitis is a common disorder. Epidemiology is a tool used for appropriate summary measures to describe how common contact dermatitis is. Epidemiology is also used to analyse whether it is more common in specific groups, and which factors are associated with the occurrence of contact dermatitis (or its subtypes) in specific populations or subgroups. Typical questions are, for example, whether nickel allergy is more common in hairdressers, and whether this contact allergy enhances the risk of occupational contact dermatitis. Epidemiologic tools are also used to evaluate the results of interventions in specific populations [1]. A classic example is the occurrence of nickel allergy in Danish women [2] and, in particular, the development of nickel allergy after regulation [3].

11.2 Measures of Disease Frequency

Basic measures of disease frequency that are used in epidemiology are *incidence* and *prevalence*. The distinction is important: all too often in publications, the term incidence is used, while prevalence is the appropriate term. For a meaningful analysis, both the measures need a denominator: the number of persons in the population from which the cases arise, i.e. the source population.

The prevalence of contact dermatitis is the number of persons with contact dermatitis at a certain point in time (point prevalence) or during a certain (usually short) period of time (period prevalence). It is likely that the prevalence of contact dermatitis at one point in time is lower than that over a longer period because symptoms

J.D. Johansen et al. (eds.), *Contact Dermatitis*,
DOI: 10.1007/978-3-642-03827-3_11, © Springer-Verlag Berlin Heidelberg 2011

11

are not continuously present, as illustrated in a Danish study [4]. In theory, the prevalence of contact dermatitis over a period of several years should be higher than the prevalence over a period of months. However, the difference may be small due to the fact that in many patients, contact dermatitis is a condition with an unfavourable prognosis and a high rate of recurrence. In addition, the accuracy of recall will decrease with time, and it is conceivable that those persons who did not have symptoms recently will more often forget to report their earlier symptoms. The number of cases with a positive patch test among all patients tested in a large clinic can be considered as the prevalence of contact sensitisation. This "clinical prevalence", is, however, difficult to interpret: usually the source population from which the cases arise is not defined, nor is its size known.

The incidence of contact dermatitis refers to the number of new cases of the same during a defined period in a specified population. The distinction with prevalence is important, because, here, an element of time (the transition from the healthy to the diseased state over time) is inserted. Commonly, the *incidence rate* is defined as the number of non-diseased persons who acquire contact dermatitis within a certain period of time, divided by the number of person-years that the subjects in this population do not have contact dermatitis. Person-years are contributed only by those who are not ill at the beginning of the study. The incidence rate is a summary measure that gives an indication of the probability of transition to morbidity (such as contact allergy) over time.

This is different from the *cumulative incidence.* The cumulative incidence is the proportion of a fixed, initially non-diseased population that acquires contact dermatitis in a specific period of time. For example, suppose that workers in an epoxy-resin factory are patch tested and examined again after a few years. The number of new cases with epoxy allergy can be determined only at the end of this follow-up period; we do not know as to when exactly contact allergy was acquired. The proportion of new cases out of this fixed population of workers is a cumulative incidence. Cumulative incidences were used in a large follow-up study on work-related hand eczema in the automobile industry [5, 6]. A similar approach, expressing the cumulative incidence in a proportion, was published in a follow-up study of 960 schoolgirls who had been patch tested for nickel allergy and examined again after 20 years [7].

The difference between the two measures of incidence is small when the proportion of people who become ill in a specific period is small, but it can be sizeable when many people become ill in a short period of time. The incidence of contact dermatitis can be measured by periodic screening to detect all new cases in the study population over a certain period of time: this approach was used to study contact allergic sensitisation in the Copenhagen region [8].

11.2.1 Source Population

The population from which the cases arise (source population) is the denominator of the measure of disease frequency (incidence or prevalence). A common feature of observational studies is the occurrence of non-responders in the population who were invited to participate in the study. In many publications, the denominator refers only to the responders. Whether generalisations can be made to the source population as a whole depends on the extent to which the non-responders were different in relevant characteristics from the source population. As a rule of thumb, response rates below 70% (some authors stipulate 75%) may give spurious results. Results originating from lower response rates are acceptable only when there is an adequate non-response analysis.

Core Message

> Contact dermatitis is a common but variable disease: symptoms accompanying the allergic state may vary in presentation or severity over time. Therefore, the term prevalence should be used judiciously, restricted to defined populations, a defined point in time and addressing a well-defined outcome.

11.3 Clinical Epidemiology

Many studies in contact dermatitis are based on populations that have been patch tested; usually this means that the participants visited a clinic or a hospital for being evaluated on having contact dermatitis. For a meaningful interpretation of such clinical epidemiological data, guidelines have been published by Uter et al. [9]. Examples of clinical epidemiological results obtained from data networks of contact dermatitis departments across the world are discussed in Chap. 54.

11.3.1 Description of (Patch Test) Patients

As a prerequisite for a meaningful interpretation of this type of clinical epidemiological findings, the denominator must be described in terms of:

- The number of subjects included (if all are not tested with all allergens of a panel of allergens, the number tested must be stated for each allergen).
- The period analysed.
- The way the allergen was patch tested (aimed testing vs. testing consecutive patients), which has an evident impact on the prevalence of contact allergy diagnosed. For example, contact allergy to Disperse Blue 106/124 was diagnosed in up to 6.7% of patients patch tested with a special textile dyes series [10], whereas the prevalence was only 1.3% in consecutively tested patients [11].
- Important demographic characteristics which may have a profound impact on the observed spectrum of contact allergy, e.g. according to the MOAHLFA index [12].

Clearly, the proportion of missing data for these items must be kept low by appropriate quality control of routine or study documentation [13].

The MOAHLFA index [14], which lists the proportions of certain demographic variables, namely M for male sex, O for occupational causation of dermatitis, A for atopy, H for hand, L for leg, F for face as affected site and the last A for the proportion of patients aged 40 and above, is an extension of the original MOHL and the later MOAHL index. Any of these factors may have a profound influence on the frequency of sensitization. For instance, a high proportion of patch test patients with lower leg dermatitis/varicose ulcers (the

"L"), will be associated with the prevalences of neomycin sulphate and lanolin contact allergy, to name a few, well above the average [13]. A high proportion of occupational contact dermatitis cases (the "O") will evidently raise the frequency of positive reactions to epoxy resin, chromate or other "occupational" allergens, depending on the spectrum of local industries. Hence, consideration of this basic demographic and clinical data will help to explain differing results from different centres [12]. Furthermore, consideration of the MOAHLFA index of the study group should put comparisons with other, dissimilar groups of patients into due perspective. With regard to the first "A", it should be mentioned that this stood for atopy in general in the MOAHL index, i.e. the presence of either atopic eczema, allergic rhinoconjuncitivitis or allergic bronchial asthma [14]. In contrast, in the MOAHLFA index, as suggested, only atopic eczema is considered because according to the current evidence there seems to be no reason to assume (1) an etiologically relevant association between contact allergy and mucosal atopic symptoms and (2) a relevant impact of the presence of these types of atopic symptoms on the indication for patch testing. Hence, the inclusion of mucosal atopic disease would render this "A" in the index less specific, while the proportion of patch tested patients with underlying previous or current atopic eczema will have some impact on the spectrum of contact allergy – due to either presumptive immunological abnormalities or disease-specific exposures to topical medicaments, ointment base ingredients, etc., similar to leg dermatitis as underlying condition.

In addition to a (standardised) description of the population characteristics as outlined above, appropriate discussion of selection processes, as far as these are known, and their potential effect on contact allergy frequencies or risk estimates should supplement the epidemiological interpretation of results. It is often a major criticism of patient-based studies (i.e. clinical epidemiology) that prevalences found in a particular group of patients are (mis-)interpreted by the authors as prevalences on a population level, which, expectedly, are usually much lower. Hence, prevalences should be put into proper perspective by delineating the recruitment process for the study subjects, e.g. specialist vs. GP referral, and specialties of the centre, like medicolegal evaluation, dermatitis due to cosmetics or a strong background of phlebology, to mention a few.

11

Core Message

> The selection process until presentation in a patch test clinic and the eventual inclusion as a patient in the study group, and the demographic and clinical characteristics of this group, namely the distribution of sex and age, occupational background and characteristic sites of dermatitis (MOAHLFA index), can have a profound impact on the allergen spectrum and should thus be described in detail.

11.3.2 Special Aspects of the Analysis of Patch Test Data

Some methods are particularly suitable for analysing patch test data, addressing issues such as a description of the reaction profile, standardisation of % positives, quantification of concomitant reactivity and adjustment for confounding factors. Due to the complexity of some research questions, however, the hints included in this chapter might not suffice. Direct consultation with biostatisticians will always be advisable. The following aspects and methods, respectively, warrant consideration when analysing and presenting patch test results, in addition to the above-mentioned adequate description of the underlying population:

- A full description of the reaction profile, including the frequency of doubtful, irritant and different grades of positive reactions, is recommended, in particular for allergens beyond the standard series.
- Proportions (%) are a very common measure of an outcome of interest, such as the proportion of irritant, doubtful and positive reactions to a certain allergen. Primarily, such proportions are descriptive of the study population. In most cases, however, researchers want to communicate these results as typical or representative of other persons or patients sharing the characteristics defining their study group. Hence, the study group is regarded as a sample. Consequently, the precision of this estimate must be addressed by supplementing the point estimate (the observed proportion) with a confidence interval (CI), usually, but not necessarily, a 95% CI. Motivating the CI from a different perspective, it could be said that empirical results, such as an observed proportion, always carry an element of chance. Hence, it may well be that upon repetition of the study under the same conditions, a slightly different proportion will be observed, especially if the sample was small (see below). The extremely useful concept of CI can be interpreted as follows: if 100 samples from a given target population were drawn, or 100 groups of patients sharing the same characteristics were assessed (or: the study repeated 100 times), the observed proportion would, in 95 (90, 99) of these 100 samples or repetitions, lie within the limits indicated by the 95% (90%, 99%) CI. The larger the study sample, the more precise the estimate will be, i.e. the narrower the CI. For example, the point estimate 10% as 10 out of 100 is accompanied by a 95% CI of 4.1–15.9, while for 100 out of 1,000, the corresponding CI is 8.1–11.9%; CIs based on the normal distribution. However, for small samples (e.g. $n < 30$), the exact CI based directly on the binomial distribution is preferable, because the normal approximation to the binomial distribution or other types of approximations do not hold good. In summary, CIs provide an indispensible measure of the precision of observed proportions. Most statistical software packages offer the calculation of a CI to a proportion. However, if less than 100 cases are analysed, the use of % to describe proportions becomes questionable, and a sample size of less than ten renders % meaningless.
- Statistical testing of proportions and rates is sometimes unnecessary. If, for instance, CIs of proportions of different subgroups do not overlap, significant difference is already evident. Otherwise, the chi-squared test can be used to statistically test for differences of proportions across two or more disjunct groups. Fisher's

exact test (or its modified versions in the case of more than two groups) is an alternative preferable in case of small samples, e.g. if any of the expected cell counts are less than five. A trend test is similar to the previous test problem, but takes the ordering of the (time) scale into account. Examples include the chi-squared test for trend or the Cochran-Armitage trend test. For instance, the prevalence of nickel allergy remained largely stable in German patch test patients during the period 1992–2001. However, a stratified analysis (see below) revealed a significant decline from 36.7 to 25.8% in the subgroup of female patients younger than 30 ($p < 0.0001$, Cochran-Armitage trend test), coinciding with the EU nickel regulation [15].

- When confounding in the comparison of sensitisation prevalences across time is suspected, for instance by a changing age composition of the patients tested and a non-negligible age-gradient of sensitisation risk, suitable strategies counteracting the confounding problem should be employed. These include (1) stratification for the levels of the confounding variable(s) – in this example, presenting separate time trend analyses for age groups – (2) (direct) standardisation of sensitisation prevalences for age (often also for gender) or (3) adjustment for the confounding factor(s) in a multifactorial analysis (for more details see Uter et al. [9].

- If (1) more than one statistical test is performed and (2) statistical hypotheses testing is intended not just to be exploratory, but to be confirmative (i.e. aiming at empirically "proving" a scientific hypothesis within the framework of predefined α[and probably β] error), the well-known problem of "multiple testing" arises, namely, spurious "significant" results. This should be counteracted by employing suitable α-adjustment techniques like Bonferroni-Holm.

- In contact allergy research, the term concordance is colloquially used to describe simultaneous (concomitant) reactions to allergens, for which there may be several causes. Beyond the original application of "chance-corrected" quantification of inter-rater agreement, the concept of concordance can be applied to describe test reactions observed during synchronous patch testing in the following situations: (1) Comparing test results obtained with different test methods, e.g. 24 vs. 48 h patch test application or otherwise different preparations of the same allergen, (2) quantifying reproducibility upon synchronous duplicate patch testing of identical allergen preparations, (3) comparing test results with mixes and any of their individual constituents and (4) comparing test reactions to allergens which are structurally related, like fragrances or para-amino compounds. A well-established measure of "chance-corrected" agreement for categorical data such as patch test results is Cohen's kappa, either as simple kappa for 2×2 contingency tables, or as weighted kappa for larger, symmetrically structured tables of ordinal data. The actual kappa value can be regarded as an estimate, and should thus be supplemented with CIs. In general, kappa values close to 0 indicate a (complete) lack of agreement beyond chance, and values close to one (almost) perfect agreement.

- Sometimes, beyond description as above, statistical analysis of paired sample results may be an issue. Examples for this include statistical testing for differences between test results obtained in the same patients with different concentrations, vehicles, exposure times, chamber sizes, etc. of an allergen or responses to allergen or irritant challenge before and after some therapeutic intervention in the same patients. For 2×2 contingency tables, McNemar's test, which is also available as an exact test based on the binomial distribution, is suitable to assess the null hypothesis of "no difference". In quadratic contingency tables larger than 2×2, the Bowker test or a generalised Cochran-Mantel-Haenszel test can be applied. For an extensive explanation, further examples and a discussion of the application of this class of statistical tests, see Gefeller et al. [16].

11

> **Core Messages**

> › Proportions, and other measures, should be supplemented with a CI to quantify their precision; a 95% CI is commonly chosen. This may help to dispel over-interpretation of results, especially with very small samples.
> › When quantifying concordance, i.e. the agreement between two related outcomes in a dependent sample, the sole consideration of observed agreement is misleading. Instead, Cohen's kappa coefficient, supplemented with CIs, should be used to describe "agreement beyond chance".
> › Statistical testing, if deemed necessary, should take design (independent vs. paired samples) and the problem of multiple testing into account.

11.4 Observational Studies

The three most important types of observational study in the epidemiology of contact dermatitis are follow-up studies, case-control studies and cross-sectional studies. Important measures of association are the *relative risk* (RR) based on incidence data, the *prevalence ratio* (PR) based on prevalence data, i.e. from cross-sectional studies, and the *odds ratio* (OR), see further below. If $p(D=1)$ is the overall probability (risk) of disease, $p(D=1|E=1)$ the probability of disease given exposure, and $p(D=1|E=0)$ the probability of disease given no exposure, and vice versa for exposure given or not disease, these important measures of association can be defined as follows:

$$\text{RR (or PR)} = \frac{p\,(D=1|E=1)}{p\,(D=1|E=0)}$$

which is equivalent to the prevalence of skin disease in the exposed, divided by that in the unexposed.

In follow-up studies, selection of subjects is based upon exposure to the factor of interest. Instead of exposure, the presence or absence of a risk factor (e.g. nickel allergy, or atopy) can also be chosen as basis for comparison. For example, the RR of getting contact dermatitis in "wet" work (relative to dry work) can be studied in a follow-up study. This implies that a population of employees performing wet work and those performing dry work is selected before the disease has developed and that they are followed over a certain

period of time. The RR is the incidence rate in persons exposed (to wet work) divided by the incidence rate among unexposed. This is a basic measure of association between exposure to wet work and contact dermatitis. Another measure of association is the *rate difference* (RD), being the difference between the risk, estimated by incidence rates, in exposed and unexposed subjects: $RD=p(D=1|E=1)-p(D=1|E=0)$. However, this difference is neither related to the prevalence of exposure nor to that of disease, making its interpretation on the population level difficult if these estimates are unknown.

For the quantification of risk on the population level, the *attributable risk* (AR) (formula 2) is commonly used, which takes into account not only individual risk (the RR), but also exposure frequency, i.e. how common a risk factor is on the population level. An application of the concept of AR to contact dermatitis research has focussed on the impact of atopy on occupational contact dermatitis [17, 18].

$$\text{AR} = \frac{p\,(D=1)-p\,(D=1|E=0)}{p\,(D=1)}$$

In case-control studies, the subjects are selected according to their disease status. Information on the past exposure of the persons with contact dermatitis (cases) and the non-diseased persons (controls) is collected. The odds of exposure among cases is compared to (divided by) the odds of exposure among control persons, arriving at the OR. Odds can be described as a probability (here: of having been exposed) divided by 1− this probability ($p/(1−p)$. The OR has a very useful property of invariance regarding the numerical value of the OR: the odds of having been exposed in the cases divided by the odds of that in the controls yield the same value as the odds of disease given exposure divided by that given no exposure – which is the measure of association of interest.

$$\text{OR} = \frac{a/c}{b/d} = \frac{a/b}{d/d} = \frac{a \cdot c}{b \cdot c}$$

$$\text{RR} = \frac{a/n_{exp}}{c/n_{non-exp}}$$

For example, when 38 cases with hand eczema (out of 97 cases) were exposed to a particular detergent and 59 were not, the exposure odds are 38:59. When the exposure odds among 94 controls are 18:76, the OR is the division of these two odds: the OR is 2.7.

	Diseased	Healthy	Exposure total
Exposed	$a = 38$	$b = 18$	$n_{(exp)}$
Non-exposed	$c = 59$	$d = 76$	$n_{(non-exp)}$
	$n_{(diseased)}$	$n_{(healthy)}$	$n_{(total)}$

This "exposure OR" approximates the RR of disease in the exposed.

A case-control study can be seen as a study among a defined population in which all diseased persons (for example those with hand eczema), and only a sample of the non-diseased persons, are studied. This design is especially efficient in the study of rare diseases, for example, positive reactions to a very uncommon allergen. In this situation, the majority of the population does not have the disease, and it is not necessary to study all non-diseased persons. For reasons of interpretability, it is necessary to make an effort to select a population of controls in such a way that they reflect the exposure distribution among the non-diseased part of the source population from which the cases originated. Case-control studies can be based on incident or prevalent cases. A study of incident cases includes as cases only those who develop the illness during a specified time period. In a case-control study of prevalent cases, existing cases of illness (e.g. persons with contact dermatitis, or persons with a specific allergy) at any point in time are selected. This approach has been chosen in population-wide study in Germany on the role of atopy [19]. Large registers of patch test data may be a good source of case-control studies.

The choice of the right controls is essential in case-control studies; non-representative controls will bias the results. This problem may easily arise from the inclusion of hospital-based controls, such as "other" dermatology patients.

In cross-sectional studies, a study population is selected regardless of exposure status or disease status (in contrast to case-control and follow-up studies). Usually, the information on exposure and disease in cross-sectional studies refers to the time of data collection. Thus, in cross-sectional studies on, for example contact dermatitis from cosmetic ingredients, it is not possible to draw conclusions with regard to the relationship between previous exposure to cosmetics and disease, because current exposure may be different from the exposure in the past which caused the disease. This problem is illustrated in a study that combines two prevalence investigations on contact sensitisation with an 8-year interval [8].

In some situations, the change of exposure status will be related to morbidity, i.e. to the fact that the person has contact dermatitis. Persons who are susceptible to the development of eczematous symptoms are often aware of this. So they may change their habits (wear gloves or use medications) to suppress symptoms. In that case, when current exposure (as opposed to past exposure) is recorded in a case-control study or a cross-sectional study, the results will show that cases use gloves or medications more often than controls. Obviously, the use of gloves is a result of being a case and not a cause ("reversed causality"). In many situations, this type of bias is less obvious. It is therefore preferable to record exposure with reference to the time prior to the first occurrence of eczematous symptoms. However, in practice, it may be difficult to obtain reliable information on past exposure in a cross-sectional setting. In follow-up studies, this poses less of a problem, because exposure is recorded before the symptoms of eczema become manifest.

11.5 Case Ascertainment

The case ascertainment refers to the methods used to let cases of contact dermatitis come to the attention of the investigator. It depends largely on the sources of data that are used, such as mortality statistics, morbidity statistics or observational studies. It may have major consequences on the magnitude of the disease frequency which one obtains. In morbidity statistics, case ascertainment usually involves registration of persons with eczema or dermatitis who fulfil additional criteria for registration, like hospital admission or sickness leave. This restriction in the definition of a "case" will probably result in selective inclusion of the more severe cases, since a large proportion of individuals suffering from contact dermatitis do not come to medical attention.

Counting the number of persons with contact dermatitis in a population requires the explicit statement of diagnostic criteria to judge whether a person is considered to have contact dermatitis or not. In many publications, diagnostic criteria for the definition of contact dermatitis are not explicitly stated, and several authors reserve this term to denote allergic contact dermatitis (ACD). Since contact dermatitis refers to eczematous symptoms due to exposure of the skin to irritant or sensitising agents, it can be considered as a subcategory of eczema. In some publications, the terms "contact dermatitis" and "eczema" (especially of the hands) are used interchangeably, assuming that irritant or sensitising agents play a role in the causation of eczema.

Nearly always, individuals who might be sensitised to a specific allergen are missed, while others are wrongly designated as cases of ACD. In order to ascertain the validity of a used instrument, for example patch testing, the terms "sensitivity", "specificity" and "predictive value" are used. Sensitivity stands for the probability that cases with an ACD (clinically relevant sensitisation to a specific allergen) are correctly diagnosed. Specificity is defined as the probability that the non-sensitised individuals are correctly diagnosed as such in this context. Besides the sensitivity and specificity of the used instruments (e.g. patch testing), the positive predictive value (PPV) is an essential measure. The PPV is the proportion of those individuals diagnosed as diseased by the used instrument (e.g. patch testing), who are actually sensitised. It should be kept in mind that the PPV is a function of the true prevalence of allergic sensitisation in the population, of the sensitivity and of the specificity, according to Bayes' formula [20]. Thus, also from a statistical point of view, it is crucial to explore the patients´ history carefully and exactly before performing patch testing: indiscriminate testing of many patients with a doubtful allergic origin of their skin problem (i.e. a low prevalence of true allergies) will lead to many cases of wrongly diagnosed contact dermatitis. In studies on contact allergy in the general population, this issue is even more important than in a clinical setting because of the lower background prevalence. From a statistical point of view, an observed increase of the prevalence of contact allergy can theoretically be explained by a decrease of the PPV over time, because of an increased awareness of allergic diseases in the population (resulting in more false positives).

In the interpretation of data on the occurrence of contact dermatitis, it is important to distinguish between sensitisation (i.e. a positive reaction in the patch test reading) and the presence of ACD ascribed to this sensitisation (clinical relevance). For example, a high prevalence of sensitisation can be found in the population for some allergens, while a low frequency of ACD due to these allergens was noticed (e.g. thiomersal, poison ivy).

This relates to another important aspect of case ascertainment, especially the ascertainment of irritant

contact dermatitis (ICD) in clinical epidemiological studies. Misclassification can easily occur when it is (erroneously) assumed that the mere absence of a positive patch test reaction implies a diagnosis of ICD. Conversely, a positive patch test reaction has to be assessed for its relevance (for a discussion on relevance, see Chap. 24) This issue can be illustrated by a (clinical) study on contact dermatitis from cutting-fluids, which carefully combined history taking, clinical pattern and relevance of patch test reactions [21].

Core Messages

> Sensitivity and specificity of the diagnostic instruments used are important. In epidemiological studies, an over estimation of prevalence can result from low sensitivity/specificity.

> Patch testing even with optimum concentration and vehicle for a given allergen is, like most diagnostic tests, neither 100% sensitive nor 100% specific. Consequently, false-positive test results must be expected especially if the true contact allergy prevalence is low, i.e. in population samples unselected for specific morbidity (suspected ACD), compared to patch test patients.

In observational studies, active case ascertainment usually involves screening of the study population by clinical examination, by questionnaire or by a combination of both. However, the frequency of cases obtained by questionnaire may be quite different from those ascertained by clinical examination. Screening of the complete study population according to standardised criteria by one or more trained dermatologists is the most reliable and therefore preferred method. But it is generally not feasible, especially in large study populations: a questionnaire that can be self-administered by the whole study population is more cost-effective, but less valid.

The problems with questionnaires have been discussed in the context of studies on hand eczema [22, 23]. However, hand eczema does not always imply contact dermatitis, and certainly not always contact allergy. In the context of questionnaires, sensitivity, specificity and PPV (as discussed above) have the same importance as in patch testing.

Given the practical limitations of a medical examination of large populations, some studies combine the validity of a clinical diagnosis with the easy applicability of a self-administered questionnaire.

In such a study, a set of three questions was developed, asking about the symptoms of hand dermatitis, their duration and whether these were recurrent [22]. The validity was evaluated among 109 nurses and compared with a medical diagnosis made by a dermatologist. A diagnosis of hand eczema, defined as "one or more symptoms, with a recurrent character, or lasting for more than 3 weeks" had a sensitivity of 100% and a specificity of 64%, resulting in a PPV of 31%. This indicates that the use of the questionnaire alone would result in a significant over estimation of the prevalence. Medical examination of only those who responded positively, to exclude false-positive cases, would, however, increase the specificity while maintaining the high sensitivity. It would reduce the screening effort by trained physicians. If the definition of hand eczema was based upon two or more symptoms with a recurrent character, or lasting for more than 3 weeks, the sensitivity remained high (80%) while the specificity increased to 89%, resulting in a PPV of 63%. When the same questionnaire, combined with a clinical examination, was applied to a different population (workers in a rubber factory), the results were quite different [23].

For current objective and past skin disorders on the face, a questionnaire was validated among employees who worked with visual display units [24]. Validation of a question on current skin symptoms has been applied in a study among farmers [25]. The use of the self-diagnosis term "hand-eczema" seems to be valid in questionnaire studies in Scandinavian countries [18]. Based on a combination of consensus and validation, an extensive set of questions (NOSQ) has been developed for use in hand-eczema studies [26].

11.6 Incidence and Prevalence of Contact Dermatitis and Contact Sensitisation

11.6.1 General Population

Morbidity statistics which provide information on the occurrence of skin diseases, or eczema or contact dermatitis, are, for example, hospitalisation records, case records from dermatology clinics and data on sickness leave and occupational diseases. As mentioned before, it is likely that these statistics mainly include the more severe cases of skin disease.

There are several publications on the number and characteristics of patients visiting dermatology clinics and/or patch testing units [27, 28]. However, no information on the incidence or prevalence of contact dermatitis can be derived from these publications, because information on the size of the source population from which the cases originated is usually lacking. It is difficult to interpret the distribution of occupations, age or sex in a patient population without knowing the distribution of these characteristics among the source population. Also, information on the type and severity of skin disease in patient populations is difficult to interpret, because of selection mechanisms that play a role before a dermatology clinic is consulted. Within a population of clinic-patients, systematic collection and registration of data can be the basis for a meaningful analysis, especially if it is on a trans-national basis (ESSCA); guidelines for publication and analysis of such data have been published [9]. When the size of the source population is known, a combination of different data sources can be made to obtain an estimate of the prevalence. Such an approach was used by combining nationwide sales of patch test materials (as an estimate of the number of persons undergoing such a test) and clinical patch test results ("CE-DUR" approach) [29, 30].

> **Core Message**
>
> › Few dermatological questionnaires have been adequately validated. Results from response rates below 70% are subject to bias, and are acceptable only if there is a rigorous non-response analysis.

> **Core Message**
>
> › Publications based on data of patients visiting dermatology clinics and/or patch testing units cannot be used to directly derive population-related incidence or prevalence estimates.

Publications that generate incidence-type data for the general population are scarce. Data from incidence studies may support and direct strategies for the prevention of contact allergy and ACD. An example is the Copenhagen Allergy Study [8]: in 1990, a random sample of 567 persons of the 15–69-year-old population living in the western part of Copenhagen County, Denmark, was patch tested in a cross-sectional study, and in 1998, a follow-up study was performed. In the follow-up study, 37 persons (12%) of the 313 patch test-negative persons in 1990 had developed one or more positive patch tests (incident contact allergy). Twenty cases (6%) of incident nickel allergy and 25 cases (8%) of incident contact allergy to one or more haptens other than nickel were found. The data indicate that female sex, young age and ear piercing (before 1990) were risk factors for developing nickel allergy. Contact sensitivity to one or more haptens was found in 16 and 19% in 1990 and 1998, respectively [31]. A third consecutive follow-up study was done in 2006; cosmetic dermatitis (defined as experiencing a redness, a rash and itching caused by exposure to cosmetics) was reported by 15% of the men and 23% of the women [32].

Information on the prevalence of hand eczema, contact sensitivity and contact dermatitis in the general population can be obtained from cross-sectional studies that were performed in recent years (Table 11.1). The aim of the Odense Adolescence Cohort Study was to assess the prevalence measures of atopic dermatitis (AD), asthma, allergic rhinitis and hand and contact dermatitis in adolescents in Odense municipality, Denmark [4, 33]. This Odense study was carried out as a cross-sectional study among 1,501 school children (age 12–16 years) and included questionnaire, interview, clinical examination and patch testing. The lifetime prevalence of hand eczema based on the questionnaire was 9%, the 1-year period prevalence was 7.3% and the point prevalence 3.2%, with a significant predominance in girls. The point prevalence of contact allergy was 15%; the most common contact allergens were nickel (8.6%) and fragrance mix (1.8%). Nickel allergy was clinically relevant in 69% and fragrance allergy in 29% of cases. A significant association was found between contact allergy and hand eczema, while no association was found between contact allergy and AD or inhalant allergy. The point prevalence of ACD was 0.7% and the lifetime prevalence was 7%.

In two other cross-sectional studies, the prevalence of hand eczema was compared between 1983 and 1996 in Swedish adults using the same questionnaire [34]. Random samples of 20,000 individuals from the population of Gothenburg, Sweden were drawn from the population register in 1983 and 1996. Data were collected with a postal questionnaire, which was identical in the two studies. The response rate was 83% in 1983 and 74% in 1996. The reported 1 year prevalence of hand eczema decreased from 12% in 1983 to 10% in 1996.

Within a population-based nested, case-control study in Germany, patch tests were performed with 25 standard allergens in 1,141 adults [19]. Additional information was obtained by a dermatological examination, a standardised interview and blood analysis. At least one positive reaction was exhibited by 40% of the subjects, with the most frequently observed reactions being that of fragrance mix (16%), nickel (13%), thimerosal (4.7%) and balsam of Peru (3.8%). Women were sensitised more often than men (50 vs. 30%), and this was also significant for fragrance mix, nickel, turpentine, cobalt chloride and thimerosal. Contact sensitisation decreased with increasing degree of occupational training. Frequency estimates for the general adult population-based on these findings were 28% for overall contact sensitisation and 11% for fragrance mix, 10% for nickel, and 3.2% for thimerosal. In this study, the sample was biased towards atopics, because 50% of the subjects exhibited allergen-specific IgE antibodies to aeroallergens by design. The clinical relevance of the patch test reactions was not assessed. A comparison with clinical data from the same catchment area (Augsburg and surrounding counties) yielded interesting hints on the selection effect due to clinical specialties – the department has a phlebological focus mirrored by high prevalences of "leg dermatitis" allergens – and differences between allergens: While the difference of contact sensitisation was little in the more common allergens such as nickel and fragrance mix, the less common allergens showed a greater difference between population-based and clinical prevalences [35].

In former decades, other cross-sectional studies were performed in The Netherlands [36, 37], Sweden [38], England [39], the United States [40] and Norway [41]. In all the studies, a geographically defined

Table 11.1 Population-based studies on incidence/prevalence of hand eczema, contact sensitisation and contact dermatitis

Reference	Country	Target population	Method of case ascertainment	n	Outcome	Measures of prevalence	Rate	Comment
Mortz et al. [33]	Denmark	12–16 years (children)	Q, I, E, patch test	1,501	Hand eczema Contact sensitivity Allergic Contact Dermatitis	Lifetime 1-year Point Point Point Lifetime	9.2% 7.3% 3.2% 15.2% 0.7% 7.2%	Cross-sectional study of high quality
Nielsen et al. [31, 67]	Denmark	15–41 years	Patch test in 1990 Patch test in 1998	290 469	Contact sensitivity in 1990 Contact sensitivity in 1998	Point in 1990 Point in 1998	15.9% 18.6%	Small sample size, low participation rates (69% and 51%)
Meding and Jarvholm [34]	Sweden	20–65 years	Q in 1983 Q in 1996	16,708 2,218	Hand eczema in 1983 Hand eczema in 1996	1-year in 1983 1-year in 1996	11.8% 9.7%	Response rate 83.5% in 1983 Response rate 73.9% in 1996
Schäfer et al. [19]	Germany	28–78 years	E, patch test	1,141	Contact sensitivity	Point	40.0%	Nested case-control study, biased target population (50% exhibited allergen-specific IgE anti-bodies to aeroallergens)
Sosted et al. [68]	Denmark	Adult population	I	4,000	Reaction to hair dye	Life time prevalence	5.3%	The 5.3% pertains to the 1,254 individuals who had ever dyed their hair
Lerbaek et al. [69]	Denmark	Twins	Q	4,128	Hand eczema	Incidence	8.8 per 1,000 PY	
Thyssen et al. [32]	Denmark	18–69 years	Q, E, patch test	4,299	Fragrance contact allergy	Point in 2006	1.6	Decrease of reactions to FM-I over the years

Q questionnaire; *I* interview; *E* clinical examination; *PY* person-years

population or a sample thereof was screened. In some of the studies, all skin disorders were recorded while others focused on eczema or hand eczema only. In most of the studies, the term "eczema" included ACD, ICD, seborrhoic eczema, nummular eczema, atopic eczema, dishydrotic eczema and unclassified eczema.

In The Netherlands, Norway and Sweden, the prevalence was higher among women, in London the prevalence was higher among men, while there was no difference between sexes in the United States. It is possible that the differences are obscured by differences in age distribution of the populations. The prevalence in women was especially high in the younger age groups.

In the United States, the prevalence of eczema seems to increase with age, while according to the publication from The Netherlands, Sweden and Norway, the prevalence seems to decrease slightly in the age groups above 50 years. The Dutch study [42] analysed the relative contribution of age and occupation to the prevalence of hand eczema and found that the relationship with age disappeared after controlling for occupation. The same phenomenon was described in a population of Australian rubber and cement industry workers: the prevalence of dermatitis was relatively high in workers under 45 years, but the age effect also disappeared after controlling for job classification [43].

Exposure to irritant or sensitising factors is considered to be the major risk factor for contact dermatitis . This exposure is common during household activities and in certain occupations. This was evident in a study, using a validated questionnaire, which compared the general population with certain occupations, and which obtained a prevalence of 5% for men and almost 11% for women [34, 37].

In conclusion, the prevalence studies strongly suggest that age and gender are not risk factors for contact dermatitis in themselves, but that these characteristics are associated with exposure in occupational and household activities. A review of the epidemiology of allergic contact sensitisation, where similar phenomena were seen concluded that the age-dependent immunological reactivity was less important than differences in exposure between age groups, and that differences in sensitisation pattern between sexes seem to be caused by different exposures [44].

Core Message

> Data from incidence studies may support and direct strategies for the prevention of contact allergy and ACD, supporting conclusions derived from clinical surveillance data. Information on the prevalence of hand eczema, contact sensitivity and contact dermatitis in the general population can be obtained from recent cross-sectional studies that demonstrate the high point and period prevalence in the general population, also in children and adolescents.

11.6.2 Incidence and Prevalence of Notified Occupational Contact Dermatitis

Occupational disease registries provide national incidence data based on the notification of occupational skin diseases and are available in many countries. Although the comparison of national data are hampered by differences across countries in reporting and the definition of occupational diseases, the average incidence rate of registered occupational contact dermatitis in some countries lies around 0.5–1.9 cases per 1,000 full-time workers per year [17, 45].

Most of the national registers combine all types of skin disease, while no distinction is made with regard to eczema or contact dermatitis. Skin diseases constitute up to 30% of all notified occupational diseases and it is estimated that eczema or contact dermatitis accounts for about 90–95% of all occupational skin diseases. Finland also keeps a register on occupational contact urticaria [46]. Some of the occupational disease statistics give a breakdown by gender and occupation or branch of industry. Most national statistics do not provide information on the actual cause of contact dermatitis and predisposing factors.

National registries are usually incomplete as a result of under-diagnosis and under-reporting of the disease. It has been estimated that the incidence of occupational skin diseases in the USA and Germany is being grossly under-estimated [47], the milder cases of skin disease not being registered at all. The extent of under-reporting is likely to differ between countries, because each country has its own system of notification and its own criteria for compensation. In the United States, occupational disease statistics are collected annually from private industries by the Bureau of Labour Statistics [48]. A detailed analysis has been made of the register of occupational diseases in Denmark [45]. In the United Kingdom, the EPIDERM project in combination with OPRA (occupational physicians reporting activity) for recording occupational dermatoses requires dermatologists in a number of centres to report confirmed or suspected cases of occupational skin disease, including the occupation of the patient concerned [1]. It is a voluntary system, and operates on the principle of simplicity, ensuring compliance. The epidemiological limitations are well recognised, but the system corrects the virtual absence of meaningful official statistics in the UK. A population-based study of occupational skin diseases in North Bavaria and the Saarland, Germany, is one of the few that can claim completeness in terms of new cases (numerator) and size of the occupational population as denominator [17, 49].

In the United Kingdom, the annual incidence of occupational contact dermatitis from dermatologist reports was 6.4 cases per 100,000 workers and 6.5 per 100,000 from reports by occupational physicians, an overall rate of 12.9 cases per 100,000 workers [44]. The highest incidence rates were seen in hairdressers [50]. Agents accounting for the highest number of ACD cases were rubber, nickel, epoxy and other resins, aromatic amines, chromium, fragrances and cosmetics and preservatives. Soaps, wet work, petroleum products, solvents and cutting oils and coolants were the most frequently cited agents in cases of irritant dermatitis [51].

In Denmark, the incidence is 17,700 cases on a workforce of about 2.6 million, i.e. about 0.8 per 1,000 per year [45]. Out of 145 grouped exposure sources, the five most frequently stated substances were detergents, water, metals, foodstuff and rubber in notified occupational skin diseases in Denmark. These substances caused approximately half of the eczema cases. The most important irritant seems to be wet work.

In Germany, occupational skin diseases excluding skin cancer are officially registered by the code "BK 5101", which is defined as "severe or recurrent skin diseases that force the discontinuation of any activity that causes or that could be causing the development,

the worsening, or the recurrence of the skin disease". In 2002, the industrial non-profit insurance institutions reported 17.848 such skin disease cases. In Northern Bavaria, Germany, a detailed population-based prospective study was performed to classify all BK 5101 cases of occupational skin diseases [49, 52–54]. From 1990 to 1999, in total 5,285 cases were recorded. In co-operation with the State Institute of Labour and Occupation, the number of all persons employed in different occupations during the same time period was collected. Since the number of employees in the different occupations was known, a population-based study was performed to investigate incidences and demographic characteristics in specific occupational groups. The estimated overall incidence was 6.7 cases per 10,000 workers per year. The highest incidence per 1,000 per year was in hairdressers (97), bakers (33) and florists (25). The induction period was very short: about 2 years in hairdressers, 3 years in the food industry and about 4 years in health service and in metalworkers. Females had a considerably higher risk to develop OCD than men. The incidence rate of contact dermatitis was the highest between the age of 15 and 24 years. In about half of all cases, a delayed-type sensitisation with occupational relevance was detected. In Fig. 11.1, the incidence rates of ICD and ACD of employees of the twelve groups with the highest risk for an occupational skin disease are presented. The population-based register in Northern Bavaria, Germany, could demonstrate a significant decline of the incidence of occupational skin disease among hairdressers between 1990 and 1999 [55]. This supports a probable "intervention effect" by legislative and preventive measures that came into effect over the last decade for hairdressers. In contrast to this, it could be demonstrated that potassium dichromate was still the most important allergen in the construction industry of Northern Bavaria; there has been no significant decline during the 1990s [49]. This contrasts with the Scandinavian countries, where the prevalence of potassium dichromate sensitisation declined following the reduction of chromate levels resulting from the addition of ferrous sulphate to cement. The impact of atopic skin diathesis on occupational contact dermatitis could be analysed by using AR estimates; almost 22% of occupational skin disease cases may be ascribed to this endogenous risk factor [56].

11

Fig. 11.1 Incidence rates (per 10,000 employees) of irritant contact dermatitis (ICD) and allergic contact dermatitis (ACD) in the 12 occupational groups with the highest risk for occupational skin diseases in North Bavaria [20]

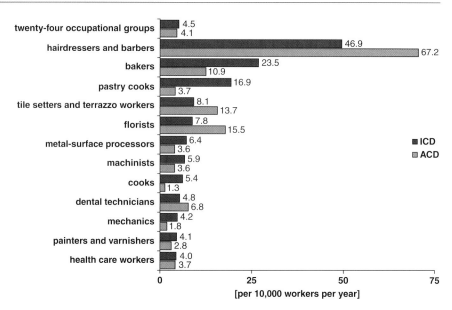

11.7 Incidence and Prevalence in Different Work Forces

Table 11.2 summarises the results of three prospective cohort studies in working populations. In the prospective Audi cohort study, 2,078 apprentices were examined at the start of their apprenticeship and systematically followed up over a 3-year period [6]. The main outcome variable was the incidences of work-related hand eczema in different apprenticeships. The 1-year cumulative incidences of hand eczema were 9.2% in metal-workers, 8.8% in other blue-collar workers and 4.6% in white-collar apprentices. The 3-year cumulative incidences of hand eczema were 15% in metalworkers,

14% in other blue-collar workers and almost 7% in white-collar apprentices. The incidence was not uni-formly distributed over the 3-year period: within the first 6 months, a high rate of hand eczema occurred, which then declined and remained steady at a lower rate over the second and the third years. Almost 10 years later, the same cohort was investigated again, showing a 29% cumulative incidence of hand eczema [5].

In a prospective cohort study of 2,352 hairdressing apprentices, there were three examinations during their 3 years vocational training [57]. The point prevalence of (mostly slight) irritant skin changes of the hands increased from 35% in the initial examination to almost 48% in the intermediate examination and to 55% in the final examination. Given a more conservative defini-tion of a case of "hand dermatitis", these estimates were almost 13, 24 and 24%, respectively. Altogether, about 34 and 15 cases of "skin changes (any degree)" and "hand dermatitis", respectively, per 100 person-years were observed during the study period. The inci-dence rate decreased in the course of the study. However, the proportion of dropouts until final follow-up was almost 52%. This study demonstrates that apprentices with skin problems leave the work force more often than healthy apprentices. A questionnaire-based retrospective cohort study among Swedish hairdressers found an incidence rate of 24/1,000 per-son-years for hand eczema, which was substantially higher than population-based controls, with most prob-lems occurring at younger age [58].

Table 11.2 Prospective cohort studies on the incidence of work-related skin complaints (hand eczema (HE), contact sensitisation and contact dermatitis) in different professions

Author/year	Country	Target population	Method of case ascertainment	n	Outcome	Measures of incidence	Rate	Comment
Funke et al. [6] Apfelbacher et al. [5]	Germany	Apprentices in the car industry	Q, I, E	2,078	HE in metalworkers (apprentices) HE in blue-collar apprentices HE in white-collar apprentices	1 year 3 years 1 year 3 years 1 year 3 years	9.2% 15.3% 8.8% 14.1% 4.6% 6.9%	Prospective cohort study of high quality, follow-up rate 98.2%
Uter et al. [57]	Germany	Hairdressing apprentices	Q, I, E	2,352	HE at the first, second and third examination during 3-year training	Point first year Point second year Point third year	12.9% 23.5% 23.9%	Prospective cohort study of high quality, high initial response rate (91.5%) but 51.8% dropouts until final follow-up
Lind et al. [58]	Sweden	Hairdressing graduates from vocational schools	Q	4,061	HE	IR	24/1,000 PYE	Variable start of follow-up: from 1970 to 1995. Incidence rate compared to general population, 2.5

Q questionnaire; *I* interview; *E* clinical examination; *PYE* person-years exposure

During the past decades, several cross-sectional studies, mostly on hand eczema, have been performed among specific occupational groups. A major problem in such studies is the healthy worker effect and the fact that a clear relationship between skin disease and work is difficult to assess retrospectively.

11.8 Special Considerations: Confounding, Atopy, Interactions and Effect Modification

Contact dermatitis is a multifactorial disease: Apart from exposure to irritating or sensitising agents, there are many factors that may influence the development of contact dermatitis, such as weather conditions including ambient humidity, psychological factors and atopic constitution. These factors may act as confounders in studies if they are not properly controlled for either in the design of the study or in the analysis. Bias of the study results, caused by confounding, occurs when a factor not adequately considered in the analysis, for example history of AD, is associated both with the exposure and with the disease of interest.

For the ascertainment of AD, diagnostic criteria and scoring systems are available [59]. Evidence has accumulated that past or present AD is a risk factor for ICD [60]. Earlier studies indicated that atopy was almost 3 times as high among patients with hand eczema as in the general population or a healthy control group. Later, it appeared that AD was particularly associated with ICD, but not with contact allergy. The proportion of subjects with sporadic or continuous hand eczema was significantly greater in those with moderate and severe AD in childhood compared with those with respiratory allergy only, or a group without atopy. In a follow-up study of hospital workers, a history of AD increased the risk of developing hand eczema threefold [61]. Population-based studies in the food industry calculated significantly greater risk of occupational contact dermatitis in employees with an atopic skin diathesis [54, 56].

Even if in epidemiological terms AD is an effect modifier, it can be argued that ICD associated with atopy is primarily an exacerbation of underlying AD. Since AD is often associated with respiratory symptoms, respiratory atopy may appear as a risk factor. The same may apply to dry skin as an expression of AD.

The problem of contact dermatitis in a particular group of patients is easy to interpret when there is a straightforward cause-effect relationship, e.g. hand eczema in a group of surgeons with a positive patch test to thiuram additives to their rubber gloves. However, the relevance of a positive patch test to very common allergens such as chromate or nickel may be difficult to assess in patients with a (contact) dermatitis that has a chronic relapsing course. As discussed above, there may be considerable (statistical) interaction between several exposure, or risk factors of interest. Elucidation of such interactions may have consequences for preventive or other public-health strategies. To illustrate this point, in Table 11.3, an example is created from the data (modified for this purpose) generated in two Scandinavian follow-up studies on hand eczema and exposure to irritants [38, 62].

In Table 11.3, the RRs of exposure to irritants on hand eczema are different according to the presence of a history of AD. There is an effect modification, meaning that the RRs of exposure to irritants are not uniform (multiplicative) in the different levels of skin-atopy: the risk of hand eczema in atopics is disproportionally increased by exposure to irritants.

The presence or absence of interactions between various factors operating on the risk of contact dermatitis (for example, the role of chromate allergy in foot eczema) has not yet been investigated in detail. As mentioned above, there are indications that such phenomena operate on nickel allergy: in the absence of signs of AD, the RR of a positive nickel patch test on

the risk of hand eczema was only 1.7 in hairdressers and only 1.1 in nurses [63]. In a German study, nickel sensitivity was not associated with an elevated risk for hand eczema. Independent risk factors were wet work, atopic skin and exposure to permanent wave. A Swedish study of a 20-year follow-up on nickel allergy noted a statistical interaction with childhood eczema (probably AD), and concluded that the risk for hand eczema is increased, but may have been over estimated previously [7, 64].

Twin studies are very helpful in separating environmental influence from genetic factors. The results are primarily attributable to twins, and to be representative for the general population, the method of recruiting twins is essential. A study on the role of genetic factors in contact allergy to nickel, based on twins with hand eczema, concluded that nickel allergy was unlikely to have a genetic basis [65]. A later study by the same group supported these findings by demonstrating that having been diagnosed with contact allergy (a positive patch test) had a negligible effect on the role of genetic factors [66].

11.8.1 Classic Articles and Monographs

In 1982, Menné et al. [2] estimated the incidence of nickel allergy by asking a large stratified sample of the female general population about skin reactions to nickel and about hand eczema. Because they were able to obtain fairly reliable age-specific prevalence-rates, they were able to calculate the incidence rates for developing nickel allergy. They were able to show a doubling of nickel allergy in all age groups. In the discussion of that publication, issues such as the relevance of a positive patch test and the question to what extent nickel allergy precedes or follows hand eczema are discussed (i.e. to what extent is nickel allergy a risk factor for hand eczema). It speculates on measures that forbid the use of nickel-releasing alloys; many years later, this measure was implemented in Europe, following an earlier implementation of this regulation in Denmark. Meanwhile, the decrease in the prevalence of nickel dermatitis after the regulation came into effect has been documented in two independent population samples of Danish women [3].

Table 11.3 Relative risks (modified) of contact dermatitis of the hands according to the level of atopic skin diathesis and exposure to irritants [38, 60, 62]

	No irritant exposure	Exposure to irritants
No atopy	1	1.5
Mild atopic dermatitis	2	4
Severe atopic dermatitis	4	12

References

1. Cherry N, Meyer JD, Adisesh A, Brooke R, Owen-Smith V, Swales C, Beck MH (2000) Surveillance of occupational skin disease: EPIDERM and OPRA. Br J Dermatol 142: 1128–1134

2. Menné T, Bogan O, Green A (1982) Nickel allergy and hand dermatitis in a stratified sample of the Danish female population: an epidemiological study including a statistic appendix. Acta Derm Venereol 62:35–41

3. Thyssen JP, Johansen JD, Menné T (2009) Nickel allergy in Danish women before and after nickel regulation. N Eng J Med 360:2259–2260

4. Mortz CG, Lauritsen JM, Bindslev-Jensen C, Andersen KE (2002) Contact allergy and allergic contact dermatitis in adolescents: prevalence measures and associations. The Odense Adolescence Cohort Study on Atopic Diseases and Dermatitis (TOACS). Acta Derm Venereol 82:352–358

5. Apfelbacher CJ, Radulescu M, Diepgen TL, Funke U (2008) Occurrence and prognosis of hand eczema in the car industry: results from the PACO follow-up study. Contact Derm 58:322–329

6. Funke U, Fartasch M, Diepgen TL (2001) Incidence of work-related hand eczema during apprenticeship: first results of a prospective cohort study in the car industry. Contact Derm 44:166–172

7. Josefson A, Färm G, Stymme B, Meding B (2006) Nickel allergy and hand eczema – a 20-year follow up. Contact Derm 55:286–290

8. Nielsen NH, Linneberg A, Menné T, Madsen F, Frolund L, Dirksen A, Jorgensen T (2002) Incidence of allergic contact sensitization in Danish adults between 1990 and 1998; the Copenhagen Allergy Study, Denmark. Br J Dermatol 147: 487–492

9. Uter W, Schnuch A, Gefeller O (2004) Guidelines for the descriptive presentation and statistical analysis of contact allergy data. Contact Derm 51:47–56

10. Uter W, Geier J, Lessmann H, Hausen BM (2001) Contact allergy to Disperse Blue 106 and Disperse Blue 124 in German and Austrian patients, 1995 to 1999. Contact Derm 44:173–177

11. Uter W, Geier J, Hausen BM (2003) Contact allergy to Disperse Blue 106/124 mix in consecutive German, Austrian and Swiss patients. Contact Derm 48:286–287

12. Schnuch A, Geier J, Uter W, Frosch PJ, Lehmacher W, Aberer W, Agathos M, Arnold R, Fuchs T, Laubstein B, Lischka G, Pietrzyk P, Rakoski J, Richter G, Rueff F (1997) National rates and regional differences in sensitization to allergens of the standard series. Population adjusted frequencies of sensitization (PAFS) in 40, 000 patients from a multicenter study (IVDK). Contact Derm 37:200–209

13. Uter W, Mackiewicz M, Schnuch A, Geier J (2005) Interne Qualitätssicherung von Epikutantest-Daten des multizentrischen Projektes "Informationsverbund Dermatologischer Kliniken" (IVDK). Dermatol Beruf Umwelt 53:107–114

14. Andersen KE, Veien NK (1985) Biocide patch tests. Contact Derm 12:99–103

15. Schnuch A, Uter W (2003) Decrease in nickel allergy in Germany and regulatory interventions. Contact Derm 49: 107–108

16. Gefeller O, Pfahlberg A, Geier J, Brasch J, Uter W (1999) The association between size of test chamber and patch test reaction: a statistical reanalysis. Contact Derm 40: 14–18

17. Dickel H, Bruckner T, Berhard-Klimt C, Koch T, Scheidt R, Diepgen TL (2002) Surveillance scheme for occupational skin disease in the Saarland, FRG: first report from BKH-S. Contact Derm 46:197–206

18. Svensson A, Lindberg M, Meding B, Sundberg K, Stenberg B (2002) Self-reported hand eczema: symptom-based reports do not increase the validity of diagnosis. Br J Dermatol 147: 281–284

19. Schäfer T, Bohler E, Ruhdorfer S, Weigl L, Wessner D, Filipiak B, Wichmann HE, Ring J (2001) Epidemiology of contact allergy in adults. Allergy 56:192–196

20. Diepgen TL, Coenraads PJ (2000) The impact of sensitivity, specificity and positive predictive value of patch testing: the more you test, the more you get? Contact Derm 42: 315–317

21. Grattan CE, English JS, Foulds IS, Rycroft RJG (1989) Cutting fluid dermatitis. Contact Derm 20:372–376

22. Smit HA, Coenraads PJ, Lavrijsen APM, Nater JP (1992) Evaluation of a self-administered questionnaire on hand dermatitis. Contact Derm 26:11–16

23. Vermeulen R, Kromhout H, Bruynzeel DP, de Boer EM (2000) Ascertainment of hand dermatitis using a symptom-based questionnaire; applicability in an industrial population. Contact Derm 42:202–206

24. Berg M, Axelson O (1990) Evaluation of a questionnaire for facial skin complaints related to work at visual display units. Contact Derm 22:71–77

25. Susitaival P, Husman L, Hollmen A, Horsmanheimo M (1995) Dermatoses determined in a population of farmers in a questionnaire-based clinical study including methodology validation. Scand J Work Environ Health 21:30–35

26. Susitaival P, Flyvholm MA, Meding B, Kanerva L, Lindberg M, Svensson A, Olafsson JH (2003) Nordic Occupational Skin Questionnaire (NOSQ-2002): a new tool for surveying occupational skin diseases and exposure. Contact Derm 49: 70–76

27. Warshaw EM, Buchholz HJ, Belsito DV et al (2009) Allergic patch test reactions associated with cosmetics: retrospective analysis of cross-sectional data from the North American Contact Dermatitis Group, 2001-2004. J Am Acad Dermatol 60:23–38

28. Wilkinson JD, Shaw S, Andersen KE, Brandao FM, Bruynzeel DP, Bruze M, Camarasa JM, Diepgen TL, Ducombs G, Frosch PJ, Goossens A, Lachapelle JM, Lahti A, Menné T, Seidenari S, Tosti A, Wahlberg JE (2002) Monitoring levels of preservative sensitivity in Europe. A 10-year overview (1991-2000). Contact Derm 46:207–110

29. Schnuch A, Uter W, Geier J, Gefeller O (2002) Epidemiology of contact allergy: an estimation of morbidity employing the clinical epidemiology and drug-utilization research (CE-DUR) approach. Contact Derm 47:32–39

30. Thyssen JP, Uter W, Scnhuch A, Linneberg A, Johansen JD (2007) 10-year prevalence of contact allergy in the general population in Denmark estimated through the CE-DUR method. Contact Derm 57:265–272

31. Nielsen NH, Linneberg A, Menné T, Madsen F, Frolund L, Dirksen A, Jorgensen T (2001) Persistence of contact allergy

among Danish adults: an 8-year follow-up study. Contact Derm 45:350–353

32. Thyssen JP, Linneberg A, Menne T, Nielsen NH, Johansen JD (2009) The prevalence and morbidity of sensitization to fragrance mix I in the general population. Br J Dermatol 161:95–101

33. Mortz CG, Lauritsen JM, Bindslev-Jensen C, Andersen KE (2001) Prevalence of atopic dermatitis, asthma, allergic rhinitis, and hand and contact dermatitis in adolescents. The Odense Adolescence Cohort Study on Atopic Diseases and Dermatitis. Br J Dermatol 144:523–532

34. Meding B, Jarvholm B (2002) Hand eczema in Swedish adults – changes in prevalence between 1983 and 1996. J Invest Dermatol 118:719–723

35. Uter W, Ludwig A, Balda BR, Schnuch A, Pfahlberg A, Schafer T, Wichmann HE, Ring J (2004) The prevalence of contact allergy differed between population-based and clinic-based data. J Clin Epidemiol 57:627–632

36. Lantinga H, Nater JP, Coenraads PJ (1984) Prevalence, incidence and course of ezema on the hands and forearms in a sample of the general population. Contact Derm 10:135–139

37. Smit HA, Burdorf A, Coenraads PJ (1993) The prevalence of hand dermatitis in different occupations. Int J Epidemiol 22:288–293

38. Meding BE, Swanbeck G (1987) Prevalence of hand eczema in an industrial city. Br J Dermatol 16:627–634

39. Rea JN, Newhouse ML, Halil T (1976) Skin diseases in Lambeth. A community study of prevalence and use of medical care. Br J Prev Soc Med 30:107–114

40. Johnson MLT, Roberts J (1978) Skin conditions and related need for medical care among persons 1–74 years. Vital Health Stat 11 (212):i-v; 1–72

41. Kavli G, Forde OH (1984) Hand dermaloses in Tromso. Contact Derm 10:174–177

42. Coenraads PJ, Nater JP, van der Lende R (1983) Prevalence of eczema and other dermaloses of the hands and arms in The Netherlands. Association with age and occupation. Clin Exp Dermatol 8:495–503

43. Varigos GA, Dunt DR (1981) Occupational dermatitis. An epidemiological study in the rubber and cement industries. Contact Derm 7:105–110

44. Menné T, Christoffersen J, Maibach HI (1987) Epidemiology of allergic contact sensitization. Monogr Allergy 21: 132–161

45. Halkier-Sorensen L (1996) Occupational skin diseases. Contact Derm 35 Suppl 1:1–120

46. Kanerva L, Toikkanen J, Jolanki R, Estlander T (1996) Statistical data on occupational contact urticaria. Contact Derm 35:229–233

47. Diepgen TL, Schmidt A (2002) Werden Inzidenz und Prävalenz berufsbedingter Hauterkrankungen unterschätzt? Arbeitsmed Sozialmed Umweltmed 37:477–480

48. BLS: Bureau of Labor Statistics http://www.bls.gov/iif/oshwc/osh/os/osh06_13.pdf. Accessed June 2009

49. Bock M, Schmidt A, Bruckner T, Diepgen TL (2003) Occupational skin disease in the construction industry. Br J Dermatol 149:1165–1171

50. Shum KW, Meyer JD, Chen Y, Cherry N, Gawkrodger DJ (2003) Occupational contact dermatitis to nickel: experience of the British dermatologists (EPIDERM) and occupational

physicians (OPRA) surveillance schemes. Occup Environ Med 60:954–957

51. Meyer JD, Chen Y, Holt DL, Beck MH, Cherry NM (2000) Occupational contact dermatitis in the UK: a surveillance report from EPIDERM and OPRA. Occup Med 50: 265–273

52. Dickel H, Kuss O, Blesius CR, Schmidt A, Diepgen TL (2001) Occupational skin diseases in Nothern Bavaria between 1990 and 1999: a population based study. Br J Dermatol 145:453–462

53. Diepgen TL (2003) Occupational skin-disease data in Europe. Int Arch Occup Environ Health 76:331–338

54. Tacke J, Schmidt A, Fartasch M, Diepgen TL (1995) Occupational contact dermatitis in bakers, confectioners and cooks. A population based study. Contact Derm 33: 112–118

55. Dickel H, Kuss O, Schmidt A, Diepgen TL (2002) Impact of preventive strategies on trend of occupational skin disease in hairdressers: population-based register study. Br Med J 324:1422–1423

56. Dickel H, Bruckner TM, Schmidt A, Diepgen TL (2003) Impact of atopic skin diathesis on occupational skin disease incidence in a working population. J Invest Dermatol 121: 37–40

57. Uter W, Pfahlberg A, Gefeller O, Schwanitz HJ (1998) Prevalence and incidence of hand dermatitis in hairdressing apprentices: results of the POSH study. Prevention of occupational skin disease in hairdressers. Int Arch Occup Environ Health 71:487–492

58. Lind ML, Albin M, Brisman J, Kronholm Diab K, Lillienberg L, Mikoczy Z, Nielsen J, Rylander L, Torén K, Meding B (2007) Incidence of hand eczema in female Swedish hairdressers. Occup Environ Med 64:191–195

59. Charman C, Chambers C, Williams H (2003) Measuring atopic dermatitis severity in controlled clinical trials: what exactly are we measuring? J Invest Dermatol 120: 932–941

60. Coenraads PJ, Diepgen TL (1998) Risk for hand eczema in employees with past or present atopic dermatitis. Int Arch Occup Environ Health 71:7–13

61. Nilsson GE, Mikaelsson B, Andersson S (1985) Atopy, occupation and domestic work as risk factors for hand eczema in hospital workers. Contact Derm 13:216–223

62. Rystedt I (1985) Hand eczema and long term prognosis in atopic dermatitis (thesis). Acta Derm Venereol (suppl) 117:1–59

63. Smit HA, van Rijssen A, Vandenbroucke J, Coenraads PJ (1994) Individual susceptibility and the incidence of hand dermatitis in a cohort of apprentice hairdressers and nurses. Scand J Work Environ Health 20:113–121

64. Josefson A, Färm G, Magnuson A, Meding B (2009) Nickel allergy as risk factor for hand eczema: population-based study. Br J Dermatol 160:828–834

65. Bryld LE, Hindsberger C, Kyvik KO, Agner T, Menné T (2004) Genetic factors in nickel allergy evaluated in a population-based female twin sample. J Invest Dermatol 123:1025–1029

66. Lerbaek A, Kyvik KO, Mortensen J, Bryld LE, Menné T, Agner T (2007–2) Heritability of hand eczema is not explained by comorbidity with atopic dermatitis. J Invest Dermatol 127:1632–1640

67. Nielsen NH, Linneberg A, Menné T, Madsen F, Frolund L, Dirksen A, Jorgensen T (2001) Allergic contact sensitization in an adult Danish population: two cross-sectional surveys eight years apart (the Copenhagen Allergy Study). Acta Derm Venereol 81:31–34

68. Sosted H, Hesse U, Menne T, Andersen KE, Johansen JD (2005) Contact dermatitis to hair dyes in a Danish adult population: an interview-based study. Br J Dermatol 153: 132–135

69. Lerbaek A, Kyvik KO, Ravn H, Menne T, Agner T (2007–1) Incidence of hand eczema in a population-based twin cohort: genetic and environmental risk factors. Br J Dermatol 157: 552–557

Skin Penetration

12

Hans Schaefer, Thomas E. Redelmeier, and Jürgen Lademann

Contents

J. Lademann (✉), H. Schaefer, and T.E. Redelmeier
Center of Applied and Cutaneous Physiology (CCP),
Department of Dermatology,
Charité - Universitätsmedizin Berlin,
Charitéplatz 1, 10117 Berlin, Germany
e-mail: juergen.lademann@charite.de

12.1 Introduction

Penetration of the skin is a key element in cutaneous reactions, be it to xenobiotics, drugs, or other compounds. The major difficulties in accurately describing percutaneous absorption are related to the size of the compartments. A topical application of a cream or ointment, for example, is routinely spread to a thickness corresponding to no greater than 10 μm.

The stratum corneum is also approximately 10 μm thick, whereas the viable epidermis, dermis, and to a greater extent, the systemic compartment represent an effective large sink where absorbed substances undergo dilution to levels that often remain undetectable to all but the most sensitive techniques. Sampling the time-dependent changes in the concentration of a compound in individual compartments is thus technically challenging. Following application:

Topical formulations may undergo radical changes in composition and structure.

Xenobiotics are in general not evenly distributed on the skin surface.

The effectiveness of the skin barrier often changes with time.

The skin barrier is influenced by the type and progression of a disease.

There is regional variation in the barrier properties of the skin.

The viable tissues themselves respond to topical contact with xenobiotics in manners that may either enhance or retard percutaneous absorption.

Drugs influence all of these processes in a more-or-less specific manner.

J.D. Johansen et al. (eds.), *Contact Dermatitis*,
DOI: 10.1007/978-3-642-03827-3_12, © Springer-Verlag Berlin Heidelberg 2011

12

In view of these facts, the description of the kinetics of penetration after topical contact with a xenobiotic is a complex affair. A number of mathematical models have been developed to describe or define the relative importance of these processes in determining the bio-availability of compounds in a target tissue [1–6].

12.2 Diffusion

Any passage into and through the skin is governed by diffusion processes. In other words, active transport mechanisms play no role in penetration. Compounds that come into contact with the skin surface migrate down the concentration gradients according to well-described laws governing the diffusion of solutes in solutions and across membranes. For a more complete derivation of relevant equations, interested readers are referred to comprehensive reviews [7, 8].

12.2.1 Fick's Laws

Diffusion of uncharged compounds across a membrane or any homogeneous barrier is described by Fick's first and second laws. The first law states that the steady-state flux of a compound (J, mol/cm/s) per unit path length (δ, cm) is proportional to the concentration gradient (ΔC) and the diffusion coefficient (D, cm^2/s):

$$J = -D(\Delta C/\Delta \delta) \tag{12.1}$$

The negative sign indicates that the net flux is in the direction of the lower concentration. This equation holds for diffusion-mediated processes in isotropic solutions under steady-state conditions. Fick's second law predicts the flux of compounds under nonsteady-state conditions. The solution to these equations depends upon defining appropriate boundary conditions [6–10]. However, regardless of whether diffusion occurs in a system under steady-state or nonsteady-state conditions, the principal factors that determine the flux of a compound between two points in an isotropic medium are the concentration gradient, the path length, and the diffusion coefficient [11].

It is worthwhile pointing out that diffusion is a highly effective transport mechanism over very short distances but not over long ones. The relationship between the

time (Δt) it takes for a molecule to transverse a path length (x) and its diffusion coefficient is governed by:

$$\Delta t = x^2 / 2D \tag{12.2}$$

For example, the diffusion coefficient for water in an aqueous solution is 2.5×10^{-5} cm^2/s, suggesting that a water molecule would traverse a 10-μm path (the equivalent of the width of the stratum corneum) in 0.4 ms. However, since diffusion depends upon the square of the distance, longer pathlengths are not efficiently traversed: a 100-μm path would take 40 ms.

This explains why xenobiotics attain high concentrations in the upper layers of the skin, i.e., in the epidermis, while serum levels after cutaneous exposure remain low. The diffusional nature of percutaneous absorption also explains the exclusion of large molecules by the intact barrier: only a small number of such molecules per square centimeter can be brought into contact with the skin surface, which then encounter multilayers consisting of low-molecular-weight lipids with corresponding narrow intermolecular spaces (see below). As a rule of thumb, the passage of proteins and polymers >50,000 Da through the horny layer barrier becomes imperceptible.

> **Core Message**
>
> › Penetration is based on passive diffusion. There is no mechanism of active transport through the horny layer barrier.

12.3 Three-Compartment Model

Although pharmacokinetic analysis of topical applications may require the description of a relatively large number of compartments, this discussion is confined to three compartments: the skin surface, the stratum corneum, and the viable tissue. In order to undergo percutaneous absorption, a compound must be released from its formulation, particulate state, solvent, etc., encounter the skin surface, penetrate the stratum corneum, diffuse through the viable epidermis into the dermis, and finally gain access to the systemic compartment through the vascular system. In addition, it may diffuse through the dermal and hypodermal layers to reach the underlying muscular tissues. Within each compartment, the compound may diffuse down its concentration gradient, bind to specific compound, or be metabolized.

12.4 The Skin Surface

12.4.1 Surface Contact

The physical forms of contact with the skin surface, i.e., dust, powders, solutions, and formulations, all differ in their physicochemical properties, and, as discussed below, this influences the kinetics of release and/or absorption. However, the principal consideration is that topical contacts represent a physically small phenomenon, significantly limited by the amount of compound that is applied to the skin surface. When a patient applies, for example, a dermatologic preparation, the layer of a semisolid formulation covering the skin is very thin, corresponding to a volume of between 0.5 and 2 mg/cm². Thicker layers are felt as "undesirable" and consciously or subconsciously rubbed or spread to larger surfaces. This restricts the amount of compound that can effectively come into contact with the skin surface to approximately 0.5–2 µg/cm² for a 1% (wt/wt) topical formulation and other contact forms.

However, even after being rubbed in, material on the skin surface does not remain homogeneous over the time frame of penetration [12]. Topical applications undergo evaporation, such that even relatively nonvolatile substances such as water are rapidly lost [13, 14]. This phenomenon is readily recognized by patients as a cooling sensation. The evaporation results in rapid concentration of nonvolatile substances on the skin surface, which may result in the formation of supersaturated "solutions" or precipitation of active ingredients. Any material also mixes with skin-surface lipids and undergoes time-dependent changes in chemical composition, as their carrier undergoes absorption. Taken together, these considerations suggest that dramatic changes in the composition and structure of form occur following surface application, which determines the subsequent bioavailability.

An additional consideration is that topical contact does not result in an even distribution over the skin surface, but the material will be deposited in crevices and appendages. This may result in a relative increase in absorption through appendages. This phenomenon may be accentuated in forms that contain particles or precipitates, since there is evidence that appropriately sized particles can rapidly penetrate along the shafts of hair follicles to a depth of up to 100–500 µm [15, 16]. Such deposits might be an important element in allergic reactions to airborne allergens such as house dust, pollen, etc.

12.5 The Skin Barrier

The primary compartment that limits the percutaneous absorption of compounds is the stratum corneum. This thin (10–20 µm) layer effectively surrounding the body represents a highly differentiated structure that determines the diffusion of compounds across the skin. The physical description of the stratum corneum has now been well documented [17], and it can be accurately characterized as "bricks," i.e., cornified cells consisting of bundled, water-insoluble proteins, embedded in a "mortar" of intercellular lipid.

The general consensus today is that the stratum corneum is a highly organized, differentiated structure. In order to participate fully in forming an effective barrier to diffusion, the biogenesis of the corneocytes as well as the synthesis and processing of the intercellular lipid must proceed in an orderly manner. Recent evidence suggests that disruption in the kinetics of skin-barrier formation by accelerating the division of the keratinocytes found in the underlying layers will lead to a disruption in the barrier properties of the skin [13, 14]. Thus the concept of dead or dying skin forming a passive barrier to diffusion is now replaced by a model of the stratum corneum as a highly differentiated structure that has unique properties particularly suited to its role in forming the skin barrier.

12.5.1 Corneocytes

Totally, 85% of the stratum corneum is protein (as a percentage of dry mass), mostly associated with cornified cells, i.e., the corneocytes. These structures contain a core of keratins surrounded by an envelope made up of cross-linked proteins [18]. The keratins may account for up to 80% of the total dry mass of the corneocytes and thus represent the most important constituents. In addition to these fibrous proteins, the core contains low-molecular-weight polar compounds such as amino acids, urocanic and pyrrolidone carboxylic acid. These compounds play a role in maintaining the hydration properties of the stratum corneum.

12

12.5.2 Intercellular Lipid

Interspersed between corneocytes, the intercellular lipid is organized into sheets, which provide the primary barrier to diffusion across the stratum corneum [19]. This lipid is located in an extracellular domain and thus is not morphologically equivalent to a cellular membrane. The lipid accounts for approximately 15% of the dry weight of the stratum corneum or 20% of the volume. It is composed of roughly equimolar mixtures of ceramides, cholesterol, and long-chain free fatty acids. There is now substantial evidence that these lipids form structures [20, 21] wherein diffusion of the lipidic substances is more than 1,000-fold less than that found in cellular membranes [22, 23]. This material property of the intercellular lipid is particularly suited to play a role as a barrier to diffusion [17].

> **Core Message**
>
> > It is the complex structure of the thin stratum corneum that limits the penetration of compounds through the horny layer barrier.

12.5.3 Appendages

A variety of appendages penetrate the stratum corneum and epidermis, facilitating thermal control and providing a protective covering. Appendages are potential sites of discontinuity in the integrity of the skin barrier. Up to the present time, no penetration of topically applied substances into the sweat glands has been observed [24]. This is understandable, because there is a continuous mass flow out of the sweat glands onto the skin surface. While in the past, it was assumed that the intercellular penetration inside the lipid layers around the corneocytes was the only penetration pathway [25–27], recent investigations demonstrated that the hair follicles can also present an efficient pathway [28–30].

The density of the hair follicles varies on different body sites from 10 to 300 follicles per square centimeter. The reservoir of the hair follicle, i.e., its volume, can achieve values of 0.2 mm³/cm² skin surface [31]. This is comparable to the reservoir of the stratum corneum, if it is taken into consideration that the stratum corneum has an average thickness between 15 and 25 μm, the topically applied substances usually being stored in the upper 25% of the horny layer.

The hair follicles offer an important target for topically applied substances, because they are surrounded by a close network of blood capillaries, which are important for drug delivery [32–34]. Additionally, they are the host of the dendritic and stem cells, which are the target structure for immunomodulation and regenerative medicine. The hair follicles possess an individual barrier structure, which is in the upper part similar to that of the stratum corneum. In the lower part, the barrier is formed by tie junctions [35]. This means that the topically applied substances which penetrate into the reservoir of the hair follicles do not automatically penetrate through the skin barrier. In contrast to the stratum corneum, the hair follicles represent a long-term reservoir for topically applied substances, where they can be stored one order of magnitude longer than in the horny layer [36, 37].

Appendages account for 0.1–1% of the area of the skin and 0.01–0.1% of the total skin volume. It can be concluded that in order to significantly influence the flux of compounds across the skin, the diffusion coefficient has to be considerably higher than that across the intercellular lipid domains or corneocytes. For this reason, it is likely that "shunt" pathways are relatively more important for molecules exhibiting relatively slow rates of percutaneous absorption and are of primary importance during early stages after topical contact. There is unequivocal proof that solid material can enter the lower lumen of the hair follicle [15]. Follicular penetration was clearly demonstrated for titanium dioxide particles [38]. Thus one has to assume that any allergenic material associated with or presented as particles can take this route, thereby bypassing the horny layer barrier. The extent to which such a passage contributes to the allergic and irritant reaction to airborne xenobiotics (pollen allergens, etc.) and to bulky proteins in general merits further investigation.

> **Core Message**
>
> > Hair follicles present sites of imperfection in the skin protection afforded by the barrier function of the horny layer. They have to be taken into consideration as a port of entry for large molecules (proteins, etc.) as well as particles carrying adsorbed allergens.

12.5.4 Pathways Across the Stratum Corneum

The relevance of the intercellular lipid domain to permeation of compounds across the stratum corneum (Fig. 12.1) is inferred from the striking relationship between the hydrophobicity of compounds and their permeability coefficients across the skin [38, 39]. This suggests that the rate-limiting step for permeation includes a hydrophobic barrier, i.e., the intercellular lipid. The observation that small polar molecules such as urea exhibit higher permeability coefficients than expected on the basis of their partition coefficient between *n*-octanol and water has been interpreted to support the presence of polar and apolar pathways [39, 40]. However, alternative single-pathway models indicate that this observation can be

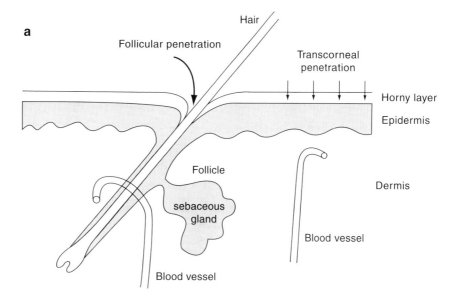

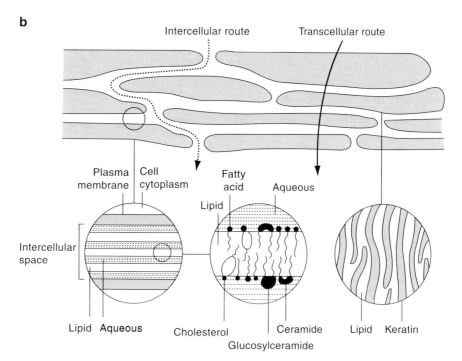

Fig. 12.1 Model of penetration pathways. (**a**) Penetration occurs via appendages that exhibit a reduced barrier to diffusion but occupy a relatively small surface area. (**b**) Permeation through the stratum corneum (transcorneal permeation) may be considered to occur through the intercellular lipid domain or through the corneocytes (transcellular route) (from ref. [17])

accounted for by considering the influence of molecular volume on the relative diffusivity of compounds in membranes [40–42]. In addition, available evidence suggests that the only continuous domain within the stratum corneum is formed by the intercellular lipid space [42, 43]. This implies that compounds penetrating the stratum corneum must pass through intercellular lipid, although it does not exclude the possibility that compounds can also enter the inner lumen of corneocytes.

There are several studies that have directly visualized the penetration pathways across the stratum corneum with electron microscopy. Osmium tetroxide vapor can be used to precipitate n-butanol that has penetrated the stratum corneum [42, 43]. Following a brief (5- or 60-s) exposure of murine or human stratum corneum, the alcohol was found enriched in the intercellular spaces (threefold), though significant levels were also found in the corneocytes. Using a different approach involving rapid freezing, water, ethanol, and cholesterol were also found preferentially concentrated in the intercellular lipid spaces [43, 44].

However, in most of these investigations, there was also significant localization of compounds in the corneocytes, more prevalent in the upper layers (stratum disjunctum). Thus, corneocytes undergoing desquamation appear to be relatively permeable, even to rather bulky ions such as mercury. There is additional evidence that other compounds can and do penetrate the corneocytes. It is well established, for example, that occlusion or immersion of the skin in a bath leads to the swelling of the corneocytes, consistent with the entry of water. Other compounds have also been localized to corneocytes, including the binding of anionic surfactants to keratins. Low-molecular-weight moisturizers such as glycerol are likely to penetrate the corneocytes and alter their water-binding capacity. Thus, the penetration of corneocytes cannot be excluded when considering percutaneous absorption pathways.

12.5.5 Inter- and Intraindividual Variation in Skin-Barrier Function

Finally, it is worthwhile considering the level of inter- and intraindividual variation in skin. The most accurate and reproducible method of measuring barrier activity is to follow transepidermal water loss (TEWL)

[44–47]. The extent of within-individual variation in this parameter has been estimated to be 8% by site and 21% from day to day. The variations between individuals are reported to be somewhat larger, ranging from 35 to 48% [47, 48]. There appears to be no significant sex- or race-dependent differences in skin-barrier activity. The skin-barrier activity of premature infants (delivered more than 3 weeks premature) has been demonstrated to be markedly impaired, whereas skin-barrier function appears normal for full-term infants. There seems to be no significant alteration in skin-barrier activity as a function of age. Better-defined differences in skin-barrier activity between different sites are observed; barrier function can be ranked as arm > abdomen > postauricular > forehead [44–47]. Undoubtedly, contact sensitization and elicitation depend on the threshold concentrations in the viable tissue, which, however, depend on quite a number of factors (surface concentration, size of contact area, antigenic potency of the allergen, number of exposures, effect of draining lymph node, vehicle, occlusion, eczematous conditions), as well as the degree and route of penetration [49, 50].

Core Message

> Thresholds for sensitization and elicitation depend on many things including the degree of penetration by allergens: potency overrules penetration.

12.6 Viable Tissue

Although the primary barrier to percutaneous absorption lies within the stratum corneum (Fig. 12.2), diffusion within the viable tissue as well as metabolism and resorption will also influence the bioavailability of compounds in, and their passage through, specific skin compartments. These processes are interrelated, and factors that increase the rate of one of these processes inevitably influence the others.

The passage of compounds from the stratum corneum into the viable epidermis results in a substantial dilution (Fig. 12.3). This reflects not only the relatively larger

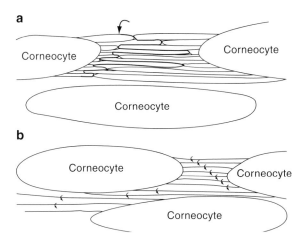

a

Corneocyte

Corneocyte

Corneocyte

b

Corneocyte

Corneocyte

Corneocyte

Fig. 12.2 Schematic representation of possible penetration pathways through the intercellular lipid domain. (**a**) Diffusion of compounds may occur along lipid lamellae (*single line*), which occasionally penetrate the stratum corneum, or (**b**) diffusion occurs across the lamellae in a mechanism that is analogous to diffusion across lipid bilayers. (**a**) The pathway is indicated by a *heavy line*; (**b**) the pathway is denoted by an *arrow* to indicate translamellar diffusion and *lines* to denote lateral-lamellar diffusion (from ref. [17])

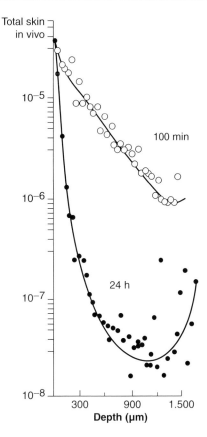

Fig. 12.3 Distribution of 8-methoxypsoralen (*8-MOP*) in the skin at the indicated time after application. At early time points, a steep nonlinear gradient is observed across the whole of the skin. At later periods, the concentration in the dermis has begun to level off (from ref. [17])

size of the epidermis as compared with the stratum corneum, but also the lower resistance to diffusion within viable tissues, corresponding approximately to that on an aqueous protein gel [47, 48]. Concentrations of 10^{-4}–10^{-6} M may be attained in the epidermis and dermis for substances that permeate readily (Fig. 12.3). Although the actual concentration gradient of a compound is influenced by both its physicochemical properties and the time of contact, the presence of a concentration gradient is visible at all times. In other words, strategies to enhance or decrease percutaneous absorption generally result in a relatively even increase or decrease in the concentration of compounds in all compartments.

Diffusion cell experiments are the standard procedure to investigate the penetration of topically applied substances through the skin barrier under in vitro conditions [51–53]. This method is well suited for the investigation of intercellular penetration. However, this method is not suited to analyze the follicular penetration. The reason for this situation is the contraction of human skin after removal in the operating theater, so that the hair follicles are closed [54]. If the excised skin is subsequently stretched to its original size, the elastic fibers between the hair follicles become stretched but not the close network of elastic fibers around them. Comparing the in vivo and in vitro storage of topically applied substances in the hair follicles, it was established that under in vivo conditions, an increase of one order of magnitude could be found in the hair follicles under in vitro conditions.

Core message

> The intercellular penetration of topically applied substances can be investigated in vitro, while the follicular penetration has to be investigated under in vivo conditions.

12

12.6.1 Skin Metabolism

The skin contains a wide range of enzymatic activities, including phase-I oxidative, reductive, hydrolytic, and phase-II conjugative reactions as well as a full complement of metabolizing enzymes [48, 49, 55, 56]. Metabolic activity is a primary consideration in the design of prodrugs and may influence the bioavailability of drugs delivered via dermatologic or transdermal formulations.

Alterations in skin metabolism have been implicated in a range of diseases including hirsutism and acne, and they may be relevant to the risk assessment of carcinogens. Metabolic processing of antigens by Langerhans cells is involved in the presentation of allergens to the immune system. Thus, metabolism in the skin compartments plays a significant role in determining the fate of a topically applied compound.

Significant cutaneous metabolism has been demonstrated for a wide variety of compounds of differing physicochemical properties, including the steroid hormones estrone, estradiol, and estriol as well as glucocorticoids, prostaglandins, retinoids, benzoyl peroxide, aldrin, anthralin, 5-fluorouracil, nitroglycerin, theophylline, and propranolol [48, 55]. It is convenient to classify metabolic reactions in terms of their cofactor dependence. Processes that require cofactors are likely to be energy-dependent and thus to be located within viable tissues. Among the best-studied examples are the interconversion of steroids (e.g., estrone and estradiol), and the oxidation of polycyclic aromatic hydrocarbons with mixed-function mono-oxygenases. Cinnamic aldehyde and cinnamic alcohol are known allergens, cinnamic aldehyde being the more potent sensitizer. It has been assumed that cinnamic alcohol is a "prohapten" that requires metabolic activation, presumably by oxidoreductase enzymes such as alcohol dehydrogenase or cytochrome P450 2E1, to the protein reactive cinnamaldehyde as hapten. In fact, such bioconversion could be demonstrated in human skin [57]. In contrast, cofactor-independent processes involve catabolism and may be located outside of viable tissues, i.e., in the transition region between the stratum corneum and stratum granulosum. The best characterized of these involve hydrolytic reactions such as those described for nonspecific ester hydrolysis. Furthermore activation can take place outside the tissue: ethoxylated nonionic surfactants were shown to be susceptible to oxidation on air exposure and to form allergenic hydroxyaldehydes. More importantly irritant components present in the oxidation mixture facilitated the penetration [58].

Metabolic activity is found in: (1) skin-surface microorganisms, (2) appendages, (3) the stratum corneum, (4) the viable epidermis, and (5) the dermis. In considering the site of the most significant metabolism, one has to take into account the relevant enzymes and their specific activity as well as their capacity relative to the size of the compartment. Thus, although the level of many enzymes is the highest in the epidermis, the relatively large size of the dermal compartment may play a significant role in determining the site of metabolism. A further consideration is that enzymes involved in cutaneous metabolism may be induced upon exposure to xenobiotics. This has been well described for various mixed-function mono-oxygenases [49, 56]. Finally, the quantitative extrapolation of results from animal models to humans is hazardous owing to the significant species differences in the metabolism of compounds.

However, despite the variety of skin-associated metabolic processes, the extent of metabolism is normally relatively modest, perhaps 2–5% of the absorbed compounds. Metabolism is limited not only by the relatively short period of time that a compound spends in the viable layers of the skin, but also by the overall level of enzyme activity. Thus, under many circumstances, the available enzymes are saturated by the level of the compound undergoing percutaneous absorption [48, 55].

Core Message

> Pure compounds are not necessarily capable of eliciting allergic reactions: metabolism before and during penetration of the skin may activate the compounds to potent allergens.

12.6.2 Resorption

Resorption, defined as the uptake of compounds by the cutaneous microvasculature, is directly related to the surface area of the exchanging capillaries as well as their blood flow. Total blood flow to the skin may vary up to 100-fold, a process primarily regulated by vascular shunts as well as by recruitment of new capillary beds [50, 55, 59, 60]. It has been estimated that, under resting conditions, only 40% of the blood flow passes via exchanging capillaries capable of acting as a sink for absorbed compounds. However, this value demonstrates considerable variation between body sites, individuals, and species [56, 61], and is influenced by disease states and environmental conditions. In particular, changes in temperature and humidity as well as the presence of vasoactive compounds may directly influence skin blood flow [57, 62].

12.6.3 The Influence of Pathologic Processes on Skin Barrier

It has been argued that the molecular weight of a compound must be under 500 Da to allow absorption through the skin [63]. This assumption is however based on a "macrophysiological" view of penetration kinetics, considering transcorneal diffusion to be the only route of entry into and through the skin. This view is contradicted by the very experience that proteins can be allergenic [49]. Two possible routes for protein penetration have to be taken into account: First, large molecules, and in fact particulate material, can enter deep into the lumen of the hair follicles, as mentioned above [39]. In that way, they reach an area that is devoid of protection by a barrier [64], surrounded by a dense population of immune-competent dendritic cells. Second, irritation is known to provoke barrier defects, thereby allowing the proteins to enter into direct contact with the viable epidermis and its immune-competent Langerhans cells [17, 49, 58, 65, 66]. Environmental factors such as low humidity are suggested to increase the number of Langerhans cells as well as favor penetration by trinitrochlorobenzene [67]. Depending on the vehicle, occlusion may increase or decrease the response when testing the allergenic potency of parabens [68].

Reduced skin-barrier function is observed for a number of pathologic conditions including ichthyosis [58–60, 69–71], psoriasis [61, 62, 72, 73], atopic dermatitis [63, 64, 74, 75], and contact dermatitis [65, 76] (Tables 12.1 and 12.2). It is generally accepted that this can be attributed to structural alterations in the stratum corneum [17]. Structural deficiencies may arise from abrasion, the extraction of lipids by solvents or strong detergents, by exposure to potent alkaline or acidic fluids and dusts, and the absence of an enzyme

Table 12.1 Excretion of triamcinolone acetonide in the urine after topical application to normal and psoriatic skin

Skin area	Applied preparation	Excretion (%)	Time (h)
Uninvolved skin	0.1% cream	0.4	72
Psoriatic skin	0.1% cream	4.3	72
Healthy skin	0.1% cream	1.4	72

Table 12.2 Barrier function as measured by transepidermal water loss (TEWL) for normal, uninvolved, and involved psoriatic skin [17]

Condition	TEWL (g/m^2/h)	Student's t test
Healthy individual	4.3 ± 1.2	NS
Uninvolved skin	6.3 ± 1.8	n.a.
Psoriatic plaque	11.5 ± 6.3	$p < 0.05$
After scale removal	29.1 ± 9.8	$p < 0.05$
Fissured plaque	20.9 ± 8.0	$p < 0.05$

NS not significant

or structural protein in the underlying viable tissues, or they may be related to the improper formation of the stratum corneum resulting from an increase in keratinocyte proliferation [46, 66], as in the case of psoriasis. A consequence of poor barrier function is a further increase in penetration by xenobiotics, which may accentuate the problem. Thus in individuals predisposed to a defective barrier, a minor perturbation may become amplified as the skin attempts to compensate by increasing keratinocyte proliferation [46, 66]. As a rule of thumb in areas devoid of a functional horny layer, the penetration by a compound is increased by a factor of 3- up to 15-fold. A further consideration is that the homeostatic mechanisms responsible for the recovery of barrier activity after perturbation may be altered in some diseases or physiologic states. For example, while the skin of elderly people exhibits normal barrier function, the recovery of barrier activity after perturbation is markedly reduced [67, 77]. This kinetic basis for reduced barrier function may also account for interindividual variation in barrier function and/or an apparently increased susceptibility of certain individuals to contact dermatitis [65, 76]. It follows that on the one hand, in skin areas with pathologically disturbed barrier function, the entrance of topical substances is accelerated and increased relative to the surrounding normal skin (targeting to the disease), while, on the other hand once an irritant has overcome the

12

barrier, it facilitates its own penetration, thereby amplifying the damage [68, 78].

> ### Core Message
>
> > Any disturbance or disorder of the barrier function facilitates penetration by allergens. This is particularly true for eczematous conditions such as atopy, psoriasis, etc.

12.6.4 Allergens

Surprisingly, little work has been published on penetration by allergens. Nickel penetrates through rubber gloves [69, 79]. However, its penetration of the skin is relatively minimal [70, 80] and depends on the vehicle [71, 81]. Occlusion enhances its penetration [72, 82]. Differences in higher penetration by squaric acid esters as compared to low penetration by squaric acid explain why the latter is a less-effective sensitizer in the sensitization therapy of alopecia areata [73, 83].

Pretreatment with topical cyclosporin appears to provoke a perturbation of the horny layer barrier and thereby enhances penetration by allergens rather than inhibiting the allergic reaction by immunosuppression [74, 84].

One has to suppose that the elicitation of allergic reactions depends largely on the individual patient's barrier function, and thus on the influence of the site of elicitation, moisture, temperature, season, and environmental and endogenous factors on the penetration by the allergen in question.

Much more work is needed to address the prevention of elicitation by restricting allergen penetration: a hypothetical reduction of such penetration by a factor of three would lower the titer, and hence the frequency and severity of allergic reactions by a factor of three as well.

Several papers address the efficiency of barrier creams in reducing penetration by allergens and irritants [46, 75–79, 85–90], demonstrating moderate to good protective capacity.

12.7 Vehicles

The influence of a carrier medium on percutaneous absorption of an incorporated substance is very complex [17]. It depends on the physicochemical interaction between a compound and its carrier as well as between the carrier and the skin surface. In very general terms, the primary factor governing the passage of a compound is its own physicochemical property, that is, its molecular size, polarity, and lipophilicity: small nonpolar and moderately lipophilic substances penetrate the best; highly polar water soluble compounds, the least. The influence of classical vehicles on the passage of these two extremes is limited [91]. The most prominent "vehicle effect" is reached either by pushing the concentration of a compound close to its solubility limits in a given carrier (thereby increasing its thermodynamic potential in favor of diffusion out of the vehicle and into the skin) or by disturbing the barrier function [92]. However, the potential of the so-called penetration enhancers is limited in practical terms, since the disturbance of the barrier function challenges the homeostatic equilibrium in the stratum corneum and provokes a counteraction in the sense of strengthening of the barrier.

> ### Core Message
>
> > The carrier acts on the barrier – it can increase or decrease the exposure to allergens.

12.8 Conclusions

The principal factors determining the kinetics of the diffusion of a xenobiotic into the skin are the physiochemical properties of the molecule. Hydrophobicity, molecular weight, and ionic charge determine the feasibility of transdermal delivery for any particular compound. The form of contact influences the kinetics largely from considerations of the thermodynamic activity of the compound. However, one should not exclude the impact of changes in the physical forms that occur following topical application. Evaporation, and changes in the structure of emulsion, dissolution in sebum, entry into the follicle, etc. may bring dramatic changes in the thermodynamic activity of the compound. Under some circumstances, this may lead to the retention of the drug on the skin surface.

The rate-limiting step for the percutaneous absorption of most compounds is its penetration through the stratum corneum. There is substantial evidence that this is related to diffusion through a tortuous path around the corneocytes within the highly structured intercellular lipid, the constituents of which exhibit diffusional properties consistent with their role in the skin barrier.

There are two penetration pathways, the intercellular penetration inside the lipid layers around the corneocytes and the follicular penetration, where the topically applied substances can pass the skin barrier [93]. The reservoir of the hair follicles is a long-term reservoir in comparison to the stratum corneum.

For skin diseases exhibiting reduced skin-barrier function, the absence of these critical structures may account for the decreased barrier activity. The progression of a disease and the inherent biological variability make predictions of percutaneous absorption for diseased skin inherently difficult. This contributes significantly to the challenges of developing topical applications of drugs as well as barrier creams.

Processes occurring in viable tissues can have a significant, although generally less-important influence on the bioavailability of compounds undergoing percutaneous absorption. It has been difficult to establish in vivo the level of skin-related metabolism of drugs undergoing percutaneous absorption.

References

1. Higuchi T (1960) Physical chemical analysis of percutaneous absorption process from creams and ointments. J Soc Cosmet Chem 11:85
2. Guy RH, Hadgraft J (1989) Mathematical models of percutaneous absorption. In: Bronaugh RL, Maibach HI (eds) Percutaneous absorption. Dekker, New York, p 13
3. Guy RH, Hadgraft J, Maibach AJ (1982) A pharmacokinetic model for percutaneous absorption. Int J Pharmaceut 11:119
4. Gupta SK et al (1993) Pharmokinetic and pharmodynamic modeling of transdermal products: in vivo methods, problems, and pitfalls. In: Shah VP, Maibach HI (eds) Topical drug bioavailability: bioequivalence and penetration. Plenum, New York, p 311
5. Kuboto K et al (1993) Percutaneous absorption: a single model. J Pharm Sci 82:450
6. Williams PL, Riviere JE (1995) A biophysically based dermatopharmokinetic compartment model for quantifying percutaneous penetration and absorption of topically applied agents. 1. Theory. J Pharm Sci 84:599
7. Jain MK, Wagner RC (eds) (1980) Introduction to biological membranes. Wiley, Toronto, p 117
8. Gennis RB (1989) Biomembranes: molecular structure and function. Springer, Berlin
9. Barry BW (1983) Dermatological formulations: percutaneous absorption. Dekker, New York

10. Scheuplein RJ (1967) Mechanism of percutaneous absorption. II. Transient diffusion and the relative importance of various routes of skin penetration. J Invest Dermatol 45:334
11. Lieb WR, Stein WD (1986) Non-stokesian nature of transverse diffusion within human red blood cell membranes. J Membr Biol 92:111
12. Brown S, Diffey BL (1986) The effect of applied thickness on sunscreen protection: in vivo and in vitro studies. Photochem Photobiol 44:509
13. Flynn GL (1993) General introduction and conceptual differentiation of topical and transdermal drug delivery systems. In: Shaw VP, Maibach HI (eds) Topical drug bioavailability: bioequivalence and penetration. Plenum, New York, p 369
14. Reifenrath WG (1995) Volatile substances. Cosmet Toil 110:85
15. Rolland A et al (1993) Site-specific drug delivery to pilosebaceous structures using polymeric microspheres. Pharm Res 10:1738
16. Rolland A (1993) Particulate carriers in dermal and transdermal drug delivery: myth or reality. In: Walters KA, Hadgraft J (eds) Pharmaceutical particulate carriers: therapeutic applications. Dekker, New York, p 1983
17. Schaefer H, Redelmeier TE (1996) Skin barrier principle of percutaneous absorption. Karger, Basel
18. Reichert U et al (1993) The cornified envelope: a key structure of terminally differentiating keratinocytes. In: Darmon M, Blumenberg M (eds) The keratinocytes. Academic, San Diego, p 107
19. Elias PM, Menon GK (1991) Structural and lipid biochemical correlates of the epidermal permeability barrier. Adv Lipid Res 24:1
20. Madison KC et al (1987) Presence of intact intercellular lipid lamallae in the upper layers of the stratum corneum. J Invest Dermatol 88:714
21. Hou SYE et al (1991) Membranes structures in normal and essential fatty acid deficient stratum corneum: characterization by ruthenium tetroxide staining and x-ray diffraction. J Invest Dermatol 96:215
22. Bouwstra JA et al (1991) Structure of human stratum corneum by small-angle x-ray scattering. J Invest Dermatol 97:1005
23. Bouwstra JA et al (1992) Structure of human stratum corneum as a function of temperature and hydration: a wide angle x-ray diffraction study. Int J Pharm 84:205
24. Shah VP et al (1974) Role of sweat in accumulation of orally administered griseofulvin in skin. J Clin Invest 53:1673
25. Cross SE et al (2007) Human skin penetration of sunscreen nanoparticles: in-vitro assessment of a novel micronized zinc oxide formulation. Skin Pharmacol Physiol 20:148
26. Godwin DA, Michniak BB (1999) Influence of drug lipophilicity on terpenes as transdermal penetration enhancers. Drug Dev Ind Pharm 25:905
27. Moser K et al (2001) Passive skin penetration enhancement and its quantification in vitro. Eur J Pharm Biopharm 52:103
28. Jacobi U et al (2005) Do follicles play a role as penetration pathways in in vitro studies on porcine skin? An optical study. Laser Phys 15:1594
29. Patzelt A et al (2008) Hair follicles, their disorders and their opportunities. Drug Discov Today 5:173

12

30. Teichmann A et al (2006) Follicular penetration: Development of a method to block the follicles selectively against the penetration of topically applied substances. Skin Pharmacol Physiol 19:216

31. Otberg N et al (2004) Variations of hair follicle size and distribution in different body sites. J Invest Dermatol 122:14

32. Gupta S et al (2001) The hair follicle as a target for gene therapy. Eur J Dermatol 11:353

33. Lademann J et al (2007) Penetration von Pollenallergenen in die Haut. Dermatologie in Beruf und Umwelt 55:127

34. Reynolds AJ et al (1999) Trans-gender induction of hair follicles. Nature 402:33

35. Oshima H et al (2001) Morphogenesis and renewal of hair follicles from adult multipotent stem cells. Cell 104:233

36. Lademann J et al (2006) Hair follicles – a long-term reservoir for drug delivery. Skin Pharmacol Physiol 19:232

37. Lademann J et al (2008) Hair follicles - An efficient storage and penetration pathway for topically applied substances. Skin Pharmacol Physiol 21:150

38. Lademann J et al (2001) Investigation of follicular penetration of topically applied substances. Skin Pharmacol Appl Skin Physiol 14:17–22

39. Flynn GL (1990) Physiochemical determinants of skin absorption. In: Gerrity TR, Henry CJ (eds) Principles of route-to-route extrapolation for risk assessment. Elsevier, New York, p 93

40. Tayar EL et al (1991) Percutaneous penetration of drugs: a quantitative structure-permeability relationship study. J Pharm Sci 80:744

41. Kastings GB et al (1987) Effect of lipid sollubility and molecular size on percutaneous absorption. In: Shroot B, Schaefer H (eds) Skin pharmakinetics, vol 1. Karger, Basel, p 138

42. Guy RH, Potts RO (1992) Structure-permeability relationships in percutaneous absorption. J Pharm Sci 81:603

43. Nemaniac MK, Elias PM (1980) In situ precipitation: a novel cytochemical technique for visualization of permeability pathways in mammalian stratum corneum. J Histol Cytochem 28:573

44. Squier CA, Lesch CA (1988) Penetration pathways of different compounds through epidermis and oral epithelial. J Oral Pathol 17:512

45. Pinnagoda J et al (1990) Guidelines for transepithelial water loss (TEWL) measurements. A report from the Standardization Group of the European Society of Contact Dermatitis. Contact Derm 22:164

46. Lavrijsen APM et al (1993) Barrier function parameters in various keratization disorders: transepithelial water loss and vascular response to hexyl nicotinate. Br J Dermatol 129:547

47. Rougier A, Lotte C (1993) Predictive approaches: I. The stripping technique. In: Shaw VP, Maibach HI (eds) Topical drug bioavailability: bioequivalence and penetration. Plenum, New York, p 163

48. Scheuplein RJ (1967) Mechanism of percutaneous absorption. II. Transient diffusion and the relative importance of various routes of skin penetration. J Invest Dermatol 45:33

49. Boukhman MP, Maibach HI (2001) Thresholds in contact sensitisation: immunologic mechanisms and experimental evidence in humans – an overview. Food Chem Tox 39:1125–1134

50. Berard F, Marty JP, Nicolas JF (2003) Allergen penetration through the skin. Eur J Dermatol 13:324–330

51. Baroli B et al (2007) Penetration of metallic nanoparticles in human full-thickness skin. J Invest Dermatol 127:1701

52. Chilcott RP et al (2002) Evaluation of barrier creams against sulphur mustard. I. In vitro studies using human skin. Skin Pharmacol Appl Skin Physiol 15:225

53. Jacobi U et al (2005) Comparison of four different in vitro systems to study the reservoir capacity of the stratum corneum. J Control Release 103:61

54. Patzelt A et al (2008) Differential stripping demonstrates a significant reduction of the hair follicle reservoir in vitro compared to in vivo. Eur J Pharm Biopharm 70:234

55. Kao J, Carver MP (1990) Cutaneous metabolism of xenobiotics. Drug Metab Rev 22:363

56. Mukhtar H, Khan WA (1989) Cutaneous cytochrome P-450. Drug Metab Rev 20:657

57. Smith CK, Moore CA, Elahi EN, Smart AT, Hotchkiss SA (2000) Human skin absorption and metabolism of the contact allergens, cinnamic aldehyde, and cinnamic alcohol. Toxical Appl Pharmacol 168:189–199

58. Bodin A, Li Ping Shao J, Nilsson LG, Karlberg AT (2001) Identification and allergenic activity of hydroxyaldehydes-a new type of oxidation product from an ethoxylated non-ionic surfactant. Contact Dermatitis 44:207–212

59. Ryan TJ (1983) Cutaneous circulation. In: Goldsmith LA (ed) Biochemistry and physiology of the skin, vol 2. Oxford University Press, New York, p 817

60. Riviere JE, Williams PL (1992) Pharmokinetic implication of changing blood flow in skin. J Pharm Sci 81:601

61. Monteiro-Riviere NA et al (1990) Interspecies and interregional analysis of the comparative histological thickness and laser Doppler blood flow measurements af five cutaneous sites in nine species. J Invest Dermatol 95:582

62. Riviere JE et al (1991) The effect of vasoactive drugs on transdermal lidocaine iontophoresis. J Pharm Sci 80:615

63. Bos JD, Meinardi MMHM (2000) The 500 Dalton rule for the skin penetration of chemical compounds and drugs. Exp Dermatol 9:165–169

64. Smith Pease CK, White IR, Basketter DA (2002) Skin as route of exposure to protein allergens. Clin Exp Dermatol 27:296–300

65. Zhai H, Maibach HI (2001) Skin occlusion and irritant and allergic contact dermatitis: an overview. Contact Dermatitis 44:201–206

66. Pedersen LK et al (2004) Augmentation of skin response by exposure to a combination of allergens and irritants – a review. Contact Dermatitis 50:265–273

67. Hosoi J et al (2000) Regulation of the cutaneous allergic reaction by humidity. Contact Dermatitis 42:81–84

68. Cross SE, Roberts MS (2000) The effect of occlusion on epidermal penetration of parabens from a commercial allergy test ointment, acetone and ethanol vehicles. J Invest Derm 115:914–918

69. Williams ML, Elias PM (1993) From basket weave to barrier: unifying concepts for the pathogenesis of the disorders of cornification. Arch Dermatol 129:626

70. Oestmann E et al (1993) Skin barrier function in healthy volunteers as assessed by transepidermal water loss and vascular response to hexyl nicotinate: intra- and inter-individual variability. Br J Dermatol 128:130

71. Blichmann CW, Serup J (1989) Reproducibility and variability of transdermal water loss measurements. Acta Derm Venereol 67:206

72. Imokawa G et al (1991) Decreased levels of ceramides in stratum corneum of atopic dermatitis: an etiologic factor in atopic dry skin? J Invest Dermatol 96:523

73. Werner Y, Linberg M (1985) Transepidermal water loss in dry and clinically normal skin in patients with atopic dermatitis. Acta Derm Venereol 65:102

74. Takenouchi M, Suzuki H, Tagami H (1986) Hydration characteristics of pathological stratum corneum: evaluation of bound water. J Invest Dermatol 87:574–576

75. Werner Y, Linberg M (1985) Transepidermal water loss in dry and clinically normal skin in patients with atopic dermatitis. Acta Derma Venereol 65:102

76. Wilhelm KP et al (1991) Effect of sodium lauryl sulfate-induced skin irritation on in vivo percutaneous absorption of four drugs. J Invest Dermatol 97:927

77. Lavrijsen APM et al (1995) Reduced skin barrier function parallels abnormal stratum corneum lipid organization in patients with lamellar ichtyosis. J Invest Dermatol 105:619

78. Fartasch M, Schnetz E, Diepgen TL (1998) Characterization of detergent-induced barrier alterations – effect of barrier cream on irritation. J Invest Dermatol 3:121–127

79. Wall LM (1980) Nickel penetration through rubber gloves. Contact Dermatitis 6:461–463

80. Kalimo K, Lammintausta K, Maki J, Teuho J, Jensen CT (1985) Nickel penetration in allergic individuals: bioavailability versus X-ray microanalysis detection. Contact Dermatitis 12:255–257

81. Fullerton A, Andersen JR, Hoelgaard A (1988) Permeation of nickel through human skin in vitro-effect of vehicles. Br J Dermatol 118:509–516

82. Fullerton A, Andersen JR, Hoelgaard A, Menne T (1986) Permeation of nickel salts through human skin in vitro. Contact Dermatitis 15:173–177

83. Sherertz EF, Sloan KB (1988) Percutaneous penetration of squaric acid and its esters in hairless mouse and human skin in vitro. Arch Dermatol Res 280:57–60

84. Surber C, Itin P, Buchner S, Maibach HI (1992) Effect of a new topical cyclosporin formulation on human allergic contact dermatitis. Contact Dermatitis 26:116–119

85. Loden M (1986) The effect of 4 barrier creams on the absorption of water, benzene, and formaldehyde into excised human skin. Contact Dermatitis 14:292–296

86. Boman A, Mellstrom G (1989) Percutaneous absorption of 3 organic solvents in the guinea pig. (III). Effect of barrier cream. Contact Dermatitis 21:134–140

87. Frosch PJ, Kurte A (1994) Efficacy of skin barrier creams (IV). The repetitive irritation test (RIT) with a set of 4 standard irritants. Contact Dermatitis 31:161–168

88. Zhai H, Maibach HI (1996) Effect of barrier creams: human skin in vivo. Contact Dermatitis 35:92–96

89. Zhai H, Maibach HI (1996) Percutaneous penetration (dermatopharmcokinetics) in evaluating barrier creams. Curr Prob Dermatol 25:193–205

90. Gawkrodger DJ, Healy J, Howe AM (1995) The prevention of nickel contact dermatitis. A review of the use of binding agents and barrier creams. Contact Dermatitis 32: 257–265

91. Hatcher ME, Plachy WZ (1993) Dioxygen diffusion in the stratum corneum: an EPR study. Biochim Biophys Acta 1149:73

92. Packer KJ, Sellwood TC (1978) Proton magnetic resonance studies of hydrated stratum corneum, part 2. Self diffusion. J Chem Soc Faraday Trans 2:1592

93. Francoeur ML, Potts RO (1988) The perturbation of stratum corneum lipids affects the diffusive but not partitioning aspects of water vapor permeability. Pharm Res 5:S130

Predictive Tests for Irritants and Allergens and Their Use in Quantitative Risk Assessment

13

David Basketter and Ian Kimber

Contents

13.1 Introduction

In this chapter, the main predictive methods, both animal and human, for the assessment of skin irritation and skin sensitisation potential are described. The principles that they embody could be transcribed to the many variants that are also available (and which for a variety of reasons may be the preferred approach for some readers). A detailed discussion of these variants is beyond the scope of this chapter; rather the reader is encouraged to apply the basic principles outlined herein to the consideration of all test methods. Whereas the panoply of assays available will serve in one way or the other to identify irritation and sensitisation hazards, it is in reality much more important to derive an estimation of the relative potency of the hazard presented, such that an appropriate risk assessment can be made and risk management measures applied. The second part of this chapter is, therefore, devoted to a consideration of the risk assessment approaches employed for chemicals known to have the capacity to irritate skin and/or sensitise skin.

13.2 Definitions

Skin sensitisation describes a state of heightened immunological reactivity for a particular chemical allergen, such that if this chemical allergen is encountered on the skin by a sensitised individual, a vigorous local immune response will be elicited, resulting in cutaneous inflammation and symptoms that are recognised clinically as allergic contact dermatitis. Skin irritation describes local damage or local trauma associated with the direct initiation of an inflammatory response and the symptoms

D. Basketter (✉)
DABMEB Consultancy Ltd, Sharnbrook,
Bedford, UK
e-mail: david.basketter@ukonline.co.uk

I. Kimber
University of Manchester, Manchester, UK

J.D. Johansen et al. (eds.), *Contact Dermatitis*,
DOI: 10.1007/978-3-642-03827-3_13, © Springer-Verlag Berlin Heidelberg 2011

13

characteristic of irritant contact dermatitis. Two important points should be made. First, that the properties of skin irritants and the potential to induce skin sensitisation are not mutually exclusive. Indeed, many chemicals display both activities and these will, at appropriate concentrations, cause both local inflammation at the site of first exposure and initiating sensitisation such that responses will be provoked subsequently, following contact with lower concentrations of the material. The possession of both irritant and sensitising properties by a chemical may have implications for the effectiveness with which skin sensitisation is induced. Second, the morphological and histopathological characteristics of allergic contact dermatitis and irritant contact dermatitis are usually inseparable. Predictive tests identify irritant or sensitising hazards (an intrinsic property) and these hazards may be scaled (e.g. by measuring relative potency). Risks to human health are then a function of the hazard, its relative potency and the extent of skin exposure.

13.3 Predictive Tests for Irritants

Human skin irritation is a more complex phenomenon than is sometimes recognised, especially by those who have devised simple tests for its assessment. The term "irritation" is deployed to embrace a broad range of skin effects, ranging (at least according to some) from immediate skin contact reactions (vide infra) through acute primary irritancy to traumiterative dermatitis that may well be chronic in nature [1]. End points considered for these responses encompass both sensory and visible effects. However, for the purposes of this chapter, the focus has been restricted to acute and cumulative irritant reactions that produce symptoms of erythema, dryness, fissuring and oedema. Methods for the assessment of immediate skin contact reactions are covered in Chap. 5. It should be noted that in vitro methods have been validated only for the purposes of regulatory hazard identification of corrosive substances (i.e. those that cause burns) and for basic category of acute irritants, and thus, they are not considered here other than to direct the reader to appropriate references [2–6].

As mentioned above, it has become possible by a variety of means to identify, without the use of animals (or humans), those chemicals that may cause a corrosive effect on skin [7]. In particular, two in vitro methods have been accepted formally as being validated for this purpose. However, these methods generally do not extend to the evaluation of lesser degrees of skin irritation, and for these other in vitro methods involving the use of 3-dimensional skin culture, systems have become more widely accepted, including recently for regulatory purposes [5]. Animal methods for the prediction of acute and cumulative skin irritation potential were first described many years ago (reviewed in [8, 9]). Most famous (notorious) among these is the rabbit skin irritation test devised by John Draize [10]. This method employs a single semi-occluded patch of undiluted chemical applied to shaved back skin (typically of three rabbits) for 4 h. Any resultant reactions are read, using a simple subjective scoring scheme, at 24, 48 and 72 h. The recovery from any induced skin irritation reaction may also be monitored. In essence, this test is now used to provide a first pass assessment of the intrinsic acute skin irritation potential (i.e. hazard) of a chemical substance, so that basic risk management measures can be implemented. This is the situation, for example, with legislation in the European Union [11] that utilises Draize test data effectively to compartmentalise chemicals into three basic categories – corrosive, irritant or unclassified. Such an approach has been largely ineffective in terms of prevention of clinical irritant contact dermatitis, since the rabbit is at best poorly predictive of human effects. Also the acute skin irritation potential measured is not an important clinical endpoint, and of course, simple categorisation hides important details/complexities and is simply no substitute for proper risk assessment. Furthermore, clinical skin irritation is more commonly associated with exposure to formulated products rather than with individual substances, and it has long been recognised that the irritant activity of a formulation cannot be predicted by a simple summation of the irritant properties of the ingredients [12].

In order to derive more useful information, other animal models have been devised for the purpose of providing a better representation of the modalities of exposure that are encountered in practise. Typically, these methods involve both exaggeration and repetition of exposure, such as with the guinea pig immersion test, or repeated dosing in a modified rabbit test [13]. In addition, investigators have made recourse to relatively uncommon laboratory species (such as the Yucatan hairless micropig) in an attempt to obtain suitable predictive systems [14]. However, in most instances these methods have either failed to gain widespread acceptance, or have fallen out of favour. Not only do they use animals, investigators have realised that it is more meaningful scientifically to conduct carefully controlled studies with human volunteers as these provide much more robust information on which to base safety assessments and risk management decisions. The generation of mild skin irritation effects in human volunteers is considered acceptable since such responses are both well tolerated and reversible. The basic principles of these methods are discussed below.

Where human skin contact with a chemical is likely, or indeed intended, and given that the necessary ethical and safety requirements (reviewed in [15]) have been met, then carefully controlled studies in humans can yield by far the most useful information for the proper evaluation of skin irritation. Where the need is for basic regulatory classification, such as in the EU, a suitable approach, the human 4 h patch test, has been well described and validated [16]. An extensive body of acute irritation data on substances tested by this method has been published [17] as has a body of information on tests for formulated products [18]. However, the real value to be derived from human testing is where the protocol is able to mirror the pattern(s) of exposure that will occur in practise. In such studies, the chemical may be tested by itself, but it is very much more common that the chemical is tested as part of the final formulation in which it is to be used. Such an approach is not only of value for the testing of cosmetic products [19], but also for many other situations. For example, in clinical trials to examine the impact of formulation on irritancy of a pharmaceutical [20], or in the evaluation of potentially irritating surfactant-based household products [21], the use of carefully optimised methodologies permits the investigator to examine irritancy in what is essentially the in-use situation. Similarly, the approach can be adapted to permit the assessment of the irritancy of materials used in an occupational setting, such as cutting fluids [22]. Human volunteers may also be of particular value in the assessment of potential protective effects of products such as barrier creams [23].

Typically, the process involved for human skin irritation studies will include the following steps:

- A scientific evaluation of the need for the investigation.
- Identification of a suitable protocol.
- Preparation of the safety dossier to support the proposed work.

- Assessment of the study by an independent ethical review committee.
- Initiation of the study by the recruitment of the participants who give fully informed written consent.
- Progression of the study through the practical phase.
- Formal reporting of the study.

All of these elements are reviewed in detail elsewhere [15, 19].

It is not appropriate to delve into detail here, but in addition to the clinical observation of skin irritation, there continues to be great progress in the objective and quantitative measurement of skin effects [24–26]. Use of tools such as these for the identification of hazards and for skin irritation risk assessment has been the subject of recent review [27, 28].

13.4 Predictive Tests for Allergens

A variety of methods is available for the identification of chemicals that have the potential to cause skin sensitisation and allergic contact dermatitis. Historically, the guinea pig has been the species of choice for toxicological evaluations of skin sensitising activity. Many guinea pig tests have been described, of which the guinea pig maximisation test (GPMT; [29]) and the occluded patch test [30] are the most widely used and most thoroughly characterised. Although guinea pig test methods vary with respect to detailed procedure, the principle in most cases is the same. Groups of animals are exposed by topical or intradermal exposure, or by a mixture of topical and intradermal exposure, to the test material. In some tests, adjuvant is also administered to enhance (maximise) immune responses provoked by the test material. Control guinea pigs receive the relevant vehicle alone, and where appropriate, adjuvant treatments. Subsequently, all animals (test and control) are exposed topically to the chemical (at the maximum concentration judged not to cause irritant effects) and the elicitation of cutaneous hypersensitivity reactions is determined as a function of challenge-induced erythema and/or oedema. Sensitising potential is judged on the basis of the frequency of specific reactions induced by challenge of treated animals. Detailed considerations of guinea

13

pig test methods, including their conduct and interpretation, are available elsewhere [31, 32]. Suffice it to say here that the better characterised guinea pig test methods have served toxicologists well, and if conducted and interpreted correctly, provide an accurate indication of likely sensitisation hazard.

Notwithstanding their proven utility, it must be recognised that guinea pig tests are not without limitations. Chief among these, in the context of this chapter, is the fact that such assays do not lend themselves to the assessment of relative potency. Some attempts have been made to modify standard guinea pig methods for the purposes of deriving dose-response relationships [33], but these have met with only limited success. The difficulties are that it is not practicable in guinea pig assays to examine in detail multiple induction concentrations of the test chemical, and even if this were to be done, an end point that comprises a subjective assessment of the frequency of responses, rather than the vigour of responses, is not well suited to determine the inherent potency of a sensitising chemical.

In the last 15 years, considerable progress has been made in characterising the immunobiological processes that result in the induction of skin sensitisation and the elicitation of allergic contact dermatitis. In parallel with this more sophisticated appreciation of the relevant cellular and molecular mechanisms, there have emerged opportunities to explore new approaches to skin sensitisation testing. Attention has been focused recently on the mouse, and two alternative approaches to hazard identification have been developed using this species. One of these, the mouse ear swelling test (MEST; [34]), is similar in principle to guinea pig methods insofar as the activity is measured on the basis of reactions induced by challenge of previously treated mice. The other approach, the local lymph node assay (LLNA; [35, 36]), is predicated upon an alternative strategy in which activity is judged as a function of responses induced in mice during the induction, rather than elicitation, phase of contact sensitisation. In this method skin sensitisers are identified as a function of their ability to provoke proliferative responses in draining lymph nodes following repeated topical exposure. In practise, skin sensitising chemicals are defined as those which, at one or more test concentrations, induce a threefold or greater increase in lymph node cell proliferation compared with concurrent vehicle-treated controls. The LLNA has been the subject of extensive evaluations and the view currently is that the method provides a reliable and robust

approach to the identification of sensitising chemicals and, as such, represents a stand-alone alternative to guinea pig assays [37].

Notwithstanding the above, as with the preceding guinea pig assays, as experience in use has accumulated with the LLNA, both the strengths and limitations have been the subject of commentary [38–41]. Particular emphasis has been placed by some on the question of the extent to which the assay may produce false positive results and this has generated a considerable body of published work [41, 42]. The key point to be emphasised is that any predictive test will be subject to a degree of both false positives and false negatives. The skill of those responsible for making assessments is that they make use of a weight of evidence approach, whether this be for regulatory decisions or for more general safety assessment. Strategies to do this are discussed in detail elsewhere [43, 44]. Even at the most fundamental level of toxicology, hazard identification, a test result rarely stands in isolation; there will be additional information available from chemical structure, from the behaviour of related chemicals, on the nature of any potential impurities arising during manufacture, of any effects arising occupationally during manufacture and so on. By bringing all of the information to bear, the imperfections inherent in any individual predictive test can be minimised.

There is interest currently in the possibility that, in addition to providing a means for identifying hazard, the LLNA may be suitable also for measurement of relative potency as a first step in the risk assessment process [45]. The use of the LLNA for this purpose appears appropriate because the available evidence indicates that the vigour of induced proliferative responses by draining lymph node cells correlates closely with the extent to which skin sensitisation will develop [46]. In practise, estimation of relative potency using the LLNA is based upon derivation by linear interpolation from the dose-response curves of an EC3 value, which has been defined as the Effective Concentration of chemical required to stimulate a threefold increase in lymph node cell proliferative activity compared with concurrent vehicle treated controls [47], (see Fig. 13.1). Experience to date indicates that the derivation in this way of an EC3 value provides a realistic, and relatively accurate and robust, measure of relative potency suitable for integration into the risk assessment process [48–50]. Further information on this aspect is given in Sect. 12.5.

The above methods are all in vivo tests. There has also been enthusiasm for the development of in vitro

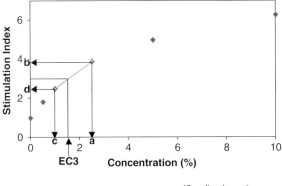

EC3 is calculated via: $c + \dfrac{(3-d) \times (a-c)}{(b-d)}$

Fig. 13.1 The derivation of the LLNA EC3 value. In the LLNA, the stimulation of proliferation in lymph nodes draining the site of application is compared to the proliferation in concurrent vehicle-treated controls. A range of test concentrations is normally used, thereby giving a dose-response curve. A stimulation index of ≥ 3 (test vs. vehicle) is indicative of a skin sensitiser. Additionally, it is possible to estimate from the dose-response curve the concentration of a sensitiser, which would give a threshold positive response

approaches to skin sensitisation testing, but although some progress has been made in the context of hazard identification [6, 51, 52], the identification of chemical structural alerts, the derivation of (quantitative) structure-activity relationships and methods based upon the in vitro assessment of cellular responses are not (yet) suitable for consideration of relative potency. Nevertheless, considerable progress is being made in respect of the development of these approaches in relation to hazard identification. Of particular interest in this respect has been the development of assays to measure the reactivity of chemicals (reviewed in [53–55]) and the detailed evaluation of an approach using a dendritic like cell line [56–59]. These methods are currently beginning the process of more formalised validation (Casati, ECVAM, personal communication, July 2009).

13.5 Quantitative Risk Assessment

In toxicology, the initial evaluation involves the identification of intrinsic properties of chemicals/formulations, including skin irritation and sensitisation hazards. However, this information, to be of any practical value, has to be placed into a real world context. Thus, where

a hazard has been identified, it must be characterised in terms of its potency and then judged in relation to the anticipated skin exposure that is likely to occur, both in normal use and in reasonably foreseeable misuse situations. These considerations form the topic of this section. Ultimately, where it is possible to make a fully quantitative risk assessment (a rare situation), there will be a prediction of the number of cases of irritation and/or sensitisation that are likely to arise.

For skin irritation, the opportunity to understand in detail the risk to man does arise. Although quantitative measures of skin irritation potency are not readily available, as mentioned above, it is possible to undertake human studies, which can provide a fairly accurate assessment of the risks presented. To achieve this, the participants in the study must comprise a representative sample of those who are likely to be exposed, and the skin exposure conditions in the study must approximate to those that are anticipated to occur in practise. In this way, the study will provide, in microcosm, a picture of what is likely to happen in use.

An important consequence of the above is that it leads to the conclusion that simple patch testing, whether single or repeated, may not necessarily provide a fair representation of the skin irritancy of a test material that will be expressed in practise. For example, it has been shown that the rank order of irritancy found under patch test conditions is not always identical to that found under more realistic use conditions [60]. This comes as no great surprise, since cumulative irritancy is a function of both the intensity of each individual skin insult and the rate of recovery there from; this concept is based on that expressed by Malten many years ago [61]. Furthermore, significant evidence of acute skin irritancy under 48 h patch test conditions on the arm has been shown to be of no relevance when a product was evaluated under exaggerated repeated open exposure conditions on the face, where it was essentially without effect [62]. However, the practical experience of toxicologists and safety evaluators is that appropriately designed human tests can be of great value in the prediction of skin irritancy in practise [8, 9, 62–64]. Also, as mentioned earlier, consideration should increasingly be given to the use of bioengineering tools for the precise measurement of skin irritation reactions, not only because they provide quantitative, objective measures, but also as they may permit very subtle levels of response to be characterised.

For skin sensitisation, it is not possible to conduct human testing in the same manner as for skin irritation,

13

not least for the obvious ethical reason that while skin irritation is a reversible phenomenon, the induction of skin sensitisation represents an irreversible (health) change for the individual. A recent commentary reviews the scientific and ethical dilemmas facing those who carry out procedures such as the human repeated insult patch test [65]. In practise, it is necessary to use the predictive methods mentioned in Sect. 12.4 to provide information on the relative potency of the potential skin sensitiser. Typically, this information on the newly identified skin sensitiser is then compared with that available for other skin sensitisers that are employed in similar exposure situations. In effect, what is being done is that the variables/unknowns associated with the relationship between skin exposure to a sensitiser of known potency, and the resultant likelihood of allergic contact dermatitis being elicited, are regarded as "constants" in the comparison of a known sensitiser in an existing use with the new sensitiser that is being used in the same situation. For example, the weak sensitising potency of cocoamidopropyl betaine (CAPB) is well understood in terms of data from predictive models. In addition, the very limited extent to which it causes clinical allergy through use in shampoos at levels up to approximately 10% is also quite well understood. Thus, were a novel material be proposed for use in shampoos, CAPB could be employed as one potential benchmark for comparison. Similarly, the much stronger sensitising potency of (chloro)methylisothiazolinone also is well understood in predictive models and in man; dose-response studies in mice, guinea pigs and man exist [66, 67]. Furthermore, there are data on acceptable and unacceptable use concentrations and product types [68]. All of these data represent a valuable source of benchmark data for use in risk assessment.

Recently, a more quantitative approach to skin sensitisation risk assessment has been promulgated. In essence, this is founded on the traditional toxicology approach of identifying a no effect level (NOEL) *in a predictive model* and then appropriate reduction of this NOEL to provide an indication *of human exposure limits* below which the adverse effect, in this case the induction of skin sensitisation, should not occur. The approach indicates safe exposure levels for individual sensitising chemicals under well-defined exposure conditions; exposure is expressed in dose per unit area and is calculated per diem. Comprehensive details of this new approach have been delineated in a short series of publications (reviewed in [69]). Given the difficulties concerning the conduct of

predictive human testing, this quantitative approach relies heavily on the direct prediction of NOELs from LLNA EC3 values, together with any other weight of evidence information. A number of publications now support the validity of this relationship [70–73]. Quantitative risk assessment for skin sensitising chemicals has been deployed to demonstrate the inappropriately high level of exposure to a preservative, methyldibromo glutaronitrile, providing an independent demonstration of the utility of the approach [74]. A generic overview of this new quantitative risk assessment strategy is outlined in (Fig. 13.2). Practical examples of its application have also been published [69, 75–77].

Use of such a quantitative approach in defining human exposure limits for sensitising chemicals relies heavily on both the accuracy and robustness of the measurement of potency in predictive models such as the LLNA. This aspect is not only mentioned in Sect. 12.4, but also demonstrated by a comparison of potency categorisations in the LLNA compared to what is understood concerning potency in man. The data in Table 13.1 (refined and corrected since the last edition of this book) display human potency categorisations based on EC3 results for over 100 chemicals. It is not only important that these predictions are accurate, but also that they are robust: such appears to be the case [48, 49]. As a further consequence, it is likely that data of this type will form the core sets of material against which in vitro alternatives ultimately will be validated [78, 79].

13.5.1 Summary and Future Perspectives

In the context of skin irritation, there is a need to define in greater detail the elements of cutaneous inflammatory reactions that are a common feature of the irritant reactions provoked by diverse chemicals (which are likely to initiate irritancy via different mechanisms). This would, in turn, create new opportunities for the development of alternative test methods and also possibly provide a rational basis for the determination of relative potency. In addition, it is vital that this knowledge takes into account the fact that it is cumulative, rather than acute, irritancy which is of importance. With respect to translating hazard characterisation into an accurate risk assessment, there is a need for an increased appreciation of the mechanistic basis for the polymorphic responses observed among exposed individuals.

Fig. 13.2 General approach to quantitative risk assessment for skin sensitisation

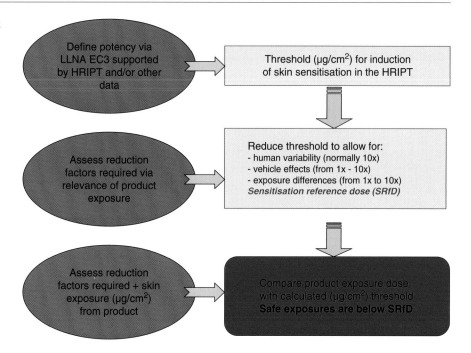

Table 13.1 Prediction of human skin sensitisation potency in the LLNA

Chemical	LLNA EC3 (%)	Human class
Oxazolone	0.003	Extreme
Methyl/ chloromethylisothiaz-olinone	0.009	Extreme
1,4-Benzoquinone	0.01	Extreme
1-Benzoylacetone	0.04	Extreme
Diphencyclopropenone	0.05	Extreme
N-Methyl-N-nitrosourea	0.05	Extreme
2,4-Dinitrochlorobenzene	0.08	Extreme
Potassium dichromate	0.08	Extreme
Cyanuric chloride	0.09	Extreme
1,4-Dihydroquinone	0.10	Strong
Glutaraldehyde	0.10	Strong
Toluene diisocyanate	0.11	Strong
Chlorpromazine	0.14	Strong
Fluorescein isothiocyanate	0.14	Strong
Hexadecyl-methanesulphonate	0.14	Strong
Maleic anhydride	0.16	Strong
p-Phenylenediamine	0.16	Strong
Dimethyl sulphate	0.19	Strong
Dodecylthiosulphonate	0.20	Strong
β-Propriolactone	0.20	Strong
Trimellitic anhydride	0.22	Strong
Benzoyl chloride	0.23	Strong
5-Methyl isoeugenol	0.30	Strong
Benzoyl peroxide	0.30	Strong
Lauryl gallate	0.30	Strong
Propyl gallate	0.32	Strong
Phthalic anhydride	0.36	Strong
2-Nitro-4-phenylenediamine	0.40	Strong
Chloramine-T	0.40	Strong
Methylisothiazolinone	0.40	Strong
2-Aminophenol	0.50	Strong
Formaldehyde	0.61	Strong
Hexahydrophthalic anhydride	0.84	Strong
Methyldibromo glutaronitrile	0.9	Moderate
Isoeugenol	1.2	Moderate

(continued)

Table 13.1 (continued)

Chemical	LLNA EC3 (%)	Human class
1-Phenyl-1,2-propanedione	1.3	Moderate
2-Hydroxyethyl acrylate	1.4	Moderate
Glyoxal	1.4	Moderate
Bisphenol A diglycidyl ether	1.5	Moderate
Vinyl pyridine	1.6	Moderate
2-Mercaptobenzothiazole	1.7	Moderate
Cinnamic aldehyde (cinnamal)	2.0	Moderate
Diethylmaleate	2.1	Moderate
Ethylenediamine	2.2	Moderate
2-Amino-6-chloro-4-nitrophenol	2.2	Moderate
3-Dimethylaminopropylamine	2.2	Moderate
Trans-2-decanal	2.5	Moderate
Zinc dimethyldithiocarbamate	2.7	Moderate
3-Aminophenol	3.2	Moderate
3-Methylisoeugenol	3.6	Moderate
3-Propylidenephthalide	3.7	Moderate
Benzylidene acetone	3.7	Moderate
Phenylacetaldehyde	4.7	Moderate
Clotrimazole	4.8	Moderate
Dipentamethylenethiuramdisulphide	5.2	Moderate
Tetramethylthiuramdisulfide	5.2	Moderate
3,4-Dihydrocoumarin	5.6	Moderate
Resorcinol	6.3	Moderate
4-Chloroaniline	6.5	Moderate
Dihydroeugenol	6.8	Moderate
1-(p-Methoxyphenyl)-1-penten-3-one	9.3	Moderate
Camphorquinone	10	Weak
Hexylcinnamal	11	Weak
Citral	13	Weak
Eugenol	13	Weak
p-Methylhydrocinnamal	14	Weak
Abietic acid	15	Weak
Hydroxymethylpentylcyclohexenecarboxaldehyde (Lyral)	17	Weak
p-tert-Butyl-α-methyl hydrocinnamal	19	Weak
Dipentamethylenethiuramtetrasulphide	21	Weak
Benzocaine	22	Weak
Cyclamen aldehyde	22	Weak
Imidazolidinyl urea	24	Weak
5-Methyl-2,3-hexanedione	26	Weak
Ethyl acrylate	28	Weak
Ethyleneglycol dimethacrylate	28	Weak
Linalool	30	Weak
Penicillin G	30	Weak
Butylglycidylether	31	Weak
3-Methyleugenol	32	Weak
Hydroxycitronellal	33	Weak
Isopropyl myristate	44	Weak
2-Ethyl butyraldehyde	60	Weak
Limonene	69	Weak
Aniline	89	Weak
1-Bromobutane	Non-sensitising	Not classified
1-Butanol	Non-sensitising	Not classified
2-Hydroxypropyl methacrylate	Non-sensitising	Not classified
4-Hydroxybenzoic acid	Non-sensitising	Not classified
6-Methyl coumarin	Non-sensitising	Not classified
Acetanisole	Non-sensitising	Not classified
Chlorobenzene	Non-sensitising	Not classified
Dextran	Non-sensitising	Not classified
Diethylphthalate	Non-sensitising	Not classified
Glycerol	Non-sensitising	Not classified

Table 13.1 (continued)

Chemical	LLNA EC3 (%)	Human class
Hexane	Non-sensitising	Not classified
Isopropanol	Non-sensitising	Not classified
Lactic acid	Non-sensitising	Not classified
Methyl salicylate	Non-sensitising	Not classified
Octanoic acid	Non-sensitising	Not classified
Tween 80	Non-sensitising	Not classified

LLNA EC3 value derived as indicated in (Fig. 13.1). The values given are representative of the published literature

Human class assignment based on the order of magnitude EC3 groups; <0.1%>extreme; 0.1–1.0>strong; 1.0–10>moderate; >10%>weak. Other classifications groupings are possible

Contact sensitisation presents rather different challenges to those of skin irritation. Real progress is being made in the development of approaches that allow robust and objective assessment of relative potency. In this regard, the utility of methods such as the LLNA needs to be evaluated further and comparisons made between experimental estimates of skin sensitising potential and what is known of allergenic activity among exposed human populations. This work also has implications for the future development of in vitro methods. To be of real value, in vitro methods must not only provide information on the presence (or absence) of sensitisation hazard, but also allow the determination of the relative potency of an identified hazard. Only in this way can in vitro tests wholly replace the use of animal models for skin sensitisation risk assessment. The strategic approach to how this can be achieved with a degree of simplicity has been published recently [80] as an attempt to populate it [81]. What remains is to populate the strategy with non-animal methods that not only identify hazard, but also provide the information necessary to calibrate allergen potency.

References

1. Maibach HI, Coenraads PJ (1995) The irritant contact dermatitis syndrome. CRC, Boca Raton
2. Basketter DA, Gerberick GF, Kimber I, Willis C (1999) The toxicology of contact dermatitis, Chapter 3. Wiley, Chichester, pp 39–56
3. Welss T, Basketter DA, Schroder KR (2004) In vitro skin irritation: facts and future. State of the art review of mechanisms and models. Toxicol In Vitro 18:231–243
4. Basketter DA, Holland G, York M (2006) Corrosive materials. In: Chew A-L, Maibach HI (eds) Handbook of irritant dermatitis. Springer, Berlin, pp 239–248
5. Basketter DA, Jones PA (2008) In vitro approaches to the assessment of skin irritation and phototoxicity of topically applied materials. In: Zhai H, Wilhelm K-P, Maibach HI (eds) Dermatotoxicology, 7th edn. CRC, Boca Raton, pp 537–546
6. Gibbs S (2009) In vitro irritation models and immune reactions. Skin Pharmacol Physiol 22:103–113
7. Lewis RW, Basketter DA (1995) Transcutaneous electrical resistance: application in predicting skin corrosives. In: Elsner P, Maibach HI (eds) Irritant dermatitis: new clinical and experimental aspects. Karger, Basel, pp 243–255
8. Simion FA (1995) In vivo models to predict skin irritation. In: van der Valk PGM, Maibach HI (eds) The irritant contact dermatitis syndrome. CRC, Boca Raton, pp 329–334
9. Patil SM, Patrick E, Maibach HI (1996) Animal, human, and in vitro test methods for predicting skin irritation. In: Marzulli FN, Maibach HI (eds) Dermatotoxicology. Taylor & Francis, Washington, pp 411–436
10. Draize JH, Woodard G, Calvery HO (1944) Methods for the study of irritation and toxicity of substances applied topically to the skin and mucous membranes. J Pharmacol Exp Ther 82:377–390
11. EC (1992) Annex to Commission Directive 92/69/EEC of 31 July 1992 adapting to technical progress for the seventeenth time Council Directive 67/548/EEC on the approximation of laws, regulations and administrative provisions relating to the classification, packaging and labelling of dangerous substances. Official Journal of the European Communities L383A:35
12. Hall-Manning TJ, Holland GH, Basketter DA, Barratt MD (1995) Skin irritation potential of mixed surfactant systems in a human 4 hour covered patch test. Allergologie 18:465
13. Marzulli FN, Maibach HI (1975) The rabbit as a model for evaluating skin irritants: a comparison of results obtained on animals and man using repeated skin exposures. Food Cosmet Toxicol 13:533–540
14. Gabard B, Treffel P, Charton-Picard F, Eloy R (1995) Irritant reactions on hairless micropig skin: a model for testing barrier creams? Curr Probl Dermatol 23:275–287
15. Walker AP, Basketter DA, Baverel M, Diembeck W, Matthies W, Mougin D, Paye M, Rothlisburger R, Dupuis J (1997) Test guidelines for assessment of skin tolerance of potentially irritant cosmetic ingredients in man. Food Chem Toxicol 35:1099–1106
16. Basketter DA, Chamberlain M, Griffiths HA, York M (1997) The classification of skin irritants by human patch test. Food Chem Toxicol 35:845–852
17. Basketter DA, York M, McFadden JP, Robinson MK (2004) Determination of skin irritation potential in the human 4-h patch test. Contact Dermat 51:1–4
18. Robinson MK, Kruszewski FH, Al-Atrash J, Blazka ME, Gingell R, Heitfeld FA, Mallon D, Snyder NK, Swanson JE, Casterton PL (2005) Comparative assessment of the acute skin irritation potential of detergent formulations using a novel human 4-h patch test method. Food Chem Toxicol 43:1703–1712
19. Walker AP, Basketter DA, Baverel M, Diembeck W, Matthies W, Mougin D, Paye M, Rothlisburger R, Dupuis J (1996) Test guideline for assessment of skin compatibility of

13

cosmetic finished products in man. Food Chem Toxicol 34:551–560

20. Prins M, Swinkels OQ, Kolkman EG, Wuis EW, Hekster YA, van der Valk PG (1998) Skin irritation by dithranol cream. A blind study to assess the role of the cream formulation. Acta Derm Venereol 78:262–265

21. Basketter DA, Gerberick GF, Kimber I, Willis C (1999) The toxicology of contact dermatitis, Chapter 4. Wiley, Chichester, pp 57–72

22. Wigger-Alberti W, Hinnen U, Elsner P (1997) Predictive testing of metalworking fluids: a comparison of 2 cumulative human irritation models and correlation with epidemiological data. Contact Dermat 36:14–20

23. Frosch PJ, Kurte A, Pilz B (1993) Efficacy of skin barrier creams. III. The repetitive irritation test (RIT) in humans. Contact Dermat 29:113–118

24. Elsner P, Berardesca E, Wilhelm K-P, Maibach HI (2002) Bioengineering of the skin: skin biomechanics, vol 5. CRC, Boca Raton

25. Fluhr J, Elsner P, Berardesca E, Maibach HI (2005) Bioengineering of the skin: water and the stratum corneum. CRC, Boca Raton

26. Wilhelm K-P, Elsner P, Berardesca E, Maibach HI (2007) Bioengineering of the skin: skin imaging and analysis. Informa Healthcare, New York

27. Charbonnier V, Paye M, Maibach HI (2008) Determination of subclinical changes of barrier function. In: Zhai H, Wilhelm K-P, Maibach HI (eds) Dermatotoxicology, 7th edn. CRC, Boca Raton, pp 561–568

28. Fluhr JW, Darlenski R, Angelova-Fischer I, Tsnkov N, Basketter DA (2008) Skin irritation and sensitization: mechanisms and new approaches for risk assessment. Part I: skin irritation. Skin Pharmacol Physiol 21:124–135

29. Magnusson B, Kligman AM (1970) Allergic contact dermatitis in the guinea pig. Charles C Thomas, Springfield, IL

30. Buehler EV (1965) Delayed contact hypersensitivity in the guinea pig. Arch Dermatol 91:171–177

31. Andersen KE, Maibach HI (1985) Contact allergy predictive tests in guinea pigs. Curr Probl Dermatol 14:263–290

32. Basketter DA, Gerberick GF, Kimber I, Willis CM (1999) Toxicology of contact dermatitis. Allergy, irritancy and urticaria. Wiley, Chichester

33. Andersen KE, Volund A, Frankild S (1995) The guinea pig maximization test with a multiple dose design. Acta Derm Venereol 75:463–469

34. Gad SC, Dunn BJ, Dobbs DW, Reilly C, Walsh RD (1986) Development and validation of an alternative dermal sensitisation test: the mouse ear swelling test (MEST). Toxicol Appl Pharmacol 84:93–114

35. Kimber I, Basketter DA (1992) The murine local lymph node assay: a commentary on collaborative studies and new directions. Food Chem Toxicol 30:165–169

36. Kimber I, Dearman RJ, Basketter DA, Ryan CA, Gerberick GF (2002) The local lymph node assay: past, present and future. Contact Dermet 47:315–328

37. Gerberick GF, Ryan CA, Kimber I, Dearman RJ, Lea LJ, Basketter DA (2000) Local lymph node assay validation assessment for regulatory purposes. Am J Cont Dermat 11:3–18

38. Vohr H-V, Jurgen AH (2005) The local lymph node assay being too sensitive? Arch Toxicol 79:721–728

39. Cockshott A, Evans P, Gerberick GF, Betts CJ, Dearman RJ, Kimber I, Basketter DA (2006) Use and abuse of the local lymph node assay: a regulatory perspective. Human Exp Toxicol 25:387–394

40. McGarry HF (2007) The murine local lymph node assay: regulatory and potency considerations under REACH. Toxicology 238:71–89

41. Kreiling R, Hollnagel HM, Hareng L, Eigler D, Lee MS, Griem P, Dreesen B, Kleber M, Albrecht A, Garcia C, Wendel A (2008) Comparison of the skin sensitizing potential of unsaturated compounds and assessed by the murine local lymph node assay (LLNA) and the guinea pig maximization test (GPMT). Food Chem Toxicol 46:1896–1904

42. Basketter DA, McFadden J, Evans P, Andersen KE, Jowsey I (2006) Identification and classification of skin sensitisers: identifying false positives and false negatives. Contact Dermat 55:268–273

43. Basketter DA (2008) Skin sensitisation: strategies for risk assessment and risk management. Brit J Dermatol 159: 267–273

44. Basketter DA, Ball N, Cagen S, Carrillo J-C, Certa H, Eigler D, Esch H, Graham C, Haux D, Kreiling R, Mehling A (2009) Application of a weight of evidence approach to analysing discordant sensitization datasets: implication for REACH. Regul Toxicol Pharmacol 55(1):90–96

45. Kimber I, Basketter DA (1997) Contact sensitisation: a new approach to risk assessment. Human Ecol Risk Assess 3:385–395

46. Kimber I, Dearman RJ (1991) Investigation of lymph node cell proliferation as a possible immunological correlate of contact sensitizing potential. Food Chem Toxicol 29: 125–129

47. Basketter DA, Lea LJ, Dickens A, Briggs D, Pate I, Dearman RJ, Kimber I (1999) A comparison of statistical approaches to derivation of EC3 values from local lymph node assay dose responses. J Appl Toxicol 19:261–266

48. Basketter DA, Andersen KE, Lidén C, van Loveren H, Boman A, Kimber I, Alanko K, Berggren E (2005) Evaluation of the skin sensitising potency of chemicals using existing methods and considerations of relevance for elicitation. Contact Dermat 52:39–43

49. Basketter DA, Gerberick GF, Kimber I (2007) The local lymph node assay EC3 value: status of validation. Contact Dermat 57:70–75

50. Van Loveren H, Cockshott A, Gebel T, Gundert-Remy U, De Jong WH, Matheson J, McGarry H, Musset L, Selgrade MK, Vickers C (2008) Skin sensitization in chemical risk assessment: report of a WHO-IPCS international workshop focusing on dose-response assessment. Regul Toxicol Pharmacol 50:155–199

51. Basketter DA, Maxwell G (2007) Identification and characterization of allergens: in vitro alternatives. Expert Rev Dermatol 2:471–480

52. Ryan CA, Kimber I, Basketter DA, Pallardy M, Gildea LA, Gerberick GF (2007) Dendritic cells and skin sensitisation: biological roles and uses in hazard identification. Toxicol Appl Pharmacol 15:384–394

53. Divkovic M, Pease CK, Gerberick GF, Basketter DA (2005) Hapten-protein binding: from theory to practical application in the in vitro prediction of skin sensitization. Contact Dermat 53:189–200

54. Natsch A, Gfeller H, Rothaupt M, Ellis G (2007) Utility and limitations of a peptide reactivity assay to predict fragrance allergens in vitro. Toxicol In Vitro 21:1220–1226

55. Gerberick GF, Aleksic M, Basketter DA, Casati S, Karlberg A-T, Kern P, Kimber I, Lepoittevin J-P, Natsch A, Ovigne J-M, Rovida C, Sakaguchi H, Schultz T (2008) Chemical reactivity measurement and the predictive identification of skin sensitisers. ATLA 36:215–242

56. Ashikaga T, Yoshida Y, Hirota M, Yoneyama K, Itagaki H, Sakaguchi H, Miyazawa M, Ito Y, Suzuki H, Toyoda H (2006) Development of an in vitro skin sensitization test using human cell lines: the human cell line activation test (h-clat). I. Optimization of the h-clat protocol. Toxicol In Vitro 20:767–773

57. Sakaguchi H, Ashikaga T, Miyazawa M, Yoshida Y, Ito Y, Yoneyama K, Hirota M, Itagaki H, Toyoda H, Suzuki H (2006) Development of an in vitro skin sensitization test using human cell lines; human cell line activation test (h-clat). 2. An inter-laboratory study of the h-clat. Toxicol In Vitro 20:774–784

58. Python F, Goebel C, Aeby P (2007) Assessment of the u937 cell line for the detection of contact allergens. Toxicol Appl Pharmacol 220:113–124

59. Sakaguchi H, Ashikaga T, Miyazawa M, Kosaka N, Ito Y, Yoneyama K, Sono S, Itagaki H, Toyoda H, Suzuki H (2009) The relationship between CD86/CD54 expression and THP-1 cell viability in an in vitro skin sensitization test–human cell line activation test (h-CLAT). Cell Biol Toxicol 25:109–126

60. Hannuksela A, Hannuksela M (1995) Irritant effects of a detergent in wash and chamber tests. Contact Dermat 32:163–166

61. Malten KE (1981) Thoughts on irritant contact dermatitis. Contact Dermat 7:238–247

62. Basketter DA, Gilpin GR, Kuhn M, Lawrence RS, Reynolds FS, Whittle E (1998) Patch tests versus use tests in skin irritation risk assessment. Contact Dermat 39:252–256

63. Basketter DA, Reynolds FS, York M (1997) Predictive testing in contact dermatitis – irritant dermatitis. In: Goh CL, Koh D (eds) Clinics in dermatology – contact dermatitis, vol 15. Elsevier, Amsterdam, pp 637–644

64. Jenkins HL, Adams MG (1989) Progressive evaluation of skin irritancy of cosmetics using human volunteers. Int J Cosmet Sci 11:141–149

65. Basketter DA (2009) The human repeated insult patch test in the 21st century: a commentary on ethics and validity. Cutan Ocul Toxicol 28:49–53

66. Chan PD, Baldwin RC, Parson RD, Moss JN, Sterotelli R, Smith JM, Hayes AW (1983) Kathon biocide: manifestation of delayed contact dermatitis in guinea pigs is dependent on the concentration for induction and challenge. J Invest Dermatol 81:409–411

67. Weaver JE, Carding CW, Maibach HI (1985) Dose response assessments of Kathon biocide. I. Diagnostic use and diagnostic threshold patch testing with sensitised humans. Contact Dermat 12:141–145

68. de Groot AC (1990) Methylisothiazolinone/methylchloroisothiazolinone (Kathon CG) allergy: an updated review. Am J Contact Dermat 1:151–156

69. Api AM, Basketter DA, Cadby PA, Cano M-F, Ellis G, Gerberick GF, Griem P, McNamee PM, Ryan CA, Safford B (2008) Dermal sensitization quantitative risk assessment (QRA) for fragrance ingredients. Regul Toxicol Pharmacol 52:3–23

70. Ryan CA, Gerberick GF, Cruse LW, Basketter DA, Lea LJ, Blaikie L, Dearman RJ, Warbrick EV, Kimber I (2000) Activity of human contact allergens in the murine local lymph node assay. Contact Dermat 43:95–102

71. Griem P, Goebel C, Scheffler H (2003) Proposal for a risk assessment methodology for skin sensitization based on sensitization potency data. Regul Toxicol Pharmacol 38:269–290

72. Schneider K, Akkan Z (2004) Quantitative relationship between the local lymph node assay and human skin sensitization assays. Regul Toxicol Pharmacol 39:245–255

73. Basketter DA, Clapp C, Jefferies D, Safford RJ, Ryan CA, Gerberick GF, Dearman RJ, Kimber I (2005) Predictive identification of human skin sensitisation thresholds. Contact Dermat 53:260–267

74. Zachariae C, Rastogi S, Devantier C, Menne T, Johansen JD (2003) Methyldibromo glutaronitrile: clinical experience and exposure-based risk assessment. Contact Dermat 48:150–154

75. Gerberick GF, Robinson MK, Felter S, White I, Basketter DA (2001) Understanding fragrance allergy using an exposure-based risk assessment approach. Contact Dermat 45:333–340

76. Basketter DA, Angelini G, Ingber A, Kern P, Menné T (2003) Nickel, chromium and cobalt in consumer products: revisiting safe levels in the new millennium. Contact Dermat 49:1–7

77. Basketter DA, Clapp CJ, Safford BJ, Jowsey IR, McNamee PM, Ryan CA, Gerberick GF (2008) Preservatives and skin sensitisation quantitative risk assessment: risk benefit considerations. Dermatitis 19:20–27

78. Gerberick GF, Ryan CA, Kern PS, Schlatter H, Dearman RJ, Kimber I, Patlewicz G, Basketter DA (2005) Compilation of historical local lymph node assay data for the evaluation of skin sensitization alternatives. Dermatitis 16:157–202

79. Kern PS, Gerberick GF, Ryan CA, Kimber I, Aptula A and Basketter DA (2009) Historical local lymph node data for the evaluation of skin sensitization alternatives: a second compilation. Dermatitis 21:8-32, accepted

80. Basketter DA, Kimber I (2009) Updating the skin sensitisation in vitro data assessment paradigm in 2009. J Appl Toxicol 29:603–611

81. Natsch A, Emter R, Ellis G (2009) Filling the concept with data: integrating data from different in vitro and in silico assays on skin sensitizers to explore the battery approach for animal-free skin sensitization testing. Toxicol Sci 107:106–121

Allergic Contact Dermatitis in Humans: Experimental and Quantitative Aspects

14

Jeanne Duus Johansen, Peter J. Frosch, and Torkil Menné

Contents

J.D. Johansen (✉)
Copenhagen University Hospital Gentofte, National Allergy
Research Centre, Department of Dermato-allergology,
Niels Andersens Vej 65, 2900 Hellerup, Denmark
e-mail: jedu@geh.regionh.dk

P.J. Frosch
Hautklinik, Klinikum Dortmund gGmbH,
Beurhausstr. 40, 44137 Dortmund, Germany
e-mail: peter.frosch@klinikumdo.de

T. Menné
Department of Dermato-allergology, Copenhagen University
Hospital Gentofte, 2900 Hellerup, Denmark

14.1 Introduction

Allergic contact dermatitis is a common and potentially disabling disease. The clinical definition of the disease is based on the history of the patient, clinical examination, patch testing, and a detailed, often repeated exposure assessment.

The literature on evaluation and standardization of the diagnostic patch test is extensive (see Chap. 24). Less effort has been focused on experimental elicitation of the disease allergic contact dermatitis. Such studies are essential for the confirmation of the diagnosis of allergic contact dermatitis in the clinical situation, and serve as an important guideline for establishing the estimates of the exposure concentrations that are safe with respect to elicitation of contact allergy in sensitized individuals.

The present chapter reviews methods for experimental allergic contact dermatitis in humans, and the most important individual and exposure-related variables for the elicitation of allergic contact dermatitis.

14.2 Individual Variation

The degree of contact allergy can be graded either according to the patch test outcome (+ to +++) or by serial dilution [1, 2] (Fig. 14.1). There is a correlation between the two grading systems, such that individuals with a +++ reaction generally react to a lower patch test concentration than those with only a + reaction [3]. The degree of contact allergy is an important individual risk factor for the development of allergic contact dermatitis. In a study of 101 patients with contact allergy to 5-chloro-2-methylisothiazol-3-one (MCI)

J.D. Johansen et al. (eds.), *Contact Dermatitis*,
DOI: 10.1007/978-3-642-03827-3_14, © Springer-Verlag Berlin Heidelberg 2011

14

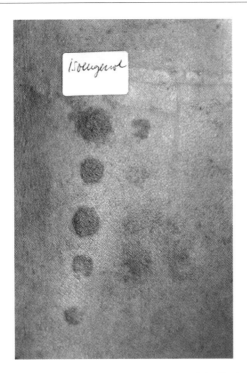

Fig. 14.1 Result of patch testing with a serial dilution of isoeugenol (2–0.008% in ethanol). The patient was highly sensitive and still showed a papular reaction at 0.125% (*upper right*)

and 2-methylisothiazol-3-one (MI), a significantly greater number of patients had a positive use test to emollients preserved with 15 ppm MCI/MI among those reacting with a positive patch test to 25 ppm than those only reacting with a positive patch test to 100 ppm [4]. Similarly, it has been shown that the degree of contact allergy is an important risk factor for perfume dermatitis in fragrance-sensitive individuals [5, 6] (Table 14.1). Rudzki et al. [7] have clearly illustrated that the numbers of patients with shoe dermatitis among chromate-sensitive individuals are greatest in those with a high degree of contact allergy.

An important observation in relation to the tendency to persistent regional dermatitis, e.g., hand eczema, is the study by Hindsen et al. [8], who demonstrated that nickel dermatitis is followed by long-lasting local hyperreactivity to nickel but not to other allergens or irritants. Similar results were obtained in a study of patients sensitized to methyldibromo glutaronitrile [9]. In the case of multiple contact allergies, as is frequently seen in patients with fragrance contact allergy, synergistic effects may result in an unpredictable propensity to react to perfumed products [10].

> **Core Message**
>
> › The degree of contact allergy is an important individual risk factor for the development of allergic contact dermatitis. Local specific hyperreactivity to an allergen at a previously exposed skin site may persist for a long time.

14.3 Exposure-Related Factors

The amount of allergen per skin surface area is the key factor that determines the risk of induction [11–13] and the same may apply for elicitation. As illustrated in Table 14.2, the exposures to MCI/MI from different sources, calculated as $\mu g/cm^2$, parallel the risk of elicitation of allergic contact dermatitis from different product types. Elicitation of allergic contact dermatitis occurs in approximately 50% of MCI/MI-sensitive individuals when exposed to a leave-on product preserved with 15 ppm MCI/MI, while elicitation with a shampoo preserved with the same amount is relatively uncommon [13].

Table 14.1 Intensity of patch test reactions to the fragrance mix and/or constituents in relation to history (*IR* Irritative reactions)

Fragrance history	?+/IR	+	++	+++	Total
Positive	13	14	39	16	82
Negative	52	25	26	0	103
Doubtful	5	14	18	2	39
Total	70	53	83	18	224

Table 14.2 Degree of MCI/MI exposure from different sources (the much lower exposure with the shampoo results from the wash-off effects)

Source	MCI/MI exposure ($\mu g/cm^2$)
Diagnostic patch test 100 ppm	3
Lotion preserved with 15 ppm	6×10^{-2}
Shampoo preserved with 15 ppm	8.7×10^{-4}

Elicitation depends not only on exposure concentration, but also on the duration of exposure. Increasing the duration of exposure to 1% *p*-phenylene-diamine (PPD) gave a proportionate increase in the number of reactors among PPD-sensitized individuals. The same effect could be obtained by increasing the PPD exposure concentration [14]. A cumulative effect of exposures has been demonstrated, so that repeating exposures cause elicitation in more individuals [14–16]. Using low concentrations of allergen means that more exposures are required to elicit a reaction than for higher concentrations, as demonstrated with the fragrance ingredient isoeugenol [15]. Repeated open exposure on the lower forearm to a solution containing 0.05% isoeugenol produced reactions in 42% of sensitized individuals within a 4-week period and in 67% at exposure to 0.2% isoeugenol. The median time until reaction was 15 days for the low and 7 days for the high concentration [15]. This and other experiments indicate that the accumulated total dose is a major determinant of the elicitation response [14, 17, 18]. Jensen et al. showed that the effect of applying a 0.04% solution of methyldibromo glutaronitrile once a day in a use test had an almost equal capability of provoking allergic contact dermatitis as application of 0.01% 4 times a day [17]. Recently, Fischer et al. in a series of studies demonstrated that allergic individuals react to lower doses, measured as dose per area per application, in a repeated open application test than in the patch test [16, 19, 20]. The accumulated doses after 1, 2, and 3 weeks of open applications gave dose-response curves that were almost identical to the data from the serial dilution patch test, when nonvolatile substances were tested (Fig. 14.2).

The matrix may influence the elicitation capacity of an allergen and the addition of irritants such as detergents has been shown to increase the clinical response to an allergen by a factor of 4–6 [21–23]. Higher doses may be needed if the allergen is volatile [20].

Skin regions differ in sensitivity. The upper arm has been shown to be more sensitive than the forehead and ventral aspect of the lower arm in use tests [24], the axilla more sensitive than the outer aspect of the upper arm [25], and recently it has been shown that the neck and face are more sensitive than the outer aspect of the upper arm [26].

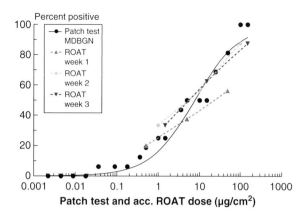

Fig. 14.2 Dose-response curve (fitted) for serial dilution patch test in 16 patients allergic to methyldibromo glutaronitile and the results of the accumulated 1-week, 2-week, 3-week repeated open application test (ROAT). The dose-response curve for the patch test and for the accumulated doses in the ROAT were not significantly different as can be seen. MDBGN: methyldibromo glutaronitrile. Reprinted with permission from Br. J. Dermatology [19]

> **Core Message**
>
> › Exposure-related factors that influence the risk of elicitation are allergen concentration (dose), duration and frequency of exposure, matrix, presence of irritants, and region of application.

14.4 Experimental Human Models

14.4.1 Serial Dilution Patch Test

A dilution series of a relevant allergen usually in ethanol, petrolatum, or water is the most used method for quantification of the elicitation response. The test is performed on the upper back similar to standard testing just with one allergen at different concentrations. The dilution steps depend on the allergen and the purpose of investigation, but usually steps of two, three, or ten are used, with a span of concentrations covering a factor 100–10,000. Thresholds are determined either as the minimal elicitation concentration (MEC) or as the maximum no effect level (NOEL).

There is a considerable interindividual variation in reactivity to an allergen, but also an intraindividual variation over time as shown for nickel-allergic patients [27]. Compiling results for groups of nickel-allergic patients, however, gives a fairly constant dose-response curve also over time [27]. At low allergen levels, the clinical response will be less pronounced: typically the reactions will become papular (Fig. 14.1). From a biological point of view, the assessment of thresholds should take these weaker responses into consideration and not rely just on diagnostic patch test criteria [28].

Serial dilution patch tests have been used to determine the optimal patch test concentration for a substance [29], as a predictor of chronic disease [30], or to obtain data of thresholds relevant for groups of sensitized individuals to be used in risk assessments and prevention [31, 32]. Data have also been subjected to a kind of meta-analysis combining results from several studies into a single dose-response curve (Fig. 14.3), which again may be used in risk assessments [31–33]. One of the results of such data analysis is that the variation between studies is limited considering that they were performed in different geographical regions and time periods.

A further standardization has been done [16, 19, 20] and it is recommended to implement dose-response elicitation data in the risk assessment routinely [34]. An equation to covert threshold data from serial dilution patch tests to thresholds at repeated open applications has been developed for nonvolatile substances

[34]. The elicitation dose is ED(ROAT) = 0.0296 × ED (patch test) for any given concentration; details are given in [34]. This means that the easier and quicker method of serial dilution patch testing may be used to predict the outcome of repeated open aplications and can be used in risk assessment.

Core Message

> Serial dilution patch tests are now standardized to an extent where they can be used more systematically in risk assessment and for the determination of safer exposure levels to substances, which has already caused outbreaks of allergic contact dermatitis.

14.4.2 The Repeated Open Application Test

Different names have been used for the repeated open application of allergens to contact-sensitized individuals, such as the usage test, provocative use test, and open patch test. The name ROAT (repeated open application test) was coined by Hannuksela and Salo [35] and has since been the generally accepted term for this procedure. The test consists of an open exposure, often with a finished product or with a well-defined vehicle containing the defined allergen at a nonirritant concentration. A 5 × 5 or 3 × 3 cm skin area on the forearm or upper arm close to the antecubital fossa is used. Application in the antecubital fossa should be avoided because the degree of natural occlusion is unpredictable. The vehicle used in the ROAT may be a finished product or patch test vehicles such as petrolatum or alcohol. Twice a day application of a 20 μL volume/9 cm² is recommended. Most ROAT studies have used an application time of 1–2 weeks. One week is undoubtedly too short, depending on the reactivity of individual patients and the hapten exposure concentration [15, 36]. In newer studies, emollients with relevant preservatives were applied on the neck and face, which have proven to be more sensitive than the upper arm [24, 37]. In one study a step-wise procedure was used with applications on the arm, neck, and face. Only in case of a negative reaction, applications were made to the next skin area [24]. Clinical tests need to take the region of application into consideration, and testing should preferably be

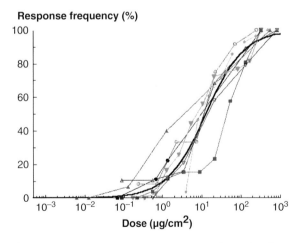

Fig. 14.3 Dose-response curves based on patch test data from eight studies of nickel allergy. The data are analyzed by logistic regression. The *black curve* represents the weighed adjusted average curve from all the studies [31]

done simulating normal exposure as closely as possible in order to avoid false-negative results.

Itching may be the first symptom in the allergic contact dermatitis reactions elicited. In a double-blind ROAT study of cinnamal, some individuals registered itching at the site of specific allergen exposure before any visible skin signs [36]; however, nonimmunologic contact urticaria may alternatively have caused these symptoms [36]. Further studies that systematically focus on this point are necessary. The morphology of the positive ROAT has given important information as to the early clinical signs of the allergic contact dermatitis reaction. The first objective sign in allergic contact dermatitis may be a follicular papular eruption, as seen from low concentrations of allergens in serial dilution patch testing (Fig. 14.1). The follicular morphology of the allergic contact dermatitis reaction is not generally recognized in textbooks, but is seen as the first clinical symptoms in ROATs done on the upper arm or neck with specific allergens [38]. The explanation for this morphology is the increased accumulation and absorption of allergens through the follicles and sweat duct orifices [39, 40]. Continued exposure may lead to infiltration and eventually vesicle formation. The morphology on the face seems to differ in the sense that uniform redness was the primary symptom in a study on formaldehyde-releasers, followed by slight infiltration like erythemateaous rosacea [38] (Fig. 14.4).

There are no generally accepted guidelines for evaluation of the ROAT. The terminology used for diagnostic patch test reading is less suitable, as early allergic reactions will be disregarded. Further, an experimental ROAT will usually be terminated before strong positive reactions comparable to ++ or +++ patch test reactions have developed. As the ROAT is usually done with nonirritant allergen concentrations and the response compared to a vehicle-treated controlled area, both the follicular reaction pattern and noninfiltrated redness represent allergic reactions and should be scored as such, in contrast to reading the occluded patch test. Johansen et al. [41] have proposed a semiquantitative reading scale for the ROAT (Table 14.3). A cut-off point for a positive reaction has in several studies been a score of five points or above [16, 19, 20, 29, 30].

Noninvasive so-called bioengineering methods are useful in the quantification of the experimental irritant response, but because of the heterogeneous and often follicular pattern of the early allergic contact dermatitis reaction, such methods are less suitable in the evaluation of the ROAT.

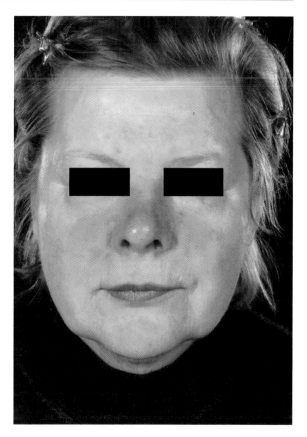

Fig. 14.4 Repeated open application done for 12 days in face with a cream containing 0.15% diazolidinyl urea in a patient allergic to formaldehyde. A positive allergic response is seen, which may resemble erythemateous rosacea. It underlines the importance of patch testing in selected cases with this diagnosis. Reprinted with permission from Contact Dermatitis [38]

Core Message

> ROATs should be continued for at least 14 days if negative. The neck and face are more sensitive than the upper arm to allergen exposure.

14.4.3 The Axillary Exposure Test

Allergens related to deodorants and textiles are relevant to the axillary region. Published research has focused on formaldehyde and fragrances. Industry has long experience of irritancy testing in the development of deodorants and antiperspirants. It is recognized that this particular skin area is problematic in relation to product development, as this moist and occluded skin

14

Table 14.3 Reading scale for repeated open application tests (ROAT) with an application area of 3×3 cm on the forearm

1. Involved area of application					
	0	1–24%	25–49%	50–89%	90–100%
	0	1	2	3	4

2. Erythema					
Involvement			Strength		
None	Spotty	Homogenous	Weak	Medium	Strong
0	1	2	1	2	3

3. Papules				Homogenous infiltration
None	<5	5–10	>10	
0	1	2	3	4

4. Vesicles				Confluent
None	<5	5–10	>10	
0	1	2	3	4

The scale is modified from [41] to fit a smaller area [29]. A positive response is defined as a score at at least five point [31], as marked in the table. It corresponds to a reaction covering at least 25% of the area with weak erythema and at least one papule, representing infiltration. Reproduced with permission from Contact Dermatitis [29]

area has a propensity to irritant reactions. When performing axillary allergen exposure studies, it is therefore always necessary to include both sensitized and nonsensitized individuals to control for irritancy.

The early morphology of the positive reactions is similar to that seen in the ROAT, with papulofollicular elements being a common feature. Studies including formaldehyde and fragrances have demonstrated lower concentration thresholds in the axillae, as compared to the skin of the upper arm and back [42, 43]. Exposure studies with standard deodorants containing cinnamal, hydroxycitronellal, or hydroxyisohexyl 3-cyclohexene-carboxaldehyde in increasing concentration illustrate a dose-response relationship in patients sensitive to the substance in question [44–46]. This type of study, combined with product analysis, clearly demonstrates the relevance of fragrance allergy in relation to deodorants. Further, it is an important step in the risk assessment process for the continued improvement of product safety.

14.4.4 The Shampoo Test

Shampoos are widely used cosmetic products with few side-effects. Reports of allergic contact dermatitis from shampoos are mainly case-based. Shampoos can cause dermatitis of the scalp, face, and neck. Cases simulating seborrheic dermatitis have been reported. The rarity of allergic contact dermatitis from shampoos is probably explained by the small degree of exposure (Table 14.2), because of allergen dilution.

In controlled exposure studies with an MCI/MI-containing shampoo including MCI/MI-sensitive individuals, Frosch et al. [47] identified cases with elicitation of exudative scalp dermatitis, facial dermatitis, and flare of hand eczema. Even if such cases are rarely reported [13], the outcome of the shampoo use test alerts the clinician to consider this possibility in the case of contact dermatitis of the scalp, face, neck, and retroauricular regions.

14.4.5 The Liquid Soap Test

Liquid soaps are a well-known cause of irritant contact dermatitis, especially at the workplace. Allergic contact dermatitis from allergens in liquid soaps is rarely documented, possibly due to the lack of adequate methods of investigation. However, a new method of testing liquid soaps has been developed [48] following clinical evidence that these types of products were involved in many cases of contact allergy to methyldibromo glutaronitrile [49–51].

Testing is performed on two identical areas of 5×10 cm at the forearms. In a blinded and randomized fashion, a soap containing the allergen in question, in this case methyldibromo glutaronitrile, is applied on one arm and an identical placebo product without the allergen on the other arm. The test site is moistened with water and two drops of soap applied. The test area is washed with the soap by moving a small water-soaked nylon sponge back and forward over the area 10 times. The soap is left for a maximum of 30 s before the skin sites are rinsed with running water and dried [48]. Applications are made twice daily for up to 4 weeks. Using this protocol it was demonstrated that 37% (7/19) of sensitized individuals gave a reaction to a liquid soap containing methyldibromo glutaronitrile in the at that time permitted concentration [48]. This was an important part of the chain of evidence that liquid soaps with methyldibromo glutaronitrile cause allergic contact dermatitis, and it also provided a new model for testing liquid soaps. The model was optimized recently, as it will often be relevant to test products with less potent allergens. In the suggested design, the skin of the lower part of each arm was pretreated with the allergen in question by patch testing with a concentration range of the allergen using 12 mm Finn chambers [9]. One month later, a use test was performed with a liquid soap containing the allergen on one arm and an identical soap without the allergen on the other arm. An increased reactivity was shown on the areas that had been pretreated with the allergen (methyldibromo glutaronitrile), while preirritated skin gave no augmented response to allergen exposure; furthermore, a control group was negative [9]. It is a design that may prove useful in assessing the risk of exposure to allergens in liquid soaps. Testing of more allergens is needed for further validation.

> **Core Message**
>
> › Models for testing allergens in liquid soaps have been developed for the purpose of risk assessment.

14.4.6 The Finger Immersion Test/ Experimental Hand Eczema

Hand eczema is a common disease and may lead to permanent disability. The diagnosis of allergic contact dermatitis on the hands is based on the outcome of patch testing and qualitative exposure assessment. In some cases, this procedure is straightforward, as for example, with rubber gloves. There is solid evidence that the rubber chemicals, thiurams, and mercaptobenzothiazole in the standard patch test series are present in rubber gloves, and are leached out during use in amounts sufficient to elicit allergic contact dermatitis [52–54]. But in many cases, when the diagnosis of allergic hand dermatitis is established, e.g., from metals, preservatives, and naturally occurring substances, the evidence is circumstantial because experimental disease models combined with quantitative exposure assessment are not developed.

There have been attempts in the past to establish such models. Hjorth and Roed Petersen [55] made provocation studies of the fingers of chefs and sandwich makers using fresh food. Christensen and Möller [56] established vesicular nickel hand eczema as part of systemic contact dermatitis.

Allenby and Basketter [57] introduced the finger immersion model. They intended to investigate whether trace amounts of nickel (0.1–1 ppm), present in some consumer products, were able to elicit allergic hand eczema. Four nickel-sensitive individuals, without previous or present hand eczema, had their thumbs immersed in a solution containing nickel (0.1–1 ppm) and sodium dodecyl sulfate (0.1–0.3%) twice daily for 10 min over 21 days. None of the volunteers developed an eczematous response. Accumulation of nickel in the fingernails was used as an objective exposure parameter (Table 14.4). Nielsen et al. [58] made a double-blind placebo-controlled finger immersion study, including 35 nickel-sensitive individuals with low-grade hand eczema (redness and scaling, but no vesicles) over 2 weeks. Finger exposure for 10 min daily to first 10 ppm and later 100 ppm nickel elicited a statistically significant flare of vesicular hand eczema in nickel-exposed patients, as compared to vehicle-exposed patients. As objective response parameters, the number of vesicles was counted and the blood flow measured by laser Doppler. Similar pilot studies have been done with chromate and cobalt [59]. The nickel concentrations in nails (Table 14.4) and skin as a consequence of experimental nickel exposure were measured [60]. A new acid wipe sampling technique of nickel, cobalt, and chromium was applied to the hands of workers in different occupations. Metals were detected in all samples and the amount of nickel was larger than that of chromium and cobalt. Fingers were

Table 14.4 Nickel in nails reflecting exposure

Type of exposure	Nickel µg/g (mean)	Reference
Occupational exposure		
None (controls)	1.19	[62]
Moderate	29.20	[62]
Heavy	123.00	[62]
Experimental exposure		
Baseline	1.58	[60]
Immersion of finger in 0.1–1 ppm	7.80	[57]
Nickel twice a day for 21 days[a]		
Immersion of finger in 10 ppm	5.50	[60]
Nickel once a day for 1 week		
Immersion of finger in 100 ppm	12.00	[60]
Nickel once a day for 1 week		

[a]Four observations

Table 14.5 Concentration threshold for reactivity to formaldehyde in formaldehyde-sensitive patients in different experimental exposure tests

Method	Threshold (ppm)	Reference
Repeated (1-week) exposure on normal skin	300 ppm	[3]
Repeated axillary exposure	150 ppm	[43]
Finn chamber patch test	150 ppm	[73]
Repeated patch testing in the same area	30 ppm	[18]
Hand eczema skin immersion (40 min) one patient	0.2 ppm	[64]

more exposed than palms. Eight-hours of exposure to nickel was calculated and was highest in locksmiths (mean $3.784 \, \mu g/cm^2$, range $1.846–5.028 \, \mu g/cm^2$) followed by carpenters, cashiers, and secretaries [61]. Combination of the knowledge from experimental studies and the quantification of nickel exposure in different industries [61, 62] will be the basis for the diagnosis of occupational hand eczema caused by nickel allergy in the future.

Moreover, perfume ingredients, e.g., hydroxycitronellal and hydroxyisohexyl 3-cyclohexene carboxaldehyde, have been tested in similar protocols with exposure concentrations equal to diluted and undiluted dish washing liquid [63]. In contrast to the studies of nickel, chromate, and cobalt, no significant difference could be found between active exposure and placebo, possibly due to the use of less potent allergens, which under normal exposure conditions would be in combination with irritants.

14.5 The Comparative Approach

Formaldehyde has been studied in different human models. Table 14.5 compares the concentration threshold for reactivity to formaldehyde in formaldehyde-sensitive patients in different experimental exposure tests. It is important to notice that some of the results are based on one or few patients. Notwithstanding this, the variation in concentration thresholds depending on exposure site and exposure condition is challenging. Horsfall [64] found a positive exposure test with 0.2 ppm formaldehyde in a patient with allergic formaldehyde dermatitis on the hands. If this observation can be confirmed, it is important for our understanding of formaldehyde hand dermatitis. While making the final risk assessment, the wide variation in elicitation concentration threshold, as illustrated for formaldehyde in Table 14.5, needs to be considered. Similar comparative data are not yet present for other allergens.

14.6 Elicitation Data Used in Prevention and Regulations

Experimental clinical exposure studies may form the basis for regulation of allergen exposure in the future. This has been the case in the regulation of nickel released from metal items designed to be in direct and prolonged skin contact. This question is relatively simple, as exposure to metal items such as jewelry, claps, buttons etc. is comparable to that in the patch test, and the evaluation can therefore be based on this technology. A number of studies have uniformly shown that metal items releasing less than $0.5 \, \mu g/cm^2$ nickel per week elicit an allergic reaction in only a few nickel-sensitive individuals [31]. This observation was the basis for the regulation of nickel exposure in Denmark and later in the EU [65]. Future studies may illustrate that the measurement of nickel in the skin, released from such items, will be a more reliable parameter than nickel released from the items in artificial sweat. Studies of nickel in nails (Table 14.4) and skin [61] measured in different industrial settings and during experimental nickel exposure illustrate that it is possible to quantify nickel exposure, even though the variation is not insignificant [56, 60–62]. Based on nickel nail concentrations, the exposure used in the experimental studies that provoked a flare of dermatitis is comparable to a moderate industrial nickel exposure. Data now exist supporting the view that nickel regulation has been an effective tool of prevention and caused a decrease in the numbers of nickel-sensitized individuals in the young part of the female population [66–68].

Exposure to chemicals from rubber gloves is analogous to nickel exposure from metal items designed to be in direct and prolonged contact with the skin. It has been shown that the amount of rubber chemicals released from rubber gloves, under the influence of synthetic sweat, is comparable to the amount of rubber chemical necessary to elicit a positive patch test [52, 53]. Such data explain why a positive patch test to thiurams is frequently relevant to exposure to rubber gloves.

Experimental exposure studies with important perfume chemicals have been made, with concentrations based on the outcome of chemical analysis of perfumed products and fine fragrances [69, 70]. In this way, it has been substantiated that the concentrations of perfume chemicals in cosmetic products and fine fragrances do not infrequently exceed those that may elicit allergic contact dermatitis in sensitized individuals. Studies of thresholds for fragrance allergens such as hydroxyisohexyl 3-cyclohexene carboxaldehyde [29, 71] and the main allergens in oak moss abs., chloroatranol [30], have formed the basis for risk assessments and recommendations for safer use concentrations for these substances.

In patients with contact allergy to more than one perfumed ingredient, combined exposure to both may lead to a synergistic eliciting effect [5]. This illustrates that a detailed knowledge of environmental exposure to well-defined allergens is needed for the performance of meaningful experimental exposure studies. The development of chemical methods in recent years to quantify exposure to metals, preservatives, plastics, fragrances, and rubber chemicals has facilitated the conduct of clinically relevant experimental exposure studies in specifically sensitized individuals. Even

though much is still to be learnt in this area, the tools now exist to define unacceptable risk based on data from contact dermatitis patients [72] and models based on elicitation data to be used in risk assessment and definitions of safe(r) exposures [32].

Core Message

> Elicitation data derived from dose-response studies have been used for preventive actions with success.

References

1. Andersen KE, Liden C, Hansen J, Volund A (1993) Dose-response testing with nickel sulphate using the TRUE test in nickel-sensitive individuals. Multiple nickel sulphate patch-test reactions do not cause an "angry back". Br J Dermatol 129:50–56
2. Menné T, Calvin G (1993) Concentration threshold of non-occluded nickel exposure in nickel-sensitive individuals and controls with and without surfactant. Contact Dermat 29: 180–184
3. Flyvholm MA, Hall BM, Agner T, Tiedemann E, Greenhill P, Vanderveken W, Freeberg FE, Menné T (1997) Threshold for occluded formaldehyde patch test in formaldehyde-sensitive patients. Relationship to repeated open application test with a product containing formaldehyde releaser. Contact Dermat 36:26–33
4. Menné T (1991) Relationship between use test and threshold patch test concentration in patients sensitive to 5-chloro-2-methyl-4-isothiazolin-3-one and 2- methyl-4-isothiazolin-3-one (MCI/MI). Contact Dermat 24:375
5. Johansen JD, Andersen KE, Menné T (1996) Quantitative aspects of isoeugenol contact allergy assessed by use and patch tests. Contact Dermat 34:414–418
6. Frosch PJ, Pilz B, Burrows D, Camarasa JG, Lachapelle JM, Lahti A, Menné T, Wilkinson JD (1995) Testing with fragrance mix. Is the addition of sorbitan sesquioleate to the constituents useful? Contact Dermat 32:266–272
7. Rudzki E, Rebandel P, Karas Z (1997) Patch testing with lower concentrations of chromate and nickel. Contact Dermat 37:46
8. Hindsen M, Bruze M (1998) The significance of previous contact dermatitis for elicitation of contact allergy to nickel. Acta Derm Venereol 78:367–370
9. Jensen CD, Johansen JD, Menné T, Andersen KE (2006) Increased retest activity by both patch and use test with methyldibromo glutaronitrile in sensitized individuals. Acta Derm Venereol Acta Derm Venereol 86(1):8–12
10. Johansen JD, Skov L, Volund A, Andersen K, Menné T (1998) Allergens in combination have a synergistic effect on the elicitation response: a study of fragrance-sensitized individuals. Br J Dermatol 139:264–270

11. Kligman AM (1966) The identification of contact allergens by human assay. 3. The maximization test: a procedure for screening and rating contact sensitizers. J Invest Dermatol 47:393–409

12. Rees JL, Friedmann PS, Matthews JN (1990) The influence of area of application on sensitization by dinitrochlorobenzene. Br J Dermatol 122:29–31

13. Fewings J, Menné T (1999) An update of the risk assessment for methylchloroisothiazolinone/methylisothiazolinone (MCI/MI) with focus on rinse-off products. Contact Dermat 41:1–13

14. Hextall JM, Alagaratnam NJ, Glendinning AK, Holloway DB, Blaikie L, Basketter DA, McFadden JP (2002) Dose–time relationship for elicitation of contact allergy to paraphenylenediamine. Contact Dermat 47:96–99

15. Andersen KE, Johansen JD, Bruze M, Frosch PJ, Goossens A, Lepoittevin JP, Rastogi S, White I, Menné T (2001) The time-dose-response relationship for elicitation of contact dermatitis in isoeugenol allergic individuals. Toxicol Appl Pharmacol 170:166–171

16. Fischer LA, Johansen JD, Menné T (2007) Nickel allergy: relationship between patch test and repeated open application test thresholds. Br J Dermatol 157:723–729

17. Jensen CD, Johansen JD, Menné T, Andersen KE (2005) Methyldibromo glutaronitrile contact allergy: effect of single versus repeated daily exposures. Contact Dermat 52:88–92

18. Jordan WPJ, Sherman WT, King SE (1979) Threshold responses in formaldehyde-sensitive subjects. J Am Acad Dermatol 1:44–48

19. Fischer LA, Johansen JD, Menné T (2008) Methyldibromo glutaronitrile allergy: relationship between patch test and repeated open application test thresholds. Br J Dermatol 159:1138–1143

20. Fischer LA, Menné T, Avnstorp C, Kasting GB, Johansen JD (2009) Hydroxyisohexyl 3-cyclohexene allergy: relationship between patch test and repeated open application test thresholds. Br J Dermatol 161(3):560–567

21. Heydorn S, Andersen KE, Johansen JD, Menné T (2003) A stronger patch test reaction to the allergen hydroxycitronellal and the irritant sodium lauryl sulfate. Contact Dermat 49:133–139

22. Pedersen LK, Haslund P, Johansen JD, Held E, Volund A, Agner T (2004) Influence of a detergent on skin response to methyldibromo glutaronitrile in sensitized individuals. Contact Dermat 50:1–5

23. Agner T, Johansen JD, Overgaard L, Volund A, Basketter D, Menné T (2002) Combined effects of irritants and allergens. Synergistic effects of nickel and sodium lauryl sulfate – in nickel sensitized individuals (1991). Contact Dermat 47: 21–26

24. Hannuksela M (1991) Sensitivity of various skin sites in the repeated open application test. Am J Contact Dermat 2:102–104

25. Johansen JD, Rastogi SC, Bruze M, Andersen KE, Frosch PJ, Dreier B, Lepoittevin JP, White IR, Menné T (1998) Deodorants: a clinical provocation study in fragrance-sensitive individuals. Contact Dermat 39:161–165

26. Zachariae C, Hall B, Cottin M, Cupferman S, Andersen KE, Menné T (2005) Experimental elicitation of contact allergy from a diazolidinyl urea-preserved cream in relation to anatomical region, exposure time and concentration. Contact Dermat 53(5):268–277

27. Hindsen M, Bruze M, Christensen OB (1999) Individual variation in nickel patch test reactivity. Am J Contact Dermat 10:62–67

28. Hansen MB, Johansen JD, Menné T (2003) Chromium allergy: significanse of both Cr(III) and Cr(VI). Contact Dermat 49:206–212

29. Frosch PJ, Pirker C, Rastogi SC, Andersen KE, Bruze M, Svedman C, Goossens A, White IR, Uter W, Giménez Arnau E, Lepoittevin JP, Menné T, Johansen JD (2005) Patch testing with a new fragrance mix detects additional patients sensitive to perfumes and missed by the current fragrance mix. Contact Dermat 52:207–215

30. Mortz CG, Lauritzen JM, Bindslev-Jensen C, Andersen KE (2002) Nickel sensitization in adolescents and association with ear piercing, use of braces and hand eczema. The Odense Adolescence Cohort Study on Atopic Diseases and Dermatitis (TOACS). Acta Derm Venereol 82:352–358

31. Johansen JD, Frosch PJ, Svedman C, Andersen KE, Bruze M, Pirker C, Menné T (2003) Hydroxyisohexyl 3-cyclohexene carboxaldehyde – known as Lyral: quantitative aspects and risk assessment of an important fragrance allergen. Contact Dermat 48:310–316

32. Johansen JD, Andersen KE, Svedman C, Bruze M, Bernard G, Giminez-Arnau E, Rastogi SC, Lepoittevin JP, Menné T (2003) Chloroatranol an extremely potent allergen hidden in perfumes – a dose-response elicitation study. Contact Dermat 49:180–184

33. Fischer LA, Menné T, Johansen JD (2005) Experimental nickel elicitation thresholds – a review focusing on occluded nickel exposure. Contact Dermat 52:57–64

34. Fischer LA, Voelund A, Andersen KE, Menné T, Johansen J (2009) The dose-response relationship between patch test and ROAT and the potential use for regulatory purposes. Contact Dermat 61(4):201–208

35. Hannuksela M, Salo H (1986) The repeated open application test (ROAT). Contact Dermat 14:221–227

36. Johansen JD, Andersen KE, Rastogi SC, Menné T (1996) Threshold responses in cinnamic-aldehyde-sensitive subjects: results and methodological aspects. Contact Dermat 34:165–171

37. Pedersen LK, Agner T, Held E, Johansen JD (2004) Methyldibromo glutaronitrile in leave-on products elicits contact allergy at low concentration. Br J Dermatol 151: 817–822

38. Zachariae C, Hall B, Cupferman S, Andersen KE, Menné T (2006) ROAT: morphology of ROAT on arm, neck and face in formaldehyde and diazolidinyl urea sensitive individuals. Contact Dermat 54(1):21–24

39. Rolland A, Wagner N, Chatelus A, Shroot B, Schaefer H (1993) Site-specific drug delivery to pilosebaceous structures using polymeric microspheres. Pharm Res 10:1738–1744

40. Vestergaard L, Clemmensen OJ, Sorensen FB, Andersen KE (1999) Histological distinction between early allergic and irritant patch test reactions: follicular spongiosis may be characteristic of early allergic contact dermatitis. Contact Dermat 41:207–210

41. Johansen JD, Bruze M, Andersen KE, Frosch PJ, Dreier B, White IR, Rastogi S, Lepoittevin JP, Menné T (1998) The repeated open application test: suggestions for a scale of evaluation. Contact Dermat 39:95–96

42. Johansen JD, Rastogi SC, Bruze M, Andersen KE, Frosch P, Dreier B, Lepoittevin JP, White I, Menné T (1998) Deodorants: a clinical provocation study in fragrance-sensitive individuals. Contact Dermat 39(4):161–165

43. Maibach HI (1983) Formaldehyde: effects on animal and human skin. In: Gibson JE (ed) Formaldehyde toxicity. Hemisphere, Washington, pp 166–174

44. Bruze M, Johansen JD, Andersen KE, Frosch PJ, Lepoittevin JP, Rastogi S, Wakelin S, White IR, Menné T (2003) Deodorants: an experimental provocation study with cinnamic aldehyde. J Am Acad Dermatol 48:194–200

45. Svedman C, Bruze M, Johansen JD, Andersen KE, Goossens A, Frosch PJ, Lepoittevin JP, Rastogi S, White IR, Menné T (2003) Deodorants: an experimental provocation study with hydroxycitronellal. Contact Dermat 48:217–223

46. Jørgensen PH, Jensen CD, Rastogi S, Andersen KE, Johansen JD (2007) Experimental elicitation with hydroxy-isohexyl-3-cyclohexene carboxaldehyde-containing deodorants. Contact Dermat 56(3):146–150

47. Frosch PJ, Lahti A, Hannuksela M, Andersen KE, Wilkinson JD, Shaw S, Lachapelle JM (1995) Chloromethylisothiazolone/methylisothiazolone (CMI/MI) use test with a shampoo on patch-test-positive subjects. Results of a multicentre double-blind crossover trial. Contact Dermat 32:210–217

48. Jensen CD, Johansen JD, Menné T, Andersen KE (2004) Methyldibromo glutaronitrile in rinse-off products causes allergic contact dermatitis: an experimental study. Br J Dermatol 150:90–95

49. Zachariae C, Rastogi S, Devantier Jensen C, Menné T, Johansen JD (2003) Methyldibromo glutaronitrile: clinical experience and expsoure-based risk assessment. Contact Dermat 48:150–154

50. Zachariae C, Johansen JD, Rastogi SC, Menné T (2005) Allergic contact dermatitis from methyldibromo glutaronitrile – clinical cases from 2003. Contact Dermat 52:6–8

51. Johansen JD, Veien NK, Laurberg G, Kaaber K, Thormann J, Lauritzen M, Avnstorp C (2005) Contact allergy to methyldibromo glutaronitrile – data from a front line network. Contact Dermat 52:138–141

52. Knudsen BB, Larsen E, Egsgaard H, Menné T (1993) Release of thiurams and carbamates from rubber gloves. Contact Dermat 28:63–69

53. Knudsen BB, Menné T (1996) Elicitation thresholds for thiuram mix using petrolatum and ethanol/sweat as vehicles. Contact Dermat 34:410–413

54. Hansson C, Bergendorff O, Ezzelarab M, Sterner O (1997) Extraction of mercaptobenzothiazole compounds from rubber products. Contact Dermat 36:195–200

55. Hjorth N, Roed-Petersen J (1976) Occupational protein contact dermatitis in food handlers. Contact Dermat 2:28–42

56. Christensen OB, Moller H (1975) External and internal exposure to the antigen in the hand eczema of nickel allergy. Contact Dermat 1:136–141

57. Allenby CF, Basketter DA (1994) The effect of repeated open exposure to low levels of nickel on compromised hand skin of nickel-allergic subjects. Contact Dermat 30:135–138

58. Nielsen NH, Menné T, Kristiansen J, Christensen JM, Borg L, Poulsen LK (1999) Effects of repeated skin exposures to low nickel concentrations – a model for allergic contact dermatitis to nickel on the hands. Br J Dermatol 141:676–682

59. Nielsen NH, Kristiansen J, Borg L, Christensen JM, Poulsen LK, Menné T (2000) Repeated exposures to cobalt and chromate on the hands of patients with hand eczema and the specific metal contact allergy. Contact Dermat 43:212–215

60. Kristiansen J, Christensen JM, Henriksen T, Nielsen NH, Menné T (1999) Determination of nickel in fingernails and forearm skin (stratum corneum). Anal Chim Acta 403:265–272

61. Lidén C, Skare L, Nise G, Vahter M (2008) Deposition of nickel, chromium, and cobalt on the skin in some occupations – assessment by acid wipe sampling. Contact Dermat 58(6):347–354

62. Peters K, Gammelgaard B, Menné T (1991) Nickel concentrations in fingernails as a measure of occupational exposure to nickel. Contact Dermat 25:237–241

63. Heydorn S, Menné T, Andersen KE, Bruze M, Svedman C, Basketter D, Johansen JD (2003) The fragrance hand immersion study – an experimental model simulating exposure for allergic contact dermatitis on the hands. Contact Dermat 48:324–330

64. Horsfall FL (1934) Formaldehyde hypersensitiveness. An experimental study. J Immunol 27:569–581

65. Liden C, Menné T, Burrows D (1996) Nickel-containing alloys and platings and their ability to cause dermatitis. Br J Dermatol 134:193–198

66. Schnuch A, Uter W (2003) Decrease in nickel allergy in Germany and regulatory interventions. Contact Dermat 49: 107–108

67. Jensen CS, Lisby S, Baadsgaard O, Volund A, Menné T (2002) Decrease in nickel sensitization in a Dansih schoolgirl population with ears pierced after implementation of a nickel-exposure regulation. Br J Dermatol 146:636–642

68. Thyssen JP, Johansen JD, Menné T, Nielsen NH, Linneberg A (2009) Nickel allergy in Danish women before and after nickel regulation. N Engl J Med 360(21):2259–2260

69. Rastogi SC, Lepoittevin JP, Johansen JD, Frosch PJ, Menné T, Bruze M, Dreier B, Andersen KE, White IR (1998) Fragrances and other materials in deodorants: search for potentially sensitizing molecules using combined GC-MS and structure activity relationship (SAR) analysis. Contact Dermat 39:293–303

70. Johansen JD, Rastogi SC, Menné T (1996) Contact allergy to popular perfumes; assessed by patch test, use test and chemical analysis. Br J Dermatol 135:419–422

71. Schnuch A, Uter W, Dickel H et al (2009) Quantitative patch and repeated open application testing in hydroxyisohexyl 3-cyclohexene carboxaldehyde sensitive patients. Contact Dermat 61(3):152–162

72. Thyssen JP, Menné T, Schnuch A, Uter W, White I, White JM, Johansen JD (2009) Acceptable risk of contact allergy in the general population assessed by CE-DUR-a method to detect and categorize contact allergy epidemics based on patient data. Regul Toxicol Pharmacol 54(2):183–187

73. Fischer T, Andersen K, Bengtsson U, Frosch P, Gunnarsson Y, Kreilgard B, Menné T, Shaw S, Svensson L, Wilkinson J (1995) Clinical standardization of the TRUE Test formaldehyde patch. Curr Probl Dermatol 22:24–30

Contents

15.1 Introduction

A diagnosis of contact dermatitis requires the careful consideration of many variables, including patient history, physical examination and various types of skin testing. A thorough knowledge of the clinical features of the skin's reactions to various contactants is important in making a correct diagnosis of contact dermatitis.

While an eczematous reaction is the most commonly encountered adverse reaction to contactants, other clinical manifestations may also be seen. These include erosions, ulcerations, urticaria, erythema multiforme, purpura, lichenoid eruptions, exanthems, erythroderma, allergic contact granuloma, lymphocytoma, sarcoidal reactions, toxic epidermal necrolysis, pigmented contact dermatitis, contact leukoderma, nodular lesions and photosensitive reactions [1–9]. Generalized symptoms have also been described in association with contact sensitivity, as documented by challenge experiments [10, 11], and contact urticaria may become anaphylactoid [12] and life-threatening [13].

The emphasis in this chapter will be on eczemas as a manifestation of contact dermatitis. Other clinical manifestations will be described in detail in Chap. 21, and hand eczema, in particular, in Chap. 19.

N.K. Veien
Dermatology Clinic, Vesterbro 99, 9000 Aalborg,
Denmark
e-mail: veien@dadlnet.dk

J.D. Johansen et al. (eds.), *Contact Dermatitis*,
DOI: 10.1007/978-3-642-03827-3_15, © Springer-Verlag Berlin Heidelberg 2011

15.2 The Medical History of the Patient

15.2.1 History of Hereditary Diseases

The family and personal history of a patient with contact dermatitis should be taken in detail, especially with regard to atopy. Patients who have suffered from severe atopic dermatitis in childhood are likely to experience irritant contact dermatitis later in life, particularly on the hands [14]. It has also been shown that hereditary factors other than atopy play a role in the development of hand eczema [15]. A history of contact urticaria, in particular on the lips and hands, due to uncooked food items is common among atopics [14]. Contact urticaria due to animal dander may aggravate atopic dermatitis of the arms and the periorbital area. It can be useful to note the results of prick tests carried out, for example, in previous attempts to discover the cause of respiratory allergy. A positive prick test to house dust mites, animal dander or pollen may correlate with the results of an atopy patch test and may be relevant as an aggravating factor in atopic dermatitis [16–18].

Patients with recurrent vesicular hand eczema are often atopic [19], and Schwanitz [20] coined the term "das atopische Palmoplantarekism" after a study of the literature and having seen 58 patients with recurrent vesicular hand eczema. Edman, however [21], found no statistical correlation between atopy and this type of hand dermatitis. Details concerning the relationship between atopy and contact sensitization are given in the Sect. 15.3.5.5.

It is unusual for a patient to have a family history of contact dermatitis. Although hereditary factors were seen to have some significance among twins with nickel allergy, these were found to be less important than environmental factors [22].

A family history of psoriasis is important as it may be difficult to distinguish psoriasis from contact dermatitis and seborrhoeic dermatitis. This is particularly true on the scalp, the face, the anogenital area and the hands. Köbner reactions on the hands of psoriasis patients can mimic irritant or allergic contact dermatitis [23]. Likewise, Köbner reactions on the hands may show a striking resemblance to hyperkeratotic hand eczema. Both psoriasis and hyperkeratotic hand eczema can be aggravated by physical trauma from, for example, the handles of tools.

15.2.2 General Medical History

Malnutrition may cause eczematous lesions in, for example, alcohol dependency [24] or in patients with acrodermatitis enteropathica or metabolic disorders like phenylketonuria. In order to make a diagnosis of systemically induced dermatitis, it is necessary to take a complete history of drug intake. Cutaneous sensitization to a drug may give rise to symmetrical dermatitis when the same drug, or a chemically related drug, is taken orally or injected (see Chaps. 17 and 38). Drug intake can also play a significant role in a number of photodermatoses.

Obesity is an important factor in the development of intertriginous dermatoses and mechanical contact dermatitis due to friction; the latter may be seen, for example, on the inner surfaces of the thighs of obese children.

Psychiatric disorders can lead to contact dermatitis caused by the compulsive clutching of keys containing nickel (Fig. 15.1) or mechanical dermatitis caused by the compulsive rubbing of the skin (Fig. 15.2).

> **Core Message**
>
> › Both family and medical history are important while making a diagnosis of contact dermatitis. Rashes seen in metabolic diseases and in obese persons may mimic contact dermatitis. Contact urticaria and irritant contact dermatitis are common in persons with current or previous atopic dermatitis.

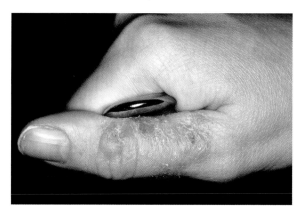

Fig. 15.1 Allergic contact dermatitis in a nickel-sensitive psychiatric patient who clutched nickel-containing keys all day

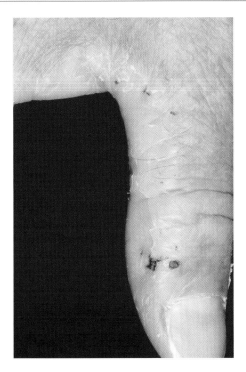

Fig. 15.2 Factitious dermatitis from compulsory rubbing of the skin of the fingers. Note the sharp delineation from normal skin

15.2.3 History of Previous Dermatitis

A firm history of previous allergic contact dermatitis from, for example, nickel, fragrances or topical medicaments would be a reason to suspect inadvertent contact with the same haptens if an otherwise unexplained eruption of contact dermatitis occurs. A history of axillary intolerance to spray deodorants is a good indication of fragrance allergy [25]. Further details on the relationship between the history of nickel allergy and atopy are given in Sect. 15.3.5.5.

A history of previous dermatitis near leg ulcers should lead to a suspicion of topical medicaments as the cause of current or possible future eruptions of dermatitis in this area or elsewhere. A history of dermatitis where adhesive tape has been applied should lead the physician to search for possible colophony sensitivity. It should be mentioned, however, that most modern adhesive tapes contain no colophony, as the adhesive substance is now usually an acrylate.

15.2.4 Time of Onset

For long-standing contact dermatitis, the exact time of onset is usually ill-defined and is not useful in establishing the final diagnosis. The cause of contact dermatitis with recent abrupt onset may be established by taking a careful history of contactants during the days immediately preceding the onset of dermatitis. The history should include occupational exposures and exposures during leisure time and while working in the home or with hobbies, as well as any changes in clothing or cosmetics, including soaps and detergents. Topical remedies used for the treatment of the dermatitis, both prescription and over-the-counter products, should be recorded, as well as any recent changes in systemic drug therapy.

15.2.5 History of Aggravating Factors

For chronic contact dermatitis, the history should include information about contactants in relation to aggravation of the dermatitis rather than to its onset. Two types of flares of chronic dermatoses should be considered: eruptions that appear suddenly and without warning, and eruptions that show seasonal variation. Seasonal variations may help to establish the type of dermatitis and possibly also the specific cause, a point that is illustrated in Fig. 15.3.

The sudden aggravation of chronic dermatitis or recurrences at short intervals may help to establish the cause of the dermatitis or, if this is not possible, those factors which aggravate it. Recurrent vesicular eczema of the hands provides a typical example of how such help can be obtained. Although a definite cause for this type of dermatitis is rarely determined, a number of factors may cause the eruption of a crop of vesicles. The time elapsing between exposure to aggravating factors and the eruption of vesicles is 1–3 days, and with proper instruction a patient is often able to recall exposures that occurred up to 3 days prior to the onset of dermatitis, and thus, identify aggravating factors.

There are certain fundamental types of dermatitis such as atopic dermatitis, seborrhoeic dermatitis, allergic contact dermatitis and irritant contact dermatitis. Possible aggravating factors include contact allergens, contact irritants (chemical, physical), contact urticaria, extreme variations in temperature, low or high humidity,

15

Fig. 15.3 Seasonal variation in dermatitis. (**a**) *Atopic dermatitis:* fluctuates, severely pruritic, improves during the summer months. (**b**) *Psoriasis:* no pruritus, slow or no fluctuations, improves during the summer months. (**c**) *Dyshidrotic eczema:* eruptive throughout the year, often especially active during the summer months. (**d**) *Occupational dermatitis:* slow improvement seen over several consecutive days away from the workplace, fades during long periods of vacation, typically during the summer months; prompt recurrence upon resumption of work. (**e**) *Photodermatoses:* sudden onset during the spring, fluctuates during the summer months, fades during late summer; there is increased sun tolerance as pigmentation and epidermal thickness increase during the summer months

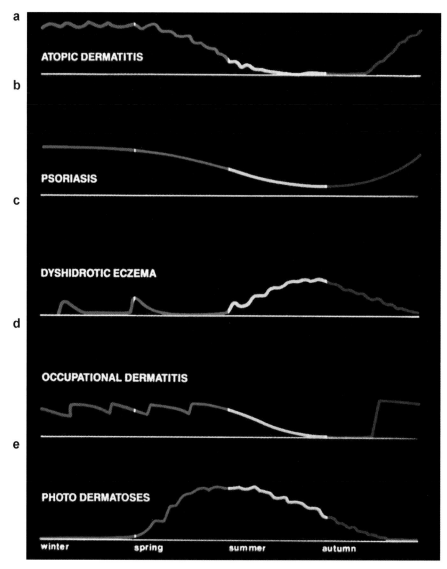

ingestion of certain foods, smoking, psychological stress, sweating, drug intake, sun exposure, infections (local and systemic), dermatophytes and yeasts, bacteria, herpes simplex virus [26, 27].

While discussing sun exposure with the patient, it should be stressed that offending ultraviolet irradiation can penetrate window glass, both in the home and in an automobile, as well as thin clothing. It should also be stressed that aggravation during outdoor activities is not necessarily related to the sun. Dermatitis in areas of the body normally exposed to the sun can also be caused by airborne irritants and allergens in dust particles, aerosols, pollen and other plant material [28]. Variations in patch test results due to meteorological conditions have been seen [29], and sun exposure may suppress immune reactions [30].

Core Message

> It is difficult for patients with persistent dermatitis to designate a precise time of onset. However, patients with chronic dermatitis may have either seasonal flares or sudden unexplained flares of dermatitis. Patients should be instructed to make note of circumstances related to sudden aggravation of their dermatitis.

15.2.6 Course of the Dermatitis

In dealing with chronic dermatoses it is important to record treatment response as well as response to the elimination of suspected causative substances. Some endogenous dermatoses like seborrhoeic dermatitis, for example, are easily suppressed by means of topical treatment, but recurrence is common. Contact dermatitis usually requires intensive treatment and recurs after discontinuation of therapy if the causative substance is not removed.

While allergic contact dermatitis usually recurs relatively quickly after re-exposure to the causative agent, irritant contact dermatitis tends to recur more slowly [31]. This difference can be useful in making the diagnosis.

The response to vacation periods and sick leave is of particular importance when occupational contact dermatitis is suspected. The result of re-exposure to the suspected causative agent is equally important.

15.2.7 Types of Symptoms

Pruritus is the fundamental symptom of irritant and allergic contact dermatitis, and in sensitized persons it usually occurs during the first day of further contact with the offending item. The intensity of symptoms varies greatly and depends on the type of dermatitis and also on various individual factors. Some persons with irritant contact dermatitis have practically no symptoms, while some adults with atopic dermatitis suffer so much from itching that it is difficult for them to sleep and carry out everyday tasks.

Subtle symptoms of insidious onset include the stinging sensation felt in some cosmetic reactions in which there is no visible physical symptom. Stinging can be caused by a number of substances and is elicited on very sensitive skin. This symptom does not necessarily represent irritancy in general [32]. Pain and burning, rather than itching, are frequent in phototoxic dermatitis like that caused by giant hogweed. A burning sensation is also common in herpes simplex and in herpes zoster. If it proves difficult to differentiate between the diagnosis of contact dermatitis and other dermatoses, a detailed description of the symptoms can be helpful.

Symptoms of contact urticaria are often noticed seconds to minutes after contact with the causative substance. Characteristically, the symptoms include stinging and smarting in addition to pruritus. Such symptoms are often caused by uncooked foods touching the perioral area or the hands or animal dander on exposed skin. In many patients, the symptoms fade quickly if the causative substance is rinsed off.

Mayonnaise preserved with sorbic acid caused an epidemic of perioral contact urticaria in a group of kindergarten children. The careful histories that were taken proved to be the most important tool in arriving at the correct diagnosis [33].

Patients who suffer from hay fever in the birch pollen season often have a history of contact urticaria of the oral mucosa caused by hazelnuts and apples due to antigens common to all three [34]. Birch pollen and grass may cause cellular immune reactions and contact dermatitis with an airborne pattern [35, 36]. An association has also been found between birch pollen allergy and reactions to apple, carrot, pear and cherry and between grass pollen and tomato and certain types of melon [37]. A careful history is, therefore, very important in the diagnostic work-up of patients with stomatitis and contact urticaria [38].

> **Core Message**
>
> ❯ Pruritus is the hallmark symptom of contact dermatitis. The intensity is variable and stinging may be more common than pruritus in cosmetic contact dermatitis. Phototoxic dermatitis is characterized by burning and smarting rather than pruritus. Contact urticaria is characterized by pruritus, burning or smarting seconds to minutes after contact with the offending substance.

15.3 Clinical Features of Eczematous Reactions

15.3.1 Acute and Recurrent Dermatitis

Spongiosis of the epidermis is one of the histological hallmarks of acute eczematous reactions. Clinically, confluence of spongiosis can lead to vesicles and even bullae [39] (see Chap. 9).

Macroscopically, vesicular response is associated with acute and recurrent contact dermatitis and is best visualized on the palms (Figs. 15.4 and 15.5), the sides of the fingers (Fig. 15.6), around the fingernails (Fig. 15.7) and on the soles of the feet. Vesicular eruptions on the palms and soles often occur simultaneously [40]. Vesicular palmar eruptions are not specific for eczema, as discussed under Differential Diagnosis.

Vesicular eruptions at other than the above-mentioned sites are uncommon. Acute dermatitis usually presents with papules, although occasionally with vesicles (Fig. 15.8) or even bullae (Fig. 15.9). The vesicular or bullous reaction may be seen in allergic as well as in irritant reactions and cannot be used to distinguish between these two types of dermatitis. A typical irritant, bullous contact dermatitis is the dermatitis seen after the application of cantharidine in the treatment of warts (Fig. 15.10).

The onset of an eczematous reaction can be more subtle. On the dorsa of the hands, the initial symptoms may be "chapping" (Fig. 15.11) [31]. Irritants may subsequently cause the chapping to progress to frank

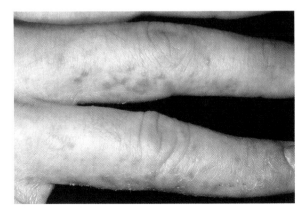

Fig. 15.6 Vesicles with inflammation on the sides of the fingers

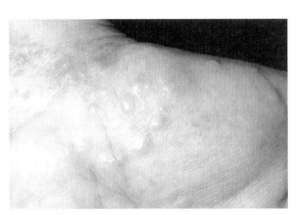

Fig. 15.4 Confluent vesicles on the palm

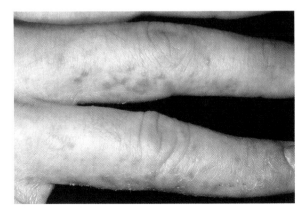

Fig. 15.7 Periungual vesicles

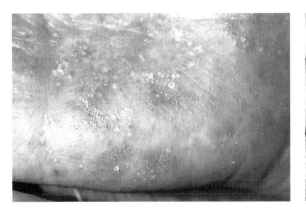

Fig. 15.5 Deep-seated vesicles on the palm

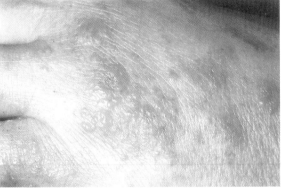

Fig. 15.8 Vesicular dermatitis on the dorsum of the hand

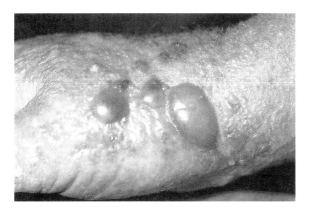

Fig. 15.9 Bullous dermatitis

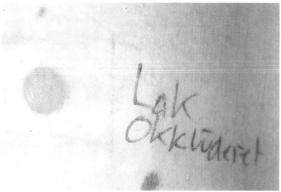

Fig. 15.12 A bullous irritant patch test reaction to a varnish

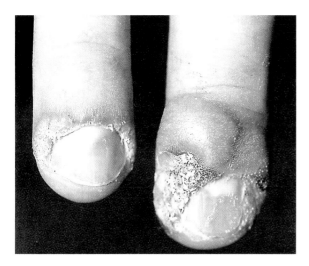

Fig. 15.10 Bullous periungual dermatitis caused by cantharidin

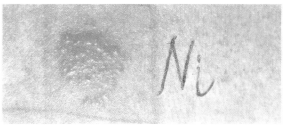

Fig. 15.13 A vesicular allergic patch test reaction to nickel

eczema. The environmental temperature and humidity are of significance for the development of dermatitis from low-grade irritants [41–44].

It is difficult to distinguish between allergic and irritant contact dermatitis. A distinction can sometimes be made at the site of "experimental" contact dermatitis, for example, a patch test site. Minimal itching occurs when a primary irritant is placed on the skin and subsequently occluded, and erythema and slight infiltration will be strictly limited to the area of the patch. Strong irritants may produce bullous or pustular reactions (Fig. 15.12), but these will also be limited to the occluded area. Similar occlusive testing with a substance to which the patient has a cellular immune reaction tends rather to give a markedly pruritic, infiltrated, papular or vesicular reaction that extends beyond the rim of the occluding disc (Fig. 15.13).

One possible explanation for this difference in the periphery of the test area may be that it is necessary to have a higher concentration of the offending substance to elicit an irritant reaction than to elicit an allergic reaction. The concentration of the substance used for a patch test will ordinarily be quite low outside the

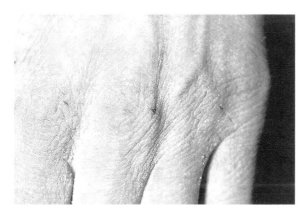

Fig. 15.11 "Chapping" on the dorsum of the hand

15

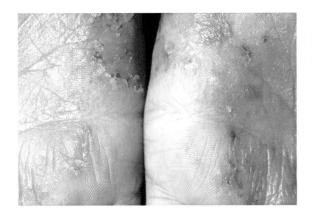

Fig. 15.14 Recurrent vesicular hand eczema mimicking chronic hand eczema. Note vesicles at the periphery of the involved area

occluded area and will, thus, be less than the amount necessary to elicit an irritant reaction, even though an allergic reaction may still occur. The recruitment of specifically sensitized cells and the ensuing release of non-specific cytokines facilitate the allergic response outside the area of direct contact.

The vesicular response is often seen as recurrent vesicular dermatitis of the palms and soles. If frequent acute eruptions occur, this type of eruption tends to take on the appearance of a chronic eczematous reaction. Careful inspection will often reveal a purely vesicular reaction, particularly at the periphery of the area of skin involved (Fig. 15.14).

15.3.2 Chronic Dermatitis

If contact with an offending item persists, chronic dermatitis may eventually develop. The characteristic features of chronic dermatitis are pruritus, lichenification, erythema, scaling, fissures and excoriations (Fig. 15.15). Histologically, spongiosis becomes less pronounced, and psoriasiform features supervene. The clinical correlate to this histological transition is lichen simplex chronicus (neurodermatitis) (Fig. 15.16).

15.3.3 Nummular (Discoid) Eczema

The term "nummular" (or "discoid") eczema is based on the morphology or coin shape of the lesions (Fig. 15.54). This type of dermatitis may be of

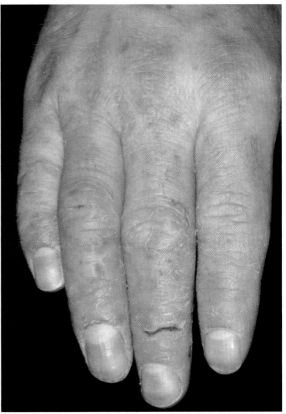

Fig. 15.15 Chronic hand eczema with fissures

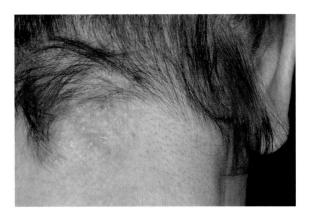

Fig. 15.16 Lichen simplex chronicus of the neck

endogenous origin and can be confused with contact dermatitis from soluble oils, irritant dermatitis from depilatory cream [45, 46] or with psoriasis. Secondary contact sensitization may occur [47].

15.3.4 Secondarily Infected Dermatitis

When, as in chronic dermatitis, the epidermal barrier is no longer intact, secondary infection can develop at the site of the dermatitis. In fact, chronic dermatitis is often the result of cumulative insults by irritants, microorganisms and allergens to which the patient has become sensitized. Frank bacterial infection of contact dermatitis is common (Fig. 15.17), and the possibility of pathogenic bacteria being present should, therefore, be considered before initiating treatment of chronic contact dermatitis.

Secondary infection should be distinguished from pustular irritant contact dermatitis caused by, for example, croton oil [48] or fluorouracil [49] and from palmo-plantar pustulosis, which typically exhibits pustules of uniform size as opposed to the varying size of the pustules in infected dermatitis (Fig. 15.18).

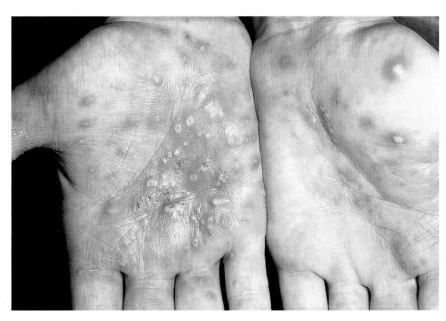

Fig. 15.17 Hand eczema with secondary bacterial infection

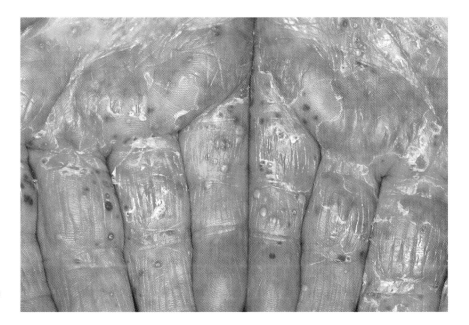

Fig. 15.18 Palmo-plantar pustulosis with uniform pustules and *brown*, dried-up lesions

15

15.3.5 Clinical Features of Contact Dermatitis in Specific Groups of Persons

The clinical features of contact dermatitis may vary among specific groups of persons.

15.3.5.1 Gender

Allergic contact dermatitis is more common among women than men. This is probably due more to exposure pattern than to gender [50]. Hand eczema is also more common among women than men [51].

15.3.5.2 Children

Children have been thought to develop allergic contact dermatitis less often than adults. However, recent literature indicates that allergic contact dermatitis is common in children. The pattern of sensitization is similar to that of adults [52–55].

Paraphenylene diamine used in so-called temporary henna tattoos is a commonly described cause of allergic contact dermatitis in children [56]. See case storey at the end of the chapter.

Epidemics of irritant contact dermatitis caused by caterpillars are particularly common among children. See the Sect. 15.4.2.3.

> **Core Message**
>
> > Children appear to develop contact dermatitis with the same frequency as adults. Babies may be an exception. The exposure pattern in children may be different from that of adults.

15.3.5.3 Elderly Persons

Elderly persons frequently develop allergic contact dermatitis from substances in topical medicaments, fragrances and balsam of Peru [57, 58]. Inflammatory reactions are more subtle in elderly persons [59], and their contact dermatitis, therefore, often has a scaly appearance and is less vesicular than in younger individuals. Dry

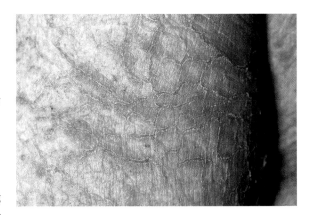

Fig. 15.19 Eczema craquelée on the lower leg

skin in combination with low humidity may in older persons cause a peculiar cracked "eczema craquelée", with inflammatory dermatitis and superficial breaks in the skin surface (Fig. 15.19).

> **Core Message**
>
> > Elderly persons often develop allergic contact dermatitis from medicaments, fragrances and balsam of Peru, as well as low-humidity dermatitis such as eczema craquelée.

15.3.5.4 Ethnicity

Black individuals and others with dark skin tend to develop hyperpigmentation and infiltration, particularly in chronic contact dermatitis, to a greater degree than those with light-coloured skin (Fig. 15.20). Contact dermatitis in dark-skinned persons frequently has the appearance of lichen simplex chronicus. The frequency of contact dermatitis or sensitive skin is probably unrelated to ethnicity [60–63]. Irritant contact dermatitis may be more common among persons of Asian descent than Caucasians [64].

15.3.5.5 Atopy

Patients with atopic dermatitis who develop allergic contact dermatitis from a given substance often react with both aggravation of their atopic dermatitis and a

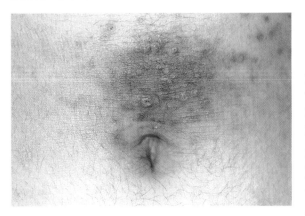

Fig. 15.20 Post-inflammatory hyperpigmentation following allergic nickel contact dermatitis

pattern of allergic contact dermatitis. There is some question as to the exact relationship between atopy and contact sensitization. It has been suggested that atopics become contact sensitized less often than non-atopics [65]. More recent investigations indicate that patients with atopic dermatitis have the same number of positive patch tests as non-atopics [66, 67].

Christophersen et al. [68] carried out a multivariate statistical analysis of various parameters in 2,166 patch-tested patients and found that nickel allergy was significantly less common among atopics than non-atopics. This difference could not be demonstrated for other common contact allergens. Since nickel is a ubiquitous environmental allergen, atopics and non-atopics are equally exposed to this allergen.

Negative nickel patch tests in patients with a history of nickel allergy have been linked to atopy [69], but no agreement has as yet been reached on the relevancy of such findings [70].

Irritant hand eczema is common among children with atopic dermatitis [71].

Core Message

> ❯ While contact allergy may be slightly less common in atopic persons than in non-atopic persons, irritant hand eczema is more common in persons with atopy. Ethnicity does not appear to play a role in contact allergy, but the exposure pattern may vary among races.

15.4 Identifying the Cause of Contact Dermatitis from the Clinical Pattern

It is often difficult to trace the substance that has caused the skin to react to contact, particularly if the patient has chronic lesions. Reactions to substances that are not a part of everyday life, such as dinitrochlorobenzene or infrequently used topical drugs, usually present little diagnostic difficulty, while the source of reactions to ubiquitous allergens like nickel and fragrances may be much more difficult to trace. Certain patterns of skin disease can, however, point in the direction of particular groups of substances, or even towards one specific causative substance.

15.4.1 Clinical Patterns Indicating General Causes of Contact Dermatitis

15.4.1.1 Contact Pattern

In the most obvious cases, an eczematous reaction is seen at the exact site of contact with the offending item. This type of reaction is frequently recognized by the patient and will commonly not be brought to the attention of a physician.

A typical example of contact-pattern dermatitis is allergic nickel contact dermatitis (Fig. 15.21). Historically, the most characteristic nickel contact sites have changed with changes in women's fashions. While, in the 1930s, most of Bonnevie's [72] patients had dermatitis at the site of contact with nickel-plated stocking suspender clasps, later the metal hooks on brassieres became a common offender. In the 1970s, sites of contact with metal buttons and studs in blue jeans became the most common sites of nickel dermatitis. At present, the earlobes, particularly if the patient has pierced ears [73], and sites of contact with nickel-plated watch bands and clasps are the most common primary sites of nickel dermatitis. A persistent patch of allergic contact dermatitis on the cheek can be caused by contact with a multi-function key on a cell phone [74]. Euro coins caused nickel dermatitis on the fingers of a taxi driver [75]. Gawkrodger et al. [76] examined 134 patients with positive patch tests to nickel and found the following prevalence of sites: palm 49%, dorsum

15

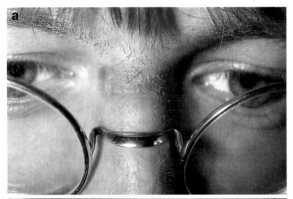

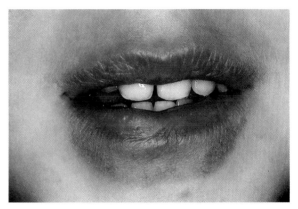

Fig. 15.22 Irritant contact dermatitis with sharp demarcation caused by lip licking

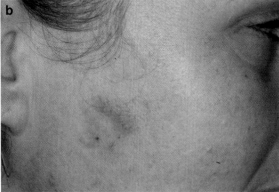

Fig. 15.21 (**a**) Allergic nickel contact dermatitis. (**b**) Allergic nickel contact dermatitis from the multi-function key in a cellular phone

of the hands 39%, wrist 22%, face 20%, arm 16%, neck 14% and periorbital area 12%.

A study carried out in Singapore showed the most common sites to be the wrist, the ears and the waist [77]. The contact pattern of nickel dermatitis is also dependent on cultural tradition and on the groups of patients studied, as well as on climatic factors. For example, sweating caused by high temperatures increases the release of nickel from nickel-plated items [78]. Nickel is also released by plasma, a fact which may explain the high rate of nickel sensitization after ear piercing [79].

In 1969, Kanan [80] described the typical site of nickel dermatitis among males in Kuwait as the sites of contact with metal studs in undergarments. Fisher [81] noted that the most common sites of nickel dermatitis in males were under blue jeans' buttons and under watchbands.

Unusual sites of nickel contact dermatitis seen by the author include a small eczematous patch at the entry site of a venepuncture needle and a patch of

eczema caused by the small nickel-plated part of a rubber stopper used to make a prosthesis airtight. Nickel dermatitis has also developed at sites of Dermojet injection [82], sites of the closure of surgical wounds with skin clips [83], and in tattoos, possibly due to contamination with nickel in red tattoo pigment [84].

Irritant contact dermatitis occurring under objects that occlude the skin, such as the metal case of a watch or a plastic watchstrap, may mimic nickel dermatitis. Repeated licking of the lips may cause irritant contact dermatitis induced by humidity and irritants in saliva. Such dermatitis is seen in areas that can be reached by the tongue (Fig. 15.22). Compulsive washing of the hands may cause irritant dermatitis on the dorsum of the hands and part of the forearms (Fig. 15.23). An older woman developed peculiar irritant dermatitis on her back due to compulsive washing with soap (Fig. 15.24).

The rubber in the elastic used in undergarments, for example brassieres, may produce characteristic patterns of dermatitis [85]. Contact-pattern dermatitis may also be caused by the chemicals in rubber used in the manufacture of shoes.

Topical medicaments may also produce eczematous contact-pattern reactions, and these often have a biphasic course. Improvement initially seen following the use of a certain medicament applied to relieve an existing problem may be followed by aggravation in the area of application.

If a contact allergen – typically a topical drug – repeatedly applied to the legs of a sensitized person results in severe dermatitis, this will tend to spread in an id-like manner to the arms and possibly to the entire

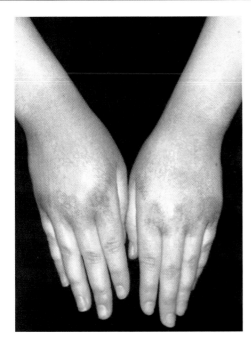

Fig. 15.23 Irritant contact dermatitis in a young girl caused by compulsive hand washing

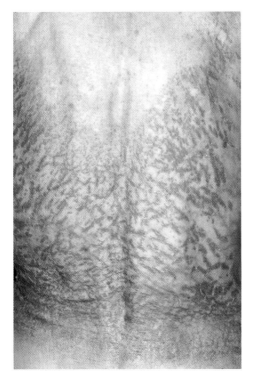

Fig. 15.24 Severe irritant contact dermatitis. This woman's husband washed her back 3 times a day with soap because he thought her itching was due to an infestation

body. This pattern of spread is also seen in severe stasis dermatitis, and it has been suggested that in patients with stasis dermatitis such spread is caused by cell-mediated autoimmunity [86, 87].

Since dermatitis caused by topical medicaments is most common in occluded areas and at sites where the skin is particularly delicate, this cause should be suspected if there is aggravation of existing dermatitis of the anogenital area, the lower leg, the ear or the eyelids [88–90].

Treatment with caustic agents may produce ulcerations at the sites of application. Severe reactions may follow the erroneous use of topical wart remedies applied to nevi on parts of the body that are normally occluded.

The computer mouse is suggested as the cause of contact dermatitis in the form of both allergic contact dermatitis [91] and as occlusive dermatitis with negative patch tests (Fig. 15.25).

Certain contact allergens can produce contact-pattern dermatitis that does not appear at the actual site of contact. Nail polish is such an allergen, and typical sites of allergic contact dermatitis caused by nail polish are the eyelids, neck and genitalia, rather than the skin around the fingernails [92].

> **Core Message**
>
> > The contact pattern of contact dermatitis depends on fashion and local traditions. Some contact allergens cause dermatitis at distant sites – eyelid dermatitis may, for example, be caused by nail polish.

15.4.1.2 Streaked Dermatitis in Exposed Areas

Dermatitis may appear in streaks if it has been caused by liquids allowed to run down the skin. Caustic substances such as those used by farmers to clean milking equipment can cause such reactions. Dermatitis caused by plant juices or the toxin from jellyfish like the Portuguese man-of-war often appears in a bizarre streaked pattern [93]. Dermatitis caused by juices from Umbelliferae is often phototoxic. Upon resolution, a streaked bullous dermatitis can be followed by marked hyperpigmentation which may last for many months (Figs. 15.26 and 15.27).

15

Fig. 15.25 Irritant or sweat retention dermatitis on the palmar side of the fingers of the right hand caused by prolonged contact with a computer mouse

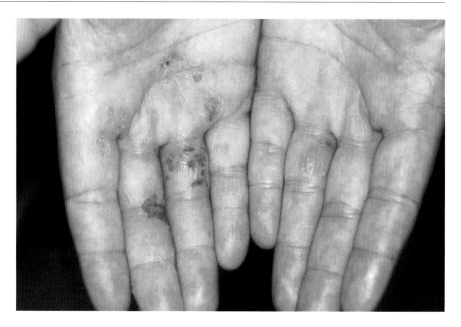

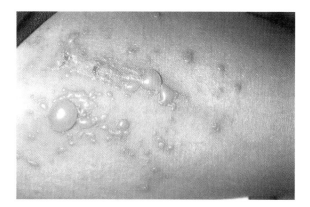

Fig. 15.26 Phototoxic dermatitis caused by giant hogweed

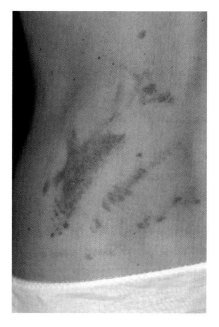

Fig. 15.27 Post-inflammatory hyperpigmentation following resolution of phototoxic dermatitis caused by plants

15.4.1.3 Airborne Contact Dermatitis

Airborne contact dermatitis may be caused by such substances as

1. Fibrous materials such as glass fibre, rock wool and grain dust, which give rise to mechanical dermatitis [94]
2. Wood and cement dust, which cause irritant reactions [95]. Wood may also sensitize
3. Dust containing particles from plants like *Parthenium hysterophorus*, ragweed or certain types of wood or medicaments to which the patient has delayed-type sensitivity [96–99]
4. Aerosols of mineral oils that cause irritant reactions.

Santos and Goossens have reviewed the causes of airborne contact dermatitis [100].

Particles of medicaments in the dust from, for example, pigsties can cause dermatitis if the patient has contact allergy to the medicament in question. Airborne contact dermatitis appears on areas of the skin where the dust or fibres can be trapped, for example on the eyelids, neck (under a shirt collar), forearms (under cuffs) or lower legs (inside trouser legs) [28, 101]. Chronic airborne contact dermatitis tends to mimic photocontact dermatitis [102]. A combination of these two forms of dermatitis may also be seen.

Dermatitis from wood dust and dust from plant particles often cause lichenified dermatitis at the sites of contact. The handling of large amounts of carbonless copy paper and laser printed paper can cause irritation of the mucous membranes of the nose and eyes and pruritus on exposed skin. In one study an increased level of plasma histamine was documented after exposure to carbonless copy paper [103].

Various cutaneous symptoms, including pruritus and paraesthesia, have been described after long-term exposure to computer screens, but few patients exhibit diagnostic skin lesions [104, 105].

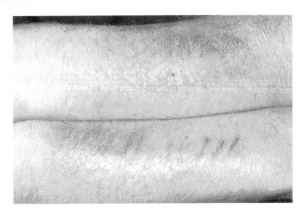

Fig. 15.28 Abrasion caused by contact with rough fibres in a sack made of jute

> ### Core Message
>
> › Airborne contact dermatitis can mimic photo contact dermatitis. Airborne contact dermatitis may be seen on exposed skin and at sites where dust is trapped under a shirt collar, shirt cuffs or trouser legs.

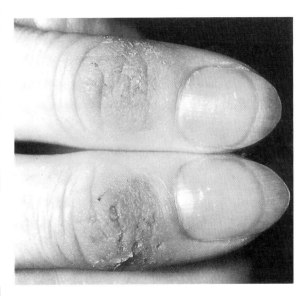

Fig. 15.29 Mechanical contact dermatitis caused by manipulation of the skin

15.4.1.4 Mechanical Dermatitis

Friction can cause both hyperkeratosis and dermatitis. Acute lesions may appear as actual abrasions of the skin (Fig. 15.28), while chronic mechanical dermatitis is often more subtle, and therefore, more difficult to diagnose. Mechanical trauma is particularly important as an occupational disorder [106, 107]. Most computer-related, occupational dermatoses are mechanical [108, 109].

The handling of large quantities of paper, for example computer printouts, may eventually lead to hyperkeratosis on the involved fingers. Eczematous dermatitis may develop after long-term, often unconscious, manipulation of the skin (Fig. 15.29). Some popular sports activities have given rise to new dermatological entities caused by physical trauma. These include "rower's rump", "jogger's nipples", "black heel", [110–112], "canyoning hand" [113] and "baseball pitcher's friction dermatitis" [114].

Mechanical dermatitis on the inner aspects of the thighs may mimic intertrigo. The treatment given to HIV-positive patients may cause "buffalo hump", and mechanical dermatitis may be seen on the hump [115]. Bizarre patterns of dermatitis and purpura may result

15

from curious cultural habits, such as coin rubbing. Unusual patterns of skin lesions can also be seen in the victims of physical or electrical torture. Cellular phone chargers caused ulcerations at the site of contact in two persons who slept on the chargers [116].

Core Message

> Mechanical contact dermatitis is a consequence of repeated physical trauma at the site of contact. Characteristic patterns of mechanical contact dermatitis are seen among participants in certain sports.

15.4.1.5 Hyperkeratotic Eczema

Symmetrical, hyperkeratotic plaques on the central parts of the palms and/or soles represent an entity that is clinically distinct from other types of eczema, because no vesicles are seen. At the onset of an eruption, this dermatitis is often pruritic, while pruritus is uncommon in chronic lesions (Fig. 15.30). Although this type of eczema is distinct from psoriasis histologically, clinically, it is difficult to distinguish from psoriasis [117]. The aetiology is unknown. The condition is most common in middle-aged men, and is very

persistent and aggravated by mechanical trauma. The condition can be treated with oral acitretin [118].

15.4.1.6 Ring Dermatitis

Dermatitis that occurs under tight-fitting jewellery, such as finger rings, can be due to allergic reactions to constituents of the jewellery. Ring finger dermatitis is significantly more common in patients who are patch test positive to gold sodium thiosulfate than in patients who do not have this contact allergy [119]. If a ring is made of relatively pure gold or of plastic, this type of eczema is most commonly due to sweat retention and the accumulation under the ring of occluded irritants from detergents (Fig. 15.31).

15.4.1.7 Follicular Reactions

Folliculitis or an acneiform appearance may develop following cutaneous contact with or the absorption of certain polyhalogenated aromatic hydrocarbons, such as dioxin, or following skin contact with crude oil or its derivatives. Exposed areas of the body are most commonly involved due to direct contact or to aerosols (Fig. 15.32), but chloracne caused by the inhalation of chlorinated compounds can appear on parts of the body which are normally covered, and oil folliculitis may occur on the thighs if a patient has worn trousers that

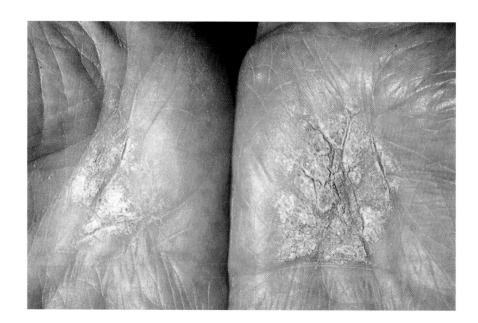

Fig. 15.30 Hyperkeratotic palmar eczema

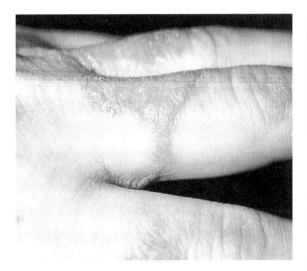

Fig. 15.31 Irritant contact dermatitis under a finger ring

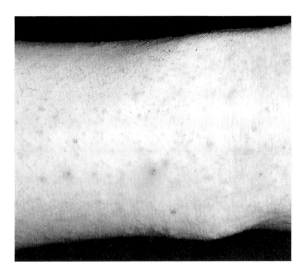

Fig. 15.32 Folliculitis caused by oil

have become soaked in oil. Pomade acne of the forehead caused by oils applied to the hair is usually found only on the forehead and the temples, while cosmetic acne is most often distributed over the entire face [120].

Allergic contact dermatitis may appear as a pustular dermatosis. Pustular reactions have been described in allergic contact dermatitis caused by mercaptobenzo-thiazoles [121]. A galvanizer was seen to have occupational contact folliculitis [122]. Pustular patch test reactions, interpreted as non-allergic, were seen in 2% of 853 persons tested with sodium tungstate. The reactions were often reproducible [123].

Core Message

> Follicular or pustular reactions are commonly due to irritant reactions to mineral oils or certain pesticides. Pustular reactions are rarely an expression of allergic contact dermatitis.

15.4.1.8 Connubial and Consort Dermatitis

Contact with rubber condoms can cause genital eczema in women. Allergic contact urticaria may occur following contact with semen, and such contact can also cause systemic symptoms and even anaphylactic reactions [124, 125]. Males can develop dermatitis of the penis after contact with contraceptive cream. Connubial dermatitis is not confined solely to the genitals, as witnessed by the fact that some women develop allergic contact dermatitis on the face after contact with a partner's aftershave lotion or other cosmetic preparations used by the sexual partner [126, 127].

15.4.1.9 Recurrent Vesicular Hand and/or Foot Dermatitis

This common pruritic dermatosis occurs as eruptions of crops of vesicles on the palms, the sides of fingers, the central part of the soles or the sides of the toes (Figs. 15.4–15.7). There may be little or no inflammation. The eruptions heal with subsequent scaling, but repeated frequent eruptions may lead to dermatitis that presents as chronic hand and/or foot eczema. Recurrent vesicular dermatitis is a non-specific clinical reaction pattern that may be caused by external agents, but it is commonly considered to be an example of an endogenous dermatosis [40, 128] (see Chap. 16). There is a statistical correlation between vesicular eruptions on the hands and tinea pedis [129].

Core Message

> Recurrent vesicular hand dermatitis is an eruptive, pruritic, vesicular, non-specific reaction pattern on palmar or plantar skin. This pattern is seen in both contact dermatitis and endogenous dermatitis.

15

15.4.1.10 Fingertip Eczema (Pulpitis)

Contact dermatitis of the fingertips, particularly on the thumb and the index and middle fingers of the non-dominant hand, is a common ailment among chefs due to their repeated contact with irritants or allergens found in plants such as garlic (Fig. 15.33). Dental technicians and dentists can also develop fingertip eczema on the same three digits – but on the dominant hand – due to contact with the acrylic substances used to make dental prostheses and plastic dental fillings [130, 131].

Pulpitis can also present as mechanical contact dermatitis in persons who handle large amounts of paper and cardboard.

Some children develop pulpitis on all ten digits. Clinically, shiny erythema, possibly with fissures, is seen. Although some children with this condition have a history of atopic dermatitis, the aetiology is unknown.

15.4.1.11 Eczema Nails

A characteristic pattern of transverse grooves and ridges may be seen in the nail plates of patients with eczema on the dorsal aspects of the fingers. There is usually also involvement or disappearance of the nail cuticle. The number of grooves on the nail often

corresponds to the number of episodes of flare of the eczema (Fig. 15.34). Subungual vesicular dermatitis under the periphery of the nail plate is less common [132]. This pattern of subungual dermatitis has been seen, however, following work with anaerobic acrylic sealants [133]. Allergic contact dermatitis from formaldehyde-based hardening resins in nail polish and acrylates used to build up artificial nails can cause severe nail damage, including irreversible nail dystrophy [134, 135].

15.4.1.12 Papular and Nodular Excoriated Lesions

Most reported cases of delayed hypersensitivity to aluminium have occurred following deposition in the dermis or subcutis of vaccines used for childhood immunizations or following hyposensitization procedures. Persistent, pruritic, excoriated, deeply infiltrated lesions at injection sites are characteristic (Fig. 15.35 and 15.36) [136–139]. Histologically, histiocytic infiltrates are characteristic, but other features may be present [140]. Intolerance to antiperspirants that contain aluminium salts has been described, but such cases appear to be rare [141].

Infiltrated papular lesions have also been seen at the sites of injection of zinc-bound insulin. The patients in

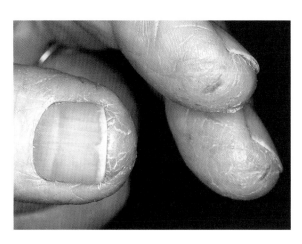

Fig. 15.33 Pulpitis caused by the handling of garlic on the thumb, index and middle fingers of the non-dominant hand of a garlic-sensitive woman

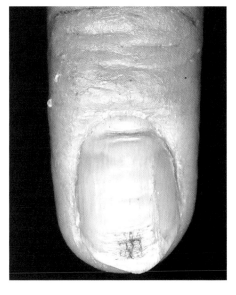

Fig. 15.34 Transverse ridges and grooves in the nail plate of a patient with eczema on the dorsal aspects of the fingers

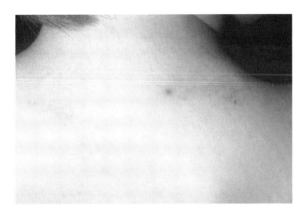

Fig. 15.35 Persistent, pruritic infiltrates following childhood immunizations in an aluminium-sensitive child

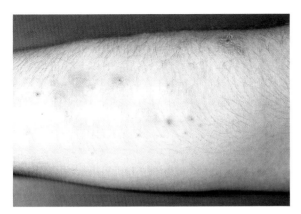

Fig. 15.36 Papular, nodular and excoriated lesions in an aluminium-sensitive person following hyposensitization with a vaccine containing aluminium

question had zinc hypersensitivity, as demonstrated by intra-cutaneous testing and lymphocyte transformation studies [142]. There have been no further reports of such cases. A similar morphology of contact sensitization is seen if tattoo pigment causes sensitization. Chromium, cobalt and mercury salts used to be common sensitizing tattoo pigments [143]. Modern tattoo pigments, however, rarely sensitize. See also the Sect. 15.5.7.

Core Message

> Pruritic, papular, excoriated infiltrates at the sites of childhood immunizations or hyposensitization injections may be due to contact allergy to aluminium – otherwise a rare sensitizer.

15.4.1.13 Contact Urticaria of the Hands and Lips

Contact urticaria should be suspected if dermatitis or intermittent urticaria is seen on the lips and/or the hands, particularly if an itching or a burning sensation has arisen seconds to minutes after contact with uncooked food items or with latex gloves (Fig. 15.37). Anaphylactic reactions may also occur. The symptoms on the hands sometimes disappear when the hands are rinsed; in some cases hand eczema develops or, more commonly, an existing hand eczema is aggravated [144–146]. This problem is particularly common among atopics. A skin application food test (SAFT) has been developed to diagnose this type of dermatitis in children [147]. Allergens in food may penetrate eczematous skin, but the same allergens usually cannot penetrate intact skin [148] (see Chap. 5).

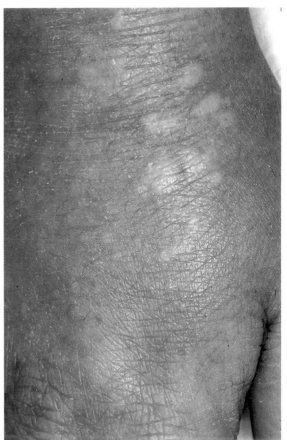

Fig. 15.37 Contact urticaria due to latex seen after a few minutes of challenge with/or exposure to latex gloves

15

15.4.1.14 Clinical Patterns of Systemically Induced Contact Dermatitis

If a substance to which a person has developed cellular immunity due to contact with the skin is subsequently ingested or otherwise absorbed, a variety of cutaneous reactions may occur (see Chap. 17) [149, 150]. Vesiculation of the hands, for example, may be seen in patients who have not previously experienced this reaction pattern. A patient who suffers from recurrent vesicular hand eczema may experience a flare of dermatitis after experimental oral challenge with the substance to which he or she is sensitive. One nickel-sensitive patient developed palmar vesicles and small bullae a few days after beginning a weight-reducing diet that called for the ingestion of vegetables rich in nickel. Nickel-sensitive patients may have dermal lesions with evidence of vasculitis, which can be reproduced by placebo-controlled oral challenge [151]. A keratotic eruption of the elbows has been described as accompanying a systemically induced dermatitis [152].

So-called secondary eruptions were noted by Calnan [153] when he described the clinical features of large groups of nickel-allergic patients. These secondary eruptions consisted of erythematous flares in skin folds such as the antecubital fossae and on the sides of the neck, the eyelids and the inner thighs. Widespread oedematous erythema in the skin folds of the anogenital area has been termed the "baboon syndrome" [154], and oedematous lesions of this type have also been observed in nickel-sensitive patients following oral challenge with nickel [155].

Sensitization from the topical application of drugs is common. If a drug to which a patient is sensitized is taken orally, a variety of reactions can be seen, ranging from recurrence of the dermatitis in its original site and reactivation of a patch test site, to widespread dermatitis. Such widespread dermatitis may be accompanied by fever and toxic epidermal necrolysis, which may be life-threatening [17, 156, 157]. Toxicoderma and fever have also been seen in gold-sensitive patients after the intramuscular injection of gold preparations [4].

Fixed drug eruption is a distinct nummular eruption occurring repeatedly in the same location after the ingestion of the drug in question [158]. The reaction may be triggered by intra-epidermal CD8+ T-cells at the site of the eruption [159].

Core Message

> The systemic administration of a hapten in contact sensitized persons can lead to a variety of symptoms such as flare-up of the current dermatitis or previous sites of contact dermatitis or previous patch test sites. Vesicular eruptions on the hands, flexural dermatitis or widespread rashes or the "baboon syndrome" may be seen.

15.4.2 Characteristic Clinical Patterns of Dermatitis Associated with Specific Substances or Types of Application

15.4.2.1 Cement Ulcerations

Caustic reactions and acute irritant contact dermatitis at the site of prolonged contact with wet cement are sometimes seen under the tops of socks or on other parts of the lower leg that are normally occluded. The alkalinity of the cement and prolonged skin contact with wet cement are the most likely causes of this dermatitis [160–162] (Fig. 15.38).

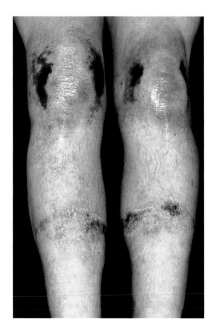

Fig. 15.38 Caustic reaction caused by cement

15.4.2.2 Pigmented Contact Dermatitis

Optical brighteners were originally described by Osmundsen and Alani [163] as the cause of severely pruritic, purpuric, allergic contact dermatitis, which caused little or no discernible change in the epidermis. In Japan, pigmented contact dermatitis is relatively common [164]. A resin commonly used in the dyeing of cotton fabrics (Naphthol AS) can cause pigmented allergic contact dermatitis, which is typically seen on the neck and upper arms [165] (see Chap. 19).

15.4.2.3 Caterpillar Dermatitis and Irritant Dermatitis from Plants and Animals

Spicules hidden among the hairs of certain caterpillars contain a toxin that can cause persistent pruritic vesicles or papules at sites of contact with the skin. This is a characteristic clinical finding among children who have played with these caterpillars [166, 167] (Fig. 15.39). Sun-worshippers may come in contact with this toxin on beaches where large numbers of such species of caterpillars have wandered in procession [168, 169]. Occupational immunologic contact urticaria has also been described [170]. Similar toxic substances are found in sea urchins and sea anemones and in various plants such as those of the *Dieffenbachia* species and in *Agave tequilana* [171]. Mechanical injuries from thorns and similar projections on plants or fish may mimic this dermatosis [172].

> ### Core Message
>
> ➤ Long-lasting, pruritic, papular and vesicular eruptions may result from contact with spicules from certain caterpillars. Children who play with caterpillars have eruptions on the hands, while forestry workers may have more widespread eruptions.

15.4.2.4 Head and Neck Dermatitis

Adults with atopic dermatitis and persistent pruritic dermatitis of the face, the sides of the neck and the

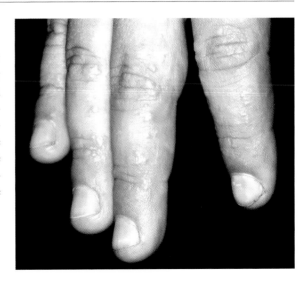

Fig. 15.39 Persistent papules and vesicles on the fingers of a child who played with a caterpillar

shoulders may have immediate-type sensitivity to the saprophytic fungus *Pityrosporum ovale* [173, 174].

15.4.2.5 Dermatitis from Transcutaneous Delivery Systems

Eczematous lesions, as well as general cutaneous reactions and systemic symptoms, sometimes occur where trans-cutaneous drug delivery systems have been applied [175, 176]. Generally speaking, such reactions are rare. Continuous percutaneous drug delivery systems are used for such drugs as clonidine, nitroglycerin, scopolamine, oestradiol, nicotine and buprenorphine [177, 178]. Studies of why the drugs applied in this manner sometimes cause cutaneous reactions have revealed that a limited number of patients have allergic contact dermatitis from the active drug or from ingredients in the delivery system itself [179–181]. Oral ingestion of the drugs in question has been seen to produce widespread dermatitis in a few patients [177].

15.4.2.6 Berloque Dermatitis

The application of perfumes on the sides of the neck may give rise to a phototoxic reaction with oedematous dermatitis and subsequent pigmentation at the exact sites of application of the perfume [182].

15

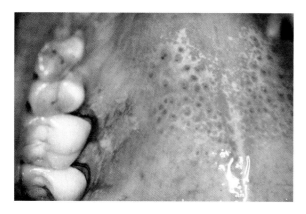

Fig. 15.40 Oral lichenoid lesions in a gold-sensitive person (courtesy of P.J. Frosch)

15.4.2.7 Stomatitis Due to Mercury or Gold Allergy

Greyish streaks, erythema or erosions on the oral mucous membranes at sites of contact with amalgam dental fillings indicate irritant or allergic contact stomatitis from the mercury in the amalgam fillings or from the gold on capped teeth (Fig. 15.40). There has been some controversy as to the use of amalgam dental fillings containing mercury. This entity is discussed in detail in the Sect. 15.6.

15.5 Regional Contact Dermatitis

The diagnosis of contact dermatitis is facilitated by a thorough knowledge of substances that characteristically cause dermatitis of specific areas of the skin. Computer analyses of the relationship between eczema sites and contact allergens have shown statistically significant correlations between, for example, nickel and cobalt and various sites on the fingers and palms, and between lanolin and the lower legs. Sensitivity to the fragrance mix was shown to correlate with dermatitis of the axillae, sensitivity to balsam of Peru with dermatitis of the face and the lower legs and sensitivity to neomycin and "caine" mix with dermatitis of the lower leg [183]. Other examples of substances that cause dermatitis in specific areas of the body are presented in the following sections.

15.5.1 Dermatitis of the Scalp

Allergic contact dermatitis of the scalp itself is surprisingly rare in view of the fact that the level of percutaneous absorption of the skin of the scalp is high compared with other areas of the body. While sensitization to leave-on products such as pomades and minoxidil does occur, dermatitis is more commonly seen on adjacent areas such as the ears, forehead and sides of the neck than on the scalp itself [184–187] (Fig 15.41).

Contact sensitizers applied to the scalp, such as thioglycolates in permanent wave solutions or dyes used to colour the hair, more frequently causes hand eczema in the persons who apply the substances than contact dermatitis in the person to whom they are applied [188]. Fifty-five patients who had their hair dyed had rather severe reactions in the face or on the scalp. All those patch tested reacted to paraphenylene diamine [189].

Contact dermatitis of the scalp may be followed by telogen effluvium [190].

Nickel in hairpins and decorative items of nickel used near the scalp may cause dermatitis at the sites of contact.

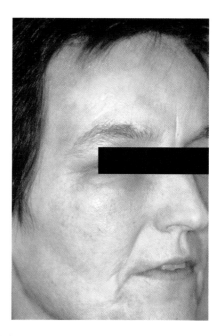

Fig. 15.41 A woman developed edematous facial dermatitis and dermatitis of the neck after having her hair dyed. She had a positive patch test to paraphenylene diamine

Rinse-off products such as shampoos may cause allergic contact dermatitis of the scalp due to surfactants, preservatives or fragrances, but such reactions are rare in view of the amounts used [191–196]. Patients who have previously become sensitized to preservatives may react to similar compounds in shampoos and other hair-care products. Methyl dibromoglutaranitril is an example of a preservative that commonly sensitizes. The use of this preservative in cosmetics has now (2009) been banned in the European Union. Bovine collagen in hair conditioners can cause contact urticaria of the scalp and face [197]. Medicated shampoos, for example those containing tar, may cause irritant contact dermatitis of the scalp or aggravation of the seborrhoeic dermatitis or psoriasis they were intended to improve.

Microorganisms like *Pityrosporum ovale* may aggravate existing diseases of the scalp, and seborrhoeic dermatitis of the scalp has been seen to improve following treatment with ketoconazole shampoo [198, 199]. Bacterial infection may aggravate atopic dermatitis of the scalp and cause folliculitis as well as exudative dermatitis.

Discoloration of the hair due to external contactants may be due to the copper salts found in swimming pool water (green colour), dithranol (anthralin) preparations used on the scalp (reddish colour) or hydroxyquinoline preparations (brownish-yellow colour). Irritant dermatitis may be seen after bleaching the hair (Fig. 15.42).

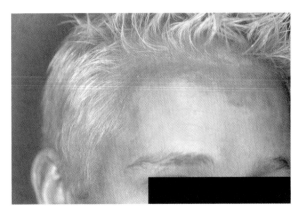

Fig. 15.42 A young man developed irritant contact dermatitis of the frontal and temporal regions after lightening his hair

---

Core Message

> Contact dermatitis caused by irritants or contact allergens applied to the scalp commonly cause dermatitis on the forehead, the ears and the neck. Hair dyes and permanent wave solutions are more often the cause than rinse-off products.

15.5.2 Dermatitis of the Face and Neck

The face and neck, like the backs of the hands, are the areas of the body most heavily exposed to the sun. These areas are, therefore, the prime targets for photocontact dermatitis. Common causes of photosensitive dermatoses were reviewed by Fotiades et al. [200]. Compositae plants and lichen are among the causes of this dermatosis [201]. In typical cases, the symptoms of this photodermatosis are burning, stinging and itching. There is a sharp delineation along the collar and no dermatitis under the chin or behind the earlobes. Less typical cases may include symptoms similar to the above but with little to be seen on physical examination. The pigmentation seen following some types of phototoxic contact dermatitis is caused by furocoumarins, and such pigmentation is in itself almost diagnostic.

Photocontact dermatitis following contact with tar products appears where drops of, for example, wood preservatives have fallen on the skin. Hyperpigmentation is more commonly seen after photocontact dermatitis caused by furocoumarins than by tar.

Photocontact dermatitis that remains undiagnosed, or which is caused by substances that are difficult to avoid, may eventually become what is known as chronic actinic dermatitis or the actinic reticuloid syndrome [202–204]. The aetiology of this entity is not clear, and airborne contact dermatitis may be a causative factor. Even when the substance causing this dermatitis has been removed, some patients remain permanently light sensitive.

The face and neck are also typical sites of airborne contact dermatitis, which in its early phases may be distinguished from photocontact dermatitis by the presence of dermatitis in sub-mental areas and behind the ears. Airborne contact dermatitis is commonly most intense where dust is trapped under the shirt collar, while light-induced dermatitis is seen only above the collar. An airborne pattern of dermatitis may be

15

caused by plants, in particular plants of the Compositae family [205–208] (Fig. 15.43), or among farm workers from fodder and cow dander [209, 210].

A typical mechanical dermatitis in this area is the classic fiddler's neck, caused by long-term contact with the chin rest on a violin [211].

Allergic contact dermatitis of the neck is commonly caused by nickel in jewellery, but jewellery made of exotic woods can also be the cause [212]. Plastics rarely cause dermatitis on the neck. Nurses in intensive-care units who wear a stethoscope for many hours a day may develop nickel dermatitis on the sides of the neck.

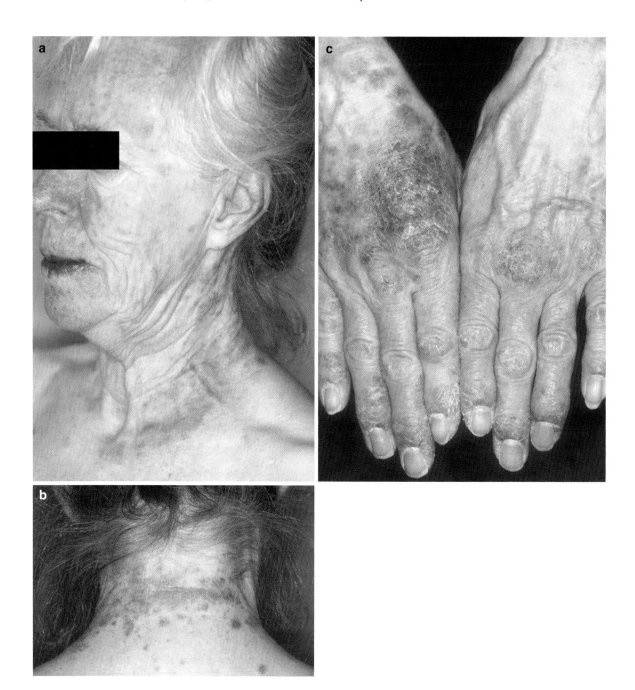

Fig. 15.43 A woman sensitive to sesquinterpene lactone developed airborne contact dermatitis of the face (**a**), neck (**b**) and dorsal aspects of the hands (**c**)

In a study by Hausen and Oestmann [213], 50% of 64 flower vendors with contact dermatitis caused by plants had dermatitis of the face. The most common causative plants were chrysanthemums, tulips and alstroemeria, while daffodils and primulas were rarely the cause.

Facial dermatitis is commonly caused by cosmetics [214]. Of 13,216 patients with contact dermatitis seen by members of the North American Contact Dermatitis Group over a 5-year period, 713 had dermatitis caused by cosmetics. Interestingly, in most cases, neither patient nor physician had suspected cosmetics as the cause of the contact dermatitis on the basis of the clinical features, and diagnoses were not made until the results of patch testing were known. 81% of the patients had dermatitis that could be described as allergic contact dermatitis; irritation accounted for the reactions of 16% of the patients, and phototoxic and photoallergic reactions each accounted for less than 1% of the reactions. Fragrances, preservatives, hair-colouring agents and permanent wave solutions accounted for most of the cases of allergic contact dermatitis seen in this study [215]. Eight men developed dermatitis of the beard area due to para-phenylenediamine in dyes for the beard [216].

In an investigation of positive patch tests to preservatives, Jacobs et al. [217] found that the face was the most commonly involved site for relevant reactions to the preservatives quaternium-15, 2-bromo-2-nitropropane-1,3-diol, imidazolidinyl urea and diazolidinyl urea. Over time, the relative frequency of allergy to quaternium-15 has decreased. Allergy to methyl dibromoglutaranitrile is, on the other hand, increasing in frequency [218]. As the use of the preservative in cosmetics has been banned in the European Union, it is expected that the frequency will decline.

The use of soap containing chromium is a rare cause of pigmented contact dermatitis of the face [219]. De-pigmentation may also be seen following the use of cosmetic products such as toothpaste containing cinnamic aldehyde (cinnamal) [220] and the use of incense [221].

Ammonium persulfate used to bleach hair is a peculiar substance in that it may produce symptoms in both the hairdresser and the customer, following either contact with the solution used to treat the hair or airborne particles of it. The substance can cause histamine release, leading to severe respiratory symptoms and urticaria. It may also produce irritant contact dermatitis and allergic reactions, which may be either immediate-type or delayed-type [222] (Fig. 15.42).

Cosmetic acne presenting as discrete poral occlusion is common. An acneiform folliculitis of the forehead known as pomade acne is occasionally seen after the long-term use of oily hair-care products [120]. A transient stinging sensation on the face, with no apparent dermatitis, following the application of cosmetic preparations is common [32]. The stinging sensation may in some cases be due to contact urticaria. Individuals with fair, freckled skin are probably more likely to develop irritation from cosmetics than others. A questionnaire study of 90 student nurses revealed contact dermatitis from cosmetics in 29, while 25 others had rhinitis caused by cosmetic preparations [223]. Sunscreen preparations may produce allergic as well as photoallergic contact dermatitis at the sites of application.

Facial dermatitis can also be caused by allergens and irritants in face masks (surgical masks, scuba-diving masks and masks worn to filter out dust or used to supply fresh air while working with dangerous substances) [224]. The contact pattern of the dermatitis characteristically follows the outline of the mask worn (Fig. 15.44). Nickel dermatitis, as illustrated in Fig. 15.21, is usually located at the site of specific contact with, for example, metal spectacle frames. The earlobe sign is a term used to describe facial dermatitis caused by substances applied to the face and neck with one hand. While there is dermatitis on the earlobe on the contralateral side of the hand used for application, the earlobe on the ipsilateral side is not involved [225].

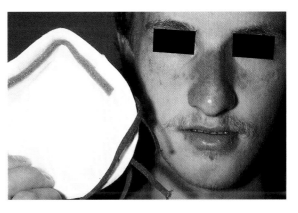

Fig. 15.44 Allergic contact dermatitis due to formaldehyde in a protective mask

15

Particular attention should be paid to three specific locations on the face and neck, as discussed below.

> **Core Message**
>
> › Photocontact dermatitis, airborne contact dermatitis and cosmetic contact dermatitis are commonly seen on the face. Sesquiterpene lactones from plants, fragrances and preservatives in cosmetics are common causes. Methyl dibromoglutaranitrile is a common contact allergen in cosmetics. This preservative is no longer used in cosmetics sold in the European Union.

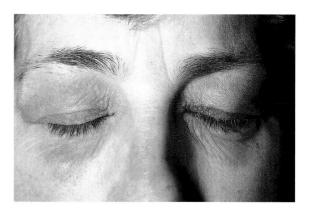

Fig. 15.45 Eyelid dermatitis

15.5.2.1 The Lips

On the lips, dermatitis may be caused both by cosmetics and food which make contact with the lips. Contact urticaria is commonly the cause when contact with certain foods results in cheilitis. The characteristic symptoms include stinging, burning, tingling and itching of the lips seconds to minutes after contact with the offending item [226]. Similar symptoms may occur on the oral mucosa. Compositae plants such as lettuce may cause cheilitis in patients sensitive to sesquiterpene lactones [227].

In series of patients tested because of lip dermatitis, common causes of the dermatitis were fragrances, lipstick ingredients and nickel [228, 229]. Series of patients sensitive to volatile oils in toothpastes, to metals and to ingredients in lipsticks have also been reported [230–234].

15.5.2.2 The Eyes and Eyelids

The skin of the eyelid is very thin and delicate. It is covered by a coat of water-fast make-up by a large proportion of the female population, and the cosmetic products used for this purpose are often based on oils considered to be irritants.

Many people rub the eyelids frequently, and substances otherwise found on the hands are thereby transported to the eyelids. The classical site of allergic contact dermatitis caused by nail varnish is the face and, in particular, the eyelids [235]. The eyelids are also a common site of airborne and systemic contact dermatitis. It is,

therefore, not surprising that eyelid dermatitis is common and that it can have a multitude of causes [66, 236–239] (Fig. 15.45). Guin [240] found that 151 of 203 patients with eyelid dermatitis had allergic contact dermatitis. Forty-six had protein contact dermatitis, 23 had atopic dermatitis and 18 had seborrhoeic dermatitis or psoriasis. Ayala et al. [241] found that 50% of 447 patients with eyelid dermatitis had allergic contact dermatitis, most commonly caused by nickel, perfume and cobalt. Twenty-one percent had irritant contact dermatitis, 14% atopic dermatitis and 6% seborrhoeic dermatitis. The very loosely bound subcutis of the eyelid makes marked oedema a characteristic feature of eyelid dermatitis.

Eyelid dermatitis has been used as a model for various enhanced patch test techniques such as patch testing on tape-stripped skin and patch testing on scarified skin. These techniques are recommended for the detection of weak sensitisers such as eye medications used for prolonged periods of time [242].

Atopic persons frequently have fissured dermatitis of the upper eyelids, probably due to mechanical irritation from rubbing the eyes and from airborne irritants such as fibres from carpets, animal hair and other sources. In patients sensitized to house dust mites and animal dander, contact urticaria on the eyelids may also be caused by these allergens.

Nickel dermatitis of the eyelids may be due to nickel in eyelid make-up or to the systemic administration of nickel, as evidenced by the flares seen after oral challenge with nickel. Shellac in mascara caused allergic contact dermatitis of the eyelids in six patients [243].

Topical ophthalmic products and preparations used in the care of contact lenses can cause contact dermatitis of the eyelids [244, 245]. Irritant contact conjunctivitis has been seen after the use of acrylic monomers found in printing inks [246], and after contact with calcium oxalate crystals from plants of the genus *Dieffenbachia* [247].

Core Message

> › Irritant eyelid dermatitis is common in atopic persons. Irritants include eyelid make-up, dust and irritants brought to the eyelid from the hands. Contact allergens include perfume and topical medicaments. Eyelid dermatitis may also be a manifestation of systemic contact dermatitis.

15.5.2.3 The Ear

There are three common causes of dermatitis of the ear. One of these is seborrhoeic dermatitis, often seen in conjunction with dermatitis of the scalp and face. This condition frequently recurs after periods of quiescence and may require long-term or intermittent treatment. Such treatment may result in sensitization and allergic contact dermatitis from topical medicaments [88–90].

A second major cause of dermatitis of the ear is objects or medicaments put into the ear. In a study involving a large number/series of patients, neomycin, framycetin and gentamicin were the most common sensitisers [248]. Corticosteroids have also caused external otitis [249]. Hairpins containing nickel used to relieve itching in the ear canal may cause allergic contact dermatitis. Matches containing chromate or phosphorus sesquisulfide may likewise cause allergic contact dermatitis of the external ear. Hearing aids rarely produce allergic contact dermatitis [250, 251], but can cause dermatitis as a result of occlusion, particularly in patients with seborrhoeic dermatitis.

The third type of dermatitis commonly found on the ear is earlobe dermatitis caused by nickel sensitization. In fact, today's most commonly described cause of nickel sensitization is earrings worn in pierced ears [73, 252]. There is sometimes a discrepancy between a history of dermatitis at sites that have been in contact with cheap jewellery and patch test results, which may be negative in spite of the repeated appearance of a rash after such jewellery is worn. One explanation for this discrepancy could be that nickel sensitization has

not actually occurred and that the dermatitis is caused by irritancy or is some other non-immunological reaction. Other possibilities are that sensitization has taken place, but that the patch test results were false negative [253]. Gold sensitization is statistically associated with ear piercing [254], and granulomatous dermatitis of the earlobe in a gold-sensitive person has been described [255]. Nickel-plated spectacle frames may cause dermatitis at the site of contact on the ear and nose, while dermatitis from plastic frames is rare [256].

Eight patients who had dermatitis on the ears had relevant positive patch tests to potassium dichromate. This substance was found in the casing of their cellular phones [257]. Dermatitis on the cheek from nickel in cellular phones is described on page 263.

Core Message

> › The ears are classic sites of allergic contact dermatitis from medicaments used to treat external otitis as well as nickel dermatitis from cheap jewellry.

15.5.3 Dermatitis of the Trunk

The principal sensitisers causing dermatitis of the trunk are

1. Nickel in brassiere straps, zippers and buttons
2. Rubber in the elastic of undergarments and other clothing (rubber items may cause contact urticaria as well as allergic contact dermatitis)
3. Fragrances used in soaps, skin-care products and detergents
4. Formaldehyde and other textile resins and dyes

Textile fibre dermatitis is usually most pronounced at sites of intense contact with the fibres and at typical sweat retention sites such as the axillary folds, the sides of the neck, the waist, the inner aspects of the thighs and the gluteal folds [258, 259]. In addition to the fibres themselves, the chemicals used to dye or improve the appearance of textiles may also cause dermatitis at the above-mentioned sites. The most common contact allergens in clothing are Disperse Dyes, in particular, Disperse Blue 106, 124, 85 and 35 [260–262]. Paraphenylene diamine may be an important marker of allergic contact dermatitis caused by textiles [263]. Nederost et al. made the point that allergens from topical medicaments can be difficult to remove from clothing using ordinary washing procedures [264]. The incidence of textile dermatitis caused by the release of formaldehyde has decreased over the past several years due to a reduction in the release of formaldehyde from fabrics [265].

New, unwashed, permanent-press sheets caused moderately pruritic of burning papules of the helices and lobes of the ears, the cheeks and the sides of the neck in 25 patients. An irritant reaction to textile resins was thought to have caused the dermatitis [266]. Irritant contact dermatitis may be caused by detergents that have not been thoroughly rinsed out of clothing after washing. Children with atopic dermatitis are particularly susceptible to irritation from detergent residues.

Mechanical dermatitis caused by rough woollen fibres and various artificial fibres is common, particularly among atopics, who may also suffer from sweat retention dermatitis on the trunk [263]. The pressure exerted by tight-fitting items of clothing such as girdles, brassieres and belts can lead to dermatitis and hyperpigmentation. Similar dermatitis may be seen from safety shoes, particularly in atopics, and from face masks in pilots and firemen.

One distinct type of mechanical dermatitis of the upper back is a patch of excoriated dermatitis seen at the site of a label in a blouse. This condition is very common among patients with atopic dermatitis, but it also occurs in adults with no history of atopic dermatitis. The label causing the dermatitis is often made of stiff artificial fibres that cause pruritus in atopic patients and others with sensitive skin [267].

Another distinct type of clothing dermatitis is seen in patients who wear undergarments that have been machine washed together with textiles containing glass fibre, for example curtains, or work clothes contaminated with rock wool or glass fibre. The fibres bound in the undergarments may cause an intensely pruritic mechanical dermatitis at the sites of contact.

Rare causes of dermatitis of the trunk include contact with the electrode jelly used for electrocardiograms, rubber in electrodes used for electrocardiograms [268], tattoo pigment used for colouring the nipple after breast reconstruction following breast cancer [269], and transcutaneous drug delivery systems and ostomi bags (see the Sect. 15.5.3.3). Brassiere paddings with propylene glycol caused allergic contact dermatitis on one patient [270].

Dermatitis under swimwear may be "seabather's eruption", a very pruritic papular dermatitis probably caused by the larvae of the sea anemone (*Edwardsiella lineata*) [271].

A papular dermatitis of the trunk of persons who bathed in hot sulphur springs was probably irritant contact dermatitis caused by sulphur or the acidity of the baths [272].

> **Core Message**
>
> › Textile dermatitis and other types of clothing dermatitis are usually seen on the trunk, particularly in areas of skin in intense contact with the item of clothing in question. Allergic contact dermatitis from detergents is rare. Mechanical contact dermatitis from rough fibres, especially labels in clothing, is common.

15.5.3.1 The Axillary Region

There are certain types of dermatitis that are peculiar to the axillary region.

In view of the extensive use of antiperspirant products containing aluminium, aluminium allergy is rare. Aluminium sensitization has been seen largely as a consequence of the injection of vaccines precipitated with aluminium hydroxide, while dermatitis elicited by aluminium in antiperspirants in uncommon.

Five of 20 patients with cosmetic dermatitis had axillary dermatitis due to the perfume in their deodorants or antiperspirants [273]. A history of axillary rash after the use of deodorant spray correlated well with fragrance allergy [25]. A similar correlation was seen between a history of a rash from scented products and fragrance allergy [274]. Fragrance dermatitis caused by deodorants and antiperspirants is characteristically seen in the entire axillary region. Dermatitis due to textile resins, on the other hand, is most intense in axillary folds and often does not affect the central area of the axilla. Dermatitis of the axillary folds caused by friction between clothes and the skin is common in patients with atopic dermatitis. It is possible that in the past the diagnosis of perfume dermatitis was obscured by the fact that a corticosteroid preparation used to suppress axillary eczema once contained perfume [275].

A form of contact dermatitis commonly seen in both the axillary and the genital area is caused by irritant reactions to chemical depilatory agents or various mechanical means of hair removal. Shaving off the pubic hair may cause pseudofolliculitis when re-growth occurs.

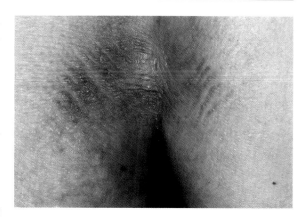

Fig. 15.46 Pressure-induced, mechanical contact dermatitis with a peculiar linear pattern ("Grandfather's disease")

Core Message

> A rash in the axillae after the use of deodorant sprays correlates well with fragrance allergy. Textile dermatitis is usually most intense in the axillary fold rather than in the central part of the axillae.

15.5.3.2 The Anogenital Region

The anogenital area is a common site of contact dermatitis [276]. This is due, among other things, to the fact that allergens and irritants can easily penetrate the delicate skin of this normally occluded area.

Age plays an important role in the development of anogenital contact dermatitis, as witnessed by the irritant contact dermatitis caused by urine and faeces during the first years of life and also in the elderly incontinent [277]. In the elderly, mechanical pressure from sitting in a fixed position can cause characteristic, striated dermatitis on the sacral area ("grandfather's disease") (Fig. 15.46). Diapers may cause mechanical dermatitis as well as irritant contact dermatitis, but they rarely cause allergic contact dermatitis. In baby girls, dermatitis at the top of the vulval folds is often considered to be evidence of dermatitis caused by diapers (W pattern) (Fig. 15.47), while dermatitis that is most intense in the vulval creases is more likely to be caused by microorganisms. "Lucky Luke" diaper dermatitis is an irritant diaper dermatitis [278].

Mothers tend to exchange disposable paper diapers for old-fashioned cloth diapers when diaper rash appears. This change is unnecessary and is, in fact, potentially harmful. A 26-week double-blind study of various diaper types used for infants with atopic

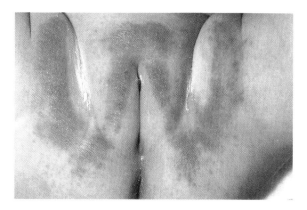

Fig. 15.47 Irritant diaper dermatitis ("W-dermatitis")

dermatitis showed that the use of disposable diapers gave rise to diaper dermatitis less often than the use of conventional cloth diapers [279].

Among sexually active individuals, connubial dermatitis may occur in the vulval area and on the penis and scrotum or even in the face [280]. One characteristic of this dermatitis is that its activity fluctuates with the sexual activity of the patient. If connubial dermatitis in the male can be relieved by the use of a condom, this suggests that it is caused by substances applied to the vulva or vagina. Such substances include spermicidal creams, jellies or suppositories, the fragrances in creams and cleansing agents and the rubber in diaphragms. Microorganisms in the vagina such as *Candida albicans* commonly cause transient balanitis in the male. Benzocaine in a condom has also been shown to cause balanitis in a man [281].

15

Vulvitis is less frequently relieved by the use of a condom. Females have been observed to suffer from contact urticaria caused by semen. This is an important entity, as anaphylactoid reactions have occurred [124, 282]. Allergic contact dermatitis from semen has also been described [283].

Pruritus vulvae may be associated with allergic contact dermatitis [284–286], while vulval vestibulitis has not been associated with relevant contact allergy [287]. Atopic dermatitis and seborrhoeic dermatitis are important endogenous causes of vulvar dermatitis [288].

Other dermatological problems associated with sexual activity include traumatic lesions such as fissures, erosions or even ulcers caused by the friction of intense sexual activity, lack of lubrication or bizarre habits. In both sexes a mechanical Köbner phenomenon may cause eruptions or aggravation of psoriasis lesions on the genitals. Lichen planus is common on the penis, and the Köbner phenomenon may delay clearing of this disease. Lichen simplex chronicus of the vulva may remain active due to sexual activity. A particular problem in males is sclerosing lymphangitis of the penile lymph vessels. This condition is commonly considered to be traumatic.

In addition to problems related to sexual activity, dermatitis on the genitals may be caused by substances normally found on the hands which have been transferred to the genitals. In males this type of dermatitis may present as allergic contact dermatitis cause, for example, by sawdust or preservatives in paints [86]. Females may develop irritant or allergic contact dermatitis of the vulva or perianal area due to contact with nail polish or from colophonium in sanitary pads [289, 290].

Widespread pruritus and dermatitis with features similar to those of systemically induced contact dermatitis have appeared following the introduction of intrauterine contraceptive devices made of copper [291]. Sensitivity to copper is unusual, and this may not be the sole explanation of these symptoms.

Another curious eruption in the anogenital and bikini area is the "baboon syndrome" described in Chap. 17.

Allergic and/or irritant contact dermatitis in the anogenital area is often caused by the topical application of various medicaments. A wide range of compounds can cause such reactions, including antifungal agents used to combat dermatophyte infections and candidiasis, haemorrhoid remedies and agents used to relieve anogenital pruritus. A characteristic pattern of dermatitis may be caused by toilet seats. This can be seen as occlusive dermatitis in atopic children or allergic contact dermatitis from disinfectants or exotic woods [292, 293]. Some of the sensitizing agents commonly used in this area of the body are benzocaine, neomycin, the hydroxyquinolines and bufexamac [294]. Recycled paper used for toilet paper may contain up to 5–10 mg nickel per kg [295].

Ingested irritants and sensitisers such as spices may cause pruritus and contact dermatitis in the perianal region [296]. The mechanism here may be the deposition of the suspected substance on perianal skin. In some situations, however, systemically induced contact dermatitis or other systemic mechanisms may be to blame, as in the case of coffee drinker's rash [297]. The anal pruritus seen after oral challenge with nickel or balsam of Peru may be due to unabsorbed substances in the faeces present in higher concentrations than those normally experienced [150].

> **Core Message**
>
> ❯ In infants and incontinent adults, the anogenital region is exposed to irritants. Irritant dermatitis may also result from intense cleansing of the area. Allergic contact dermatitis from topical medicaments is common in the perianal region.

15.5.3.3 Stoma Dermatitis

Excretions from a stoma may cause dermatitis when irritant substances come into contact with skin, which is not suited for such contact. Incorrectly attached ostomy bags may be responsible. Leakage from ileostomies is potentially the most irritating, as the faeces are rather liquid and may contain enzymes and other irritants that would normally be degraded during passage through the colon and rectum [298, 299]. The materials used for the stoma appliances themselves, or their adhesive surfaces, are today so well researched and carefully selected that they rarely cause sensitization or irritation [300]. An important exception was noted by Beck et al. [301] who discovered low molecular weight epoxy resin in a type of ostomy bag that sensitized six patients. A similar patient was described by Mann et al. [302].

Dermatological problems in connection with the use of ostomy bags may also be due to sweat retention in the area of the stoma or under the bag itself if this makes direct contact with the skin [303]. Rothstein [304] has provided a detailed review of the problems associated with stoma care and their management.

> **Core Message**
>
> ❯ Stoma dermatitis is more commonly due to ill-fitting ostomy bags with leakage of intestinal content or to sweat retention than to allergic contact dermatitis.

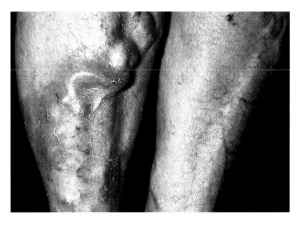

Fig. 15.48 Early stasis dermatitis

15.5.4 Dermatitis of the Legs

Dermatitis of the thighs may be clinically characterized by patches of eczema at sites where pockets make contact with the skin. Persons who normally carry nickel-plated items, "strike-anywhere" matches containing phosphorus sesquisulfide or matches with heads containing chromium in their pockets may suffer from dermatitis of the thighs. Follicular dermatitis on the anterior aspects of the thighs is a typical consequence of wearing trousers that have become soaked with splashing cutting oil or caked with oil rubbed off the hands.

Thirty-three patients developed allergic contact dermatitis to a modified colophonium derivative in an epilating agent used on the legs [305].

The dermatitis occasionally seen on the stump of a femur amputee has several possible causes. Among the most common are friction and pressure exerted on specific skin areas due to an ill-fitting prosthesis or insufficient tissue under the distal tip of the femur bone. In such situations there may also be trophic disturbance of the skin overlying the bone. Irritant contact dermatitis and dermatitis due to sweat retention under the prosthesis may also occur, even when it fits well [306].

Allergic contact dermatitis may be caused by materials in the prostheses themselves or by substances used under them [306–308].

Dermatitis at the site of, or in close proximity to, varicose veins is an early indication of stasis dermatitis (Fig. 15.48). This type of dermatitis tends to become

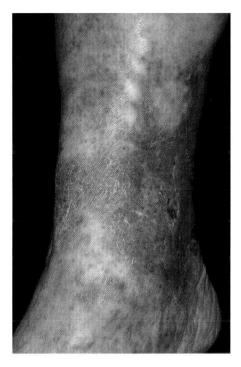

Fig. 15.49 Chronic stasis dermatitis surrounding a small leg ulcer

chronic, and eventually the pattern of dermatitis becomes less characteristic (Fig. 15.49). Trophic disturbance, often aggravated by the oedema of the lower leg typical of patients with varicose veins, is probably an aetiological factor. Patients with stasis dermatitis may develop venous leg ulcers.

The chronicity of leg ulcers and stasis dermatitis, in combination with the occlusive bandages applied to afflicted legs, makes this area a rival to the anogenital

15

region as the most common site of allergic contact dermatitis caused by topical medicaments [309–311]. Unless a short course of treatment can be anticipated, the selection of agents for the topical treatment of stasis dermatitis should be made with emphasis on substances that rarely sensitize.

Of 1,270 patients with leg ulcers, 106 patients had positive patch tests to colophonium and/or ester gum resin. Had ester gum resin not been used for testing, the diagnosis of 47 patients would not have been based on a relevant positive patch test [312].

Stocking dermatitis is seen in those areas with the most intense contact with stockings or socks [313]. Rubber dermatitis due to the elastic in men's socks occurs in a limited area of the lower legs, while nylon stocking dermatitis may appear on the medial aspects of the thighs as well as in the popliteal fossae and on the feet. Shoe dermatitis may mimic stocking dermatitis on the feet, and mercaptobenzothiazole and colophonium leached from shoes has been shown to accumulate in socks [314, 315]. Children with atopic dermatitis often develop irritant contact dermatitis from synthetic fibres in tights (panty hose), wool in leggings or rubber chemicals in the shin protectors used by football players. Obese children, in particular, may also develop friction dermatitis on the medial aspects of the thighs.

> **Core Message**
>
> > The lower leg is a prime site of allergic contact dermatitis from topical medicaments, particularly in leg ulcer patients. Textile dermatitis may be seen under socks and on the thighs. Detergents and mineral oils in work clothes may cause irritant dermatitis.

15.5.5 Dermatitis of the Feet

Dermatitis of the feet presents with specific characteristic clinical patterns at, for example, the points of shoe contact, primarily on the dorsal aspects of the feet and toes and on the sides of the feet. This dermatitis rarely appears on the sides of the toes or in the plantar flexure creases of the toes. Rubber chemicals, in particular mercaptobenzothiazole, glues such as *p*-tert-butylphenol-formaldehyde and chromates, are commonly the cause of allergic footwear dermatitis [316–320]. Seventeen

men who wore the same type of socks at work developed foot dermatitis caused by basic red 46 in the socks [321]. Frictional dermatitis on the dorsal aspects of the toes, usually on the big toes, may be seen in children with atopic dermatitis.

One type of dermatitis that is specific to children is juvenile plantar dermatosis. Although the aetiology of this dermatitis is unknown, friction and pressure probably play significant roles in the pathogenesis, as illustrated in Fig. 15.50 [322–324]. In this patient the dermatitis appeared only on the weight-bearing aspects of the soles. There are two characteristic morphologies of plantar dermatoses in addition to juvenile plantar dermatitis. These are recurrent, pruritic, vesicular plantar dermatitis and hyperkeratotic eczema.

15.5.5.1 Recurrent, Pruritic, Vesicular, Plantar Dermatitis

This dermatitis consists of crops of vesicles in the central part of the sole and sometimes also on the sides of the toes.

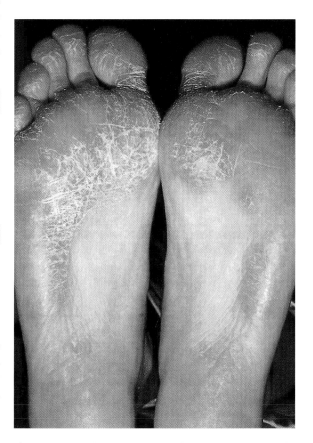

Fig. 15.50 Juvenile plantar dermatosis in pressure areas on the soles

If frequent eruptions occur, this dermatitis may appear to be a chronic eczematous condition. This plantar eruption is less common than an eruption of similar morphology that appears on the hands. It is not usually possible to identify the aetiology of the dermatitis, although it has been reproduced by oral challenge with metal salts in some patients with positive patch tests to the same substances, and even in some patch test negative patients [40].

15.5.5.2 Hyperkeratotic Plantar Eczema

Hyperkeratotic eczema consists of well-demarcated plaques of hyperkeratosis, often with painful fissures (Fig. 15.51). It is commonly associated with similar lesions on the palms. For further details, see the Sect. 15.5.5.2.

Core Message

> Allergic contact dermatitis on the feet may be due to dichromates in leather, to rubber chemicals and glue in shoes or to dyes in socks.

15.5.6 Dermatitis of the Arms

There are two main sites of dermatitis of the arms. One is the antecubital fossa, which is a typical site of sweat retention dermatitis, atopic dermatitis and secondary nickel dermatitis. The other is the forearm, to which hand dermatitis frequently spreads. Eczema of the forearm with no involvement of the hands can be seen in

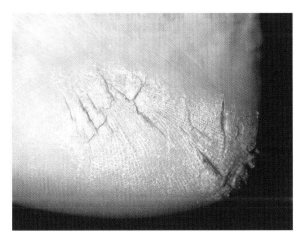

Fig. 15.51 Fissured, hyperkeratotic eczema on a heel

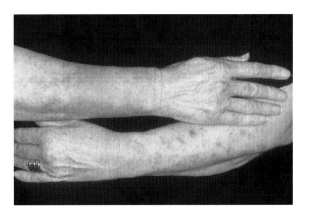

Fig. 15.52 Allergic contact dermatitis on the arms caused by the preservative MCl/Ml (methylchloroisothiazolinone/methylisothiazolinone or Kathon CG) in an emollient

occupational eczema caused by dust, detergents, isocyanate laquer [325] and the juices of meat and fish. Isothiazolinones caused allergic contact dermatitis of the forearms of one patient (Fig. 15.52).

Tattoos are commonly placed on the upper arm. Modern tattoo pigments rarely sensitize. Patchy Red 904A and DC 99060 each caused allergic contact dermatitis in one tattooed person [326, 327].

15.5.7 Contact Stomatitis

The metals and plastics used in dentistry may cause allergic contact stomatitis. Erythema, lichen planus-like lesions and erosion and ulceration of the oral mucosa have been linked to mercury allergy elicited by mercury in amalgam dental fillings and to gold [328–336]. Greyish streaks on the buccal mucosa at the sites of contact with amalgam dental fillings in patients who have positive patch tests to mercury salts certainly suggest a causative relationship (Fig. 15.53). The relationship is less clear if the oral lesions are not directly in contact with metals in the mouth [337, 338].

Of a group of 67 patients with atrophic-erosive oral lichen planus, 17% had positive patch tests to mercury compounds, compared with 8% of a reference group [339]. In another group of 29 patients with similar symptoms, 18 patients (62%) had contact allergy to mercury compared with 3.2% of a control group. For three of the patients, the symptoms disappeared after removal of all amalgam dental fillings [340]. Sensitization to mercury and systemic toxicity of amalgam dental restorations are subjects that are still open to discussion [341].

15

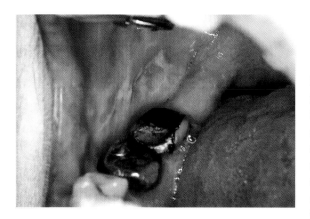

Fig. 15.53 Lichen planus-like stomatitis adjacent to amalgam dental fillings in a mercury-sensitive person

It has been suggested that dental braces made of steel and containing nickel, cobalt and/or chromium are sometimes responsible for systemic contact dermatitis [342, 343]. In view of the common use of dental plates and their intense contact with the oral mucosa, sensitization to such plates is rare [344]. A man sensitive to budesonide developed stomatitis when he inhaled budesonide for his seasonal respiratory symptoms [345]. Dental technicians who manufacture the uncured dental plates may, however, become sensitized to the acrylic materials they handle.

Flavourings added to toothpaste may also cause contact stomatitis. Common causes of contact stomatitis and cheilitis have been reviewed by Fisher [346] and Chan and Mowad [347]. Foodstuffs rarely cause allergic contact stomatitis, but contact urticaria of the oral mucosa caused by food is common. Sonnex et al. [348] described a patient with contact stomatitis from coffee. The term "oral allergy syndrome" has been proposed to describe immediate-type reactions that include irritation of the oral mucosa shortly after the ingestion of certain foods [37]. Cross-sensitivity between pollen and food allergens may precipitate such symptoms. The burning mouth syndrome is a poorly understood entity that may be caused by a number of factors including systemic diseases, psychological stress and, occasionally, contact sensitivity [349].

Core Message

> Lichen planus-like greyish streaks on the bucal mucosa adjacent to dental fillings can be caused by mercury or gold in the fillings. Stomatitis from acrylates in dental prostheses is rare.

15.5.8 Dermatitis Caused by Items Within the Body

Implanted items such as pacemakers have been blamed for widespread pruritic dermatitis and for eczema and bullous eruptions on the skin overlying them. The aetiology of such dermatitis is uncertain, but traces of metals, and in some cases epoxy resin, released from the case of the pacemaker have been suggested as a cause of these rare reactions [350, 351]. Copper intrauterine devices have been blamed for similar types of dermatitis [291], as have metal orthodontic braces [342].

Nickel wiring left in the tissues following surgery may give rise to dermatitis of the skin overlying these tissues or to vesicular hand eczema. Such dermatitis has also been seen in sensitized individuals whose fractures have been set with metal plates and screws, and in a patient who had shrapnel fragments left in the tissues [352].

Artificial hip joints are now primarily of the metal-to-plastic type and rarely give rise to allergic reactions [352].

Widespread dermatitis and vesicular hand eczema have been seen in patients who have swallowed coins containing nickel. The dermatitis faded when the coins were removed [353].

The tattoo pigments used today rarely lead to sensitization, but one study described a granulomatous reaction in a tattoo caused by aluminium [354], and Patchy Red 904A caused allergic contact dermatitis in one patient [326].

Metals in the oral cavity are dealt with in the Sect. 15.5.7.

15.6 Differential Diagnosis

Two main groups of diseases should be considered in the differential diagnosis when dealing with possible contact dermatitis, namely

1. Other types of eczema
2. Non-eczematous dermatoses that have clinical features similar to those of contact dermatitis

Atopic dermatitis may have a number of features in common with contact dermatitis, and contact dermatitis is commonly superimposed on atopic dermatitis. One example of this is "head and neck dermatitis", which has already been described as a contact urticaria reaction caused by *Pityrosporum ovale*.

Lichen simplex chronicus (neurodermatitis) and nummular eczemas are morphological terms used to describe eczema which may be endogenous, the nummular eczema often with superimposed bacterial infection (Fig. 15.54). Lichen simplex chronicus may be mechanically aggravated by, for example, rubbing a foot on the eczematous plaque (Fig. 15.55) [44]. The patch testing of 48 patients with discoid eczema gave 16 relevant reactions, but this was not reproduced by other studies. There is some evidence of a connection between discoid eczema and alcohol-dependence [355].

Seborrhoeic dermatitis is usually so characterized that it presents no diagnostic difficulty but, when there is facial and anogenital involvement, seborrhoeic dermatitis can be difficult to distinguish from contact dermatitis and psoriasis. The term sebopsoriasis has been

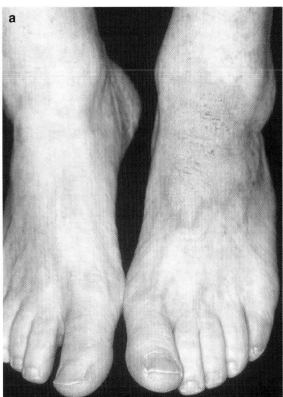

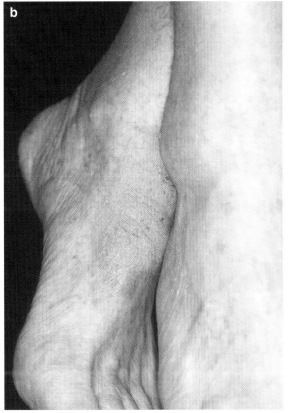

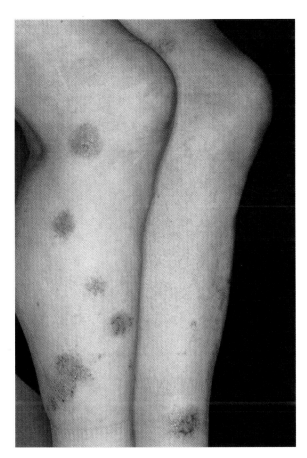

Fig. 15.54 Nummular eczema on the lower leg

Fig. 15.55 Lichen simplex chronicus of the left ankle (**a**) maintained by rubbing the right heel against the area of dermatitis (**b**)

15

coined to describe dermatitis with features of both psoriasis and seborrhoeic dermatitis [356, 357]. Low-
humidity dermatoses may have clinical features similar
to those of seborrhoeic dermatitis of the face [43] and
may also mimic lichen simplex chronicus of the lower
leg [358]. Eczematous eruptions associated with rare
metabolic diseases such as acrodermatitis enteropathica, other zinc deficiency syndromes or phenylketonuria may also mimic contact dermatitis.

Pityriasis alba may be mistaken for contact dermatitis, but is morphologically characteristic with dry patches
of eczema on the cheeks and/or upper arms followed
by post-inflammatory hyperpigmentation (Fig. 15.56).
Asteatotic eczema is seen mainly in elderly persons due
to xerosis of the skin. Hailey-Hailey disease, as well as
intertrigo, may mimic contact dermatitis and acrodermatitis continua. Acrodermatitis continua, hallopeau
and palmo-plantar pustulosis may have clinical features
similar to those of contact dermatitis.

Most cases of psoriasis and hyperkeratotic eczema are
easily recognized as distinct entities, but psoriasis on the
hands may be difficult to distinguish from contact dermatitis (Fig. 15.57). Koebner-induced psoriasis at the site of
nickel contact in a nickel-sensitive person is another difficult differential diagnosis. Occasionally, patients with psoriasis may have relevant positive patch tests [359, 360].

Collagenoses such as lupus erythematosus of the
palms may have eczematous features similar to those
of contact dermatitis.

It calls for a high degree of suspicion to make a correct diagnosis of Norwegian scabies, which, clinically,
can mimic contact dermatitis.

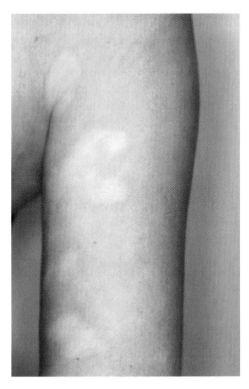

Fig. 15.56 Pityriasis alba of the upper arm with central post-
inflammatory hypopigmentation and discrete dermatitis at the
periphery of the lesions

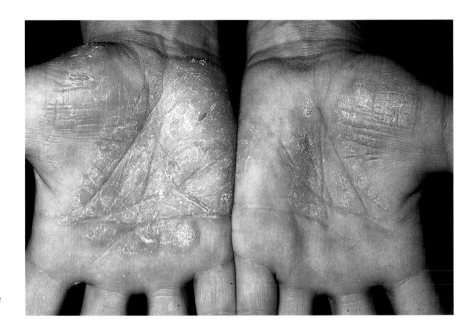

Fig. 15.57 Psoriasis on the
hands

Another important differential diagnosis is dermatophytosis, particularly when there is involvement of the feet or when *T. rubrum* has infected the skin of the hands (Fig. 15.58). The diagnostic problems increase if the dermatophytosis has been treated with topical steroids. Dermatophytids on the fingers resulting from plantar dermatophytosis are clinically indistinguishable from vesicles associated with other causes, such as systemic contact dermatitis [128]. This supports the view that a vesicular eruption of the fingers is a non-specific reaction pattern which may have a number of different causes. Examples are lichen planus [361], cutaneous T-cell lymphoma [362] and bullous pemphigoid (Fig. 15.59). Palmar lichen planus can also have a striking resemblance to hand eczema (Fig. 15.60).

Dysplasias such as actinic keratoses and in situ tumours such as from Bowen's disease may mimic contact dermatitis (Fig. 15.61).

A diagnosis of contact dermatitis cannot be made by means of histological examination of a biopsy specimen. Nonetheless, a biopsy may be a useful tool in making this diagnosis, as it will enable the exclusion of a number of the above-mentioned diseases that have specific histological features.

Core Message

> Contact dermatitis may be mimicked by other types of dermatitis such as seborrhoeic dermatitis, atopic deramtitis and nummular dermatitis. Tinea, particularly in the face or perianal regions, is an important differential diagnosis together with Bowen's disease, in particular on the fingers.

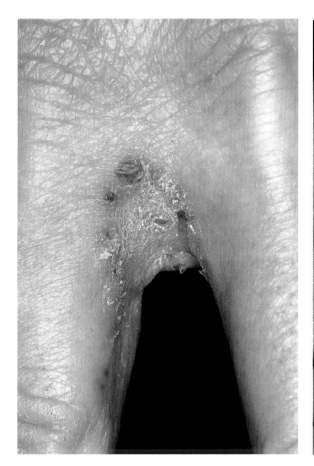

Fig. 15.58 Dermatophyte infection on a finger web

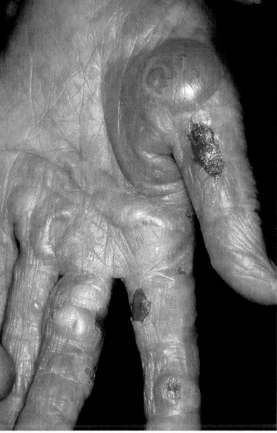

Fig. 15.59 Bullous pemphigoid presenting with vesicular and bullous lesions on the hands

15

Fig. 15.60 Lichen planus of the palms

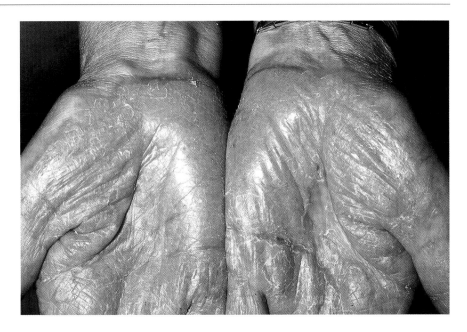

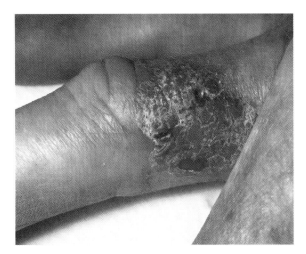

Fig. 15.61 Bowen's disease on a finger

15.7 Case Reports

15.7.1 Case Report 1

A 47-year-old woman had worked as a flower vendor in a supermarket for 15 years. She was seen because she had developed dermatitis on her hands and forearms, particularly on the right side (Fig. 15.62).

Patch testing with the European Standard Series showed a ++reaction to primin.

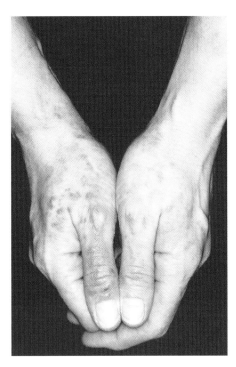

Fig. 15.62 Allergic contact dermatitis caused by *Primula obconica*, mostly on the right hand

While discussing the relevance of this test, she remembered that a different type of primula had been introduced in the store where she worked.

She brought a plant to our clinic, and we identified it as *Primula obconica* (Fig. 15.63). A close-up of a

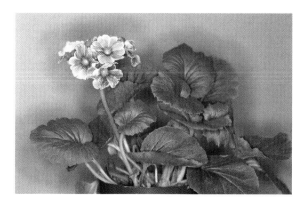

Fig. 15.63 *Primula obconica*

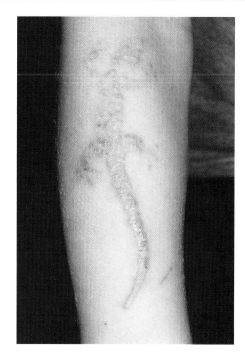

Fig. 15.65 Allergic contact dermatitis on the forearm of one of 5-year-old twin boys after a temporary, black "Henna" tattoo

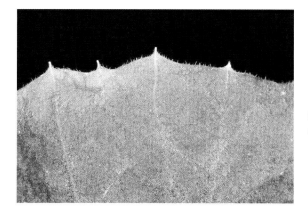

Fig. 15.64 Tiny spicules on a leaf of *Primula obconica*

leaf of this plant shows the spicules that contain primin (Fig. 15.64).

Comment: Most positive patch tests to primin are seen in older women, and the reaction is most often of past relevance. A low-allergenic *Primula obconica* has been developed, and contact allergy to primin should become a thing of the past.

15.7.2 Case Report 2

A family of four had a 1-week vacation in Turkey. After their return, 5-year-old twin sons developed intense dermatitis at the sites of temporary tattoos they had made during the holiday (Figs. 15.65 and 15.66). Both the boys had positive patch tests to paraphenylene diamine. One of the boys subsequently developed an id-like eruption on the trunk (Fig. 15.67a). Curiously, the eruption was seen on areas of the skin

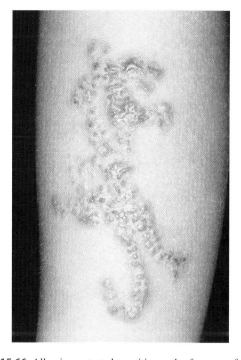

Fig. 15.66 Allergic contact dermatitis on the forearm of the other twin

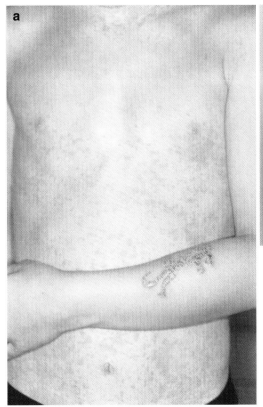
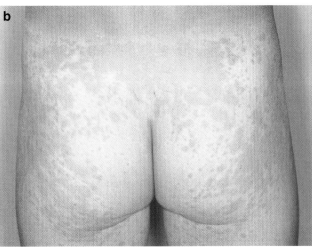

Fig. 15.67 The twin in Fig. 15.66 developed an id-like eruption on the trunk (**a**). The eruption was most predominant on skin that was not exposed to the sun (**b**)

that had not been exposed to the sun (Fig. 15.67b). The eruption became so intense that a short course of systemic steroid was necessary to suppress the symptoms.

Comment: It is well known that the colours used to make temporary, so-called Henna tattoos, often contain paraphenylene diamine. In this case, twins became sensitized to paraphenylene diamine, and one of them developed a widespread id-like eruption.

References

1. Armstrong DKB, Walsh MY, Dawson JF (1997) Granulomatous contact dermatitis due to gold earrings. Br J Dermatol 136:776–778
2. Khamaysi Z, Bergman R, Weltfriend S (2000) Positive patch test reactions to allergens of the dental series and the relation to the clinical presentations. Contact Dermat 55:216–218
3. Evans AV, Banerjee P, McFadden JP, Calonje E (2003) Lymphomatoid contact dermatitis to para-tertyl-butyl phenol resin. Clin Exp Dermatol 28:272–273
4. Blum R, Baum HP, Ponnighaus M, Kowalzick L (2003) Sarcoidal allergic contact dermatitis due to palladium following ear piercing [In German]. Hautarzt 54:160–162
5. Werchniak AE, Schwarzenberger K (2004) Poison ivy: an underreported cause of erythemamultiforme. J Am Acad Dermatol 51:S159–S160
6. Gueraa L, Rogkakou A, Massacane P, Gamalero C, Compalati E, Zanella C, Scordamaglia A, Canonica WG, Passalacqua G (2007) Role of contact sensitization in chronic urticaria. J Am Acad Dermatol 56:88–90
7. Ghosh S, Mukhopadhyay S (2009) Chemical leucoderma: a clinico-aetiological study of 864 cases in the perspective of a developing country. Br J Dermatol 160:40–47
8. Saitta P, Cohen D, Brancaccio R (2009) Contact leukoderma from para-phenylenediamine. Dermatitis 20:56–57
9. Wedgeworth EK, Banerjee P, White IR (2009) Linear lichenified nodules in a case of thiuram allergy. Contact Dermat 60:181–182
10. Möller H, Ohlsson K, Linder C, Björkner B, Bruze M (1998) Cytokines and acute phase reactants during flare-up of contact allergy to gold. Am J Contact Dermat 9:15–22
11. Möller H, Björkner B, Bruze M (1996) Clinical reactions to systemic provocation with gold sodium thiomalate in patients with contact allergy to gold. Br J Dermatol 135:423–427
12. Krecisz B, Kiec-Swierczynska PK, Chomiczewska D, Palcynski C (2009) Cobalt-induced anaphylaxis, contact

urticaria, and delayed allergy in a ceramics decorator. Contact Dermat 60:173–174

13. Van der Meeren HLM, Van Erp PEJ (1986) Life-threatening contact urticaria from glove powder. Contact Dermat 14: 190–191

14. Rystedt I (1985) Hand eczema and long-term prognosis in atopic dermatitis. (Dissertation) Department of Occupational Dermatology, National Board of Occupational Safety and Health and Karolinska Hospital. Karolinska Institute, Stockholm

15. Lerbæk A (2007) Epidemiological and clinical studies on hand eczema in a opulation-based twin sample. (Dissertation) University of Copenhagen, Denmark

16. Darsow U, Vieluf D, Ring J (1999) Evaluating the relevance of aeroallergen sensitization in atopic eczema with the atopy patch test: a randomized, double-blind multicenter study. J Am Acad Dermatol 40:187–193

17. Darsow U, Laifaoui J, Kerschenlohr K, Wollenberg A, Przybilla B, Wüthrich B, Borelli S Jr, Giusti F, Seidenari S, Drzimalla K, Simon D, Disch R, Borelli S, Devillers AC, Oranje AP, De Raeve L, Hachem JP, Dangoisse C, Blondeel A, Song M, Breuer K, Wulf A, Werfel T, Roul S, Taieb A, Bolhaar S, Bruijnzeel-Koomen C, Brönnimann M, Braathen LR, Didierlaurent A, André C, Ring J (2004) The prevalence of positive reactions in the atopy patch test with aeroallergens and food allergens in subjects with atopic eczema: a European multicenter study. Allergy 59: 1318–1325

18. Pónyai G, Hidvégi B, Németh I, Sas A, Temesvári E, Kárpáti S (2008) Contact and aeroallergens in adulthood atopic dermatitis. J Eur Acad Dermatol Venerol 22:1346–1355

19. Thelin I, Agrup G (1985) Pompholyx – a one year series. Acta Derm Venereol (Stockh) 65:214–217

20. Schwanitz HJ (1986) Das Atopische Palmoplantarekzem. Springer, Berlin, Heidelberg, New York

21. Edman B (1988) Palmar eczema: a pathogenetic role for acetylsalicylic acid, contraceptives and smoking? Acta Derm Venereol (Stockh) 68:402–407

22. Menné T (1983) Nickel allergy. (Dissertation) University of Copenhagen, Denmark

23. Ancona A, Fernandez-Diez J, Bellamy C (1986) Occupationally induced psoriasis. Derm Beruf Umwelt 34: 71–73

24. Rothenborg HW, Andersen HB (1993) Alcohol and skin disorders. J Eur Acad Dermatol Venereol 2:113–120

25. Johansen JD, Andersen TF, Kjoller M, Veien N, Avnstorp C, Andersen KE, Menné T (1998) Identification of risk products for fragrance contact allergy: a case-referent study based on patients' histories. Am J Contact Dermat 9: 80–86

26. Linneberg A, Nielsen NH, Menné T, Madsen F, Jørgensen T (2003) Smoking might be a risk factor for contact allergy. J Allergy Clin Imunol 111:980–984

27. Niemeier V, Nippesen M, Kupfer J, Schill WB, Gieler U (2002) Psychological factors associated with hand dermatoses: which subgroup needs additional psychological care? Br J Dermatol 146:1031–1037

28. Dooms-Goosens AE, Debusschere KM, Gevers DM et al (1986) Contact dermatitis caused by airborne agents. J Am Acad Dermatol 15:1–11

29. Hegewald J, Uter W, Kränke B, Schnuch A, Pfahlberg A, Gefeller O (2008) Meteorological conditions and the diag-

nosis of occupationally related contact sensitizations. Scand J Work Environ Health 34:316–321

30. Veien NK, Hattel T, Laurberg G (1992) Is patch testing a less accurate tool during the summer months? Am J Contact Dermat 3:35–36

31. Malten KE (1981) Thoughts on irritant contact dermatitis. Contact Dermat 7:238–247

32. Frosch PJ, Kligman AM (1977) A method for appraising the stinging capacity of topically applied substances. J Soc Cosmet Chem 28:197–209

33. Clemmensen O, Hjorth N (1982) Perioral contact urticaria from sorbic acid and benzoic acid in a salad dressing. Contact Dermat 8:1–6

34. Andersen KE, Løwenstein H (1978) An investigation of the possible immunological relationship between allergen extracts from birch pollen, hazelnut, potato and apple. Contact Dermat 4:73–79

35. Murphy GM, Rycroft RJG (1989) Allergic contact dermatitis from silver birch pollen. In: Frosch PJ, Dooms-Goosens A, Lachapelle J-M, Rycroft RJG, Scheper RJ (eds) Current topics in contact dermatitis. Springer, Berlin, Heidelberg, New York, pp 146–148

36. Koh D, Goh CL, Tan HTW, Ng SK, Wong WK (1997) Allergic contact dermatitis from grasses. Contact Dermat 37:32–34

37. Amlot PL, Kemeny DM, Zachary C, Parkes P, Lessor MH (1987) Oral allergy syndrome (OAS): symptoms of IgE-mediated hypersensitivity to foods. Clin Allergy 17:33–42

38. Hofmann A, Burks AW (2008) Pollen food syndrome: update on the allergens. Curr Allergy Asthma Rep 8:413–417

39. Ackerman AB (1978) Histological diagnosis of inflammatory skin diseases. Lea and Febiger, Philadelphia, p 863

40. Veien NK (2009) Acute and recurrent vesicular hand dermatitis. Dermatol Clin 27:337–353

41. Frosch PJ (1989) Irritant contact dermatitis. In: Frosch PJ, Dooms-Goosens A, Lachapelle J-M, Rycroft RJG, Scheper RJ (eds) Current topics in contact dermatitis. Springer, Berlin, Heidelberg, New York, pp 385–403

42. Rothenborg HW, Menné T, Sjølin K-E (1977) Temperature dependent primary irritant dermatitis from lemon perfume. Contact Dermat 3:37–48

43. Rycroft RJG (1985) Low humidity and microtrauma. Am J Ind Med 8:371–373

44. Rycroft RJG (1987) Low-humidity occupational dermatoses. In: Gardner AW (ed) Current approaches to occupational health, 3rd edn. Wright, Bristol, pp 1–13

45. Hellgren L, Mobacken H (1969) Nummular eczema – clinical and statistical data. Acta Derm Venereol (Stockh) 49:189–196

46. Le Coz C-J (2002) Contact nummular (discoid) eczema from depilating cream. Contact Dermat 46:111–112

47. Krupa Shankar DS, Shrestha S (2005) Relevance of patch testing in patients with nummular dermatitis. Indian J Dermatol Venereol Leprol 71:406–408

48. Torinuki W, Tagami H (1987) Pustular irritant dermatitis due to croton oil. Acta Derm Venereol (Stockh) 68:257–260

49. Sevadjian CM (1985) Pustular contact hypersensitivity to fluorouracil with rosacealike sequelae. Arch Dermatol 121: 240–242

50. Modjtahedi BS, Modjtahedi SP, Maibach HI (2004) The sex of the individual as a factor in allergic contact dermatitis. Contact Dermat 50:53–59

51. Zug KA, McGinley-Smith D, Warshaw EM, Taylor JS, Rietschel RL, Maibach HI, Belsito DV, Fowler JF Jr, Storrs FJ, DeLeo VA, Marks JG Jr, Mathias CGT, Pratt MD, Sasseville D (2008) Contact allergy in children referred for patch testing. Arch Dermatol 144:1329–1336

52. Hammonds LM, Hall VC, Yiannias JA (2009) Allergic contact dermatitis in 136 children patch tested between 2000 and 2006. Int J Dermatol 48:271–274

53. Hogeling M, Pratt M (2008) Allergic contact dermatitis in children: the Ottawa hospital patch testing clinic experience, 1996 to 2006. Dermatitis 19:86–89

54. Lee PW, Elsaie ML, Jacob SE (2009) Allergic contact dermatitis in children: common allergens and treatment: a review. Curr Opin Pediatr 21:491–498

55. Wolf R, Wolf D, Matz H, Orion E (2003) Cutaneous reactions to temporary tattoos. Dermatol Online J 9:3

56. Balato A, Balato N, De Costanzo L, Ayala F (2008) Contact sensitization of older patients in an academic department in Naples, Italy. Dermatitis 19:209–212

57. Uter W, Geier J, Pfahlberg A, Effendy I (2002) The spectrum of contact allergy in elderly patients with and without lower leg dirmatitis. Dermatology 204:266–272

58. Nedorost ST, Stevens SR (2001) Diagnosis and treatment of allergic skin disorders in the elderly. Drugs Aging 18:827–835

59. Berardesca E, Maibach HI (1988) Contact dermatitis in blacks. Dermatol Clin 6:363–368

60. Jourdain R, De Lacharrière O, Bastien P, Maibach HI (2002) Ethnic variations in self-perceived sensitive skin: epidemiological survey. Contact Dermat 46:162–169

61. Deleo VA, Taylor SC, Belsito DV, Fowler JF Jr, Fransway AF, Maibach HI, Marks JG Jr, Mathias CG, Nethercott JR, Pratt MD, Reitschel RR, Sherertz EF, Storrs FJ, Taylor JS (2002) The effect of race and ethnicity on patch test results. J Am Acad Dermatol 46:S107–S112

62. Modjtahedi SP, Maibach HI (2002) Ethnicity as a possible endogenous factor in irritant contact dermatitis: comparing the irritant response among Caucasians, blacks, and Asians. Contact Dermat 47:272–278

63. Robinson MK (2002) Population differences in acute skin irritation responses. Race, sex, age, sensitive skin and repeat subject comparisons. Contact Dermat 46:86–93

64. Jones HE, Lewis CW, McMarlin SL (1973) Allergic contact sensitivity in atopic patients. Arch Dermatol 107:217–222

65. Mortz CG, Lauritsen JM, Bindslev-Jensen C, Andersen KE (2002) Contact allergy and allergic contact dermatitis in adolescents: prevalence measures and associations. The Odense Adolescence Cohort Study on Atopic Diseases and Dermatitis (TOACS). Acat Derm Venereol 82:352–358

66. Buckley DA, Basketter DA, Kan-King-Yu D, White IR, White JL, McFadden JP (2008) Atopy and contact allergy to fragrance: allergic reactions to the fragrance mix I (the Larsen mix). Contact Dermat 59:220–225

67. Christophersen J, Menné T, Tanghøj P, Andersen KE, Brandrup F, Kaaber K, Osmundsen PE, Thestrup-Pedersen K, Veien NK (1989) Clinical patch test data evaluated by multivariate analysis. Contact Dermat 21:291–299

68. Möller H, Svensson A (1986) Metal sensitivity: positive history but negative test indicates atopy. Contact Dermat 14:57–60

69. Todd DJ, Burrows D, Stanford CF (1989) Atopy in subjects with a history of nickel allergy but negative patch tests. Contact Dermat 21:129–133

70. Dotterud LK, Falk ES (1995) Contact allergy in relation to hand eczema and atopic diseases in north Norwegian schoolchildren. Acta Paediatr 84:402–406

71. Bonnevie P (1939) Aethiologie und Pathogenese der Eczemkrankheiten. (Dissertation) Nyt Nordisk, Copenhagen

72. Larsson-Stymne B, Widström L (1985) Ear piercing – a cause of nickel allergy in schoolgirls? Contact Dermat 13:289–293

73. Thyssen JP, Johansen JD, Zachariae C, Menné T (2008) The outcome of dimethylglyoxime testing in a sample of cell phones in Denmark. Contact Dermat 59:38–42

74. Sánchez-Pérez J, Ruís-Genao GD, Río I, García Diez A (2003) Taxi driver's occupational allergic contact dermatitis from nickel in euro coins. Contact Dermat 48:340–341

75. Gawkrodger DJ, Vestey JP, Wong W-K, Buxton PK (1986) Contact clinic survey of nickel-sensitive subjects. Contact Dermat 14:165–169

76. Moorthy TT, Tan GH (1986) Nickel sensitivity in Singapore. Int J Dermatol 25:307–309

77. Hemingway JD, Molokhia MM (1987) The dissolution of metallic nickel in artificial sweat. Contact Dermat 16:99–105

78. Emmett EA, Risby TH, Jiang L, Sk N, Feinman S (1988) Allergic contact dermatitis to nickel: bioavailability from consumer products and provocation threshold. J Am Acad Dermatol 19:314–322

79. Kanan MW (1969) Contact dermatitis in Kuwait. J Kuwait Med Assoc 3:129–144

80. Fisher AA (1985) Nickel dermatitis in men. Cutis 35:424–426

81. De Corres LF, Garrastazu MT, Soloeta R, Escayol P (1982) Nickel contact dermatitis in a blood bank. Contact Dermat 8:32–37

82. Oakley AMM, Ive FA, Car MM (1987) Skin clips are contraindicated when there is nickel allergy. J R Soc Med 80:290–291

83. Corazza M, Zampio MR, Montanari A, Pagnoni A, Virgili A (2002) Lichenoid reaction from a permanent red tatto: has nickel a possible aetiologic role? Contact Dermat 46:114–115

84. Moritz K, Sesztak-Greinecker G, Wantke F, Götz M, Jarisch R, Hemmer W (2007) Allergic contact dermatitis due to rubber in sports equipment. Contact Dermat 57:131–132

85. Kasteler JS, Petersen MJ, Vance JE, Zone JJ (1992) Circulating activated T lymphocytes in autoeczematization. Arch Dermatol 128:795–798

86. Cunningham MJ, Zone JJ, Petersen MJ, Green JA (1986) Circulating activated (DR-positive) T lymphocytes in a patient with autoeczematization. J Am Acad Dermatol 14:1039–1041

87. Warshaw EM, Furda LM, Maibach HI, Rietschel RL, Fowler JF Jr, Belsito DV, Zug KA, DeLeo VA, Marks JC Jr, Mathias CGT, Pratt MD, Sasseville D, Storrs FJ, Taylor JS (2008) Anogenital dermatitis in patients referred for patch testing. Restrospecitve analysis of cross-sectional data from the North American Contact Dermatitis Group, 1994–2004. Arch Dermatol 144:749–755

88. Feser A, Plaza T, Vogelgsang L, Mahler V (2008) Periorbital dermatitis – a recalcitrant disease: causes and differential diagnoses. Br J Dermatol 159:858–863

89. Smart V, Alavi A, Coutts P, Fierheller M, Coelho S, Holness L, Sibbald RG (2008) Contact allergens in persons with leg ulcers: a Canadian study in contact sensitization. Int J Low Extrem Wounds 7:120–125

90. Goossens A, Blondeel S, Zimerson E (2002) Resorcinol monobenzoate: a potential sensitizer in a computer mouse. Contact Dermat 47:235

91. Avnstorp C, Hamann K (1981) Neglelakeksem. Ugeskr Laeger 143:2504–2505

92. Burnett JW, Calton GJ (1987) Jellyfish envenomation syndromes updated. Ann Emerg Med 16:1000–1005

93. Dosman HDJ, JA Li KYR et al (1986) Questionnaire survey of pruritus and rash in grain elevator workers. Contact Dermat 14:170–175

94. Saary MJ, House RA, Holness DL (2001) Dermatitis in a particleboard manufacturing facility. Contact Dermat 44:325–330

95. Beck MH, Hausen BM, Dave VK (1984) Allergic contact dermatitis from *Machaerium scleroxylum* Tul. (Pao ferro) in a joinery shop. Clin Exp Dermatol 9:159–166

96. Ippen H, Wereta-Kubek M, Rose U (1986) Haut- und Schleimhautreaktionen durch Zimmerpflanzen der Gattung Dieffenbachia. Dermatosen 34:93–101

97. Hausen BM (1982) Häufigkeit und Bedeutung toxischer und allergischer Kontaktdermatitiden durch *Machaerium scleroxylum* Tul. (Pao ferro), einem Ersatzholz für Palisander (*Dalbergia nigra* All.). Hautarzt 33:321–328

98. Møller NE, Nielsen B, von Würden K (1986) Contact dermatitis to semisynthetic penicillins in factory workers. Contact Dermat 14:307–311

99. Santos R, Goossens A (2007) An update on airborne contact dermatitis: 2001-2006. Contact Dermat 57:353–360

100. Karlberg AT, Gafvert E, Meding B, Stenberg B (1996) Airborne contact dermatitis from unexpected exposure to rosin (colophony). Rosin sources revealed with chemical analyses. Contact Dermat 35:272–278

101. Hjorth N, Roed-Petersen J, Thomsen K (1976) Airborne contact dermatitis from Compositae oleoresins simulating photodermatitis. Br J Dermatol 95:613–619

102. LaMarte FP, Merchant JA, Casale TB (1988) Acute systemic reactions to carbonless copy paper associated with histamine release. JAMA 260:242–243

103. Berg M (1988) Skin problems in workers using visual display terminals. Contact Dermat 19:335–341

104. Berg M, Lonne-Rahm SB, Fischer T (1998) Patients with visual display unit-related facial symptoms are stingers. Acta Derm Venereol 78:44–45

105. McMullen E, Gawkrodger DJ (2006) Physical friction is under-recognized as an irritant that can cause or contribute to contact dermatitis. Br J Dermatol 154:154–156

106. Gambichler T, Uzun A, Boms S, Altmeyer P, Altemüller E (2008) Skin conditions in instrumental musicians: a self-reported survey. Contact Dermat 58:217–222

107. Wintzen M, Van Zuuren EJ (2003) Computer-related skin diseases. Contact Dermat 48:241–243

108. García-Morales I, García Bravo B, Camacho Martínez F (2003) Occupational contact dermatitis caused by a personal-computer mouse mat. Contact Dermat 49:172

109. Powell FC (1994) Sports dermatology. J Eur Acad Dermatol Venereol 3:1–15

110. Tomecki KJ, Mikesell JF (1987) Rower's rump. J Am Acad Dermatol 16:890–891

111. Kanerva L (1998) Knuckle pads from boxing. Eur J Dermatol 8:359–361

112. Descamps V, Peuchal X (2002) "Canyoning hand": a new recreational hand dermatitis. Contact Dermat 47:363–364

113. Inue S, Yamamoto S, Ikegami R, Ozawa K, Itami S, Yoshikawa K (2002) Baseball pitcher's friction dermatitis. Contact Dermat 47:176–177

114. Sullivan JR, Rachlis A, Phillips E (2003) "Buffalo-hump" dermatitis: a hat trick of antiretroviral side-effects. Contact Dermat 48:169–170

115. Kato A, Shoji A, Aoki N (2003) Very-low-voltage electrical injuries caused by cellular-phone chargers. Contact Dermat 49:168–169

116. Hersle K, Mobacken H (1982) Hyperkeratotic dermatitis of the palms. Br J Dermatol 107:195–202

117. Thestrup-Pedersen K, Andersen KE, Menné T, Veien NK (2001) Treatment of hyperkeratotic dermatitis of the palms (eczema keratoticum) with oral acitretin. A single-blind, placebo-controlled study. Acta Derm Venereol 81:353–355

118. Sabroe RA, Sharp LA, Peachey RDG (1996) Contact allergy to gold sodium thiosulfate. Contact Dermat 34:345–348

119. Plewig G, Fulton JE, Kligman AM (1970) Pomade acne. Arch Dermatol 101:580–584

120. Pecegueiro M, Brandao M (1984) Contact plantar pustulosis. Contact Dermat 11:126–127

121. Andersen KE, Sjølin KE, Solgard P (1989) Actuce irritant contact folliculitis in a galvanizer. In: Frosch PJ, Dooms-Goossens A, Lachapelle J-M, Rycroft RJG, Scheper RJ (eds) Current topics in contact dermatitis. Springer, Berlin, Heidelberg, New York, pp 417–418

122. Rystedt I, Fischer T, Lagerholm B (1983) Patch testing with sodium tungstate. Contact Dermat 9:69–73

123. Freeman S (1986) Woman allergic to husband's sweat and semen. Contact Dermat 14:110–112

124. Poskitt BL, Wojnarowska FT, Shaw S (1995) Semen contact urticaria. J R Soc Med 88:108P–109P

125. Held JL, Ruszkowski AM, Deleo VA (1988) Consort contact dermatitis due to oak moss. Arch Dermatol 124:261–262

126. Bernedo N, Audicana MT, Uriel O, Velasco M, Gastraminza G, Fernández E, Muñoz D (2004) Allergic contact dermatitis from cosmetics applied by the patient's girlfriend. Contact Dermat 50:252–253

127. Veien NK, Hattel T, Laurberg G (1994) Plantar *Trichophyton rubrum* infections may cause dermatophytids on the hands. Acta Derm Venereol (Stockh) 74:403–404

128. Bryld LE, Agner T, Menné T (2003) Relation between vesicular eruptions on the hands and tinea pedis, atopic dermatitis and nickel allergy. Acta Derm Venereol 83:186–188

129. Rustemeyer T, Frosch PJ (1996) Occupational skin diseases in dental laboratory technicians. (I). Clinical picture and causative factors. Contact Dermat 34:125–133

130. Delaney TZ, Donnelly AM (1996) Garlic dermatitis. Australas J Dermatol 37:109–110

131. Rycroft FJG, Baran R (1984) Occupational abnormalities and contact dermatitis. In: Baran R et al (eds) Diseases of the nails. Blackwell, London, pp 267–287

132. Mathias CGT, Maibach HI (1984) Allergic contact dermatitis from anaerobic acrylic sealants. Arch Dermatol 120:1202–1205

133. Cronin E (1982) "New" allergens of clinical importance. Semin Dermatol 1:33–41

134. Foti C, Cassano N, Conserva A, Vena GA (2003) Irritant paronychia with onychodystrophy caused by cyanoacrylate nail glue. Contact Dermat 49:274–275

15

135. Veien NK, Hattel T, Justesen O, Nørholm A (1986) Aluminium allergy. Contact Dermat 15:295–297
136. Kaaber K, Nielsen AO, Veien NK (1992) Vaccination granulomas and aluminium allergy: course and prognostic factors. Contact Dermat 26:304–306
137. Netterlid E, Hindsén M, Bjork J, Ekqvist S, Günder N, Henricson KÅ, Bruze M (2009) There is an association between contact allergy to aluminium and persistent subcutaneous nodules in children undergoing hyposensitization therapy. Contact Dermat 60:41–49
138. Bergfors E, Trollfors B, Inerot A (2003) Unexpectedly high incidence of persistent itching odules and delayed hypersensitivity to aluminium in children after the use of adsorbed vaccines from a single manufacturer. Vaccine 22:64–69. Erratum in: Vaccine (2004) 22:1586
139. Culora GA, Ramsay AD, Theaker JM (1996) Aluminium and injection site reactions. J Clin Pathol 49:844–847
140. Fischer T, Rystedt I (1982) A case of contact sensitivity to aluminium. Contact Dermat 8:343
141. Feinglos MN, Jegasothy BV (1979) "Insulin" allergy due to zinc. Lancet 1:122–124
142. Cronin E (1980) Contact dermatitis. Churchill Livingstone, Edinburgh
143. Hjorth N, Roed-Petersen J (1976) Occupational protein contact dermatitis in food handlers. Contact Dermat 2: 28–42
144. Chan EF, Mowad C (1998) Contact dermatitis to foods and spices. Am J Contact Dermat 9:71–79
145. Kanerva L, Toikkanen J, Jolanki R, Estlander T (1996) Statistical data on occupational contact urticaria. Contact Dermat 35:229–233
146. Oranje AP, Van Gysel D, Mulder PG, Dieges PH (1994) Food-induced contact urticaria syndrome (CUS) in atopic dermatitis: reproducibility of repeated and duplicate testing with a skin provocation test, the skin application food test (SAFT). Contact Dermat 31:314–318
147. Iliev D, Wuthrich B (1998) Occupational protein contact dermatitis with type I allergy to different kinds of meat and vegetables. Int Arch Occup Environ Health 71:289–292
148. Menné T, Veien N, Sjølin K-E, Maibach HI (1994) Systemic contact dermatitis. Am J Contact Dermat 5:1–12
149. Veien NK (1989) Systemically induced eczema in adults. Acta Derm Venereol (Stockh) Suppl 147. Dissertation, University of Copenhagen, Denmark
150. Veien NK, Krogdahl A (1989) Is nickel vasculitis a clinical entity? In: Frosch PJ, Dooms-Goossens A, Lachapelle J-M, Rycroft RJG, Scheper RJ (eds) Current topics in contact dermatitis. Springer, Berlin, Heidelberg, New York, pp 172–177
151. Kaaber K, Sjølin KE, Menné T (1983) Elbow eruptions in nickel and chromate dermatitis. Contact Dermat 9:213–216
152. Calnan CD (1956) Nickel dermatitis. Br J Dermatol 68:229–236
153. Andersen KE, Hjorth N, Menné T (1984) The baboon syndrome: systemically-induced allergic contact dermatitis. Contact Dermat 10:97–100
154. Christensen OB (1981) Nickel allergy and hand eczema in females. Dissertation, University of Lund, Malmö
155. Lechner T, Grytzmann B, Bäurle G (1987) Hämatogenes allergisches Kontaktekzem nach oraler Gabe von Nystatin. Mykosen 30:143–146
156. Bernard P, Rayol J, Bonnafoux A et al (1988) Toxidermies apres prise orale de pristinamycine. Ann Dermatol Venereol 115:63–66
157. Shiohara T (2009) Fixed drug eruption: pathogenesis and diagnostic tests. Curr Opin Allergy Clin Immunol 9:316–321
158. Mizukawa Y, Yamazaki Y, Shiohara T (2008) In vivo dynamics of intraepidermal CD8+ T cells and CD4+ T cells during the evolution of fixed drug eruption. Br J Dermatol 158:1230–1238
159. Rycroft RJG (1980) Acute ulcerative contact dermatitis from Portland cement. Br J Dermatol 102:487–489
160. Rycroft RJG (1980) Acute ulcerative contact dermatitis from ready mixed cement. Clin Exp Dermatol 5:245–247
161. Koch P (1996) Brulures, necroses et ulcerations cutanees dues au ciment, au beton premixe et a la chaux. Huit cas. Ann Dermatol Venereol 123:832–836
162. Osmundsen PE, Alani MD (1971) Contact allergy to an optical whitener, "CRY", in washing powders. Br J Dermatol 85:61–66
163. Valsecchi R, de Landro A, Pansera B, Cainelli T (1995) Pigmented contact dermatitis. Contact Dermat 33:70–71
164. Hayakawa R, Matsunaga K, Kojima S, Kaniwa M, Nakamura A (1985) Naphthol AS as a cause of pigmented contact dermatitis. Contact Dermat 13:20–25
165. Gottschling S, Meyer S, Dill-Mueller D, Wurm D, Gortner L (2007) Outbreak report of airborne caterpillar dermatitis in a kindergarten. Dermatology 215:5–9
166. Balit CR, Geary MJ, Russell RC, Isbister GK (2004) Clinical effects of exposure to the White-stemmed gum moth (*Chelepteryx collesi*). Emerg Med Australas 16:74–81
167. Maier SW, Kinaciyan T, Krehan H, Cabaj A, Schopf A, Honigsmann H (2003) The oak processionary caterpillar as the cause of an epidemic airborne disease: survey and analysis. Br J Dermatol 149:990–997
168. Artola-Bordás F, Arnedo-Pena A, Romeu-Garcia MA, Bellido-Blasco JB (2008) Outbreak of dermatitis caused by pine processionary caterpillar (*Thaumetopoea pityocampa*) in schoolchildren. An Sist Sanit Navar 31:289–293
169. Vega J, Vega JM, Moneo I, Armentia A, Caballero ML, Miranda A (2004) Occupational immunologic contact urticaria from pine processionary caterpillar (*Thaumetopoea pityocampa*): experience in 30 cases. Contact Dermat 50: 60–64
170. Salinas ML, Ogura T, Soffchi L (2001) Irritant contact dermatitis caused by needle-like calcium oxalate crystals, raphides, in *Agave tequilana* among workers in tequila distilleries and agave plantations. Contact Dermat 44: 94–96
171. Modi GM, Doherty CB, Katta R, Orengo IF (2009) Irritant contact dermatitis from plants. Dermatitis 20:63–78
172. Darabi K, Hostetler SG, Bechtel MA, Zirwas M (2009) The role of Malassezia in atopic dermatitis affecting the head and neck of adults. J Am Acad Dermatol 60:125–136
173. Mayser P, Kupfer J, Nemetz D, Schäfer U, Nilles M, Hort W, Gieler U (2006) Treatment of head and neck dermatitis with ciclopiroxolamine cream – results of a double-blind, placebo-controlled study. Skin Pharmacol Physiol 19: 153–158
174. Maibach HI (1987) Oral substitution in patients sensitized by transdermal clonidine treatment. Contact Dermat 16: 1–8

175. Harai Z, Sommer I, Knobel B (1987) Multifocal contact dermatitis to nitroderm TTS 5 with extensive postinflammatory hypermelanosis. Dermatologica 174:249–252

176. Holdiness MR (1989) A review of contact dermatitis associated with transdermal therapeutic systems. Contact Dermat 20:3–9

177. Carmichael AJ (1994) Skin sensitivity and transdermal drug delivery. A review of the problem. Drug Saf 10: 151–159

178. Weickel R, Frosch PJ (1986) Kontaktallergie auf Glyceroltrinitrat (Nitroderm TTS). Hautarzt 37:511–512

179. Wilson DE, Kaidbey K, Boike SC, Jorkasky DK (1998) Use of topical corticosteroid pretreatment to reduce the incidence and severity of skin reactions associated with testosterone transdermal therapy. Clin Ther 20:299–306

180. Hulst KV, Amer EP, Jacobs C, Dewulf V, Baeck M, Vallverdú RMP, Giménez-Arnau A, Tennstedt D, Goossens A (2008) Allergic contact dermatitis from transdermal buprenorphine. Contact Dermat 59:366–369

181. Zaynoun ST, Aftimos BA, Tenekjian KK, Kurban AK (1981) Berloque dermatitis – a continuing cosmetic problem. Contact Dermat 7:111–116

182. Edman B (1985) Sites of contact dermatitis in relationship to particular allergens. Contact Dermat 13:129–135

183. Näher H, Frosch PJ (1987) Contact dermatitis to thioxolone. Contact Dermat 17:250–251

184. Tosti A, Guerra L, Bardazzi F (1991) Contact dermatitis caused by topical minoxidil: case reports and review of the literature. Am J Contact Dermat 2:56–59

185. Ebner H, Müller E (1995) Allergic contact dermatitis from minoxidil. Contact Dermat 32:316

186. Friedman ES, Friedman PM, Coen DE, Washenik K (2002) Allergic contact dermatitis to topical minoxidil solution: etiology and treatment. J Am Acad Dermatol 46: 309–312

187. Storrs FJ (1984) Permanent wave contact dermatitis: contact allergy to glyceryl monothioglycolate. J Am Acad Dermatol 11:74–85

188. Søsted H, Agner T, Andersen KE, Menné T (2002) 55 cases of allergic reactions to hair dye: a descriptive, consumer complaint-based study. Contact Dermat 47:299–303

189. Tosti A, Piraccini BM, van Neste DJ (2001) Telogen effluvium after allergic contact dermatitis of the scalp. Arch Dermatol 137:187–190

190. Andersen KE, Roed-Petersen J, Kamp P (1984) Contact allergy related to TEA-PEG-3 cocamide sulfate and cocamidopropyl betaine in a shampoo. Contact Dermat 11: 192–193

191. Pérez RG, Aguirre A, Ratón JA, Eizaguirre X, Díaz-Pérez JL (1995) Positive patch tests to zinc pyrithione. Contact Dermat 32:118–119

192. Brand R, Delaney TA (1998) Allergic contact dermatitis to cocamidopropylbetaine in hair shampoo. Australs J Dermatol 39:121–122

193. Nielsen NH, Menné T (1997) Allergic contact dermatitis caused by zinc pyrithione associated with pustular psoriasis. Am J Contact Dermat 8:170–171

194. Fowler JF, Fowler LM, Hunter JE (1997) Allergy to cocamidopropyl betaine may be due to amidoamine: a patch test and product use test study. Contact Dermat 37: 276–281

195. Fowler JF Jr, Zug KM, Taylor JS, Storrs FJ, Sherertz EA, Sasseville DA, Rietschel RL, Pratt MD, Mathias CGT, Marks JG, Mailbach HI, Fransway AF, Deleo VA, Belsito DV (2004) Allergy to cocamidopropyl betaine and amidoamine in North America. Dermatitis 15:5–6

196. Pasche-Koo F, Claeys M, Hauser C (1996) Contact urticaria with systemic symptoms caused by bovine collagen in a hair conditioner. Am J Contact Dermat 7:56–58

197. Dobrev H, Zissova L (1997) Effect of ketoconazole 2% shampoo on scalp sebum level in patients with seborrhoeic dermatitis. Acta Derm Venereol (Stockh) 77:132–134

198. Peter RU, Richarz-Barthauer U (1995) Successful treatment and prophylaxis of scalp seborrhoeic dermatitis and dandruff with 2% ketoconazole shampoo: results of a multicentre, double-blind, placebo-controlled trial. Br J Dermatol 132:441–445

199. Fotiades J, Soter NA, Lim HW (1995) Results of evaluation of 203 patients for photosensitivity in a 7.3-year period. J Am Acad Dermatol 33:597–602

200. Beach RA, Pratt MD (2009) Chronic actinic dermatitis: clinical cases, diagnostic workup, and therapeutic management. J Cutan Med Surg 13:121–128

201. Frain-Bell W, Lakshmipathi T, Rogers J, Willock J (1974) The syndrome of chronic photosensitivity dermatitis and actinic reticuloid. Br J Dermatol 91:617–634

202. Russell SC, Dawe RS, Collins P, Man I, Ferguson J (1998) The photosensitivity dermatitis and actinic reticuloid syndrome (chronic actinic dermatitis) occurring in seven young atopic dermatitis patients. Br J Dermatol 138:496–501

203. Healy E, Rogers S (1995) Photosensitivity dermatitis/actinic reticuloid syndrome in an Irish population: a review and some unusual features. Acta Derm Venereol (Stockh) 75:72–74

204. Goulden V, Wilkinson SM (1998) Patch testing for Compositae allergy. Br J Dermatol 138:1018–1021

205. Machet L, Vaillant L, Callens A, Demasure M, Barruet K, Lorette G (1993) Allergic contact dermatitis from sunflower (Helianthus annuus) with cross-sensitivity to arnica. Contact Dermat 28:184–200

206. Hausen BM (1996) A 6-year experience with compositae mix. Am J Contact Dermat 7:94–99

207. Paulsen E, Søgaard J, Andersen KE (1998) Occupational dermatitis in Danish gardeners and greenhouse workers (III). Compositae-related symptoms. Contact Dermat 38:140–146

208. Mahajan VK, Sharma VK, Kaur I, Chakrabarti A (1996) Contact dermatitis in agricultural workers: rôle of common crops, fodder and weeds. Contact Dermat 35:373–374

209. Mahler V, Diepgen TL, Heese A, Peters K-P (1998) Protein contact dermatitis due to cow dander. Contact Dermat 38: 47–48

210. Moreno JC, Gata IM, Garcia-Bravo B, Camacho FM (1997) Fiddler's neck. Am J Contact Dermat 8:39–42

211. Hausen BM (1997) Allergic contact dermatitis from a wooden necklace. Am J Contact Dermat 8:185–187

212. Hausen BM, Oestmann G (1988) Untersuchungen über die Häufigkeit berufsbedingter allergischer Hauterkrankungen auf einem Blumengrossmarkt. Dermatosen 36:117–124

213. Schnuch A, Szliska C, Uter W (2009) Facial allergic contact dermatitis. Data from the IVDK and review of literature. Hautarzt 60:13–21

214. Adams RM, Maibach HI (1985) A five-year study of cosmetic reactions. J Am Acad Dermatol 13:1062–1069

15

215. Hsu TS, Davis MD, el-Azhary R, Corbett JF, Gibson LE (2001) Beard dermatitis due to para-phenylenediamine use in Arabic men. J Am Acad Dermatol 44:867–869

216. Jacobs M-C, White IR, Rycroft RJG, Taub N (1995) Patch testing with preservatives at St John's from 1982 to 1993. Contact Dermat 33:247–254

217. Wilkinson JD, Shaw S, Andersen KE, Brandao FM, Buynzeel DP, Bruze M, Camarasa JM, Diepgen TL, Ducombs G, Frosch PJ, Goossens A, Lachappelle JM, Lahti A, Menné T, Seidenari S, Tosti A, Wahlberg JE (2002) Monitoring levels of preservative sensitivity in Europe. A 10-year overview (1991–2000). Contact Dermatitis 46:207–210. Comment in: Contact Dermatitis 2002 46:189–190

218. Mathias CGT (1982) Pigmented cosmetic dermatitis from contact allergy to a toilet soap containing chromium. Contact Dermat 8:29–31

219. Mathias CGT, Maibach HI, Conant MA (1980) Perioral leukoderma simulating vitiligo from use of a toothpaste containing cinnamic aldehyde. Arch Dermatol 116:1172–1173

220. Hayakawa R, Matsunaga K, Arima Y (1987) Depigmented contact dermatitis due to incense. Contact Dermat 16:272–274

221. Fisher AA, Dooms-Goossens A (1976) Persulfate hair bleach reactions. Arch Dermatol 112:1407–1409

222. Guin JD, Berry VK (1980) Perfume sensitivity in adult females. J Am Acad Dermatol 3:299–302

223. Brandrup F, Hansen NS, Schultz K (1987) Ansigtseksem fremkaldt af gummi i åndedraetsvaern. Ugeskr Laeger 149:968

224. Rotstein E, Rotstein H (1997) The ear-lobe sign: a helpful sign in facial contact dermatitis. Australas J Dermatol 38:215–216

225. Hannuksela M, Lahti A (1977) Immediate reactions to fruits and vegetables. Contact Dermat 3:79–84

226. Paulsen E (1996) Compositae-dermatitis på Fyn. (Dissertation), Odense University, Odense

227. Zug KA, Kornik R, Belsito DV, DeLeo VA, Fowler JF Jr, Maibach HI, Marks JG Jr, Mathias CG, Pratt MD, Rietschel RL, Sasseville D, Storrs FJ, Taylor JS, Warshaw EM, North American Contact Dermatitis Group (2008) Patch-testing North American lip dermatitis patients: data from the North American Contact Dermatitis Group, 2001 to 2004. Dermatitis 19:202–208

228. Schena D, Fantuzzi F, Girolomoni G (2008) Contact allergy in chronic eczematous lip dermatitis. Eur J Dermatol 18:688–692

229. Downs AMR, Lear JT, Sansom JE (1998) Contact sensitivity in patients with oral symptoms. Contact Dermat 39:258–259

230. Goldsmith PC, White IR, Rycroft FJG, McFadden JP (1995) Probable active sensitization to tixocortol pivalate. Contact Dermat 33:429–430

231. Serra-Baldrich E, Puig LL, Arnau AG, Camarasa JG (1995) Lipstick allergic contact dermatitis from gallates. Contact Dermat 32:359–372

232. Niinimäki A (1995) Spice allergy. Acta Univ Oul D 357 (Dissertation), University of Oulu, Finland

233. Lavy Y, Slodownik D, Trattner A, Ingber A (2009) Toothpaste allergy as a cause of cheilitis in Israeli patients. Dermatitis 20:95–98

234. Liden C, Berg M, Farm G, Wrangsjo K (1993) Nail varnish allergy with far-reaching consequences. Br J Dermatol 128:57–62

235. Rietschel RL, Warshaw EM, Sasseville D, Fowler JF, LeLeo VA, Belsito DV, Taylor JS, Storrs FJ, Mathias CG, Maibach HI, Marks JG, Zug KA, Pratt M, North American Contact Dermatitis Group (2007) Common contact allergens associated with eyelid dermatitis: data from the North American Contact Dermatitis Group 2003-2004 study period. Dermatitis 18:78–81

236. Amin KA, Belsito DV (2006) The aetiology of eyelid dermatitis: a 10-year retrospective analysis. Contact Dermat 55:280–285

237. Karlberg AT, Gafvert E, Meding B, Stenberg B (1996) Airborne contact dermatitis from unexpected exposure to rosin (colophony). Rosin sources revealed with chemical analyses. Contact Dermat 35:272–278

238. Herbst RA, Uter W, Pirker C, Geier J, Frosch PJ (2004) Allergic and non-allergic periorbital dermatitis: patch test results of the Information Network of the Departments of Dermatology during a 5-year period. Contact Dermat 51:13–19

239. Guin JD (2002) Eyelid dermatitis: experience in 203 cases. J Am Acad Dermatol 47:755–765

240. Ayala F, Fabbrocini G, Bacchilega R, Berardesca E, Caraffini S, Corazza M, Flori ML, Francalanci S, Guarrera M, Lisi P, Santucci B, Schena D, Suppa F, Valsecchi R, Vincenzi C, Balato N (2003) Eyelid dermatitis: an evaluation of 447 patients. Am J Contact Dermat 14:69–74

241. Frosch PJ, Weickel R, Schmitt T, Krastel H (1988) Nebenwirkungen von opthalmologischen Externa. Z Hautkr 63:126–136

242. Le Coz C-J, Leclere J-M, Arnoult E, Raison-Peyron N, Pons-Guiraud A, Vigan M (2002) Allergic contact dermatitis from shellac in mascara. Contact Dermat 46:149–152

243. Grundmann H, Wozniak K-D, Tost M (1981) Zum allergischen Kontakteksem im Lid- und Augenbereich. Folia Ophthalmol 6:258–261

244. Valsecchi R, Imberti G, Martino D, Cainelli T (1992) Eyelid dermatitis: an evaluation of 150 patients. Contact Dermat 27:143–147

245. Nethercott JR (1978) Skin problems associated with multifunctional acrylic monomers in ultraviolet curing inks. Br J Dermatol 98:541–551

246. Ottosen C-O, Irgens-Møller L (1984) Øjenskader kan skyldes stueplanten Dieffenbachia. Ugeskr Laeger 146:3927–3928

247. Millard TP, Orton DI (2004) Changing patterns of contact allergy in chronic inflammatory ear disease. Contact Dermat 50:83–86

248. Wilkinson SM, Bech MH (1993) Hypesensitivity to topical corticosteroids in otitis externa. J Laryngol Otol 107:597–599

249. Lear JT, Sandhu G, English JSC (1998) Hearing aid dermatitis: a study in 20 consecutive patients. Contact Dermat 38:212–238

250. Sood A, Taylor JS (2004) Allergic contact dermatitis from hearing aid materials. Dermatitis 15:48–50

251. Nielsen NH, Menné T (1993) Nickel sensitization and ear piercing in an unselected Danish population. Glostrup Allergy Study. Contact Dermat 29:16–21

252. Kieffer M (1979) Nickel sensitivity: relationship between history and patch test reaction. Contact Dermat 5: 398–401

253. Nakada T, Iijima M, Nakayama H, Maibach HI (1997) Role of ear piercing in metal allergic contact dermatitis. Contact Dermat 36:233–236

254. Armstrong DK, Walsh MY, Dawson JG (1997) Granulomatous contact dermatitis due to gold earrings. Br J Dermatol 136:776–778

255. Carlsen L, Andersen KE, Egsgaard H (1986) Triphenyl phosphate allergy from spectacle frames. Contact Dermat 15:274–277

256. Seishima M, Yama Z, Oda M (2003) Cellular phone dermatitis with chromate allergy. Dermatology 207:48–50

257. Hatch KL, Maibach HI (1985) Textile fiber dermatitis. Contact Dermat 12:1–11

258. Hatch KL, Maibach HI (1986) Textile chemical finish dermatitis. Contact Dermat 14:1–13

259. Ryberg K, Isaksson M, Gruvberger B, Hindsén M, Zimerson E, Bruze M (2006) Contact allergy to textile dyes in southern Sweden. Contact Dermat 54:313–321

260. Lazarov A (2004) Textile dermatitis in patients with contact sensitization in Israel: a 4-year prospective study. J Eur Acad Dermatol Venereol 18:531–537

261. Brookstein DS (2009) Factors associated with textile pattern dermatitis caused by contact allergy to dyes, finishes, foams, and preservatives. Dermatol Clin 27:309–322, vi–vii

262. Ryberg K, Goossens A, Isaksson M, Gruvberger B, Zimerson E, Nilsson F, Björk J, Hindsén M, Bruze M (2009) Is contact allergy to disperse dyes and related substances associated with textile dermatitis? Br J Dermatol 160:107–115

263. Nedorost S, Kessler M, McCormick T (2007) Allergens retained in clothing. Dermatitis 18:212–214

264. Scheman AJ, Carroll PA, Brown KH, Osburn AH (1998) Formaldehyde-related textile allergy: an update. Contact Dermat 38:332–336

265. Tegner E (1985) Sheet dermatitis. Acta Derm Venereol (Stockh) 65:254–257

266. Veien NK, Hattel T, Laurberg G (1992) Can "label dermatitis" become "creeping neurotic excoriations"? Contact Dermat 27:272–273

267. Corazza M, Maranini C, La Malfa W, Virgili A (1998) Unusual suction-like contact dermatitis due to ECG electrodes. Acta Derm Venereol (Stockh) 78:145–159

268. Goossens A, Verhamme B (2002) Contact allergy to permanent colorants used for tattooing a nipple after breast reconstruction. Contact Dermat 47:250

269. Lamb SR, Ardley HE, Wilkinson SM (2003) Contact allergy to propylene glycol in brassiere padding inserts. Contact Dermat 48:224–225

270. Freudenthal AR, Joseph PR (1993) Seabather's eruption. N Engl J Med 329:542–544

271. Sun C-C, Sue M-S (1995) Sulfur spring dermatitis. Contact Dermat 32:31–34

272. Larsen WG (1977) Perfume Dermatitis. Arch Dermatol 113:623–626

273. Johansen JD, Andersen TF, Veien N, Avnstorp C, Andersen KE, Menné T (1997) Patch testing with markers of fragrance contact allergy. Do clinical tests correspond to patients' self-reported problems? Acta Derm Venereol (Stockh) 77:149–153

274. Larsen WG (1979) Allergic contact dermatitis to the perfume in Mycolog cream. J Am Acad Dermatol 1: 131–133

275. Bauer A, Geier J, Elsner P (2000) Allergic contact dermatitis in patients with anogenital complaints. J Reprod Med 45:649–654

276. Longhi F, Carlucci G, Bellucci R, di Girolamo R, Palumbo G, Amerio P (1992) Diaper dermatitis: a study of contributing factors. Contact Dermat 26:248–252

277. Di Landro A, Greco V, Valsecchi R (2002) "Lucky Luke" contact dermatitis from diapers with negative patch tests. Contact Dermat 46:48–49

278. Seymour JL, Keswick BH, Haifin JM, Jordan WP, Milligan MC (1989) Clinical effects of diaper types on the skin of normal infacts and infants with atopic dermatitis. J Am Acad Dermatol 17:988–997

279. de Groot AC, Frosch PJ (1997) Adverse reactions to fragrances. A clinical review. Contact Dermat 36:57–86

280. Muratore L, Calogiuri G, Foti C, Nettis E, Di Leo E, Vacca A (2008) Contact allergy to benzocaine in a condom. Contact Dermat 59:173–174

281. Poskitt BL, Wojnarowska FT, Shaw S (1995) Semen contact urticaria. J R Soc Med 88:108P–109P

282. Guillet G, Dagregorio G (2004) Seminal fluid as a missed allergen in vulvar allergic contact dermatitis. Contact Dermat 50:318–319

283. Haverhoek E, Reid C, Gordon L, Marshman G, Wood J, Selva-Nayagam P (2008) Prospective study of patch testing in patients with vulval pruritus. Australs J Dermatol 49:80–85

284. Utas S, Ferahbas A, Yildiz S (2008) Patients with vulval pruritus: patch test results. Contact Dermat 58:296–298

285. Nardelli A, Degreef H, Goossen A (2004) Contact allergic reactions of the vulva: a 14-year review. Dermatitis 15: 131–136

286. Nunns D, Ferguson J, Beck M, Mandal D (1997) Is patch testing necessary in vulval vestibulitis? Contact Dermat 37:87–89

287. Crone AM, Stewart EJ, Wojnarowska F, Powell SM (2000) Aetiological factors in volvar dermatitis. J Eur Acad Dermatol Venereol 14:181–186

288. Lazarov A (1999) Perianal contact dermatitis caused by nail lacquer allergy. Am J Contact Dermat 10:43–44

289. Lauerma AI (2001) Simultaneous immediate and delayed hypersensitivity to chlorhexidine digluconate. Contact Dermat 44:59–60

290. Romaguera C, Grimalt F (1981) Contact dermatitis from a copper-containing intrauterine contraceptive device. Contact Dermat 7:163–164

291. Lembo S, Panariello L, Lemo C, Ayala F (2008) Toilet contact dermatitis. Contact Dermat 59:59–60

292. Ezzedine K, Rafii N, Heenen M (2007) Lymphomatoid contact dermatitis to an exotic wood: a very harmful toilet seat. Contact Dermat 57:128–130

293. Frosch PJ, Raulin C (1987) Kontaktallergie auf Bufexamac. Hautarzt 38:331–334

294. Blecher P, Korting HC (1992) Irritative und allergologische Aspekte der Verwendung Altpapier-haltiger Hygienepapiere im Analbereich. Dermatosen 40:30–34

15

295. Vermaat H, Smienk F, Rustemeyer T, Bruynzeel DP, Kirtschig G (2008) Anogenital allergic contact dermatitis, the role of spices and flavour allergy. Contact Dermat 59: 233–237

296. Veien NK, Hattel T, Justesen O, Nørholm A (1987) Dermatoses in coffee drinkers. Cutis 40:421–422

297. Ratliff CR, Conovan AM (2001) Frequency of peristomal complications. Ostomy Wound Manage 47:26–29

298. Lyon CC, Smith AJ, Griffiths CE, Beck MH (2000) The spectrum of skin disorders in abdominal stoma patients. Br J Dermatol 143:1248–1260

299. Martin JA, Hughes TM, Stone NM (2005) Peristomal allergic contact dermatitis – case report and review of the literature. Contact Dermat 52:273–275

300. Beck MH, Burrows D, Fregert S, Mendelsohn S (1985) Allergic contact dermatitis to epoxy resin in ostomy bags. Br J Surg 72:202–203

301. Mann RJ, Stewart E, Peachey RDG (1983) Sensitivity to urostomy pouch plastic. Contact Dermat 9:80–81

302. Rietschel RL, Fowler JF Jr (eds) Fisher's contact dermatitis, 6th edn. BC Decker, Hamilton, pp 373–374

303. Rothstein MS (1986) Dermatologic considerations of stoma care. J Am Acad Dermatol 15:411–432

304. Goossens A, Armingaud P, Avenel-Audran M, Begon-Bagdassarian I, Constandt L, Giordano-Labadie F, Girardin P, Coz CJLE, Milpied-Homsi B, Nootens C, Pecquet C, Tennstedt D, Vanhecke E (2002) An epidemic of allergic contact dermatitis due to epilating products. Contact Dermat 46:67–70

305. Lyon CC, Kulkarni J, Zimeson E, Van Ross E, Beck MH (2000) Skin disorders in amputees. J Am Acad Dermatol 42:501–507

306. van Ketel WG (1977) Allergic contact dermatitis of amputation stumps. Contact Dermat 3:50–61

307. Komamura H, Foi T, Inui S, Yoshikawa K (1997) A case of contact dermatitis due to impurities of cetyl alcohol. Contact Dermat 36:44–46

308. Jankicevic J, Vesic S, Vukicevic J, Gajic M, Adamic M, Pavlovic MD (2008) Contact sensitivity in patients with venous leg ulcers in Serbia: comparison with contact dermatitis patients and relationship to ulcer duration. Contact Dermat 58:32–36

309. Barbaud A, Collet E, Le Coz CJ, Meaume S, Gillois P (2009) Contact allergy in chronic leg ulcers: results of a multicentre study carried out in 423 patients and proposal for an updated series of patch tests. Contact Dermat 60:279–287

310. Machet L, Couhe C, Perrinaud A, Hoarau C, Lorette G, Vaillant L (2004) A high prevalence of sensitization still persists in leg ulcer patients: a retrospective series of 106 patients tested between 2001 and 2002 and a meta-analysis of 1975-2003 data. Br J Dermatol 150:929–935

311. Salim A, Shaw S (2001) Recommendation to include ester gum resin when patch testing patients with leg ulcers. Contact Dermat 44:34–60

312. Hausen BM, Schulz KH (1984) Strumpffarben-Allergie. Dtsch Med Wochenschr 109:1469–1475

313. Rietschel RL (1984) Role of socks in shoe dermatitis. Arch Dermatol 120:398

314. Bugnet LD, Sanchez-Politta S, Sorg O, Piletta P (2008) Allergic contact dermatitis to colophonium-contaminated socks. Contact Dermat 59:127–128

315. Warshaw EM, Schram SE, Belsito DV, LeLeo VA, Fowler JF Jr, Maibach HI, Marks JG Jr, Mathias CG, Pratt MD, Rietschel RL, Sasseville D, Storrs FJ, Taylor JS, Zug KA (2007) Shoe allergens: retrospective analysis of cross-sectional data from the North American Contact Dermatitis Group, 2001-2004. Dermatitis 18:191–202

316. Nardelli A, Taveirne M, Drieghe J, Carbonez A, Degreef H, Goossens A (2005) The relation between the localization of foot dermatitis and the causative allergens in shoes: a 13-year retrospective study. Contact Dermat 53:201–206

317. Castanedo-Tardan MP, Gelpi C, Jacob SE (2008) Allergic contact dermatitis to Crocs™. Contact Dermat 58: 248–249

318. Saha M, Srinivas CR, Shenoy SD, Balachandran C, Acharya S (1993) Footwear dermatitis. Contact Dermat 28: 260–264

319. Trattner A, Farchi Y, David M (2003) Shoe contact dermatitis in Israel. Am J Contact Dermat 14:12–14

320. Opie J, Lee A, Frowen K, Fewings J, Nixon R (2004) Foot dermatitis caused by the textile dye Basic Red 46 in acrylic blend socks. Contact Dermat 49:297–303

321. Möller H (1972) Atopic winter feet in children. Acta Derm Venereol (Stockh) 52:401–405

322. Jones SK, English JSC, Forsyth A, Mackie RM (1987) Juvenile plantar dermatosis: an 8-year follow-up of 102 patients. Clin Exp Dermatol 12:5–7

323. Chougule A, Thappa DM (2008) Patterns of lower leg and foot eczema in South India. Indian J Dermatol Venereol Leprol 74:458–461

324. Frick M, Isaksson M, Björkner B, Hindsén M, Pontén A, Bruze M (2003) Occupational allergic contact dermatitis in a company manufacturing boards coated with isocyanate lacquer. Contact Dermat 48:255–260

325. Bhardwaj SS, Brodell RT, Taylor JS (2003) Red tattoo reactions. Contact Dermat 48:236–237

326. Greve B, Chytry R, Raulin C (2003) Contact dermatitis from red tattoo pigment (quinacridone) with secondary spread. Contact Dermat 49:265–266

327. Raap U, Stiesch M, Reh H, Kapp A, Werfel T (2009) Investigation of contact allergy to dental metals in 206 patients. Contact Dermat 60:339–343

328. Laeijendecker R, Dekker SK, Burger PM, Mulder PG, Van Joost T, Neumann MH (2004) Oral lichen planus and allergy to dental amalgam restorations. Arch Dermatol 140: 1434–1438

329. Torgerson RR, Davis MD, Bruce AJ, Farmer SA, Rogers RS 3rd (2007) Contact allergy in oral disease. J Am Acad Dermatol 57:315–321

330. Hosoki M, Bando E, Asaoka K, Takeuchi H, Nishigawa K (2009) Assessment of allergic hypersensitivity to dental materials. Biomed Mater Eng 19:53–61

331. Koch P (1998) Orale lichenoide Läsionen. Auslösung durch exogene Faktoren? Dermatosen 46:196–201

332. von Mayenburg J, Frosch PJ, Fuchs T, Aberer W, Bäurle G, Brehler R, Busch R, Gaber G, Hensel O, Koch P, Peters K-P, Rakoski J, Rueff F, Szliska C (1996) Mercury and amalgam sensitivity. Possible clinical manifestations and sources of contact sensitization. Dermatosen 44:213–221

333. Räsänen L, Kalimo K, Laine J, Vainio O, Kotiranta J, Pesola I (1996) Contact allergy to gold in dental patients. Br J Dermatol 134:673–677

334. Bruze M, Edman B, Björkner B, Möller H (1994) Clinical relevance of contact allergy to gold sodium thiosulfate. J Am Acad Dermatol 31:579–583

335. Wong L, Freeman S (2003) Oral lichenoid lesions (OLL) and mercury in amalgam fillings. Contact Dermat 48:74–79

336. Östman P-O, Anneroth G, Skoglund A (1996) Amalgam-associated oral lichenoid reactions. Clinical and histologic changes after removal of amalgam fillings. Oral Surg Oral Med Oral Pathol Oral Radiol Endod 81:459–465

337. Laine J, Kalimo K, Happonen R-P (1997) Contact allergy to dental restorative materials in patients with oral lichenoid lesions. Contact Dermat 36:141–146

338. Mobacken H, Hersle K, Sloberg K, Thilander H (1984) Oral lichen planus: hypersensitivity to dental restoration material. Contact Dermat 10:11–15

339. Finne K, Göransson K, Winckler L (1982) Oral lichen planus and contact allergy to mercury. Int J Oral Surg 11:236–239

340. Burrows D (1989) Mischievous metals – chromate, cobalt, nickel and mercury. Clin Exp Dermatol 14:266–272

341. Veien NK, Borchorst E, Hattel T, Laurberg G (1994) Stomatitis or systemically-induced contact dermatitis from metal wire in orthodontic materials. Contact Dermat 30:210–213

342. Pigatto PD, Guzzi G (2004) Systemic contact dermatitis from nickel associated with orthodontic appliances. Contact Dermat 50:100–101

343. Hensten-Pettersen A (1989) Nickel allergy and dental treatment procedures. In: Maibach HI, Menné T (eds) Nickel and the skin: immunology and toxicology. CRC, Boca Raton, pp 195–205

344. Garcia AP, Tovar V, de Barrio M, Villanueva A, Tornero P (2008) Contact allergy to inhaled budesonide. Contact Dermat 59:60–61

345. Fisher AA (1987) Reactions of the mucous membrane to contactants. Clin Dermatol 5:123–136

346. Chan EF, Mowad C (1998) Contact dermatitis to foods and spices. Am J Contact Dermat 9:71–79

347. Sonnex TS, Dawber RPR, Ryan TJ (1981) Mucosal contact dermatitis due to instant coffee. Contact Dermat 7:298–300

348. Guerra L, Vincenzi C, Peluso AM, Tosti A (1993) Role of contact sensitizers in the burning mouth syndrome. Am J Contact Dermat 4:154–157

349. Peters MS, Schroeter AL, Van Hale VM, Braodbent JC (1984) Pacemaker contact sensitivity. Contact Dermat 11:214–218

350. Romaguera C, Grimalt F (1981) Pacemaker dermatitis. Contact Dermat 7:333

351. Schuh A, Lill C, Hönle W, Effenberger H (2008) Prevalence of allergic reactions to implant materials in total hip and knee arthroplasty. Zentralbl Chir 133:292–296

352. Lacroix J, Morin CL, Collin P-P (1979) Nickel dermatitis from a foreign body in the stomach. J Pediatr 95:428–429

353. McFadden N, Lyberg T, Hensten-Pettersen A (1989) Aluminium-induced granulomas in a tattoo. J Am Acad Dermatol 20:903–908

354. Fleming C, Parry E, Forsyth A, Kemmett D (1997) Patch testing in discoid eczema. Contact Dermat 36:261–264

355. Janniger CK, Schwartz RA (1995) Seborrhoeic dermatitis. Am Fam Physician 52(149–155):159–160

356. Kerl H, Pachinger W (1979) Psoriasis: odd varieties in the adult. Acta Derm Venereol (Stockh) Suppl 87:90–94

357. Veien NK, Hattel T, Laurberg G (1997) Low-humidity dermatosis from car heaters. Contact Dermat 37:138

358. Clark AR, Sherertz EF (1998) The incidence of allergic contact dermatitis in patients with psoriasis vulgaris. Am J Contact Dermat 9:96–99

359. Heule F, Tahapary GJM, Bello CR, van Joost Th (1998) Delayed-type hypersensitivity to contact allergens in psoriasis. A clinical evaluation. Contact Dermat 38:78–82

360. Feuerman EJ, Ingber A, David M, Weissman-Katzenelson V (1982) Lichen ruber planus beginning as a dyshidrosiform eruption. Cutis 30:401–404

361. Jakob T, Tiemann M, Kuwert C, Abeck D, Mensing H, Ring J (1996) Dyshidrotic cutaneous T-cell lymphoma. J Am Acad Dermatol 34:295–297

Clinical Aspects of Irritant Contact Dermatitis

16

Peter J. Frosch and Swen Malte John

Contents

P.J. Frosch
Hautklinik, Klinikum Dortmund gGmbH,
Beurhausstr. 40, 44137 Dortmund, Germany
e-mail: peter.frosch@klinikumdo.de

S.M. John
Department of Dermatology, Environmental Medicine and
Health Theory, University of Osnabrueck, Sedanstrasse 115,
49069 Osnabrück, Germany
e-mail: sjohn@uos.de

16.1 Definition

Irritant contact dermatitis may be defined as a nonallergic inflammatory reaction of the skin to an external agent. The acute type comprises two forms, the irritant reaction and acute irritant contact dermatitis, and usually has only a single cause. In contrast, the chronic form, cumulative insult dermatitis, is a multifactorial disease in most cases. Toxic chemicals (irritants) are the major cause, but mechanical, thermal, and climatic effects are important contributory cofactors. The clinical spectrum of irritant contact dermatitis is much wider than that of allergic contact dermatitis and ranges from slight scaling of the stratum corneum, through redness, whealing, and deep caustic burns, to an eczematous condition indistinguishable from allergic contact dermatitis. Acute forms of irritant contact dermatitis may be painful and may be associated with sensations such as burning, stinging, or itching. Individual susceptibility to irritants is extremely variable.

Core Message

> Irritant contact dermatitis is caused by chemicals which damage skin structures in a direct nonallergic way. The clinical picture is extremely variable and ranges from chemical burns to chronic irritant forms, often indistinguishable from allergic contact dermatitis.

16.2 Clinical Picture

The morphology of cutaneous irritation varies widely and depends on the type and intensity of the irritant(s).

J.D. Johansen et al. (eds.), *Contact Dermatitis*,
DOI: 10.1007/978-3-642-03827-3_16, © Springer-Verlag Berlin Heidelberg 2011

Based on clinical criteria we may distinguish the following types:

Chemical burns
Irritant reactions
Acute irritant contact dermatitis
Chronic irritant contact dermatitis (cumulative insult dermatitis)

Folliculitis, acneiform eruptions, miliaria, pigmentary alterations, alopecia, contact urticaria, and granulomatous reactions may result from irritancy to chemicals (Table 16.1, Fig. 16.1), but in the following, only the first four types, clinically the most important, will be discussed in detail.

16.2.1 Chemical Burns

Highly alkaline or acid materials can cause severe tissue damage even after short skin contact. Painful erythema develops at exposed sites, usually within minutes, and is followed by vesiculation and formation of necrotic eschars (Figs. 16.2–16.7). Occasionally, intense whealing can be observed in the erythematous phase due to toxic degranulation of mast cells (Fig. 16.7). The shape of lesions is bizarre and "artificial" in most cases and does not follow the usual pattern of known dermatoses. This is an important hallmark in differentiating accidental and self-inflicted lesions from genuine skin disease (Figs. 16.3, 16.8, and 16.9). In accidents, the clothing may cause a sharp border due to its protective effect (e.g., explosion of liquids in containers).

Strong acids and alkalis are the major causes of chemical burns (Fig. 16.10). The halogenated acids are particularly dangerous because they may lead to deep continuous tissue destruction even after short skin contact (Fig. 16.2). Holes in protective gloves may result in serious injuries with scar formation. Caustic chemicals are also often trapped by clothing and footwear, resulting in deep ulceration down to the subcutaneous tissue, whereas other, open, areas are less severely affected because of the possibility of rapid removal (Fig. 16.4).

It is important to realize that a number of other chemicals, including dusts and solids, may also cause severe necrotic lesions after prolonged skin contact, particularly under occlusion (cement, amine hardeners, etc.). If the concentration of the irritant is low or contact time short, multiple lesions can develop (Fig. 16.11).

Table 16.1 Clinical effects of chemical irritants (adapted from [112])

Ulcerations	Strong acids (chromic, hydrofluoric, nitric, hydrochloric, sulfuric) Strong alkalis (especially calcium oxide, calcium hydroxide, sodium hydroxide, sodium metasilicate, sodium silicate, potassium cyanide, trisodium phosphate) Salts (arsenic trioxide, dichromates) Solvents (acrylonitrile, carbon disulfide) Gases (ethylene oxide, acrylonitrile)
Folliculitis and acneiform lesions	Arsenic trioxide Fiberglass (Fig. 16.1) Oils and greases Tar Asphalt Chlorinated naphthalenes Polyhalogenated biphenyls
Miliaria	Occlusive clothing and dressing Adhesive tape Aluminum chloride
Hyperpigmentation	Any irritant (especially phototoxic agents such as psoralens, tar, asphalt) Metals (inorganic arsenic, silver, gold, bismuth, mercury)
Hypopigmentation	p-tert-Amylphenol p-tert-Butylphenol Hydroquinone Monobenzyl ether of hydroquinone p-tert-Catechol 3-Hydroxyanisole 1-tert-Butyl-3, 4-catechol
Alopecia	Borax Chloroprene dimers
Urticaria	Chemicals (dimethylsulfoxide) Cosmetics (sorbic acid) Animals Foods Plants Textiles Woods
Granulomas	Silica Beryllium Talc

Core Message

> Chemical burns result from strong acids or alkalis. Halogenated acids are particularly dangerous. Severe tissue damage may result even after short contact. Typical is the initial painful whitening and edema of the skin, followed by deep necrosis and scarring.

16.2.2 Irritant Reactions

Irritants may produce cutaneous reactions that do not meet the clinical definition of "dermatitis." In English-speaking countries the term "dermatitis" is held to be

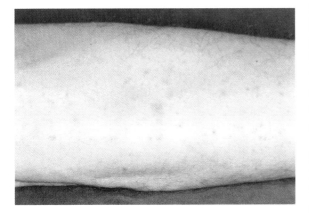

Fig. 16.1 Glass fiber dermatitis. Severe itchy small papules on the forearms of a teacher who isolated his roof with glass wool from a do-it-yourself store without any protection

synonymous with "eczema" by most authors, though this can be disputed. The diagnosis "acute irritant reaction" is thus increasingly used if the clinical picture is monomorphic rather than polymorphic and characterized by one or more of the following signs: scaling (including the initial stage of "dryness"), redness (starting with faint follicular spots, up to dusky red areas with hemorrhages), vesicles (blisters), pustules, and erosions (follicular and planar). Severe cutaneous damage reaching down to dermal structures should be termed a "chemical burn" (German: *Verätzung*, French: *cautérisation*). In practice, some overlap will exist which may result in a variable clinical picture, particularly when the course over time is followed (Table 16.6).

Chemicals which can cause irritant reactions are listed in Table 16.2, and typical clinical effects are shown in Figs. 16.12–16.13 and 16.15. The substances are mainly "mild irritants," i.e., ones that do not cause a severe skin reaction on short contact (<1 h). The resulting skin lesion may vary with the type of exposure, body region, and individual susceptibility (Figs. 16.14 and 16.12).

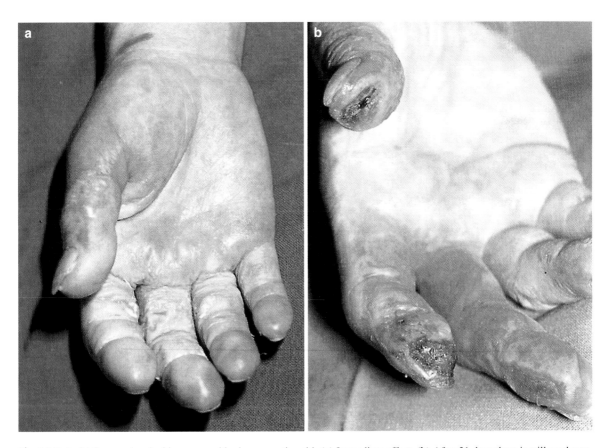

Fig. 16.2 (**a**, **b**) Severe chemical burn caused by bromoacetic acid. (**a**) Immediate effect. (**b**) After 21 days there is still erythema, edema, and deep necrotic lesions

16

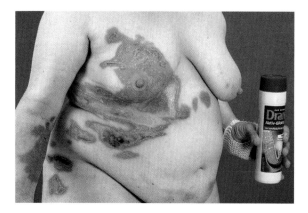

Fig. 16.3 Severe chemical burns from a sewage cleaner applied by a dement patient for relief of itching. Note the undamaged area of the nipple

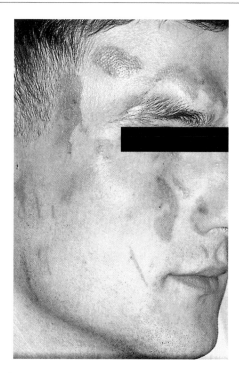

Fig. 16.5 Brown–yellow staining and superficial epidermal damage induced by splashes of nitric acid. Note the streaky pattern

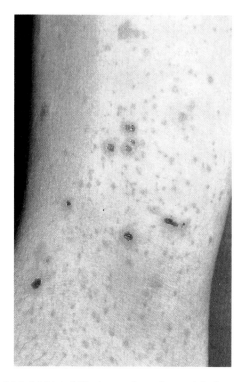

Fig. 16.4 Multiple follicular papules and necrotic lesions on the arm of a factory worker caused by sodium hydroxide trapped in the clothes after the explosion of a container

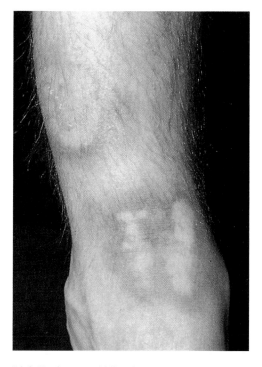

Fig. 16.6 Erythema and blistering on the lower leg caused by undiluted isothiazolinone (Kathon WT) trapped in the rubber boot of a machinist adding the biocide to cutting oil

---

Core Message

> An irritant reaction is monomorphous (ery-thema, wheals, papules, pustules) and often experimentally induced.

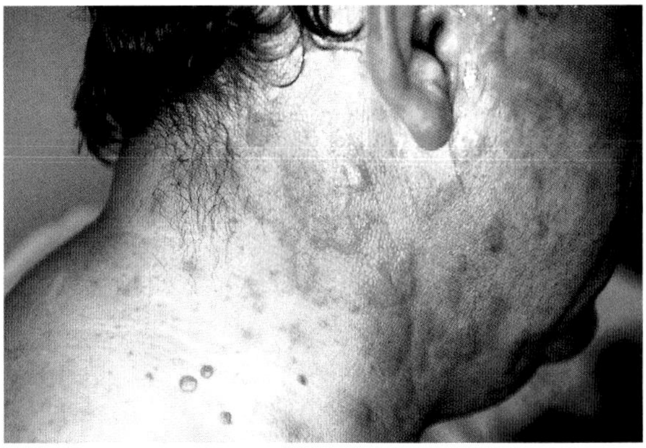

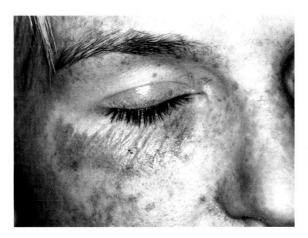

Fig. 16.7 Urticarial plaques 20 min after contact with concentrated phenol (explosion of a container)

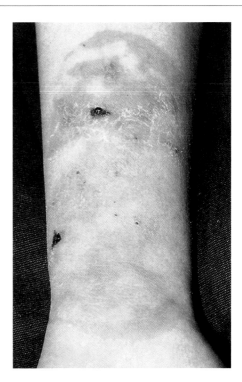

Fig. 16.9 Artifactual dermatitis with erythema, scaling, and crusting in a psychotic patient caused by rubbing in a harsh floor cleanser. Typical of an artifact is the sharp demarcation

Fig. 16.8 Acute chemical burn with sharply demarcated erythema and superficial erosions due to a concentrated acid (most likely hydrochloric acid); pH in the lesion was 1.2, in the adjacent areas 5.4. This artifactual dermatitis was seen in a car mechanic who claimed for legal compensation

16.2.3 Acute Irritant Contact Dermatitis

The clinical appearance of acute irritant contact dermatitis is very variable and it may even be indistinguishable from the allergic type. There are numerous reports in the literature of even experienced dermatologists being misled into an initial assumption of allergic contact dermatitis, which later, after a careful workup, turned out to be "only irritation." (Fig. 16.16).

Most instructive is the report by Malten et al. [1] on hexanediol diacrylate. A UV-cured paint used in a door factory contained hexanediol diacrylate, which caused an epidemic of papular and burning, rather than itching, dermatitis among the workers. Retrospectively, it is clear that the irritant contact dermatitis did not show the typical

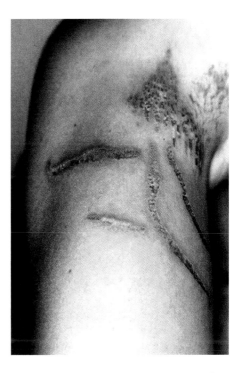

Fig. 16.10 Deep ulcerations with scar formation after contact with a jellyfish when bathing in the Mediterranean Sea

16

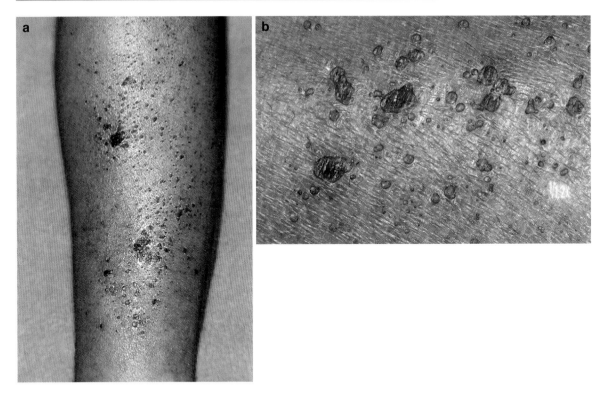

Fig. 16.11 (**a**, **b**) Multiple small chemical burns due to cement dust on the arms of a mason. The lesions appeared when freshly set plaster was roughened with a sharp instrument

polymorphic picture of contact allergy, with the synchronous presence of macules, papules, and vesicles. These lesions developed one after another over the course of a few days (metachronic polymorphism). Malten et al. used the term "delayed irritation" for this type of cutaneous irritancy. In the meantime, it has also been reported with other diacrylates [2] and various other substances [3].

Delayed irritation may be more common than so far generally thought. Further substances causing it are listed in Table 16.3. Irritant patch test reactions to benzalkonium chloride may be papular and increase in intensity with time [4–6]. On the normal skin surrounding psoriatic plaques, dithranol causes redness and edema, which may become very severe on the legs with venous stasis.

Calcipotriol frequently causes delayed irritation after several applications. Although redness and edema dominate, papules and vesicles may develop and mimic contact allergy. The latter has been verified only in rare cases, requiring patch testing with serial dilutions, repeated open application, and, if possible, repeat of those procedures at a later stage [7]. Diclofenac gel is now widely used for the treatment of solar keratoses. In

patients with sensitive skin, a severe irritant dermatitis may develop within a few days, clinically indistinguishable from allergic contact dermatitis (Fig. 16.17a). Imiquimod applied for the treatment of superficial basal cell carcinoma or actinic keratoses is also producing severe inflammatory reactions. It is often so fierce that the patient discontinues the treatment and the physician thinks of an allergic contact dermatitis (Fig. 16.17b).

A series of cases with chemical burns due to bromide was reported [8]. Small vesicles and bullae, or erythematous patches followed by hyperpigmentation, developed 2–5 days after exposure to bromine in the face and neck region of workers exposed to bromine vapors or liquids [8]. Bromine is used for gasoline additives, agricultural chemicals, flame retardants, dyes, photographic and pharmaceutical chemicals, bleaching of pulp and paper, etc.

The model irritants sodium lauryl sulfate (SLS) and nonanoic acid have been used in many patch test studies as a "positive control." Using detailed visual scoring, and particularly with bioengineering methods (transepidermal water loss, skin blood flow, skin surface contour),

Table 16.2 Common irritants which are important causes of occupational dermatitis (adapted from [288–290])

Water and its additives	(Salts and oxides of calcium, magnesium, and iron)
Skin cleansers	Soaps, detergents, "waterless cleansers," and additives (sand, silica)
Industrial cleaning agents	Detergents, surface-active agents, sulfonated oils, wetting agents, emulsifiers, enzymes
Alkalis	Soap, soda, ammonia, potassium and sodium hydroxides, cement, lime, sodium silicate, trisodium phosphate, and various amines
Acids	Severe irritancy (caustic): sulfuric, hydrochloric, nitric, chromic, and hydrofluoric acids Moderate irritancy: acetic, oxalic, and salicylic acids
Oils	Cutting oils with various additives (water, emulsifiers, antioxidants, anticorrosive agents, preservatives, dyes, and perfumes) Lubricating and spindle oils
Organic solvents	White spirit, benzene, toluene, trichloroethylene, perchloroethylene, methylene chloride, chlorobenzene Methanol, ethanol, isopropanol, propylene glycol Ethyl acetate, acetone, methyl ethyl ketone, ethylene glycol monomethyl ether, nitroethane, turpentine, carbon disulfide Thinners (mixtures of alcohols, ketones, and toluene)
Oxidizing agents	Hydrogen peroxide, benzoyl peroxide, cyclohexanone peroxide, sodium hypochlorite
Reducing agents	Phenols, hydrazines, aldehydes, thioglycolates
Plants	Citrus peel and juice, flower bulbs, garlic, onion, pineapple, pelargonium, iris, cucumbers, buttercups, asparagus, mustard, barley, chicory, corn Various plants of the spurge family (Euphorbiaceae), Brassicaceae family (Cruciferae) and Ranunculaceae family (for further details see [291])
Animal products	Pancreatic enzymes, bodily secretions
Miscellaneous irritants	Alkyl tin compounds and penta-, tetra-, and trichlorophenols (wood preservatives) Bromine (in gasoline, agricultural chemicals, paper industry, flame retardant) Methylchloroisothiazolinone and methylisothiazolinone (irritant at high concentrations during production or misuse) Components of plastic processing (formaldehyde, phenol, cresol, styrene, di-isocyanates, acrylic monomers, diallyl phthalate, aliphatic and aromatic amines, epichlorohydrin) Metal polishes Fertilizers Propionic acid (preservative in animal feed) Rust-preventive products Paint removers (alkyl bromide) Acrolein, crotonaldehyde, ethylene oxide, mercuric salts, zinc chloride, chlorine

it can be demonstrated that the intensity of reaction may increase over time (48 h vs. 96 h), at least within a certain low concentration range [9, 10]. Furthermore, data from right to left comparisons showed good reproducibility. The traditional view in patch testing that reactions that fade after 48 h are necessarily irritant, rather than allergic, has to be discarded.

Irritation due to tretinoin develops usually after a few days and is characterized by mild to fiery redness, followed by large flakes of stratum corneum. The dermatitis is burning rather than itching. The skin becomes sensitive to touch and to water (Fig. 16.18).

Acute irritant contact dermatitis includes other well-known entities such as irritation from adhesive tapes (Fig. 16.19), diaper dermatitis [11], perianal dermatitis [12], and airborne irritant contact dermatitis due to dusts and vapors (Table 16.4, Fig. 16.20). A long list of airborne irritants that caused a dermatitis, which initially was often thought to be allergic, has been compiled and recently updated (Table 16.5) [13–15].

Cosmetics are not infrequently the cause of mild irritant contact dermatitis on the face, particularly the eyelids, where contact allergy has to be excluded by appropriate patch and use testing [16].

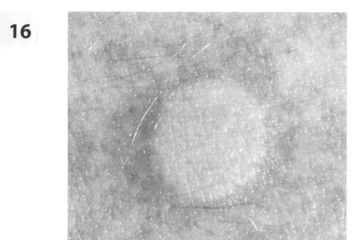

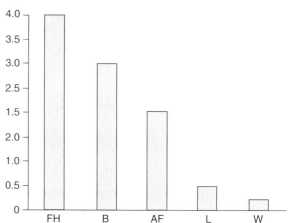

Fig. 16.14 Regional variation in cutaneous reactivity to the irritant *DMSO*. The whealing response is most intense in the facial region and least on the palms of the hands (*AF* Antecubital fossa; *B* upper back; *FH* forehead; *L* lower leg; *W* wrist)

Fig. 16.12 Marked whealing induced by the application of undiluted dimethylsulfoxide (*DMSO*) in a cup for 5 min

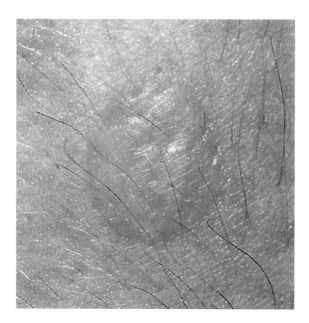

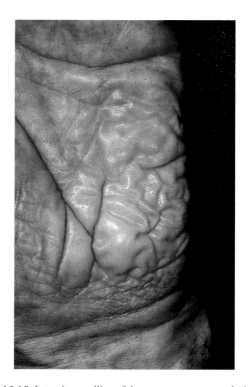

Fig. 16.13 Superficial blister after the application of 0.1% cantharidin in acetone for 24 h

Reaction to prostheses of the limbs (Fig. 16.21) or hearing aids are often not allergic but irritant. Perianal dermatitis is primarily due to fecal enzymes, but in patients taking pancreatic enzymes as supplements, this may provoke a severe spreading dermatitis, even with vulvodynia [17]. It has also been described in

Fig.16.15 Intensive swelling of the stratum corneum and edema caused by undiluted DMSO applied for 12 h under a dressing. DMSO was used as an "antidote" after the patient had accidentally pricked himself with the needle of a syringe containing a cytostatic drug [287]

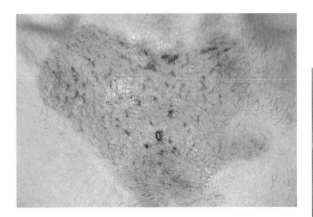

Fig. 16.16 Acute irritant contact dermatitis with acneiform features in a patient with severe acne vulgaris. Initially thought to be caused by the prescribed topical medications (benzoyl peroxide washing solution, clindamycin gel), it turned out to be due to an epilating wax, which the patient applied once weekly

Table 16.3 Substances causing delayed irritancy. The peak of intensity may show a crescendo pattern more typical of contact allergens

Benzalkonium chloride
Benzoyl peroxide
Bis (2-chloroethyl) sulfide
Bromine
Butanediol diacrylate
Calcipotriol
Dichlor (2-chlorovinyl) arsine
Diclofenac
Dithranol
Epichlorhydrin
Ethylene oxide
Hexanediol diacrylate
Nonanoic acid
Octyl gallate
Podophyllin
Propane sulfone
Propylene glycol
Sodium lauryl sulfate
Tetraethylene glycol diacrylate
Tretinoin

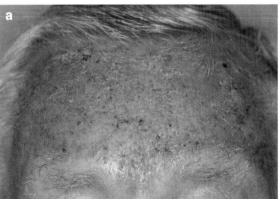

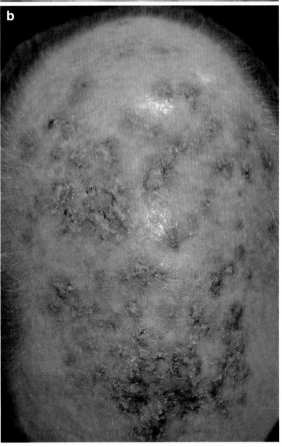

Fig. 16.17 Acute irritant contact dermatitis on the forehead 1 week after the application of diclofenac gel (twice daily) for the treatment of actinic keratoses. (**a**) The patient had skin type I and very sensitive skin all his life. Patch testing with diclofenac gel as well as a repetitive open application test on the forearm for 1 week was negative. Severe inflammatory reaction by imiquimod after only four applications for the treatment of actinic keratoses (**b**). The dermatitis may mimic an allergic contact dermatitis

16

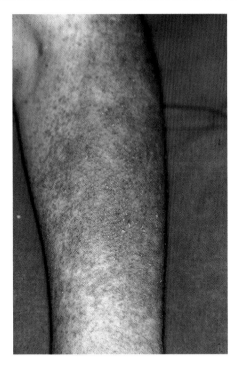

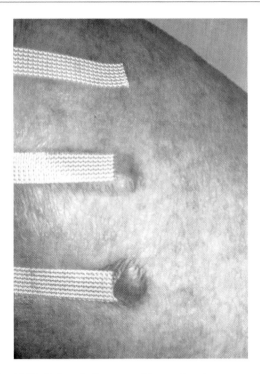

Fig. 16.18 Acute irritant contact dermatitis with erythema, papules, and scaling after 2 weeks of application of a cream containing tretinoin and urea for follicular hyperkeratosis. Patch testing was negative

Fig. 16.19 Bullous lesions caused by tension along tape strips for the closure of a surgical wound. There was no dermatitis; patch testing with the tape was negative

patients taking danthron laxatives, converted in the colon to the well-known irritant dithranol.

Dermatitis at the borders of a stoma (fecal or urinary) is frequently seen and in most cases nonallergic (Fig. 16.22) [18]. The same is true for inflamed margins of wounds treated with synthetic hydrocolloid dressings. However, allergic reactions to the adhesives may occur [19].

Table 16.4 Dermatoses where irritants play a major role in the pathogenesis

Hand eczema
Cosmetic dermatitis
Eyelid eczema
Reactions to therapeutics
Tape irritation
Diaper dermatitis
Perianal and stoma dermatitis
Asteatotic eczema
"Status eczematicus"
Juvenile plantar dermatosis
Photoirritation
Plant dermatitis
Reactions to wool and textiles
Contact urticaria
Subjective irritation ("stinging")
Airborne irritant contact dermatitis

Depending on individual susceptibility and intensity of exposure to the irritant(s), the dermatitis may be more acute or more chronic

Core Message

> Acute irritant contact dermatitis is often indistinguishable from allergic contact dermatitis. It may be a diagnosis by exclusion after careful patch testing. In practice, the most common causes are cosmetics, reactions to therapeutics (e.g., for acne, psoriasis) and adhesive tapes. Further examples are diaper, perianal, and stoma dermatitis.

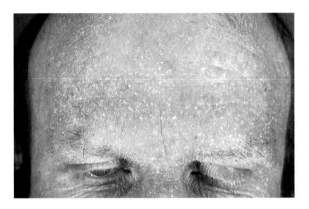

Fig. 16.20 Airborne irritant contact dermatitis with slight erythema and scaling caused by irritating stone dust (lime and chalk)

Table 16.5 Causes of airborne contact dermatitis

Plants, natural resins, and wood allergens	*Acacia melanoxylon* (Australian blackwood) *Alstroemeria* (tulipalin A) Anethole *Apium graveolens* *Apuleia leiocarpa* wood (Brazilian wood) Atranorin (metabolite of oak moss) *Bowdichia nitida* (sucupira, South-American wood) Champignon mushroom Citrus fruits (lemon essential oils) *Coleus* plant Colophonium and pine dust Compositae (Asteraceae) *Dalbergia latifolia* Roxb (East-Indian rosewood) *Dendranthema morifolium* *Entandrophragma cylindricum* Essential oils *Fraxinus americanus* (a domestic wood) *Frullania* (liverwort) Garlic *Helianthus annuus* (sunflower) Iroko (*Chlorophora excelsa*, West-African hard wood) Lichens *Machaerium acutiforium* (Bolivian rosewood, a tropical wood) *Machaerium scleroxylon* (Santos rosewood. pao ferro) *Panthenium hyserophorus* *Primula obconica* Soybean
	Tea tree oil Tropical woods (e.g., framire) Wild plants (*Anthemis nobilis, Sisymbrium officinale*)
Plastics, rubbers, glues	Acrylates Aziridine derivates Benzoyl peroxide Diaminodiphenylmethane Dibutylthiourea Epoxy acrylates Epoxy resin (and amines) Formaldehyde and formaldehyde resins isocyanates (diphenyl-methane-4, 4-diisocyanate) Isophoronediamine Triglycidyl isocyanurate Unsaturated polyester resin
Metals	Arsenic salts Chromate (potassium dichromate) Cobalt Gold Mercury Nickel
Industrial and pharmaceutical chemicals	Albendazole(antihelminthic agent) 2-Aminophenyldisulfide 2-Aminothiophenol Apomorphine Benzalkonium chloride Bis-(aminopropyl)-laurylamine Budesonide Cacodylic acid Cefazolin Chloroacetamide Chlorprothixene Chlorothalonil Color developers Didecyldimethylammonium chloride Difencyprone Di-isopropyl carbodi-imide DOPPI Ethylenediamine FADCP Famotidine and intermediates Hydroxylammonium chloride Isoflurane Isothiazolinones Metaproterenol Methyl red (dye) Nicergoline Ortho-chlorobenzylidenemalonitrile Paracetamol Phosphorus sesquisulfide Phthalocyanine pigments Propacetamol Pyritinol (and pyritinol hydrochloride)

(continued)

16

Table 16.5 (continued)

Pesticides and animal feed additives	Carbamates (fungicides)
	Cobalt (animal feed additive)
	Dyrene
	Ethoxyquin (antioxidant in animal feed)
	Olaquindox
	Oxytetracycline hydrochloride (animal feed antibiotic)
	Penicillin (animal feed antibiotic)
	Pyrethrum
	Spiramycin (animal feed antibiotic)
	tetrachloroacetophenone (insecticide)
	Tylosin (animal feed antibiotic)
Miscellaneous	Cigarettes and matches
	Tyrophagus putrescentiae
	Pig epithelia
	Penicillium
	Cladosporium

Listed are reports on allergic contact dermatitis, irritant contact dermatitis, photoallergic reactions, contact urticaria, erythema-multiforme-like eruption, pigmented contact dermatitis, and various eruptions (adapted from [13, 14, 292–294])

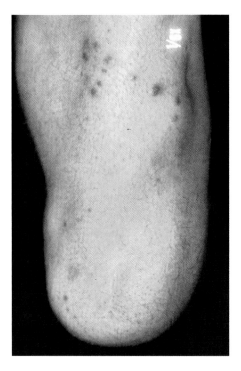

Fig. 16.21 Acneiform lesions and erythema on an amputated leg due to occlusion of the prosthesis. Extensive patch testing was negative

Various irritants have been tested under experimental conditions and it has been shown that a wide range of lesions can be produced by varying the dose and mode of exposure (Table 16.6).

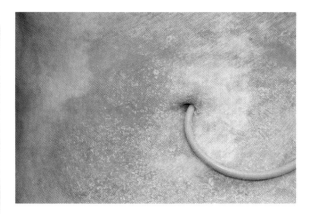

Fig. 16.22 Irritant dermatitis around a ureter catheter in a patient with metastasized ovarial carcinoma. The dermatitis was due to urinary leakage and various adhesive dressings

The reaction's intensity depends on numerous exogenous and endogenous factors. Under experimental conditions a full range of lesions may be produced with the same irritant by varying its dose. In this table, the most typical skin changes are given as observed frequently after more or less "normal" exposure. Most irritants can produce severe bullous reactions if applied under occlusion at high concentration for 24 h. For further details, see [5, 20–25]. The irritant potential of water after repetitive short contact or long continuous exposure has been underestimated in the past [26]. Warner et al. have shown by ultrastructural studies that water directly disrupts stratum corneum lipid lamellar bilayers even after a 4-h occlusion phase [27]. Effects are similar to those induced by surfactants [28].

16.2.4 Chronic Irritant Contact Dermatitis

Other terms synonymous with chronic irritant contact dermatitis include "cumulative insult dermatitis," "traumiterative dermatitis," and "wear and tear dermatitis" (German: *Abnutzungsdermatose, chronisch degeneratives Ekzem*). Although never clearly defined, this diagnosis applies to an eczematous condition that persists for a considerable time period (minimum 6 weeks) and for which careful diagnostic investigation has failed to demonstrate an allergic cause. Taking a detailed history usually reveals the dermatitis to be caused by repetitive contact with water, detergents, organic solvents, irritant foods, or other known mild to moderate irritants.

Table 16.6 Materials causing irritant reactions on human skin

Irritant	Cutaneous reaction
Water	Dryness, erythema, scaling, wrinkling ("immersion foot")
Detergents (anionic), soaps	Dryness, erythema, scaling, fissuring, (rarely vesicles)
Tretinoin, benzoyl peroxide dithranol, calcipotriol, diclofenac	Dryness, erythema, scaling
Benzalkonium chloride (and other cationic detergents)	Erythema, pustules (rarely delayed reactions) with papules
Dimethylsulfoxide	Erythema, whealing (strong)
Methyl nicotinate	Erythema, whealing (weak)
Capsaicin	Erythema, vesiculation
Sodium hydroxide	Erythema, erosions (follicular initially)
Lactic acid	Erythema, whealing
Nonanoic acid	Erythema, scaling
Croton oil	Erythema, pustules, purulent bullae
Kerosene	As croton oil
Cantharidin	Erythema, bullae
Metal salts (mercury chloride, cobalt chloride, nickel sulfate, potassium dichromate)	Erythema, pustules, purulent bullae
Formic acid	Erythema, superficial blistering (removal of stratum corneum)
Xylene	Dryness, erythema
Toluene	Dryness, erythema, purpura

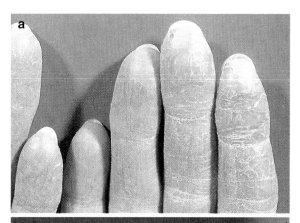

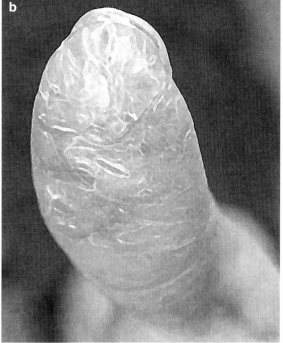

Fig. 16.23 (**a**, **b**) Chronic irritant contact dermatitis (cumulative insult dermatitis). (**a**) Housewife's eczema due to wet work and a number of irritants. (**b**) Close-up view of the thumb

The prime localization is on the hands ("housewives' eczema"). In a fully developed case, redness, infiltration, and scaling with fissuring are seen all over the hands (Fig. 16.23). The dermatitis includes the fingers, initially starting in the webs, but spreading later to the sides and backs of the hands and finally including the palmar aspect. This is frequently observed in hairdressers [29] (Fig. 16.24a–c). The volar aspect of the wrist is usually unaffected, in contrast to allergic or atopic hand eczema. Occasionally, there is a nummular pattern on the backs of the hands (Fig. 16.25). If there is extensive occupational contact with moderate irritants (organic solvents, detergents), the dermatitis may be limited to those fingers with most exposure. Friction is a further contributing factor and plays an important part in determining the localization of the dermatitis

[30–33]. Hyperkeratosis of the fingertips was observed in nearly half of the shoemakers in the sole-cutting department as a reaction to the continuous trauma of working with leather [34].

The hallmark of chronic irritant contact dermatitis may be the absence of vesicles and the predominance of dryness and chapping, and a number of studies on hand eczema have confirmed that vesiculation is less frequent in the irritant type than in allergic and atopic types [35–38]. However, the diagnosis is often complicated by so-called hybrids, where there is a combination of irritancy and contact allergy, or of irritancy and atopy, or even all three [38, 39]. For further information see

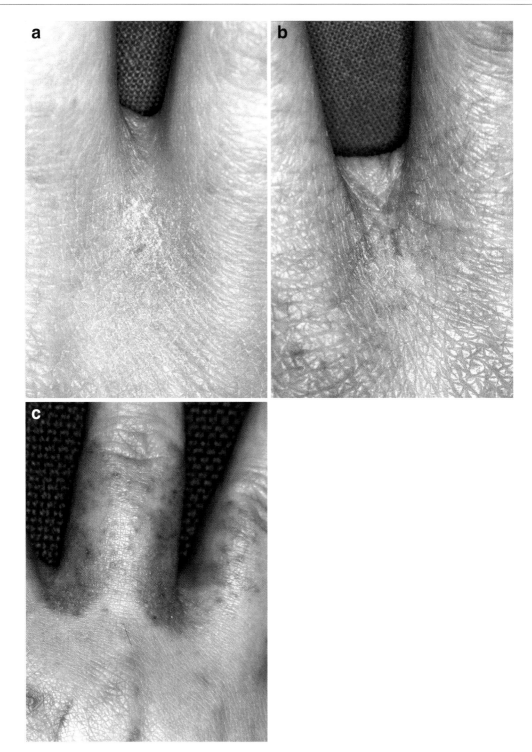

Fig. 16.24 (**a–c**) Characteristic sequence of events in the development of irritant hand dermatitis due to unprotected wet work in the hairdressing trade (17-year-old female apprentice): initial mild interdigital scaling (**a**), gradual onset of erythema, lichenification, superficial fissures (**b**), marked erythema, vesicles, deep fissures, and erosions (**c**)

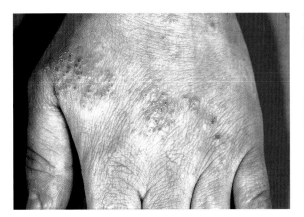

Fig. 16.25 Chronic irritant contact dermatitis of the nummular type on the back of the hand of a housewife

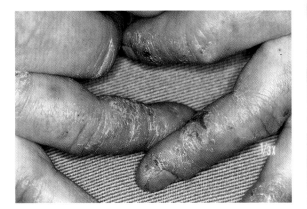

Fig. 16.26 Chronic irritant contact dermatitis on the fingers from metalworking fluids in a metalworker polishing small objects

Table 16.7 High-risk occupations for chronic irritant (cumulative insult) contact dermatitis (adapted from [80])

Baker
Butcher
Canner
Caterer
Cleaner
Cook
Construction worker
Dental assistant or technician
Fisherman
Florist
Hairdresser
Health care worker
Horticulture and nursery gardening
Machinist
Masseur
Mechanic
Metalworker (surface processor)
Motor mechanic
Nurse (hospitals and nursing homes for elderly)
Painter
Pastry cook
Printer
Shoemaker
Tile setter and terrazzo worker

Chap. 20, a recent monograph on hand eczema [40] and some pertinent recent original publications [41–45].

Dermatitis due to metalworking fluids is irritant in most cases and shows a variable morphological pattern (Fig. 16.26). Some workers exhibit only dryness and scaling of the hands, whereas others develop an itchy nummular type of dermatitis spreading to the forearms and sometimes other exposed body regions. The correct diagnosis can often be made only after careful patch testing and reexposure to the work environment [46].

In atopic hand eczema, irritant factors often play a major role in the pathogenesis. It is sometimes a matter of definition whether these cases are diagnosed primarily as atopic or irritant contact dermatitis.

High-risk occupations for chronic irritant contact dermatitis are listed in Table 16.7, and the major irritants in various occupations are summarized in Table 16.8.

> ## Core Message
>
> › Chronic irritant contact dermatitis is most frequently localized on the hands. Usually, several chemical irritants are involved and cumulate together with climatic and mechanical factors to low-grade damage over months. Redness, scaling, and fissures on the back of the hands, between fingers or on the most exposed parts of the hands are prominent clinical signs. Lack of itching and slow aggravation after resuming work are typical. However, the diagnosis is often difficult, requires careful patch testing and a follow-up. Furthermore, combined forms with a contact allergy may exist.

Table 16.8 List of irritants in various occupations (based on [112, 288, 289, 295])

Occupation	Irritants
Agricultural workers	Pesticides, artificial fertilizers, disinfectants and cleansers for milking utensils, petrol, diesel oil, plants, animal secretions
Artists	Solvents used for cleansing and degreasing, soaps and detergents, paint removers
Bakers and pastry makers	Soaps and detergents, oven cleaners, fruit juices, acetic, ascorbic and lactic acid, enzymes
Bartenders	Wet work, soaps and detergents, fruit juices, alcohol
Bathing attendants	Wet work, soaps and detergents, free or combined chlorine/bromine
Bookbinders	Glue, solvents
Building workers	Cement, chalk, hydrochloric and hydrofluoric acids, wood preservatives, glues
Butchers	Soaps and detergents, wet work, spices, meat, entrails
Canning and food industry workers and fruit juices	Soaps and detergents, wet work, brine, syrup, vegetables and vegetable juices, fruit and fruit juices, fish, meat, crustaceans
Carpenters, cabinet makers	French polish, solvents, glues, cleansers, wood preservatives
Chemical and pharmaceutical workers	Soaps and detergents, wet work, solvents, numerous other irritants that industry are specific for each workplace
Cleaners	Wet work, detergents, solvents
Coal and other miners	Oil, grease, cement, powdered limestone
Cooks, catering industry	Soaps and detergents, wet work, vegetable and fruit juices, spices, fish, meat, crustaceans, dressing, vinegar
Dentists and dental technicians	Soaps and detergents, wet work, soldering, fluxes, adhesives, acrylic monomers, solvents
Dyers	Solvents, oxidizing and reducing agents, hypochlorite, hair removers
Electricians, electronics industry	Soldering flux, metal cleaners, epoxy resin hardeners
Fishermen	Wet work, oils, petrol fish, crustaceans, entrails
Floor layers	Detergents, solvents, cement, adhesives
Florists, gardeners, plant growers	Manure, fertilizers, pesticides, irritating plants and plant parts
Foundry workers	Cleansers, oils, phenol-formaldehyde and other resins
Hairdressers and barbers	Soap, wet work, shampoos, permanent wave liquids, bleaching agents
Histology technicians	Solvents, formaldehyde
Hospital workers	Soaps and detergents, wet work, hand creams, disinfectants, quaternary ammonium compounds
Housework	Soaps and detergents, wet work, cleaners, polishes, food
Jewelers	Acids and alkalis for metal cleaning, polishes, soldering fluxes, rust removers, adhesives
Laundry workers	Detergents, wet work, bleaches, solvents, stain removers
Masons	Cement, chalk, acids
Mechanics	Detergents, hand cleansers, degreasers, lubricants, oils, cooling system fluids, battery acid, soldering flux, petrol, diesel oil
Metalworkers	Hand cleansers, cutting and drilling oils, solvents
Office workers	Ammonia from photocopy paper, carbonless copy paper

Table 16.8 (continued)

Occupation	Irritants
Painters	Solvents, emulsion paints, paint removers, organic tin compounds, hand cleanser
Photographers	Alkalis, acids, solvents, oxidizing and reducing agents
Plastic industry workers	Solvents, acids, oxidizing agents, styrene, di-isocyanates, acrylic monomers, phenols, formaldehyde, diallyl phthalate, ingredients in epoxy resin systems
Plating industry workers	Acids, alkalis, solvents, detergents
Plumbers	Wet work, hand cleansers, oils, soldering flux
Printers	Solvents, hand cleansers, acrylates in radiation-curing printing lacquers and inks
Radio and television repairers	Organic solvents, metal cleansers, soldering fluxes
Roofers	Tar, pitch, asphalt, solvents, hand cleansers
Rubber workers	Talc, zinc stearate, solvents
Shoemakers	Solvents, polishes, adhesives, rough leather
Shop assistants	Detergents, vegetables, fruit, fish, meat
Tanners	Wet work, acids, alkalis, oxidizing and reducing agents, solvents, proteolytic enzymes
Textile workers	Solvents, bleaching agents, detergents
Veterinarians	Soaps and detergents, hypochlorite, cresol, entrails, animal secretions
Welders	Oils, metal cleansers, degreasing agents
Woodworkers	Detergents, solvents, oils, wood preservatives

16.3 Case Report

A 28-year-old teacher developed a mild dermatitis on the back of both hands, on the finger webs, and on the finger tips of the right hand. There were slight redness, scaling, and fissures on the right thumb and index finger. The dermatitis started about 4 months after she gave birth to her first child. For 10 years, she had slight rhinitis in early spring, but had never suffered from atopic eczema. Skin testing revealed positive prick test to birch and hazelnut pollens. Patch testing with the standard series, vehicle/emulsifier series, preservatives and corticosteroid series showed a 2+ reaction to thiomersal and a doubtful reaction to thiuram mix (day 3 reading). In order to determine the clinical relevance of these reactions, she reported upon focused questioning to have had several vaccinations without adverse effects. After the hand dermatitis had started she frequently wore rubber gloves during housework; occasionally she noticed slight itching, particularly when using them for more than 1 h.

Diagnosis: Chronic irritant contact dermatitis of hands. Allergic rhinitis. Contact allergy to thiomersal and possibly to thiuram mix.

Treatment and course: The patient was advised to avoid harsh detergents and long exposures to water and other known irritants (information leaflet for hand eczema). Bland emollients without fragrance were to be applied several times daily. She was told that she probably had a rubber allergy and should therefore use vinyl gloves. The thiomersal sensitization was of no current relevance but could become important in the future (eye makeup, eye drops).

Comment: If the contact allergy to thiuram were certain, a combined form of hand eczema would exist in this case (irritant and contact allergic). The use of fragrance-free skin care products was recommended prophylactically to prevent further sensitizations common in patients with chronic hand eczema.

16.3.1 Special Forms of Irritation

16.3.1.1 Climatic Factors

Low outdoor temperatures and low humidity may cause dryness and scaling on the hands and face, and

16

later on also on other body regions. Erythema is usually absent, but may be prominent in more severe conditions with fissures or nummular eczema-like lesions ("eczema craquelée"). Living or working in overheated dry rooms will further aggravate the process, which has also been termed "low-humidity dermatosis" [47]. Office workers and outdoor occupations of various types are predisposed. Aircraft personnel suffer frequently from dry skin due to the low air humidity in airplanes on long flights [48]. Atopics are more easily affected than nonatopics. In a retrospective analysis of 29,000 patients who attended a contact dermatitis clinic in London, a diagnosis of physical irritant contact dermatitis was made in 1.15% of all patients. The most common cause was low humidity due to air-conditioning, which caused dermatitis of face and neck in office workers due to drying out of the skin [49].

Meteorological factors (dry and cold weather) can contribute to the pathogenesis of irritant hand dermatitis in wet work professions [50]. Some authors found increased irritability to standard irritants such as SLS, even of skin not directly exposed to weather conditions during the winter season in bioengineering studies [51–53]. Thus, it is no surprise that there is also a seasonal variation in allergy patch test results: the likelihood of weak, i.e., "false-positive" reactions is increased. This will particularly be the case for those allergens that are also marginal irritants [54–58].

Thermal injury can be very subtle and lead to an itchy eczematous plaque on the lower legs of car drivers in the winter ("car heater dermatitis," Fig. 16.27), [59].

16.3.1.2 Aggravation of Endogenous Dermatoses by Friction and Occlusion

Shoes, helmets, and other garments or carried equipment can lead to circumscribed lesions that may mimic allergic contact dermatitis. This is primarily seen in patients with a past or present atopic dermatitis or psoriasis (*Köbner phenomenon*) [60]. Typical cases are shown in Figs. 16.28–16.30. Friction, heat, and occlusion are triggering factors for the manifestation of the endogenous disease in previously nonaffected regions. The sharp demarcation often suggests an allergic contact dermatitis, which must always be excluded by adequate testing. On the other hand, psoriasis can be due to contact allergy to rubber gloves [61], but may also result solely from irritation, particularly in hospital personnel wearing gloves frequently [62, 63]. Several studies have shown that gloves impair skin barrier function and can further damage primarily irritated skin [63–65]. However, as yet, there is still conflicting evidence [66–68]. A recent review summarizes the effects of occlusion on irritant and allergic contact dermatitis [69]: barrier function is decreased; the effect of irritants and contact allergens is increased, particularly on compromised skin; hydrocolloid patches that absorb water can decrease the irritant reaction caused by the occlusive agent itself; and occlusion does not significantly delay barrier repair in humans. Similar findings have recently been obtained with semipermeable polyethylenegylcol membranes (Sympatex®), which have been shown to even accelerate barrier repair following SLS-irritation. As individuals affected by hand dermatitis frequently start to use gloves only after initial irritant lesions, this

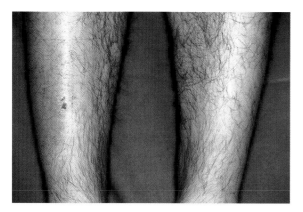

Fig. 16.27 Car heater dermatitis in a salesman due to frequent long car driving. The hot air stream came from the center of the car and induced redness and scaling only on the directly exposed right leg

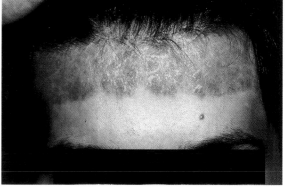

Fig. 16.28 Psoriatic lesions on the forehead due to a tightly fitting safety helmet. Patch testing was negative – the patient had only minor psoriatic lesions on the extremities

Fig. 16.29 Nonallergic frictional dermatitis from safety boots in a coal miner with mild atopic dermatitis on the neck and flexures. Hyperhidrosis visible between the toes was certainly a cofactor in this case

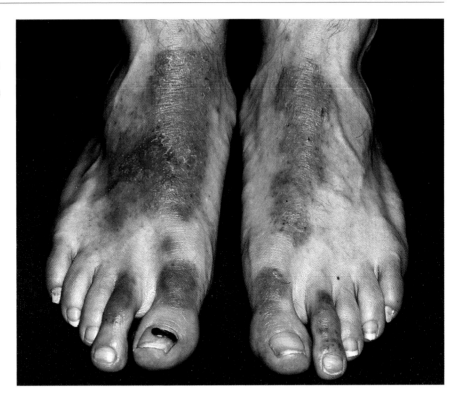

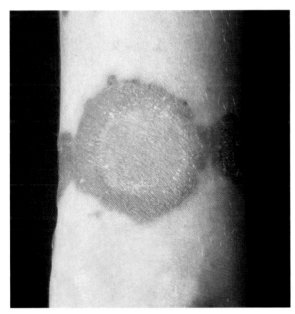

Fig. 16.30 Psoriasis, Köbner effect by stainless steel watch on left wrist. Note the small adjacent psoriatic plaque. Patch test was negative

might be an interesting option for future glove or underglove materials [66]. Tests with such gloves have demonstrated a high degree of user acceptance; however, the lack of resistance to chemicals remains a problem [70].

The ubiquitous usage of the computer mouse has led to reports of low-grade frictional irritant dermatitis and formation of calluses [71, 72]. Contact allergy to plastic materials present in the mouse or in the pad has also been observed [73]. In view of the high number of users worldwide these side-effects are apparently very rare.

16.4 Epidemiology

Hard data on the incidence of irritant contact dermatitis are still very limited. In many studies on contact dermatitis no clear distinction is made between irritant and allergic types. The source population is also often either ill-defined or highly selected (patients attending a contact dermatitis clinic, for example), and cases of slight cutaneous irritation where medical attention is not sought are therefore missed. Recent data are presented and discussed in detail in Chap. 11. Some studies are, however, worthy of note in this context.

In Denmark, the compensation paid for occupational skin diseases was analyzed by Halkier-Sørensen [74]. Skin diseases represented 36% of all compensated cases and were closely followed by musculoskeletal disorders. For irritant eczema (59%) a total of

DKr 102,671,567 was paid in comparison to allergic eczema (41%), DKr 71,147,070.

In a large multicenter prospective study on reactions caused by cosmetics, Eiermann et al. [75] found irritancy to account for 16% of 487 cases of contact dermatitis due to cosmetics. Over a time period of 40 months, approximately 179,800 patients were seen by 11 dermatologists and 8,093 patients were tested for contact dermatitis. In all, 487 cases (6%) were caused by cosmetics, the majority of them (407) being due to contact allergy. The authors pointed out that during the course of the study irritation was more frequently diagnosed once the physicians had been mentally "sensitized" to this type of reaction. When the adverse effects of 253 cosmetics and toiletries as reported to the Swedish Medical Products Agency were analyzed, 90% were eczematous reactions. Of these, 70% were classified as allergic and 30% as irritant [76]. The number of reports for the years 1989–1994 appears to be small and can be explained by underreporting.

In Heidelberg, Germany, a retrospective study of 190 cases of hand dermatitis revealed the following distribution of diagnoses: atopic dermatitis 40%, chronic irritant contact dermatitis 27%, allergic contact dermatitis 23%, and various other diseases 10% [37]. The 50 patients with chronic irritant hand dermatitis (without clinical or laboratory signs of atopy) came from typical high-risk occupations: housework, nursing, hairdressing, and cleaning.

Bäurle et al. [35, 36] studied 683 patients with hand eczema in Erlangen, Germany. They considered 24.2% to suffer from chronic irritant contact dermatitis, 15.8% from allergic contact dermatitis, and 38.5% from atopic hand dermatitis.

Meding [38] made an extensive study of hand eczema in Gothenburg, an industrial city in southern Sweden. When a questionnaire was sent out to 20,000 inhabitants, the point prevalence of hand eczema was determined to be 5.4% (1-year period prevalence 11%). Females outnumbered males by 2:1. The distribution of the three main diagnoses in her panel of 1,585 patients who were investigated further was: 35% irritant contact dermatitis, 22% atopic hand dermatitis, and 19% allergic contact dermatitis. The author pointed out that, due to careful clinical examination, a considerable number of mild cases of irritant contact dermatitis were recognized, hence the relatively high figure for irritant contact dermatitis. In this study, the most harmful exposures turned out to be to "unspecified

chemicals," water, detergents, dust, and dry dirt. For irritant contact dermatitis of the hand, a significantly higher period prevalence was found in people doing service work (15.4%; even higher in hairdressers), medical and nursing work, and administrative work (11.8%). The lowest prevalence was found in female computer operators (3.2%).

For dental personnel in Finland, exact figures on the incidence rates per 10,000 workers were published recently [77]. The incidence rates for irritant contact dermatitis as reported in the years 1982–1994 varied between 11 and 21 per 10,000, while there was a sharp increase in the rate of allergic cases (26–79 respectively) due to the extensive use of acrylates. Detergents, wet and dirty work, plastic chemicals, and antimicrobials were considered to be the major irritants. In a German study on 55 dental technicians suffering from moderate to severe occupational dermatitis, allergic contact dermatitis was diagnosed in 63.6% and irritant contact dermatitis in 23.6% [78].

Paulsen [79] studied 253 gardeners in Odense (Denmark) and found irritant occupational contact dermatitis in 59%. Plants were the most commonly involved irritants (Compositae, Primulaceae, Araceae, Euphorbiaceae, Eraliaceae, Geraniaceae), but pesticides and rubber gloves must also be considered.

Based on the clinical criteria used by dermatologists, slight chronic irritant contact dermatitis of the hands may affect nearly 100% of exposed persons in certain occupations, such as food processing, fishing, hairdressing, construction, or veterinary medicine. In the metal industry, at least 50% of dermatoses due to cutting oils are of the irritant type (see Chaps. 36 and 42). Most workers do not seek medical attention, because the effect is not serious and is accepted as "normal" in that occupation.

The most accurate figures on the incidence of irritant and allergic contact dermatitis as a cause of occupational disease have been generated in Northern Bavaria (Germany) by Diepgen's group [80–82]. The data are based on all workers' compensation claims reported to the register of occupational skin diseases in the years from 1990 to 1999. Incidence rates were calculated for 24 occupational groups using the known number of insured employees in those professions. Of 5,285 patients, an occupational skin disease was diagnosed in 59% after careful diagnostic procedures including extensive patch testing. This amounted to an incidence rate of 4.5 patients per 10,000 workers for irritant contact dermatitis and 4.1 patients for 10,000 workers for allergic contact dermatitis. The highest incidence of irritant contact dermatitis rates were found in hairdressers (46.9 per 10,000 workers per year), bakers (23.5 per 10,000 workers per year), and pastry cooks (16.9 per 10,000 workers per year); at the same time, irritant contact dermatitis was the main diagnosis of occupational skin disease in pastry cooks (76%), cooks (69%), food processing industry workers and butchers (63%), mechanics (60%), and locksmiths and automobile mechanics (59%). The results of a questionnaire showed frequent skin contact with detergents (52%), disinfectants (24%), and acidic and alkaline chemicals (24%) in the workplace.

In a patch test clinic of Kansas City (Kansas, USA) a retrospective analysis between 1994 and 1999 was performed [83]. Of the 437 patients who underwent patch testing, 25% had occupational skin disease. Allergic contact dermatitis was diagnosed in 60% of the patients and irritant contact dermatitis in only 34%. Healthcare professionals, machinists, and construction workers accounted for nearly half of all the patients with occupational skin disease. Nickel sulfate, glutaraldehyde, and thiuram mix were the most common allergens. The authors emphasize the importance of patch testing and particularly an extension of the very limited number of materials officially available in the USA in order not to miss cases of occupational contact allergy. Thus, as other authors have pointed out, the investigator's knowledge of allergens and irritants at the workplace and the quality of allergological workup, including the patient's own materials which might reveal the decisive allergen, are of utmost importance, and influence the ratio of irritant contact dermatitis to allergic contact dermatitis [81, 83–93].

Core Message

> In general, irritant contact dermatitis is more frequent than allergic contact dermatitis. High-risk professions are nursing, hairdressing, food processing, construction work, and handling of plants. Water, detergents, dust, and dry dirt are the most common causes. Water-soluble cutting oils are the major culprit for occupational dermatitis in the metal industry. Figures on prevalence are extremely variable due to differences in the spectrum of irritants, working conditions, and protective measures. Furthermore, the observed frequency depends on the type of population studied and the quality of diagnostic workup.

16.5 Pathogenesis

A number of factors have now been identified as being involved in the pathogenesis of irritant contact dermatitis, particularly of the chronic cumulative type [94–99]. These can be divided into exogenous and endogenous factors (Table 16.9).

16.5.1 Exogenous Factors

Table 16.9 lists the numerous exogenous factors influencing the irritant response. These include the type of chemical, the mode of exposure, and the body site, but the most important are the inherent toxicity of the chemical for human skin and its penetration.

Agner et al. [100] have studied the penetration of human skin by SLS using an in vitro model. Different formulations of SLS applied to the skin for 24 h (aqueous solution and gels) were studied, but irrespective of the vehicle used permeation of SLS into the recipient phase was poor. Results were compared to in vivo patch testing in 12 subjects. Approximately, 70% of SLS applied in aqueous solution was released from the patch test system. Release from gels was poorer. Good agreement was found between the in vivo results and the in vitro model. No correlation was found between the amount of SLS left in the filter disc and the strength of the clinical reaction in vivo.

Table 16.9 Exogenous and endogenous factors influencing the irritant response of human skin

Exogenous factors	Endogenous factors
Type of irritant (chemical structure, pH)	Individual susceptibility to irritant(s)
Amount of irritant penetrating (solubility, time of application)	Primary hyperirritable ("sensitive") skin
Body site	Atopy (particularly atopic dermatitis)
Body temperature	Inability to develop hardening
Mechanical factors (pressure, friction, abrasion)	Secondary hyperirritability (status eczematicus)
Climatic conditions (temperature, humidity, wind speed)	Racial factors
	Age
	Sensitivity to UV light

Apart from strong acids and alkalis, it is not possible to predict the irritant potential of a chemical on the basis of its molecular structure as, to a certain extent, can be done for contact allergens (Chaps. 4 and 13). The pH is not strictly correlated with irritancy, as studies with detergents, alkaline soaps, and α-hydroxy acids have shown [101–104]. However, in a study with 12 basic compounds, a positive correlation was found between increasing dissociation constant (pKa) and skin irritation capacity on human volunteers, measured either visually or by reflectance spectroscopy [105]. Compounds with low pKa induced vasoconstriction whereas high values generated vasodilation. Disruption of barrier was minimal with these irritants except mecamylamine.

Prediction of the irritation potential is even more difficult if one deals with formulated products containing many and sometimes ill-defined chemicals. Instructive is the report of Fischer and Bjarnason [106] on an epidemic outbreak of skin symptoms after a new class of diesel oil ("green diesel") had been marketed in Sweden. Initially thought to be a problem of contact allergy related to the added dyes, it turned out to be irritant contact dermatitis. The new "lighter" diesel oils are considered to be "friendlier" to the environment due to a lower concentration of aromatic compounds and low sulfur content. But these features caused more cutaneous irritation than the old types with high sulfur levels and a high degree of aromatic compounds, as careful studies on human volunteers including the use of laser Doppler perfusion imaging revealed. Paradoxically, the authors conclude, "what is good for the environment is not always good for the skin."

The intensity of the resulting irritation depends greatly on the body region. The face and the postauricular and genital regions are particularly sensitive skin areas, a major reason being a reduced barrier and the abundance of "holes" in the skin (sweat ducts and hair follicles) [107]. Figure 16.14 shows the large regional variation in reactivity to the solvent dimethylsulfoxide (DMSO), which causes toxic degranulation of mast cells [108]. Cua et al. [109] studied the reactivity to SLS in ten body regions: the thigh had the highest sensitivity and the palm the lowest.

Important but frequently unrecognized cofactors of irritant reactions are mechanical, thermal, and climatic influences. Rough sheets have produced facial dermatitis in babies, and rough tabletops and paper have aggravated hand dermatitis in post office workers [31,

110]. In a cohort of 111 office apprentices, the point prevalence of irritant or atopic eczema of the hands was 18.9% in the initial and 25% in the final examination after 3 years [111]. Handling of paper, particularly carbonless copy paper, and low relative humidity were considered to be the major causative factors, in agreement with other reports [112, 113].

In an epidemiological study on 246 shoemakers in five different factories, the prevalence of occupational contact dermatitis was found to be 14.6%:8.1% irritant contact dermatitis and 6.5% allergic contact dermatitis. Solvents, adhesives, varnishes, and mechanical forces were considered to be the major irritants [34].

One detergent caused an epidemic in hospital kitchen workers, mainly because it was used at too high a temperature [114]. The influence of the temperature of two different detergents was studied in a hand/forearm immersion test [115].

Cold windy climates produce drying of the skin due to the reduced capacity of the stratum corneum to retain water at lower temperatures. The condition is aggravated by frequent bathing or showering and the use of soaps and detergent bars. An eczema-like picture is seen in elderly persons. In a wash study, hard water with a higher content of calcium was found to be more irritating than soft water [116]. The type of water also had an influence on soap deposition to the skin. On the other hand, in hot humid climates, sweating and friction may induce a clothing dermatitis, which seems to be a contact allergy. Elevated plaques with a sharp margin followed by scaling, fissures, and hyperpigmentation, associated with various types of garment closely apposed to the skin, were observed in a series of Indian patients [117]. Most patients reported mild burning or stinging and some had developed the condition several times only in the hot summer months.

16.5.2 Endogenous Factors

Relevant endogenous factors include atopy and skin sensitivity. A number of studies from Scandinavia, such as those by Nilsson et al. [118], Rystedt [119] and Lammintausta and Kalimo [120], have confirmed the supposition of experienced clinicians that previous or current atopic dermatitis is a risk factor for the development of hand eczema in occupations involving wet work. Further confirmation came from a large study of 1,600 hand eczema patients in Erlangen, Germany [35, 36], and one in Osnabrueck, Germany [121]. It is important to point out that, on the basis of these studies, persons with a history of hay fever and/or bronchial asthma do not show a markedly increased risk of developing hand eczema in comparison to non-atopic controls. However, in Meding's study [38] there was a statistically significant but weak correlation between hand eczema and atopic mucosal symptoms.

Persons with atopic dermatitis in childhood often have dry skin for the rest of their lives. Histologically, dry skin shows some similarities to subclinical eczema. Clinically, overt irritation may therefore be precipitated more easily by a number of irritant factors.

Using SLS patch testing for 24 h and measuring transepidermal water loss, Löffler and Effendy [122] found enhanced skin susceptibility only in individuals with active dermatitis. Subjects with a history of past atopic dermatitis or rhinoconjunctivitis/asthma were not more sensitive. However, this experimental design might not reliably predict the actual conditions in most occupations, where there is repetitive low-dose irritancy over a long time.

If clinical signs of an atopic skin diathesis are carefully evaluated this can be of help in estimating the risk of occupational irritant contact dermatitis. In a study on bakers and confectioners in Germany, a significant correlation was found between a high score (>10 points on the Erlangen atopy score) and the development of hand dermatitis [123]. Other studies of high-risk professions have not corroborated such a correlation; two reviews summarize the complexity of this issue [124, 125]. Differences in methodology account in part for the discrepancies in results.

The protein filaggrin plays an important role in the structure and the hydration of the stratum corneum. Recently, two studies have shown that loss-of-function polymorphisms in the filaggrin gene are associated with an increased susceptibility to chronic irritant contact dermatitis [126–130]. The interindividual differences in the inflammatory response of the skin have been linked to gene polymorphisms of interleukin-1alpha and tumor necrosis factor (TNF)-alpha. As the methods are not invasive for the patient (tape stripping of the stratum corneum, buccal mucosa swabs for DNA sampling) identification of persons at high-risk for irritant contact dermatitis may be possible one day, if further studies will confirm this.

16.5.3 Sensitive (Hyperirritable) Skin

Individuals with sensitive, hyperirritable skin do exist [131]. This may be due to a genetic predisposition, independent of atopy. Racial differences in cutaneous irritability have been well documented [20, 108, 132, 133]. Blacks in general have less irritable skin than whites of northern (Celtic) extraction. This view has been challenged by using noninvasive techniques such as transepidermal water loss (TEWL) measurements. A higher susceptibility to SLS has been found in blacks compared to whites [134]. Similarly, a greater sensitivity to SLS was reported in Hispanic skin than in white skin [135]. However, in a recent study with a dishwashing liquid as irritant, the skin of African Americans was less sensitive than the skin of Caucasians [136]. This conclusion was based on the clinical evaluation of threshold response, reflectance confocal microscopy, and TEWL measurements.

It has been shown that subjects with light skin complexions (types 1 and 2) not only have high UVB sensitivity but also skin that is hyperirritable to chemicals in general [137]. Hyperirritable skin can also develop secondarily during the course of hand or leg eczema. Status eczematicus and "angry back syndrome" fall into this category. There is evidence that secondary (acquired) hyperirritability in a subgroup of patients may persist even months and years after a previous eczema has healed [66, 138, 139].

In a recent study on human volunteers, it was demonstrated that previous chronic irritant contact dermatitis sites to SLS showed hyperreactivity compared to normal skin even after the tenth week postinduction [140]. This phenomenon is not rarely seen in patients with persistent postoccupational dermatitis (PPOD) – the dermatitis continues even after all occupational causative factors are eliminated [141, 142].

The cause of hyperirritable skin is still unknown. Apart from the mentioned genetic links to filaggrin and cytokine expression, there is good evidence so far that a thin and/or permeable stratum corneum plays a key role. Based on Fick's law of penetration, the thickness of the stratum corneum influences the flux of the penetrating chemical. Weigand et al. [133] have shown that the stratum corneum of blacks has more cell layers on average than that of whites. This group also found that the buoyant density of black stratum corneum was higher, which may indicate a more compact barrier. Marks' group was able to demonstrate a relationship between the minimal irritancy dose for dithranol and the mean corneocyte surface area: the smaller the corneocyte area, the lower the irritancy threshold [143]. They also found a positive correlation between the minimal blistering time with ammonium hydroxide and the skin surface contour. This was also true for other irritants.

Regional variations in irritability are related to differences in keratinization and to the density of transepidermal shunts allowing penetration (sweat ducts, hair follicles). The intercellular lipids of the stratum corneum play an important part in the barrier function of the skin, as has been shown by a number of investigators [144–148]. Based on recent reports, it seems that the ceramides and glycosylceramides may be the key elements in storage of water in the stratum corneum. In animals fed a diet free of essential fatty acids, administering linoleic acid either topically or systemically has been shown to improve the stratum corneum barrier [146]. There is also some clinical evidence that this may have an effect in humans, but therapeutic trials with linoleic acid or ceramide-containing medicaments in atopic eczema and dry skin have not been encouraging [149].

Ceramides in the stratum corneum are also considered to be important in the regulation of the skin barrier. Inverse correlations were found between baseline ceramide 6 I and the 24-h erythema score for SLS 3%, between ceramide 1 and 24-h TEWL, and between ceramide 6II and 72-h TEWL for SLS 3% [150]. These findings suggest that low levels of ceramides may determine a proclivity to SLS-induced irritation.

Individuals with hyperirritable skin are also more reactive when tested on scarified or stripped skin, i.e., after the removal of the stratum corneum, the major rate-limiting factor for penetration [151]. This is also the basis for the assumption that these individuals may release more inflammatory mediators or may be more reactive to them in comparison to normal or hyporeactive skin [137, 152].

Using noninvasive bioengineering methods, it has been possible to demonstrate that female skin is more reactive to the anionic detergent SLS in the premenstrual phase than in the remainder of the menstrual cycle [153]. In general, however, females do not seem to have more sensitive skin than males [5, 154]. Rather, it is assumed that females are exposed more frequently to potential irritants than males (household products, cosmetics) and are therefore more prone to develop irritant contact dermatitis, of both acute and chronic types. Accordingly, in a recent large multicenter study in 5,971 individuals, male sex was a weak but significant risk factor for a clinically positive reaction to 0.25% and 0.5% SLS [58].

Cutaneous irritability is influenced by age. There is now increasing evidence that, for several compounds, percutaneous penetration in the old age group is less than in the young [155, 156]. In one study, susceptibility to detergents was found to increase with age, whereas the pustulogenic effect of croton oil decreased [157]. The same group found no difference with the irritants thymoquinone and croton aldehyde. In another study with SLS, the old age group showed significantly less reactivity than young adults [109]. This was quantified by visual scoring and measurements of TEWL. TEWL in the elderly is usually lower than in the young, which might be related to the latter group having a better stratum corneum barrier against water [158]. Grove et al. [159] studied different irritants in young and old cohorts. With ammonium hydroxide, blistering occurred more rapidly in older persons. Histamine, DMSO, 48/80, chloroform, methanol, lactic acid, and ethyl nicotinate induced stronger (visual) reactions in the younger cohort. A comparison of cumulative irritation (7.5% SLS on 5 days consecutively, open application) revealed delayed and decreased reaction of older compared to younger skin and recovery appeared to be prolonged [160]. Further details on population differences regarding skin structure, physiology, and susceptibility to irritants are given in recent reviews [161–164]. See also Chap. 30.

The phenomenon of "hardening" has been less studied, despite its common occurrence in many occupations [165]. The skin becomes slightly erythematous and hyperkeratotic from daily contact with a mild irritant, and high concentrations of the irritant can then be tolerated. If the hardening stimulus stops, the skin shows desquamation and reactivity returns to its previous level. Hardening can be induced by SLS. It seems to be an irritant-specific phenomenon because reactivity to other irritants may even be increased [166]. The subject has been recently reviewed [167].

Core Message

> Individuals with primary (endogenous) sensitive skin react to many but not all irritants more strongly compared to individuals with "tough" skin. So far, no single test can identify these persons or predict their reactivity to a certain (new) irritant.

16.6 Diagnostic Tests and Experimental Irritant Contact Dermatitis

The diagnostic tests used to quantify a patient's susceptibility to irritants are [9, 20, 24, 52, 137, 168]:

> Alkali resistance (sodium hydroxide).
> Ammonium hydroxide.
> Dimethylsulfoxide.
> Threshold response to various irritants (SLS, nonanoic acid, benzalkonium chloride, kerosene, croton oil, anthralin).
> Lactic acid stinging.
> Minimal erythema dose of UVB light.
> Measurement of TEWL.

None is really so simple and reliable that it can be used clinically on a large scale, and the diagnostic value of the older tests such as Burckhardt's alkali resistance test has been overestimated, particularly with regard to their capacity to distinguish between allergic and irritant eczema.

Recently, a quick NaOH-challenge as a routine irritant patch test in occupational dermatology (swift modified alkali resistance test (SMART)) was suggested [138, 139]. The test comprises a 0.5 M NaOH-challenge for only 2 × 10 min with intermediate biophysical measurements (TEWL) and a clinical assessment. It also incorporates a 0.9% NaCl-control. This test has recently been validated in two cohorts of 1,111 individuals with former occupational dermatoses (now healed). Performed on the volar forearm, it was helpful to detect constitutional risks, namely atopic skin. It showed an almost fivefold increased chance of a positive reaction in the forearm in atopics, and a threefold increased chance on the back of the hand [138]. Comparing skin reactivity to SMART on the forearm and the back of the hand simultaneously (differential irritation test, DIT), the study confirmed that in general, the back of the hand is relatively robust, even in skin-sensitive individuals. However, there is a minority of ca. 10% of patients who formerly suffered from hand eczema where the normal hierarchy of skin sensitivity to NaOH is absent, and an isolated hyperreactivity of the back of the hand occurs [66]. The authors claim that this a priori paradoxical constellation – which is not to be found in healthy controls – provides strong evidence for a persistent acquired hyperirritability after previous eczema. Some patients with healed irritant contact dermatitis complain of experiencing ongoing increased skin sensitivity. However, in many of these cases the clinician cannot identify any skin impairment. The DIT is an approach to objectify the phenomenon of subclinical secondary cutaneous hyperreactivity.

The results indicate that there may be pertinent options associated with epicutaneous NaOH-challenges [169–171]. An interesting aspect as to why NaOH may be a candidate for a predictive patch test in occupational dermatology is that the major cause of occupational dermatoses – "wet work" – alkalinizes the skin (dilution and exhausting of buffer-systems [172]). This occupational hazard may be mimicked by the test. The vital importance of a physiological, *acidic* pH for barrier homeostasis, especially for the formation of the lamellar lipid bilayer system, was demonstrated [173].

Nevertheless, the topic of predictive testing remains controversial. The diagnostic methods listed, however, are very useful in determining threshold responses to various irritants. Subjects with increased reactivity to one or more irritants can be identified and various influences such as the effect of repeated UVB exposure, the cumulative effects of mild irritants, or the protective effects of "barrier" creams can be quantified. Using these techniques, Frosch [20] demonstrated that in a normal population with healthy skin, the proportion of subjects with hyperirritable skin was 14%; 25% were regarded as "hypoirritable" and 61% as "normal." The distinction between the three groups was made by the use of cluster analysis, a statistical method that can compare and validate a number of criteria in one subject. Although some individuals seem to have hyperirritable skin per se, one finds that the correlation between some irritants is rather weak if a large number of irritants of very different chemical structure are used. In one study, we found a good correlation between the responses to sodium hydroxide, ammonium hydroxide, and water-soluble irritants, but a very weak and insignificant one between SLS and lipid-soluble irritants such as croton oil and kerosene [137]. As early as 1968, Björnberg showed that one might not necessarily be able to predict the reactivity to one irritant on the basis of reactivity to another irritant [5].

Recently, the model irritant SLS has been studied extensively [122, 174, 175, 296]. Concentrations vary from 0.5 to 2.5% usually applied with small or large Finn chambers for 24 h. Then most Caucasian subjects will develop an erythema of different intensity. Reactions are rarely severe and, even if a blistering reaction does occur, healing is swift and rarely followed by pigmentary changes. Basketter's group [175–177] has developed a 4-h test with large Hill Top chambers (25 mm diameter, 0.1 mL). With a concentration gradient of 0.1–20%, the threshold of erythema is determined, rather than a visual grading of intensity. Using this technique, they could not find any significant differences in a population of six different skin types (typing according to complexion and UVB sensitivity). Neither did they find differences between atopics and nonatopics. This suggests that short-term relatively high dosing of an irritant such as SLS cannot detect subtle differences in the susceptibility to cumulative insults over a longer period of time. On the other hand, this test is of value in providing a positive control for studies with other irritants for comparative reasons. According to an EU guideline, the irritancy potential of new chemicals must be assessed, avoiding animal tests whenever possible [52, 178–183]. For predictive testing of irritants and quantitative risk assessment, see also Chap. 13 of this book and a monograph [184].

The measurement of the baseline TEWL may be a useful indicator of reactivity to irritants. After 3 weeks of treatment with SLS, TEWL showed significant linear correlation with pretreatment TEWL values [185]. This supported an earlier study [186]. However, when a single 24-h occlusive SLS application was employed, no correlation was found [187].

16.7 Action of Irritants and Inflammatory Mediators

In contrast to contact allergy, the basic inflammatory mechanisms of irritants have been less studied; but recently, new pathogenetic concepts have begun to emerge [125, 188, 189]. As irritants are very diverse in chemical structure, pH, penetration, and other features, they are generally assumed to have very different modes of action in the skin. However, some basic initial mechanisms seem to be fairly common to the early events in the elicitation of acute and chronic irritant contact dermatitis, e.g., the release of the proinflammatory mediators interleukin-1 (IL-1) and tumor necrosis factor alpha (TNF-α) following any kind of barrier perturbation, regardless of whether chemically or mechanically induced. Furthermore, for SLS-induced irritation, the role of heat-shock proteins [190]

and oxidative stress [191] has recently been demonstrated. The body of evidence is growing, to enable skin irritation research to move on from the descriptive level to the assessment of the underlying cascade of pathogenetic events, which seem to be pivotally influenced by multiple genetic polymorphisms. These recent findings may provide the crucial key to explaining the as yet enigmatic great interindividual variability in irritant susceptibility, including the enhanced irritant response in atopics [125].

The reader is referred to Chaps. 3, 4, 6, 9, and 10 of this volume, recent reviews, and some pertinent original publications [39, 108, 130, 184, 185, 192–211].

16.8 Quantification of the Irritant Response (Bioengineering Techniques)

A very worthwhile approach in the study of cutaneous toxicity is the use of noninvasive methods to quantify the irritant response. This rapidly expanding research area is reviewed in Chap. 30. Many groups are now using evaporimeters to measure TEWL [103, 186], and laser flow meters can quantify blood flow using the Doppler principle [22, 118, 212, 213]. Both the techniques are quite sensitive, and measurements can be made in minutes without damaging the skin or requiring a biopsy.

Limitations of these instruments have been demonstrated: very high rates of TEWL, as well as very intense hyperemia due to venous stasis may be evaluated inaccurately by these instruments [51]. Despite this, they are very useful in attempts to measure objectively the degree of skin damage, and have been successfully used to measure the toxic effects of surfactants and organic solvents, singly or in combination ("tandem application" [214–217]). Recently, several groups assessed the protective function of barrier creams [218–224].

The quantification of increased cutaneous irritability has proven to be helpful for the interpretation of weak or query reactions to contact allergens as allergic or irritant; that is why recent recommendations were made to include SLS 0.25 and 0.5% – applied for 24 or 48 h on the back – in routine allergy patch testing [54, 55, 58, 225].

Lammintausta et al. [226] have shown that subjects with increased susceptibility to stinging have more vulnerable skin than those with no increased susceptibility to stinging. After applying various irritants, they found a greater increase in blood flow and TEWL in "stingers" than in "nonstingers." These differences in cutaneous reactivity were not detected on clinical examination. This supports the view that the measurement of skin functions is worthwhile and should be promoted in future studies, even though recent studies could not corroborate marked differences in cutaneous irritability between stingers and nonstingers (see below).

Studying the dose–response relationship for SLS in humans, Agner and Serup [9] found measurement of TEWL to be the method best suited overall for the quantification of patch test results, whereas colorimetry was found to be the least sensitive of the methods tested. Wilhelm et al. [227] quantified the cutaneous response to six concentrations of SLS using visual scores, skin color reflectance, TEWL and laser Doppler flow (LDF) measurements. All noninvasive techniques were more sensitive than the human eye in detecting irritation by the lowest concentration of SLS (0.125%). TEWL showed the highest discriminating power and the best correlation with visual scores. Change in total color (ΔE^*) correlated better than redness (Δa^*) to the SLS dose applied and visual score, whereas Δa^* correlated better with TEWL and LDF than ΔE^*.

Ultrasound A-mode scanning was found to be a promising method for the quantification of the inflammatory response, being consistently more sensitive than the measurement of skin color. Wahlberg has successfully used the LDF technique in assessing the irritant response to organic solvents [23], and van der Valk and coworkers [103, 104] have used evaporimetry in a series of studies quantifying the irritant potential of various detergents. Pinnagoda et al. [186] have described a repetitive exposure test for 3 weeks on human forearm skin using SLS. Baseline TEWL before exposure to the irritant correlated with the resulting cumulative irritancy caused by the detergent. The authors concluded that baseline TEWL might be a valuable predictor of cutaneous irritability.

The topic, however, remains controversial [125]. Unlike some laboratory studies, in a number of recent field studies of high-risk professions, such as hairdressers [228–230], metal workers [169], and nurses [229], it could not be proven that baseline TEWL and other baseline bioengineering parameters are relevant predictors of occupational dermatitis, and even preemployment irritation tests were not or only poorly predictive [169, 230]. At the workplace, there are many complex interacting factors apart from preemployment barrier function that influence the likelihood of the development of occupational skin disease. Obviously, one factor of

particular importance is the individual motivation to employ skin protection measures. As could be shown for hairdressers' apprentices, even atopics could reduce their risks of suffering an occupational dermatosis by 50% if they continuously used skin protection [231].

Core Message

> Today, the measurement of TEWL is the most frequently used procedure for quantifying impaired function of the stratum corneum. Clinically invisible subtle damage, e.g., by detergents, is reliably detected by an increase in TEWL.

16.9 Therapy and Prevention

The reader is referred to Chaps. 42, 46, and 47 which provide many details on this important subject.

In the acute stage of irritant contact dermatitis, topical corticosteroids are indicated. If there is deep tissue destruction or signs of bacterial infection, systemic corticosteroids and antimicrobial agents should be administered. Long-term administration of potent corticosteroids is dangerous because of the risk of atrophy and impairment of the stratum corneum [232]. The anti-inflammatory effect of corticosteroids against various irritants is weak or nonexistent. The effect depends on the potency of the corticosteroid and the mode of application (before or after the irritant, single or repetitive application, topical, or systemic administration). This explains the discrepant results reported in the literature [233–235].

Recent studies have revealed that even short-term glucocorticoid treatment – down to 3 days of clobetasol – compromises both barrier permeability and stratum corneum integrity [236, 237]. Therefore, anti-inflammatory agents with less adverse effects are needed. A topical calcineurin inhibitor such as tacrolimus has been shown to be efficacious in the treatment of chronic occupational hand dermatitis, although randomized controlled studies are still necessary [238].

Dental laboratory technicians are frequently affected by occupational skin disease due to multiple irritants and allergens [78, 239]. In a controlled clinical trial, two popular commercial barrier creams and two moisturizers containing urea and beeswax respectively were evaluated in a total of 192 technicians [240]. Every technician used one barrier cream (several applications during work) and one moisturizer applied at home at least once daily for 4 weeks each with a wash-out period of 2 weeks in between. The sequence barrier cream – moisturizer, and vice versa, was randomized in two single, blind cross-over designs for both the combinations. The skin condition was evaluated on a clinical score by a dermatologist at regular intervals and TEWL was measured on the back of the hand and on the forearm. Both the moisturizers were assessed as "good" or "very good" in 77–98% and superior to both the barrier creams (58–67% respectively). Regarding TEWL, both the moisturizers proved to be significantly more effective than the barrier creams. The acceptance of the products was high. The results demonstrate the high value of skin care after work.

In a controlled study on 39 nurses a prevention model was evaluated and compared to regular work [241]. In the prevention model, the use of hand alcohol instead of soap and water in disinfection procedures when the hands were not visibly dirty was followed; furthermore, the use of gloves in wet activities such as patient washing to prevent the hands from becoming wet and visibly dirty was mandatory. After 3 weeks, the prevention model was found to be beneficial and less damaging to the stratum corneum as assessed by the measurements of TEWL, even though the time of occlusion by wearing gloves more frequently had increased. The group of Löffler demonstrated in a series of studies that alcohol as disinfectant is much less irritating than previously thought; acceptance of a skin care program is high, if the health personnel attend training lessons [242–244].

In all cases of chronic irritant contact dermatitis a systematic approach on a wide front must be undertaken. Potential irritants in the work and home environments must be identified and, whenever possible, eliminated (replacement by other less irritant substances, reduction of exposure, use of protective gloves, etc.). Skin cleansing should be as mild as possible (liquid detergents based on alkylether sulfates or sulfosuccinate esters, avoiding organic solvents and hard brushes or other abrasives). Several methods have been described recently for irritancy ranking of detergents. The one-time patch test provides orienting data that must be compared to the results of immersion or wash tests, which better simulate the in-use situation [245–248].

Corneosurfametry involves superficial biopsy of the stratum corneum with cyanoacrylate, exposure to detergents, and measuring the absorbed toluidine/fuchsin dye by colorimetry. Harsh surfactants considerably increase the staining of the corneocytes. With this technique detergents can be evaluated regarding mildness [152, 249]. Furthermore, subjects with self-perceived sensitive skin showed an increased reactivity in this assay when compared to individuals with normal skin who had not experienced any adverse reaction to detergents, wool, or rough textile objects in the past. This suggests that these sensitive subjects could have a weakened resistance of their stratum corneum to surfactants.

Interestingly, the application of ionized water (mineral water, CO_2-enriched water) seems to be beneficial in the treatment of irritant contact dermatitis and may accelerate barrier recovery [250, 251], possibly due to a change of pH to an acidic milieu.

Regular application of bland emollients to counteract desiccation should be encouraged. Several groups have shown in elegant experiments that the application of skin moisturizers improves repair mechanisms [252, 253]. Forearm immersion in SLS and measurement of TEWL seems to be the most discriminating procedure [174, 254]. For further information there are helpful reviews [255, 256]. The use of barrier creams remains controversial. Few well-controlled clinical studies have been conducted (for review [219, 257]). In a model called the repetitive irritation test (RIT), designed for guinea pigs as well as for human volunteers, Frosch and coworkers [220, 258] were able to demonstrate large differences in efficacy among commercial products. While some were quite effective in suppressing the irritation of SLS, sodium hydroxide, and lactic acid, others were not, or even aggravated the irritation. In a similar model, Zhai et al. [259] found several commercial formulations that were effective against irritation by SLS – although to a variable degree – but all failed against a mixture of ammonium hydroxide and urea. A modified version of the RIT was recently evaluated in a multicenter study showing remarkable differences in various dermatological emollients. Interlaboratory differences were present but the ranking of the formulations stayed the same [223].

The value of phototherapy for chronic cases of eczema has been well established. Results with portable UVB lamps permitting home treatment for hand eczema are encouraging [260, 261].

If all measures fail, the diagnosis of an irritant contact dermatitis must be reevaluated: atopy may be the dominant cause or contact allergy (e.g., to preservatives, fragrances, or corticosteroids) may be preventing recovery. Recent studies have shown synergistic effects of irritants and allergens [262, 263]. The realistic combined exposure to irritants and allergens at the workplace can lead to augmentation of the cutaneous response. Mechanisms for a changed response involve immunological effects and enhanced penetration. Low levels of sensitization may thus become clinically relevant. As chronic contact dermatitis is commonly a multifactorial disease, psychological factors and lack of compliance by the patient must also be kept in mind. The value of "eczema schools" has now been well established [264, 265]. If patients in high-risk occupations are trained in detail as how to avoid irritant and allergic factors in their job, the prognosis improves considerably [111, 266–270]. This special education must start early with apprentices before dangerous habits are accepted [231, 271]. Training seminars highly benefit from the didactic experience of pedagogues focusing on health education and prevention (in Germany a relatively new university degree "Gesundheitspädagoge" [health educationalist] [270] – see also Chap. 47).

> **Core Message**
>
> > The most important therapeutic approach in the treatment of irritant contact dermatitis is the identification of causative chemicals and climatic as well as mechanical factors. Mild forms may be sufficiently controlled by the regular use of emollients/ moisturizers. Severe relapsing forms require corticosteroids, calcineurin inhibitors, UV treatment, and the attendance at "eczema schools." In such cases, it is not rare for the causative activity to be completely abandoned, particularly if the patient's compliance is low.

16.10 Neurosensory Irritation ("Stinging")

While the subjective hallmark of allergic cutaneous reactions is often an unbearable pruritus, many irritants cause painful sensations described as burning, stinging or smarting. We may distinguish two types of reactions regarding the time course: (1) immediate-type stinging, and (2) delayed-type stinging.

16.10.1 Immediate-Type Stinging

A few chemicals cause painful sensations within seconds of contact with normal intact skin. Best known is a mixture of chloroform and methanol (1:1). Depending on the body region and, to some extent, on individual susceptibility, a sharp pain develops within a few seconds or a few minutes of exposure. This phenomenon has been used for the assessment of the cutaneous barrier, which mainly resides in the stratum corneum [20, 272]. On the volar forearm of healthy white subjects, discomfort is experienced after an average exposure time of 47 s (range 13–102 s). The irritant mixture is applied in abundant quantity in a small plastic cup (8 mm diameter). Regional differences in sensitivity can easily be documented (mastoid region – upper back – forearm – palmar region; in order of decreasing sensitivity). Once they have started, subjective reactions to chloroform:methanol increase in intensity within seconds to such an extent that the irritant must be removed in order to avoid torturing the subject. The pain abates quickly, with some individual differences. In most cases only faint erythema is visible for a short duration. Rarely, superficial necrosis of the epidermis is seen in "tough" subjects who endure the pain for a longer exposure of several minutes.

Undiluted ethanol (95%) causes a short-lasting sharp stinging sensation in most individuals in sensitive skin regions (face and neck, genital area). If the skin has slight abrasions, e.g., due to shaving, this phenomenon is experienced by everybody. The immediate type of stinging can also be observed with strong caustic chemicals, primarily acids in irritant concentrations. Typical of these agents is that severe cutaneous damage is nearly always associated with the subjective reaction. The latter is the warning signal of imminent somatic destruction if exposure is continued.

16.10.2 Delayed-Type Stinging

When a sunscreen containing amyldimethyl-p-aminobenzoic acid (ADP, Padimate) was marketed on a wide scale in Florida, many users experienced disagreeable stinging or burning after application. The discomfort usually occurred 1 or 2 min after application and intensified over the next 5–10 min.

Attempts to remove the sunscreen by washing brought no relief. The pain slowly abated over the next half hour. Objective signs of irritation did not develop. The condition was primarily experienced on the face after sweating and contact with salt water [273].

This is a typical example of the phenomenon of delayed-type stinging, which can be induced by a number of substances. Frosch and Kligman [101] were the first to study this systematically on human skin. The key observation was that this type of discomfort is not experienced by everybody but only by certain "stingers." A panel of subjects can be screened for stingers by the application of 5% aqueous lactic acid to the nasolabial fold after the induction of profuse sweating in a sauna. Stinging is scored on an intensity scale of 0–3 (severe) at 10 s, 2.5 min, 5 min, and 8 min. A subject is regarded a stinger if he or she complains of severe (3+) discomfort between 2.5 and 8 min.

In the *stinging assay,* the material to be evaluated is applied to the cheek of preselected sensitive subjects after intensive sweating has been induced. The stinging score of a material is the mean score of three readings taken at 2.5, 5.0, and 8.0 min. Substances with average scores falling between 0.4 and 1.0 are arbitrarily regarded as having "slight" stinging potential, the range 1.1–2.0 signifies "moderate" stinging, and the range 2.1–3.0 indicates "severe" stinging. The immediate, and in most cases transient, type of stinging is identified by questioning the subject 10 s after the application of the material. Thus, the subjective tolerance of a cosmetic or topical drug can be evaluated under exaggerated test conditions on subjects with increased sensitivity.

Although a very subjective and seemingly unreliable method, this stinging assay has stood the test of time and proven valuable in screening various agents for subjective discomfort. The existence of the stinging phenomenon was, however, frequently disputed because signs of objective irritation are missing and there is no method of validation. In Table 16.10 are listed several substances with which this phenomenon has been observed for years. Among them are the sunscreens ADP and 2-ethoxyethyl-p-methoxycinnamate, the insect repellent *N*, *N*-diethyltoluamide, the solvent propylene glycol (undiluted), and dermatological therapeutics such as salicylic acid, aluminum chloride, benzoyl peroxide, and crude coal tar. The intensity of

stinging depends on the concentration of the agent and its vehicle. For further details, the reader is referred to the original publication, to a review [101, 274], and to recent publications [275–277].

Based on extensive experience with this test, Soschin and Kligman [274] found the classification of a substance to be more reliable if the cumulative score in a 12-member panel is used:

> <10: Insignificant stinging potential in normal use.
> 11–24: Modest stinging potential, creating a problem for persons with sensitive skin.
> >25: Definite stinging potential, certain to be "troublesome"

These authors confirmed that stingers have a higher susceptibility to a number of diverse chemical irritants and have a history of "sensitive" skin due to reactions to toiletries and cosmetics. Stingers also usually suffer from generalized dry skin in winter time, and persons with a past history of atopic dermatitis of the face usually sting severely.

The eye area is the most sensitive portion of the entire face. Certain eye-shadows may pass the stinging test on the nasolabial fold but produce subjective discomfort upon regular use. Therefore, eye cosmetics should be tested in this region to assure optimal compatibility.

16.10.3 Pathogenesis of Stinging and Influencing Factors

The pathogenesis of the stinging phenomenon remains uncertain, although it clearly involves the excitation of the sensory nerve endings. The fact that these are more abundant around hair follicles may explain why the stinging threshold is lowest on the face, particularly on the cheek and nasolabial fold. Sweating and increase in body temperature might further enhance the penetration of the sting-inducing agent.

Initially, it was thought that stingers were primarily females with a fair complexion and very sensitive (hyperirritable) skin. Further experience on larger panels of subjects failed to confirm this with regard to the fair complexion: dark-skinned individuals can be stingers, too. However, Lammintausta et al. provided evidence

Table 16.10 Agents causing subjective reactions of the skin in the form of stinging or burning (from [101])

Stinging type	Agent	Concentration
Immediate-type stinging	Chloroform	50% Ethanol
	Methanol	100%
	Ethanol (primarily on abraded skin)	100%
	Strong acids	
	Hydrochloric acid	1% Water
	Trichloracetic acid	5% Water
	Weak acids	
	Ascorbic, acetic, citric and sorbic acids	5% Water
	Retinoic acid	0.05% Ethanol
Delayed-type stinging		
Slight stinging	Benzene	1% Ethanol
	Phenol	1% Ethanol
	Salicylic acid	5% Ethanol
	Resorcinol	5% Water
	Phosphoric acid	1% Water
	Aluminum chloride	30% Water
	Zirconium hydroxychloride	30% Water
Moderate stinging	Sodium carbonate	15% Water
	Trisodium phosphate	5% Water
	Propylene glycol	100%
	Propylene carbonate	100%
	Propylene glycol diacetate	100%
	Dimethylacetamide	100%
	Dimethylformamide	100%
	Dimethylsulfoxide	100%
	Diethyltoluamide (Deet)	50% Ethanol
	Dimethyl phthalate	50% Ethanol
	Benzoyl peroxide	5% Grease-free washable lotion base
Severe stinging	Crude coal tar	5% Dimethylformamide
	Lactic acid	5% Water
	Phosphoric acid	3.3% Water
	Hydrochloric acid	1.2% Water
	Sodium hydroxide	1.3% Water
	Amyldimethyl-*p*-aminobenzoic acid (Escalol 506)	5% Ethanol
	2-Ethoxyethyl-p-methoxy-cinnamate (Giv-Tan FR)	2% Ethanol

The *immediate type of stinging* develops after short exposure (seconds or minutes) and abates quickly after removal of the irritant. The *delayed-type of stinging* builds up over a certain time period, does not disappear quickly after removal of the causative agent, and is experienced only by predisposed individuals ("stingers")

that hyperirritability is associated with the stinging phenomenon [226]. The repeated application of the anionic detergent SLS to the skin of the upper back damaged the stratum corneum barrier in stingers more than in nonstingers. This was quantified by visual scoring and measurements of TEWL. Furthermore, in the facial region of stingers lactic acid produced an increase in blood flow recognized by the laser Doppler technique but not with the naked eye. Subjects who did not experience stinging with lactic acid showed less or no change in blood flow.

Issachar et al. [278] measured the blood flow induced by methyl nicotinate, applying a computer-assisted Doppler perfusion image technique. Significant differences were found between stingers and nonstingers. Reactors to lactic acid also showed an increased response to methyl nicotinate as early as 5 min after application, and for 30 min afterwards, though the duration of inflammation in these two groups was the same. This suggests an increased penetration of (water-soluble) substances and a higher vascular reactivity in subjects who are susceptible to neurosensory irritation.

However, when irritant reactions are assessed only visually without the use of bioengineering equipment, the differences in reactivity between stingers and nonstingers were very small or nonexistent. This is the conclusion of a series of experiments conducted by Basketter and coworkers [279]. For DMSO, methyl nicotinate, and cinnamic aldehyde, there was no difference in the response of stingers and nonstingers. In contrast, for benzoic acid and *trans*-cinnamic acid, both the mean intensity of erythema and its spread were greater in the panelists graded as stingers. It was confirmed that a high reactivity to one urticant was not predictive of high reactivity to the other urticants [280]. There was no significant difference in the reactivity of males and females.

Measurement of the pH on the face revealed no difference before but after the application of lactic acid. Stingers showed a sharp decrease and a slight, but persistent over 30 min, increase in pH [281]. Nonstingers had a similar pattern but the pH values remained lower and it took longer to regain the values before lactic acid application. This finding may be explained by the differences in penetration and neutralization of the acid on the skin surface.

Seidenari et al. [282] studied 26 Caucasian women with sensitive skin by their own assessment and with high scores in the lactic acid stinging test. Furthermore a wash test with a harsh soap was undertaken. Several baseline biophysical parameters were used: TEWL, capacitance, pH, sebum, and skin color measurements. The skin of sensitive subjects was described as less subtle, less hydrated, and more erythematous and telangiectatic with respect to the skin of normal subjects. A trend towards an increase in TEWL, pH, and colorimetric $a*$ values, and a decrease in capacitance, sebum, and colorimetric $L*$ values was observable. However, significances were only present for capacitance and $a*$ values.

Wu et al. recently reported similar findings in 50 healthy Chinese volunteers, who underwent a modified lactic acid stinging test with 3 and 5% aqueous solutions of lactic acid and biophysical measurements (TEWL, capacitance). Again, there was only a trend but no statistically significant association between lactic acid stinging test score and TEWL increase [283].

Blacks develop stinging less frequently than whites. This is Frosch and Kligman's experience as well as that of Weigand and Mershon [132] when evaluating the tear gas *o*-chlorobenzylidene malononitrile.

It is a common clinical observation that skin care products and topical medicaments frequently cause stinging sensations in patients with atopic dermatitis. This symptom often worsens during stress. In a recent Swedish study of 25 patients with atopic dermatitis various neuroimmune mechanisms were studied [284]. In the 16 patients who developed stinging to lactic acid the following differences compared to the nine nonstingers were found: in stingers, the papillary dermis had an increased number of mast cells, vasoactive intestinal polypeptide-positive fibers, and a tendency to a higher number of substance P-positive nerve fibers, but a decrease of calcitonin gene-related peptide fibers. The stingers had a tendency to lower salivary cortisol. Finally, there is now evidence that the stinging phenomenon is linked to neuroimmunological mechanisms and that chronic stress may be an aggravating factor.

A set of experiments has elucidated further factors influencing delayed-type stinging [101]. They can be summarized as follows:

> Stinging is markedly reduced after the inhibition of sweating.
> Prior damage to the skin increases stinging (sunburn, tape stripping, chemical irritation by detergents).
> The intensity of stinging is dose-dependent with regard to concentration and frequency of application.

> The vehicle plays an important role (solutions in ethanol or propylene glycol are more effective than fatty ointments).
> There are marked regional differences: the intensity of stinging decreases in the order nasolabial fold >cheek >chin >retroauricular region >forehead; scalp, back, and arm are virtually unreactive in respect of stinging.

The correlation of stinging with irritancy is inconsistent. With the α-hydroxy acids a positive correlation was found (pyruvic >glycolic >tartaric >lactic acid) [101]. pH did not account for the differences in either stinging or irritancy. Laden [285] also found that acids of the same pH could have quite different stinging capacities. The esters of *p*-aminobenzoic acid are examples of divergent action with regard to irritancy and stinging. A stinging ester such as ADP was found to be nonirritating on scarified skin, while an irritating one (glyceryl-*p*-aminobenzoic acid) was nonstinging.

Strong irritants (undiluted kerosene, benzalkonium chloride) may cause severe blistering reactions if applied under occlusion for 24 h, and yet they do not induce delayed- or immediate-type stinging.

In summary, our knowledge about the stinging phenomenon is still very limited [286]. Stinging undoubtedly exists and causes considerable discomfort in susceptible persons. They may as a result discontinue the use of a cosmetic or a medicament prescribed by a dermatologist.

Core Message

> The immediate type of stinging (e.g., as induced by alcohol) develops after exposure and abates quickly within seconds or minutes. The delayed-type of stinging builds up over a certain time, does not disappear after removal of the causative agent, occurs frequently in the face when sweating, and is experienced primarily by predisposed individuals ("stingers"). These individuals can be identified by a positive response to 5% lactic acid. They are often fair-skinned, have a history of "sensitive" or "dry" skin and reveal an atopic background. Neuroimmunological mechanisms are probably involved.

16.11 Suggested Reading

1. Björnberg A (1968) Skin reactions to primary irritants in patients with hand eczema. Isacsons, Göteborg

The first careful prospective hand eczema study: 100 patients with active hand eczema, 50 patients with hand eczema healed for at least 3 months, 20 patients with active hand eczema and eczematous lesions elsewhere on the body, and 100 healthy control persons were investigated with a series of irritants applied open or under occlusion (NaOH, SLS, benzalkonium chloride, hydrochloric acid, croton oil, mercury bichloride, phenol, trichloracetic acid, etc.). Patients with atopic and dyshidrotic eczema were excluded. The main conclusions were as follows. A constitutional increase in skin reactivity to primary irritants was not present in patients with hand eczema. A general increase in skin reactivity to primary irritants was found in patients with an active eczematous process ("status eczematicus"). The alkali tests were judged to be of no value in the diagnosis of "alkali eczema" and "occupational eczema." It is not possible to predict the intensity of skin reaction to one irritant by knowing the strength of a reaction to another irritant.

These observations still hold true after many years. The use of one or several irritants as a preemployment test to judge a predisposition to eczema has no scientific basis.

2. Frosch PJ, Kligman AM (1977) A method for appraising the stinging capacity of topically applied substances. J Soc Cosmet Chem 28:197–209

Subjective discomfort such as smarting or prolonged stinging known for decades was studied in a systematic way for the first time. The phenomenon does not occur in everybody but is frequent in so-called stingers. These individuals are identified by the application of 5% lactic acid to the cheek after induction of profuse sweating in a sauna. Stinging is scored on a 0 to 3+ scale at various intervals up to 8 min. Numerous substances causing delayed-type of stinging have been identified (propylene glycol, diethyltoluamide, benzoyl peroxide, coal tar, amyldimethyl-*p*-aminobenzoic acid, etc.). There is no correlation between the stinging capacity of a material and its irritancy.

Most cosmetics are now routinely tested for stinging in volunteers before marketing. Various modifications of the original stinging assay have been described in order to increase its reliability.

References

1. Malten KE, den Arend JACJ, Wiggers RE (1979) Delayed irritation: hexanediol diacrylate and butanediol diacrylate. Contact Dermatitis 5:178–184
2. Nethercott JR, Gupta S, Rosen C, Enders LJ, Pilger CW (1984) Tetraethylene glycol diacrylate. A cause of delayed cutaneous irritant reaction and allergic contact dermatitis. J Occup Med 26:513–516
3. Lovell CR, Rycroft RCG, Williams DMJ, Hamlin J (1985) Contact dermatitis from the irritancy (immediate and delayed) and allergenicity of hydroxypropyl acrylate. Contact Dermatitis 12:117–118
4. Basketter DA, Marriott M, Gilmour NJ, White IR (2004) Strong irritants masquerading as skin allergens: the case of benzalkonium chloride. Contact Dermatitis 50:213–217
5. Björnberg A (1968) Skin reactions to primary irritants in patients with hand eczema. Isacsons, Göteborg
6. Bruynzeel DP, van Ketel WG, Scheper RJ, von Blomberg-van der Feier BME (1982) Delayed time course of irritation by sodium lauryl sulfate: observations on threshold reactions. Contact Dermatitis 8:236–239
7. Frosch PJ, Rustemeyer T (1999) Contact allergy to calcipotriol does exist. Contact Dermatitis 40:66–71
8. Kim IH, Seo SH (1999) Occupational chemical burns caused by bromine. Contact Dermatitis 41:43
9. Agner T, Serup J (1990) Sodium lauryl sulphate for irritant patch testing – a dose-response study using bioengineering methods for determination of skin irritation. J Invest Dermatol 95:543–547
10. Reiche L, Willis C, Wilkinson J, Shaw S, de Lacharièrre O (1998) Clinical morphology of sodium lauryl sulfate (SLS) and nonanoic acid (NAA) irritant patch test reactions at 48 h and 96 h in 152 subjects. Contact Dermatitis 39:240–243
11. Atherton DJ (2004) A review of the pathophysiology, prevention and treatment of irritant diaper dermatitis. Curr Med Res Opin 20:645–649
12. Kügler K, Brinkmeier T, Frosch PJ, Uter W (2005) Anogenital dermatoses – allergic and irritative causative factors. Analysis of IVDK data and review of the literature. J Dtsch Dermatol Ges 3:979–986
13. Dooms-Goossens AE, Debusschere KM, Gevers DM, Dupre KM, Degreef HJ, Loncke JP, Snaauwaert JE (1986) Contact dermatitis caused by airborne agents. J Am Acad Dermatol 15:1–10
14. Huygens S, Goossens A (2001) An update on airborne contact dermatitis. Contact Dermatitis 44:1–6
15. Santos R, Goossens A (2007) An update on airborne contact dermatitis: 2001-2006. Contact Dermatitis 57:353–360
16. Feser A, Plaza T, Vogelsang L, Mahler V (2008) Periorbital dermatitis-a recalcitrant disease: causes and differential diagnoses. Br J Dermatol 159:858–863
17. Lyon CC, Yell J, Beck MH (1998) Irritant contact dermatitis from pancreatin exacerbating vulvodynia. Contact Dermatitis 38:362
18. Zimmaro Bliss D, Zehrer C, Savik K, Thayer D, Smith G (2006) Incontinence-associated skin damage in nursing home residents: a secondary analysis of a prospective, multicenter study. Ostomy Wound Manage 52:46–55

19. Timmer-de Mik L, Toonstra J (2008) Allergy to hydrocol-loid dressings. Contact Dermatitis 58:124–125

20. Frosch PJ (1985) Hautirritation und empfindliche Haut. Grosse, Berlin

21. Jackson EM, Goldner R (eds) (1990) Irritant contact dermatitis. Dekker, New York

22. Wahlberg JE (1984) Skin irritancy from alkaline solutions assessed by laser Doppler flowmetry. Contact Dermatitis 10:111

23. Wahlberg JE (1989) Assessment of erythema: a comparison between the naked eye and laser Doppler flowmetry. In: Frosch PJ, Dooms-Goossens A, Lachapelle JM, Rycroft RJG, Scheper RJ (eds) Current topics in contact dermatitis. Springer, Berlin, pp 549–553

24. Wahlberg JE, Lindberg M (2003) Nonanoic acid – an experimental irritant. Contact Dermatitis 49:117–123

25. Willis CM, Stephens CJM, Wilkinson JD (1988) Experimentally-induced irritant contact dermatitis. Contact Dermatitis 18:20–24

26. Tsai TF, Maibach HI (1999) How irritant is water? An overview. Contact Dermatitis 41:311–314

27. Warner RR, Stone KJ, Boissy YL (2003) Hydration disrupts human stratum corneum ultrastructure. J Invest Dermatol 120:275–284

28. Warner RR, Boissy YL, Lilly NA, Spears MJ, McKillop K, Marshall JL, Stone KJ (1999) Water disrupts stratum corneum lipid lamellae: damage is similar to surfactants. J Invest Dermatol 113:960–966

29. Frosch PJ, Rustemeyer T (2000) Hairdresser's eczema. In: Menné T, Maibach HI (eds) Hand eczema, 2nd edn. CRC Press, Boca Raton, pp 195–207

30. Gollhausen R, Kligman AM (1985) Effects of pressure on contact dermatitis. Am J lnd Med 8:323–328

31. Menné T (1983) Frictional dermatitis in post-office workers. Contact Dermatitis 9:172–173

32. Menné T, Hjorth N (1985) Frictional contact dermatitis. Am J Ind Med 8:401–402

33. McMullen E, Gawkrodger DJ (2006) Physical friction is under-recognized as an irritant that can cause or contribute to contact dermatitis. Br J Dermatol 154:154–156

34. Mancuso G, Reggiani M, Berdondini RM (1996) Occupational dermatitis in shoemakers. Contact Dermatitis 34:17–22

35. Bäurle G, Hornstein OP, Diepgen TL (1985) Professionelle Handekzeme und Atopie. Dermatosen 33:161–165

36. Bäurle G (1986) Handekzeme. Studie zum Einfluß von konstitutionellen und Umweltfaktoren auf die Genese. Schattauer, Stuttgart

37. Kühner-Piplack B (1987) Klinik und Differentialdiagnose des Handekzems. Eine retrospektive Studie am Krankengut der Universitäts-Hautklinik Heidelberg 1982–1985. Thesis, Ruprecht-Karls-University, Heidelberg

38. Meding B (1990) Epidemiology of hand eczema in an industrial city. Acta Derm Venerol (Stockh) (suppl) 153:1–43

39. Rietschel RL (1990) Diagnosing irritant contact dermatitis. In: Jackson EM, Goldner R (eds) irritant contact dermatitis. Dekker, New York, pp 167–171

40. Menné T, Maibach HI (eds) (2000) Hand eczema, 2nd edn. CRC, Boca Raton, FL

41. Veien NK, Hattel T, Laurberg G (2008) Hand eczema: Causes, course, and prognosis I. Contact Dermatitis 58:330–334

42. Veien NK, Hattel T, Laurberg G (2008) Hand eczema: Causes, course, and prognosis II. Contact Dermatitis 58:335–339

43. Warshaw EM, Ahmed RL, Belsito DV, DeLeo VA, Fowler JF Jr, Maibach HI, Marks JG Jr, Toby Mathias CG, Pratt MD, Rietschel RL, Sasseville D, Storrs FJ, Taylor JS, Zug KA (2007) Contact dermatitis of the hand: cross-sectional analyses of North American Contact Dermatitis Group Data, 1994-2004. J Am Acad Dermatol 57:301–314

44. Cvetkovski RS, Zachariae R, Jensen H, Olsen J, Johansen JD, Agner T (2006) Prognosis of occupational hand eczema: a follow-up study. Arch Dermatol 142:305–311

45. Hald M, Agner T, Blands J, Veien NK, Laurberg G, Avnstorp C, Menné T, Kaaber K, Kristensen B, Kristensen O, Andersen KE, Paulsen E, Thormann J, Sommerlund M, Nielsen NH, Johansen JD (2009) Clinical severity and prognosis of hand eczema. Br J Dermatol 160:1229–1236

46. De Boer EM, van Keitel WG, Bruynzeel DP (1989) Dermatoses in metal workers. I. Irritant contact dermatitis. Contact Dermatitis 20:212–218

47. Rycroft RJG, Smith WD (1980) Low humidity occupational dermatoses. Contact Dermatitis 6:488–492

48. Leggat PA, Smith DR (2006) Dermatitis and aircrew. Contact Dermatitis 54:1–4

49. Morris-Johns R, Robertson SJ, Ross JS et al (2002) Dermatitis caused by physical irritants. Br J Dermatol 147:270–275

50. Uter W, Gefeller O, Schwanitz HJ (1998) An epidemiological study of the influence of season (cold and dry air) on the occurrence of irritant skin changes of the hands. Br J Dermatol 138:266–272

51. Agner T, Serup J (1989) Seasonal variation of skin resistance to irritants. Br J Dermatol 121:323–328

52. Basketter DA, Griffiths HA, Wang XM, Wilhelm KP, McFadden J (1996) Individual, ethnic and seasonal variability in irritant susceptibility of skin: the implications for a predictive human patch test. Contact Dermatitis 35: 208–213

53. Löffler H, Happle R (2003) Influence of climatic conditions on the irritant patch test with sodium lauryl sulphate. Acta Derm Venereol (Stockh) 83:338–341

54. Brasch J, Schnuch A, Geier J, Aberer W, Uter W (2004) Iodopropynylbutyl carbamate 0.2% is suggested for patch testing of patients with eczema possibly related to preservatives. Br J Dermatol 151:608–615

55. Geier J, Uter W, Pirker C, Frosch PJ (2003) Patch testing with the irritant sodium lauryl sulfate (SLS) is useful in interpreting weak reactions to contact allergens as allergic or irritant. Contact Dermatitis 48:99–107

56. Uter W, Geier J, Land M, Pfahlberg A, Gefeller O, Schnuch A (2001) Another look at seasonal variation in patch test results. A multifactorial analysis of surveillance data of the IVDK. Information Network of Departments of Dermatology. Contact Dermatitis 44:146–152

57. Uter W, Hegewald J, Pfahlberg A, Pirker C, Frosch PJ, Gefeller O (2003) The association between ambient air conditions (temperature and absolute humidity), irritant sodium lauryl sulfate patch test reactions and patch test reactivity to standard allergens. Contact Dermatitis 49: 97–102

58. Uter W, Geier J, Becker D, Brasch J, Löffler H (2004) The MOAHLFA index of irritant sodium lauryl sulfate reactions: first results of a multicentre study on routine sodium lauryl sulfate patch testing. Contact Dermatitis 51:259–262

59. Veien NK, Hattel T, Laurberg G (1997) Low-humidity dermatosis from car heaters. Contact Dermatitis 37:138
60. Moroni P, Cazzaniga R, Pierini F, Panella V, Zerboni R (1988) Occupational contact psoriasis. Dermatosen 36: 163–164
61. Hill VA, Ostlere LS (1998) Psoriasis of the hands köbnerizing in contact dermatitis. Contact Dermatitis 39:194
62. Gawkrodger DJ, Lloyd MH, Hunter JAA (1986) Occupational skin disease in hospital cleaning and kitchen workers. Contact Dermatitis 15:132–135
63. Ramsing DW, Agner T (1996) Effect of glove occlusion on human skin (II). Long-term experimental exposure. Contact Dermatitis 34:258–262
64. Wrangsjö K, Osterman K, van Hage-Hamsten M (1994) Glove-related skin symptoms among operating theatre and dental care unit personnel. Contact Dermatitis 30:102–107
65. Kwon S, Campbell LS, Zirwas MJ (2006) Role of protective gloves in the causation and treatment of occupational irritant contact dermatitis. J Am Acad Dermatol 55:891–896
66. John SM (2006) Primary and acquired sensitive skin. In: Berardesca E, Fluhr J, Maibach HI (eds) The sensitive skin syndrome. Taylor & Francis, New York, pp 129–147
67. Wetzky U, Bock M, Wulfhorst B, John SM (2009) Short- and long-term effects of single and repetitive glove occlusion on the epidermal barrier. Arch Dermatol Res 301: 595–602
68. Bock U, Dahmer K, Wulfhorst B, John SM (2009) Semipermeable glove membranes. Effects on skin barrier repair following SLS-irritation. Contact Dermatitis 61: 276–280
69. Zhai H, Maibach HI (2001) Skin occlusion and irritant and allergic contact dermatitis: an overview. Contact Dermatitis 44:201–206
70. Wulfhorst B, Schwanitz HJ, Bock M (2004) Optimizing skin protection with semipermeable gloves. Dermatitis 15:184–191
71. Kanerva L, Estlander T, Jolanki R (2000) Occupational contact dermatitis caused by personal-computer mouse. Contact Dermatitis 43:362–363
72. Tanaka M, Fujimoto A, Kobayashi S et al (2001) Keyboard wrist pad. Contact Dermatitis 44:253–254
73. Capon F, Cambie MP, Clinard F, Bernardeau K, Kalis B (1996) Occupational contact dermatitis caused by computer mice. Contact Dermatitis 35:57–58
74. Halkier-Sørensen L (1998) Occupational skin disease: reliability and utility of the data in the various registers; the course from notification to compensation and the costs. Contact Dermatitis 39:71–78
75. Eiermann HJ, Larsen W, Maibach HI, Taylor JS (1982) Prospective study of cosmetic reactions: 1977–1980. J Am Acad Dermatol 6:909–917
76. Berne B, Boström Å, Grahnén AF, Tammela M (1996) Adverse effects of cosmetics and toiletries reported to the Swedish Medical Products Agency 1989–1994. Contact Dermatitis 34:359–362
77. Kanerva L, Lahtinen A, Toikkanen J, Forss H, Estlander T, Susitaival P, Jolanki R (1999) Increase in occupational skin diseases of dental personnel. Contact Dermatitis 40:104–108
78. Rustemeyer T, Frosch PJ (1996) Occupational skin diseases in dental laboratory technicians. I. Clinical picture and causative factors. Contact Dermatitis 34:125–133
79. Paulsen E (1998) Occupational dermatitis in Danish gardeners and greenhouse workers (II.) Etiological factors. Contact Dermatitis 38:14–19
80. Dickel H, Kuss O, Schmidt A, Kretz J, Diepgen TL (2002) Importance of irritant contact dermatitis in occupational skin disease. Am J Clin Dermatol 3:283–289
81. Dickel H, John SM (2003) Ratio of irritant contact dermatitis in occupational skin disease. J Am Acad Dermatol 49:361–362
82. Diepgen TL (2003) Occupational skin disease data in Europe. Int Arch Occup Environ Health 76:331–338
83. Kucenic MJ, Belsito DV (2003) Occupational allergic contact dermatitis is more prevalent than irritant contact dermatitis: a 5-year study. J Am Acad Dermatol 49: 360–361, authors' reply 362
84. Dickel H, Kuss O, Blesius CR, Schmidt A, Diepgen TL (2001) Occupational skin diseases in Northern Bavaria between 1990 and 1999: a population-based study. Br J Dermatol 145:453–462
85. Frosch PJ, Pilz B, Peiler D, Dreier B, Rabenhorst S (1997) Die Epikutantestung mit patienten-eigenen Produkten. In: Plewig G, Przybilla B (eds) Fortschritte der praktischen Dermatologie und Venerologie. Springer, Berlin, pp 166–181
86. Geier J, Uter W, Lessmann H, Frosch PJ (2004) Patch testing with metal-working fluids from the patient's workplace. Contact Dermatitis 51:172–179
87. Jolanki R, Estlander T, Alanko K, Kanerva L (2000) Patch testing with a patient's own material handled at work. In: Kanerva L, Elsner P, Wahlberg JE, Maibach HI (eds) Handbook of occupational dermatology, vol 47. Springer, Berlin, pp 375–383
88. Menné T, Dooms-Goossens A, Wahlberg JE, White IR, Shaw S (1992) How large a proportion of contact sensitivities are diagnosed with the European Standard series? Contact Dermatitis 26:201–202
89. Uter W, Balzer C, Geier J, Schnuch A, Frosch PJ (2005) Ergebnisse der Epikutantestung mit patienteneigenen Parfums, Deos und Rasierwässern. Dermatol Beruf Umwelt 53:25–36
90. Belsito DV (2005) Occupational contact dermatitis: etiology, prevalence, and resultant impairment/disability. J Am Acad Dermatol 53:303–313
91. Diepgen TL, Andersen KE, Brandao FM, Bruze M, Bruynzeel DP, Frosch P, Goncalo M, Goossens A, Le Coz CJ, Rustemeyer T, White IR, Agner T (2009) European Enviromental and Contact Dermatitis Research Group. Hand eczema classification: a cross-sectional, multicentre study of the aetiology and morphology of hand eczema. Br J Derm 160:353–358
92. Meding B, Wrangsjö K, Järvholm B (2005) Fifteen-year follow-up of hand eczema: persistence and consequences. Br J Dermatol 152:975–980
93. Agner T, Andersen KE, Brandao FM, Bruze M, Bruynzeel DP, Frosch P, Goncalo M, Goossens A, Le Coz CJ, Rustemeyer T, White IR, Diepgen TL (2008) EECDRG. Hand eczema severity and quality of life: a crosssectional, multicentre study of hand eczema patients. Contact Dermatitis 59:43–47
94. Fleming MG, Bergfeld WF (1990) The etiology of irritant contact dermatitis. In: Jackson EM, Goldner R (eds) Initant contact dermatitis. Dekker, New York, pp 41–66
95. Gehse M, Kändler-Stürmer P, Gloor M (1987) Über die Bedeutung der Irritabilität der Haut für die Entstehung des berufsbedingten allergischen Kontaktekzems. Dermatol Monatsschr 173:400–404
96. Kligman AM (1979) Cutaneous toxicity: an overview from the underside. Curr Probl Dermatol 7:1–25

97. Landman G, Farmer ER, Hood AF (1990) The pathophysiology of irritant contact dermatitis. In: Jackson EM, Goldner R (eds) Irritant contact dermatitis. Dekker, New York, pp 67–77

98. Malten KE (1981) Thoughts on irritant contact dermatitis. Contact Dermatitis 7:238–247

99. Rietschel RL (1989) Persistent maleic acid irritant dermatitis in the guinea pig. In: Frosch PJ, Dooms-Goossens A, Lachapelle JM, Rycroft RJG, Scheper RJ (eds) Current topics in contact dermatitis. Springer, Berlin, pp 429–434

100. Agner T, Fullerton A, Broby-Johnson U, Batsberg W (1990) Irritant patch testing: penetration of sodium lauryl sulphate into human skin. Skin Pharmacol 3:213–217

101. Frosch PJ, Kligman AM (1977) A method for appraising the stinging capacity of topically applied substances. J Soc Cosmet Chem 28:197–209

102. Frosch PJ, Kligman AM (1979) The soap chamber test: a new method for assessing the irritancy of soaps. J Am Acad Dermatol 1:35–41

103. Van der Valk PGM, Crijns MC, Nater JP, Bleumink E (1984) Skin irritancy of commercially available soap and detergent bars as measured by water vapour loss. Dermatosen 32:87–90

104. Van der Valk PGM, Nater JP, Bleumink E (1984) Skin irritancy of surfactants as assessed by water vapor loss measurements. J Invest Dermatol 82:291–293

105. Nangia A, Andersen PH, Berner B, Maibach HI (1996) High dissociation constants (pKa) of basic permeants are associated with in vivo skin irritation in man. Contact Dermatitis 34:237–242

106. Fischer T, Bjarnason B (1996) Sensitizing and irritant properties of 3 environmental classes of diesel oil and their indicator dyes. Contact Dermatitis 34:309–315

107. Feldman RJ, Maibach HI (1967) Regional variations in percutaneous absorption of 14 C cortisol in man. J Invest Dermatol 48:181–185

108. Frosch PJ, Duncan S, Kligman AM (1980) Cutaneous biometrics 1: the DMSO test. Br J Dermatol 102:263–274

109. Cua AB, Wilhelm KP, Maibach HI (1990) Cutaneous sodium lauryl sulfate irritation potential: age and regional variability. Br J Dermatol 123:607–613

110. Dahlquist I, Fregert S (1979) Skin irritation in newborns. Contact Dermatitis 5:336

111. Uter W, Pfahlberg A, Gefeller O, Schwanitz HJ (1998) Hand eczema in a prospectively-followed cohort of office-workers. Contact Dermatitis 38:83–89

112. Adams RM (1999) Occupational skin disease, 3rd edn. Saunders, Philadelphia

113. Rycroft RJG (1986) Occupational dermatoses among office personnel. Occup Med State Art Rev 1:323–328

114. Rothenborg HW, Menné T, Sjolin KE (1977) Temperature dependent primary irritant dermatitis from lemon perfume. Contact Dermatitis 3:37–48

115. Clarys P, Manou I, Barel AO (1997) Influence of temperature on irritation in the hand/forearm immersion test. Contact Dermatitis 36:240–243

116. Warren R, Ertel KD, Bartolo RG, Levine MJ, Bryant PB, Wong LF (1996) The influence of hard water (calcium) and surfactants on irritant contact dermatitis. Contact Dermatitis 35:337–343

117. Ramam M, Khaitan BK, Singh MK, Gupta SD (1998) Frictional sweat dermatitis. Contact Dermatitis 38:49

118. Nilsson E, Mikaelsson B, Andersson S (1985) Atopy, occupation and domestic work as risk factors for hand eczema in hospital workers. Contact Dermatitis 13:216–223

119. Rystedt I (1985) Atopic background in patients with occupational hand eczema. Contact Dermatitis 12:247–254

120. Lammintausta K, Kalimo K (1981) Atopy and hand dermatitis in hospital wet work. Contact Dermatitis 7:301–308

121. Uter W, Pfahlberg A, Gefeller O, Schwanitz HJ (1998) Risk factors for hand dermatitis in hairdressing apprentices. Dermatosen 46:151–158

122. Löffler H, Effendy I (1999) Skin susceptibility of atopic individuals. Contact Dermatitis 40:239–242

123. Bauer A, Bartsch R, Stadeler M, Schneider W, Grieshaber R, Wollina U, Gebhardt M (1998) Development of occupational skin diseases during vocational training in baker and confectioner apprentices: a follow-up study. Contact Dermatitis 39:307–311

124. Gallacher G, Maibach HI (1998) Is atopic dermatitis a predisposing factor for experimental acute irritant contact dermatitis? Contact Dermatitis 38:1–4

125. Tupker R (2003) Prediction of irritancy in the human skin irritancy model and occupational setting. Contact Dermatitis 49:61–69

126. de Jongh CM, Khrenova L, Verberk MM, Calkoen F, van Dijk FJ, Voss H, John SM Kezic S (2008) Loss of-function polymorphisms in the filaggrin gene are associated with an increased susceptibility to chronic irritant contact dermatitis: a case-control study. Br J Dermatol 159:621–627

127. Giwercman C, Lerbaek A, Bisgaard H, Menné T (2008) Classification of atopic hand eczema and the filaggrin mutations. Contact Dermatitis 59:257–260

128. de Jongh CM, Khrenova L, Kezic S, Rustemeyer T, Verberk MM, John SM (2008) Polymorphisms in the interleukin-1 gene influence the stratum corneum interleukin-1 α concentration in uninvolved skin of patients with chronic irritant contact dermatitis. Contact Dermatitis 58: 263–268

129. Molin S, Vollmer S, Weiss EH, Ruzicka T, Prinz JC (2009) Filaggrin mutations may confer susceptibility to chronic hand eczema characterized by combined allergic and irritant contact dermatitis. Br J Dermatol 161:801–807

130. de Jongh CM, John SM, Bruynzeel DP, Caloen F, van Duk FJ, Khrenova L, Rustemeyer T, Verberk MM, Kezic S (2008) Cytokine gene polymorphisms and susceptibility to chronic irritant contact dermatitis. Contact Dermatitis 58: 269–277

131. Marriott M, Holmes J, Peters L, Cooper K, Rowson M, Basketter DA (2005) The complex problem of sensitive skin. Contact Dermatitis 53:93–99

132. Weigand DA, Mershon MM (1970) The cutaneous irritant reaction to agent o- chlorobenzylidene malononitrile (CS). II. Quantitation and racial influence in human subjects. Edgewood Arsenal Technique no 4332

133. Weigand DA, Haygood C, Gaylor JR (1974) Cell layers and density of negro and caucasian stratum corneum. J Invest Dermatol 62:563–568

134. Berardesca E, Maibach HI (1988) Racial differences in sodium lauryl sulphate induced cutaneous irritation: black and white. Contact Dermatitis 18:65–70

135. Berardesca E, Maibach HI (1988) Sodium-lauryl-sulphate-induced cutaneous irritation: comparison of white and hispanic subjects. Contact Dermatitis 19:136–140

136. Astner S, Burnett N, Rius-Diaz F, Doukas AG, González S, Gonzalez E (2006) Irritant contact dermatitis induced by a common household irritant: a noninvasive evaluation of ethnic variability in skin response. J Am Acad dermatol 54:458–465

137. Frosch PJ, Wissing C (1982) Cutaneous sensitivity to ultraviolet light and chemical irritants. Arch Dermatol Res 272:269–278

138. John S, Uter W (2005) Meteorological influence on NaOH irritation varies with body site. Arch Derm Res 296:320–326

139. John SM, Schwanitz HJ (2006) Functional skin testing: the SMART-procedures. In: Chew A-L, Maibach HI (eds) Handbook of irritant dermatitis. Springer, Berlin, pp 211–221

140. Choi JM, Lee JY, Cho BK (2000) Chronic irritant contact dermatitis: recovery time in man. Contact Dermatitis 42:264–269

141. Sajjachareonpong P, Cahill J, Keegel T, Saunders H, Nixon R (2004) Persistent post-occupational dermatitis. Contact Dermatitis 51:278–283

142. Apfelbacher CJ, Radulescu M, Diepgen TL, Funke U (2008) Occurrence and prognosis of hand eczema in the car industry: results from the PACO follow-up study (PACO II). Contact Dermatitis 58:322–329

143. Hamami I, Marks R (1988) Structural determinants of the response of the skin to chemical irritants. Contact Dermatitis 18:71–75

144. Downing DT, Stewart ME, Wertz PW, Colton SW, Abraham W, Strauss JS (1987) Skin lipids: an update. J Invest Dermatol 88:2s–62s

145. Elias PM, Brown BE, Zoboh VA (1980) The permeability barrier in essential fatty acid deficiency: evidence for a direct role for linoleic acid in barrier function. J Invest Dermatol 74:230–233

146. Elias PM (1985) The essential fatty acid deficient rodent: evidence for a direct role for intercellular lipid in barrier function. In: Maibach HI, Lowe N (eds) Models in dermatology, vol 1. Karger, Basel, pp 272–285

147. Landmann L (1985) Permeabilitätsbarriere der Epidermis. Grosse, Berlin (Grosse Scripta 9)

148. Wertz PW, Miethke MC, Long SA, Strauss JS, Downing DT (1985) The composition of the ceramides from human stratum corneum and from comedones. J Invest Dermatol 84:410–412

149. Bamford JTM, Gibson RW, Renier CM (1985) Atopic eczema unresponsive to evening primrose oil (linoleic and gammalinolenic acids). J Am Acad Dermatol 13:959–965

150. Di Nardo A, Sugino K, Wertz P, Ademola J, Maibach HI (1996) Sodium lauryl sulfate (SLS) induced irritant contact dermatitis: a correlation study between ceramides and in vivo parameters of irritation. Contact Dermatitis 35:86–91

151. Willers P (1984) Die Bedeutung der Hornschicht für die Irritabilität der Haut. Thesis, Westfälische Wilhelms University, Münster

152. Goffin V, Piérard-Franchimont C, Piérard G (1996) Sensitive skin and stratum corneum reactivity to household cleaning products. Contact Dermatitis 34:81–85

153. Agner T, Damm P, Skouby SO (1991) Menstrual cycle and skin reactivity. J Am Acad Dermatol 24:566–570

154. Lammintausta K, Maibach HI (1987) Irritant reactivity in males and females. Contact Dermatitis 17:276–280

155. Roskos KV, Maibach HI, Guy RH (1989) The effect of aging on percutaneous absorption in man. J Pharmacokinet Biopharm 17:617–630

156. Rougier A, Lotte C, Corcuff P, Maibach HI (1988) Relationship between skin permeability and corneocyte size according to anatomic site, age, and sex in man. J Soc Cosmet Chem 39:15–26

157. Coenraads PJ, Bleumink E, Nater JP (1975) Susceptibility to primary irritants. Age dependance and relation of contact allergic reactions. Contact Dermatitis 1:177–181

158. Wilhelm KP, Maibach HI (1993) The effect of aging on the barrier function of human skin evaluated by in vivo transepidermal water loss measurement. In: Frosch PJ, Kligman AM (eds) Noninvasive methods for the quantification of skin functions. Springer, Berlin, pp 181–189

159. Grove GL, Duncan S, Kligman AM (1982) Effect of ageing on the blistering of human skin with ammonium hydrxide. Br J Dermatol 107:393–400

160. Schwindt DA, Wilhelm KP, Miller DL, Maibach HI (1998) Cumulative irritation in older and younger skin: a comparison. Acta Derm Venereol (Stockh) 78:279–283

161. Berardesca E, Maibach HI (2003) Ethnic skin: overview of structure and function. J Am Acad Dermatol 48 (suppl):S139–S142

162. Hicks SP, Swindells KJ, Middelkamp-Hup MA, Sifakis MA, Gonzalez E, Gonzalez S (2003) Confocal histopathology of irritant contact dermatitis in vivo and the impact of skin color (black vs white). J Am Acad Dermatol 48:727–734

163. Robinson MK (1999) Population differences in skin structure and physiology and the susceptibility to irritant and allergic contact dermatitis: implications for skin safety testing and risk assessment. Contact Dermatitis 41:65–79

164. Swindells K, Burnett N, Ruis-Diaz F, Gonzalez E, Mihm MC, Gonzalez S (2004) Reflectance confocal microscopy may differentiate acute allergic and irritant contact dermatitis in vivo. J Am Acad Dermatol 50:220–228

165. Wulfhorst B (2000) Skin hardening in occupational dermatology. In: Kanerva L, Elsner P, Wahlberg J, Maibach H (eds) Handbook of occupational dermatology. Springer, Berlin, pp 115–121

166. McOsker DE, Beck LW (1967) Characteristics of accomodated (hardened) skin. J Invest Dermatol 48:372–383

167. Watkins SA, Maibach HI (2009) The hardening phenomenon in irritant contact dermatitis: an interpretative update. Contact Dermatitis 60:123–130

168. Frosch PJ, Kligman AM (1977) Rapid blister formation in human skin with ammonium hydroxide. Br J Dermatol 96:461–473

169. Berndt U, Hinnen U, Iliev D, Elsner P (1999) Is occupational irritant contact dermatitis predictable by cutaneous bioengineering methods? Results of the Swiss metalworkers' eczema study (PROMETES). Dermatology 198:351–354

170. Kolbe L, Kligman AM, Stoudemayer T (1998) The sodium hydroxide erosion assay: a revision of the alkali resistance test. Arch Derm Res 290:382–387

171. Wilhelm KP, Pasche F, Surber C, Maibach HI (1990) Sodium hydroxide- induced subclinical irritation. A test for evaluating stratum corneum barrier function. Acta Derm Venereol (Stockh) 70:463–367

172. Grunewald AM, Gloor M, Gehring W, Kleesz P (1995) Damage to the skin by repetitive washing. Contact Dermatitis 32:225–232

16

173. Hachem J, Crumrine D, Fluhr J (2003) pH directly regulates epidermal permeability barrier homeostasis, and stratum corneum integrity/cohesion. J Invest Dermatol 121:345–353

174. Held E, Agner T (1999) Comparison between 2 test models in evaluating the effect of a moisturizer on irritated human skin. Contact Dermatitis 40:261–268

175. McFadden JPP, Wakelin SH, Basketter DA (1998) Acute irritation thresholds in subjects with Type I-Type VI skin. Contact Dermatitis 38:147–149

176. Basketter DA, Miettinen J, Lahti A (1998) Acute irritant reactivity to sodium lauryl sulfate in atopics and non-atopics. Contact Dermatitis 38:253–256

177. Robinson MK, Perkins MA, Basketter DA (1998) Application of a 4-h human patch test method for comparative and investigative assessment of skin irritation. Contact Dermatitis 38:194–202

178. Basketter DA, Whittle E, Chamberlain M (1994) Identification of irritation and corrosion hazards to skin: an alternative strategy to animal testing. Food Chem Toxicol 32:539–542

179. Basketter DA, Whittle E, Griffiths HA, York M (1994) The identification and classification of skin irritation hazard by human patch test. Food Chem Toxicol 32:769–775

180. Basketter DA, Chamberlain M, Griffiths HA, York M (1997) The classification of skin irritants by human patch test. Food Chem Toxicol 35:845–852

181. EC Annex to Commission Directive 92/69/EEC of 31 July 1992 adapting to technical progress for the seventh time Council Directive 67/548/EEC on the approximation of laws, regulations and administrative provisions relating to the classification, packaging and labelling of dangerous substances. Official J Eur Commun L383A: 35 (1992)

182. Judge MR, Griffiths HA, Basketter DA, White IR, Rycroft RJG, McFadden JP (1996) Variation in response of human skin to irritant challenge. Contact Dermatitis 34:115–117

183. York M, Griffiths HA, Whittle E, Basketter DA (1996) Evaluation of human patch test for the identification and classification of skin irritation potential. Contact Dermatitis 34:204–212

184. Basketter D, Gerberick F, Kimber I, Willis C (1999) Toxicology of contact dermatitis. Wiley, Chichester

185. Wilhelm KP, Saunders JC, Maibach HI (1990) Increased stratum corneum turnover induced by subclinical irritant dermatitis. Br J Dermatol 122:793–798

186. Pinnagoda J, Tupker RA, Coenraads PJ, Nater JP (1989) Prediction of susceptibility to an irritant response by transepidermal water loss. Contact Dermatitis 20:341–346

187. Wilhelm KP, Maibach HI (1990) Susceptibility to SLS-induced irritant dermatitis: relation to skin pH, TEWL, sebum concentration, and stratum corneum turnover time. J Am Acad Dermatol 23:122–124

188. Elias PM, Wood LC, Feingold KR (1999) Epidermal pathogenesis of inflammatory dermatoses. Am J Contact Dermat 10:119–126

189. Willis CM (2002) Variability in responsiveness to irritants: thoughts on possible underlying mechanisms. Contact Dermatitis 47:267–271

190. Boxman IL, Hensbergen PJ, van der Schors RC, Bruynzeel DP, Tensen CP, Ponec M (2002) Proteomic analysis of skin irritation reveals the induction of HSP27 by sodium lauryl sulphate in human skin. Br J Dermatol 146:777–785

191. Willis CM, Britton LE, Reiche L, Wilkinson JD (2001) Reduced levels of glutathione S-transferases in patch test reactions to dithranol and sodium lauryl sulphate as demonstrated by quantitative immunocytochemistry: evidence for oxidative stress in acute irritant contact dermatitis. Eur J Dermatol 11:99–104

192. Barr RM, Brain SC, Camp RD, Cilliers J, Greaves MW, Al M, Misch K (1984) Levels of arachidonic acid and its metabolites in the skin in human allergic and irritant contact dermatitis. Br J Dermatol 111:23–28

193. Cumberbatch M, Dearman RJ, Groves RW, Antanopoulos C, Kimber I (2002) Differential regulation of epidermal Langerhans cell migration by interleukins (IL)-1alpha and IL-1beta during irritant and allergen-induced cutaneous immune responses. Toxicol Appl Pharmacol 182: 126–135

194. Frosch PJ, Czarnetzki BM (1987) Surfactants cause in vitro chemotaxis and chemokinesis of human neutrophils. J Invest Dermatol 88:52s–55s

195. Imokawa G, Mishima Y (1981) Cumulative effect of surfactants on cutaneous horny layers. Contact Dermatitis 7:65–71

196. Kucharekova M, Hornix M, Ashikaga T et al (2003) The effect of the PDE-4 inhibitor (cipamfylline) in two human models of irritant contact dermatitis. Arch Dermatol Res 295:29–32

197. Larsen CG, Ternowitz T, Larsen EG, Thestrup-Pedersen K (1989) ETAF/interleukin 1 and epidermal lymphocyte chemotactic factor in epidermis overlying an irritant patch test. Contact Dermatitis 20:335–340

198. Li LF, Fiedler VC, Kumar R (1998) Down-regulation of protein kinase C isoforms in irritant contact dermatitis. Contact Dermatitis 38:319–324

199. Nickoloff BJ (1988) The role of gamma interferon in cutaneous trafficking of lymphocytes with emphasis on molecular and cellular adhesion events. Arch Dermatol 124:1835–1843

200. Oxholm AM, Oxholm P, Avnstorp C, Bendtzen K (1991) Keratinocyte-expression of interleukin-6 but not of tumour necrosis factor-alpha is increased in the allergic and the irritant patch test reaction. Acta Derm Venereol (Stockh) 71:93–98

201. Patrick E, Burkhalter A, Maibach HI (1987) Recent investigations of mechanisms of chemically induced skin irritation in laboratory mice. J Invest Dermatol 88:24s–31s

202. Prottey C (1978) The molecular basis of skin irritation. In: Breuer MM (ed) Cosmetic science, vol 1. Academic, London, pp 275–349

203. Reilly DM, Green MR (1999) Eicosanoid and cytokine levels in acute skin irritation in response to tape strip-ping and capsicain. Acta Derm Venereol (Stockh) 79:187–190

204. Smith HR, Basketter DA, McFadden JP (2002) Irritant dermatitis, irritancy and its role in allergic contact dermatitis. Exp Dermatol 27:138–146

205. Van der Valk PGM, Maibach HI (eds) (1996) The irritant contact dermatitis syndrome. CRC Press, Boca Raton

206. Wallengren J, Larsson B (2001) Nitric oxide participates in prick test and irritant patch test reactions in human skin. Arch Derm Res 293:121–125

207. Carter EL, O'Herrin S, Woolery C, Jack Longley B (2008) Epidermal stem cell factor augments the inflammatory response in irritant and allergic contact dermatitis. J Invest Dermatol 128:1861–1863

208. Törmä H, Lindberg M, Berne B (2008) Skin barrier disruption by sodium lauryl sulfate-exposure alters the expressions of involucrin, trasglutaminase 1, profilaggrin, and kallikreins during the repair phase in human skin in vivo. J Invest Dermatol 128:1212–1219

209. de Jongh CM, Lutter R, Verberk MM, Kezic S (2008) Differential cytokine expression in skin after single and repeated irritation by sodium lauryl sulfate. Exp Dermatol 16:1032–1040

210. Meller S, Lauerma AI, Kopp FM, Winterberg F, Anthoni M, Müller A, Gombert M, Haahtela A, Alenius H, Rieker J, Dieu-Nosjean MC, Kubitza RC, Gleichmann E, Ruzicka T, Zlotnik A, Homey B (2007) inflammation: memory T cells make the difference. J Allergy Clin Immunol 119:1470–1480

211. Bonneville M, Chavagnac C, Vocanson M, Rozieres A, Benetiere J, Pernet I, Denis A, Nicolas JF, Hennino A (2007) Skin contact irritation conditions the development and severity of allergic contact dermatitis. J Invest Dermatol 127:1430–1435

212. Blanken R, van der Valk PGM, Nater JP (1986) Laser-Doppler flowmetry in the investigation of irritant compounds on human skin. Dermatosen 34:5–9

213. Nilsson GE, Otto U, Wahlberg JE (1982) Assessment of skin irritancy in man by laser Doppler flowmetry. Contact Dermatitis 8:401–406

214. Fluhr JW, Bankova L, Fuchs S, Kelterer D, Schliemann-Willers S, Norgauer J, Kleesz P, Grieshaber R, Elsner P (2004) Fruit acids and sodium hydroxide in the food industry and their combined effect with sodium lauryl suphate: controlled in vivo tandem irritation study. Br J Dermatol 151:1039–1048

215. Kappes UP, Goritz N, Wigger-Alberti W, Heinemann C, Elsner P (2001) Tandem application of sodium lauryl sulfate and n-propanol does not lead to enhancement of cumulative skin irritation. Acta Derm Venereol (Stockh) 81:403–405

216. Wigger-Alberti W, Krebs A, Elsner P (2000) Experimental irritant contact dermatitis due to cumulative epicutaneous exposure to sodium lauryl sulphate and toluene: single and concurrent application. Br J Dermatol 143:551–556

217. Wigger-Alberti W, Spoo J, Schliemann-Willers S, Klotz A, Elsner P (2002) The tandem repeated irritation test: a new method to assess prevention of irritant combination damage to the skin. Acta Derm Venereol (Stockh) 82:94–97

218. Elsner P, Wigger-Alberti W (2003) Skin-conditioning products in occupational dermatology. Int Arch Occup Environ Health 76:351–354

219. Frosch PJ, Kurte A, Pilz B (1993) Biophysical techniques for the evaluation of skin protective creams In: Frosch PJ, Kligman AM (eds) Noninvasive methods for the quantification of skin functions. Springer, Berlin, pp 214–222

220. Frosch PJ, Kurte A (1994) Efficacy of skin barrier creams. IV. The repetitive irritation test (RIT) with a set of four standard irritants. Contact Dermatitis 31:161–168

221. Schliemann-Willers S, Wigger-Alberti W, Elsner P (2001) Efficacy of a new class of perfluoropolyethers in the prevention of irritant contact dermatitis. Acta Derm Venereol (Stockh) 81:392–394

222. Schliemann-Willers S, Wigger-Alberti W, Kleesz P, Grieshaber R, Elsner P (2002) Natural vegetable fats in the prevention of irritant contact dermatitis. Contact Dermatitis 46:6–12

223. Schnetz E, Diepgen TL, Elsner P, Frosch PJ, Klotz AJ, Kresken J, Kuss O, Merk H, Schwanitz HJ, Wigger-Alberti W, Fartasch M (2000) Multi-centre study for the development of an in vivo model to evaluate the influence of topical formulations on irritation. Contact Dermatitis 42:336–343

224. Spoo J, Wigger-Alberti W, Berndt U, Fischer T, Elsner P (2002) Skin cleansers: three test protocols for the assessment of irritancy ranking. Acta Derm Venereol (Stockh) 82:13–17

225. Löffler H, Pirker C, Aramaki J, Frosch PJ, Happle R, Effendy I (2001) Evaluation of skin susceptibility to irritancy by routine patch testing with sodium lauryl sulfate. Eur J Dermatol 11:416–419

226. Lammintausta K, Maibach HI, Wilson D (1988) Mechanisms of subjective (sensory) irritation. Dermatosen 36:45–49

227. Wilhelm KP, Surber C, Maibach HI (1989) Quantification of sodium lauryl sulfate irritant dermatitis in man: comparison of four techniques: skin color reflectance, transepidermal water loss, laser Doppler flow measurement and visual scores. Arch Dermatol Res 281:293–295

228. John SM, Uter W, Schwanitz HJ (2000) Relevance of multiparametric skin bioengineering in a prospectively-followed cohort of junior hairdressers. Contact Dermatitis 43:161–168

229. Smit HA, van Rijssen A, Vandenbrouke JP, Coenrads PJ (1994) Susceptibility to and incidence of hand dermatitis in a cohort of apprentice hairdressers and nurses. Scand J Work Environ Health 20:113–121

230. Smith HR, Armstrong DK, Holloway D, Whittam L, Basketter DA, McFadden JP (2002) Skin irritation thresholds in hairdressers: implications for the development of hand dermatitis. Br J Dermatol 146:849–852

231. Uter W (1999) Epidemiologie und Prävention von Handekzemen in Feuchtberufen am Beispiel des Friseurhandwerks. Universitätsverlag Rasch, Osnabrück

232. Frosch PJ (1985) Human models for quantification of corticosteroid adverse effects. In: Maibach HI, Lowe NJ (eds) Models in dermatology, vol 2. Karger, Basel, pp 5–15

233. Anveden I, Kindberg M, Andersen KE, Bruze M, Isaksson M, Lidén C, Sommerlund M, Wahlberg JE, Wilkinson JD, Willis CM (2004) Oral prednisone suppresses allergic but not irritant patch test reactions in individuals hypersensitive to nickel. Contact Dermatitis 50:298–303

234. Levin C, Zhai H, Bashir S, Chew AL, Anigbogu A, Stern R, Maibach H (2001) Efficacy of corticosteroids in acute experimental irritant contact dermatitis? Skin Res Technol 7:214–218

235. Ramsing DW, Agner T (1995) Efficacy of topical corticosteroids on irritant skin reactions. Contact Dermatitis 32:293–297

236. Kao JS, Fluhr JW, Man M-Q, Fowler AJ, Hachem J-P, Crumrine D, Ahn SK, Brown BE, Elias PM, Feingold KR (2003) Short-term glucocorticoid treatment compromises both permeability barrier homeostasis and stratum corneum integrity: inhibition of epidermal lipid synthesis accounts for functional abnormalities. J Invest Dermatol 120:456–464

237. Kolbe L, Kligman AM, Schreiner V, Stoudemayer T (2001) Corticosteroid-induced atrophy and barrier impairment measured by non-invasive methods in human skin. Skin Res Technol 7:73–77

238. Schliemann S, Kelterer D, Bauer A, John SM, Schindera I, Wehrmann W, Elsner P (2008) Tacrolimus in the treatment of occupationally-induced chronic hand dermatitis. Contact Dermatitis 58:299–306

239. Peiler D, Rustemeyer T, Pflug B, Frosch PJ (2000) Allergic contact dermatitis in dental laboratory technicians. II. Major allergens and their clinical relevance. Dermatosen 48:48–54

240. Frosch PJ, Peiler D, Grunert V (2003) Wirksamkeit von Hautschutzprodukten im Vergleich zu Hautpflegeprodukten bei Zahntechnikern – eine kontrollierte Feldstudie. JDDG 1:547–557

241. Jungbauer FHW, van der Harst JJ, Groothoff JW, Coenraads PJ (2004) Skin protection in nursing work: promoting the use of gloves and hand alcohol. Contact Dermatitis 51:135–140

242. Löffler H, Kampf G, Schmermund D, Maibach HI (2007) How irritant is alcohol? Br J Dermatol 157:74–81

243. Slotosch CM, Kampf G, Löffler H (2007) Effects of disinfectants and detergents on skin irritation. Contact Dermatitis 57:235–241

244. Stutz N, Becker D, Jappe U, John SM, Ladwig A, Spornraft-Ragaller P, Uter W, Löffler H (2009) Nurses' perceptions of the benefits and adverse effects of hand disinfection: alcohol-based hand rubs vs. hygienic handwashing: a multicentre questionnaire study with additional patch testing bei the German Contact Dermatitis Research Group. Br J Dermatol 160:565–572

245. English JSC, Ratcliffe J, Williams HC (1999) Irritancy of industrial hand cleansers tested by repeated open application on human skin. Contact Dermatitis 40:84–88

246. Paye M, Gomes G, Zerweck CR, Piérard GD, Grove GL (1999) A hand immersion test under laboratory-controlled usage conditions: the need for sensitive and controlled assessment methods. Contact Dermatitis 40: 133–138

247. Tupker RA, Bunte EE, Fidler V, Wiechers JW, Coenraads PJ (1999) Irritancy ranking of anionic detergents using one-time occlusive, repeated occlusive and repeated open tests. Contact Dermatitis 40:316–322

248. Wigger-Alberti W, Fischer T, Greif C, Maddern P, Elsner P (1999) Effects of various grit-containing cleansers on skin barrier function. Contact Dermatitis 41:136–140

249. Piérard GE, Goffin V, Herrmanns-Lê T, Arrese JE, Piérard-Franchimont C (1995) Surfactant induced dermatitis. A comparison of corneosurfametry with predicitve testing on human and reconstructed skin. J Am Acad Dermatol 33:462–469

250. Bock M, Schürer NY, Schwanitz HJ (2004) Effects of CO_2-enriched water on barrier recovery. Arch Derm Res 296:163–168

251. Yoshizawa Y, Kitamura K, Kawana S, Maibach HI (2003) Water, salts and skin barrier of normal skin. Skin Res Technol 9:31–33

252. Halkier-Sørensen L, Thestrup-Pedersen K (1993) The efficacy of a moisturizer (Locobase) among cleaners and kitchen assistants during everyday exposure to water and detergents. Contact Dermatitis 29:1–6

253. Lodén M (1997) Barrier recovery and influence of irritant stimuli in skin treated with a moisturizing cream. Contact Dermatitis 36:256–260

254. Hannuksela A, Hannuksela M (1996) Irritant effects of a detergent in wash, chamber and repeated open application tests. Contact Dermatitis 34:134–137

255. Held E (2002) Prevention of irritant skin reactions in relation to wet work. Thesis, University of Copenhagen

256. Zhai H, Maibach HI (1998) Moisturizers in preventing irritant contact dermatitis: an overview. Contact Dermatitis 38:241–244

257. Goh CL, Gan SL (1994) Efficacies of a barrier cream and an afterwork emollient cream against cutting fluid dermatitis in metal workers. A prospective study. Contact Dermatitis 31:176–180

258. Frosch PJ, Pilz B (1994) Hautschutz für Friseure – die Wirksamkeit von zwei Hautschutzprodukten gegenüber Detergentien im repetitiven Irritationstest. Dermatosen 42:199–202

259. Zhai H, Willard P, Maibach HI (1999) Putative skin-protective formulations in preventing and/or inhibiting experimentally-produced irritant and allergic contact dermatitis. Contact Dermatitis 41:190–192

260. Bayerl C, Garbea A, Peiler D, Rzany B, Allgäuer T, Kleesz P, Jung EG, Frosch PJ (1999) Pilotstudie zur Therapie des beruflich bedingten Handekzems mit einer neuen tragbaren UVB-Bestrahlungseinheit. Aktuel Dermatol 25:302–305

261. Sjövall P, Christensen OB (1994) Treatment of chronic hand eczema with UV-B Handylux in the clinic and at home. Contact Dermatitis 31:5–8

262. Agner T, Johansen JD, Overgaard L, Volund A, Basketter D, Menné T (2002) Combined effects of irritants and allergens. Contact Dermatitis 47:21–26

263. Pedersen LK, Johansen JD, Held E, Agner T (2004) Augmentation of skin response by exposure to a combination of allergens and irritants – a review. Contact Dermatitis 50:265–273

264. Agner T, Held E (2002) Skin protection programmes. Contact Dermatitis 46:253–256

265. Weisshaar E, Radulescu M, Bock M et al (2005) Hautschutzseminare zur sekundären Individualprävention bei Beschäftigten in Gesundheitsberufen: erste Ergebnisse nach über 2-jähriger Durchführung. JDDG 3:33–38

266. Funke U, Diepgen T, Fartasch M (1996) Risk-group-related prevention of hand eczema at the workplace. Curr Probl Dermatol 25:123–132

267. Itschner L, Hinnen U, Elsner P (1996) Prevention of hand eczema in the metal-working industry. Risk awareness and behaviour of metal worker apprentices. Dermatology 193:226–229

268. Kalimo K, Kautiainen H, Niskanen T, Niemi L (1999) "Eczema school" to improve compliance in an occupational dermatology clinic. Contact Dermatitis 41:315–319

269. Schwanitz HJ, Uter W, Wulfhorst B (eds) (1996) Neue Wege zur Prävention – Paradigma Friseurekzem. Rasch, Osnabrück

270. John SM (2008) Occupational skin diseases: options for multidisciplinary networking in preventive medicine. GMS Ger Med Sci 6:Doc07 (Online-Publikation: http://www.egms.de/en/gms/2008-6/000052.shtml)

271. Jungbauer FHW, van der Vleuten P, Groothoff JW, Coenraads PJ (2004) Irritant hand dermatitis: severity of disease, occupational exposure to skin irritants and preventive measures 5 years after initial diagnosis. Contact Dermatitis 50:245–251

272. Klaschka F (1979) Arbeitsphysiologie der Hornschicht in Grundzügen. In: Marchionini A (ed) Jadassohns Handbuch der Haut- und Geschlechtskrankheiten. Ergänzungswerk, vol 1, part 4A. Springer, Berlin, pp 153–261

273. Parrish JA, Pathak MA, Fitzpatrick TB (1975) Facial irritation due to sunscreen products (letter to the editor). Arch Dermatol 111:525

274. Soschin D, Kligman AM (1982) Adverse subjective reactions. In: Kligman AM, Leyden JJ (eds) Safety and efficacy of topical drugs and cosmetics. Grune and Stratton, New York, pp 377–388

275. Kerr AC, Niklasson B, Dawe RS, Escoffier AM, Krasteva M, Sanderson B, Ferguson J (2009) A double-blind, randomized assessment of the irritant potential of sunscreen chemical dilutions used in photopatch testing. Contact Dermatitis 60:203–209

276. Agin PP, Ruble K, Hermansky SJ, McCarthy TJ (2008) Rates of allergic sensitization and irritation to oxybenzone-containing suscreen products: a quantitative meta-analysis of 64 exaggerated use studies. Photodermatol Photoimmunol Photomed 24:211–217

277. Lee E, An S, Choi D, Moon S, Chang I (2007) Comparison of objective and sensory skin irritations of several cosmetic preservatives. Contact Dermatitis 56:131–136

278. Issachar N, Gall Y, Borrel MT, Poelman MC (1998) Correlation between percutaneous penetration of methyl nicotinate and sensitive skin, using laser Doppler imaging. Contact Dermatitis 39:182–186

279. Coverly J, Peters L, Whittle E, Basketter DA (1998) Susceptibility to skin stinging, non-immunologic contact urticaria and acute skin irritation; is there a relationship? Contact Dermatitis 38:90–95

280. Basketter DA, Wilhelm KP (1996) Studies on non-immune contact reactions in an unselected population. Contact Dermatitis 35:237–240

281. Issachar N, Gall Y, Borell MT, Poelman MC (1997) pH measurements during lactic acid stinging test in normal and sensitive skin. Contact Dermatitis 36:152–155

282. Seidenari S, Francomano M, Mantovani L (1998) Baseline biophysical parameters in subjects with sensitive skin. Contact Dermatitis 38:311–315

283. Wu Y, Wang X, Zhou Y, Tan Y, Chen D, Chen Y, Ye M (2003) Correlation between stinging, TEWL and capacitance. Skin Res Technol 9:90–93

284. Lonne-Rahm S, Berg M, Mrin P, Nordlind K (2004) Atopic dermatitis, stinging, and effects of chronic stress: a pathocausal study. J Am Acad Dermatol 51:899–905

285. Laden K (1973) Studies on irritancy and stinging potential. J Soc Cosmet Chem 24:385–393

286. Villarama C, Maibach HI (2005) Sensitive skin and transepidermal water loss. In: Fluhr J, Elsner P, Berardesca E, Maibach HI (eds) Bioengineering and the skin. CRC Press, Boca Raton, pp 135–141

287. Pilz B, Löffler T, Frosch PJ (1994) Toxische Dermatitis durch Dimethylsulfoxid (DMSO) als Antidot gegen Epirubicin. Dermatosen 42:204–209

288. Bruze M, Emmett EA (1990) Occupational exposures to irritants. In: Jackson EM, Goldner R (eds) Irritant contact dermatitis. Dekker, New York, pp 81–106

289. Fregert S (1981) Manual of contact dermatitis, 2nd edn. Munksgaard, Copenhagen

290. Rycroft RJG (1998) The principal irritants and sensitizers. In: Rook A, Wilkinson DS, Ebling FJG, Champion RH, Burton JL, Burns DA, Breathnach SM (eds) Textbook of dermatology, 6th edn. Blackwell, Oxford, pp 821–860

291. Epstein WL (1990) House and garden plants. In: Jackson EM, Goldner R (eds) Irritant contact dermatitis. Dekker, New York, pp 127–165

292. Lachapelle JM, Mahmoud G, Vanherle R (1984) Anhydrite dermatitis in coal miners. Contact Dermatitis 11:188–189

293. Lensen G, Jungbauer F, Goncalo M, Coenraads PJ (2007) Airborne irritant contact dermatitis and conjunctivitis after occupational exposure to chlorothalonil in textiles. Contact Dermatitis 57:181–186

294. Ermertcan AT, Oztürkcan S, Sahin MT, Bilaç C, Bilaç DB (2007) Acute irritant contact dermatitis due to 'apium graveolens. Contact Dermatitis 57:122–123

295. Cronin E (1980) Contact dermatitis. Churchill Livingston, Edinburgh

296. Aramaki J, Effendy I, Happle R, Kawana S, Löffler C, Löffler H (2001) Which bioengineering assay is appropriate for irritant patch testing with sodium lauryl sulfate? Contact Dermatitis 45:286–290

Systemic Contact Dermatitis

17

Niels K. Veien and Torkil Menné

Contents

N.K. Veien (✉)
Dermatology Clinic, Vesterbro 99, 9000 Aalborg,
Denmark
e-mail: veien@dadlnet.dk

T. Menné
University of Copenhagen, Gentofte Hospital,
Niels Andersen Vej 65, 2900 Hellerup, Denmark

17.1 Introduction

Systemic contact dermatitis may occur in persons with contact sensitivity when these persons are exposed to the hapten orally, transcutaneously, intravenously, or by inhalation. The entity can present with clinically characteristic features or be clinically indistinguishable from other types of contact dermatitis. Contact sensitization to ubiquitous haptens is common. In a Danish population-based study, 15.2% reacted to one or more of the haptens in the European standard patch test series [1]. Many of these haptens can be presented to the immune system by a systemic route. The total number of individuals at risk of developing systemic contact dermatitis is therefore large.

The first description of systemic contact dermatitis can probably be ascribed to the pioneering British dermatologist, Thomas Bateman [2]. His description of the mercury dermatitis called eczema rubrum is similar to what we today describe as the "baboon syndrome": "Eczema rubrum is preceded by a sense of stiffness, burning, heat and itching in the part where it commences, most frequently the upper and inner surface of the thighs and about the scrotum in men, but sometimes it appears first in the groin, axillae or in the bends of the arms, on the wrists and hands or on the neck."

In this century, the systemic spread of nickel dermatitis to areas other than the sites of contact was described by Schittenhelm and Stockinger in Kiel in 1925 [3]. After patch testing nickel-sensitive workers with nickel sulfate, they observed dermatitis and flares in former areas of contact dermatitis even when there was no current contact with nickel items in these areas. The literature on systemic contact dermatitis is now comprehensive. Reviews include Cronin [4], Fisher [5], Menné et al. [6], Veien et al. [7], and Nijhawan et al. [8].

J.D. Johansen et al. (eds.), *Contact Dermatitis*,
DOI: 10.1007/978-3-642-03827-3_17, © Springer-Verlag Berlin Heidelberg 2011

17

17.2 Clinical Features

The clinical features of systemic contact dermatitis are summarized in Table 17.1.

A causal relationship between systemic administration of the hapten and these clinical manifestations is most easily documented in persons sensitized to medicaments. For such persons, the exposure to the hapten can be controlled. This is less feasible for persons sensitized to, for example, ubiquitous metals.

Flare-up reactions at former sites of dermatitis or previously positive patch test sites after systemic administration of the hapten raise a suspicion of systemic contact dermatitis [9–11]. A flare at a previously positive patch test site following ingestion of the

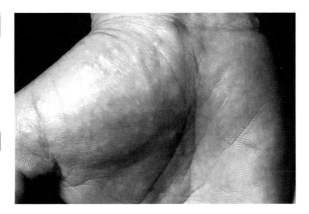

Fig. 17.1 Vesicular eruption in the thenar region after oral challenge with 4 mg nickel

hapten is a fascinating and specific sign of systemic contact dermatitis. Such reactions may be caused by medicaments and are also sometimes seen in experimental oral provocation studies. This symptom is hapten specific and can be seen years after the original patch testing [12, 13].

Vesicular hand eczema (Fig. 17.1) [14] is a pruritic eruption on the palms, volar aspects and sides of the fingers, around the nails, and occasionally on the plantar aspects of the feet with deep-seated vesicles and sparse or no erythema. If the periungual area is involved, transverse ridging of the fingernails can be a consequence. Vesicular hand eczema is a common disease, often with unknown etiology. It may have the appearance of chronic hand eczema if frequent vesicular eruptions occur, and the dermatitis does not clear completely between eruptions. Crops of vesicles may be seen at the periphery of an area of dermatitis. This type of hand eczema may be a symptom of systemic contact dermatitis.

A flare-up of dermatitis in the elbow and the knee flexures is a common symptom of systemic contact dermatitis. Such flares are difficult to distinguish from the early lesions of atopic dermatitis [15].

The "baboon syndrome" (Fig. 17.2) [16] is a characteristic, although rare, clinical manifestation of systemic contact dermatitis. It is a well-demarcated eruption on the buttocks, in the genital area, and in a V-shape on the inner thighs, of a color ranging from dark-violet to pink. It may occupy the whole area or only part of it. Nakayama et al. [17] described the same

Table 17.1 Clinical aspects of systemic contact dermatitis

Dermatitis in areas of previous exposure
Flare-up of previous dermatitis
Flare-up of previously positive patch test sites
Dermatitis on previously unaffected skin
Vesicular hand eczema
Flexural dermatitis
Baboon syndrome
Maculopapular rash (toxicoderma)
Vasculitis-like lesions
General symptoms
Headache
Malaise
Arthralgia
Diarrhea and vomiting
Fever

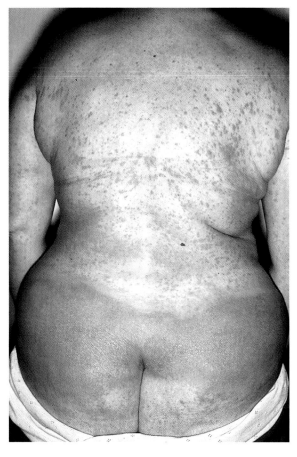

Fig. 17.2 Baboon syndrome in a balsam of Peru-sensitive patient after the use of suppositories that contained balsam of Peru

17.3 Mechanism

Based on human and animal experiments, it appears that both the humoral and the cellular immune systems are activated in systemic contact dermatitis. The histopathology of flare-up reactions is similar to that seen in ordinary contact dermatitis, while the accumulation of neutrophils in the baboon syndrome suggests that circulating immune complexes play a role [7].

Flares at sites of previous dermatitis or previously positive patch test sites are probably caused by specifically sensitized T-cells, either resting at the site or homing to the area after specific hapten exposure [13, 23, 24]. A reduction of CD_4+ cells, CD_4+ CD45Ro+, and CD_8+ cells was seen in the peripheral blood of nickel-sensitive women after oral challenge with nickel. The oral challenge induced maturation of naive T-cells into memory cells. Memory cells were seen particularly in the intestinal mucosa [25].

A reduction of the number of CLA+ $CD_{45}Ro+ CD_3+$ and CLA+ $CD_{45}Ro+ CD_8+$, but not CLA+ $CD_{45}Ro+$ CD_4+ cells was seen in the peripheral blood of nickel-sensitive patients after oral challenge with nickel [26].

CD_4+ T-cell clones reacted to cobalt but not to nickel in a patient following the removal of a cobalt-containing metal joint prosthesis [27].

Flexural eczema, vesicular hand eczema, the baboon syndrome, and toxicoderma may be caused by nonspecific cytokine release [28]. Möller et al. [20] recorded a significant increase of cytokines such as IL-ra, IFN-8, TNF-α, TNF-RI, IL-6, and acute phase reactants during systemic contact reactions to gold. In a patient with systemic contact dermatitis from prednisolone, elevated serum values of the interleukins 5, 6, and 10 were seen [29].

In a study of 42 patients with systemic contact dermatitis from *Toxicodendron*, it was suggested that a

clinical features as mercury exanthema. In mercury-sensitive patients, the baboon syndrome may also be seen in connection with acute generalized exanthematous pustulosis [18].

A nonspecific, maculopapular rash (toxicoderma) is often seen in systemic contact dermatitis. General symptoms such as headache and malaise are rarely seen in sensitized individuals following oral provocation with gold and medicaments. In patients sensitive to neomycin [9] and chromate [19], oral provocation with the hapten can cause nausea, vomiting, and diarrhea. A few patients have complained of arthralgia. Systemic administration of gold in gold-sensitized individuals has led to toxicoderma and slight fever [20, 21]. Malaise, leukocytosis, and pyrexia have also been seen in patients with systemic contact dermatitis from mercury [22].

17

toxic rather than a specific immune reaction might be responsible [30].

Antigen-specific tolerance to nickel has been demonstrated in guinea pigs [31]. Flares of dermatitis are frequently seen in clinical hyposensitization experiments when the hapten is given orally. Six of twenty parthenium-sensitive patients had to stop oral hyposensitization therapy due to aggravation of their dermatitis [32].

A parthenium-sensitive patient inhaled fresh plant material and experienced pruritus and a flare of dermatitis after 8–10 h [33].

Two patients with chrysanthemum dermatitis were successfully hyposensitized using chrysanthemum juice for 21 days. Aggravation of the dermatitis was seen initially in both patients. The patients remained clear of dermatitis for more than 2 years [34].

Mak et al. [35] speculated that the common use of chrysanthemum tea in Asia could induce tolerance and explain why contact allergy to composita plants is less common in Asia than in Europe.

In one corticosteroid contact-sensitized person, oral intake of corticosteroids was suspected to cause temporary anergy in the skin after the intake had caused a generalized eruption [36].

> **Core Message**
>
> › The mechanism of systemic contact dermatitis includes both specifically sensitized T-cells and nonspecific cytokine release. The latter could explain nonspecific symptoms such as flexural dermatitis and the baboon syndrome.

17.4 Medicaments

Most diagnosed cases of systemic contact dermatitis have occurred as a consequence of systemic exposure to medicaments in specifically contact-sensitized individuals. Such cases were common in the early era of the use of antibiotics, when drugs like streptomycin and penicillin were given both topically and systemically.

Medicaments known to cause systemic contact dermatitis are summarized in Chap. 35 and in [7]. Many case reports are available, and while the list illustrates the wide range of possibilities, it is not complete. Any

Table 17.2 Routes of sensitization to medicaments

Use as a topical medicament (particularly in leg ulcer patients)
Leaking of the medicament to the epidermis from various sites of intravenous injection
Occupational exposure
Eye drops
Suppositories
Intravesical installation
Injection of medicaments, middle ear, surgical wounds, and intraperitoneal injection
Cross-reactivity

drug is probably capable of causing systemic contact dermatitis if cutaneous sensitization precedes systemic exposure. In this context, the opposite sequence of events should be kept in mind, as it is not uncommon that a drug reaction can be diagnosed later by patch testing (Chap. 35).

Table 17.2 shows how contact sensitization to medicaments may result in systemic contact dermatitis. Contact sensitization is most commonly caused by the use of topical antibiotics in the treatment of leg ulcers, but the less common exposures outlined in Table 17.2 should be kept in mind. In a controlled study, Isaksson [37] showed that some budesonide-sensitive patients react to the inhalation of budesonide. Inhalation of budesonide caused angioedema in one contact-sensitized person [38, 39]. Occupational exposure to drugs is seen in the pharmaceutical industry, as well as among health care professionals such as nurses, who administer tablets or give injections. Among those with occupational contact with medicaments, veterinarians have a high frequency of contact allergy to medicaments. Systemic contact dermatitis can be caused by the cross-reactivity of certain medicaments. Corticosteroids can cause anaphylactoid-like reactions [40].

> **Core Message**
>
> › Drugs used both topically and systemically may cause systemic contact dermatitis either as a flare-up of dermatitis in previous areas of dermatitis or as a widespread rash.

17.5 Metals

17.5.1 Nickel

Shittenhelm and Stockinger [3] observed the spread of nickel dermatitis after cutaneous exposure to nickel. Many patients with severe suspender dermatitis in the 1950s and 1960s had widespread dermatitis, with vesicular hand eczema and flexural dermatitis similar to that seen in systemic contact dermatitis [41, 42]. Systemic exposure from the absorption of nickel in the area of the dermatitis was thought to explain the clinical picture. Recently, it has been documented that avoidance of prolonged skin contact with nickel-releasing alloys results in a statistically significant decrease in the frequency of hand eczema in nickel-sensitive individuals [43]. It has also been shown that following the adoption in Denmark of a regulation prohibiting the use of nickel in clothing or jewellery, a previously identified statistical association between nickel sensitivity and hand eczema no longer exists [44].

The study of orally provoked flare-ups of nickel dermatitis was pioneered by Christensen and Möller [10], followed up by Kaaber et al. [45, 46] and Veien et al. [47] In a double-blind study, Christensen and Möller [10] provoked 12 nickel-sensitive individuals with an oral dose of 5.6 mg nickel. Nine of the 12 patients reacted with systemic contact dermatitis after an average of 8 h. These patients had the symptoms listed in Table 17.1, in particular, vesicular hand eczema (Fig. 17.2). The results of this study have been repeated and confirmed by several authors [6, 13]. The evidence for immunological specificity includes flare-up reactions at previous nickel contact sites, for example, under metal spectacle frames (Fig. 17.3). Such a reaction was seen under previous sites of suspender nickel dermatitis in a woman who had not used garter belts containing nickel for over 30 years (Fig. 17.4). Vasculitis-like lesions may also be seen (Fig. 17.5).

The above-mentioned studies illustrate that few patients react to a dose of less than 0.5 mg nickel given as a single oral dose, while the majority of patients react to a dose of 5 mg or more. Dose response in nickel-sensitive patients has been demonstrated in two studies in which 0.3–4 mg and 1 or 3 mg nickel, respectively, was used for oral challenge [48, 49]. Systemic nickel dermatitis has been seen following accidental intravenous exposure to micrograms of nickel [50–52].

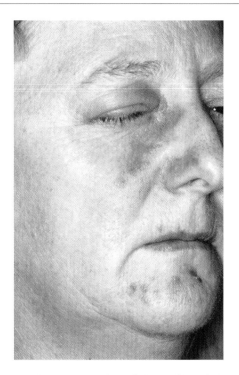

Fig. 17.3 Edematous eruption of the eyelid and dermatitis where spectacle frames touched the facial skin after oral challenge with 2.5 mg nickel

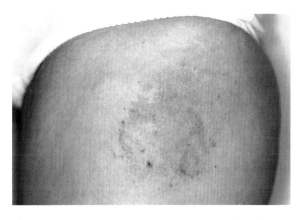

Fig. 17.4 A plaque of dermatitis on the upper thigh in a 64-year-old woman after oral challenge with 2.5 mg nickel. As a young girl she had suspender dermatitis on the thighs from nickel in garter belts. She had not worn a garter belt for 30 years

A neurostimulator with exposed stainless steel caused widespread dermatitis in a nickel-sensitive woman [53]. Nickel released from dental braces [54–56] and from older types of orthopedic prostheses can cause systemic nickel dermatitis and/or loosening of the prostheses [57, 58].

17

Fig. 17.5 Following a placebo-controlled challenge with 2.5 mg nickel, this nickel-sensitive patient developed discrete, very pruritic, vasculitis-like lesions on the forearms and thighs

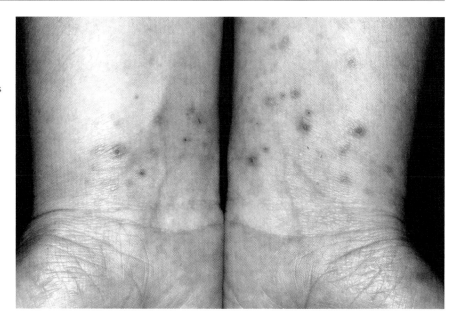

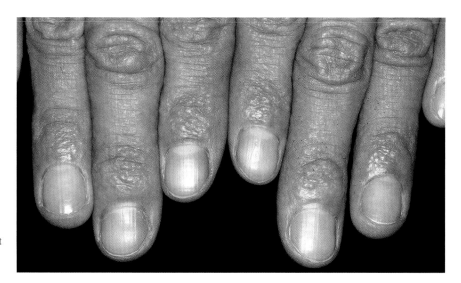

Fig. 17.6 Symmetrical vesicular dermatitis of the periungual area in a nickel-sensitive person a few days after beginning treatment for alcohol-dependence with disulfiram (Antabuse)

The daily ingestion of nickel from food varies from 150 to 500 µg and depends both on the type of food and the production environment for the individual foodstuff. Foods with high nickel content include whole-grain flour, oats, soybeans, legumes, shellfish, nuts, licorice, and chocolate [59]. Some complementary and alternative remedies may be a source of ingested nickel [60]. Nickel may be leached from cooking utensils [61]. The amount of nickel absorbed depends upon the concurrent intake of other foodstuffs such as proteins and alcohol. Chelating medicaments can interfere with nickel absorption and metabolism, and in that way, provoke systemic contact dermatitis. This has been well described for Antabuse (Fig. 17.6) [46].

Dietary intervention is indicated for nickel-sensitive patients with vesicular hand eczema or more widespread systemic contact dermatitis, if the elimination of nonoccupational as well as occupational nickel exposure does not improve or clear the dermatitis.

Dietary restriction following the guidelines by Veien et al. [62] should be followed for 1–2 months, and the outcome at that time should determine whether dietary restriction should be continued. Clinical studies suggest that approximately one-fourth of selected patients benefit from prolonged dietary treatment [63, 64]. Theoretically, 10% of the most nickel-sensitive persons could benefit from diet treatment [65]. A combination of diet treatment and short courses of disulfiram helped 10 of 11 nickel-sensitive patients compared with 1 of 10 in a control group [66].

> **Core Message**
>
> › A flare-up of dermatitis at a previously positive patch tests site or widespread eruptions may be seen after placebo-controlled oral challenge with nickel.

17.5.2 Chromium and Cobalt

Cobalt and chromium salts can provoke systemic contact dermatitis [6, 67]. Dose response studies with chromium suggest a range from 0.05 to 14.2 mg potassium dichromate given as a single oral dose is appropriate. Chromium picolinate given as a nutritional supplement caused systemic contact dermatitis in one person [68]. Only one study has been made of cobalt-sensitive individuals. Four of six cobalt-sensitive patients with vesicular hand eczema had a flare of the dermatitis after placebo-controlled oral challenge with 1 mg cobalt given as 4.75 mg cobalt chloride [69]. The removal of chromium and cobalt releasing dental braces or dietary restrictions may help individual patients. A diet low in cobalt has recently been presented [70].

17.5.3 Gold

Following the introduction of routine testing with gold sodium thiosulfate, a frequency of up to 10% positive reactions have been seen among consecutively patch-tested patients. Systemic contact dermatitis from gold in patients with rheumatoid arthritis treated with gold salts is probably common, as indicated by both clinical and experimental experience [71–74].

17.5.4 Mercury

Widespread eruptions, erythema-multiforme-like eruptions and the baboon syndrome, have been described in mercury-sensitive patients exposed to systemic mercury. Exposure can be from the vapors released from a broken thermometer, from homeopathic drugs, or the drilling of amalgam dental fillings [18, 22, 75–78].

> **Core Message**
>
> › Mercury-sensitive persons exposed to mercury vapors from a broken thermometer may develop baboon syndrome.

17.6 Other Contact Allergens

Most clinical and experimental studies of systemic contact dermatitis deal with either metals or medicaments, but important anecdotal evidence suggests that systemic contact dermatitis may be caused by certain plants, spices, and preservatives [79].

Kligman [80] attempted to hyposensitize persons with Rhus dermatitis by giving increasing oral doses of the allergen. Half of the moderately to severely sensitive patients developed either pruritus or a rash. Ten percent of the patients experienced flares of their dermatitis at sites of previously healed contact dermatitis. Flare-ups of vesicular hand eczema and erythema multiforme were rare. Perianal pruritus occurred in 10% of the highly sensitive individuals. Severe systemic contact dermatitis has been described in Rhus-sensitive patients who had eaten cashew nuts [81]. This reaction was explained by an allergen in cashew nut shells that cross-reacts with urishiols in poison ivy [82]. Raw cashew nuts in a pesto sauce caused systemic contact dermatitis [83].

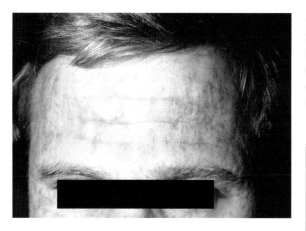

Fig. 17.7 Facial dermatitis in a baker sensitive to balsam of Peru after oral challenge with 1 g balsam of Peru

Systemic contact dermatitis has been seen in patients sensitive to *Myroxylon Pereirae* (balsam of Peru), which contains naturally occurring flavors. Hjorth [84] observed systemic contact dermatitis in balsam of Peru-sensitive patients who had eaten flavored ice cream and orange marmalade. Veien et al. [85] challenged 17 patients sensitive to balsam of Peru with an oral dose of 1 g of balsam of Peru. Ten patients reacted to balsam of Peru and one to a placebo (Fig. 17.7).

Eight of 102 patients sensitive to balsam of Peru reacted to coniferous benzoate and benzyl alcohol. All eight had systemic contact dermatitis. Three had hand eczema, and three had widespread dermatitis [86].

In other studies, reduction of the dietary intake of balsams has been shown to improve the dermatitis of more than half of selected patients who were sensitive to balsam of Peru [87–89].

> **Core Message**
>
> › Patients with contact sensitivity to balsam of Peru may develop systemic contact dermatitis from spices and other flavorings. Open studies indicate that diet treatment may be helpful.

Members of the Compositae family of plants commonly cause allergic contact dermatitis. Systemic contact dermatitis in this group of patients is easily overlooked [90]. Sesquiterpene lactones are found in food and herbal remedies containing laurel, chamomile, and goldenrod [91–94]. One of four patients with contact allergy to lettuce had a flare of vesicular hand dermatitis after oral challenge with lettuce, and one of ten reacted to feverfew [90].

> **Core Message**
>
> › Herbal remedies such as laurel, chamomile, and goldenrod contain sesquiterpene lactones and may cause systemic contact dermatitis in sensitized persons.

Garlic tablets caused a flare of vesicular hand eczema in a 58-year-old man with a positive patch test to garlic. A double-blind oral challenge was positive, and the dermatitis resolved when the garlic tablets were discontinued [95]. Periorbital and flexural dermatitis were seen in another garlic-sensitive person after the ingestion of garlic [96].

The antioxidant butylated hydroxyanisole (BHA), used both in cosmetics and foods, can cause systemic contact dermatitis [97] as can the preservatives sorbic acid [98–100] and propylene glycol [101].

Systemically aggravated contact dermatitis has been caused by aluminum in toothpaste in children sensitized to aluminum in vaccines [102].

17.7 Risk Assessment-Oriented Studies

While the risk of systemic contact dermatitis from drugs can be assessed, it is more difficult to carry out similar studies on ubiquitous contact allergens such as metals and naturally occurring flavors. In spite of intensive research on the significance of orally ingested nickel in nickel-sensitive individuals, we are unable to give firm advice concerning the oral dose that would represent a risk for the wide range of nickel-sensitive individuals. Many variables, such as the route of administration, bioavailability, individual sensitivity to nickel, interaction with naturally occurring amino acids, and interaction with medicaments, must be considered. A number of as yet unknown factors could influence nickel metabolism. Furthermore, immuno-logical reactivity to nickel can change with time [13] and can be influenced by sex hormones and the development of tolerance [103, 104]. It is important to recognize that this area of research is extremely complex and that much well-controlled research is still needed.

> **Core Message**
>
> › Systemic contact dermatitis in nickel-sensitive patients is complex. Reactions may vary with individual sensitivity to nickel, bioavailability, interaction with other food items, or medicaments. Reactions may also be influenced by sex hormones and the development of tolerance.

Well-controlled oral challenge studies can be carried out with medicaments in sensitized individuals. The beta-adrenergic blocking agent alprenolol is a potent contact sensitizer. Ekenvall and Forsbeck [105] identified 14 workers employed in the pharmaceutical industry who were contact sensitized to this compound. Oral challenge with a therapeutic dose (100 mg) led to a flare-up in one worker who developed pruritus and widespread dermatitis.

The preservative Merthiolate (thimerosal) is widely used in sera and vaccines. Förström et al. [106] investigated 45 Merthiolate contact-sensitive persons to evaluate the risk of a single therapeutic dose of 0.5 mL of a 0.01% Merthiolate solution given subcutaneously. Only one of the 45 patients developed a systemic contact dermatitis reaction. Aberer [107] did not observe any reactions in a similar study involving 12 patients.

Maibach [108] studied a group of patients who had discontinued the use of transdermal clonidine because of dermatitis. Of 52 patients with positive patch tests to clonidine, 29 were challenged orally with a therapeutic dose of the substance. Only one patient reacted with a flare-up at the site of the original dermatitis.

Propylene glycol is used as a vehicle in topical medications and cosmetics and as a food additive. Propylene glycol is both a sensitizer and an irritant. Hannuksela and Förström [109] challenged ten contact-sensitized individuals with 2–15 mL propylene glycol. Eight reacted with exanthema 3–16 h after the ingestion.

The overall impression of these studies is that systemic contact dermatitis in patients sensitized to a particular medicament is rare when the same patients are exposed to a therapeutic systemic dose of the medicament. Gold may constitute an exception to this general impression.

> **Core Message**
>
> › Although systemic contact dermatitis to medicaments given in therapeutic doses is probably rare in relation to the number of patients treated, there are many case reports of such reactions.

17.8 Diagnosis

Systemic contact dermatitis can occur in patients who are contact sensitized to a particular hapten if these patients are then systemically exposed to the same hapten or to break-down products such as formaldehyde, a break-down of aspartame [110].

The number of persons who will actually react to systemic exposure depends on the dose administered. In the case of nickel, whether or not a patient reacts to systemic exposure may also depend on the strength of the patch test reaction and the time that has elapsed since patch testing [49].

According to the available literature, particularly from experimental nickel challenge studies and challenge studies with medicaments, a relatively high dose of the hapten is needed to produce systemic contact dermatitis. The number of patients with systemic contact dermatitis seen in clinical practice is low compared to the number of patients with allergic and irritant contact dermatitis [111]. In spite of the fact that systemic contact dermatitis is relatively rare, it is important to identify this type of reaction to provide optimal management of the individual patient. The diagnosis rests on the history of the patient, patch testing and oral challenge, and elimination studies. Severe reactions are unusual. Anaphylactic reactions following the administration of corticosteroids have been described [40].

17

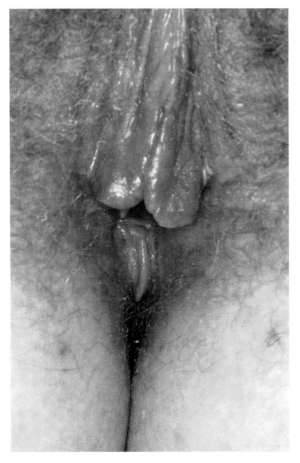

Fig. 17.8 Edematous anogenital dermatitis in a nickel-sensitive patient prior to initiation of a low-nickel diet

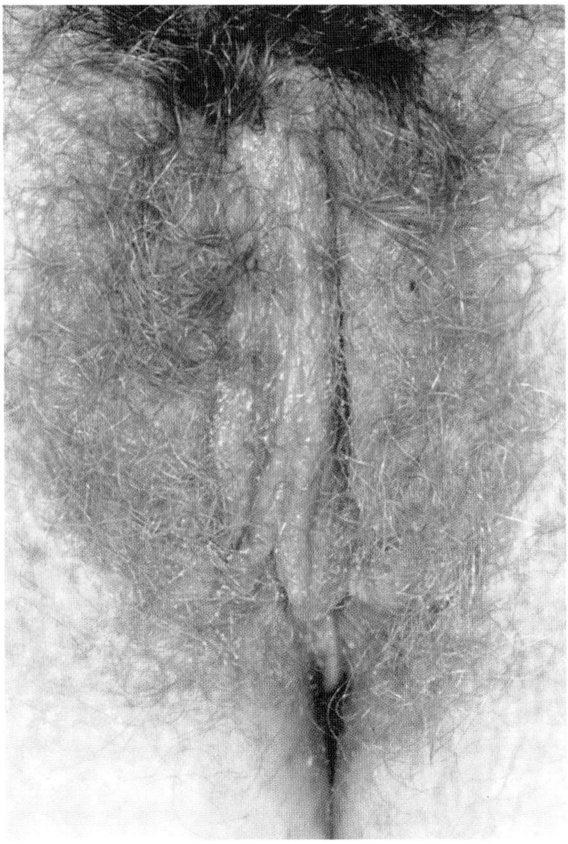

Fig. 17.9 The same patient as in Fig. 17.8 after 2 months on a low-nickel diet

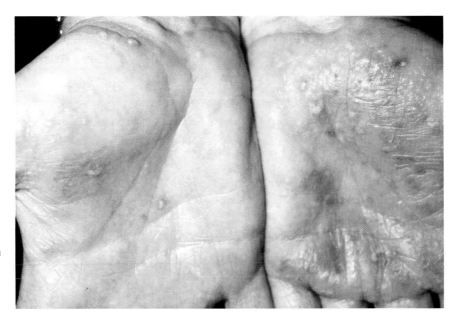

Fig. 17.10 An acute eruption of vesicular hand eczema after a weight-reducing diet that included food items with a high nickel content

Fig. 17.11 The same patient as in Fig. 17.10. The dermatitis faded after she was instructed to follow a low-nickel diet

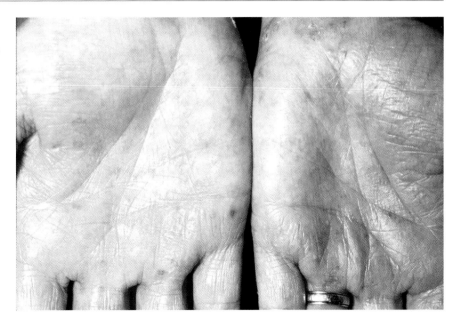

17.9 Case Reports

17.9.1 Case Report 1

A 37-year-old woman had severe anogenital dermatitis for 3 years (Fig. 17.8). She had previously been treated by her gynecologist who had found no explanation for the dermatitis.

The result of various topical treatments was unsatisfactory. Patch testing showed a ++reaction to nickel. She had no memory of rashes under cheap jewellery or other nickel items.

Placebo-controlled oral challenge with 2.5 mg nickel produced a severe flare of her anogenital dermatitis after 2 days. The flare lasted more than a week. She was instructed to follow a low-nickel diet, and after 2 months the dermatitis was quiescent (Fig. 17.9).

Two years later the woman was seen again. The current problem was very pruritic perianal dermatitis. She was again advised to reduce the nickel intake in food, and after 2 months, the dermatitis had practically cleared. She admitted that on both occasions she had eaten lots of chocolate, known to contain significant amounts of nickel.

17.9.2 Case Report 2

A 43-year-old woman was seen because of an acute eruption of vesicular hand eczema (Fig. 17.10). She was known to have nickel allergy, and the eruption had occurred after 1 week on a weight-reducing diet. Many of the food items included in this diet were high in nickel content. She was instructed in how to avoid food items with a high content of nickel, and the dermatitis faded (Fig. 17.11).

References

1. Nielsen NH, Linneberg A, Menné T, Madsen F, Frølund L, Dirksen A, Jørgensen T (2001) Allergic contact sensitization in an adult Danish population: two cross-sectional surveys eight years apart. Acta Derm Venereol (Stockh) 81:31–34
2. Shelley WB, Crissey JT (1970) Thomas bateman. In: Shelley WB, Crissey JT (eds) Classics in clinical dermatology. Thomas, Illinois, p 22
3. Schittenhelm A, Stockinger W (1925) Über die Idiosynkrasie gegen Nickel (Nickel-krätze) und ihre Beziehung zur Anaphylaxie. Z Ges Exp Med 45:58–74
4. Cronin E (1980) Reactions to the systemic absorption of contact allergens in: contact dermatitis. Churchill Livingstone, London, pp 26–29

5. Fisher AA (1986) Systemic contact-type dermatitis. In: Fisher AA (ed) Contact dermatitis. Lea and Febiger, Philadelphia, pp 119–131

6. Menné T, Veien NK, Sjølin K-E, Maibach HI (1994) Systemic contact dermatitis. Am J Contact Dermat 5:1–12

7. Veien NK, Menné T, Maibach HI (2008) Systemic contact dermatitis. In: Zhai H, Wilhelm K-P, Maibach HI (eds) Dermatotoxicology, 7th edn. CRC, Boca Raton, pp 139–153

8. Nijhawan RI, Molenda M, Zirwas MJ, Jacob SE (2009) Systemic contact dermatitis. Dermatol Clin 27:355–364

9. Ekelund A-G, Möller H (1969) Oral provocation in eczematous contact allergy to neomycin and hydroxyquinolines. Acta Derm Venereol 49:422–426

10. Christensen OB, Möller H (1975) External and internal exposure to the antigen in the hand eczema of nickel allergy. Contact Derm 1:136–141

11. Menné T, Weisman K (1984) Hämatogenes Kontakteksem nach oraler Gabe von Neomycin. Der Hautarzt 35:319–320

12. Christensen OB, Lindström C, Löfberg H, Möller H (1981) Micromorphology and specificity of orally induced flare-up reactions in nickel-sensitive patients. Acta Derm Venereol 61:505–510

13. Hindsén M (1998) Clinical and experimental studies in nickel allergy. Dissertation, Malmö

14. Veien NK (2009) Acute and recurrent vesicular hand dermatitis. Dermatol Clin 27:337–353

15. Wintzen M, Donker AS, van Zuuren EJ (2003) Recalcitrant atopic dermatitis due to allergy to Compositae. Contact Derm 48:87–88

16. Andersen KE, Hjorth N, Menné T (1984) The baboon syndrome: systemically induced allergic contact dermatitis. Contact Derm 10:97–101

17. Nakayama H, Niki F, Shono M, Hada S (1983) Mercury exanthem. Contact Derm 9:411–417

18. Lerch M, Bircher AJ (2004) Systemically induced allergic exanthem from mercury. Contact Derm 50:349–353

19. Kaaber K, Veien NK (1977) The significance of chromate ingestion in patients allergic to chromate. Acta Derm Venereol 57:321–323

20. Möller H, Ohlsson K, Linder C, Björkner B, Bruze M (1998) Cytokines and acute phase reactants during flare-up of contact allergy to gold. Am J Cont Derm 9:15–22

21. Möller H, Gjörkner B, Bruze M et al (1999) Laser Doppler perfusion imaging for the documentation of flare-up in contact allergy to cold. Contact Derm 41:131

22. Vena GA, Foti C, Grandolfo M, Angelini G (1994) Mercury exanthem. Contact Derm 31:214–216

23. Scheper RJ, von Blomberg B, GH BD, van Dinther A, Vos A (1983) Induction of local memory in the skin. Role of local T cell retention. Clin Exp Immunol 51:141–151

24. Yamashita N, Natsuaki M, Sagamis S (1989) Flare-up reactions on murine contact hypersensitivity. I. Description of an experimental model: rechallenge system. Immunology 67:365–369

25. Di Gioacchino M, Boscolo P, Cavallucci E, Verna N, Di Stefano F, Di Sciascio M, Masci S, Andreassi M, Sabbioni E, Angelucci D, Conti P (2000) Lymphocyte subset changes in blood and gastrointestinal mucosa after oral nickel challenge in nickel-sensitized women. Contact Derm 43:206–211

26. Jensen CS, Lisby S, Larsen JK, Veien NK, Menné T (2004) Characterization of lymphocyte subpopulations and cytokine

profiles in peripheral blood of nickel-sensitive individuals with systemic contact dermatitis after oral nickel exposure. Contact Derm 50:31–38

27. Thomssen H, Hoffmann B, Schank M, Hohler T, Thabe H, Meyer zum Buschenfelde KH, Marker-Hermann E (2001) Cobalt-specific T lymphocytes in synovial tissue after an allergic reaction to a cobalt alloy joint prosthesis. J Rheumatol 28:1121–1128

28. Möller H, Ohlsson K, Linder C, Björkner B, Bruze M (1999) The flare-up reactions after systemic provocation in contact allergy to nickel and gold. Contact Derm 40: 200–204

29. Yawalka N, Hari Y, Helbling A, von Gregerz S, Kappeler A, Braathen LR, Pichler WJ (1998) Elevated serum levels of interleukins 5, 6 and 10 in a patient with drug-induced exanthem caused by systemic corticosteroids. J Am Acad Dermatol 39:790–793

30. Oh S-H, Haw C-R, Lee M-H (2003) Clinical and immunologic features of systemic contact dermatitis from ingestion of Rhus (Toxicodendron). Contact Derm 48:251–254

31. Van Hoogstraten IMW, Boden D, von Blomberg ME, Kraal G, Scheper RJ (1992) Persistent immune tolerance to nickel and chromium by oral administration prior to cutaneous sensitization. J Invest Dermatol 99:607–611

32. Handa S, Sahoo B, Sharma VK (2001) Oral hyposensitization in patients with contact dermatitis from Parthenium hysterophorus. Contact Derm 44:279–282

33. Mahajan VK, Sharma NL, Sharma RC (2004) Parthenium dermatitis: is it a systemic contact dermatitis or an airborne contact dermatitis? Contact Derm 51:231–234

34. Mori Y, Son S, Murakami K et al (2000) Two cases of chrysanthemum dermatitis – successful oral tolerance induction using chrysanthemum juice. Environ Dermatol 7:223–229

35. Mak RKH, White IR, White JML, McFadden JP, Goon AJT (2007) Lower incidence of sesquiterpene lactone sensitivity in a population in Asia versus a population in Europe: an effect of chrysanthemum tea? Contact Derm 57:163–164

36. Thong H-Y, Yokota M, Chan H, Maibach HI (2008) Possible anergy after generalized orally elicited allergic contact dermatitis to corticosteroid. Contact Derm 58:126–128

37. Isaksson M (2000) Clinical and experimental studies in corticosteroid contact allergy (Dissertation). Department of Dermatology, University Hospital, Malmö, Sweden

38. Pirker C, Misic A, Frosch PJ (2003) Angioedema and dysphagia caused by contact allergy to inhaled budesonide. Contact Derm 49:77–79

39. Isaksson M (2007) Systemic contact allergy to corticosteroids revisited. Contact Derm 57:386–388

40. Vidal C, Tomé S, Fernándex-Redondo V, Tato F (1994) Systemic allergic reactions to corticosteroids. Contact Derm 31:273–274

41. Calnan CD (1956) Nickel dermatitis. Br J Dermatol 68: 229–236

42. Marcussen PV (1957) Spread of nickel dermatitis. Dermatologica 115:596–607

43. Kalimo K, Lammintausta K, Jalava J, Niskanen T (1997) Is it possible to improve the prognosis in nickel contact dermatitis? Contact Derm 37:121–124

44. Nielsen NN, Linneberg A, Menné T, Madsen F, Frolund L, Dirksen A, Jørgensen T (2002) The association between contact allergy and hand eczema in 2 cross-sectional surveys 8 years apart. Contact Derm 47:71–77

45. Kaaber K, Veien NK, Tjell JC (1978) Low nickel diet in the treatment of patients with chronic nickel dermatitis. Br J Dermatol 98:197–201
46. Kaaber K, Menné T, Tjell JC, Veien N (1979) Antabuse treatment of nickel dermatitis. Chelation – a new principle in the treatment of nickel dermatitis. Contact Derm 5:221–228
47. Veien NK, Hattel T, Justesen O, Nørholm A (1987) Oral challenge with nickel and cobalt in patients with positive patch tests to nickel and/or cobalt. Acta Derm Venereol 67: 321–325
48. Jensen CS, Menné T, Lisby S, Kristiansen J, Veien NK (2003) Experimental systemic contact dermatitis from nickel: a dose-response study. Contact Derm 49:124–132
49. Hindsen M, Bruze M, Christensen OB (2001) Flare-up reactions after oral challenge with nickel in relation to challenge dose and intensity and time of previous patch test reactions. J Am Acad Dermatol 44:616–623
50. Stoddard JC (1960) Nickel sensitivity as a cause of infusious reaction. Lancet 2:741–742
51. Smeenk G, Teunissen PC (1977) Allergische reacties op nikkel uit infusietoedieningssystemen. Ned Tijdschr Geneeskd 121:4–9
52. Olerud JE, Lee MY, Ulvelli DA, Goble GJ, Babb AL (1984) Presumptive nickel dermatitis from hemodialysis. Arch Dermatol 120:1066–1068
53. Nosbaum A, Rival-Tringali AL, Barth X, Damon H, Vital-Durand D, Claudy A, Faure M (2008) Nickel-induced systemic allergic dermatitis from a sacral neurostimulator. Contact Derm 59:319–320
54. Veien NK, Borchorst E, Hattel T, Laurberg G (1994) Stomatitis or systemically induced contact dermatitis from metal wire in orthodontic materials. Contact Derm 30:210–213
55. Kerosuo H, Kanerva L (1997) Systemic contact dermatitis caused by nickel in a stainless steel orthodontic appliance. Contact Derm 36:112–113
56. Mancuso G, Berdondini RM (2002) Eyelid dermatitis and conjunctivitis as sole manifestations of allergy to nickel in an orthodontic appliance. Contact Derm 46:245
57. Wilkinson JD (1989) Nickel allergy and orthopaedic prostheses. In: Maibach HI, Menné T (eds) Nickel and the skin. Immunology and toxicology. CRC, Boca Raton, pp 188–193
58. Antony FC, Dudley W, Field R, Holden CA (2003) Metal allergy resurfaces in failed hip endoprostheses. Contact Derm 48:49–50
59. Veien NK, Menné T (1990) Nickel contact allergy and a nickel-restricted diet. Semin Dermatol 9:197–205
60. De Medeiros LM, Fransway AF, Taylor JS, Wyman M, Janes J, Fowler JF Jr, Rietschel RL (2008) Complementary and alternative remedies: an additional source of potential systemic nickel exposure. Contact Derm 58:97–100
61. Berg T, Petersen A, Pedersen GA, Petersen J, Madsen C (2000) The release of nickel and other trace elements from electric kettles and coffee machines. Food Addit Contam 17:189–196
62. Veien NK, Hattel T, Laurberg G (1993) Low nickel diet: an open, prospective trial. J Am Acad Dermatol 29:1002–1007
63. Veien NK, Hattel T, Justesen O, Nørholm A (1985) Dietary treatment of nickel dermatitis. Acta Derm Venereol 65: 138–142
64. Antico A, Soana R (1999) Chronic allergic-like dermatopathies in nickel-sensitive patients. Results of dietary restrictions and challenge with nickel salts. Allergy Asthma Proc 20:235–242
65. Jensen CS, Menné T, Johansen JD (2006) Systemic contact dermatitis after oral exposure to nickel: a review with a modified meta-analysis. Contact Derm 54:79–86
66. Sharma AD (2006) Disulfiram and low nickel diet in the management of hand eczema: a clinical study. Indian J Dermatol Venereol Leprol 72:113–118
67. Veien NK, Hattel T, Laurberg G (1994) Chromate-allergic patients challenged orally with potassium dichromate. Contact Derm 31:137–139
68. Fowler JF Jr (2000) Systemic contact dermatitis caused by oral chromium picolinate. Cutis 65:116
69. Veien NK, Hattel T, Laurberg G (1995) Placebo-controlled oral challenge with cobalt in patients with positive patch test to cobalt. Contact Derm 33:54–55
70. Stuckert J, Nedorost S (2008) Low-cobalt diet for dyshidrotic eczema patients. Contact Derm 59:361–365
71. Wichs IP, Wong D, McCullagh RB, Fleming A (1988) Contact allergy to gold after systemic administration of gold for rheumatoid arthritis. Ann Reum Dis 47:421–422
72. Möller H, Björkner B, Bruze M (1996) Clinical reactions to provocation with gold sodium thiomalate in patients with contact allergy to gold. Br J Dermatol 135:423–427
73. Möller H, Larsson Å, Björkner B, Bruze M, Hagstam Å (1996) Flare up of contact allergy sites in a gold-treated rheumatic patient. Acta Derm Venereol 76:55–58
74. Möller H, Svensson Å, Björkner B, Bruze M, Lindroth Y, Marthorpe R, Theander J (1997) Contact allergy to gold and gold therapy in patients with rheumatoid arthritis. Acta Derm Venerol 77:370–373
75. Nakayama H, Shono M, Hada S (1984) Mercury exanthem. J Am Acad Dermatol 11:137–139
76. Audicana M, Bernedo N, Gonzalex I, Munoz D, Fernandez E, Gastaminza G (2001) An unusual case of baboon syndrome due to mercury present in a homeopathic medicine. Contact Derm 45:185
77. Adachi A, Horikawa T, Takashima T et al (2000) Mercury-induced nummular dermatitis. J Am Acad Dermatol 43: 383–385
78. Garcia-Menaya JM, Cordobés-Durán C, Bobadilla P, Lamilla A, Moreno I (2008) Baboon syndrome: 2 simultaneous cases in the same family. Contact Derm 58: 108–109
79. Veien NK (1997) The role of ingested food in systemic allergic contact dermatitis. Clin Dermatol 15:547–555
80. Kligman AM (1958) Hyposensitization against rhus dermatitis. Arch Dermatol 78:47–72, 93
81. Ratner JH, Spencer SK, Grainge JM (1974) Cashew nut dermatitis. Arch Dermatol 110:921–923
82. Kligman AM (1958) Cashew nut shell oil for hyposensitization against rhus dermatitis. Arch Dermatol 78:359–363
83. Hamilton TK, Zug KA (1998) Systemic contact dermatitis to raw cashew nuts in a pesto sauce. Am J Contact Dermat 9:51–54
84. Hjorth N (1965) Allergy to balsams. Spectrum Int 7:97–101
85. Veien NK, Hattel T, Justesen O, Nørholm N (1985) Oral challenge with balsam of Peru. Contact Derm 12: 104–107
86. Hausen BM (2001) Rauchen, Süssigkeiten, Perubalsam – ein Circulus vitiosus? Akt Dermatol 27:136–143

87. Veien NK, Hattel T, Laurberg G (1996) Can oral challenge with balsam of Peru predict possible benefit from a low-balsam diet? Am J Contact Dermat 7:84–87

88. Salam TN, Fowler JF Jr (2001) Balsam-related systemic contact dermatitis. J Am Acad Dermatol 45:377–381

89. Pfutzner W, Thomas P, Niedermeier A, Pfeiffer C, Sander C, Przybilla B (2003) Systemic contact dermatitis elicited by oral intake of balsam of Peru. Acta Derm Venereol 83:294–295

90. Oliwiecki S, Beck MH, Hausen BM (1991) Compositae dermatitis aggravated by eating lettuce. Contact Derm 24:318–319

91. Dooms-Goossens A, Bubelloy R, Degreef H (1990) Contact and systemic contact-type dermatitis to spices. Dermatol Clin 8:89–93

92. Rodríguez-Serna M, Sánchez-Motilla MM, Ramón R, Aliaga A (1998) allergic and systemic contact dermatitis from *Matricaria chamomilla* tea. Contact Derm 39:192–193

93. Schatzle M, Agathos M, Breit R (1998) Allergic contact dermatitis from goldenrod (*Herba solidaginis*) after systemic administration. Contact Derm 39:271–272

94. Rycroft RJG (2003) Recurrent facial dermatitis from chomomile tea. Contact Derm 48:229

95. Barden AD, Wilkinson SM, Bech MH, Chalmers RJG (1994) Garlic induced systemic contact dermatitis. Contact Derm 30:299–300

96. Pereira F, Hatia M, Cardoso J (2002) Systemic contact dermatitis from diallyl disulfide. Contact Derm 46:124

97. Roed-Petersen J, Hjorth N (1976) Contact dermatitis from antioxidants. Br J Dermatol 94:233–241

98. Gierdano-Labadil F, Pech-Ormieres C, Bazex J (1996) Systemic contact dermatitis from sorbic acid. Contact Derm 34:61–62

99. Raison-Peyron N, Meynadier JM, Meynadier J (2000) Sorbic acid: an unusual cause of systemic contact dermatitis in an infant. Contact Derm 43:247–248

100. Dejobert Y, Delaporte E, Piette F, Thomas P (2001) Vesicular eczema and systemic contact dermatitis from sorbic acid. Contact Derm 45:291

101. Lowther A, McCormick T, Nedorost S (2008) Systemic contact dermatitis from propylene glycol. Dermatitis 19: 105–108

102. Veien NK, Hattel T, Laurberg G (1993) Systemically aggravated contact dermatitis caused by aluminium in tooth paste. Contact Derm 28:199–200

103. Bonamonte D, Foti C, Antelmi AR, Biscozzi AM, Naro ED, Fanelli M, Loverro G, Angelini G (2005) Nickel contact allergy and menstrual cycle. Contact Derm 52: 309–313

104. White JML, Goon ATJ, Jowsey IR, Basketter DA, Mak RKH, Kimber I, McFadden JP (2007) Oral tolerance to contact allergens: a common occurrence? A review. Contact Derm 56:247–254

105. Ekenvall L, Forsbeck M (1978) Contact eczema produced by a beta-adrenergic blocking agent (alprenolol). Contact Derm 4:190–194

106. Förström L, Hannuksela M, Kousa M, Lehmuskallio E (1980) Merthiolate hypersensitivity and vaccines. Contact Derm 6:241–245

107. Aberer W (1991) Vaccinations despite thiomersal sensitivity. Contact Derm 24:6–10

108. Maibach HI (1987) Oral substitution in patients sensitized by transdermal clonidine treatment. Contact Derm 16:1–9

109. Hannuksela M, Förström L (1978) Reactions to peroral propylene glycol. Contact Derm 4:41–45

110. Hill AM, Belsito DV (2003) Systemic contact dermatitis of the eyelids caused by formaldehyde derived from aspartame? Contact Derm 49:258–259

111. Veien NK, Hattel T, Justensen O, Nørholm A (1987) Diagnostic procedures for eczema patients. Contact Derm 17:35–40

Phototoxic and Photoallergic Reactions

18

Margarida Gonçalo

Contents

M. Gonçalo
Clinic of Dermatology, Coimbra University Hospital,
University of Coimbra, Praceta Mota Pinto,
3000-175 Coimbra, Portugal
e-mail: mmgoncalo@netcabo.pt

18.1 Introduction

Phototoxicity and photoallergy are different expressions of an abnormal skin reaction from the exposure to light, usually enhanced by endogenous or exogenous substances that are selectively activated by solar radiation.

It can occur with artificial light sources (sun lumps used for aesthetic or therapeutic purposes or ultraviolet (UV) sources in occupational settings), but mostly occurs on sun exposure. From the solar spectrum that reaches the earth, UV radiation, and particularly UVA (320–400 nm), is responsible for most cases of photosensitivity. Even though some chromophores absorb in the UVB (290–320 nm) and UVB is more energetic, UVA penetrates the skin more deeply and, particularly for systemic chromophores, this is certainly the most important spectrum for inducing photodermatosis [1]. Only exceptional reports have a well-documented exogenous photosensitivity exclusively from UVB [2].

Photosensitivity from topical agents, once frequent and often associated with persistent reactions to light, is now becoming rare [3, 4], as the main topical photosensitizers are removed from the market, or maybe photosensitivity is underreported or underdiagnosed [5]. On the other hand, and even though sun avoidance is recommended in those exposed to known photosensitizers, new drugs are reported to have photosensitizing properties, eventually associated with late problems.

Therefore, photosensitivity is still a problem and a field on intense research. New photosensitizers are reported as a cause of skin disease, whereas others are used for phototherapy. Studies are still being undertaken on the mechanisms and chromophores responsible for diseases associated with photosensitivity, such as HIV infection [6, 7].

J.D. Johansen et al. (eds.), *Contact Dermatitis*,
DOI: 10.1007/978-3-642-03827-3_18, © Springer-Verlag Berlin Heidelberg 2011

18

18.2 General Mechanisms of Photosensitivity

Normal skin has several molecules that are activated upon sun exposure and undergo chemical reactions – the chromophores – which are important for our survival under the sun and necessary for our life. An example is 7-dehydrocholesterol which, upon activation by UVB, forms provitamin D3 necessary for Vitamin D synthesis.

Photosensitivity develops when an abnormal chromophore, or a normal chromophore in exaggerated amounts, is present in the skin. When excited by a photon, these molecules suffer changes within the molecule itself, often also within neighboring molecules, in a cascade of events that result in skin damage and inflammation. This can occur through the direct molecular modification (isomerization, breaking of double bounds, oxidation) or production of free radicals, dependent or not on oxygen, which modify unsaturated lipids of cell membranes, aromatic amino acids of proteins, or DNA or RNA bases of nucleic acids. If the repair mechanisms do not act immediately, there is damage and/or death of skin cells and inflammatory mediators are produced (prostaglandins, IL-1, 6, 8, other cytokines, and chemokines) with consequent skin lesions – this is briefly the mechanism of phototoxicity [1]. In some circumstances, the energy of the photon can be used by the chromophore to transform itself into a new molecule (photoproduct) or to bind an endogenous peptide and, therefore, form a hapten or an allergen that can be recognized by the skin immune system. In these cases, photoallergy may develop with a sensitization phase and effector phase similar to allergic contact dermatitis (see Chap. 8 for more details).

Apart from the capacity to generate free radicals responsible for phototoxicity, several phototoxic substances, such as psoralens, chlorpromazine, and fluorquinolones, have shown to induce chromosomal damage in the presence of UVR. Both in vitro and animal studies have shown they are photomutagenic and photoimmunosuppressive, with consequent implications in photocarcinogenesis [8–12]. Epidemiological studies and recent reports are showing this may also be significant for humans. In 1999, the group of Przybilla showed an association between actinic keratosis and the use of potentially photosensitizing chemicals [13]. More recent data tend to confirm an increased risk in patients on long-term PUVA treatments [14] and, also

in those exposed to fluorquinolones, diuretics [15], and voriconazole [16].

The chromophore responsible for the photosensitive reaction can be an endogenous molecule, like a porphyrin that accumulates in the skin due to an inborn metabolic error, or it can be an exogenous molecule that is applied on the skin or reaches the skin through the systemic circulation. In many diseases, the chromophore has been identified, but there are many idiopathic photodermatoses for which the main chromophore is still unknown. Some resemble exogenous photoallergic reactions, like "Lucite Estivale Bénigne," polymorphic light eruption, or chronic actinic dermatitis, whereas others have very typical clinical patterns, like hydroa vacciniforme or actinic prurigo. Also, as sunscreens are widely used to prevent skin lesions in these photodermatoses, these patients frequently develop allergic or photoallergic contact dermatitis to UV filters [3, 4], thereby associating the effect of endogenous and exogenous chromophores.

In some patients, photosensitivity develops because of a deficiency in the capacity to repair UV aggression, due to a genetic problem (xeroderma pigmentosum, Bloom's syndrome) or a transient imbalance of antioxidant skin defense (in pellagra due to reduced levels of niacin in diet or alcohol consumption), or because the natural mechanisms of skin protection are deficient (vitiligo, albinism) [1, 17].

Core Message

> UV activation of an endogenous or an exogenous skin chromophore can induce an inflammatory reaction (phototoxicity) or a T-cell-mediated reaction (photoallergy).

18.2.1 Phototoxicity vs. Photoallergy

In theory, it is easy to differentiate photoallergy, a T-cell-mediated hypersensitivity reaction to an allergen formed upon UV exposure, from phototoxicity, that represents an exaggerated inflammatory response to the sun enhanced by an exogenous chromophore. Classically, photoallergy develops only in a limited number in individuals, needs previous sensitization but is extensive to cross-reactive chemicals, is subject to flare-ups, is not dependent on the dose of the exogenous chromophore and needs low UV exposure, appears as eczema that can spread to nonexposed sites, and on skin biopsy, there is mainly spongiosis as in eczema. Phototoxicity is more frequent and considered to develop in every individual, as long as enough photosensitizer and sun exposure are present; it occurs even on a first and single contact, with no flare-ups or cross-reactions; and appears mainly as well-demarcated erythema exclusively on sun-exposed areas (mimicking sunburn); and on histology, apoptotic keratinocytes (sunburn cells) are abundant (Table 18.1).

But, even though there are typical aspects of these two polar types of photosensitivity, some molecules may induce both phototoxic and photoallergic dermatitis. Although rare, this can occur with plant furocoumarins (*Ruta graveolans, Ficus carica, Umbeliferae*) or during photochemotherapy, as individuals become reactive to very low concentrations of psoralens [18]. Also, for mainly phototoxic drugs like promethazine and lomefloxacin, a few patients develop photoallergy, reacting to very low doses of the drug or sun exposure [19–21]. Most probably, as occurs with contact allergens that have an inherent "irritant" potential to awaken the innate immune system necessary to promote the sensitization process [22], photoallergens are photoactive molecules with some inherent phototoxicity, which may be the "danger signal" necessary to initiate the sensitizing process.

Although it is considered that photoallergy does not occur on a first contact due to the need for previous sensitization, this may not be necessary if you have already been sensitized by contact to a similar molecule. This occurs in patients who are allergic to thiomersal, namely to its moiety thiosalicylic acid, who develop photosensitivity to piroxicam on the first intake of the drug. Upon UVA irradiation, piroxicam is photodecomposed into a molecule very similar antigenically and structurally to thiosalicylic acid, responsible for piroxicam photoallergy [23–25].

Phototoxicity is considered to occur in every patient as long as enough chromophore and sun are present at the same time, but there is also individual susceptibility to phototoxicity from drugs and phytophotodermatitis, even though the parameters that characterize this susceptibility are not precisely known.

Therefore, and although, in theory, we can separate these two mechanisms – phototoxicity and photoallergy, there is often an overlap between both.

18.3 Clinical Patterns of Photosensitivity

The clinical patterns of photosensitive disorders are sometimes very typical, like phytophotodermatitis, acute exaggerated sunburn from exposure to a phototoxic

Table 18.1 Distinction between phototoxicity and photoallergy

	Phototoxicity	Photoallergy
Frequency	High	Low
Latency period/sensitization	No	Yes
Doses of UV/photosensitizer	High	Low
Cross-reactions	No	Yes
Morphology of lesions	Sunburn, polymorphic	Eczema, erythema multiforme
Sharp limits	Yes	No
Covered areas	Not involved	Possibly involved
Resolution	Quick	May recur, persistent reactors
Residual hyperpigmentation	Yes	No
Histology	Sunburn cells	Eczema
Pathomechanism	DNA/cell damage ROS/inflammation	Type IV hypersensitivity Photoproduct

ROS reactive oxygen species

drug, and, among some idiopathic photodermatoses, hydroa vacciniforme and xeroderma pigmentosum. But, sometimes, the diagnosis or even the suspicion of photosensitivity is not so obvious. It is the example of acute or chronic eczematous skin lesions, extending to covered areas, with a less well-established relation with sun exposure (often a regular exposure), like in chronic actinic dermatitis or in photoaggravation of rosacea or lupus erythematosus by sunscreens.

The clinical manifestations of photosensitivity are very polymorphic (Table 18.2), extending from urticaria through eczema or subacute lupus erythematosus up to vitiligo-like lesion or squamous cell carcinomas [14, 16, 19].

In some cases, exposure to sun induces immediate reactions, like in solar urticaria, but the appearance of skin lesions may be delayed 1 or 2 days, as in photoallergic contact dermatitis or systemic photoallergy, several days or weeks, as in pseudoporphyria or subacute lupus erythematosus, or even years, as in photocarcinogenesis enhanced by a long exposure to the sun and photoactive drugs.

Localization of the lesions in photosensitivity from a topical agent draws the area of application and concomitant sun exposure. But localization and distribution of lesions may be more peculiar extending to areas of accidental contact, as in a contra-lateral limb (kissing faces of the legs) or areas of inadvertent spread by the hands or other contaminated objects [26]. Also, as some topical drugs are absorbed through the skin (NSAIDs), the distribution of the lesions can be similar to systemic photosensitivity. This is usually very typical, as the reaction frequently involves, in a symmetric distribution, all exposed areas of the face, the V-shaped area of the neck, and upper chest, dorsum of the hands and forearms. Shaded areas are spared, namely the upper eyelids, upper lip, deep wrinkles (Fig. 18.1), retroauricular areas, submandibular area (Fig. 18.2), and areas covered by the beard or hair, and the large body folds, like axillae, groins, finger webs, and to all the areas covered by clothing or other accessories (watch strip, shoes). This allows a distinction from airborne dermatitis where the allergen in the environment can localize in these shaded areas and induce skin lesions, without the need for sun exposure.

In exceptional cases where sun exposure is asymmetric, this pattern can be different, as in car drivers who only expose the left arm. Sometimes, in systemic photosensitivity, the lower lip is mainly or almost exclusively involved, because of its higher exposure and, most probably, because of the lower thickness of the corneal layer, which is one of the main defenses against solar radiation [27–29].

Table 18.2 Clinical patterns of photosensitivity

Predominant in phototoxicity	Predominant in photoallergy
Exaggerated "sunburn"	Urticaria of sun exposed area
Pseudoporphyria	Acute or subacute eczema
Photoonycholysis	Cheilitis
Hyperpigmentation	Erythema multiform-like
Hypopigmentation (vitiligo-like lesions)	Lichenoid reactions
Pellagra like-reactions Telangiectasia Purpura	Subacute or chronic lupus erythematosus
Actinic keratosis and squamous cell carcinoma	

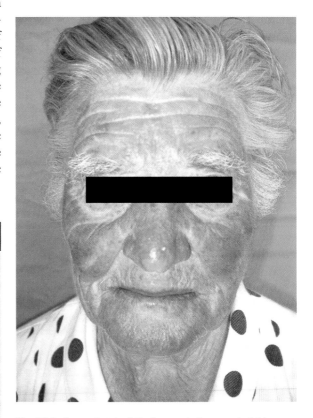

Fig. 18.1 Acute phototoxicity from amiodarone, mimicking sunburn and sparing the deep wrinkles

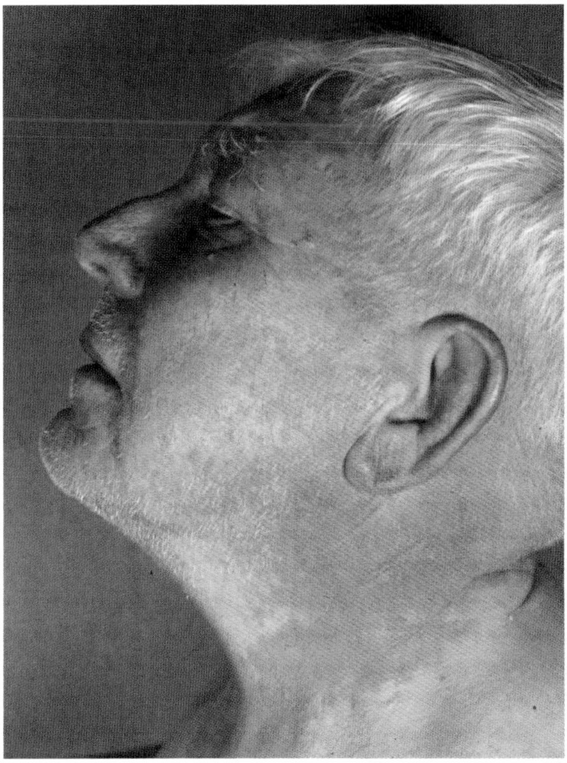

Fig. 18.2 Acute eczema from systemic piroxicam, sparing the submandibular shaded area

---

Core Message

> Phototoxic reactions present mainly as an exaggerated sunburn, but may be very polymorphic and difficult to distinguish from photoallergy.

18.3.1 Acute Manifestations of Photosensitivity

18.3.1.1 Immediate Reactions

Apart from idiopathic solar urticaria, for which a chromophore is not identified, urticaria as a manifestation of photosensitivity from an exogenous substance has been rarely described with 5-aminolevulinic acid, used in photodynamic therapy [30], with oxybenzone [31, 32] and chlorpromazine [33]. Nevertheless for some drugs, like amiodarone and benoxaprofen (already removed from the market), immediate prickling and burning with transient erythema may occur as a manifestation of photosensitivity [14].

18.3.1.2 Acute Phototoxicity, Mimicking Sunburn

The main acute clinical manifestation of phototoxicity is a well-demarcated acute erythema or edema with prickling and burning, eventually progressing to bullae with skin pain, which develops within 12–24 h of sun exposure. This gives rise to large sheets of epidermal detachment within the next days and can resolve with residual hyperpigmentation. This is similar to exaggerated sunburn (Fig. 18.1), and eventually, can also be associated with systemic symptoms like fever.

18.3.1.3 Acute Photoallergic Eczema

Photoallergy occurs usually as a pruritic eczematous reaction of the sun exposed areas, with irregular limits, often extending to covered areas. It develops more than 24–48 h after sun exposure, and not on a first contact. This resolves, like in acute eczema, with desquamation and no hyperpigmentation. Distribution of lesions is usually symmetric in systemic photosensitivity and shaded areas are also protected but not as sharply as in phototoxicity (Fig. 18.2).

In the more intense photoallergic reactions, typical or atypical target lesions, characteristic of erythema multiforme and with histopathology of erythema multiforme, can occur in association with the eczematous plaques, mainly at its limits or at distant sites, as was described for ketoprofen [34, 35]

In some cases, a systemic photosensitizer can induce a photodistributed erythema multiforme or toxic epidermal necrolysis, as described with paclitaxel [36], naproxen [37] and clobazam [38].

18.3.2 Subacute Manifestations of Photosensitivity

Other less frequent clinical patterns develop with a delay of days/weeks after exposure to the photosensitizer and the sun, or rarely acutely. These patterns that

18

evoke mainly a phototoxic reaction are pseudoporphyria, photoonycholysis, hyper or hypopigmentation, telangiectasia, and purpura.

18.3.2.1 Pseudoporphyria

Pseudoporphyria with chronic skin fragility and flaccid bullae on noninflamed sun-exposed skin, occasionally with later milia formation, mimicking porphyria cutanea tarda on clinical and histopathology (bullae formation below the lamina densa), was described initially for nalidixic acid, furosemide, and naproxen, predominantly in children [14, 39] and, more recently, for ciprofloxacin [40], celecoxib [41, 42], voriconazole [28, 43], and imatinib [44]. This may represent a typical phototoxic reaction where the drug, as the chromophore, has a similar mechanism of inducing the phototoxic reaction (singlet oxygen) as the uroporphyrin in the hereditary disease [14, 39].

18.3.2.2 Photoonycholysis

Photoonycholysis, with a half moon distal onycholysis of one or several nails, is a typical pattern of phototoxicity and often the single manifestation of this reaction. It appears late (2–3 weeks after drug intake and sun exposure), may be preceded by pain in the nail apparatus, and occurs mainly with tetracyclines (demethylchlortetracyclie or doxycycline) [45], psoralens, and fluorquinolones [46]. There is no definite explanation for the single involvement of the nail: the nail bed is relatively unprotected from sunlight, contains less melanin, the nail plate may work as a lens, and the inflammatory reaction induces detachment of the nail plate from the nail bed [45–47].

18.3.2.3 Dyschromia

Hyperpigmentation that follows mainly an acute phototoxic reaction is frequently due to the residual melanocytic hyperpigmentation, and is very typical in phytophotodermatitis, or after lichenoid reactions, e.g., from phenothiazines (Fig. 18.3).

In rare occasions, like those induced by flutamide, vitiliginous lesions with sharp limits occur after the acute photosensitive reaction [48, 49].

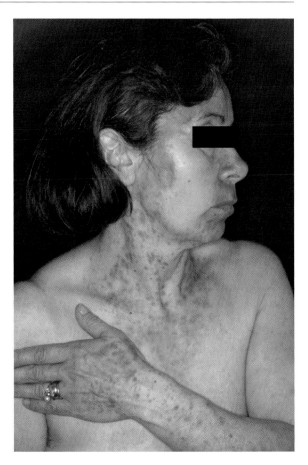

Fig. 18.3 Lichenoid lesions and pigmentation in the photoexposed areas in a patient taking thioridazine for several months

Hyperpigmentation, or more precisely dyschromia, may occur from the accumulation of the drug or drug metabolites in the dermis, namely from amiodarone, minocycline, and phenothiazines [50, 51]. Apart from acute photosensitivity reaction that occurs more frequently, a smaller percentage of patients on amiodarone, mainly those with lower phototypes, develop a golden-brown, slate gray, or bluish color on sun-exposed areas. This discoloration develops later and persists much longer than residual melanocytic hyperpigmentation [14, 50] (Fig. 18.4).

18.3.2.4 Other Clinical Patterns

Telangiectasia as a manifestation of photosensitivity has been reported with calcium channel blockers [52] and the telangiectatic pattern of photoaging with lesions mainly in the lateral folds of the neck, sparing the shaded

Fig. 18.4 Chronic phototoxicity in a patient on a long-term treatment with minocycline. Note the lichenification, with ectropion and the brownish pigmentation (**a**) and onycholysis in all his fingers (**b**). Photoonycholysis can occur as an isolated manifestation of photosensitivity

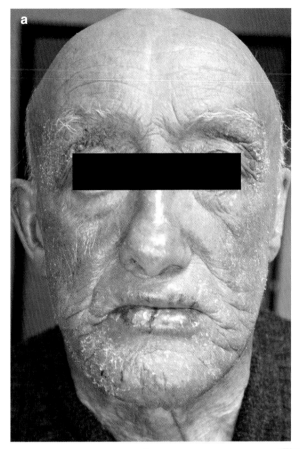

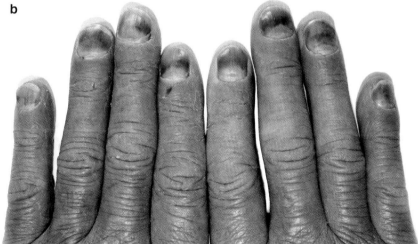

skin under the chin, is frequently observed in patients chronically exposed to photoactive drugs. In rare cases, petechial purpura with sharp limits on shaded areas was described with ciprofloxacin [53].

Pellagra is associated with the prolonged use of isoniazid, which consumes niacin for its metabolization, and pellagroid reactions were reported with anticancer agents such as 6-mercaptopurin and 5-fluoruracil.

18.3.3 Delayed and Late Effects of Photosensitivity

18.3.3.1 Lupus Erythematosus

Cases of lupus erythematosus, both subacute and chronic, have been attributed to the exposure to exogenous drugs/allergens and the sun. Most patients have anti-Ro auto-antibodies, the hallmark of photosensitivity in lupus erythematosus. Lesions develop weeks or months after exposure on the exposed areas of face, neck, upper chest, and arms, as erythematosus and scaling annular lesions typical of subacute lupus erythematosus or, more rarely, chronic lesions on the face or V of the neck [14]. This was described initially for thiazide diuretics, calcium channel blockers, ACE inhibitors [54], terbinafine [55], and recently from the anticancer taxanes, paclitaxel, and docetaxel [36, 56]. The drugs may enhance UV-induced expression of the Ro antigen on the surface of keratinocytes, interfere with apoptosis or cytokine production, thereby promoting photosensitivity and the development of skin lesions in susceptible individuals [54].

18.3.3.2 Chronic Actinic Dermatitis

Chronic actinic dermatitis, more common in older men, can present as a photosensitive eczema or, more frequently, like a long-lasting chronic eczema with a brown–gray hyperpigmentation, skin edema, lichenification that resemble its lymphomatoid variant, the actinic reticuloid (Fig. 18.4). Also, on histology, large activated lymphocytes in the dermis mimic lymphoma. Lesions are localized on photoexposed areas (face, sides and back of the neck, upper chest, and dorsum of the hands and forearms) and are aggravated by sun exposure; even this may not be very apparent because of the small amounts of UV necessary to aggravate the lesions. The hallmark of this disease is the extreme photosensitivity to UVB (reduced MED) and, often, also UVA and visible light [7, 57].

In many cases, these patients have previously suffered from an idiopathic photodermatosis, a chronic photodermatitis or, more frequently, from an airborne allergic contact dermatitis from perfumes, sesquiterpene lactones from Compositae, or colophony from conifers, and in its evolution, they become extremely photosensitive even with no further exposure to an exogenous chromophore or allergen. An autoantigen (DNA or RNA modified by plant products or another autoantigen) may have been formed during the acute reaction or, may be the regular UV-induced immunosuppression did not work correctly and individuals were sensitized to this new autoantigen and developed a reaction similar to allergic contact dermatitis [17, 57].

18.3.3.3 Enhancement of Photocarcinogenesis

Recent reports are documenting the relation between exposure from photoactive molecules and increasing incidence of actinic keratosis or squamous cell carcinoma, in a parallel of what was observed with long time therapeutic exposure to PUVA. Apart from psoralens, naproxen, chlorpromazine, and the fluorquinolones, particularly lomefloxacin, also have the capacity to induce DNA aggression upon UV exposure, in vitro, and to increase epidermal neoplasia in animals [8, 9]. This concern may have to be taken into account, namely as severe photosensitivity associated with skin cancer has been observed with voriconazole [16] and ciprofloxacin (personal experience) and epidemiological studies seem to correlate exposure to photoactive drugs and an increase in the risk of developing actinic keratoses, nonmelanoma skin cancer and, even, malignant melanoma [13, 15]. Also, photoaging may be enhanced by the exposure to topical or systemic photosensitizers.

> **Core Message**
>
> > On a long term, skin exposure to photoactive substances may enhance photocarcinogenesis.

18.4 Main Topical and Systemic Photosensitizers

There is a large and increasing list of photoactive molecules to which we can be exposed to in our daily life and which can induce photosensitivity. But there has been increasing concern on the evaluation of the phototoxic potential, particularly of cosmetics and consumer products, and very important photosensitizers have been eliminated or highly reduced in our ambience. These "historical" photosensitizers are musk ambrette and natural bergamot oil, removed by the perfume industry; the sunscreen isopropyldibenzoylmethane, withdrawn in 1994; the antibiotic olaquindox, a swine feed additive banned in 1998 by the European Commission [58]; and the halogenated salicylanilides removed from disinfectants and hygiene products in most countries since 1976. Nevertheless, even though some products are not available in Europe, they can be "imported" from other countries and induce photosensitivity [58, 59].

In most reports, the main topical photosensitizers are the UV filters [3, 60, 61], which represent 56–80% of the cases diagnosed by photopatch testing [3, 62–64]. Furocoumarins from plants are an important source of photosensitivity, mainly in more sunny countries. Drugs are, by far, the most frequent photosensitizers in Southern Europe [62, 64–66].

18.4.1 UV Filters

Due to the increased awareness of the sun damaging effects, sunscreens are used in large amounts and UV filters are also present in cosmetics, like moisturizing and facial creams, lipstick, nail varnish, shampoos, and other hair products. Apart from protecting the skin and hair from solar aggression, they are intended to prevent the degradation of the product by the sun and, therefore, increase its shelf half life. But, happily, concurrent with this high use, adverse skin reactions from UV filters are not reported so frequently [3]. In recent studies, positive photopatch tests or photoaggravated reactions to UV filters occurred in 5.7–12% of a total of about 2,400 patients tested [4, 62, 64–67].

The newer UV filters – Mexoryl SX (terephtalydene dicamphor sulfonic acid), Tinosorb M (methylene-*bis*-benzotriazolyl tetramethylbutylphenol or bisoctrizole), and Tinosorb S (bis-ethylhexyloxyphenol methoxyphenyl triazine) – are photostable molecules and, in mixtures of several sunscreens, are able to stabilize older photo labile UV filters, like butyl methoxydibenzoylmethane and cinnamates. Therefore, they seem to be more efficient in protecting the skin from the harmful effects of UVR [68] and eventually in reducing photoallergic dermatitis, even from the other UV filters. Apparently, a single case of photoallergy was reported from Mexoryl SX [60] with no cases of photoallergy from Tinosorb M or S. There are only very rare cases of allergic contact dermatitis from the surfactant decylglucoside that is used to solubilize the active molecule of Tinosorb M [69, 70].

The other UV filters have been responsible for allergic contact and/or photocontact dermatitis, or photoaggravated contact dermatitis [4]. In the 50s and 60s, PABA (*p*-aminobenzoic acid) was responsible for many cases of allergic and photoallergic contact dermatitis (4% of the population in an American study) [68] and, therefore, since then it was seldom used. Nevertheless, a very recent case of photoallergic contact dermatitis was published [59].

In the studies from the 70s till the end of the 90s, most frequent photosensitizers are the UVA filters, oxybenzone (benzophenone 3), and isopropyldibenzoylmethane [31, 63, 64, 67, 71]. At present, the latter is not produced anymore, and the other dibenzoylmethane on the market, butyl methoxydibenzoylmethane, is not such a potent photosensitizer. Many reactions previously reported were probably due to a cross-reaction [71].

Oxybenzone, still the most used UV filter, is being replaced in many sunscreens. Those sunscreens having a concentration higher than 0.5% must print a warning on the label. Nevertheless, in this setting or as a common ingredient in cosmetics, oxybenzone is still the most frequently used UV filter responsible for positive photopatch tests [4, 60, 64, 67]. Rarely, it can also induce contact photocontact urticaria or anaphylaxis [32]. Sulisobenzone (benzophenone 4) and mexenone (benzophenone 10) induce allergic or photoallergic contact dermatitis less frequently [64, 72, 73]. Another concern on oxybenzone, and the other benzophenones, is related to its percutaneous absorption and its environmental spread, which may be harmful due to its potential estrogen-like effects [74].

Cinnamates, namely isoamyl-*p*-methoxycinnamate and ethylhexyl-*p*-methoxycinnamate, and 4-methylbenzylidene camphor, phenylbenzimidazole sulfonic acid, drometrizole trisiloxane (Mexoryl XL) and octyl dimethyl PABA (Padimate O) are also regularly responsible for cases of photoallergy [3, 4, 62, 64, 66, 67]. Other UVB filters, namely the salicylates (octylsalicilate and homosalate) and octocrylene are seldom reported to cause allergic or photoallergic contact dermatitis [75, 76], except in an Italian study where octocrylene was the most frequent UV filter responsible for photopatch test reactions [66].

18

Core Message

> UV filters in sunscreens or cosmetics are the main cause of photoallergic contact dermatitis.

18.4.2 Plants Causing Phytophotodermatitis

Photoactive furocoumarins, e.g., bergapten, 5- and 8-methoxypsoralen, run in the sap of several plants, in variable amounts, as a protection against fungus and insects. Since the antiquity, these substances have been used in folk Medicine (vitiligo) and, more recently, in photochemotherapy (PUVA), and the aromatic oils rich in furocoumarins were used by the cosmetic industry in tanning oils and perfumes. As enhancement of skin pigmentation is known to be a marker for DNA aggression, the use of tanning oils has been considerably reduced, and the natural bergamot oil responsible for "Berloque dermatitis" from perfumes is no more used [77].

Dermatitis can also occur from inadvertent contact with these plants, both during recreation or in an occupational setting, e.g., rural workers or gardeners who harvest fruits or vegetables (parsnip, figs) or cut bushes and weeds (common rue – *Ruta graveolans* – burning bush – *Dictamus albus* – or fig trees – *Ficus carica*) [77, 78], or barmen who squeeze and peal lime (*Citrus aurantifolia*) and other citrus fruits to prepare cocktails in the sunny weather [77, 79, 80] (Fig. 18.5).

The most typical pattern of phytophotodermatitis was described by Oppenheim in 1934 – *dermatosis bullosa*

striata pratensis. Linear streaks, corresponding to the contact with the damaged leaves of the plant, begin within 24–48 h with prickling erythema and, later, painful vesicles and bullae (Fig. 18.6). All these gradually give rise to long-lasting linear hyperpigmentation, which, sometimes, allows a retrospective diagnosis [80].

Another pattern is the "strimmer dermatitis" with a diffuse involvement as the sap of the plant is sprayed all over by the string trimmer [77]. Children who play in nature were more prone to this dermatitis and, very particularly, those making trumpets or pea shooters from the hollow stems of the giant hogweed (*Heracleum mantegazzianum*) developed blisters around their mouth [77]. Very occasionally, the ingestion of these plants can induce systemic photosensitivity as in the cases of celery, parsnip, or infusions of St. John's wort (*Hypericum perforatum L.*) used to treat depression [77, 81].

Plants rich in furocoumarins causing phytophotodermatitis occur all over the globe and belong mainly to the families of Umbelliferae, Rutacea, and Moracea (Table 18.3).

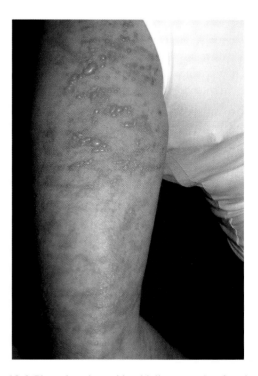

Fig. 18.6 Phytophotodermatitis with linear streaks of erythema and bullae in the arms of a patient who had been cutting a fig tree during a sunny afternoon

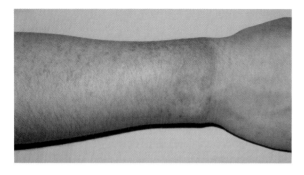

Fig. 18.5 Residual pigmentation in the forearms in a barman who had been squeezing limes and lemons for cocktails, during an outdoor summer festival (note limit due to glove protection)

Table 18.3 Main agents causing exogenous photosensitivity

Sunscreens

Benzophenones: oxybenzone, sulisobenzone, mexenone

Dibenzoylmethanes: butyl methoxydibenzoylmethane

Cinnamates: isoamyl-*p*-methoxycinnamate, ethylhexyl methoxycinnamate

PABA and analogs: *p*-aminobenzoic acid; padimate O

Other: 4-methylbenzylidene camphor, phenylbenzimidazole sulfonic acid, octocrylene, drometrizole trisiloxane

Plants (main Families in Europe)

Umbelliferae: *Ammi majus*, *Apium graveolens* (celery), *Pastinaca sativa* (parsnip), *Petroselinum crispum* (parsley), *Heracleum mantegazzianum* (giant hogweed)

Rutacea: Citrus spp, *Citrus aurantica v. bergamia* (bergamot), *Citrus aurantifolia* (lime), *Citrus limon* (lemon), *Ruta graveolans* (common rue), *Dictamus albus* (burning bush)

Moracea: *Ficus carica* (fig)

Drugs (see details in Table 18.4)

"Historical" photosensitizers[a]

Perfumes: musk ambrette, bergamot oil

Halogenated salicylanilides: tetrachlorsalicylanilide, trichlorocarbanilide, tribromsalicylanide

Sunscreens: isopropyldibenzoylmethane, PABA

Antibiotics: olaquindox

Dyes: eosin, acridine orange, acriflavin

[a]Although "historical," some still induce photoallergic contact dermatitis

---

Core Message

> *Dermatosis bullosa striata pratensis,* with linear lesions that regress with hyperpigmentation, is a phototoxic dermatitis from psoralen rich plants.

18.4.3 *Photosensitive Drugs*

According to the results of the photopatch series in Southern European countries, drugs are by far the main cause of exogenous photoallergy, whereas in the Northern countries sunscreens occupy the first rank as photosensitizers [62, 64–66]. This may be due to different prescription habits or because NSAIDs, the main drugs responsible for positive photopatch tests, were not regularly included in most photopatch test series.

Drugs used systemically, applied topically, or handled in an occupational setting can induce photosensitivity. Carprofen, a NSAID no more used in humans, induced photoallergic contact dermatitis in workers who manufacture the drug for animals [82, 83]. Also, we observed cases of photosensitivity in nurses and family members who had to smash the tablets of chlorpromazine to give to their patients or relatives [62].

Antimicrobials, particularly tetracyclines, fluorquinolones, sulfonamides, and some antifungals (voriconazole, griseofulvin), NSAIDs, phenothiazines, and cardiovascular drugs are mainly responsible for systemic photosensitivity. After topical application, NSAIDs are by far the most frequent cause [62, 64–66].

Core Message

> Topical NSAIDs (ketoprofen) and systemic antibiotics (fluorquinolones, tetracyclines) can induce photoallergic contact dermatitis or systemic photosensitivity.

18.4.3.1 Antimicrobials

Systemic tetracyclines, particularly doxycycline and minocycline, are highly phototoxic and induce photoonycholysis and pseudoporphyria and, the latter can also induce a bluish persistent pigmentation [51, 52] (Fig. 18.4).

The fluorquinolones induce phototoxic reactions, in some cases presenting as pseudoporphyria [40], as initially described for the first quinolone antibiotic, nalidixic acid [51], or as purpura in a case by ciprofloxacin [53]. Phototoxicity is particularly important and frequent (4–15% of treated patients) with fleroxacin, lomefloxacin, sparfloxacin, and pefloxacin and less frequent with ciprofloxacin, norfloxacin, ofloxacin, and enoxacin [14]. This can be reduced with drug intake by the end of the day, to reduce drug concentrations in the circulation and in the skin during the midday. Photoallergy has also been reported with lomefloxacin [20, 21] and enoxacin [51], sometimes with cross-reaction to other fluorquinolones (ciprofloxacin and flerofloxacin) [84, 85]. Experimental studies proved the photoallergenicity of fluorquinolones, with positive lymphocyte stimulation tests and drug specific Th1 cells that recognize skin cells combined with UV-irradiated ofloxacin [86]. The fluorquinolones also photosensitize DNA and may be photomutagenic and photocarcinogenic [8]. We had the opportunity to observe a patient on long-term ciprofloxacin therapy for multiresistant tuberculosis, who developed photosensitivity and highly aggressive squamous cell carcinomas on the face.

Sulphonamide antibacterials, as well as sulfa-drug analogs (thiazidic diuretics, hypoglycemic sulfonylureas, and celecoxib) and dapsone (diamidiphenylsulfone), have been reported to cause photosensitivity within the spectrum both of UVB and UVA [51, 87, 88], but this side effect is not so frequent with the most currently used cotrimoxazole (trimethoprim/sulfamethoxazole) [14, 51].

Griseofulvin is a known phototoxic drug and can aggravate lupus erythematosus, as the more recent antifungal, terbinafine, which also induced subacute lupus erythematosus in patients with anti-Ro antibodies [55]. Another antifungal, still from a different chemical group, voriconazole, has recently been reported to cause severe photosensitivity [7] and was considered responsible for skin cancer [16, 28, 43].

18.4.3.2 Nonsteroidal Anti-Inflammatory Drugs

Benoxaprofen marketed between 1980 and 1982 called the attention to photosensitivity from this class of drugs. Thereafter, all the other arylpropionic derivatives (carprofen, naproxen, suprofen, tiaprofenic acid, ketoprofen, ibuprofen) and NSAIDs from other groups (azapropazone, diclofenac, piroxicam, fenilbutazone, celecoxib, benzydamine, etofenamate) have been shown to cause photosensitivity [39].

Most topically applied NSAIDs are absorbed through the skin and cause distant lesions, resembling systemic photosensitivity. Benzydamine, widely used in the oral or genital mucosa, causes photosensitivity at distant sites [89], eventually after systemic absorption [29, 65] and, when used in the mouth, can induce cheilitis and chin dermatitis as a manifestation of photoallergy [29, 62].

Although not the most sold, ketoprofen and piroxicam cause most cases of photosensitivity [62, 64, 65, 90]. Contrary to most other drugs, these NSAIDs cause photoallergy with very particular patterns of cross-reactivity.

Ketoprofen

Ketoprofen, particularly when used topically, is responsible for severe photoallergic reactions [7, 91], often with edema, bullae or erythema multiform, extending well beyond the area of application [34, 35, 92], due to contamination of the hands or other personal objects or due to systemic absorption [92]. Reactions may recur on sun exposure with no apparent further drug application [34, 91], but they do not fulfill the criteria for the diagnosis of persistent photosensitivity. Some may be explained by persistence of the drug in the skin (at least 17 days) [92] by contact with previously contaminated objects, even after washing [26], or from exposure to cross-reactive chemicals [34].

Although such a high frequency might suggest phototoxicity, the clinical pattern with erythema multiform, positive lymphocyte stimulation tests with ketoprofen photomodified cells, animal studies with the absence of phototoxic potential [93], the capacity to photosensitize and transfer photoallergy by T-cells, both CD4 and CD8 exhibiting chemokine receptors for Th1 and Th2, in vitro activation and maturation of antigen-presenting cells by ketoprofen and UVA, [35, 94, 95], and characterization of a stable photoproduct – 3-ethyl-benzophenone [34, 96] – highly support a photoallergic reaction.

Cross-reactions occur between arylpropionic acid derivatives that share the benzophenone radical, namely tiaprofenic acid and suprofen, and are not extensive to naproxen or ibuprofen. As that radical is common to the benzophenone UV filters, cross-reactions are common with sunscreens containing mainly oxybenzone [96]. A similar structure is present in the systemic hypolipemic agent, fenofibrate, that also induces systemic photosensitivity with cross-reactions with ketoprofen [62] and patients taking fenofibrate have a higher risk for severe photoallergic contact dermatitis from Ketoprofen [91, 96].

These patients have a higher reactivity, in patch tests, to balsam of Peru and perfume mix I, particularly cinnamic aldehyde [34, 97], still not completely explained.

Analogs of ketoprofen, piketoprofen, and dexketoprofen also cause photosensitivity with cross-reactivity to ketoprofen [98, 99].

Piroxicam

Piroxicam is a well-known photosensitizer, with the first report of photosensisitivty dating from 1983. Although there was some enigma to explain this photosensitivity at the beginning [100], soon a relation was established with contact sensitivity to thiomersal [101, 102], more precisely to thiosalicylic acid [24], one of the sensitization moieties most frequently responsible for contact allergy to thiomersal [103]. Actually, upon low UVA irradiation, piroxicam decomposes and gives rise to a photoproduct structurally similar to thiosalicylic acid, UVA-irradiated solutions of piroxicam induce positive patch tests in thiosalicylic allergic patients [24, 39, 103, 104], animals sensitized by thiosalicylic acid develop photosensitivity from piroxicam, and their lymphocytes are stimulated both by thiosalicylic acid and by piroxicam, in the presence of UVA [25].

Photoallergy from piroxicam can occur both from topical application and systemic use and, although it is becoming less frequent, probably because of the replacement of this NSAIDs by the newer drugs [23], it is still observed in Southern Europe [29, 64–66].

Systemic photosensitivity usually occurs within 24–48 h after the first drug intakes, as the individuals have been previously been sensitized though thiomersal. It can present as an acute eczema involving diffusely the whole face (Fig. 18.2) or, often, as scattered erythematosus papules and vesicles on the face and dorsum of the hands and dyshidrosis [19, 23, 105, 106]

These patients do not react, neither on photopatch nor on drug rechallenge, to tenoxicam, meloxicam, or lornoxicam, as these oxicams do not share the thiosalicylate moiety [24, 107]. Nevertheless, it is important to remember that cross-reactivity between piroxicam and these oxicams occurs regularly in fixed drug eruption [108, 109].

18.4.3.3 Other Drugs as Photosensitizers

Phenothiazines used systemically (chlorpromazine and thioridazine) can induce photosensitivity, often with a lichenoid pattern and with residual pigmentation [52] (Fig. 18.3). Promethazine, still being used as a topical antipruritic, at least in Portugal, Greece, and Italy [62, 66, 110], and its analog chlorproethazine, which is being marketed in France as Neuriplege® cream for muscle pain (Genevrier, Antibes, France)

are frequent causes of photoallergic contact dermatitis in these countries [111, 112].

The list of drugs causing photosensitivity is very large and always increasing; therefore, whenever a patient has a photosensitive eruption a systematic inquiry for drugs should be carefully conducted (Table 18.4). The complementary methods for its diagnosis, photopatch testing and photoprovocation, will be the object of Chap. 29.

Table 18.4 Main drugs causing exogenous photosensitivity

Antimicrobials
Tetracyclines (doxycycline, minocycline)
Sulphonamides (sulfamethoxazole)
Fluoroquinolones (lomefloxacin[a], ciprofloxacin[a])
Voriconazole, griseofulvin
Efavirenz
Nonsteroidal anti-inflammatory drugs (NSAIDs)
Arylpropionic acids
Ketoprofen,[b] tiaprofenic acid,[a] suprofen, naproxen, ibuprofen, ibuproxam, carprofen
Piroxicam[c]
Benzydamine,[a] etofenamate[d]
Azapropazone, diclofenac, fenilbutazone, indometacine
Phenothiazines
Chlorpromazine, thioridazine
Promethazine[a], chlorproethazine
Antidepressants
Clomipramine, imipramine, sertraline
Cardiovascular drugs
Amiodarone, quinidine
Furosemide and thiazide diuretics
Anticancer agents
Paclitaxel, 5-fluoruracil, dacarbazine, methotrexate
Miscellaneous
Flutamide, sulfonylureas
Fenofibrate, simvastatin

[a]Although phototoxic, can induce photoallergic reactions
[b]Induce photoallergic and allergic contact dermatitis
[c]Induces mainly systemic photoallergy
[d]Induces mainly allergic contact dermatitis

18.5 Conclusions

Phototoxic and photoallergic reactions are still a frequent problem, with a highly polymorphic clinical presentation. Responsible agents vary according to the geographical areas, and along the years, as new photosensitizers come into the market whereas others are abandoned. Therefore, we must be highly alert to suspect the involvement of an exogenous chromophore in a photosensitive patient, to conduct the questionnaire in this sense, and to proceed to further complementary tests to prove such a diagnosis and, consequently, advise the patient concerning further eviction of the photosensitizer and related chemicals.

References

1. Hawk J (1999) Photodermatology, 1st edn. Oxford University Press, Oxford
2. Fujimoto N, Danno K, Wakabayashi M et al (2009) Photosensitivity with eosinophilia due to ambroxol and UVB. Contact Derm 60:110–113
3. Darvay A, White I, Rycroft R et al (2001) Photoallergic contact dermatitis is uncommon. Br J Dermatol 145:597–601
4. Bryden A, Moseley H, Ibbotson S et al (2006) Photopatch testing of 1115 patients: results of the U.K. multicentre photopatch study group. Brit J Dermatol 155:737–747
5. Zeeli T, David M, Trattner A (2006) Photopatch tests: any news under the sun? Contact Derm 55:305–307
6. Bilu D, Mamelak A, Nguyen R et al (2004) Clinical and epidemiologic characterization of photosensitivity in HIV-positive individuals. Photoderm Photoimmunol Photomed 20:175–183
7. Béani J (2009) Les photosensibilisations graves. Ann Dermatol Vénéreol 136:76–83
8. Urbach F (1997) Phototoxicity and possible enhancement of photocarcinogenesis by fluorinated quinolone antibiotics. J Photochem Photobiol B 37:169–170
9. Klecak G, Urbach F, Urwyler H (1997) Fluoroquinolone antibacterials enhance UVA-induced skin tumors. J Photochem Photobiol B 37:174–181
10. Marrot L, Belaïdi J, Jones C et al (2003) Molecular responses to photogenotoxic stress induced by the antibiotic lomefloxacin in human skin cells: from DNA damage to apoptosis. J Invest Dermatol 121:596–606
11. Lhiaubet-Vallet V, Bosca F, Miranda M (2009) Photosensitized DNA damage: the case of fluoroquinolones. Photochem Photobiol 85:861–868
12. Müller L, Kasper P, Kersten B, Zhang J (1998) Photochemical genotoxicity and photochemical carcinogenesis – two sides of a coin? Toxicol Lett 102–103:383–387
13. Placzek M, Eberlein-König B, Przybilla B (1999) Association between actinic keratoses and potentially photosensitizing drugs. N Engl J Med 341:1474–1475
14. Ferguson J (1999) Drug and chemical photosensitivity. In: Hawk's photodermatology, 1st edn. Oxford University Press, Oxford, pp 155–169
15. Jensen A, Thomsen H, Engebjerg M et al (2008) Use of photosensitising diuretics and risk of skin cancer: a population based case-control study. Br J Cancer 99:1522–1528
16. McCarthy K, Playforf E, Looke D, Whitby M (2007) Severe photosensitivity causing multifocal squamous cell carcinomas secondary to prolonged voriconazole therapy. Clin Inf Dis 44:e55–e56
17. Lim H, Hawk J (2008) Photodermatosis. In: Bolognia JL, Jorizzo JL, Rapini RP (eds) Dermatology, 2nd edn. Elsevier, Philadelphia
18. Karimian-Teherani D, Kinaciyan T, Tanew A (2008) Photoallergic contact dermatitis from Heracleum giganteum. Photoderm Photoimmunol Photomed 24:99–101
19. Gonçalo M (1998) Explorations dans les photo-allergies médicamenteuses. In: GERDA (eds) Progrès en Dermato-Allergologie. John Libbey Eurotext. Nancy, France, pp 67–74
20. Oliveira H, Gonçalo M, Figueiredo A (1996) Photosensitivity from lomefloxacin. A clinical and photobiological study. Photoderm Photoimmunol Photomed 16:116–120
21. Kurumajin Y, Shono M (1992) Scarified photopatch testing in lomefloxacin photosensitivity. Contact Derm 26:5–10
22. Neves B, Cruz M, Francisco V et al (2008) Differential modulation of CXCR4 and CD40 protein levels by skin sensitizers and irritants in the FSCD cell line. Toxicol Lett 177:74–82
23. Serra D, Gonçalo M, Figueiredo A (2008) Two decades of cutaneous adverse drug reactions from piroxicam. Contact Derm 58:S35
24. Gonçalo M, Figueiredo A, Tavares P et al (1992) Photosensitivity to piroxicam: absence of cross-reaction with tenoxicam. Contact Derm. 27:287–290
25. Hariva T, Kitamura K, Osawa J, Ikezawa Z (1993) A cross-reaction between piroxicam-photosensitivity and thiosalicylate hypersensitivity in lymphocyte proliferation test. J Dermatol Sci 5:165–174
26. Hindsén M, Isaksson M, Persson L et al (2004) Photoallergic contact dermatitis from ketoprofen induced by drug-contaminated personal objects. J Am Acad Dermatol 50:215–219
27. Due E, Wulf H (2006) Cheilitis – the only presentation of photosensitivity. JEADV 20:766–767
28. Auffret N, Janssen F, Chevalier P et al (2006) Photosensibilisation au voriconazole. Ann Dermatol Vénéreol 133:330–332
29. Canelas M, Cravo M, Cardoso J et al (2008) Dermatite de contacto fotoalérgica à benzidamina – Estudo de 8 casos. Trab Soc Port Dermatol Venereol 66:35–40
30. Kerr A, Ferguson J, Ibbotson S (2007) Acute phototoxicity with urticarial features during topical 5-aminolaevulinic acid photodynamic therapy. Clin Exp Dermatol 32:201–202
31. Collins P, Ferguson J (1994) Photoallergic contact dermatitis to oxybenzone. Br J Dermatol 131:124–129
32. Spijker G, Schuttelaar M, Barkema L et al (2008) Anaphylaxis caused by topical application of a sunscreen containing benzophenone-3. Contact Derm 59:248–249
33. Lovell C, Cronin E, Rhodes E (1986) Photocontact urticaria from chlorpromazine. Contact Derm 14:290–291
34. Devleeschouwer V, Roelandts R, Garmyn M, Goossens A (2008) Allergic and photoallergic contact dermatitis from

ketoprofen: results of (photo) patch testing and follow-up of 42 patients. Contact Derm 58:159–166

35. Izu K, Hino R, Isoda H et al (2008) Photocontact dermatitis to ketoprofen presenting with erythema multiforme. Eur J Dermatol 18:710–713

36. Cohen P (2009) Photodistributed erythema multiforme: paclitaxel-related, photosensitive conditions in patients with cancer. J Drugs Dermatol 8:61–64

37. Mansur A, Aydingöz J (2005) A case of toxic epidermal necrolysis with lesions mostly on sun-exposed skin. Photoderm Photoimmunol Photomed 21:100–102

38. Redondo V, Vicente J, España A et al (1996) Photo-induced toxic epidermal necrolysis caused by clobazam. Br J Dermatol 135:999–1002

39. Figueiredo A (1994) Fotossensibilidade aos anti-inflamatórios não esteróides. Estudo fisiopatológico. Doctoral Thesis, Coimbra

40. Schmutz J, Barbaud A, Tréchot P (2008) Ciprofloxacin and pseudoporphyria. Ann Dermatol Vénéreol 135(11):804

41. Cummins R, Wagner-Weiner L, Paller A (2000) Pseudoporphyria induced by celecoxib in a patient with juvenile rheumatoid arthritis. J Rheumatol 27:2938–2940

42. Schmutz J, Barbaud A, Tréchot P (2006) Pseudoporphyria and coxib. Ann Dermatol Vénéreol 133:213

43. Tolland J, McKeown P, Corbett J (2007) Voriconazole-induced pseudoporphyria. Photoderm Photoimmunol Photomed 23: 29–31

44. Timmer-de Mik L, Kardaun S, Krammer M et al (2009) Imatinib-induced pseudoporphyria. Clin Exp Dermatol 34(6):705–707

45. Passier A, Smits-van Herwaarden A, van Puijenbroek E (2004) Photo-onycholysis associated with the use of doxycycline. BMJ 329:265

46. Baran R, Juhlin L (2002) Photoonycholysis. Photoderm Photoimmunol Photomed 18:202–207

47. Gregoriou S, Karagiorga T, Stratigos A et al (2008) Photoonycholysis caused by olanzapine and aripiprazole. J Clin Psychopharmacol 28:219–220

48. Gonçalo M, Domingues J, Correia O, Figueiredo A (1999) Fotossensibilidad a Flutamida. Boletim Informativo del GEIDC 29:45–48

49. Vilaplana J, Romaguera C, Azón A, Lecha M (1990) Flutamide photosensitivity-residual vitiliginous lesions. Contact Derm 38:68–70

50. Ammoury A, Michaud S, Paul C et al (2008) Photodistribution of blue-gray hyperpigmentation after amiodarone treatment. Molecular characterization of amiodarone in the skin. Arch Dermatol 144:92–96

51. Vassileva S, Matev G, Parish L (1998) Antimicrobial photosensitive reactions. Arch Intern Med 158:1993–2000

52. Ferguson J (2002) Photosensitivity due to drugs. Photoderm Photoimmunol Photomed 18:262–269

53. Urbina F, Barrios M, Sudy E (2006) Photolocalized purpura during ciprofloxacin therapy. Photoderm Photoimmunol Photomed 22:111–112

54. Sontheimer R, Henderson C, Grau R (2008) Drug-induced subacute cutaneous lupus erythematosus: a paradigm for bedside-to-bench patient-oriented translational clinical investigation. Arch Dermatol Res 301:65–70

55. Farhi D, Viguier M, Cosnes A et al (2006) Terbinafine-induced subacute cutaneous lupus erythematosus. Dermatology 212: 59–65

56. Chen M, Crowson A, Woofter M et al (2004) Docetaxel (taxotere) induced subacute cutaneous lupus erythematosus: report of 4 cases. J Rheumatol 31:818–820

57. Hawk J (2004) Chronic actinic dermatitis. Photoderm Photoimmunol Photomed 20:312–314

58. Emmert B, Schauder S, Palm H et al (2007) Disabling work-related persistent photosensitivity following photoallergic contact dermatitis from chlorpromazine and olaquindox in a pig breeder. Ann Agric Environ Med 14:329

59. Waters A, Sandhu D, Lowe G, Ferguson J (2009) Photocontact allergy to PABA: the need for continuous vigilance. Contact Derm 60:172–173

60. Schauder S, Ippen H (1997) Contact and photocontact sensitivity to sunscreens. Review of a 15-year experience and of the literature. Contact Derm 37:221–232

61. Sheuer E, Warshaw E (2006) Sunscreen allergy: a review of epidemiology, clinical characteristics, and responsible allergens. Dermatitis 17:3–11

62. Cardoso J, Canelas M, Gonçalo M, Figueiredo A (2009) Photopatch testing with an extended series of photoallergens. A 5-year study. Contact Derm 60:314–319

63. Bakkum R, Heule F (2002) Results of photopatch testing in Rotterdam during a 10-year period. Br J Dermatol 146: 275–279

64. Leonard F, Adamski H, Bonnevalle A et al (2005) Étude prospective multicentrique 1991-2001 de la batterie standard des photopatch-tests de la Société Française de Photodermatologie. Ann Dermatol Vénéreol 132:313–320

65. La Cuadra-Oyanguren J, Pérez-Ferriols A, Lecha-Carralero M et al (2007) Results and assessment of photopatch testing in Spain: towards a new standard set of photoallergens. Actas Dermosifiliogr 98:96–101

66. Pigatto P, Guzzi G, Schena D et al (2008) Photopatch tests: an Italian multicentre study from 2004 to 2006. Contact Derm 59:103–108

67. Berne B, Ros A (1998) 7 years experience of photopatch testing with sunscreen allergens in Sweden. Contact Derm 38:61–64

68. Lowe N (2006) An overview of ultraviolet radiation, sunscreens and photo-induced dermatosis. Dermatol Clin 24:9–17

69. Andersen K, Goossens A (2006) Decyl glucoside contact allergy from a sunscreen product. Contact Derm 54:349–350

70. Andrade P, Gonçalo M, Figueiredo A (2009) Allergic contact dermatitis to decyl glucoside in Tinosorb M. Contact Derm 62:119–120

71. Gonçalo M, Ruas E, Figueiredo A, Gonçalo S (1995) Contact and photocontact sensitivity to sunscreens. Contact Derm 33:278–280

72. Hughes T, Stone N (2007) Benzophenone 4: an emerging allergen in cosmetics and toiletries? Contact Derm 56:153–156

73. Torres V, Correia T (1991) Contact and photocontact allergy to oxybenzone and mexenone. Contact Derm 25:126–127

74. Kunz P, Fent K (2006) Estrogenic activity of UV filter mixtures. Toxicol Appl Pharmacol 15:86–99

75. Singh M, Beck M (2007) Octyl salicylate: a new contact sensitivity. Contact Derm 56(1):48

76. Madan V, Beck M (2005) Contact allergy to octocrylene in sunscreen with recurrence from passive transfer of a cosmetic. Contact Derm 53:241–242

77. Lovell C (2000) Phytophotodermatitis. In: Avalos J, Maibach HI (eds) Dermatological botany. CRC Press, Boca Raton, pp 51–65

18

78. Gonçalo S, Correia C, Couto J, Gonçalo M (1989) Contact and photocontact dermatitis from Ruta chalepensis. Contact Derm 21:200–201

79. Wagner A, Wu J, Hansen R et al (2002) Bullous phytophotodermatitis associated with high natural concentrations of furanocoumarins in limes. Am J Contact Derm 13:10–14

80. Gonçalo M (2004) Dermatitis por plantas y maderas. Em: Conde-Salazar Gómez L, Ancona-Alayón A (eds) Dermatologia professional. Aula Médica Ediciones, Madrid, pp 193–210

81. Schempp C, Müller K, Winghofer B et al (2002) St. John's wort (Hypericum perforatum L.). A plant with relevance for dermatology. Hautarzt 53:316–321

82. Kerr A, Muller F, Ferguson J, Dawe R (2008) Occupational carprofen photoallergic contact dermatitis. Br J Dermatol 159:1303–1308

83. Walker S, Ead R, Beck M (2006) Occupational photoallergic contact dermatitis in a pharmaceutical worker manufacturing carprofen, a canine nonsteroidal anti-inflammatory drug. Br J Dermatol 154:551–577

84. Kimura M, Kawada A (1998) Photosensitivity induced by lomefoxacin with cross-photosensitivity to ciprofloxacin and fleroxacin. Contact Derm 38:130

85. Correia O, Delgado L, Barros M (1994) Bullous photodermatosis after lomefloxacin. Arch Dermatol 130:808–809

86. Tokura Y, Seo N, Fujie M, Takigawa M (2001) Quinolone-photoconjugated major histocompatibility complex class II-binding peptides with lysine are antigenic for T cells mediating murine quinolone photoallergy. J Invest Dermatol 117:1206–1211

87. Kar B (2008) Dapsone-induced photosensitivity: a rare clinical presentation. Photoderm Photoimmunol Photomed 24:270–271

88. Yazici A, Baz K, Ikizoglu G et al (2004) Celecoxib-induced photoallergic drug eruption. Int J Dermatol 43:459–461

89. Lasa Elgezua O, Gorrotxategi P, Gardeazabal Gracia J et al (2004) Photoallergic hand eczema due to benzydamine. Eur J Dermatol 14:69–70

90. Diaz R, Gardeazabal J, Manrique P et al (2006) Greater allergenicity of topical ketoprofen in contact dermatitis confirmed by use. Contact Derm 54:239–243

91. Veyrac G, Paulin M, Milpied B et al (2002) Bilan de l'enquête nationale sur les effets indésirables cutanés do kétoprofène gel enregistrés entre le 01/09/1996 et le 31/08/2000. Thérapie 57:55–64

92. Sugiura M, Hayakawa R, Kato Y et al (2000) 4 cases of photocontact dermatitis due to ketoprofen. Contact Derm 43:16–19

93. Lee B, Choi Y, Son W et al (2007) Ketoprofen: experimental overview of dermal toxicity. Arch Toxicol 81:743–748

94. Imai S, Atarashi K, Ikesue K et al (2005) Establishment of murine model of allergic photocontact deermatitis to ketoprofen and characterization of pathogenic T cells. J Dermatol Sci 41:127–136

95. Hino R, Orimo H, Kabashima K (2008) Evaluation of the photoallergic potential of chemicals using THP-1 cells. J Dermatol Sci 52:140–143

96. LeCoz C, Bottlaender A, Scrivener J et al (1998) Photocontact dermatitis from ketoprofen and tiaprofenic acid: cross-reactivity study in 12 consecutive patients. Contact Derm 38:245–252

97. Pigatto P, Bigardi A, Legori A et al (1996) Cross reactions in patch testing and photopatch testing with ketoprofen, tiaprofenic acid and cinnamic aldehyde. Am J Contact Derm 7:220–223

98. Asensio T, Sanchis M, Sánchez P et al (2008) Photocontact dermatitis because of oral dexketoprofen. Contact Derm 58:59–60

99. Fernández-Jorge B, Buján J, Paradela S, Mazaira M, Fonseca E (2008) Consort contact dermatitis from piketoprofen. Contact Derm 58:113–115

100. Lunggren B (1989) The piroxicam enigma. Photodermatology 6:151–154

101. Cirne de Castro J, Vale E, Martins M (1989) Mechanism of photosensitive reactions induced by piroxicam. J Am Acad Dermatol 20:706–707

102. Cirne de Castro J, Freitas J, Brandão F, Themido R (1991) Sensitivity to thimerosal and photosensitivity to piroxicam. Contact Derm 24:187–192

103. Gonçalo M, Figueiredo A, Gonçalo S (1996) Hypersensitivity to thimerosal: the sensitizing moiety. Contact Derm 34:201–203

104. Ikezawa Z, Kitamura K, Osawa J, Hariva T (1992) Photosensitivity to piroxicam is induced by sensitization to thimerosal and thiosalicylate. J Invest Dermatol 98:918–920

105. Varela P, Amorim I, Massa A, Sanches M, Silva E (1998) Piroxicam-beta-cyclodextrin and photosensitivity reactions. Contact Derm 38:229

106. Youn J, Lee H, Yeo U, Lee Y (1993) Piroxicam photosensitivity associated with vesicular hand dermatitis. Clin Exp Dermatol 18:52–54

107. Trujillo M, Barrio M, Rodríguez A et al (2001) Piroxicam-induced photodermatitis. Cross-reactivity among oxicams. A case report. Allergol et Immunopathol 29:133–136

108. Gonçalo M, Oliveira H, Fernandes B etal (2002) Topical provocation in fixed drug eruption from nonsteroidal anti-inflammatory drugs. Exog Dermatol 1:81–86

109. Oliveira H, Gonçalo M, Reis J, Figueiredo A (1999) Fixed drug eruption to piroxicam. Positive patch tests with cross-sensitivity to tenoxicam. J Dermatol Treat 10:209–212

110. Katsarou A, Makris M, Zarafonitis G et al (2008) Photoallergic contact dermatitis: the 15-year experience of a tertiary reference center in a sunny Mediterranean city. Int J Immunopathol Pharmacol 21:725–727

111. Barbaud A, Collet E, Martin S et al (2001) Contact sensitization to chlorproéthazine can induce persistent light reaction and cross photoreactions to other phenothiazines. Contact Derm 44:373

112. Kerr A, Woods J, Ferguson J (2008) Photocontact allergic and phototoxic studies of chlorproethazine. Photoderm Photoimmunol Photomed 24:11–15

Pigmented Contact Dermatitis and Chemical Depigmentation

Hideo Nakayama

Contents

H. Nakayama
Nakayama Dermatology Clinic, Shinyo-CK Building 6F, 3-3-5,
Kami-Ohsaki, Shinagawa-ku, 141-0021 Tokyo, Japan
e-mail: nakayamadermatology@eos.ocn.ne.jp

19.1 Hyperpigmentation Associated with Contact Dermatitis

19.1.1 Classification

Hyperpigmentation associated with contact dermatitis is classified into three categories: (1) hyperpigmentation due to incontinentia pigmenti histologica; (2) hyperpigmentation due to an increase in melanin in the basal layer cells of the epidermis, i.e., basal melanosis; and (3) hyperpigmentation due to slight hemorrhage around the vessels of the upper dermis, resulting in an accumulation of hemosiderin, such as in the Majocchi–Schamberg dermatitis.

It is easy to understand that when the grade of contact dermatitis is more severe, or its duration longer, the secondary hyperpigmentation following dermatitis is more prominent. However, the first type mentioned above, incontinentia pigmenti histologica, often occurs without showing any positive manifestations of dermatitis, such as marked erythema, vesiculation, swelling, papules, rough skin, or scaling. Therefore, patients may complain only of a pigmentary disorder, even though the disease is entirely the result of allergic contact dermatitis. Hyperpigmentation caused by incontinentia pigmenti histologica has often been called a lichenoid reaction, since the presence of basal liquefaction degeneration, the accumulation of melanin pigment, and the mononuclear cell infiltrate in the upper dermis are very similar to the histopathological manifestations of lichen planus. However, compared with typical lichen planus, hyperkeratosis is usually milder, hypergranulosis and saw-tooth-shape acanthosis are lacking, hyaline bodies are hardly seen, and the band-like massive infiltration with lymphocytes and histiocytes is lacking.

J.D. Johansen et al. (eds.), *Contact Dermatitis*,
DOI: 10.1007/978-3-642-03827-3_19, © Springer-Verlag Berlin Heidelberg 2011

A lichenoid reaction is considered to be a scaled-down type-IV allergic reaction of the lichen planus type, based on positive patch test reactions in patients and negative reactions in controls, as in ordinary allergic contact dermatitis.

An increase in melanin pigment in keratinocytes is noted after allergic contact dermatitis, presumably caused by hyperfunction of melanocytes, but the same phenomenon is also seen with irritant contact dermatitis. When sodium lauryl sulfate, a typical skin irritant, was repeatedly applied on the forearms of Caucasians, the number of epidermal melanocytes was observed to almost double, suggesting hyperplasia, hypertrophy, and increased function [1].

The pathological processes involved in the third form of hyperpigmentation with contact dermatitis and purpuric dermatitis, have not yet been clarified. Shiitake mushroom, very commonly eaten in Asia, has been known to produce a transient urticarial dermatitis with severe itching, which results in a purpuric scratch effect when insufficiently cooked. This is thought to be due to toxic substances in the mushroom unstable to heat, and the pigmentation due to purpura is not caused by hypersensitivity [2]. As with other forms of dermatitis, accompanying capillary fragility results in purpura. Some cases are associated with contact hypersensitivity to rubber components or textile finishes, but in many cases the causes are not known.

19.1.2 Pigmented Contact Dermatitis

19.1.2.1 History and Causative Agents

Core Message

> Pigmented contact dermatitis on the covered area cannot be cured by the application of corticosteroid ointments, even though it is a result of contact allergens from textiles, soaps, or washing powders for textile. Successive contact of small amount of allergens makes destruction of basal layer cells of the epidermis result in the melanin accumulation in the upper dermis for a long time. Finding out the contact allergens and their avoidance for a long time is necessary for the treatment.

Pigmented contact dermatitis was first reported by Osmundsen in Denmark in 1969. In 8 months he had 120 patients, seven of whom showed a pronounced and bizarre hyperpigmentation. In four of these seven cases, contact dermatitis preceded the hyperpigmentation, while the other three did not notice any signs of dermatitis, such as itching or erythema, before the pigmentation appeared [3, 4].

Hyperpigmentation, with or without dermatitis, was located mostly in covered areas, such as the chest, back, waist, arms, neck, and thighs. After a patient wanted to conceal the pigmentation by wearing long sleeves and a high-neck sweater, which she washed with a washing powder every day, the hyperpigmentation extended from the neck and axillae to all over the neck, chest, and arms. The hyperpigmentation was brown, slate-colored, grayish-brown, reddish-brown, bluish-brown, etc., according to the case, and often had a reticulate pattern. The histopathology of the pigmentation showed incontinentia pigmenti histologica.

Patch tests with the standard series current at that time gave no information as to the causative allergens. However, Osmundsen noticed that the patients had used washing powders that contained a new optical whitener, Tinopal or CH3566 (Table 19.1). This was one of numerous optical whiteners that became available at that time to make textiles "whiter than white." Patch tests with CH3566 1% pet. finally explained the pigmentary disorder, as they showed strong positive reactions in the patients and negative results in the controls. The pigmentation was persistent, but the dermatitis that often preceded hyperpigmentation was observed to disappear following the elimination of washing powders that contained CH3566. Fortunately, the identification of the causative chemical was made rapidly, and the widespread usage of CH3566 was avoided in time.

Pigmented contact dermatitis is rare in Caucasians, but not uncommon in Mongoloids. The next pigmented contact dermatitis was reported by Ancona-Alayón et al. in Mexico [5]. Among 53 workers handling azo dyes in a textile factory, 12 developed a spotted hyperpigmentation without pruritus, and 18 suffered from hyperpigmentation to a lesser extent. This new occupational skin disorder appeared 4 months after the introduction of a new dyeing process of azo-coupling on textiles, and most of the patients had contact with azo dyes on weaving machines. Hyperpigmentation varied from a bizarre dark pigmentation to a streaky milder pigmentation of the neck, arms, face, and in exceptional cases, covered areas.

Table 19.1 The main contact sensitizers producing secondary hyperpigmentation

Name	Chemical structure	Purpose	Patch test concentration and base
Tinopal CH3566		Optical whitener in washing powder	1% pet.
Naphthol AS		Dye for textile	1% pet.
Benzyl salicylate		Fragrance	5% - 1% pet.
Hydroxycitronellal		Fragrance	5% - 1% pet.
D & C Red 31 (Brilliant lake red R)		Pigment for cosmetics	1% pet.
Phenyl-azo-2-naphthol (PAN)		Impurity	0.1% pet.
D & C Yellow 11		Pigment for cosmetics	0.1% pet.
Ylang-ylang oil	(main sensitizer, dehydrodiisoeugenol)	Fragrance, incense	5% pet.
Jasmin absolute	Main sensitizers not yet identified	Fragrance	10% - 5% pet.
Synthetic sandalwood	Main sensitizers not yet identified	Fragrance	10% pet.
Cinnamic alcohol	CH=CHCH$_2$OH	Fragrance	1% pet.
Musk ambrette		Fragrance, incense	5% cream
Biocheck 60®	C$_{12}$H$_{25}$-NH-C-NH-HCl $\quad\quad\quad$ $\overset{\|}{NH}$	Pesticide for textiles	0.2% aq.
PPP-HB		Textile finish	5% eth.

(*continued*)

Table 19.1 (continued)

Name	Chemical structure	Purpose	Patch test concentration and base
Impurity of commercial Cl, Blue 19 (Brilliant Blue®)	Main sensitizers not yet identified	Dye	5% eth.
Mercury compounds	Hg^{2+}	Bactericides	0.05% aq. or pet. (not with aluminum chambers)
Nickel (sulfate)	Ni^{2+}	Metal products	5% aq. or pet.
Chromate (K dichromate)	Cr^{6+}	Leather, foundation	0.5% aq. or pet.

Histopathological examination of the pigmentary disorder showed spongiosis, irregular acanthosis, edema of the dermis, pericapillary lymphocytic infiltration, basal liquefaction degeneration, and incontinentia pigmenti histologica. Melanocyte proliferation at the affected sites was also noted.

Patch tests showed that 24 of the 53 workers were positive to Naphthol AS 5% in water, while the other 29, as well as ten controls, were negative to Naphthol AS. The dermatoses disappeared after the dyeing process was changed so that the workers did not directly touch Naphthol AS, an azo dye coupling agent.

In the early 1980s, pigmented contact dermatitis due to Naphthol AS appeared in central Japan, but this time it was not occupational. A textile factory manufacturing flannel nightwear, a traditional Japanese garment called yukata, economized on water for washing the products after the process of azo-coupling using Naphthol AS. This modification of production resulted in the appearance of pigmented contact dermatitis of the covered areas of skin of people living in the districts where the products were distributed and worn. Kawachi et al. [6] and Hayakawa et al. [7] reported such cases, and the hyperpigmentation was mainly located on the back and neck. The factory was said to have improved the washing process and the materials quickly, but the presence of such cases indicates that whenever the textile industry uses Naphthol AS and, at the same time, economizes on water for washing the products, there must be a risk of producing pigmented contact dermatitis of the covered areas. According to Hayakawa et al. [7], the amount of Naphthol AS detected in the patients' nightwear was 4,900–8,700 ppm, a considerable amount. A case due to Naphthol AS in a pillow case was later reported [8].

In 1984, the city of Tokyo decided to investigate new textile finishes that seemed to have produced contact dermatitis of the covered skin areas, including pigmented contact dermatitis (Fig. 19.1). On the basis of information about the textile finishes that actually came into contact with the patients' skin or were very commonly used, 115 chemicals were finally chosen and patch tested. The test materials included 50 dyes of all colors, 13 whiteners, 5 fungicides, 32 resin components, 13 softening agents, and 15 other miscellaneous textile finishes, which were widely used at that time by the textile industry in Japan. They were chosen from approximately 1,200 textile finishes, either imported or produced in Japan. They were checked for their solubility in water, ethanol, acetone, etc., diluted to 5% (except bactericides, fungicides, and other pesticides for textiles that were diluted to 1%), and then applied to dry paper disks 8 mm in diameter, to make dry allergen-containing disks named "instant patch test allergens." They were peeled off silicon-treated covering paper before use.

The results obtained from five hospitals in and around Tokyo revealed that several new contact sensitizers were responsible for producing textile dermatitis and secondary hyperpigmentation. These textile finishes included Biochek 60, a very toxic fungicide that seemed also to have acted as a sensitizer, a phosphite polymer of pentaerythritol and hydrogenated bisphenol A (PPP-HB), impurities in a dye CI Blue 19 (or Brilliant Blue R), and mercury compounds [9].

The research on these 115 chemicals was performed in the five hospitals on 80–101 persons, among whom 51–62 were patients suffering from textile contact dermatitis, and the rest, 29–39, were controls with atopic

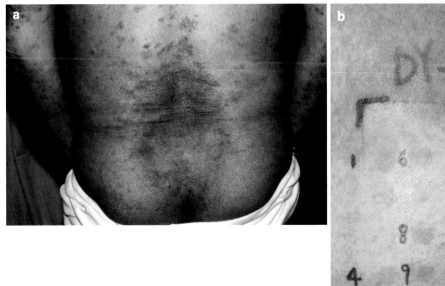
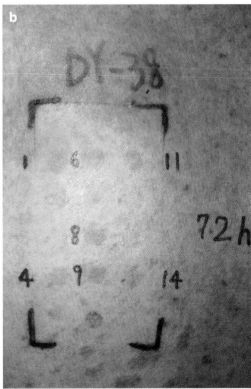

Fig. 19.1 Pigmented contact dermatitis (**a**) in a 67-year-old man who was sensitized by several textile finishes, including commercial grade *red* and *brown* dyes and fungicides (**b**)

dermatitis and dermatitis due to causes other than textiles. Among those with textile contact dermatitis, 27–33 had pigmented contact dermatitis. Such cases had been deliberately chosen for patch testing because the investigators hoped to find out the causative contact sensitizers producing such hyperpigmentation. Of these pigmented contact dermatitis patients, nine showed positive reactions suggestive of an allergy to Biochek 60 and one to several textile finishes. The results were rather disappointing, but they did show that it is not easy to discover the contact sensitizers producing pigmented contact dermatitis from contact with textile finishes. The discoveries of CH3566 and Naphthol AS can be regarded as having been important and valuable. Pigmented contact dermatitis due to blue dyes, Blue 106, and 124 was reported by Kovacevic et al. in 2001 [10].

Besides the above-mentioned textile finishes, rubber components can also produce dermatitis resulting in hyperpigmentation, mainly around the waist. Sometimes in such cases the pigmentation is not due to incontinentia pigmenti histologica, but to purpura (see Sect. 19.1.4). Thus far, only cases of pigmented contact dermatitis in

which causative allergens were found have been reported. Causes other than contact sensitivity have not yet been well investigated, except for friction melanosis which is described in Sect. 19.1.2.2.

19.1.2.2 Differential Diagnosis

Differential diagnosis of pigmented contact dermatitis due to washing powder or textile components includes Addison's disease, friction melanosis, amyloidosis cutis, drug eruption, atopic dermatitis with pigmentation and dermatitis, and secondary hyperpigmentation due to dental metal sensitivity (dental metal eruption).

Friction melanosis was frequently seen in Japan in the 1970s and 1980s, the disease consisting of dark brown or black hyperpigmentation unaccompanied by dermatitis or itching [11]. Friction melanosis occurred predominantly on the skin over or along bones, such as the clavicles, ribs, scapulae, spine, knees, and elbows. The color and distribution of friction melanosis sometimes lead to confusion with pigmented contact dermatitis. The disease, however, is produced by patients vigorously rubbing the skin with a hard nylon towel or nylon brush every day when bathing. Patch testing with various contact allergens failed to demonstrate allergens that seemed to be correlated with the disease. It was Tanigaki et al. [12] in 1983 who pointed out the causative association of rubbing with a nylon towel or brush, and the disease has gradually decreased since this hazard has become known to the public.

The use of nylon towels or brushes for washing the skin should, therefore, be checked before the diagnosis of pigmented contact dermatitis due to textiles is made. If the dark hyperpigmentation of the skin over bones gradually fades and disappears after the use of nylon towels or brushes is discontinued and patients change their mode of washing to a milder technique, the diagnosis of friction melanosis should be considered. Curiously, the histopathology of friction melanosis shows incontinentia pigmenti histologica, which is a characteristic feature of pigmented contact dermatitis. However, liquefaction degeneration of basal layer cells of the epidermis is not present [11].

Another skin disorder to be distinguished is skin amyloidosis, especially lichen amyloidosus or papular amyloidosis. It is possible that a small amount of amyloid, which can be demonstrated by Dylon staining, is found in lichenoid tissue reactions, probably because amyloid in the upper dermis is considered to be derived from degenerate epidermal cells produced by epidermal inflammation. Special staining with Congo red or thioflavine T and electron-microscopic study of the skin specimen are also helpful in the differential diagnosis.

19.1.2.3 Prevention and Treatment

It is essential to avoid the use of textiles and washing powders containing strong contact sensitizers, in order to prevent contact dermatitis and pigmented contact dermatitis of the skin areas that come into contact with the fabric and washing powders or softening agents that remain on them even after rinsing. There are, however, many textile finishes available today, with more than 1,200 commercial finishes being sold to the textile industry, and unfortunately their components are mainly secret. The purity of dyes is, in general, very low and some of the many impurities are allergenic.

For example, the very commonly used CI Blue 19 (or Brilliant Blue R) turned out to be allergenic and caused some patch-test-positive cases of pigmented contact dermatitis in 1985 [9]. Purified CI Blue 19, in contrast, never produced positive patch test reactions at the same 5% concentration.

The experiences accumulated in the past show that when entirely new textile finishes are introduced to the textile industry, the minimum safety evaluation tests such as LD50, Ames test, and skin irritation test should be performed, and their sensitization potential should be investigated by a research team including dermatologists. Strong contact sensitizers can be detected by several experimental procedures using animals. Although animal experiments are now the subject of ethical scrutiny in connection with such investigations, they are yet to indicate if the irritability and allergenicity of textile finishes are to be adequately investigated.

The textile industry should cooperate with dermatologists when pigmented contact dermatitis has once occurred, by immediately informing them of the components of the chemical finishes of the textile suspected to have caused the disease, and a precise study of impurities and quality control in the factory should also be performed. Shortening of the washing process should be strictly refrained, otherwise surplus dyes, their impurities, and other chemical finishes may remain and produce a problem.

When a causative allergen is discovered, the solution of pigmented contact dermatitis is not difficult [4, 5, 7]. However, when causative allergens are not identified, the solution of the pigmentary disorder is usually very difficult. In 1985, in Japan, a new strategy for the treatment of both recurrent textile dermatitis and pigmented contact dermatitis was introduced. Based on the research project for finding out contact sensitizers and irritants in textiles [9], underwear – with only four or five kinds of textile finishes that showed no evidence of positive reactions in patients with contact dermatitis, pigmented contact dermatitis, atopic dermatitis, and healthy controls – was put into mass production and became available. This is a measure to prevent the patients coming into contact with the responsible allergen in ordinary underwear again, and keeps the patients out of range of the responsible allergens.

Such allergen-free underwear for patients is called allergen-controlled wearing apparel (ACW) and has successfully counteracted pigmented contact dermatitis.

The idea was inspired by the success of allergen-controlled cosmetics in 1970, which is discussed later (see Sect. 19.1.3). It is not surprising that persistent secondary hyperpigmentation disappears only very slowly when the causative contact allergens are completely eliminated from the patient's environment for a long period, as the hyperpigmentation is considered to be brought about by frequent and repeated contact with a very small amount of contact sensitizer in the textile or washing material. Patients were requested to use allergen-free soaps and allergen-eliminated washing materials for their clothing at the same time, so that their skin was not contaminated by the responsible allergens in ordinary soaps and washing materials. Matsuo et al. reported several cases in which this treatment was successful [13, 14].

Even though cases are very rare, pigmented contact dermatitis can also occur following systemic contact dermatitis. In a 50-year-old man, for example, recurrent and persistent dermatitis accompanied diffuse secondary hyperpigmentation. The use of corticosteroid ointments, oral antihistamines, and allergen-free soaps did not improve the condition at all. A patch test with nickel sulfate 5% aq. showed a strong positive reaction, with a focal flare of most of the original skin lesion. This implied not only that the patient was sensitive to nickel, but also that only a few hundred parts per million of nickel ions absorbed from the patch test site into the bloodstream were enough to provoke an allergic reaction over a wide area of the site of the original skin lesions. This observation led to a search for a source of nickel ions in the patient, and five nickel alloys were subsequently found in the patient's oral cavity. He agreed to eliminate these nickel crowns, as they turned out to have been acting as cathodes, attracting an electric current of 1–3 mA at 100–200 mV. According to Faraday's law of electrolysis, cations elute from the cathode in proportion to the amount of electric current passing into the cathode.

The complete elimination of nickel-containing alloys from his oral cavity and their substitution with gold alloys, which did not contain any nickel at all, resulted in complete cure of the dermatitis and secondary hyperpigmentation in 3 months, and there has never been any recrudescence of the disease. The patient's pigmented contact dermatitis had been kept going for a long period by metal allergens continuously supplied from his own oral cavity [15].

19.1.3 Pigmented Cosmetic Dermatitis

19.1.3.1 Signs

> **Core Message**
>
> › Pigmented cosmetic dermatitis is caused by the same mechanism as pigmented contact dermatitis of the covered area; however, the causative allergens are quite different: a number of cosmetic allergens. Patch test of cosmetic series allergens is recommended, and continual and exclusive usage of allergen-controlled cosmetics and soaps cures the disease.

The most commonly seen hyperpigmentation due to contact dermatitis in the history of dermatology must be the pigmented cosmetic dermatitis, which affected the faces of Oriental women [16]. Innumerable patients with this pigmentary disorder presented in the 1960s and 1970s in Japan, and similar patients were also seen in Korea, India, Taiwan, China, and the USA.

The signs of pigmented cosmetic dermatitis are diffuse or reticular, black or dark brown hyperpigmentation of the face, which cannot be cured by the use of corticosteroid ointments or the continuous ingestion of vitamin C. The border of pigmented cosmetic dermatitis is not sharp, as in lichen planus or melasma, and it is not spot-like as in nevus of Ota tardus bilateralis.

Slight dermatitis is occasionally seen with hyperpigmentation, or dermatitis may precede hyperpigmentation. In contrast to Addison's disease, pigmented cosmetic dermatitis does not show any systemic symptoms such as weakness, fatigue, and emaciation. Laboratory findings such as full blood count, liver function tests, daily urinary excretion of 17-ketosteroid and 17-hydroxy corticosteroid, and serum immunoglobulins and electrolytes are normal in the majority of patients with pigmented cosmetic dermatitis [16].

Histopathological examination of pigmented cosmetic dermatitis shows basal liquefaction degeneration of the epidermis and incontinentia pigmenti histologica. The epidermis may be mildly acanthotic; however, it is sometimes atrophic, presumably the effect of frequently applied corticosteroid ointments for the treatment of itchy

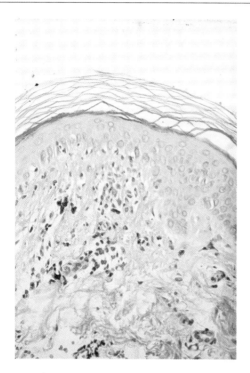

Fig. 19.2 Histopathology of a typical lichenoid reaction, with incontinentia pigmenti histologica of pigmented cosmetic dermatitis. The epidermis shows mild atrophy, and occasional liquefaction degeneration in the basal layer of the epidermis has dropped melanin pigments into the upper dermis. Note that the cellular infiltration in the upper dermis is not as dense as in lichen planus

dermatitis of the face. Cellular infiltrates of lymphocytes and histiocytes are seen perivascularly, as are often seen in ordinary allergic contact dermatitis (Fig. 19.2).

In some cases, the dark brown or black hyperpigmentation is also seen on skin other than on the face. The neck, chest, and back can be involved and, in a few exceptional cases, hyperpigmentation may extend to the whole body. In these cases, the allergens cinnamic alcohol and its derivatives sensitize the patients first to cosmetics and then provoke allergic reactions to soaps, domestic fabric softeners, and food, all of which sometimes contain cinnamic derivatives. The ingestion of 1 g cinnamon sugar from a cup of tea in a supermarket was enough to provoke a mild focal flare of dermatitis at the sites of diffuse reticular black hyperpigmentation of the whole body in one reported case [17]. When one of the common potent sensitizers producing pigmented cosmetic dermatitis, D & C Red 31 (Japanese name R-219), was discovered, a focal flare of dermatitis at the site of facial hyperpigmentation was occasionally noted by patch testing 5% R-219 in petrolatum. These findings show that the allergen could provoke the dermatitis not only by contact with the skin surface, but also from within the skin, by allergens transported via blood vessels, just as allergic contact dermatitis can be provoked by the administration of small amounts of nickel or drugs.

19.1.3.2 Causative Allergens

The term "pigmented cosmetic dermatitis" was introduced in 1973 for what had previously been known as melanosis faciei feminae when the mechanism (type IV allergy), most of the causative allergens, and successful treatment with allergen control for this miserable pigmentary disorder were clarified for the first time [18, 19]. The name was adopted by modifying Osmundsen's designation pigmented contact dermatitis, for the disease caused by CH3566 on the trunk.

Historically, the first description of the disease goes back to 1948, when Japanese dermatologists encountered this peculiar pigmentary disorder for the first time, and were greatly embarrassed as to diagnosis. Bibliographical surveys showed that Riehl's melanosis, described in 1917 [20], seemed probable, because World War II had ended just 3 years before the investigation. Subsequently, the disease was erroneously called Riehl's melanosis for almost 30 years in Asian countries. Riehl's melanosis, however, was a dark brown hyperpigmentation observed during World War I in Caucasian men, women, and children, when food was extremely scarce and the patients had to surivive on decayed corn and weed crops instead of normal food. Besides hyperpigmentation of the face, ears, and scalp, there were nodules and, histopathologically, dense cellular infiltration was present in the dermis. Cosmetics could be excluded as a cause because during World War I it was not possible for all these people, especially the men and children, to have used cosmetics before they contracted the disease. Riehl could not discover the true cause of this pigmentary disorder, but suspected the role of the abnormal wartime diet [20]. Riehl's melanosis disappeared when World War I ended, when normal food was available again, to reappear for a short period in France during the German occupation in World War II, when food became scarce yet again.

Consequently, Riehl's melanosis, a wartime melanosis having no relationship to cosmetic allergy, should not be confused with pigmented cosmetic dermatitis, which affected many Asian women in peacetime for many years. In 1950, Minami and Noma [21] designated the disease melanosis faciei feminae, and recognized the disease as a new entity. The causation was not known for many years. However, Japanese dermatologists gradually became aware of the role of cosmetics in this hyperpigmentation. First, it occurred only in those women, and very exceptionally men, who used cosmetics and, secondly, even though the bizarre brown hyperpigmentation was so conspicuous, the presence of slight, recurrent, or preceding dermatitis was observed. The problem for the dermatologists at that time was that the components of cosmetics were completely secret, and the kinds of cosmetic ingredients were too many (more than 1,000) for their allergenicity to be evaluated.

Finally, in 1969, a research project was set up to identify the causative allergens from 477 cosmetic ingredients by patch and photopatch testing. It was a new idea, because melanosis faciei feminae had been regarded as a metabolic disorder rather than a type of contact dermatitis. This was 7 years before Finn chambers became available; therefore, small patch test plasters of 10.2 cm with six disks 7 mm in diameter (Miniplaster) were put into production to enable 48–96 samples to be patch tested at 1 time on the backs of volunteer control subjects and patients. Many cosmetic ingredients, adjusted to nonirritant concentrations with the cooperation of 30–40 volunteers, were subsequently patch and photopatch tested in the patients. Results for each ingredient were obtained from 172 to 348 patients, including 79–121 with melanosis faciei feminae. Statistical evaluation brought to light a number of newly discovered contact sensitizers among the cosmetic ingredients, mainly fragrance materials and pigments, including jasmine absolute, ylang-ylang oil, cananga oil, benzyl salicylate, hydroxycitronellal, sandalwood oil, artificial sandalwood, geraniol, geranium oil, D & C Red 31, and Yellow No. 11 [16, 18, 19, 22].

Other rare causations of pigmented cosmetic dermatitis include fragrances, musk ambrette (Fig. 19.3), musk moskene [23], a pigment Orange F2G [24], and diisostearyl maleate in the lipsticks.

19.1.3.3 Treatment

The above-mentioned research project at the same time included a plan to produce soaps (acylglutamate) and cosmetics for the patients from whom the causative allergens had been completely eliminated, as even those who suffered from severe and bizarre hyperpigmentation

usually could not accept abandoning their use of cosmetics to remove this pigmentary disorder. Patch testing with a series of 30 standard cosmetic ingredients to find the allergens causing the disease [25], followed by the exclusive use of soaps and cosmetics that were completely allergen-free for such patients, designated the allergen control system and produced dramatic effects. Around 1970, most textbooks of dermatology in Japan said that melanosis faciei feminae was very difficult to cure and that the causation was unknown. However, after allergen control was introduced, the disease became completely curable. Table 19.2 shows the effect of allergen control in 165 cases reported to the American Academy of Dermatology in 1977, and also the long-term follow-up results of allergen control obtained by Watanabe after 3–11 years (mean, 5 years). In 50 cases of pigmented cosmetic dermatitis cured by allergen control (i.e., patch test with 30 cosmetic series patch test allergens [26] followed by the exclusive use of allergen-free soaps and cosmetics, Acseine® in Japan and Hong Kong), there were, on average, 2.5 allergens for each patient. It usually required 1–2 years for a patient to regain normal nonhyperpigmented facial skin (Figs. 19.3 and 19.4). Contamination with ordinary soaps and cosmetics was the most influential and decisive factor inhibiting therapy, because such ordinary daily necessities contained the allergens that were producing the disease. The patients were therefore requested to visit the dermatologist once a month to be checked for improvement, and were persuaded every time to avoid such contamination, including products used in beauty parlors [16, 27].

In 1979, Kozuka [26] discovered a new contact sensitizer, phenylazo-2-naphthol (PAN), as an impurity in

Table 19.2 Effect of allergen-controlled cosmetics on pigmented cosmetic dermatitis patients

	Nakayama et al. 1977	Watanabe 1989 [27]
Total	165	53
Complete cure	52	40
Almost complete cure	21	0
Remarkable improvement	51	13
Improvement	22	0
Not Effective	19	0
Follow-up	3 months to 5 years	3–11 years (mean 5 years)

Fig. 19.3 Diffuse and reticular type of pigmented cosmetic dermatitis in a 56-year-old woman (**a**). Patch test revealed a clear positive reaction to musk ambrette, a fragrant material, tested at 5% in a cream. In this case, the positive reaction was obtained without UV-A irradiation, and therefore, the reaction was not photoallergy, but ordinary contact allergy (**b**). Hyperpigmentation could not be cured by the application of corticosteroid ointments; however, it was completely cured by the exclusive usage of allergen-free cosmetics and soaps for 2 years. (**c**) shows complete cure was still maintained after 6 years of (**a**)

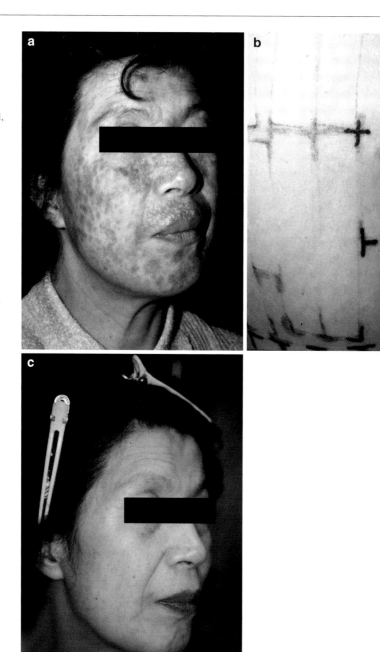

commercial supplies of D & C Red 31. Its sensitizing ability and ability to produce secondary hyperpigmentation were as great as those of Yellow No. 11 and, therefore, many industries began to eliminate or considerably decrease the amount of PAN and Yellow No. 11 in their products. The legal partial restriction of Red No. 31 and Yellow No. 11 by the Japanese government and the voluntary restriction by cosmetic companies of the use of allergenic fragrances, bactericides, and pigments resulted in a remarkable decrease in pigmented cosmetic dermatitis after 1980. One of the reasons for the proposal to change the name from "melanosis faciei feminae" to "pigmented cosmetic dermatitis" [18] was that the latter name makes it easier for the patients to

Fig. 19.4 Pigmented cosmetic dermatitis in a 43-year-old woman, caused by contact hypersensitivity to jasmine absolute (**a**). Jasmine absolute 10% in petrolatum produced reactions (site 1) which were still positive even on the eighth day of the patch test (**b**). The exclusive use of soaps and cosmetics that did not contain common and rare cosmetic sensitizers cleared the persistent dermatitis with pigmentation completely after 1 year and 8 months of use (**c**)

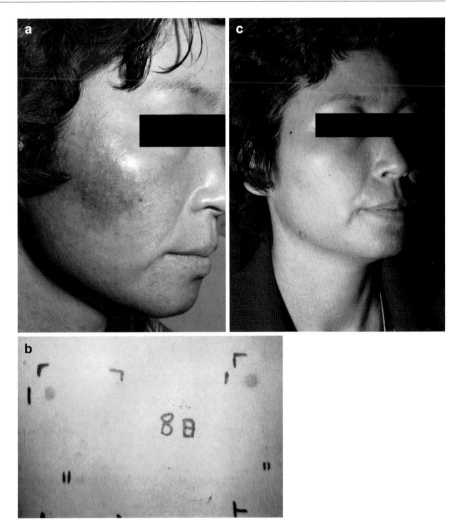

understand the causation of the disease and, at the same time, for industry to recognize the danger of cosmetics in producing such disastrous pigmentary disorders through contact sensitization. The disease was still present in the 2000s [28, 29], and the newer allergens included metal ions present in various cosmetics from containers and mixers for production. It is necessary for dermatologists to recognize the importance of cosmetic allergens in producing hyperpigmentation.

19.1.4 Purpuric Dermatitis

In 1886, Majocchi described purpura annularis telangiectodes and, 4 years later, Schamberg described a progressive pigmentary dermatitis, which is now well known as Schamberg's disease. The pigmentation in this dermatitis is due to the intradermal accumulation of hemosiderin, the predominant sites being the legs and thighs. Later, Gougerot and Blum described a similar dermatosis as pigmented purpuric lichenoid dermatitis.

The disease was rare but most often occurred in middle-aged or elderly men. However, when a similar disease occurred in many British soldiers during World War II, especially in those who sweated freely or experienced friction when wearing khaki shirts or woolen socks, with severe pruritus, dermatitis, and pigmentation due to purpura, dermatologists became aware that some textile finishes must have been responsible for the disease [30, 31]. Patch tests and use tests revealed that a blend of vegetable oils and oleic acid seemed to have been responsible.

In 1968, Batschvarov and Minkov [32] reported that rubber components such as *N*-phenyl-*N*´-isopropyl-*p*-phenylenediamine (IPPD), *N*-phenyl-b-naphthylamine (PNA), 2-mercaptobenzothiazole (MBT), and dibenzo-thiazole disulfide (DBD), i.e., derivatives of p-phenylene-diamine, naphthylamine, and benzothiazoles, were the allergens responsible for a purpuric dermatitis around the waist underneath the elastic of underwear. A similar pig-mented dermatitis was recognized in the shoulders, breasts, groins, and thighs. The capillary resistance (Rumpel-Leede) test was positive in all 23 cases studied. Similar test results were obtained in a smaller proportion of patients with the khaki dermatitis mentioned above. In Bulgaria, over 600 patients were recorded, and the neces-sity for dermatologists to investigate contact allergens in textiles to solve the problem of purpuric dermatitis of covered areas of skin was stressed [32]. A dye, blue 85, was reported as a causation in 1988 [33]. A case due to a textile finish of socks is demonstrated (Fig. 19.5).

19.1.5 "Dirty Neck" of Atopic Eczema

Core Message

> Today, there are many evidences that house dust mites are one of the most important causations of severe atopic dermatitis patients. Suffering from this dermatitis for many years often leads to reticular dark brown hyperpigmentation of the neck, i.e., the dirty neck. Finding out the worsening factors of each case by patch test and RAST, and the active removal of these factors, if necessary even house dust mites, by measur-ing the mite fauna of the patients' homes, is recommended.

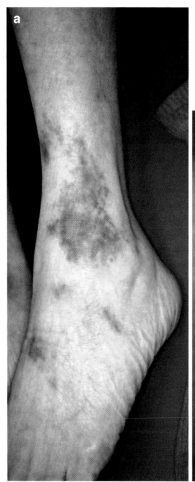
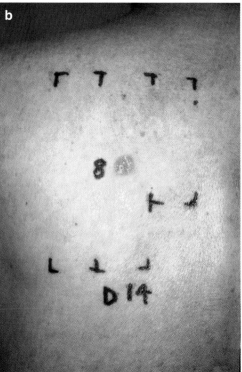

Fig. 19.5 Reticular brown hyperpigmentation of pigmented purpuric lichenoid dermatitis on an 80-year-old male (**a**). Biopsy showed marked hemorrhage around capillaries of the upper dermis, along with the cellular infiltrates composed of lymphocytes and histiocytes. Patch test revealed strong contact hypersensitivity to paratertia-rybutyl phenolformaldehyde resin at 1% petrolatum (**b**). It had been (site 8) positive from D2 to D14 and confirmative patch test was again strongly positive. Exposure to the contact allergen was considered to have been from the textile finishes of his socks. The exclusive usage of well-washed white cotton socks gradually improved the dermatitis. Complete blood count (CBC) and liver function test results were normal. This case indicates the importance of patch test of textile finishes, if possible, for the treatment of this pigmentary disorder

Atopic dermatitis has been increasing in incidence in many countries, and approximately 1.7–2% of moderate or severe atopic dermatitis patients suffer from reticular dark brown or dark purple pigmentation of the neck. It has been called "dirty neck" [34, 35]. Atopic dermatitis is a multifactorial disease with increased serum IgE in 70–80% of moderate or severe cases, and also shows an aspect of contact hypersensitivity to house dust mites [36–38], metals [39], and other environmental substances.

The elevation of serum IgE in patients with moderate or severe atopic dermatitis up to 2,000 or even to 20,000 IU/mL is peculiar, since with bronchial asthma, rhinitis, conjunctivitis, and urticaria, only rarely does the level of IgE exceed 1,000 IU/mL [40]. However, it is certain that some 20–30% of moderate or severe atopic dermatitis patients do not show any rise in serum IgE levels; therefore, one explanation for this controversy is that atopic dermatitis has two aspects of immunity for the production of eczema: first, IgE-mediated allergy resulting in spongiosis [41], and second, cell-mediated allergic contact dermatitis [42, 43].

The so-called dirty neck is, histologically, a moderate dermatitis composed of slight acanthosis, lymphocyte, and histiocyte infiltration around the vessels in the upper dermis, and incontinentia pigmenti histologica. The reticular pattern of "dirty neck" resembles macular amyloidosis; however, amyloid is usually negative according to Congo red stain, and only a small amount of amyloid was detected by electron microscopy [34]. The pigmentation and configuration are also similar to pigmented cosmetic dermatitis morphologically; however, the most commonly detected contact allergens with severe atopic dermatitis including "dirty neck" were not previously described cosmetic allergens, but frequently house dust mite components [36, 37]. Today, a test to demonstrate mite contact hypersensitivity is possible using a commercially sold patch test reagent Dermatophagoides Mix® (Chemotechnique, Sweden) in a Finn chamber. House dust mite proteins such as Der 1–7 have been known as sensitizers, and recently α-acaridial, a component of a house dust mite Tyrophagus putrescentiae, turned out to be a primary sensitizer [44]. Active sensitization was observed by the patch test of α-acaridial at 5–0.5% in petrolatum, and the positive reactions in the appearance of prurigo were maintained for 1–11 months. It is amazing that such a strong contact sensitizer is present in house dust mites.

The treatment of "dirty neck" is not easy. When the mite fauna were investigated by a new methylene blue agar method in the homes of atopic dermatitis patients, and environmental improvements were made to decrease the mite numbers to fewer than 20/m² at 20 s aspiration using a 320-W cleaner, 88% of severe atopic dermatitis patients showed considerable improvement in their severe dermatitis when they were followed up for 1–2 years [45]. The statistically significant effect of house dust mite elimination with controls in atopic dermatitis was also reported by Tan et al. [46]. The "dirty neck," however, was difficult to cure even with this method, and it can be regarded as the last symptom to improve for atopic dermatitis (Fig. 19.6).

19.2 Depigmentation from Contact with Chemicals

19.2.1 Mechanism of Leukoderma Due to Chemicals

There are at least three kinds of mechanism producing leukoderma from contact with chemicals:

- Leukoderma due to selective destruction of melanocytes.
- Leukomelanoderma or photoleukomelanoderma due to pigment blockade.
- Hypopigmentation due to reduction of melanin synthesis.

Allergic contact dermatitis and irritant contact dermatitis can both produce a secondary leukoderma, which is almost impossible to differentiate from idiopathic vitiligo. The incidence is low, except for certain phenol derivatives and catechols, which produce a much higher incidence in workers who frequently come into contact with them (Table 19.3).

Monobenzyl ether of hydroquinone (MBEH) has been known to be a cause of occupational vitiligo since the 1930s [47], the main source of contact having been rubber, in which it is used as an antioxidant to prevent degeneration. The use of MBEH in the rubber industry today is rare, as it had a long history of causing occupational leukoderma by destroying melanocytes. Instead, MBEH came to be used as a bleaching agent for melanotic skin, being used to treat diseases such as

19

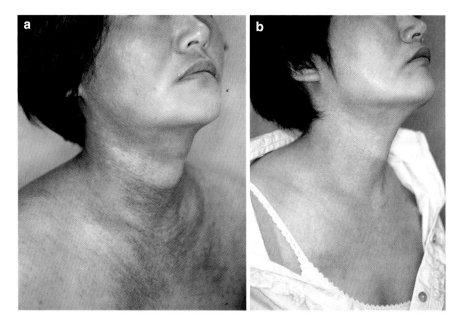

Fig. 19.6 A severe case of atopic dermatitis of a 28-year-old woman had resulted in "dirty neck" for almost 10 years (**a**). The generalized severe eczema could not be sufficiently controlled by corticosteroid ointments; therefore, among her multiple allergens, mite and metal were selected for elimination to obtain improvement. First, mite fauna was investigated in her home followed by environmental improvement to efficiently decrease Dermatophagoides. Second, she was hypersensitive to stannic (tin) derivatives; therefore, dental metals containing stannic were all eliminated and replaced by other metals to which she was not hypersensitive. Tacrolimus ointment has been used as an antisymptomatic treatment recently. Generalized severe eczema disappeared after the above-mentioned allergen elimination, then "dirty neck" slowly disappeared in 4 years, as the last symptom of this case (**b**)

melasma and solar lentigo and by dark-skinned people for cosmetic purposes. However, as its toxic effect on melanocytes was too strong, the treatment often resulted in a mottled pattern of leukoderma (confetti-like depigmentation), which was worse than simple hyperpigmentation, and produced problems [48].

Historically, the next chemical to produce leukoderma by contact was 4-tert-butylcatechol (PTBC), known since the 1970s [49, 50]. Approximately half of the 75 workers in a tappet assembly plant in the United States were reported to have various grades of leukoderma from daily occupational contact with PTBC. Four severe cases reported in 1970 by Gellin et al. [47] initially had itchy erythematous reactions at the sites of contact, then developed sharply outlined or confluent leukoderma on the face, scalp, hands, fingers, forearms, etc. The patients were all Caucasians.

Patch tests revealed that 0.1% PTBC in acetone produced positive reactions in three of these four cases, one of whom later developed leukoderma at the site of the patch test. However, an exposure test with 1% PTBC in the assembly oil, carried out with occlusion of the forearms in six volunteers, failed to produce leukoderma artificially. Animal tests revealed that PTBC was an irritant, producing erythema and necrosis in albino rabbits, and a bleaching test with 10% PTBC in black guinea pigs resulted in depigmentation of the black skin, both macroscopically and histologically, from the loss of pigment in the epidermis and hair follicles.

At almost the same time, at the beginning of the 1970s, occupational contact leukoderma due to p-tert-butylphenol (PTBP) began to be recognized. The incidence of vitiligo vulgaris in the general population was considered to be less than 1%. Therefore, the presence of several cases of vitiligo, located mainly on exposed areas of skin, in the same factory of 20–30 workers alerted dermatologists to the fact that the depigmentation was an occupational dermatosis [51]. PTBP is contained in cobblers' glues, shoes cemented with rubber glues, resins, industrial oils, paints, adhesives, bactericides, plasticizers for cellulose acetate, and printing inks [51–54].

The changes produced by PTBP are similar to those caused by p-tert-butylcatechol, and can occur with or

Table 19.3 Chemicals producing leukoderma or hypopigmentation on contact

Hydroquinone	
Monobenzyl ether of hydroquinone	
p-*tert*-butylcatechol (PTBC)	
p-*tert*-butylphenol (PTBP)	
Kojic acid (hypopigmentation only)	
Catechol	
Monomethyl ether of hydroquinone (MMEH)	
Alstroemeria components (tulipalin A)	
Squaric acid dibutylester	
Cerium oxide	CeO$_2$

without sensitization. Kahn [52] and Romaguera et al. [55] reported patients who were apparently sensitized to PTBP with positive reactions on a closed patch test with 1% PTBP.

Hydroquinone is an excellent depigmenting agent for clinical treatment of various pigmentations [56]. However, it may rarely produce leukoderma that is similar to vitiligo vulgaris [57, 58]. The mechanism of the hypopigmentation caused by hydroquinone is thought to be decreased formation of melanosomes and destruction of the membranous organelles in the melanocytes, thereby causing degeneration of melanocytes [59].

These historically accumulated cases of contact leukoderma caused by phenol derivatives indicate that selective toxicity of these chemicals to melanocytes is the main cause of leukoderma, judging from the degeneration of melanocytes, the irritation often noted, and the fact that sensitization is not always demonstrated.

Another hazard of using hydroquinone as a bleaching agent is ochronosis, especially when it is used at high concentrations (e.g., 3.5–7.5%) [60]. Ochronosis means "yellow disease," and black Africans suffer

19

from hyperpigmentation of the face due to the degeneration of elastic fibers caused by this topical agent [61]. Therefore, the use of hydroquinone as a bleaching agent by blacks should be advised carefully, and high concentrations are not recommended.

19.2.2 Contact Leukoderma Caused Mainly by Contact Sensitization

Very rarely, allergic contact dermatitis produces a secondary depigmentation similar to vitiligo. A gardener was reported to have developed secondary leukoderma after allergic contact dermatitis due to Alstroemeria [62], and when squaric acid dibutylester was used for immunotherapy in a 26-year-old male with alopecia areata, depigmentation over the whole scalp was reported after repeated contact dermatitis produced by nine courses of treatment. Regrowth of hair was also noted [63]. A herbicide, Carbyne R, and cerium oxide have also been reported to produce contact hypersensitivity and secondary leukoderma [64, 65].

References

1. Papa CM, Kligman AM (1965) The behavior of melanocytes in inflammation. J Invest Dermatol 45:465–474
2. Nakamura T (1977) Toxicoderma caused by "Shiitake", lentinus edodos (in Japanese). Rinsho-Hifuka 31:65–68
3. Osmundsen PE (1969) Contact dermatitis due to an optical whitener in washing powders. Br J Dermatol 81:799–803
4. Osmundsen PE (1970) Pigmented contact dermatitis. Br J Dermatol 83:296–301
5. Ancona-Alayón A, Escobar-Márques R, González-Mendoza A et al (1976) Occupational pigmented contact dermatitis from Naphthol AS. Contact Dermat 2:129–134
6. Kawachi S, Kawashima T, Akiyama J et al (1985) Pigmented contact dermatitis due to dyes from nightgown (in Japanese). Hifuka No Rinsho 27(91–92):181–187
7. Hayakawa R, Matsunaga K, Kojima S et al (1985) Naphthol AS as a cause of pigmented contact dermatitis. Contact Dermat 13:20–25
8. Osawa J, Takekawa K, Onuma S, Kitamura K, Ikezawa Z (1997) Pigmented contact dermatitis due to Naphthol AS in a pillow case. Contact Dermat 37:37–38
9. Nakayama H, Suzuki A (1985) Investigation of skin disturbances caused by the chemicals contained in daily necessities, part 1. On the ability of textile finishes to produce dermatitis (in Japanese). Tokyo-To Living Division Report. pp 1–27
10. Kovacevic Z, Kränke B (2001) Pigmented purpuric contact dermatitis from Disperse Blue 106 and 124 dyes. J Am Acad Dermatol 45:456–458
11. Takayama N, Suzuki T, Sakurai Y et al (1984) Friction melanosis (in Japanese). Nishinihon Hifuka (West Japan Dermatol) 46:1340–1345
12. Tanigaki T, Hata S, Kitano M et al (1983) On peculiar melanosis occuring on the trunk and extremities (in Japanese). Rinsho Hifuka 37:347–351
13. Matsuo S, Nakayama H, Suzuki A (1989) Successful treatment with allergen controlled wearing apparel of textile dermatitis patients (in Japanese). Hifu 31(Suppl 6):178–185
14. Nakayama H (1989) Allergen control, an indispensable treatment for allergic contact dermatitis. Dermat Clin 8:197–204
15. Nakayama H (1987) Dental metal and allergy (in Japanese). Jpn J Dent Assoc 40:893–903
16. Nakayama H, Matsuo S, Hayakawa K et al (1984) Pigmented cosmetic dermatitis. Int J Dermatol 23:299–305
17. Matsuo S, Nakayama H (1984) A case of pigmented dermatitis induced by cinnamic derivatives (in Japanese). Hifu 26:573–579
18. Nakayama H (1974) Perfume allergy and cosmetic dermatitis (in Japanese). Jpn J Dermatol 84:659–667
19. Nakayama H, Hanaoka H, Ohshiro A (1974) Allergen controlled system. Kanehara Shuppan, Tokyo, pp 1–42
20. Von Riehl G (1917) Über eine eigenartige Melanose. Wien Klin Wochenschr 30:780–781
21. Minami S, Noma Y (1950) Melanosis faciei feminae (in Japanese). Dermatol Urol 12:73–77
22. Nakayama H, Harada R, Toda M (1976) Pigmented cosmetic dermatitis. Int J Dermatol 15:673–675
23. Hayakawa R, Hirose O, Arima Y (1991) Pigmented contact dermatitis due to musk moskene. J Dermatol 18(7): 420–424
24. Jolanki R, Kanerva L, Estlander T (1987) Organic pigments in plastics can cause allergic contact dermatitis. Acta Derm Venereol Suppl (Stockh) 134:95–97
25. Nakayama H (1983) Cosmetic series patch test allergens, types 19 to 20 (in Japanese, with English abstract). Fragrance Journal, Tokyo, pp 1–121
26. Kozuka T, Tashiro M, Sano S et al (1979) Brilliant Lake Red R as a cause of pigmented contact dermatitis. Contact Dermat 5:294–304
27. Watanabe N (1989) Long term follow-up of allergen control system on patients with cosmetic dermatitis (in Japanese). Nishinihon Hifuka 51:113–130
28. Gonçalo S, Sil J, Gonçalo M, Polares Batista A (1991) Pigmented photoallergic contact dermatitis from musk ambrette. Contact Dermat 24:229–231
29. Trattner A, Hodak E, David M (1999) Screening Patch tests for pigmented contact dermatitis in Israel. Contact Dermat 40:155–157
30. Greenwood K (1960) Dermatitis with capillary fragility. Arch Dermatol 81:947–952
31. Twiston Davies JH, Neish Barker A (1944) Textile dermatitis. Br J Dermatol 56:33–43
32. Batschvarov B, Minkov DM (1968) Dermatitis and purpura from rubber in clothing. Trans St John's Hosp Dermatol Soc 54:178–182
33. Van der Veen JPW, Neering H, DeHaan P et al (1988) Pigmented purpuric clothing dermatitis due to Disperse Blue 85. Contact Dermat 19:222–223

34. Humphreys F, Spencer J, McLaren K, Tidman MJ (1996) An histological and ultrastructural study of the dirty neck appearance in atopic eczema. Clin Exp Dermatol 21:17–19
35. Manabe T, Inagaki Y, Nakagawa S et al (1987) Ripple pigmentation of the neck in atopic dermatitis. Am J Dermatopathol 9:301–307
36. Nakayama H (1995) The role of the house dust mite in atopic eczema. Practical contact dermatitis. McGraw-Hill, New York, pp 623–630
37. Vincenti C, Trevisi P, Guerra L, Lorenzi S, Tosti A (1994) Patch testing with whole dust mite bodies in atopic dermatitis. Am J Contact Dermat 5:213–215
38. Sakurai M (1996) Results of patch tests with mite components in atopic dermatitis patients (in Japanese with English abstract). Allergy 45:398–408
39. Shanon J (1965) Pseudoatopic dermatitis, contact dermatitis due to chrome sensitivity simulating atopic dermatitis. Dermatologica 131:118–190
40. Okudaira H (1997) Atopic diseases and house dust mite allergens (in Japanese with English abstract). Hifu 39 (Suppl 19):45–51
41. Bruynzeel-Koomen C VanWichen, DF TJ et al (1986) The presence of IgE molecules on epidermal Langerhans cells in patients with atopic dermatitis. Arch Dermatol Res 278: 199–205
42. Imayama S, Hashizume T, Miyahara H et al (1992) Combination of patch test and IgE for dust mite antigens differences 130 patients with atopic dermatitis into four groups. J Am Acad Dermatol 27:531–538
43. Rawle FC, Mitchell EB, Platts-Mills TAE (1984) T cell responses to major allergen from the house dust mite Dermatophagoides pteronyssinus antigen P1: comparison of patients with asthma, atopic dermatitis, and perennial rhinitis. J Immunol 44:195–201
44. Nakayama H, Kumei A (2003) House dust mite – an important causation of atopic dermatitis. SP World 31:13–20
45. Kumei A (1995) Investigation of mites in the house of atopic dermatitis (AD) patients, and clinical improvements by mite elimination (in Japanese with English abstract). Allergy 44:116–127
46. Tan BB, Weald D, Strickland I, Friedmann PS (1996) Double-blind controlled trial of effect of housedust-mite allergen avoidance on atopic dermatitis. Lancet 347: 15–18
47. Oliver EA, Schwartz L, Warren LH (1939) Occupational leukoderma: preliminary report. J Am Med Assoc 113: 927–928
48. Yoshida Y, Usuba M (1958) Monobenzyl ether of hydroquinone leukomelanodermia (in Japanese). Rinsho Hifuka Hinyokika 12:333–338
49. Gellin GA, Possik PA, Davis IH (1970) Occupational depigmentation due to 4-tertiarybutyl catechol (TBC). J Occup Med 12:386–389
50. Gellin GA, Maibach HI, Mislazek MH, Ring M (1979) Detection of environmental depigmenting substances. Contact Dermat 5:201–213
51. Malten KE, Sutter E, Hara I, Nakajima T (1971) Occupational vitiligo due to paratertiary butylphenol and homologues. Trans St John's Hosp Dermatol Soc 57:115–134
52. Kahn G (1970) Depigmentation caused by phenolic detergent germicides. Arch Dermatol 102:177–187
53. Malten KE (1967) Contact sensitization caused by p-tert-butylphenol and certain phenolformaldehyde-containing glues. Dermatologica 135:54–59
54. Malten KE (1975) Paratertiary butylphenol depigmentation in a consumer. Contact Dermat 1:180–192
55. Romaguera C, Grimalt F (1981) Occupational leukoderma and contact dermatitis from paratertiary-butylphenol. Contact Dermat 7:159–160
56. Arndt KA, Fitzpatrick TB (1965) Topical use of hydroquinone as a depigmenting agent. J Am Med Assoc 194: 965–967
57. Frenk E, Loi-Zedda P (1980) Occupational depigmentation due to a hydroquinone-containing photographic developer. Contact Dermat 6:238–239
58. Kersey P, Stevenson CJ (1981) Vitiligo and occupational exposure to hydroquinone from servicing self-photographing machines. Contact Dermat 7:285–287
59. Jimbow K, Obata H, Pathak M, Fitzpatrick TB (1974) Mechanism of depigmentation by hydroquinone. J Invest Dermatol 62:436–449
60. Findlay GH (1982) Ochronosis following skin bleaching with hydroquinone. J Am Acad Dermatol 6:1092–1093
61. Hoshaw RA, Zimmerman KG, Menter A (1985) Ochronosis-like pigmentation from hydroquinone bleaching creams in American Blacks. Arch Dermatol 121:105–108
62. Björkner BE (1982) Contact allergy and depigmentation from alstromeria. Contact Dermat 8:178–184
63. Valsecchi R, Cainelli T (1984) Depigmentation from squaric acid dibutyl ester. Contact Dermat 10:108
64. Brancaccio RR, Chamales MH (1977) Contact dermatitis and depigmentation produced by the herbicide carbyne. Contact Dermat 3:108–109
65. Rapaport MJ (1982) Depigmentation with cerium oxide. Contact Dermat 8:282–283

Hand Eczema

20

Tove Agner

Contents

20.1 Epidemiology

20.1.1 Frequency

The occurrence of hand eczema depends on basal characteristics such as age, sex, atopy and occupation in the population, which is investigated. In a Swedish study, the self-reported 1-year prevalence of hand eczema in the general population was 11.8% in 1983 and had decreased to 9.7% in 1996 [1, 2]. The crude incidence rate of self-reported hand eczema in individuals aged 20–65 years has been reported to be 5.5–8.5 cases per 1,000 person-years [3, 4]. The incidence of hand eczema is high among young people. In school children, the 1-year prevalence of hand eczema was reported to be 7.3% for children aged 12–16 years and 10.0% for children aged 16–19 years, respectively [5, 6]. Early onset of hand eczema is frequent, and in around one third of cases, onset of hand eczema occurs before the age of 20 [4].

20.1.2 Risk Factors

Hand eczema may often take a chronic course with a tendency to frequent relapses. A history of earlier hand eczema is a major indication of vulnerable skin, predisposing the individual for development of hand eczema. Even short episodes of eczema may predict a tendency to future disease, and the most important risk factor for the development of hand eczema seems to be previous episodes of hand eczema earlier in life [7]. Atopic dermatitis is another major predictive factor, and considerably increased risk for the development of hand eczema in persons with previous or current atopic

T. Agner
Department of Dermatology, University of Copenhagen,
Bispebjerg Hospital, Bispebjerg Bakke 23,
2400 Copenhagen NV, Denmark
e-mail: t.agner@dadlnet.dk

J.D. Johansen et al. (eds.), *Contact Dermatitis*,
DOI: 10.1007/978-3-642-03827-3_20, © Springer-Verlag Berlin Heidelberg 2011

20

dermatitis is well established. In a population study, a history of childhood eczema was found to be more important for the development of hand eczema than other risk factors such as female sex and occupational exposure [8]. The prevalence of hand eczema in adults reporting moderate and severe atopic dermatitis in childhood was 25% and 41%, respectively [9], and a long-term follow-up study confirmed that more than 40% of patients attending the Karolinska Hospital in Stockholm for atopic dermatitis in childhood had developed hand eczema when re-examined 25 years later [10]. In a population-based survey including 15,000 people, 42% of those who reported childhood eczema stated positively that they had hand eczema at some time [11]. The importance of mucosal atopy for the development of hand eczema is not fully agreed, but it is a significantly less essential risk factor than atopic dermatitis [4, 9, 12, 13]. Although the frequency of atopic dermatitis has been increasing over the last decades, the prevalence of hand eczema has, however, slightly decreased between 1983 and 1996 in Swedish adults (from 11.8 to 9.7, [2]). The decrease in the prevalence of hand eczema could be an effect of an increased focus on preventive measures for occupational diseases during the last decades.

Hand eczema occurs more frequently in females than in males [1, 8, 14–16], the female/male-ratio being 1.8/1 [4]. Females are traditionally more exposed to wet work than males, and many jobs involving extensive wet work, e.g. hairdressing, health care work, catering and cleaning, are usually female-jobs. Generally, females report more hand washings per day than males [4, 11], and they may often have more domestic irritant skin exposure, including cooking and child caring. No sex-related difference in skin susceptibility to irritants has been reported from experimental studies [17]. In a recent population-based twin study, female sex was confirmed to be a risk factor for the development of hand eczema, but when nickel allergy and wet work were included as co-variates in the analysis, the effect of gender was no longer statistically significant [18]. This clearly indicates that the high frequency of hand eczema in females compared to males is caused by different exposures.

Recent findings point to the fact that the increased risk for adult women to develop hand eczema is present in the age group 20–29 years only, in which the incidence rate is doubled as compared to males, while no increased risk for women is present beyond the age of 30 [4]. An increased amount of wet work in young

females is most likely to explain this pattern [4]. Female preponderance among hand eczema patients has, however, also been reported in school pupils, probably due to increased frequency of atopic dermatitis and nickel allergy among females in the study population [5].

Contact allergy, and especially nickel allergy, is generally accepted to be a risk factor for the development of hand eczema [18–20]. The interaction between nickel allergy and hand eczema was analysed by Menné et al., who found it to be "both ways" [21]: Compared with non-nickel-sensitive females, those who had become nickel sensitised ran an increased risk of developing hand eczema, and those who had first developed hand eczema ran an increased risk of developing nickel allergy later [21]. This association has been confirmed in more recent studies [5, 11, 18, 19]; however, it was recently reported that contact allergy to nickel in childhood did not seem to increase the prevalence of hand eczema later in life [22]. In two cross-sectional studies examining the prevalence of hand eczema and contact allergy of the general population in Copenhagen performed before and after nickel exposure regulation in Denmark, the first study in 1990 found a significant association between nickel allergy and a history of hand eczema in women, while the second study in 1998 could not find this association [23]. This is probably due to the diminished nickel exposure after nickel legislation was introduced [24] and is an interesting example of how regulations and legislation as preventive measures may diminish the risk for contact allergy and subsequently for hand eczema. Tobacco and alcohol have been debated as risk factors for hand eczema. No clear association was found between prevalence of hand eczema and smoking or alcohol [3, 25].

20.1.3 Validity of Self-Reported Hand Eczema

Much information about occurrence and risk factors for hand eczema is based on questionnaires asking either risk groups or the general population about clinical signs of previous and present hand eczema. Naturally, this way of obtaining information is not as precise as an objective assessment by a dermatologist. The validity of self-reported hand eczema depends on the type of population investigated and has been evaluated in several studies. It is generally agreed that self-reported prevalence of hand eczema underestimates the true prevalence [26]. A simple question as "do you have hand eczema?" had higher sensitivity and specificity than more complex symptom-based questions, since it is difficult for individuals to identify skin signs compatible with the clinical diagnosis of hand eczema [27]. Standardised questions for occupational hand eczema have been developed, providing more standardised data [28].

20.2 Aetiology and Morphology

> **Core Message**
>
> › A precise diagnosis is necessary for optimal treatment and prevention.

The most common aetiology for hand eczema is irritant contact dermatitis (35%), followed by atopic hand eczema (22%) and allergic contact dermatitis (19%), while endogenous forms as vesicular eczema and hyperkeratotic eczema only constitute a minor group [1, 29].

It is important to realise that the aetiology of hand eczema cannot be determined from the clinical manifestations, and that different etiological diagnoses cannot be distinguished by clinical pattern [30, 31]. Although a clinical presentation with numerous vesicles may indicate an allergic contact dermatitis, and a chronic, scaly appearance may lead to a suspicion of irritant contact dermatitis, these clinical signs may in some cases be misleading, and omission of a full diagnostic programme cannot be justified. Until now there has been no general agreement on classification of hand eczema, but recently a proposal for this has been published [32].

> **Core Message**
>
> › Morphology may not be related to aetiology.

20.2.1 Allergic Contact Dermatitis

> **Core Message**
>
> › Patients with hand eczema lasting for more than one month should be patch tested.

A positive patch test with relevance to the current hand eczema may be expected to occur in less than 1/3 of all cases of hand eczema. Contact sensitisation may be the primary cause of hand eczema, or may be a complication to irritant or atopic hand eczema. Number of positive patch tests has been reported to correlate positively with the duration of hand eczema, indicating that longstanding hand eczema may often be complicated with sensitisation [33]. The most common contact allergies in patients with hand eczema are nickel, cobalt, fragrance-mix, balsam of Peru and colophony [1]. Contact sensitivity, especially to nickel, but also to other allergens, is generally considered to be a risk factor for the development of hand eczema [5, 21, 33] and the risk increases with increasing strength of contact allergy [18, 19]. The importance of metal allergy for flare-up of hand eczema was underlined in experimental studies of hand eczema in patients with metal allergy. Exposure to even very low doses of the metal caused a flare-up in the sensitised patients, but not in controls [34, 35]. Allergic nickel contact dermatitis seems to be caused mainly by environmental, and only to a lesser degree, by genetic factors [36].

Recent papers also indicate that fragrance allergy can be a common and relevant problem in patients with hand eczema, since perfumes are often present in consumer products to which the hands are exposed [37]. Formaldehyde allergy was also found to be of significance for patients with hand eczema [38], and more recently, sensitisation to methyldibromo glutaronitrile was frequently found to be relevant in patients with hand eczema [39].

20.2.2 Irritant Contact Dermatitis

Irritant contact dermatitis is the most common cause of hand eczema [29]. In an epidemiological population-based study, irritant factors were found to play either a primary or an additional role in 73% of all cases of hand eczema [40]. The most common exposure to cause irritant contact dermatitis on the hands is wet work, at the working place or at home. Young women are of special risk for this type of hand eczema, since this group has an increased frequency of occupational exposure to wet work, and at the same time, has a significant domestic exposure.

Children below 4 years of age in the family and lack of dishwashing machine have been demonstrated

20

as separate and significant risk factors for hand eczema [13]. The level of pre-existing skin irritation and barrier disruption is important for the skin susceptibility to further irritation. Detergents have a significant ability to harm the barrier function of the skin, which can be quantified as an increased transepidermal water loss. This explains that wet work is in a majority of cases a complicating factor, since the disturbed barrier function leads to an increased penetration of irritants, allergens and bacteria. Combined effects of irritants and allergens may change the threshold value for elicitation of allergic contact dermatitis, either by immunological effects or by enhanced penetration of allergen [41]. Elicitation thresholds for allergens may be considerably influenced by the simultaneous exposure.

In a population-based twin study hereditary risk factors were found to play a significant part in the development of hand eczema in the general population, when no extreme environmental exposure exists [14]. Recently, it was concluded that this heretability is not explained by co-morbidity with atopic eczema [42]. This hereditary risk factor could only partly be explained by atopic dermatitis or contact allergy, and a separate genetic risk factor, independent of atopic dermatitis and contact allergy, is suggested to be of importance for the development of irritant contact dermatitis of the hands [18, 19].

20.2.3 Atopic Dermatitis

Persons with atopic dermatitis have a significantly increased risk for the development of hand eczema when exposed to irritants at work or at home [43]. Preventive measures are taken to inform young people with atopic dermatitis to avoid a profession including wet or dirty work or food handling. Hand eczema in atopics often takes a chronic course, and change of job seems to improve the prognosis less for atopics than for others [10]. The cellular immunity in atopics is decreased, and allergic contact dermatitis seems to occur in a smaller number of patients with past or present atopic disease than in non-atopics [44]. Positive patch tests, often related to topical treatments, are however, sometimes found in atopics, and patch testing should be performed as in other patients with hand eczema. It has traditionally been the clinical

impression that involvement of the dorsal hand surfaces and the volar wrist may suggest atopic dermatitis to be a contributing aetiological factor [45], but this was not confirmed in a recent study on classification of hand eczema [32]. Recently, with the identification of null mutations within the gene encoding the key epidermal protein filaggrin, a breakthrough in the genetics of atopic eczema has been achieved [46]. Filaggrin is an essential component in keratinocyte differentiation and has also been attributed a regulatory role for natural moisturising factors. A possible association between the variant alleles and chronic hand eczema has been studied. While Lerbaek et al. [47] were not able to find an association to hand eczema or contact allergy, other studies have supported that nonfunctional mutations in the filaggrin gene may contribute to manifestation of a chronic hand eczema subtype [48, 49].

20.2.4 Contact Urticaria

Contact urticaria on the hands may in a chronic phase imitate eczema, so that this entity cannot be recognised from the clinical examination only. Skin prick tests or RAST tests are necessary to identify contact urticaria, which on the hands are most often found after occupational exposure either to latex gloves or to food. Contact urticaria on the hands has an increased frequency in atopics.

20.2.5 Endogenous Forms

20.2.5.1 Vesicular Hand Eczema (Pompholyx)

Vesicular hand eczema is a clinical manifestation of hand eczema with an uncertain aetiology [50, 51]. Preceded by itching, a vesicular eruption occurs on the palmar aspects of fingers and hand, interdigitally and sometimes in the periungual area. Infections and allergic contact dermatitis should be excluded. A relationship to atopic dermatitis, to tinea pedis and to nickel allergy has been suspected. In a recent study an association to tinea pedis was statistically confirmed, while no association with atopy or nickel allergy could be established [19].

20.2.5.2 Hyperkeratotic Eczema

Hyperkeratotic dermatitis of the palms is a clinically characteristic entity that occurs mainly in individuals above the age of 40. Hyperkeratosis is present symmetrically in the palms, fissures are common, while vesicles are not found. It may, however, be preceded by an initial vesicular stage. Although hard manual labour may be a risk factor for hyperkeratotic hand eczema, no such thing can be identified in the majority of cases [52, 110]. The differential diagnosis to psoriasis may sometimes be difficult, but widespread lesions are not found in hyperkeratotic eczema. Also in case of a clinically typical hyperkeratotic hand eczema patch testing should be performed, since the clinical pattern may sometimes be misleading, or a complicating contact allergy may be identified (Tables 20.1 and 20.2).

20.3 Severity Assessment

Disease severity is not only important in clinical studies, but also in the clinical work to monitor the effect of treatment. Different scoring systems have been developed, evaluated and found useful [53–55]. However, the patient and the doctor may assess severity quite different from each other, indicating that other parameters than just clinical severity should be supported during treatment of the disease [56, 57].

20.4 Occupational Hand Eczema

Skin diseases constitute up to 30% of all occupational diseases. The most common work-related dermatosis is contact dermatitis, for which the annual incidence is reported to be 12.9 per 100,000 workers [58, 59].

Core Message

> ❯ Hand eczema is one of the most commonly recognised occupational diseases and also one of the most expensive in workers compensation.

Table 20.1 Diagnosis of hand eczema

Medical history

  Questions:

    Previous episodes of hand eczema

    Atopic dermatitis (previous or current)

    Psoriasis

Exposures

  Domestic

  Occupational

  Leisure time

Clinical examination

  Assessment of severity

  Assessment of morphology

    Localisation

    Extension

    Hyperkeratotic

    Vesicular eczema

Patch testing

Should be performed in all patients with hand eczema lasting for more than 1 months. In case of positive patch test reactions:

  Present relevance? (exposure assessment)

  Past relevance?

  Unknown relevance?

Based on the examination above, one or more of the following diagnoses should be reached

  Irritant contact dermatitis

    Occupational

    Non-occupational

  Allergic contact dermatitis (or allergic contact urticaria)

    Occupational

    Non-occupational

  Atopic dermatitis

  Endogenous dermatitis (hyperkeratotic, vesicular)

(Several aetiological factors may often be included in the diagnosis, e.g. irritant contact dermatitis and atopic dermatitis, or allergic contact dermatitis and irritant contact dermatitis)

Occupational contact dermatitis is most often located on the hands. The true incidence for occupational hand eczema varies from one region to another, dependent on industrialisation and workplaces in the region. Legal aspects regarding occupational hand eczema and workers' compensation influence the frequency by which the cases are reported to the authorities, and the

Table 20.2 Treatment and prevention of hand eczema

Allergen and irritant avoidance

Exposure assessment

Substitution of products causing irritation (domestic and occupational)

Substitution of products causing elicitation of allergy (domestic and occupational)

Personal protection

Avoidance of wet work

Avoidance of dirty work and mechanical irritation of the skin of the hands

Information

Skin protection programme

Expectations – what can be done and what is the prognosis

Notification of possible occupational cases

Treatment

Basic treatment (skin care programme and moisturisers)

Topical therapy (topical corticosteroids being the most frequently used treatment)

Systemic therapy (limited to severe cases)

Physical therapy (UVA, UVB, PUVA)

true number of cases may very well be much higher than the reported and/or recognised number. The cost for the society is high, including workers' compensation, sick leave, retraining and costs to health services. In addition to being a burden for the individual, the disease is expensive for the society since it most often affects young people and is a predictor of long-term sick leave and unemployment [60].

Occupational hand eczema is more often due to irritant than to allergic contact dermatitis [61, 62]. Frequent harmful occupational exposures were reported to be unspecified chemicals, water and detergents, dust and dry dirt [63]. In a recent Danish study the highest number of occupational hand eczema was found among health care workers [62]. A large number of hand eczema cases have been reported among cleaners and in people with wet work in hospitals [33, 63, 64], and a high incidence is also found in the metal working industry [65]. High numbers were also reported among factory workers, cleaners, kitchen workers/cooks and hairdressers. The highest relative risk of eczema per employee was found for bakers [62]. Bakers were reported to have a threefold increased risk of hand eczema as compared to the background population,

due to exposure to dough and wet work [66]. A high relative risk was also reported for hairdressers, dental surgery assistants and kitchen workers/cooks. Common for occupations with high risk of occupational hand eczema is exposure to wet work, which has also been identified as a risk factor for the development of hand eczema. Many female-dominated occupations involve extensive wet work (health care workers, hair dressers, catering). Focus on the prevention of hand eczema within this area would be a benefit for the workers as well as for the society, due to a reduction in economical cost.

Also, metal workers have an increased risk for the development of hand eczema. In a prospective study the 3-year cumulative incidence of hand eczema in metal workers was 15.3% as compared to 6.9% in "white collar-workers" [67]. A study of metal worker trainees found that apart from atopic dermatitis, other major risk factors for the development of hand eczema were mechanical factors as well as chemical irritants, and insufficient amount of recovery time [68]. Frequent causes for occupational allergic contact dermatitis are allergy to metals, rubber, biocides and fragrances.

Cases of occupational hand eczema should be reported to the authorities as work-related disease. For further information on legal aspects of occupational contact dermatitis within different countries see Chap. 50.

20.5 Prognosis

Hand eczema is a long-lasting disease, and although treatment may improve eczema, it rarely clears completely over a short time span [69, 70]. A mean duration of 11.6 years was reported [1], 12.0 and 9.9 years for allergic and irritant contact dermatitis, respectively, while atopic hand eczema was reported to have a duration of 16.3 years. Another study reported 41% of cases to be healed when re-examined after 3 years [33]. Hand eczema may often lead to sick leave, and the mean total sick leave time for hand eczema patients was reported to be 4 weeks [71]. In a 15-year follow-up of hand eczema patients, far reaching consequences, including sick leave, pension or change of occupation, was reported in 5% [72]. In a cohort of patients with occupational hand eczema, sick leave for more than 5 weeks owing to the eczema was reported by 19.9%. It is generally agreed that high degree of severity and sick leave is often related to atopic hand eczema, as well as to low socioeconomic status and greater age [73, 74]. Earlier studies have reported a higher degree of severity in patients with allergic contact dermatitis as compared to irritant contact dermatitis on the hands, as measured by symptom duration, sick leave and extent of involvement [71, 75–77]. New data, however, indicate that this has changed. A recent study reports occupational irritant contact dermatitis to be more strongly associated with severe hand eczema than allergic contact dermatitis [78], and in a recent Danish study on occupational hand eczema, a substantially greater severity among those with occupational irritant contact dermatitis was found [112]. This alteration in risk factors for severity is probably explained by regulation of exposure to allergens, e.g. nickel and chromate, in the society over the last decades, which has reduced the risk for allergic contact dermatitis. With respect to loss of job, having a food-related occupation appears to be associated with increased risk of loss of job (Skoet et al. 2004b).

It is generally assumed that a long lack-time before diagnosis and treatment of hand eczema leads to a poor prognosis, and new data support this hypothesis [79].

Considering the severe consequences of having hand eczema, it is evident that prevention of the disease should be promoted.

20.6 Treatment (Table 20.3)

Three important steps in the treatment of hand eczema are

- To ensure that the patient understands the precise diagnosis (e.g. allergic or irritant contact dermatitis) and its consequences.
- To teach the patient good skin care habits.
- To initiate an effective medical treatment (topical, systemical and physical therapies).

Understanding the diagnosis improves the prognosis for the patient [80, 81], and is necessary to ensure compliance. Making the patient understand the importance of avoiding skin contact with allergens in case of allergic contact dermatitis may be a time-consuming procedure, and several consultations may often be necessary.

Table 20.3 Skin protection programme for workers in wet occupations

Use gloves when starting wet work tasks
Protective gloves should be used when necessary, but as short time as possible
Protective gloves should be intact and clean and dry inside
When protective gloves are used for more than 10 min cotton gloves should be worn underneath
Wash your hands in lukewarm water. Rinse and dry your hands thoroughly after washing
Avoid frequent hand wash unless the hands are visibly dirty. Instead use disinfectants based on alcohol
Do not wear finger rings at work
Apply moisturisers on your hands during the working day. Select a fragrance-free, lipid-rich moisturiser
Moisturisers should be applied all over the hands, including the webs, finger tips and dorsal aspects
Take care when doing domestic work. Use protective gloves for dish washing and insulating gloves in the winter

The message that the patient needs to understand is often quite complex, and it is a challenge for the dermatologist to keep the information as simple and practical as possible. Independent of the diagnosis, the patient should be instructed in good skin care habits. Written information and video programmes may be helpful. Reports on eczema schools for patients with hand eczema are few, and more experience is needed [82].

An extremely important aspect of treatment of hand eczema is the use of moisturisers. Topically applied lipids improve skin barrier function, and the effect of the moisturiser corresponds with the amount of lipids in the product [83]. Recently, it was investigated whether moisturisers containing skin-related lipids were more effective than petrolatum-based creams in patients with chronic hand eczema, and advantage of the skin-related lipids for the treatment of contact dermatitis could not be demonstrated [84]. Since use of moisturisers may sometimes be neglected or looked upon as being "not important" by the patients, it is necessary that the dermatologist underlines the significance of moisturisers, and helps the patient to select an effective and acceptable moisturiser. Males seem to be less familiar with the use of topical treatments than females, and especially in this group the importance of moisturisers should be underlined [113]

20

Topical corticosteroids are still the core treatment for hand eczema [85], and 51% of patients with hand eczema reported use of topical steroids [71]. Few studies are, however, available about efficacy and side effects when used as long-term treatment. Nine weeks treatment with mometasone furoate was reported to clear 80% of cases, and maintenance therapy 3 times weekly for 36 weeks did not cause any significant side effects [86]. However, the chronicity of the disease increases the risk for side effects due to long-term treatment with topical corticosteroids. Use of topical steroids under occlusion for short periods, i.e. 1 h a day for few weeks, may be helpful for hyperkeratotic eczema, but increases the risk for side effects considerably. When the eczema continues in spite of treatment, the possibility of contact allergy to topical corticosteroids should be considered.

Tacrolimus or pimecrolimus may be suitable treatments for some types of hand eczema, but more experience with these preparations is needed [87–89].

A recent prospective open multicentre study indicated that topical tacrolimus might be an efficacious treatment option for chronic occupational hand eczema [90]. In severe cases systemic treatment with immunosuppressants such as cyclosporine, azathioprine or methotrexate may sometimes be necessary, but randomised controlled trials on these treatments for hand eczema are not available. Acitretin is an effective treatment for keratotic hand eczema [91]. Recently, alitretinoin has been introduced on the market, and in a randomised controlled study design it was shown that this drug was well tolerated, and clear or almost clear hands were achieved in almost half of the patients [92].

Botulinum toxin has been used in the treatment of vesicular eczema [93]. Physical treatment either with PUVA therapy or UVB may be considered, and UVA-1 treatment was recently advocated for vesicular eczema [94]. Grenz rays have traditionally been used particularly for the treatment of hyperkeratotic hand eczema [95], although this is today, due to its potential carcinogenic side effects, widely replaced by newer treatments.

To compare the efficacy of different medical treatments for hand eczema, randomised controlled trials are needed. In clinical trials subgroups of hand eczema should be identified [32], and the evaluation should comprise objective assessment of the eczema as well as self-assessment by the patients. Instruments for self-assessment are available either as VAS-score or health-related quality of life [96] or self-assessment of severity by a photo guide [97].

20.7 Prevention

Since hand eczema is a disease that may often become chronic, is a burden for the patient and is a great cost to the society, prevention is obviously an attractive alternative. Prevention should aim mainly at exposure, but knowledge about endogenous risk factors should also be taken into account.

20.7.1 Regulation of Threshold Values for Allergens

Exposure to allergens in sufficiently high concentrations on the skin to cause sensitisation is decisive for the development of allergic contact dermatitis on the hands. Regulation of allergen exposure either by legislation on threshold values or regulations on precautions in handling of allergenic products reduces allergen exposure and subsequently reduces the frequency of allergic contact dermatitis. One example of this is the nickel exposure regulation, of which a positive effect has been documented [23]; other examples are regulation of chromate in cement, and recently, prohibition of the preservative methyldibromo glutaronitrile in cosmetics.

20.7.2 Identification of Risk Groups

Previous or current atopic dermatitis is, as already mentioned, a significant endogenous risk factor for the development of hand eczema, and counselling about avoiding wet and dirty occupations should be given to atopics already in childhood. A separate genetic risk factor, independent of atopic dermatitis, has recently been suggested to be of importance for the development of irritant contact dermatitis of the hands [18], but further studies are needed to confirm this hypothesis.

Exposure to wet work is a special risk factor for the development of hand eczema, and to achieve the optimal effect of preventive efforts, the focus for prevention should aim at reducing wet exposure.

20.7.3 Skin Protection

Protection of the hands is essential for the prevention of hand eczema and is a fundamental aspect in the treatment of hand eczema. Effects of protective measures such as use of moisturisers and gloves have mostly been documented in laboratory studies with experimentally damaged skin [98]. An intervention programme for people working in wet occupations has been developed, based on results from experimental studies, and its effectiveness was documented in an intervention study [59].

Use of gloves in wet work has generally been recommended and accepted as an important preventive measure. Compliance with this recommendation is good in some, but far from all jobs [99]. Although the protective effect of gloves should not be doubted, gloves may sometimes be the cause of hand eczema. Protective rubber gloves may cause irritant contact dermatitis due to increased sweating or allergic contact dermatitis due to contact sensitisation to rubber additives, or they may cause contact urticaria due to immediate natural rubber latex allergy [100–102]. The diagnostic work to be done when suspecting glove-related dermatitis includes exposure assessment (how many hours a day), as well as patch test for rubber additives and skin prick test or RAST test for latex.

20.8 Quality of Life

Not surprisingly, hand eczema has been demonstrated to have a negative impact on quality of life to the same degree as psoriasis or asthma [25, 73]. Females seem to report a higher degree of discomfort than males [16, 103]. Also, psychological factors may have a significant impact on the disease [104], although no significant increase in frequency of depression has been reported [105]. Chronic hand eczema has also been reported to cause sexual dysfunction [106]. Subjects diagnosed by patch testing more than 36 months after disease onset seem to have worse QoL scores than those diagnosed earlier, and hand eczema seems to be as equally impairing for quality of life as generalised eczema [107, 108, 111].

20.9 Differential Diagnosis

In most cases of hand eczema the diagnosis does not provide any difficulties, but there are some pitfalls that should be avoided. A diagnosis often to be mistaken for hand eczema is dermatomycosis, which should always be expected when hand eczema is limited to one hand. Psoriasis is more difficult to differentiate from hand eczema, but sharply demarcated extension of the lesions should raise the suspicion. Scabies in the hand and porphyria cutanea tarda may also sometimes mimic hand eczema, the latter being localised to the dorsal side of the hands [109].

References

1. Meding B (1990) Epidemiology of hand eczema in an industrial city. Acta Derm-Venereol 153 (Suppl):1–43
2. Meding B, Järvholm B (2002) Hand eczema in Swedish adults: changes in prevalence between 1983 and 1996. J Invest Dermatol 118:719–723
3. Lerbaek A, Kyvik KO, Ravn H, Menné T, Agner T (2007) Incidence of hand eczema in a population-based twin cohort: genetic and environmental risk factors. Br J Dermatol 157(3):552–557
4. Meding B, Jarvholm B (2004) Incidence of hand eczema – a polulation-based retrospective study. J Invest Dermatol 122:873–877
5. Mortz CG, Lauritsen JM, Bindslev-Jensen C, Andersen KE (2001) Prevalence of atopic dermatitis, asthma, allergic rhinitis, and hand and contact dermatitis in adolescents. The Odense adolescence cohort study on atopic diseases and dermatitis. Br J Dermatol 144:523–532
6. Yngveson M, Svensson Å, Isacsson Å (1998) Prevalence of self-reported hand dermatosis in upper secondary school pupils. Acta Derm-Venereol 78:371–374
7. Nilsson E, Back O (1986) The importance of anamnestic information of atopy, metal dermatitis and earlier hand eczema for development of hand dermatitis in women in wet hospital work. Acta Derm Venereol 66:45–50
8. Meding B, Swanbeck G (1990) Predictive factors for hand eczema. Contact Derm 23:154–161
9. Rystedt I (1985) Long term follow-up in atopic dermatitis. Acta Derm Venereol Suppl (Stockh) 114:117–120
10. Rystedt I (1985) Work-related hand eczema in atopics. Contact Derm 12:164–171
11. Meding B, Lidén C, Berglind N (2001) Self-diagnosed dermatitis in adults – results from a population survey in Stockholm. Contact Derm 45:341–345
12. Holm JO, Veierod MB (1994) An epidemiological study of hand eczema. II. Prevalence of atopic diathesis in hairdressers, compared with a control group of teachers. Acta Derm Venereol Suppl 187:12–14

13. Nilsson E, Mikaelsson B, Andersson S (1985) Atopy, occupation and domestic work as risk factors for hand eczema in hospital workers. Contact Derm 13:216–233

14. Bryld LE, Agner T, Kyvik KO, Brøndsted L, Hindsberger C, Menné T (2000) Hand eczema in twins: a questionnaire investigation. Br J Dermatol 142:298–305

15. Coenraads PJ, Nater JP, van der Lende R (1983) Prevalence of eczema and other dermatoses of the hands and arms in the Netherlands. Association with age and occupation. Clin Exp Dermatol 8:495–503

16. Meding B (2000) Differences between the sexes with regard to work-related skin disease. Contact Derm 43:65–71

17. Agner T (1992) Noninvasive measuring methods for the investigation of irritant patch test reactions. Acta Derm Venereol (Stockh) Suppl. 173:1–26

18. Bryld LE, Hindsberger C, Kyvik KO, Agner T, Menné T (2003) Risk factors influencing the development of hand eczema in a population-based twin sample. Br J Dermatol 149(6):1214–1220

19. Bryld LE, Agner T, Menné T (2003) Relation between vesicular eruptions on the hands and tinea pedis, atopic dermatitis and nickel allergy. Acta Derm Venereol 83:186–188

20. Mortz CG, Lauritsen JM, Bindslev-Jensen C, Andersen KE (2002) Contact allergy and allergic contact dermatitis in adolescents: prevalence measures and associations. The Odense Adolescent Cohort Study on Atopic Diseases and Dermatitis. Acta Derm Venereol 82:352–358

21. Menné T, Borgan Ø, Green A (1982) Nickel allergy and hand dermatitis in a stratified sample of the Danish female population: an epidemiological study including a statistic appendix. Acta Derm-Venereol 62:35–41

22. Josefson A, Färm G, Stymne B, Meding B (2006) Nickel allergy and hand eczema–a 20-year follow up. Contact Derm 55(5):286–290

23. Nielsen NH, Linneberg A, Menné T, Madsen F, Frolund L, Dirksen A, Jørgensen T (2002) The association between contact allergy and hand eczema in two cross-sectional surveys 8 years appart. Contact Derm 47:71–77

24. Danish Ministry of the Environment. Statutory Order no. 472, 27 June, 1989

25. Meding B, Alderling M, Albin M, Brisman J, Wrangsjö K (2008) Does tobacco smoking influence the occurrence of hand eczema. Br J Dermatol 160(3):514–518. Epub 2008 Nov 25

26. Meding B, Barregard L (2001) Validity of self-reports of hand eczema. Contact Derm 45:99–103

27. Svensson A, Lindberg M, Meding B, Sundberg K, Stenberg B (2002) Self-reported hand eczema: symptombased reports do not increase the validity of diagnosis. Br J Dermatol 147:281–284

28. Susitaival P, Flyvholm MA, Meding B, Kanerva L, Lindberg M, Svensson A, Olafsson JH (2003) Nordic Occupational Skin Questionnaire (NOSQ-2002): a new tool for surveying occupational skin diseases and exposures. Contact Derm 49:70–76

29. Veien NK, Hattel T, Laurberg G (2008) Hand eczema: causes, course, and prognosis I. Contact Derm 58(6): 330–334

30. Kang YC, Lee S, Ahn SK, Choi EH (2002) Clinical manifestations of hand eczema compared by etiological classification and irritation reactivity to SLS. J Dermatol 29:477–483

31. Magina S, Barros MA, Ferreira JA, Mesquita-Guimaraes J (2003) Atopy, nickel sensitivity, occupation, and clinical patterns in different types of hand eczema. Am J Contact Dermat 14(2):63–68

32. Diepgen TL, Andersen KE, Brandao FM, Bruze M, Bruynzeel DP, Frosch P, Gonçalo M, Goossens A, Le Coz CJ, Rustemeyer T, White IR, Agner T; European Environmental and Contact Dermatitis Research Group (2009) Hand eczema classification: a cross-sectional, multicentre study of the aetiology and morphology of hand eczema. Br J Dermatol 160(2):353–358

33. Lammintausta K, Kalimo K, Havu VK (1982) Occurrence of contact allergy and hand eczema in hospital wet work. Contact Derm 8:84–90

34. Nielsen NH, Menné T, Kristiansen J, Christensen JM, Borg L, Poulsen LK (1999) Effects of repeated skin exposure to low nickel concentrations: a model for allergic contact dermatitis to nickel on the hands. Br J Dermatol 141:676–682

35. Nielsen NH, Kristiansen J, Borg L, Christensen JM, Poulsen LK, Menné T (2000) Repeated exposures to cobalt or chromateon the hands of the patients with hand eczema and contact allergy to that metal. Contact Derm 43:212–215

36. Bryld LE, Hindsberger C, Kyvik KO, Agner T, Menné T (2004) Genetic factors in nickel allergy evaluated in a population-based female twin sample. J Invest Dermatol 123(6):1025–1029

37. Heydorn S, Johansen JD, Andersen KE, Bruze M, Svedman C, White I, Basketter DA, Menné T (2003) Fragrance allergy in patients with hand eczema. Contact Derm 48:317–323

38. Cronin E (1991) Formaldehyde is a significant allergen in women with hand eczema. Contact Derm 25:276–282

39. Zachariae C, Rastogi S, Devantier C, Menné T, Johansen J (2003) Methyldibromo glutaronitrile: clinical experience and exposure based risk assessment. Contact Derm 48:150–154

40. Lantinga H, Nater JP, Coenraads PJ (1984) Prevalence, incidence and course of eczema on the hands and forearms in a sample of the general population. Contact Derm 10: 135–139

41. Pedersen LK, Johansen JD, Held E, Agner T (2004) Augmentation of skin response by exposure to a combination of allergens and irritants – a review. Contact Derm 50:265–273

42. Lerbaek A, Kyvik KO, Mortensen J, Bryld LE, Menné T, Agner T (2007) Heritability of hand eczema is not explained by comorbidity with atopic dermatitis. J Invest Dermatol 127(7):1632–1640

43. Coenraads PJ, Diepgen TL (1998) Risk for hand eczema in employees with past or present atopic dermatitis. Int Arch Occup Environ Health 71:7–13

44. Rystedt I (1985) Atopic background in patients with occupational hand eczema. Contact Derm 12:247–254

45. Simpson EL, Thompson MM, Hanifin JM (2006) Prevalence and morphology of hand eczema in patients with atopic dermatitis. Dermatitis 17(3):123–127

46. Palmer CN, Irvine AD, Terron-Kwiatkowski A et al (2006) Common loss-of-function variants of the epidermal barrier protein filaggrin are a major predisposing factor for atopic dermatitis. Nat Genet 38:441–446

47. Lerbaek A, Bisgaard H, Agner T, Ohm Kyvik K, Palmer CN, Menné T (2007) Filaggrin null alleles are not associated with hand eczema or contact allergy. Br J Dermatol 157(6):1199–1204

48. de Jongh CM, Khrenova L, Verberk MM, Calkoen F, van Dijk FJ, Voss H, John SM, Kezic S (2008) Loss-of-function polymorphisms in the filaggrin gene are associated with an increased susceptibility to chronic irritant contact dermatitis: a case-control study. Br J Dermatol 159(3):621–627

49. Molin S, Vollmer S, Weiss EH, Ruzicka T, Prinz JC (2009) Filaggrin mutations may confer susceptibility to chronic hand eczema characterized by combined allergic and irritant contact dermatitis. Br J Dermatol 161:801–807

50. Guillet MH, Wierzbicka E, Guillet S, Dagregorio G, Guillet G (2007) A 3-year causative study of pompholyx in 120 patients. Arch Dermatol 143(12):1504–1508

51. Menné T, Hjorth N (1985) Pompholyx: dyshidrotic eczema. Semin Dermatol 2:5

52. Hersle K, Mobacken H (1982) Hyperkeratotic dermatitis of the palms. Br J Dermatol 107:195

53. Coenraads PJ, Van der Walle H, Thestrup-Petersen K, Ruzicka T, Dreno B, De La Loge C, Viala M, Querner S, Brown T, Zultak M (2005) Construction and validation of a photographic guide for assessing severity of chronic hand dermatitis. Br J Dermatol 152(2):296–301

54. Dulon M, Skudlik C, Nübling M, John SM, Nienhaus A (2009) Validity and responsiveness of the Osnabrück Hand Eczema Severity Index (OHSI): a methodological study. Br J Dermatol 160(1):137–142

55. Held E, Skøt R, Johansen JD, Agner T (2005) The hand eczema severity index (HECSI): a scoring system for clinical assessment of hand eczema. A study of inter- and intra-observer reliability. Br J Dermatol 152(2):302–307

56. Cvetkovski RS, Jensen H, Olsen J, Johansen JD, Agner T (2005) Relation between patients' and physicians' severity assessment of occupational hand eczema. Br J Dermatol 153:596–600

57. van Coevorden AM, van Sonderen E, Bouma J, Coenraads PJ (2006) Assessment of severity of hand eczema: discrepancies between patient- and physician-rated scores. Br J Dermatol 155(6):1217–1222

58. Cherry N, Meyer JD, Adisesh A (2000) Surveillance of occupational skin disease: EPIDERM and OPRA. Br J Dermatol 142:1128–1134

59. Held E, Mygind K, Wolff C, Gyntelberg F, Agner T (2002) Prevention of work-related skin problems: an intervention study in wet work employees. Occup Environ Med 59:556–561

60. Leino-Arjas P, Liira J, Mutanen P (1999) Predictors and consequences of unemployment among construction workers: prospective cohort study. BMJ 4:600–605

61. Halkier-Sorensen L (1996) Occupational skin diseases. Contact Derm 35:1–120

62. Skoet R, Olsen J, Mathiesen B, Iversen L, Johansen JD, Agner T (2004) A survey of occupational hand eczema in Denmark. Contact Derm 51(4):159–166

63. Meding B, Swanbeck G (1990) Occupational hand eczema in an industrial city. Contact Derm 22:13–23

64. Flyvholm MA, Bach B, Rose M, Jepsen KF (2007) Self-reported hand eczema in a hospital population. Contact Derm 57(2):110–115

65. Apfelbacher CJ, Radulescu M, Diepgen TL, Funke U (2008) Occurrence and prognosis of hand eczema in the car industry: results from the PACO follow-up study (PACO II). Contact Derm 58(6):322–329

66. Meding B, Wrangsjo K, Brisman J, Jarvholm B (2003) Hand eczema in 45 bakers – a clinical study. Contact Derm 48:7–11

67. Funke U, Fartasch M, Diepgen TL (2001) Incidence of work-related hand eczema during apprenticeship: first results of a prospective cohort study in the car industry. Contact Derm 44:166–172

68. Berndt U, Hinnen U, Iliev D, Elsner P (2000) Hand eczema in metalworker trainees – an analysis of risk factors. Contact Derm 43:327–332

69. Hald M, Agner T, Blands J, Veien NK, Laurberg G, Avnstorp C, Menné T, Kaaber K, Kristensen B, Kristensen O, Andersen KE, Paulsen E, Thormann J, Sommerlund M, Nielsen NH, Johansen JD (2009) Clinical severity and prognosis of hand eczema. Br J Dermatol 160(6):1229–1236

70. Veien NK, Hattel T, Laurberg G (2008) Hand eczema: causes, course, and prognosis II. Contact Derm 58(6):335–339

71. Meding B, Swanbeck G (1990) Consequences of having hand eczema. Contact Derm 23:6–14

72. Meding B, Wrangsjö K, Järvholm B (2005) Fifteen-year follow-up of hand eczema: persistence and consequences. Br J Dermatol 152(5):975–980

73. Cvetkovski RS, Zachariae R, Jensen H, Olsen J, Johansen JD, Agner T (2006) Prognosis of occupational hand eczema: a follow-up study. Arch Dermatol 142(3):305–311

74. Lerbaek A, Kyvik KO, Ravn H, Menné T, Agner T (2008) Clinical characteristics and consequences of hand eczema – an 8-year follow-up study of a population-based twin cohort. Contact Derm 58(4):210–216

75. Adiesh A, Meyer JD, Cherry NM (2002) Prognosis and work absence due to occupational contact dermatitis. Contact Derm 46:273–279

76. Fregert S (1975) Occupational dermatitis in a 10-year material. Contact Derm 1:96–107

77. Menné T, Bachmann E (1979) Permanent disability from skin diseases. Dermatosen 27:37–42

78. Jungbauer FH, Van Der Vleuten P, Groothoff JW, Coenraads PJ (2004) Irritant hand dermatitis: severity of disease, occupational exposure to skin irritants and preventive measures 5 years of initial diagnosis. Contact Derm 50(4):245–251

79. Hald M, Agner T, Blands J, Johansen JD; Danish Contact Dermatitis Group. Delay in medical attention to hand eczema: a follow-up study. Br J Dermatol. 2009 Dec; 161(6):1294–1300.

80. Agner T, Flyvholm MA, Menné T (1999) Formaldehyde allergy: a follow-up study. Am J Contact Dermat 10(1):12–17

81. Holness DL, Nethercott JR (1991) Is a worker's understanding of their diagnosis an important determinant of outcome in occupational contact dermatitis? Contact Derm 25(5):296–301

82. Kalimo K, Kautiainen H, Niskanen T, Niemi L (1999) Eczema school to improve compliance in an accupational dermatology clinic. Contact Derm 41:315–319

83. Held E, Agner T (2001) Effect of moisturizers on skin susceptibility to irritants. Acta Derm Venereol 81(2):104–107

84. Kucharekova M, Van De Kerkhof PC, Van Der Valk PG (2003) A randomized comparison of an emollient containing skinrelated lipids with a petrolatum-based emollient as adjunct in the treatment of chronic hand eczema. Contact Derm 48:293–299

85. Veien NK, Menné T (2003) Treatment of hand eczema. Skin Therapy Lett 8(5):4–7

86. Veien NK, Olholm Larsen P, Thestrup-Pedersen K, Schou G (1999) Long-term, intermittent treatment of chronic hand eczema with mometasone furoate. Br J Dermatol 140(5): 882–886

87. Schnopp C, Remling R, Mohrenschlager M, Weigl L, Ring J, Abeck D (2002) Topical tacrolimus (FK506) and mometasone furoate in treatment of dyshidrotic palmar eczema: a randomized, observer-blinded trial. J Am Acad Dermatol 46(1):73–77

88. Thaci D, Steinmeyer K, Ebelin M, Scott G, Kaufmann R (2003) Occlusive treatment of chronic hand dermatitis with pimecrolimus cream 1% results in low systemic exposure, is well tolerated, safe ans effective. Dermatology 207: 37–42

89. Thelmo MC, Lang W, Brooke E, Osborne BE, McCarty MA, Jorizzo JL, Fleischer A Jr (2003) An open-label pilot study to evaluate the safety and efficacy of topically applied tacrolimus ointment for the treatment of hand and/or foot eczema. J Dermatolog Treat 14(3):136–140

90. Schliemann S, Kelterer D, Bauer A, John SM, Skudlik C, Schindera I, Wehrmann W, Elsner P (2008) Tacrolimus ointment in the treatment of occupationally induced chronic hand dermatitis. Contact Derm 58(5):299–306

91. Thestrup-Pedersen K, Andersen KE, Menné T, Veien NK (2001) Treatment of hyperkeratotic dermatitis of the palms (eczema keratoticum) with oral acitretin. A single-blind placebo-controlled study. Acta Derm Venereol 81(5):353–355

92. Ruzicka T, Lynde CW, Jemec GB, Diepgen T, Berth-Jones J, Coenraads PJ, Kaszuba A, Bissonnette R, Varjonen E, Holló P, Cambazard F, Lahfa M, Elsner P, Nyberg F, Svensson A, Brown TC, Harsch M, Maares J (2008) Efficacy and safety of oral alitretinoin (9-cis retinoic acid) in patients with severe chronic hand eczema refractory to topical corticosteroids: results of a randomized, double-blind, placebo-controlled, multicentre trial. Br J Dermatol 158(4):808–817

93. Swartling C, Naver H, Lindberg M, Anveden I (2002) Treatment of dyshidrotic hand dermatitis with intradermal botulinum toxin. J Am Acad Dermatol 47(5):667–671

94. Polderman MC, Govaert JC, le Cessie S, Pavel S (2003) A double-blind placebo-controlled trial of UVA-1 in the treatment of dyshidrotic eczema. Clin Exp Dermatol 28: 584–587

95. Lindelof B, Wrangsjo K, Lidén S (1987) A double-blind study of Grenz ray therapy in chronic eczema of the hands. Br J Dermatol 117(1):77–80

96. Wallenhammar LM, NyfjallM, Lindberg M, Meding B (2004) Health-related quality of life and hand eczema – a comparison of two instruments, including factor analysis. J Invest Dermatol 122:1381–1389

97. Hald M, Veien NK, Laurberg G, Johansen JD (2007) Severity of hand eczema assessed by patients and dermatologists using a photographic guide. Br J Dermatol 156(1):77–80

98. Coenraads P, Diepgen TL (2003) Problems with trials and intervention studies on barrier creams and emollients at the workplace. Int Arch Occup Environ Health 76:362–366

99. Wrangsjo K, Wallenhammar LM, Ortengren U, Barregard L, Andreasson H, Bjorkner B, Karlsson S, Meding B (2001) Protective gloves in Swedish dentistry: use and side effects. Br J Dermatol 145:32–37

100. Ramsing DW, Agner T (1996) Effect of glove occlusion on human skin. (I). short-term experimental exposure. Contact Derm 34(1):1–5

101. Ramsing DW, Agner T (1996) Effect of glove occlusion on human skin (II). Long-term experimental exposure. Contact Derm 34(4):258–262

102. Strauss RM, Gawkrodger DJ (2001) Occupational contact dermatitis in nurses with hand eczema. Contact Derm 44:293–296

103. Agner T, Andersen KE, Brandao FM, Bruze M, Bruynzeel DP, Frosch P, Gonçalo M, Goossens A, Le Coz CJ, Rustemeyer T, White IR, Diepgen TL, EECDRG (2008) Hand eczema severity and quality of life: a cross-sectional, multicentre study of hand eczema patients. Contact Derm 59(1):43–47

104. Niemeier V, Nippesen M, Kupfer J, Schill WB, Gieler U (2002) Psychological factors associated with hand dermatoses: which subgroups needs additionally care? Br J Dermatol 146:1031–1037

105. Cvetkovski RS, Zachariae R, Jensen H, Olsen J, Johansen JD, Agner T (2006) Quality of life and depression in a population of occupational hand eczema patients. Contact Derm 54(2):106–111

106. Ergün M, Türel Ermertcan A, Oztürkcan S, Temelta G, Deveci A, Dinç G (2007) Sexual dysfunction in patients with chronic hand eczema in the Turkish population. J Sex Med 4(6):1684–1690

107. Kadyk DL, McCarter K, Achen F, Belsito DV (2003) Quality of life in patients with allergic contact dermatitis. J Am Acad Dermatol 49:1037–1048

108. Skoet R, Zachariae R, Agner T (2003) Contact dermatitis and quality of life: a structured review of the literature. Br J Dermatol 149(3):452–456

109. Sommer S, Wilkinson SM (2004) Porphyria cutanea tardamasquerading as chronic hand eczema. Acta Derm Venereol 84:170–171

110. Menné T (2000) Hyperkeratotic dermatitis of the palms. In: Menné T, Maibach HI (eds) Hand eczema. CRC press, Boca Raton

111. Moberg C, Alderling M, Meding B (2009) Hand eczema and quality of life: a population-based study. Br J Dermatol 161:397–403

112. Cvetkovski RS, Rothman KJ, Olsen J, Mathiesen B, Iversen L, Johansen JD, Agner T (2005) Relation between diagnoses on severity, sick leave and loss of job among patients with occupational hand eczema. Br J Dermatol 152(1):93–98

113. Noiesen E, Munk MD, Larsen K, Høyen M, Agner T. Gender differences in topical treatment of allergic contact dermatitis. Acta Derm Venereol. 2009;89(1):79–81

Protein Contact Dermatitis

21

An Goossens and Cristina Amaro

Contents

21.1 Introduction

Protein contact with the skin can be associated with two major clinical conditions: immunological contact urticaria (ICU) and protein contact dermatitis (PCD).

In 1976, *Hjorth and Roed-Petersen* [1] reported a particular form of contact dermatitis in Danish food handlers, which they called "protein contact dermatitis". Most patients suffered from eczema of the hands and forearms. The development of an immediate-type, IgE-mediated allergy to the proteinaceous material is a common feature of both CU and PCD [2, 3]. However, in contrast to CU, the latter presents as a chronic dermatitis with acute flares appearing within a few minutes following contact with the causal proteins. Patch tests are usually negative and the diagnosis is confirmed by a positive prick test with the offending agent. Sometimes specific IgE antibodies can be found.

Over the years, numerous agents have been added to an ever-expanding list of causes, most often occupation-induced. Some extensive reviews on the subject have recently been published [4, 5]. This chapter reviews the pathogenesis, clinical pictures and the proteins causing PCD, most of which are responsible for occupation-related skin problems, i.e. fruits, vegetables, spices, plants and woods, grains, enzymes and animals.

21.2 Clinical Features

The most frequent clinical presentation of PCD is a chronic or recurrent eczema. It may be manifested just as a fingertip dermatitis (Fig. 21.1) or extend to hands, wrists and arms. An urticarial or vesicular exacerbation can be noted in a few minutes after contact with the causal

A. Goossens (✉)
Department of Dermatology, University Hospital,
Katholieke Universiteit Leuven, 3000 Leuven, Belgium
e-mail: an.goossens@uz.kuleuven.ac.be

C. Amaro
Department of Dermatology, Hospital de Curry Cabral,
Rua da Beneficência, nº 8, 1069-166 Lisbon, Portugal

J.D. Johansen et al. (eds.), *Contact Dermatitis*,
DOI: 10.1007/978-3-642-03827-3_21, © Springer-Verlag Berlin Heidelberg 2011

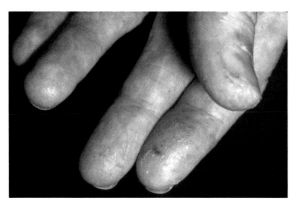

Fig. 21.1 Fingertip protein contact dermatitis in a cook

protein on previously affected skin. Some cases of chronic paronychia were considered a variety of PCD, with redness and swelling of the proximal nail fold, for example, after handling food [6] and natural rubber latex [7].

As for ICU, the allergen characteristics influence the co-existence of extra-cutaneous symptoms: if it is volatile, allergic rhino-conjunctivitis or asthma may accompany the skin manifestations, as it occurs with bakers who are in continuous contact with flour [8]. Even contact anaphylaxis may accompany PCD, such as with chicory [9], which emphasizes the role of airborne exposure. Abdominal pain, diarrhoea and the "oral allergy syndrome" may occasionally develop when the allergen comes in contact with the oro-pharyngeal mucosa [2], the latter particularly in an atopic context.

> **Core Message**
>
> › The most frequent clinical presentation of PCD is a chronic or recurrent eczema on the fingertips. An urticarial or vesicular exacerbation can be noted in a few minutes after contact with the causal protein on previously affected skin.

21.3 Causes [2, 4, 5] (Tables 21.1–21.3)

Classically, the protein sources are divided into four main groups: group 1: fruits, vegetables, spices, plants and woods; group 2: animal proteins; group 3: grains and group 4: enzymes. Taking into account the nature of the causal proteins, a wide variety of jobs can be affected [2, 4, 5].

Table 21.1 Fruits, vegetables, spices, plants, woods [4]

Almond
Asparagus
Banana
Bean
Bishop's weed
Caraway
Carrot
Castor bean
Cauliflower
Celery
Chicory
Chives
Chrysanthemum
Coriander
Cress
Cucumber
Cumin
Curry
Dill
Eggplant
Endive
Fig
Garlic
Gerbera
Green pepper
Hazelnut
Hedge mustard
Horseradish
Kiwi
Lemon
Lettuce
Melon
Mushroom
Natural rubber latex
Olive
Onion
Orange

Table 21.1 (continued)

Papaw skin

Paprika

Parsley

Parsnip

Peach

Peanuts

Pear

Pecan nuts

Pineapple

Potato

Ruccola

Sapele wood

Spathe flowers

Spinach

Tomato

Walnut

Watercress

Weeping fig

Yucca

Table 21.2 Proteins having caused immunological CU and/or PCD: animal derived [4]

Amniotic fluid

Amphibian serum

Blood

Cow

Horse

Lamb

Pig

Brains

Cockroach

Frog

Dairy products

Cheddar

Cheese

Cheese products

Emmental

Milk:cow

Milk:dog

Parmesan

Dander/epithelium

Cow

Giraffe

Egg yolk

Gut: pig

Hydrolyzed collagen

Liver

Calf/Ox

Chicken

Lamb

Locust

Meat

Cow

Chicken

Frog

Horse

Lamb

Pork

Mesenteric fat: pig

Parasites

Anisakis simplex

Placenta: calf

Saliva: cow

Seafood

Abalone

Angler fish

Baby squid

Clam

Codfish

Crab

Cuttlefish

Dory

(*continued*)

Table 21.2 (continued)

Fish mix

Fluke

Haddock

Herring

Horse mackerel

Lobster

Mackerel

Mussel

Oyster

Perch

Plaice

Prawn

Rainbow trout

Red mullet

Salmon

Scampi

Sea bream

Sea eel

Shellfish

Shrimp

Sole

Tuna fish

White fish

Whitebait

Whiting

Seminal fluid: dog

Skin

Chicken

Turkey

Wool: ewe

Worms/larvae

Calliphora vomitoria

Lumbrinereis impatientis

Midge larvae

Nereis diversicolor

Table 21.3 Proteins having caused immunological CU and/or PCD: grains and enzymes [4]

Grains	Enzymes
Barley	Cellulase
Chapatti [17]	Glucoamylase
Cornstarch	Papain
Oat	Protease
Rye	Xylanase
Wheat	α-amylase

Some of the suspected proteins are not yet clearly identified; reports of extremely rare, or even isolated cases (without epidemiologic value) may have contributed to this situation. This is in contrast to, for example, natural rubber latex, a serious occupational hazard in the past two decades in health care workers, in particular. Indeed, several allergenic proteins have been identified, for which tools for both in vitro and in vivo diagnosis are still being developed (e.g. [10]). Although CU is the commonest reported form of natural rubber latex allergy, there are also a few cases of PCD.

Food handlers, cooks, housewives and caterers are at risk from fruits, vegetables and spices. Typical localizations can be observed as with garlic and onion, affecting only the first, third and fourth fingers of the non-dominant hand.

Plants are known to cause immediate skin and mucosal symptoms among gardeners, greenhouse workers, florists, plant caretakers and researchers.

Proteins of animal origin constitute the largest group: they can cause problems in slaughterhouse workers and butchers, but veterinarians are also at great risk of CU or PCD from amniotic or seminal fluid, blood and saliva having their origin in obstetric procedures or daily contact with the animals.

Geographic differences, reflecting countries' costumes, have become evident. In statistical data from Finland, cow dander persists as a major cause of occupational disease among farmers, as previously reported [11]. Finnish farmers' exposure to cow dander is extremely high, as cows are kept inside for most of the year.

Animal keepers can be affected in multiple contexts, though. Recently also, a case of PCD from a ferret was reported [12].

Case reports of laboratory workers suffering from skin and respiratory symptoms following contact with insects have also been published. Cockroaches have provoked CU, dermatitis, rhinitis and asthma. ICU and also PCD due to locusts is an occupational hazard well known to professional entomologists or breeders.

Numerous fish or seafood species, as well as fishing bait maggots (*Nereis diversicolor, Calliphora vomitoria, Chironomus thummi thummi* and *Lumbrinereis impatientis*) have been described in relation to fisherman and fishing for leisure time.

Different grains and enzymes are known to cause PCD, sometimes accompanied by respiratory problems in bakers. Moreover, the use of hydrolysed proteins and extracts derived from grains such as soy, oat and wheat has been debated, particularly in atopic subjects [13, 14].

penetration of the proteins. Since the demonstration of IgE receptors on the epidermal Langerhans cells, it has been speculated that these cells could be responsible for a delayed IgE-mediated reaction, a similar process to that of atopic dermatitis [2, 4, 5].

Homologies between proteins are now known to explain the cross-reactivity described in certain sources, i.e. natural rubber latex and fruits, and the mugwort-spice syndrome, a form of pollen-related food allergy due to cross-reactivity of epitopes, and a subset of perioral syndrome and PCD with cross-reactivity between profilin in birch pollen, apple and peach. Interestingly, in several of the reported clinical cases multiple allergens were implicated. Along with structural homologies, probably, this also reflects a priming factor to the subsequent allergic process.

> **Core Message**
>
> › PCD is most often occupation-related and may be caused by proteins from fruits, vegetables, spices, plants, woods, grains, enzymes and animals (Tables 21.1–21.3).

> **Core Message**
>
> › The pathogenesis of ICU and PCD reflects a type I hypersensitivity reaction, mediated by allergen-specific IgE in a previously sensitized individual.

21.4 Pathogenesis

The occupations involved may be associated with pre-existing dermatitis, i.e. atopic dermatitis, for which associations have been noted in about 50% of the cases [2], as well as irritant contact dermatitis, physical damage (burns, wounds), chemical damage (detergents and other penetration enhancers), increased hydration (excessive hand washing) and occluded skin (e.g. wearing gloves). All such causes of reduced stratum corneum barrier integrity may indeed facilitate high molecular weight proteins to penetrate into the skin.

The pathogenesis of ICU and PCD reflects a type I hypersensitivity reaction, mediated by allergen-specific IgE in a previously sensitized individual.

The exact patho-physiological mechanism in PCD is still unclear. Several authors have reported a combination of type I and IV allergic skin reactions, the latter supported by positive delayed patch tests, while this association has been difficult to prove in most cases. Negative patch testing on intact skin does not necessarily mean that a type IV reaction is not involved though: false-negative results might be due to insufficient

21.5 Diagnostic Tests

Tests for immediate IgE-mediated allergy are of paramount importance when CU or PCD are investigated and reactions appear within 20 min. Skin prick tests with fresh material or commercial reagents are the gold standard [2, 4, 5]. Histamine and physiological saline are used as the positive and negative controls, respectively.

Open testing (quite similar to the Skin Application Food Test or SAFT), which has been mentioned only in the diagnosis of food allergy in atopic children can be helpful, but is generally negative unless the substance is applied on damaged or eczematous skin (where it even may cause a vesicular reaction). Sometimes a rubbing test (gentle rubbing with the material) on intact or lesional skin might be indicated, if an open test is negative. Scratch and scratch-patch testing (scratch-chamber test) [15] may be useful as well , but carry a higher risk of false-positive reactions and the latter lacks sensitivity compared to prick testing (Fig. 21.2). As mentioned above, patch tests in PCD are usually negative.

21

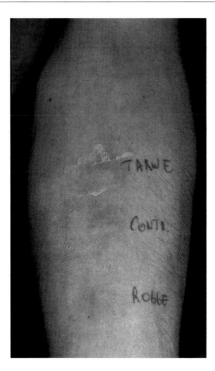

Fig. 21.2 Immediate positive scratch tests to wheat (tarwe) and rye (rogge) in a baker (nowadays prick tests are standard)

If there is a suspicion of any kind of serious extracutaneous symptoms, tests should be done with the necessary precautions and resuscitation facilities should be adequately available.

Measurement of specific IgE in serum (e.g. radioallergosorbent-RAST) is useful for some of the known proteins. Indeed, as mentioned above, many of the protein allergens have not yet been identified.

The basophil activation test is a relatively new procedure: it is based on the demonstration of a membrane protein marker that appears following exposure to allergens and can be particularly interesting when assessing reactions to rare allergens, for which routine diagnostic tests, such as the measurement of specific IgE antibodies, are not available. It has been shown to be a useful technique for the study of PCD, although disagreement with specific IgE analysis may occur [16].

> **Core Message**
>
> › Skin prick tests with fresh material or commercial reagents are the gold standard. Readings need to be performed within 20 min (with positive and negative controls).

21.6 Differential Diagnosis

It should be kept in mind that the same substance can originate different clinical pictures by distinct mechanisms.

An allergic contact dermatitis (ACD) to low molecular weight allergens should be ruled out as the major cause of the eczematous clinical picture [2]. Both PCD and ACD can however occur simultaneously: for example, PCD from proteins in onion and garlic and ACD from diallyldisulfide present in them.

Last but not the least, atopic and irritant contact dermatitis have to be considered in the differential diagnosis.

21.7 Conclusion

Macromolecules can penetrate the skin and cause immunological, urticarial or eczematous clinical pictures, which seem to share a common pathogenic mechanism of a type I immediate reaction, making prick testing the gold standard method for diagnosis. A large number of causes have been documented, plant or animal derived, flours or enzymes, grouped in ever-expanding lists of occupational sources.

PCD is a recognized problem particularly in the food industry; however, the domestic setting also needs to be taken into consideration, for example, with garlic, and as has recently been shown, with chapatti flour in Asian housewives [17].

Infrequent clinical features may not be recognized if they are not properly investigated, and new potent protein allergen sources need to be kept in mind. Indeed, new social habits will probably open new pathways for other allergens, such as the growing consumption of raw and smoked fish due to the influence of Japanese cuisine, or natural remedies such as the widespread use of alternative herbal products. Moreover, processed chemical or enzymatic proteins can also become a hazard, such as protein hydrolysates in cosmetics.

Extensive studies on the incidence and follow-up of latex allergy in health care workers were of utmost importance and resulted in specific guidelines that succeeded in reducing its incidence in high-risk populations within the medical field. In time, other occupational groups might need to be targeted as well, providing new opportunities for starting potential prevention programmes.

References

1. Hjorth N, Roed-Petersen J (1976) Occupational protein contact dermatitis in food handlers. Contact Derm 2:28–42

2. Janssens V, Morren M, Dooms-Goossens A, Degreef H (1995) Protein contact dermatitis: myth or reality? Br J Dermatol 132:1–6

3. Doutre M (2005) Occupational contac urticaria and protein contact dermatitis. Eur J Dermatol 15:419–424

4. Amaro C, Goossens A (2008) Immunological occupational contact urticaria and contact dermatitis from proteins: a review. Contact Derm 58:67–75

5. Levin C, Warshaw E (2008) Protein contact dermatitis: allergens, pathogenesis, and management. Dermatitis 19:241–251

6. Tosti A, Guerra L, Morelli R, Bardazzi F, Fanti R (1992) Role of foods in the pathogenesis of chronic paronychia. J Am Acad Dermatol 27:706–710

7. Kanerva L (2000) Occupational protein contact dermatitis and paronychia from natural rubber latex. J Eur Acad Dermatol Venereol 14:504–506

8. Morren M, Janssens V, Dooms-Goossens A, Hoeyveld E, Cornelis A, De Wolf-Peeters C, Heremans A (1993) α-Amylase, a flour additive: an important cause of protein contact dermatitis in bakers. J Am Acad Dermatol 29:723–728

9. Willi R, Pfab F, Huss-Marp J, Buters JTM, Zilker T, Behrendt H, Ring J, Darsow U (2009) Contact anaphylaxis and protein contact dermatitis in a cook handling chicory leaves. Contact Derm 60:226–227

10. Wagner S, Bublin M, Hafner C, Kopp T, Allwardt D, Seifert U, Arif SA, Scheiner O, Breiteneder H (2007) Generation of allergen-enriched protein fractions of hevea brasiliensis latex for in vitro and in vivo diagnosis. Int Arch Allergy Immunol 143:246–254

11. Hannuksela M (2006) Contact dermatitis, 4th edn. Springer, Berlin, pp 345–348

12. Splingard B (2008) A new case of face eczema: the ferret. Contact Derm 58 (suppl):74

13. Boussault P, Léauté-Labrèze C, Saubusse E, Maurice-Tison S, Perromat M, Roul S, Sarrat A, Taïeb A, Boralevi F (2007) Oat sensitization in children with atopic dermatitis: prevalence, risks and associated factors. Allergy 62:1251–1256

14. Goujon-Henry C, Hennino A, Nicolas J-F (2008) Do we have to recommend not using oat-containing emollients in children with atopic dermatitis? Letter to the editor. Allergy 63:781–782

15. Niinimäki A (1987) Scratch-chamber tests in food handler dermatitis. Contact Derm 16:11–20

16. González-Muñoz M, Gómez M, Alday E, Del Castillo A, Moneo I (2007) Occupational protein contact dermatitis to chicken meat studied by flow cytometry. Contact Derm 57:62–63

17. Davies E, Orton D (2009) Contact urticaria and protein contact dermatitis to chapatti flour. Contact Derm 60:113–114

Noneczematous Contact Reactions

22

Anthony Goon and Chee-Leok Goh

Contents

A. Goon (✉) and C.-L.Goh
National Skin Center, 1 Mandalay Road,
Singapore 308205, Republic of Singapore
e-mail: anthonygoon@nsc.gov.sg

22.1 Introduction

Cutaneous contact reactions may present as noneczematous eruptions. Several noneczematous eruptions resulting from contact reaction have been described. The exact mechanisms of these eruptions are unknown. It is important for the clinician to recognize these noneczematous contact reactions as often the cause can be confirmed by simple patch testing and unnecessary investigations into systemic diseases can be avoided. Contact reactions manifesting as noneczematous eruptions include the following:

- Erythema multiforme-like eruption (urticarial papular and plaque eruption [UPPE]).
- Pigmented purpuric eruption.
- Lichen planus-like or lichenoid eruption.
- Bullous eruption.
- Papular and nodular eruption.
- Granulomatous eruption.
- Pustular eruption.
- Erythematous and exfoliative eruption.
- Scleroderma-like eruption.
- Pigmented contact dermatitis.
- Lymphomatoid contact dermatitis.
- Vascular-occlusive contact dermatitis.

22.2 Erythema Multiforme-Like Reaction (Urticarial Papular and Plaque Eruptions)

This is an important contact reaction as it is often mistaken for erythema multiforme from various systemic causes. Several contact allergens including metals, topical medicaments, woods, and industrial chemicals have

J.D. Johansen et al. (eds.), *Contact Dermatitis*,
DOI: 10.1007/978-3-642-03827-3_22, © Springer-Verlag Berlin Heidelberg 2011

22

Table 22.1 Reported causes of UPPE

Woods and plants	
Dalbergia nigra (Brazilian rosewood)	*Toxicodendron radicans* (poison ivy)
Machaerium scleroxylon (pao ferro)	*Primula obconica*
Eucalyptus saligna (gum)	*Artemisia vulgaris* (common mugwort)
Topical medicaments	
Ethylenediamine	Nitroglycerin
Pyrrolnitrin	Tea tree oil
Sulfonamide	Nitrogen mustard
Promethazine	Proflavine
Balsam of Peru	Diphencyprone
Diaminodiphenylmethane	Sulfanilamide
Clioquinol (Vioform)	Furazolidone
Mafenide acetate	Nifuroxime
Mefenesin	Scopolamine hydrobromide
Econazole	*Alpinia galanga*
Vitamin E	
Metals and chemicals	
Nickel	Trinitrotoluene
Cobalt	Dimethoate
Eumulgin L	Epoxy resin
9-Bromofluorene precursors	*p*-Chlorobenzene sulfonylglycolic acid nitrile
Phenylsulfone derivatives	*p*-Phenylenediamine bisphenol A
1,2-ethanedithiol	Costus resinoid
Formaldehyde	Laurel oil
Trichloroethylene	

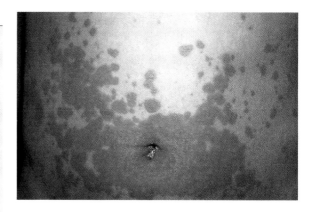

Fig. 22.1 Erythema multiforme-like eruption (UPPE) from contact allergy to trinitrotoluene. Note urticarial papular and plaque eruption

Clinical features: The characteristic presentation is usually an urticarial eruption about 1–14 days after an episode of allergic contact dermatitis. The primary site may be eczematous but becomes urticarial within a few days. This will be followed by erythematous urticarial papular and/or plaque eruptions (Fig. 22.1) around the primary contact site. The eruption often also appears at distant sites. This lasts longer than the primary eczematous lesion and tends to persist after the clearance of the initial dermatitis. The lesions are usually pruritic.

Patch test: Contact allergy to the allergens can be confirmed by a positive patch test. The patch test reactions are eczematous and often vesicular or bullous, but may occasionally be urticarial.

Histology: The histology of these lesions does not show the classical changes of erythema multiforme. The epidermis is either normal or shows mild spongiosis with upper dermal edema and a mild perivascular lymphohistiocytic infiltrate. Vacuolar degeneration of the basal cells is rarely present. There are no epidermal necrosis or interface infiltration, as are present in erythema multiforme (Fig. 22.2).

22.2.1 Differentiation from Classical Erythema Multiforme

Besides the occasional target-like lesions, the morphology, clinical course, and history of erythema multiforme-like eruptions of contact allergy are not

been reported to cause "erythema multiforme-like" eruptions (see Table 22.1). In these reports the allergic nature of the reactions can be confirmed by positive patch test reactions. These eruptions have been described as "target-like," "erythematovesicular," and "urticarial" by different authors. In Asian countries such reactions have been reported to be due to contact allergy to proflavine and trinitrotoluene.

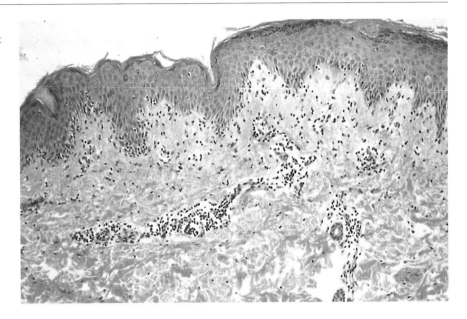

Fig. 22.2 Histology of a UPPE lesion from the patient in Fig. 22.1. Mild upper dermal edema and lympho-histiocytic infiltrates with normal epidermis. Note absence of changes typical of erythema multiforme

characteristic of classical erythema multiforme. Lesions of erythema multiforme tend to have an acral distribution, appear in crops, and are almost all target-like. The term "UPPE" of contact allergy was suggested to describe such an eruption [1]. UPPE will be used synonymously with erythema multiforme-like eruption in the rest of this chapter.

The exact mechanism of UPPE is unknown. The eruption appears to represent an allergic immune complex reaction. The allergens are probably absorbed percutaneously, causing an allergic contact dermatitis with concurrent immune complex reaction.

22.2.2 Causes

Allergens reported to cause erythema multiforme-like eruptions include (a) woods and plants, (b) topical medications, and (c) metals and chemicals. Table 22.1 lists the known causes of UPPE.

Woods and Plants

Tropical woods, including Brazilian rosewood (*Dalbergia nigra*), pao ferro (*Machaerium scleroxylon*), and *Eucalyptus saligna,* have been reported to cause occupational UPPE in three carpenters [2]. Patients wearing wooden bracelets and pendants made from *Dalbergia nigra* and hobbyists handling pao ferro wood have been reported to develop UPPE. The specific chemical antigen in Brazilian rosewood is the quinone, R-4-methoxy-dalbergione. The antigen in pao ferro is R-3,4-dimethoxy-dalbergione [3]. Plants reported to cause UPPE include poison ivy (*Toxicodendron radicans*), primula (*Primula obconica*), mugwort (*Artemesia vulgaris*), and *Compositae* weeds.

Topical Medicaments

Ethylenediamine, pyrrolnitrin, sulphonamide, promethazine, balsam of Peru, diaminodiphenylmethane, and clioquinol (Vioform) have been reported as the contact allergens responsible for such eruptions. Some of the patients reported had vasculitic or purpuric lesions. Other implicated medicaments include a cream containing mafenide acetate, mephenesin (Fig. 22.3), econazole, vitamin E, nitroglycerin patches, tea tree oil, and topical nitrogen mustard. In Asia, proflavine has been reported to cause purpuric contact dermatitis and UPPE when applied to abrasions.

UPPE due to diphencyprone was also described in a patient who received the sensitizer as immunotherapy for plane warts on the face.

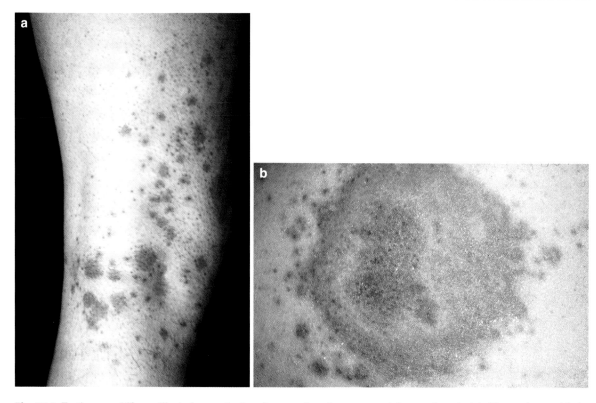

Fig. 22.3 Erythema multiforme-like lesions on the leg after use of an ointment containing mephenesin (**a**). The patch test with the active ingredient was strongly positive (**b**) (courtesy of P.J. Frosch)

Medicaments that are applied to mucosae are rapidly absorbed systemically and may enhance the skin and systemic sensitization process. UPPE occurred in a patient who applied sulfanilamide cream for vulvovaginitis; she had a positive patch test reaction to the sulfanilamide cream and also developed UPPE after ingesting sulfanilamide. UPPE was also described in contact allergy to furazolidone- and nifuroxine-containing suppositories in another patient. A flare-up of the eruption developed when she was patch tested to the suppository. UPPE was also reported from contact allergy to eye drops. Two case reports of Stevens-Johnson syndrome from contact allergy to sulfonamide-containing eye drops were described. Another patient developed UPPE from scopolamine hydrobromide eyedrops; his eruption recurred on rechallenge to the eye drops. There has also been a case of localized contact dermatitis and subsequently generalized erythema multiforme-like eruptions after topical *Alpinia galanga*, which is also a popular spice in Southeast Asian cuisines.

Metals and Chemicals

Metals: UPPE may be a manifestation of contact allergy to some metals and industrial chemicals. Calnan first described UPPE in the secondary spread of nickel dermatitis [4]. Cook reported UPPE in a 13-year-old girl following allergic contact dermatitis from nickel and cobalt in the metal studs of her jeans. A similar eruption was reported in a garment worker who developed nickel dermatitis on her hands from nickel-plated scissors; she had a vesiculopapular patch test reacting to nickel salt, and during patch testing her hand dermatitis and UPPE reappeared. UPPE was also reported in a patient with nickel dermatitis due to a metallic necklace.

Noneczematous urticarioid dermatitis involving the axillae from contact allergy to Eumulgin L (cetearyl alcohol) in deodorant has been reported. Patch test to the emulsifier was strongly positive.

Laboratory Chemicals: UPPE from laboratory chemicals was first described by Cavendish in 1940 in a student who developed recurrent eruptions after 9-bro-mofluorene exposure. During patch testing, one of the control patients became sensitized to the chemical and developed UPPE 13 days after the patch test [5]. Powell also reported a student with a similar eruption due to 9-bromofluorene and, similarly, one control patient became sensitized to the chemical [6]. De Feo also described how, out of 250 chemistry students, 24 developed localized acute contact eczema followed by generalized UPPE, while synthesizing 9-bromofluorene in the laboratory. They had positive patch tests to the chemical [7]. Roed-Petersen reported a chemistry student who developed UPPE on the exposed skin from a phenyl sulphone derivative which he was synthesizing. He had a strong positive reaction to the compound [8].

Tjiu et al. reported on a 22-year-old female chemistry student who developed widespread erythema multiforme-like lesions after local contact with 1,2-eth-anedithiol. The patient had a positive patch test to 1,2-ethanedithiol [9].

Industrial chemicals: Several industrial chemicals have been suspected to cause UPPE. Nethercott et al. reported UPPE in four workers handling printed circuit boards. Liver involvement was documented in three of the workers. Two of the workers had a positive reaction to formaldehyde and formaldehyde was implicated as the cause of the eruptions [10]. Phoon et al. described five workers who developed UPPE and Stevens-Johnson syndrome after exposure to trichloroethylene in an electronics factory. Three workers had hepatitis and one died of hepatic failure. A patch test to trichloroethylene on one worker was negative. The eruption was suspected to be due to a hypersensitivity reaction to trichloroethylene from percutaneous and/or transrespiratory absorption of trichloroethylene [11].

UPPE was also reported in a worker with allergic contact dermatitis from trinitrotoluene; the patient had a strong eczematous patch test reaction to trinitrotoluene [12]. It was recently reported in a warehouseman allergic to dimethoate, an organophosphorus insecticide and acaricide [13]. Other industrial chemicals include epoxy resin and *p*-chlorobenzene sulfonylglycolic acid nitrile.

Others: More recently, there have been reports of UPPE due to *p*-phenylenediamine in henna tattoos, rubber gloves, cutting oil, costus resinoid, and laurel oil.

Core Message

> A persistent erythema multiforme-like reaction may occur after an episode of allergic contact dermatitis from woods and plants, medicaments, metals, and chemicals. The histology of these lesions does not show the classical changes of epidermal necrosis or interface infiltration, which are present in erythema multiforme.

22.3 Pigmented Purpuric Eruption

Contact allergy may present as a purpuric eruption. The eruption is usually asymptomatic, macular, and purpuric, with or without preceding itch or erythema (Fig. 22.4). The purpuric eruption then becomes brownish and fades away. The exact mechanism of the reaction is unknown.

Allergic contact dermatitis to isopropyl-*N*-phenyl-*p*-phenylenediamine (IPPD) in rubber clothing [14], rubber boots [15], rubber diving suits, elasticized shorts, rubberized support bandages [16], and rubberized

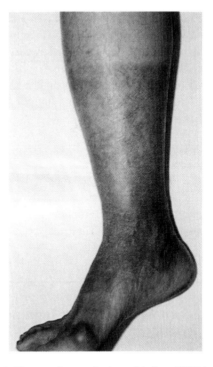

Fig. 22.4 Pigmented purpuric dermatitis from IPPD in rubber boots

22

brassieres [17] have been reported to cause contact purpuric eruptions.

Allergic contact dermatitis from *p*-phenylenedi-
amine after handling black hats has been reported to be
associated with a purpuric eruption. Raw wool was
also reported to cause a contact purpuric eruption.

Contact allergy to balsam of Peru and proflavine in
medicaments, and the azo dye Disperse Blue 85 in
naval uniforms, may also manifest as a purpuric eruption. More recently, contact allergy to the azo dyes,
Disperse Blue 106 and Disperse Blue 124, has been
reported to cause progressive pigmented purpura.

An acute nonpruritic eruption with focal purpura
from contact allergy to 5% benzoyl peroxide in acne
gel has been reported. Patch tests with benzoyl peroxide in petrolatum and the acne gel containing benzoyl
peroxide produced similar reactions. Alterations of the
capillary endothelium included obliteration of the
lumina with perivascular mononuclear cell infiltrates,
with no epidermal alterations in the histology [18].

Emla cream, a topical anesthetic, has been reported
to cause toxic purpuric contact reactions [19]. Four
patients were reported to develop toxic purpuric reaction 30 min after Emla application before the treatment
of molluscum contagiosum. Patch tests with Emla and
its individual ingredients were negative. The authors
concluded that the purpuric reaction was not of an
allergic nature. Possibly, it was caused by a toxic effect
on the capillary endothelium [19].

The sap of *Agave americana*, a popular ornamental
plant, has been reported to cause purpuric irritant
contact dermatitis.

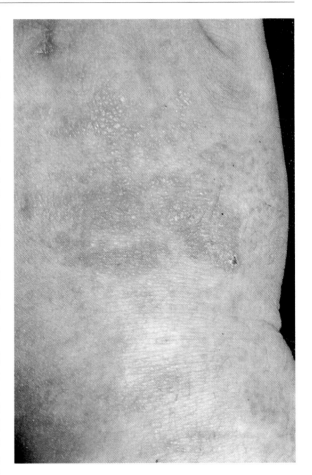

Fig. 22.5 Lichenoid eruption on the back of the hand from a
color developer (CD 4) (courtesy of P. Frosch)

> ### Core Message
>
> › Contact reactions from black rubber, dyes, and
>   medicaments may present as usually asymp-
>   tomatic macular purpuric eruptions that become
>   brownish and fade away. These may be allergic,
>   toxic, or irritant in nature.

22.4 Lichen Planus-Like or Lichenoid Eruption

Lichenoid eruptions mimicking lichen planus may be a
manifestation of allergic contact dermatitis to some
color developers. The eruptions present as itchy dusky
or violaceous papules or plaques on areas of skin
exposed to the allergen (Fig. 22.5). The hands and forearms are commonly affected sites. Unlike idiopathic
lichen planus, the skin lesions clear within a few weeks
upon cessation of contact with the causative allergen.

Several color developers have been reported to cause
such eruptions (Fig. 22.6). Kodak CD2 (4-*N, N*-diethyl-2
methyl-phenylenediamine monohydrochloride), Kodak
CD3 (4-(*N*-ethyl-N-2-methanesulphonylaminoethyl)-
2-methyl-phenylenediamine sesquisulphate monohydrate), Agfa TSS(4-amino-*N*-diethylaniline sulfate),
Ilford MI 210(*N*-ethyl-*N*(5-hydroxy-amyl) *p*-phe-
nylenediamine hydrogen sulfate), and Kodak CD4
(2-amino-5-*N*-ethyl-*N*-(β-hydroxyethyl)-aminotoluene
sulfate) are reported allergens [20]. Mandel reported
that 9 out of 11 workers with contact allergy to color
developer showed lichen planus-like eruptions [21],
but Fry reported a lower rate of 7 out of 20 patients, the
remainder presenting with eczematous reactions [22].

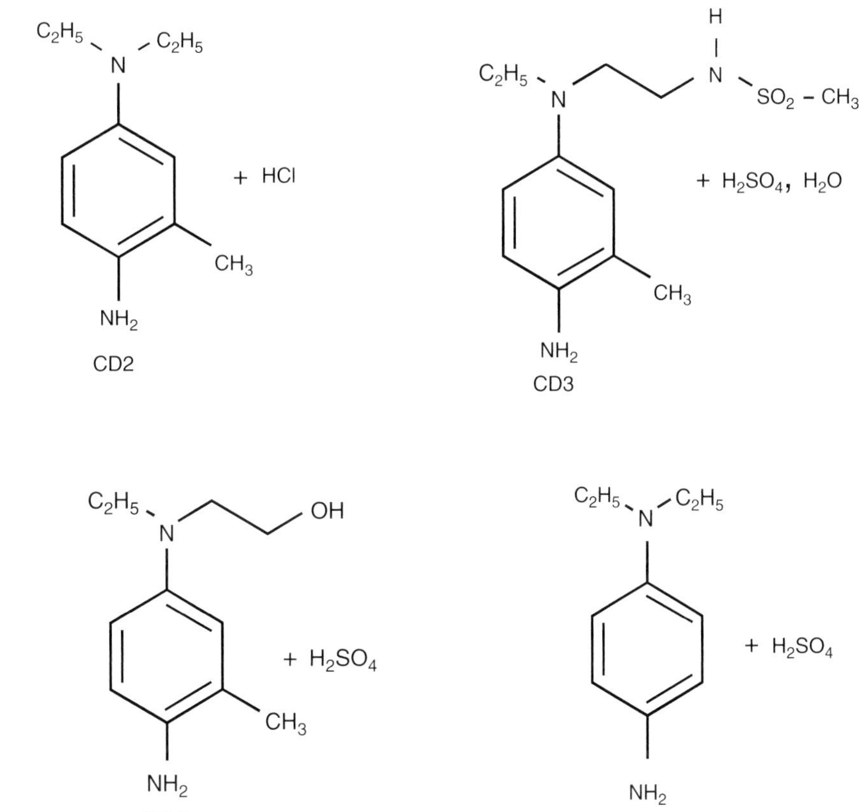

Fig. 22.6 Contact sensitizing color developers

22.4.1 Histology

The histology of lichen planus-like eruptions from color developers may show features compatible with lichen planus or a nonspecific chronic superficial perivascular dermatitis. Some reports indicate that the histology in the majority of patients shows changes compatible with lichen planus [23], but others indicate that a nonspecific chronic dermatitis change is more common [21]. In Fry's report, out of seven patients with lichenoid lesions biopsied, one showed changes of eczema, two showed lichenoid dermatitis, and two showed lichen planus changes [22].

22.4.2 Mechanism

There is controversy about the etiology of the lichen planus-like eruption from color developers. Lichenoid eruptions may be due to direct contact with the chemicals on the skin producing allergic contact dermatitis, but may also represent eruptions resulting from systemic absorption of the allergen [22]. A combination of both mechanisms may be responsible.

Other allergens reported to cause lichenoid eruptions include metallic copper and mercury from dental amalgam. These patients presented with lichen planus-like lesions on the buccal mucosa. Both had positive patch test reactions to the respective allergen. Oral lichen planus-like lesions have also been reported from gold and cinnamal. Nickel salts were also reported to cause lichenoid dermatitis. Lembo et al. reported a chronic lichenoid eruption in a schoolboy from aminoglycoside-containing creams. Biopsy showed a band-like mononuclear upper dermal infiltrate. Patch tests showed a lichenoid reaction to neomycin. A lichenoid reaction has also been reported to epoxy resin.

More recently, other contact allergens reported to cause lichenoid eruptions include para-substituted

22

amino-compounds in temporary henna tattoos and parthenium hysterophorus.

> **Core Message**
>
> > Lichenoid eruptions clinically and histologically resembling lichen planus may be due to allergic contact dermatitis from color developers, metals, aminoglycosides, epoxy resin, and other agents.

22.5 Bullous Eruption

Contact allergy to cinnamon produced bullous eruptions in a female in Singapore after she used cinnamon powder to treat scars on her lower limbs [24]. The morphology and histology of the eruption resembled bullous pemphigoid. However, direct immuno-fluorescent studies were negative. Patch test showed a strong positive reaction to the cinnamon powder, cinnamic aldehyde and cinnamic alcohol. Her eruption was attributed to the latter allergens present in the cinnamon powder. The exact mechanism of the cell-mediated hypersensitivity reaction is unknown.

Contact allergy to nickel and its oral ingestion has also been reported to cause dyshidrosiform pemphigoid.

Bullous irritant reactions may also occur upon the application of cantharidin, a vesicant produced by beetles in the order Coleoptera, which has a long history in both folk and traditional medicine.

> **Core Message**
>
> > Bullous contact allergic reactions have been reported from cinnamon and nickel, while bullous contact irritant reactions may be due to vesicants from Coleoptera beetles.

22.6 Nodular and Papular Eruption

Contact allergy to gold is known to cause chronic papular and nodular skin eruptions. Such eruptions tend to be on the earlobes of sensitized individuals after the wearing of pierced-type gold earrings. The eruptions characteristically persist for months after the patients have avoided contact with metallic gold [25]. Patch test reactions to gold and gold salts in these patients are usually strongly positive. In some patients, the positive reactions to gold salts tend to be indurated and persist for months. Occasionally, the patch test may evoke an infiltrative lymphoblastic reaction which persists for months [25]. The histology of these eruptions or its patch test reaction usually shows a dense lymphomonocytic infiltrate mimicking mycosis fungoides, but mycosis fungoides cells are absent. The cellular infiltrate consists mainly of suppressor/cytotoxic T-cells [26]. Dental amalgam allergy was reported to cause a nodular eruption mimicking oral carcinoma.

> **Core Message**
>
> > Chronic papular and nodular skin eruptions due to gold may sometimes last for months. A nodular eruption due to dental amalgam allergy may mimic oral carcinoma.

22.7 Granulomatous Eruption

Skin injury from zirconium, silica, magnesium, and beryllium may cause granulomas. Some reactions are usually due to a delayed-type allergic reaction that can be confirmed by patch testing, while others are nonallergic reactions.

Zicornium granuloma was first reported to be a manifestation of allergic contact dermatitis from zirconium compounds in deodorants [27]. Clinically, the granulomatous eruptions appear 4–6 weeks after applying the zirconium compounds and are usually confined to the area of application, e.g., the axillae. Eczema is usually present, but pruritus is minimal. Patients with the eruptions have associated positive patch test reactions to zirconium compounds. The histology shows epithelioid cells and may be indistinguishable from sarcoidosis. Allergic granulomatous eruptions were also reported in sensitized patients who use zirconium compounds to treat rhus dermatitis.

Cutaneous granulomas may also occur following immunization with vaccines containing aluminum hydroxide in such patients having positive patch tests to aluminum chloride and/or aluminum Finn Chambers. In one series of 21 children, the granulomas of 11 improved with time [28].

Chromium and mercurial pigments in tattoos can produce allergic granulomatous reactions. Mercury (red cinnabar, mercury sulfide-red pigment), chromium (chromium oxide powder-green pigment), cobalt (cobaltous aluminate-blue pigment), and cadmium (cadmium sulfide-yellow pigment) are known causative agents. An unknown substance in purple tattoo pigment has also been reported to cause a granulomatous reaction. Granulomatous reactions may be preceded by or associated with eczematous reactions (Fig. 22.7). The lesions are usually nonpruritic. Histology shows typical granulomas. These patients usually have positive patch test reactions to the respective metallic salts.

A young woman developed persistent nodules at sites of ear piercing with gold earrings, and patch testing demonstrated a positive allergic response to gold sodium thiosulfate. Histological examination of the nodules demonstrated a prominent sarcoidal-type granulomatous tissue reaction. This is in contrast to the previous reports of lymphocytoma cutis type histology and was associated with the occurrence of epithelioid granulomata at the site of a strongly positive and long-lasting patch test reaction [29].

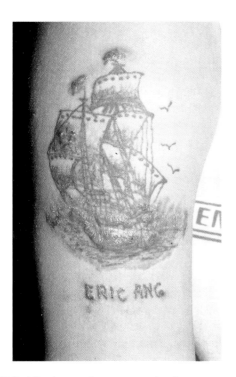

Fig. 22.7 Allergic granulomatous reaction from mercury pigment (*red*) and cobalt pigment (*blue*). Note overlying eczematous reactions

Contact orofacial granulomatosis has been reported to be caused by delayed hypersensitivity to gold and mercury. Sarcoidal allergic contact dermatitis due to palladium following ear piercing and exudative granulomatous reactions to hyaluronic acid (Hylaform) has also been reported. Granulomatous contact dermatitis due to propolis has been described in a patient with a cutaneous nodule below the nose accompanied by marked regional lymphadenopathy. Ear piercing with titanium alloy and palladium has also been reported to cause granulomatous reactions.

> **Core Message**
>
> › Granulomatous skin reactions from zirconium, silica, magnesium, beryllium, metallic tattoo pigments, and gold may mimic sarcoidosis or lymphocytoma cutis.

22.8 Pustular Eruption

Metallic salts, e.g., nickel, copper, arsenic, and mercury salts, have been reported to cause transient sterile pustular reactions [30]. These reactions have also been reported following contact allergy to black rubber [31]. The significance of such pustular reactions remains speculative. Stone and Johnson explained that such reactions may represent an enhanced reaction of prior inflammation rather than an irritant or allergic reaction [32]. Atopics are predisposed to such reactions [33]. Wahlberg and Maibach believe that such reactions are usually irritant in nature, but may also be a manifestation of allergic reactions [34].

Allergic contact dermatitis from a nitrofurazone-containing cream manifested as a pustular eruption. Subcorneal pustular eruption may also be a manifestation of allergy to trichloroethylene. Pustular allergic contact dermatitis from topical minoxidil has also been reported.

22.9 Erythematous and Exfoliative Eruption

Some industrial chemicals, e.g., trichloroethylene and methyl bromide, appear to cause characteristic localized or generalized erythema with or without a papulo-vesicular eruption followed by exfoliation. The skin lesions usually take several weeks to clear. In most of the cases, the skin reaction was believed to be a toxic or allergic reaction from percutaneous or mucosal absorption of the chemicals. The allergic mechanism may be confirmed in some cases by a positive patch test reaction to trichloroethylene and trichloroethanol (its metabolite).

22.9.1 Trichloroethylene

Generalized erythema followed by exfoliation resulting from exposure to trichloroethylene was first described by Schwartz et al. [35] and later by Bauer and Rabens [36]. The reaction was believed to be due to a systemic sensitization to trichloroethylene.

Conde-Salazar et al. reported a patient who developed a generalized erythema and sub-corneal pustular eruption from a cutaneous hypersensitivity reaction to trichloroethylene [37]. The allergic reaction was confirmed by a positive erythematous scaly patch test reaction to 5% trichloroethylene. The patient also reacted systemically to a cutaneous challenge test made by exposing his leg to an environment saturated with trichloroethylene. Nakayama et al. also described generalized erythema and exfoliation with mucous membrane ulceration in a patient from cutaneous exposure to trichloroethylene. The patient had positive patch test reactions to trichloroethylene and trichloroethanol (a metabolite of trichloroethylene) [38]. The patient's skin eruption continued to appear after the cessation of exposure to trichloroethylene. The prolonged duration of the eruption was believed to be due to the slow release of accumulated trichloroethylene and its metabolites in the patient's fatty tissue.

Cutaneous reaction to inhaled trichloroethylene can also cause a characteristic skin eruption consisting of localized erythematous xerotic plaques, which become parched and fissured [39].

22.9.2 Methyl Bromide

Exposure to methyl bromide was described as causing sharply demarcated erythema with vesiculation in six fumigators [40]. Plasma bromide levels in these patients after exposure strongly suggested percutaneous absorption of methyl bromide. The lesions were more prominent on the skin that was relatively moist or subject to mechanical pressure, such as the axillae, groins, and abdomen. Histologically, the early skin lesions showed keratinocytes, necrosis, severe upper dermal edema and bullae, and diffuse dermal neutrophilic infiltration. The skin eruptions were believed to be due to the direct toxic effect of methyl bromide as an alkylating agent.

> **Core Message**
>
> › Localized or generalized erythema with or without a papulo-vesicular eruption followed by exfoliation may be due to a toxic or allergic reaction from percutaneous or mucosal absorption of chemicals. This reaction may persist for weeks.

22.10 Scleroderma-Like Eruption

Solvents have been reported as predisposing or eliciting factors in some patients with scleroderma-like eruptions [41]. The pathogenic mechanism is unknown. Solvents implicated include aromatic hydrocarbon solvents, such as benzene, toluene, and white spirit, and aliphatic hydrocarbons, such as naphtha, n-hexane, and hexachloroethane. Unlike chlorinated hydrocarbons, these hydrocarbons do not produce multisystem disease resembling vinyl chloride disease. The associated scleroderma and morphoea-like sclerosis is usually limited to the skin of the hands and feet, where direct contact took place, but occasionally may be widespread.

In 1972, Texier et al. [42] reported atrophic sclerodermoid patches following phytonadione injections. Intradermal testing with phytonadione gave positive results in 50% of patients. The clinical findings are indistinguishable from those of morphoea [43]. Histology shows dense sclerosis of the reticular dermis and subcutaneous fat and a lymphocytic inflammatory infiltrate. The pathogenesis is unknown. A possible immune mechanism has been suggested. Pang et al. reported a cutaneous reaction to intradermal phytomenadione challenge in a patient with sclerodermoid plaques, which had persisted more than 10 years after subcutaneous phytomenadione injections. Positive intradermal test produced persistent erythematous indurated plaque at the test site for more than 5 months, suggesting a marked cutaneous hypersensitivity to the drug. Serial biopsies of the test site showed transition from spongiotic eczematous features initially to inflammatory morphoea-like histology over a 5-month period [44].

> ## Core Message
>
> › Aromatic and aliphatic hydrocarbons may be associated with scleroderma-like eruptions, but do not produce multisystem disease. The sclerosis is usually limited to the sites of contact, but may occasionally be widespread.

22.11 Pigmented Contact Dermatitis

Pigmented contact dermatitis is a characteristic allergic contact dermatitis reaction manifesting as macular pigmentation on sites of contact. Patients often observe brownish to gray pigmentation on the face after using cosmetics containing azo dyes (as contaminants) [45] or fragrances [46]. Optical whiteners have been reported to cause similar reactions. Characteristically, female patients present with patchy macular pigmentation mimicking melasma. Patients may experience slight erythema and itch before the onset of pigmentation. Unlike melasma, the pigmentation clears upon avoiding the causative allergen. The allergic nature of the skin lesion can be confirmed by patch testing with the incriminated allergens.

An outbreak of pigmented contact dermatitis was reported in Japan in the 1970s. Fragrances and Sudan I (an impurity in Brilliant Lake Red) were the causative allergens. In Asian countries, pigmented contact dermatitis from fragrances in cosmetics and Sudan I have also been reported. The source of these contact allergens is usually cosmetics which are produced by small-time cosmetic manufacturers where there is little product quality control. Another common cause of pigmented contact dermatitis is seen in Hindu women who present with pigmentation on their midforehead due to allergens (usually Sudan I) in the red dye applied to their forehead for cultural reasons.

More recently, reported causes of pigmented contact dermatitis include ricinoleic acid in lipsticks causing pigmented contact cheilitis, topical minoxidil, *p-tert*-butylphenol formaldehyde resin used as an adhesive in a watch strap, and dipentaerythritol fatty acid ester in a lipstick.

An entire chapter of this textbook has been devoted to pigmented contact dermatitis, where it will be covered in greater detail.

22.12 Lymphomatoid Contact Dermatitis

Lymphomatoid contact dermatitis refers to the relatively little-known phenomenon of allergic contact dermatitis producing histological features suggestive of cutaneous T-cell lymphoma. The skin lesions were mainly localized to areas in contact with the allergen and resolved with avoidance. This condition was first reported in 1976 by Orbaneja et al. [47]. The histology is characterized by a superficial band-like T-cell infiltrate, which resembles early-stage mycosis fungoides. The density of infiltrate exceeds that seen in allergic contact dermatitis, and atypical lymphocytes are present. This reaction has been reported to be caused by nickel, gold, isopropyl-diphenylenediamine, cobalt naphthenate, ethylenediamine dihydrochloride, *p*-phenylenediamine, *p-tertyl*-butyl phenol resin, and teak.

A second type of lymphomatoid contact dermatitis had been reported by Ecker and Winkelmann in 1981 [48], where patients had erythroderma resembling actinic reticuloid associated with positive patch test findings. However, most other authors contended that this latter group does not fit into the original description of lymphomatoid contact dermatitis.

Before diagnosing lymphomatoid contact dermatitis, an exhaustive investigation to exclude lymphoma may be necessary. There has been a report of a patient treated for "pseudolymphoma of the eyelids, lymphomatoid contact dermatitis type, induced by topical eye treatments," who later developed T-cell prolymphocytic leukemia 6 years after initial remission [49].

22

> **Core Message**
>
> › Allergic contact dermatitis producing histological features suggestive of cutaneous T-cell lymphoma can occur in areas in contact with various chemical allergens. The skin lesions usually resolve with avoidance. Further investigations to exclude lymphoma may be prudent.

22.13 Vascular-Occlusive Contact Dermatitis

A 75-year-old man presented with purpuric papulonecrotic lesions on his back 2 days after applying a spray containing the nonsteroidal anti-inflammatory drug, fepradinol [50]. Patch tests showed strong positive reactions to the spray as well as fepradinol 0.1, 1, and 2% eth., while 30 controls tested negative to fepradinol at the same concentrations. The histology of his lesions showed a thrombotic vasculopathy with epidermal necrosis without related leucocytoclastic vasculitis. This is the first reported case of vascular-occlusive contact dermatitis.

References

1. Goh CL (1989) Urticarial papular and plaque eruption. A manifestation of allergic contact dermatitis. Int J Dermatol 28:172–176
2. Holst R, Kirby J, Magnusson B (1976) Sensitization to tropical woods giving erythema multiforme-like eruptions. Contact Derm 2:295–296
3. Hausen BM (1981) Woods injurious to human health. De Gruyter, Berlin, p 59
4. Calnan CD (1956) Nickel dermatitis. Br J Dermatol 68:229–232
5. Cavendish A (1968) A case of dermatitis from 9 bromofluorene and a peculiar reaction to a patch test. Br J Dermatol 52:155–164
6. Powell EW (1968) Skin reactions to 9-bromofluorene. Br J Dermatol 80:491–496
7. De Feo CP (1966) Erythema multiforme bullosum caused by 9-bromofluorene. Arch Dermatol 94:545–551
8. Roed-Petersen J (1975) Erythema multiforme as an expression of contact dermatitis. Contact Derm 1:270–271
9. Tjiu JW, Chu CY, Sun CC (2004) 1, 2-Ethanedithiol-induced erythema multiforme-like contact dermatitis. Acta Derm Venereol 84:393–396
10. Nethercott JR, Albers J, Gurguis S et al (1982) Erythema multiforme exudativum linked to the manufacture of printed circuit boards. Contact Derm 3:314–322
11. Phoon WH, Chan MOY, Rajan VS et al (1984) Stevens-Johnson syndrome associated with occupational exposure to trichloroethylene. Contact Derm 10:270–276
12. Goh CL (1988) Erythema multiforme-like eruption from trinitrotoluene allergy. Int J Dermatol 27:650–651
13. Schena D, Barba A (1992) Erythema-multiforme-like contact dermatitis from dimethoate. Contact Derm 27:116–117
14. Batchvaros B, Minkow DM (1968) Dermatitis and purpura from rubber in clothing. Trans St John's Hosp Derm Soc 54:73–78
15. Calnan CD, Peachey RDG (1971) Allergic contact purpura. Clin Allergy 1:287–290
16. Fisher AA (1974) Allergic petechial and purpuric rubber dermatitis. The PPPP syndrome. Cutis 14:25–27
17. Romaguera C, Grimalt F (1977) PPPP syndrome. Contact Derm 3:103
18. van Joost T, van Ulsen J, Vuzevski VD, Naafs B, Tank BA (1990) Purpuric contact dermatitis to benzoyl peroxide. J Am Acad Dermatol 22:359–361
19. de Waard van der Spek FB, Oranje AP (1997) Purpura caused by Emla is of toxic origin. Contact Derm 36:11–13
20. Goh CL, Kwok SF, Rajan VS (1984) Cross sensitivity in colour developers. Contact Derm 10:280–285
21. Mendel EH (1960) Lichen planus-like eruption caused by a colourfilm developer. Arch Dermatol 70:516–519
22. Fry L (1965) Skin disease from colour developers. Br J Dermatol 77:456–461
23. Buckley WR (1958) Lichenoid eruptions following contact dermatitis. Arch Dermatol 78:454–457
24. Goh CL, Ng SK (1988) Bullous contact allergy from cinnamon. Dermatosen 36:186–187
25. Monti M, Berti E, Cavicchini S, Sala F (1983) Unusual cutaneous reaction after gold chloride patch test. Contact Derm 9:150–151
26. Iwatsuki K, Yamada M, Takigawa M, Inoue K, Matsumoto K (1987) Benign lymphoplasia of the earlobes induced by gold earrings: immunohistologic study on the cellular infiltrates. J Am Acad Dermatol 16:83–88
27. Rubin L (1956) Granulomas of axillae caused by deodorants. JAMA 162:953–955
28. Kaaber K, Nielsen AO, Veien NK (1992) Vaccination granulomas and aluminium allergy: course and prognostic factors. Contact Derm 26:304–306
29. Armstrong DK, Walsh MY, Dawson JF (1997) Granulomatous contact dermatitis due to gold earrings. Br J Dermatol 136:776–778
30. Fisher AA, Chargin L, Fleischmayer R et al (1959) Pustular patch test reactions. Arch Dermatol 80:742–752
31. Schoel VJ, Frosch PJ (1990) Allergisches Kontaktekzem durch Gummiinhaltsstoffe unter dem Bild einer Pustulosis palmaris. Dermatosen 38:178–180
32. Stone OJ, Johnson DA (1967) Pustular patch test-experimentally induced. Arch Dermatol 95:618–619
33. Hjorth N (1977) Diagnostic patch testing. In: Marzulli F, Maibach HI (eds) Dermatoxicology and pharmacology. Wiley, New York, p 344
34. Wahlberg JE, Maibach HI (1981) Sterile cutaneous pustules – a manifestation of primary irritancy? J Invest Dermatol 76:381–383

35. Schwartz L, Tulipan L, Birmingham A (1947) Occupational diseases of the skin, 3rd edn. Lea and Febiger, Philadelphia, p 771
36. Bauer M, Rabens SF (1977) Trichloroethylene toxicity. Int J Dermatol 16:113–116
37. Conde-Salazar L, Guimaraens D, Romero LV, Yus ES (1983) Subcorneal pustular eruption and erythema from occupational exposure to trichloroethylene. Contact Derm 9:235–237
38. Nakayama H, Bobayashi M, Takahashi M, Ageishi Y, Takano T (1988) Generalized eruption with severe liver dysfunction associated with occupational exposure to trichloroethylene. Contact Derm 19:48–51
39. Goh CL, Ng SK (1988) A cutaneous manifestation of trichloroethylene toxicity. Contact Derm 18:59–60
40. Hezemans-Boer M, Toonstra J, Meulenbelt J, Zwaveling JH, Sangster B, van Vloten WA (1988) Skin lesions due to exposure to methyl bromide. Arch Dermatol 124:917–921
41. Walder BK (1983) Do solvents cause scleroderma? Int J Dermatol 22:157–158
42. Texier L, Gautheir Y, Gauthier O et al (1972) Hypodermite sclerodermiforme lombo-fessiere induite par des injections de vitamine K1 et de Fer 300. Bull Soc Fr Dermatol Syphil 79:499–500
43. Rommel A, Saurat JH (1982) Hypodermite fessiere sclerodermiforme et injections de vitamine K1 a la naissance. Ann Pediatr 29:64–66
44. Pang BK, Munro V, Kossard S (1996) Pseudoscleroderma secondary to phytomenadione (vitamin K1) injections: Texier's disease. Aust J Dermatol 37:44–47
45. Kozuka T, Tashiro M, Sano S, Fujimoto K, Nakamura Y, Hashimoto S, Nakaminami G (1979) Brilliant Lake Red R as a cause of pigmented contact dermatitis. Contact Derm 5:297–304
46. Ippen H, Tesche S (1971) Freund's pigmented photodermatitis. ("Berloque-dermatitis", "eau de cologne-pigmentation"). Hautarzt 22:535–536
47. Orbaneja JG, Diez LI, Lozano JL, Salazar LC (1976) Lymphomatoid contact dermatitis: a syndrome produced by epicutaneous hypersensitivity with clinical features and a histopathologic picture similar to that of mycosis fungoides. Contact Derm 2:139–143
48. Ecker RI, Winkelmann RK (1981) Lymphomatoid contact dermatitis. Contact Derm 7:84–93
49. Braun RP, French LE, Feldmann R, Chavaz P, Saurat JH (2006) Cutaneous pseudolymphoma, lymphomatoid contact dermatitis type, as an unusual cause of symmetrical upper eyelid nodules. Br J Dermatol 155:633–634
50. Santos-Briz A, Antunez P, Munoz E, Moran M, Fernandez E, Unamuno P (2004) Vascular-occlusive contact dermatitis from fepradinol. Contact Derm 50:44–46

Respiratory Symptoms from Fragrances and the Link with Dermatitis

23

Jesper Elberling

Contents

J. Elberling
The Danish Research Centre for Chemical Sensitivities,
Department of Dermato-allergology, Gentofte Hospital,
University of Copenhagen, Denmark
e-mail: jeel@geh.regionh.dk

23.1 Introduction

Fragrances are added to commercial products in order to deliver a pleasing scent or mask an unpleasant scent. In exceptions, the function of adding a fragrance is to deliver an unpleasant scent, like mercaptan, which is added to natural gas to warn in case of a gas leak.

More than 2,000 fragrance chemicals are used by the perfume industry and a fragranced product can contain up to several hundred chemicals. Fragrances are present in most cosmetics and toiletries and are added to various consumer products, e.g. fabric softeners, detergents, cleaning agents, polishes, air fresheners, candles, plastic articles, fuels, paints, cat litter, animal sprays, treated textiles, cars and children's toys. It appears that scent marketing is a developing industry wherein fragrances are also added to stores and products with the purpose of enhancing sales. Consequently, exposure to fragrances is an everyday occurrence for most people.

Inhalation of fragrances may stimulate the olfactory and trigeminal systems. Olfactory and trigeminal receptors relay messages to the brain using the first and fifth cranial nerve respectively. Olfaction is essential for food selection, social interactions and avoidance of danger such as gas leaks, smoke or spoiled food. Trigeminal receptors are responsible for sensing irritation or pungency of chemicals in order to protect the organism against injury. Signals from fragrances can be purely olfactory or both olfactory and trigeminal. Generally, olfactory receptors respond to chemicals at lower concentrations than trigeminal receptors, but both the neuronal pathways are important for our ability to characterise the inspired air, and protect the organism against potential damage [1, 2].

Brain imaging studies have shown that olfactory stimuli are processed by the limbic system; amygdale

23

and piriform cortex, orbitofrontal-, inferior insular, and anterior cingulate cortex. Trigeminal stimulation, on the other hand, predominantly engages insular cortex, the dorsal portion of anterior cingulate, a minor portion of primary somatosensory cortex, brainstem, thalamus and cerebellum [3].

It is well established that skin exposure to fragrances implies a risk of allergic contact sensitisation as well as contact urticaria, but it is less documented as to what extent inhalation of fragrances implies a health hazard in the general population or in particular subgroups [4–8]. Nevertheless, fragrances are associated with respiratory symptoms such as upper airway irritation, breathing problems and cough in many individuals [9–11]. Even though the pathophysiological mechanisms of such symptoms are unclear and no effective treatments of the symptoms have been documented, the symptoms are noteworthy as they severely affect many individuals and often coincide with asthma and dermatitis.

> **Core Message**
>
> › A fragrance may act as a purely olfactory, or both an olfactory and trigeminal stimulating agent. Generally, olfactory receptors respond to chemicals at lower concentrations than trigeminal receptors, but both the pathways are important for our ability to characterise the inspired air and protect the organism against potential damage.

23.2 Localisation, Prevalence and Severity

The frequently reported adverse symptoms include dry, itching or watery eyes, nasal irritation, congestion and sneezing, as well as mouth and throat irritation, shortness of breath and cough. Generally, ocular and nasal symptoms are reported more frequently than respiratory symptoms at other locations [9–11]. Population-based studies measuring fragrance-related respiratory symptoms are limited in number [10] and prevalence estimates of the affected individuals varies a lot depending on the applied questionnaire and investigated populations [9–18]. Most population-based

studies on symptoms related to inhalation of chemicals are limited in their ability to link exposure to fragrances with specific respiratory symptoms or to distinguish clinically important from clinically unimportant symptoms [9, 11–18]. Prevalence rates may be over or under-estimated by selection procedures and lack of internationally standardised and linguistic validated questionnaires.

In a Danish suburban population-based questionnaire study of 6,000 randomly selected 18–69 year-old individuals [9], 45% reported annoyance attributed to the inhalation of at least one of the 11 common chemicals. Twenty seven percent of the respondents declared that it was not just the smell of the chemicals they disliked and stated that they were actually bothered by symptoms. At least one respiratory symptom was reported by 24%, and the most frequently reported symptoms in both the sexes were nasal symptoms together with headache. Others wearing perfume, aftershave or deodorant were the commonest cause of symptoms, reported by 15% of all respondents and influenced the choice of personal hygiene products, the way of cleaning at home and to a lesser degree, the choice of shopping places, in most cases. In 3.5% of the population, the symptoms from fragrances and other chemicals had more severe consequences for the social and occupational life [9]. The above given prevalences are in accordance with other studies [10–18] when different severity dimensions are taken into account [9]. Thus, most fragrance-related respiratory symptoms reported in general populations are mild, but across different populations, approximately 0.5–4% are more severely affected by symptoms.

> **Core Message**
>
> › Symptoms from the upper airways are dominating and the symptoms are for the most part mild. Severe symptoms affect between 0.5 and 4% across different populations.

23.3 Epidemiological Associations

Individuals with asthma often report upper airway irritation and asthma-like symptoms following exposure to fragrances in their everyday environments [10, 19, 20].

In contradistinction to asthma, individuals with positive skin prick tests to common aeroallergens do not report fragrance-related respiratory symptoms more frequently than others [10], not even when the severity of the symptoms is taken into account.

Interestingly, individuals with hand eczema and/or contact allergy report fragrance-related respiratory symptoms 2–4 times more frequently than others, independent of asthma, skin prick test reactivity to common aeroallergens, sex and psychological vulnerability [21]. Further, the symptoms are also associated with atopic dermatitis [20]. The co-occurrence of fragrance-related symptoms with the dermatological conditions could not be ascribed to a general increased tendency to report symptoms, as individuals with atopic dermatitis, hand eczema or contact allergy did not report pollen-related respiratory symptoms more frequently than other persons [20].

Fragrance-related respiratory symptoms are also reported frequently by individuals who are psychologically vulnerable [21]. Psychological vulnerability has been associated with upper dyspepsia and irritable bowel syndrome [22, 23], and predict prolonged pain after lumbar spine surgery and cholecystectomy [24–26].

Fragrance-related respiratory symptoms are reported to be more frequent among women, as opposed to men [10, 20]. This gender difference could reflect a biological difference, cultural differences where men underreport, or more severe responses in women than men e.g. a heavier exposure in women to fragrance chemicals from personal cosmetic usage or other unidentified risk factors. It has been speculated whether the higher oestrogen level in women could play a role, as oestrogens may act directly on receptors expressed on sensory neurons and trigeminal ganglia. To support this suggestion, the cough threshold measured by the inhaled capsaicin is significantly lower in healthy women compared to healthy men [27].

Core Message

> ❭ Fragrance-related respiratory symptoms are frequently reported in general populations and co-occur regularly with asthma, contact dermatitis and atopic dermatitis.

23.4 Pathophysiology

The mechanisms by which fragrance chemicals induce respiratory symptoms at exposure levels tolerated by most individuals are unclear, but may theoretically involve immunological, sensory and psychological mechanisms.

23.4.1 Immunological Mechanisms

Individuals with fragrance contact allergy report fragrance-related respiratory symptoms more frequently than others [21]. In one of the two published case reports on occupational asthma to fragrances [28, 29], a positive patch test to fragrance chemicals was found, and bronchial obstruction was elicited subsequently after a fragrance provocation [28]. Contact allergy is a cell-mediated and non-immediate hyper-sensitivity reaction, wherein dermatitis in sensitised individuals usually develops hours after exposure to an allergen. It is therefore difficult to explain immunologically as to how fragrance chemicals in sensitised individuals can induce immediate respiratory symptoms upon inhalation. Hypothetically, fragrance chemicals can induce IgE-mediated allergy, but unlike proteins, chemicals must combine with larger carrier molecules in order to induce an IgE-mediated immune response [30]. In a review on chemicals causing allergic sensitisation of the respiratory tract resulting in occupational asthma [30], no fragrances are listed as chemical allergens. Nevertheless, anaphylaxis has been reported in one case after spraying perfume in the eyes [31], but evidence of fragrance-specific IgE was not provided. Thus non-immunological mechanisms are also possible since mast cell deregulation can be achieved by a variety of other stimuli than IgE e.g. anaphylaxotoxins C5a and C3a, neuropeptides such as substance P and engagement of toll-like receptors [32]. To support this view, it has been demonstrated in vitro that fragrances induce a concentration-dependent non-IgE mediated basophil histamine release [33] both in healthy volunteers and eczema patients with fragrance-related respiratory symptoms. In a population-based study, even severe fragrance-related respiratory symptoms were not associated with positive skin prick tests to common aeroallergens [10]. Asthma can be suspected in individuals who experience symptoms from strong smells

[34]. Although a decline in lung function upon fragrance inhalation has been reported in individuals with severe and/ or occupational asthma [28, 29, 35], fragrance-related symptoms in individuals with mild to moderate asthma is not attributable to bronchial obstruction [36]. Despite reporting by mild–moderate asthmatics that exposure to fragranced products triggers ocular and respiratory symptoms, no changes in ocular redness or nasal mucosal swelling were elicited by a 30 min of exposure to fragranced aerosols [19].

Taken together, IgE-mediated allergy to fragrance cannot be ruled out as a possible mechanism. However, since fragrance-specific IgE has never been proven, this mechanism may be involved only in extremely rare cases. In the vast majority of individuals with even severe fragrance-related respiratory symptoms, the mechanism of action is most probably different from that which mediates contact or IgE-mediated allergy.

23.4.2 Sensory Mechanisms

Sensory neurones play important roles in response to chemical stimulation by activating airway defensive reflexes such as nasal congestion, sneezing, mucous production or cough [37, 38]. Inhalation of irritants may activate sensory reflexes [37, 39, 40] and eventually evoke neurogenic inflammation [41]. Based on the inhalation studies with capsaicin (the pungent and odourless component in hot chilli pepper), Millqvist et al. have suggested that hyper-reactivity of airway sensory neurones underlie chemical- and fragrance-related cough and asthma-like symptoms [42]. Inhalation of capsaicin stimulates the afferent C-fibres and Aδ-fibres in the airways [39] and triggers the cough reflex in a dose-dependent manner [43]. It is important to note that capsaicin does not act as a bronchoconstrictor agent in humans. Increased cough responses induced by capsaicin is associated with fragrance-related symptoms in asthmatic, non-asthmatic and non-allergic patients [36, 42]. In eczema patients with fragrance-related symptoms, lower, but not upper, respiratory symptoms were associated with increased capsaicin cough responsiveness, independent of positive patch test to fragrances [44]. The association between fragrance-related respiratory symptoms and capsaicin-induced sensory hyper-reactivity is significant, but it does not provide evidence that fragrances act as sensory irritants in individuals with increased capsaicin sensitivity. The main controversy in this context is that provocational studies with fragrances have not convincingly been able to demonstrate that patients with fragrance-related respiratory symptoms actually are more sensitive (at a peripheral level) to fragrance exposure [19, 45–47]. Thus, sensitisation to fragrances at a more central level could be suspected [48].

Fragrance-related respiratory symptoms are frequently reported by individuals with multiple chemical sensitivity (MCS) [49], a non-allergic multi-symptom disorder, that may imply a dysfunction of the central nervous system [3, 48, 50], wherein exposure to certain chemicals and fragrances are perceived as injurious. As mentioned above, the heat and acid-sensitive capsaicin receptors are important nociceptors providing pain perceptions in response to potentially damaging stimuli [1, 51]. In this context, it has been suggested that a violent exposure to chemical odours may trigger plastic changes in the central nervous system (CNS) followed by enhanced central reactions to exposure levels below the normal threshold for the manifestation of a toxic response. Such potential changes in the CNS would be comparable to those involved in the transition from an acute pain episode to the development of a persistent pathological pain state and abnormal increases in pain sensitivity [52]. In accordance with this hypothesis, positron emission tomography (PET) activation studies with several odorants found that individuals with MCS showed a reduced rather than enhanced activation of cerebral regions processing odour signals with hyper-activation of the anterior cingulate and hypo-activation of the olfactory circuits which could reflect harm avoidance of chemical odours [3]. Similarly, plastic changes in the central nervous system may, to some extent, explain fragrance-related respiratory symptoms.

23.4.3 Psychological Mechanisms

Psychological factors may affect fragrance-related respiratory symptoms [21]. In a study of healthy individuals, where beliefs about the nature of a chemical exposure was systematically modified, individuals who were given a harmful bias reported significantly more health symptoms and more intense odour and irritation during exposure than did individuals who were induced with a neutral or healthful bias [53]. Such observations have, together with the inability to provoke symptoms (below odour thresholds) among chemically sensitive individuals, led to suggestions of a predominant psychological or behavioural basis for symptoms related to inhalation of chemical odours [54]. Although there are good indications that psychological factors, to a certain degree, influence individuals with symptoms from inhalation of chemicals, no trials have yet provided evidence of the efficacy of psychological interventions in order to treat such symptoms [55].

> **Core Message**
>
> › There are no indications that fragrance-related respiratory symptoms in the vast majority are caused by immunological hyper-sensitivity reactions. Instead, sensory mechanisms at a peripheral receptor level as well as more central mechanisms at the level of sensory signal processing may influence.

23.5 Genetic and Environmental Factors

The heritability of respiratory symptoms related to perfume has been estimated in a population-based twin study of 4,128 twin individuals. An increased familial occurrence of fragrance-related respiratory symptoms was found with 35% of the phenotypic variation attributable to additive genetic effects and 65% due to individual specific environmental effects [20]. About 40% of the correlation found between fragrance-related respiratory symptoms and atopic dermatitis could be attributed to genes shared between these two traits [20]. This is interesting since atopic dermatitis also influences the development of asthma and hand eczema [56, 57]. The co-occurrence of fragrance-related respiratory symptoms with hand eczema, contact allergy and asthma was not attributable to shared genetic factors [20]. An alternative explanation for the observed associations is that the intrinsic environment related to tissue inflammation in otherwise susceptible individuals increases the sensitivity to inhaled fragrances [20]. This could be due to mechanisms at a peripheral level, for example, those possibly involved in bronchial sensory hyper-reactivity, suggested in patients with lower respiratory symptoms related to fragrances [42], or it could

involve an abnormal central processing of sensory odour signals, as suggested in patients with multiple chemical sensitivities [3, 48].

> **Core Message**
>
> › Fragrance-related respiratory symptoms are influenced by environmental factors and also by additive genetic factors of which some genes seems to be shared with atopic dermatitis.

23.6 Conclusion

Fragrance-related respiratory symptoms are frequently reported in general populations and co-occur regularly in patients with asthma, contact dermatitis and atopic dermatitis. The symptoms are especially influenced by environmental factors and also by additive genetic factors of which some genes seems to be shared with atopic dermatitis. There are no indications that fragrance-related respiratory symptoms in the vast majority are caused by immunological hyper-sensitivity reactions. Instead, sensory mechanisms may influence the symptoms, but it is not clarified as to what extent these involve mechanisms at a peripheral level, a central level or a combination.

So far, no validated methods or objective measurements have been established to verify the symptoms, neither has documentation of effective treatments. Besides, to acknowledge patients with annoying respiratory symptoms related to fragrances, the pragmatic approach when meeting these patients could be to reduce inflammation in patients where asthma and/or eczema co-occur.

23.7 Case Report with a Typical Treatment Strategy

A 45-year-old woman working as a chief secretary in a pharmaceutical company developed nasal irritation, sore throat and head ache provoked by a colleague's use of perfume over a 6-months period.

The symptoms began after a damp damage at the office which had been thoroughly repaired. In the same period, she also developed nasal symptoms and headache from her own use of fragranced cleaning agents and cosmetics.

23

The patient had no history of asthma or allergic rhinitis, but a previous history of nickel allergy and hand eczema without eruption for several years. She appeared sound and intelligent and had no history of psychiatric illness.

All laboratory measurements were within normal limits. Skin prick test with a standard panel of aeroallergens and her colleague's perfume; Opium®, parfum (Yves Saint Laurent, Paris, France) were negative. Patch testing with the European standard test series showed ++ positive reaction to Nickel and erythema without infiltration i.e. not a positive test to Fragrance Mix I.

The patient was advised to totally avoid, whenever possible, fragranced products in her environment.

After some time, a cautious stepwise exposure to various lightly scented products could be tried.

Initially, treatment with oral antihistamine daily was prescribed with a moderate improvement. After 3 weeks, nasal steroids were prescribed, but terminated after 1 month because of no additional effect.

23.8 Diagram Summarising the Current View on the Pathogenesis of Respiratory Symptoms from Fragrance Exposure

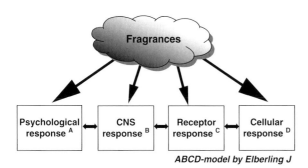

ABCD-model by Elberling J

[A]Emotional and/or cognitive response to fragrance exposure e.g. anxiety or attention bias.
[B]Abnormal processing of sensory fragrance signals in the biological brain e.g. cortical reorganisation.
[C]Olfactory and/or somatosensory/trigeminal responses to fragrances e.g. sensory hyper-reactivity.
[D]Cytokine release in response to fragrance exposure in skin and airways e.g. histamine.

The horizontal arrows in the ABCD-model imply that abnormal response to fragrances in one modality may increase abnormal responses to fragrances in relative modalities.

References

1. Finger TE, Silver WL, Restrepo D (2000) The neurobiology of taste and smell, 2nd edn. Wiley-Liss, New York
2. Paustenbach DJ, Gaffney SH (2006) The role of odor and irritation, as well as risk perception, in the setting of occupational exposure limits. Int Arch Occup Environ Health 79:339–342
3. Hillert L, Musabasic V, Berglund H, Ciumas C, Savic I (2007) Odor processing in multiple chemical sensitivity. Hum Brain Mapp 28:172–182
4. Nimmermark S (2004) Odour influence on well-being and health with specific focus on animal production emissions. Ann Agric Environ Med 11:163–173
5. Steinemann AC (2008) Fragranced consumer products and undisclosed ingredients. Environ Impact Asses Rev doi:10 1016/j eiar 2008 05 002 2008
6. Ezendam J (2007) Immune effects of respiratory exposure to fragrance chemicals; RIVM Report 340301001. Ref Type: Report
7. Farrow A, Taylor H, Northstone K, Golding J (2003) Symptoms of mothers and infants related to total volatile organic compounds in household products. Arch Environ Health 58:633–641
8. Elberling J, Linneberg A, Mosbech H, Dirksen A, Menne T, Nielsen NH, Madsen F, Frolund L, Johansen JD (2005) Airborne chemicals cause respiratory symptoms in individuals with contact allergy. Contact Derm 52:65–72
9. Berg ND, Linneberg A, Dirksen A, Elberling J (2008) Prevalence of self-reported symptoms and consequences related to inhalation of airborne chemicals in a Danish general population. Int Arch Occup Environ Health 81:881–887
10. Elberling J, Linneberg A, Dirksen A, Johansen JD, Frolund L, Madsen F, Nielsen NH, Mosbech H (2005) Mucosal symptoms elicited by fragrance products in a population-based sample in relation to atopy and bronchial hyper-reactivity. Clin Exp Allergy 35:75–81
11. Johansson A, Bramerson A, Millqvist E, Nordin S, Bende M (2005) Prevalence and risk factors for self-reported odour intolerance: the Skovde population-based study. Int Arch Occup Environ Health 78:559–564
12. Baldwin CM, Bell IR, O'Rourke MK, Lebowitz MD (1997) The association of respiratory problems in a community sample with self-reported chemical intolerance. Eur J Epidemiol 13:547–552
13. Caress SM, Steinemann AC (2005) National prevalence of asthma and chemical hypersensitivity: an examination of potential overlap. J Occup Environ Med 47:518–522
14. Carlsson F, Karlson B, Orbaek P, Osterberg K, Ostergren PO (2005) Prevalence of annoyance attributed to electrical equipment and smells in a Swedish population, and relationship with subjective health and daily functioning. Public Health 119:568–577
15. Hunter PR, Davies MA, Hill H, Whittaker M, Sufi F (2003) The prevalence of self-reported symptoms of respiratory disease and community belief about the severity of pollution from various sources. Int J Environ Health Res 13:227–238

16. Kreutzer R, Neutra RR, Lashuay N (1999) Prevalence of people reporting sensitivities to chemicals in a population-based survey. Am J Epidemiol 150:1–12

17. Meggs WJ, Dunn KA, Bloch RM, Goodman PE, Davidoff AL (1996) Prevalence and nature of allergy and chemical sensitivity in a general population. Arch Environ Health 51:275–282

18. Caress SM, Steinemann AC (2009) Prevalence of fragrance sensitivity in the American population. J Environ Health 71:46–50

19. Opiekun RE, Smeets M, Sulewski M, Rogers R, Prasad N, Vedula U, Dalton P (2003) Assessment of ocular and nasal irritation in asthmatics resulting from fragrance exposure. Clin Exp Allergy 33:1256–1265

20. Elberling J, Lerbaek A, Kyvik K, Hjelmborg J (2009) A twin study of respiratory symptoms related to perfume. Int J Hyg Environ Health. doi:10.1016/j.ijheh.2009.05.001

21. Elberling J, Linneberg A, Mosbech H, Dirksen A, Frolund L, Madsen F, Nielsen NH, Johansen JD (2004) A link between skin and airways regarding sensitivity to fragrance products? Br J Dermatol 151:1197–1203

22. Kay L, Jorgensen T, Jensen KH (1995) Irritable colon among 30-60-year old subjects. A cohort study of 4581 Danes. Ugeskr Laeger 157:3476–3480

23. Kay L, Jorgensen T (1995) Upper dyspepsia in persons aged 50 to 60 years. Results from a 5-year follow-up population study in Glostrup. Ugeskr Laeger 157:2574–2578

24. Thorvaldsen P, Sorensen EB (1990) Psychological vulnerability as a predictor for short-term outcome in lumbar spine surgery. A prospective study (Part II). Acta Neurochir (Wien) 102:58–61

25. Jess P, Jess T, Beck H, Bech P (1998) Neuroticism in relation to recovery and persisting pain after laparoscopic cholecystectomy. Scand J Gastroenterol 33:550–553

26. Jorgensen T, Teglbjerg JS, Wille-Jorgensen P, Bille T, Thorvaldsen P (1991) Persisting pain after cholecystectomy. A prospective investigation. Scand J Gastroenterol 26: 124–128

27. Dicpinigaitis PV, Rauf K (1998) The influence of gender on cough reflex sensitivity. Chest 113:1319–1321

28. Baur X, Schneider EM, Wieners D, Czuppon AB (1999) Occupational asthma to perfume. Allergy 54:1334–1335

29. Jensen OC, Petersen I (1991) Occupational asthma caused by scented gravel in cat litter boxes. Ugeskr Laeger 153:939–940

30. Isola D, Kimber I, Sarlo K, Lalko J, Sipes IG (2008) Chemical respiratory allergy and occupational asthma: what are the key areas of uncertainty? J Appl Toxicol 28: 249–253

31. Lessenger JE (2001) Occupational acute anaphylactic reaction to assault by perfume spray in the face. J Am Board Fam Pract 14:137–140

32. Galli SJ, Nakae S, Tsai M (2005) Mast cells in the development of adaptive immune responses. Nat Immunol 6: 135–142

33. Elberling J, Skov PS, Mosbech H, Holst H, Dirksen A, Johansen JD (2007) Increased release of histamine in patients with respiratory symptoms related to perfume. Clin Exp Allergy 37:1676–1680

34. Bateman ED, Hurd SS, Barnes PJ, Bousquet J, Drazen JM, FitzGerald M, Gibson P, Ohta K, O'Byrne P, Pedersen SE, Pizzichini E, Sullivan SD, Wenzel SE, Zar HJ (2008) Global strategy for asthma management and prevention: GINA executive summary. Eur Respir J 31:143–178

35. Kumar P, Caradonna-Graham VM, Gupta S, Cai X, Rao PN, Thompson J (1995) Inhalation challenge effects of perfume scent strips in patients with asthma. Ann Allergy Asthma Immunol 75:429–433

36. Millqvist E, Lowhagen O (1998) Methacholine provocations do not reveal sensitivity to strong scents. Ann Allergy Asthma Immunol 80:381–384

37. Bryant B, Silver WL (2000) Chemestesis: the common chemical sense. In: Finger TE, Silver WL, Restrepo D (eds) The neurobiology of taste and smell. Wiley-Liss, New York, pp 73–100

38. Lee LY, Pisarri TE (2001) Afferent properties and reflex functions of bronchopulmonary C-fibers. Respir Physiol 125:47–65

39. Belvisi MG (2003) Sensory nerves and airway inflammation: role of A delta and C-fibres. Pulm Pharmacol Ther 16:1–7

40. Sanico AM, Atsuta S, Proud D, Togias A (1997) Dose-dependent effects of capsaicin nasal challenge: in vivo evidence of human airway neurogenic inflammation. J Allergy Clin Immunol 100:632–641

41. Barnes PJ (2001) Neurogenic inflammation in the airways. Respir Physiol 125:145–154

42. Millqvist E, Bende M, Lowhagen O (1998) Sensory hyper-reactivity–a possible mechanism underlying cough and asthma-like symptoms. Allergy 53:1208–1212

43. Midgren B, Hansson L, Karlsson JA, Simonsson BG, Persson CG (1992) Capsaicin-induced cough in humans. Am Rev Respir Dis 146:347–351

44. Elberling J, Dirksen A, Johansen JD, Mosbech H (2006) The capsaicin cough reflex in eczema patients with respiratory symptoms elicited by perfume. Contact Derm 54: 158–164

45. Elberling J, Duus JJ, Dirksen A, Mosbech H (2006) Exposure of eyes to perfume: a double-blind, placebo-controlled experiment. Indoor Air 16:276–281

46. Millqvist E, Lowhagen O (1996) Placebo-controlled challenges with perfume in patients with asthma-like symptoms. Allergy 51:434–439

47. Millqvist E, Bengtsson U, Lowhagen O (1999) Provocations with perfume in the eyes induce airway symptoms in patients with sensory hyperreactivity. Allergy 54:495–499

48. Yunus MB (2008) Central sensitivity syndromes: a new paradigm and group nosology for fibromyalgia and overlapping conditions, and the related issue of disease versus illness. Semin Arthritis Rheum 37:339–352

49. Labarge XS, McCaffrey RJ (2000) Multiple chemical sensitivity: a review of the theoretical and research literature. Neuropsychol Rev 10:183–211

50. Winder C (2002) Mechanisms of multiple chemical sensitivity. Toxicol Lett 128:85–97

51. Szallasi A, Blumberg PM (1999) Vanilloid (Capsaicin) receptors and mechanisms. Pharmacol Rev 51:159–212

52. Rainville P, Bushnell MC, Duncan GH (2001) Representation of acute and persistent pain in the human CNS: potential implications for chemical intolerance. Ann NY Acad Sci 933:130–141

53. Dalton P (1999) Cognitive influences on health symptoms from acute chemical exposure. Health Psychol 18:579–590

23

54. Das-Munshi J, Rubin GJ, Wessely S (2006) Multiple chemical sensitivities: a systematic review of provocation studies. J Allergy Clin Immunol 118:1257–1264

55. Das-Munshi J, Rubin GJ, Wessely S (2007) Multiple chemical sensitivities: review. Curr Opin Otolaryngol Head Neck Surg 15:274–280

56. Dold S, Wjst M, von ME, Reitmeir P, Stiepel E (1992) Genetic risk for asthma, allergic rhinitis, and atopic dermatitis. Arch Dis Child 67:1018–1022

57. Meding B, Swanbeck G (1989) Epidemiology of different types of hand eczema in an industrial city. Acta Derm Venereol 69:227–233

Patch Testing

24

Magnus Lindberg and Mihaly Matura

Contents

M. Lindberg (✉)
Department of Dermatology, University Hospital Örebro,
701 85 Örebro, Sweden
e-mail: magnus.lindberg@orebroll.se

M. Matura
Unit of Occupational and Environmental Dermatology,
Institute of Environmental Medicine, Karolinska Institutet,
17176 Stockholm, Sweden

24.1 Introduction

24.1.1 The Purpose of Patch Testing

Patch testing is a well-established method of diagnosing contact allergy – a delayed type of hypersensitivity (type IV reaction). Patients with a history and clinical picture of contact dermatitis are reexposed to the suspected allergens under controlled conditions to verify the diagnosis. Contact allergy

J.D. Johansen et al. (eds.), *Contact Dermatitis*,
DOI: 10.1007/978-3-642-03827-3_24, © Springer-Verlag Berlin Heidelberg 2011

can also be a complicating factor in other skin conditions. Thus, testing patients with hand (dyshidrotic, hyperkeratotic), arm, face, or leg eczema (stasis dermatitis), testing of other types of eczema (atopic, seborrheic dermatitis, nummular eczema), including patients with chronic psoriasis, vulval disorders, or drug reactions (Chap. 26), is sometimes indicated, especially when they are recalcitrant to the prescribed treatment and the dermatologist suspects contact allergy to prescribed topical medicaments and their vehicles. Apart from its use to confirm a suspected allergic contact dermatitis, the patch test procedure can also be used before recommending alternative medicaments, skin care products, cosmetics, gloves, etc. in a particular patient. If the patient does not react to the alternatives tested, it is unlikely that he or she will react to the products in ordinary use.

Early classic publications on patch testing are reviewed in Chap. 1. More recent, often-quoted guidelines are presented by Malten et al. [1], Fregert [2] and Bandmann and Wohn [3]. Several studies (e.g., [4–6]) have shown that detailed patch testing is beneficial for patients and that it improves their quality of life (QoL). However, it has also been claimed that random patch testing with a baseline series should be discouraged due to low pretest probability [7]. When performing patch testing, it has to be remembered that the patch test is a biological provocation test, and as such, the outcome is dependent on multiple factors including the test system and test material, the biological/functional status of the tested person, and the knowledge and experience of responsible dermatologist [8]. Most of these aspects will be discussed in this chapter.

Core Message

> Indications for patch testing:

- – Cases of contact dermatitis
- – Other types of eczema and dermatoses, where a superimposed contact allergy is suspected, particularly if recurrent and non-responsive to treatment
- – Suspected contact allergy to topical medicaments and their vehicles
- – "Predictive testing" of alternative products such as gloves, skin care products, medicaments

---

24.1.2 Standardization

The first patch tests according to the present principles were carried out in 1895 [9] but were preceded by some preliminary experiments [10] (see Chap. 1). During the last few decades, much effort has been put into standardization of allergens, vehicles, concentrations, patch test materials, tapes, and the scoring of test reactions, and the method used today is considered accurate and reliable. A series of papers has demonstrated the reproducibility of patch test results regarding different techniques, over time and between individuals [11–27]. Standardization has facilitated comparisons of contact allergy frequency in and between clinics, geographical areas, and areas with various degrees of industrialization, but some questions still remain, especially concerning the reading and scoring of test reactions. This will be discussed in detail below.

24.1.3 Bioavailability

To obtain optimal bioavailability of a hapten one can influence the following five variables:

- Intrinsic penetration capacity
- Concentration, dose
- Vehicle
- Occlusivity of patch test system and tape
- Exposure

Since it is desirable to remove all test strips at the same time – usually at day 2 (48 h) – 4 factors remain and can be varied and optimized by the manufacturers of patch test materials and allergen preparations and by the dermatologist responsible for the testing. The penetration capacity can depend upon the salts used; for example, there is a big difference between the penetration of nickel achieved by nickel sulfate and nickel chloride [28]. The higher penetration of nickel from the chloride is probably explained by the partition skin/vehicle of the salts, when applied in the same vehicle in equimolar concentration and under occlusion.

24.2 Test Systems

One can distinguish two test systems: the original one, where the allergens, patches, and tapes are supplied separately, and the ready-to-use system, where only a covering material has to be removed before the test is applied.

24.2.1 Original System (Allergen–Patch–Tape)

24.2.1.1 Patches

Some of the patch test units available are depicted in Fig. 24.1. In Finn chamber (Epitest, Finland) the test area is circular and in van der Bend (van der Bend, The Netherlands) and IQ chambers (Chemotechnique Diagnostic, Sweden) they are square. The latter is claimed to facilitate distinguishing allergic from irritant reactions (IR), since an irritant reaction tends to look square, while an allergic reaction tends to look round [1]. Based on a comparative study with ordinary (8 mm) and large (12 mm) Finn chambers, it was found that the larger chambers may be useful for the detection of weak sensitization to some contact allergens [29, 30]. However, the larger chambers are usually recommended for experimental studies when testing for irritancy. Finn chambers are made of aluminum. Polypropylene-coated chambers are available for use when the test substance is believed to react with or be affected by aluminum, e.g., when testing with acrylates.

24.2.1.2 Allergens

The standard patch test allergens available on the market, can, according to the suppliers' product catalogs, be considered chemically defined and pure. However, the dermatologist responsible for patch testing is recommended repeatedly to request the manufacturers to provide the results of chemical analyses. For example, in a recent publication on patch testing with disperse dyes it was demonstrated that the test preparation contained impurities [31]. The test preparations are presented in plastic syringes or bottles of inert material to prevent degradation or other chemical changes due to air, humidity, and light. The suppliers' recommendations on storage must be followed in order to minimize these risks. It is suspected that several of the contact allergies reported earlier were due to impurities or degradation products [32]. It has not been possible to confirm the allergenic potential of some claimed "allergens."

24.2.1.3 Vehicles

Each allergen almost certainly has its own optimal vehicle; it is improbable that just one vehicle (e.g., petrolatum) could be optimal for all allergens. White petrolatum is the most widely used vehicle, but its general reliability can be questioned. It gives good occlusion, keeps the allergens stable, and is inexpensive. On the other hand, it can retain the allergen (see Sect. 24.5.6.1), irritate the skin, and has even been reported to cause allergic skin reactions [33]. Liquid vehicles such as water and solvents (acetone, ethanol, methyl ethyl ketone) are recommended since they facilitate penetration of the skin, but they also have some drawbacks. Solvents may evaporate, which does not favor exact dosing, and most test solutions must be freshly prepared. Liquid vehicles are used mainly when testing chemicals and products brought by patients (see Sect. 24.13), and in research projects. By using buffer solutions for acid and alkaline products, the test concentration can be raised [34]. A filter paper must be used for liquid allergen preparations when using Finn chambers. Modern vehicles are hydrophilic gels (cellulose derivatives), used, for example, in the TRUE test (Mekos, Denmark, see Sect. 24.2.2) [35]. When using more sophisticated vehicles containing salicylic acid, anionic detergents, solvents, and others than those mentioned above (e.g., dimethylsulfoxide, DMSO), alkalis, etc. to increase penetration (see Sect. 24.1.3), an extra patch with the vehicle, as is, must be applied to exclude the possibility that the vehicle is irritant. Since the number of test sites is limited, these vehicles cannot be recommended for routine use. However, they might be valuable where the standard preparation has given a negative reaction but the clinical impression of an allergic contact dermatitis remains.

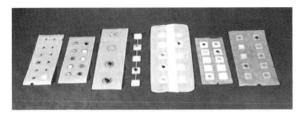

Fig. 24.1 Figure one shows different test systems. From *left* to *right*: TRUE Test (the first strip), Finn chambers, ordinary (diameter 8 mm) and large (diameter 12 mm), van der Bend square chambers with and without tape, IQ ultra and IQ chamber. Different test preparations applied for illustration (photo by Gunnel Hagelthorn)

24

> › White petrolatum is used as the vehicle in the majority of patch test preparations. However, in cases of unexpected, negative patch test results alternative vehicles have to be considered.

24.2.1.4 Concentrations

In textbooks on contact dermatitis and patch testing, and in suppliers' catalogs, the concentration of an allergen is given as a percentage. In one catalog, molality (M) is given together with percentage (weight/weight), and in the TRUE Test, concentration is given in milligrams or micrograms per square centimeter. The traditional method of presenting concentrations as a percentage is simple and probably practical, but has been questioned [36, 37], as we do not know if this means weight/weight, volume/volume, volume/weight, or weight/volume. Using Finn chambers for patch testing, the recommended amount of petrolatum preparation is 20 mg to obtain an optimal dose of allergens [38]. When comparing substances and in research projects, it is the dose, the number of molecules delivered, that is of interest [39]. The concentration of Ni ions is 20.9% in nickel sulfate ($NiSO_4 \cdot 7H_2O$) compared to 24.7% in nickel chloride ($NiCl_2 \cdot 6H_2O$) [40]. Thus in comparative studies with these salts it is essential to use the same molality [41].

> **Core Message**

> › Test concentrations should preferably be expressed as weight per area, e.g., milligrams or micrograms per square centimeter (mg/cm^2, $\mu g/cm^2$).

24.2.1.5 Tapes

Previously, most tapes were based on colophony and could cause severe and lasting reactions in patients for whom such a sensitivity was not anticipated. By introducing modern acrylate-based adhesive tapes, the problem with colophony reactions has been eliminated. However, acrylate-based adhesive tapes might

also cause skin reactions. Few studies targeted the question of whether the etiology is irritant in nature because of acrylic acid residues in the tape (personal communication) or because of contact allergy to some culprits not identified up till now, e.g., antioxidants, acrylate monomers [42]. Contact urticaria from acrylic acid has also been reported [43]. In cases where loosening can be anticipated (oily or hairy skin, sweating, high humidity), some reinforcing tapes are recommended. Methods for studies on conformability and irritancy of tapes have been published [44, 45].

24.2.1.6 Application of Test Preparations to the Patches

Commercial test preparations – allergens in petrolatum and kept in syringes – are applied directly into the test chambers, or onto the filter paper disks of the other patches (Fig. 24.2a) and a small amount, "a snake" (approximately 7 mm long), of the mixture is applied across the diameter of the disk. The orifice of the syringe is adjusted to facilitate this. In order to obtain an optimal dose of allergens applied at patch testing the recommended amount of petrolatum preparation is 20 mg in Finn chambers [38]. Liquid test preparations are preferably applied via a digital pipette with disposable plastic tips to allow exact dosing (15 µL calculated for ordinary Finn chambers) (Fig. 24.2b).

24.2.1.7 Suppliers

The catalogs from the suppliers contain lists of test preparations in alphabetical order, allergens in the European and International baseline series, tables of mixes, and lists of screening series. The catalogs also contain information on the occurrence of allergens and cross-reactivity, as well as some service items such as test sheets, guides to patch testing, skin markers, questionnaires, and advice to patients. There are several suppliers on the market, e.g., Allergy EAZE system (www.allergyeaze.com), Chemotechnique Diagnostics (www.chemotechnique.se), Trolab, Hermal (www.hermal.de).

24.2.2 Ready-to-Use Systems

In the ready-to-use patch test system, all necessary material is prepared in advance, and the dermatologist, nurse,

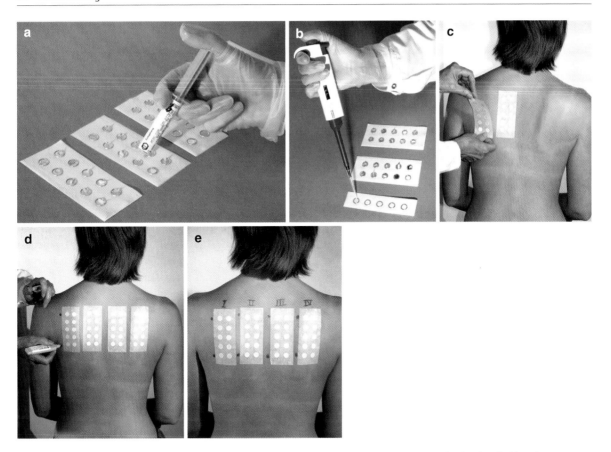

Fig. 24.2 Patch testing. (**a, b**) Application of allergens to test patches (**a**) allergen in petrolatum, (**b**) allergen in liquid test preparation using digital pipette with disposable tip). (**c**) Application of patch tests on the *upper back*. (**d**) Marking the test area. (**e**) Test applied to the *upper back* (photo by Gunnel Hagelthorn)

or technician only has to remove the covering material, apply the test strips, and mark. In the TRUE Test system [35] the allergens are incorporated in hydrophilic gels and the patches are 9 mm by 9 mm (Fig. 24.1). At present, this system is commercially available with 28 allergens (Mekos, www.mekos.dk). Some comparative studies have been carried out with TRUE Test vs. Finn chambers [20–24], demonstrating good concordance. The accuracy, reliability, simplicity, and costs of the ready-to-use system must be balanced by the costs, including personnel, of the original systems (see Sect. 24.2.1).

24.2.3 Some Practical Suggestions

24.2.3.1 Storage

The allergens should be kept in a cool, dark place (refrigerator) to minimize degradation. Those diluted in liquids (water, solvents) should be kept in dark bottles. Allergens should be renewed according to their expiry dates.

24.2.3.2 Sequence of Allergens

Adjust the sequence of the allergens so that those frequently causing strong, cross, or concomitant reactions are not adjacent. In a study [46] using the TRUE Test system, it was found that positive tests to nickel did not intensify reactions to dichromate (distance 1, 3, and 7 cm between the patches) while another [47] concluded that substances with a tendency to cross-reaction or co-sensitizing substances should be tested distant from one another, thus preventing the occurrence of false-positive results. The order given in the product catalogs of the suppliers can usually be followed.

24.2.3.3 Testing in Pregnancy

We usually do not test pregnant women. There are no indications that the minute amounts of allergens absorbed in patch testing could influence the fetus, but in cases of miscarriage or deformity, it is natural to blame several things, including medical investigations.

24.2.3.4 Test Sites

The preferred site is the upper back. For a small number of allergens, for example at retesting, the outer aspect of the upper arm is also acceptable. False-negative test results can be obtained when testing on the lower back or on the volar forearms (see Sect. 24.5.6.1).

24.2.3.5 Removal of Hair

On hairy areas of the back it is difficult to get acceptable skin contact, and for this reason clipping is recommended. Do not shave! However, a combination of clipping, petrolatum, and tapes sometimes contributes to the irritation seen, which makes reading somewhat difficult.

24.2.3.6 Degreasing of Test Site

In cases of oily skin, gentle treatment with ethanol or other mild solvents is recommended. The solvent must evaporate before the test strips are applied.

24.2.3.7 Application of Test Strips

Test strips should be applied from below with mild pressure to remove air pouches, followed by some moderate strokes with the back of the hand to improve adhesion [48] (Fig. 24.2c).

24.2.3.8 Skin Markers

Several solutions, inks, or marking pens are available [2, 48, 49] (Fig. 24.2d, e). If test strips with constant distance between the disks are used, only two marks are needed.

24.2.3.9 Positive Control

To exclude hyporeactivity, an impaired inflammatory response, and the possibility that the test patches do not adhere properly, sodium lauryl sulfate and nonanoic acid have been suggested as positive controls [50–53].

24.2.3.10 Instructions

We have found it valuable to inform our patients the aim of the test; about avoidance of showers, wetting the test site, irradiation, and excessive exercise; and about symptoms such as itch, loosening of patches, and late reactions. Examples of such written instructions and guidelines for patients are available [1, 49].

24.2.3.11 Reading

The light should be good (side lighting may be of help) and adjustable. A magnifying lamp or lens is often helpful. To facilitate reading, most test systems have a special reading plate with punched-out holes corresponding to the test sites.

24.3 Allergens

24.3.1 Numbers

There are 4,350 chemicals described that can cause allergic contact dermatitis [54], and data on new ones are published every year.

24.3.2 Screening Series

To evaluate the significance of special exposures – mainly occupational – a number of screening series are available (Table 24.1). They are compiled from the experience gathered from test clinics and from the literature [55]. Newly defined allergens are added regularly. However, there is a need for caution while using screening series. Older allergens are not always removed in the same way as new are added. Furthermore, it is not certain that a specific screening

Table 24.1 Examples of commercially available screening series

Antioxidants	Bakery	Corticosteroids	Cosmetics
Cutting oils	Dental materials	Disinfectants	Epoxy
Fragrance, flavors	Hairdressing	Industrial biocides	Isocyanate
Medicaments	Metal compounds	Nails – artificial	Oil and cooling fluid
Photographic chemicals	Plants	Plastic and glues	Photoallergens
Printing	Preservatives	Rubber additives	Shoe
Textile colors and finish			

series covers the exposure situation of the patient under investigation. Using screening series can thus give a false sense of security. It is important to evaluate the actual skin exposure situation and choose the correct allergens (including the patients own material) for testing.

24.3.3 Variations Concerning Concentration and Vehicle

Slight differences in recommendations on concentrations and vehicles can be found in catalogs and textbooks on contact dermatitis and patch testing [2, 49, 56–58]. There are thus no ultimate test preparations that are optimal in all clinics or geographical areas. Patch and tape occlusion, humidity, temperature and other climatic factors (see also below Sect. 24.7.4), local experience, and tradition can motivate deviations from these recommendations. Test concentrations for children are presented in Chap. 45. In an ideal case, the concentration of a test preparation offered in catalogs are based on tests of several thousand patients and must be considered very useful guidelines when setting up and running a patch test clinic. However, it is not always the case when uncommon allergens are used. In determining the optimal test concentration for an allergen or a test mixture, it is important to have a high enough patch test concentration to ensure detection of cases of contact allergy, while minimizing the risk of adverse events such as irritation or active sensitization. The fact that this is the so-called maximal nonirritant concentration does not exclude the possibility that a minority of patients tested might still react to these concentrations with an irritative response. Due to decreased bioavailability of chemicals and the local immunology of the healthy skin at the test sites, it requires that the optimal

test concentration of a chemical is usually several times higher than usage concentrations in chemical products. (e.g., Neomycin is tested at 20% pet., although the usual concentration in locally applied products is 0.5%).

24.4 Baseline Series

The allergens of the baseline series (previously called standard series) are discussed in Chap. 31. The present European baseline series contains both single allergens and mixes. Balsam of Peru, colophony, and lanolin are examples of natural mixes, where much effort has been spent identifying the allergens [59–62]. The basic idea of using mixes instead of single allergens is to save time and space. Also, the patients are tested with a number of closely related substances, among others, rubber chemicals. The screening capacity of the baseline series is thereby greatly increased. However, the value of these mixes is sometimes questioned [63]. It is difficult to find an optimal concentration for each allergen in a common vehicle (usually petrolatum) and to determine whether the allergens metabolize or interact to potentiate or decrease reactivity [64, 65]. At our clinic we use the mixes for screening purposes, positive cases being retested with the ingredients. Not unusually, these tests are negative and we then have to ask ourselves whether the initial reaction was an expression of irritancy and/or whether the ingredients have interacted. The opposite has also been noticed. The patient may be negative to a particular mix, but react when retested with its ingredients. The advantages and disadvantages of using a baseline series of patch tests were discussed by Lachapelle and Maibach [66]. They pointed out that it can be considered a limited technical tool, representing one of the pieces of a puzzle, to be combined with other means of diagnosis, and that it

24

also compensates for anamnestic failures. The allergens of the baseline series are presented in detail in Chap. 31 and the test concentrations in Chap. 56.

24.4.1 Deciding What to Include in the Baseline Series

The original baseline series was based on the experience of the members of the International Contact Dermatitis Research Group (ICDRG) and mirrored the findings and current situation in different parts of Europe and the United States. The series is evaluated regularly by national and international contact dermatitis groups. In these ways, the baseline series continually changes in composition and in the total number of substances included. Today, the use of patch test data bases plays an important role in this process (see Chap. 54). The new allergens introduced are often preservatives. 5-Chloro-2-methylisothiazol-3-one (MCI) plus 2-methylisothiazol-3-one (MI) can be mentioned as a typical example. The first cases were observed in Southern Sweden in 1980 [67] and isothiazolinone then became an almost universal allergen, with local epidemics in Finland, The Netherlands, Italy, and Switzerland [68]. It was included in the Swedish baseline series in 1985 and in the European baseline series in 1988 [69]. A scheme [70] for the identification of new contact allergens includes the following:

Clinical

- Positive patch test reaction to a product
- Test with ingredients of the product
- Serial dilution test to define a threshold of sensitivity
- Control tests for irritancy
- Cross-reactivity – equimolar concentrations
- Use tests – repeated open application test (ROAT), provocative use test (PUT)

Experimental

- Structural formula
- Chemical analyses – test material, product, purity, stability
- Animal testing – allergenic potency, cross-reactivity pattern

Table 24.2 Results of a serial dilution test with nickel sulfate in a patient who previously reacted to 5.0% (+++)

Dilution step (%)	Score
1.0	+++
0.3	++
0.1	+
0.03	+
0.01	A few papules
0.003	?
0.001	–
0.0003	–

The choice of patch test concentrations is initially decided by the dermatologist studying a suspected allergen in an index case of contact dermatitis. Most allergens are tested in the concentration range of 0.01–10%, and by analogy with similar chemicals, the dermatologist will probably start within this range and then continue with a serial dilution test (Table 24.2). The threshold of sensitivity defined must be checked for irritancy by tests in controls [70]. If these control tests are negative, information on the case and on the test preparation, where allergen, concentration, and vehicle are stated, will be published as scientific reports and also disseminated to suppliers of patch test allergens. An instructive example of the procedure of defining a new allergen – the preservative iodopropynyl butylcarbamate – was recently presented [71, 72]. The issue is further discussed in Sect. 24.13.3. Nowadays, following local epidemics, conference reports, and communications in scientific journals, several patch test clinics may choose to include a newly identified allergen in their baseline series to investigate the frequency in their geographical area. If the initial reports can be confirmed and the allergen is present in many and various products, it is then recommended for inclusion in the baseline series [73].

24.5 Reading and Evaluation of Patch Tests

The diagnosis allergic contact dermatitis is based on patch testing and quantitative and qualitative exposure assessment. The frequency of patch testing in national health care systems varies considerably around the world. Patch testing is a medical technology that has developed over the last 100 years and is now of major significance in the evaluation and classification of dermatitis. In cases of allergic contact dermatitis, a clear outcome of the patch test can be obtained in most cases with a significant impact on clinical diagnosis and prognosis. Difficulties in discriminating weak allergic and IR will undoubtedly occur. Such gray zones need to be handled by supplementary tests such as dose-response, serial dilution, and ROATs and in the final conclusion related to the clinical history. Reading of patch tests is based on morphological criteria only. Reading of a patch test, as with all other tests in medicine, is a question of strictly following defined criteria. The interpretation of test results and the relevance depend on a global evaluation including the history of the patient, clinical observations, and exposure assessment.

24.5.1 Reading: When and How

The reading should be done by the dermatologist him- or herself, after adequate training.

24.5.1.1 Exposure Time

Most authors advocate an exposure time of 48 h.

24.5.1.2 Reading When?

Wherever possible, it was strongly recommended that two readings be carried out, the first after removal of the patches (usually day 2–3) and the second 2–5 days later [74]. In a study, paired readings on days 4 and 7 were found to be more reliable than those on days 2 and 4 [75]. The readings must be related to the exposure times (see Sect. 24.5.1.1). In our practice we use an exposure time of 48 h (i.e., removal of patches at day 2) with readings at day 3 (D3) and day 7 (D7). If the patches are removed at the dermatologist's clinic or office, it is possible to check that they have adhered properly and the marking is adequate. However, this procedure must be balanced by the great(er) value of later readings for the patients (see below). One should wait at least 15–30 min after the removal, since the combination of allergen, vehicle, patches, and tape causes a transient increase in skin blood flow, a sign of irritation [76]. At later readings, it is possible to record which reactions have turned negative and which reactions have become apparent and/or increased (crescendo) or decreased (decrescendo) in intensity. When day 2 and day 3/4 readings are performed, it is not mandatory but common to observe an increase in intensity of an allergic patch test reaction. However, due to the longer time between reading on day 3 and 7, the decrescendo phenomenon in such settings should not be interpreted as a sign of an irritative response. From studies with repeated readings, it is obvious that the same patch test preparation can produce lost as well as found reactions [77, 78]. Neomycin, corticosteroids, and gold are often-quoted examples of allergens with late appearance ("slow" allergens) while others (fragrance mix, Balsam of Peru) are classified as "early" allergens. When readings were carried out on days 2, 3, and 7, 3 and 8.2% respectively of the reactions first appeared on day 7 [79, 80]. However, some of the positive late reactions proved negative when retested [79]. Long-lasting reactions persisting weeks or months after the initial readings are increasingly attended [81]. However, the clinical significance is not yet settled.

24.5.1.3 Compromise

Multiple readings are thus highly justified and the importance of readings beyond day 2 is stressed [82]. If practical or geographical circumstances permit only one reading, the present accepted compromise is at day 3 (72 h), i.e., 24 h after the removal of the patches. However, in recent papers [83, 84], it was stated that a single reading on day 4 would have been most useful. Patients are instructed to report any late reactions. Options and recommendations concerning multiple readings are presented in Table 24.3. Options three to six enable discrimination between crescendo and decrescendo reactions. When comparing options three and four – both with three visits – we slightly prefer option four since it gives an opportunity to do a late reading (day 5/7).

The value of repeated readings must be balanced by the discomfort, costs, and practical problems (e.g., travel) the repeated visits will cause the patients. However, it is our firm belief that repeated readings will increase the accuracy of our only method of establishing contact allergy.

24

Table 24.3 Multiple readings – options and recommendations

Option	Number of visits	Day 0 application	Day 2 removal, reading	Day 3/4 reading	Day 5/7 reading	Comment
1	2	×	×			Not recommended
2	2	×	Removal by patient	×		Fair-good
3	3	×	×	×		Good
4	3	×	×		×	Good
5	3	×	Removal by patient	×	×	Better
6	4	×	×	×	×	Best

Core Message

> Late-appearing positive patch test reactions can appear for most allergens and are common for some. These reactions are missed if only early readings are carried out. Multiple readings are thus encouraged and if one wants to restrict the number of visits to three we consider that an exposure time of 48 h and readings at day 3 and day 5/7 is most valuable.

Table 24.4 Recording of patch test reactions according to the International Contact Dermatitis Research Group (ICDRG) [36]

?+	Doubtful reaction; faint erythema only
+	Weak positive reaction; erythema, infiltration, possibly papules
++	Strong positive reaction; erythema, infiltration, papules, vesicles
+++	Extreme positive reaction; intense erythema and infiltration and coalescing vesicles
−	Negative reaction
IR	Irritant reactions of different types
NT	Not tested

24.5.2 Recording of Test Reactions

The common method of recording patch test reactions, recommended by the ICDRG [2], is presented in Table 24.4. These recommendations are followed worldwide and are referred to in most scientific reports. Typical examples are shown in Fig. 24.3. However, this recording system is somewhat simplified and not all types of reaction fit this outline. While experienced patch testers rarely disagree concerning the reading of the obvious irritant (IR), ++ and +++ reactions, the reading of the +? and + reactions and some of the IR may cause difficulties. Just recently, it was demonstrated that the knowledge of the test substance and its nature as an allergen, might be a bias in the interpretation of weaker test reactions [85]. For documentation of patch test results, it is recommended that forms be used with space for additional notes on the morphological appearance of the test reactions. It should be mentioned that some investigators record any changes from normal skin and others might ignore a very weak follicular reaction and record it as negative. Especially, when repeated readings are taken, or lesser-known or new substances have been applied, it is essential to follow the appearance and disappearance of the various components of the reactions. Pictures can be of value for documentation and it has been suggested that digital images can be used for continious medical education and in mulicentre networks [86]. However, they can not yet replace our traditional aids for inspection and palpation in clinical day to day testing. Instruction and supervision by an experienced patch tester is recommended for the *novice*. Each test site should be inspected and palpated and daily readings in selected cases would enable her/him to follow the dynamics of test reactions.

24.5.3 Interpretation of Reactions at Test Sites

A reaction at a test site merely indicates some kind of change compared to adjacent, nontested skin: it is not synonymous with "allergic" or "relevant"! Some important and somewhat controversial issues on the interpretation of patch test reactions will now be discussed.

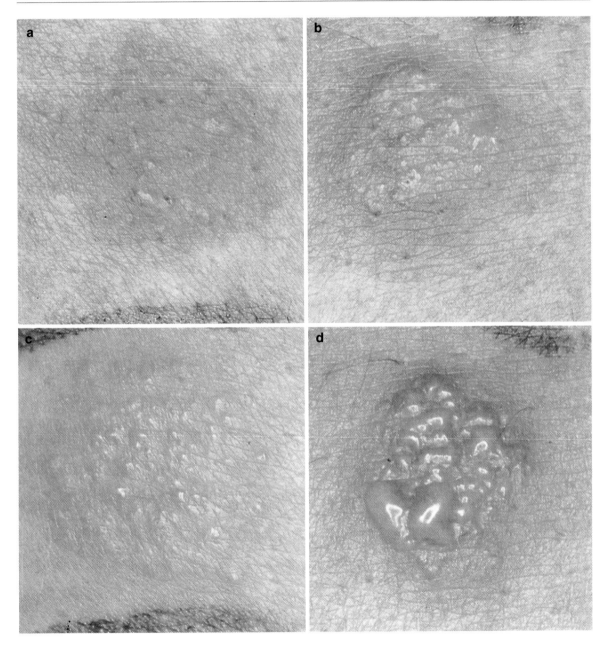

Fig. 24.3 Allergic patch test reactions (all day 3) of increasing intensity. (**a**) + Reaction to nickel sulfate; (**b**) still a + reaction to *para*-phenylenediamine (*PPDA*); (**c**) ++ reaction to PPDA; (**d**) +++ reaction to PPDA (courtesy of P.J. Frosch)

Core Message

> Patch test reactions should be recorded according to the scheme presented in Table 24.4. Repeated readings would enable the reader – especially when under training – to follow the appearance and disappearance of various components of a reaction. A reaction at a test site merely indicates some kind of change compared to adjacent, nontested skin: it is not synonymous with "allergic" or "relevant." Patch testing and especially patch test reading should preferably be performed by dermatologists who have a long experience with this technique.

24

24.5.3.1 Discrimination Between Allergic and Irritant Reactions

To distinguish allergic (Fig. 24.3) reactions from irritant (Fig. 24.4) reactions on morphological grounds alone is difficult. IR are said [1, 48, 56] to be characterized by fine wrinkling ("silk paper"), erythema, and superficial papules in follicular distribution, petechiae, pustules, bullae, and necrosis and with minimal infiltration. Typical examples are shown in Fig. 24.4. Extension beyond the defined area exposed to the allergen is used to discriminate between allergic and IR [1]. Fisher [49] frankly states: "there is no morphological way of distinguishing a weak irritant patch test from a weak allergic test." Examples are benzalkonium chloride and MCI/MC, where there has been some discussion concerning the somewhat peculiar features of the test reactions. In Table 24.2 the results from a serial dilution test with nickel sulfate are shown. At dilution step 5 (0.01%), a few papules have been recorded, and in this case, we know that the reaction is relevant and that this patient is highly sensitive. However, if "a few papules" are noticed in another patient, where only *one* concentration of an allergen has been applied, the interpretation is much more difficult. Usually, we have to repeat the test and probably raise the concentration and/or carry out a serial dilution test.

24.5.3.2 Ring-Shaped Test Reactions

The somewhat peculiar ring-shaped test reactions (the "edge effect"), observed with – among other allergens – formaldehyde and MCI/MC in liquid vehicles, are in most cases an expression of contact allergy [87]. A special type can be seen with corticosteroids where the margins of the positive test are red, whereas the central area is whitish.

24.5.3.3 Ultrastructure

For distinguishing between allergic and irritant patch test reactions, traditional light or electronic microscopy has been of minimal help (see Chap. 10). Studies with monoclonal antibodies and newer molecular techniques have not yet provided methods for clinical use to separate the two types of patch test reactions.

24.5.3.4 Doubtful and One Plus Reactions

When vesicles are present there is rarely any discussion of the allergic nature of the reaction, but the presence or absence of papules is more controversial [66, 88]. However, observed +? and + reactions may cause difficulties. As can be seen from Table 24.4, "possibly papules" is included in the + reaction. This expression can be interpreted in different ways: to be classified as a one plus (+) reaction – is erythema plus infiltration enough? What about erythema and papules, but no infiltration? According to Cronin [56], + is a palpable erythema. Historically, the reading criteria for +? and + have not developed in parallel in all geographical areas. These differences in the interpretation of the objective skin changes explain some of the differences seen between departments and geographical areas. When such a weak reaction (+? or +) has been obtained we recommend – as discussed in Sect. 24.5.3.1, discrimination between allergic and IR – repeating the test, increasing the concentration by a factor 3, 5 or 10, and carrying out serial dilution (Table 24.2) and use tests (see below). Consensus on the denomination and interpretation of doubtful and weak reactions would be of great value and would facilitate comparisons between clinics and geographical areas.

> **Core Message**
>
> ❯ Doubtful (+?) and weak test reactions (+) are hard to interpret. In those cases repeating the test, increasing the test concentration, serial dilution tests, or Use tests are recommended.

24.5.3.5 Cross-Sensitivity

A cross-sensitivity occurs when a person who has initially been sensitized to an allergen (the primary allergen) reacts to a second allergen he or she has never been exposed to (the secondary allergen). The compounds involved are usually chemically similar. Cross-reaction, in the strict sense, means: a T-cell clone, selected by a peptide modified by the primary allergen, is activated by a peptide modified by the secondary allergen. Primary and secondary allergens have to be

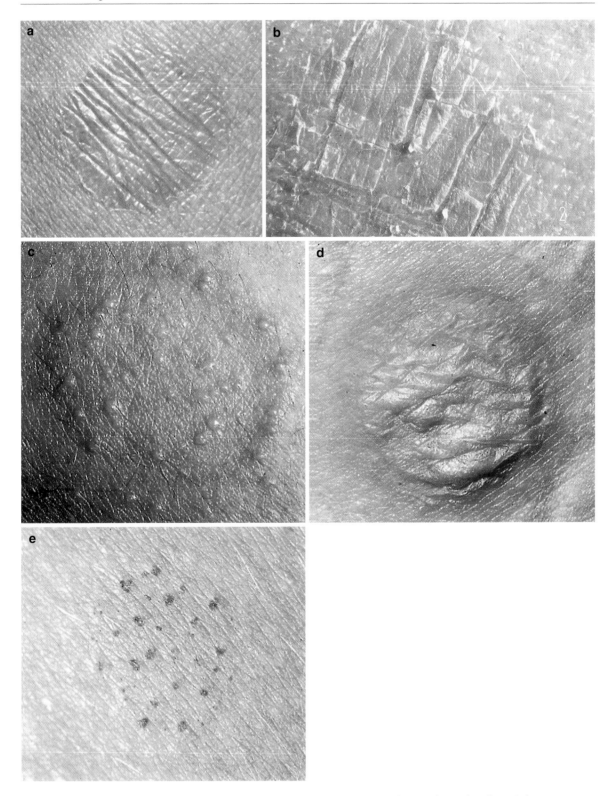

Fig. 24.4 (**a**, **b**) Irritant reactions. (**a**) Soap effect: typical irritant reaction with glistening of the stratum corneum after a 2-day exposure to a 1% solution of toilet soap. (**b**) Irritant reaction with redness and scaling after repetitive application of an 8% soap solution over 4 days (soap chamber test according to Frosch and Kligman). (**c**) Redness and pustules after a 1-day exposure to 80% croton oil. (**d**) Full blister after applying undiluted kerosene for 1 day. (**e**) Follicular crusts after a 15-min application of 2% sodium hydroxide. The photograph was taken 1 day after the induction of follicular erosions (courtesy of P.J. Frosch)

24

different. As we have limited knowledge on T-cell receptor level, a broader cross-sensitization term is often used by dermatologists for the clinical situation when a patient reacts to two or more chemically similar substances simultaneously. For most of the cases, it is almost impossible to know for certain what the primary sensitizer was, as humans may have been exposed earlier to substances they now apparently "cross-react" to. Besides "real" cross-reactivity, different factors such as concomitant sensitization, skin metabolism, impurities, different epitopes on an allergen might explain clinical observations when in patients who have become sensitized to one substance, an allergic contact dermatitis can be provoked or worsened by several other related substances. A patient positive to *para*-phenylendiamine not only reacts to the dye itself, but also to immunochemically related substances that have an amino group in the *para* position, e.g., azo compounds, local anesthetics, and sulfonamides. When studying cross-reactivity it is essential to use pure test compounds [32].

24.5.4 Relevance

Evaluating the relevance of a reaction is the most difficult and intricate part of the patch test procedure, and is a challenge to both dermatologist and patient. The dermatologist's skill, experience, and curiosity are crucial factors. For standard allergens, detailed lists that present the occurrence of each in the environment are available. The patient and the dermatologist should study the lists together, in order to judge the relevance of a positive patch test reaction, in relation to the exposure, site, course, and relapses of the patient's current dermatitis. A positive test reaction can also be explained by a previous, unrelated episode of contact dermatitis (past relevance). Sometimes, the relevance of a positive reaction remains unexplained ("unexplained positive") until the patient brings a package or bottle where the allergen in question is named on the label. In other cases, chemical analyses demonstrate the presence of the allergen, or the manufacturer finally – after many inquiries – admits that the offending substance is present in the product. Methods for increasing the accuracy of the relevance of positive patch test reactions were recently presented [63, 89]. See also below, Sect. 24.10. In cosmetics, skin care products, detergents, paints, cutting fluids, glues, etc., it is common that new ingredients are

added or replace previous ones, but the product keeps its original trade name. Alternatively, well-known allergens are included in new products but with other fields of application than the original. To discover the cause of the patient's dermatitis the dermatologist must sometimes be obstinately determined! The relative importance of different exogenous and endogenous factors to a given case of dermatitis might be hard to evaluate.

> **Core Message**
>
> › Evaluating the relevance of positive test reactions is the most difficult and intricate part of the test procedure and in this process the dermatologist's skill, experience, and curiosity are crucial factors. Clinical examination, repeated checking of history and exposure, Use tests, chemical analyses, and work-site visits ("the patient's chemical environment") can be of great help.

24.5.5 False-Positive Test Reactions

A false-positive reaction is a positive patch test reaction in the absence of contact allergy [90]. The most common causes can be summarized as follows:

1. Too high a test concentration for that particular patient
2. Impure or contaminated test preparation
3. The vehicle is irritant (especially solvents and sometimes petrolatum)
4. Excess of test preparation applied
5. The test substance, usually as crystals, is unevenly dispersed in the vehicle
6. Influence from adjacent test reactions (see above Sect. 24.2.3.2)
7. Current or recent dermatitis at test site
8. Current dermatitis at distant skin sites
9. Pressure effects of tapes, mechanical irritation of solid test materials, furniture and garments (brassiere)
10. Adhesive tape reactions
11. The patch itself has caused the reactions

Some are self-evident and can be predicted and monitored by the dermatologist carrying out patch testing, while others cannot.

24.5.5.1 The Compromise (Item 1)

While the current recommendations on allergen concentrations in relation to vehicle, patch, and tapes are based on long experience, they are nevertheless a compromise! The general problem is that if you lower the concentration to avoid irritancy you will also lose some cases that will be of special occupational and medicolegal importance. Well-known examples are dichromate, formaldehyde, tars, fragrance mix, and, previously, carba mix. It is probably better to have a (weak) false-positive reaction than a false-negative reaction because at least with a potentially false-positive reaction, one is *alerted* to the possibility of allergy, which one can then confirm or deny, whereas with a false-negative reaction, one is never alerted at all and may altogether miss a true allergy. Therefore, most dermatologists seem to prefer the higher concentrations of these marginal irritants, even though they know that nonspecific reactions from them are not uncommon.

Core Message

> Current recommendations on allergen concentrations in relation to vehicles, patches, and tapes are based on long experience but are nonetheless a compromise. If you lower the concentration to avoid irritancy you will also lose some cases. It is probably better to have a weak false-positive reaction than a false-negative reaction because the dermatologist is then alerted.

24.5.5.2 Excited-Skin Syndrome: "Angry Back" (Items 7 and 8)

Patients with current eczema may show cutaneous hyperirritability which can cause problems in patch testing. In the excited-skin syndrome, the presence of a strong positive reaction will influence the reactivity at adjacent test sites. When more than one site shows a

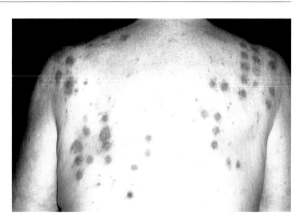

Fig. 24.5 Patients with multiple sensitizations do exist. This leg ulcer patient was allergic to numerous allergens. The strong reactions have been reproduced and were clinically relevant (wool wax alcohols, propylene glycol, parabens, PPDA, MCI/MI, imidazolidinyl urea, thimerosal, thiuram mix, triamcinolone acetonide, amcinonide, and bufexamac) (courtesy of P.J. Frosch)

reaction, this phenomenon must be considered, and retesting of the items one at a time is the usual recommendation (Fig. 24.5). On the basis of Björnberg's [91] important observations, we have always avoided patch testing a patient with current eczema and labile skin, and the excited-skin syndrome is seldom seen in our latitudes [92]. There is extensive literature on this syndrome [93, 94].

24.5.5.3 The Patch (Item 11)

After receiving intradermal allergen extracts due to pollen allergy, a few patients will develop sensitivity to aluminum. They will then react to an Al-test as well as to Finn chambers. Mercury-containing test preparations can react with aluminum, but nowadays plastic-coated Finn chambers are available.

24.5.6 False-Negative Test Reactions

24.5.6.1 Common Causes

A false-negative reaction is a negative patch test reaction in the presence of contact allergy [90]. The most common causes can be summarized as follows:

24

1. Insufficient penetration of the allergen.

   (a) Too low a test concentration for that particular patient

   (b) The test substance is not released from the vehicle or retained by the filter paper

   (c) Insufficient amount (dose) of test preparation applied; patch test concentration lower than declared [95]

   (d) Insufficient occlusion

   (e) Duration of contact too brief – the test strip has fallen off or slipped

   (f) The test was not applied to the recommended site – the upper back

2. Failure to perform delayed readings; e.g., neomycin and corticosteroids are known to give delayed reactions (see Table 24.3).

3. The test site has been treated with corticosteroids or irradiated with UV or Grenz rays.

4. Systemic treatment with corticosteroids or immunomodulators.

5. Allergen is not in active form, insufficiently oxidized (oil of turpentine, rosin compounds, d-limonene), or degraded.

6. Compound allergy.

Some of them are self-evident and can be predicted and monitored by the dermatologist, while others cannot. Examples of the latter category may arise in the following situations: when testing has been carried out in a refractory or "anergic" phase [93]; when the test does not reproduce the clinical exposure to reach the critical elicitation level (multiple applications), where some adjuvant factors are present (sweating, friction, pressure, damaged skin); or penetration at the test site (see Sect. 24.1.3) is lower than that of clinical exposure (eyelids, axillae). The differential diagnoses of photoallergy and contact urticaria should also be considered. Skin hyporeactivity in relation to patch testing was recently reviewed [96] and it was pointed out that the failure to elicit a response might be due to a faulty immune response, a defective inflammatory response, or both. The defective inflammatory response can be evaluated by using a positive control, such as the irritant sodium lauryl sulfate [52] or nonanoic acid [50].

24.5.6.2 Compound Allergy (Item 6)

The term "compound allergy" is used to describe the condition in patients who are patch test positive to formulated products, usually cosmetic creams or topical medicaments, but are test negative to all the ingredients tested individually [97]. This phenomenon can sometimes be explained by the irritancy of the original formulation, but in some cases, it has been demonstrated that reactivity was due to a combination of the ingredients to form reaction products [98, 99]. Another reason might be that the ingredients were patch tested at the usage concentrations, which are too low for many allergens (e.g., MCI/MI, neomycin). Pseudocompound allergy, due to faulty patch testing technique, is likely to be commoner than true compound allergy. In previous publications [100, 101], several proven or possible compound allergens were listed. The formation of allergenic reaction products can take place within the product ("chemical allergenic reactions") and probably also metabolically in the skin ("biological allergenic reactions") [100]. The topic remains the subject of continuing debate [102, 103]. False-positive and false-negative reactions have been reviewed [63].

24.6 Ethnic and Climatic Considerations

Problems and recommendations for patch testing at different climatic environments and in oriental and black populations were recently reviewed [66].

24.7 Effect of Medicaments and Irradiation on Patch Tests

24.7.1 Corticosteroids

Treatment of test sites with topical corticosteroids [104] can give rise to false-negative reactions (see Sect. 24.5.6.1). Testing a patient on oral corticosteroids always creates uncertainty. The problem was studied 25–30 years ago [105–107] by comparing the intensity of test reactions before and during treatment with corticosteroids (20–40 mg prednisone). Diminution and disappearance of test reactions were noted in several cases, but not regularly. These findings have been interpreted as allowing us to test patients on oral doses equivalent to 20 mg of prednisone without missing any important allergies. However, the test reactions studied were strong (+++), and fairly weak (+) and questionable reactions were not evaluated. In a recent study [108] patch testing with serial dilution tests with nickel, it was found that the total number of positive nickel patch tests decreased significantly when the patients were on 20 mg prednisone compared to on placebo. The threshold concentration to elicit a patch test reaction increased and the overall degree of reactivity to nickel shifted toward weaker reactions. In clinical practice, we prefer to defer testing until the patient's dermatitis has cleared although successful testing during concomitant low-dose prednisone use have been reported [109]. When testing a patient with labile skin there is also the risk of excited-skin syndrome [93]. In selected cases, where one or two allergens are strongly suspected, we choose to test for these only, even if the patient is on oral corticosteroids. However, when the dermatitis has cleared, we repeat the test with the whole series to relieve our uncertainty.

24.7.2 Antihistamines

In one study [106], the antihistamine mebhydrolin napadisylate did not influence reactivity, while in another [110] a decrease in intensity was seen in 6 out of 17 patients after cinnarizine had been administered for 1 week. Oral loratadine was found to reduce patch test reactions, evaluated clinically and echographically [111]. These results also give the dermatologist a feeling of some uncertainty. We perform patch testing without discontinuation of antihistamine treatment. However, this contraindication is not universally accepted [112].

24.7.3 Immunomodulators

Topical cyclosporine inhibits test reactions in humans and animal models [113–115]. As yet, there is no comparison of test reactions in allergic patients before and during treatment with orally or parenterally administered cytostatic agents.

24.7.4 Irradiation

It has been shown that irradiation with UVB [116] and Grenz rays [117, 118] reduced the number of Langerhans cells and the intensity of patch test reactions in humans. Repeated suberythema doses of UVB depressed reactivity even at sites shielded during the exposures. This indicates a systemic effect of UVB [116]. Experiments to clarify the mechanism behind these observations have been carried out on experimental animals, but their relevance to humans is not finally settled [119, 120].

24.7.5 Seasonal Variations

Seasonal variations in patch test reactivity is not fully explored. In Israel, negative patch test reactivity was found among 55% in winter and 70% in summer among tested patients [121]. In a German study [122], formaldehyde exhibited a distinct increase in questionable or irritant as well as weak positive reactions associated with dry, cold weather. In a more recent German study [123], it was concluded that ambient temperature and humidity and sodium lauryl sulfate reactivity independently contribute information on individual irritability at the time of patch testing. We recommend avoidance of patch testing on severely tanned persons and that a minimum of 4 weeks after heavy sun exposure should be allowed before testing. At our clinic, we refrain from testing during July and August.

24.8 Complications

Reported complications of patch testing are listed below. However, most can be predicted and avoided:

1. Patch test sensitization
2. IR from nonstandard allergens or products, brought by the patient
3. Flare of previous or existing dermatitis due to percutaneous absorption of the allergen
4. Subjective complaints
5. Depigmentation, e.g., phenols

24

6. Pigmentation, sometimes after sunlight exposure of test sites
7. Scars, keloids
8. Granulomas from beryllium, zirconium
9. Anaphylactoid reactions or shock from, e.g., neomycin, bacitracin (regarding penicillin, see below)
10. Infections (bacteria, virus)

24.8.1 Patch Test Sensitization (Item 1)

By definition, a negative patch test reaction followed by a flare-up after 10–20 days, and then a positive reaction after 3 days at retesting, means that sensitization was induced by the patch test procedure. Recently, this definition has been questioned [124]. It was suggested that it is more common than believed that a late patch test reaction is a delayed immune response rather than a active patch test sensitization. The evaluation of late patch test reactions must be done carefully also including past and present skin exposure. There is a small risk of active sensitization from the baseline series and common examples are *para*-phenylenediamine, primula extracts and, in recent years, isothiazolinone [67], acrylates [125], and a bleach accelerator (PBA-1) [126]. The risk, however, is an extremely low one when the testing is carried out according to internationally accepted guidelines.

It must be emphasized that the overall risk–benefit equation of patch testing patients is much in favor of the benefit.

24.8.2 Subjective Complaints (Item 4)

Subjective complaints, e.g., fever, fatigue, indisposition, vomiting, headache, dizziness, etc., were more often reported on the day of test application compared to the day of reading, however, with one exception – itch on the back [127]. This itch can mainly be related to positive patch test reactions and irritation from adhesive tapes. However, 10–15% of patients with positive test reactions, but without itch, reported complaints such as tiredness, feeling unwell, headache, shakiness, and light-headedness [128]. Of the patients without complaints on the day of application, 36% later reported complaints other than itch [129].

24.8.3 Penicillin (Item 9)

Penicillin can give rise to anaphylactoid reactions or shock and is therefore not recommended for routine patch testing (see also Chap. 40).

24.9 Open Tests

24.9.1 Open Test

"Open test" and "use test" (see Sect. 24.10) are sometimes used as synonyms and no clear-cut definitions seem to exist. Open testing usually means that a product, as is or dissolved in water or some solvent (e.g., ethanol, acetone, ether), is dropped onto the skin and allowed to spread freely. No occlusion is used. An open test is recommended as the first step when testing poorly defined or unknown substances or products, such as those brought by the patient (paints, glues, oils, detergents, cleansing agents based on solvents, etc.). The test site should be checked at regular intervals during the first 30–60 min after application, especially when the history indicates immediate reactions or contact urticaria (see Chap. 26). A second reading should be done at 3–4 days. The usual test site is the volar forearm, but this is less reactive than the back or the upper arms. A negative open test can be explained by insufficient penetration, but indicates that one dares to go on with an occlusive patch test.

24.9.2 Semi-Open Test

This method was introduced by Goossens [130] and is mainly used for products – brought by the patients – with suspected irritant properties due to solvents or emulsifiers, e.g., detergents, shampoos, paints, resins, varnishes, glues, waxes, cooling fluids, pharmaceuticals, and cosmetics. The product (solution or suspension) is applied with a cotton swab as is in a small amount (about 15 μL) to an area of 2×2 cm. After complete drying it is covered with acrylate tape for 2 days. The site is checked for contact urticaria and at days 2 and 4 for signs of contact eczema.

24.10 Use Tests

24.10.1 Purpose

The original (provocative) use (or usage) tests (PUT) were intended to mimic the actual use situation (repeated open applications) of a formulated product such as a cosmetic, a shampoo, an oil or a topical medicament. A positive result supported the suspicion that the product had caused the patient's dermatitis. The primary goal was not to clarify the nature (allergic or irritant) of the dermatitis – just to reproduce it!

Nowadays, these tests are increasingly used to evaluate the clinical significance of the ingredient(s) of a formulated product previously found reactive by ordinary patch testing. The concentration of the particular ingredient can be so low that one may wonder whether the positive patch test reaction can explain the patient's dermatitis.

24.10.2 Repeated Open Application Test

The ROAT in a standardized form was introduced by Hannuksela and Salo [131]. Test substances, either commercial products, as is, or special test substances (e.g., patch test allergen) are applied twice daily for 7 days to the outer aspect of the upper arm, antecubital fossa, or back skin (scapular area). The size of the test area is not crucial: a positive result may appear on a 1×1-cm area 1–2 days later than on a larger area. The amount of test substance should be approximately 0.1 mL to a 5×5-cm area and 0.5 mL to a 10×10-cm area [132, 133]. A positive response – eczematous dermatitis – usually appears on days 2–4 (Fig. 24.6), but it is recommended to extend the applications up to 3 weeks in order not to miss late-appearing reactions

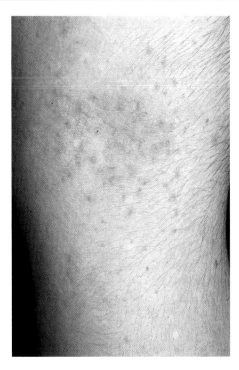

Fig. 24.6 A positive ROAT on the third day in a patient allergic to iso-eugenol (courtesy of P.J. Frosch)

[134–136]. A refined scheme for scoring of ROAT reactions has recently been presented [137]. The patient is told to stop the application of the test substance(s) when he or she notices a reaction [131].If a ROAT is carried out with a formulated product, the observed reaction may be due to allergy to an ingredient, but irritancy from other ingredients cannot be excluded. At our clinic, we therefore use two coded samples – one containing the allergen and the other without it. We instruct the patient to apply one product to the left arm and the other to the right arm, according to a special protocol where the treatments and any observed reaction can be noted. If there is a reaction only at the test site where the allergen-containing product has been applied, we consider the initial patch test reaction relevant. On the other hand, we interpret reactions of the same intensity on both arms as an expression of irritancy. The value of ROAT has been verified in cases with positive, negative, or questionable reactions at initial patch testing [134, 135, 138–140] and in animal studies [136], and it was pointed out that Use testing has significant potential in refinement of the evidence-based diagnosis of clinical relevance [141].

24.11 Noninvasive Techniques

To reduce the well-known interindividual variation when scoring patch test reactions, several attempts have been made to introduce objective bioengineering techniques for assessment. Erythema and skin color can be assessed by laser Doppler flowmetry (LDF), skin reflectance, and colorimeters, and edema with calipers, ultrasound, and electrical impedance. The advantages and limitations of these methods have been reviewed [142]. These sophisticated techniques cannot replace visual assessment and palpation of test sites by the dermatologist, but are valuable in research work [143]. The topic is further reviewed in Chap. 30. A significant correlation between visual scoring of patch test reactions and LDF values was claimed by Staberg et al. [144]. The method discriminated between negative and positive reactions, but failed to quantify strong positive reactions. However, in a recent guideline from the standardization group of the European Society of Contact Dermatitis, it was stated that laser Doppler perfusion imaging does not directly distinguish between allergic and irritant patch test reactions [145]. It has also been shown that the combination of allergen, vehicle, patch, and tape will cause a transient increase in skin blood flow, even in healthy subjects [75]. An increase was noticed for 1–2 days after the removal of the patches, without causing any visual changes. Skin blood flow must be increased three to four times before the naked eye can detect an erythema [146].

24.12 Quality Control of Test Materials

24.12.1 Identification and Purity

As pointed out above (see Sect. 24.2.1.2), the dermatologist is recommended to obtain protocols of chemical analyses and data on purity from suppliers of test preparations. Some dermatologists have the laboratory facilities to check the information presented, but most just have to accept it. Especially when "new" allergens are detected, in cases of unexpected multiple reactivity or suspected cross-reactivity, detailed information on purity, chemical identification, and stability of the allergen is indispensable [32]. Some mixes, such as fragrance mix, contain emulsifiers (sorbitan sesquioleate), and a correct retest with the ingredients of a mix should thus include the individual fragrances as well as the emulsifier.

24.12.2 Test Preparations Under the Microscope

Light microscope examination (magnification 100–400) of commercial test preparations with petrolatum as vehicle is usually disappointing. Crystals [147–149] or globules [150] of different size are seen and one wonders how this influences the bioavailability of the allergen. However, in one comparative study no difference in reactivity was found [151]. In the TRUE Test, the allergens are incorporated in hydrophilic gels and are evenly distributed [35].

24.12.3 Fresh Samples

In cases of unexpected negative test reactions, the items listed in Sect. 24.5.6.1, common causes should be considered. If the case remains unsolved, it is suggested that a fresh sample of the allergen be purchased from a different supplier.

24.12.4 Adhesive Tapes

A significant development in tape quality has taken place [44, 152] (see also above Sect. 24.2.1.5).

24.13 Tests with Unknown Substances

24.13.1 Warning!

A word of warning: totally unknown substances or products should never be applied to human skin! Scarring, necrosis, keloids, pigmentation, depigmentation, systemic effects following percutaneous absorption, and any other complications listed earlier can appear and the dermatologist may be accused of malpractice.

24.13.2 Strategy

When patients bring suspected products or materials from their (work) environment, we recommend that adequate product safety data sheets, lists of ingredients, etc.

be requested from the manufacturer so that a general impression of the product, ingredients, concentrations, intended use, etc. can be formed. There are usually one or two ingredients that are of interest as suspected allergens, while the rest are well-known substances of proven innocuousness for which detailed information is available. For substances or products where skin contact is unintentional and the dermatitis is a result of misuse or accident, detailed information from the manufacturer is required before any tests are initiated.

24.13.3 Test or Not?

The next step is to look for the suspected allergens. If they are available from suppliers of patch test allergens, one can rely on the choice of vehicle and concentration. If one suspects that impurities or contaminants have caused the dermatitis, this can only be discovered via samples of the ingredient from the manufacturer. If it is an entirely new substance, where no data on toxicity, etc. are available, the patient and dermatologist have to decide how to find an optimal test concentration and vehicle, and to discuss the risk of complications. To minimize the risk, one can start with an open test and, if this is negative, continue with occlusive patch testing. Most allergens are tested in the concentration range of 0.01–10%, and we usually start with the lowest and raise the concentration when the preceding test is negative. A very practical method is to apply 0.01 and 0.1% for 1 day in a region where the patient can easily remove the patch her- or himself (upper back or upper arm). If severe stinging or burning occurs, he or she should be instructed to remove it immediately. If the test is negative, the concentration can be raised to 1%. Occasionally, the likely irritant or sensitization potential of a chemical may be such that starting with concentrations of 0.001 and 0.01% is advisable, increasing to 0.1% if negative. If the test is positive in the patient, one has to demonstrate in unexposed controls that the actual test preparation is nonirritant [70]. Otherwise, the observed reaction in the particular patient does not prove allergenicity. It is important to check the pH of products before testing. When testing the products brought by the patient, it is essential to use samples from the actual batch to which the patient has been exposed, and also when testing, for example, cutting fluids, unused products must be tested for comparison. When testing with dilutions, one runs the risk of overlooking true allergens by using overdiluted materials. See also Chap. 57, section on solid products and extracts. When a solid product is suspected (textiles, rubber, plants, wood, paper etc.), these can usually be applied as is. Rycroft [90] recommends that the material be tested as wafer-thin, regular-sided, smooth sheets (e.g., rubber) or as finely divided particulates (e.g., woods). A transient so-called pressure effect is sometimes seen when testing with solids. Plants and woods and their extracts constitute special problems, due to variations in the quantity of allergens produced and their availability on the surface. Extracts for testing can be obtained by placing the product or sample in water, synthetic sweat, ethanol, acetone or ether, and heating to 40–50°C. Ultra sound bath can be used for facilitating the extraction process. False reactions to nonstandardized patch tests have been reviewed by Rycroft [90]. Patch testing with thin-layer chromatograms has been found valuable for products such as textiles, plastics, food, plants, perfumes, drugs, and grease [153].

24.13.4 Cosmetics and Similar Products

For most products with intended use on normal or damaged skin (cosmetics, skin care products, soap, shampoos, detergents, topical medicaments, etc.), detailed predictive testing and clinical and consumer trials have been performed. The results can usually be obtained from the manufacturer. For this category of products, open tests and Use tests probably give more information than an occlusive patch test on the pathogenesis of the patient's dermatitis. Suggestions on concentrations and vehicles can be found in textbooks [49, 56].

24.14 The Future

This chapter concludes with the following list of hopes and needs for the future:

- Diversified vehicles to obtain optimal bioavailability of allergens.
- Statements in suppliers' catalogs on the purity and stability of individual allergens.

24

- Consensus on the reading, scoring, interpretation, and relevance of weak test reactions.
- Objective assessment of test reactions.
- Further standardization of Use tests.
- Irritancy from test preparations – refinement of predictive methods.
- Systemic treatment with immunomodulators and antihistamines – influence on patch test reactivity.
- Influence on patch test reactivity due to seasonal variation, latitude, temperature, and humidity.

Acknowledgement Professor Jan Wahlberg (1932–2005) conceived this chapter for the first to the fourth edition. This edition is dedicated to him in memory of his scientific impact in this field. His devotion to science may serve as a stimulus to the young generation.

References

1. Malten KE, Nater JP, van Ketel WG (1976) Patch testing guidelines. Dekker and van de Vegt, Nijmegen
2. Fregert S (1981) Manual of contact dermatitis, 2nd edn. Munksgaard, Copenhagen
3. Bandmann HJ, Dohn W (1967) Die Epicutantestung. Bergmann, Munich
4. Rajagopalan R, Anderson R (1997) Impact of patch testing on dermatology-specific quality of life in patients with allergic contact dermatitis. Am J Contact Dermat 8:215–221
5. Thomson KF, Wilkinson SM, Sommer S, Pollock B (2002) Eczema: quality of life by body site and the effect of patch testing. Br J Dermatol 146:627–630
6. Woo PN, Hay IC, Ormerod AS (2003) An audit of the value of patch testing and its effect on quality of life. Contact Dermatitis 48:244–247
7. Van der Valk PGM, Devos SA, Coenraads P-J (2003) Evidence-based diagnosis in patch testing. Contact Dermatitis 48:121–125
8. Mowad CM (2006) Patch testing: pitfalls and performance. Curr Opin Allergy Clin Immunol 6:340–344
9. Jadassohn J (1896) Zur Kenntnis der medikamentösen Dermatosen, Verhandlungen der Deutschen Dermatologischen Gesellschaft. Fünfter Congress, Raz, 1895. Braunmuller, Vienna, p 106
10. Foussereau J (1984) History of epicutaneous testing: the blotting-paper and other methods. Contact Dermatitis 11:219–223
11. Fischer TI, Hansen J, Kreilgård B, Maibach HI (1989) The science of patch test standardization. Immunol Allergy Clin North Am 9:417–443
12. Belsito DV, Storrs FJ, Taylor JS, Marks JG Jr, Adams RM, Rietschel RL, Jordan WP, Emmett EA (1992) Reproducibility of patch tests: a United States multi-centre study. Am J Contact Dermat 3:193–200
13. Breit R, Agathos M (1992) Qualitätskontrolle der Epikutantestung – Reproduzierbarkeit im Rechts-Links-Vergleich. Hautarzt 43:417–421
14. Bousema MT, Geursen AM, van Joost T (1991) High reproducibility of patch tests. J Am Acad Dermatol 24:322–323
15. Lachapelle JM, Antoine JL (1989) Problems raised by the simultaneous reproducibility of positive allergic patch test reactions in man. J Am Acad Dermatol 21:850–854
16. Macháčková J, Seda O (1991) Reproducibility of patch tests. J Am Acad Dermatol 25:732–733
17. Lindelöf B (1990) A left versus right side comparative study of Finn Chamber™ patch tests in 220 consecutive patients. Contact Dermatitis 22:288–289
18. Stransky L, Krasteva M (1992) A left versus right side comparative study of Finn Chamber patch tests in consecutive patients with contact sensitization. Dermatosen 40:158–159
19. Brasch J, Henseler T, Aberer W, Bäuerle G, Frosch PJ, Fuchs T, Fünfstück V, Kaiser G, Lischka GG, Pilz B, Sauer C, Schaller J, Scheuer B, Szliska C (1994) Reproducibility of patch tests. A multicenter study of synchronous left-versus right-sided patch tests by the German Contact Dermatitis Research Group. J Am Acad Dermatol 31:584–591
20. Gollhausen R, Przybilla B, Ring J (1989) Reproducibility of patch test results: comparison of True test and Finn Chamber test. In: Frosch PJ, Dooms-Goossens A, Lachapelle JM, Rycroft RJ, Scheper RJ (eds) Current topics in contact dermatitis. Springer, Berlin, pp 524–529
21. Lachapelle J-M, Bruynzeel DP, Ducombs G, Hannuksela M, Ring J, White IR, Wilkinson J, Fischer T, Billberg K (1988) European multicenter study of the True test™. Contact Dermatitis 19:91–97
22. Ruhnek-Forsbeck M, Fischer T, Meding B, Pettersson L, Stenberg B, Strand A, Sundberg K, Svensson L, Wahlberg JE, Widström L, Wrangsjö K, Billberg K (1988) Comparative multi-center study with True test™ and Finn Chamber® patch test methods in eight Swedish hospitals. Acta Derm Venereol (Stockh) 68:123–128
23. Stenberg B, Billberg K, Fischer T, Nordin L, Pettersson L, Ruhnek-Forsbeck M, Sundberg K, Swanbeck G, Svensson L, Wahlberg JE, Widström L, Wrangsjö K (1989) Swedish multicenter study with True test, panel 2. In: Frosch PJ, Dooms-Goossens A, Lachapelle JM, Rycroft RJ, Scheper RJ (eds) Current topics in contact dermatitis. Springer, Berlin, pp 518–523
24. Wilkinson JD, Bruynzeel DP, Ducombs G, Frosch PJ, Gunnarsson Y, Hannuksela M, Ring J, Shaw S, White IR (1990) European multicenter study of TRUE test, panel 2. Contact Dermatitis 22:218–225
25. Ale SI, Maibach HI (2004) Reproducibility of patch test results: a concurrent right-versus-left study using TRUE test ™. Contact Dermatitis 50:304–312
26. Bourke JF, Batta K, Prais L, Abdullah A, Foulds IS (1999) The reproducibility of patch tests. Br J Dermatol 140:102–105
27. Schiessl C, Wolber C, Strohal R (2004) Reproducibility of patch tests: comparison of identical test allergens from different commercial sources. Contact Dermatitis 50:27–30

28. Fullerton A, Rud Andersen J, Hoelgaard A, Menné T (1986) Permeation of nickel salts through human skin in vitro. Contact Dermatitis 15:173–177

29. Brasch J, Szliska C, Grabbe J (1997) More positive patch test reactions with larger test chambers? Contact Dermatitis 37:118–120

30. Gefeller O, Phahlberg A, Geier J, Brasch J, Uter W (1999) The association between size of test chamber and patch test reaction: a statistical reanalysis. Contact Dermatitis 40:14–18

31. Ryberg K, Gruvberger B, Zimerson E, Isaksson M, Persson L, Sörensen Ö, Goossens A, Bruze M (2008) Chemical investigations of disperse dyes in patch test preparations. Contact Dermatitis 58:199–209

32. Fregert S (1985) Publication of allergens. Contact Dermatitis 12:123–124

33. Dooms-Goossens A, Degreef H (1983) Contact allergy to petrolatums I. Sensitizing capacity of different brands of yellow and white petrolatums. Contact Dermatitis 9:175–185

34. Bruze M (1984) Use of buffer solutions for patch testing. Contact Dermatitis 10:267–269

35. Fischer T, Maibach H (1989) Easier patch testing with TRUE test. J Am Acad Dermatol 20:447–453

36. Magnusson B, Blohm S-G, Fregert S, Hjorth N, Høvding G, Pirilä V, Skog E (1966) Routine patch testing II. Acta Derm Venereol (Stockh) 46:153–158

37. Benezra C, Andanson J, Chabeau C, Ducombs G, Foussereau J, Lachapelle JM, Lacroix M, Martin P (1978) Concentrations of patch test allergens: are we comparing the same things? Contact Dermatitis 4:103–105

38. Bruze M, Isaksson M, Gruvberger B, Frick-Engfeldt M (2007) Recommendation of appropriate amounts of petrolatum preparation to be applied at patch testing. Contact Dermatitis 56:281–285

39. Bruze M (1986) Sensitizing capacity of 2-methylol phenol, 4-methylol phenol and 2, 4, 6-trimethylol phenol in the Guinea Pig. Contact Dermatitis 14:32–38

40. Wall LM, Calnan CD (1980) Occupational nickel dermatitis in the electroforming industry. Contact Dermatitis 6:414–420

41. Wahlberg JE (1996) Nickel: the search for alternative, optimal and non-irritant patch test preparations. Assessments based on laser Doppler flowmetry. Skin Res Technol 2:136–141

42. Widman TJ, Oostman H, Storrs FJ (2008) Allergic contact dermatitis from medical adhesive bandages in patients who report having a reaction to medical bandages. Dermatitis 19:32–37

43. Daecke C, Schaller S, Schaller J, Goos M (1993) Contact urticaria from acrylic acid in Fixomull tape. Contact Dermatitis 29:216–217

44. Tokumura F, Ohyama K, Fujisawa H, Matsuda T, Kitazaki Y (1997) Conformability and irritancy of adhesive tapes on the skin. Contact Dermatitis 37:173–178

45. Fischer T, Dahlén Å, Bjkarnason B (1999) Influence of patch-test application tape on reactions to sodium lauryl sulphate. Contact Dermatitis 40:32–37

46. Brasch J, Kreilgård B, Henseler T, Aberer W, Fuchs T, Pfluger R, Hoeck U, Gefeller O (2000) Positive nickel patch tests do not intensify positive reactions to adjacent patch tests with dichromate. Contact Dermatitis 43:144–149

47. Duarte I, Lazzarini R, Buense R (2002) Interference of the position of substances in an epicutaneous patch test battery with the occurrence of false-positive results. Am J Contact Dermat 13:125–132

48. Fischer T, Maibach HI (1986) Patch testing in allergic contact dermatitis: an update. Semin Dermatol 5:214–224

49. Fisher AA (1986) Contact dermatitis, 3rd edn. Lea and Febiger, Philadelphia

50. Wahlberg JE, Maibach HI (1980) Nonanoic acid irritation – a positive control at routine patch testing? Contact Dermatitis 6:128–130

51. Wahlberg JE, Wrangsjö K, Hietasalo A (1985) Skin irritancy from nonanoic acid. Contact Dermatitis 13:266–269

52. Geier J, Uter W, Pirker C, Frosch PJ (2003) Patch testing with the irritant sodium lauryl sulphate (SLS) is useful in interpreting weak reactions to contact allergens as allergic or irritant. Contact Dermatitis 48:99–107

53. Wahlberg JE, Lindberg M (2003) Nonanoic acid – an experimental irritant. Contact Dermatitis 49:117–123

54. De Groot AC (2008) Patch testing. Test concentrations and vehicles for 4350 chemicals, 3rd edn. Wapserveen, The Netherlands

55. Kanerva L, Elsner P, Wahlberg JE, Maibach HI (2000) Handbook of occupational dermatology. Springer, Berlin

56. Cronin E (1980) Contact dermatitis. Churchill Livingstone, London

57. Adams RM (1990) Occupational skin disease, 2nd edn. Saunders, Philadelphia

58. Foussereau J, Benezra C, Maibach HI (1982) Occupational contact dermatitis. Clinical and chemical aspects. Munksgaard, Copenhagen

59. Hjorth N (1961) Eczematous allergy to balsams. Allied perfumes and flavouring agents. Munksgaard, Copenhagen

60. Takano S, Yamanaka M, Okamoto K, Saito F (1983) Allergens of lanolin: parts I and II. J Soc Cosmet Chem 34:99–125

61. Fregert S, Dahlquist I, Trulsson L (1984) An attempt to isolate and identify allergens in lanolin. Contacts Dermat 10:16–19

62. Karlberg A-T (1988) Contact allergy to colophony. Chemical identifications of allergens, sensitization experiments and clinical experiences. Thesis, Karolinska Institute, Stockholm, Sweden

63. Alé SI, Maibach HI (2002) Scientific basis of patch testing. Dermatol Beruf Umwelt 50:43–50; 91–96;131–133

64. Hansson C, Agrup G (1993) Stability of the mercaptobenzothiazole compounds. Contact Dermatitis 28:29–34

65. Bergendorff O, Hansson C (2001) Stability of thiuram disulfides in patch test preparations and formation of asymmetric disulfides. Contact Dermatitis 45:151–157

66. Lachapelle J-M, Maibach HI (2003) Patch testing, prick testing. A practical guide. Springer, Berlin

67. Björkner B, Bruze M, Dahlquist I, Fregert S, Gruvberger B, Persson K (1986) Contact allergy to the preservative Kathon® CG. Contact Dermatitis 14:85–90

68. de Groot AC (1988) Adverse reactions to cosmetics. Thesis, Rijksuniversiteit Groningen, The Netherlands

69. Andersen KE, Burrows D, Cronin Dooms-Goossens A, Rycroft RJG, White IR (1988) Recommended changes to baseline series. Contact Dermatitis 19:389–390

70. Wahlberg JE (1998) Identification of new allergens and non-irritant patch test preparations. Contact Dermatitis 39: 155–156

71. Bryld LE, Agner T, Rastogi SC, Menné T (1997) Idopropynyl butylcarbamate: a new contact allergen. Contact Dermatitis 36:156–158

72. Schnuch A, Geijer J, Brasch J, Uter W (2002) The preservative iodoproponyl butylcarbamate: frequence of allergic reactions and diagnostic considerations. Contact Dermatitis 46:153–156

73. Bruze M, Condé-Salazar L, Goossens A, Kanerva L, White I (1999) Thoughts on sensitizers in a standard patch test series. Contact Dermatitis 41:241–250

74. Rietschel R, Adams RM, Maibach HI, Storrs FJ, Rosenthal LE (1988) The case for patch test readings beyond day 2. J Am Acad Dermatol 18:42–45

75. MacFarlane AW, Curley RK, Graham RM, Lewis-Jones MS, King CM (1989) Delayed patch test reactions at days 7 and 9. Contact Dermatitis 20:127–132

76. Wahlberg JE, Wahlberg ENG (1987) Quantification of skin blood flow at patch test sites. Contact Dermatitis 17: 229–233

77. Geier J, Gefeller O, Wiechmann K, Fuchs T (1999) Patch test reactions at D4, D5 and D6. Contact Dermatitis 40: 119–126

78. Dickel H, Taylor JS, Evey P, Merk HF (2000) Delayed readings of a standard screening patch test tray: frequency of "lost", "found", and "persistent" reactions. Am J Contact Dermat 11:213–217

79. Saino M, Rivara P, Guarrera M (1995) Reading patch tests on day 7. Contact Dermatitis 32:312

80. Jonker MJ, Bruynzel DP (2000) The outcome of an additional patch-test reading on days 6 or 7. Contact Dermatitis 42:330–335

81. Bygum A, Andersen KE (1998) Persistent reactions after patch testing with TRUE Test™ panels 1 and 2. Contact Dermatitis 38:218–220

82. Uter WJC, Geier J, Schnuch A (1996) Good clinical practice in patch testing: readings beyond day 2 are necessary: a confirmatory analysis. Am J Contact Dermat 7:231–237

83. Shehade SA, Beck MH, Hiller VF (1991) Epidemiological survey of baseline series patch test results and observations on day 2 and day 4 readings. Contact Dermatitis 24: 119–122

84. Todd DJ, Handley J, Metwali M, Allen GE, Burrows D (1996) Day 4 is better than day 3 for a single patch test reading. Contact Dermatitis 34:402–404

85. Uter W, Frosch PJ, Becker D, Schnuch A, Pfahlberg A, Gefeller O (2009) Are we biased when reading a doubtful patch test reaction to a 'clear-cut' allergen such as the thiuram mix? Contact Dermatitis 60:234–235

86. Uter W, Becker D, Schnauch A, Gefeller O, Frosch PJ (2007) The validity of rating patch test reactions based on digital images. Contact Dermatitis 57:337–342

87. Lachapelle JM, Tennstedt D, Fyad A, Masmoudi ML, Nouaigui H (1988) Ring-shaped positive allergic patch test reactions to allergens in liquid vehicles. Contact Dermatitis 18:234–236

88. Bruze M, Isaksson M, Edman B, Björkner B, Fregert S, Möller H (1995) A study on expert reading of patch test reactions: inter-individual accordance. Contact Dermatitis 32:331–337

89. Lachapelle J-M (1997) A proposed relevance scoring system for positive allergic patch test reactions: practical implications and limitations. Contact Dermatitis 36:39–43

90. Rycroft RJG (1986) False reactions to nonstandard patch tests. Semin Dermatol 5:225–230

91. Björnberg A (1968) Skin reactions to primary irritants in patients with hand eczema. An investigation with matched controls. Thesis, Sahlgrenska Sjukhuset, Gothenburg, Sweden

92. Andersen KE, Lidén C, Hansen J, Vølund Å (1993) Dose-response testing with nickel sulphate using the TRUE test in nickel-sensitive individuals. Multiple nickel sulphate patch-test reactions do not cause an 'angry back'. Br J Dermatol 129:50–56

93. Bruynzeel DP, Maibach HI (1990) Excited skin syndrom and the hyporeactive state: current status. In: Menné T, Maibach HI (eds) Exogenous dermatoses: environmental dermatitis. CRC, Boca Raton, FL, pp 141–150

94. Cockayne SE, Gawkrodger DJ (2000) Angry back syndrome is often due to marginal irritants: a study of 17 cases seen over 4 years. Contact Dermatitis 43:280–282

95. Kanerva L, Estlander T, Jolanki R, Alanko K (2000) False-negative patch test reactions due to a lower concentration of patch test substance than declared. Contact Dermatitis 42: 289–291

96. Koehler AM, Maibach HI (2000) Skin hyporeactivity in relation to patch testing. Contact Dermatitis 42:1–4

97. Kelett JK, King CM, Beck MH (1986) Compound allergy to medicaments. Contact Dermatitis 14:45–48

98. Aldridge RD, Main RA (1984) Contact dermatitis due to a combined miconazole nitrate/hydrocortisone cream. Contact Dermatitis 10:58–60

99. Smeenk G, Kerckhoffs HPM, Schreurs PHM (1987) Contact allergy to a reaction product in Hirudoid® cream: an example of compound allergy. Br J Dermatol 116: 223–231

100. Bashir SJ, Maibach HI (1997) Compound allergy. An overview. Contact Dermatitis 36:179–183

101. Bashir SJ, Kanervaq L, Jolanki R, Maibach HI (2000) Occupational and non-occupational compound allergy. In: Kanerva L, Elsner P, Wahlberg JE, Maibach HI (eds) Handbook of occupational dermatology. Springer, Berlin, pp 351–355

102. McLelland J, Shuster S, Matthews JNS (1991) "Irritants" increase the response to an allergen in allergic contact dermatitis. Arch Dermatol 127:1016–1019

103. McLelland J, Shuster S (1990) Contact dermatitis with negative patch tests. Br J Dermatol 122:623–630

104. Sukanto H, Nater JP, Bleumink E (1981) Influence of topically applied corticosteroids on patch test reactions. Contact Dermatitis 7:180–185

105. O'Quinn SE, Isbell KH (1969) Influence of oral prednisone on eczematous patch test reactions. Arch Dermatol 99: 380–389

106. Feuerman E, Levy A (1972) A study of the effect of prednisone and an antihistamine on patch test reactions. Br J Dermatol 86:68–71

107. Condie MW, Adams RM (1973) Influence of oral prednisone on patch-test reactions to Rhus antigen. Arch Dermatol 107:540–543

108. Anveden I, Lindberg M, Andersen KE, Bruze M, Isaksson M, Lidén C, Sommerlund M, Wahlberg J, Wilkinson J,

Willis C (2004) Oral prednisone suppresses allergic but not irritant patch test reactions in individuals hypersensitive to nickel. Contact Dermatitis 50:298–303

109. Olupona T, Scheinman P (2008) Successful patch testing despite concomitant low-dose prednisone use. Dermatitis 19:117–118

110. Lembo G, Presti ML, Balato N, Ayala F, Santoianni P (1985) Influence of cinnarizine on patch test reactions. Contact Dermatitis 13:341–343

111. Motolese A, Ferdani G, Manzini BM, Seidenari S (1995) Echographic evaluation of patch test inhibition by oral anti-histamine. Contact Dermatitis 32:251

112. Elston D, Licata A, Rudner E, Trotter K (2000) Pitfalls in patch testing. Am J Contact Dermat 11:184–188

113. Aldridge RD, Sewell HF, King G, Thomson AW (1986) Topical cyclosporin A in nickel contact hypersensitivity: results of a preliminary clinical and immunohistochemical investigation. Clin Exp Immunol 66:582–589

114. Nakagawa S, Oka D, Jinno Y, Takei Y, Bang D, Ueki H (1988) Topical application of cyclosporine on guinea pig allergic contact dermatitis. Arch Dermatol 124:907–910

115. Biren CA, Barr RJ, Ganderup GS, Lemus LL, McCullough JL (1989) Topical cyclosporine: effects on allergic contact dermatitis in guinea pigs. Contact Dermatitis 20:10–16

116. Sjövall P (1988) Ultraviolet radiation and allergic contact dermatitis. An experimental and clinical study. Thesis, University of Lund, Sweden

117. Lindelöf B, Lidén S, Lagerholm B (1985) The effect of grenz rays on the expression of allergic contact dermatitis in man. Scand J Immunol 21:463–469

118. Ek L, Lindelöf B, Lidén S (1989) The duration of Grenz ray-induced suppression of allergic contact dermatitis and its correlation with the density of Langerhans cells in human epidermis. Clin Exp Dermatol 14:206–209

119. Cruz PD (1996) Effects of UV light on the immune system: answer to five basic questions. Am J Contact Dermat 7:47–52

120. Tie C, Golomb C, Taylor JR, Strelein JW (1995) Suppressive and enhancing effects of ultraviolet B radiation on expression of contact hypersensitivity in man. J Invest Dermatol 104:18–22

121. Ingber A, Sasson A, David M (1998) The seasonal influence on patch test reactions is significant in Israel. Contact Dermatitis 39:318–319

122. Uter W, Geier J, Land M, Phahlberg A, Gefeller O, Schnauch A (2001) Another look at seasonal variation in patch test results. Contact Dermatitis 44:146–152

123. Uter W, Hegewald J, Phahlberg A, Pirker C, Frosch PJ, Gefeller O (2003) The association between ambient air conditions (temperature and absolute humidity), irritant sodium lauryl sulphate patch test reactions and patch test reactivity to standard allergens. Contact Dermatitis 49:97–102

124. Gawkrodger DJ, Paul L (2008) Late patch test reactions: delayed immune response appears to be more common than active sensitization. Contact Dermatitis 59:185–187

125. Kanerva L, Estlander T, Jolanki R (1988) Sensitization to patch test acrylates. Contact Dermatitis 18:10–15

126. Lidén C, Boman A, Hagelthorn G (1982) Flare-up reactions from a chemical used in the film industry. Contact Dermatitis 8:136–137

127. Inerot A, Möller H (2000) Symptoms and signs reported during patch testing. Am J Contact Dermat 11:49–52

128. Kunkeler L, Bikkers SCE, Bezemer PD, Bruynzeel DP (2000) (Un)usual effects of patch testing? Br J Dermatol 143:582–586

129. Kamphof WG, Kunkeler L, Bikkers SCE, Bezemer PD, Bruynzeel DP (2003) Patch-test-induced subjective complaints. Dermatology 207:28–32

130. Dooms-Goossens A (1995) Patch testing without a kit. In: Guyin JD (ed) Practical contact dermatitis. McGraw-Hill, New York, pp 63–74

131. Hannuksela M, Salo H (1986) The repeated open application test (ROAT). Contact Dermatitis 14:221–227

132. Hannuksela M (1991) Sensitivity of various skin sites in the repeated open application test. Am J Contact Dermat 2:102–104

133. Hannuksela A, Niinimäki A, Hannuksela M (1993) Size of the test area does not affect the result of the repeated open application test. Contact Dermatitis 28:299–300

134. Johansen JD, Andersen KE, Rastogi SC, Menné T (1996) Threshold responses in cinnamic-aldehyde-sensitive subjects: results and methodological aspects. Contact Dermatitis 34:165–171

135. Johansen JD, Andersen KE, Menné T (1996) Quantitiative aspects of isoeugenol contact allergy assessed by use and patch tests. Contact Dermatitis 34:414–418

136. Wahlberg JE, Färm G, Lidén C (1997) Quantification and specificity of the repeated open application test (ROAT). Acta Derm Venereol (Stockh) 77:420–424

137. Johansen JD, Bruze M, Andersen KE, Frosch PJ, Dreier B, White IR, Rastogi S, Lepoittevin JP, Menné T (1997) The repeated open application test: suggestions for a scale of evaluation. Contact Dermatitis 39:95–96

138. Flyvholm M-A, Hall BM, Agner T, Tiedemann E, Greenhill P, Vanderveken W, Freeberg FE, Menné T (1997) Threshold for occluded formaldehyde patch test in formaldehyde-sensitive patients. Contact Dermatitis 36:26–33

139. Tupker RA, Schuur J, Coenraads PJ (1997) Irritancy of antiseptics tested by repeated open exposures on the human skin, evaluated by non-invasive methods. Contact Dermatitis 37:213–217

140. Färm G (1998) Repeated open application tests (ROAT) in patients allergic to colophony – evaluated visually and with bioengineering techniques. Acta Derm Venereol (Stockh) 78:130–135

141. Nakada T, Hostynek JJ, Maibach HI (2000) Use tests: ROAT (repeated open application test)/PUT (provocative use test): an overview. Contact Dermatitis 43:1–3

142. Berardesca E, Maibach HI (1988) Bioengineering and the patch test. Contact Dermatitis 18:3–9

143. Bjarnason B, Flosadottir E, Fischer T (1999) Objective non-invasive assessment of patch tests with the laser Doppler perfusion scanning technique. Contact Dermatitis 40:251–260

144. Staberg B, Klemp P, Serup J (1984) Patch test responses evaluated by cutaneous blood flow measurements. Arch Dermatol 120:741–743

145. Fullerton A, Stucker M, Wilhelm K-P, Wårdell K, Anderson C, Fischer T, Nilsson GE, Serup J (2002) Guidelines for visualization of cutaneous blood flow by laser Doppler perfusion imaging. Contact Dermatitis 46: 129–140

146. Wahlberg JE (1989) Assessment of erythema: a comparison between the naked eye and laser Doppler flowmetry.

24

In: Frosch PJ, Dooms-Goossens A, Lachapelle JM, Rycroft RJ, Scheper RJ (eds) Current topics in contact dermatitis. Springer, Berlin, pp 549–553

147. Wahlberg JE (1971) Vehicle role of petrolatum. Acta Derm Venereol (Stockh) 51:129–134

148. Vanneste D, Martin P, Lachapelle JM (1980) Comparative study of the density of particles in suspension for patch testing. Contact Dermatitis 6:197–203

149. Fischer T, Maibach HI (1984) Patch test allergens in petrolatum: a reappraisal. Contact Dermatitis 11:224–228

150. Mellström GA, Sommar K, Wahlberg JE (1992) Patch test preparations of metallic mercury under the microscope. Contact Dermatitis 26:64–65

151. Karlberg A-T, Lidén C (1988) Comparison of colophony patch test preparations. Contact Dermatitis 18:158–165

152. Magnusson B, Hersle K (1966) Patch test methods. III. Influence of adhesive tape on test response. Acta Derm Venereol (Stockh) 46:275–278

153. Bruze M, Frick M, Persson L (2003) Patch testing with thin-layer chromatograms. Contact Dermatitis 48:278–279

Atopy Patch Testing with Aeroallergens and Food Proteins

25

Ulf Darsow and Johannes Ring

Contents

25.1 Introduction

Atopy patch test (APT) means an epicutaneous patch test with allergens known to elicit IgE-mediated reactions, and the evaluation of eczematous skin lesions after 24–72 h [1]. This test was developed as a diagnostic tool for characterizing patients with aeroallergen-triggered atopic eczema (AE, atopic dermatitis), a chronic inflammatory skin disease [2]. Patients with AE in the meaning of the WAO definition [3], formerly called "extrinsic" type, have evidence for elevated levels of total and/or allergen-specific immunoglobulin E (IgE), frequently directed against aeroallergens (e.g., house dust mite) and food allergens. These allergens produce flares in some patients with AE, but not in all sensitized individuals. Apart from the long-standing clinical reports and experience on single cases, flares can be experimentally induced, as has been shown with bronchial house dust mite exposure [4]. Although the percentage of aeroallergen-responsive eczema cases in the total eczema population is not known, a recent German population-based panel study established a significant association of eczema severity and the regional grass pollen count in a subgroup of 46% of children with eczema investigated for seasonal changes [5]. The association was stronger in children sensitized to grass pollen. Among the allergens found to be relevant in AE, aeroallergens and food allergens (in children) are most important. Therapeutical consequences of the diagnosis of allergy are based upon avoidance strategies; thus the relevance of (often multiple) IgE-mediated sensitizations in patients with AE for the skin disease has to be evaluated. In spite of these clinical aspects, the role of allergy in eliciting and maintaining the eczematous skin lesions was controversial, partially due to a lack of specificity of the

U. Darsow (✉)
Department of Dermatology and Allergy Biederstein,
Biedersteiner Strasse 29, 80802 München, Germany
e-mail: ulf.darsow@lrz.tu-muenchen.de

J. Ring
Department of Dermatology and Allergy Biederstein,
Technische Universität München,
Munich, Germany

J.D. Johansen et al. (eds.), *Contact Dermatitis*,
DOI: 10.1007/978-3-642-03827-3_25, © Springer-Verlag Berlin Heidelberg 2011

25

classic tests for IgE-mediated hypersensitivity, skin prick test, and measurement of specific serum IgE. Studies in this field are difficult due to the influence of remarkable placebo effects and other interfering allergens like animal dander or food. Consequently, a close look on the investigated population and inclusion criteria applied is mandatory to interpret seemingly contradictory outcomes [6].

Mite allergen in the epidermis of patients with AE under natural conditions [7], as well as in APT sites [8], has been demonstrated in proximity to Langerhans cells. In APT biopsies, T-cell populations have been characterized [9]. These T-cells showed a characteristic TH2 (T helper cell subpopulation) secretion pattern initially, whereas after 24 h a TH1 pattern was predominant. This same pattern is also found in chronic lesions of AE. Langerhans cells in the skin express IgE receptors of three different classes [10–12]. In addition, a Birbeck granule negative, non-Langerhans dendritic cell population with an even higher IgE-receptor expression than the Langerhans cell, the so-called inflammatory dendritic epidermal cell (IDEC) [13], has been demonstrated in freshly induced APT lesions, a phenomenon that occurred in both "intrinsic" and "extrinsic" patients [14]. This might explain IgE-associated activation of allergen-specific T-cells, finally leading to eczematous skin lesions in the APT (Fig. 25.1) [15, 16]. According to the results of Langeveld-Wildschut et al., the positive APT reaction requires the presence of epidermal IgE⁺ CD1a⁺ cells [17].

Core Message

> Aeroallergens are relevant triggers of AE. The APT, an epicutaneous patch test with allergens known to elicit IgE-mediated reactions and the evaluation of eczematous skin lesions after 24–72 h, was developed as diagnostic tool for characterizing patients with aeroallergen-triggered AE. Positive APT reactions are associated with allergen-specific T-cell responses.

Early studies describing experimental patch testing with aeroallergens were published in 1937 by Rostenberg and Sulzberger [18] and 1982 by Mitchell et al. [19]; the methods and results since showed wide variations. Potentially irritating procedures like skin abrasion [8, 20], tape stripping [21, 22], and sodium lauryl sulfate application [9] were used to enhance allergen penetration. No clear-cut correlations to skin prick test or specific IgE measurements could be obtained and the sensitivity and specificity of experimental APTs with regard to clinical history remained unclear. For better standardization we performed APT on nonlesional, nonabraded, untreated skin during remission [1, 23]. The results were compared for vehicle and dose of allergen in the preparations used. It was shown that healthy controls and patients with respiratory atopy without a history of eczema do not react in

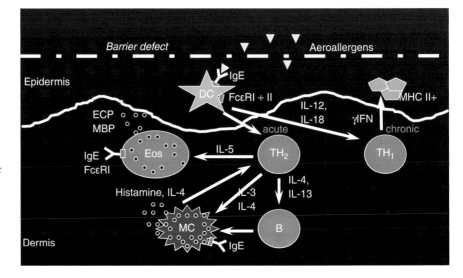

Fig. 25.1 Proposed pathophysiology of aeroallergen-triggered atopic eczema. *DC* dendritic cell (Langerhans cell, inflammatory dendritic epidermal cell); *FceR* IgE receptor; *Eos* eosinophil granulocyte; *TH* T-cell populations; *B* B cell; *MC* mast cell

the APT [23] or with a lower frequency and intensity of APT reactions to whole body mite extract compared to patients with AE [24]. Sensitivity and specificity of different diagnostic procedures were calculated [25].

25.2 APT Methods and Influence on Reactions

Table 25.1 summarizes the methods for APT resulting from methodological studies [14, 25–28]: APT with significant correlations to clinical parameters like allergen-specific IgE or patients history are today performed with a very similar technique to conventional patch tests for the diagnosis of classical contact allergy. Exclusion criteria (use of antihistamines, systemic and in loco topical steroids: 1 week, calcineurin antagonists: probably 1 week, UV radiation: 3 weeks, acute eczema flare) and the possibility of contact urticaria should be considered. Epicutaneous tests with lyophilized allergens, e.g., from house dust mite (*Dermatophagoides pteronyssinus, D. pter.*), cat dander, grass pollen, are performed with a petrolatum vehicle (including a vehicle control). Patients should be in a state of remission of their eczema; the patch test is applied in large Finn Chambers for 48 h on their back on nonabraded and uninvolved skin. Any potentially irritating methods of skin barrier disruption like tape stripping of the skin should be avoided. In several studies, nonatopic volunteers and patients suffering from allergic rhinoconjunctivitis only presented no

Table 25.1 Atopy patch test methods resulting from methodological studies [14, 25–28]

Allergen-specific individual history, eczema pattern, and routine diagnosis skin prick test and specific IgE

Patients in remission phase of eczema

Atopy patch test:

Lyophilized aeroallergens (house dust mite, cat dander, grass, and birch pollen)

Allergen doses: 5.000–7.000 PNU/g or 200 IR/g

Vehicle: petrolatum, large finn chambers

Application for 48 h on clinically uninvolved, not pretreated back skin (no tape stripping, no antiinflammatory pretreatment)

Evaluation after 48 and 72 h according to ETFAD key[a]

[a]See Table 25.5

Table 25.2 Intraindividual reproducibility of different APT models

Reproducibility of positive APT reactions at different time points			
Patch test	*n*	Time (months)	Reproducible
APT petrolatum[a]	20	6–12	18
D. pter., grass and birch pollen, no tape stripping			
APT petrolatum[b]	16	12–24	15
D. pter., cat, grass, and birch pollen, no tape stripping			
APT aqueous[c]	5	6	5
D. pter., 10× tape stripping			

[a,b]Own data
[c]From [17]

positive APT reactions with the methods described in Table 25.1. The reproducibility of different APT methods is high, if the test is performed on the back (Table 25.2). Allergens in petrolatum elicited twice as many APT reactions as allergens in a hydrophilic vehicle [23]. High allergen-specific IgE in serum is not a prerequisite for a positive APT, but patients with *D.pter.*-positive APT showed in 62% a corresponding positive skin prick test and in 77% a corresponding elevated specific IgE. In other allergens, the concordance was even higher. Allergen concentrations of 500, 3,000, 5,000, and 10,000 PNU (protein nitrogen units)/g in petrolatum were comparatively used in 57 patients [26]. It was shown that the percentage of patients with clear-cut positive reactions was significantly higher in patients with eczematous skin lesions in air-exposed areas (69%) as compared to patients without this predictive pattern (39%; $p=0.02$). A case report of a patient is given with Fig. 25.2. In the first group, the maximum reactivity was nearly reached with 5,000 PNU/g. The data from a randomized, double-blind multicenter trial, involving 253 adult patients and 30 children with AE, were used to calculate a suitable APT allergen dosage [25]. The optimal allergen doses were in the range of 5,000–7,000 PNU/g. For children, lower allergen concentrations seem possible. Simultaneously tested, the allergen doses of 7,000 PNU/g and 200 IR/g (biological unit; Index réactif) of the most important aeroallergens in Europe showed comparable concordance with the patients' history, suggesting clinical relevance in another study in 50 patients with AE. Results of a placebo-controlled 2 weeks in loco pretreatment study with 1% pimecrolimus [28] suggest that this calcineurin

25

Fig. 25.2 Case report

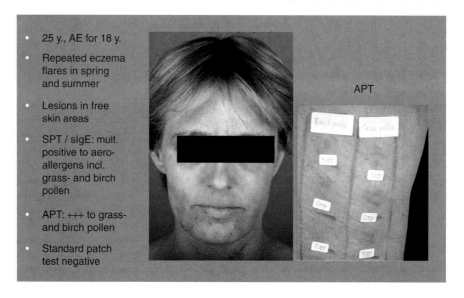

- 25 y., AE for 18 y.
- Repeated eczema flares in spring and summer
- Lesions in free skin areas
- SPT / sIgE: mult. positive to aero-allergens incl. grass- and birch pollen
- APT: +++ to grass- and birch pollen
- Standard patch test negative

APT

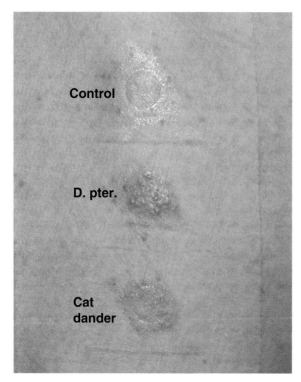

Fig. 25.3 APT reactions to different allergens after removal of Finn Chambers after 48 h. Clear-cut eczematous appearance with infiltration and spreading papules, partially with a follicular pattern. Control: petrolatum

Table 25.3 Summary of principal study results for aeroallergen APT [14, 25–27]

Controls: no positive reaction (nonatopic/rhinoconjunctivitis only)
Vehicle: petrolatum better than hydrogel
Allergen concentration >1,000 PNU/g; 7,000 PNU/g gave "optimal results" in adults
Biologically standardized allergens: 200 IR/g
Atopic eczema in uncovered skin areas: associated with higher frequency of positive APT
Seasonal eczema flares (Summer): positive grass pollen APT
APT correlates with clinical history

> **Core Message**
>
> › See Table 25.1.

antagonist can suppress the intensity of APT reactions. An example of a positive APT reaction to a biologically standardized allergen preparation is shown in Fig. 25.3. The clinical outcome of the methods studies is summarized in Table 25.3.

The standardization of aeroallergen APT is still more advanced than food patch testing; in Europe the efforts are coordinated in the European Task Force on Atopic Dermatitis (ETFAD), the eczema task force of the EADV. The ETFAD study in six European Countries ($n = 314$) showed again that house dust mite (*D. pter.*) most often elicited positive APT reactions, followed by pollen allergens (Table 25.4) [29]. This study also investigated food extract preparations in petrolatum. To date, food APT are performed with unstandardized fresh food preparations with conflicting results.

Table 25.4 Positive test results and patients' history of allergen-associated eczema flare

	SPT (%)	sIgE (%)	APT (%)	History (%)	Hx-concordance (%)
Aeroallergens					
D. pter.	56	56	39	34	57
Birch pollen	49	53	17	20	61
Grass pollen	57	59	15	31	64
Cat dander	44	46	10	30	62
Food allergens					
Egg white	25	19	11	7	77
Wheat flour	16	38	10	3	78
Celery	20	30	9	1	79

Frequency of positive APT reactions is lower than that of positive IgE-mediated sensitizations. Patients' allergen-specific history of eczema flares after allergen exposure was obtained prospectively. $n = 314$, 24 % children ≤10 years. *SPT* skin prick test ≥3 mm; *sIgE* specific IgE ≥0.35 kU/L; *APT* atopy patch test ≥ +; Hx-concordance, allergen-specific concordance of APT result and clinical history. Data from [29]

25.3 Evaluation of APT Reactions

Usually, APT reactions are read after 48 and 72 h. In patients with contact urticaria, a wheal and flare reaction may be seen after 30 min. Most reactions are visible and palpable at 48 h, sometimes with decrescendo to 72 h. After tape stripping followed by allergen application, there are more early reactions visible. Clear-cut positive reactions should be distinguished from negative or questionable ones understanding the fact that only reactions showing papules or at least some degree of infiltration were correlated with clinical relevance. A consensus APT reading key for describing the intensity of APT reactions was developed and published [30]. Following its use in a multicenter trial in six European countries, ETFAD proposed 2003 a simplified version given in Table 25.5.

Table 25.5 ETFAD key for the grading of positive APT reactions (modified from [30])

–	Negative
?	Only erythema, questionable
+	Erythema, infiltration
++	Erythema, few papules
+++	Erythema, many or spreading papules
++++	Erythema, vesicles

ETFAD European Task Force on Atopic Dermatitis

However, clinically meaningful APT results were also obtained with the ICDRG key for conventional patch testing [23, 25].

> **Core Message**
>
> › APT is read according to ETFAD (or ICDRG) guidelines, see Table 25.5.

25.4 Predictors, Sensitivity and Specificity of APT

As long as no "gold standard" of provocation for aeroallergen allergy in AE exists, the history of allergen-specific exacerbation is used as a parameter for clinical relevance. A study compared outcome of the APT with a seasonal history of "summer eruption" of AE in 79 patients [27]. Significantly higher frequencies of positive grass pollen APT reactions (with two methods used) occurred in patients with a corresponding history of exacerbation of skin lesions during the grass pollen season of the previous year (75% with positive APT). Patients without this history showed significantly lower APT reactivity (16% with positive APT; $p < 0.001$).

Core Message

> The APT specificity exceeded the specificity of the classic tests of IgE-mediated hypersensitivity, which was 0.33 for skin prick test and specific IgE measurement by radioallergosorbent test (RAST). On the other hand, the sensitivity of the classical methods was higher (0.92 for RAST, and 1.0 for skin prick test, Table 25.6).

Table 25.7 Logistic regression model: predictors of a positive APT reaction (from [25]), highest significance on top of table

Positive reactions are associated with
Increased specific serum IgE
Positive skin prick test reaction
Allergen-specific corresponding history
Increased total IgE
Long eczema duration
Rhinoconjunctivitis (grass pollen)

In two multicenter studies with up to five aeroallergens, the predictors of a positive APT reaction were investigated (Table 25.7) [25, 29]. Sensitivity and specificity of the APT in these studies are also shown in Table 25.6. It has to be kept in mind that at least for a nonseasonal aeroallergen, the history may be unreliable, thereby limiting the precision of such calculations like in Table 25.6. For most allergens, a significant association of APT and specific IgE could be demonstrated.

Table 25.6 Sensitivity and Specificity of different test procedures with regard to clinical history: the APT shows a higher specificity than classical tests for IgE-mediated hypersensitivity with regard to the allergen-specific history

Test	Sensitivity (%)[a]	Specificity (%)[a]
Different grass pollen preparations, $n=79$		
Skin prick	100	33
sIgE	92	33
APT	75	84
European multicenter study $n=314$, four allergens		
Skin prick	68–80	50–71
sIgE	72–84	52–69
APT	14–45	64–91
German multicenter study $n=253$, three allergens		
Skin prick	69–82	44–53
sIgE	65–94	42–64
APT	42–56	69–92

Studies used different allergen standardizations. Data from [25, 27, 29]

[a]Depending on allergen, with regard to a clinical history with eczema flares in pollen season or after direct contact with allergen

Problems like irrelevant positive or spreading APT reactions may occur in patients undergoing APT during an eczema flare, or if methods of abrasion of the stratum corneum are used. The issue of pharmacological influence on APT still holds many unanswered questions [28]. As the standardization of the high molecular weight allergens has some specific problems, a commercial provider of test substances with reproducible quality and major allergen content is desirable. However, to date, such allergen preparations are still not easily available. Even more problems with allergen standardization are known for food APT.

25.5 APT with Food Proteins

The APT with food is still an experimental method, but the available standardized food challenge protocols allowed the evaluation of the clinical relevance of food APT reactions to a certain degree. Often, native foods like hen's egg, wheat flour, cow's milk, or soy products were applied in 12 mm aluminum test chambers for 24 or 48 h on the patient's skin. Majamaa et al. [31] investigated 142 children under 2 years with suspected cow's milk allergy. In 50% the oral provocation test was positive (22 immediate-type reactions). Of these patients, 26% had an increased corresponding specific IgE, 14% a positive skin prick test, and 44% a positive APT with cow's milk. In this age group, most positive APT reactions were seen without corresponding positive skin prick test results. Further investigations by Isolauri and Turjanmaa [32] showed an interesting association between the clinical pattern of the reaction and the result of skin prick test and APT. They also suggested to perform skin prick test and APT simultaneously to increase the precision of diagnosis. In the investigated group of children (2–36 months) with AE, the skin prick test with cow's milk was positive in 67% of cases with *immediate*-type reactions in the oral challenge, mostly accompanied by negative APT. On the other hand, a positive APT was seen in 89% of cases with *delayed eczematous* reaction, whereas in these cases the skin prick test was mostly negative.

An association of positive APT (with native preparations of cow's milk, hen's egg, wheat flour, and soy) with eczema flares following oral provocation was described by Niggemann et al. [33, 34]. Roehr et al. [35] calculated for the APT with these native foods a sensitivity of 47–89% and a specificity of 86–96% with regard to the result of the oral provocation. The positive predictive value of the diagnostic method could be increased to 94–100% when positive skin prick tests, elevated specific IgE, and a positive APT were combined for these calculations. Own investigations in a multicenter study in six European countries using an APT with food preparations in petrolatum ([29] Table 25.4) showed a concordance of APT result and clinical history of 77% (hen's egg), 78% (wheat flour), and 79% (celery). The specificity of this APT was 91% with regard to a predictive clinical history, but the sensitivity was only 30–33% ($n = 314$). More recently, the authors of initially optimistic studies [33–35] point to the fact that most oral food challenges cannot be replaced by their native food patch tests [36].

An IgE-mediated sensitization. Interestingly, 7% of the tested patients, who would be labeled as "intrinsic type" of AE according to Wüthrich's definition [37], show a sensitization in the APT. A similar finding of positive APT reactions in subjects without sIgE to *Dermatophagoides* was described by Seidenari et al. and Manzini et al. [38, 39]. Also, eight of twelve "intrinsic" AE patients were shown to react to a partially purified whole mite APT preparation [40]. Similar results have been obtained by APT with *Malassezia sympodialis* antigen [41]. House-dust-mite-specific antibodies of the IgG4 subtype, as well as a rapid influx of IDEC in the APT lesions, have been reported in two otherwise "intrinsic" AE patients [42]. However, the mechanism of these "intrinsic" APT reactions remains hypothetical to date, but a T-cell-mediated mechanism without IgE involvement seems probable.

> **Core Message**
>
> › With regard to the recently proposed novel nomenclature for allergy by the European Academy of Allergy and Clinical Immunology [3], these cases may be diagnosed as "non-IgE-associated (nonatopic) eczema" or "T-cell-mediated eczema."

> **Core Message**
>
> › Contradicting results of different studies are obvious, especially for the sensitivity of unstandardized food APT; further clinical studies for standardization and patient group selection for food APT are necessary. Food provocation tests are currently not replaced by APT.

25.6 APT and Atopic Eczema "Intrinsic Type"

A sensitization detected by APT, which is supposedly T-cell-mediated, may be even more relevant for the clinical course of AE than the demonstration of

25.7 Outlook

The current state of APT is summarized and critically discussed in a recent ETFAD/EAACI position paper [43]. Accordingly, the indications for APT are summarized in Table 25.8. The APT with *aeroallergens* may provide an especially important diagnostic tool in two patient subgroups: In patients with an air-exposed eczema distribution pattern, positive APT reactions occurred at lower allergen doses compared with other patients with eczema. Patients with an aeroallergen-specific history had significantly more positive APT reactions.

25

Table 25.8 ETFAD/EAACI position paper: APT indications

Consensus APT indications

Suspicion of aeroallergen symptoms without proof of positive specific IgE and/or a positive skin prick test

Severe and/or persistent atopic eczema with unknown trigger factors

Multiple IgE sensitizations without proven clinical relevance in patients with eczema

---

Core Message (see also Table 25.8)

> The lower sensitivity but higher specificity of the APT compared to skin prick test or RAST favors the notion that the classical tests may have some value as screening tests, specificity may be added by the APT. The APT does not replace the classical methods of diagnosis of IgE-mediated allergy.

Questions remain open concerning the clinical relevance of positive APT results in patients with a negative history and discordant negative skin prick tests or RAST, since no gold standard exists for the provocation of eczematous skin lesions in aeroallergen-triggered AE [43]. These questions may only be answered by controlled studies using specific provocation and elimination procedures in patients with positive and negative APT results. However, this does not argue against the clinical use by allergists at this time point, since one has to keep in mind that in many classical contact allergens the standardization and evaluation efforts have been less systematic. Still, these allergens are used for routine diagnosis in patch test clinics. Appropriate allergen-specific avoidance strategies are recommended in patients showing positive APT reactions [44]. Future indications for food APT may be found in clinical studies on eosinophilic esophagitis [45].

25.8 Classic Article

Tanaka Y, Tanaka M, Anan S, Yoshida H (1989) Immunohistochemical studies on dust mite antigen in positive reaction site of patch test. Acta Derm Venereol (Stockh) suppl 144:93–96.

Eczematous reactions could be induced by patch testing with mite antigens in patients with AE. Using an immuno-double-labeling technique, authors demonstrated that many mite antigen-bearing Langerhans cells are visible in the epidermis in the early stage of the APT reaction. Twenty-four hours later, these cells were observed only in the deep dermis. Immunoelectron microscopically, it was found that the mite antigens were trapped by macrophages, which were in contact with lymphocytes. Many IgE-positive dendritic cells bearing mite antigen were seen in positive APT sites.

One of the first and most often cited studies suggests IgE-mediated contact hypersensitivity to mite antigens in the pathogenesis of AE. These observations still hold true and are also discussed with regard to the allergen specificity of APT reactions, which was later corroborated by others.

References

1. Ring J, Kunz B, Bieber T, Vieluf D, Przybilla B (1989) The "atopy patch test" with aeroallergens in atopic eczema. J Allergy Clin Immunol 82:195
2. Ring J, Przybilla B, Ruzicka T (eds) (2006) Handbook of atopic eczema, 2nd edn. Springer, Berlin
3. Johansson SGO, Bieber T, Dahl R, Friedmann PS, Lanier BQ, Lockey RF, Motala C, Ortega Martell JA, Platts-Mills TAE, Ring J, Thien F, Van Cauwenberge P, Williams HC (2004) Revised nomenclature for allergy for global use: Report of the Nomenclature Review Committee of the World Allergy Organization, October 2003. J Allergy Clin Immunol 113:832–836
4. Tupker R, DeMonchy J, Coenraads P, Homan A, van der Meer J (1996) Induction of atopic dermatitis by inhalation of house dust mite. J Allergy Clin Immunol 97:1064–1070
5. Krämer U, Weidinger S, Darsow U, Möhrenschlager M, Ring J, Behrendt H (2005) Seasonality in symptom severity influenced by temperature or grass pollen: results of a panel study in children with eczema. J Invest Dermatol 124:514–523
6. Holm L, Ohman S, Bengtsson A, van Hage-Hamsten M, Scheynius A (2001) Effectiveness of occlusive bedding in the treatment of atopic dermatitis – a placebo-controlled trial of 12 months duration. Allergy 56:152–158
7. Maeda K, Yamamoto K, Tanaka Y, Anan S, Yoshida H (1992) House dust mite (HDM) antigen in naturally occurring lesions of atopic dermatitis (AD): the relationship between HDM antigen in the skin and HDM antigen-specific IgE antibody. J Derm Sci 3:73–77
8. Gondo A, Saeki N, Tokuda Y (1986) Challenge reactions in atopic dermatitis after percutaneous entry of mite antigen. Br J Dermatol 115:485–493
9. Eyerich K, Huss-Marp J, Darsow U, Wollenberg A, Forster S, Ring J, Behrendt H, Traidl-Hoffmann C (2008) Pollen grains

induce a rapid and biphasic eczematous immune response in atopic eczema patients. Int Arch Allergy Immunol 145:213–223

10. Bieber T, Rieger A, Neuchrist C, Prinz JC, Rieber EP, Boltz-Nitulescu G, Scheiner O, Kraft D, Ring J, Stingl G (1989) Induction of FCeR2/CD23 on human epidermal Langerhans-Cells by human recombinant IL4 and IFN. J Exp Med 170:309–314

11. Bieber T, de la Salle H, Wollenberg A, Hakimi J, Chizzonite R, Ring J, Hanau D, de la Salle C (1992) Human epidermal Langerhans cells express the high affinity receptor for immunoglobulin E (Fc epsilon RI). J Exp Med 175:1285–1290

12. Wollenberg A, de la Salle H, Hanau D, Liu FT, Bieber T (1993) Human Keratinocytes release the endogenous ß-galactoside-binding soluble lectin εBP which binds to Langerhans cells where it modulates their binding capacity for IgE glycoforms. J Exp Med 178:777–785

13. Wollenberg A, Kraft S, Hanau D, Bieber T (1996) Immunomorphological and ultrastructural characterization of Langerhans cells and a novel, inflammatory dendritic epidermal cell (IDEC) population in lesional skin of atopic eczema. J Invest Dermatol 106:446–453

14. Kerschenlohr K, Decard S, Przybilla B, Wollenberg A (2003) Atopy patch test reactions show a rapid influx of inflammatory dendritic epidermal cells (IDEC) in extrinsic and intrinsic atopic dermatitis patients. J Allergy Clin Immunol 111:869–874

15. van Reijsen FC, Bruijnzeel-Koomen CAFM, Kalthoff FS (1992) Skin-derived aeroallergen-specific T-cell clones of Th2 phenotype in patients with atopic dermatitis. J Allergy Clin Immunol 90:184–192

16. Sager N, Feldmann A, Schilling G, Kreitsch P, Neumann C (1992) House dust mite-specific T cells in the skin of subjects with atopic dermatitis: frequency and lymphokine profile in the allergen patch test. J Allergy Clin Immunol 89:801–810

17. Langeveld-Wildschut EG, Bruijnzeel PLB, Mudde GC, Versluis C, Dijk AG Van Ieperen-Van, Bihari IC, Knol EF, Thepen T, Bruijnzeel-Koomen CAFM, van Reijsen F (2000) Clinical and immunologic variables in skin of patients with atopic eczema and either positive or negative atopy patch test reactions. J Allergy Clin Immunol 105:1008–1016

18. Rostenberg A, Sulzberger MD (1937) Some results of patch tests. Arch Dermatol 35:433–454

19. Mitchell E, Chapman M, Pope F, Crow J, Jouhal S, Platts-Mills T (1982) Basophils in allergen-induced patch test sites in atopic dermatitis. Lancet I:127–130

20. Norris P, Schofield O, Camp R (1988) A study of the role of house dust mite in atopic dermatitis. Br J Dermatol 118:435–440

21. van Voorst Vader PC, Lier JG, Woest TE, Coenraads PJ, Nater JP (1991) Patch tests with house dust mite antigens in atopic dermatitis patients: methodological problems. Acta Derm Venereol (Stockh) 71:301–305

22. Bruijnzeel-Koomen C, van Wichen D, Spry C, Venge P, Bruijnzeel P (1988) Active participation of eosinophils in patch test reactions to inhalant allergens in patients with atopic dermatitis. Br J Dermatol 118:229–238

23. Darsow U, Vieluf D, Ring J (1995) Atopy patch test with different vehicles and allergen concentrations – an approach to standardization. J Allergy Clin Immunol 95:677–684

24. Seidenari S, Giusti F, Pellacani G, Bertoni L (2003) Frequency and intensity of responses to mite patch tests are lower in non atopic subjects in respect to patients with atopic dermatitis. Allergy 58:426–429

25. Darsow U, Vieluf D, The APT study group (1999) Evaluating the relevance of aeroallergen sensitization in atopic eczema with the atopy patch test: a randomized, double-blind multicenter study. J Am Acad Dermatol 40:187–193

26. Darsow U, Vieluf D, Ring J (1996) The atopy patch test: an increased rate of reactivity in patients who have an air-exposed pattern of atopic eczema. Br J Dermatol 135: 182–186

27. Darsow U, Behrendt H, Ring J (1997) Gramineae pollen as trigger factors of atopic eczema – evaluation of diagnostic measures using the atopy patch test. Br J Dermatol 137: 201–207

28. Weissenbacher S, Traidl-Hoffmann C, Eyerich K, Katzer K, Bräutigam M, Loeffler H, Hofmann H, Behrendt H, Ring J, Darsow U (2006) Modulation of atopy patch test and skin prick test by pretreatment with 1% pimecrolimus cream. Int Arch Allergy Immunol 140:239–244

29. Darsow U, Laifaoui J, Bolhaar S, Bruijnzeel-Koomen CAFM, Breuer K, Wulf A, Werfel T, Brönnimann M, Braathen LR, Dangoisse C, Blondeel A, Song M, Didierlaurent A, André C, Drzimalla K, Simon D, Disch R, Borelli S, Elst L, Devilliers A, Oranje AP, de Raeve L, Reiser K, Wollenberg A, Przybilla B, Roul S, Taieb A, Seidenari S, Wüthrich B, Ring J (2004) The prevalence of positive reactions in the atopy patch test with aeroallergens and food allergens in subjects with atopic eczema: a European multicenter study. Allergy 59:1318–1325

30. Darsow U, Ring J (2000) Airborne and dietary allergens in atopic eczema: a comprehensive review of diagnostic tests. Clin Exp Dermatol 25:544–551

31. Majamaa H, Moisio P, Holm K, Kautiainen H, Turjanmaa K (1999) Cow's milk allergy: diagnostic accuracy of skin prick test and specific IgE. Allergy 54:346–351

32. Isolauri E, Turjanmaa K (1996) Combined skin prick and patch testing enhances identification of food allergy in infants with atopic dermatitis. J Allergy Clin Immunol 97:9–15

33. Niggemann B, Reibel S, Wahn U (2000) The atopy patch test – a useful tool for the diagnosis of food allergy in children with atopic dermatitis. Allergy 55:281–285

34. Niggemann B, Reibel S, Roehr CC, Felger D, Ziegert M, Sommerfeld C, Wahn U (2001) Predictors of positive food challenge outcome in non-IgE-mediated reactions to food in children with atopic dermatitis. J Allergy Clin Immunol 108:1053–1058

35. Roehr CC, Reibel S, Ziegert M, Sommerfeld C, Wahn U, Niggemann B (2001) Atopy patch tests, together with determination of specific IgE levels, reduce the need for oral food challenges in children with atopic dermatitis. J Allergy Clin Immunol 107:548–553

36. Mehl A, Rolinck-Werninghaus C, Staden U, Verstege A, Wahn U, Beyer K, Niggemann B (2006) The atopy patch test in the diagnostic workup of suspected food-related symptoms in children. J Allergy Clin Immunol 118:923–929

37. Schmid-Grendelmeier P, Simon D, Simon HU, Akdis CA, Wüthrich B (2001) Epidemiology, clinical features, and immunology of the "intrinsic" (non-IgE-mediated) type of atopic dermatitis (constitutional dermatitis). Allergy 56: 841–849

38. Seidenari S, Manzini BM, Danese P, Giannetti A (1992) Positive patch tests to whole mite culture and purified mite extracts in patients with atopic dermatitis, asthma, and rhinitis. Ann Allergy 69:201–206

39. Manzini BM, Motolese A, Donini M, Seidenari S (1995) Contact allergy to dermatophagoides in atopic dermatitis patients and healthy subjects. Contact Derm 33:243–246

40. Ingordo V, D'Andria G, D'Andria C, Tortora A (2002) Results of atopy patch tests with house dust mites in adults with "intrinsic" and "extrinsic" atopic dermatitis. J Eur Acad Dermatol Venereol 16:450–454

41. Johansson C, Sandstrom MH, Bartosik J, Sarnhult T, Christiansen J, Zargari A, Back O, Wahlgren CF, Faergemann J, Scheynius A, Tengvall Linder M (2003) Atopy patch test reactions to Malassezia allergens differentiate subgroups of atopic dermatitis patients. Br J Dermatol 148:479–488

42. Kerschenlohr K, Decard S, Darsow U, Ollert M, Wollenberg A (2003) Clinical and immunologic reactivity to aeroallergens in 'intrinsic' atopic dermatitis patients. J Allergy Clin Immunol 111:195–197

43. Turjanmaa K, Darsow U, Niggemann B, Rancé F, Vanto T, Werfel T (2006) EAACI/GA2LEN position paper: present status of the atopy patch test – position paper of the Section on Dermatology and the Section on Pediatrics of the EAACI. Allergy 61:1377–1384

44. Darsow U, Wollenberg A, Simon D, Taïeb A, Werfel T, Oranje A, Geimetti C, Svensson A, Deleuran M, Calza AM, Giusti F, Lübbe J, Seidenari S, Ring J (2010) for the European Task Force on Atopic Dermatitis / EADV Eczema Task Force. ETFAD / EADV Eczema Task Force 2009 position paper on diagnosis and treatment of atopic dermatitis. J Eur Acad Dermatol Venereol 24:317–328

45. Spergel JM, Brown-Whitehorn T, Beausoleil JL, Shuker M, Liacouras CA (2006) Predictive values for skin prick test and atopy patch test for eosinophilic esophagitis. J Allergy Clin Immunol 119:509–511

Patch Testing in Adverse Drug Reactions

26

Margarida Gonçalo and Derk P. Bruynzeel

Contents

M. Gonçalo (✉)
Clinic of Dermatology, Coimbra University Hospital,
University of Coimbra, Praceta Mota Pinto,
3000-175 Coimbra, Portugal
e-mail: mmgoncalo@netcabo.pt

D.P. Bruynzeel
Burg. Dedelstraat 42, 1391 GD Abcoude,
The Netherlands

26.1 Introduction

26.1.1 Definition and Types of Cutaneous Adverse Drug Reactions

A CADR is a skin eruption induced by drugs, systemic or topical drugs, used in adequate doses and in the correct indications. CADRs are a frequent problem in Dermatology, but their incidence is not exactly known; 1–5% of inpatients experience such a reaction and it is a frequent cause of consultation in Dermatology [1–5]. Most CADRs are mild, but about 20% can be severe and require hospitalization, for example, in patients with drug hypersensitivity syndrome/drug reaction with eosinophilia and systemic symptoms (DRESS) and toxic epidermal necrolysis which, apart from the skin, have involvement of other organs [5].

Considering its pathomechanism, CADRs can be divided into several types. Most cases belong to type A and C, predictable and chemical, which represent an exaggerated pharmacologic activity of the drug, such as cheilitis from isotretinoin, or xerosis and papulo-pustulo-follicular reactions from inhibitors of epidermal growth factor receptor [6]. They can be enhanced by modification of drug bioavailability due to drug interactions, reduced metabolization, or elimination, especially in genetically susceptible individuals. Type D includes late (delayed) reactions, such as teratogenesis or carcinogenesis, and type E results from end-of-dose reactions [7]. Type B reactions are idiosyncratic, unexpected, unpredictable, and among these, many are due to immune reactions induced by the drug [5] (Table 26.1).

J.D. Johansen et al. (eds.), *Contact Dermatitis*,
DOI: 10.1007/978-3-642-03827-3_26, © Springer-Verlag Berlin Heidelberg 2011

26

Table 26.1 Main types of adverse drug reactions, according to its mechanism [7]

Type of adverse reaction	Mechanisms
A – Augmented	Exaggerated pharmacologic activity of the drug
B – Bizarre[a]	Idiosyncratic, unpredictable, usually immune-mediated
C – Chemical	Chemical or pharmacological effect of drug
D – Delayed	Reactions occurring late, related mainly with carcinogenesis or teratogenesis
E – End-of-dose	Reaction to drug suspension

[a]These are the ones that will be dealt with in this chapter

26.1.2 Main Clinical Patterns of Immune-Mediated CADRs

Systemic exposure to drugs can sensitize the individual and lead to a wide variety of CADRs or drug eruptions. Some reactions are not specifically induced by a drug, such as a maculopapular exanthema, urticaria or angioedema, lichenoid reaction, or subacute lupus erythematosus. Other patterns are almost exclusively induced by drugs (>90%), such as Stevens–Johnson syndrome, toxic epidermal necrolysis, fixed drug eruption, and acute generalized exanthematous pustulosis [5, 8].

According to their time course, drug eruptions can be divided into immediate reactions, occurring within minutes to 1–2 h of drug intake, and delayed reactions that occur several hours, days or up to 6 weeks after drug exposure. Immediate reactions present as urticaria, angioedema, or anaphylaxis, whereas for delayed reactions the clinical spectrum is much wider: maculopapular eruptions (the most frequent reaction pattern) (Fig. 26.1), exfoliative erythroderma, acute generalized exanthematous pustulosis (Fig. 26.2), localized fixed drug eruptions, Stevens–Johnson syndrome (Fig. 26.3), toxic epidermal necrolysis (Fig. 26.4), other bullous reactions mimicking pemphigus vulgaris or bullous pemphigoid, vasculitis, and lupus erythematosus [9].

Topically applied drugs may cause contact dermatitis reactions or photosensitive contact dermatitis. Topical sensitization and subsequent systemic exposure may induce skin reactions similar to systemic drug eruptions (maculopapular exanthema) [10] or patterns more typical of a systemic contact dermatitis,

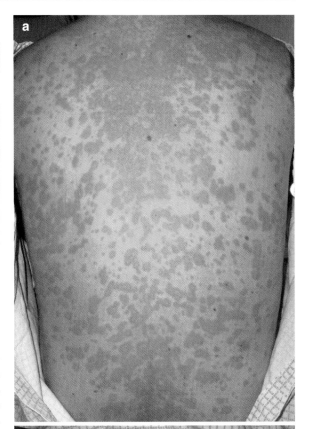

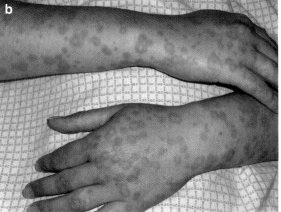

Fig. 26.1 Generalized maculopapular exanthema from amoxicillin that developed on the ninth day of therapy, with symmetric lesions on the trunk (**a**) and targetoid lesions on the hands and forearms (**b**). This patient had positive patch tests with amoxicillin and ampicillin at 1 and 10% pet. and negative tests with penicillin G, dicloxacillin, and several cefalosporins

such as acrovesicular dermatitis, the "baboon syndrome" (see Chap. 17), or Symmetrical drug-related intertriginous and flexural exanthema (SDRIFE) [11, 12]. It is clear that in these situations patch testing can be of great help as a diagnostic tool [11].

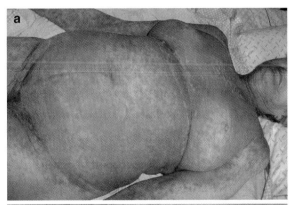

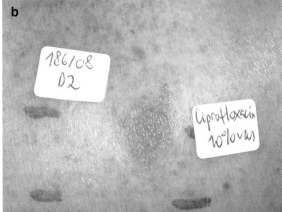

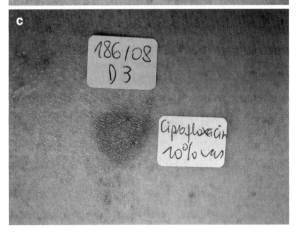

Fig. 26.2 Acute generalized exanthematous pustulosis from ciprofloxacin, on the third day of evolution, with coalescent pustules on erythema, predominating on the main body folds (**a**). Patch tests were positive with ciprofloxacin at 10% pet. and also norfloxacin and lomefloxacin. The erythemato-vesicular reaction at D2 (**b**) changed into a pustular reaction at D3 (**c**). Histopathology showed an intraepidermal spongiform pustule as in the acute eruption

In patients with drug eruptions without previous contact sensitization, patch testing can also induce specific positive reactions, but the sensitivity of this

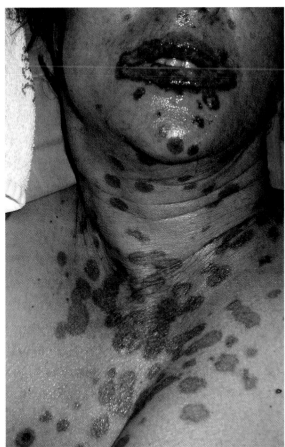

Fig. 26.3 Stevens–Johnson syndrome from lamotrigine, an antiepileptic drug frequently responsible for this clinical reaction pattern, particularly in children. Note the typical oral involvement, with erosion of the whole semimucosa of the lower lip

test is much lower than in allergic contact dermatitis [13, 14]. The value of patch testing in CADRs has not always been appreciated, but there is growing interest in this field. It is a safe method and results can be very rewarding, as positive test results can be very useful to confirm drug imputability established on clinical grounds. Patch testing can also be helpful for studying cross-reactions and understanding pathomechanisms involved in drug eruptions [15].

Core Message

› Drug eruptions are adverse skin reactions caused by a drug used in normal doses. They present with a very wide variety of clinical patterns.

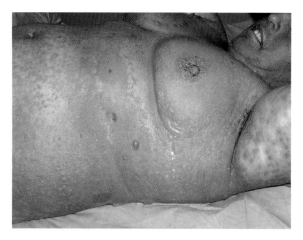

The pseudo-allergic (anaphylactoid) reactions, including urticaria induced by acetylsalicylic acid and other nonsteroidal anti-inflammatory drugs (NSAIDs) and angioedema induced by angiotensin conversing enzyme inhibitors (ACEi), are examples of nonimmunological reactions mimicking a true (type I) allergic reaction. The most plausible explanation for these reactions is a nonspecific release of histamine and other mast cell and basophil mediators without the participation of IgEs or a reduced capacity to metabolize kinins, with consequent accumulation of the potent vasodilator bradykinin [24].

Fig. 26.4 Toxic epidermal necrolysis/Lyell's syndrome induced by carbamazepine. Note confluent flaccid bullae on the trunk, already with a few areas of epidermal detachment, and atypical target lesions in the arms. Although this is not frequent, this patient had positive patch tests to carbamazepine, which on histology had skin apoptosis of the whole epidermis, such as in the acute eruption of the toxic epidermal necrolysis

26.1.3 Pathomechanisms Involved in Immune-Mediated Drug Eruptions

In most CADRs of the type B there is involvement of the immune system. Either antibodies or T-cells with their specific receptor recognize the drug, or a metabolite, or any of these combined with a peptide or with an autologous cell. These drug reactions can be classified according to the immunological reaction types of Gell and Coombs (see Chap. 3), but often it is not one isolated immunological mechanism that is responsible for the event: combinations of type I and IV hypersensitivity exist [16] and even more complex mechanisms can be involved [5, 17]. Genetic susceptibility is also important, as in cases of toxic epidermal necrolysis and Stevens–Johnson syndrome from allopurinol and carbamazepine and, particularly, in abacavir hypersensitivity syndrome, where HLA-B*5701 pretesting has significantly reduced this severe adverse reaction [18, 19].

Immediate reactions involve mainly drug-specific IgE and mast cell and basophil degranulation [20], whereas delayed reactions after systemic drug exposure depend mainly on type IV hypersensitivity reactions, with previous T-cell sensitization [21, 22]. By the clinical pattern and time course, we can suspect which mechanisms can be involved, but sometimes it is not possible [23].

26.1.4 T-Cell Involvement in Drug Eruptions

Apart from allergic contact dermatitis and systemic contact dermatitis, delayed type IV hypersensitivity has been documented in maculopapular exanthema, in drug hypersensitivity syndrome/DRESS, in acute generalized exanthematous pustulosis, in the localized fixed drug eruption, and in the more extended bullous reactions in a continuum from Stevens–Johnson syndrome to toxic epidermal necrolysis [9]. These reactions usually begin within 7–21 days on the first exposure, but rechallenge is usually accelerated, positive with lower dose and more severe, suggesting specific immune sensitization. In the skin biopsies of the CADR there is mainly a dermo-epidemal infiltration of activated T-cells, some of which specifically recognize the drug or one of its metabolites. And, apart from the skin, drug-specific T-cells have been isolated from the blood or blister fluid during the acute reaction and also, later, from skin biopsies of positive patch tests [9, 25–28]. As previously referred, the clinical presentation of these CADRs is very heterogeneous, even though there are data to support the involvement of delayed type hypersensitivity mechanisms [5]. Apart from other individual circumstances, this heterogeneity very probably depends on different pathways of drug recognition by the immune system and on the subtypes of effector T-cells. Although there is little knowledge on which cells participate in the process of drug presentation during the sensitization phase, the drug, a metabolite or both, can be recognized by the TCR combined with HLA molecules, either class I, class II, or both, with or without previous processing by the antigen presenting cell [29]. There are many studies on the effector T-cells (Th1, Th2, Tcit) and on the main cytokines and chemokines involved in the final reaction (IFN-gama, IL-8, IL-5, eotaxin, TNF-alfa, Fas) [22, 30]. Recently, subtypes of type IV hypersensitivity have been defined in the participation of CADR [22, 31]. A Th1 pattern with IFN-gama production, considered a type IVa hypersensitivity, is mainly involved in allergic contact dermatitis and maculopapular exanthema. Type IVb involves mainly a Th2 response, with IL-5 and eotaxin production and, consequently, eosinophil recruitment and activation. Actually, there is eosinophil infiltration in the dermis in maculopapular exanthema, and systemic eosinophilia is one of the criteria for drug hypersensitivity syndrome/DRESS [17, 32, 33]. In acute generalized exanthematous pustulosis, T-cells isolated from the blood and the skin produce high amounts of the chemokine CXCL8 (IL-8) and GM-CSF, with consequent preferential neutrophil recruitment that is responsible for the epidermal spongiform pustule typical of this CADR (type IVd hypersensitivity) [34, 35]. Type IVc, with predominant T-cell cytotoxic activity, is involved at a lower level in maculopapular exanthems, but is very pronounced in Stevens–Johnson syndrome and toxic epidermal necrolysis, where keratinocyte apoptosis is the hallmark of the reaction [22, 36, 37]. Fixed drug eruptions are also typical T-cell-mediated reactions, with a special localization pattern and a very particular retention of drug-specific T-cells in lesional areas. These resting T-cells are activated very shortly after topical or systemic drug exposure, and produce high amounts of IFN-gama and cytotoxic mediators (TNF-alfa and Fas), but precocious infiltration of regulatory T-cells (Tregs) seems to prevent its evolution to the more severe bullous reactions [38, 39]. Delayed type hypersensitivity is also involved in some photosensitive drug reactions, mainly in those with an eczematous pattern [40–42].

Therefore, the participation of drug-specific T-cells in several drug eruptions other than allergic contact dermatitis makes patch testing suitable for their study. Nevertheless, the rate of negative reactions is much higher, as mechanisms other than T-cell-derived hypersensitivity are involved, often in a more complex interplay with other systemic inflammatory reactions (viral infections, autoimmune diseases). Also in some CADRs, very probably, the allergen is not the drug itself, but a systemic metabolite and, although skin metabolism is quite efficient, some drugs are not metabolized by skin cells [43]. And there are certainly other reasons, not completely understood, to explain many negative patch tests.

> ### Core Message
>
> ❯ Many delayed drug eruptions are T-cell-mediated and, therefore, patch testing can be adequate in their study.

26.2 The Workup in the Diagnosis of an Immune-Mediated CADR

26.2.1 Clinical Diagnosis and Drug Imputation

The diagnosis of a drug eruption is easier if we are facing a clinical pattern typical of a CADR, such as a fixed drug eruption, a toxic epidermal necrolysis, or a generalized exanthematous pustulosis. In nonspecific skin reactions patterns, a particular workup has to be done to exclude other causes for the rash, such as a viral infection in maculopapular exanthema or a non-drug allergen in acute urticaria or angioedema. In these situations, the diagnosis of drug eruption can be a diagnosis of exclusion.

In severe CADR, such as toxic epidermal necrolysis, DRESS, and acute generalized exanthematous pustulosis, complementary tests are needed to evaluate the degree of systemic involvement.

At the time of diagnosis, it is extremely important to identify the culprit drug. In most CADRs, improvement depends on the drug suspension and prognosis depends mainly on an early drug withdrawal.

Imputation of the culprit drug is performed mainly on clinical grounds, based on extrinsic and intrinsic criteria. Extrinsic criteria include all previous reports of such a CADR. Intrinsic criteria are mainly based on the chronology and clinical characteristics of the adverse event: the clinical pattern of the eruption, its chronological relation with the initiation and suspension of the drug, and information on previous drug exposure, with or without reaction (accidental rechallenge) [44]. No single complementary test can replace a good characterization of these parameters. But, even

Table 26.2 Main CADRs and the most adequate skin test according to each clinical pattern

CADR pattern	Expected free interval	Most adequate test to perform	
		In vivo	In vitro
Urticaria/angioedema anaphyalxis	Minutes to 1 h	Prick, i.d.[a] Oral challenge[b]	IgE (RAST/CAP) Basophil activation
Maculopapular exanthema	7–21 days 2 days[c]	Patch, i.d.[a] Oral challenge	LST/LTT
Drug hypersensitivity/DRESS	3–6 weeks	Patch, i.d.[d]	LST/LTT[e]
Acute generalized exanthematic pustulosis	2–3 days	Patch	LST/LTT
Stevens–Johnson syndrome Toxic epidermal necrolysis	7–21 days 2 days[c]	Patch	LST/LTT
Fixed drug eruption	6–24 h	Lesional testing	
Systemic photosensitivity	2 days	Photopatch test Oral photoprovocation	

[a]Perform i.d. tests only if prick or patch tests are negative

[b]Not adequate in cases of anaphylaxis or severe angioedema

[c]On drug reintroduction

[d]i.d. is not advised, on a first basis, due to a possible severe reaction

[e]LST/LTT (lymphocyte stimulation or transformation tests) are often negative during the acute phase of DRESS

in the cases where very accurate data are available, the imputability or causality index for a single drug can be very low: many patients who develop a CADR are on multiple drugs; any drug can induce a drug eruption; different drugs can induce the same clinical pattern of drug eruption; and, the interval between drug initiation and development of the CADR can vary widely (6 h up to 6 weeks), even considering only delayed reactions (Table 26.2).

26.2.2 Complementary Tests to Confirm Drug Imputation

Drug reintroduction is considered the more definitive test for confirming the culprit drug, but it does not always reproduce the skin reaction [45, 46]; it is time-consuming when several drugs are suspected and it is contraindicated in severe reactions, such as toxic epidermal necrolysis or drug hypersensitivity syndrome/DRESS [45]. Therefore, complementary clinical and laboratory investigations have to be conducted in order to try to confirm, or deny, an imputable drug.

Laboratory tests, such as specific IgE or basophil activation, are used for the study of immediate reactions,

and lymphocyte transformation tests (LTT) or lymphocyte stimulation tests (LST) are used for studying mainly delayed hypersensitivity reactions [47]. They can help in the diagnosis, with the advantage of being an in vitro method that, in some circumstances, can be performed during the acute phase. Nevertheless, these tests are not available for most drugs, procedures are not standardized, results are inconsistent with undetermined sensitivity and specificity, and therefore, they are not performed on a routine basis [23, 47].

Skin testing can be used later, after the resolution of the CADR. It is important to choose the most adequate skin test, according to the reaction pattern, even though this is not always so straight. (Table 26.2) Tests with immediate readings, such as prick, scratch, or intradermal (i.d.) tests, are advised for immediate reactions such as urticaria and angioedema, whereas tests with delayed readings, such as the patch test, are mainly recommended for delayed skin reactions, e.g., eczematous reactions, maculopapular exanthema, erythroderma, drug hypersensitivity syndrome/DRESS, acute generalized exanthematous pustulosis, fixed drug eruption, Stevens–Johnson syndrome, and toxic epidermal necrolysis [15, 48]. Prick and i.d. tests with late readings, performed when patch tests are negative, may increase the effectiveness of skin testing. In two separate studies these tests improved the diagnosis by about 10% in nonimmediate reactions from aminopenicillins and synergistins [49, 50]. Commercial material for i.d. testing is not available for most drugs and, therefore, it has to be prepared, on a patient basis, in a sterilized setting, which is not always feasible. Moreover, in case of positive results, it may be difficult to use controls to evaluate the specificity of the reaction. Also, it is recommended to perform i.d. testing in a hospital setting, particularly in the study of severe CADRs [51].

When positive, in vitro or in vivo tests can be of help in confirming which drug was responsible for the CADR, but, on the contrary, these tests are very seldom able to exclude the involvement of a drug.

26.3 Patch Testing in CADRs

26.3.1 The General Value of Patch Testing

Patch testing in the study of drug eruptions has been performed for many years, but not as a systematic investigation in large multicenter investigational studies. There are a few studies with a relative large number of patients patch tested with drugs [13, 51, 52] and they include a wide variety of patterns of drug eruptions. Nevertheless, the inclusion criteria are quite different and the imputability/causality index for the drugs studied (very probable/probable/possible) is not known in most cases. Also, as there are so many patterns and so many responsible drugs, it is difficult to ascertain the patch test reactivity and its real value (sensitivity and negative predicative value) in the many different settings.

While considering a wide range of drug eruptions, the frequency of positive tests varies from 7.5 to 54% [13, 14, 51–54]. Apart from patient selection, patch test reactivity depends mainly on the clinical pattern of the drug eruption and the drugs involved [51–54].

Patch tests are mostly positive in eczematous eruptions, systemic contact dermatitis, maculopapular, exanthema, and erythroderma, and particularly, in more severe reactions [12, 14, 20, 51, 53, 55] (Table. 26.3).

In acute generalized exanthematous pustulosis there are many reports with positive patch tests, but with a few cases each [8, 26, 34, 35, 55–59]. In their study, Wolkenstein et al. found 50% of positive tests (7+out of the 14 patients tested) [60]. In this CADR, patch tests can show a pustular reaction with an epidermal spongiform pustule on skin biopsy, as in the acute reaction [26, 35, 56, 61] (Fig. 26.2b, c).

Table 26.3 Patch test results according to the type of eruption (adapted from Osawa et al. [52] Barbaud et al. [51] and Lamminatausta and Kortekangas-Savolainen [13])

CADR pattern	Number positive tests/number patients tested (%)			
	Osawa et al. [52] ($n=197$)	Barbaud et al. [51] ($n=72$)	Lammintausta et al. [13] ($n=826$)	Other studies
Maculopapular	10/72 (14)	16/27 (59)	81/785 (10.3)	33/61 (54) [14]
Erythroderma	8/15 (53)	5/7 (71)		
Eczematous	9/17 (53)	3/9 (33)		
Erythema multiforme	6/29 (21)			
Lichenoid	2/11 (18)			
Photosensitivity		4/4[a] (100)	2/12 (16.7)	
Fixed eruptions	2/6 (33)	0/3	8/28 (28.6)	26/30 (87) [68]
Urticaria/angioedema		2/18 (11)		
AGEP				7/14 (50) [60]
SJS/TEN				2/22 (9) [60]
Miscellaneous	15/47 (32)	1/6[b] (17)		
Total	62/197 (31)	31/72 (43)	101/826 (12.2)	

[a]Photopatch test

[b]Positive test in acute generalized exanthematous pustulosis

26

In DRESS, patch tests are often positive with aba-cavir [19, 62, 63] and antiepileptics, particularly car-bamazepine [17, 64, 65] (Fig. 26.5). Patch test reactivity is much lower, below 10%, in Stevens–Johnson syndrome or toxic epidermal necrolysis [55, 60]. In some occasions histopathology of the patch test can also reproduce the full thickness epidermal apoptosis, such as in the acute reaction.

Fixed drug eruptions are unique in the persistence of drug-specific T-cells in residual skin lesions, so we can expect to find positive tests on the these lesions, in a high percentage of cases [66–68], particularly, in fixed drug eruptions from NSAIDs [66, 69, 70] (Fig. 26.6). Alanko found as many as 26 positive tests out of 30 (87%) [68].

In photosensitive eruptions, when it is not a clearly phototoxic reaction, photopatch tests can be rewarding in the study of systemic photosensitivity as in photoallergic contact dermatitis [41, 42, 71, 72]. Piroxicam [40, 73–77], ketoprofen [71, 78], the fluorquinolones [42, 79, 80], and flutamide [81, 82] are examples of drugs that frequently elicit positive photopatch tests.

The reactivity of patch testing also depends on the culprit drug. Carbamazepine induces positive patch tests in more than 70% of the cases of delayed drug eruptions [51, 65, 83–86] (Fig. 26.5). High reactivity is also observed with tetrazepam [35, 51, 87–89], abacavir [19, 62, 63, 90], aminopenicillins [13, 20, 91], cefa-losporins [13, 92], synergistines [50], cotrimoxazole [14]

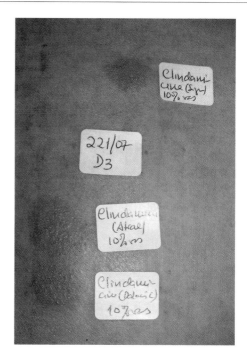

Fig. 26.6 Positive patch tests with clindamycin, the pure substance tested at 10% in pet (*upper test*), with identical results when testing with the smashed content of the pills of clindamycin from two different brands (Dalacin C® and Clindamicina Atral®), both prepared at 10% in pet (*lower reactions*)

clindamycin [13, 93–95], (Fig. 26.7) diltiazem [14, 96–98], heparin derivatives [14, 99, 100], corticosteroids [101–103], pseudoephedrine [104], and hydroxyzine [14, 105, 106]. Nevertheless, contrary to the most regularly referred rate of 30–40% of positive reactions to betalac-tam antibiotics [51], in a recent review by Blanca et al., the rate of positive reactions was much lower (2.6%) [20], which is probably due to a different patient selection (Table 26.4).

The list of drugs reported to elicit positive patch or photopatch test reactions is increasing every day, as this method is increasingly being used in the diagnosis of drug eruptions.

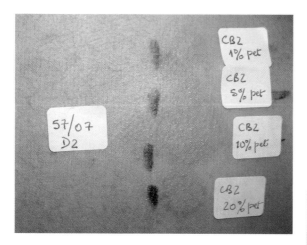

Fig. 26.5 Positive reactions to carbamazepine tested at several concentrations (1–20% pet) in a patient with a severe exanthema in the context of a DRESS (drug reaction with eosinophilia and systemic symptoms). In this severe drug reaction it is advised to test carbamazepine only at 1% pet

---

Core Message

> Patch tests are more frequently positive in maculopapular exanthema, acute generalized exanthematous pustulosis, and fixed drug eruptions.

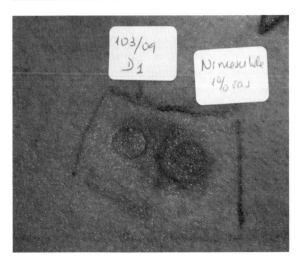

Fig. 26.7 Lesional testing in a residual pigmented lesion of fixed drug eruption. Positive reaction with the NSAID, nimesulide, tested at 1% pet, presenting as erythema and infiltration. Note the negative reaction to another NSAID, tested at the *left* side, confirming the specific nature of the reaction

26.3.2 Patch Test Technique

It can take weeks before skin reactivity can be evaluated properly by patch testing. Thus, it is advisable to wait several weeks after the rash has gone to perform patch tests. It is not known exactly how long, but 6 weeks after complete resolution of the CADR is usually advised [15, 107]. Also, we do not know for how long skin sensitivity persists. Although some reactions are lost, many patients tested after 10 years still react positively [49]. Therefore, it is usually recommended to patch test within 6 weeks to 6 months [15].

Patch testing is performed in the generally accepted way on the back, as in the study of allergic contact dermatitis. In particular cases, as in fixed eruptions, reactivity occurs only in skin areas where the skin reaction has occurred [66, 108, 109]. The application time is usually 2 days, but occasionally it can be convenient to remove tests at D1 [49]. Readings are performed at D2 and at D3 or D4, and scored negative to 3+, according to the ICDRG guidelines.

In fixed drug eruptions, test materials are applied in duplicate: on an inactive, residual lesion and on the normal back skin, which serves as a negative control. The residual pigmentation is a useful marker to indicate the area to apply the test. Tests are usually applied for 1 day, with occlusion, as in patch testing. Readings are performed at D1 and D2, or at D3 if previously negative [66]. As sometimes positive reactions are seen only in the first 24 h, Alanko [68] prefers an open test, which makes observations possible during this period.

Table 26.4 Patch test results in delayed CADR, according to the culprit drug

Culprit drug	Number positive reactions/number of patients tested (%)							
Betalactam antibiotics	4/24	(29)	[53]					
Amoxicillin	10/247	(4)	[13]	7/17	(41.2)	[51]		
Cefalosporins	12/220	(4.1)	[13]					
Pristinamycin	7/8	(87)	[51]	17/20	(85)	[13]		
Trimethoprim	10/163	(6.2)	[13]					
Cotrimoxazole	4/140	(2.9)	[13]					
Clindamycin	12/63	(19)	[13]	5/33	(15)	[94]	8/26 (31)[a]	
Aciclovir	2/8	(25)	[45]					
Abacavir							7 [63][b]	
Carbamazepine	6+/7	(86)	[53]	13/17	(76.5)	[64]		
Diltiazem	3/9	(33.3)	[13]	7/13	(54)	[98]		
Allopurinol	1/10	(10)	[13]	0/19		[64]		
Pseudoephedrine	5/16	(31.2)	[13]					
Piroxicam (Photo)	75/82	(91.4)	[73]					

[a]Personal data
[b]One study with seven positive patch tests [63]

A reaction is regarded as positive, if it occurs only in the residual lesion, and when clear erythema is visible for at least 6 h. Often there is erythema with infiltration (Fig. 26.6), eczema, or a bullous reaction that mimics the histopathology and clinical pattern of the acute fixed drug eruption [66, 70]. The reaction occurs exclusively in the area of application of the test or reactivation of the whole residual lesion can occur [66].

In systemic drug photosensitivity photoepicutaneous patch tests are performed, as in photoallergic contact dermatitis, using mainly UVA irradiation, at a dose of 5 J/cm^2 [41, 110, 111] (see Chap. 29).

26.3.3 Material for Patch Testing with Drugs

26.3.3.1 Patch Testing with Pure Drugs

In recent years, with the increasing interest in patch testing in drug eruptions, several firms that prepare allergens for the study of contact allergy are also producing standardized drug allergens with the pure active products. Of course, there is only a very limited number of drug allergens and every drug can induce a CADR. Nevertheless, the list includes drugs more frequently responsible for delayed CADRs: antibiotics, antiepileptic, NSAIDs, and some isolated drugs (Table 26.5). No controls are needed for these allergens, as many patients, who have been exposed to the drug with no reaction and, also nondrug exposed subjects, have been tested with no reaction.

This makes patch testing with drugs simple, allows testing several drugs at the same time and, particularly, testing with analogous chemicals to study cross-reactions and find possible replacement drugs. Actually, these studies have shown very interesting data on patterns of cross-reactivity that may be very informative for the patient and the doctor.

But, these commercialized drug allergens might be improved, as it is not known yet if the most correct concentrations or the most adequate vehicles are being used. Recommended concentrations are usually between 1 and 20% of the pure chemical, doses that are usually higher than in the study of allergic contact dermatitis. But for drugs, such as carbamazepine, low concentration, 1% or even below, can be enough [86, 112] (Fig. 26.5). Increasing concentration above 1 or 5%

pet. does not always increase patch test reactivity, as shown for carbamazepine and amoxicillin [49, 112]. For the 20% concentration, carbamazepine, hydrochlorotiazide, propanolol, sulphametoxazol, and thrimetoprim did not evoke reactions either when tested in 200 volunteers [1], or in previously exposed patients [65]. Although reactivation of the CADR during patch testing is exceptional [65] [114], in the case of a severe drug eruption, it is advisable to start with lower concentrations [15].

Also, there is not enough data on the best vehicle to perform patch testing. Most chemicals react when prepared in petrolatum, but in some cases water, ethanol, or acetone may be more adequate, as in the case of estradiol [10], or DMSO may be necessary to solubilize cotrimoxazole and its constituents [55, 113].

26.3.3.2 Patch Testing with Drugs Used by the Patient

If the pure drug is not available, which is often the case, patch testing can be done with the drug used by the patient, either a tablet, a capsule, or the solution for oral, i.v., or i.m. use. The amount of active drug in a tablet varies and can be very low. Therefore, it is preferable to use the content of a capsule or the powder for parenteral use, which usually have more active drug. This powder, or the fine powder obtained from smashing the pill after removing the external coating, can be diluted in petrolatum and water, or other vehicles, in a way to have the active drug in the final concentration at 10% (Fig. 26.7). If the concentration of the active drug is too low, it is recommended to prepare the smashed powder of the pill at 30% [15]. Of course, in this method, the final concentration of the active drug can vary a lot, but 30% is the highest concentration to obtain a homogenous preparation [15].

When tests are positive with these preparations, it is recommended to have serial dilutions and it is obligatory to test, at least, ten controls, preferably previously exposed individuals who have given their informed consent.

When tests have been done with pure chemicals, it can also be worthwhile to perform tests with the filler materials and the original drug preparation. In principle, reactions to the "inert" filler substances and additives are possible, but in practice they are rare [114–117].

Table 26.5 Commercially available drug allergens for patch testing

Group of drugs	Drug allergen	Concentration vehicle (% pet)	Company
Antibiotics	Penicillin G, potassium salt	10	CD
	Ampicillin	5	MT
	Amoxicillin trihydrate	10	CD
	Dicloxacillin sodium salt hydrate	10	CD
	Cefradine	10	CD
	Cefalexin	10	CD
	Cefotaxim sodium salt	10	CD
	Doxycyclin monohydrate	10	CD
	Minocycline hydrochloride	10	CD
	Erythromycin base	10	CD MT
	Spiramycin base	10	CD
	Clarithromycin	10	CD
	Pristinamycin	10	CD
	Cotrimoxazole	10	CD
	Norfloxacine	10	CD
	Ciprofloxacine hydrochloride	10	CD
	Clindamycin phosphate	10	CD
Antiepileptics	Carbamazepine	1	CD
	Hydantoin	10	CD
NSAIDs	Acetylsalicylic acid	10	CD MT
	Diclofenac sodium salt	1	CD Bi MT
	Ketoprofen	1	CD Bi Mt
	Naproxen	5	Bi MT
	Piroxicam	1	CD Bi MT
	Acetaminophen	10	CD Bi
	Ibuprofen	10	CD Bi MT
Miscellaneous	Acyclovir	10	CD
	Hydrochlorothiazide	1 and 10	CD
	Diltiazem hydrochloride	10	CD
	Captopril	5[a]	CD

CD chemotechnique diagnostics, Malmö Sweden

MT Martí Tor, Dermatitis de Contacto, Barcelona, Spain

Bi Bial Aristégui, Bilbao, Spain

[a]Doubtful reactions may occur with this concentration

26.3.4 Safety of Patch Testing

The risk of reactivation of the drug eruption is very low [14, 118], even in serious delayed CADRs [64], but it has been occasionally reported with acyclovir, pseudoephedrin, pristinamycin [51], and carbamazepine, particularly when testing with the powder of the pills [119].

Serious immediate reactions evoked by patch testing are rare and have been described mainly in the study of anaphylaxis [120–122], particularly with penicillins, neomycin, or bacitracin. For safety reasons, it is practical to observe the patient for approximately half an hour after application of the test material.

The risk of patch testing is considerably lower compared with i.d. tests. Thus, the patch test is a good test to start with. If negative and, for the particular patient, it is important to prove the causality of the drug, the study can continue with the sequential use of prick, scratch, and i.d. tests with a delayed reading [15]. If all are negative, as a next step, a provocation test can be performed in a hospital setting, except if there is a contraindication, namely, a previous severe reaction, such as DRESS or toxic epidermal necrolysis, or the involvement of drugs as antiepileptics or salazosulfapyridine [45].

Another adverse patch test effect is sensitization by patch testing; this is rarely seen, even with penicillins [123].

26.3.5 Specificity of Patch Test Reactions

Positive patch test reactions, performed according to the recommendations [15], have been shown to be highly specific. Histopathology of drug patch tests is often analogous to the acute reaction [61, 124] and some T-cells that infiltrate the skin, in the patch test, specifically recognize the drug [25–28, 34]. Actually, drug-specific T-cells, with phenotypic and functional characteristics similar to those isolated from the blood or the skin during the acute phase of the CADR, have been isolated from positive patch tests with several drugs, such as amoxicillin, carbamazepine, lamotrigine, sulfonamides, fluorquinoles, and tetrazepam [25–28, 34, 35].

Patch testing with pure drugs or with low concentrations of the commercial products rarely yields false positive reactions. But, occasionally, constituents of the excipient of the commercial drug can cause false positive reactions due to irritation or low pH or they can induce a nonrelevant positive patch test reaction in a previously contact sensitized patient [114]. Such false positive results have been observed with the powder of the pills of spironolactone (Aldactone®), colchicine, captopril (Lopril®), cloroquine (Nivaquine®), celecoxib (Celebrex®) tested at 30% pet, and with omeprazole (Mopral®) tested at 30% aq. [14, 55, 114].

False-negative reactions can be expected due to technical problems of the patch tests (low concentration or wrong vehicle, deficient skin penetration, wrong timing for performing patch testing), but there are certainly many other explanations for the absence of skin reactivity on patch testing: the responsible hapten is a drug metabolite that is not formed in the skin, the CADR is not an immune reaction or not dependent on the delayed hypersensitivity or, apart from drug exposure, concomitant factors (viral infection or concomitant drugs) are necessary for enhancing drug hypersensitivity [91].

For cotrimoxazol and acyclovir, patch tests in petrolatum are often negative, and DMSO or other penetration enhancers may be necessary to have positive patch tests. There is, for the moment, no explanation for the negative patch tests to allopurinol in delayed CADRs, presumed to be immune-mediated, even when there is a positive accidental rechallenge. Although there is one report of a positive test in the study by Lammintausta and KorteKangas-Savolainen [13], in our experience, with more than 30 patients now, we did not observe a positive patch test with allopurinol, using low or high concentrations (1–20%), petrolatum or ethanol as excipient, with or without tape stripping, or even using one of its metabolites (8-oxypurinol) in different concentrations and vehicles [125].

26.3.6 Evaluating Cross-Reactivity on Patch Testing

Cross-reactivity observed among drugs in CADRs can be studied at the patch test level with very interesting results.

It has been shown, in maculopapular exanthema, that amoxicillin and ampicillin always cross-react [54, 112], and this cross-reactivity is neither often extensive to benzilpenicillin or carbopenens [20], nor to cefalosporins except, eventually, cefalexin [126]. A similar pattern is usually confirmed by oral challenge [20, 49]. There is also frequent cross-reactivity among the cefalosporins and the fluorquinolones [30] and between pristinamycin and virginiamycin [50]. On the other hand, absence of cross-reactions between tetrazepam and other benzodiazepines, particularly diazepam, was confirmed by patch testing and oral provocation [89, 127].

Cross-reactions in fixed drug eruptions were also found among different sulfonamides, among the three piperazine derivatives (hydroxyzine, cetirizine, and levocetirizine) [128], and oxicams (tenoxicam and piroxicam) [66, 70]. This pattern of cross-reactivity between piroxicam and tenoxicam, observed in all cases of fixed drug eruptions studied, does not occur in other patterns of CADR from oxicams. In patients with photosensitivity from piroxicam, tenoxicam is safe, as shown by photopatch testing and drug challenge [40, 66].

Another particular pattern of cross reaction was shown in photopatch tests between the arylpropionic NSAIDs, ketoprofen, suprofen, and tiaprofenic acid in photoallergic contact dermatitis, and the lipid lowering agent, fenofibrate, in systemic photosensitivity [111, 129].

Unfortunately, there is not always correlation between cross-reactivity in patch testing and oral provocation, as in patients who react only to carbamazepine in the patch test, but do not tolerate other aromatic antiepileptics [65].

> **Core Message**
>
> > Patch tests with drugs are specific and can be important to study relevant cross-reactions between drugs.

26.4 Conclusions: Interpretation of Patch Test Results

Patch tests results in the study of drug eruptions should be interpreted very carefully.

A positive test, using nonstandardized products, has to be checked in controls to exclude false positive reactions. A true positive test can be regarded as a sign of immunological reactivity of the patient and should be taken seriously, if compatible with the history. Readministration of the drug should be avoided as it can again elicit an adverse reaction, usually, a more severe one.

A negative test result does not exclude hypersensitivity or an adverse drug reaction. The test method might not be adequate due to another pathomechanism,

the bioavailability of the test material might have been insufficient, the wrong drug may have been tested (history and drug records can be surprisingly inaccurate), or the right drug may have been tested but the allergen could be a metabolite. Thus, a negative test result does not allow a definitive conclusion.

If necessary, other tests have to be performed, such as prick, scratch and intradermal skin tests or a challenge (provocation) test [48]. In vitro tests for IgE (RAST) exist for some drugs, as well as lymphocyte stimulation/transformation tests. However, these tests are rarely available or performed on a routine basis and their sensitivity and specificity has yet to be precisely evaluated.

In conclusion, although many suspected patients have negative reactions, it remains worthwhile to perform patch tests in patients with delayed CADRs. They can confirm a clinical imputability and avoid an eventual drug reintroduction with more severe consequences. In very particular cases, they can also give important information on cross-reacting drugs.

> **Core Message**
>
> > It is worthwhile to perform patch tests in individual patients with a suspected drug eruption.

26.5 Classic Articles and Monographs

Barbaud A, Gonçalo M, Bruynzeel D, Bircher A (2001) Guidelines for performing skin tests with drugs in the investigation of cutaneous adverse drug reactions. Contact Derm 45:321–328.

In detail is described how to perform skin tests in CADRs. The presented guidelines are proposed by the Working party of the European Society of Contact Dermatitis for the study of skin testing in investigating CADRs.

Kauppinen K, Alanko K, Hannuksela M, Maibach H (eds) (1998) Skin reactions to drugs. CRC, Bocca Raton

This book gives extensive information on cutaneous adverse reactions and challenge tests, how to perform skin tests and in whom.

Pichler WJ (ed) (2007) Drug hypersensitivity. Karger AG, Basel

This book gives an extensive overview on the pathomechanisms of especially type 4 allergy involvement in adverse drug reactions.

26

References

1. Bruynzeel D, Maibach H (1998) Patch testing in systemic drug eruptions. In: Kaupinen K, Alanko K, Hannuksela M, Maibach H (eds) Skin reactions to drugs. CRC, Boca Raton, pp 97–109

2. Roujeau J (1997) Drug induced skin reactions. In: Grobb JJ, Stern RS, Mac Kie RM, Weinstock WA (eds) Epidemiology, causes and prevention of skin diseases. Blackwell, Oxford

3. Bigby M (2001) Rates of cutaneous reactions to drugs. Arch Dermatol 137:765–770

4. Fiszenson-Alabala F, Auzerie V, Mahe E et al (2003) A 6-month prospective survey of cutaneous drug reactions in a hospital setting. Br J Dermatol 149:1018–1022

5. Roujeau J (2005) Clinical heterogeneity of drug hypersensitivity. Toxicology 209:123–129

6. Lacouture M, Melosky D (2007) Cutaneous reactions to anticancer agents targeting the epidermal growth factor receptor: a dermatology – oncology perspective. Skin Therapy Lett 12:1–5

7. Friedmann P (2003) Mechanisms in cutaneous drug hypersensitivity. Clin Exp Allergy 33:861–872

8. Halevy S (2009) Acute generalized exanthematous pustulosis. Curr Opin Allergy Clin Immunol 9:322–328

9. Gonçalo M, Bruynzeel D (2008) Mechanisms in cutaneous drug hypersensitivity reactions. In: Marzulli FN, Maibach HI (eds) Dermatotoxicology, 7th edn. CRC, Boca Raton, pp 259–268

10. Gonçalo M, Oliveira H, Monteiro C et al (1999) Allergic and systemic contact dermatitis from estradiol. Contact Derm 40:58–59

11. Veien N, Menné T, Maibach H (2008) Systemic contact-type dermatitis. In: Marzulli FN, Maibach HI (eds) Dermatotoxicology, 7th edn. CRC, Boca Raton, pp 139–153

12. Hausermann P, Harr T, Bircher A (2004) Baboon syndrome resulting from systemic drugs: is there strife between SDRIFE and allergic contact dermatitis syndrome? Contact Derm 51:297–310

13. Lammintausta K, KorteKangas-Savolainen O (2005) The usefulness of skin tests to prove drug hypersensitivity. Br J Dermatol 152:968–974

14. Barbaud A (2005) Drug patch testing in systemic cutaneous drug allergy. Toxicology 209:209–216

15. Barbaud A, Gonçalo M, Bircher A, Bruynzeel D (2001) Guidelines for performing skin tests with drugs in the investigation of cutaneous adverse drug reactions. Contact Derm 45:321–328

16. Bruynzeel D, Von Blomberg-Van der Flier M, Scheper R et al (1985) Allergy for penicillin and the relevance of epicutaneous tests. Dermatologica 171:429–434

17. Elzagallaai A, Knowles S, Rieder M et al (2009) Patch testing in the diagnosis of anticonvulsivant hypersensitivity syndrome. A systematic review. Drug Safety 32:391–408

18. Phillips E, Mallal S (2009) HLA and drug-induced toxicity. Curr Opin Mol Ther 11:231–242

19. Phillips E, Mallal S (2009) Successful translation of pharmacogenetics into the clinic: the abacavir example. Mol Diagn Ther 13:1–9

20. Blanca M, Romano A, Torres M et al (2009) Update on the evaluation of hypersensitivity reactions to betalactams. Allergy 64:183–193

21. Hari Y, Frutig-Schnyder K, Hurni M et al (2001) T cell involvement in cutaneous drug eruptions. Clin Exp Allergy 31:1398–1408

22. Pichler W (2003) Delayed drug hypersensitivity reactions. Ann Intern Med 139:683–693

23. Pichler W, Tilch J (2004) The lymphocyte transformation test in the diagnosis of drug hypersensitivity. Allergy 59:809–820

24. Bircher A (1999) Drug-induced urticaria and angioedema caused by non-IgE mediated pathomechanisms. Eur J Dermatol 9:657–663

25. Yawalkar N, Hari Y, Frutig K et al (2000) T cells isolated from positive epicutaneous test reactions to amoxicillin and ceftriaxone are drug specific and cytotoxic. J Invest Dermatol 115:647–652

26. Britschgi M, Steiner U, Schmid S et al (2001) T-cell involvement in drug-induced acute generalized exanthematic pustulosis. J Clin Invest 107:1433–1441

27. Kuechler P, Britschgi M, Schmid S et al (2004) Cytotoxic mechanisms in different forms of T-cell-mediated drug allergies. Allergy 59:613–622

28. Naisbitt D (2004) Drug hypersensitivity reactions in the skin: understanding mechanisms and the development of diagnostic and predictive tests. Toxicology 194: 179–196

29. Pichler W (2002) Pharmacological interactions of drugs with antigen-specific immune receptors: the p-i concept. Curr Opin Allergy Clin Immunol 2:301–305

30. Schmid D, Depta J, Pichler W (2006) T cell-mediated hypersensitivity to quinolones: mechanisms and cross-reactivity. Clin Exp Allergy 36:59–69

31. Posadas S, Pichler W (2007) Delayed drug hypersensitivity reactions: new concepts. Clin Exp Allergy 7:898–999

32. Choquet-Kastylevsky G, Intrator L, Chenal C et al (1998) Increased levels of interleukin-5 are associated with the generation of eosinophilia in drug-induced hypersensitivity syndrome. Br J Dermatol 139:1026–1032

33. Kardaun S, Sidoroff A, Valleyrie-Allanore L et al (2007) Variability in the clinical pattern of cutaneous side-effects of drugs with systemic symptoms: does a DRESS syndrome really exist? Br J Dermatol 156:609–612

34. Britschgi M, Pichler W (2002) Acute generalized exanthematous pustulosis. Role of cytotoxic T cells in pustule formation: a clue to neutrophil-mediated processes orchestrated by T cells. Curr Opin Allergy Clin Immunol 2: 325–331

35. Thomas E, Bellón T, Barranco P et al (2008) Acute generalized exanthematous pustulosis due to tetrazepam. J Investig Allergol Clin Immunol 18:119

36. Nassif A, Bensussan A, Boumsell L et al (2004) Toxic epidermal necrolysis: effector cells are drug specific cytotoxic T cells. J Allergy Clin Immunol 114:1209–1215

37. Nassif A, Moslehi H, Le Gouvello S et al (2004) Evaluation of the potential role of cytokines in toxic epidermal necrolysis. J Invest Dermatol 123:850–855

38. Shiohara T, Mizukawa Y, Teraki Y (2002) Pathophysiology of fixed drug eruption: the role of skin-resident T cells. Curr Opin Allergy Clin Immunol 2:317–323

39. Mizukawa Y, Yamazaki Y, Shiohara T (2008) In vivo dynamics of intraepidermal CD8+ T cells and CD4+ T cells during the evolution of fixed drug eruption. Br J Dermatol 158:1230–1238

40. Gonçalo M, Figueiredo A, Tavares P et al (1992) Photosensitivity to piroxicam: absence of cross reaction with tenoxicam. Contact Derm 27:287–290

41. Gonçalo M (1998) Exploration dans les photo-allergies médicamenteuses. In: GERDA. Progrès en Dermato-Allergologie. John Libbey Eurotext, Nancy, pp 67–74

42. Oliveira H, Gonçalo M, Figueiredo A (1996) Photosensitivity from lomefloxacine. A clinical and photobiological study. Photoderm Photoimmunol Photomed 16:116–120

43. Griem P, Wulferink M, Sachs B et al (1998) Allergic and autoimmune reactions to xenobiotics: how do they arise? Immunol Today 19:133–141

44. Moore N, Biour M, Paux G et al (1985) Adverse drug reaction monitoring: doing it the French way. Lancet 9:1056–1058

45. Lammintausta K, KorteKangas-Savolainen O (2005) Oral challenge in suspected cutaneous adverse drug reactions. Acta Derm Venerol 85:491–496

46. Alanko K, Kaupinnen K (1998) Diagnosis of drug eruptions: clinical evaluation and drug challenge. In: Kauppinen K, Alanko K, Hannuksela M, Maibach H (eds) Skin reactions to drugs. CRC, Boca Raton, pp 75–79

47. Merk H (2005) Diagnosis of drug hypersensitivity: lymphocyte transformation test and cytokines. Toxicology 209: 217–220

48. Hannuksela M (1998) Skin testing in drug hypersensitivity. In: Kauppinen K, Alanko K, Hannuksela M, Maibach H (eds) Skin reactions to drugs. CRC, Boca Raton

49. Torres M, Sánchez-Sabaté E, Alvarez J et al (2004) Skin test evaluation in non-immediate allergic reactions to penicillins. Allergy 59:219–224

50. Barbaud A, Tréchot P, Weber-Muller F et al (2004) Drug skin tests in cutaneous adverse drug reactions to pristinamycin: 29 cases with a study of cross-reactions between synergistins. Contact Derm 50:22–26

51. Barbaud A, Reichert-Penetrat S, Tréchot P et al (1998) The use of skin testing in the investigation of cutaneous adverse drug reactions. Br J Dermatol 139:49–58

52. Osawa J, Naito S, Aihara M et al (1990) Evaluation of skin test reactions in patients with non-immediate type drug eruptions. J Dermatol 17:235–239

53. Barbaud A (2002) Tests cutanés dans l'investigation des toxidermies: de la physiopathologie aux résultats des investigations. Thérapie 57:258–262

54. Gonçalo M, Fernandes B, Oliveira H, Figueiredo A (2000) Epicutaneous patch testing in drug eruptions. Contact Derm 42:S22

55. Barbaud A (2009) Skin testing in delayed reactions to drugs. Immunol Allergy Clin North Am 29:517–535

56. Sidoroff A, Halevy S, Bavinck J et al (2001) Acute generalized exanthematous pustulosis (AGEP) – a clinical reaction pattern. J Cutan Pathol 28:113–119

57. Buettiker U, Keller M, Pichler W et al (2006) Oral prednisolone induced acute generalized exanthematous pustulosis due to corticosteroids of group A confirmed by epicutaneous testing and lymphocyte transformation tests. Dermatology 213:40–43

58. Schmid S, Kuechler P, Britschgi M et al (2002) Acute generalized exanthematous pustulosis. Role of cytotoxic T cells in pustule formation. Am J Pathology 161:2079–2086

59. Gonçalo M, Figueiredo A, Poiares-Baptista A (1991) Pustulose exantemática aguda generalizada. Dois casos clínicos e revisão da literatura. Med Cut ILA 19:81–85

60. Wolkenstein P, Chosidow O, Fléchet M et al (1996) Patch testing in severe cutaneous adverse drug reactions, including Stevens–Johnson syndrome and toxic epidermal necrolysis. Contact Derm 35:234–236

61. Serra D, Mariano A, Gonçalo M, Figueiredo A (2009) Acute exanthematic pustulosis, psoriasis and drugs. In Proceedings of 10th International Congress of Dermatology-ICD. Prague

62. Hughes C, Foisy M, Dewhurst N et al (2008) Abacavir hypersensitivity reaction: an update. Ann Pharmacother 42:387–396

63. Phillips E, Sullivan J, Knowles S, Shear N (2002) Utility of patch testing in patients with hypersensitivity syndromes associated with abacavir. AIDS 16:2223–2225

64. Santiago F, Gonçalo M, Vieira R et al (2010) Epicutaneous patch testing in the diagnosis of drug hypersensitivity syndrome (DRESS). Contact Derm 62(1):47–53

65. Santiago F, Gonçalo M, Brites M et al (2008) Drug hypersensitivity syndrome (DRESS): what patch tests can reveal us. Contact Derm 58:S17

66. Gonçalo M, Oliveira H, Fernandes B et al (2002) Topical provocation in fixed drug eruption from nonsteroidal anti-inflammatory drugs. Exogenous Dermatol 1:81–86

67. Lee A (1998) Topical provocation in 31 cases of fixed drug eruption: change of causative drugs in 10 years. Contact Derm 38:258–260

68. Alanko K (1994) Topical provocation of fixed drug eruption. A study of 30 patients. Contact Derm 31:25–27

69. Robalo-Cordeiro M, Gonçalo M, Fernandes B et al (2000) Positive lesional patch tests in fixed drug eruptions from nimesulide. Contact Derm 43:307

70. Oliveira H, Gonçalo M, Reis J, Figueiredo A (1999) Fixed drug eruption to piroxicam. Positive patch tests with cross-sensitivity to tenoxicam. J Dermatolog Treat 10:209–212

71. Devleeschouwer V, Roelandts R, Garmyn M, Goossens A (2008) Allergic and photoallergic contact dermatitis from ketoprofen: results of (photo) patch testing and follow-up of 42 patients. Contact Derm 58:159–166

72. Asensio T, Sanchis M, Sánchez P, Vega J, Garcia J (2008) Photocontact dermatitis because of oral dexketoprofen. Contact Derm 58:59–60

73. Serra D, Gonçalo M, Figueiredo A (2008) Two decades of cutaneous adverse drug reactions from piroxicam. Contact Derm 58:S35

74. Vasconcelos C, Magina S, Quirino P, Barros M, Mesquita-Guimarães J (1997) Cutaneous drug reactions to piroxicam. Contact Derm 39:145

75. Varela P, Amorim I, Massa A et al (1998) Piroxicam-beta-cyclodextrin and photosensitivity reactions. Contact Derm 38:229

76. Youn J, Lee H, Yeo U, Lee Y (1993) Piroxicam photosensitivity associated with vesicular hand dermatitis. Clin Exp Dermatol 18:52–54

77. Figueiredo A, Fontes Ribeiro C, Gonçalo S et al (1987) Piroxicam-induced photosensitivity. Contact Derm 17:73–79

78. Hindsén M, Zimerson E, Bruze M (2006) Photoallergic contact dermatitis from ketoprofen in Southern Sweden. Contact Derm 54:150–157

79. Kurumajin Y, Shono M (1992) Scarified photopatch testing in lomefloxacin photosensitivity. Contact Derm 26:5–10

80. Kimura M, Kawada A (1998) Photosensitivity induced by lomefoxacin with cross-photosensitivity to ciprofloxacin and fleroxacin. Contact Derm 38:130

81. Vilaplana J, Romaguera C, Azón A, Lecha M (1998) Flutamide photosensitivity-residual vitiliginous lesions. Contact Derm 38:68–70

82. Martín-Lázaro J, Buján J, Arrondo A et al (2004) Is photopatch testing useful in the investigation of photosensitivity due to flutamide? Contact Derm 50:325–326

83. Alanko K (1993) Patch testing in cutaneous reactions caused by carbamazepine. Contact Derm 29:254–247

84. Camarasa J (1985) Patch test diagnosis of exfoliative dermatitis due to carbamazepine. Contact Derm 12:49

85. Puig L, Nadal C, Fernández-Figueras M, Alomar A (1996) Carbamazepine-induced drug rashes: diagnostic value of patch tests depends on clinico-pathologic presentation. Contact Derm 34:435–437

86. Silva R, Machado A, Brandão M, Gonçalo S (1982) Patch test diagnosis in carbamazepine erythroderma. Contact Derm 45:283–284

87. Camarasa J, Serra-Baldrich E (1990) Tetrazepam allergy detected by patch test. Contact Derm 22:246

88. Sánchez-Morillas L, Laguna-Martínez J, Reaño-Matos M et al (2008) Systemic dermatitis due to tetrazepam. J Investig Allergol Clin Immunol 18:404–406

89. Pirker C, Misic A, Brinkmeier T, Frosch P (2002) Tetrazepam drug sensitivity – usefulness of the patch test. Contact Derm 47:135–138

90. Shear N, Milpied B, Bruynzeel D, Phillips E (2009) A review of drug patch testing and implications for HIV clinicians. AIDS 22:999–1007

91. Renn C, Straff W, DorfMüller A et al (2002) Amoxicillin-induced rash in young adults with infectious mononucleosis: demonstration of drug specific reactivity. Br J Dermatol 147:1166–1170

92. Gonzalo-Garijo M, Rodríguez-Nevado I, Argila D (2006) Patch tests for diagnosis of delayed hypersensitivity to cephalosporins. Allergol et Immunopathol 34:39–41

93. Canelas M, Cardoso J, Gonçalo M, Figueiredo A (2008) Patch tests in the study of cutaneous drug reactions in erysipelas. Contact Derm 58:S18

94. Seitz C, Bröcker E, Trautmann A (2009) Allergy diagnostic testing in clindamycin-induced skin reactions. Int Arch Allergy Immunol 149:246–250

95. Lammintausta K, Tokola R, Kalimo K (2002) Cutaneous adverse reactions to clindamycin: results of skin testing and oral exposure. Br J Dermatol 146:643–648

96. Gonzalo-Garijo M, Pérez Calderón R, Argila Fernandéz-Durán D, Rangel Mayoral J (2005) Cutaneous reactions due to diltiazem and cross reactivity with other calcium channel blockers. Allergol et Immunopathol 33:328–340

97. Sousa-Basto A, Azenha A, Duarte M, Pardal-Oliveira F (1993) Generalized cutaneous reaction to diltiazem. Contact Derm 29:44–45

98. Lachapelle J, Tennstedt D (1998) Les tests épicutanés dans les txidermies médicamenteuses. In: Progrès en Dermato-Allergologie. John Libbey Eurotext, Nancy, pp 57–66

99. Scherer K, Tsakiris D, Bircher A (2008) Hypersensitivity reactions to anticoagulant drugs. Curr Pharm Des 14:2863–2873

100. Koch P (2003) Delayed-type hypersensitivity skin reactions due to heparins and heparinoids. Tolerance of recombinant hirudins and of the new synthetic anticoagulant fondaparinux. Contact Derm 49:276–280

101. Isaksson M, Persson L (1998) Contact allergy to hydrocortisone and systemic contact dermatitis from prednisolone with tolerance of betamethasone. Am J Contact Dermat 9:136–138

102. Whitmore S (1995) Delayed systemic allergic reactions to corticosteroids. Contact Derm 32:193–198

103. Beck M, Marot L, Nicolas J et al (2009) Allergic hypersensitivity to topical and systemic corticosteroids: a review. Allergy 64:978–994

104. Barranco P, Rodríguez A, de Barrio M et al (2004) Sympathomimetic drug allergy: cross-reactivity study by patch test. Am J Clin Dermatol 5:351–355

105. Dalmau J, Serra-Baldrich E, Roé E et al (2006) Skin reaction to hydroxyzine (Atarax): patch test utility. Contact Derm 54:216–217

106. Ash S, Scheman A (1997) Systemic contact dermatitis to hydroxyzine. Am J Contact Dermat 8:2–5

107. Bruynzeel D, Van Ketel W (1989) Patch testing in drug eruptions. Semin Dermatol 8:196–203

108. Barbaud A, Tréchot P, Reichert-Penetrat S et al (2001) The usefulness of patch testing on the previously most severely affected site in a cutaneous adverse drug reaction to tetrazepam. Contact Derm 44:259–260

109. Klein C, Trautmann A, Zillikens D, Bröcker E (1995) Patch testing in an unusual case of toxic epidermal necrolysis. Contact Derm 33:448–449

110. Bruynzeel D, Ferguson J, Andersen K et al (2004) Photopatch testing: a consensus methodology for Europe. JEADV 18:679–682

111. Cardoso J, Canelas M, Gonçalo M, Figueiredo A (2009) Photopatch testing with an extended series of photoallergens. A 5-year study. Contact Derm 60:314–319

112. Gonçalo M, Coelho S, Figueiredo A (2006) Ascertaining patch test concentration in cutaneous adverse drug reactions to aminopenicillins and carbamazepine. J Invest Dermatol 126:S67

113. Özkaya-Bayazit E, Bayazit H, Özmarmagan G (1999) Topical provocation in 27 cases of cotrimoxazole-induced fixed drug eruption. Contact Derm 41:185–189

114. Barbaud A, Tréchot P, Reichert-Penetrat S et al (1999) Relevance of skin tests with drugs in investigating cutaneous adverse drug reactions. Contact Derm 45:265–268

115. Verecken P, Birringer C, Knitelius A et al (1998) Sensitisation to benzyl alcohol: a possible cause of "corticosteroid allergy". Contact Derm 38:106

116. Shmunes E (1984) Allergic dermatitis to benzyl alcohol in an injectable solution. Arch Dermatol 120:1200–1201

117. Schäfer T, Enders F, Przybilla B (1995) Sensitization to thimerosal and previous vaccination. Contact Derm 32:114–116

118. Mashiah J, Brenner S (2003) A systemic reaction to patch testing for the evaluation of acute generalized exanthematous pustulosis. Arch Dermatol 139:1181–1183
119. Vaillant L, Camenen I, Lorette G (1989) Patch testing with carbamazepine: reinduction of an exfoliative dermatitis. Arch Dermatol 125:299
120. Pietzcker F, Kuner V (1975) Anaphylaxie nach epicutanem Ampicillin-Test. Z Hautkr 50:437–440
121. Maucher O (1972) Anaphylaktische Reaktionen beim Epicutantest. Hautartz 23:139–140
122. Jonker M, Bruynzeel D (2003) Anaphylactic reaction by patch testing with diclofenac. Contact Derm 49:114–115
123. Van Ketel W (1975) Patch testing in penicillin allergy. Contact Derm 1:253–254
124. Barbaud A, Bene M, Schmutz J et al (1997) Role of delayed cellular hypersensitivity and adhesion molecules in maculopapular rashes induced by amoxycillin. Arch Dermatol 133:481–486
125. Vieira R, Gonçalo M, Figueiredo A (2004) Patch testing with allopurinol and oxypurinol in drug eruptions. Contact Derm 50:156
126. Schiavino D, Nucera E, de Pasquale T et al (2006) Delayed allergy to aminopenicillins: clinical and immunological findings. Int J Immunopathol Pharmacol 19:831–840
127. Barbaud A, Girault P, Schmutz J et al (2009) No cross-reactions between tetrazepam and other benzodiazepines: a possible chemical explanation. Contact Derm 61: 53–56
128. Cravo M, Gonçalo M, Figueiredo A (2007) Fixed drug eruption to cetirizine with positive lesional patch tests to the three piperazine derivatives. Int J Dermatol 46:760–762
129. LeCoz C, Bottleander A, Scrivener J et al (1998) Photocontact dermatitis from ketoprofen and tiaprofenic acid: cross-reactivity study in 12 consecutive patients. Contact Derm 38:245–252

Allergens Exposure Assessment

27

Birgitta Gruvberger, Magnus Bruze, Sigfrid Fregert, and Carola Lidén

Contents

B. Gruvberger (✉), M. Bruze and S. Fregert
Department of Occupational and Environmental Dermatology,
University Hospital, SE-205 02 Malmö, Sweden
e-mail: birgitta.gruvberger@med.lu.se
e-mail: sigtrid.fregert@bredband.net

C. Lidén
Unit of Occupational and Environmental Dermatology,
Institute of Environmental Medicine, Karolinska Institutet,
Box 210, SE-171 77 Stockholm, Sweden
e-mail: carola.liden@ki.se

27.1 Spot Tests and Chemical Analyses

Birgitta Gruvberger
Magnus Bruze
Sigfrid Fregert

27.1.1 Introduction

Many allergens are widely used in both environmental and occupational products. In many cases, it is difficult to know all the ingredients of a product since most products are not sufficiently labelled. To diagnose and prevent allergic contact dermatitis, the demonstration of allergens in the products from the patient´s environment is important. Chemical analysis of a product can make it possible to demonstrate the presence or absence of known allergens. Simple spot tests or documented analytical methods such as thin-layer chromatography (TLC), high-performance liquid chromatography (HPLC), gas chromatography (GC), atomic absorption spectrophotometry (AAS) and inductively coupled plasma –mass spectrometry (ICP-MS) can be used. Moreover, with chemical methods, the purity of a substance can be checked and new allergens can be isolated and identified. Advanced methods such as mass spectrometry (MS), nuclear magnetic resonance spectroscopy (NMR) and infrared spectrophotometry (IR) are often required to identify isolated allergens.

In this chapter, some principal chemical methods and some examples of chemical methods for dermatological applications are described.

J.D. Johansen et al. (eds.), *Contact Dermatitis*,
DOI: 10.1007/978-3-642-03827-3_27, © Springer-Verlag Berlin Heidelberg 2011

27

27.1.2 pH Measurement

Acidic and, particularly, alkaline products play a significant role in the development of irritant contact dermatitis and in chemical skin burns [1]. It is important to determine the degree of acidity or alkalinity in a product suspected of causing skin problems in order to avoid false-positive diagnoses of allergic contact dermatitis.

pH determinations are relevant only in water-based products/solutions. A universal pH paper is usually satisfactory for clinical work. A few drops of the solution/emulsion to be investigated are applied on the pH paper. The resulting colour is compared with the colour scale on the package of the pH paper. pH paper moistened with water can be applied to solid objects to demonstrate residual acidic or alkaline solution on the object. For accurate determination of the pH in a solution, a pH meter is necessary.

27.1.3 Spot Tests

Spot tests can be used to demonstrate both inorganic and organic compounds [2, 3]. A specific reagent may react with a specific substance to give a specific colour and thus indicate the occurrence of the specific substance. However, other substances can disturb the chemical reaction and the specific colour can be difficult to identify. A discoloured sample can contain the investigated substance. To confirm its presence and quantify the substance, more sophisticated methods are required.

To demonstrate nickel ions released from metal objects a spot test is commonly used.

27.1.4 Thin-Layer Chromatography

Chromatography is a general term applied to a variety of separation techniques based upon the sample partitioning between a moving phase, which can be a gas or a liquid, and a stationary phase, which may be either a liquid or a solid.

In TLC, the stationary phase consists of an inert absorbent, e.g., silica gel. The stationary phase covers the surface of a glass plate. The moving phase constitutes an eluting solvent. The sample to be analysed is dissolved in a low-boiling solvent and a small amount is applied near the bottom of the plate. The plate is placed in a closed vessel containing a small amount of the eluting solvent. The eluent is drawn up to the top of the plate owing to the capillary forces. Substances with high affinity to the stationary phase will move slower than substances with a low affinity. When the eluent has almost reached the top of the plate, the plate is removed from the glass vessel and dried. To detect the spots on the plate they must be made visible. UV-absorbing substances can be detected by irradiating the plate with a UV lamp. Some substances may react with various reagents applied to the plates, giving visible compounds. The R_F-value for a substance is the ratio between the distance travelled by the substance and the distance travelled by the eluent. To investigate if a sample contains a specific substance (reference), the reference is applied beside the sample on the plate. If the sample contains a substance with the same R_F-value as the reference, it will indicate that the substance and the reference may be identical. However, more chromatographic methods are required to confirm this.

27.1.5 Gas Chromatography

A gas chromatograph consists of an injector, a column and a detector. In GC, the mobile phase constitutes a carrier gas, e.g., nitrogen or helium, and the stationary phase is a non-volatile liquid on a solid support or on the walls of the column. The most common supports are inert porous materials. The sample, dissolved in an organic solvent, is injected into the column and heated. The components evaporate and the gas carries the components through the column. Depending on the molecular weight of the components and the polar interactions between them and the stationary phase, they will be retarded. Detectors with different sensitivity for specific compounds are available on the market. A flame ionisation detector (FID) is a common device that detects most organic components passing through the column. The organic compounds are readily pyrolyzed when introduced into a hydrogen-air flame, and ions are produced in the process. The signals are recorded as peaks on a chromatogram.

To identify the substances in a sample, it is often necessary to use several columns with different stationary phases that give the substances different retention times. GC combined with a mass spectrometer often makes it possible to identify unknown substances.

27.1.6 High-Performance Liquid Chromatography

In HPLC, the eluent is pumped through the column under high pressure in a closed system. In an isocratic system, the composition of the mobile phase is the same throughout the analysis. In a gradient system, at least two pumps are used, delivering varying amounts of different eluents. In this manner, the composition of the mobile phase can be changed during the analysis. The sample, dissolved in the mobile phase, is injected into the HPLC. The components of the sample pass through the column to the detector at different speeds. The most common detector is a UV detector. A refractive index (RI) detector can be used to detect components that do not absorb UV radiation. In some cases, derivatization can be used by adding a UV-absorbing substance which will react with the component to give a new component detectable by UV. The signals from the detector are registered as a chromatogram. A variety of columns of both non-polar and polar types are available on the market. Columns containing polar groups are used in straight-phase HPLC and columns with non-polar groups are used in reversed-phase HPLC.

The HPLC technique can be employed for both analytical and preparative purposes. In preparative HPLC, larger amounts of a sample can be injected, and fractions containing various components can be separated and collected for further analyses and/or patch testing.

27.1.7 Atomic Absorption Spectrophotometry

AAS is one of the most common methods to identify and quantify small amounts of metals in both organic and inorganic materials. The method relies on the absorption of light by atoms. The atoms can absorb light, but only at certain wavelengths corresponding to the energy requirements of the particular atoms. The successful operation of an atomic absorption spectrophotometer lies in generating a supply of free, un-combined atoms in the ground state and exposing this atom population to light at the characteristic absorption wavelength. The atomization process consists of heating a solution to a temperature that is sufficient to dissociate the compound. The thermal energy required can be supplied by a flame (air-acetylene) or by a flameless technique (graphite furnace). For quantitative measurements, the sample must be compared with standard solutions of known concentrations.

27.1.8 UV-VIS Spectrophotometry

With a UV-VIS spectrophotometer, substances that absorb light in the ultraviolet and visible regions can be detected. The substance is dissolved in a solvent with a low UV absorption and placed in the light beam in the spectrophotometer. The absorbance is plotted as a function of the wavelengths. An absorption curve often includes both maximum/maxima and minimum/minima. Many substances have characteristic absorption curves in the UV-VIS region and this information can be useful to identify substances.

A UV detector is most commonly used in HPLC.

27.1.9 Infrared Spectrophotometry

IR is used especially to identify organic substances. Nearly all molecules containing covalent bonds will show some degree of selective absorption in the infrared region. Various functional groups in a molecule give specific patterns of peaks in an IR spectrum, which can be used to identify, for example, amino groups, carbonyl groups and nitro groups. Transparent samples such as plastic films can be analyzed without processing. Other samples can be mixed with potassium bromide and pressed into a tablet. The IR spectra can be compared with reference spectra.

27.1.10 Mass Spectrometry

Mass spectrometry (MS) is used especially to determine the molecular weights and structures of organic substances. Pure substances can be analyzed directly, while components in products have to be separated before analysis. GC is often combined with an MS (GC-MS). The gas flow containing separated components is introduced directly into the mass spectrometer. In the MS, ions are generated by collision of rapidly moving electrons with the molecules of the gas. The ions are separated in an electromagnetic field according to their mass-to-charge ratio. The result of the analysis is demonstrated in a mass spectrum, showing the relative intensities of the ions formed. Fragmentation of a substance into smaller ions is very common. This fragmentation pattern is unique for each compound and gives valuable information about the chemical structure.

27.1.11 Inductively Coupled Plasma-Mass Spectrometry

Inductively coupled plasma-mass spectrometry (ICP-MS) is a technique where the ICP is used as the ion source for MS. The ions are separated according to their mass and charge, and measured individually. The major attractiveness of ICP-MS is its exceptional sensitivity combined with high analysis speed. For most elements, ICP-MS offers detection limits which are better than those of graphite furnace AA.

27.1.12 Nuclear Magnetic Resonance Spectroscopy

Using nuclear magnetic resonance spectroscopy (NMR) together with MS and/or IR analysis, it is often possible to elucidate the molecular structures of unknown substances.

The NMR technique is based on the absorption of energy by the sample to be analyzed. The sample is placed in a strong magnetic field that will affect the atoms in the sample. The nucleus can absorb energy from an additionally applied radio pulse when the frequency of the pulse matches that of the oscillating nucleus. The absorption is recorded by the instrument.

The atom most commonly studied is hydrogen (^{1}H-NMR). An NMR spectrum consists of absorption peaks from which information on functional groups

and relative number of hydrogen atoms can be retrieved. Other atoms that can be studied are carbon 13, fluorine 19 and phosphorus 31.

Many reports have been published concerning chemical methods for detecting various allergens. In Table 27.1, the methods applied to allergens in the European standard test series are shown. Chemical methods for identifying and/or quantifying miscellaneous sensitizers are shown in Table 27.2.

27.1.13 Common Chemical Methods Used by Dermatologists

27.1.13.1 Detection of Nickel Ions Released from Metal Objects

Nickel is most commonly detected by using the dimethylglyoxime test [4]. A few drops each of dimethylglyoxime 1% in ethanol and ammonia 10% in water are applied to a cotton-tipped applicator, which is rubbed against the metal object to be investigated. Dimethylglyoxime reacts with nickel ions in the presence of ammonia, giving a pink–red salt (Fig. 27.1). Coins known to contain nickel can be used to test the reagent and to observe the pink–red colour.

The sensitivity of the test can be enhanced by pretreatment of the surface of the object with a solution of artificial sweat and by heating. This test is proposed by the European Committee for Standardization [5].

The method is very simple and can be used, for example, by dermatologists and nickel-allergic individuals to detect nickel release from various metal objects.

27.1.13.2 Detection of Hexavalent Chromium (Chromate)

The chromium spot test is valid only for hexavalent chromium. Sym-diphenylcarbazide reacts with chromate and dichromate ions in the presence of sulphuric acid, giving a red–violet colour.

Reagents: (1) Sym-diphenylcarbazide 1% w/v in ethanol (must be prepared immediately before the investigation). (2) Sulphuric acid 1 mol/L. Reference: Solutions of potassium chromate 2.0, 1.0, 0.5 and 0.25 µg chromate/mL.

Table 27.1 Literature references of chemical methods for allergens in the European standard series

Allergen	Spot test	TLC	HPLC	GC	AAS/ICP-MS	UV-VIS
Potassium dichromate					[38–45]	[39, 43, 46]
4-Phenylenediamine base			[21]			
Thiuram mix			[47, 48]	[49]		
Neomycin sulphate						
Cobalt chloride					[38, 41, 44, 45]	
Benzocaine		[50–52]	[51, 52]			
Nickel sulphate	[4, 5, 53, 54]				[41, 44, 45, 55–58]	
Quinoline mix						
Colophony			[59–62]	[59, 61, 63, 64]		
Parabens			[65–67]			
N-isopropyl-N-phenyl-4-phenylenediamine			[68]	[68]		
Wool wax alcohols						
Mercapto mix		[69]	[48, 69–71]	[69, 71]		
Epoxy resin		[6, 72, 74]	[72–75]			
Myroxylon pereirae (balsam of Peru)			[76]			
4-tert-Butylphenol formaldehyde resin			[71, 77]			
Mercaptobenzothiazole		[69, 71]	[48, 69, 71, 78]	[69, 71]		
Formaldehyde	[7, 8, 79–82]		[80, 83–85, 122]			[8]
Fragrance mix			[86]	[87, 88]		
Sesquiterpene lactone mix						
Quaternium 15			[89] (Kreilgård 1996, Pharmacia Research Hilleröd Denmark, personal communication)			
Primin						
Methylchloroisothiazolinone/methylisothiazolinone			[90, 91]			
Budesonide			[92]			
Tixocortol-21-pivalate			[92]			
Methyldibromoglutaronitrile			[89, 93, 94]			
Fragrance mix 2			[86]			
Hydroxyisohexyl 3-cyclohexene carboxaldehyde			[86]			

TLC thin-layer chromatography; *HPLC* high-performance liquid chromatography; *GC* gas chromatography; *AAS* atomic absorption spectrophotometry; *ICP-MS* inductively coupled plasma-mass spectrometry; *UV-VIS* ultraviolet-visible spectrophotometry

Table 27.2 Literature references of chemical methods for miscellaneous sensitizers

Sensitizer	Spot test	TLC	HPLC	GC	AAS	UV-VIS
Various acrylates				[95]		
Alkyl thioureas		[96]	[96, 97]			
Allyl glycidyl ether			[98]			
p-Aminobenzoic acid		[50, 51]	[51, 52]			
Amyl p-dimethylaminobenzoate			[51, 52]			
Bithionol		[50]				
2-Bromo-2-nitropropane-1,3-dioll			[89, 99, 100]			
Buclosamide		[50]				
Chlorhexidine acetate/gluconate		[50]				
Chlorpromazine hydrochloride		[50]				
Diazolidinyl urea			[89, 101]			
Dichlorophene		[50]				
Diglycidylether of bisphenol F			[102]			
Dimethyloldimethylhydantoin			[89, 103]			
Diphenhydramine chloride		[50]				
Diphenylmethane-4,4´-diisocyanate			[104]			
Diphenylthiourea		[105]	[105, 106]			
Disperse dyes		[107, 108]	[107, 108]			
Dithiocarbamates		[109]	[48, 78, 109]			
Ethyl-4-bis(hydroxypropyl)aminobenzoate		[51]	[51, 52]			
Ethylene thiourea		[105, 110]	[110]			
2-Ethylhexyl p-dimethylaminobenzoate		[51]	[51, 52]			
Fentichlor		[50]				
Various fragrances				[86, 111–113]		
Glyceryl p-aminobenzoate		[51]	[51, 52]			
Hexachlorophene		[50]				
Hydrocortisone-17-butyrate			[92]			
Imidazolidinyl urea			[67, 89]			
d-Limonene				[114, 115]		
6-methylcoumarin		[50]				

Table 27.2 (continued)

Sensitizer	Spot test	TLC	HPLC	GC	AAS	UV-VIS
Moskene		[116]	[116]			
Musk ambrette		[116]	[116, 117]			
Musk ketone		[116]	[116]			
Musk tibetine		[116]	[116]			
Musk xylene		[116]	[116]			
Phenol formaldehyde resin			[118]			
Phenylisothiocyanate			[106]			
Promethazine hydrochloride	[50]					
Tetrachlorosalicylanilide	[50]					
Thiourea	[50]					
Tinuvin P			[119–121]	[119]		
Tribromosalicylanilide	[50]					
Trichlorocarbanilide	[50]					
Triclosan	[50]					

TLC thin-layer chromatography; *HPLC* high-performance liquid chromatography; *GC* gas chromatography; *AAS* atomic absorption spectrophotometry; *UV-VIS* ultraviolet-visible spectrophotometry

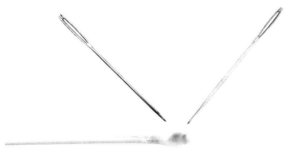

Fig. 27.1 Detection of nickel ions released from sewing needles. A few drops each of dimethylglyoxime 1% in ethanol and ammonia 10% in water were applied to the cotton-tipped applicator, which was rubbed against the needles. The *pink–red colour* of the cotton indicates the presence of nickel ions

Chromate on the Surface of a Solid Object

A few drops each of reagent I and II are applied to a cotton swab. The cotton swab is thereafter rubbed against the surface of the object for 1 min. If chromate is present a red–violet colour appears.

Chromate in Solutions

To a sample of approximately 10 mL, a few drops each of reagent I and II are added. If chromate is present a red–violet colour appears (Fig. 27.2).

Chromate in Powders Insoluble in Water (E.g. Cement)

Five grams of cement is mixed with 10 mL of water for some minutes. The mixture is then filtered and the filtrate is handled as for chromate in solutions. Iron ions can interfere with the reagent and give discoloured solutions.

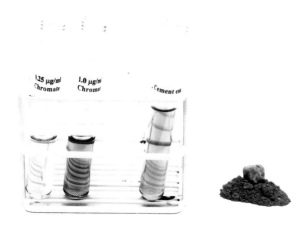

Fig. 27.2 Detection of chromate in cement. A few drops of the reagents were added to the reference solutions and to the cement extract. The *red–violet* colour of the extract indicates the presence of chromate in the investigated cement

27.1.13.3 Detection of Epoxy Resin Based on Bisphenol A

The most common epoxy resin of the bisphenol A type is diglycidyl ether of bisphenol A resin (DGEBA-R). This epoxy resin contains oligomers of various molecular weights (e.g., 340, 624, 908, 1,024). Since DGEBA with a molecular weight of 340 is a strong sensitizer, a chemical method to detect the sensitizer in various types of products is important. There is a simple TLC method to demonstrate the oligomers [6].

Demonstration of epoxy resin of bisphenol A type (Fig. 27.3a) requires the following:

Material: TLC plates (silica gel 60, F 254). Eluent: chloroform/acetonitrile 90/10 (v/v). Spray reagents: sulphuric acid 1 mol/L. Anisaldehyde in methanol 2.5% (v/v). Standard: 1% (w/v) epoxy resin of bisphenol A type in acetone containing low mol.-wt. (340, 624, 908, etc.) oligomers. Extraction solution: acetone/methanol (90/10 v/v) or ethanol. Procedure: The sample to be investigated is dissolved in the extraction solution. Solid samples are extracted at room temperature or in an ultrasonic bath. The required extraction time is dependent on the amount of low molecular epoxy resin in the sample. The

extract is evaporated to a volume of a few millilitres before being applied to the plate. The standard solution, 2–5 μL (20–50 μg), is deposited with a capillary pipette on a TLC plate. A similar volume of the sample is applied beside the standard. Since the concentration of the epoxy resin in the sample is often unknown, it is advisable to apply double and triple amounts of the sample on the same plate. The plate is eluted in a tank lined with filter paper saturated with the eluent. The plate is air-dried and sprayed with sulphuric acid until just moist and then sprayed lightly with anisaldehyde. After being heated in an oven at 110°C for 10 min, the oligomers are visible as violet spots with oligomer 340 at the top, followed by 624 (Fig. 27.3b). If the sample contains unhardened low molecular weight epoxy resin, the oligomers 340, 624 and 908 can be identified with the same R_F values as the oligomers in the standard.

Fillers and pigments in the sample can disturb the analysis. In such cases, special treatment of the sample may be required.

27.1.13.4 Detection of Formaldehyde

Formaldehyde is a gas that dissolves easily in water-based products. Small amounts may be released from many preservatives, and many water-based products may thus contain formaldehyde. Two simple methods are frequently used to identify formaldehyde in various types of products.

Chromotropic Acid Method

Reagent: 40 mg of chromotropic acid is dissolved in 10 mL of concentrated sulphuric acid (freshly prepared). Standard solutions: A concentrated water solution of formaldehyde (35%) is diluted to 100 μg/mL and refrigerated (stock solution). Standard solutions containing 2.5, 10, 20 and 40 μg formaldehyde/mL are prepared. The standard solutions should be refrigerated and freshly prepared every week.

Approximately, 0.5 g of the sample is placed in a 25-mL glass jar with a ground-glass stopper. One mL

Fig. 27.3 TLC analysis of epoxy resin based on bisphenol A. (**a**) Small amounts of the reference solution and the extract of the product to be investigated were applied on the plate before eluting in a tank. After spraying with the reagents and heating in an oven, the oligomers are visible as violet spots. (**b**) Product containing diglycidyl ether of bisphenol A (DGEBA)

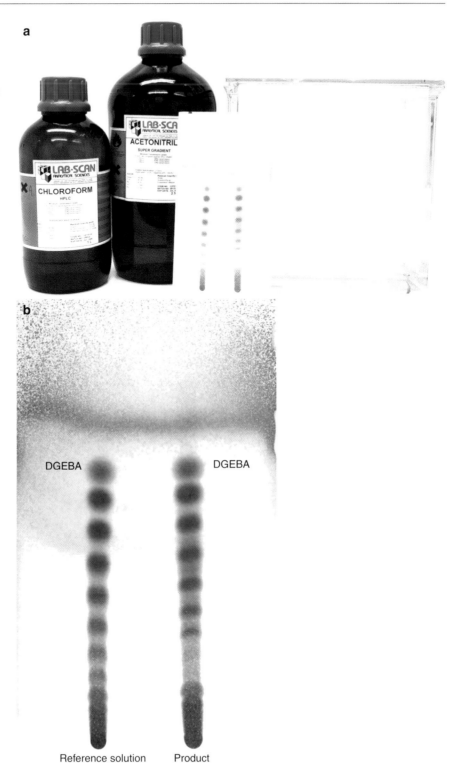

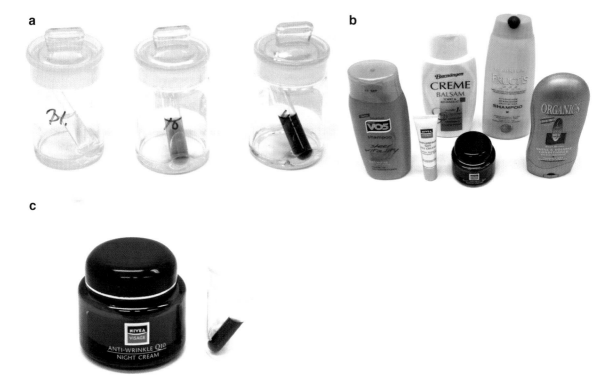

Fig 27.4 Detection of formaldehyde with the chromotropic acid method. *Violet colour* of the reagent indicates the presence of formaldehyde. (**a**) A blank and two standard solutions of formaldehyde. (**b**) Products to be analyzed. (**c**) A leave-on product containing formaldehyde

of each standard solution and 1 mL water (blank) is placed in separate glass jars. 0.5 mL of the reagent is added to small glass tubes and then placed individually in the glass jars containing the sample, the standards and the blank, respectively. The jars are kept in the dark and observed after 1 and 2 days. A violet reagent indicates the presence of formaldehyde (Fig. 27.4a–c).

This method is based on a chemical reaction of chromotropic acid and free formaldehyde evaporated from the sample/standards [7]. However, other aldehydes and ketones can also react with chromotropic acid giving colours that can interfere with the violet.

With the chromotropic acid method, a rough estimation of the concentration of formaldehyde can be obtained by comparing the intensity of the sample colour with those of the standards.

Acetylacetone Method

Reagent: 15 g ammonium acetate, 0.2 mL acetylacetone and 0.3 mL glacial acetic acid are dissolved in water to make 100 mL. The solution should be refrigerated and freshly prepared every week.

Standard solutions: From the stock solution of formaldehyde (100 µg/mL), standards containing 2.5, 10, 20 and 40 µg formaldehyde/mL are prepared. The standard solutions should be refrigerated and freshly prepared every week.

Approximately, 0.5 g of the sample is placed in a glass jar with ground-glass stopper. Ointments and other fat products should be emulsified with a few drops of formaldehyde-free emulsifier such as Triton X-100. One mL of each standard solution and 1 mL water (blank) is added to separate glass jars. To each glass jar, 2.5 mL of the reagent solution is added and the jar is then shaken. The jars are heated at 60°C for 10 min. A yellow mixture indicates the presence of formaldehyde. If the concentration of formaldehyde is high, the yellow will already appear before heating. The intensity of the yellow can be compared with that of the standards to estimate the content of formaldehyde in the sample.

If the sample to be analyzed is coloured, an extraction procedure with 1-butanol can be performed, as described by Fregert et al. [8]. Quantification of the content can be performed using a UV-VIS spectrophotometer [8].

27.1.14 Summary

To diagnose and prevent allergic contact dermatitis, it is important to demonstrate allergens in products from the patient´s environment. With various chemical methods, it is possible to demonstrate the presence or absence of known allergens in products and to isolate and identify new allergens. However, chemical methods have limitations, and false-positive as well as false-negative results can be obtained, especially when simple methods are used.

> **Core Message**
>
> › Chemical analysis of a product can make it possible to demonstrate the presence of known allergens. This knowledge can be used in the assessment of the clinical relevance of atopic dermatitis.
> › Release of nickel ions from various metal objects can be demonstrated by a simple spot test.
> › Water-soluble chromate can be demonstrated by a spot test.

27.2 Skin Exposure Assessment

Carola Lidén

27.2.1 Introduction

Contact allergens, skin irritants and other hazardous substances can come into contact with the skin, but there is little experience on how to measure the dose deposited on the skin. Solid materials, solutions, vapours, gases, and particles may contaminate the skin by direct contact, indirect contact or airborne exposure. Exposure may be intended or unintended, voluntary or accidental, known or unknown, visible or invisible, etc.

Occupational hygiene has traditionally been concerned mainly with exposure by inhalation. Skin exposure to pesticides and some organic solvents has been an exception, due to the importance of skin absorption for their toxic effects (see Chap. 47). During recent years, there has been increasing attention to exposure by skin contact; however, it is still mainly focused on exposure causing systemic effects, rather than dermatitis and other local effects. The EC Dermal Exposure Network (DEN) and the EU RISKOFDERM projects have made efforts to increase knowledge in the area. A review of dermal exposure data in EU workplaces is given in [9]. The hands were found to be the most contaminated parts of the body, which is not a surprise to experts in occupational dermatology and contact dermatitis.

A conceptual model of the process leading to uptake via the dermal route has been postulated [10]. A method for structured, semi-quantitative dermal exposure assessment (DREAM) has been developed [11]. The method consists of an inventory and an evaluation part. It can be used in occupational hygiene and epidemiological studies. A European Standardisation project (CEN/TC 137) has produced a technical report for guidance on a strategy for the evaluation of dermal exposure in workplaces [12].

27.2.2 Techniques for the Assessment of Skin Exposure

A brief review of techniques which may be useful in the assessment of skin exposure to contact allergens, skin irritants and other skin-hazardous substances is given.

27.2.2.1 Fluorescent Tracer Technique

The fluorescent tracer technique has often been used for the assessment of skin exposure to pesticides [13–17] (see Chap. 47). The technique has also been applied for the assessment of skin exposure to dental acrylates (Fig. 27.5) and paint, and the assessment of efficacy in the application of hand disinfectants.

In brief, a fluorescent tracer is dissolved or mixed in the preparation of interest, e.g., a pesticide. Different fluorescent tracers have been used (e.g. Uvitex OB, Tinopal CBS-X, Calcofluor and riboflavin). Some of them are used as laundry whitener. After the work process to be assessed has been carried out, the body surface, clothes, gloves and possibly, the surrounding surfaces and equipment are illuminated with UV light in a darkened room, preferably under standardized conditions. The contaminated areas are, thus, visualized. A video camera, together with a computer programme for image analysis, may be used for the recording and analysis of the area and intensity of contamination. Documentation and evaluation may also be performed in a less sophisticated manner, depending on conditions, resources and needs of the investigation.

The fluorescent tracer technique may be used for qualitative or quantitative assessment of skin exposure [18]. As the contamination is visualized, the method may be used, and have a great impact on training workers, to minimize contamination of skin surfaces. Other applications may be to identify the sources of contamination, improve risk assessment, and follow-up intervention. A comparison was made between the assessment of skin exposure by the fluorescent tracer technique and by using a rinsing method. Good agreement was found between the methods [19].

27.2.2.2 Removal Techniques

Among the most frequently used methods for sampling chemicals deposited on the skin are removal techniques, e.g. different washing methods and tape stripping.

Washing, Rinsing and Wiping

Different washing techniques have been much used in studies of skin exposure to pesticides, as reviewed in [20]. The methods may also be used for skin irritants and contact allergens. Recent studies have been carried out to study the deposition of hair dye substances on the hands of hairdressers and the contamination of surfaces [21, 22]. Sampling was carried out by *bag rinsing*. The hands are shaken in plastic bags containing a borate buffer in 10% ethanol, before and after work.

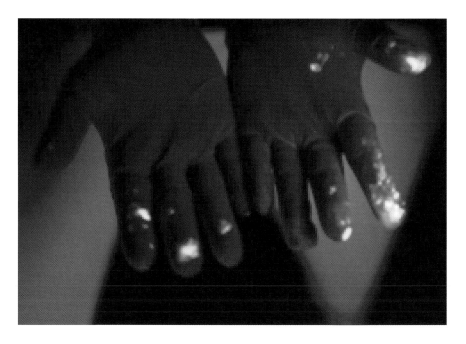

Fig. 27.5 Contamination of protective gloves with dental acrylates, visualized by the fluorescence tracer technique (courtesy of A. Boman)

Table 27.3 Method development for skin exposure assessment – some examples

Substance	Sampling	Analytical method	Result	References
Multifunctional acrylates	Tape stripping	GC	The first tape strip removed 94% of tripropylene glycol diacrylate (TPGDA); 89% of UV resin	[31]
Jet fuel (naphtalene)	Tape stripping	GC-MS	The first two tape strips removed 70% of the applied dose	[30]
Metal working fluid	Bag rinsing with 20% isopropanol	LC-MS	Recovery efficiency 55% in general for alkanolamines	[23]
Hair dye substances	Bag rinsing with borate buffer in 10% ethanol	HPLC	Sampling efficiency 70–90%	[21]
Nickel	Tape stripping	ICP-MS	Adsorption studied by 20 strips	[33]
Nickel, chromium, cobalt	Acid wipe sampling with 1% nitric acid	ICP-MS	Sampling efficiency >90%	[24]
Particles	Vacuuming	Light microscopy, XRF	Sampling efficiency 95–100%	[29]
Particles	Tape stripping	Light microscopy, XRF	The first 2 strips removed 99.8%	[29]

GC gas chromatography; *GC-MS* gas chromatography with mass spectrometry; *HPLC* high-performance liquid chromatography; *ICP-MS* inductively coupled plasma-mass spectrometry; *XRF* X-ray fluorescence

The hands of more than 50% of the hairdressers studied were contaminated by the permanent hair dyes analyzed (Tables 27.3 and 27.4). A bag rinsing method using 20% isopropanol has been developed for the assessment of skin exposure to alkanolamines in metal working fluids [23] (Table 27.3).

Studies have been carried out to study the deposition of nickel, chromium and cobalt on the hands of cashiers, locksmiths, carpenters and office employees. Sampling was performed by wipe-washing defined areas on the hands by a novel method (*acid wipe sampling*) with dilute nitric acid (1%) before and after work [24–26]. It was shown that substantial amounts of nickel are deposited on the hands of locksmiths, cashiers and carpenters (Tables 27.3 and 27.4). Acid wipe sampling has very high sampling efficiency, much higher than a finger immersion technique using water [27]. Acid wipe sampling is suitable also for other metals.

When sampling by washing, rinsing or wiping, it is essential to consider the choice of the materials used (soap, solvent, wipe, plastic bag, etc.). They may interfere with skin absorption or chemical analysis.

Sampling efficiency and sampling strategy are important factors for the outcome. By washing and rinsing, the chemicals deposited on large areas may be sampled. By wipe-washing, the mass per area unit, e.g. $\mu g/cm^2$, may be calculated, which is of high relevance when considering contact allergy.

Tape Stripping

Tape stripping, by stripping up to 20 times, is often used in dermatology for studies of different processes in the stratum corneum. Tape stripping has been applied also for sampling in the assessment of skin exposure to acrylates, jet fuel, nickel, resin acids and particles (Tables 27.3 and 27.4) [28–32]. Stripping up to 3 times may also be done. Tape stripping, by several strippings, has been used for studies of how nickel is adsorbed in the skin (Table 27.3) [33]. Such an application may be referred to as biomonitoring. Different types of tapes have been used, depending on the substance of interest and the analytical procedure used.

Table 27.4 Examples of skin exposure assessment by different technique in the occupational setting

Exposure	Sampling	Analytical method	Dose on skin (mean value); (number of subjects or samples)	References
Metalworking fluid	Whole-body oversuits, sampling gloves	HPLC, ICP-AES	Boron in suit: 62 $\mu g/cm^2/h$ ($n=31$) gloves: 2,900 $\mu g/cm^2/h$ ($n=7$)	[36]
Electroplating fluid	Whole-body oversuits, sampling gloves	PXRF	Ni, Cr, Cu and Zn in suit: 37 $\mu g/cm^2/h$ ($n=26$) In gloves: 190 $\mu g/cm^2/h$ ($n=25$)	[36]
Permanent hair dyes in hairdressers	Bag rinsing	HPLC	PPD: 22–939 nmol/hand ($n=33$); exposure by dye application, cutting newly-dyed hair, from background exposure	[22]
UV-curable acrylates in furniture industry	Tape stripping	GC	Tripropylene glycol diacrylate (TPGDA): 30.4 $\mu g/10\ cm^2/$ work shift ($n=36$)	[32]
Nickel in different occupations (2 h work)	Acid wipe sampling	ICP-MS	Locksmiths ($n=3$): 3.8; carpenters ($n=4$): 0.9; cashiers ($n=6$): 0.8; office workers ($n=4$): 0.2 $\mu g/cm^2/8$ h	[25]

GC gas chromatography; *HPLC* high-performance liquid chromatography; *ICP-MS* inductively coupled plasma-mass spectrometry; *PXRF* portable X-ray fluorescence

Vacuuming

Vacuuming may be used for sampling particles deposited on skin. A suction sampler was constructed for this purpose and it was used in method development in an exposure chamber (Table 27.3) [29]. Comparisons were made with results from tape stripping and patch sampling, confirming good agreement. The suction sampler allows for dust sampling from large areas of skin.

27.2.2.3 Surrogate Skin Sampling

In skin exposure assessment, the concept of surrogate skin is used for a medium used to collect chemicals deposited on the sampler, as a surrogate for the skin surface. The technique has been much used in the assessment of skin exposure to pesticides ([34], review in [35]), and also to assess skin exposure to metal working fluids and electroplating fluid (Table 27.4) [36]. Whole-body oversuits, gloves and patches applied in different locations on the body are used as samplers. They may be made of cotton or other fabric, filter paper, aluminium foil or other material. After exposure, the substance is extracted and analyzed; oversuits may be sectioned before analysis.

27.2.2.4 Assessment by Observation

Assessment of skin exposure to wet work has been performed by continuous observation and registration of exposure events on hand-held computer [37]. The method was initially developed for the validation of a questionnaire on exposure to water, and it is useful for the assessment of frequency and accumulated duration of skin exposure to chemicals, wet work and protective gloves, etc.

27.2.2.5 Biomonitoring

Common biomonitoring has little use in the assessment of skin exposure to contact allergens and skin irritants. In the future, tape stripping and micro-dialysis may, however, be used more for this purpose.

27.2.3 Analytical Methods

See Sect. 27.1, Tables 27.3 and 27.4, and the publications referred to above for a broad range of analytical methods suitable for contact allergens.

27.2.4 Application of Results

There is a great need for further development and application of methods for the assessment of skin exposure to contact allergens, skin irritants and other skin-hazardous substances. The application of solid methods for skin exposure assessment will increase the understanding of skin contamination, the dose–effect relationship and the possibilities for prevention. The results may be used in risk assessment, in setting occupational dermal exposure limits and limits for chemicals in products, and in follow-up after intervention by exposure control. Skin exposure assessment may, in the future, be applied in the evaluation of patients with contact dermatitis.

Core Message

> Assessment of skin exposure to contact allergens, skin irritants and other skin-hazardous substances is a new research area. It will help us to understand skin exposure and dose–effect relationships better and improve risk assessment and prevention of contact dermatitis.

References

1. Bruze M, Gruvberger B, Fregert S (2006) Chemical skin burns. In: Chew A, Maibach HI, Lepoittevin JP (eds) Irritant dermatitis. Springer, Berlin, pp 53–61
2. Feigl F, Anger V (1966) Spot tests in organic analysis, 7th edn. Elsevier, Amsterdam
3. Feigl F, Anger V (1972) Spot tests in inorganic analysis, 6th edn. Elsevier, Amsterdam
4. Fisher's Contact Dermatitis (1995) eds Rietschel RL, Fowler JF Jr 4th edn. Williams & Wilkins, Baltimore, pp 857–857
5. European Committee for Standardisation (CEN) (2002) Screening tests for nickel release from alloys and coatings in items that come in direct and prolonged contact with the skin. CR: 12471
6. Fregert S, Trulsson L (1978) Simple methods for demonstration of epoxy resin of bisphenol A type. Contact Dermatitis 4:69–72
7. Dahlquist I, Fregert S, Gruvberger B (1980) Reliability of the chromotropic acid method for qualitative formaldehyde determination. Contact Dermatitis 6:357–358
8. Fregert S, Dahlquist I, Gruvberger B (1984) A simple method for detection of formaldehyde. Contact Dermatitis 10:132–134
9. Rajan-Sithamparanadarajah R, Roff M, Delgado P et al (2004) Patterns of dermal exposure to hazardous substances in European Union workplaces. Ann Occup Hyg 48: 285–297
10. Schneider T, Vermeulen R, Brouwer DH et al (1999) Conceptual model for assessment of dermal exposure. Occup Environ Med 56:765–773
11. Van Wendel-de-Joode B, Brouwer DH, Vermeulen R et al (2003) DREAM: a method for semi-quantitative dermal exposure assessment. Ann Occup Hyg 47:71–87
12. European Committee for Standardisation (CEN) (2006) Workplace exposure–measurement of dermal exposure– principles and methods. CEN/TS 15279:2006
13. Aragón A, Blanco L, López L et al (2004) Reliability of a visual scoring system with fluorescent tracers to assess dermal pesticide exposure. Ann Occup Hyg 48:601–606
14. Aragón A, Blanco LE, Funez A et al (2006) Assessment of dermal pesticide exposure with fluorescent tracer: a modification of a visual scoring system for developing countries. Ann Occup Hyg 50:75–83
15. Blanco LE, Aragón A, Lundberg I et al (2005) Determinants of dermal exposure among Nicaraguan subsistence farmers during pesticide applications with backpack sprayers. Ann Occup Hyg 49:17–24
16. Cohen Hubal EA, Suggs JC, Nishioka MG et al (2005) Characterizing residue transfer efficiencies using a fluorescent imaging technique. J Expo Anal Environ Epidemiol 15:261–270
17. Fenske RA (1988) Visual scoring system for fluorescent tracer evaluation of dermal exposure to pesticides. Bull Environ Contam Toxicol 41:727–736
18. Cherrie JW, Brouwer DH, Roff M et al (2000) Use of qualitative and quantitative fluorescence techniques to assess dermal exposure. Ann Occup Hyg 44:519–522
19. Roff M, Wheeler J, Baldwin P (2001) Comparison of fluorescence and rinsing methods for assessing dermal exposure. Appl Occup Environ Hyg 16:319–322 ta troligen bort ref
20. Brouwer DH, Boeniger MF, van Hemmen J (2000) Hand wash and manual skin wipes. Ann Occup Hyg 44:501–510
21. Lind M-L, Boman A, Surakka J et al (2004) A method for assessing occupational dermal exposure to premanent hair dyes. Ann Occup Hyg 48:533–539
22. Lind M-L, Boman A, Sollenberg J et al (2004) Occupational dermal exposure to permanent hair dyes among hairdressers. Ann Occup Hyg 49(49):473–480
23. Henriks-Eckerman ML, Suuronen K, Jolanki R et al (2007) Determination of occupational exposure to alkanolamines in metal-working fluids. Ann Occup Hyg 51:153–160
24. Lidén C, Skare L, Lind B et al (2006) Assessment of skin exposure to nickel, chromium and cobalt by acid wipe sampling and ICP-MS. Contact Dermatitis 54:233–238
25. Lidén C, Skare L, Nise G et al (2008) Deposition of nickel, chromium, and cobalt on the skin in some occupations— assessment by acid wipe sampling. Contact Dermatitis 58:347–354
26. Lidén C, Skare L, Vahter M (2008) Release of nickel from coins and deposition onto skin from coin handling— comparing euro coins and SEK. Contact Dermatitis 59: 31–37
27. Staton I, Ma R, Evans N et al (2006) Dermal nickel exposure associated with coin handling and in various occupational settings: assessment using a newly developed finger immersion method. Br J Dermatol 154:658–664

28. Eriksson K, Hagström K, Axelsson S et al (2008) Tape-stripping as a m ethod for measuring dermal exposure to resin acids during wood pellet production. J Environ Monit 10:345–352

29. Lundgren L, Skare L, Lidén C (2006) Measuring dust on skin with a small vacuuming sampler—a comparison with other sampling techniques. Ann Occup Hyg 50:95–103

30. Mattorano DA, Kupper LL, Nylander-French LA (2004) Estimating dermal exposure to jet fuel (naphthalene) using adhesive tape strip samples. Ann Occup Hyg 48:139–146

31. Nylander-French LA (2000) A tape-stripping method for measuring dermal exposure to multifunctional acrylates. Ann Occup Hyg 44:645–651

32. Surakka J, Lindh T, Rosén G et al (2000) Workers' dermal exposure to UV-curable acrylates in the furniture and parquet industry. Ann Occup Hyg 44:635–644

33. Hostýnek JJ, Dreher F, Nakada T et al (2001) Human stratum corneum adsorption of nickel salts. Investigation of depth profiles by tape stripping in vivo. Acta Derm Venereol Suppl (Stockh) 212:11–18

34. OECD (1997) Guidance document for the conduct of studies of occupational exposure to pesticides during agricultural application. Environment, health and safety publications series on testing and assessment, no 9

35. Soutar A, Semple S, Aitken RJ et al (2000) Use of patches and whole body sampling for the assessment of dermal exposure. Ann Occup Hyg 44:511–518

36. Roff M, Bagon DA, Chambers H et al (2004) Dermal exposure to electroplating fluids and metalworking fluids in the UK. Ann Occup Hyg 48:209–217

37. Anveden I, Lidén C, Alderling M et al (2006) Self-reported skin exposure – validation of questions by observation. Contact Dermatitis 55:186–191

38. Fregert S, Gruvberger B (1972) Chemical properties of cement. Berufsdermatosen 20:238–248

39. Hansen MB, Menné T, Johansen JD (2006) Cr(III) and Cr(VI) in leather and elicitation of eczema. Contact Dermatitis 54:278–282

40. Ingber A, Gammelgaard B, David M (1998) Detergents and bleaches are sources of chromium contact dermatitis in Israel. Contact Dermatitis 38:101–104

41. Julander A, Hindsén M, Skare L et al (2009) Cobalt-containing alloys and their ability to release cobalt and cause dermatitis. Contact Dermatitis 60:165–170

42. Lachapelle JM, Lauwerys R, Tennstedt D et al (1980) Eau de Javel and prevention of chromate allergy in France. Contact Dermatitis 6:107–110

43. Nygren O, Wahlberg JE (1998) Speciation of chromium in tanned leather gloves and relapse of chromium allergy from tanned leather samples. Analyst 123:935–937

44. Summer B, Fink U, Zeller R et al (2007) Patch test reactivity to a cobalt-chromium-molybdenum alloy and stainless steel in metal-allergic patients in correlation to the metal ion release. Contact Dermatitis 57:35–39

45. Tandon R, Aarts B (1993) Chromium, nickel and cobalt contents of some Australian cements. Contact Dermatitis 28:201–205

46. Wass U, Wahlberg JE (1991) Chromated steel and contact allergy. Recommendation concerning a "threshold limit value" for the release of hexavalent chromium. Contact Dermatitis 24:114–118

47. Bergendorff O, Hansson C (2001) Stability of thiuram disulfides in patch test preparations and formation of asymmetric disulfides. Contact Dermatitis 45:151–157

48. Bergendorff O, Persson C, Hansson C (2006) High-performance liquid chromatography analysis of rubber allergens in protective gloves used in health care. Contact Dermatitis 55:210–215

49. Knudsen BB, Larsen E, Egsgaard H et al (1993) Release of thiurams and carbamates from rubber gloves. Contact Dermatitis 28:63–69

50. Bruze M, Fregert S (1983) Studies on purity and stability of photopatch test substances. Contact Dermatitis 9:33–39

51. Bruze M, Fregert S, Gruvberger B (1984) Occurrence of para-aminobenzoic acid and benzocaine as contaminants in sunscreen agents of para-aminobenzoic acid type. Photodermatology 1:277–285

52. Bruze M, Gruvberger B, Thulin I (1990) PABA, benzocaine, and other PABA esters in sunscreens and after-sun products. Photodermatol Photoimmunol Photomed 7: 106–108

53. Lidén C, Johnsson S (2001) Nickel on the Swedish market before the Nickel Directive. Contact Dermatitis 44:7–12

54. Lidén C, Röndell E, Skare L et al (1998) Nickel release from tools on the Swedish market. Contact Dermatitis 39:127–131

55. Andersen KE, Nielsen GD, Flyvholm M-A et al (1983) Nickel in tap water. Contact Dermatitis 9:140–143

56. Bang Pedersen N, Fregert S, Brodelius P et al (1974) Release of nickel from silver coins. Acta Derm Venereol (Stockh) 54:231–234

57. European Committee for Standardization (CEN) (1998) Reference test method for release of nickel from products intended to come into direct and prolonged contact with the skin. EN 1811

58. Fischer T, Fregert S, Gruvberger B et al (1984) Contact sensitivity to nickel in white gold. Contact Dermatitis 10: 23–24

59. Bergh M, Menné T, Karlberg A-T (1994) Colophony in paper-based surgical clothing. Contact Dermatitis 31: 332–333

60. Ehrin E, Karlberg A-T (1990) Detection of rosin (colophony) components in technical products using an HPLC technique. Contact Dermatitis 23:359–366

61. Karlberg A-T, Gäfvert E, Meding B et al (1996) Airborne contact dermatitis from unexpected exposure to rosin (colophony). Contact Dermatitis 35:272–278

62. Sadhra S, Gray CN, Foulds IS (1997) High-performance liquid chromatography of unmodified rosin and its application on contact dermatology. J Chromatogr B Biomed Sci Appl 24(700):101–110

63. Karlberg A-T, Magnusson K (1996) Rosin components identified in diapers. Contact Dermatitis 34:176–180

64. Karlberg A-T, Gäfvert E, Lidén C (1995) Environmentally friendly paper may increase risk of hand eczema in rosin-sensitive persons. J Am Acad Dermatol 33:427–432

65. Rastogi SC, Schouten A, de Kruijf N et al (1995) Contents of methyl-, ethyl-, propyl-, butyl-, and benzylparaben in cosmetic products. Contact Dermatitis 32:28–30

66. Seventh Commission Directive 96/45/EC of 2 July 1996 relating to methods of analysis necessary for checking the composition of cosmetics products

67. Sottofattori E, Anzaldi M, Balbi A et al (1998) Simultaneous HPLC determination of multiple components in a commercial cosmetic cream. J Pharm Biomed Anal 18:213–217

68. Kaniwa M-A, Isama K, Nakamura A et al (1994) Identification of causative chemicals of allergic contact dermatitis using a combination of patch testing in patients and chemical analysis. Application to cases from industrial rubber products. Contact Dermatitis 30:20–25

69. Kaniwa M-A, Momma J, Ikarashi Y et al (1992) A method for identifying causative chemicals of allergic contact dermatitis using a combination of chemical analysis and patch testing in patients and animal groups: application to a case of rubber boot dermatitis. Contact Dermatitis 27:166–173

70. Hansson C, Bergendorff O, Ezzelarab M et al (1997) Extraction of mercaptobenzothiazole compounds from rubber products. Contact Dermatitis 36:195–200

71. Kaniwa M-A, Isama K, Nakamura A et al (1994) Identification of causative chemicals of allergic contact dermatitis using a combination of patch testing in patients and chemical analysis. Application to cases from rubber footwear. Contact Dermatitis 30:26–34

72. Fregert S, Meding B, Trulsson L (1984) Demonstration of epoxy resin in stoma pouch plastic. Contact Dermatitis 10(2):106

73. Hansson C (1994) Determination of monomers in epoxy resin hardened at elevated temperature. Contact Dermatitis 31:333–334

74. Jenkinson HA, Burrows D (1987) Pitfalls in the demonstration of epoxy resins. Contact Dermatitis 16:226–227

75. Le Coz CJ, Coninx D, Van Rengen A et al (1999) An epidemic of occupational contact dermatitis from an immersion oil for micros in laboratory personnel. Contact Dermatitis 40:77–83

76. Oxholm A, Heidenheim M, Larsen E et al (1990) Extraction and patch testing of methylcinnamate, a newly recognized fraction of balsam of peru. Am J Contact Dermatitis 1:43–46

77. Avenel-Audran M, Goossens A, Zimerson E et al (2003) Contact dermatitis from electrocardiograph-monitoring electrodes: role of p-tert-butylphenol-formaldehyde resin. Contact Dermatitis 48:108–111

78. Depree GJ, Bledsoe A, Siegel PD (2005) Survey of sulphur-containing rubber accelerator levels in latex and nitrile exam gloves. Contact Dermatitis 53:107–113

79. Blom G (1959) Formaldehyde contact dermatitis. Acta Derm Venereol 39:450–453

80. Gryllaki-Berger M, Mugny Ch, Perrenoud D et al (1992) A comparative study of formaldehyde detection using chromotropic acid, acetylacetone and HPLC in cosmetics and household cleaning products. Contact Dermatitis 26: 149–154

81. Sheretz EF (1992) Clothing dermatitis: practical aspects for the clinician. Am J Contact Dermatitis 3:55–64

82. Stonecipher MR, Sherertz EF (1993) Office detection of formaldehyde in fabric: assessment of methods and update on frequency. Am J Contact Dermatitis 4:172–174

83. Bergendorff O, Ezzelarab M, Wallengren J et al (1994) Airborne contact dermatitis from formaldehyde released from heated plastic polymers. Am J Contact Dermatitis 5:223–225

84. Karlberg A-T, Skare L, Lindberg I et al (1998) A method for quantification of formaldehyde in the presence of formaldehyde donors in skin-care products. Contact Dermatitis 38:20–28

85. Second Commission Directive 82/434/EEC, Annex IV, Identification and determination of free formaldehyde

86. Villa C, Gambaro R, Mariani E et al (2007) High-performance liquid chromatographic method for the simultaneous determination of 24 fragrance allergens to study scented products. J Pharm Biomed Anal 44:775–762

87. Rastogi SC (1995) Analysis of fragrances in cosmetics by gas chromatography-mass spectrometry. J High Resol Chromatogr 18:653–658

88. Rastogi SC, Johansen JD, Menné T (1996) Natural ingredients based cosmetics. Content of selected fragrance sensitizers. Contact Dermatitis 34:423–426

89. Gruvberger B, Bruze M, Tammela M (1998) Preservatives in moisturizers on the Swedish market. Acta Derm Vernerol (Stockh) 78:52–56

90. Gruvberger B, Persson K, Björkner B et al (1986) Demonstration of Kathon CG® in some commercial products. Contact Dermatitis 15:24–27

91. Rastogi SC (1990) Kathon CG and cosmetic products. Contact Dermatitis 22:155–160

92. Isaksson M, Gruvberger B, Persson L et al (2000) Stability of corticosteroid patch test preparations. Contact Dermatitis 42:144–148

93. Rastogi SC, Johansen SS (1995) Comparison of high-performance liquid chromatographic methods for the determination of 1, 2-dibromo-2, 4-dicyanobutane in cosmetic products. J Chromatogr A 692:53–57

94. Rastogi SC, Zachariae C, Johansen JD et al (2004) Determination of methyldibromoglutaronitrile in cosmetic products by high-performance liquid chromatography with electrochemical detection. Method validation. J Chromatogr 26:1031:315–317

95. Henriks-Eckerman M-L, Kanerva L (1997) Gas chromatographic and mass spectrometric purity analysis of acrylates and methacrylates used as patch test substances. Am J Contact Dermatitis 8:20–23

96. Kerre S, Devos L, Verhoeve L et al (1996) Contact allergy to diethylthiourea in a wet suit. Contact Dermatitis 35: 176–178

97. Bergendorff O, Persson CM, Hansson C (2004) HPLC analysis of alkyl thioureas in an orthopaedic brace and patch testing with pure ethylbutylthiourea. Contact Dermatitis 51:273–277

98. Dooms-Goossens A, Bruze M, Buysse L et al (1995) Contact allergy to allyl glycidyl ether present as an impurity in 3-glycidyloxypropyltrimethoxysilane, a fixing additive in silicone and polyurethane resins. Contact Dermatitis 33:17–19

99. Guthrie WG (1984) Analysis of bronopol in water-based lotion. Provisional HPLC method. The Boots Company PLC, Nottingham

100. Wang H, Provan GJ, Helliwell K (2002) Determination of bronopol and its degradation products by HPLC. J Pharm Biomed Anal 29:387–392

101. Williams RO III, Mahaguna V, Sriwongjanya M (1997) Determination of diazolidinyl urea in a topical cream by high-performance liquid chromatography. J Chromatogr B Biomed Sci Appl 29;696:303–306

102. Pontén A, Zimerson E, Sörensen Ö et al (2004) Chemical analysis of monomers in epoxy resins based on bisphenol F and A. Contact Dermatitis 50:289–297

103. Schouten A, Vermeulen M (1994) The determination of dimethyloldimethylhydantoin (DMDMH) in cosmetic products. TNO Nutrition and Food Research report V 94.608

27

104. Frick M, Zimerson E, Karlsson D et al (2004) Poor correlation between stated and found concentrations of diphenylmethane-4, 4′-diisocyanate in petrolatum patch test preparations. Contact Dermatitis 51:73–78

105. Meding B, Baum H, Bruze M et al (1990) Allergic contact dermatitis from diphenylthiourea in Vulkan heat retainers. Contact Dermatitis 22:8–12

106. Fregert S, Trulsson L, Zimerson E (1982) Contact allergic reactions to diphenylthiourea and phenylisothiocyanate in PVC adhesive tape. Contact Dermatitis 8:38–42

107. Ryberg K, Gruvberger B, Zimerson E et al (2008) Chemical 9nvestigations of disperse dyes in patch test preparations. Contact Dermatitis 58:199–209

108. Uter W, Hildebrandt S, Geier J et al (2007) Current test results in consecutive patients with, and chemical analysis of, disperse blue(DB) 106, DB 124, and the mix of DB 106 and 124. Contact Dermatitis 57:230–234

109. Kaniwa M-A, Isama K, Nakamura A et al (1994) Identification of causative chemicals of allergic contact dermatitis using a combination of patch testing in patients and chemical analysis. Application to cases from rubber gloves. Contact Dermatitis 31:65–71

110. Bruze M, Fregert S (1983) Allergic contact dermatitis from ethylene thiourea. Contact Dermatitis 9:208–212

111. Gimenez-Arnau A, Gimenez-Arnau E, Serra-Baldrich E et al (2002) Principles and methodology for identification of fragrance allergens in consumer products. Contact Dermatitis 47:345–352

112. Rastogi SC, Johansen JD, Frosch P et al (1998) Deodorants on the European market: quantitative chemical analysis of 21 fragrances. Contact Dermatitis 38:29–35

113. Rastogi SC, Lepoittevin J-P, Johansen JD et al (1998) Fragrances and other materials in deodorants: search for potentially sensitizing molecules using combined GC-MS and structure activity relationship (SAR) analysis. Contact Dermatitis 39:293–303

114. Karlberg A-T, Dooms-Goossens A (1997) Contact allergy to oxidized *d*-limonene among dermatitis patients. Contact Dermatitis 36:201–206

115. Karlberg A-T, Magnusson K, Nilsson U (1992) Air oxidation of *d*-limonene (the citrus solvent) creates potent allergens. Contact Dermatitis 26:332–340

116. Bruze M, Edman B, Niklasson B et al (1985) Thin layer chromatography and high pressure liquid chromatography of musk ambrette and other nitromusk compounds including photopatch studies. Photodermatology 2:295–302

117. Bruze M, Gruvberger B (1985) Contact allergy to photoproducts of musk ambrette. Photodermatology 2:310–314

118. Bruze M, Persson L, Trulsson L et al (1986) Demonstration of contact sensitizers in resins and products based on phenol-formaldehyde. Contact Dermatitis 14:146–154

119. Arisu K, Hayakawa R, Ogino Y et al (1992) Tinuvin P® in a spandex tape as a cause of clothing dermatitis. Contact Dermatitis 26:311–316

120. Björkner B, Niklasson B (1997) Contact allergy to the UV absorber Tinuvin P in a dental restorative material. Am J Contact Dermatitis 8:6–7

121. Niklasson B, Björkner B (1989) Contact allergy to the UV-absorber Tinuvin P in plastics. Contact Dermatitis 21:330–334

122. Benassi CA, Semenzato A, Bettero A (1989) High-Performance Liquid Chromatographic determination of free formaldehyde in cosmetics. J Chromatogr 464:387–393

Skin Tests for Immediate Hypersensitivity

28

Carsten Bindslev-Jensen

Contents

C. Bindslev-Jensen
Department of Dermatology and Allergy Centre,
Odense University Hospital, 5000 Odense, Denmark
e-mail: carsten.bindslev-jensen@ouh.regionsyddanmark.dk

28.1 Introduction

Testing for immediate allergic reactions (type 1 allergy) can be divided into in vivo and in vitro test procedures. The commercially available in vitro test systems primarily determine the presence of specific IgE molecules directed against epitopes on the allergenic protein; either direct (ImmunoCap, Phadia, www.phadia.com) or by using circulating basophil leucocytes as solid phase (HR-Test, Copenhagen, www.reflab.dk) (reviewed in [24]).

In vivo testing for immediate hypersensitivity works by studying the result in the skin of the release of histamine and other mediators from skin mast cells by bringing an allergen in contact with the cells in situ. This can be done by injecting the allergen (most often a protein) into the skin (skin prick test (SPT), intracutaneous (or intradermal) test (ICT)), or in case of damaged skin (e.g., atopic dermatitis) by direct application enabling allergen contact with the mast cell by diffusion through the broken skin barrier (skin application food test (SAFT), open application test (OAT), scratch-patch test (S-P)) [4, 5, 9, 11, 16, 18, 19, 26, 30] (Table 28.1).

Skin testing for immediate hypersensitivity serves as a very useful tool in the diagnostic workup of a suspected allergic patient, but it is mandatory to bear in mind that the tests measure *sensitization* and not clinical disease (Table 28.2). Any positive (or negative) outcome of skin testing must, therefore, always be correlated to patient's case history, and in unclear cases, be followed by challenge with the suspected allergen in the relevant organ. Therefore, the skin test used must ideally be as sensitive as possible (i.e., the risk of false negative test should be negligible), whereas the specificity of the test is less important because it mainly relies on the clinician's knowledge in the field especially on exposure, test procedures, and cross-sensitization.

J.D. Johansen et al. (eds.), *Contact Dermatitis*,
DOI: 10.1007/978-3-642-03827-3_28, © Springer-Verlag Berlin Heidelberg 2011

Table 28.1 Skin tests for immediate hypersensitivity

Test method	Indication	Advantage	Disadvantage
SPT with standardized (commercial) extracts	Routine Skin testing. First choice when available	Standardized extracts with established sensitivity	Many relevant allergens not available
SPT with unstandardized extracts	Suspicion of immediate reaction to an allergen, where standardized extracts of established quality are not available	Any water soluble allergen can be used. Readily available and relevant to the patient	Unstandardized extraction procedures. Often need for including controls for testing
Prick–prick method	A variant of SPT with unstandardized extracts especially for use with solid allergens	As above	As above
Intracutaneous test	Should only be used in SPT negative patients and with sterile test material	Higher sensitivity	Lower specificity Difficult to perform and read. Risk of systemic reaction
Scratch-patch test	Should not be used		
Open application test	Contact urticaria	Both high and low molecular weight substances can be tested	Unstandardized
SAFT	Suspicion of food allergy in children <3 years of age	No skin puncture needed	Should only be used in children with atopic dermatitis in specialized clinics
Atopy patch test	See Chap. 25		

Table 28.2 Testing for immediate hypersensitivity

Case history ↓	Selection of test substances (exposure)
Skin Prick Test Standard Panel skin prick test with relevant material ↓	Depending on exposure and type of allergen (e.g, testing for pollen allergy in gardeners, birch pollen allergy in suspected latex allergy) Evaluation of cross-sensitization
(Intracutaneous test) ↓	Only selected cases especially suspected drug allergy, where is SPT negative
In vitro testing ↓	Depending on nature of reaction and availability Measurement of specific IgE, basophil histamine release
Organ challenge	If a clear cut diagnosis has not been established

28.2 Skin Prick Testing

The principle of the method relies on bringing a small volume of allergen (approximately 5–10 nL) into contact with the skin mast cells by puncturing the skin with a special needle, a lancet (Fig. 28.1). A positive reaction is thereby elicited by the release of histamine and other mediators over a period of 15–20 min giving rise to a classical *wheal and flare* reaction in the skin. The released mediators (mainly histamine) are only present in the wheal, whereas the flare reaction is neuronally mediated [20].

SPT is the normal standard procedure for skin testing in case of suspected immediate reaction to an allergen.

28.2.1 Material for Testing

In some cases, standardized extracts for SPT are commercially available. This holds true for many major inhalant allergens together with some food, drugs, and insects (see www.alk-abello.com, www.stallergenes.

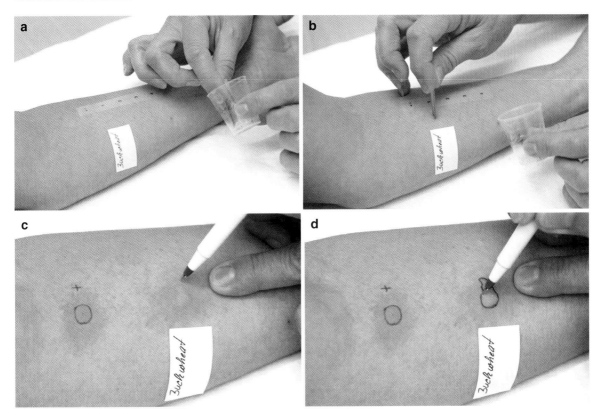

Fig. 28.1 Skin prick test (prick–prick technique) with a freshly prepared solution of allergen (buckwheat). The lancet is dipped into the solution (**a**) whereafter the skin is punctured (**b**). Fifteen minutes later, the wheal area (**c**) is outlined with a filter tip pen (**d**). The positive control is also demonstrated in (**c, d**)

com, www.hal-allergy.com, and others). In all other cases, nonstandardized, often freshly prepared material can be used. Since in many cases, potential allergens are destroyed by processing (e.g., heating), it is normally wise to use the least processed, but clinically relevant raw material for testing. There are, however, also examples of increased allergenicity by processing (e.g., roasting peanuts [22]).

A special issue to be evaluated is the possibility of cross-sensitization, meaning that sensitization to one species also gives rise to positive SPT when testing with other species, drugs, or chemicals with the same or closely related allergens – examples are positive SPT to shrimp in patients sensitized to house dust mites [1], positive SPT to fresh apple peel in birch pollen allergic patients [19], or positive SPT to amoxicillin in a penicillin V positive patient [2]. Families of allergens are listed at www.meduniwien.ac.at/allergens/allfam/.

Since almost all allergens giving rise to type 1 reactions are water soluble, addition of 0.9% NaCl is normally sufficient for dissolving dry raw material (e.g.,

flour), whereas other raw materials (e.g., plants) contain sufficient water to enable transferral of allergenic material from the material to the skin by first pricking the material with the lancet and thereafter puncturing the skin with the same needle (the prick–prick method, see later). The added volume of saline should be as small as possible but standardized, ensuring that the solubility product for the allergens in question is exceeded every time.

Many materials contain different parts with different allergen content (insects, plant leaves, plant flowers, plant pollen); the most relevant part(s) should be selected for testing.

Some items are toxic to skin mast cells (plant toxins, lectins, and many others) or act as direct histamine liberators (morfin, radiocontrastmedia [4, 21]), or may even contain histamine (venoms, extracts for skin testing [31]). The so-called irritative reactions, which by definition are nonimmunologic in nature, are contained in the above reactions, and it is therefore always necessary to include normal controls when testing with unstandardized material in order to ascertain a possible allergic reaction in the patient.

With due respect to the above, all nontoxic or non-infectious material can be used for SPT, as long as the allergens are water soluble.

Some drugs and chemicals (e.g., penicillin, chemicals, or chlorhexidine) act as haptens and will therefore only elicit a positive SPT when coupled to a carrier molecule (e.g., albumin) [7, 26, 27]. This coupling may take place in vivo since chlorhexidine in saline can elicit a positive SPT [7]. Further, the immune system may recognize metabolic products of a substance given orally and not the parent compound – this is normally the case with penicillin, and therefore, commercially available preparations of penicillin metabolites have been developed [25].

Finally, serial dilutions of the allergen enable investigations of relative sensitivity of a given patient, but this procedure is time-consuming and most often restricted to allergen standardization procedures [24].

As obvious from the above, the selection of the relevant material for testing is the crucial point in SPT.

Table 28.3 Reading of skin reactions

False positive reaction	False negative reaction
Dermographism	Insufficient raw material (e.g., frozen green pea)
Active skin diseases at site of testing	Allergens in test material labile (e.g., apple)
Test material contains irritative or toxic components	Insufficient extraction procedure (e.g., gliadins in wheat)
Patient sensitized but not clinically allergic	Drugs (antihistamines, neuroleptics, SSRI's especially mirtazapine, high dose systemic glucocorticoid)
Cross-sensitization – i.e., positive skin reaction to a substance immunologically related to the culprit substance, but without clinical significance (e.g., positive skin prick test to birch pollen in a latex sensitized individual)	

Since the tests measure sensitization and not clinical disease or relevance, "false positive" means in this context in relation to clinical disease

28.2.2 Procedure

SPT is normally performed on the volar part of the forearm, but other areas may be used [6]. High potency local steroids may in some cases interfere with the test result; more important are, however, the suppression of the wheal (and flare) by a number of drugs (Table 28.3), which should be discontinued before testing. SPT can be performed in all age groups from infancy [12].

It is important always to include a positive (histamine) and a negative control (saline or saline/glycerol) in order to avoid false negative or false positive reactions (Table 28.2).

When using standardized, commercially available allergens, single testing is routinely sufficient, but in case of nonstandardized material, testing in duplicate is advisable.

A drop of the allergen – or dissolved allergen material – is placed on the forearm; the skin is penetrated through the drop with the lancet and the wheal and flare reaction measured 15 min later. In case of material of considerable size (e.g., meat) the allergens are transferred from the material to the patient skin on the tip of the lancet (the prick–prick method). Normally, a

standard battery of the most relevant local allergens is always used (standard battery [10]), supplemented with material (foods, plants, drugs, chemicals) relevant to the patient's case history.

28.2.3 Reading of SPT

For routine use, outlining of the wheal size 15 min after application by a filter tip pen is sufficient. For documentation purposes, the size of the wheal is transferred to paper by the use of adhesive tape.

Wheal size can be measured by measuring the largest diameter plus the diameter perpendicular hereto divided by 2 or planimetry [23].

Normally, in adults and older children a positive SPT is defined as a wheal with a largest diameter above 3 mm. If the negative controls elicit a small reaction, the diameter hereof should be taken into account, but in most cases, a measurable reaction to the negative control renders the whole SPT inconclusive, and the patient should be investigated by in vitro technique. Here, specific IgE is the first choice when available, but in many cases, for example, plants, food, or drugs, a validated IgE-test is not available, and in these cases histamine release from basophils can be used, since this technique only requires blood from the patient and the relevant allergen, *as is*.

As mentioned, a positive SPT denotes sensitization to the allergen, but gives no direct evidence for an eventual clinical relevance or disease per se. A positive reaction must, therefore, always be correlated to case history including exposure, and an evaluation for cross-sensitization should also be performed in order to pinpoint the primary sensitizer.

Besides the local itching, SPT is very rarely accompanied by other side effects, and thus comprises an easy, reproducible, and safe test procedure. Systemic reactions including anaphylaxis have, however, been described especially to food, and facilities for resuscitation should, therefore, be readily available [15].

28.3 Intracutaneous (or Intradermal) Test

Intracutaneous testing serves as the second choice of skin testing in vivo and should be restricted to cases, where SPT is negative. This is due to the fact that ICT is technically much more difficult to perform in a standardized and reproducible way, is more painful to the patient, and carries a higher risk of elicitation of a systemic reaction [5, 11, 26].

28.3.1 Material for Testing

Besides injection of autologous serum in the diagnosis of autoimmune urticaria [8], only sterile material should be used for ICT, and therefore, the test is mostly used with water soluble drugs [3].

28.3.2 Procedure

In intracutaneous testing with allergens, a small volume (50 or 100 μL) of diluted allergen is injected with a 25 gauge needle intradermally (Fig. 28.2). Correct injection technique results in a small raised papule on the skin surface, from which the wheal develops over a period of 20–30 min. As positive control, histamine 50 or 100 μM is used with saline as negative control. As is the case for SPT, a positive ICT is elicited by the release of histamine and other mediators from the mast cell giving rise to a *wheal and flare* reaction (Fig. 28.2).

In contrast to SPT, both the initial papule and the elicited wheal are outlined with a filter tip pen. A standardized read out system for ICT has not been developed, but normally a ICT is considered positive when the diameter of the wheal is double the length of the initial papule and surrounded by a typical flare (Fig. 28.2). There is agreement that ICT is more sensitive than SPT, but larger published series on reproducibility, sensitivity, and specificity are lacking.

28.4 Scratch-Patch Test (S-P)

In this technique, the skin barrier is broken by linear scratching with a needle or lancet whereafter the allergen is applied directly upon the scratched skin, most often held in place by a Finn chamber. As mentioned previously, the water soluble allergens then diffuse through the broken skin to the skin mast cells eliciting a wheal and flare reaction. S-P has no obvious advantages over SPT, is difficult to perform in a standardized and reproducible way, and is therefore not recommended for routine use [19].

28.5 Skin Application Food Test

This procedure has the potential benefit of avoiding direct penetration of the skin with a needle or a lancet, which is an obvious advantage when testing children below the age of three [17]. The disadvantage is that it can best be done in damaged skin (atopic dermatitis) and outside specialized clinics perform with a low reproducibility compared to SPT. SAFT is basically an elicitation of contact urticaria by direct application of the suspected allergen (most often foods) in a Finn chamber onto the skin, thereby mimicking a patch test, but only applied for 10–30 min. Positive reactions are scored from 2 (erythema), 3 (edema and erythema within the area of the chamber), and 4 (edema and erythema outside the area of chamber), where 3 and 4 are considered positive. In one small comparative study in

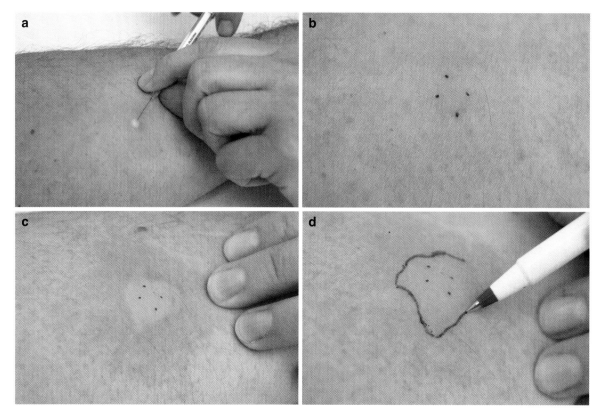

Fig. 28.2 Intracutaneous testing. 50 μL of test material is carefully injected intradermally giving rise to a small wheal (**a**). The border of the lesion is marked with a filtertip pen (**b**) and the arising wheal read after 15 min (**c**, **d**)

children with egg allergy, several systemic reactions were elicited by SAFT and combined with the low reproducibility of testing in duplicate in the same study [9]; the test should be confined to specialized clinics with routine in this test procedure.

28.6 Open Application Test

The OAT utilizes direct application of a suspected allergen (both high molecular weight allergens like meat in food handlers or chefs or low molecular weight substances such as sorbic or ascorbic acid in patients with atopic dermatitis) on the skin [13, 14]. The test is useful when investigating both immunological and nonimmunological contact urticaria, but has never been compared to SPT in controlled trials and a standardized test procedure is also lacking. OAT can be used when SPT are negative and the suspicion high, but care should be taken to avoid systemic reactions.

28.7 Atopy Patch Testing

This procedure utilizing type 1 allergens in patch testing with reading both immediately and after prolonged application will be dealt with in Chap. 25.

28.8 Conclusions

Skin testing for immediate type allergy is a very useful tool, but care has to be taken on both the technique applied and on the interpretation of positive or negative results. For routine testing, SPT should be the standard test applied, except for investigations of suspected drug allergy, where ICTs should also be included. It is important always to consider delayed reactions also combining testing for type 1 and type IV allergy when appropriate [28, 29]. Since skin testing evaluates sensitization and not clinical disease, it should be supplemented with in vitro testing and/or organ challenge in dubious cases in order to ascertain clinical relevance of the test result.

References

1. Ayuso R, Reese G, Leong-Kee S et al (2002) Molecular basis of arthropod cross-reactivity: IgE-binding cross-reactive epitopes of shrimp, house dust and cockroach tropomyosins. Int Arch Allergy Immunol 129(1):38–48

2. Blanca M, Romano A, Torres MJ et al (2009) Update on the evaluation of hypersensitivity reactions to betalactams. Allergy 64(2):183–193

3. Bousquet PJ, Demoly P, Romano A et al (2009) Pharmacovigilance of drug allergy and hypersensitivity using the ENDA-DAHD database and the GALEN platform. The Galenda project. Allergy 64(2):194–203

4. Brockow K, Romano A, Aberer W et al (2009) Skin testing in patients with hypersensitivity reactions to iodinated contrast media – a European multicenter study. Allergy 64:234–241

5. Calabria CW, Hagen L (2008) The role of intradermal skin testing in inhalant allergy. Ann Allergy Asthma Immunol 101(4):337–347

6. Dreborg S (1989) The skin prick test in the diagnosis of atopic allergy. J Am Acad Dermatol 21(4 pt 2):820–821

7. Garvey LH, Kroigaard M, Poulsen LK et al (2007) IgE-mediated allergy to chlorhexidine. J Allergy Clin Immunol 120(2):490–515

8. Grattan CE, Wallington TB, Warin RP et al (1986) A serological mediator in chronic idiopathic urticaria – a clinical, immunological and histological evaluation. Br J Dermatol 114(5):583–590

9. Hansen TK, Host A, Bindslev-Jensen C (2004) An evaluation of the diagnostic value of different skin tests with egg in clinical egg-allergic children having atopic dermatitis. Pediatr Allergy Immunol 15:428–434

10. Heinzerling L, Frew AJ, Bindslev-Jensen C et al (2005) Standard prick testing and sensitization to inhalant allergens across Europe – a survey from the GALEN network. Allergy 60(10):1287–1300

11. Henzgen M, Ballmer-Weber BK, Erdmann S et al (2008) Skin testing with food allergens. Guideline of the German Society of Allergology and Clinical Immunology (DGAKI), the Physicians' Association of German Allergologists (ADA) and the society of Pediatric Allergology (GPA) together with the Swiss Society of Allergology. J Dtsch Dermatol Ges 6(11):983–988

12. Kjaer HF, Eller E, Host A et al (2008) The prevalence of allergic diseases in an unselected group of 6-year old children. The DARC birth cohort study. Pediatr Allergy Immunol 19(8):737–745

13. Lahti A (1980) Non-immunologic contact urticaria. Acta Derm Venereol Suppl (Stockh) 91:1–49

14. Lahti A (1986) Contact urticaria to plants. Clin Dermatol 4(2):127–136

15. Liccardi G, D'Amato G, Canonica GW et al (2006) Systemic reactions from skin testing: literature review. J Investig Allergol Clin Immunol 16(2):75–78

16. Oppenheimer J, Nelson HS (2006) Skin testing. Ann Allergy Asthma Immunol 96(2 suppl):6–12

17. Oranje AP (1991) Skin provocation test (SAFT) based on contact urticaria: a marker of dermal food allergy. Curr Probl Dermatol 20:228–231

18. Oranje AP, Van Gysel D, Mulder D et al (1994) Food-induced contact urticaria syndrome (CUS) in atopic dermatitis: reproducibility of repeated and duplicate testing with skin provocation test, the skin application food test (SAFT). Contact Dermatitits 31(5):314–318

19. Osterballe M, Scheller R, Skov PS et al (2003) Diagnostic value of scratch-chamber test, skin prick test, histamine release and specific IgE in birch-allergic patients with oral allergy syndrome to apple. Allergy 58(9):950–953

20. Petersen LJ, Mosbech H, Skov PS (1996) Allergen-induced histamine release in intact human skin in vivo assessed by skin microdialysis technique: characterization of factors influencing histamine releasability. J Allergy Clin Immunol 97(2):672–679

21. Petersen LJ, Skov PS (1995) Methacholine induces wheal-and-flare reactions in human skin but does not release histamine in vivo as assessed by the skin microdialysis technique. Allergy 50(12):976–980

22. Pomés A, Butts CL, Chapman MD (2006) Quantification of Ara h 1 in peanuts: why roasting makes a difference. Clin Exp Allergy 36(6):824–830

23. Poulsen LK, Liisberg C, Bindslev-Jensen C et al (1993) Precise area determination of skin-prick tests: validation of a scanning device and software for a personal computer. Clin Exp Allergy 23(1):61–68

24. Poulsen LK (2001) In vivo and in vitro techniques to determine the biological activity of food allergens. J Chromatogr B 756:41–55

25. Romano A, Viola M, Bousquet PJ et al (2007) A comparison of the performance of two penicillin reagent kits in the diagnosis of β-lactam hypersensitivity. Allergy 62:53–58

26. Romano A, Demoly P (2007) Recent advances in the diagnosis of drug allergy. Curr Opin Allergy Clin Immunol 7:299–303

27. Tarvainen K, Jolanki R, Estlander T et al (1995) Immunologic contact urticaria du to airborne methylhexahydrophthalic and methyltetrahydrophthaltic anhydrides. Contact Dermatitis 32(4):204–209

28. Thormann H, Paulsen E (2008) Contact urticaria to common ivy (*Hedera helix* cv. 'Hester') with concomitant immediate sensitivity to the labiate family (Lamiaceae) in a Danish gardener. Contact Dermatitis 59:179–180

29. Usmani N, Wilkinson SM (2007) Allergic skin disease: investigation of both immediate- and delayed-type hypersensitivity is essential. Clin Exp Allergy 37:1541–1546

30. De Waard-van Der Spek FB, Elst EF, Mulder PG et al (1998) Diagnostic tests in children with atopic dermatitis and food allergy. Allergy 53(11):1087–1091

31. Williams PB, Nolte H, Dolen WK et al (1992) The histamine content of allergen extracts. J Allergy Clin Immunol 89(3):738–745

Photopatch Testing

29

Margarida Gonçalo

Contents

29.1 Introduction

Photopatch testing combines the techniques of two subspecialties in Dermatology, patch testing for allergic contact dermatitis and phototesting for photodermatology. Due to difficulties in having both technologies together (a patch test clinic and an UV irradiation source), or because photoallergic contact dermatitis is uncommon [1], this technique is not so widely performed. In a survey by Lehmann in the beginning of 2000, only a few dozens of clinics in Europe were performing photopatch testing and only two centres tested more than 50 patients/year [2].

Also, in photopatch testing, apart from the inherent temporal and regional variability of skin reactivity, many variables have to be dealt with: allergen concentrations and vehicles, test series and reading of test results from allergic contact dermatitis, UV source, UV spectrum, UV irradiance and UV dose reaching the skin from photodermatology, and, then, the common final interpretation of test results. Therefore, there has been some difficulty in standardizing procedures. But, photodermatologists and contact dermatologists met in Amsterdam, in 2002 and 2007, and agreed upon a consensus methodology, allergen series and interpretation of test results [2]. Also, thereafter, several studies are being performed in order to strengthen and improve this consensus methodology [3–5].

> **Core Message**
>
> › Photopatch testing is probably underused and photoallergic contact dermatitis is presumed to be uncommon.

M. Gonçalo
Clinic of Dermatology, Coimbra University Hospital,
University of Coimbra, Praceta Mota Pinto,
3000-175 Coimbra, Portugal
e-mail: mmgoncalo@netcabo.pt

J.D. Johansen et al. (eds.), *Contact Dermatitis*,
DOI: 10.1007/978-3-642-03827-3_29, © Springer-Verlag Berlin Heidelberg 2011

29.2 Indications for Performing Photopatch Tests

29.2.1 Main Indication

The primary indication for photopatch testing is to confirm a diagnosis of photoallergic contact eczema / photoallergy and find the responsible allergen. It can also contribute to distinguish photoallergic from phototoxic reactions, although this is not always easy. This distinction may be important as photoallergic reactions are usually more severe, with increasing intensity on further exposures, with the possibility of progressing to persistent photosensitivity and reactivity to cross-reactive chemicals. Therefore, recognizing and avoiding the allergen is crucial for the prognosis of the dermatitis.

Clinical manifestations of photosensitivity are very polymorphic, sometimes with difficulty in distinguishing photoallergy from phototoxicity – acute or chronic eczema, urticarial, lichenoid and pigmented reactions, erythema multiforme, exaggerated sunburn, etc. (see Chap. 18 for details). In photosensitivity from systemic agents, lesions are usually localized on a symmetrical distribution, on the face, neck, V-area of the upper chest, forearms, back of the hands and legs, whereas in photoallergic contact dermatitis, lesions occur in the areas of concomitant application of a photosensitizer and UV exposure (Fig. 29.1a, b). But there are less obvious patterns of photoallergy: the eczematous reactions, sometimes associated with targetoid lesions of erythema multiforme, can also involve some shaded areas [6]; the allergen may, inadvertently, be transported by hands to areas other than the one of primary application, as for ketoprofen (ectopic dermatitis) [6–8]; only part of the exposed skin may be involved, e.g. cheilitis as a manifestation of photoallergy from a systemic photosensitizer [9] or cheilitis and chin dermatitis from a mouth wash containing benzydamine [10]; sometimes lesions spare the area of application and occur at a distance, as in the case of hand dermatitis from using a vaginal wash containing benzydamine [11] and connubial photoallergic contact dermatitis can also occur [7, 12, 13] (Fig. 29.1a, b).

Also, the relation to sunlight exposure may not be so evident for the patient, as most reactions do not occur immediately on sun exposure, some involve non-exposed areas or have an asymmetric distribution, namely in car drivers who expose mainly one arm/forearm.

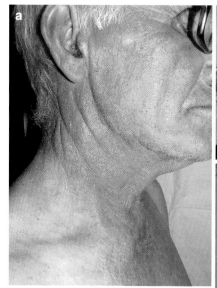
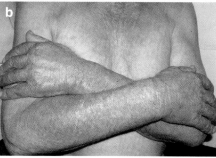
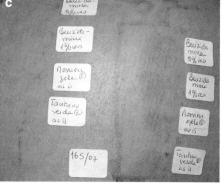

Fig. 29.1 (**a**, **b**) Chronic photoallergic contact dermatitis from benzydamine contained in Momem gele®, which the patient applied regularly to his wife. The distribution of lesions is similar to systemic photosensitivity, probably due to systemic transcutaneous absorption of the NSAID. (**c**) Positive photopatch tests to benzydamine at 1 and 5% pet. irradiated with 5 J/cm² of UVA and to the drugs containing the drug (Tantum verde® and Momem gele®) (*right side*), with negative reactions in the left, non-irradiated area

Core Message

> Photopatch testing is mainly indicated for the study of photoallergic contact dermatitis/photoallergy, but many other patients may benefit from photopatch testing.

29.2.2 Other Indications for Photopatch Testing

Apart from patients with suspected photoallergic contact eczema / photoallergy, others can also benefit from this study, namely any patient with a dermatitis that mainly affects the exposed sites (Table 29.1).

Photopatch testing may be important to distinguish an airborne allergic contact dermatitis from photosensitivity. Both involve the face, neck, V-area of the upper chest, dorsum of the hands, forearms and the legs, and even though shaded and hairy areas, e.g. upper eyelid, retroauricular folds and submandibular area, are classically spared in photosensitivity and involved in airborne dermatitis, this difference is not always so evident [7]. Also, photoallergic contact dermatitis can occur from an airborne allergen, as olaquindox, present in pig feeds [14].

Facial dermatitis, suspected to be cosmetic dermatitis, can be due to a photosensitizer in a cosmetic, e.g. UV filters, which are frequently responsible for allergic and photoallergic contact dermatitis in cosmetics

Table 29.1 Indications for performing photopatch tests

Photoallergic contact dermatitis
Photosensitive eczematous eruptions
Any dermatitis predominant on exposed sites (suspected airborne dermatitis)
Facial dermatitis (suspected cosmetic dermatitis)
Skin intolerance to sunscreens
Idiopathic photodermatosis (chronic actinic dermatitis, polymorphic light eruption) or diseases with chronic photosensitivity (atopic dermatitis, lupus erythematosus), with worsening of photosensitivity or no response to adequate therapy
Systemic drug photosensitivity
Dermatitis suspected from a phototoxic substance, when occurring with a low UV dose and slight contact

[15–18]. Facial, hair and nail cosmetics usually contain UV filters, both to prevent photoaging and skin cancer in the users and also to photostabilize the product and increase its shelf life.

UV filters, both in cosmetics and sunscreens, are the main cause of photoallergic contact dermatitis (Fig. 29.2a). Therefore, any suspicion of skin intolerance to a sunscreen deserves photopatch testing. Patients with idiopathic photodermatoses (chronic actinic dermatitis, polymorphic light eruption) or other types of chronic photosensitivity (photosensitive atopic dermatitis, lupus erythematosus) are particularly prone to develop photoallergic contact dermatitis from UV filters, as they use sunscreens daily to prevent photosensitivity [1, 16, 17]. Therefore, this is another indication to perform photopatch testing, most particularly when these patients present with an eczematous reaction or there is an unexpected cutaneous response to therapy.

In the investigation of photosensitivity, when the patient refers exposure to a known phototoxic agent, particularly if it occurs with a slight sun exposure or little contact with the phototoxic substance, photopatch testing may also reveal photoallergy. Photoallergy to psoralens can develop during PUVA therapy or from contact with plants containing psoralens [19]. These patients react to very low concentrations of psoralen (down to 0.0001%) in the photopatch test [20] or, both in the patch and photopatch test, therefore, associating both allergic and photoallergic contact dermatitis [21, 22]. Also, for known phototoxic drugs like promethazine, chlorpromazine, benzydamine, lomefloxacin and tiaprofenic acid, cases of photoallergy have been diagnosed by photopatch testing [23, 24].

In patients with photosensitivity from systemic agents, particularly drugs, photopatch testing has shown to be positive in several instances [10, 25–27], namely for piroxicam [28–32], ketoprofen and carprofen [26], fenofibrate [10, 31], lomefloxacin (Fig. 29.3) [23, 24, 33], ciprofloxacin [24], flutamide [34, 35], carbamazepine [27] and efavirenz [36], among others. Nevertheless, in this setting, photopatch tests are more frequently negative and the study has to proceed with other tests. Systemic photoprovocation (irradiation of a small area of the normal back skin with increasing doses of UVA (1–5 J/cm^2) and/or UVB after drug intake) and the determination of the minimal erythema dose (MED) in UVB and UVA, before and after exposure to the drug, can be important to confirm the participation of the drug in the photosensitive reaction [26, 37].

29

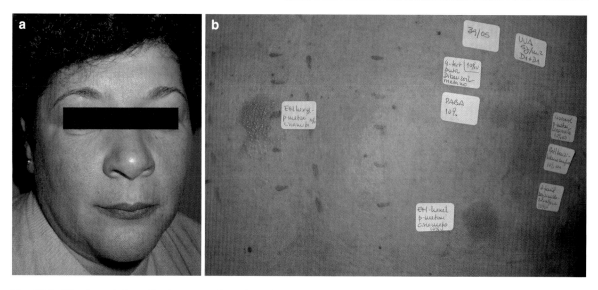

Fig. 29.2 Allergic and photoallergic contact dermatitis of the face from sunscreens (**a**), with positive patch tests to ethylhexyl methoxycinnamate (equal reaction score in the irradiated and non-irradiated areas), and positive photopatch tests to the other UV filters, namely butilmetoxydibenzoylmethane, PABA, iso-amyl-*p*-metoxycinnamate, methylbenzyliden camphor and phe-nylbenzimidazol sulphonic acid (1+ or 2+ reactions, only in the irradiated set of allergens, on the *right*) (**b**)

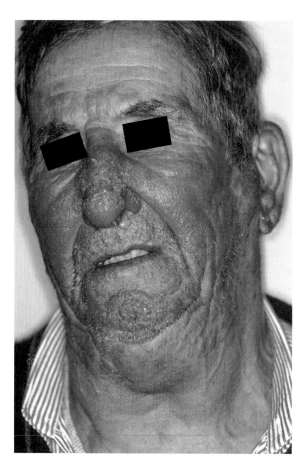

Fig. 29.3 Photoallergic reaction from oral lomefloxacin, with positive photopatch tests to lomefloxacin

Even though all these are indications for photopatch testing, this procedure is not performed very frequently; it certainly is underused, both in Europe and in the rest of the world [2, 31]. This and, eventually, a wrong choice of photoallergens may explain the presumed low prevalence of photoallergy [1, 38]. But, in a recent Italian study, photoallergic contact dermatitis represented 10% of all photodermatosis [31], which probably means that this is not such a rare problem, at least in geographical areas with high sun exposure.

29.3 Photopatch Testing Technique

29.3.1 How to Perform Photopatch Tests

A standardized amount of the allergens, diluted on the most convenient vehicle, is applied on the chambers as for patch testing, e.g. 15, 20 and 25 µL for liquids, respectively in Finn Chambers® (Epitest Ltd Oy, Tuusula, Finland), van der Bend Chambers® (van der Bend, Brielle, the Netherlands) and large IQ chambers (Chemotechnique Diagnostics, Malmö, Sweden), and 20 mg for petrolatum in 8 mm Finn Chambers®, which correspond to a string across the chamber or a small pile in the middle [39, 40]. For photopatch testing, two equal sets of allergens are prepared and applied on symmetrical areas of the back, avoiding the central vertebral groove. Occlusion is best maintained for 2 days, but the variation of results is not very significant in case patches are removed after 1 day, the usual procedure in photodermatology units as it is the time to read photo tests performed simultaneously [3].

A first reading should be performed after removing the patches to detect contact reactions present before irradiation. Then, while one set is shield from light with a UV opaque material, the other is irradiated with 5 J/cm^2 of UVA.

A reading within 30 min after irradiation should be performed, in order to detect immediate urticarial reactions.

At least one other reading should be performed 2 or 3 days after irradiation (D3/D4), to evaluate allergic reactions and detect new photoallergic reactions (Table 29.2).

29.3.2 When to Perform Photopatch Tests

Photopatch testing should be performed, whenever possible, when there are no active lesions. How long after their resolution is not known, but it is advised at least 2 weeks after stopping a local or systemic steroid [2]. If it is not possible, at least the back has to be clear of lesions, but more false positive reactions can be expected.

As that for patch testing, it is not adequate to perform photopatch testing after sunburn or after an important sun exposure on the back. The immunosuppressive effect of UV light is known for the sensitization phase of allergic contact dermatitis and although not so well studied, this effect may be extensive to the elicitation phase [41]. Therefore, due to transient modifications of the antigen presenting capacity of the skin induced by UV, it is probably advised to postpone the tests, for 3–4 weeks, after sunburn.

29.3.3 Irradiation Source and UV Dose

The dose of 5 J/cm^2 of UVA, tolerated by most individuals, including those with lower phototypes, is now consensual. Irradiation with 10 J/cm^2, or more, is responsible for more phototoxic reactions. Some photoallergic reactions occur after 1–2 J/cm^2 of UVA but false negatives might occur with this low UV dose [42].

There are several possible sources for UV irradiation, as long as the spectrum is broad-band UVA (320–400 nm), and a dose of 5 J/cm^2 delivered at the skin surface can be adequately measured. Usually fluorescent UV lamps are used, like those used for PUVA therapy (both for whole body or hand and feet irradiation). They emit a reproducible and stable-wide UVA spectrum and are easily accessible.

For regular photopatch testing monochromator is not adequate. Also, UVB lamps are not used on a regular basis. Most photopatch test results occur also with UVA, even if the photoallergen absorbs mainly in UVB, as sulfonamides and diphenhydramine [7]. Only in exceptional cases UVB irradiation was needed to prove photosensitivity, like in a case of systemic photosensitivity from ambroxol [43]. But, probably, there

Table 29.2 Timings for occlusion, irradiation and reading of photopatch tests

Procedure	D0	D1	D2	D3	D4	D5/6
A	Apply two sets of allergens		Remove allergens Irradiate UVA			
			Reading 1 (a,b)	Reading 2 (optional)	Reading 3	Reading 4 (optional)
B	Apply two sets of allergens	Remove allergens Irradiate UVA				
		Reading 1 (a,b)	Reading 2 (optional)	Reading 3	Reading 3/4	Reading 4 (optional)

Two accepted procedures, type A, used most frequently in contact dermatitis clinics and type B, mainly in photodermatology units
Reading 1 includes a reading before and another immediately after irradiation (a,b)
Reading 2 is optional. Its main interest is to distinguish crescendo from decrescendo reactions, considered respectively photoallergic and phototoxic
Reading 3 is the most important. It is usually performed at D4 (procedure A), but can be done either at D3 or D4 in procedure B
Reading 4 is optional, but could be interesting to detect late reactions and, also, to evaluate crescendo or decrescendo reactions

are not enough data on the regular photopatch testing with UVB [44].

Core Message

> Photopatch tests are irradiated with 5 J/cm^2 of UVA, or 50–75% of the MED in patients with UVA photosensitivity.

29.3.4 Photopatch Testing in Particular Cases (Immunosuppression and Photosensitivity)

It is usually advised not to test patients on immunosuppressive drugs, but it may not be possible to stop them, as in patients under immunosuppression for solid organ transplantation. Photopatch tests can be positive in this setting but, of course, more false negative reactions can be expected. If the patient is under transient treatment with corticosteroids, it is advised to wait, at least, 2 weeks after its suspension or to its reduction to a dose equivalent to10 mg prednisolone/day.

A similar problem may arise when photopatch testing HIV-positive patients with severe immunosuppression. Nevertheless, these patients still develop contact hypersensitivity reactions [45] and patch and photopatch tests can be positive independent of the CD4 count. In a recent case of efavirenz photosensitivity, photopatch tests were positive in a patient with a high number of circulating viral copies and with a very low CD4 cell count (56 CD4/μL) [36].

In these settings, a positive test can be validated, but no definite conclusion can be taken on negative photopatch tests.

When testing a UVA photosensitive patient, like a patient with chronic actinic dermatitis, it is better to evaluate the threshold of reactivity to UV beforehand, that is perform phototests to evaluate MED. Irradiation for the phototests can be done, on Day 0, simultaneous with the application of the patches. Then, after reading the phototests and determining the MED (Day1), choose only a dose of 50–75% of the MED for irradiating the photopatch tests. In the interpretation of the test results, more false positive results can be expected, as when testing patients with active lesions elsewhere.

29.4 Reading and Interpretation of Test Results

29.4.1 Timing of the Readings

Readings have, obligatorily, to be performed immediately before and after UV irradiation, and 2 or 3 days after the irradiation. Some variability on the timing of the readings is admitted and has to do with the occlusion time and, consequently, the day of irradiation (procedure A and B – see Table 29.2).

After irradiation, it would be interesting to perform readings for 3 or more consecutive days. It could evaluate the crescendo or decrescendo pattern interpreted, respectively, as a photoallergic or phototoxic pattern, but this is not practical. Moreover, this crescendo/decrescendo pattern has been questioned and is not uniformly consistent with these two mechanisms of photosensitive reactions [46].

Readings performed before and immediately after UV irradiation (D1 or, preferably D2) are necessary, respectively, to record reactions present before irradiation (contact allergy) and those that appear immediately thereafter.

The most important obligatory reading for evaluating delayed photoallergic reactions is performed 2 or 3 days after irradiation (D3, D4 or D5). This interval is necessary for the development of the T-cell-mediated hypersensitivity reaction to the new photoproduct formed during UV irradiation. In this reading, it is important to compare reactions in the irradiated and non-irradiated panel of allergens, to distinguish contact allergy (positive in both sets) from photoallergy (positive only in the irradiated set) (Table 29.3). At this time, irradiated areas contiguous to those of allergen application are used as a control for evaluating skin reactivity to UVA with no allergen. Reaction in this control area may occur in chronic actinic dermatitis or another photosensitive dermatosis or if the patient is, inadvertently, taking a systemic photosensitive drug (amiodarone, chlorpormazine or thioridazine, fluorquinolone, NSAID, fenofibrate, etc.).

29.4.2 Scoring of the Reactions

Reactions should be scored according to the International Contact Dermatitis Research Group (ICDRG), as

Table 29.3 Interpretation of photopatch test results

| Reading 1 | | Reading 2 | | Reading 3[a] | | Test results | Interpretation of positive reactions |
No UV	UVA	No UV	UVA	No UV	UVA		
–	–	–	+ to +++	–	+ to +++	+ Photopatch test	Photoallergy or phototoxicity
+	+	++	++	++	++	+ Patch test	Contact allergy
+	+	+	++ or +++	+	++ or +++	Photo-aggravated + patch test	Photo-augmented contact allergy/or allergic+photoallergic contact dermatitis
++	++	++	– or +	++	– or +	Photo-inhibition[b]	

[a]Optional
[b]The meaning of this type of reaction is not completely understood

"–" (negative), "+?" (doubtful, only with faint erythema), "+" to "+++" (faint to strongly positive reactions, namely with erythema, infiltration and possibly papules for 1+, erythema, infiltration, papules and possibly vesicles for 2+ and erythema, infiltration and coalescent vesicles or a bulla for 3+), "IR" (irritant), and NT (not tested) [2].

Core Message

> A photopatch test is positive when the reaction to the allergen occurs only in the irradiated set of allergens. Most often, on a single reading, it is not possible to distinguish definitively photoallergy from phototoxicity.

29.4.3 Interpretation of Test Results: Allergy or Photoallergy

A photopatch test is positive when it occurs only in the irradiated set of allergens. When 2+ or 3+ reactions are observed interpretation is easy, but a doubtful or weak 1+ reaction occurring only in the irradiated area can be more difficult to interpret. It can be due to the additional effect of UV irradiation on a subclinical allergic or irritant patch test [4].

When reading immediately after irradiation, an urticarial reaction to an allergen exclusively in the irradiated area can be due to immediate hypersensitivity, as in photoallergic contact urticaria, which has been described with oxybenzone [47] and chlorpromazine [48].

A transient macular erythema that regresses within 24 h, sometimes with residual hyperpigmentation, attributed to phototoxicity, occurs very occasionally with NSAIDs (benoxaprofen and tiaprofenic acid), promethazine and some UV filters [5, 46, 49, 50].

When reading 1 or more days after irradiation, if an allergen reacts on both sets of tests, with a similar intensity, this is contact dermatitis, allergic or irritant. Probably, at D2, when removing the patches, this reaction was already present (Fig. 29.2b).

When a reaction, graded as 1+ to 3+, occurs only in the irradiated set of allergens it is a positive photopatch test (Fig. 29.1c and 29.2b). A simple observation does not discriminate definitively between a phototoxic and a photoallergic reaction. In a phototoxic reaction, the test is usually more uniform, with erythema, sometimes with infiltration and with sharp limits, and tends to regress more quickly (peak intensity by 24 h), and this reaction occurs in a high percentage of individuals tested under the same circumstances. A typical photoallergic reaction is more pruritic, with papules or vesicles, which sometimes goes beyond the strict area of contact with the allergen, and tends to increase in intensity with a peak in 48 or 72 h after irradiation. Another argument to support photoallergy is the absence of this reaction in control patients and maintenance of the positive reaction with serial dilutions of the allergen and with lower UV doses of irradiation. Spongiotic dermatitis with no sunburn cells, on histology, also suggests photoallergy.

Other combinations of reactions can occur, namely negative reactions on both sides, irritant reactions on both sides, eventually with photo-augmentation (photo-augmented irritation, probably not relevant), a photo-augmented or photo-aggravated allergic contact reaction or a photo-inhibited or photo-suppressed allergic contact reaction (Table 29.3).

By definition, a photo-aggravated allergic contact reaction is considered when, in the irradiated set, it is graded with at least one "+" more than in the non-irradiated site. This can occur with contact allergens that also have some photoactive potential, like etofenamate, ketoprofen, UV filters and perfumes [7]. It can represent the association of allergic and photoallergic contact dermatitis or a photo-augmentation of contact allergy [4].

Photo-inhibition or photo-suppression, with reduction in the intensity or complete suppression of an allergic contact reaction on the irradiated site, is seldom observed. This may not be relevant or it can be due to UV-induced immunosuppression or variability of the cutaneous response in different areas of the back [4].

Also, in the interpretation of the results, it is important to have in mind a possible technical error, namely with inadvertent UV exposure in the set of allergens that was supposed to be shielded.

29.4.4 Relevance of Positive Reactions

To determine reaction relevance, a good detailed questionnaire with recent and past history has to be done very carefully with the patient. Positive reactions may explain the present dermatitis (current relevance) or be due to a past exposure, with or without lesions, representing past or old relevance or, simply, previous exposure [2].

Also, it is important to know that many photoallergens cross-react with contact allergens or other photoallergens, which can explain some positive reactions. Photoallergy to ketoprofen is associated with positive photopatch tests to other NSAIDs of the arylpropionic acid group that share the benzophenone moiety (tiaprofenic acid and suprofen), to benzophenone UV filters, mostly oxybenzone, to the UV filter octocrylene, and to the lipid lowering drug, fenofibrate [6, 8]. More frequently, these patients also have positive photopatch tests to fentichlor [51] and positive patch tests to balsam of Peru and fragrance mix I, probably due to the similarity to cinnamic aldehyde [52]. Fluorquinolones can cross-react within the group (lomefloxacin, ciprofloxacin) [23], like the phenothiazines used as neuroleptics (chloropromazine and thioridazine), topical antihistamines (promethazine) or muscle relaxants

(chlorproethazine) [53]. Positive photopatch tests to piroxicam occur in patients with previous contact allergy to thiomersal and its moiety thiosalicylic acid [10, 54]. Therefore, in the rare situations of a negative photopatch test to piroxicam and a very typical history of photoallergic contact dermatitis or systemic photoallergy from this drug, a positive patch test to thiosalicylic acid (0.1% pet.) can be a good indication that piroxicam was responsible [32, 55].

Core Message

> › The recommended Basic tray of allergens for photopatch testing has to be dynamic. At present, it is recommended to include UV filters and some NSAIDs, namely ketoprofen. Regional additions are necessary to adapt it to the population habits.

29.5 Allergens for Photopatch Testing (Basic and Additional Series)

The allergens used in photopatch testing are very different from centre to centre, but there is usually a common group of allergens responsible for most positive reactions. Therefore, for detecting the most common allergens and comparing results among centres, a recommended basic list of photoallergens should be used for regular photopatch testing [2], with the additions of regionally prevalent allergens [10, 16, 31, 56, 57] (Table 29.4).

A photoallergen basic tray of allergens has to be dynamic and subject to temporal changes (additions and removals). Along the last decades, the main allergens responsible for photoallergic contact dermatitis were identified and removed from the market, therefore, they became "historical" photoallergens and, for the moment, they have no place in a basic tray of photoallergens. These are musk ambrette, prohibited in perfumes, the UVA filter isopropyl-dibenzoylmethane, withdrawn in 1994, the antibiotic olaquindox, a swine feed additive banned, in 1998, by the European Commission [14], and the halogenated salicylanilides, removed from disinfectants and hygiene products in most countries, since 1976.

On the other hand, as new UV filters have been introduced in the market – Mexoryl SX (terephtalydene

Table 29.4 Allergens for photopatch testing, to be included in a basic tray (*) and in an extended tray for photopatch testing, according to geographical variations (⁺) and for aimed testing

INCI/INN	CAS	Vehicle
UV filters		
*Butyl methoxydibenzoylmethane/avobenzone	70356-09-1	10% pet.
*Benzophenone-3/oxybenzone	131-57-7	10% pet.
*Benzophenone-4/sulisobenzone	4065-45-6	2% pet.
*Ethylhexyl methoxycinnamate	71617-10-2	10% pet.
*Isoamyl-*p*-methoxycinnamate	71617-10-2	10% pet
*PABA/*p*-aminobenzoic acid	150-13-0	10% pet.
*Octyl dimethyl PABA	21245-02-3	10% pet.
*4-methylbenzylidene camphor	27503-81-7	10% pet.
*Phenylbenzimidazole sulfonic acid	27503-81-7	10% pet.
⁺Benzophenone-10/mexenone	1641-17-4	10% pet.
⁺Homosalate	8045-71-4	5% pet.
⁺Octyl salicylate/2-ethylhexyl salicylate	118-60-5	10% pet.
⁺Octocrylene/ethyl-hexyl-cyano-diphenylacrylate	6197-30-4	10% pet.
⁺Octyltriazone/ethylhexyl triazone	88122-99-0	10% pet.
⁺Drometrizole trisiloxane (Mexoryl XL)	155633-54-8	10% pet.
Terepthalylidene dicamphor sulphonic acid (Mexoryl SX)[a]	92761-26-7	10% H$_2$0
Bis-ethylhexyloxyphenol methoxyphenol triazine (Tinosorb S)[a]	187393-00-6	10% pet.
Methylene-*bis*-benzotriazolyl tetramethylbutylphenol(Tinosorb M)[a]	103597-45-1	10% pet.
Diethylamino hydroxybenzoyl hexyl benzoate (Uvinul A Plus)[a]	302776-68-7	10% pet.
Disodium phenyl dibenzimidazole tetrasulfonate(NeoheliopanAP)[a]	180898-37-7	10% pet.
Diethylhexyl butamido triazone (Uvasorb HEB)[a]	154702-15-5	10% pet.
Drugs		
*Ketoprofen	22161-86-0	1% pet.
⁺Diclofenac sodium	15307-79-6	5% pet.
⁺Ibuprofen	15687-27-1	5% pet.
⁺Naproxen	22204-53-1	5% pet.
⁺Etofenamate	30544-47-9	2% pet.
⁺Piroxicam	36322-90-4	1% pet.
⁺Benzydamine	642-72-8	1-5% pet.
⁺Chlorpromazine	50-53-3	0.1% pet.
⁺Promethazine	60-87-7	0.1% pet.
Other allergens		
Fentichlor	97-24-5	1% pet.
Bithionol	97-18-7	1% pet.

(continued)

Table 29.4 (continued)

INCI/INN	CAS	Vehicle
Hexachlorophene	70-30-4	1% pet.
6-Methylcoumarin	92-48-8	1% pet.
Quinine sulphate	6119-70-6	1% pet.
Diphenhydramine	58-73-1	1% pet.
"Historical" photoallergens		
Tetrachlorosalicylanilide/benzamide	1154-59-2	0.1% pet.
Tribromosalicylanilide/tribromsalan	1322-38-9	1% pet.
5-Bromochlorosalicylanilide	3679-64-9	1% pet.
Triclocarban	101-20-2	1% pet.
Olaquindox	23696-28-8	1% pet.
Musk ambrette	83-66-9	5% pet.
Isopropyl-dibenzoylmethane	63250-25-9	10% pet

INCI international nomenclature of cosmetic ingredients; *INN* international nonproprietary names; *CAS* chemical abstracts service
[a]New UV filters that may be included in a photopatch test series, mainly for research purposes

dicamphor sulfonic acid), Tinosorb M (methylene-*bis*-benzotriazolyl tetramethylbutylphenol), Tinosorb S (*bis*-ethylhexyloxyphenol methoxyphenyl triazine), Uvinul A Plus (diethylamino hydroxybenzoyl hexyl benzoate), Neoheliopan AP (disodium phenyl dibenzimidazole tetrasulfonate) and Uvasorb HEB (diethylhexyl butamido triazone), it may be adequate to add some of these molecules to a photopatch test tray [5], even though they are more photostable and, for the moment, there are no or very few references to contact dermatitis [58, 59].

29.5.1 UV Filters in the Basic and Additional Tray for Photopatch Testing

In most studies, including those from outside Europe [60, 61], UV filters are the most frequent photoallergens. In European studies they were responsible for 5.6–80% of the positive photopatch tests or photoaggravated reactions and, when considering all patients tested, positive photopatch reactions to UV filters occurred in 5.7–21.8% [10, 15, 16, 31, 56, 57, 62]. Therefore, UV filters have to be the main constituents of a photoallergen series [2, 16], even though, which ones can be a subject of discussion. It is consensual to

include, in a basic series, the following UV filters: the benzophenones, oxybenzone and sulizobenzone, the dibenzoylmethane, butyl methoxydibenzoylmethane, the cinnamates, isoamyl-*p*-methoxycinnamate and ethylhexyl methoxycinnamate, *p*-aminobenzoic acid and its analogue, octyl-dimethylPABA, 4-methylbenzylidene camphor and phenylbenzimidazole sulfonic acid. The recommended concentration for testing these molecules is 10% pet. (equal to the maximum allowed concentration for most UV filters in sunscreens), except for benzophenone 4/sulizobenzone for which 2% pet. is advised [5]. Other UV filters that have been responsible for photoallergic reactions can be tested in an extended series, namely mexenone (benzophenone 10), octocrylene, drometrizole trisiloxane, homosalate, ethylhexyl salicilate and ethyl hexyl triazone [56, 63–65]. At present, the newer UV filters are being, prospectively, evaluated in an European multicentre photopatch study to decide, whether or not, to include in a photopatch test tray. (Table 29.4)

29.5.2 Drugs in the Basic and Additional Tray for Photopatch Testing

With the wide use of topical NSAIDs and their frequent responsibility in cases of photoallergic contact dermatitis, some of them quite severe, it is also mandatory to include some of these molecules in a basic photopatch test series. The most important candidate is ketoprofen [2, 6, 8, 66, 67], which is the most frequent photoallergen in recent Italian, French and Spanish studies [31, 56, 57] and also quite frequent in Belgium and Sweden [6, 66]. Other NSAIDs, recently proposed to be included in the basic series, as naproxen, diclofenac and ibuprofen [2], are not so frequently responsible for photoallergy.

Apart from a basic series, recommended for all photopatch tests, regionally prevalent allergens should be added adequately [10, 16, 31, 56, 57]. This is the example of drugs used more frequently in some countries where they are responsible for a large number of photoallergic reactions, namely the NSAID piroxicam, used both topically and by systemic administration, in Portugal, Spain and Italy [10, 31, 57], benzydamine, used as a topical NSAID or a mouth or vaginal wash, in Portugal and Spain [10, 12, 57], the topical antihistamine, promethazine, widely used in Portugal and Greece [10, 68] or its analogue chlorproethazine, used in France as a muscle relaxant [53, 56] or the neuroleptic chlorpromazine that can induce photoallergic contact dermatitis in health care workers or relatives of patients who smash the pills before administration [10, 69].

29.5.3 Other Allergens for Photopatch Testing

Also, we must take into account the "historical" photosensitizers. Some are not available anymore, like musk ambrette and isopropyl-dibenzoylmethane, and, therefore, it is not probable that new cases of photoallergy are diagnosed. On the other hand, other "historical" photoallergens, like olaquindox and halogenated salicylanilides, are still used in countries outside Europe, and some "imported" products can be responsible for new cases of photoallergy [14]. Occasional relevant reactions are still found with other halogenated antimicrobials, like fentichlor and bithionol [31, 70], but they occur more often in patients with photoallergy from other causes, like that from ketoprofen [51, 66]. The photosensitizer, 6-methylcumarin, an ingredient of perfumes not allowed in Europe, was recently responsible for facial pigmentation in a patient

from Thailand [71]. PABA, which was frequently responsible for photoallergic contact dermatitis in the 60s and therefore was almost completely removed from sunscreens, was responsible for a recent case of photoallergic contact dermatitis from a sunscreen market in the UK until recently [72]. Therefore, these historical allergens can still be used in aimed photopatch testing.

Also, it is important to photopatch test patient's own products, namely cosmetics, sunscreens, drugs or occupational material. New or hidden photoallergens may be discovered in these products. Even though there is an increased concern on pretesting the phototoxic/photoallergic potential of new cosmetics, UV filters and drugs before the introduction in the market, there is always the chance of finding a new photoallergen.

> **Core Message**
>
> › It can be important to photopatch test with patient's own products, e.g. cosmetics, sunscreens, drugs, etc.

29.6 Conclusions

Although there is still some variation in the procedures and, particularly, in allergens used for photopatch testing, we are nearer to standardization which will allow a more regular use of this procedure and comparison of results between centres. As we have shown, the technique is not so difficult to perform and probably many more patients, than those with typical photoallergic contact dermatitis, can benefit from it.

It is important to publish regularly the results of multicentre studies to know the more prevalent photoallergens and cross-reactive substances in order to take measures to reduce their expression in the market, as has occurred with the "historical" photoallergens. Local or regional studies are also important to adapt photopatch test trays to the population that is the object of the study.

If we perform this technique more often, under standardized procedures, we may, probably, get to the conclusion that photoallergy and, particularly, photoallergic contact dermatitis, is not so uncommon.

29

References

1. Darvay A, White I, Rycroft R et al (2001) Photoallergic contact dermatitis is uncommon. Br J Dermatol 145:597–601
2. Bruynzeel D, Ferguson J, Andersen K et al (2004) Photopatch testing: a consensus methodology for Europe. J Eur Acad Dermatol Venereol 18:679–682
3. Batchelor R, Wilkinson S (2006) Photopatch testing – a retrospective review using the 1 day and 2 day irradiation protocols. Contact Dermatitis 54:75–78
4. Beattie P, Traynor N, Woods J et al (2004) Can a positive photopatch test be elicited by subclinical irritancy or allergy plus suberythemal UV exposure? Contact Dermatitis 51:235–240
5. Kerr A, Niklasson B, Dawe R et al (2009) A double-blind, randomized assessment of the irritant potential of sunscreen chemical dilutions used in photopatch testing. Contact Dermatitis 60:203–209
6. Devleeschouwer V, Roelandts R, Garmyn M, Goossens A (2008) Allergic and photoallergic contact dermatitis from ketoprofen: results of (photo) patch testing and follow-up of 42 patients. Contact Dermatitis 58:159–166
7. Goossens A (2004) Photoallergic contact dermatitis. Photoderm Photoimmunol Photomed 20:121–125
8. LeCoz C, Bottlaender A, Scrivener J et al (1998) Photocontact dermatitis from ketoprofen and tiaprofenic acid: cross-reactivity study in 12 consecutive patients. Contact Dermatitis 38:245–252
9. Due E, Wulf H (2006) Cheilitis – the only presentation of photosensitivity. J Eur Acad Dermatol Venereol 20:766–767
10. Cardoso J, Canelas M, Gonçalo M, Figueiredo A (2009) Photopatch testing with an extended series of photoallergens. A 5-year study. Contact Dermatitis 60:314–319
11. Lasa Elgezua O, Gorrotxategi P, Gardeazabal Gracia J et al (2004) Photoallergic hand eczema due to benzydamine. Eur J Dermatol 14:69–70
12. Canelas M, Cravo M, Cardoso J et al (2008) Dermatite de contacto fotoalérgica à Benzidamina – Estudo de 8 casos. Trab Soc Port Dermatol Venereol 66:35–40
13. Fernández-Jorge B, Buján J, Paradela S et al (2008) Consort contact dermatitis from piketoprofen. Contact Dermatitis 58:113–115
14. Emmert B, Schauder S, Palm H et al (2007) Disabling work-related persistent photosensitivity following photoallergic contact dermatitis from chlorpromazine and olaquindox in a pig breeder. Ann Agric Environ Med 14:329–333
15. Berne B, Ros A (1998) 7 years experience of photopatch testing with sunscreen allergens in Sweden. Contact Dermatitis 38:61–64
16. Bryden A, Moseley H, Ibbotson S et al (2006) Photopatch testing of 1115 patients: results of the U.K. multicentre photopatch study group. Brit J Dermatol 155:737–747
17. Gonçalo M, Ruas E, Figueiredo A (1995) Contact and photocontact sensitivity to sunscreens. Contact Dermatitis 33:278–280
18. Schauder S, Ippen H (1997) Contact and photocontact sensitivity to sunscreens. Review of a 15-year experience and of the literature. Contact Dermatitis 37:221–232
19. Karimian-Teherani D, Kinaciyan T, Tanew A (2008) Photoallergic contact dermatitis from Heracleum giganteum. Photoderm Photoimmunol Photomed 24:99–101
20. Ljunggren B (1977) Psoralen photoallergy caused by plant contact. Contact Dermatitis 3:85–90
21. Gonçalo S, Correia C, Couto J, Gonçalo M (1989) Contact and photocontact dermatitis from Ruta chalepensis. Contact Dermatitis 21:200–201
22. Möller H (1990) Contact and photocontact allergy to psoralens. Photoderm Photoimmunol Photomed 7:43–44
23. Oliveira H, Gonçalo M, Figueiredo A (1996) Photosensitivity from lomefloxacine. A clinical and photobiological study. Photoderm Photoimmunol Photomedicine 16:116–120
24. Kimura M, Kawada A (1998) Photosensitivity induced by lomefloxacin with cross-photosensitivity to ciprofloxacin and fleroxacin. Contact Dermatitis 38:130
25. Barbaud A, Gonçalo M, Bircher A, Bruynzeel D (2001) Guidelines for performing skin tests with drugs in the investigation of cutaneous adverse drug reactions. Contact Dermatitis 45:321–328
26. Gonçalo M (1998) Explorations dans les photo-allergies médicamenteuses. In: GERDA (eds) Progrès en Dermato-Allergologie. John Libbey Eurotext, Nancy, pp 67–74
27. Lee A, Joo H, Chey W, Kim Y (2001) Photopatch testing in seven cases of photosensitive drug eruptions. Ann Pharmacother 35:1584–1587
28. Gonçalo M, Figueiredo A, Tavares P et al (1992) Photosensitivity to piroxicam: absence of cross-reaction with tenoxicam. Contact Dermatitis 27:287–290
29. Varela P, Amorim I, Massa A et al (1998) Piroxicam-beta-cyclodextrin and photosensitivity reactions. Contact Dermatitis 38:229
30. Barbaud A, Reichert-Penetrat S, Tréchot P et al (1998) The use of skin testing in the investigation of cutaneous adverse drug reactions. Br J Dermatol 139:49–58
31. Pigatto P, Guzzi G, Schena D et al (2008) Photopatch tests: an Italian multicentre study from 2004 to 2006. Contact Dermatitis 59(2):103–108
32. Serra D, Gonçalo M, Figueiredo A (2008) Two decades of cutaneous adverse drug reactions from piroxicam. Contact Dermatitis 58:35
33. Kurumajin Y, Shono M (1992) Scarified photopatch testing in lomefloxacin photosensitivity. Contact Dermatitis 26:5–10
34. Gonçalo M, Domingues J, Correia O, Figueiredo A (1999) Fotossensibilidad a flutamida. Boletim Informativo del GEIDC 29:45–48
35. Vilaplana J, Romaguera C, Azón A, Lecha M (1990) Flutamide photosensitivity-residual vitiliginous lesions. Contact Dermatitis 38:68–70
36. Yoshimoto E, Konishi M, Takahashi K et al (2004) The first case of efavirenz-induced photosensitivity in a Japanese patient with HIV infection. Intern Med 43:630–631
37. Murphy G (2004) Investigation of photosensitive disorders. Photoderm Photoimmunol Photomed 20:305–311
38. Zeeli T, David M, Trattner A (2006) Photopatch tests: any news under the sun? Contact Dermatitis 55:305–307
39. Shaw D, Zhai H, Maibach H, Niklasson B (2002) Dosage considerations in patch testing with liquid allergens. Contact Dermatitis 47:86–90
40. Bruze M, Isaksson M, Gruvberger B, Frick-Engfeldt M (2007) Recommendation of appropriate amounts of petrolatum preparation to be applied at patch testing. Contact Dermatitis 56:281–285

41. Stoebner P, Rahmoun M, Ferrand C et al (2006) A single sub-erythematous exposure of solar-simulated radiation on the elicitation phase of contact hypersensitivity induces IL-10-producing T-regulatory cells in human skin. Exp Dermatol 15:615–624

42. Duguid C, O'Sullivan D, Murphy G (1993) Determination of threshold UV-A elicitation dose in photopatch testing. Contact Dermatitis 29:192–194

43. Fujimoto N, Danno K, Wakabayashi M et al (2009) Photosensitivity with eosinophilia due to ambroxol and UVB. Contact Dermatitis 60:110–113

44. Avenel-Audrun M (2009) Photopatch testing. Ann Dermatol Vénéreol 136:626–629

45. Curr N, Nixon R (2006) Allergic contact dermatitis to basic red 46 occurring in an HIV-positive patient. Australas J Dermatol 47:195–197

46. Neumann N, Holzle E, Lehmann P et al (1994) Patterns analysis of photopatch test reactions. Photoderm Photoimmunol Photomed 16:65–73

47. Collins P, Ferguson J (1994) Photoallergic contact dermatitis to oxybenzone. Br J Dermatol 131:124–129

48. Lovell C, Cronin E, Rhodes E (1986) Photocontact urticaria from chlorpromazine. Contact Dermatitis 14:290–291

49. Gonçalo M, Figueiredo A (1992) Photopatch testing with non-steroidal anti-inflammatory drugs. In: Proceedings of the First European Symposium of Contact Dermatitis, Brussels, pp 25

50. Neumann N, Holzle E, Plewig G et al (2000) Photopatch testing: the 12-year experience of the german, austrian and swiss photopatch test group. J Am Acad Dermatol 42:183–192

51. Durbize E, Vigan M, Puzenat E et al (2003) Spectrum of cross-photosensitization in 18 consecutive patients with contact photoallergy to ketoprofen: associated photoallergies to non-benzophenone-containing molecules. Contact Dermatitis 48:144–149

52. Pigatto P, Bigardi A, Legori A et al (1996) Cross reactions in patch testing and photopatch testing with ketoprofen, tiaprofenic acid and cinnamic aldehyde. Am J Contact Dermatitis 7:220–223

53. Barbaud A, Collet E, Martin S et al (2001) Contact sensitization to chlorproéthazine can induce persistent light reaction and cross photoreactions to other phenothiazines. Contact Dermatitis 44:373

54. Hariva T, Kitamura K, Osawa J, Ikezawa Z (1993) A cross-reaction between piroxicam-photosensitivity and thiosalicylate hypersensitivity in lymphocyte proliferation test. J Dermatol Sci 5:165–174

55. Gonçalo M, Figueiredo A, Gonçalo S (1996) Hypersensitivity to thimerosal: the sensitizing moiety. Contact Dermatitis 34: 201–203

56. Leonard F, Adamski H, Bonnevalle A et al (2005) Étude prospective multicentrique 1991-2001 de la batterie standard des photopatch-tests de la Société Française de Photodermatologie. Ann Dermatol Vénéreol 132:313–320

57. La Cuadra-Oyanguren J, Pérez-Ferriols A, Lecha-Carralero M et al (2007) Resultdos y evaluación del fotoparche en España: hacia una nueva batería estándar de fotoalergenos. Actas Dermosifiliogr 98:96–101

58. Andersen K, Goossens A (2006) Decyl glucoside contact allergy from a sunscreen product. Contact Dermatitis 54: 349–350

59. Andrade P, Gonçalo M, Figueiredo A (2010) Allergic contact dermatitis to decyl glucoside in Tinosorb M. Contact Dermatitis 62:119–120

60. Rodríguez E, Valbuena M, Rey M, Porras de Quintana L (2006) Causal agents of photoallergic contact dermatitis diagnosed in the national institute of dermatology of Colombia. Photoderm Photoimmunol Photomed 22:189–192

61. Scalf L, Davis M, Rohlinger A, Connolly S (2009) Photopatch testing of 182 patients: a 6-year experience at the Mayo Clinic. Dermatitis 20:44–52

62. Bakkum R, Heule F (2002) Results of photopatch testing in Rotterdam during a 10-year period. Br J Dermatol 146: 275–279

63. Singh M, Beck M (2007) Octyl salicylate: a new contact sensitivity. Contact Dermatitis 56:48

64. Madan V, Beck M (2005) Contact allergy to octocrylene in sunscreen with recurrence from passive transfer of a cosmetic. Contact Dermatitis 53:241–242

65. Torres V, Correia T (1991) Contact and photocontact allergy to oxybenzone and mexenone. Contact Dermatitis 25:126–127

66. Hindsén M, Zimerson E, Bruze M (2006) Photoallergic contact dermatitis from ketoprofen in Southern Sweden. Contact Dermatitis 54:150–157

67. Diaz R, Gardeazabal J, Manrique P et al (2006) Greater allergenicity of topical ketoprofen in contact dermatitis confirmed by use. Contact Dermatitis 54:239–243

68. Katsarou A, Makris M, Zarafonitis G et al (2008) Photoallergic contact dermatitis: the 15-year experience of a tertiary reference center in a sunny Mediterranean city. Int J Immunopathol Pharmacol 21:725–727

69. Horio T (1975) Chlorpromazine photoallergy. Coexistence of immediate and delayed type. Arch Dermatol 111: 1469–1471

70. Jeanmougin M, Menciet J, Dubertret L (1992) Contact fentichlor photoallergy from soap for handwashing. Ann Dermatol Vénéreol 119:983–985

71. Vachiramon V, Wattanakrai P (2005) Photoallergic contact sensitization to 6-methylcoumarin in poikiloderma of Civatte. Dermatitis 16:136–138

72. Waters A, Sandhu D, Lowe G, Ferguson J (2009) Photocontact allergy to PABA: the need for continous vigilance. Contact Dermatitis 60(3):172–173

Noninvasive Techniques for Quantification of Contact Dermatitis

30

Jørgen Serup

Contents

30.1 Introduction

History and clinical examination are the main tools of clinical dermatologists. Inspection of the skin is rapid, and the lateral extension and severity of a dermatitis are easily assessed. The disadvantage is that this method is, essentially, subjective. As a research tool, it is open to bias and is, thus, difficult to use. With punch biopsy and microscopy, detailed information about the layers of the skin and their involvement with dermatitis is obtained; however, a punch usually represents only a very small fraction of diseased skin, and processing and staining are a kind of desirable artifact. The result still has a subjective element, which is related to the pathologist's examination.

Information and knowledge are not simply a matter of high magnification and fine detail. In the dermatological armamentarium, there is an area between clinical evaluation and sophisticated technique, where noninvasive bioengineering techniques may be relevant. Bioengineering techniques offer (1) noninvasiveness and in vivo information, with instant results; (2) objective assessment (quantitation or imaging as a basis for computerized analysis); (3) choice of body region and site of examination, with only a few limitations, depending on technique; and (4) the same site can be studied by different techniques, and follow-up examinations can be performed to study the spontaneous course and effect of treatment, without interfering with the subject being studied.

30.2 Prerequisites and Planning of Study by Noninvasive Techniques

Various devices for the noninvasive evaluation of the skin have become available. It is straightforward to put a probe on the skin and get a reading on a digital

J. Serup
Department of Dermatology D41, Bispebjerg Hospital,
2400 Copenhagen, NV, Denmark
e-mail: JS16@bbh.hosp.dk

J.D. Johansen et al. (eds.), *Contact Dermatitis*,
DOI: 10.1007/978-3-642-03827-3_30, © Springer-Verlag Berlin Heidelberg 2011

30

display. Generally, variation and inconclusiveness are more likely to be attributable to the way in which devices are used, rather than to inaccuracy of the equipment. Before a study based on bioengineering methods is conducted, the essentials of the method need to be known, and a number of questions must be asked. These include the following:

> What information is expected?
> What is the most relevant variable to be measured, and which variables serve for description, comparison, support, or exclusion?
> What is the expected time course of variables, and when should measurements be performed?
> Are variables expected to develop linearly or not?
> What are the ranges of variables in relation to the expected phenomenon or structure being studied, including interindividual and intraindividual variation and dependence of anatomical site, sex, and age?
> What function or structure is actually being tested?
> What is the measuring area, and if small, should more recordings be taken and averaged to overcome local site variation?
> Are recordings with the equipment reproducible, and is the accuracy acceptable relative to variables being measured and their expected range?
> What are the measuring standards and calibration procedures?
> Are there environmental standards and calibration procedures?
> Are there environmental influences, including season, and a need for special laboratory room facilities?
> Is preconditioning of the individual necessary before testing?
> What precludes measurements from being performed?
> Does the researcher or technician have both the training and sufficient practical experience to conduct the study?

As in any other research field, the results depend essentially on the ratio between signal and noise, where noise means sources of variation, some predictable and others unknown. At the moment, the success of studies based on noninvasive techniques depends mainly on the training of the researcher and appropriate planning, with an emphasis on proper control of predictable sources of variation.

30.3 Review of Noninvasive Techniques Relevant to the Study of Contact Dermatitis

The essentials of skin structure and function as a basis for bioengineering studies were reviewed in the past by Frosch and Kligman [1] and more recently by Goldsmith [2] and Serup and Jemec [3]. Various monographs about bioengineering methods and their technical principles and applications have appeared [3–7]. Previously, bioengineering and the patch test were summarized [8].

Several noninvasive techniques were used in the past to study contact dermatitis, often prototypes or laboratory equipment. Some techniques, such as polysulfide rubber replica, are simple and can be used directly, while others are complicated, and validation, multiplication, and commercialization are needed before they can attract general interest. This introduction deals mainly with techniques that are available and can be practiced in a variety of laboratories.

30.3.1 Changes in the Skin Surface

A change of color and skin surface is central to the visual assessment of contact dermatitis. The color of the skin, including erythema, can be measured by two different principles: (1) spectrophotometric scanning, using wavelengths of 400–800 nm and measurements of absorbency and reflectance; and (2) tristimulus analysis of reflected flash light. Spectrophotometric scanning has proven to be of little practical use because the broad melanin absorption band overlaps with the hemoglobin band, and because nonspecific optical phenomena of the skin, related to scaling and scattering, influence recordings significantly.

However, devices that measure the hemoglobin band specifically and express erythema as an index of hemoglobin relative to melanin have appeared; if they are of technically high precision, these devices are useful [9].

The alinear perception of color by the human eye and brain is in the range 400–800 nm, with the most sensitive range of detection being between 500 and 600 nm, corresponding to the color of blood and, therefore, redness. Equipment based on tristimulus analysis of reflected light and the Commission International d'Eclairage

(CIE) takes this alinearity of the eye into account and expresses any color in a three-dimensional system (Fig. 30.1), with green–red ($a*$), yellow–blue ($b*$), and L axes, where $L*$ expresses brightness [10]. In erythema, $a*$ increases, $L*$ decreases, and $b*$ is unaltered [11]. Tristimulus devices are convenient and rapid to operate.

The contour of the skin surface, with scales, papules, vesicles, etc., can be studied by clinical photography and various replica techniques. The main difficulty of close-up photography is that the flashgun light, after scattering within the skin, is reflected back to the camera lens from different layers of the skin with different microstructures and under different angles from the same structure. Skin surface pictures become much sharper if the surface is coated and transmission and scattering are eliminated. If immersion oil is applied and the optical effects of the surface are thus eliminated, dermal structures, such as blood vessels, may be seen. Reflections from the surface may also be avoided by using polarized light. In clinical photography, the film and copy process are also subject to variation between batches, with significant influences on the photograph [12]. Today, digital photography is taking over. This allows sophisticated image analysis of color and surface structures of clinical relevance. Using polysulfide rubber imprint material, 30° incident light, and a stereomicroscope surface, the finer details are clearly illustrated,

since the flexible rubber material is not transparent. Replicas are cheap and simple and can be stored and evaluated blind and in batches under routine laboratory conditions. Replicas can also be used as a basis for advanced quantification by the stylus method and computerized image analysis [13]. A tape method, representing a development of the sticky slide technique for harvesting stratum corneum material, is commonly employed. This is useful for quantitative evaluation of the scaling and hyperkeratosis of dermatitis [14].

30.3.2 Epidermal Hydration and Water Barrier Function

Although invisible, the water barrier of the skin is very often damaged in dermatitis, affecting the biology of the epidermis and the clinical manifestations. Hydration of the skin surface can be measured by electrical methods [15, 16]. The construction of the detector and the technical specifications determine the layer of the epidermis that is measured. The contour of the skin and the size and shape of the detector determine the electrical contact and influence the results. If the detector is small, more measurements need to be taken and averaged to minimize local site variation. The conductance measurer described by Tagami [16] measures very superficially, and the Corneometer of Courage and Khazaka, based on electrical capacitance, is able to measure more deeply in the epidermis [17, 18]. The compartment of the epidermis that is able to bind water is only small, and diffusional equilibrium between stratum corneum and ambient air takes place quickly, i.e., within 10 min [19]. Following occlusion, the biology of the epidermis changes, and equilibrium with ambient air takes longer, i.e., after 24 h of occlusion, 30 min, or longer. Thus, when skin surface hydration is being measured, the skin should be uncovered for a predetermined period before the recordings. The temperature and humidity of the laboratory also need to be kept within certain limits.

The parameter of transepidermal water loss (TEWL) expresses diffusional water loss through the skin and is of major importance in irritant reactions to detergents. Various closed-chamber methods have been used in the past; however, these were cumbersome and interfered with the spontaneous TEWL parameter. The method of open-chamber water vapor evaporation and gradient estimation, as described by Nilsson [20] and

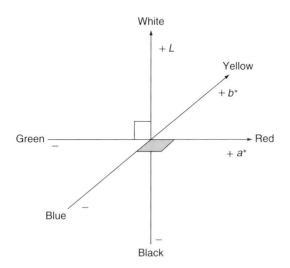

Fig. 30.1 The Commission International d'Eclairage (*CIE*) color system, which is essentially constructed to substitute for the human eye, taking the alinearity of color perception into account. Each color has its position in a three-dimensional coordinate system, with two horizontal axes for color and a vertical axis for brightness

30

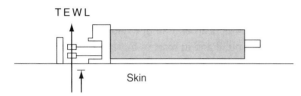

TEWL

Skin

Fig. 30.2 Open-chamber probe for the measurement of the TEWL. Pairs of sensors (hygrosensors coupled with thermistors) mounted in the chamber at different levels above the skin for the determination of the humidity gradient in the chamber, representing the flux of water out of the skin, or the TEWL

Spencer [21], is widely used. The water vapor pressure gradient is measured with sensors (Fig. 30.2) at two different levels above the skin, and then the TEWL is calculated [20, 21]. Proper preconditioning and good control of the measuring conditions are essential for accurate recordings. Sources of variation were reviewed and guidelines were given by the standardization group of the European Society of Contact Dermatitis (ESCD) [22]. The water barrier of the skin does not resemble a filter or membrane within the skin, but, instead, a gradient across the skin, including a 10-mm layer of ambient air. Thus, the environment is part of the water barrier, and changes in temperature and humidity influence the passage of water out of the skin, and also the skin surface's hydration. Eccrine sweating is, in most body regions, less important, except after physical activity, when it has the capacity to increase manifold. Environmental changes related to the seasons also need to be considered [23].

dermatitis is to image lateral temperature gradients, which may give detailed information about inflammation and crusting of patch test reactions [7, 24, 25].

The *vasodilatation* of inflammation and the increase in blood flow are often measured by laser Doppler flowmetry [6]. A variety of equipment is available. The tone of the cutaneous vasculature is normally in a relatively contracted condition, and it may be difficult to monitor vasoconstriction, such as blanching, due to corticosteroids. A 30-fold increase in flow may be seen in dermatitis; however, in advanced inflammation, the edema may compress vessels, and the degree of inflammatory activity may be underestimated. As compared with other methods, laser Doppler flowmetry is both sensitive and discriminative. Recently, laser Doppler scanners have been developed. With this method, the mapping of, for example, the hyperperfusion of a patch reaction is possible (Fig. 30.3). Site variation in patch test reactions is major. With the scanner, the average hyperperfusion is easily calculated. The vasculature and its tone are in a state of dynamic balance, and factors such as mental stress and noise instantly influence the flow. Thus, both preconditioning and measuring conditions need to be considered.

Measurement of the *edema* of inflammatory reactions may be carried out with skin-fold calipers and high-frequency ultrasound (Fig. 30.4). Calipers inevitably compress the edema, and it is unclear what layer of the skin is being included in the fold and measured. With ultrasound, high frequency and broad bandwidth are

30.3.3 Parameters of Inflammation

Vasodilatation and edema formation are the essential features of inflammation. Blood flow has been extensively studied, while edema formation has been comparatively overlooked.

The use of the skin surface's temperature as a measure of inflammatory activity is more or less obsolete in contact dermatitis. In normal skin, the temperature varies within narrow limits. In dermatitis, vasodilatation tends to increase the temperature toward the core temperature, but evaporation, crusting, and scaling tend to decrease the temperature. Skin surface temperature can be measured by contact methods, including cholesteric crystal sheets, and by infrared nontouch methods. The main application of contact thermography in contact

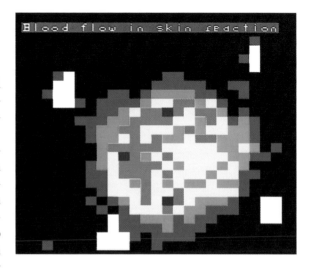

Fig. 30.3 Laser Doppler scanning. Irritant reaction to sodium lauryl sulfate (*SLS*). *Red* is high perfusion, *blue* is low. *White pixels* represent markings made on the skin with black ink

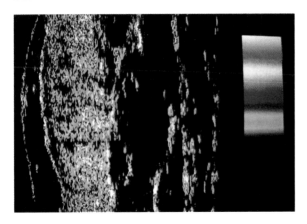

Fig. 30.4 High-frequency B-mode scanning of a 2+ allergic reaction to nickel, obtained with Dermascan C. A plastic membrane from the probe chamber is seen over the skin. Underneath the epidermis, an echolucent band of edema formation appears, with projections along the hair follicles and sebaceous glands. *White* and *blue* represent strong ultrasound reflections, *yellow* and *red* moderate, and *green* weak reflections. Subcutaneous fat is minimally echogenic and is shown in *black*, as is the coupling medium between the ultrasound transducer and the skin surface with the plastic membrane

needed. Transducers of 20 MHz have provided a good compromise between the needs of resolution and depth of the viewing field. With A-mode scanners, the thickness of dermatitis skin can be measured and the increase in thickness representing the edema formation calculated [26]. With B-mode and C-mode scanners, cross-sectional imaging of the skin is possible [27]. In vivo distances, areas, volume, and structure analysis are possible with the use of computerized analysis. Ultrasound shows that inflammatory edema develops mainly in the papillary dermis, where it propagates and results in an echolucent band, which can be measured and followed during the different stages of the inflammatory process (Fig. 30.4). Education and training are needed in order to perform ultrasound examination, as in any other specialty. Generally, methods assessing static features, such as structure and dimension, are less vulnerable to measuring conditions and are easier to standardize compared to methods based on functions.

30.4 Allergic Contact Dermatitis

Erythema, edema, papules, and vesicles are the well-known manifestations of acute allergic contact dermatitis that are read in diagnostic patch testing. Using noninvasive techniques, the same manifestations can be quantified. In strong reactions, bullae, erosions, and crusts may appear. Once elicited, it is held that the cascade of events follows essentially the same course. In the chronic-stage, hyperkeratosis and scaling are often prominent. Unlike the situation in irritant contact dermatitis, allergic reactions have been relatively seldom studied by noninvasive techniques in the past.

Study of the skin surface contour by polysulfide rubber replica shows that counts of papules and vesicles correlate with clinical readings, and doubtful reactions may be divided into those with sporadic papules and those without, but with an impression from the margin of the test chamber instead [28].

Studies of skin color and allergic contact dermatitis have not appeared. It is likely that weak and moderate reactions can be ranked, but in strong reactions, changes of the physical character of the skin surface are likely to influence the optical properties and create variation.

Epidermal hydration and TEWL depend very much on the clinical state of the dermatitis. In chronic dermatitis with scaling, the conductance is decreased due to a reduced water-binding capacity, in contrast to TEWL, which is increased [29]. The value of conductance measurements seems to lie not in the grading of early-stage dermatitis, but in the assessment of chronic stages and documentation of healing. Decreased conductance and increased TEWL are very common in long-lasting dermatitis, irrespective of its origin. Nevertheless, increased TEWL is not a primary event in allergic reactions; rather, the water barrier becomes progressively damaged during the first few days, as inflammation develops [30].

The surface temperature of acute allergic reactions is increased; however, if vesicles and bullae leaving crusts appear, the temperature pattern of the surface may be irregular, with decreased temperature corresponding to the crusts [24, 25, 31]. Increased temperature may persist for a period after visible changes have disappeared [7].

Allergic reactions to nickel show increased blood flow as measured by laser Doppler flowmetry, and positive, doubtful, and negative reactions can be distinguished [32]. However, the positive reactions may be difficult to rank. Probably, the inflammatory response has an initial stage dominated by vasodilation and a more advanced stage dominated by edema formation, which compresses the vasculature. Allergic patch test reactions and irritant reactions to sodium lauryl sulfate (SLS) show an increase of blood flow at the same level [33].

30

Ultrasound measurement of skin thickness and the edema of allergic patch test reactions show progressive thickening of the skin as the clinical reaction increases [26, 27, 34]. With ultrasound, strong reactions can also be graded. The edema formation of allergic reactions is more severe as compared with irritant reactions after SLS, matched with respect to the strength of the reactions clinically [26]. With ultrasound B-mode scanning, an echolucent band is seen in the papillary dermis immediately underneath the epidermis, representing more advanced edema and swelling of the outer dermis (Fig. 30.4) [27]. It is a general feature that the inflammation of contact dermatitis involves mainly the papillary dermis, which is more easily distended than the reticular dermis under the influence of the pressure of edema. Such changes cannot be evaluated by routine histology, since histological processing is highly intrusive to tissue water, which is extracted and replaced by lipophilic media prior to embedding in paraffin.

30.5 Irritant Contact Dermatitis

Irritant contact dermatitis is not a uniform disease entity; each irritant exerts its particular noxious effects on the skin, and each occupation has its special set of risk substances and mode of physical contact [35]. Obviously, this creates diversity in the manifestations of irritancy and the way in which it is best assessed. Moreover, reactions are dependent on age, body region, menstrual phase, skin complexion, and skin type, including sensitivity to sunlight, etc. Thus, control of a great number of variables is a prerequisite.

A number of substances and test procedures were evaluated in the past by Björnberg [36] and more recently by Frosch [37]. Monographs on irritant contact dermatitis and TEWL have been published by van der Valk [38], Pinnagoda [39], and Tupker [40]. Irritancy and laser Doppler flowmetry were studied by de Boer [41], and Agner has studied irritancy by various methods, including replica, thermography, TEWL, laser Doppler flowmetry, colorimetry, high-frequency ultrasound, and conductance [42].

The change in color in the direction of redness as elicited by the irritant SLS is characterized by an increase in a^*, a minor decrease in L^*, and unchanged b^*, as measured according to the CIE system [11]. Colorimeters based on the CIE system and tristimulus color analysis are especially suited to a busy routine and for situations in which preconditioning is difficult.

Colorimetry appears accurate for the distinction of positive reactions from negative reactions; however, colorimetry is less precise for a more differentiated ranking of redness, depending on the irritant being studied [42, 43]. A major reason why the grading of redness can be difficult is that the vasodilatation of inflammation, as mentioned above, does not run linearly, but fades out as the edema progresses. Moreover, microanatomical changes in the skin surface of strong reactions influence the optical properties of the skin nonspecifically, with consequences for the measurement of color. In chronic dermatitis, hyperkeratosis and scaling may influence colorimeter measurements.

The skin surface contour changes depending on the irritant and the time of examination, as demonstrated by studies with polysulfide rubber replica [44]. SLS has become the preferred experimental irritant. Some irritants induce a papular pattern, and others, a nonpapular pattern. Propanol, which is used as a vehicle for nonanoic acid, is itself irritant and changes the skin relief.

The skin surface hydration of irritant contact dermatitis is the result of damage to the cutaneous water barrier induced by the irritant on the one hand, resulting in increased water vapor pressure in and over the stratum corneum, and by the formation of crusts, hyperkeratosis, and scales on the other, resulting in reduced water-binding capacity and decreased stratum corneum hydration. Already in the acute stage of dermatitis, most irritants exert a noxious effect, with a decrease of electrical conductance and capacitance, depending on the specific irritant and its ability to coagulate the skin surface, while increased hydration is found only in some individuals and mainly from the detergent SLS [18]. In chronic-stage contact dermatitis, the electrical measurements are decreased almost without exception [29]. Due to the variable structure and pathophysiology of acute irritant reactions, electrical methods have not been found to be very useful for the grading of irritancy [43].

Measurement of the TEWL and the damage to the water barrier have proven to be important for the characterization of irritant effects on skin elicited by detergents [38–40, 42]. Studies using mainly SLS as a model detergent have demonstrated that the TEWL measurement is more accurate than other methods, such as laser Doppler flowmetry, colorimetry, and ultrasound, for the grading of this irritant [39, 40, 42, 43, 45]. Impairment of the water barrier and increase of the TEWL are found not only in the acute stage of dermatitis, but also in chronic stages, with hyperkeratosis and scaling [29]. The difficulty with TEWL is that a number of prerequisites with respect to preconditioning and laboratory conditions need to be fulfilled for measurements to be accurate, as described by the standardization group [21]. It must be stressed again that different irritants act differently on the skin, and experiences obtained with detergents cannot be uncritically extended to any other substance [35, 44, 45]. The use of TEWL to detect sensitive skin and predict the occupational risk of irritant contact dermatitis is described below.

Skin-surface temperature, as mentioned above, is not an accurate measure of the inflammatory activity of irritant contact dermatitis. However, thermographic imaging of skin-surface temperature gradients demonstrates that some reactions to irritants are cold, due to the formation of a temperature-insulating crusting, while others are warm [24, 25, 31]. Different skin-surface temperature patterns appear during the course of irritant reactions, and such patterns may be followed using thermographic methods and compared with allergic reactions.

Laser Doppler flowmetry has been used extensively for the evaluation of irritant contact dermatitis [41, 42, 46]. Experiments with SLS and laser Doppler flowmetry have demonstrated a dose-response relationship [41–43, 45, 46], and the method has proven to be valuable for the quantification of irritant reactions and their inflammatory component. In the evaluation of reactions elicited by SLS, laser Doppler flowmetry with monochannel equipment is less accurate than TEWL and ultrasound measurements [43, 45]. However, with modern laser scanners, the precision is substantially improved (Fig. 30.3). As noted above, the edema of strong reactions may compress the vasculature and influence the flow. Also, changes in the skin surface, such as vesicles, bullae, crusts, hyperkeratosis, and scaling, may influence the optics of the skin and the laser signal. Using probes covering a small surface area only, averaging of three or more recordings is necessary to overcome local site variation in the cutaneous blood supply. The laser Doppler method registers the total blood flow, and recordings are easily influenced by the measuring conditions, such as talking, breathing, noise, and mental stress. Thus, preconditioning and laboratory conditions need to be carefully controlled.

30.5.1 Edema

High-frequency (20 MHz) ultrasound measurement of skin thickening and edema formation has been used in numerous studies of SLS irritant reactions [26, 27, 42,

43, 45], and a dose-response relationship has been demonstrated. For the evaluation of SLS reactions in which damage of the water barrier is prominent, ultrasound has a level of accuracy in between those of TEWL and laser Doppler flowmetry [43, 45]. In types of reactions with less pronounced damage to the water barrier, ultrasound is probably more accurate. The cross-sectional ultrasound image of contact dermatitis has been relatively seldom studied to date. However, inflammatory edema of the skin does not expand it in a uniform way. Edema extends mainly in the more soft and pliable papillary dermis, and an echolucent band is seen by ultrasound [27]. Ultrasound has the advantage in that structure is studied, and preconditioning and laboratory conditions are, therefore, not critical. Its disadvantage is that training in this special technique is necessary.

30.5.2 Sensitive Skin and Hyperirritable Skin

During his or her lifetime, almost every person experiences a dermatitis on some occasion, and skin sensitivity represents a spectrum of reactivity. On the basis of reactivity to SLS, Frosch and Kligman defined a group of people who suffer more constantly from irritant contact dermatitis [47]. A skin type with high basal TEWL reacts more strongly to SLS, and this may be used to predict occupational risk [39, 40, 42, 48], although prognostic and epidemiological studies gave no convincing confirmation of this. Sensitive skin was also found to be more sensitive to light; more fair, with a higher L^* and lower b^* according to colorimetry, and thinner, according to ultrasound. These findings may indicate a more profound structural and functional inferiority of sensitive skin, including deviations in both the epidermis and the dermis [42, 49]. However, skin sensitivity is not simply a constant, but it also changes with age, menstrual cycle, season of the year, etc. – factors which interfere and overlap, and may occasionally create the preconditions for an irritant contact dermatitis to appear [23, 50]. All of these variables need to be taken into account whenever skin sensitivity is evaluated by noninvasive techniques, and when the determination of risk factors or dynamic testing by provocation with a standard noxious agent, such as SLS, is performed.

Patients with active hand dermatitis and young patients with atopic dermatitis have hyperirritable skin and react more strongly to SLS, while reactivity in chronic or healed eczema and in adult atopy and hand

30

dermatitis is normal [51–53]. Thus, whenever groups of patients are studied by noninvasive techniques, they need to be clearly defined clinically. Extensive guidelines on provocative and sensibility testing with SLS were published by the standardization group of the ESCD [54].

30.6 Urticarial Wheals

Wheals or hives are very dynamic lesions with rapid changes during the initial 30 min when a triple response develops (Fig. 30.5). Thus, in the measurement of

wheals, the timing of the recordings needs to be precise and relevant.

Laser Doppler flowmetry of wheals shows an increase of blood flow in both the center and the flare of the wheal. The edema formation interferes with the vasculature, and measurements in the flare are more suitable for the distinction of the strength of the reaction after different concentrations of histamine [55, 56].

Ultrasound examination of histamine wheals shows that the wheal is initially globoid, and at a diameter of about 5 mm, it extends laterally in the skin and becomes more flat [27, 57]. With ultrasound, the thickness and volume of wheals can be measured.

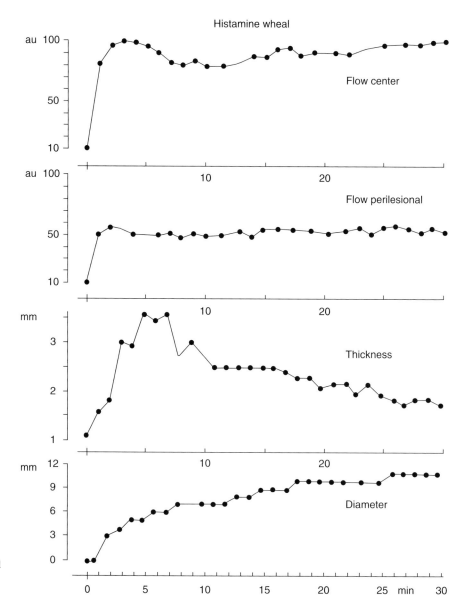

Fig. 30.5 Histamine wheal followed for 30 min with laser Doppler flowmetry (center and perilesional flare), ultrasound measurement of wheal thickness, and measurement of mean diameter

Ultrasound cross-sectional imaging shows that the edema of wheal reactions propagates mainly laterally in the skin of the papillary dermis, which is more easily distended [27]. At the same time, this explains the formation of pseudopodia. Van Neste developed the noninvasive measurement of wheal reactions into a useful method for the quantification of the effect of antihistamines [56, 58–60].

Wheal reactions to dimethylsulfoxide have been studied by TEWL, conductance, ultrasound skin thickness, and laser Doppler measurements, and all the methods were concluded to be suitable for the quantification of responses, except for laser Doppler flowmetry, due to the influence of edema on the vasculature [61].

References

1. Frosch PJ, Kligman AM (eds) (1993) Noninvasive methods for the quantification of skin functions. Springer, Berlin
2. Goldsmith LA (ed) (1983) Biochemistry and physiology of the skin. Oxford University, New York
3. Serup J, Jemec G (eds) (1995) Handbook of non-invasive methods and the skin. CRC, Boca Raton
4. Agache P, Humbert P (eds) (2004) Measuring the skin. Springer, Berlin
5. Berardesca E, Elsner P, Wilhelm K-P, Maibach HI (eds) (1995) Bioengineering of the skin: methods and instrumentation. CRC, Boca Raton
6. Wilhelm K-P, Elsner P, Berardesca E, Maibach HI (eds) (1997) Bioengineering of the skin: skin surface imaging and analysis. CRC, Boca Raton
7. Elsner P, Barel AO, Berardesca E, Gabard B, Serup J (eds) (1998) Skin bioengineering techniques and applications in dermatology and cosmetology. Karger, Basel
8. Berardesca E, Maibach HI (1988) Bioengineering and the patch test. Contact Derm 18:3–9
9. Diffey BL, Oliver RJ, Farr PM (1984) A portable instrument for quantifying erythema induced by ultraviolet radiation. Br J Dermatol 111:663–672
10. Robertson AR (1977) The CIE 1976 color difference formulas. Color Res Appl 2:7–11
11. Serup J, Agner T (1990) Colorimetric quantification of erythema – a comparison of two colorimeters (Lange Micro Color and Minolta Chroma Meter CR-200) with a clinical scoring scheme and laser-Doppler flowmetry. Clin Exp Dermatol 15:267–272
12. Slue WE (1989) Photographic cures for dermatologic disorders. Arch Dermatol 125:960–962
13. Grove GL, Grove MJ (1989) Objective methods for assessing skin surface topography noninvasively. In: Leveque J-L (ed) Cutaneous investigation in health and disease. Dekker, New York
14. Serup J, Winther A, Blichmann C (1989) A simple method for the study of scale pattern and effects of a moisturizer: qualitative and quantitative evaluation by D-Squame tape compared with parameters of epidermal hydration. Clin Exp Dermatol 14:277–282
15. Leveque J-L, de Rigal J (1983) Impedance methods for studying skin moisturization. J Soc Cosmet Chem 34:419–428
16. Tagami H (1989) Impedance measurement for evaluation of the hydration state of the skin surface. In: Leveque J-L (ed) Cutaneous investigation in health and disease. Dekker, New York, pp 79–111
17. Blichmann C, Serup J (1988) Assessment of skin moisture. Measurement of electrical conductance, capacitance and transepidermal water loss. Acta Derm Venereol (Stockh) 68:284–290
18. Agner T, Serup J (1988) Comparison of two electrical methods for measurement of skin hydration. An experimental study on irritant patch test reactions. Bioeng Skin 4:263–269
19. Stender IM, Blichmann C, Serup J (1990) Effects of oil and water baths on the hydration state of the epidermis. Clin Exp Dermatol 15:206–209
20. Nilsson GE (1977) Measurement of water exchange through skin. Med Biol Eng Comput 15:209–218
21. Spencer TS (1990) Transepidermal water loss: methods and applications. In: Rietschel RL, Spencer TS (eds) Methods for cutaneous investigation. Dekker, New York, pp 191–217
22. Pinnagoda J, Tupker RA, Agner T, Serup J (1990) Guidelines for transepidermal water loss (TEWL) measurement. A report from the standardization group of the European Society of Contact Dermatitis. Contact Derm 22:164–178
23. Agner T, Serup J (1989) Seasonal variation of skin resistance to irritants. Br J Dermatol 121:323–328
24. Agner T, Serup J (1988) Contact thermography for assessment of skin damage due to experimental irritants. Acta Derm Venereol (Stockh) 68:192–195
25. Baillie AJ, Biagioni PA, Forsyth A, Garioch JJ, McPherson D (1990) Thermographic assessment of patch-test responses. Br J Dermatol 122:351–360
26. Serup J, Staberg B (1987) Ultrasound for assessment of allergic and irritant patch test reactions. Contact Derm 17:80–84
27. Serup J (1992) Ten years' experience with high-frequency ultrasound examination of the skin: development and refinement of technique and equipment. In: Altmeyer P, Hoffman K (eds) Ultrasound in dermatology. Springer, Berlin, pp 41–54
28. Peters K, Serup J (1987) Papulo-vesicular count for the rating of allergic patch test reactions. A simple technique based on polysulfide rubber replica. Acta Derm Venereol (Stockh) 67:491–495
29. Blichmann C, Serup J (1987) Hydration studies on scaly hand eczema. Contact Derm 16:155–159
30. Serup J, Staberg B (1987) Differentiation of allergic and irritant reactions by transepidermal water loss. Contact Derm 16:129–132
31. Serup J (1987) Contact thermography – towards the Sherlock Holmes magnifying glass for solving allergic and irritant patch test reactions? Contact Derm 17:61–62
32. Staberg B, Serup J (1984) Patch test responses evaluated by cutaneous blood flow measurements. Arch Dermatol 120:741–743
33. Staberg B, Serup J (1988) Allergic and irritant skin reactions evaluated by laser Doppler flowmetry. Contact Derm 18:40–45
34. Serup J, Staberg B, Klemp P (1984) Quantification of cutaneous oedema in patch test reactions by measurement of

skin thickness with high-frequency pulsed ultrasound. Contact Derm 10:88–93

35. Willis CM, Stephens CJM, Wilkinson JD (1989) Epidermal damage induced by irritants in man. A light and electron microscopy study. J Invest Dermatol 93:695–700

36. Bjørnberg A (1968) Skin reactions to primary irritants in patients with hand eczema. An investigation with matched controls. Thesis, Oscar Isacson, Göteborg

37. Frosch P (1985) Hautirritation und empfindliche Haut. Grosse, Berlin

38. van der Valk PGM (1983) Water vapour loss measurements on human skin. Thesis, State University Hospital, Gröningen

39. Pinnagoda J (1990) Transepidermal water loss. Its role in the assessment of susceptibility to the development of irritant contact dermatitis. Thesis, State University Hospital, Gröningen

40. Tupker RA (1990) The influence of detergents on the human skin. A study on factors determining the individual susceptibility assessed by transepidermal water loss. Thesis, State University Hospital, Gröningen

41. De Boer EM (1989) Occupational dermatitis by metalworking fluids. An epidemiological study and an investigation on skin irritation using laser Doppler flowmetry. Thesis, Vrije University, Amsterdam

42. Agner T (1991) Noninvasive measuring methods for the investigation of irritant contact dermatitis. Thesis, University of Copenhagen

43. Agner T, Serup J (1990) Sodium lauryl sulphate for irritant patch testing. A dose response study using bioengineering methods for determination of skin irritation. J Invest Dermatol 95:543–547

44. Agner T, Serup J (1987) Skin reactions to irritants assessed by polysulfide rubber replica. Contact Derm 17:205–211

45. Agner T, Serup J (1990) Individual and instrumental variations in irritant patch-test reactions – clinical evaluation and quantification by bioengineering methods. Clin Exp Dermatol 15:29–33

46. Bircher AJ, Guy RH, Maibach HI (1990) Laser-Doppler blood flowmetry. Skin pharmacology and dermatology. In: Shepherd AP, Öberg PÅ (eds) Laser-Doppler blood flowmetry. Kluwer, Boston, pp 141–174

47. Frosch PJ, Kligman AM (1982) Recognition of chemically vulnerable and delicate skin. In: Frost PH, Horwith SN (eds) Principles of cosmetics for the dermatologist. Mosby, St Louis, pp 287–296

48. Murahata RI, Crowe DM, Roheim JR (1986) The use of transepidermal water loss to measure and predict the irritation response to surfactants. Int J Cosmet Sci 8: 225–231

49. Frosch P, Wissing C (1982) Cutaneous sensitivity to ultraviolet light and chemical irritants. Arch Dermatol Res 272: 269–278

50. Agner T, Damm P, Skouby SO (1991) Menstrual cycle and skin reactivity. J Am Acad Dermatol 24:566–570

51. Werner Y, Lindberg M (1985) Transepidermal water loss in dry and clinically normal skin in patients with atopic dermatitis. Arch Dermatol Res 65:102–105

52. Agner T (1991) Skin susceptibility in uninvolved skin of hand eczema patients and healthy controls. Br J Dermatol 125:140–146

53. Agner T (1990) Susceptibility to sodium lauryl sulphate in patients with atopic dermatitis and controls. Acta Derm Venereol (Stockh) 71:296–300

54. Tupker RA, Willis C, Berardesca E, Lee CH, Fartasch M, Agner T, Serup J (1997) Guidelines on sodium lauryl sulfate (SLS) exposure tests. A report from the Standardization Group of the European Society of Contact Dermatitis. Contact Derm 37:53–69

55. Serup J, Staberg B (1985) Quantification of weal reactions with laser Doppler flowmetry. Comparative blood flow measurements of the oedematous centre and the perilesional flare of skin-prick histamine weals. Allergy 40: 233–237

56. Van Neste D (1991) Skin response to histamine: reproducibility study of the dry skin prick test method and of the evaluation of microvascular changes with laser Doppler flowmetry. Acta Derm Venereol (Stockh) 71:25–28

57. Serup J (1984) Diameter, thickness, area, and volume of skin-prick histamine weals. Allergy 39:359–364

58. Van Neste D, Ghys L, Antoine JL, Rihoux JP (1989) Pharmacological modulation by cetirizine and atropine of the histamine- and methacholine-induced wheals and flares in human skin. Skin Pharmacol 2:93–102

59. Van Neste D (1990) Skin response to histamine dry skin prick test: influence of duration of the skin prick on clinical parameters and on skin blood flow monitoring. J Dermatol Sci 1:435–439

60. Leroy T, Tasset C, Valentin B, Van Neste D (1998) Comparison of the effects of cetirizine and ebastine on the skin response to histamine iontophoresis monitored with laser Doppler flowmetry. Dermatology 197:146–151

61. Agner T, Serup J (1989) Quantification of the DMSO response, a test for assessment of sensitive skin. Clin Exp Dermatol 14:214–217

Part VI

Allergic Contact Dermatitis Related to Specific Exposures

Allergens from the European Baseline Series

31

Klaus E. Andersen, Ian R White, and An Goossens

Contents

K.E. Andersen (✉)
Department of Dermatology and Allergy Centre, Odense University Hospital, University of Southern Denmark, 5000 Odense, Denmark
e-mail: keandersen@health.sdu.dk

I.R. White
Department of Cutaneous Allergy, St John's Institute of Dermatology, St. Thomas' Hospital, London SE1 7EH, UK

A. Goossens
Department of Dermatology, University Hospital KU Leuven, 3000 Leuven, Belgium

31.1 Introduction

The distinction between allergic and irritant contact dermatitis is based on a patient's history and clinical features, in combination with diagnostic patch testing. This test procedure is indicated in the investigation of long-standing cases of contact dermatitis and should also be used to exclude contact allergy as a complicating factor in stubborn cases of other eczematous diseases, such as atopic dermatitis, stasis eczema, seborrheic dermatitis, and vesicular hand eczema. A patch test is the cutaneous application of a small amount of the suspected allergen in a suitable concentration and vehicle. The test site, usually the back, is covered with an occlusive dressing for 2 days.

J.D. Johansen et al. (eds.), Contact Dermatitis,
DOI: 10.1007/978-3-642-03827-3_31, © Springer-Verlag Berlin Heidelberg 2011

The skin condition, vehicle and concentration, volume of the test substance, size of the test chamber, test site, application time, and the number of readings influence the result, and frequent errors are possible [1–4] (see Chap. 24). Proper performance and interpretation of this bioassay require considerable training and experience.

Patch testing is routinely performed by applying a baseline series of the most frequently occurring contact allergens and those contact allergens that may be missed without routine screening. The choice of test concentration is based on patch test experience such that there is a minimum number of irritant reactions and a maximum of clinically explicable allergic positive reactions. Test concentrations are generally expressed in percentages. This can be misleading, since the molecular weight of allergens can be very different. A better way of expressing concentration would be both the percentage and molality (m = number of moles per 1,000 g of solvent or vehicle) [5]. In the TRUE test® the concentrations are given in microgram per square centimeter.

An experienced contact dermatologist will be able to guess correctly the clinically relevant contact allergen in some patients, based on the history and the clinical appearance of the eczema. This guess is more likely to be correct for common allergens, such as nickel (50–80%), and less likely to be correct for less common allergens (<10%) [6, 7]. This failure to guess correctly explains the general acceptance of the use of a baseline series in the evaluation of all patients suspected of having a contact dermatitis.

Supplementary tests with skin care products, cosmetics, topical drugs, gloves, properly diluted working materials, and extra allergens selected on the basis of patient history and known exposures, are often required in order to determine the nature of the patient's suspected contact dermatitis. The baseline series was previously named the "standard series," but this term has been deselected because a "standard series" is not sufficient to diagnose the patient´s all clinically important contact allergies. The European standard series detected approximately 75–80% of all contact allergies in a multicenter European study in 1992 [8]. The TRUE test® Panel 1 & 2 detected relevant contact allergies in about 77% of consecutively patch tested ezcema patients at Kansas Medical Center, but 52% of the patients had supplementary contact allergies of importance not identified by the TRUE test® panels [9]. So, the yield of a screening series testing depends on the extent of the series, which may vary from country to country.

The baseline series is dynamic and subject to regular changes depending on population exposures and prevalence of contact allergy [10, 11] (Table 31.1). Among the major patch test material companies, Hermal, Chemotechnique, and Brial supply with some modifications in the baseline series, as recommended by the European Society of Contact Dermatitis (ESCD), and Mekos supplies TRUE Test Panel 1–3, which, in the collection and preparation of the allergens, differ from the ESCD baseline series on several positions, as seen in Table 31.1. The baseline series can be extended to include allergens of local importance to specific departments. The frequency of allergic contact sensitization to the allergens of the standard series varies from study to study, depending on the composition of the study population. Comparison of the frequencies in different populations is valid only when the results are standardized with respect to confounding factors, such as age, sex, presence of atopy, presence of diseased skin, and occupational exposure – the MOAHLFA index, indicating the frequency of occurrence of males, occupational dermatitis, atopy, hand dermatitis, leg ulcers or stasis dermatitis, facial dermatitis, and age above 40 years [12–14]. Moreover, when evaluating multicenter patch test studies, the patch test application time, the amount of the allergens applied on the chambers, the reading time, and the reading scale should as well be taken into account [15].

31.2 Nickel

Nickel is a metal which is used in a large number of alloys and chemical compounds. Only iron, chromium, and lead are produced in larger amounts. Nickel is ubiquitous in the environment and constitutes about 0.008% of the Earth's crust. Humans are constantly exposed, though in variable amounts [16]. Nickel is the most common contact allergen in children and adults [17, 18]. Metallic nickel (only after corrosion), as well as nickel salts, gives rise to contact allergy. The corrosiveness of sweat, saliva, and other body fluids to nickel and nickel alloys is of primary importance [19].

Nickel is the most common allergen in the standard series and the most common cause of allergic contact dermatitis, particularly in women. The frequency of nickel allergy in women is 3–10 times higher than in men [17, 20]. This gender difference is traditionally explained by increased exposure in women, due to

Table 31.1 The current European baseline patch test series from Trolab Hermal and Chemotechnique, and the contact allergens available from TRUE Test Panel 1–3. The patch test concentrations are shown

	Trolab Hermal[a]	Chemotechnique[a]	TRUE test[b] ($\mu g/cm^2$)
Potassium dichromate	0.5% pet.	0.5% pet.	23
Neomycin sulfate	20% pet.	20% pet.	230
Thiuram mix	1% pet.	1% pet.	25
p-phenylenediamine free base	1% pet.	1% pet.	90
Cobalt chloride	1% pet.	1% pet.	20
Benzocaine	5% pet.	5% pet.	
Formaldehyde	1% aq.	1% aq.	180
Colophony (colophonium)	20% pet.	20% pet.	850
Clioquinol	5% pet.	5% pet.	
Balsam of Peru (*Myroxylon pereirae*)	25% pet.	25% pet.	800
N-isopropyl-*N*-phenyl-para-phenylenediamine (IPPD)	0.1% pet.	0.1% pet.	
Wool alcohols (lanolin alcohol)	30% pet.	30% pet.	1,000
Mercapto mix	1% pet.	2% pet.	75
Epoxy resin	1% pet.	1% pet.	50
Paraben mix	16% pet.	16% pet.	1,000
para-Tertiary-butylphenol-formaldehyde resin (PTBP resin)	1% pet.	1% pet.	40
Fragrance mix	8% pet.	8% pet.	430
Quaternium-15	1% pet.	1% pet.	100
Nickel sulfate	5% pet.	5% pet.	200
Cl+Me-isothiazolinone[c]	0.01% aq.	0.01% aq.	4
Mercaptobenzothiazole	2% pet.	2% pet.	75
Primin	0.01% pet.	0.01% pet.	
Sesquiterpene lactone mix	0.1% pet.	0.1% pet.	
Budesonide	0.1% pet.	0.01% pet.	1
Tixocortol pivalate	1% pet.	0.1% pet.	3
Methyldibromo glutaronitrile	0.3% pet.	0.5% pet.	
Hydroxyisohexyl 3-cyclohexene carboxaldehyde	5% pet.	5% pet.	
Fragrance mix II		14% pet.	
Caine mix			630
Quinoline mix			190
Black-rubber mix			75
Carba mix			250
Thimerosal			8
Ethylenediamine			50

(*continued*)

Table 31.1 (continued)

	Trolab Hermal[a]	Chemotechnique[a]	TRUE test[b] ($\mu g/cm^2$)
Hydrocortisone-17-butyrate			20
Diazolidinyl urea			550
Imidazolidinyl urea			600

aq. water; *pet.* petrolatum

[a]Hermal and Chemotechnique offer more than these allergens

[b]TRUE allergens for a Panel 3 are under development

[c]Methylchloroisothiazolinone/methylisothiazolinone

direct skin contact with nickel-releasing metal, such as in jewelry, wristwatches, and clothing accessories. Wet work at home and exposure in certain occupational groups with a majority of women, such as hairdressers, cleaners, and food service workers, are also associated with the increased frequency of nickel allergy in women [21, 22]. An important endogenous factor related to allergic contact sensitization to nickel seems to be loss-of-function mutations in the filaggrin gene, which are associated with skin barrier diseases such as ichthyosis vulgaris and atopic eczema [23]. The incidence of nickel allergy in women has increased until the most recent decade, and has reached a plateau of around 15–20%, depending on the source of reference [18, 20, 24]. The incidence of nickel allergy in Denmark is now decreasing in the younger age group, probably due to the fact that nickel regulation was implemented in Denmark in 1992 [25]. The most common cause of sensitization is thought to be ear piercing [17, 26], even in men [27]. The clinical pattern of nickel dermatitis is described in the classic paper of Calnan and Wells [28]. The primary sites of dermatitis develop as a result of direct skin contact with nickel-releasing metal. The secondary sites are unrelated to direct skin contact. A systemic contact dermatitis may develop in particularly sensitive patients through oral intake through foods. The systemic contact dermatitis is symmetrical and often includes the neck and face, eyelids, elbow flexures and forearms, hands, inner thighs, anogenital region, and may be generalized [29]. Flare-up reactions of previous nickel patch test sites may occur. The systemic allergic nickel dermatitis is hapten-specific and with a clear dose–response relationship. Immunological investigations in nickel-sensitive individuals whose dermatitis flared after oral nickel provocation showed that CD8+ "memory", CLA+ T lymphocytes, and T lymphocytes with a type 2 cytokine profile are involved in the development of systemic nickel dermatitis [30]. The doses used experimentally have been much larger than the normal daily dietary nickel intake, which varies between 0.1 and 0.5 mg nickel, and the induction of systemic nickel dermatitis from daily dietary nickel intake remains controversial [31–34]. However, nickel-sensitive patients with vesicular hand eczema worsened after an oral challenge with nickel in water and with a diet naturally high in nickel [35]. Nickel absorption and retention in the body is highly dependent on food intake and fasting, but nickel toxicokinetics is the same in nickel-allergic women and age-matched controls [36].

The relationship between nickel allergy and hand eczema is also controversial. It is evident that allergic dermatitis of the hands occurs as a result of contact with solubilized nickel and takes place more rapidly if the patient has preexisting irritant hand eczema [37]. Hand eczema is more common in nickel-sensitized women than in the general population [38, 39]. However, a Swedish study in men [27] did not reveal a higher frequency of hand eczema among metal-sensitive subjects, nor in individuals with pierced ears, compared to a nonsensitized group. A recent Swedish population-based study of 369 women patch tested 20 years ago found a doubled risk for hand eczema in nickel-positive women without a history of childhood eczema, but the most important risk factor for hand eczema was childhood eczema.[40]. Recent Danish studies have shown contradictory results. Mortz et al. [17] found a significant association between hand eczema and nickel allergy in a population of unselected adolescents, and Bryld et al. found the same in a population-based twin sample [41, 42]. However, when the analysis was limited to twins with vesicular hand eczema, there was no association [41].

Other conundrums about nickel allergy remain unsolved; for instance, the question of whether nickel allergy renders a person, even with normal skin, more vulnerable to irritant contact dermatitis. It would appear that it can [43], but atopic dermatitis is the major risk factor to the development of hand eczema [35, 40,

42, 44]. A survey of 368 nickel-sensitive subjects attempted to determine the overall importance of nickel as an occupational allergen and it was found in about 23% of the cases to function as a secondary occupational allergen, in conjunction with other factors [21].

The incidence of allergy in men, even in those with earrings, is lower than in females, the cause not being clear. Some experimental studies claim that women are more easily sensitized than men [45]. A more likely explanation for the fewer nickel-allergic men may be less exposure from wet work and less skin contact with nickel-releasing jewelry.

Certainly, in nickel allergy, one can see patterns of dermatitis which are unusual for contact dermatitis; for instance, on the palmar aspects of the fingers and the adjacent palm. This can sometimes be explained by local contact, as exemplified by allergic nickel contact dermatitis caused by mobile telephones releasing nickel [46]. It is to be expected that a solid such as metal will produce a different distribution of dermatitis compared to liquids and detergents. However, intensive handling of nickel coins in a controlled experiment did not provoke allergic contact hand eczema in nickel-sensitive individuals [47].

There is no method of desensitization, but it is possible to produce immune tolerance in animals fed with nickel prior to attempted sensitization, and this has been confirmed in humans. Adolescents who have dental braces (causing ingestion of nickel) prior to ear piercing develop much less nickel allergy [17, 48]. This is clearly not a practical method of solving the problem. Oral administration of nickel sulfate, 5.0 mg once a week for 6 weeks in nickel-allergic patients, lowered the degree of contact allergy significantly, as measured by the patch test reactions before and after nickel administration [49].

There is little doubt that metal plates on bones can initiate a dermatitis, which occurs particularly over the areas of the plate [50, 51], but it is now well accepted that nickel allergy is not a contraindication to a metal hip of stainless steel or vitallium type. There is no convincing evidence that these sensitize or exacerbate a preexisting dermatitis, or lead to rejection of the hip [52].

Nickel allergy was not claimed to increase the risk of developing other allergies [53, 54]. However, nickel allergy is often associated with reactivity to other metals. This seems, in most cases, to be caused by multiple exposure and sensitization and not cross-reactivity [55], and may simply be due to the fact that these metals are commonly associated. It is difficult to obtain pure compounds and most of these metals are contaminated

with another. On the other hand, Moss et al. [56] suggested that the acquisition of sensitivity to one allergen might predispose to the acquisition of another unrelated sensitivity – based on a statistical analysis of patch test data from 2,200 consecutive patients and experimental sensitization using dinitrochlorobenzene (DNCB). Further, guinea pigs sensitized to nickel were found to be more easily sensitized to cobalt [57], and it has been shown that lymphocytes with monoclonal sensitivity to nickel will react to palladium and copper, but not with cobalt [58]. Nickel is an intriguing contact allergen, and some cases of nickel patch test reactivity may be unspecific, as nickel, in analogy to superantigens, may directly link to the T-cell receptor (TCR) and major histocompatibility complex (MHC) in a peptide-independent manner. However, nickel requires human histocompatibility leukocyte antigen (HLA)-determined TCR amino acids [59].

The dimethylglyoxime (DMG) test, which is used to detect nickel release from metal surfaces, is accurate to about 10 ppm ($0.001\% = 2.1$ μg Ni/g) and is a good routine test to eliminate metals as a source of nickel which may be causing allergy. However, metals containing lower amounts can still produce an exacerbation of nickel dermatitis, and, therefore, the DMG test cannot be relied upon absolutely to rule out a piece of metal as the cause of a patient's dermatitis [60, 61]. The release of nickel from stainless steel is minimal and is directly correlated with its sulfur content, since sulfur affects corrosion resistance, and, hence, also the release of nickel [62]. Experimental studies have shown that nickel-sensitive patients rarely react following repeated exposures to levels below 10 ppm nickel [63]. An experimental study comparing the elicitation thresholds for patch testing and repeated open application tests (ROAT) with nickel in nickel-allergic individuals showed that the elicitation threshold for patch test is higher than that for ROAT (per application), but when the ROAT applications are accumulated until a positive reaction is obtained, then the thresholds are appproximately the same [64].

The EU nickel directive aimed at the prevention of nickel allergy covers metal items in direct contact with skin, piercing materials, and requirements on resistance to wear (Council Directive 94/27/EC, OJ No. L 188 of 22.7.94). The nickel release threshold is 0.5 μg/cm^2/week, and a European standard for testing nickel release from articles intended to come in prolonged and direct skin contact has been adopted.

The nickel directive seems to be effective, as a significant decrease in the frequency of nickel allergy in

31

Denmark is reported in the age group of 0–18 years [25, 65], and in Germany, in patients below 31 years of age [66].

The standard patch test concentration of nickel sulfate in Europe is 5% pet. or 200 $\mu g/cm^2$ in the TRUE test. In the USA, 2.5% pet. is recommended. Follicular and irritant reactions may occur and complicate clinical interpretation. A problem in patch testing is that, depending on the questioning procedure, 15–50% of those who give a clear history of reaction to metal jewelry, which strongly suggests nickel allergy, do not react [33, 67]. The reason for this is not clear. It does not appear to be due to a fault in the test reagent, or method of testing, as other salts, for instance, nickel chloride, or intradermal (ID) testing will increase the positive yield by a very small amount [68]. Nickel contact allergy does not seem to be associated with atopic dermatitis [69, 70]. Positive nickel sulfate patch tests are, in general, very reproducible [71, 72]. However, the individual variation in nickel patch test threshold reactivity between one test session and another with a dilution series among nickel-sensitive patients may be considerable [73].

31.3 Chromium

It is probably more accurate to use the term "chromate," because chromium is unique in that the metal itself does not sensitize, but, rather, its salts. Both hexavalent (Cr^{6+}) and trivalent (Cr^{3+}) chromium salts may cause allergic contact dermatitis. Trivalent chromium salts are less soluble and penetrate the skin poorly, binding with proteins on the surface skin, while hexavalent chromium is readily soluble and penetrates the skin easily but binds poorly with proteins. It is thought that hexavalent chromium penetrates the skin and is then reduced enzymatically to trivalent chromium, which combines with protein as the hapten. Using standard patch test techniques, Fregert and Rorsman [74] showed that, if the concentration of trivalent chromium is high enough, and the exposure time sufficiently prolonged, positive patch tests will also result. However, the evidence would suggest that, at a cellular level, the body develops an allergy to both hexavalent and trivalent chromium [75, 76]. Recent clinical dose–response patch test experiments using volunteer chromate allergic patients showed that the calculated minimal elicitation threshold (MET)

giving a positive patch test reaction in 10% of the patients was 0.18 $\mu g/cm^2$ (6 ppm.) for Cr(III) and 0.03 $\mu g/cm^2$ (1 ppm) for Cr(VI) [77]. The frequency of patch test positives to chromate on routine patch testing varies considerably from region to region. In Denmark, about 2% of consecutively tested eczema patients have chromate allergy [78], much less than in neighboring countries such as Germany and England, where the frequency of chromate allergy ranges from 3.1 to 10.5% [20, 79]. Where higher rates are reported, some irritant reactions may be included. It is difficult to compare these results unless the patient materials are examined for confounding factors, such as age, sex, atopy, occupational dermatitis, site of dermatitis, etc. Cement has been considered as the main cause of chromate allergy. All authorities agree that cement dermatitis is decreasing in incidence, and increasing evidence indicates that this may be partly due to the introduction of ferrous sulfate in cement in some countries in order to reduce the levels of hexavalent chromium [80–83]. However, the decline in cement dermatitis may also result from other factors, such as automation and prefabrication processes in the construction industry [84, 85]. A remarkable observation is the fact that chromate allergy was common among construction workers employed at the Channel Tunnel project, in which normal cement was used [86]. In contrast, only a few workers developed cement dermatitis during the construction of the Great Belt tunnel and bridge in Denmark, a project of a comparable size [78]. In Denmark, legislation has, since 1981, regulated the concentration of hexavalent chromate in ready-to-use cement, and, since 2003, a similar legislation has been adopted in the EU, making it illegal to sell cement and cement products containing more than 2 ppm hexavalent chromium. Recent epidemiological investigations support this legislation, since chromate sensitization among construction workers in Northern Bavaria, Germany was still common throughout the 1990s, without the declining frequency seen in Scandinavian countries, where the addition of ferrous sulfate to cement had been practiced since the 1980s [87]. Chromate allergy is more common in male than in female eczema patients, due to the occupational exposure in male-dominated occupations, such as building and machine industry [20]. This has changed in Denmark since introduction of the legislation limiting the content of hexavalent chromate in cement. Now, chromate allergy is more common in female patients, probably caused by chrome-tanned leather in gloves and shoes [65].

There are many causes of chromate allergy other than cement, including chrome-tanned leather, anti-rust paint, timber preservatives, the wood pulp industry, ash either from burnt wood in general or matches with chromate in the match head, coolants and machine oils, galvanizing, defatting solvents, brine added to yeast residues, welding, the dye industry (due to either a dye, a reducing agent, or a mordant), printing, glues, foundry sand, boiler linings, television work (ammonium bichromate to produce cross-linking of light-sensitive polyvinyl alcohol), magnetic tapes (chromium dioxide), solutions used to facilitate tire fitting, chromium plating, hardeners and resins in the aircraft industry, preservatives used in milk testing, bleaches, and detergents. An extensive list of the possible sources of contact allergy is in Table 31.2. Of these sources, many are rare and one-off contacts. Cement, by far, still remains the commonest source of chromate allergy, followed by welding, chrome tanning, leather, pigments, and chrome plating. The relevance of a positive chromate patch test may be difficult to ascertain. More detailed information can be obtained in references [76] and [88]. Allergic chromate dermatitis is often widespread and persistent, and may appear in a nummular eczema pattern [89]. However, if the patient carefully aims to avoid contact with chromate-containing products, the chromate dermatitis often clears [90]. A change of occupation may be beneficial in some cases, but it does not ensure the healing of the dermatitis. Substitution for the chromate-containing products is often possible for leather gloves, shoes, and printing material, among others. The occasionally seen persistent nature of chromate dermatitis is not clear. It may be due to chromate remaining in the skin for a long time, or it may require minute quantities of chromate to flare up a contact allergy, and minute quantities of an amount similar to that in cement are found in many everyday objects, such as paper, soil, ash, etc. Recent clinical experimental exposure studies in volunteer patients have revealed that the vast majority of sensitized individuals fail to react to levels of chromate below 10 ppm under realistic exposure conditions [63, 91]. Clinical experiments with leather exposure in volunteer chromate allergic patients have shown that there is no clear-cut relationship between the measured content of chromium III and VI and the elicitation of dermatitis. Extended exposure for up to 2 weeks caused dermatitis in patients who had negative ordinary patch

Table 31.2 Industrial exposure to chromium is possible during contact with the following compounds or work procedures (from [90])

Analytic standards reagents
Anticorrosion agents
Batteries
Catalysts (for hydrogenation, oxidation, and polymerization)
Ceramics
Corrosion inhibitors
Chromate surface treatments
Drilling muds
Electroplating and anodizing agents
Engraving
Explosives
Fire retardants
Magnetic tapes
Milk preservatives
Paints and varnishes
Paper
Photography
Roofing
Surgical sutures
Tanning leather
Textile mordants and dyes
Television screens
Wood preservatives

tests to the leather sample [92]. It has been suggested that dermatitis can be aggravated in those allergic to chromate by oral ingestion, but this remains unproven and has not received the attention that the same theory has received in nickel allergy [93].

Chromium is an essential element in the body, especially for glucose metabolism.

Potassium dichromate 0.5% pet. is the standard dilution for testing. However, this percentage can produce an irritant reaction, which may explain the wide difference in dichromate allergy reported throughout the world. It has been suggested that 0.25% would be more accurate, but while this produces fewer reactions, it does miss some true dichromate allergies [94]; the same applies to a dilution of 0.375% [95].

The patch test concentration in the TRUE Test system is 23 μg/cm². The closeness of irritant concentration to that to detect contact allergy is a problem in assessing the true incidence of chromate allergy and in diagnosing individual patients. Meteorological conditions such as cold and dry weather may affect patch test reactivity to metal salts causing an increase in irritant and doubtful reactions which may falsely be regarded as weak allergic reactions [95]. A practical solution to improve the clinical evaluation may be to repeat the patch test to see if the reaction is reproducible.

31.4 Cobalt

Today, more than 75% of the world's production of cobalt is used in the manufacture of alloys. It is also an integral and necessary component of vitamin B12. Meats, fruits, vegetables, and cereals are major sources of vitamin B12, and, thus, of cobalt [63].

A positive patch test to cobalt often occurs in association with a positive test to nickel or chromate, more particularly, nickel, although the pattern may be different in males and females [96, 97]. However, cobalt allergy without nickel allergy may occur in about 30% of the cases [98]. The association between nickel and cobalt allergy is explained by the metals being commonly present in alloys and products so that considerable contact with nickel means a correspondingly high contact with cobalt, and, hence, a corresponding possibility of sensitization to both [99]. Cobalt containing hard metal alloys may be a clinically relevant source of cobalt contact dermatitis. Experiments with alloys released cobalt up to 290 g/cm²/week in artificial sweat. Patch tests with discs of the alloys caused positive test reactions in a number of previously patch tested cobalt allergic patients [100]. The importance of cobalt exposure for maintaining allergic hand dermatitis in sensitized individuals is questionable, as patients who immersed a finger in a cobalt salt solution containing 200 mg/L for 10 min daily for 2 weeks failed to develop a flare of hand eczema [101].

The importance of metal sensitivity in patients with orthopedic implants is still a matter of debate. Even if the number of clinically relvant cases is low [52], recent expriments have shown that allergy to cobalt – and other metal salts – may be clinically important as source of pain, ostolysis, dislocation, or loosening in patients with failed metal-on-metal hip prostheses and peri-implant

T-lymphotycic inflammation [102]. Experimental studies in guinea pigs have shown that concomitant nickel and cobalt patch test reactivity is due to multiple sensitizations rather than cross-reactivity [103]. However, a positive test to cobalt occurs 20 times more frequently in those allergic to nickel than in those not allergic, and a person with a +++ nickel positive patch test is 50 times more likely to have +++ positive cobalt reaction [104]. Rystedt and Fischer [105] reported 7% positive patch tests in 4,034 eczema patients, and of these, 50 were isolated cobalt reactions.

Cases of allergy due to contact with nonmetal sources, such as cobalt naphthenate, oleate, and cobalt-2-ethylhexanoate used as dryers for varnishes, paints, and printing inks, or as a contact catalyst in polyester resin systems [106], an oxidizing agent in automobile exhaust controls, in electroplating, and in the rubber tire industry have been reported. Exposure and allergy to cobalt has also occurred in wet alkaline clay in pottery and china plants; the latter may be due to porcelain dyes. Cobalt is often added to animal feeds, and due to this,dermatitis has been described. Cobalt and chromate are still prominent allergens in construction workers in Germany [107], although the cobalt content in cement is low. Cobalt chloride was the third most frequently occurring contact allergen among construction workers with occupational eczema, after chromate and epoxy resin [87]. It is often difficult to identify the source of a single positive cobalt patch test; that is, one with a negative nickel test. However, most of these patients are probably allergic to jewelry, as with nickel.

Cobalt chloride 1% pet. is the standard dilution for patch testing, and the concentration in the TRUE Test is 20 μg/cm². Cobalt reactions may appear late [108], and cobalt may also be an irritant, giving rise to false-positive reactions of a spotty nature ("poral") associated with a toxic effect on the eccrine acrosyringium [109].

31.5 Fragrance Mix I & II

Fragrance and flavor substances are organic compounds with characteristic, usually pleasant, odors [110]. They are ubiquitous and are used in perfumes and perfumed products and are found not only in cosmetics, but also in detergents, fabric softeners, and other household products where fragrance may be used to mask unpleasant odors from raw materials. Flavors

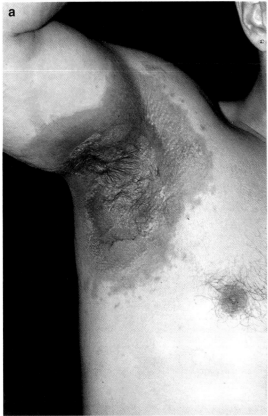

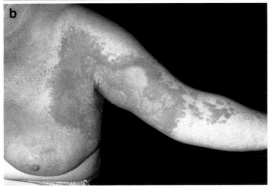

Fig. 31.1 Contact allergy to fragrances in deodorants can be very severe: formation of large blisters (**a**) and erythema-multiforme-like lesions with spreading (**b**) (courtesy of P.J. Frosch)

are used in foods, beverages, and dental products. Common clinical features of fragrance contact dermatitis are shown in Fig. 31.a, b.

Axillary dermatitis.
Dermatitis of the face and neck.
Well-circumscribed patches in areas where perfumes are dabbed on (wrists, behind the ears) and (aggravation of) hand eczema.

Depending on the degree of sensitivity, the severity of dermatitis may range from mild to severe with dissemination. Airborne and connubial contact dermatitis occurs. There is a possible association between fragrance allergy and hand eczema [111]. Other less frequent adverse reactions to fragrances are: photocontact dermatitis, contact urticaria, irritation, and pigmentary disorders [112].

Evaluation of fragrance allergy may be difficult. A complete fragrance compound consists of 10 to more than 300 basic ingredients, selected from about 3,000 materials (http://ec.europa.eu/enterprise/cosmetics/html/cosm_inci_index.htm), which can be divided into the following:

1. Natural products isolated from various parts of plants, e.g., blossoms, buds, fruit, peel, seeds, leaves, bark, wood, roots, or from resinous exudates.
2. Synthetic fragrance chemicals.
3. Animal products and their extracts such as ambergris from the sperm whale, tonkin musk from the testes of musk deer, castoreum from beaver glands, beeswax absolute from beeswax, and civet from the glands of the civet cat. These are now mostly replaced by blends of fragrance chemicals.

Because of the difficulties in testing with individual fragrances, two fragrance screening mixtures for patch testing have been developed to increase the ability to detect fragrance allergy [113, 114].

The first mixture, fragrance mix I was developed in the late 1970s and consists of eight ingredients [113] making up a total of 8% in petrolatum. The eight ingredients are each at a concentration of 1%: Amyl cinnamal; Cinnamal; Cinnamyl alcohol; Eugenol; *Evernia prunastri* (oak moss); Geraniol; Hydroxycitronellal; Isoeugenol.

The fragrance mix I from hermal and chemotechnique contains sorbitan sesquioleate as an emulsifier. This fragrance mix I has been shown to be a valuable screening agent for fragrance dermatitis: most reactions have been caused by oak moss (Fig. 31.2), isoeugenol, and cinnamal. The test concentration in the TRUE test is 430 µg/cm^2.

The second fragrance mix was officially included in the baseline series in 2008 [115]. The Fragrance mix II consists of six ingredients, which have been shown to be frequent allergens in multicentre studies [114, 116]. The six ingredients are: hydroxyisohexyl 3-cyclohexene carboxaldehyde 2.5%, citral 1.0%, farnesol 2.5%, coumarin 2.5%, citronellol 0.5%, and α-hexyl cinnamal 5%. This gives a Fragrance mix II of 14% in pet.[116]. In case of a positive reaction to the Fragrance mix II, the individual ingredients are tested in the double concentration to compensate for the effect of the mixture. The most important individual allergen is hydroxyisohexyl 3-cyclohexene carboxaldehyde, which is tested separately as part of the baseline series [114]. Fragrance mix II is not yet available in TRUE Test .

Between one-third and half of patients with a positive patch test to Fragrance mix II do not react to Fragrance mix I [114, 117], so both the mixtures are necessary in the screening of fragrance allergy. Frosch et al. reported that contact allergy to Fragrance mix II was found in 2.9% of the patients and that 1/3 of the patients reacting to Fragrance mix II were negative to Fragrance mix I [114, 116]. Still, cases may be overlooked if additional screening is not made with the scented products used by the patients and further fragrance allergens [118, 119].

In most centers, fragrances allergy ranks second only to nickel as the most common contact allergen, with a response rate of 6–11% to Fragrance mix I and 2.1–4.6% to Fragrance mix II in dermatological patients [118, 120](Fig. 31.3). In recent years, a decreasing trend is seen in the frequency of allergy to Fragrance mix I [120–122]. This is counterbalanced by additional cases detected by the Fragrance mix II.

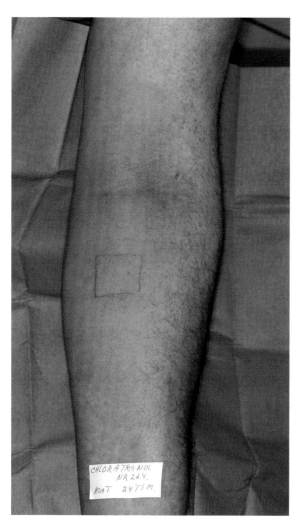

Fig. 31.2 Strongly positive ROAT to 5 ppm chloratranol solution in ethanol 1 day after one application of two drops in a male patient with oak moss allergy

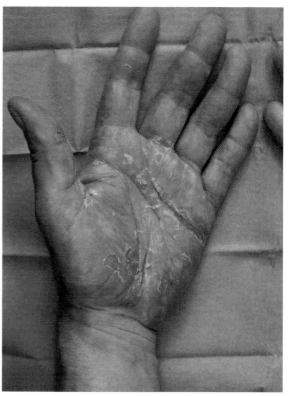

Fig. 31.3 Forty-year-old man with long-lasting hand eczema and strong allergic reactions to fragrance mix and balsam of Peru. Eczema cleared completely after the elimination of skin contact with perfumed products

Fragrance allergy is more common among women than men due to greater exposure, though the differences are small [112, 121, 123] and may increase with age [124]. Clinical studies have shown a highly significant association between reporting a history of visible skin symptoms from using scented products and a positive patch test to the fragrance mixes (Fig. 31.4) [114, 125]. Provocation studies with perfumes and deodorants have also shown that fragrance-mix-positive eczema patients often react to use tests with the products, and subsequent chemical analysis of such products has detected significant amounts of one or more fragrance mix ingredients, confirming the relevance of positive patch tests to fragrance mix in these patients [116, 126, 127].

False-positive and false-negative reactions to the mix are common. Marginal reactions may, in some cases, be regarded as irritant, while in other cases, retesting with the ingredients of the mix may reveal positive patch tests to one or more of them. To avoid false-negative reactions, ingredient testing is necessary, but evaluation of the patch test results may be difficult, because it appears that patch tests in perfume-sensitive patients with fragrance allergens in combination give additive responses compared to patch tests with the allergens separately [128]. Thus, it is important to test patients with their own products.

Evaluation of perfume allergy within Europe is being eased by the mandatory listing, on the ingredients label, of the fragrance mix substances present in cosmetics and detergents (together with other household products), if present at 10 ppm or more in a finished leave-on cosmetic product, or 100 ppm or more in a rinse-off product.

α-Isomethyl ionone; Amyl cinnamal*; Amylcinnamyl alcohol; Anisyl alcohol;Benzyl alcohol; Benzyl benzoate; Benzyl cinnamate; Benzyl salicylate; Butylphenyl methylpropional(lilial); Cinnamal*; Citral**; Citronellol**; Coumarin**; d-Limonene; Eugenol*; Hydroxycitronellal*; Isoeugenol*; Farnesol**; Geraniol; *Hexyl cinnamal**; Hydroxyisohexyl-3-cyclohexene carboxaldehyde (Lyral)**; Linalool; Methyl heptine carbonate; 2-(4-*tert*-butylbenzyl) propionaldehyde3-methyl-4-(2,6,6-tri-methyl-2-cyclohexen1-yl)-3-buten-2-one; Evernia prunastri** (oak moss) (*Present in Fragrance mix I; **present in Fragrance mix II).

31.6 Hydroxyisohexyl 3-Cyclohexene Carboxaldehyde (Lyral®)

Hydroxyisohexyl 3-cyclohexene carboxaldehyde is the INCI name for a synthetic fragrance ingredient better known under some of its trade names such as Lyral® or Kovanol® [129] (Scheme 31.1).

It is one of the six ingredients of Fragrance mix II [130]. It is in itself a frequent allergen and is therefore also included in the baseline series as an indvididual allergen [115]. Hydroxyisohexyl 3-cyclohexene carboxaldehyde is tested in 2.5% as part of the Fragrance mix II and in 5% in pet., when tested as an individual allergen [115, 130]. Hydroxyisohexyl 3-cyclohexene carboxaldehyde was first identified as an allergen by De Groot in one case, where the causative product was a deodorant [131]. Later investigations made by Frosch have established hydroxyisohexyl 3-cyclohexene carboxaldehyde as a frequent allergen and often of clinical relevance [117, 129, 130, 132, 133]. In an

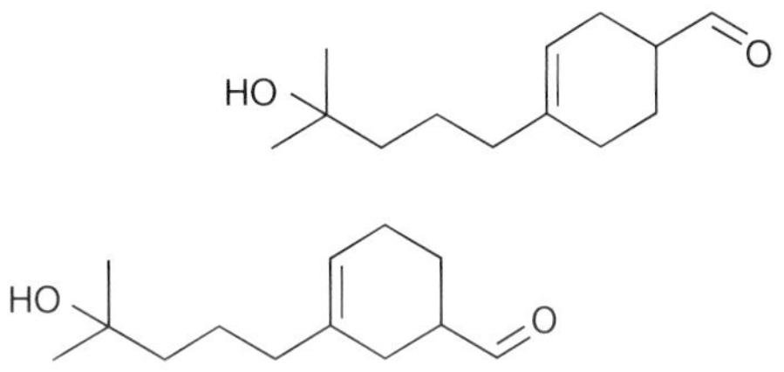

Fig. 31.4 Severe long-standing cheilitis in a patient allergic to isoeugenol present in her lipstick (courtesy of P.J. Frosch)

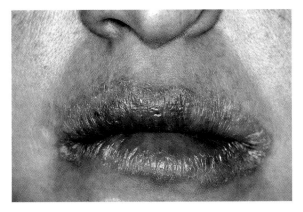

Scheme 31.1 Hydroxyisohexyl 3-cyclohexene carboxaldehyde

investigation of fragrance allergy in 1,855 eczema patients recruited from different clinics in Europe, a positive reaction to hydroxyisohexyl 3-cyclohexene carboxaldehyde 5% in pet. was found in 2.7% of the patients. A history of fragrance intolerance was found in 80% of these patients, significantly more than among those positive to Fragrance mix I [129].

Hydroxyisohexyl 3-cyclohexene carboxaldehyde is a widely used fragrance ingredient. It has been detected in 72% of 25 popular fine fragrances [134], 53% of 73 deodorants on the European market [135], and named on the label of 29% of 300 cosmetic and household products found on the retail market in UK [136]. It seems that allergy to hydroxyisohexyl 3-cyclohexene carboxaldehyde especially is related to the use of deodorants [118, 120, 137].

In spite of the attempt by fragrance industry to limit the use of hydroxyisohexyl 3-cyclohexene carboxaldehyde, the incidence of contact allergy to the substance has been unaffected [138].

31.7 Balsam of Peru

Balsam of Peru (INCI name: *Myroxylon pereirae*) is the natural resinous balsam which exudes from the trunk of the Central American tree *Myroxylon pereirae* after scarification of the bark. It consists of essential oil and resin and is, thus, of the oleoresin type. The composition varies and standardization is based on physical characteristics and the identification of some major chemical constituents. Balsam of Peru contains 30–40% resins of unknown composition, while the remaining 60–70% consist of well-known chemicals: benzyl benzoate, benzyl cinnamate, cinnamic acid, benzoic acid, vanillin, farnesol (which is also increasingly being used in deodorants) [139], and nerolidol. In a series of 93 patients with contact allergy to balsam of Peru, reactions were seen, in decreasing order, to the following components: cinnamic alcohol, cinnamic acid, coniferyl alcohol, benzoic acid, cinnamyl cinnamate, eugenol, resorcinol monobenzoate, coniferyl alcohol, and benzyl alcohol [140]. Many perfumes and flavorings contain components either identical to, or cross-reacting with, materials contained in balsam of Peru and other natural resins. Positive patch tests with one or more of these substances may be an indication of perfume allergy. In medicinal preparations, balsam of Peru is still used for its dermatological effects. Some chemicals present in balsam of Peru and similar resinous substances may also have antimicrobial effects and be used as preservatives.

The early epidemiology of perfume allergy is based on Hjorth's [141] classic monograph on balsam of Peru. It gave positive reactions in 4.0% of males and 4.0% of females in a Danish epidemiological study consisting of 2,166 eczema patients [142]. However, the importance of balsam of Peru as a marker for perfume allergy shows wide variation [120–122, 125] Because of its sensitizing properties, crude balsam of Peru has been banned by the International Fragrance Association from use as a fragrance compound since 1982. Extracts and distillates of balsam of Peru are still used up to a maximum level of 0.4% in consumer products [143]. Patients with contact allergy to balsam of Peru may react to these extracts and distillates and thus have a relevant fragrance allergy. Neither balsam of Peru nor the extracts and distillates are covered by the mandatory labelleling of certain fragrance ingredients on cosmetics.

Contact allergy to balsam of Peru is also relevant to leg ulcer patients [144, 145]. Immediate reactions to patch tests with balsam of Peru occur. Systemic contact dermatitis-type reactions, like aggravation of vesicular hand dermatitis following ingestion of related compounds, has been reported in previously sensitized patients [32, 146–148], but the benefits of a flavor-avoidance diet may not be obvious [146]. Balsam of Peru 25% pet. is the standard dilution for patch testing, and 800 $\mu g/cm^2$ in the TRUE Test.

31.8 Colophonium

Colophony (rosin) (INCI name: colophonium) is a widespread, naturally occurring material that is the residue from the distillation of the volatile oil from the oleoresin obtained from trees of the *Pinaceae* family. Its chemical composition is complex and variable depending on the manufacturing process, geographical area, and storage conditions. There exist three kinds namely gum rosin from the tops of living trees, the resin being distilled to yield turpentine oil and the gum resin residue; wood rosin, a distillate from pine tree stumps; and tall oil rosin, a byproduct from pine wood pulp [see 149, for a review].

In a 5-year retrospective study involving 16,210 consecutive eczema patients, 4.5% were allergic to it [150]. Beside contact eczema, it may also cause type I hypersensitivity [149] and photosensitivity [149, 151].

Colophonium is composed of about 90% resin acids and 10% neutral substances, among which the resin acids i.e., abietic acid and dehydroabietic acid, and their oxidized derivatives have been identified as important allergens [152, 153], the latter also present in fragrance materials such as *Evernia furfuracea* or tree moss growing on pine trees [154], and as contaminants in *Evernia prunastri* or oak moss growing on oak trees [154–156].

Concomitant and/or cross-reactions between colophonium (rosin), Myroxylon pereirae resin (balsam of Peru), propolis, oil of turpentine, wood tar, pine resin, spruce resin [157], sesquiterpene lactone mix [158], and Compositae plant extracts occur, often in the context of a fragrance allergy [159–166]. Paulsen et al. have shown that positive reactions to colophonium and Compositae plant extracts, as well as to essential oils were based on cross-reactivity rather than concomitant sensitization to common allergens, although the presence of terpenes [158] in some of these materials explain this phenomenon only partly. Colophonium and Compositae mix may thus act as important markers of fragrance allergy [167].

Exposure to colophonium and its derivatives [149] is likely during both work and leisure hours (Table 31.3). In cosmetics, colophonium occurs in depilatories, tonics, dressing and hair grooming aids, make-up, mascara, and hair products. In pharmaceutical products, it is used in topical medicaments, including surgical paints [168] and Chinese herbal medicine [169]. Colophonium allergy from adhesives has been known for nearly a century, and when strong adhesive effects are needed as in footwear [170–172] and wound dressings [173], colophonium or its derivatives may still be used.

Furthermore, their presence has also been detected in paper, including no carbon required (NCR) paper [174], as well as in diapers [175] and sanitary pads [176]. In the modern electronics industry, the use of colophony as a fluxing agent in assembly work may be the cause of hand [177] and airborne facial [178] dermatitis. Airborne dermatitis may also result from exposure to sawdust – even associated with leukoderma [179] – cutting oils [180], and even jewelry [181] (Fig. 31.5).

The allergenicity of colophonium can be reduced by chemical modification, i.e., by hydrogenation of the nonaromatic double bonds in the resin, which minimizes

Table 31.3 Products commonly containing colophony or colophony derivatives

Adhesives	Paper
Chewing gums	Polishes
Cleansing agents	Printing inks
Cosmetics	Rosin (used by, e.g., violinists, sportmen)
Cutting fluids[a]	Soldering flux
Dentistry products	Surface coatings
Glues (shoes!)	Ulcer bandages
Insulating tapes	Varnishes
Ostomy appliances	Wood wool
	Wound dressings

[a]Tall oil containing abietic acid may be added

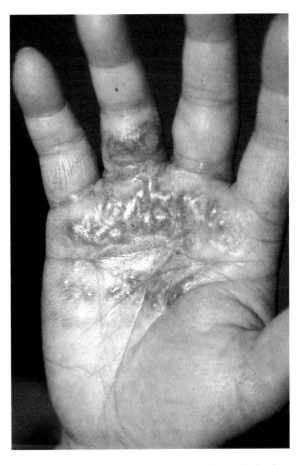

Fig. 31.5 Severe allergic contact dermatitis from colophonium in a Chinese balsam (courtesy of A. Goossens)

the content of easily oxidized acids of the abietic type [182]. A mixture of unmodified Chinese and Portuguese gum rosin is used in the baseline standard series at a concentration of 20% pet. [183], although the optimal patch test material still needs to be defined [184, 185]. In the TRUE test, the concentration is 850 µg/cm². Indeed, if the patient's history indicates heavy exposure to rosin, additional testing with other types of gum rosin and also tall oil rosin may be indicated. If negative responses are still obtained, the possibility of sensitivity to components of modified rosin must be considered [184], since tests with unmodified rosin (in the baseline series) are most often negative in patients who react to modified-rosin derivatives, the latter probably being stronger sensitizers [173, 185, 186].

31.9 Neomycin

Neomycin is a widely used aminoglycoside antibiotic produced from *Streptomyces fradiae*. Aminoglycosides such as neomycin, in particular, and also framycetin and gentamycin have been identified as the most important contact allergens among topical drugs [187–189], for which positive reactions are usually found only on the second patch test reading.

The frequency of neomycin sensitivity varies from clinic to clinic depending to a large extent on local referral and prescription habits [20]. In a series of 40,000 consecutive eczema patients, the patch test results of which were published in 1997, 1–6% had neomycin contact allergy. This is comparable to the results obtained in a study by the EECDRG concerning 26,210 consecutive eczema patients tested in 10 different centers [150] in which the frequency was 3%, with individual frequencies varying from 1.6 to 7.7%.

The patients particularly at risk of neomycin sensitivity appear to be those with chronic and recurrent dermatitis in skin areas where occlusion or bandaging is prone to occur or is used, respectively, as in stasis dermatitis, and also those with otitis externa [190, 191] and perianal eczema. Occupational contact dermatitis as well as systemic reactions may occur.

The diagnosis of neomycin allergy may be difficult because the dermatitis is not vesicular or bullous, but, instead, often appears as an aggravation or simply chronicity of a preexisting dermatitis. It is instructive to note that the therapeutic concentration of neomycin is often

0.5%, while the patch test concentration is 20% in petrolatum. The neomycin concentration in the TRUE Test is 230 µg/cm². Even at this concentration (and in this vehicle) [192], some positives may be missed; the positive neomycin patch test appears late, after 3–4 days in many cases, and there are many interindividual variations.

The cross-sensitization pattern of neomycin is complex. Cross-sensitivity occurs, although not with the same frequency, between neomycin, amikacin, arbekacin, dibekacin, framycetin, gentamycin, isepamicin, kanamycin, paromomycin, ribostamycin, sisomycin, spectinomycin, and tobramycin [193].

31.10 Benzocaine (Ethylaminobenzoate)

Local anesthetics of the *p*-aminobenzoic acid derivatives (benzocaine, procaine, tetracaine) are thought to have strong sensitizing potential, but are less used currently (Scheme 31.2).

Benzocaine is a common sensitizer in patch test clinic patients as was demonstrated by the 1996–1998 North American Contact Dermatitis Group (NACDG) compilation of over 3,400 patch tested patients, revealing an incidence of up to 2% type IV sensitivity to benzocaine [194], similar to the findings in Europe [150]. In the States, this percentage has risen to 3.5% in some centers [195]. Occupational cases have been reported in health-care-personnel dealing with topical anesthesia.

Positive reactions are mainly due to cross-reactivity with *para*-amino compounds such as *para*-aminobenzoic acid and *para*-phenylenediamine (PPD); parabens have also been put forward in this regard although it is thought to be extremely rare [196]. Indeed, to evaluate the rate of cross-reactivity between parabens, PPD, and benzocaine in a population of patients patch tested in a hospital-based contact dermatitis clinic, Turchin

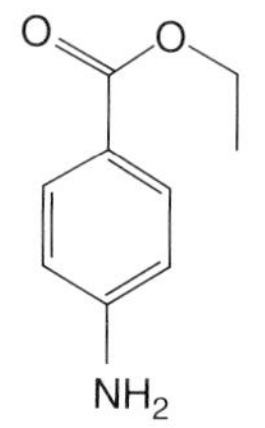

Scheme 31.2 4-Aminobenzoic acid ethyl ester

et al (Canada) performed a retrospective analysis of 4,368 patients consecutively patch tested between July 1989 and June 2005. The study confirmed that the rate of cross-reactions to parabens in PPD- and benzocaine-positive patients combined was 2%. The authors concluded that although this cross-reaction rate was significant in the tested population, it was still falling within the previously reported rates [197]. Benzocaine, being an ester-type local anesthetic, cross-reacts with other esters; however, according to Warshaw et al. [195], in their study, cross-reactivity patterns were not consistent with structural groups. However, in general, benzocaine-sensitive individuals can safely use amide-derivatives such as lidocaine (lignocaine).

According to Sidhu et al. [198] and in agreement with other studies [195, 199, 200], benzocaine (5% petrolatum) alone is inadequate to detect allergic reactions to local anesthetics. Therefore, inclusion of a "caine mix" in the baseline series consisting of benzocaine, tetracaine HCl, and dibucaine HCl (each 5% pet.) was recommended. The TRUE test includes a caine mix containing benzocaine, dibucaine hydrochloride, and tetracaine hydrochloride (5:1:1) 630 μg/cm². Indeed, in the States, dibucaine, an amide anesthetic, was the second most frequent allergen found among these substances. Moreover, in order to detect more patients sensitive to topical anesthetics, testing with all relevant anesthetics is recommended [200, 201] since cross-sensitivity is not consistent [195].

31.11 Clioquinol

Synonyms for clioquinol are: chinoform, chloroiodo-quine, cliochinolum, iodochlorhydroxyquin, iodochlor-rhydroxyquinoline, and 5-chloro-7-iodoquinolin-8-ol (Scheme 31.3).

Because of manufacturing problems, clioquinol 5% pet. replaced the quinoline mix in the European baseline

series. The mix contained a mixture of clioquinol and chlorquinaldol [202]. Both the substances have antibacterial and antifungal activity, and are commonly used in creams and ointments to treat skin conditions in which an antiinfective agent is required. In such preparations, a concentration of 3% is usual, and they are often combined with a topical corticosteroid. Clioquinol has been used orally. Chlorquinaldol is 5,6-dichloro-2-methylquinolin-8-ol. These quinolines are not potent allergens. Cross-reactions between clioquinol and chlorquinaldol are not common, and clioquinol is the more important one of the two allergens. The acquisition of allergic sensitivity to them does not generally cause a marked worsening of eczema, and, when combined with a topical corticosteroid, the steroid will cause some suppression of the inflammatory response. Although Cronin [203] found that no particular pattern of eczema predisposed to clioquinol sensitivity, it may be more common in relation to stasis dermatitis and otitis externa [190, 204]. Geographical variation in the incidence depends on the types of products locally available and the type of patient being investigated. The prevalence of contact allergy to clioquinol is about 0.7% [205]. The oral administration of either clioquinol or chlorquinaldol has resulted in a generalized eruption in individuals allergic to these compounds [206–208]. A recurrent drug eruption due to clioquinol has been reported [209]. An immediate-type reaction occurred in a woman intolerant of oral quinine when clioquinol was applied topically [210]; a quinoline ring is common to both. It may cause contact urticaria on patch testing [211]. In patients tested consecutively to both quinoline mix and clioquinol, it was found that clioquinol alone missed 34% of the patients reacting to quinoline mix [202]. However, in three patients believed to have been sensitized previously to clioquinol, a spectrum of reactions to other halogenated hydroxyquinolines was recorded [212]. Irritant reactions to clioquinol-containing products have also been described, particularly when used in sensitive skin areas, such as the perineum [213, 214].

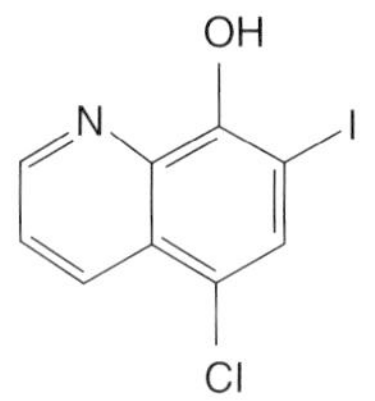

31.12 Wool Wax Alcohols (Lanolin)

Lanolin is a natural product from sheep fleece and consists of a complex mixture of esters and polyesters of high-molecular-weight alcohols and fatty acids. The composition varies from time to time and from place to

Scheme 31.3 Clioquinol

place. Wool wax alcohols (INCI name: lanolin alcohol) are a complex mixture of esters of alcohols and fatty acids derived from the hydrolysis of the oily, waxy fraction of sheep fleece. The general incidence of lanolin allergy in consecutively tested eczema patients is around 2–3% [215, 216] and has decreased over the years [216]. Lanolin and wool wax alcohols are weak allergens and experimental sensitization cannot be achieved in humans and animals [217].

The use of lanolin extends from topical preparations to industrial lubricants, polishes, anticorrosives, printing inks, leather-and textile finishes, and paper constituents. The literature on contact allergy to lanolin has been extensively reviewed [218].

Lanolin allergy is uncommon on normal skin, occurs [219], albeit rarely, with cosmetic usage and is most common when applied to leg ulcers [220] and other diseased skin as in the anogenital area. Because of the rarity of lanolin sensitization when applied to normal skin, every positive patch test to wool wax alcohols and lanolin should be verified to determine if it represents an allergy or nonspecific reactivity (e.g., the excited skin syndrome) [221].

To detect contact allergy cases, wool wax alcohols at a concentration of 30% pet are tested in the baseline series, and the concentration in the TRUE Test is 1,000 µg/cm². Other derivatives have also been tested, among them hydrogenated lanolin and Amerchol L-101 (mineral oil and lanolin alcohol), the latter having been found to be an additional marker for lanolin sensitivity [222]. However, irritant reactions with this compound are not excluded either [221].

31.13 Paraben Mix

The most widely used preservatives in foods, drugs, and cosmetics are the parabens (alkyl esters of *p*-hydroxybenzoic acid) [223]. Parabens were present in 58 of 67 skin creams (87%) analyzed chemically in Denmark [224] (Scheme 31.4).

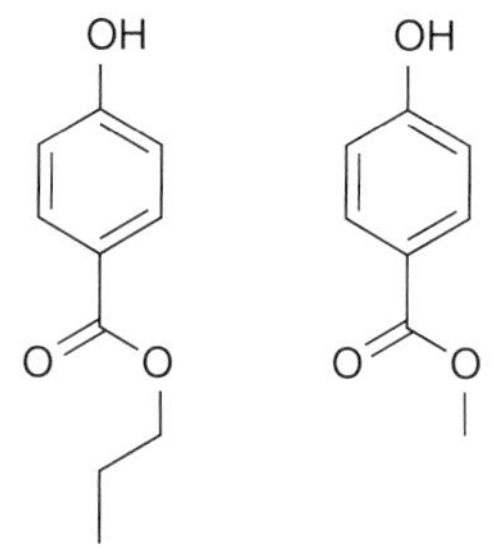

This group of preservatives has been used for more than 60 years and includes methyl-, ethyl-, propyl-, and butylparaben (INCI names). They are also marketed under a number of trade names for use in non-cosmetic products, i.e., Solbrol, Tegosept, Betacide, Bonomold, Chemoside, Nipagin, and Propagin. The parabens are most often used in combination due to

Scheme 31.4 Propylparaben and methylparaben

their different solubility and action spectrum. They are less efficient against gram-negative bacteria; therefore, parabens are often used in cosmetic products in combination with other biocides. The vast majority of the cosmetics registered at the FDA contain parabens and the use concentration is usually in the range of 0.1–0.8%. Cross-reactions between the four paraben esters methyl-, ethyl-, propyl- ,and butylparaben are common, but exceptions can occur. The paraben mix used to contain these four esters plus benzylparaben. Benzylparaben has been removed because it is no longer allowed for use in cosmetics and drugs as it is suspected to be a carcinogen. Further, butylparaben is now in discredit because of estrogenic effects in animal models; however, the clinical implications of this suspicion has not yet been determined [225]. A recent final report on the safety assessment of parabens as used in cosmetic products concluded that they are very safe to use. The expert panel considered both products containing single parabens and multiple parabens, and infant exposures separately from adult exposures. The estimated Margin of Safety (MOS) ranged from 3,000 to 6,000 for infants and from 840 to 1,690 for adults. Further, these estimates were considered to be very conservative [226]. This is a safety margin which is hard to match for most cosmetic ingredients.

In diagnostic patch testing, Menné and Hjorth [227] found that approximately 1.0% of more than 8,000 eczema patients tested were sensitized. Similar frequencies are reported in other large-scale patch test studies [228–230]. The frequency of positive reactions has been remarkably constant over many years [229]. In spite of the extensive use of parabens, it must be regarded as a very safe preservative in topical products and allergic contact dermatitis, as it is relatively rare. In animal experiments, they also seem to be weak allergens; propylparaben was not able to show any sensitization in a guinea pig maximization test [231].

Clinical experience shows that the incidence of paraben sensitization in healthy persons is small, and agrees with the impression that occasional cases of paraben sensitivity occur and are important to the particular patient's welfare [232]. Cosmetics seems to be an uncommon source of paraben sensitization. Clinical experience shows that patients with chronic dermatitis are at risk, particularly patients with stasis dermatitis and leg ulcers [233, 234]. Fisher coined the term "paraben paradox," denoting the fact that many leg ulcer patients with a paraben allergy tolerate paraben-preserved cosmetics on healthy skin [235, 236]. In spite of the low frequency of paraben contact allergy, it is important to keep the allergen in the standard series, since it is difficult to verify the suspicion of the existence of paraben allergy. Often, the sufferers are patients with long-lasting dermatitis that do not get better under normal treatment and skin care. If the allergen is not included in the standard battery series, the diagnosis will be missed.

Fisher et al. [232] and Schorr [237] assumed that repeated topical application of low concentrations of parabens in medicaments or cosmetics could cause sensitization, while Hjorth and Trolle-Lassen [238] stated that higher concentrations were necessary for the majority of cases. They reported a 1% incidence of paraben sensitivity, suggesting that this was due to the frequent use of topical antifungal agents containing up to 5% paraben (Amycen) in Denmark. Cross-reactions have been described to other para compounds, such as benzocaine, PPD, and sulfonamides, but they are rare [239]. It has been reported that paraben-sensitive patients may experience flares of dermatitis from parabens in food and systemic medicaments [240–242]. Placebo-controlled oral challenge with methyl-p-hydroxybenzoate in 14 paraben-sensitive patients was negative in 11, doubtful in one, and two had a flare of dermatitis. However, subsequent low-paraben diet had no effect on the dermatitis [243]. Immediate-type reactions (both systemic and contact urticaria) from parabens have been reported, but are very rare and not related to paraben-induced allergic dermatitis [244, 245].

In the European baseline series, the parabens are tested as a mix of 4% of methyl-, ethyl-, propyl-, and butylparaben, a total of 16% pet., and in the TRUE Test, the concentration is 1,000 µg/cm² (Table 31.1). In Menné and Hjorth's study [227], two-thirds of the patients reacting to the mix showed positive reactions to one or more of the individual esters. Multiple patch test reactivity is probably due to cross-sensitization, but concomitant sensitization to individual esters is a possibility because the esters are often used in combination. Patch testing with products preserved with parabens is often negative in paraben-sensitized patients, because the paraben concentration is too low to elicit dermatitis on normal skin, even under occlusive conditions.

The final details of the paraben story remain to be elucidated. Except for high concentration (i.e., >1%) drug use and application to leg ulcers, the parabens are rare contact sensitizers. Combined with the extensive chronic toxicity data available on their systemic effects, these compounds set the standard for relative safety that new preservatives will have difficulty matching. Technical and microbiological considerations sometimes make alternative preservatives necessary. As development and elicitation of contact allergy is dose dependent, the level of preservative concentration in a product should also be evaluated to avoid over preservation with the subsequent increased risk of causing allergic reactions [246] However, the paraben mix is important in the standard series, because paraben allergy is difficult to detect from the history or clinical appearance of dermatitis.

31.14 Formaldehyde

Formaldehyde is a ubiquitous and potent sensitizer, industrially, domestically, and medically. Lowering its usage concentration to 30 ppm could decrease the cases of allergy observed [247]. Formaldehyde exposure is difficult to estimate because the chemical – besides being manufactured, imported, and used as such – is incorporated into a large variety of products and reactants in many chemical processes, including formaldehyde releasers, polymerized plastics, metal-working fluids, medicaments, fabrics, cosmetics, and detergents (Table 31.4) [248]. Therefore, the detection of the formaldehyde content by chemical analysis, such as the closed container diffusion method as proposed by Karlberg et al., would be interesting for the prevention of recurrence of allergic contact dermatitis in formaldehyde-allergic patients [249]. Shampoos may contain formaldehyde, but because they are quickly diluted and washed off, only exquisitely formaldehyde-sensitive consumers develop dermatitis on the scalp and face from them. However, hairdressers may get hand dermatitis from similar products due to

Table 31.4 Formaldehyde uses and exposure

Clothing, wash and wear, crease-resistant clothing
Medications: wart remedies, anhidrotics
Antiperspirants
Preservative in cosmetics
Photographic paper and solutions
Paper industry
Disinfectants and deodorizers
Cleaning products
Polishes
Paints and coatings
Printing etching materials
Tanning agents
Dry cleaning materials
Chipboard production
Mineral wool production
Glues
Phenolic resins and urea plastics in adhesives and footwear
Fish meal industry
Smoke from wood, coal, and tobacco (relevance is controversial)

their more intense exposure, and it is important to be aware of the fact that formaldehyde-releasing preservatives in cosmetics and topical drugs may elicit allergic contact dermatitis in formaldehyde-sensitive consumers [250, 251].

Formaldehyde dermatitis from textiles is rare today because the manufacturers have improved the fabric finish treatment and have reduced the amount of formaldehyde residues in new clothing. Garments made from 100% acrylic, polyester, linen, silk, nylon, and cotton are generally considered to be formaldehyde free [252, 253]. Formaldehyde sensitivity is not necessarily accompanied by a simultaneous sensitivity to formaldehyde resins and formaldehyde releasers, and vice versa [254, 255]. Fifty-three percent of formaldehyde-sensitive patients tested in a UK multicentre study were positive to 1 or more of the 4 formaldehyde releasers tested: quaternium-15, imidazolidinyl urea, diazolidinyl urea, and 2-bromo-2-nitropropane-1,3-diol [229]. Indeed, some of the formaldehyde releasers might act as prohaptens. It depends on the exposure conditions

and the actual release of formaldehyde. The frequency of formaldehyde-positive patch tests in consecutive eczema patients is around 2–3% [20, 230, 256].

Inexplicable positive patch test reactions frequently occur where no clinical relevance is found. A deeper search, however, might often reveal it. Hidden sources of formaldehyde at home may be a cause of hand eczema in some women with formaldehyde allergy. Occupational formaldehyde allergy is quite common and occurs in metal workers, hairdressers, masseurs, and workers using protective creams, detergents, and liquid soaps. Seventeen samples of metal working fluid concentrates were analyzed for formaldehyde and detected in all samples in concentrations ranging between 0.002 and 1.3%, and the content of total formaldehyde was not declared in any of the safety data sheets [257]. In a Finnish retrospective study of occupational formaldehyde allergy, reactivity to formaldehyde releasers without formaldehyde allergy was rare [258] In certain cases, the positive patch test should be confirmed by a repeated test and a use test, since false-positive reactions may occur; this may explain as to why about one-third of allergies reported to formaldehyde and its releasers can be lost on repeated patch testing, although a lack of reproducibility in patch testing might also account for this phenomenon [259, 260]. In a detailed clinical experiment, the eliciting closed patch test threshold concentration was 10,000 ppm formaldehyde in 10 of 20 formaldehyde-sensitive individuals, 9 reacted to 5,000 ppm, 3 reacted to 1,000 ppm, 2 reacted to 500 ppm, and 1 reacted to 250 ppm (Fig. 31.6). Positive reactions were not observed in nonoccluded patch tests with a dilution series from 25 to 10,000 ppm, or in a ROAT with a leave-on cosmetic product containing a formaldehyde releaser (an average of 300 ppm formaldehyde) [261]. Thus, the threshold concentration for occluded patch test to formaldehyde in formaldehyde-sensitive patients seems to be around 250 ppm.

A follow-up study of 57 formaldehyde-sensitive eczema patients interviewed and examined 1–5 years after initial diagnosis showed that many of the patients were still exposed to formaldehyde-containing products. However, those who paid attention to their allergy had significantly fewer exacerbations of dermatitis than those who did not, and there was a trend that severe eczema was found more often in patients still exposed to formaldehyde. This study also showed that formaldehyde is widely distributed in the environment and is difficult to avoid, because many finished

Fig. 31.6 Lowest formaldehyde concentration giving positive reactions in occluded patch testing, compared to the strength of the reactions in diagnostic patch testing (10,000 ppm) among 19 formaldehyde-sensitive eczema patients (from [261])

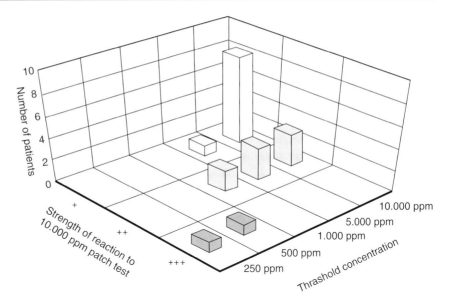

products may contain small amounts of formaldehyde. It may not appear on the label though, as formaldehyde can be present in raw materials that may be released during storage and use [262]. It is a challenge to inform and train formaldehyde-allergic patients how to best avoid exposure to formaldehyde and formaldehyde releasers because there are so many sources in the environment [263].

Immediate reactions from formaldehyde may also occur, both of presumably allergic and nonallergic nature [264–266].

Formaldehyde releasers used as preservatives in cosmetics and technical products are often concealed by a multitude of trade names or synonyms [267]. The epidemiology of formaldehyde sensitization requires reevaluation. Most early studies utilized irritant patch test concentrations. The current recommended patch test concentration is 1% aq. [268], and the TRUE Test contains 180 μg/cm^2.

31.15 Quaternium-15

Quaternium-15 is a quaternary ammonium salt that conforms to the formula (Scheme 31.5):

It is a formaldehyde releaser used chiefly as a cosmetic preservative, and it is also an antistatic agent [269].

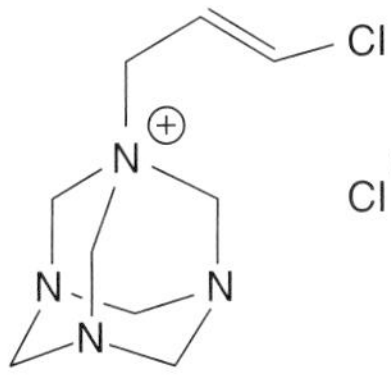

Scheme 31.5 Quaternium-15

Formaldehyde releasers are in widespread usage in industry, household products, and cosmetics. They are marketed under a multitude of trade names. Chemically, they are linear or cyclic reversible polymers of formaldehyde, and formaldehyde is formed in different amounts, depending mainly on temperature and pH.

Quaternium-15 has several synonymous names: Dowicil 200, 100, and 75, CoSept 200, Preventol D1, 1-(3-chloroallyl)-3,5,7-triaza-1-azonia – adamantane chloride, chloroallyl methanamine chloride, *N*-(3-chlorallyl)-hexamine chloride, chlorallyl methenamine chloride. Formaldehyde is released in small amounts and formaldehyde-sensitive patients may react simultaneously to this preservative [270]. However, quaternium-15 sensitivity may also be directed towards the entire molecule. Allergic contact dermatitis from a formaldehyde-releasing agent may, thus, be due to the entire molecule, to formaldehyde, or to both [229, 255, 271]. Positive quaternium-15 patch tests are often of

31

clinical relevance [272]. In about 50% of the cases, simultaneous reactivity is seen to formaldehyde [260]. The usual preservative concentration of 0.1% releases about 100 ppm free formaldehyde and this concentration can elicit dermatitis in the axillae in formaldehyde-sensitive patients [273].

The repeated use of lotions and creams with this preservative may provoke dermatitis by mild irritation from the vehicles and subsequent sensitivity to the preservative. Sensitive patients should request cosmetics without formaldehyde releasers, even though some alternative formaldehyde releasers might be tolerated due to reduced formaldehyde production. Full cosmetic ingredients labeling, as that required today, makes it easy to avoid the use of specific ingredients in sensitized subjects [274]. However, because of the many different formaldehyde-releasing preservatives on the market, it is difficult for many patients to read and comprehend the list of ingredients on cosmetic products and safety data sheets for industrial products [263]. Occupational contact dermatitis due to quaternium-15 is extremely uncommon; two cases of hand dermatitis in hairdressers, one case of nail dystrophy in an engineer, and a case of periorbital and hand dermatitis from an electrode gel in an electroencephalogram technician, and airborne dermatitis from a photocopier toner containing quaternium-15 have been reported [275–278]. The frequency of positive reactions varies from country to country, possibly due to variations in the frequency of use [228–230]. Quaternium 15 is an important allergen for hand eczema [279]. The patch test concentration is 1% pet. and 100 μg/cm^2 in the TRUE Test.

31.16 Methylchloro- and Methylisothiazolinone (MCI/MI)

The isothiazolinones (5-chloro-2-methyl-4-isothiazolin-3-one and 2-methyl-4-isothiazolin-3-one, 3:1 ratio by weight) are the active ingredients in Kathon CG (Rohm and Haas, Philadelphia), a cosmetic preservative. The INCI-adopted names for the active chemicals are MCI/MI, and they appear in the preservative in the ratio of 3:1 (Scheme 31.6).

Isothiazolinones are used extensively as effective biocides to preserve the water content of cosmetics, toiletries, household, and industrial products, such as metalworking fluids, water-based paints (Fig. 31.5), cooling

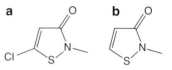

Scheme 31.6 Methylchloroisothiazolinone and methylisothiazolinone

Table 31.5 Biocides containing methylchloroisothiazolinone/methylisothiazolinone. Some of these products may also contain other ingredients

Kathon CG	Metat GT
Kathon DP	Metatin GT
Kathon 886 MW	Mitco CC 31 L
Kathon LX	Mitco CC 32 L
Kathon WT	Special Mx 323
Acticide	Parmetol DF 35
Algucid CH 50	Parmetol DF 12
Amerstat 250	Parmetol A 23
Euxyl K 100	Parmetol K 50
Fennosan IT 21	Parmetol K 40
GR 856 Izolin	Parmetol DF 18
Grotan TK 2	P 3 Multan D
Grotan K	Piror P 109
Mergal K 7	

tower water, latex emulsions, and for slime control in paper mills [280]. Also, other isothiazolinone derivatives, such as 2-methyl-4,5 trimethylene-4-isothiazolin-3-one (MTI) and 2-octyl-4-isothiazolin-3-one (Skane M8) are used as biocides for paints and latex emulsions [281, 282].

Isothiazolinones are marketed under many brand names (Table 31.5) [283], which make it easy to overlook the presence of these chemicals in the formulations. Approximately 25% of all cosmetic products and toiletries – in particular, rinse-off products – in the Netherlands in the late 1980s contained Kathon CG and synonymous preservatives [280]. A Danish study examined the content of MCI/MI in registered chemical products for occupational use in 2005 and compared with similar data from 2002. It appeared that the use of MCI/MI increased considerably in water-based paint and laquers while it decreased for toiletries and cosmetics.

Some of the change may be explained be changes in registration practice [284]. The frequent registration of MCI/MI in water-based paints and lacquers may be a possible explanation for the relatively high and stable frequency of positive patch tests to MCI/MI [229].

MCI/MI is a strong sensitizer in guinea pig allergy tests, and when tested separately, MCI is stronger than MI [231, 285]. Multiple reports have documented a varying and, in some countries in the late 1980s, an increasing incidence of allergic contact dermatitis from these chemicals, probably explained by increased exposure [286]. Over the last 15 years, the incidence of MCI/MI contact allergy has remained around 2.0–2.5% of consecutively tested eczema patients in Europe [230]. A retrospective survey in Finland encompassing about 9,000 consecutively tested patients showed a decrease in MCI/MI patch test positivity from 2.4% during the period 1995–1997 to 1.3% during the period 2000–2002, probably a reflection of changed exposure from cosmetics [287]. MI alone has appeared as a preservative for use in cosmetics, glues, and paints and has caused an outbreak of occupational contact dermatitis in a paint factory [288] (Fig. 31.7).

MCI/MI is an important allergen for the hands and the face, and it may also cause urticaria [289, 290] and airborne contact dermatitis [291–293]. The airborne MCI/MI dermatitis may appear in the face of sensitized individuals who stay in newly painted rooms, and the diagnosis is easily missed unless specifically considered [291–293]. In cosmetic products, the permissible level of MCI/MI is 15 ppm, and it appears that this concentration in rinse-off products is rather safe, since most subjects previously sensitized to MCI/MI tolerated the use of a shampoo preserved with MCI/MI for 2 weeks [294]. In leave-on products, a maximum concentration of 7.5 ppm is recommended. A double-blind, placebo-controlled, dose–response ROAT in MCI/MI sensitive volunteers and controls showed that both time and exposure dose determines the outcome of the ROAT with an elicitation threshold for MCI/MI in the proximity of 2 ppm [295].

Patch test reactions to MCI/MI may show unusually sharp borders and can still be true allergic reactions. The patch test concentration is 100 ppm aq. This is the best compromise, as higher concentrations (200–300 ppm) may produce irritation and patch test sensitization [280, 296]. On the other hand, 100 ppm may, in some cases, perhaps give false-negative test results on normal back skin in patients with an isothiazolinone-induced aggravation of hand dermatitis. A use test is helpful in doubtful cases of allergy. Due to the activity of isothiazolinones on the skin, it is imperative that exact dosing be used when isothiazolinones are used for patch testing. In the TRUE Test, the concentration is 4 $\mu g/cm^2$. Patch testing with products preserved with MCI/MI is often negative in sensitized patients, while a use test may be positive. With regard to the prevention of chemical burns and allergic contact dermatitis from higher concentrations, addition of sodium bisulfite seems to have the capacity to "deactivate" the MCI/MI mixture [297]. There is no cross-sensitization between MCI/MI and two other isothiazolinones, benzisothiazolinone (Proxel) and octyl-isothiazolinone (Kathon 893, Skane M8) [298]. Patients sensitized to MI also react to MCI while the opposite is not obligatory [299].

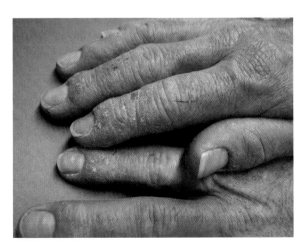

Fig. 31.7 Painter with occupational hand eczema and contact allergy to Bronopol and Kathon CG used as preservatives in water-based paints

31.17 Para-phenylenediamine

PPD is a colorless compound that acts as a primary intermediate in hair dyes. It is oxidized by hydrogen peroxide and then polymerized to a color within the hair by a coupler (such as resorcinol). In Europe, it is now permitted in amounts of up to 4% free base in hair dyes before the addition of peroxide. This equates to 2% as the maximum use dilution (Scheme 31.7).

Most cases of contact allergy to PPD occur from contact with hair dyes, in either the consumer or the hairdresser [300]. It is one of the substances most

31

Scheme 31.7 *para*-Phenylenediamine

useful in the initial patch test screening of hairdressers with dermatitis [301]. A weighted average prevalence was 4.6% among 21 515 patients tested in European clinics. PPD sensitization occurred more often in centers located in Central and Southern Europe than in Scandinavian centers. The overall proportion of positive patch test reactions to PPD that were registered as being of either current or "past" relevance was high (weighted average 53.6 and 20.3%, respectively). Consumer hair dyeing was the most prominent cause of PPD sensitization (weighted average 41.8%). Furthermore, occupational hair dye exposure (10.6%) and cross-sensitization to textile dyes (12.6%) were frequently reported. [302]. The information network of the Departments of Dermatology in Germany (IVDK) reported that PPD was the fifth most common allergen (4.8%) in 40,000 patients, again with considerable geographical variation in frequency, ranging from 2.8 to 7.1% [20]. A review of published literature containing PPD patch test data showed that the median prevalence among dermatitis patients was 4.3% in Asia, 4% in Europe, and 6.2% in North America. A widespread increase in the prevalence of PPD sensitization was observed among Asian dermatitis patients [303]. Many cases of PPD allergy are seen in men from the Indian subcontinent who are resident in the United Kingdom, due to the fact that they dye their hair and beard.

PPD is an important occupational allergen in hairdressers in relation to hand dermatitis. In this group, sensitization may be facilitated by irritation of the hands from wetness, shampoos, and perming lotions. The most important measures to reduce the risk of allergic reactions from hair dyes include, besides improved products, effective removal of excess hair dye formulation from newly dyed hair, the use of protective gloves, and adequate education and information. A multicenter German study of hairdressers with hand dermatitis showed that the prevalence of contact allergy to PPD dropped from 26.6 to 17.2% between 1995 and 2002 [304]. Among a series of 40

hairdressers with a known contact allergy to PPD, none reacted to a new generation of hair dyes containing FD&C and D&C colors, which suggests a possible safer alternative [305].

In consumers, allergic contact dermatitis caused by PPD can be severe [306], with edema of the face, scalp, and ears that may be clinically mistaken for angioedema [307]. Although its use is illegal in Europe, active sensitization to PPD has been increasingly observed from its use as a skin paint in so-called *temporary tattoos* when *black henna* is used [308, 309].

PPD often gives rise to strong patch test reactions in sensitive patients. The reactions may appear after a very short patch test application time. In six of 16 PPD-sensitive patients, 15 min exposure to 1% PPD was sufficient to elicit an eczematous reaction [310]. Patients with PPD allergy may show cross-reactions with benzocaine, procaine, sulfonamides and PABA sunscreens, azo and aniline dyes, anthraquinone, antihistamines, and the rubber antioxidant 4-isopropylamino-diphenylamine [311]. However, Cronin did not find that any of 47 hairdressers positive to PPD reacted to the PPD–rubber mix [312]. Cross-reactions to other related hair dyes, such as *p*-toluenediamine, *p*-aminodiphenylamine, 2,4-diaminoanisole, and *p*-aminophenol are seen. Also, cross-reactivity between azo dyes and *para*-amino compounds are common. Seidenari et al. [313] studied 236 consecutively tested dermatitis patients sensitized to at least one of six azo textile dyes. Cosensitizations to PPD were present in most subjects sensitized to *p*-aminoazobenzene (75%) and Disperse Orange 3 (66%), while the following gave lower rates of cosensitization; Disperse Yellow 3 (36%), Disperse Red 1 (27%), and Disperse Blue 124 (only 16%) [313]. Apart from the hands and face, the neck and axilla were the most frequently involved skin sites in these patients. Cross-sensitizations between azo dyes and *para*-amino compounds can partly be explained on the basis of structural affinities or metabolic conversion in the skin [314]. Further, clinical experiments in selected patients with contact allergy to para-group haptens have shown that patch test reactivity to oxidizable aromatic haptens depends on the amount of freshly reduced substance, the rate of oxidation on the skin, and, therefore, the quantity of reactive intermediates, such as quinones [315]. This cross-reactivity pattern may explain the difficulty in finding the relevance of some PPD positives. Immediate-type hypersensitivity to PPD, with urticarial reactions, including anaphylaxis have been reported [316, 317]. PPD base

1% pet. was replaced by PPD dihydrochloride 0.5% pet. in the standard series in 1984. There was a general impression that this led to fewer positives. A multicenter trial showed that the dihydrochloride missed some true positives, and so, it was replaced in 1988 by PPD free base 1% pet. [94]. The TRUE Test contains 90 μg/cm². PPD is not present in the baseline series used in Germany, because the risk of active sensitization is considered to be unacceptable [318], a decision which is arguable.

31.18 Thiuram Mix

The thiuram mix used in the baseline series contains the following four compounds, each at a dilution of 0.25%.

Tetraethylthiuram disulfide (TETD, disulfiram), tetramethylthiuram disulfide (TMTD), tetramethylthiuram monosulfide (TMTM), and dipentamethylenethiuram disulfide (PTD). The concentration in the TRUE Test is 25 μg/cm² (Scheme 31.8):

These chemicals are accelerating agents used in the vulcanization of rubber. They increase the rate of crosslinking by sulfur between the hydrocarbon chains of the uncured rubber and may also donate some sulfur to the reaction. In the fully cured product, unreacted accelerators remain. Over time, some of these may migrate onto the surface of the finished article, together with other rubber chemicals. By thorough washing with hot water of thin rubber items, such as latex-dipped gloves or condoms, it is possible to leach out most of these thiuram residues.

The use of thiurams is ubiquitous in the rubber industry. The compounds are encountered in rubbers for both industrial and domestic use. Different manufacturers have preferences for the particular thiurams that they use for particular applications. This fact may explain geographical variations in the incidence of sensitivity to components of the mix [319]. Gloves are the most common cause of rubber dermatitis, and the allergen is usually a thiuram [320, 321]. Rubber glove dermatitis is important in the health care setting [322], where an increase in thiuram allergy in health care workers with hand dermatitis has been reported [323]. Release of thiuram from rubber gloves into synthetic sweat may vary between brands [324]. Thiuram sensitivity is more common in women than in men. Foot dermatitis, particularly in children, may be caused by the rubber in shoes [325]. Construction workers also constitute a risk group regarding the development of rubber allergy due to frequent use of gloves and boots [326].

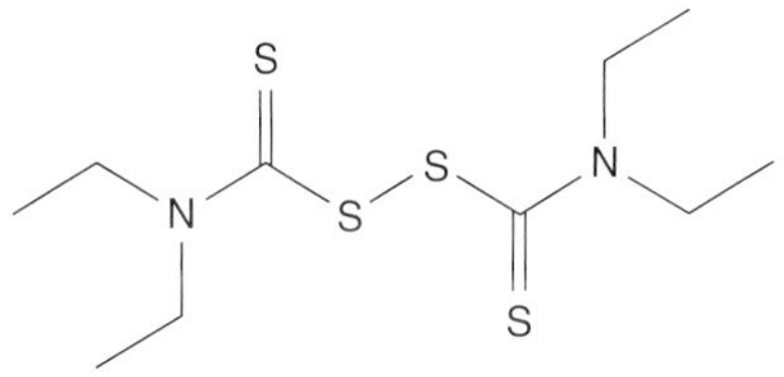

An allergic contact dermatitis from a thiuram in rubber often has no clear clinical pattern, and, in a glove dermatitis, the classical distribution of the eczematous reaction may not be present. This classical pattern consists of a diffuse eczema over the back of the hands and a band of eczema to the midforearm at the level of the cuff of the glove. Rubber sensitivity is often clinically significant for eczema.

In individuals who are sensitive to thiurams, the use of vinyl gloves, shoes with leather or polyurethane soles, and clothing elasticated with elastane (a polyurethane elastomer) may be required where indicated to reduce personal exposure to the allergens.

Thiurams have found wide use as fungicides, particularly for agricultural purposes, and also for such applications in wallpaper adhesives and paints. They have also been used in animal repellents. TETD has been used in scabicidal soap. TETD, when administered systemically, causes inhibition of the enzyme aldehyde dehydrogenase. On taking an alcoholic drink, there is a build-up of acetaldehyde, which causes skin irritation, erythema, and urticaria. In the form of Antabuse®, TETD is used to treat alcohol dependence. Topical exposure to TETM and oral intake of alcohol has caused a similar toxic reaction, as has the taking of Antabuse and topical exposure to alcohol in toiletries [327–330]. TETD has been used to treat vesicular hand eczema in nickel-sensitive individuals [331]. A widespread eczematous reaction may develop after systemic administration of TETD to previously sensitized individuals [332, 333].

The carbamates (as the caraba mix) are no longer included in the European baseline series of contact allergens [94, 334]. It was shown that the majority of individuals who gave an allergic reaction to carba mix (diphenylguanidine, zinc dibutyl dithiocarbamate, zinc diethyl dithiocarbamate) also reacted to the thiuram mix. The thiuram mix is, therefore, a good

Scheme 31.8 TETD

detector of rubber sensitivity to this group of rubber chemicals, to which they are chemically similar – although a concomitant sensitization cannot always be excluded, since rubber gloves usually contain more than one accelerator [334]. However, a more extensive series of rubber components may be useful in selected risk groups of dermatitis patients with significant exposure to rubber in an industrial setting [335].

Both the thiuram mix and the carba mix may cause false-positive patch test results [321, 336]. The carba mix produced gave irritant reactions, which were frequently misinterpreted.

31.19 Mercapto Mix and Mercaptobenzothiazole

The mercapto mix contains the following four compounds, each at a concentration of 0.5% pet.:

2-mercaptobenzothiazole (MBT), N-cyclohexyl-2-benzothiazyl sulfenamide (CBS), 2,2-dibenzothiazyl disulfide (MBTS), and Morpholinyl mercaptobenzothiazole MMBT (Scheme 31.9).

Mercaptobenzothiazole is tested alone at a concentration of 2% pet. The TRUE Test includes MBT 75 µg/cm^2 and MBS, MBTS, and CBS (1:1:1) 75 µg/cm^2 in two separate patches. These chemicals are present in many rubbers, to which they are added as accelerators before vulcanization takes place (see Sect. 31.18), and, like thiurams, are ubiquitous in rubber products. The majority of individuals who react to the mix react to MBT if tested to the individual components of the mix, and it is, therefore, not possible to identify the primary allergen. Fregert [337] observed that benzene with a thiazole ring and a thiol group in the two position was required for cross-sensitization to occur.

According to Cronin [338], gloves or shoes have probably sensitized women who react to MBT, but, in men, the sensitization is mainly from footwear, in which MBT is one of the most important allergens [339]. Among the numerous other sources of contact with rubbers containing MBT are rubber handles, masks, elastic bands, tubing, elasticated garments, artificial limbs [340], and even cosmetic sponges [341]. MBT may be present in a variety of nonrubber products, including cutting oils, greases, coolants, antifreezes, fungicides, adhesives, and veterinary medicaments [342].

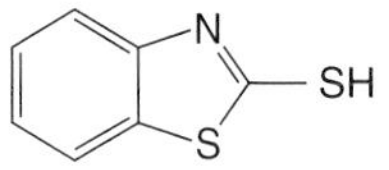

In 32,475 consecutive tested patients attending European clinics, 327 patients were positive to the mix or MBT, or both. Two hundred and sixty one were positive to the mix and 254 to MBT. MBT was negative in 73 patients who were positive to the mix. If the mix had not been in the standard series, on an average, 22% of patients allergic to a mercapto-compound would have been missed; for MBT, this would have been, on an average, 20%. All clinics would have missed a significant number of positive reactions if both compounds had not been tested. Therefore, it has been concluded that both the mercapto mix and MBT are required in the baseline series [343].

The mercapto mix used in North America does not contain MBT, which is tested separately at 1% pet., the concentration of the remaining three allergens being 0.33%. On reviewing the sensitivity of patch test material, the German Contact Dermatitis Research Group (DKG) has recommended testing with the components of the mercapto mix when there is a reaction to either the mix or MBT itself [344]. Analysis of the stability of the mercaptobenzothiazole compounds has shown that the so-called cross-sensitivity reported for this group may be the result of chemical interaction resulting in one main hapten in the presence of reducing sulfhydryl compounds [345].

31.20 N-Isopropyl-N-Phenyl-p-Phenylenediamine (IPPD)

IPPD 0.1% pet. replaced, in the baseline series, the black-rubber mix, which contained the following three compounds in pet.:

IPPD, phenylisopropyl-p-phenylenediamine, 4-isopropylamino-diphenylamine: 0.1% N-phenyl-N-cyclohexyl-p-phenylenediamine (CPPD): 0.25% N,N-diphenyl-p-phenylenediamine (DPPD): 0.25% (Scheme 31.10).

Scheme 31.9 MBT

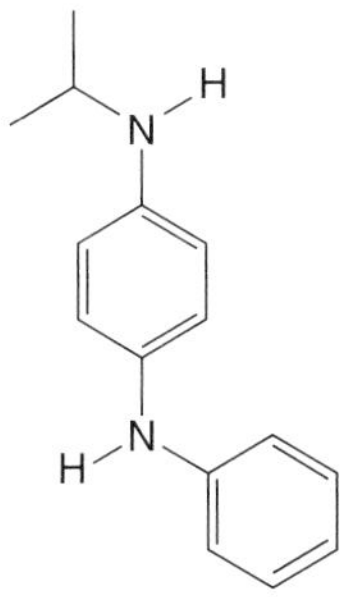

Scheme 31.10 IPPD

Although IPPD was the most important allergen in the black-rubber mix, by testing only with IPPD in the standard series, approximately 10% of allergy to these industrial rubber chemicals may escape detection [346]. The TRUE Test includes IPPD, CPPD, and DPPD (2:5:5) 75 μg/cm^2. With time, vulcanized rubber gradually reacts with atmospheric oxygen and ozone to crack and crumble, a process known as perishing. To reduce this effect, antioxidants and antiozonants may be added before vulcanization, particularly to those rubbers intended for heavy and stressful uses, such as in tires and industrial applications. A number of antiozonant types are available, but those based on the derivatives of p-phenylenediamine (PPD derivatives, staining antidegradants) are in common use [347]. The chemicals used as antiozonants are not related in use to p-phenylenediamine, which is a hair dye. IPPD was established as a contact allergen in heavy-duty rubber goods when Bieber and Foussereau [348] reported nine cases, including four men who had occupational contact with tires.

Manufacturers of rubber chemicals have attempted to produce an antiozonant with the desired technical properties of IPPD, but having a reduced potential for inducing sensitization. A substitute that has been proposed for IPPD is N-(1,3-dimethylbutyl)-N-phenyl-p-phenylenediamine (DMPPD), which was claimed to have a lower potential for inducing cutaneous sensitization and, as a result, has replaced IPPD and some of its derivatives in many applications. However, in practice, it has been noted that individuals who are allergic to IPPD usually react to DMPPD on patch testing [349]. Herve-Bazin et al. [350] evaluated 42 tire handlers who were IPPD-sensitive and found that all 15 who were also tested to DMPPD reacted to it. Guinea-pig maximization test performed independently by this group showed DMPPD to be a more potent allergen than IPPD

in this animal model. DMPPD was not present in the standard series mix.

In factories where IPPD continues to be used as an antiozonant, no significant excess of allergic reactions to it was found [351]; this may be related to the considerably improved hygiene in rubber factories and automation in recent years. The hand dermatitis induced by hypersensitivity to PPD-derived antiozonants often has a palmar distribution, because this is the usual area of skin contact with rubbers most likely to contain these agents. Clinically, a PPD-derivative hand dermatitis can look endogenous. The prognosis of such a PPD-derivative hand dermatitis can be adversely affected by allowing chronic exposure to the offending allergen and may cause the dermatitis to persist after avoidance of further contact. IPPD has been shown to be an important occupational allergen for construction workers and farmers [107, 352]. Although PPD-derived antiozonants are commonly present in rubbers for heavy-duty applications, they may also be present in other rubbers. Examples of these include squash balls, scuba masks [353], motorcycle handles [354], boots [355, 356], watch straps [357], rubber bracelets [358], eyelash curlers [359], spectacle chains [360], and orthopedic bandages [361]. A purpuric contact dermatitis has been described in some individuals sensitive to IPPD. The dermatitis was summarized by Fisher [362] as being pruritic, petechial, and purpuric. The reaction is usually localized to the area of skin contact, but may also be widespread. Purpuric patch tests to IPPD have been reported. A lichenoid contact dermatitis from IPPD has been observed [363], although the histological features of the reaction were those of a lichenified dermatitis.

31.21 Epoxy Resin

Some 95% of all epoxy resins consist of a glycidyl ether group formed by the reaction of bisphenol A with epichlorohydrin. Theoretically, there are many different chemical compositions that can be used to make an epoxy resin. Along with the resin itself, there are fillers, pigments, plasticizers, reactive diluents, and solvents, and these compounds are then mixed with a hardening/curing agent that polymerizes the resin (Scheme 31.11).

Epichlorohydrin/bisphenol A epoxy resin can vary in molecular weight from 340 to much larger polymers, the latter having much less sensitizing capacity [364]. Epoxy

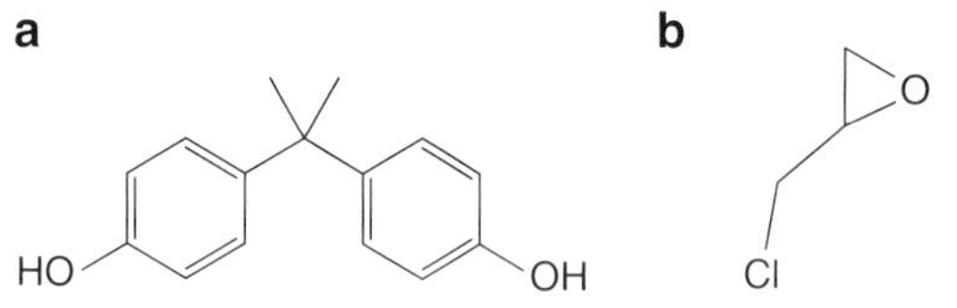

31

a

b

Scheme 31.11 Bisphenol A, epichlorohydrin polymer

resins are used as adhesives (also in shoes!); in paints requiring hardness and durability, for instance in ships; in electrical insulation; as an additive to cement for quick bonding and strength; as well as in fiber glass (e.g., in boats) and for impregnating carbon fiber cloth [365] used in situations of stress and heat, such as aeroplanes. Epoxy resin has also been reported to be the cause of occupational contact dermatitis in the production of skis [366], in a windmill factory [367], and more recently, related to sports such as bowling [368], and golf [369]. An unexpected source of epoxy allergy, epoxy compounds present in an immersion oil, caused a worldwide epidemic among laboratory technicians performing microscopy some years ago[see 370, for a review].

Epoxy resin systems are important sensitizers and are very often responsible for occupational airborne dermatitis. However, other dermatological conditions have also been associated with epoxy resin, reactive diluents, or other components, i.e., vitiligo [371] and lichenoid reactions [372]. IgE-mediated reactions are also known occupational hazards [373, 374].

In the baseline series, it is the epoxy resin of the bisphenol A type that is tested (1% pet). The TRUE Test contains 50 μg/cm^2.In a retrospective study in 26,210 consecutively tested patients the frequency was 1.3% [375], A negative patch test to epoxy resin does not mean that the patient is not allergic to the epoxy product that they have been using for the following reasons: (a) there may be some other epoxy resin in the compound; (b) they may be allergic to some other compound in the resin, for instance dyes, fillers, plasticizers, etc. (uncommon); (c) or they may be allergic to the hardener. If epoxy allergy is suspected, it is very important to test for other types of epoxy resins such as bisphenol F-based resins [376, 377], dimethacrylated epoxy resins, which are used extensively in dental composite resins [e.g., 378], UV-cured inks [379], which have become important allergens, as well as other epoxy systems [380]. Attempts have been made to improve the diagnostics of contact allergy to epoxy resin systems [381]. Moreover, the specific compounds used by the patients

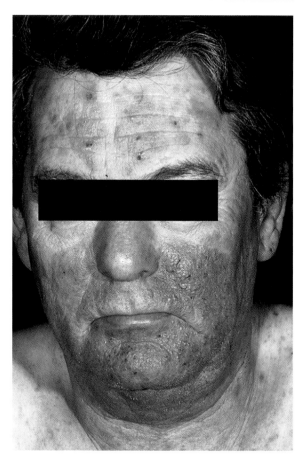

Fig. 31.8 Airborne contact dermatitis from epoxy resin in a patient who frequently repaired models (airplanes, ships) in his toy shop. He wore glasses due to presbyopia, explaining the sparing of the ocular region (courtesy of P.J. Frosch)

should also be tested, but extreme care must be taken to avoid primary sensitization [370] (Fig. 31.8).

Hardeners cannot be contained in the standard series, because, although 95% of epoxy resins are one particular chemical, very many different hardeners are used. Both epoxy resins and hardeners can be irritant – also in patch testing – as well as sensitizing, although isolated contact allergy to hardeners without an allergy to epoxy resins is rare. Here too, patch testing with the hardeners to which the patients have been exposed may be advisable in order to detect the allergen [382].

Many patients give a positive patch test to epoxy resin without any obvious contact with uncured epoxy resin. It may be that the source of sensitization is contact with the so-called cured epoxy, which may contain pockets of uncured resin. Fregert and Trulsson [383] have suggested that chemical tests may be of value in demonstrating uncured resin. There are two tests for epoxy resin, one a simple color reaction, which is not specific for uncured resin, the other thin-layer chromatography, which is specific.

Finally, some others have observed a relationship between epoxy resin and fragrance allergy, the reason for which is not yet clear [384, 385].

31.22 *Para-Tertiary*-Butylphenol-Formaldehyde Resin

Para-tertiary-butylphenol-formaldehyde resin (PTBP resin) is made by reacting the substituted phenol *p-tert*-butylphenol with formaldehyde. It is a useful adhesive that sticks rapidly, is durable and pliable, and has high strength at raised temperatures. Because of its flexibility, it is used in shoe construction and in leather goods. It is also used in other contact adhesives such as those used in laminating surfaces and in the rubber industry for bonding rubber to rubber and rubber to metal [386]. These contact adhesives based on PTBP resins are often formulated with neoprene (a synthetic rubber), which provides the initial bonding until the resin cures (Scheme 31.12).

PTBP resins have commonly been reported as causes of both occupational and nonoccupational allergic contact dermatitis. The first occupational cases were described in individuals making or repairing shoes [387] who developed hand eczema, but PTBP resins are also among the most important allergens in those who wear shoes containing this adhesive [387–389].

There are, however, many other occupational sensitizing sources to PTBP resin, such as adhesives for fixing rubber weather-strip car-door seals in place in car assembly plants [390] and finishes for glass wool causing airborne dermatitis [391]. PTBP resin in athletic tape has been reported as an occupational sensitization source in female athletes in Japan [392]. Nonoccupational

sources of hypersensitivity to PTBP resin include an adhesive of the pads of a derotation brace and a finishing agent in a raincoat fabric [393], leather watchstraps glued with the adhesive [394], some brands of plastic fingernail adhesive [395], as well as domestic PTBP resin adhesives [396]. It may also be present on adhesive labels [397], even in the adhesive dressing used to secure an intravenous canula [398]. Other sensitization sources include items, such as a wetsuit [399], a knee brace [400], a limb prosthesis [401, previously reported in 1985, 402], and electrodes [403]. Also religious practices may be involved [404].

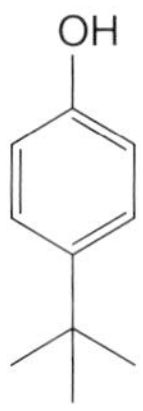

The frequency of PTBP-resin sensitivity reported by the Information Network of Departments of Dermatology in Germany was 0.9% in 40,000 patients [20] and 1.3% in a recent study by the EECDRG of 26,210 consecutively tested eczema patients [375].

There are many allergens in PTBP resin, including low-, medium-, and high-molecular-weight fractions, for which the pattern of reactivity differs among patients hypersensitive to the resin [405], but PTBP itself is a rare allergen (as is formaldehyde in the resin). *Para-tert*-butylcatechol (PTBC), a potent sensitizer used in paint manufacture and in the rubber and plastics industries [406], was found to be present in some PTBP-F-resins and to cross-react with a strong allergenic monomer present in the resin [407]. This explains the statistically significant overrepresentation of simultaneous patch test reactions to PTBP resin and PTBC in contact dermatitis patients [406].

In a polychloroprene/PTBP resin adhesive that caused an allergic contact dermatitis, the allergens were found to be 2-hydroxy-5-*tertiary*-butyl benzyl alcohol and a condensate of 4-*para-tertiary*-butylphenol molecules joined by methylene bridges [408]. In a case of contact allergy to a phenolic resin used as tackifier in a marking pen, the patient reacted to PTBP resin in the standard series and to 2-hydroxy-5-*tert*-butyl benzylalcohol and 2,6-bis(hydroxymethyl)-4-*tert*-butylphenol identified in the phenolic resin [409]. Depigmentation of the skin caused by PTBP and other substituted phenols has been reported to occur in workers manufacturing the chemical when exposure has been excessive. Exceptionally, nonoccupational sources were also concerned, for example, in shoes and bindi adhesives [410, 411], and such depigmentation can occur without any accompanying skin irritation. Also, noneczematous pigmented [412] and lymphomatoid [413] contact dermatitis have been described.

Scheme 31.12 PTBP

The patch test concentration of PTBP resin is 1% pet. It has been pointed out, however, that patch testing with PTBP resin is not sufficient to detect allergy to phenol-formaldehyde resins based on phenols other than *para-tertiary*-butyl phenol [414]. The TRUE Test contains 45 μg/cm².

31.23 Primin

Primin or 2-methoxy-6-*n*-pentyl-*p*-benzoquinone is the major allergen in *Primula* dermatitis (Scheme 31.13).

Primin is included in the European standard series because it is an important allergen in certain countries, e.g., in Northern Europe. The frequency of positive primin patch tests in European clinics varies from 0.1 to 1.2% of consecutively tested eczema patients. The vast majority of patch test positive patients are women. Florists, nursery workers, and housewives are particularly at risk when exposed to primula plants. Primin sensitization seems to be relatively more common in elderly patients [415], and primin allergy may be difficult to suspect, because the patients may not be aware of contact with the plant. It is recommended to show color photos of the plant as a routine procedure in cases where there are positive patch test reactions to primin [416–418].

However, the sensitization rate is so low in some countries, for example, the USA, that it is not incorporated into the local baseline series [419]. Contact allergy to primin is also decreasing in Northern Europe and it is debated if it should be kept in the baseline series [420, 421]. However, if you don´t test with it you might miss important cases.

Primula obconica, which has round leaves covered with fine hairs, is the usual culprit, but other species of *Primula* may cause dermatitis. *Primula auricula, P. vulgaris*, and *P. forrestii* have been reported to cause dermatitis [422], and it may be more frequent than previously recorded. On the other hand, primin-free *P. obconica* has

been introduced into the European market, and it mimics the allergenic variety in color and appearance [423].

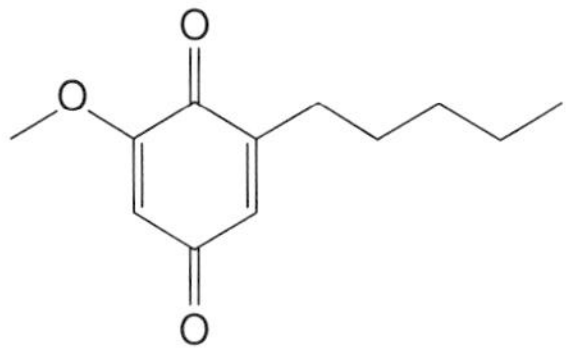

Primin is a powerful sensitizer contained in the fine hairs, and the content varies with the season, hours of sunshine, and the care of the plant [418, 424]; the primin content is highest in warm summer and lowest during winter [424]. Besides primin, another potential allergen is also present in primula, i.e., miconidin, which is biogenetically related to primin [425, 426]. Primin may be emitted to the surrounding air from intact plants and plant parts, and may be a source of airborne contact dermatitis [427].

In *Primula* dermatitis, lesions are often arranged in linear streaks and most often appear on exposed skin. The parts most often affected are the eyelids, cheeks, chin, neck, fingers, hands, and arms. Sometimes, severe reactions, such as erythema-multiforme-like lesions [428] and photodermatitis have been observed [429]. Other plants and woods containing quinones may show cross-reactivity with primin [430].

The patch test concentration is 0.01% pet. Testing with synthetic primin is preferable to an extract of the plant for various reasons: standardization, decreased risk of active sensitization, avoidance of irritant or false-positive reactions, and seasonal variation in the allergenicity of the plant [431, 432]. Testing may invoke flare reactions. However, we should take into account that testing with primin alone might miss allergy to the plant itself [418, 421, 433].

31.24 Sesquiterpene Lactone Mix (SL Mix)

The SL mix contains the following three SLs in pet.:
Alantolactone 0.033%, Dehydrocostus lactone 0.033%, and Costunolide 0.033% (Scheme 31.14).

The SL mix was developed by Ducombs et al. [434]. These SLs are contact allergens present in Compositae plants (syn. Asteraceae), which constitute one of the largest plant families in the world. More than 200 of the ~25,000 known Compositae species have caused allergic contact dermatitis. The Compositae family includes many of the common weeds, milfoil, yarrow (*Achillea millefolium* L.), tansy (*Tanacetum vulgare* L.), mugwort (*Artemisia vulgaris* L.), wild chamomile [*Chamomilla recutita* (L.) Rauschert], and feverfew [*Tanacetum parthenium* (L.) Schultz-Bip.] – and many

Scheme 31.13 Primin

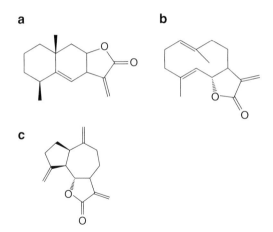

Scheme 31.14 Alantolactone, dehydrocostus lactone, and costunolide

cultivated garden flowers, such as chrysanthemum (*Chrysanthemum indicum* L.), marguerite, ox-eye daisy (*Leucanthemum vulgare* L.), marigold (*Calendula officinalis* L.), goldenrod (*Solidago virgaurea* L.), African marigolds (*Tagetes*), and sunflowers (*Helianthus annuus* L.). The edible types of Compositae include ordinary lettuce [435, 436], endive, and artichoke [437]. Cross-sensitivity between Compositae plants is common [437–439]. The SL mix detected about 65% of Compositae-allergic patients in a Danish investigation comprising of more than 4,000 consecutively tested eczema patients [164]. The remaining cases were diagnosed by testing with the Hausen Compositae mix and other Compositae extracts [440].

The Compositae are the most frequent cause of occupational allergic plant dermatitis in gardeners and greenhouse workers in Denmark, and important sensitizers are chrysanthemums, marguerite, daisies, and lettuce [441]. Besides localized eczema, most often hand eczema, caused by direct contact between the skin and the plants, the Compositae may give rise to a more widespread dermatitis localized to light- and air-exposed skin areas causing suspicion toward an airborne contact dermatitis [442, 443]. Recently, it has been shown in clinical experiments that airborne particles containing the SL, parthenolide, are released from the Compositae plant, feverfew, and some feverfew-allergic patients react to minute amounts of allergen present in the particles Testing with a dilution series of parthenolide showed positive reactions down to 8.1 ng per patch in selected patients [444]. Emission of terpenes from feverfew plants have been documented, and these

terpenes have elicited positive reactions only in few Compositae-sensitive patients [445]. Seasonal variation in the severity of the eczema with summer exacerbation is frequently seen [446, 447]. A number of patients have had localized eczema, particularly hand eczema, for a number of years when it suddenly turns into a widespread dermatitis one summer [443]. The duration of exposure as well as a history of childhood eczema or hay fever, seems to be significant risk factors for the development of Compositae-related symptoms [441, 448]. Compositae sensitivity may also predispose to photosensitivity [449]. Many Compositae-sensitive patients have multiple contact allergies. The high prevalence of other contact allergies in Compositae gardeners may reflect the impact of strongly allergenic SLs [450]. They may also be responsible for severe systemically induced skin eruptions [451]. The allergens are present in all parts of the plant and also in dead plant material and dust. The SL mix reveals about 60–70% of all cases of Compositae contact allergy and it is important to supplement testing with the plants in suspicion and ether extracts of Compositae plants, such as the Hausen Compositae mix [440, 441, 452]. Paulsen et al. [441] found that, among gardeners, the Compositae extract mix detected twice as many of the sensitized as the SL mix. However, the Compositae mix seems to be more irritating and the overall detection rate with the two mixes was still not higher than 76% in the group of gardeners. The detection rate of both mixes was raised to 93% in the series of consecutive eczema patients [164]. It has been claimed that the Compositae mix 6% pet. may cause patch test sensitization [453, 454], and a reduced concentration of extracts in the mix has been proposed. However, this also reduced the sensitivity of the mix [455]. Late-appearing reactivation patch reaction to Compositae allergens is also documented in previously sensitized patients, and this phenomenon should be differentiated from patch test sensitization [164]. The mixes have their limitations and the importance of aimed patch testing in persons with specific exposures is emphasized. The addition of parthenolide, the main allergen in feverfew, to the existing SL mix did not turn out to be of great value, although it was a fairly good screen on its own, detecting 75% of the cases positive to the SL mix [456]. Therefore, the creation of another SL mix might be appropriate. Further, it is important to emphasize that the content of allergenic SLs in plants may vary from season to season and from area to area. A European multicenter patch test study with the SL mix in 11 clinics showed 1% of patients as positive in more than 10,000 consecutively tested patients, three-quarters of which were of current or old relevance. The prevalence varied between 0.1 and 2.7% in different centers; it was highest in areas with pot flower and cut plant industries. More than one-third were positive to perfume and/or colophony, possibly reflecting cross-reactivity [457]. SL sensitization is in one report significantly lower and less severe in the Asian compared with the European population. The induction of oral tolerance through the ingestion of chrysanthemum tea was suggested as a plausible, though unproven, explanation. [458]. The SL mix is nonsensitizing and nonirritating.

31.25 Budesonide

The glucocorticoid budesonide is an epimeric mixture of the α- and β-propyl forms of 16α, 17α-butylidenedioxy-11-β,21-dihydroxypregna-1,4-diene-3,20-dione. It has been used topically (0.025% in a cream or ointment) in the treatment of various skin disorders, but is more often used by inhalation in the management of asthma in the form of a metered aerosol, a dry powder inhaler, or a nebulized solution, and as a nasal spray for the prophylaxis and treatment of allergic rhinitis [459]. It is also used in rectal preparations to treat inflammatory bowel diseases (Scheme 31.15).

Beginning in 1986, several publications appeared reporting budesonide-containing aerosols and sprays as the cause of eczematous eruptions, sometimes associated with endonasal complaints, with, in a few cases, indications for both type I and IV allergic mechanisms [for a review see 460]. Although reactions to inhalation products occur, they still seem to be infrequent relative to the large scale of their use and, in most cases, they are secondary to sensitization via skin

application of budesonide or a cross-reacting corticosteroid. However, subjects, not themselves treated by aerosols containing this corticosteroid, but taking care or living together with patients who use them regularly because of a chronic respiratory infection, seem to get sensitized by airborne exposure and/or present clinical signs of airborne contact dermatitis [461].

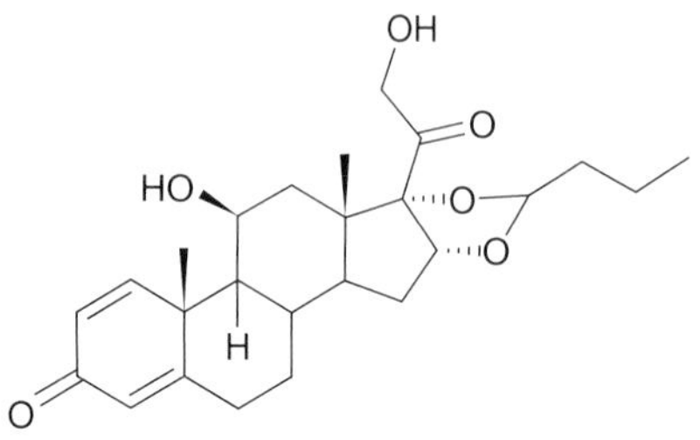

Budesonide has been recognized as an important screening agent for the detection of contact allergy of corticosteroids of group B (acetonides) [462] and of group D2 (the labile prodrug esters), which is due to the acetal function in budesonide, with its R and S diastereoisomers, the R-sensitive subjects reacting to group B, the S-sensitive ones to group D2 corticosteroids [463]. Budesonide contact allergy has been detected in 1.0–1.5% of consecutively tested dermatitis patients [464].

The question on the optimal patch test preparation has been debatable. While petrolatum works well for tixocortol pivalate and budesonide, ethanol was the vehicle used to test all other corticosteroid molecules [465, 466]. Concerning the optimal patch test concentration, there are not enough comparative studies to provide a definitive answer, but the results obtained comparing different patch test concentrations [467], favor the 0.01% dilution. The concentration in TRUE test is 1 μg/cm² and gives reactions comparable to petrolatum-based patch test preparation [468]. With respect to the reliability and adverse effects of the patch test, irritant reactions are not common. Reactions such as blanching, reactive vasodilation, and "edge" effects often occur and are the result of the intrinsic pharmacological characteristics of the corticosteroid, which also influence the patch test readings that should be performed not only on D3 or 4 but also on D7 [469].

31.26 Tixocortol Pivalate

The glucocorticoid tixocortol pivalate is 11β, 17α-dihydroxy-21-mercaptopregn-4-ene-3,20-dione 21-pivalate. It is used in buccal, nasal, throat, and rectal preparations [470], but not in the treatment of skin diseases (Scheme 31.16).

The initial reports of allergic reactions caused by mucosal application of tixocortol pivalate came from France [471]. The occasional, almost immediate occurrence of such reactions (1–2 days) after the initiation of therapy indicated the possibility of an already

Scheme 31.15 Budesonide

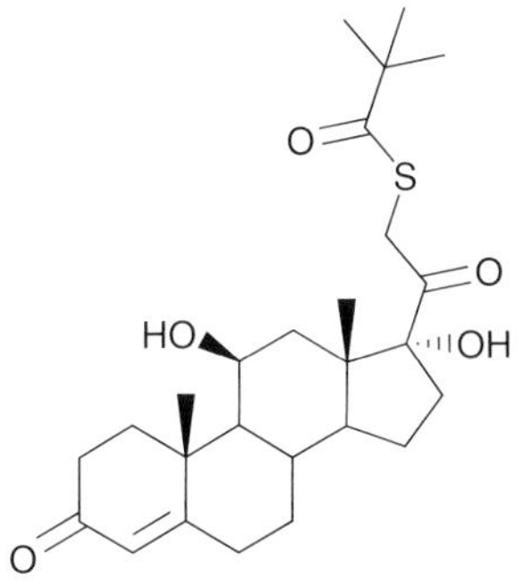

Scheme 31.16 Tixocortol pivalate

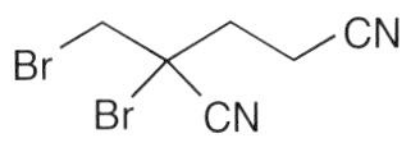

Scheme 31.17 Methyldibromo glutaronitrile

existing corticosteroid allergy [472], an hypothesis that has later been confirmed [462], and which resulted in the use of tixocortol pivalate as a marker for group A corticosteroids (e.g., hydrocortisone and derivatives) [473]. Primary sensitization due to mucosal preparations, however, are, of course, not excluded. Tixocortol pivalate allergy has been detected in 0.9–4.4% of consecutive dermatitis patients [464, 474, 475].

With respect to the vehicle, equivalent patch test results were found for both ethanol and petrolatum, but petrolatum is the vehicle commonly used [465]. Based on a study performed by the EECDRG [464], testing with 0.1% in petrolatum has been recommended; however, in selected cases, where tixocortol pivalate is strongly suspected and testing with the routine concentration is negative, additional testing with 1.0% in petrolatum should be done [469]. The concentration in the TRUE test is 3 μg/cm^2. Tixocortol pivalate does not produce irritant patch test reactions, and similar to budesonide, late readings should be performed.

31.27 Methyldibromo Glutaronitrile

In the mid 1980s, the preservative methyldibromoglutaronitrile (MDBGN) (CAS no 35691-65-7) was approved for use in cosmetic products at a maximum concentration of 0.1% in both leave-on and rinse-off cosmetics except for sunscreen products, in which MDBGN was not allowed to exceed a concentration of 0.025% (Scheme 31.17).

MDBGN was effective at low in-use concentrations, and animal tests indicated that the preservative was a weak sensitizer [476, 477] These attributes were favorable and MDBGN gradually became more

widespread throughout the 1990s in household, industrial products, and cosmetics in particular.

The preservative was marketed as Euxyl K400 (Schülke & Mayr, Hamburg, Germany), a combination of MDBGN and phenoxyethanol (1:4), which is a weak sensitizer. Methyldibromo glutaronitrile is the INCI name and it is synonymous with 1,2-dibromo-dicyanobutane. However, dermatological clinics in Europe found increasing numbers of eczema patients sensitized to the chemical [478–481]. In 2001, patch test data from 16 European clinics showed an increasing average frequency of sensitivity to MDBGN in eczema patients from 0.7% in 1991 to 3.5% in 2000 [482] MDBGN was introduced to the European baseline series in 2005 [483] Based on the frequency data, a change in the Cosmetics Directive was made in 2005 banning the use of MDBGN in stay-on products, and later also in rinse-off products. The effect of this regulation is already evident [484, 485], and this is a prime example of primary prevention. Clinical experimental studies in MDBGN-sensitive volunteer patients have documented the importance of repeated short-term exposures, as frequent hand washing with MDBGN-containing liquid soap could be a significant cause of sensitization and elicitation of allergic contact dermatitis to this preservative [486]. Further, reduction of the concentration in the product did not reduce the elicitation capacity if the number of exposures increased equivalently [487]. The patch test concentration is 0.5% in petrolatum based on the consideration of the rates of contact allergy, doubtful and irritant reactions, as well as information on clinical relevance represented by the results of a ROAT [483]. However, others have recommended 0.2% as the optimal patch test concentration due to increased number of false-positive reactions at 0.5% [488].

31.28 Ethylenediamine (No Longer Included in the Baseline Series)

When patch testing, 1% pet. is the standard test concentration. The concentration in the TRUE test is 50 μg/cm^2. Allergy to this compound is the commonest

31

by far in the United States and Belgium, where MycologR cream, a preparation containing neomycin, nystatin, and triamcinolone, is widely used. A similar preparation – Tri-Adcortyl® cream has been used in Britain till January 2009. Ethylenediamine functions as a stabilizer in the cream formulation. The corresponding ointment does not contain it as a stabilizer.

Ethylenediamine has other uses, and dermatitis due to it has been described in the following sources – floor polish remover [489], epoxy hardener, and coolant oil [490–492]. Its use has also been described in a number of other industries, rubber, dyes, insecticides, and synthetic waxes. Occupational dermatitis has been reported in nurses and a laboratory technician working with theophylline and aminophylline [493, 494].

There is a potential problem with systemic administration in those sensitized, either with drugs which contain ethylenediamine, for instance aminophylline, or with drugs chemically related to it, including various antihistamines, among which are hydroxyzine hydrochloride and its active metabolite ceterizine, piperazine, and cyclizine [495–498]. Cases with generalized erythroderma have been described in patients who have become allergic to piperazine in local applications, who received piperazine phosphate to treat worms [499]. Patients seldom, if ever, become sensitized through systemic administration and problems arise only in those already sensitized, who receive the drugs, and it is surprising how few reactions occur considering the number of patients sensitized. Immediate-type reactions have also been reported [500]. Few patients become sensitized through contact in industry, and ethylenediamine is a rare sensitizer outside the local application which contains it.

References

1. Wahlberg JE, Elsner P, Kanerva L, Maibach HI (2003) Management of positive patch test reactions. Springer, Berlin
2. Rietschel RL, Fowler JF (2008) Fisher's contact dermatitis, 6th edn. BC Dekker, Hamilton
3. Kanerva L, Elsner P, Wahlberg JE, Maibach HI (2000) Handbook of occupational dermatology. Springer, Berlin
4. Brasch J, Szlinka C, Grabbe J (1997) More positive patch test reactions with larger test chambers? Contact Dermatitis 37:118–120
5. Benezra C, Andanson J, Chabeau C, Ducombs G, Foussereau J, Lachapelle JM, Lacroix M, Martin P (1978) Concentrations of patch test allergens: are we comparing the same things? Contact Dermatitis 4:103–105
6. Cronin E (1972) Clinical prediction of patch test results. Trans St John's Hosp Dermatol Soc 58:153–162
7. Podmore P, Burrows D, Bingham EA (1984) Prediction of patch test results. Contact Dermatitis 11:283–284
8. Menné T, Dooms-Goossens A, Wahlberg JE, White IR, Shaw S (1992) How large a proportion of contact sensitivities are diagnosed with the European standard series? Contact Dermatitis 26:201–202
9. Saripalli YV, Achen F, Belsito DV (2003) The detection of clinically relevant contact allergens using a standard screening tray of twenty-three allergens. J Am Acad Dermatol 49:65–69
10. Bruynzeel DP, Andersen KE, Camarasa JG, Lachapelle J-M, Menné T, White IR (1995) The European standard series. European Environmental and Contact Dermatitis Research Group (EECDRG). Contact Dermatitis 33:145–148
11. Bruynzeel DP, Diepgen TL, Andersen KE, Brandão FM, Bruze M, Frosch PJ, Goossens A, Lahti A, Mahler V, Maibach HI, Menné T, Wilkinson JD, European Environmental and Contact Dermatitis Research Group (2005) Monitoring the European standard series in 10 centres 1996-2000. Contact Dermatitis 53:146–149
12. Smith HR, Wakelin SH, McFadden JP, Rycroft RJ, White IR (1999) A 15-year review of our MOAHLFA index. Contact Dermatitis 40:227–228
13. Uter W, Geier J, Schnuch A (1999) The MOAHLFA index in 17 centers of the Information Network of Departments of Dermatology (IVDK) over 6 years. Contact Dermatitis 41(6):343–344
14. Uter W, Gefeller O, Geier J, Schnuch A (2008) Changes of the patch test population (MOAHLFA index) in long-term participants of the Information Network of Departments of Dermatology, 1999-2006. Contact Dermatitis 59:56–57
15. Andersen KE (1998) Multicentre patch test studies: are they worth the effort. Contact Dermatitis 38:222–223
16. Grandjean P, Nielsen GD, Andersen O (1989) Human nickel exposure and chemobiokinetics. In: Maibach HI, Menne T (eds) Nickel and the skin: immunology and toxicology. CRC, Boca Raton, pp 9–34
17. Mortz CG, Lauritsen JM, Bindslev-Jensen C, Andersen KE (2002) Nickel sensitization in adolescents and association with ear piercing, use of dental braces and hand eczema. The Odense Adolescence Cohort Study on Atopic Diseases and Dermatitis (TOACS). Acta Derm Venereol (Stockh) 82:359–364
18. Nielsen NH, Linneberg A, Menne T, Madsen F, Frolund L, Dirksen A, Jorgensen T (2001) Allergic contact sensitization in an adult Danish population: two cross-sectional surveys eight years apart (the Copenhagen Allergy Study). Acta Derm Venereol 81:31–34
19. Morgan LG, Flint GN (1989) Nickel alloys and coatings: release of nickel. In: Maibach HI, Menne T (eds) Nickel and the skin: immunology and toxicology. CRC, Boca Raton, pp 45–54
20. Schnuch A, Geier J, Uter W, Frosch PJ, Lehmacher W, Aberer W, Agathos M, Arnold R, Fuchs T, Laubstein B, Lischka G, Pietrzyk PM, Rakoski J, Richter G, Rueff F (1997) National rates and regional differences in sensitization to

allergens of the standard series. Population-adjusted frequencies of sensitization (PAFS) in 40, 000 patients from a multicenter study (IVDK). Contact Dermatitis 37: 200–209

21. Shah M, Lewis FM, Gawkrodger DJ (1998) Nickel as an occupational allergen. A survey of 368 nickel-sensitive subjects. Arch Dermatol 134:1231–1236

22. Shum KW, Meyer JD, Chen Y, Cherry N, Gawkrodger DJ (2003) Occupational contact dermatitis to nickel: experience of the British dermatologists (EPIDERM) and occupational physicians (OPRA) surveillance schemes. Occup Environ Med 60:954–957

23. Novak N, Baurecht H, Schäfer T, Rodriguez E, Wagenpfeil S, Klopp N, Heinrich J, Behrendt H, Ring J, Wichmann E, Illig T, Weidinger S (2008) Loss-of-function mutations in the filaggrin gene and allergic contact sensitization to nickel. J Invest Dermatol 128:1430–1435

24. Marks JG Jr, Belsito DV, DeLeo VA, Fowler JF Jr, Fransway AF, Maibach HI, Mathias CG, Pratt MD, Rietschel RL, Sherertz EF, Storrs FJ, Taylor JS, North American Contact Dermatitis Group (2003) North American Contact Dermatitis Group patch-test results, 1998 to 2000. Am J Contact Dermat 14:59–62

25. Thyssen JP, Johansen JD, Menne T, Nielsen NH, Linneberg A (2009) Nickel allergy in Danish women before and after nickel regulation. N Engl J Med 360:2259–2260

26. Larsson-Stymne B, Widström L (1985) Ear piercing – a cause of nickel allergy in schoolgirls? Contact Dermatitis 13:289–293

27. Meijer C, Bredberg M, Fischer T, Widstrom L (1995) Ear piercing, and nickel and cobalt sensitization, in 520 young Swedish men doing compulsory military service. Contact Dermatitis 32:147–149

28. Calnan CD, Wells GC (1956) Suspender dermatitis and nickel sensitivity. Br Med J 4978:1265–1268

29. Andersen KE, Hjorth N, Menne T (1984) The baboon syndrome: systemically-induced allergic contact dermatitis. Contact Dermatitis 10:97–100

30. Jensen CS, Lisby S, Larsen JK, Veien NK, Menne T (2004) Characterization of lymphocyte subpopulations and cytokine profiles in peripheral blood of nickel-sensitive individuals with systemic contact dermatitis after oral nickel exposure. Contact Dermatitis 50:31–38

31. Jensen CS, Menne T, Lisby S, Kristiansen J, Veien NK (2003) Experimental systemic contact dermatitis from nickel: a dose-response study. Contact Dermatitis 49: 124–132

32. Veien N (1989) Systemically induced eczema in adults. Acta Derm Venereol Suppl (Stockh) 147:1–58

33. Burrows D (1988) The Prosser White oration 1988. Mischievous metals – chromate, cobalt, nickel and mercury. Clin Exp Dermatol 14:266–272

34. Santucci B, Manna F, Cristaudo A, Cannistraci C, Capparella MR, Picardo M (1990) Serum concentrations in nickel-sensitive patients after prolonged oral administration. Contact Dermatitis 22:253–256

35. Nielsen GD, Jepsen LV, Jorgensen PJ, Grandjean P, Brandrup F (1990) Nickel-sensitive patients with vesicular hand eczema: oral challenge with a diet naturally high in nickel. Br J Dermatol 122:299–308

36. Nielsen GD, Soderberg U, Jorgensen PJ, Templeton DM, Rasmussen SN, Andersen KE, Grandjean P (1999) Absorption and retention of nickel from drinking water in relation to food intake and nickel sensitivity. Toxicol Appl Pharmacol 154: 67–75

37. Wilkinson DS, Wilkinson JD (1989) Nickel allergy and hand eczema. In: Maibach HI, Menne T (eds) Nickel and the skin: immunology and toxicology. CRC, Boca Raton, pp 133–163

38. Menne T, Holm NV (1983) Hand eczema in nickel-sensitive female twins. Genetic predisposition and environmental factors. Contact Dermatitis 9:289–296

39. Menne T, Borgan O, Green A (1982) Nickel allergy and hand dermatitis in a stratified sample of the Danish female population: an epidemiological study including a statistic appendix. Acta Derm Venereol (Stockh) 62:35–41

40. Josefson A, Färm G, Magnuson A, Meding B (2009) Nickel allergy as risk factor for hand eczema: a population-based study. Br J Dermatol 160:828–834

41. Bryld LE, Agner T, Menne T (2003) Relation between vesicular eruptions on the hands and tinea pedis, atopic dermatitis and nickel allergy. Acta Derm Venereol (Stockh) 83: 186–188

42. Bryld LE, Hindsberger C, Kyvik KO, Agner T, Menne T (2003) Risk factors influencing the development of hand eczema in a population-based twin sample. Br J Dermatol 149:1214–1220

43. van der Burg CK, Bruynzeel DP, Vreeburg KJ, von Blomberg BM, Scheper RJ (1986) Hand eczema in hairdressers and nurses: a prospective study. I. Evaluation of atopy and nickel hypersensitivity at the start of apprenticeship. Contact Dermatitis 14:275–279

44. Mortz CG, Lauritsen JM, Bindslev-Jensen C, Andersen KE (2001) Prevalence of atopic dermatitis, asthma, allergic rhinitis, and hand and contact dermatitis in adolescents. The Odense Adolescence Cohort Study on Atopic Diseases and Dermatitis. Br J Dermatol 144:523–532

45. Rees JL, Friedmann PS, Matthews JN (1989) Sex differences in susceptibility to development of contact hypersensitivity to dinitrochlorobenzene (DNCB). Br J Dermatol 120:371–374

46. Wöhrl S, Jandl T, Stingl G, Kinaciyan T (2007) Mobile telephone as new source for nickel dermatitis. Contact Dermatitis 56:113

47. Zhai H, Chew AL, Bashir SJ, Reagan KE, Hostynek JJ, Maibach HI (2003) Provocative use test of nickel coins in nickel-sensitized subjects and controls. Br J Dermatol 149: 311–317

48. Van Hoogstraten IM, Andersen KE, von Blomberg BM, Boden D, Bruynzeel DP, Burrows D, Camarasa JG, Dooms-Goossens A, Kraal G, Lahti A (1991) Reduced frequency of nickel allergy upon oral nickel contact at an early age. Clin Exp Immunol 85:441–445

49. Sjovall P, Christensen OB, Moller H (1987) Oral hyposensitization in nickel allergy. J Am Acad Dermatol 17:774–778

50. Thomas RH, Rademaker M, Goddard NJ, Munro DD (1987) Severe eczema of the hands due to an orthopaedic plate made of Vitallium. Br Med J Clin Res Ed 294:106–107

51. Wilkinson JD (1989) Nickel allergy and orthopedic prosthesis. In: Maibach HI, Menne T (eds) Nickel and the skin: immunology and toxicology. CRC, Boca Raton, pp 187–193

31

52. Gawkrodger DJ (2003) Metal sensitivities and orthopaedic implants revisited: the potential for metal allergy with the new metal-on-metal joint prostheses. Br J Dermatol 148: 1089–1093

53. Lammintausta K, Kalimo K (1987) Do positive nickel reactions increase nonspecific patch test reactivity? Contact Dermatitis 16:160–163

54. Paramsothy Y, Collins M, Smith AG (1988) Contact dermatitis in patients with leg ulcers. The prevalence of late positive reactions and evidence against systemic ampliative allergy. Contact Dermatitis 18:30–36

55. Liden C, Wahlberg JE (1994) Cross-reactivity to metal compounds studied in guinea pigs induced with chromate or cobalt. Acta Derm Venereol (Stockh) 74:341–343

56. Moss C, Friedmann PS, Shuster S, Simpson JM (1985) Susceptibility and amplification of sensitivity in contact dermatitis. Clin Exp Immunol 61:232–241

57. Lammintausta K, Pitkanen OP, Kalimo K, Jansen CT (1985) Interrelationship of nickel and cobalt contact sensitization. Contact Dermatitis 13:148–152

58. Moulon C, Vollmer J, Weltzien HU (1995) Characterization of processing requirements and metal cross-reactivities in T cell clones from patients with allergic contact dermatitis to nickel. Eur J Immunol 25:3308–3315

59. Gamerdinger K, Moulon C, Karp DR, Van Bergen J, Koning F, Wild D, Pflugfelder U, Weltzien HU (2003) A new type of metal recognition by human T cells: contact residues for peptide-independent bridging of T cell receptor and major histocompatibility complex by nickel. J Exp Med 197:1345–1353

60. Menne T, Brandup F, Thestrup-Pedersen K, Veien NK, Andersen JR, Yding F, Valeur G (1987) Patch test reactivity to nickel alloys. Contact Dermatitis 16:255–259

61. Kanerva L, Sipilainen-Malm T, Estlander T, Zitting A, Jolanki R, Tarvainen K (1994) Nickel release from metals, and a case of allergic contact dermatitis from stainless steel. Contact Dermatitis 31:299–303

62. Haudrechy P, Mantout B, Frappaz A, Rousseau D, Chabeau G, Faure M, Claudy A (1997) Nickel release from stainless steels. Contact Dermatitis 37:113–117

63. Basketter DA, Angelini G, Ingber A, Kern PS, Menné T (2003) Nickel, chromium and cobalt in consumer products: revisiting safe levels in the new millennium. Contact Dermatitis 49:1–7

64. Fischer LA, Johansen JD, Menné T (2007) Nickel allergy: relationship between patch test and repeated open application test thresholds. Br J Dermatol 157:723–729

65. Johansen JD, Menne T, Christophersen J, Kaaber K, Veien N (2000) Changes in the pattern of sensitization to common contact allergens in Denmark between 1985–1986 and 1997–1998, with a special view to the effect of preventive strategies. Br J Dermatol 142:490–495

66. Schnuch A, Geier J, Lessmann H, Uter W (2003) Decrease in nickel sensitization in young patients–successful intervention through nickel exposure regulation? Results of IVDK, 1992–2001. Hautarzt 54:626–632

67. Kieffer M (1979) Nickel sensitivity: relationship between history and patch test reaction. Contact Dermatitis 5: 398–401

68. Moller H, Svensson A (1986) Metal sensitivity: positive history but negative test indicates atopy. Contact Dermatitis 14:57–60

69. Uter W, Pfahlberg A, Gefeller O, Geier J, Schnuch A (2003) Risk factors for contact allergy to nickel – results of a multifactorial analysis. Contact Dermatitis 48:33–38

70. Mortz CG, Lauritsen JM, Bindslev-Jensen C, Andersen KE (2002) Contact allergy and allergic contact dermatitis in adolescents: prevalence measures and associations. The Odense Adolescence Cohort Study on Atopic Diseases and Dermatitis (TOACS). Acta Derm Venereol (Stockh) 82:352–358

71. Memon AA, Friedmann PS (1996) Studies on the reproducibility of allergic contact dermatitis. Br J Dermatol 134: 208–214

72. Andersen KE, Liden C, Hansen J, Volund A (1993) Dose-response testing with nickel sulfate using the TRUE test in nickel-sensitive individuals. Multiple nickel sulfate patch-test reactions do not cause an 'angry back'. Br J Dermatol 129:50–56

73. Hindsen M, Bruze M, Christensen OB (1999) Individual variation in nickel patch test reactivity. Am J Contact Dermat 10:62–67

74. Fregert S, Rorsman H (1964) Allergy to trivalent chromium. Arch Dermatol 90:4–6

75. Burrows D (1984) The dichromate problem. Int J Dermatol 23:215–220

76. Burrows D (1983) Chromium: metabolism and toxicity. CRC, Boca Raton

77. Hansen MB, Johansen JD, Menne T (2003) Chromium allergy: significance of both Cr(III) and Cr(VI). Contact Dermatitis 49:206–212

78. Zachariae CO, Agner T, Menne T (1996) Chromium allergy in consecutive patients in a country where ferrous sulfate has been added to cement since 1981. Contact Dermatitis 35: 83–85

79. Olsavszky R, Rycroft RJ, White IR, McFadden JP (1998) Contact sensitivity to chromate: comparison at a London contact dermatitis clinic over a 10-year period. Contact Dermatitis 38:329–331

80. Avnstorp C (1989) Prevalence of cement eczema in Denmark before and since addition of ferrous sulfate to Danish cement. Acta Derm Venereol (Stockh) 69:151–155

81. Avnstorp C (1989) Follow-up of workers from the prefabricated concrete industry after the addition of ferrous sulphate to Danish cement. Contact Dermatitis 20:365–371

82. Roto P, Sainio H, Reunala T, Laippala P (1996) Addition of ferrous sulfate to cement and risk of chromium dermatitis among construction workers. Contact Dermatitis 34:43–50

83. Turk K, Rietschel RL (1993) Effect of processing cement to concrete on hexavalent chromium levels. Contact Dermatitis 28:209–211

84. Goh CL, Gan SL (1996) Change in cement manufacturing process, a cause for decline in chromate allergy? Contact Dermatitis 34:51–54

85. Wong SS, Chan MT, Gan SL, Ng SK, Goh CL (1998) Occupational chromate allergy in Singapore: a study of 87 patients and a review from 1983 to 1995. Am J Contact Dermat 9:1–5

86. Irvine C, Pugh CE, Hansen EJ, Rycroft RJ (1994) Cement dermatitis in underground workers during construction of the Channel Tunnel. Occup Med Oxf 44:17–23

87. Bock M, Schmidt A, Bruckner T, Diepgen TL (2003) Occupational skin disease in the construction industry. Br J Dermatol 149:1165–1171

88. Burrows D, Adams RM, Flint GN (1999) Metals. In: Adams RM (ed) Occupational skin disease, 3rd edn. Saunders, Philadelphia, pp 395–433

89. Thormann J, Jespersen NB, Joensen HD (1979) Persistence of contact allergy to chromium. Contact Dermatitis 5:261–264

90. Lips R, Rast H, Elsner P (1996) Outcome of job change in patients with occupational chromate dermatitis. Contact Dermatitis 34:268–271

91. Fowler JFJ, Kauffman CL, Marks JG Jr, Proctor DM, Fredrick MM, Otani JM, Finley BL, Paustenbach DJ, Nethercott JR (1999) An environmental hazard assessment of low-level dermal exposure to hexavalent chromium in solution among chromium-sensitized volunteers. J Occup Environ Med 41:150–160

92. Hansen MB, Menne T, Johansen JD (2006) Cr(III) and Cr(VI) in leather and elicitation of eczema. Contact Dermatitis 54:278–282

93. Kaaber K, Veien N (1977) The significance of chromate ingestion in patients allergic to chromate. Acta Derm Venereol (Stockh) 57:321–323

94. Andersen KE, Burrows D, Cronin E, Dooms Goossens A, Rycroft RJ, White IR (1988) Recommended changes to standard series. Contact Dermatitis 19:389–390

95. Burrows D, Andersen KE, Camarasa JG, Dooms-Goossens A, Ducombs G, Lachapelle JM, Menne T, Rycroft RJ, Wahlberg JE, White IR et al (1989) Trial of 0.5% versus 0.375% potassium dichromate. European Environmental and Contact Dermatitis Research Group (EECDRG). Contact Dermatitis 21:351

96. Schafer T, Bohler E, Ruhdorfer S, Weigl L, Wessner D, Filipiak B, Wichmann HE, Ring J (2001) Epidemiology of contact allergy in adults. Allergy 56:1192–1196

97. Kanerva L, Jolanki R, Estlander T, Alanko K, Savela A (2000) Incidence rates of occupational allergic contact dermatitis caused by metals. Am J Contact Dermat 11:155–160

98. Edman B (1985) Sites of contact dermatitis in relationship to particular allergens. Contact Dermatitis 13:129–135

99. Basketter DA, Briatico-Vangosa G, Kaestner W, Lally C, Bontinck WJ (1993) Nickel, cobalt and chromium in consumer products: a role in allergic contact dermatitis? Contact Dermatitis 28:15–25

100. Julander A, Hindsén M, Skare L, Lidén C (2009) Cobalt-containing alloys and their ability to release cobalt and cause dermatitis. Contact Dermatitis 60:165–170

101. Nielsen NH, Kristiansen J, Borg L, Christensen JM, Poulsen LK, Menne T (2000) Repeated exposures to cobalt or chromate on the hands of patients with hand eczema and contact allergy to that metal. Contact Dermatitis 43:212–215

102. Thomas P, Braathen LR, Dörig M, Auböck J, Nestle F, Werfel T, Willert HG (2009) Increased metal allergy in patients with failed metal-on-metal hip arthroplasty and peri-implant T-lymphocytic inflammation. Allergy 64:1157–1165

103. Wahlberg JE, Liden C (2000) Cross-reactivity patterns of cobalt and nickel studied with repeated open applications (ROATS) to the skin of guinea pigs. Am J Contact Dermat 11:42–48

104. van Joost T, van Everdingen JJ (1982) Sensitization to cobalt associated with nickel allergy: clinical and statistical studies. Acta Derm Venereol (Stockh) 62:525–529

105. Rystedt I, Fischer T (1983) Relationship between nickel and cobalt sensitization in hard metal workers. Contact Dermatitis 9:195–200

106. Anavekar NS, Nixon R (2006) Occupational allergic contact dermatitis to cobalt octoate included as an accelerator in a polyester resin. Australas J Dermatol 47:143–144

107. Uter W, Ruhl R, Pfahlberg A, Geier J, Schnuch A, Gefeller O (2004) Contact allergy in construction workers: results of a multifactorial analysis. Ann Occup Hyg 48:21–27

108. Geier J, Gefeller O, Wiechmann K, Fuchs T (1999) Patch test reactions at D4, D5 and D6. Contact Dermatitis 40: 119–126

109. Storrs FJ, White CR Jr (2000) False-positive "poral" cobalt patch test reactions reside in the eccrine acrosyringium. Cutis 65:49–53

110. Bauer K, Garbe D, Surburg H (1990) Common fragrance and flavor materials. VCH Verlagsgesellschaft mbH, Weinheim

111. Heydorn S, Menne T, Johansen JD (2003) Fragrance allergy and hand eczema – a review. Contact Dermatitis 48:59–66

112. de Groot AC, Frosch PJ (1997) Adverse reactions to fragrances: a clinical review. Contact Dermatitis 36:57–86

113. Larsen WG (1977) Perfume dermatitis. A study of 20 patients. Arch Dermatol 113:623–627

114. Frosch PJ, Pirker C, Rastogi SC, Andersen KE, Bruze M, Svedman C, Goossens A, White IR, Uter W, Arnau EG, Lepoittevin JP, Menné T, Johansen JD (2005) Patch testing with a new fragrance mix detects additional patients sensitive to perfumes and missed by the current fragrance mix. Contact Dermatitis 52:201–215

115. Bruze M, Andersen KE, Goossens A (2008) Recommendation to include fragrance mix 2 and hydroxyisohexyl 3-cyclohexene carboxaldehyde (Lyral®) in the European Baseline patch test series. Contact Dermatitis 58:129–133

116. Frosch PJ, Rastogi SC, Pirker C, Brinkmeier T, Andersen KE, Bruze M, Svedman C, Goossens A, White IR, Uter W, Arnau EG, Lepoittevin JP, Johansen JD, Menné T (2005) Patch testing with a new fragrance mix – reactivity to the single constituents and chemical detection in relevant cosmetic products. Contact Dermatitis 52:216–225

117. Geier J, Brasch J, Schnuch A, Lessmann H, Pirker C, Frosch PJ, For the Information Network of Departments of Dermatology (IVDK)and the German Contact Dermatitis Research Group (DKG) (2002) Lyral has been included in the patch test standard series in Germany. Contact Dermatitis 46(5):295–297

118. Uter W, Geier J, Schnuch A, Frosch PJ (2007) Patch test results with patients' own perfumes, deodorants and shaving lotions: results of the IVDK 1998-2002. J Eur Acad Dermatol Venereol 21(3):374–379

119. Matura M, Sköld M, Börje A, Andersen KE, Bruze M, Frosch P, Goossens A, Johansen JD, Svedman C, White IR, Karlberg AT (2005) Selected oxidized fragrance terpenes are common contact allergens. Contact Dermatitis 52(6): 320–328

120. Nardelli A, Carbonez A, Ottoy W, Drieghe J, Goossens A (2008) Frequency of and trends in fragrance allergy over a 15-year period. Contact Dermatitis 58(3):134–141

121. Thyssen JP, Carlsen BC, Menné T, Johansen JD (2008) Trends of contact allergy to fragrance mix I and Myroxylon pereirae among Danish eczema patients tested between 1985 and 2007. Contact Dermatitis 59(4):238–244

122. Schnuch A, Lessmann H, Geier J, Frosch PJ, Uter W, IVDK (2004) Contact allergy to fragrances: frequencies of sensitization from 1996 to 2002. Results of the IVDK. Contact Dermatitis 50(2):65–76

123. Katsarou A, Kalogeromitros D, Armenaka M, Koufou V, Davou E, Koumantaki E (1997) Trends in the results of patch testing to standard allergens over the period 1984–1995. Contact Dermatitis 37:245–246

124. Buckley DA, Rycroft RJ, White IR, McFadden JP (2003) The frequency of fragrance allergy in patch-tested patients increases with their age. Br J Dermatol 149:986–989

125. Johansen JD, Andersen TF, Veien N, Avnstorp C, Andersen KE, Menné T (1997) Patch testing with markers of fragrance contact allergy. Do clinical tests correspond to patients' self-reported problems? Acta Derm Venereol (Stockh) 77:149–153

126. Johansen JD, Rastogi SC, Menné T (1996) Contact allergy to popular perfumes; assessed by patch test, use test and chemical analysis. Br J Dermatol 135:419–422

127. Johansen JD, Rastogi SC, Bruze M, Andersen KE, Frosch P, Dreier B, Lepoittevin JP, White IR, Menné T (1998) Deodorants: a clinical provocation study in fragrance-sensitive patients. Contact Dermatitis 39:161–165

128. Johansen JD, Skov L, Vølund AA, Andersen KE, Menné T (1998) Allergens in combination have a synergistic effect on the elicitation response: a study of fragrance-sensitized individuals. Br J Dermatol 139:264–270

129. Frosch PJ, Johansen JD, Menné T, Rastogi SC, Bruze M, Andersen KE, Lepoittevin JP, Giménez Arnau E, Pirker C, Goossens A, White IR (1999) Lyral is an important sensitizer in patients sensitive to fragrances. Br J Dermatol 141(6):1076–1083

130. Frosch PJ, Pirker C, Rastogi SC, Andersen KE, Bruze M, Svedman C, Goossens A, White IR, Uter W, Arnau EG, Lepoittevin JP, Menné T, Johansen JD (2005) Patch testing with a new fragrance mix detects additional patients sensitive to perfumes and missed by the current fragrance mix. Contact Dermatitis 52(4):207–215

131. de Groot AC (1987) Contact allergy to cosmetics: causative ingredients. Contact Dermatitis 17(1):26–34

132. Frosch PJ, Pilz B, Andersen KE, Burrows D, Camarasa JG, Dooms-Goossens A, Ducombs G, Fuchs T, Hannuksela M, Lachapelle JM et al (1995) Patch testing with fragrances: results of a multicenter study of the European Environmental and Contact Dermatitis Research Group with 48 frequently used constituents of perfumes. Contact Dermatitis 33(5): 333–342

133. Johansen JD, Frosch PJ, Svedman C, Andersen KE, Bruze M, Pirker C, Menné T (2003) Hydroxyisohexyl 3-cyclohexene carboxaldehyde- known as Lyral: quantitative aspects and risk assessment of an important fragrance allergen. Contact Dermatitis 48(6):310–316

134. Rastogi SC, Johansen JD, Bossi R (2007) Selected important fragrance sensitizers in perfumes-current exposures. Contact Dermatitis 56(4):201–204

135. Rastogi SC, Johansen JD, Frosch P, Menné T, Bruze M, Lepoittevin JP, Dreier B, Andersen KE, White IR (1998) Deodorants on the European market: quantitative chemical analysis of 21 fragrances. Contact Dermatitis 38(1):29–35

136. Buckley DA (2007) Fragrance ingredient labelling in products on sale in the U.K. Br J Dermatol 157(2):295–300

137. Jørgensen PH, Jensen CD, Rastogi S, Andersen KE, Johansen JD (2007) Experimental elicitation with hydroxy-isohexyl-3-cyclohexene carboxaldehyde-containing deodorants. Contact Dermatitis 56(3):146–150

138. Braendstrup P, Johansen JD, Danish Contact Dermatitis Group (2008) Hydroxyisohexyl 3-cyclohexene carboxaldehyde (Lyral) is still a frequent allergen. Contact Dermatitis 59(3):187–188

139. Goossens A, Merckx L (1997) Allergic contact dermatitis from farnesol in a deodorant. Contact Dermatitis 37: 179–180

140. Hausen BM (2001) Contact allergy to balsam of Peru. II. Patch test results in 102 patients with selected balsam of Peru constituents. Am J Contact Dermat 12:93–102

141. Hjorth N (1961) Eczematous allergy to balsams, allied perfumes and flavouring agents. Munksgaard, Copenhagen

142. Christophersen J, Menné T, Tanghoj P, Andersen KE, Brandrup F, Kaaber K, Osmundsen PE, Thestrup-Pedersen K, Veien NK (1989) Clinical patch test data evaluated by multivariate analysis. Contact Dermatitis 21:291–297

143. Api AM (2006) Only Peru Balsam extracts or distillates are used in perfumery. Contact Dermatitis 54:179

144. Barbaud A, Collet E, Le Coz CJ, Meaume S, Gillois P (2009) Contact allergy in chronic leg ulcers: results of a multicentre study carried out in 423 patients and proposal for an updated series of patch tests. Contact Dermatitis 60(5):279–287

145. Saap L, Fahim S, Arsenault E, Pratt M, Pierscianowski T, Falanga V, Pedvis-Leftick A (2004) Contact sensitivity in patients with leg ulcerations: a North American study. Arch Dermatol 140(10):1241–1246

146. Niinimaki A (1995) Double-blind placebo-controlled peroral challenges in patients with delayed-type allergy to balsam of Peru. Contact Dermatitis 33:78–83

147. Salam TN, Fowler JF Jr (2001) Balsam-related systemic contact dermatitis. J Am Acad Dermatol 45:377–381

148. Pfutzner W, Thomas P, Niedermeier A, Pfeiffer C, Sander C, Przybilla B (2003) Systemic contact dermatitis elicited by oral intake of Balsam of Peru. Acta Derm Venereol (Stockh) 83:294–295

149. Downs AMR, Sansom JE (1999) Colophony allergy: a review. Contact Dermatitis 41:305–310

150. Bruynzeel DP, Diepgen TL, Andersen KE, Brandão FM, Bruze M, Frosch PJ, Goosssens A, Lahti A, Mahler V, Maibach HI, Menné T, Wilkinson JD (2005) Monitoring the European Standard series in 10 centres: 1996-2000. Contact Dermatitis 53:146–149

151. Kuno Y, Kato M (2001) Photosensitivity from colophony in a case of chronic actinic dermatitis associated with contact allergy from colophony. Acta Derm Venereol 81:442–443

152. Karlberg AT, Bohlinder K, Boman A, Hacksell U, Hermansson J, Jacobsson S, Nilsson JL (1988) Identification of 15-hydroperoxyabietic acid as a contact allergen to Portuguese colophony. J Pharm Pharmacol 40:42–47

153. Karlberg AT (1991) Air oxidation increases the allergenic potential in of tall oil rosin. Colophony contact allergens also identified in tall oil rosin. Am J Contact Dermatitis 2:43–49

154. Schnuch A, Geier J, Uter W, Frosch PJ (2002) Another look on allergies to fragrances: frequencies of sensitisation to the fragrance mix and its constituents. Results from the IVDK. Exogenous Dermatol 1:231–237

155. Johansen JD, Heydorn S, Menné T (2002) Oak moss extracts in the diagnosis of fragrance contact allergy. Contact Dermatitis 46:157–161

156. Lepoittevin JP, Meschkat E, Huygens S, Goossens A (2000) Presence of resin acids in "Oakmoss" patch test material: a source of misdiagnosis? J Invest Dermatol 115:129–130

157. Hjorth N (1961) Allergy to balsams, allied perfumes and flavouring agents. Munksgaard, Copenhagen

158. Paulsen E, Andersen KE, Brandão FM, Bruynzeel DP, Ducombs G, Frosch PJ, Goossens A, Lahti A, Menné T, Shaw S, Tosti A, Wahlberg JE, Wilkinson JD, Wrängsjö K (1999) Routine patch testing with the sesquiterpene lactone mix in Europe: a 2-year experience (a multicentre study of the EECDRG). Contact Dermatitis 40:72–76

159. Wöhrl S, Hemmer W, Focke M, Götz M, Jarisch R (2001) The significance of fragrance mix, balsam of Peru, colophony and propolis as screening tools in the detection of fragrance allergy. Br J Dermatol 145:268–273

160. Thomson KF, Wilkinson SM (2000) Allergic contact dermatitis to plant extracts in patients with cosmetic dermatitis. Br J Dermatol 142:84–88

161. Simpson EL, Law SV, Storrs FJ (2004) Prevalence of botanical extract allergy in patients with contact dermatitis. Dermatitis 15:67–72

162. Paulsen E (2002) Contact sensitization from Compositae-containing herbal remedies and cosmetics. Contact Dermatitis 47:189–198

163. Thune P, Sandberg M (1987) Allergy to lichen and Compositae compounds in perfumes. Investigations on the sensitizing, toxic and mutagenic potential. Acta Derm Venereol Suppl (Stockh) 134:87–89

164. Paulsen E, Andersen KE, Hausen BM (2001) An 8-year experience with routine SL mix patch testing supplemented with Compositae mix in Denmark. Contact Dermatitis 45: 29–35

165. Paulsen E, Andersen KE, Brandão FM et al (1999) Routine patch testing with sesquiterpene lactone mix in Europe: a 2-year experience. A multicentre study of the EECDRG. Contact Dermatitis 40:72–76

166. Geier J, Hausen BM (2000) Epikutantestung mit dem Kompositen-Mix. Ergebnisse einer Studie der Deutschen Kontaktallergie-Gruppe (DKG) und des Informationsverbundes Dermatologischer Kliniken (IVDK). Allergologie 23:334–341

167. Paulsen E, Andersen KE (2005) Colophonium and Compositae mix as markers of fragrance allergy: cross-reactivity between fragrance terpenes, colophonium and compositae plant extracts. Contact Dermatitis 53:285–291

168. Reichert-Pénétrat S, Barbaud A, Pénétrat E, Granel F, Schmutz J-L (2001) Allergic contact dermatitis from surgical paints. Contact Dermatitis 45:116–117

169. Li LF, Wang J (2002) Patch testing in allergic contact dermatitis caused by topical Chinese herbal medicine. Contact Dermatitis 47:166–168

170. Saha M, Srinivas CR, Shenoy SD, Balachandrar C, Acharya S (1993) Footwear dermatitis. Contact Dermatitis 28:260–264

171. Lyon CC, Tucker SC, Gäfvert E, Karlberg A-T, Beck MH (1999) Contact dermatitis from modified rosin in footwear. Contact Dermatitis 41:102–110

172. Strauss RM, Wilkinson SH (2002) Shoe dermatitis due to colophonium used as leather tanning or finishing agent in Portuguese shoes. Contact Dermatitis 47:59

173. Pereira TM, Flour M, Goossens A (2007) Allergic contact dermatitis from modified colophonium in wound dressings. Contact Dermatitis 56:5–9

174. Lange-Ionescu S, Bruze M, Gruvberger B, Zimerson E, Frosch P (2000) Kontaktallergie durch kohlefreies Durchschlagpapier. Derm Beruf Umwelt 48:183–187

175. Karlberg A-T, Magnusson K (1996) Rosin components identified in diapers. Contact Dermatitis 34:176–180

176. Kanerva L, Rintala H, Henriks-Eckerman K, Engström K (2001) Colophonium in sanitary pads. Contact Dermatitis 44:59–60

177. Färm G (1996) Contact allergy to colophony and hand eczema. A follow-up study of patients with previously diagnosed contact allergy to colophony. Contact Dermatitis 34:93–100

178. Karlberg A-T, Gäfvert E, Meding B, Stenberg B (1996) Airborne contact dermatitis from unexpected exposure to rosin (colophony). Contact Dermatitis 35:272–278

179. Kumar A, Freeman S (1999) Leukoderma following occupational allergic contact dermatitis. Contact Dermatitis 41:94–98

180. Corazza M, Borghi A, Virgili A (2004) A medicolegal controversy due to a hidden allergen in cutting oils. Contact Dermatitis 50:254–255

181. Agarwal S, Gawkrodger DJ (2002) Occupational allergic contact dermatitis to silver and colophonium in a jeweler. Am J Contact Dermatitis 13:74

182. Karlberg A-T, Boman A, Nilsson JLG (1988) Hydrogenation reduces the allergenicity of colophony. Contact Dermatitis 19:22–29

183. Karlberg A-T, Gäfvert E (1996) Isolated colophony allergens as screening substances for contact allergy. Contact Dermatitis 35:201–207

184. Sadhra S, Foulds IS, Gray CN (1998) Oxidation of resin acids in colophony (rosin) and its implications for patch testing. Contact Dermatitis 39:58–63

185. Gäfvert E, Bordalo O, Karlberg A-T (1996) Patch testing with allergens from modified rosin (colophony) discloses additional cases of contact allergy. Contact Dermatitis 35:290–298

186. Hausen BM, Mohnert J (1989) allergy due to colophony. (V) Patch test results with different types of colophony and modified-colophony products. Contact Dermatitis 20: 295–301

187. Morris SD, Rycroft RJG, White IR, Wakelin SH, McFadden JP (2002) Comparative frequency of patch test reactions to topical antibiotics. Br J Dermatol 146: 1047–1051

188. Mirshahpanah P, Maibach HI (2007) Relationship of patch test positivity in a general versus an eczema population. Contact Dermatitis 56:125–130

189. Menezes de Pádua CA, Uter W, Schnuch A (2007) Contact allergy to topical drugs: prevalence in a clinical setting and estimation of frequency at the population level. Pharmacoepidemiol Drug Saf 16:377–384

190. van Ginkel CJ, Bruintjes TD, Huizing EH (1995) Allergy due to topical medications in chronic otitis externa and chronic otitis media. Clin Otolaryngol 20:326–328

191. Hillen U, Geier J, Goos M (2000) Kontaktallergien bei Patienten mit Ekzemen des äusseren Gehörgangs. Hautarzt 51:239–243

192. Bjarnason B, Flosadóttir E (2000) Patch testing with neomycin sulfate. Contact Dermatitis 43:295–302
193. Kimura M, Kawada A (1998) Contact sensitivity induced by neomycin with cross-sensitivity to other aminoglycoside antibiotics. Contact Dermatitis 39:148–150
194. Marks JG, Belsito DV, DeLeo VA et al (2000) North American Contact Dermatitis Group Patch Test results, 1996-1998. Arch Dermatol 136:272–273
195. Warshaw EM, Schram SE, Belsito DV, DeLeo VA, Fowler JF, Maibach HI, Marks JG, Mathias CGT, Pratt MD, Rietzchel RL, Sasseville D, Storrs FJ, Taylor JS, Zug KA (2008) Patch-test reactions to topical anesthetics: retrospective analysis of cross-sectional data, 2001-2004. Dermatitis 19:81–85
196. Gail H, Kaufmann R, Kalservan CM (1996) Adverse reactions to local anesthetics: analysis of 197 cases. J Allergy Clin Immunol 97:933–937
197. Turchin I, Moreau L, Warshaw E, Sasseville D (2006) Cross-reactions among parabens, para-phenylenediamine, and benzocaine: a retrospective analysis of patch testing. Dermatitis 17:192–195
198. Sidhu SK, Shaw S, Wilkinson J (1999) A 10-year retrospective study on benzocaine allergy in the United Kingdom. Am J Contact Dermatitis 10:57–61
199. Wilkinson JD, Andersen KE, Lahti A, Rycroft RJG, Shaw S, White I (1990) Preliminary patch testing with 25% and 15% "caine" mixes. Contact Dermatitis 22:244–245
200. Beck MH, Holden A (1988) Benzocaine an unsatisfactory indicator of topical local anaesthetic sensitization for the U.K. Br J Dermatol 118:91–94
201. Van Ketel WG, Bruynzeel DP (1991) A "forgotten" topical anaesthetic sensitizer: butyl aminobenzoate. Contact Dermatitis 25:131–132
202. Agner T, Menné T (1993) Sensitivity to clioquinol and chlorquinaldol in the quinoline mix. Contact Dermatitis 29:163
203. Cronin E (1980) Contact dermatitis. Churchill Livingstone, Edinburgh, p 219
204. Goh CL, Ling R (1998) A retrospective epidemiology study of contact eczema among the elderly attending a tertiary dermatology referral centre in Singapore. Singapore Med J 39:442–446
205. Morris SD, Rycroft RJ, Wakelin SH, McFadden JP (2002) Comparative frequency of patch test reactions to topical antibiotics. Br J Dermatol 146:1047–1051
206. Ekelund A, Möller H (1969) Oral provocation in eczematous contact allergy to neomycin and hydroxy-quinolines. Act Derm Verereol (Stockh) 49:422–426
207. Skog E (1975) Systemic eczematous contact-type dermatitis induced by iodochlorhydroxyquin and chloroquine phosphate. Contact Dermatitis 1:187
208. Silvestre JF, Alfonso R, Moragón M, Ramón R, Botella R (1998) Systemic contact dermatitis due to norfloxacin with a positive patch test to quinoline mix. Contact Dermatitis 39:83
209. Janier M, Vignon MD (1995) Recurrent fixed drug eruption due to clioquinol. Br J Dermatol 133:1013–1034
210. Simpson JR (1974) Reversed cross-sensitisation between quinine and iodochlorhydroxyquinoline. Contact Dermatitis Newslett 15:431
211. Katsarou A, Armenaka M, Ale I, Koufou V, Kalogeromitros D (1999) Frequency of immediate reactions to the European standard series. Contact Dermatitis 41:276–279
212. Allenby CF (1965) Skin sensitisation to remederm and cross-sensitisation to hydroxyquinoline compounds. Br Med J ii:208–209
213. Kero M, Hannuksela M, Sothman A (1979) Primary irritant dermatitis from topical clioquinol. Contact Dermatitis 5:115–117
214. Beck MH, Wilkinson SM (1994) A distinctive irritant contact reaction to Vioform (clioquinol). Contact Dermatitis 31:54–55
215. Bruynzeel DP, Diepgen TL, Andersen KE, Brandão FM, Bruze M, Frosch PJ, Goosssens A, Lahti A, Mahler V, Maibach HI, Menné T, Wilkinson JD (2005) Monitoring the European Standard series in 10 centres: 1996-2000. Contact Dermatitis 53:146–152
216. Warshaw EM, Nelsen DD, Maibach HI, Marks JG, Zug KA, Taylor JS, Rietschel RL, Fowler JF, Mathias CG, Ptatt MD, Sasseville D, Storrs FJ, Belsito DV, DeLeo VA (2009) Positive patch test reactions to lanolin: cross-sectional data from the North American Contact Dermatitis Group, 1994 to 2006. Dermatitis 20:79–88
217. Kligman AM (1983) Lanolin allergy: crisis or comedy. Contact Dermatitis 9:99–107
218. Lee B, Warshaw E (2008) Lanolin allergy: history, epidemiology, responsible allergens and management. Dermatitis 19:63–72
219. Schnuch A, Szliska C, Uter W (2009) Facial allergic contact dermatitis. Data from the IVDK and review of the literauture. Hautarzt 60:13–21
220. Machet L, Couhé C, Perrinaud A, Hoarau C, Lorette G, Vaillant L (2004) A high prevalence of sensitization still persists in leg ulcer patients: a retrospective series of 106 patients tested between 2001 and 2002 and a meta-analysis of 1975-2003 data. Brit J Dermatol 150:929–935
221. Wakelin SH, Smith H, White IR, Rycroft RJG, Mc Fadden JP (2001) A retrospective analysis of contact allergy to lanolin. Brit J Dermatol 145:28–31
222. Matthieu L, Dockx P (1997) Discrepancy in patch test results with wool wax alcohols and Amerchol-L101®. Contact Dermatitis 36:150–151
223. Rastogi SC, Schouten A, de Kruijf N, Weijland JW (1995) Contents of methyl-, ethyl-, propyl-, butyl- and benzylparaben in cosmetic products. Contact Dermatitis 32:28–30
224. Rastogi SC (2000) Analytical control of preservative labelling on skin creams. Contact Dermatitis 43:339–343
225. Harvey PW, Everett DJ (2004) Significance of the detection of esters of p-hydroxybenzoic acid (parabens) in human breast tumours. J Appl Toxicol 24:1–4
226. Anonymous (2008) Final amended report on the safety assessment of Methylparaben, Ethylparaben, Propylparaben, Isopropylparaben, Butylparaben, Isobutylparaben, and Benzylparaben as used in cosmetic products. Int J Toxicol 27(suppl 4):1–82
227. Menné T, Hjorth N (1988) Routine patch testing with paraben esters. Contact Dermatitis 19:189–191
228. Schnuch A, Geier J, Uter W, Frosch PJ (1998) Patch testing with preservatives, antimicrobials and industrial biocides. Results from a multicentre study. Br J Dermatol 138:467–476
229. Jong CT, Statham BN, Green CM, King CM, Gawkrodger DJ, Sansom JE, English JS, Wilkinson SM, Ormerod AD, Chowdhury MM (2007) Contact sensitivity to preservatives

in the UK, 2004-2005: results of multicentre study. Contact Dermatitis 57:165–168

230. Wilkinson JD, Shaw S, Andersen KE, Brandao FM, Bruynzeel DP, Bruze M, Camarasa JM, Diepgen TL, Ducombs G, Frosch PJ, Goossens A, Lachapelle JM, Lahti A, Menne T, Seidenari S, Tosti A, Wahlberg JE (2002) Monitoring levels of preservative sensitivity in Europe. A 10-year overview (1991–2000). Contact Dermatitis 46:207–210

231. Andersen KE, Volund A, Frankild S (1995) The guinea pig maximization test – with a multiple dose design. Acta Derm Venereol (Stockh) 75:463–469

232. Fisher AA, Pascher F, Kanof NB (1971) Allergic contact dermatitis due to ingredients of vehicles. A "vehicle tray" for patch testing. Arch Dermatol 104:286–290

233. Gallenkemper G, Rabe E, Bauer R (1998) Contact sensitization in chronic venous insufficiency: modern wound dressings. Contact Dermatitis 38:274–278

234. Praditsuwan P, Taylor JS, Roenigk HH Jr (1995) Allergy to Unna boots in four patients. J Am Acad Dermatol 33:906–908

235. Fisher AA (1973) The paraben paradox. Cutis 12:830–832

236. Fisher AA (1979) Paraben dermatitis due to a new medicated bandage: the "paraben paradox". Contact Dermatitis 5:273–274

237. Schorr WF (1968) Paraben allergy. A cause of intractable dermatitis. JAMA 204:859–862

238. Hjorth N, Trolle-Lassen C (1963) Skin reactions to ointment bases. Trans St John's Hosp Dermatol Soc 49:127–140

239. Maucher OM (1974) Beitrag zur Kreuz-oder Kopplingsallergie zur parahydroxybenzoe-säure-ester. Berufsdermatosen 22:183–187

240. Fisher AA (1975) Letter: paraben-induced dermatitis. Arch Dermatol 111:657–658

241. Carradori S, Peluso AM, Faccioli M (1990) Systemic contact dermatitis due to parabens. Contact Dermatitis 22:238–239

242. Sánchez-Pérez J, Diez MB, Pérez AA, Jiménez YD, Diez G (2006) Allergic and systemic contact dermatitis to methylparaben. Contact Dermatitis 54:117–118

243. Veien NK, Hattel T, Laurberg G (1996) Oral challenge with parabens in paraben-sensitive patients. Contact Dermatitis 34:433

244. Henry JC, Tschen EH, Becker LE (1979) Contact urticaria to parabens. Arch Dermatol 115:1231–1232

245. Nagel JE, Fuscaldo JT, Fireman P (1977) Paraben allergy. JAMA 237:1594–1595

246. Lundov MD, Moesby L, Zachariae C, Johansen JD (2009) Contamination versus preservation of cosmetics: a review on legislation, usage, infections, and contact allergy. Contact Dermatitis 60:70–78

247. Flyvholm MA, Menne T (1992) Allergic contact dermatitis from formaldehyde. A case study focussing on sources of formaldehyde exposure. Contact Dermatitis 27:27–36

248. Feinman SE (1988) Formaldehyde sensitivity and toxicity. CRC, Boca Raton

249. Karlberg AT, Skare L, Lindberg I, Nyhammar E (1998) A method for quantification of formaldehyde in the presence of formaldehyde donors in skin-care products. Contact Dermatitis 38:20–28

250. Zachariae C, Hall B, Cottin M, Cupferman S, Andersen KE, Menné T (2005) Experimental elicitation of contact allergy from a diazolidinyl urea-preserved cream in relation to

anatomical region, exposure time and concentration. Contact Dermatitis 53:268–277

251. Isaksson M, Gruvberger B, Goon AT, Bruze M (2006) Can an imidazolidinyl urea-preserved corticosteroid cream be safely used in individuals hypersensitive to formaldehyde? Contact Dermatitis 54:29–34

252. Adams RM, Fisher AA (1986) Contact allergen alternatives: 1986. J Am Acad Dermatol 14:951–969

253. Scheman AJ, Carroll PA, Brown KH, Osburn AH (1998) Formaldehyde-related textile allergy: an update. Contact Dermatitis 38:332–336

254. Ford GP, Beck MH (1986) Reactions to Quaternium-15, Bronopol and Germall 115 in a standard series. Contact Dermatitis 14:271–274

255. Anderson BE, Tan TC, Marks JG Jr (2007) Patch-test reactions to formaldehydes, bioban, and other formaldehyde releasers. Dermatitis 18:92–95

256. Christophersen J, Menne T, Tanghoj P, Andersen KE, Brandrup F, Kaaber K, Osmundsen PE, Thestrup-Pedersen K, Veien NK (1989) Clinical patch test data evaluated by multivariate analysis. Danish Contact Dermatitis Group. Contact Dermatitis 21:291–299

257. Henriks-Eckerman ML, Suuronen K, Jolanki R (2008) Analysis of allergens in metalworking fluids. Contact Dermatitis 59:261–267

258. Aalto-Korte K, Kuuliala O, Suuronen K, Alanko K (2008) Occupational contact allergy to formaldehyde and formaldehyde releasers. Contact Dermatitis 59:280–289

259. Uter W, Geier J, Land M, Pfahlberg A, Gefeller O, Schnuch A (2001) Another look at seasonal variation in patch test results. A multifactorial analysis of surveillance data of the IVDK. Information Network of Departments of Dermatology. Contact Dermatitis 44:146–152

260. Kang KM, Corey G, Storrs FJ (1995) Follow-up study of patients allergic to formaldehyde and formaldehyde releasers: retention of information, compliance, course, and persistence of allergy. Am J Contact Dermat 6:209–215

261. Flyvholm MA, Hall BM, Agner T, Tiedemann E, Greenhill P, Vanderveken W, Freeberg FE, Menne T (1997) Threshold for occluded formaldehyde patch test in formaldehyde-sensitive patients. Relationship to repeated open application test with a product containing formaldehyde releaser. Contact Dermatitis 36:26–33

262. Agner T, Flyvholm MA, Menne T (1999) Formaldehyde allergy: a follow-up study. Am J Contact Dermat 10:12–17

263. Noiesen E, Munk MD, Larsen K, Johansen JD, Agner T (2007) Difficulties in avoiding exposure to allergens in cosmetics. Contact Dermatitis 57:105–109

264. Maurice F, Rivory JP, Larsson PH, Johansson SG, Bousquet J (1986) Anaphylactic shock caused by formaldehyde in a patient undergoing long-term hemodialysis. J Allergy Clin Immunol 77:594–597

265. Orlandini A, Viotti G, Magno L (1988) Anaphylactoid reaction induced by patch testing with formaldehyde in an asthmatic. Contact Dermatitis 19:383–384

266. Andersen KE, Maibach HI (1984) Multiple application delayed onset contact urticaria: possible relation to certain unusual formalin and textile reactions? Contact Dermatitis 10:227–234

267. de Groot AC, Flyvholm M, Lensen G, Menne T, Coenraads P-J (2009) Formaldehyde releasers: relationship to

31

formaldehyde contact allergy. Contact allergy to formaldehyde and inventory of formaldehyde releasers. Contact Dermatitis 61:63–85

268. Trattner A, Johansen JD, Menne T (1998) Formaldehyde concentration in diagnostic patch testing: comparison of 1% with 2%. Contact Dermatitis 38:9–13

269. Anonymous (1997) International cosmetic ingredients dictionary and handbook, 7th edn. The Cosmetic, Toiletry, and Fragrance Association, Washington

270. Dickel H, Taylor JS, Bickers DR, Merk HF, Bruckner TM (2003) Multiple patch-test reactions: a pilot evaluation of a combination approach to visualize patterns of multiple sensitivity in patch-test databases and a proposal for a multiple sensitivity index. Am J Contact Dermat 14:148–153

271. Kranke B, Szolar-Platzer C, Aberer W (1996) Reactions to formaldehyde and formaldehyde releasers in a standard series. Contact Dermatitis 35:192–193

272. Maouad M, Fleischer AB Jr, Sherertz EF, Feldman SR (1999) Significance-prevalence index number: a reinterpretation and enhancement of data from the North American contact dermatitis group. J Am Acad Dermatol 41: 573–576

273. Jordan WP Jr, Sherman WT, King SE (1979) Threshold responses in formaldehyde-sensitive subjects. J Am Acad Dermatol 1:44–48

274. Boffa MJ, Beck MH (1996) Allergic contact dermatitis from quaternium-15 in Oilatum cream. Contact Dermatitis 35:45–46

275. Tosti A, Piraccini BM, Bardazzi F (1990) Occupational contact dermatitis due to quaternium-15. Contact Dermatitis 23:41–42

276. Marren P, de Berker D, Dawber RP, Powell S (1991) Occupational contact dermatitis due to quaternium-15 presenting as nail dystrophy. Contact Dermatitis 25:253–255

277. Finch TM, Prais L, Foulds IS (2001) Occupational allergic contact dermatitis from quaternium-15 in an electroencephalography skin preparation gel. Contact Dermatitis 44: 44–45

278. Zina AM, Fanan E, Bundino S (2000) Allergic contact dermatitis from formaldehyde and quaternium-15 in photocopier toner. Contact Dermatitis 43:241–242

279. Warshaw EM, Ahmed RL, Belsito DV, DeLeo VA, Fowler JF Jr, Maibach HI, Marks JG Jr, Toby Mathias CG, Pratt MD, Rietschel RL, Sasseville D, Storrs FJ, Taylor JS, Zug KA, North American Contact Dermatitis Group (2007) Contact dermatitis of the hands: cross-sectional analyses of North American Contact Dermatitis Group Data, 1994-2004. J Am Acad Dermatol 57:301–314

280. de Groot AC, Weyland JW (1988) Kathon CG: a review. J Am Acad Dermatol 18:350–358

281. Burden AD, O'Driscoll JB, Page FC, Beck MH (1994) Contact hypersensitivity to a new isothiazolinone. Contact Dermatitis 30:179–180

282. Mathias CG, Andersen KE, Hamann K (1983) Allergic contact dermatitis from 2-n-octyl-4-isothiazolin-3-one, a paint mildewcide. Contact Dermatitis 9:507–509

283. Bjorkner B, Bruze M, Dahlquist I, Fregert S, Gruvberger B, Persson K (1986) Contact allergy to the preservative Kathon CG. Contact Dermatitis 14:85–90

284. Flyvholm MA (2005) Preservatives in registered chemical products. Contact Dermatitis 53:27–32

285. Bruze M, Fregert S, Gruvberger B, Persson K (1987) Contact allergy to the active ingredients of Kathon CG in the guinea pig. Acta Derm Venereol 67:315–320

286. Bruze M, Dahlquist I, Fregert S, Gruvberger B, Persson K (1987) Contact allergy to the active ingredients of Kathon CG. Contact Dermatitis 16:183–188

287. Hasan T, Rantanen T, Alanko K, Harvima RJ, Jolanki R, Kalimo K, Lahti A, Lammintausta K, Lauerma AI, Laukkanen A, Luukkaala T, Riekki R, Turjanmaa K, Varjonen E, Vuorela AM (2005) Patch test reactions to cosmetic allergens in 1995–1997 and 2000–2002 in Finland–a multicentre study. Contact Dermatitis 53:40–45

288. Thyssen JP, Sederberg-Olsen N, Thomsen JF, Menné T (2006) Contact dermatitis from methylisothiazolinone in a paint factory. Contact Dermatitis 54:322–324

289. de Groot AC (1997) Vesicular dermatitis of the hands secondary to perianal allergic contact dermatitis caused by preservatives in moistened toilet tissues. Contact Dermatitis 36:173–174

290. Gebhardt M, Looks A, Hipler UC (1997) Urticaria caused by type IV sensitization to isothiazolinones. Contact Dermatitis 36:314

291. Schubert H (1997) Airborne contact dermatitis due to methylchloro- and methylisothiazolinone (MCI/MI). Contact Dermatitis 36:274

292. Bohn S, Niederer M, Brehm K, Bircher AJ (2000) Airborne contact dermatitis from methylchloroisothiazolinone in wall paint. Abolition of symptoms by chemical allergen inactivation. Contact Dermatitis 42:196–201

293. Hunter KJ, Shelley JC, Haworth AE (2008) Airborne allergic contact dermatitis to methylchloroisothiazolinone/methylisothiazolinone in ironing water. Contact Dermatitis 58:183–184

294. Frosch PJ, Lahti A, Hannuksela M, Andersen KE, Wilkinson JD, Shaw S, Lachapelle JM (1995) Chloromethylisothiazolone/methylisothiazolone (CMI/MI) use test with a shampoo on patch-test-positive subjects. Results of a multicentre double-blind crossover trial. Contact Dermatitis 32:210–217

295. Zachariae C, Lerbaek A, McNamee PM, Gray JE, Wooder M, Menné T (2006) An evaluation of dose/unit area and time as key factors influencing the elicitation capacity of methylchloroisothiazolinone/methylisothiazolinone (MCI/MI) in MCI/MI-allergic patients. Contact Dermatitis 55:160–166

296. Farm G, Wahlberg JE (1991) Isothiazolinones (MCI/MI): 200 ppm versus 100 ppm in the standard series. Contact Dermatitis 25:104–107

297. Gruvberger B, Bruze M (1998) Can chemical burns and allergic contact dermatitis from higher concentrations of methylchloroisothiazolinone/methylisothiazolinone be prevented? Am J Contact Dermat 9:11–14

298. Geier J, Schnuch A (1996) No cross-sensitization between MCI/MI, benzisothiazolinone and octylisothiazolinone. Contact Dermatitis 34:148–149

299. Isaksson M, Bruze M, Gruvberger B (1998) Cross-reactivity between methylchloroisothiazolinone/methylisothiazolinone, methylisothiazolinone, and other isothiazolinones in workers at a plant producing binders for paints and glues. Contact Dermatitis 58:60–62

300. Guerra L, Bardazzi F, Tosti A (1992) Contact dermatitis in hairdressers' clients. Contact Dermatitis 26:108–111

301. Holness DL, Nethercott JR (1990) Epicutaneous testing results in hairdressers. Am J Contact Dermatitis 1: 224–234

302. Thyssen JP, Andersen KE, Bruze M et al (2009) p-Phenylenediamine sensitization is more prevalent in central and southern European patch test centres than in Scandinavian: results from a multicentre study. Contact Dermatitis 60:314–319

303. Thyssen JP, White JML (2008) Epidemiological data on consumer allergy to p-phenylenediamine. Contact Dermatitis 59:327–343

304. Uter W, Lessmann H, Geier J, Schnuch A (2003) Contact allergy to ingredients of hair cosmetics in female hairdressers and clients – an 8-year analysis of IVDK data. Contact Dermatitis 49:236–240

305. Fautz R, Fuchs A, van der Walle H, Henny V, Smits L (2002) Hair dye-sensitized hairdressers: the cross-reaction pattern with new generation hair dyes. Contact Dermatitis 46:319–324

306. Sosted H, Rastogi SC, Andersen KE, Johansen JD, Menne T (2004) Hair dye contact allergy: quantitative exposure assessment of selected products and clinical cases. Contact Dermatitis 50:344–348

307. Sosted H, Agner T, Andersen KE, Menné T (2002) 55 cases of allergic reactions to hair dye: a descriptive, consumer complaint-based study. Contact Dermatitis 47:299–303

308. Wakelin SH, Creamer D, Rycroft RJG, White IR, McFadden JP (1998) Contact dermatitis from paraphenylenediamine used as a skin paint. Contact Dermatitis 39:92–93

309. Nawaf AM, Joshi A, Nour-Eldin O (2003) Acute allergic contact dermatitis due to para-phenylenediamine after temporary henna painting. J Dermatol 30:797–800

310. McFadden JP, Wakelin SH, Holloway DB, Basketter DA (1998) The effect of patch duration on elicitation of para-phenylenediamine contact allergy. Contact Dermatitis 39:79–81

311. Herve-Bazin B, Gradiski D, Duprat P, Marignac B, Foussereau J, Cavelier C, Bieber P (1977) Occupational eczema from N-isopropyl-N′-phenyl-paraphenylenediamine (IPPD) and N-dimethyl-1, 3-butyl-N′-phenylparaphenylenediamine (DMPPD) in tyres. Contact Dermatitis 3:1–15

312. Cronin E (1980) Contact dermatitis. Churchill Livingstone, Edinburgh, p 137

313. Seidenari S, Mantovani L, Manzini BM, Pignatti M (1997) Cross-sensitizations between azo dyes and para-amino compound. A study of 236 azo-dye-sensitive subjects. Contact Dermatitis 36:91–96

314. Goon AT, Gilmour NJ, Basketter DA, White IR, Rycroft RJ, McFadden JP (2003) High frequency of simultaneous sensitivity to Disperse Orange 3 in patients with positive patch tests to para-phenylenediamine. Contact Dermatitis 48:248–250

315. Picardo M, Cannistraci C, Cristaudo A, De Luca C, Santucci B (1990) Study on cross-reactivity to the para group. Dermatologica 181:104–108

316. Edwards EK Jr, Edwards EK (1984) Contact urticaria and allergic contact dermatitis caused by paraphenylenediamine. Cutis 34:87–88

317. Wong GA, King CM (2003) Immediate-type hypersensitivity and allergic contact dermatitis due to para-phenylenediamine in hair dye. Contact Dermatitis 48:166

318. Hillen U, Jappe U, Frosch PJ, Becker D, Brasch J, Lilie M, Fuchs T, Kreft B, Pirker C, Geier J, German Contact Dermatitis Research Group (2006) Late reactions to the patch-test preparations para-phenylenediamine and epoxy resin: a prospective multicentre investigation of the German Contact Dermatitis Research Group. Br J Dermatol 154:665–670

319. Cronin E (1980) Contact dermatitis. Churchill Livingstone, Edinburgh, pp 716–745

320. Estlander T, Jolanki R, Kanerva L (1994) Allergic contact dermatitis from rubber and plastic gloves. In: Mellström G, Wahlberg JE, Maibach HI (eds) Protective gloves for occupational use. CRC, Boca Raton, pp 221–240

321. Geier J, Lessmann H, Uter W, Schnuch A (2003) Occupational rubber glove allergy: results of the Information Network of Departments of Dermatology (IVDK), 1995–2001. Contact Dermatitis 48:39–44

322. Nettis E, Assennato G, Ferrannini A, Tursi A (2002) Type I allergy to natural rubber latex and type IV allergy to rubber chemicals in health care workers with glove-related skin symptoms. Clin Exp Allergy 32:441–447

323. Gibbon KL, McFadden JP, Rycroft RJ, Ross JS, White IR (2001) Changing frequency of thiuram allergy in healthcare workers with hand dermatitis. Br J Dermatol 144:347–350

324. Knudsen BB, Larsen E, Egsgaard H, Menné T (1993) Release of thiurams and carbamates from rubber gloves. Contact Dermatitis 28:63–69

325. Cockayne SE, Shah M, Messenger AG, Gawkrodger DJ (1998) Foot dermatitis in children: causative allergens and follow-up. Contact Dermatitis 38:203–206

326. Conde-Salazar L, del-Rio E, Guimaraens D, Gonzalez Domingo A (1993) Type IV allergy to rubber additives: a 10-year study of 686 cases. J Am Acad Dermatol 29: 176–180

327. Frosch PJ, Born CM, Schultz R (1987) Kontaktallergien auf Gumini-, Operations- und Vinylhandschuhe. Hautarzt 38:210–217

328. Gold S (1966) A skinful of alcohol. Lancet 2:1417

329. Stole D, King LE Jr (1980) Disulfiram-alcohol skin reaction to beer-containing shampoo. J Am Med Assoc 244:2045

330. Rebandel P, Rudzki E (1996) Secondary contact sensitivity to TMTD in patients primarily positive to TETD. Contact Dermatitis 35:48

331. Kaaber K, Menné T, Veien N, Hougaard P (1983) Treatment of dermatitis with Antabuse; a double blind study. Contact Dermatitis 9:297–299

332. Gamboa P, Jauregui I, Urrutia I, Antepara I, Peralta C (1993) Disulfiram-induced recall of nickel dermatitis in chronic alcoholism. Contact Dermatitis 28:255

333. van Hecke E, Vermander F (1984) Allergic contact dermatitis by oral disulfiram. Contact Dermatitis 10:254

334. Logan RA, White JR (1988) Carbamix is redundant in the patch test series. Contact Dermatitis 18:303–304

335. Holness DL, Nethercott JR (1997) Results of patch testing with a special series of rubber allergens. Contact Dermatitis 36:207–211

336. Geier J, Gefeller O (1995) Sensitivity of patch tests with rubber mixes. Results of the Information Network of Departments of Dermatology from 1990 to 1993. Am J Contact Dermatitis 6:143–149

337. Fregert S (1969) Cross-sensitivity pattern of 2-mercaptobenzothiazole (MBT). Acta Derm Venereol (Stockh) 49:45–48

338. Cronin E (1980) Contact dermatitis. Churchill Livingstone, Edinburgh, pp 734–735
339. Mancuso G, Reggiani M, Berdondini RM (1996) Occupational dermatitis in shoemakers. Contact Dermatitis 34:17–22
340. Condè-Salazar L, Llinas Volpe MG, Guimaraens D, Romero L (1988) Allergic contact dermatitis from a suction socket prosthesis. Contact Dermatitis 19:305–306
341. Maibach HI (1996) Possible cosmetic dermatitis due to mercaptobenzothiazole. Contact Dermatitis 34:72
342. Taylor JS (1986) Rubber. In: Fisher AA (ed) Contact dermatitis, 3rd edn. Lea and Febiger, Philadelphia, p 623
343. Diepgen TL, Bruynzeel DP, Andersen KE et al (2006) Mercaptobenzothiazole or the mercapto-mix: which should be in the standard series. Contact Dermatitis 55:36–38
344. Geier J, Uter W, Schnuch A, Brasch J, German Contact Dermatitis Research Group (DKG); Information Network of Departments of Dermatology (IVDK) (2002) Diagnostic screening for contact allergy to mercaptobenzothiazole derivatives. Am J Contact Dermat 13:66–70
345. Hansson C, Agrup G (1993) Stability of the mercaptobenzothiazole compounds. Contact Dermatitis 28:29–34
346. Menné T, White IR, Bruynzeel DP, Goossens A (1992) Patch test reactivity to the PPD-black-rubber-mix (industrial rubber chemicals) and individual ingredients. Contact Dermatitis 26:354
347. Fisher AA (1991) The significance of a positive reaction to the "black rubber mix". Am J Contact Dermatitis 2: 141–142
348. Bieber MP, Foussereau J (1968) Role de deux amines aromatiques dans l'allergie au caoutchouc; PBN et 4010 NA, amines anti-oxydantes dans l'industrie du pneu. Bull Soc Franc Dermatol Syphilogr 75:63–67
349. Hansson C (1994) Allergic contact dermatitis from N-(1, 3-dimethylbutyl)-N′-phenyl-p-phenylenediamine and from compounds in polymerized 2, 2, 4- trimethyl-1, 2-dihydroquinoline. Contact Dermatitis 30:114–115
350. Herve-Bazin B, Gradiski D, Marignac B, Foussereau J (1977) Occupational eczema from N-isopropyl-N′-phenylparaphenylenediamine (IPPD) and N-dimethyl-1, 3-butyl-N′-phenylparaphenylenediamine (DMPPD) in tyres. Contact Dermatitis 3:1–15
351. White IR (1988) Dermatitis in rubber manufacturing industries. Dermatol Clin 6:53–59
352. Rademaker M (1998) Occupational contact dermatitis among New Zealand farmers. Australas J Dermatol 39:164–167
353. Tuyp E, Mitchell JC (1983) Scuba diver facial dermatitis. Contact Dermatitis 9:334–335
354. Goh CL (1987) Hand dermatitis from a rubber motorcycle handle. Contact Dermatitis 16:40–41
355. Ho VC, Mitchell JC (1985) Allergic contact dermatitis from rubber boots. Contact Dermatitis 12:110–111
356. Nishioka K, Murata M, Ishikawa T, Kaniwa M (1996) Contact dermatitis due to rubber boots worn by Japanese farmers, with special attention to 6-ethoxy-2, 2, 4-trimethyl-1, 2-dihydroquinoline (ETMDQ) sensitivity. Contact Dermatitis 35:241–245
357. Romaguera C, Aguirre A, Diaz Perez JL, Grimalt F (1986) Watch strap dermatitis. Contact Dermatitis 14:260–261
358. Lodi A, Chiarelli G, Mancini LL, Coassini A, Ambonati M, Crosti C (1996) Allergic contact dermatitis from a rubber bracelet. Contact Dermatitis 34:146
359. McKenna KE, McMillan C (1992) Facial contact dermatitis due to black rubber. Contact Dermatitis 26:270–271
360. Conde-Salazar L, Guimaraens D, Romero LV, Gonzalez MA (1987) Unusual allergic contact dermatitis to aromatic amines. Contact Dermatitis 17:42–44
361. Carlsen L, Andersen KE, Egsgaard H (1987) IPPD contact allergy from an orthopedic bandage. Contact Dermatitis 17:119–121
362. Fisher AA (1984) Purpuric contact dermatitis. Cutis 33:346, 349, 351
363. Ancona A, Monroy F, Fernandes-Diez J (1982) Occupational dermatitis from IPPD in tyres. Contact Dermatitis 8:91–94
364. Fregert S, Thorgeirsson A (1977) Patch testing with low molecular oligomers of epoxy resin in humans. Contact Dermatitis 3:301–303
365. Burrows D, Campbell H, Fregert S, Trulsson L (1984) Contact dermatitis from epoxy resins, tetraglycidyl-4, 4-methylene dianiline and O-diglycidyl pthalate in composite material. Contact Dermatitis 11:80–83
366. Jolanki R, Tarvainen R, Tatar T, Estlander T, Henricks-Eckerman M-L, Mustakallio KK, Kanerva L (1996) Occupational dermatoses from exposure to epoxy resin compounds in a ski factory. Contact Dermatitis 38:299–301
367. Pontén A, Carstensen O, Rasmussen K, Gruvberger B, Isaksson M, Bruze M (2004) Epoxy-based production of wind turbine rotor blades: occupational dermatoses. Contact Dermatitis 50:329–338
368. Amado A, Taylor S (2008) Contact dermatitis in the bowling pro shop. Dermatitis 19:334–338
369. Isaksson M, Möller H, Pontén A (2008) Occupational allergic contact dermatitis from epoxy resin in a golf club repairman. Dermatitis 19:30–32
370. Kanerva L, Jolanki R, Estlander T (2001) Active sensitization by epoxy in Leica immersion oil. Contact Dermatitis 44:194–219
371. Jappe U, Geier J, Hausen BM (2005) Contact vitiligo following a strong patch test reaction to trigycidyl-p-aminophenol in an aircraft industry worker: case report and review of the literature. Contact Dermatitis 53:89–92
372. Beliauskiene A, Sabaliauskas G, Valiukevicienne S (2008) Lichenoid dermatitis caused by contact allergy to epoxy resin. Contact Dermatitis 58(suppl):76
373. Stutz N, Hertl M, Löffler H (2008) Anaphylaxis caused by contact urticaria because of epoxy resins: an extraordinary emergency. Contact Dermatitis 58:307–309
374. Hannu T, Frilander H, Kauppi P, Kuuliala O, Alanko K (2009) IgE-mediated occupational asthma from epoxy resin. Int Arch Allergy Immunol 148:41–44
375. Bruynzeel DP, Diepgen TL, Andersen KE, Brandão FM, Bruze M, Frosch PJ, Goosssens A, Lahti A, Mahler V, Maibach HI, Menné T, Wilkinson JD (2005) Monitoring the European Standard series in 10 centres: 1996-2000. Contact Dermatitis 53:146–149
376. Géraut C, Seroux D, Dupas D (1989) Allergie cutanée aux nouvelles résines époxydiques. Arch Mal Prof 50:187–188
377. Pontén A, Zimerson E, Bruze M (2004) Contact allergy to the isomers of diglycidyl ether of bisphenol F. Acta Derm Venereol 84:12–17
378. Koch P (2003) Allergic contact dermatitis from BIS-GMA and epoxy resins in dental bonding agents. Contact Dermatitis 49:104–105

379. Kanerva L, Estlander T, Jolanki R, Alanko K (2000) Occupational allergic contact dermatitis from 2, 2-bis [4-(2-hydroxy-3-acryloxypropoxy) phenyl] propane (epoxy diacrylate) in ultraviolet-cured inks. Contact Dermatitis 43:56–59

380. Jolanki R, Estlander T, Kanerva L (2001) 182 patients with occupational allergic epoxy contact dermatitis over 22 years. Contact Dermatitis 44:121–123

381. Geier J, Lessmann H, Hillen U, Jappe U, Dickel H, Koch P, Frosch PJ, Schnuch A, Uter W (2004) An attempt to improve diagnostics of contact allergy due to epoxy resin systems. First results of the multicentre study EPOX 2002. Contact Dermatitis 51:263–272

382. Kanerva L, Jolanki R, Estlander T (1998) Occupational epoxy dermatitis with patch test reactions to multiple hardeners including tetraethylenepentamine. Contact Dermatitis 38:299–301

383. Fregert S (1988) Physicochemical methods for detection of contact allergens. Dermatol Clin 6:97–104

384. Pontén A, Björk C, Carstensen O, Gruvberger B, Isaksson M, Rasmussen K, Bruze M (2004) Associations between contact allergy to epoxy resin and fragrance mix. Acta Derm Venereol 84:151–152

385. Andersen KE, Christensen LP, Völund A, Johansen JD, Paulsen E (2009) Association between positive patch tests to epoxy resin and fragrance mix I ingredients. Contact Dermatitis 60:155–157

386. van der Willingen AH, Stolz E, van Joost T (1987) Sensitisation to phenol formaldehyde in rubber glue. Contact Dermatitis 16:291–292

387. Foussereau J, Cavelier C, Selig D (1976) Occupational eczema from para-tertiairy-butylphenol formaldehyde resins: a review of the sensitising resins. Contact Dermatitis 2:254–258

388. Freeman S (1997) Shoe dermatitis. Contact Dermatitis 36:247–251

389. Rani Z, Hussain L, Hazoon TS (2003) Common allergens in shoe dermatitis: our experience in Lahore, Pakistan. Int J Dermatol 42:605–607

390. Engel HO, Calnan CD (1966) Resin dermatitis in a car factory. Br J Ind Med 23:62–66

391. Wollina U (2002) Contact sensitisation to para-tertiairy-butylphenol-formaldehyde resin possibly due to glass wool exposure. Exogenous Dermatol 1:265

392. Shono M, Ezoe K, Kaniwa M, Ikarashi Y, Kojima S, Nakamura A (1991) Allergic contact dermatitis from para-tertiary-butylphenol-formaldehyde resin (ptbp-fr) in athletic tape and leather adhesive. Contact Dermatitis 24:281–288

393. Hayakawa R, Ogino Y, Suzuki M, Kaniwa M (1994) Allergic contact dermatitis from para-tertiary-butylphenol-formaldehyde resin (ptbp-f-r). Contact Dermatitis 30:187–188

394. Mobacken H, Hersle K (1976) Allergic contact dermatitis caused by para-tertiary butylphenol-formaldehyde resin in watch straps. Contact Dermatitis 2:59

395. Rycroft RJG, Wilkinson JD, Holmes R, Hay RJ (1980) Contact sensitization to p-tertiary butylphenol (PTBP) resin plastic nail adhesive. Clin Exp Dermatol 5:441–445

396. Moran M, Martin-Pascual A (1978) Contact dermatitis to para-tertiary-butylphenol formaldehyde. Contact Dermatitis 4:372–373

397. Dahlquist I (1984) Contact allergy to paratertiary butylphenol formaldehyde resin in an adhesive label. Contact Dermatitis 10:54

398. Burden AD, Lever RS, Morley WN (1994) Contact hypersensitivity induced by p-tert-butylphenol-formaldehyde resin in an adhesive dressing. Contact Dermatitis 31:276–277

399. Nagashima C, Tomitaka-Yagami A, Matsunaga K (2003) Contact dermatitis due to para-tertiary-butylphenol-formaldehyde resin in a wetsuit. Contact Dermatitis 49:267–268

400. Bredlich RO, Gall H (1998) Generalisiertes allergisches Kontaktekzem durch Kniebandagen. Dermatosen Beruf Umwelt 46:125–128

401. Sood A, Taylor J, Billock JN (2003) Contact dermatitis to a limb prosthesis. Am J Contact Dermatitis 14:169–171

402. Romaguera C, Grimalt F, Vilaplana J (1985) Paratertiairy butylphenol formaldehyde resin in prosthesis. Contact Dermatitis 12:174

403. Avenel-Audran M, Goosssens A, Zimerson E, Bruze M (2003) Contact dermatitis from electrocardiograph-monitoring electrodes: role of Contact dermatitis due to p-tert-butylphenol-formaldehyde resin. Contact Dermatitis 48:108–111

404. Feit NE, Weinberg JM, DeLeo VA (2004) Cutaneous disease and religious practice: case of allergic dermatitis to tefillin and review of the literature. Int J Dermatol 43:886–888

405. Zimerson E, Bruze M (2002) Low-molecular-weight contact allergens in p-tert-butylphenol-formaldehyde resin. Am J Contact Dermatitis 13:190–197

406. Zimmerson E, Bruze M, Goossens A (1999) Simultaneous p-tert-butylphenol-formaldehyde resin and p-tert-butylcatechol contact allergies in man and sensitizing capacities of p-tert-butylphenol and p-tert-butylcatechol in guinea pigs. JOEM 41:23–27

407. Zimerson E, Bruze M (1999) Demonstration of the contact sensitizer p-tert-butylcatechol in p-tert-butylphenol-formaldehyde resin. Am J Contact Dermatitis 10:2–6

408. Schubert H, Agatha G (1979) Zur Allergennatur der paratert Butylphenolformaldehydharze. Dermatosen Beruf Umwelt 27:49–52

409. Hagdrup H, Egsgaard H, Carlsen L, Andersen KE (1994) Contact allergy to 2-hydroxy-5-tert-butyl benzylalcohol and 2, 6-bis(hydroxymethyl)-4-tert-butylphenol, components of a phenolic resin used in a marking pen. Contact Dermatitis 31:154–156

410. Bajaj AK, Gupta SC, Chatterju AK (1990) Contact depigmentation from free paratertiary-butylphenol in bindi adhesive. Contact Dermatitis 22:99–102

411. Malten KE, Rath R, Pastors PMH (1983) Para-tert-Butylphenol Formaldehyde and other causes of Shoe Dermatitis. Dermatosen Beruf Umwelt 31:149–153

412. Özkaja-Bayazit N, Büjükbabani N (2001) Non-eczematous pigmented interface dermatitis from para-tertiairy-butylphenol formaldehyde resin in a watchstrap adhesive. Contact Dermatitis 44:45–46

413. Evans AV, Banerjee P, Mc Fadden JP, Calonje E (2003) Lymphomatoid contact dermatitis to para-tertyl-butylphenol resin. Clin Exp Dermatol 28:272–273

414. Bruze M (1987) Contact dermatitis from phenol-formaldehyde resins. In: Maibach HI (ed) Occupational and industrial dermatology, 2nd edn. Year Book Medical, Chicago, pp 430–435

415. Piaserico S, Larese F, Recchia GP, Corradin MT, Scardigli F, Gennaro F, Carriere C, Semenzato A, Brandolisio L, Peserico A, Fortina AB, North-East Italy Contact Dermatitis Group (2004) Allergic contact sensitivity in elderly patients. Aging Clin Exp Res 16:221–225

416. Paulsen E (1994) Primula eczema – well-known and overlooked. Ugeskr Laeger 156:1147–1148

417. Britton JE, Wilkinson SM, English JS, Gawkrodger DJ, Ormerod AD, Sansom JE, Shaw S, Statham B (2003) The British standard series of contact dermatitis allergens: validation in clinical practice and value for clinical governance. Br J Dermatol 148:259–264

418. Christensen LP (2000) Primulaceae. In: Avalos J, Maibach HI (eds) Dermatologic botany. CRC, Boca Raton, pp 201–235

419. Mowad CM (1998) Routine testing for *Primula obconica*: is it useful in the United States? Am J Contact Dermat 9:231–233

420. Zachariae C, Engkilde K, Johansen JD, Menné T (2007) Primin in the European standard patch test series for 20 years. Contact Dermatitis 56:344–346

421. Connolly M, Mc Cune J, Dauncey E, Lovell CR (2004) *Primula obconica*–is contact allergy on the decline? Contact Dermatitis 51:167–171

422. Aplin CG, Lovell CR (2001) Contact dermatitis due to hardy Primula species and their cultivars. Contact Dermatitis 44:23–29

423. Christensen LP, Larsen E (2000) Primin-free *Primula obconica* plants available. Contact Dermatitis 43:45–46

424. Hjorth N (1967) Seasonal variations in contact dermatitis. Acta Derm Venereol (Stockh) 47:409–418

425. Hausen BM (1978) On the occurrence of the contact allergen primin and other quinoid compounds in species of the family of primulaceae. Arch Dermatol Res 261:311–321

426. Paulsen E, Christensen LP, Andersen KE (2006) Miconidin and miconidin methyl ether from *Primula obconica* Hance: new allergens in an old sensitizer. Contact Dermatitis 55:203–209

427. Christensen LP, Larsen E (2000) Direct emission of the allergen primin from intact *Primula obconica* plants. Contact Dermatitis 42:149–153

428. Virgili A, Corazza M (1991) Unusual primin dermatitis. Contact Dermatitis 24:63–64

429. Ingber A (1991) Primula photodermatitis in Israel. Contact Dermatitis 25:265–266

430. Krebs M, Christensen LP (1995) 2-methoxy-6-pentyl-1, 4-dihydroxybenzene (miconidin) from *Primula obconica*: a possible allergen? Contact Dermatitis 33:90–93

431. Fregert S, Hjorth N, Schulz KH (1968) Patch testing with synthetic primin in persons sensitive to *Primula obconica*. Arch Dermatol 98:144–147

432. Tabar AI, Quirce S, Garcia BE, Rodriguez A, Olaguibel JM (1994) Primula dermatitis: versatility in its clinical presentation and the advantages of patch tests with synthetic primin. Contact Dermatitis 30:47–48

433. Dooms-Goossens A, Biesemans G, Vandaele M, Degreef H (1989) Primula dermatitis: more than one allergen? Contact Dermatitis 21:122–124

434. Ducombs G, Benezra C, Talaga P, Andersen KE, Burrows D, Camarasa JG, Dooms-Goossens A, Frosch PJ, Lachapelle JM, Menne T et al (1990) Patch testing with the "sesquiterpene lactone mix": a marker for contact allergy to Compositae and other sesquiterpene-lactone-containing plants. A multicentre study of the EECDRG. Contact Dermatitis 22:249–252

435. Hausen BM, Andersen KE, Helander I, Gensch KH (1986) Lettuce allergy: sensitizing potency of allergens. Contact Dermatitis 15:246–249

436. Oliwiecki S, Beck MH, Hausen BM (1991) Compositae dermatitis aggravated by eating lettuce. Contact Dermatitis 24:318–319

437. Paulsen E (1992) Compositae dermatitis: a survey. Contact Dermatitis 26:76–86

438. Paulsen E, Andersen KE, Hausen BM (2001) Sensitization and cross-reaction patterns in Danish Compositae-allergic patients. Contact Dermatitis 45:197–204

439. Nandakishore T, Pasricha JS (1994) Pattern of cross-sensitivity between 4 Compositae plants, *Parthenium hysterophorus, Xanthium strumarium, Helianthus annuus* and *Chrysanthemum coronarium*, in Indian patients. Contact Dermatitis 30:162–167

440. Hausen BM (1996) A 6-year experience with compositae mix. Am J Contact Dermat 7:94–99

441. Paulsen E, Sogaard J, Andersen KE (1998) Occupational dermatitis in Danish gardeners and greenhouse workers (III). Compositae-related symptoms. Contact Dermatitis 38:140–146

442. Fitzgerald DA, English JS (1992) Compositae dermatitis presenting as hand eczema. Contact Dermatitis 27:256–257

443. Paulsen E, Andersen KE (1993) Compositae dermatitis in a Danish dermatology department in 1 year (II). Clinical features in patients with Compositae contact allergy. Contact Dermatitis 29:195–201

444. Paulsen E, Christensen LP, Andersen KE (2007) Compositae dermatitis from airborne parthenolide. Br J Dermatol 156:510–515

445. Paulsen E, Christensen LP, Andersen KE (2002) Do monoterpenes released from feverfew (Tanacetum parthenium) plants cause airborne Compositae dermatitis? Contact Dermatitis 47:14–18

446. Wrangsjo K, Ros AM, Wahlberg JE (1990) Contact allergy to Compositae plants in patients with summer-exacerbated dermatitis. Contact Dermatitis 22:148–154

447. Paulsen E, Andersen KE, Hausen BM (1993) Compositae dermatitis in a Danish dermatology department in one year (I). Results of routine patch testing with the sesquiterpene lactone mix supplemented with aimed patch testing with extracts and sesquiterpene lactones of Compositae plants. Contact Dermatitis 29:6–10

448. Paulsen E, Otkjær A, Andersen KE (2008) Sesquiterpene lactone dermatitis in the young: is atopy a risk factor? Contact Dermatitis 59:1–6

449. Murphy GH, White IR, Hawk JL (1990) Allergic airborne contact dermatitis to Compositae with photosensitivity – chronic actinic dermatitis in evolution. Photodermatol Photoimmunol Photomed 7:38–39

450. Paulsen E (1998) Occupational dermatitis in Danish gardeners and greenhouse workers (II). Etiological factors. Contact Dermatitis 38:14–19

451. Mateo MP, Velasco M, Miquel FJ, de la Cuadra J (1995) Erythema-multiforme-like eruption following allergic contact dermatitis from sesquiterpene lactones in herbal medicine. Contact Dermatitis 33:449–450

452. Goulden V, Wilkinson SM (1998) Patch testing for Compositae allergy. Br J Dermatol 138:1018–1021
453. Kanerva L, Estlander T, Alanko K, Jolanki R (2001) Patch test sensitization to Compositae mix, sesquiterpene-lactone mix, Compositae extracts, laurel leaf, Chlorophorin, Mansonone A, and dimethoxydalbergione. Am J Contact Dermat 12: 18–24
454. Wilkinson SM, Pollock B (1999) Patch test sensitization after use of the Compositae mix. Contact Dermatitis 40:277–278
455. Bong JL, English JS, Wilkinson SM; British Contact Dermatitis Group (2001) Diluted Compositae mix versus sesquiterpene lactone mix as a screening agent for Compositae dermatitis: a multicentre study. Contact Dermatitis 45:26–28
456. Orion E, Paulsen E, Andersen KE, Menne T (1998) Comparison of simultaneous patch testing with parthenolide and sesquiterpene lactone mix. Contact Dermatitis 38:207–208
457. Paulsen E, Andersen KE, Brandao FM, Bruynzeel DP, Ducombs G, Frosch PJ, Goossens A, Lahti A, Menne T, Shaw S, Tosti A, Wahlberg JE, Wilkinson JD, Wrangsjo K (1999) Routine patch testing with the sesquiterpene lactone mix in Europe: a 2-year experience. A multicentre study of the EECDRG. Contact Dermatitis 40:72–76
458. Mak RK, White IR, White JM, McFadden JP, Goon AJ (2007) Lower incidence of sesquiterpene lactone sensitivity in a population in Asia versus a population in Europe: an effect of chrysanthemum tea? Contact Dermatitis 57: 163–164
459. Reynolds JEF (1993) Martindale, the extra pharmacopoeia, 30th edn. The Pharmaceutical Press, London, p 726
460. Dooms-Goossens A (1995) Allergy to inhaled corticosteroids: a review. Am J Contact Dermatitis 6:1–3
461. Baeck M, Goossens A (2009). Patients with airborne sensitization/contact dermatitis from budesonide-containing aerosols "by proxy" Contact Dermatitis 6:1–8
462. Lepoittevin J-P, Drieghe J, Dooms-Goossens A (1995) Studies in patients with corticosteroid contact allergy. Understanding cross-reactivity among different steroids. Arch Dermatol 131:31–37
463. Goossens A, Matura M, Degreef H (2000) Reactions to corticosteroids: some new aspects regarding cross-sensitivity. Cutis 65:43–46
464. Isaksson M, Andersen KE, Brandão FM, Bruynzeel DP, Camarasa JG, Diepgen T, Ducombs G, Frosch PJ, Goossens A, Lahti A, Menné T, Rycroft RJG, Seidenari S, Shaw S, Tosti A, Wahlberg J, White IR, Wilkinson JD (2000) Patch testing with corticosteroid mixes in Europe. A multicentre study of The EECDRG. Contact Dermatitis 42:27–35
465. Wilkinson SM, Beck MH (1996) Corticosteroid hypersensitivity: what vehicle and concentration? Contact Dermatitis 34:305–308
466. Isaksson M, Beck MH, Wilkinson SM (2002) Comparative testing with budesonide in petrolatum and ethanol in a standard series. Contact Dermatitis 47:123–124
467. Isaksson M, Andersen KE, Brandão FM, Bruynzeel DP, Camarasa JG, Diepgen T, Ducombs G, Frosch PJ, Goossens A, Lahti A, Menné T, Rycroft RJG, Seidenari S, Shaw S, Tosti A, Wahlberg J, White IR, Wilkinson JD (2000) Patch testing with budesonide in serial dilutions. A multicentre study of the EECDRG. Contact Dermatitis 42:352–354
468. Andersen KE, Paulsen E (2009) Concordance of patch test results with four new TRUE test allergens compared with the same allergens from chemotechnique. Contact Dermatitis 60:59
469. Isaksson M, Brandão FM, Bruze M, Goossens A (2000) Recommendations to include budesonide and tixocortol pivalate in the European standard series. Contact Dermatitis: 43:41–42
470. Reynolds JEF (1993) Martindale, the extra pharmacopoeia, 30th edn. The Pharmaceutical Press, London, p 739
471. Boujnah-Khouadja A, Brandle I, Reuter G, Foussereau J (1984) Allergy to 2 new corticoid molecules. Contact Dermatitis 11:83–87
472. Dooms-Goossens A, Verschaeve H, Degreef H, Van Berendoncks J (1986) Contact allergy to hydrocortisone and tixocortol pivalate: problems with the detection of corticosteroid sensitivity. Contact Dermatitis 14:94–102
473. Lauerma AI (1991) Screening for corticosteroid contact sensitivity. Comparison of tixocortol pivalate, hydrocortisone-17-butyrate, and hydrocortisone. Contact Dermatitis 24:123–130
474. Burden AD, Beck MH (1992) Contact hypersensitivity to topical corticosteroids. Br J Dermatol 127:497–500
475. Lutz ME, el-Azhary RA, Gibson LE, Fransway AF (1998) Contact hypersensitivity to tixocortol pivalate. J Am Acad Dermatol 38:691–695
476. Bruze M, Gruvberger B, Agrup G (1988) Sensitization studies in the guinea pig with the active ingredients of Euxyl K 400. Contact Dermatitis 18:37–39
477. Hausen BM (1993) The sensitizing potency of Euxyl K 400 and its components 1, 2-dibromo-2, 4-dicyanobutane and 2-phenoxyethanol. Contact Dermatitis 28:149–153
478. de Groot AC, de Cock PA, Coenraads PJ et al (1996) Methyldibromoglutaronitrile is an important contact allergen in the Netherlands. Contact Dermatitis 34:118–120
479. van Ginkel CJ, Rundervoort GJ (1995) Increasing incidence of contact allergy to the new preservative 1, 2-dibromo-2, 4-dicyanobutane (methyldibromoglutaronitrile). Br J Dermatol 132:918–920
480. Tosti A, Vincenzi C, Trevisi P et al (1995) Euxyl K 400: incidence of sensitization, patch test concentration and vehicle. Contact Dermatitis 33:193–195
481. Vigan M, Brechat P (1996) Sensitization to Euxyl K400: a prospective study in 1217 patients. Eur J Dermatol 6: 175–177
482. Wilkinson JD, Shaw S, Andersen KE et al (2002) Monitoring levels of preservative sensitivity in Europe. A 10-year overview (1991–2000). Contact Dermatitis 46:207–210
483. Bruze M, Goossens A, Gruvberger B, ESCD; EECDRG (2005) Recommendation to include methyldibromo glutaronitrile in the European standard patch test series. Contact Dermatitis 52:24–28
484. Jong CT, Statham BN, Green CM et al (2007) Contact sensitivity to preservatives in the UK, 2004–2005: results of multicentre study. Contact Dermatitis 57:165–168
485. Johansen JD, Veien N, Laurberg G, Avnstorp C, Kaaber K, Andersen KE, Paulsen E, Sommerlund M, Thormann J, Nielsen NH, Vissing S, Kristensen O, Kristensen B, Agner T, Menné T (2008) Decreasing trends in methyldibromo glutaronitrile contact allergy–following regulatory intervention. Contact Dermatitis 59:48–51

31

486. Jensen CD, Johansen JD, Menne' T, Andersen KE (2004) Methyldibromoglutaronitrile in rinse-off products causes allergic contact dermatitis: an experimental study. Br J Dermatol 150:90–95

487. Jensen CD, Johansen JD, Menne' T, Andersen KE (2005) Methyldibromo glutaronitrile contact allergy: effect of single versus repeated daily exposure. Contact Dermatitis 52: 88–92

488. Schnuch A, Kelterer D, Bauer A, Schuster Ch, Aberer W, Mahler V, Katzer K, Rakoski J, Jappe U, Krautheim A, Bircher A, Koch P, Worm M, Löffler H, Hillen U, Frosch PJ, Uter W (2005) Quantitative patch and repeated open application testing in methyldibromo glutaronitrile-sensitive patients. Contact Dermatitis 52:197–206

489. English JS, Rycroft RJ (1989) Occupational sensitization to ethylenediamine in a floor polish remover. Contact Dermatitis 20:220–221

490. Chieregato C, Vincenzi C, Guerra L, Farina P (1994) Occupational allergic contact dermatitis due to ethylenediamine dihydrochloride and cresyl glycidyl ether in epoxy resin systems. Contact Dermatitis 30:120

491. Crow KD, Peachey RD, Adams JE (1978) Coolant oil dermatitis due to ethylenediamine. Contact Dermatitis 4: 359–361

492. Angelini G, Meneghini CL (1977) Dermatitis in engineers due to synthetic coolants. Contact Dermatitis 3:219–220

493. Dias M, Fernandes C, Pereira F, Pacheco A (1995) Occupational dermatitis from ethylenediamine. Contact Dermatitis 33:129–130

494. Dal Monte A, de Benedictis E, Laffi G (1987) Occupational dermatitis from ethylenediamine hydrochloride. Contact Dermatitis 17:254

495. Stingeni L, Caraffini S, Agostinelli D, Ricci F, Lisi P (1997) Maculopapular and urticarial eruption from cetirizine. Contact Dermatitis 37:249–250

496. Walker SL, Ferguson JE (2004) Systemic allergic contact dermatitis due to ethylenediamine following administration of oral aminophylline. Br J Dermatol 150:594

497. Ash S, Scheman AJ (1997) Systemic contact dermatitis to hydroxyzine. Am J Contact Dermat 8:2–5

498. Isaksson M, Ljunggren B (2003) Systemic contact dermatitis from ethylenediamine in an aminophylline preparation presenting as the baboon syndrome. Acta Derm Venereol 83(1):69–70

499. Price ML, Hall Smith SP (1984) Allergy to piperazine in a patient sensitive to ethylenediamine. Contact Dermatitis 10:120

500. de la Hoz B, Perez C, Tejedor MA, Lazaro M, Salazar F, Cuevas M (1993) Immediate adverse reaction to aminophylline [see comments]. Ann Allergy 71:452–454

Cosmetics and Skin Care Products[1]

32

Jonathan M.L. White, Anton C. de Groot, and Ian R. White

Contents

J.M.L. White (✉)
Department of Cutaneous Allergy, St John's Institute of
Dermatology, St Thomas' Hospital, London SE1 7EH, UK

A.C. de Groot
acdegroot publishing, Schipslootweg 5,
8351, HV Wapserveen, The Netherlands

I.R. White
Department of Cutaneous Allergy, St John's Institute of
Dermatology, St. Thomas' Hospital, London SE1 7EH, UK

32.1 What are Cosmetics?

In European legislation, a "cosmetic product" is any substance or preparation intended to be placed in contact with the various external parts of the human body (epidermis, hair system, nails, lips, and external genital organs) or with the teeth and the mucous membranes of the oral cavity with a view exclusively, or mainly, to cleaning them, perfuming them, changing their appearance, and/or correcting body odors, and/or protecting them, or keeping them in good condition (Cosmetics Directive 76/768/EEC; article 1) (http://eur-lex.europa.eu/LexUriServ/LexUriServ.do?uri=CONSLEG:1976L0768:20080424:EN:PDF).

The definition of a cosmetic includes the following:

Soap, shampoo, toothpaste, cleansing and moisturizing cream for regular care, color cosmetics (such as eye shadow, lipstick, nail varnish, hair colorant, and styling agents), fragrance products (such as deodorant, aftershave, and perfume), and ultraviolet light (UV light) screening preparations.

32.2 Epidemiology of Side Effects from Cosmetics

32.2.1 The General Population

Everyone uses cosmetics and, given the enormous volume of sales and the range of products available, there is remarkably little information available on the incidence of

---

[1]In this chapter, the nomenclature used is according to the International Nomenclature of Cosmetic Ingredients (INCI), as required for ingredient labeling in Europe.

J.D. Johansen et al. (eds.), *Contact Dermatitis*,
DOI: 10.1007/978-3-642-03827-3_32, © Springer-Verlag Berlin Heidelberg 2011

32

adverse reactions to them. Most individuals who experience an adverse reaction to a cosmetic have a mild reaction and simply change to another product. Only rarely is an adverse reaction reported to a manufacturer, unless discomfort is marked or significant. In Europe, the industry is required to record adverse reactions reported to it and make the register available to the appropriate "competent authority". Individuals are also unlikely to present to a dermatologist for evaluation, unless the adverse reaction is severe, as in the case of contact allergy to a hair dye, where it is persistent, or when the connection between the product and the eruption has not been made.

The cosmetic scientist has access to several thousand substances for incorporation into cosmetics. The European Commission publishes an indicative, but not exhaustive, list of general ingredients and fragrance substances, which used to be known as the Inventory but is now called "CosIng" [1]. Many of these ingredients have had a long and established use, and are recognized as being safe or having a favorable toxicological profile. Some substances, however, pose a significant risk of causing adverse reactions, and , little is known about the safety of these other substances. Regulatory aspects are discussed in Chap. 52.

In the general population, a questionnaire survey of 1,022 individuals in the United Kingdom found 85 people (8.3%) who claimed to have experienced an adverse reaction related to the use of a cosmetic [2]. Of these 85 individuals, 44 were patch tested and in 11 (1.1%), a significant reaction to a cosmetic ingredient was obtained. In The Netherlands, a survey of 982 individuals attending beauticians found 254 (26%) who claimed to have experienced an adverse reaction to a cosmetic [3]. Evaluation of 150 cases of this group by patch testing demonstrated ten individuals, 1% of the total, with an allergic reaction attributable to a cosmetic ingredient. These and other studies give an idea of the proportion of the population who may have experienced an allergic contact reaction to a cosmetic ingredient at some time. An estimated 1% is allergic to fragrances [4] and 2–3% are allergic to substances that may be present in cosmetics and toiletries [5].

32.2.2 Patients Seen by Dermatologists

Detailed information is available regarding the prevalence of contact allergy to some cosmetic ingredients among individuals who have been patch tested as an investigation for their dermatitis (of whatever type). The European baseline series of contact allergens includes the following substances that may be used in cosmetics: fragrance mix I, *Myroxylon pereirae* (balsam of Peru – not used as such in cosmetics, but included as an indicator of fragrance sensitivity), formaldehyde, quaternium-15, methylchloroisothiazolinone (and) methylisothiazolinone (MCI/MI), parabens, lanolin (wool alcohols), colophonium (colophony), and *p*-phenylenediamine. Many centers also routinely test with the preservatives methyldibromo glutaronitrile (no longer permitted in cosmetic products in Europe), imidazolidinyl urea, and diazolidinyl urea, and some include iodopropynyl butylcarbamate and others. A European study of the frequency of hypersensitivity to some of these agents in a patch-tested population totaling 20,791 individuals showed the incidence of reactions as listed in Table 32.1 [5]. Of dermatological patients patch tested for suspected allergic contact dermatitis, about 10% are allergic to cosmetic ingredients [5].

Women are more at risk of acquiring hypersensitivity to cosmetic ingredients than men, due to their greater product use. Variability in the frequency of reactions reported is partially attributable to different patient selection between centers. True temporal and geographical variations in the frequency of hypersensitivity to cosmetic ingredients occur because of differences in ingredient use. These differences involve marketing strategies, local product preference, and preferred ingredient usage by manufacturers. There may be some effect of ethnicity on contact allergy, perhaps due to targetted marketing of cosmetic items to different ethnic groups. Formaldehyde and formaldehyde-releasing preservative contact allergy

Table 32.1 Frequency of reactions (mean from all centers and range) to cosmetic ingredients in the baseline series ($n=20,791$) [5]

Substance	Mean (%)	Range (%)
Fragrance mix	7.0	6.4–9.4
Myroxylon pereirae (Balsam of Peru)	5.8	4.0–6.7
Colophonium (colophony)	3.4	1.7–4.7
p-Phenylenediamine	2.8	0.3–4.9
Lanolin (wool alcohols)	2.8	1.2–3.9
Formaldehyde	2.2	1.4–5.2
Parabens	1.1	0.5–2.6
Quaternium-15	0.9	0.3–2.2

[6] are reported to be lower in African–Americans than Whites and *p*-phenylenediamine contact allergy higher [6, 7]. Additionally, changes in legislation, recommendations on ingredient use, and availability are further important factors. Dillarstone [8] has pointed out the phasic nature of the prevalence of contact allergy to preservatives that results from these latter factors.

32.3 Clinical Picture

Sometimes, allergic contact dermatitis from cosmetic products can easily be recognized. Examples include reactions to deodorant, eye shadow, perfume dabbed behind the ears or on the wrist, and lipstick. In more than half of all cases, however, the diagnosis of cosmetic allergy is not clinically suspected [9]. This is particularly the case with preservative allergy.

The clinical picture of allergic cosmetic dermatitis depends on the type of products used (and, consequently, the sites of application), exposure, and the patient's sensitivity. Usually, a cosmetic contains only weak allergens or stronger ones present at low dilution, and the dermatitis resulting from cosmetic allergy is mild: erythema, minimal edema, desquamation, and papules. Weeping vesicular dermatitis rarely occurs, although some products, especially the permanent hair dyes, may cause fierce reactions, notably on the face, ears, and scalp. Allergic reactions on the scalp may be seborrhoeic dermatitis-like with (temporary) hair loss.

Contact allergy to fragrances may resemble an endogenous eczema [10]. Lesions in the skin folds may be mistaken for atopic dermatitis. Dermatitis due to perfumes or toilet water may be "streaky." Allergy to tosylamide/formaldehyde resin in nail polish may affect the fingers [11], but most allergic reactions are located on the eyelids, in and behind the ears, on the neck (resembling seborrhoeic dermatitis), and sometimes around the anus or vulva. Eczema of the lips and the perioral region (cheilitis) [12] may be caused by toothpastes [13], notably from the flavors contained therein [14], and also from lipsticks and lip balms.

The face itself is frequently involved, and often the dermatitis is limited to the face and/or eyelids. Other sites of predilection for cosmetic dermatitis are the neck, arms, and hands. However, all parts of the body may be involved. Most often, the cosmetics have been applied to previously healthy skin (especially the face), nails, or hair. However, allergic cosmetic dermatitis may be caused by products used on previously damaged skin, for example, to treat or prevent dry skin of the arms and legs or irritant or atopic hand dermatitis.

32.4 The Products Causing Cosmetic Allergy

Most allergic reactions are caused by those cosmetics that remain on the skin: "stay-on" or "leave-on" products such as skin care products (moisturizing and cleansing creams, lotions, milks, tonics), hair cosmetics (notably hair dyes), nail cosmetics (nail varnish), deodorants and other perfumes, and facial and eye make-up products [15–17]. "Rinse-off" or "wash-off" products, such as soap, shampoo, bath foam, and shower foam, less commonly induce or elicit contact allergic reactions. This is explained by the dilution of the product (and, consequently, of the [potential] allergen) under normal circumstances of use, and because the product is removed from the skin by rinsing after a short period. An exception to this general rule was allergy to a fraction in some commercial grades of the surfactant cocamidopropyl betaine, which caused reactions to shampoo in consumers and occupational dermatitis in hairdressers, and to shower gels [18–20].

Trends in cosmetic usage, e.g., the expansion of the cosmetic market for men and the targeting of products specifically for children, may influence the situation.

32.5 The Allergens

Although there are numerous publications on contact allergy to the ingredients of cosmetics, the systematic investigation of the allergens in such products has been rare [9, 17]. Fragrances and preservatives are the most common causative ingredients in allergic cosmetic dermatitis. Other important allergens are the hair color *p*-phenylenediamine (and related permanent dyes), the nail varnish resin tosylamide/formaldehyde resin [21], and uncommonly to UV filters, lanolin, and other substances.

32.5.1 Fragrances

Adverse reactions to fragrances in perfumes and in fragranced cosmetic products include allergic contact dermatitis, irritant contact dermatitis, photosensitivity, immediate contact reactions (contact urticaria), and pigmented contact dermatitis [22]. Reviews of the adverse effects of fragrances (and essential oils) are available [16, 23]. The history of fragrances has been well described [24, 25].

Considering the enormous use of fragrances, the frequency of contact allergy to them is relatively small. In absolute numbers, however, fragrance allergy is common. In a group of 90 student nurses, 12 (13%) were shown to be fragrance allergic [26]. In a group of 567 unselected individuals aged 15–69 years, 6 (1.1%) were shown to be allergic to fragrances, as evidenced by a positive patch test reaction to fragrance mix I [4]. In a large normal population from Thailand, 2.5% of the study group tested positive to fragrance mix I [27]. In dermatitis patients seen by dermatologists, the prevalence of contact allergy to fragrances is between 6 and 14% [28]; only nickel allergy occurs more frequently. When tested with ten popular perfumes, 6.9% of female eczema patients proved to be allergic to them [29] and 3.2–4.2% were allergic to fragrances from perfumes present in various cosmetic products [30].

When patients with suspected allergic cosmetic dermatitis are investigated, fragrances are identified as the most frequent allergens, not only in perfumes, aftershaves and deodorants, but also in other cosmetic products not primarily used for their smell [21, 31]. Occupational contact with fragrances is rarely significant [16]. Fragrance allergy appears to increase with age [32].

Contact allergy to fragrances usually causes dermatitis of the hands, face, and/or axillae. Patients appear to become sensitized to fragrances, particularly from the use of deodorant sprays and/or perfumes, and to a lesser degree, from cleansing agents, deodorant sticks, or hand lotions [33]. Thereafter, eczema may appear or be worsened by contact with other fragranced products: cosmetics, toiletries, household products, industrial contacts, and flavorings in food and drinks.

Over 100 fragrance chemicals have been identified as allergens [16]. Most reactions have been identified as the substances in the fragrance mix I, and of these,

Evernia prunastri (oak moss), isoeugenol, and cinnamal are the main sensitizers. Most recently, hydroxyisohexyl 3-cyclohexene carboxaldehyde (Lyral®) has been identified as an important fragrance allergen [34]. An exhaustive review of fragrance allergens is available [35] and was the tool used by the European Commission in evaluating the need for the introduction of fragrance ingredient labeling.

Contact allergy to a particular product or chemical is established by means of patch testing. A perfume may contain as many as 200 or more individual ingredients. This makes the diagnosis of perfume allergy by patch test procedures complicated. Fragrance mix I (sometimes known as the perfume mix) was introduced as a screening tool for fragrance sensitivity in the late 1970s [36]. It contains eight commonly used fragrance substances: amyl cinnamal, cinnamyl alcohol, cinnamal, *Evernia prunastri* (oak moss), eugenol, geraniol, hydroxycitronellal and isoeugenol.

Between 6 and 14% [28] of patients routinely tested for suspected allergic contact dermatitis react to it. It has been estimated that this mix detects 70–80% of all cases of fragrance sensitivity; this may be an overestimation, as it was positive in only 57% of patients who were allergic to popular commercial fragrances [29]. Testing with the components of the mix is required when a positive reaction to the mix is found. Occasionally, a component of the mix may be positive when tested individually, but not when tested in the mix itself.

Although Fragrance mix I remains an extremely important tool for the detection of cases of contact allergy to fragrances, it is far from ideal: it misses 20–30% of relevant reactions or more, and may cause both false-positive (i.e., a "positive" patch test reaction in a non-fragrance allergic individual) and false-negative reactions (i.e., no patch test reaction in an individual who is actually allergic to one or more of the ingredients of the mix). The routine testing with hydroxyisohexyl 3-cyclohexene carboxaldehyde (Lyral®) and Fragrance mix II (now in the European baseline series) developed by Frosch et al [37] improves the rate of detection.

In addition to patch testing, another useful test in cases of doubt (for example, with weakly positive patch test reactions, which are difficult to interpret) is the repeated open application test (ROAT; see below).

The finding of a positive reaction to the fragrance mix should be followed by a search for its relevance, i.e., is fragrance allergy the cause of the patient's current or previous complaints, or does it at least contribute to it? Between 50 and 65% of all positive patch test reactions to the mix are relevant. There is a highly significant association between the occurrence of self-reported visible skin symptoms to scented products earlier in life and a positive patch test to the fragrance mix, and most fragrance-sensitive patients are aware that the use of scented products may cause skin problems [38].

For Fragrance mix I or II-positive patients with concomitant positive reactions to perfumes or scented products, interpretation of the reaction as relevant is highly likely. For such patients, the incriminated cosmetics very often contain fragrances present in the mix and, thus, the fragrance mix appears to be a good reflection of actual exposure [39]. Indeed, one or more of the ingredients of the mix are present in nearly all deodorants [40], popular prestige perfumes [29], perfumes used in the formulation of other cosmetic products [30], and natural-ingredient-based cosmetics [41], often at levels high enough to cause allergic reactions [42, 43]. Thus, fragrance allergens are ubiquitous and virtually impossible to avoid if perfumed cosmetics are used.

Correlation with the clinical picture is occasionally lacking; some patients can tolerate perfumes and fragranced products without problems [16] despite a seemingly positive patch test to the mix. This may sometimes be explained by irritant (false-positive) patch test reactions. Alternative explanations include the absence of relevant allergens in those products or a concentration in the product too low to elicit clinically visible allergic contact reactions.

Determination of relevance has now been made easier by ingredients listing of well-recognized fragrance allergens when present at 10 ppm or more in leave-on cosmetic products and at 100 ppm or more in rinse-off products: amyl cinnamal, cinnamyl alcohol, cinnamal, *Evernia prunastri* (oak moss), *Evernia furfuracea* (tree moss), eugenol, geraniol, hydroxycitronellal, isoeugenol, alpha-isomethyl ionone, amylcinnamyl alcohol, anisyl alcohol, benzyl alcohol, benzyl benzoate, benzyl cinnamate, benzyl salicylate, citral, citronellol, coumarin, d-limonene, farnesol, hexyl cinnamal, hydroxyisohexyl 3-cyclohexene carboxaldehyde, butylphenyl methylpropional, linalool, methyl heptine carbonate

The fragrance chemicals that must be labeled are under review.

32.5.2 Preservatives

Preservatives are added to water-containing cosmetics to inhibit the growth of nonpathogenic and pathogenic microorganisms, which may cause degradation of the product or be harmful to the consumer. After fragrances, they are the most frequent cause of allergic cosmetic dermatitis. Important review articles on the earlier aspects of preservative allergy have been published [44–46]. A review on various aspects of preservatives in cosmetics including legislation, usage, infections, and contact allergy was recently published [47]. It should be appreciated that though the use of diazolidinyl urea and imidazolidinyl urea is largely restricted to cosmetics, the preservatives discussed here are also applied to numerous noncosmetic products and processes.

32.5.2.1 Methylchloroisothiazolinone (and) Methylisothiazolinone

Methylchloroisothiazolinone (and) methylisothiazolinone (MCI/MI) is a preservative system containing, as active ingredients, a mixture of methylchloroisothiazolinone and methylisothiazolinone. The most widely used commercial product contains 1.5% active ingredients; the methylchloroisothiazolinone moiety is the prime allergenic fraction. This highly effective preservative remains an important cosmetic allergen in most European countries. Allergic reactions on the face to cosmetics preserved with MCI/MI can have unusual clinical presentations that are very similar to seborrheic dermatitis and other dermatoses [48]. MCI/MI is tested at 100 ppm in water in the European standard series, although testing at 200 ppm may detect more cases of sensitization [49]. Currently, MCI/ MI is primarily used in rinse-off cosmetic products at low concentrations between 3 and 15 ppm, which infrequently leads to the induction or elicitation of contact allergy [50]. As a consequence, prevalence rates in Europe are static but are still between 2 and 2.5% of patch tested individuals [51–55], which is comparable to USA levels [56]. Methylisothiazolinone itself is now permitted as a cosmetic preservative; it is, however, a much weaker allergen than methylchloroisothiazoline.

32

32.5.2.2 Methyldibromo Glutaronitrile

Methyldibromo glutaronitrile (synonym: 1,2-dibromo-2,4-dicyanobutane) is a preservative that has been widely used in cosmetics and toiletries. It was thought to be a suitable alternative to the MCI/MI, but, unfortunately, soon proved to be a frequent cause of contact allergy to cosmetics [57]. Prevalence rates of sensitization in patients routinely investigated for suspected allergic contact dermatitis rose from 0.7% in 1990 to 3.5% in 2000 in 16 centers in Europe [55] and were 11.7% in the United States [58]. In a recent NACDG study, the frequency of sensitization was 5.8% (tested as methyldibromo glutaronitrile/phenoxyethanol 2.5% pet) [56]. Between 23 and 75% of positive patch test reactions were considered to be relevant.

There is some controversy as to the optimal patch test concentration. A 0.3% preparation is often used, but clinically relevant reactions may be missed [59] and 0.5% may be preferable [60].

In Europe, the use of methyldibromo glutaronitrile since 2004 was only permitted in rinse-off products at a maximum concentration of 0.1%. However, following accumulated evidence of the role of rinse-off products in contact allergy to methyldibromo glutaronitrile, in 2007 its use was prohibited in these products also. This regulatory intervention resulted in a significantly decreasing trend in the frequency of positive patch tests to methyldibromo glutaronitrile in Denmark (4.6% in 2003, 2.6% in 2007) *and* in the percentages of current relevant reactions [61]. Increasing awareness of the problem probably led cosmetic manufacturers to use the preservative less commonly, as frequencies of sensitization even before regulatory restrictions tended to decrease [51].

32.5.2.3 Formaldehyde

Formaldehyde is a frequent and potent sensitizer and ubiquitous allergen, with numerous noncosmetic sources of contact. Because of this, the cosmetic industry uses small but effective concentrations, and its use is restricted almost exclusively to rinse-off products. In recent years, it has largely been replaced by other preservatives such as MCI/MI and the formaldehyde-releasers. Currently, the frequency of sensitization to formaldehyde remains at a stable and relatively low level of around 2–3% in most (European) countries in the general patch test population. In the USA, however, rates of 8–9% are the rule rather than the exception [56, 62] The literature on formaldehyde allergy has been reviewed [62].

32.5.2.4 Formaldehyde Donors

Formaldehyde donors are preservatives that, in the presence of water, release formaldehyde. Therefore, cosmetics preserved with such chemicals will contain free formaldehyde; the amount depending on the preservative used, its concentration, the pH of the product, its age, and the other ingredients of the cosmetic [63]. The antimicrobial effects of formaldehyde donors are probably related to formaldehyde release for the most part, but may also be intrinsic properties of the parent molecules. Formaldehyde donors used in cosmetics and toiletries include quaternium-15, imidazolidinyl urea, diazolidinyl urea, 2-bromo-2-nitropropane-1,3-diol, and DMDM hydantoin. Quaternium-15 releases the largest amounts of formaldehyde, followed by diazolidinyl urea, DMDM hydantoin, and imidazolidinyl urea. 2-Bromo-2-nitropropane-1,3-diol releases little formaldehyde [63]. Contact allergy to formaldehyde donors may be due either to the preservative itself or to formaldehyde sensitivity [45, 46]. There is a clear relationship between positive patch test reactions to formaldehyde-releasers and formaldehyde contact allergy: 15% of all reactions to 2-bromo-2-nitropropane-1,3-diol and 40–60% of the reactions to the other releasers are caused by a reaction to the formaldehyde in the test material. There is only fragmented data on the amount of free formaldehyde in cosmetics preserved with formaldehyde donors. However, all releasers (with the exception of 2-bromo-2-nitropropane-1,3-diol, for which adequate data are lacking) can – in the right circumstances of concentration and product composition – release >200 ppm formaldehyde, which may result in allergic contact dermatitis. Whether this is actually the case in any particular product cannot be decided solely on the basis of ingredient labeling. Thus, patients allergic to formaldehyde should avoid stay-on cosmetics preserved with quaternium-15, diazolidinyl urea, DMDM hydantoin, or imidazolidinyl urea [63]. Approximately, one in every five cosmetic products contains a formaldehyde-releasers, both in the USA and in Europe [64]. The literature on formaldehyde-releasers in cosmetics has been recently reviewed [63, 65].

32.5.3 Quaternium-15

There are major differences in the frequencies of sensitization to quaternium-15 between the USA and Europe. In the studies from the USA, frequencies of sensitization have ranged from 7.1 to 9.6% (mean 8.8%) [65–67]. In the European studies, prevalences were consistently lower, ranging from 0.6 to 1.9% (mean 1.1%) [52–54, 65]. This may partly be explained by the use of a 2% patch test substance in the USA vs. 1% in Europe. Also, about half of all reactions to quaternium-15 are due to concomitant formaldehyde allergy, which is much more frequent in the USA. Relevance was established or considered to be "probable" in 29–90% of the positive patch test reactions [65].

32.5.4 Imidazolidinyl Urea

In the USA, frequencies of sensitization to the preservative have ranged from 1.3 to 3.3% (mean 2.7%). Frequencies of sensitization in Europe were consistently lower and ranged from 0.3 to 1.4% (mean 0.7%) [65]. Relevance was established or considered to be "probable" in 21–90% of the positive patch test reactions [65]. Cross-reactions to and from the structurally related diazolidinyl urea may be observed [65]. The chemistry of imidazolidinyl urea has been reviewed [68].

32.5.5 Diazolidinyl Urea

Diazolidinyl urea is the most active member of the imidazolidinyl urea group, and case reports of cosmetic allergy from diazolidinyl urea have been published since 1988 [69]. Routine testing in the USA has revealed frequencies of sensitization ranging from 2.4 to 3.7% (mean 3.1%) [65–67]. In the few studies performed in European countries, prevalences were consistently lower, ranging from 0.5 to 1.4% (mean 1%) [65]. Relevance was established or considered to be "probable" in 24–75% of the positive patch test reactions [65]. Cross-reactions to and from imidazolidinyl urea occur [69]. Diazolidinyl urea appears to be a stronger sensitizer than imidazolidinyl urea. The chemistry of diazolinyl urea has been reviewed [68].

32.5.6 2-Bromo-2-Nitropropane-1,3-Diol (Bronopol)

In the USA, frequencies of sensitization to this formaldehyde-releaser have ranged from 2.1 to 3.3% (mean 2.8%) [65–67]. In studies performed in European countries, prevalence rates were consistently lower, ranging from 0.4 to 1.2% (mean 0.9%) [65]. Relevance was established or considered to be "probable" in 7–80% of the positive patients [65]. Because interaction with amines and amides can result in the formation of nitrosamines or nitrosamides, suspected carcinogens, there is restriction in the formulations that may contain this preservative.

32.5.7 DMDM Hydantoin

In the United States, frequencies of sensitization to this preservative have ranged from 0.5 to 3.4%, but were usually in the 1.3–2.5% range (mean 2%). Relevance was established or considered to be "probable" in 15–86% of the positive patch test reactions [65–67]. In Europe, no routine testing has been performed with DMDM hydantoin recently.

32.5.7.1 Parabens

The paraben esters (methyl, ethyl, propyl, butyl) are widely used preservatives in cosmetic products. Parabens have had an unwarranted reputation as sensitizers. However, most cases of paraben sensitivity are caused by topical medicaments applied to leg ulcers or stasis dermatitis. Routine testing in the European standard series yields low prevalence rates of sensitization between 0.5 and 1.2% [52–55] and 1.2% in the USA [56]. At the usual concentration of 0.1–0.3% in cosmetics, parabens rarely cause adverse reactions. The parabens have been reviewed [70].

32.5.7.2 Iodopropynyl Butylcarbamate

This preservative was popular in many skin care and hair care products, and contact allergy to it from cosmetic use has been reported [71, 72]. The recommended patch test concentration, based on an analysis of concurrent testing with several dilutions, is 0.2%, though 0.1% is also used [56]. The current frequency of sensitization in the USA is 0.5% [56]. Because of concerns about the bioavailability of iodine, there has been considerable reduction in the use of iodopropynyl butylcarbamate in cosmetics.

32.5.7.3 Miscellaneous Preservatives

Preservatives used in cosmetics that have occasionally caused allergy include benzyl alcohol [73], chloroacetamide, chloroxylenol [74], chlorphenesin [75], phenoxyethanol, and triclosan [76, 77].

32.5.8 Tosylamide/Formaldehyde Resin

Contact allergy to the main allergen in nail varnish, tosylamide/formaldehyde resin, is common [11, 78–82]. Up to 6.6% of women habitually or occasionally using nail cosmetics and presenting with dermatitis are allergic to it [78], and the prevalence in patients routinely tested in the United States was 1.6% [28]. Eighty percent of all reactions are observed as a dermatitis of the face and neck, with many cases manifesting as an eyelid dermatitis. Occasionally, other parts of the body are involved, including the thighs, the genitals, and the trunk; generalized dermatitis is rare. Periungual dermatitis may be far more common (60%) than previously thought [11]. Desquamative gingivitis was the sole manifestation in a compulsive nail-biter [83]. Partner ("connubial") dermatitis has been observed. Other, but rarely reported, allergens in nail lacquers include formaldehyde, nitrocellulose [84], polyester resin, phthalates, and o-toluenesulfonamide [79, 80].

Important sociomedical consequences of nail varnish allergy have been reported [11]. Allergic patients should stop using nail varnishes or use varnishes free from tosylamide/formaldehyde resin. However, some products claiming not to contain the resin may still do so [85]. Also, such nail varnishes may contain other sensitizers, such as methyl acrylate and epoxy resin [86]. Useful review articles on adverse reactions to nail cosmetics [87, 88] and sculptured nails [89] are available.

32.5.9 p-Phenylenediamine and Related Hair Dyes

p-Phenylenediamine and related hair dyes are very common and important sensitizers. Safer permanent dyes with a lower risk of contact allergy, but with the same technical qualities, are not yet available. Many cases of sensitization were reported in the 1930s, and sensitization was considered so great a hazard that the use of p-phenylenediamine in hair dyes was prohibited in several countries. Currently, its incorporation in cosmetic products is allowed in the European Union up to a maximum concentration of 4% (as free base; until 2009 it was 6%)), which equates, after mixing with the oxidizing agent, to 2%, the maximum level to which the consumer is now exposed.

p-Phenylenediamine remains an important cause of cosmetic allergy, with a 6.8% prevalence rate of sensitization in routinely tested patients in the United States [28]. The incidence of p-phenylenediamine allergy is increasing [90]. In normal (nonpatch test) populations, the incidence of sensitization is reported as 2.7% [27]. The clinical features of hair dye allergy are discussed in Chap. 34.

These oxidation dyes are also an occupational hazard for hairdressers and beauticians [91]. The chemistry of, and adverse reactions to, oxidation coloring agents have been reviewed [92]. Semipermanent and temporary dyes rarely cause allergic cosmetic dermatitis.

32.5.10 Cocamidopropyl Betaine

Cocamidopropyl betaine is an amphoteric surfactant, which is widely present in shampoos and bath products, such as bath and shower gels [18–20]. Residues in some commercial grades, dimethylaminopropylamine [93] and cocamidopropyl dimethylamine [94], were responsible for prevalence rates of sensitization to cocamidopropyl betaine in a range from 3.7 to 5% [93, 95, 96]. Due to its presence in shampoos, cocamidopropyl betaine was an important occupational hazard to hairdressers. Consumers became sensitized to shampoos and a variety of other hygiene products, such as liquid shower soaps and facial cleansers [93]. Since the allergenic fractions were removed, the problem has disappeared; however, there are reports of high rates of sensitization in patch test populations in China [97].

32.5.11 UV Filters

Ultraviolet light filters (UV filters) are used in sunscreens to protect the consumer from harmful UV irradiation from the sun and are also incorporated in some cosmetics, notably facial skin care products, to inhibit UV photo-degradation of the product and protect the skin of the user. The main classes of sunscreens are PABA and its esters (amyl dimethyl, glyceryl, octyl dimethyl), cinnamates, salicylates, anthranilates, benzophenones, and dibenzoyl-methanes [98]. The latter have become very popular, since they absorb mainly the UVA range (315–400 nm).

The most frequent adverse reaction to sunscreen preparations is irritation, which occurs in over 15% of users [99]. UV filters have also been identified as allergens and photoallergens, but such reactions are uncommon. Patients who regularly use sunscreens because they suffer from chronic actinic dermatitis may have an increased risk for developing allergic side effects to sunscreens [100]. (Photo)allergic reactions can easily be overlooked, as the resulting dermatitis may be interpreted by the patient or consumer as a failure of the product to protect against sunburn or as worsening of the (photo)dermatosis for which the sunscreen was used.

Currently, the most frequent cause of (photo)contact allergy to UV filters is benzophenone-3 (oxybenzone) [101]. Cross-reactions between benzophenones appear to be rare [102]. Some UV filters are reported to have caused (photo)contact allergy [15, 98, 102–105] and these are discussed further in Chap. 29.

32.5.12 Lanolin and Derivatives

Lanolin and lanolin derivatives are used extensively in cosmetic products as emollients and emulsifiers. However, the majority of individuals have been sensitized by using topical pharmaceutical preparations containing lanolin, especially for treating varicose ulcers and stasis dermatitis (a similar situation to that of parabens) [106].

Additionally, many "positive" patch test reactions are not reproducible [107]. Thus, it appears that the currently used test allergen (30% wool wax alcohols) may cause false-positive, irritant, patch test reactions [107, 108]. Possibly, the same applies to the lanolin derivative Amerchol® L-101, which is often used in addition to patch testing [109].

The presence of lanolin or its derivatives in cosmetics may cause cosmetic dermatitis in lanolin-sensitive individuals, but the risk of sensitization from using such products is small [110]. In the general population, contact allergy to lanolin is considered to be rare [107, 108]. Its prevalence in North America seems to be decreasing [111].

32.5.13 Glyceryl Thioglycolate

Glyceryl thioglycolate, a waving agent used in acid permanent waving products, occasionally sensitizes consumers [112], but it is usually an occupational hazard for the hairdresser [91]. Patients allergic to glyceryl thioglycolate infrequently react to ammonium thioglycolate, also a contact allergen, used in "hot" permanent wave procedures.

32.5.14 Propylene Glycol

Propylene glycol is widely used in dermatologic and nondermatologic topical formulations, including cosmetics, as well as in numerous other products, including food [113–115]. Propylene glycol may cause irritant contact dermatitis, allergic contact dermatitis, nonimmunologic immediate contact reactions, and subjective or sensory irritation [113].

Allergic contact dermatitis is uncommon and its clinical significance has been overestimated. In earlier studies, higher concentrations of propylene glycol may have induced many irritant patch test reactions. Currently, a concentration of 1–10% [115] is advised in order to avoid such irritation, but cases of contact allergy are probably missed as a result (false-negative reactions). A diagnosis of allergic contact dermatitis should never be made on the basis of one positive patch test alone. Testing should be repeated after several weeks. In addition, repeat tests with serial dilutions down to 1% propylene glycol helps in discriminating between irritant responses and true allergic ones. ROATs and/or provocative use tests (PUT) can be conducted to verify the allergic basis of a positive patch test result.

32

32.5.15 Antioxidants

Antioxidants are added to cosmetics to prevent the deterioration of unsaturated fatty acids and are an occasional cause of cosmetic allergy [9, 17], though the actual prevalence may be underestimated [116]. Antioxidants that have caused cosmetic allergy include BHA (butylated hydroxyanisole) [116], BHT (butylated hydroxytoluene) [116], *t*-butylhydroquinone [116, 117], gallates (dodecyl, octyl, propyl) [118], tocopherol (vitamin E), and its esters [119, 120].

32.5.16 Miscellaneous Allergens

Examples of other, infrequent causes of cosmetic allergy include oleamidopropyl dimethylamine [121], cetearyl alcohol [122], maleated soya bean oil [123], dicapryl maleate [124], diisostearyl malate [125], triethanolamine, and methyl glucose dioleate, castor oil [126], ricinoleates [127], polyvinylpyrrolidone (PVP) eicosene copolymer [128], PVP triacontene copolymer [129], polyoxyethylene lauryl ether [130], tetrahydroxypropyl ethylenediamine, 1,3-butylene glycol [131], shellac [132], phthalic anhydride/trimellitic anhydride/glycols copolymer [133], colophonium [134], propolis [135], colors [136], and botanicals [137].

The depigmenting agent kojic acid is reported as an allergen in Japan [138].

A comprehensive literature survey on cosmetic allergy has been published [15, 139].

32.6 Diagnostic Procedures

The diagnosis of cosmetic allergy should be strongly suspected in any patient presenting with dermatitis of the face, eyelids, lips, and neck [15, 140]. Cosmetic allergic dermatitis may develop on previously healthy skin of the face or on already damaged skin (irritant contact dermatitis, atopic dermatitis, seborrhoeic dermatitis, allergic contact dermatitis from other sources). Also, dermatitis of the arms and hands may be caused or worsened by skin care products used to treat or prevent dry skin, irritant, or atopic dermatitis. Patchy dermatitis on the neck and around the eyes is suggestive of cosmetic allergy from nail varnish or hardeners. More widespread problems

may be caused by ingredients in products intended for general application to the body. Hypersensitivity to other products, such as deodorants, usually causes a reaction localized to the site of application. A thorough history of cosmetic usage should always be obtained.

When the diagnosis of cosmetic allergy is suspected, patch tests should be performed to confirm the diagnosis and identify the sensitizer. Only in this way can the patient be counseled about their future use of cosmetic (and other) products, and the prevention of recurrence of dermatitis from cosmetic or noncosmetic sources. Patch tests should be performed with the European (or other national) baseline series, a "cosmetics series" containing established cosmetic allergens, and the products used by the patient.

The European baseline series contains a number of cosmetic allergens and "indicator" allergens including colophonium, *Myroxylon pereirae* (balsam of Peru), fragrance mixes I and II, formaldehyde, quaternium-15, methylchloroisothiazolinone (and) methylisothiazolinone, lanolin, and *p*-phenylenediamine.

Although the patient's products should always be tested (for test concentrations, see Chap. 57), patch testing with cosmetics has problems. Both false-negative and false-positive reactions occur frequently. False-negative reactions are due to the low concentration of some allergens and the usually weak sensitivity of the patient. Classic examples of false-negative reactions have occurred with methylchloroisothiazolinone (and) methylisothiazolinone [141, 142] and parabens sensitivity. False-positive reactions may occur with any cosmetic product, but especially with products containing detergents or surfactants, such as shampoos, soaps, and bath and shower products. As a consequence, these products must be diluted (1% in water) before testing. Even then, mild irritant reactions are observed frequently, and of course, the (necessary) dilution of these products may result in false-negative results in patients actually allergic to them. Testing such products is, therefore, highly unreliable.

In many cases, testing with the European baseline series, suspected products, and a cosmetics screening series will establish the diagnosis of cosmetic allergy and identify one or more contact allergens. The label on the incriminated product will indicate whether or not the product actually contains the allergen(s). If not, the possibility of a false-positive reaction to the product should be suspected. The test should be repeated and/or control tests on nonexposed individuals should be performed. If an allergy is confirmed, an ingredient not included in the European series or the cosmetics screening series may be responsible. In such cases, the manufacturer should be asked for samples of the ingredients, and these can be tested on the patient after proper dilution [143].

In certain cases, an allergy to cosmetics is strongly suspected, but patch testing remains negative. In such patients, ROAT and/or usage tests can be performed. In the ROAT, the product is applied twice daily for a maximum of 14 days to the same area of skin over the antecubital fossa. A negative reaction after 2 weeks indicates that sensitivity is highly unlikely and cautious application to the implicated area may be attempted. This procedure should be performed with all suspected products, except detergent-containing cosmetics, such as soap, shampoo, and shower products.

During the usage test, the use of all cosmetic products is stopped until the dermatitis has disappeared. The cosmetics are then reintroduced as normally used, one at a time, with an interval of 3 days for each product, until a reaction develops. Photopatch testing should be performed whenever photoallergic cosmetic dermatitis is suspected. When all tests remain negative, the possibility of seborrheic dermatitis (scalp, eyelids, face, axillae, trunk), atopic dermatitis (all locations), irritant contact dermatitis (also from cosmetic products), and allergic contact dermatitis from other sources should be considered.

32.7 Ingredient Labeling in the European Union

Cosmetic ingredient labeling (introduced voluntarily in the United States in the 1970s) was a constant demand of European dermatologists for years. On 1 January 1997, the sixth Amendment to the Cosmetics Directive (76/768/EEC) in Europe became effective. This directive requires all cosmetic products marketed in the European Union to display their ingredients on the outer package or, in certain cases, in an accompanying leaflet, label, tape, or tag. The primary purpose of ingredient labeling is to allow dermatologists to identify specific ingredients that cause allergic responses in their patients, and to enable such patients to avoid cosmetic products containing the substances to which they are allergic.

The mandatory nomenclature used throughout the European Union for labeling is the International Nomenclature of Cosmetic Ingredients (INCI), based on the American Cosmetic, Toiletry, and Fragrance Association (CTFA) system. Most CTFA terms have been retained unchanged. However, all colorants are listed as color index (CI) numbers, except hair dyes, which have INCI names. Plant ingredients are declared as genus/species names using the Linnaean system. The source of information on ingredients is the European Inventory [1] published by the European Commission. Provided are the INCI names (in alphabetical order), CAS number, EINECS/ELINCS numbers, chemical/IUPAC names, and functions.

Patients allergic to certain ingredients of cosmetics must be supplied with the INCI names of their allergens; otherwise, they may fruitlessly seek for well-known names such as Kathon® CG, oxybenzone, balsam of Peru, Amerchol® L-101, dibromodicyanobutane, or orange oil.

Dermatologists must be familiar with the INCI nomenclature. However, the relevant names are sometimes difficult to find, but a list of substances that can be present in cosmetics and have been described as allergens has been generated and their names [CTFA, Merck Index, names provided by the producers of commercially available allergens (e.g., Chemotechnique, Trolab), "common names," and commonly used trade names] compared with those of the INCI [144].

References

1. The European Commission's Inventory of Ingredients http://ec.europa.eu/enterprise/cosmetics/cosing/
2. Consumers' Association (1979) Reactions of the skin to cosmetics and toiletry products. Consumers' Association, London
3. de Groot AC, Beverdam EG, Ayong CT, Coenraads PJ, Nater JP (1988) The role of contact allergy in the spectrum of adverse effects caused by cosmetics and toiletries. Contact Derm 19:195–201
4. Nielsen NH, Menné T (1992) Allergic contact sensitization in an unselected Danish population. Acta Derm Venereol (Stockh) 72:456–460
5. de Groot AC (1990) Labelling cosmetics with their ingredients. Br Med J 300:1636–1638
6. De Leo VA, Taylor SC, Belsito DV, Fowler JF, Fransway AF, Maibach HI, Marks JG, Mathias CGT, Nethercott JR, Pratt MD, Reitschel RR, Sherertz EF, Storrs FJ, Taylor JS (2002) The effect of race and ethnicity on patch test results. J Am Acad Dermatol 46:S107–S112

7. Dickel H, Taylor JS, Evey P, Merk HF (2001) Comparison of patch test results with a standard series among white and black racial groups. Am J Contact Dermat 12:77–82

8. Dillarstone A (1997) Letter to the editor. Contact Derm 37:190

9. Adams RM, Maibach HI (1985) A five-year study of cosmetic reactions. J Am Acad Dermatol 13:1062–1069

10. Meynadier J-M, Raison-Peyron N, Meunier L, Meynadier J (1997) Allergie aux parfums. Rev Fr Allergol 37:641–650

11. Lidén C, Berg M, Färm G, Wrangsjö K (1993) Nail varnish allergy with far-reaching consequences. Br J Dermatol 128:57–62

12. Ophaswongse S, Maibach HI (1995) Allergic contact cheilitis. Contact Derm 33:365–370

13. Sainio EL, Kanerva L (1995) Contact allergens in toothpastes and a review of their hypersensitivity. Contact Derm 33:100–105

14. Skrebova N, Brocks K, Karlsmark T (1998) Allergic contact cheilitis from spearmint oil. Contact Derm 39:35

15. de Groot AC, Weyland JW, Nater JP (1994) Unwanted effects of cosmetics and drugs used in dermatology, 3rd edn. Elsevier, Amsterdam

16. de Groot AC, Frosch PJ (1997) Adverse reactions to fragrances. A clinical review. Contact Derm 36:57–86

17. de Groot AC, Bruynzeel DP, Bos JD, van der Meeren HLM, van Joost T, Jagtman BA, Weyland JW (1988) The allergens in cosmetics. Arch Dermatol 124:1525–1529

18. de Groot AC (1997) Cocamidopropyl betaine: a "new" important cosmetic allergen. Dermatosen 45:60–63

19. de Groot AC, van der Walle HB, Weyland JW (1995) Contact allergy to cocamidopropyl betaine. Contact Derm 33:419–422

20. de Groot AC (1997) Contact allergens – what's new? Cosmetic dermatitis. Clin Dermatol 15:485–492

21. Berne B, Boström Å, Grahnén AF, Tammela M (1996) Adverse effects of cosmetics and toiletries reported to the Swedish Medical Product Agency 1989–1994. Contact Derm 34:359–362

22. de Groot AC, Frosch PJ (1998) Fragrances as a cause of contact dermatitis in cosmetics: clinical aspects and epidemiological data. In: Frosch PJ, Johansen JD, White IR (eds) Fragrances: beneficial and adverse effects. Springer, Berlin, pp 66–75

23. Frosch PJ, Johansen JD, White IR (eds) (1998) Fragrances: beneficial and adverse effects. Springer, Berlin

24. Guin JD (1982) History, manufacture, and cutaneous reactions to perfumes. In: Frost P, Horwitz SW (eds) Principles of cosmetics for the dermatologist. Mosby, St. Louis pp 111–129

25. Scheinman PL (1996) Allergic contact dermatitis to fragrance: a review. Am J Contact Dermat 7:65–76

26. Guin JD, Berry VK (1980) Perfume sensitivity in adult females. A study of contact sensitivity to a perfume mix in two groups of student nurses. J Am Acad Dermatol 3: 299–302

27. White JML, Gilmour NJ, Jeffries D, Duangdeeden I, Kullavanijaya P, Basketter DA, McFadden JP (2007) A general population from Thailand: incidence of common allergens with emphasis on para-phenylenediamine. Clin Exp Allergy 37:1848–1853

28. Marks JG Jr, Belsito DV, DeLeo VA, Fowler JF Jr, Fransway AF, Maibach HI, Mathias CGT, Nethercott JR, Rietschel RL, Sheretz EF, Storrs FJ, Taylor JS (1998) North American Contact Dermatitis Group patch test results for the detection of delayed-type hypersensitivity to topical allergens. J Am Acad Dermatol 38:911–918

29. Johansen JD, Rastogi SC, Menné T (1996) Contact allergy to popular perfumes; assessed by patch test, use test and chemical analysis. Br J Dermatol 135:419–422

30. Johansen JD, Rastogi SC, Andersen KE, Menné T (1997) Content and reactivity to product perfumes in fragrance mix positive and negative eczema patients. A study of perfumes used in toiletries and skin-care products. Contact Derm 36:291–296

31. Dooms-Goossens A, Kerre S, Drieghe J, Bossuyt L, Degreef H (1992) Cosmetic products and their allergens. Eur J Dermatol 2:465–468

32. Buckley DA, Rycroft RJ, White IR, McFadden JP (2003) The frequency of fragrance allergy in patch-tested patients increases with their age. Br J Dermatol 149:986–989

33. Johansen JD, Andersen TF, Kjøller M, Veien N, Avnstorp C, Andersen KE, Menné T (1998) Identification of risk products for fragrance contact allergy: a case-referent study based on patients' histories. Am J Contact Dermat 9:80–86

34. Frosch PJ, Johansen JD, Menne T, Rastogi SC, Bruze M, Andersen KE, Lepoittevan JP, Gimenez Arnau E, Pirker C, Goossens A, White IR (1999) Lyral is an important sensitizer in patients sensitive to fragrances. Br J Dermatol 141:1076–1083

35. The Scientific Committee on Cosmetic Products and Non-Food Products intended for Consumers (1999) Concerning Fragrance Allergy in Consumers. Available at http://europa.eu.int/comm/health/ph_risk/committees/sccp/documents/out98_en.pdf

36. Nethercott JR, Larsen WG (1997) Contact allergens – what's new? Fragrances. Clin Dermatol 15:499–504

37. Frosch PJ, Pirker C, Rastogi SC, Andersen KE, Bruze M, Svedman C, Goossens A, White IR, Uter W, Arnau EG, Lepoittevin JP, Menné T, Johansen JD (2005) Patch testing with a new fragrance mix detects additional patients sensitive to perfumes and missed by the current fragrance mix. Contact Derm 52:207–215

38. Johansen JD, Andersen TF, Veien N, Avnstorp C, Andersen KE, Menné T (1997) Patch testing with markers of fragrance contact allergy. Do clinical tests correspond to patients' self-reported problems? Acta Derm Venereol (Stockh) 77:149–153

39. Johansen JD, Rastogi SC, Menné T (1996) Exposure to selected fragrance materials. A case study of fragrance-mix-positive eczema patients. Contact Derm 34:106–110

40. Rastogi SC, Johansen JD, Frosch PJ, Menné T, Bruze M, Lepoittevin JP, Dreier B, Andersen KE, White IR (1998) Deodorants on the European market: quantitative chemical analysis of 21 fragrances. Contact Derm 38:29–35

41. Rastogi S, Johansen JD, Menné T (1996) Natural ingredients based cosmetics. Content of selected fragrance sensitizers. Contact Derm 34:423–426

42. Johansen JD, Andersen KE, Menné T (1996) Quantitative aspects of iso-eugenol contact allergy assessed by use and patch tests. Contact Derm 34:414–418

43. Johansen JD, Andersen KE, Rastogi SC, Menné T (1996) Threshold responses in cinnamic-aldehyde-sensitive subjects: results and methodological aspects. Contact Derm 34:165–171

44. Fransway AF (1991) The problem of preservation in the 1990s. I. Statement of the problem, solution(s) of the industry, and the current use of formaldehyde and formaldehyde-releasing biocides. Am J Contact Dermat 2:6–23

45. Fransway AF, Schmitz NA (1991) The problem of preservation in the 1990s. II. Formaldehyde and formaldehyde-releasing biocides: incidences of cross-reactivity and the significance of the positive response to formaldehyde. Am J Contact Dermat 2:78–88

46. Fransway AF (1991) The problem of preservation in the 1990s. III. Agents with preservative function independent of formaldehyde release. Am J Contact Dermat 2:145–174

47. Lundov MD, Moesby L, Zachariae C, Johansen JD (2009) Contamination versus preservation of cosmetics: a review on legislation, usage, infections, and contact allergy. Contact Derm 60:70–78

48. Morren MA, Dooms-Goossens A, Delabie J, De Wolf-Peeters C, Marien K, Degreef H (1992) Contact allergy to isothiazolinone derivatives: unusual clinical presentations. Dermatology 184:260–264

49. Davies E, Orton D (2009) Identifying the optimal patch test concentration for methylchloroisothiazolinone and methylisothiazolinone. Contact Derm 60:288–289

50. Frosch PJ, Lahti A, Hannuksela M, Andersen KE, Wilkinson JD, Shaw S, Lachapelle JM (1995) Chloromethylisothiazolone/methylisothiazolinone (CMI/MI) use test with a shampoo on patch-test-positive subjects. Results of a multicentre double-blind crossover trial. Contact Derm 32:210–217

51. Jong CT, Statham BN, Green CM et al (2007) Contact sensitivity in the UK, 2004-2005: results of multicentre study. Contact Derm 57:165–168

52. Bruynzeel DP, Diepgen TL, Andersen KE, EECDRG et al (2005) Monitoring the European Standard Series in 10 centres 1996-2000. Contact Derm 53:146–152

53. Uter W, Hegewald J, Aberer W et al (2005) The European standard series in 9 European countries, 2002/2003 – first results of the European Surveillance System on Contact Allergies. Contact Derm 53:136–145

54. Uter W, The ESSCA writing group (2008) The European Surveillance System of Contact Allergies (ESSCA): results of patch testing the standard series, 2004. JEADV 22:174–181

55. Wilkinson JD, Shaw S, Andersen KE et al (2002) Monitoring levels of preservative sensitivity in Europe. A 10-year overview (1991-2000). Contact Derm 46:207–210

56. Zug KA, Warshaw EM, Fowler JF Jr et al (2009) Patch-test results of the North American Contact Dermatitis Group 2005-2006. Dermatitis 20:149–160

57. de Groot AC, van Ginkel CJW, Weyland JW (1996) Methyldibromo glutaronitrile (Euxyl K 400): an important "new" allergen in cosmetics. J Am Acad Dermatol 35:743–747

58. Jackson JM, Fowler JF (1998) Methyldibromoglutaronitrile (Euxyl K400): a new and important sensitizer in the United States? J Am Acad Dermatol 38:934–937

59. Isaksson M, Gruvberger B, Bruze B (2007) Repeated open application tests with methyldibromoglutaronitrile in dermatitis patients with and without hypersensitivity to methyldibromoglutaronitrile. Dermatitis 18:203–207

60. Bruze M, Gruvberger B, Goossens A, Hindsén M, Pontén A (2005) Allergic contact dermatitis from methyldibromoglutaronitrile. Dermatitis 16:80–86

61. Johansen JD, Veien N, Laurberg G et al (2008) Decreasing trends in methyldibromo glutaronitrile contact allergy – following regulatory intervention. Contact Derm 59:48–51

62. De Groot AC, Flyvholm M-A, Lensen G, Menné T, Coenraads P-J (2009) Formaldehyde releasers: relationship to formaldehyde contact allergy. I Contact allergy to formaldehyde and inventory of formaldehyde-releasers. Contact Derm 61:63–85

63. de Groot AC, White IR, Flyvholm M-A, Lensen GJ, Coenraads P-J (2010) Formaldehyde-releasers: relationship to formaldehyde contact allergy. II. Formaldehyde-releasers used in cosmetics Part 2. Patch test relationship to formaldehyde contact allergy, experimental provocation tests, amount of formaldehyde released and assessment of risk to consumers allergic to formaldehyde. Contact Dermat 62:18–31

64. De Groot AC, Veenstra M (2010) Formaldehyde releasers in cosmetics in the USA and in Europe. Contact Derm 62:221–224

65. de Groot AC, White IR, Flyvholm M-A, Lensen G, Coenraads P-J (2010) Formaldehyde-releasers: relationship to formaldehyde contact allergy. II Formaldehyde-releasers used in cosmetics. Part 1. Characterization, frequency and relevance of sensitization, and frequency of use in cosmetics. Contact Derm 62:2–17

66. Davis MD, Scalf LA, Yiannias JA et al (2008) Changing trends and allergens in the patch test standard series. A Mayo Clinic 5-year retrospective review, January 1, 2001, through December 31, 2005. Arch Dermatol 144:67–72

67. Pratt MD, Belsito DV, DeLeo VA et al (2004) North American Contact Dermatitis Group patch-test results, 2001-2002 study period. Dermatitis 15:176–183

68. Lehmann SV, Hoeck U, Breinholdt J, Olsen CE, Kreilgaard B (2006) Characterization and chemistry of imidazolidinyl urea and diazolidinyl urea. Contact Derm 54:50–58

69. de Groot AC, Bruynzeel DP, Jagtman BA, Weyland JW (1988) Contact allergy to diazolidinyl urea (Germall II). Contact Derm 18:202–205

70. Cashman AL, Warshaw EM (2005) Parabens. A review of epidemiology, structure, allergenicity, and hormonal properties. Dermatitis 16:57–66

71. Brasch J, Schnuch A, Geier J, Aberer W, Uter W, German Contact Dermatitis Research Group; Information Network of Departments of Dermatology (2004) Iodopropynylbutyl carbamate 0.2% is suggested for patch testing of patients with eczema possibly related to preservatives. Br J Dermatol 151:608–615

72. Natkunarajah J, Osborne V, Holden C (2008) Allergic contact dermatitis to iodopropynyl butylcarbamate found in a cosmetic cleansing wipe. Contact Derm 58:316–317

73. Curry EJ, Warshaw EM (2005) Benzyl alcohol allergy: importance of patch testing with personal products. Dermatitis 16:203–208

74. Berthelot C, Zirwas MJ (2006) Allergic contact dermatitis to chloroxylenol. Dermatitis 17:156–159

75. Wakelin SH, White IR (1997) Contact dermatitis from chlorphenesin in a facial cosmetic. Contact Derm 37:138–139

76. Campbell L, Zirwas MJ (2006) Triclosan. Dermatitis 17:204–207

77. Robertshaw H, Leppard B (2007) Contact dermatitis to triclosan in toothpaste. Contact Derm 57:383–384

78. Tosti A, Guerra L, Vincenzi C, Piraccini BM, Peluso AM (1993) Contact sensitization caused by toluene sulfonamide-formaldehyde resin in women who use nail cosmetics. Am J Contact Dermat 4:150–153

79. Hausen BM (1994) Nagellackallergie. HG Z Hautkr 69: 252–262

80. Hausen BM, Milbrodt M, Koenig WA (1995) The allergens of nail polish (I). Allergenic constituents of common nail polish and toluenesulfonamide-formaldehyde resin (TS-F-R). Contact Derm 33:157–164

81. Giorgini S, Brusi C, Francalanci S, Gola M, Sertoli A (1994) Prevention of allergic contact dermatitis from nail varnishes and hardeners. Contact Derm 31:325–326

82. Kardorff B, Fuchs M, Kunze J (1995) Kontaktallergien auf Nagellack. Aktuel Dermatol 21:349–352

83. Staines KS, Felix DH, Forsyth A (1998) Desquamative gingivitis, sole manifestation of tosylamide/formaldehyde resin allergy. Contact Derm 39:90

84. Castelain M, Veyrat S, Laine G, Montastier C (1997) Contact dermatitis from nitrocellulose in a nail varnish. Contact Derm 36:266–267

85. Hausen BM (1995) A simple method of determining TS-F-R in nail polish. Contact Derm 32:188–190

86. Kanerva L, Lauerma A, Jolanki R, Estlander T (1995) Methyl acrylate: a new sensitizer in nail lacquer. Contact Derm 33:203–204

87. Rosenzweig R, Scher RK (1993) Nail cosmetics: adverse reactions. Am J Contact Dermat 4:71–77

88. Barnett JM, Scher RK (1992) Nail cosmetics. Int J Dermatol 31:675–681

89. Kanerva L, Lauerma A, Estlander T, Alanko K, Henriks-Eckerman M-L, Jolanki R (1996) Occupational allergic contact dermatitis caused by photobonded sculptured nails and a review of (meth) acrylates in nail cosmetics. Am J Contact Dermat 7:109–115

90. McFadden JP, White IR, Frosch PJ, Søsted H, Johansen JD, Menné T (2007) Allergy to hair dye. Br Med J 334:220

91. Conde-Salazar L, Baz M, Guimaraens D, Cannavo A (1995) Contact dermatitis in hairdressers: patch test results in 379 hairdressers. Am J Contact Dermat 6:19–23

92. Marcoux D, Riboulet-Delmas G (1994) Efficacy and safety of hair-coloring agents. Am J Contact Dermat 5:123–129

93. Pigatto PD, Bigardi AS, Cusano F (1995) Contact dermatitis to cocamidopropylbetaine is caused by residual amines: relevance, clinical characteristics, and review of the literature. Am J Contact Dermat 6:13–16

94. Fowler JF, Fowler LM, Hunter JE (1997) Allergy to cocamidopropyl betaine may be due to amidoamine: a patch test and product use test study. Contact Derm 37:276–281

95. Fowler JF Jr (1993) Cocamidopropyl betaine: the significance of positive patch test results in twelve patients. Cutis 52:281–284

96. Angelini G, Foti C, Rigano L, Vena G (1995) 3-Dimethylaminopropylamine: a key substance in contact allergy to cocamidopropylbetaine? Contact Derm 32:96–99

97. Li LF (2008) A study of the sensitization rate to cocamidopropyl betaine in patients patch tested in a university hospital of Beijing. Contact Derm 58:24–27

98. Funk JO, Dromgoole SH, Maibach HI (1995) Sunscreen intolerance. Contact sensitization, photocontact sensitization, and irritancy of sunscreen agents. Dermatol Clin 13:473–481

99. Foley P, Nixon R, Marks R, Frowen K, Thompson S (1993) The frequency of reactions to sunscreens: results of a longitudinal population-based study on the regular use of sunscreens in Australia. Br J Dermatol 128:512–518

100. Bilsland D, Ferguson J (1993) Contact allergy to sunscreen chemicals in photosensitivity dermatitis/actinic reticuloid syndrome (PD/AR) and polymorphic light eruption. Contact Derm 29:70–73

101. Darvay A, White IR, Rycroft RJG, Jones AB, Hawk JLM, McFadden JP (2001) Photoallergic contact dermatitis is uncommon. Br J Dermatol 145:597–601

102. Manciet JR, Lepoittevin JP, Jeanmougin M, Dubertret L (1994) Study of the cross-reactivity of seven benzophenones between themselves and with fenofibrate. Nouv Dermatol 13:370–371

103. Pons-Guiraud A, Jeanmougin M (1993) Allergie et photoallergie de contact aux crèmes de photoprotection. Ann Derm Venereol (Stockh) 120:727–731

104. Gonçalo M, Ruas E, Figueiredo A, Gonçalo S (1995) Contact and photocontact sensitivity to sunscreens. Contact Derm 33:278–280

105. Theeuwes M, Degreef H, Dooms-Goossens A (1992) Para-aminobenzoic acid (PABA) and sunscreen allergy. Am J Contact Dermat 3:206–207

106. Wilson CI, Cameron J, Powell SM, Cherry G, Ryan TJ (1997) High incidence of contact dermatitis in leg-ulcer patients – implications for management. Clin Exp Dermatol 16:250–261

107. Nachbar F, Korting HC, Plewig G (1993) Zur Bedeutung des positiven Epicutantests auf Lanolin. Dermatosen 41:227–236

108. Kligman AM (1998) The myth of lanolin allergy. Contact Derm 39:103–107

109. Matthieu L, Dockx P (1997) Discrepancy in patch test results with wool wax alcohols and Amerchol L-101. Contact Derm 36:150–151

110. Wolf R (1996) The lanolin paradox. Dermatology 192: 198–202

111. Warshaw EM, Nelsen DD, Maibach HI, Marks JG, Zug KA, Taylor JS, Rietschel RL, Fowler JF, Mathias CG, Pratt MD, Sasseville D, Storrs FJ, Belsito DV, De Leo VA (2009) Positive patch test reactions to lanolin: cross-sectional data from the north american contact dermatitis group, 1994 to 2006. Dermatitis 20:79–88

112. Guerra L, Bardazzi F, Tosti A (1992) Contact dermatitis in hairdressers' clients. Contact Derm 26:108–111

113. Funk JO, Maibach HI (1994) Propylene glycol dermatitis: re-evaluation of an old problem. Contact Derm 31:236–241

114. Aberer W, Fuchs T, Peters KP, Frosch PJ (1993) Propylenglykol: kutane Nebenwirkungen und Testmethodik. Dermatosen 41:25–27

115. Wahlberg JE (1994) Propylene glycol: search for a proper and nonirritant patch test preparation. Am J Contact Dermat 5:156–159

116. White IR, Lovell CR, Cronin E (1984) Antioxidants in cosmetics. Contact Derm 11:265–267

117. Le Coz CJ, Schneider G-A (1998) Contact dermatitis from tertiary-butylhydroquinone in a hair dye, with cross-sensitivity to BHA and BHT. Contact Derm 39:39–40

118. Serra-Baldrich E, Puig LL, Gimenez Arnau A, Camarasa JG (1995) Lipstick allergic contact dermatitis from gallates. Contact Derm 32:359–360

119. Parsad D, Saini R, Verma N (1997) Xanthomatous reaction following contact dermatitis from vitamin E. Contact Derm 37:294

120. Wyss M, Elsner P, Homberger H-P, Greco P, Gloor M, Burg G (1997) Follikuläres Kontaktekzem auf eine Tocopherol-linoleat-haltige Körpermilch. Dermatosen 45:25–28

121. Foti C, Rigano L, Vena GA, Grandolfo M, Liguori G, Angelini G (1995) Contact allergy to oleamidopropyl dimethylamine and related substances. Contact Derm 33:132–133

122. Tosti A, Vincenzi C, Guerra L, Andrisano E (1996) Contact dermatitis from fatty alcohols. Contact Derm 35:287–289

123. le Coz CJ, Lefebvre C (2000) Contact dermatitis from maleated soybean oil: last gasps of an expiring cosmetic allergen. Contact Derm 43:118–119

124. Laube S, Davies MG, Prais L, Foulds IS (2002) Allergic contact dermatitis from medium-chain triglycerides in a moisturizing lotion. Contact Derm 47:171

125. Guin JD (2001) Allergic contact cheilitis from di-isostearyl malate in lipstick. Contact Derm 44:375

126. le Coz CJ, Ball C (2000) Recurrent allergic contact dermatitis and cheilitis due to castor oil. Contact Derm 42:114–115

127. Magerl A, Heiss R, Frosch PJ (2001) Allergic contact dermatitis from zinc ricinoleate in a deodorant and glyceryl ricinoleate in a lipstick. Contact Derm 44:119–121

128. le Coz CJ, Lefebvre C, Ludmann F, Grosshans E (2000) Polyvinylpyrrolidone (PVP)/eicosene copolymer: an emerging cosmetic allergen. Contact Derm 43:61–62

129. Stone N, Varma S, Hughes TM, Stone NM (2002) Allergic contact dermatitis from polyvinylpyrrolidone (PVP)/1-triacontene copolymer in a sunscreen. Contact Derm 47:49

130. Kimura M, Kawada A (2000) Follicular contact dermatitis due to polyoxyethylene laurylether. J Am Acad Dermatol 42:879–880

131. Diegenant C, Constandt L, Goossens A (2000) Allergic contact dermatitis due to 1, 3-butylene glycol. Contact Derm 43:234–235

132. Le Coz CJ, Leclere JM, Arnoult E, Raison-Peyron N, Pons-Guiraud A, Vigan M, Members of Revidal-Gerda (2002) Allergic contact dermatitis from shellac in mascara. Contact Derm 46:149–152

133. Moffitt DL, Sansom JE (2002) Allergic contact dermatitis from phthalic anhydride/trimellitic anhydride/glycols copolymer in nail varnish. Contact Derm 46:236

134. Batta K, Bourke JF, Foulds IS (1997) Allergic contact dermatitis from colophony in lipsticks. Contact Derm 36:171–172

135. Hausen BM, Wollenweber E, Senff H, Post B (1987) Propolis allergy (I). Origin, properties, usage and literature review. Contact Derm 17:163–170

136. Guin JD (2003) Patch testing to FD&C and D&C dyes. Contact Derm 49:217–218

137. Kiken DA, Cohen DE (2002) Contact dermatitis to botanical extracts. Am J Contact Dermat 13:148–152

138. Nakagawa M, Kawai K, Kawai K (1995) Contact allergy to kojic acid in skin care products. Contact Derm 32:9–13

139. de Groot AC (1988) Adverse reactions to cosmetics. Thesis, State University of Groningen

140. De Groot AC (1998) Fatal attractiveness: the shady side of cosmetics. Clin Dermatol 16:167–179

141. de Groot AC, Weyland JW (1988) Kathon CG: a review. J Am Acad Dermatol 18:350–358

142. de Groot AC (1990) Methylisothiazolinone/methylchloroisothiazolinone (Kathon CG) allergy: an updated review. Am J Contact Dermat 1:151–156

143. De Groot AC (2009) Patch testing. Test concentrations and vehicles for 4350 allergens, 3rd edn. Acdegroot, Wapserveen

144. de Groot AC, Weijland JW (1997) Conversion of common names of cosmetic allergens to the INCI nomenclature. Contact Derm 37:145–150

Fragrances

33

Jeanne Duus Johansen and Jean-Pierre Lepoittevin

Contents

J.D. Johansen (✉)
Copenhagen University Hospital Gentofte, National Allergy
Research Centre, Department of Dermato-allergology,
Niels Andersens Vej 65, 2900 Hellerup, Denmark
e-mail: jedu@geh.regionh.dk

J.-P. Lepoittevin
Institut le Bel, Labo. Dermatochimie,
4, rue Blaise Pascal, 67070 Strasbourg Cedex, France
e-mail: jplepoit@unistra.fr

33.1 Introduction

The applications of fragrances are numerous and contact may be difficult to avoid, even if one wishes. Fragrances are used in all kinds of cosmetics and toiletries, in cleansing agents, air fresheners, over-the-counter topical pharmaceutical products, toys and textiles, and in industrial settings. Many fragrance ingredients are also used as flavors in food and some are naturally occurring in spices. Fragrance products are used in aromatherapy, may be contained in herbal remedies, and in some regions, natural fragrance products are used as topical medicaments for their antiseptic properties. Fragrances are capable of neutralizing unpleasant odors. They are added to products to produce a pleasant scent, add special character to the product, or as functional ingredients, e.g., providing antibacterial effects.

33.2 Fragrance Ingredients

The International Fragrance Association (IFRA) defines fragrance ingredients as any basic ingredient used in the manufacture of fragrance materials for its odorous, odor enhancing, or blending properties (www. ifraorg.org). A fragrance ingredient may be a chemically defined substance or a natural product.

Natural fragrance products are obtained by processing material from fragrance-producing plants. The fragrance can be present in almost any part of the plant and is obtained by pressing or steam distillation to give essential oils or by organic solvent extraction to give concretes and absolutes [1]. The content and consistency of the naturals depend on climatic and soil

J.D. Johansen et al. (eds.), *Contact Dermatitis*,
DOI: 10.1007/978-3-642-03827-3_33, © Springer-Verlag Berlin Heidelberg 2011

33

conditions for the plant, as well as many other factors, which make it very difficult, if not impossible, to fully standardize the contents and quality of the end product.

The volatile fragrance product obtained from plants usually contains numerous ingredients. The characteristic odor of the fragrance product may be due either to a particular ingredient, or in the case of a complex composition, the blending of a number of ingredients [2]. Oak moss absolute contains at least 250 ingredients and has several odor-determining agents [3], while clove oil contains up to 80% eugenol, which is the determining odor agent [4].

Previously, also animal secretions, such as musk from deer and ambergris from the sperm whale, were used as the basis for the production of natural fragrance ingredients. These are now replaced by blends of fragrance chemicals.

Originally, all perfumes were composed of natural products, but with the scientific and technical developments in the first half of the nineteenth century, chemists were able to identify the odor-determining major ingredients of natural fragrance materials. Following this development, industrial production of synthetic fragrance materials began. The synthesized ingredients are often nature-identical chemicals, that is, imitations of naturally occurring substances; however, also, the production of entirely new chemicals takes place.

Based on information from industry, it is estimated that about 2,500 different fragrance ingredients are in use.

> **Core Message**
>
> › Two thousand five hundred (2,500) fragrance ingredients are in current use for compounding perfumes. The ingredients are natural extracts of plant products, nature-identical, or entirely synthetic chemicals.

33.3 The Fragrance Formula

A fragrance formula consists of a mixture of 10–300 or more different fragrance ingredients, naturals, and/or chemicals. The fragrance formula is incorporated into the end product, e.g., a cosmetic. Some cosmetic products are used primarily for their scent, such as perfumes, eau de cologne, and aftershaves. These products

consist mainly of fragrance ingredients diluted with alcohol/water. A perfume usually contain 15–30% fragrance ingredients, a cologne about 3–5%, a deodorant 1%, a cream 0.4%, and undiluted soaps 0.5–2% [5].

The creation of a perfume, the fragrance formula, is regarded as an art. In designing a perfume, components from different odor families and of different volatilities are combined to form an esthetic whole. The most volatile ingredients are called top notes, usually fruity and spicy, which is followed by the heart note, built up by floral accords, forming the most essential part of the perfume; the long-lasting materials are known as the bottom notes. These include woody, moss-like, and sweet vanilla-like ingredients [6]. The basic pattern and principal structure of perfumes have not changed dramatically throughout the history of perfumery. The difference lies in the quality and availability of the raw materials and a different way of compounding [7].

33.4 Chemistry

Fragrance ingredients are organic compounds and must be volatile to be perceived. Therefore, in addition to the nature of the functional groups and the molecular structure of a substance, the molecular mass is an important factor. Molecular masses of about 200 occur relatively frequently [4]; further, many of the fragrance ingredients are lipophilic in nature and, thus, have good penetration abilities, even of intact skin [8].

A fragrance formula is a mixture of molecules with very different physico-chemical properties; allergens may be formed in the mixture, e.g., by oxidation [7, 9, 10] or in the skin by metabolism [11]. The mixture of molecules may result in interactions during skin penetration, skin metabolism, and epitope formation [8]. These interactions may lead to a change in sensitization and elicitation potential [12–14], effects, which, as yet, have only been seldom investigated.

33.5 Fragrance Contact Allergens

Allergenic fragrance ingredients have been identified by predictive assays in humans [15] and animals [16]. Due to the high number of fragrance ingredients in use, structure activity relationship (SAR) analysis has been employed to identify potential allergens, e.g., in deodorants [17]. Testing a series of individual aldehydes in the animal assay, local lymph node assay (LLNA), and combining these results with reactivity and lipophilicity parameters has developed further quantitative SARs (QSARs). Equations derived from these QSARs allow improvement of the predictions made based on chemical structure alone of new aldehydes [16, 18]. However, most clinically relevant knowledge comes from patch testing eczema patients with fragrance ingredients suspected of causing allergic reactions. In this way, the first screening test for fragrance contact allergy was designed [19], an approach followed by others [20–30]. This first true screening test for fragrance allergy, called the fragrance mix (FM I), was composed in the late 1970s by Larsen [19]. It consists of a mixture of eight ingredients: seven chemicals and a natural extract with the addition of an emulsifier (Table 33.1). Among the ingredients of FM I, the natural oak moss absolute (INCI: evernia prunastri) has, for some years, been the top ranked, usually followed by isoeugenol, cinnamal, and/or hydroxycitronellal. In recent multinational studies, additional important allergens have been identified [23–27]. Among these are both chemicals, such as hydroxyisohexyl 3-cyclohexene carboxaldehyde (HICC) [31], farnesol, citral, α-hexylcinnamic aldehyde [23], as well as natural extracts, such as ylang ylang oil, lemongrass oil, narcissus absolute, sandalwood oil, and jasmine absolute [24]. The following sections are comments on selected fragrance chemicals and naturals of special interest.

Table 33.1 Ingredients of fragrance mix I (FM I) and fragrance mix II (FM II)

Fragrance ingredients, INCI name (chemical name)	Concentration % in mixture
FM I	
α-Amyl cinnamal (α-amylcinnamicaldehyde)	1
Cinnamal (cinnamic aldehyde)	1
Cinnamyl alcohol (cinnamic alcohol)	1
Eugenol (eugenol)	1
Geraniol (geraniol)	1
Hydroxycitronellal (hydroxycitronellal)	1
Isoeugenol (isoeugenol)	1
Evernia prunastri (oak moss absolute)	1
Emulsifier	
Sorbitan sesquioleate	5
FM II	
Hydroxyisohexyl 3-cyclohexene carboxaldehyde	2.5
Citral	1.0
Farnesol	2.5
Citronellol	0.5
α-Hexyl cinnamal	5.0
Coumarin	2.5

For FM I, each ingredient is tested at the same concentration in FM I as individually, except sorbitan sesquioleate, which is individually tested at 20% in petrolatum, while the individual test concentration for FM II is the double as in the mix see Table 33.5

33.5.1 Fragrance Chemicals

Cinnamal (chemical name cinnamic aldehyde) is a strong allergen [15] and has, for many years, been a top-ranking fragrance allergen [32, 33], though recently a decline in reactions has been seen [34]. Cinnamal is the main component of cinnamon oil. It is also used as a flavoring and is described as an occupational allergen in bakers on a case basis [35, 36]. Cinnamal was found labeled in 7% of 243 cosmetic products in an investigation in UK, most often in women's perfumes [37]. The chemically related substance, cinnamyl alcohol, seems to be converted in the skin to cinnamal [11, 38] and exposure may be of relevance in those allergic to

cinnamal. Isoeugenol is a strong allergen [15]. It caused contact allergy in 1.7% of 2,261 consecutively tested eczema patients in a European multicenter study [39]. It is found in many cosmetic products and may be present in relatively high concentrations, especially in colognes and similar products [40]. There seems to be no relation between the metabolism of eugenol, which is also a constituent of fragrance mix, and isoeugenol [41, 42]. Isoeugenol is restricted to 0.02% in cosmetic products in the Cosmetic Directive (ec.europa.eu/enterprise/cosmetics/cosing) Despite this, an increasing trend has been found in isoeugenol allergy from 2001 to 2005 [40]. Patients with isoeugenol contact allergy may react to esters of isoeugenol [43], which is commonly used in cosmetics [44]. Hydroxycitronellal is classified as a relatively weak allergen based on its inherent properties; [45] even so, it is one of the top ranking causes of fragrance contact allergy. It is widely used in cosmetic products, both perfumes and deodorants, and often in relatively high concentrations. It is restricted to 1% in cosmetic products according to the Cosmetic Directive.

Hydroxyisohexyl 3-cyclohexene carboxaldehyde (Lyral®) has been used for many years without restrictions. It is related to hydroxycitronellal and has probably been used as a substitute in many cases as hydroxycitronellal was restricted [46]. The use concentrations have generally been very high; more than 3.0% in perfumes have been reported [46]. A series of systematic investigations have shown that hydroxyisohexyl 3-cyclohexene carboxaldehyde is one of the most frequent allergens, giving positive reactions in 1–2.7% of consecutively patch-tested patients in Europe [22, 23, 26, 31, 33].

It seems that allergy to hydroxyisohexyl 3-cyclohexene carboxaldehyde is especially related to exposures from deodorants [47–49]. A voluntary restiction of 1.5% hydroxyisohexyl 3-cyclohexene carboxaldehyde in cosmetics was made in 2003 by IFRA, and in 2007 this was changed to various concentrations from 0.11 to 1.5% depending on the product type. The incidence of contact allergy to hydroxyisohexyl 3-cyclohexene carboxaldehyde has remained unaffected [50].

Farnesol is both used as a fragrance ingredient and as a biocide, e.g., in deodorants [51]. It has been shown to cause allergy in 0.9–1.1% of patients consecutively patch tested by the German Information Network of Departments of Dermatology (IVDK) [33, 52]. Those positive to farnesol were characterized by being young females and having hands and face more often affected than patients negative to farnesol [52]. Probably, many cases of deodorant contact allergy due to farnesol have been missed in the past, as most of the patients reacting to farnesol are negative to the fragrance mix [36, 52].

Citral is a relatively weak allergen, which also has irritant properties. It has a steep dose-response curve [53] and has been shown to be of possible significance in patients with long-term chronic hand eczema, which may be due to its combined allergenic and irritant effects [53, 54]. The irritant properties of citral have been shown to be temperature dependent [55]. In European multicenter studies, 0.7–1.1% of consecutively tested eczema patients gave a positive reaction to citral 2% [23, 26].

Coumarin is the subject of several studies and case investigations [23, 56]. It has been reported to cause reactions in 0.4% of consecutively tested patients [57] and also gave rise to positive reactions in 0.3% of patients in a European multicenter study [23]. Impurities have been blamed for the sensitizing effect [58, 59].

> **Core Message**
>
> › Hydroxyisohexyl 3-cyclohexene carboxaldehyde (Lyral®) has, for a number of years, been one of the most frequent causes of contact allergy to fragrance ingredients

33.5.2 Oxidation Products

d-Limonene is obtained as a byproduct from the citrus juice industry. Peal oil from the skins of citrus fruits contains normally more than 95% d-limonene. It is used as a fragrance ingredient, but also has many other applications. In itself, it is not a sensitizer or a very weak one, but rapidly oxidizes when in contact with air [7]. Antioxidants such as butylated hydroxytoluene (BHT) are, therefore, often added to commercial products. However, once the antioxidant is consumed, the oxidation starts immediately. The allergens formed are mainly hydroperoxides [60], with strong sensitizing potential [7]. Testing consecutive patients in different clinics with oxidized d-limonene gave positive results in 0.3–6.5% of cases [61]. A patch test concentration of 6% in pet. of oxidized linalool has been suggested as optimal [9].

Similar findings have been obtained for linalool, another terpene [62, 63]. This emphasizes the need for testing with the chemicals that are in the products and not just what was originally added. Patch test material of the oxidized forms of linalool and limonene are currently being developed . In terms of prevention, expiry dates taking autooxidation into consideration will help solve the problem.

Geraniol, an ingredient of FM I, is also a terpene. The oxidation process follows two paths in which hydroperoxide, as for other terpenes, is formed, and in addition, the aldehydes geranial and neral [10]. Autooxidation greatly influences the sensitizing effect of geraniol, which becomes a potent allergen [10].

> ## Core Message
>
> ❯ Strong allergens are formed by autooxidation of d-limonene, linalool, and geraniol. This can probably be extended to other terpenes. If patch testing is done with nonoxidized material, false-negative results may be expected.

33.5.3 Fragrance Naturals

Oak moss absolute is derived from the lichen *Evernia prunastri*. It has been used as a basic ingredient and a fixative in many perfumes. It is a constituent of the fragrance mix and is a top-ranking allergen when the single ingredients are tested [34, 64]. A systematic search of the allergens in the extract has been performed. A bio-guided fractionation procedure was used based on the testing of patients sensitized to oak moss absolute with fractions of the natural in question. This was combined with chemical analysis and SAR analysis to ultimately identify the allergens in oak moss absolute [3]. Several allergens were identified, and among these, chloroatranol, atranol, and methyl-β-orcinol carboxylate gave the most reactions. These allergens are formed during the processing of the lichen (for details, please see Chap. 5). Chloroatranol and atranol have been further studied and are shown to be strong allergens and potent elicitors, giving reactions at extremely low levels [58]. An explanation of the high rates of sensitization to oak moss absolute was found by assessing exposure. Chloroatranol and/or atranol were found in 87% of 31 investigated products, mostly perfumes [65].

Based on these investigations, the Scientific Committee on Consumer Products (SCCP) advisory to the EU Commission has published an opinion that neither chloroatranol nor atranol should be present in consumer products. Attempts have been made to remove chloroatranol and atranol down to a level of 100 ppm of each in the concentrate. IFRA recommended that a maximum of 0.1% oak moss absolute is used in a finished product, which will give a maximum level of 0.1 ppm of these allergens in the product. Patch testing of the chemically modified oak moss absolute with a low level of chloroatranol and atranol still gave positive patch test reactions in 8 out of 14 patients with a known allergy to oak moss absolute [66]. The SCCP has recommended a further assessment of the safety.

Ylang ylang oil is produced by steam distillation of the flowers of *Cananga odorata*. Four grades are produced, which differ in odor, price, and composition. Ylang ylang oil is a major cause of allergic contact dermatitis in Asian countries, where it is frequently followed by hyperpigmentation [67]. In a European multicenter study including 1,606 patients, ylang ylang oils of grades I and II were tested and gave a positive patch test reaction in 2.6 and 2.5% of patients, respectively, with the highest frequency in London, possibly due to the city's large Asian population; detailed information can be found in a paper by Frosch et al. [24].

Lemongrass oil, narcissus absolute, jasmine absolute, geranium oil bourbon, spearmint oil, sandalwood oil, lavender oil, and others have also been reported as frequent sensitizers [24, 27–29, 67] (Table 33.2).

It was recently shown that natural lavendel oil offers no protection against autooxidation and is as allergenic as a synthetic lavender scent composed of the three main terpenes present in lavendel oil [68].

Table 33.2 Patch test reactions to selected natural ingredients [24, 27–30]

Ingredient	$n=1,606$ [24][a] (%)	$n=218$ [27][b] (%)	$n=178$ [28][c] (%)
Ylang ylang oil I	2.6		
Ylang ylang oil II	2.5		
Lemongrass oil	1.6		
Narcissus abs.	1.3		
Jasmine abs.	1.2		16.9
Sandalwood oil	0.9		
Patchouli oil	0.8		
Spearmint oil	0.8		5.0
Dwarf pine needle oil	0.7		
Cedarwood oil	0.6		
Peppermint oil	0.6		
Clove bud oil		19.3	
Lavender oil		2.8	
Eucalyptus oil		1.8	
Geranium oil bourbon			8.4

[a] Consecutively tested patients

[b, c] Selected patients with fragrance sensitivity

33

Myroxylon pereirae (MP) (balsam of Peru) is derived from the sap of a tree, MP, and is composed of 250 constituents, of which 189 are known structurally [69]. MP has been used in topical medicaments, such as wound treatment, for its antibacterial properties [70], but also as a flavor and perfume ingredient. In many countries, the use of MP in topical medicaments has been discontinued due to its sensitizing properties; however, it may still occur in herbal and natural products [71]. The crude form of MP has been banned from use in perfumes by IFRA since 1982; however, extracts and destillates of MP are still used in perfumes [72]. It is likely that these can cause allergic reactions in MP sensitized individuals. MP has been in the standard series since its first edition and is still causing many reactions [64], even though a decline has been seen in some countries [73].

Colophony (rosin) is a resin obtained from different species of coniferous trees. It is a complex mixture of resin acids and natural substances. Its composition varies with the species from which it is obtained and also depends on the recovery processes and storage conditions [74]. Unmodified colophony is known to cause contact allergy. The main allergenic components are oxidized resin acids formed on exposure to air. The allergenicity can be changed by chemical modification, e.g., it can be decreased by hydrogenation, while other kinds of modifications may enhance the allergenicity [74]. Colophony has many applications and has also been used as a fragrance ingredient. The use of unmodified colophony in perfumes was banned in 1992 by IFRA; however, it is unknown if modified forms of colophony are used in perfumes.

An extensive review has been published listing fragrance ingredients, chemicals, and natural products identified in the available literature as allergens in clinical studies of groups of patients or single cases; [75] about 100 chemicals and a similar number of natural products are in these lists.

Core Message

> The main allergens in the natural extract oak moss absolute (INCI: *evernia prunastri*) have been identified as chloroatranol and atranol, which elicit contact allergy at very low levels. A ban on those ingredients in cosmetics has been proposed.

33.6 Epidemiology of Fragrance Contact Allergy

Frequencies of sensitization to perfume ingredients were previously difficult to estimate due to the lack of a reliable test substance to screen for this allergy, but it was regarded as a common condition [76]. MP was shown by Hjorth to be a marker of contact allergy to fragrances in the 1960s [70], and later the FM I was developed, which enabled assessment of the problem [19]. A second fragrance mix was officaly included in the baseline serie in 2008 [77].

Contact allergy to fragrance ingredients as identified with FM I is seen in all geographical regions of the industrialized world [25, 78–80]. Studies of the general population show that about 2% of adolescents and 1–4% of adults have contact allergy to FM I [73, 81–84], depending on the age group of investigation.One-third of 12- to 16-year-old children had, at the time of diagnosis, symptoms of their allergy, as did half of the adult population [81, 82]. In a recent study from Poland 7.3% of 7-year-old children were patch test positive to FM I and none among a sample of 16-year-olds [156].

An estimation based on the sales of patch test materials in Germany and patient data showed that 1.8–4.2% of the German population is sensitized to FM I amounting to 1.4–3.4 million people in the German population of 82 million inhabitants [85]. A decreasing trend in FM I allergy has been seen in eczema patients since 1998 [48, 64, 86] and has now been confirmed among younger women of the general population [73]. Comparing the results from three cross-sectional studies done in a sample of the general population in 1990, 1998, and 2006, it was shown that the prevalence of FM I and MP contact allergy followed an inverse V-pattern among women aged 18–41 years, increasing from 1990 to 1998 and then decreasing to a level of 2.3 % with a postive reaction to FM I in 2006 [73]. This was followed by a decreasing trend in MP allergy. No significant changes were seen in men or in other age groups [73]. In 2006, FM I allergy was still significantly associated with reporting cosmetic dermatitis and use of health care [73]. No data from testing FM II in the general population exist, yet.

In adults with contact eczema undergoing patch testing, FM I and FM II are some of the the most frequent causes of contact allergy. In multicenter investigations in Europe covering the period of 1996–2000, 9.7% of adult eczema patients reacted to the FM I, and in a different investigation from 2002 to 2003 6.7% reacted to FM I [87, 88]; the data from the North American Contact Dermatitis Group from 2005 to 2006 showed that 11.5% of consecutive patients tested gave a positive reaction to FM I [89]. Among Thai eczema patients, the frequency of positive reaction to FM I was 20.7% [90]. The FM II gives positive reactions in 2.9–4.6% of consecutively tested eczema patients [25, 91].

The frequency of fragrance allergy in patch-tested patients increases with age; [92, 93] nevertheless, FM I is also among the top ranking allergens in children with eczema [94, 95], and cases down to 2 years of age have been reported, even though it is rare [92]. In eczema patients, the female: male ratio of FM I allergy is usually 2:1 [34, 64, 96], while in the general population, especially in the younger years, a more equal sex distribution is seen [81]. It has been suggested that patients with current or past atopic dermatitis has reduced rates of contact allergy to fragrance allergens with dietary exposures such as cinnamic compounds, as a sign of oral tolerance, compared to those with cutanous exposure only such as evernia prunastri [97].

In accordance with the decrease in FM I, a chemical analysis of ten prestige perfumes showed that fewer FM allergens were present in newly launched perfumes in comparison with perfumes manufactured more than 10 years ago [98]. MP has shown a similar downward trend in some countries [73]. However, in Germany MP surpassed the FM I in frequency in 2002 [64]. This may be a reminder that the use of other allergenic fragrance compounds, structurally similar to ingredients in MP, may have increased [64]. Certainly, high frequencies of contact allergy to natural extracts such as ylang ylang oil and jasmine absolute have been demonstrated [24, 27, 28] and, in addition, a number of chemicals not included in FM I and II may be of importance [23, 27–29, 99]. Thus, the epidemiology of fragrance contact allergy is only partly displayed by the results from testing with FM I and II, which should be borne in mind both in assessing the size of the problem on a community level and in the diagnostic workup of the individual patient.

33.7 Clinical Aspects

Allergic contact dermatitis may develop as itchy eczematous patches where perfume has been applied, usually behind the ears, on the neck, the upper chest,

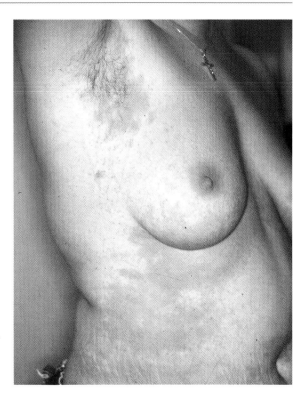

Fig. 33.1 Allergic contact dermatitis from perfume in deodorant (courtesy of N. Veien)

and sometimes the elbow flexures and wrists [76]. Another typically presenting feature is a bilateral axillary dermatitis caused by perfume in deodorants; if the reaction is severe, it may spread to other areas of the body [76] (Fig. 33.1). It is not always that such patients will consult a dermatologist, but a history of such first-time symptoms have been shown to be statistically significantly related to the diagnosis of perfume allergy by FM I in eczema patients [100].

Facial eczema is a classical manifestation of fragrance allergy from the use of different fragranced cosmetic products [30, 48, 101, 102]. In men, after-shave lotion may cause a eczematous eruption of the beard area and adjacent part of the neck [76] (Fig. 33.2) and men using wet shaving opposed to dry have been shown to have an increased risk of being fragrance-allergic [103].

Data from St Johns in London in 1980s showed that perfumes and deodorants were the most frequent sources of sensitization in women, and aftershave lotions and deodorants were usually the most responsible in men [76]. More recent investigations have confirmed that this is still the case [40, 47, 104–108].

33

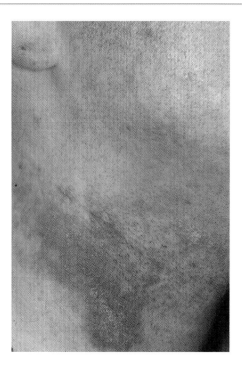

Fig. 33.2 Allergic contact dermatitis from perfume in aftershave (courtesy of N. Veien)

Primary hand eczema or aggravation of hand eczema can be caused by contact to fragranced products, as seen in occupational settings [109]. Also, a significant relationship between hand eczema and fragrance contact allergy has been found in some studies based on patients investigated for contact allergy [110–112]. However, hand eczema is a multifactorial disease and the clinical significance of fragrance contact allergy in chronic hand eczema is controversial. A review on the subject has been published by Heydorn et al. [109].

Pigmented contact dermatitis has been described in Japan as a manifestation of contact allergic reaction to a range of contact allergens, e.g., ylang ylang oil and jasmine absolute [67]. The pigmentation disappears or improves upon avoidance.

Systemic contact dermatitis may occur in selected cases. The phenomenon that patients, sensitized by skin contact, react with a rash to oral intake of flavored food has especially been described in conjunction with MP sensitivity [71, 113–115]. In general, the problem is to quantify exposure and determine the relevance to chronic eczema. Systemic contact dermatitis is the subject of a separate chapter in this book.

Core Message

> Deodorants and perfumes/aftershaves are frequent sources of fragrance allergy.

33.8 Exposure to Fragrance Allergens

33.8.1 Consumer Products

Exposure may be by direct skin contact, and the longer the time of contact, the higher the risk of sensitization and elicitation, even though the frequency of applications also plays a role. The most significant nonoccupational exposure is from cosmetics products. Chemical analysis of more than 150 different cosmetic products has shown that the fragrance mix ingredients occur widely and, in some products, in high concentrations (Table 33.3). Isoeugenol was found in 24% of products in a concentration of between <0.001 and 0.34% [5]. Hydroxyisohexyl 3-cyclohexene carboxaldehyde (Lyral®) has been shown to be widely distributed in cosmetic products and, in particular, in high concentrations of 3% or more in fine fragrances [31, 46, 116], as well as in many deodorants. Natural-ingredient-based cosmetic perfumes have been shown to contain fragrance allergens to the same degree or more than ordinary products [117], which perhaps is not so surprising, since most fragrance ingredients and, thus, allergens are nature-identical. Children's products may also contain fragrance allergens; however, in an investigation of 25 children's products, the fragrance mix ingredients were either not present or present in fairly low concentrations [118]. The highest levels of FM I-allergens were found in perfumes and extreme levels were seen in a toy perfume [118]. Chemical analysis of 59 household products showed that the most commonly detected fragrance allergen was limonene, which was found in 78% of products, followed by linalool in 61% and citronellol in 47% [119], while the ingredients of the fragrance mix were found less frequently than expected from the analysis of cosmetic products. Some of the investigated household products were also for occupational use. In a British study, exposure to fragrance allergens was

Table 33.3 Exposure assessment of fragrance allergens in cosmetics and household products by chemical analysis and information from the industry

Ingredient	Prestige perfumes, n=10[a]; n=NG[b]; n=31[c]; [40][a]; [46][b]; [58][c]		Natural-ingredient-based perfumes n=22 [117]		Deodorants n=73 [155]		Household products n=59 [119]	
	In % of analyzed products	Concentration range (ppm)	In % of analyzed products	Concentration range (ppm)	In % of analyzed products	Concentration range (ppm)	In % of analyzed products	Concentration range (ppm)
α-Amyl cinnamal	30[a]	300–6,900	36	1,940–30,390	31	1–617	8	NQ
Cinnamal	0[a]		0		17	1–424	3	NQ
Cinnamyl alcohol	60[a]	300–7,900	14	890–21,010	39	6–1,169	2	NQ
Eugenol	90[a]	400–8,900	36	350–22,890	57	1–2,355	27	32–349
Geraniol	90[a]	800–4,800	63	NQ	76	1–1,178	41	53–1,758
Hydroxycitronellal	90[a]	2,500–11,900	23	1,350–60,440	50	1–1,023	12	15–140
Isoeugenol	70[a]	500–3,400	9	270–1,390	29	1–458	5	NQ
Lyral	46[b]	32,000 (mean)	ND		53	1–1,874	10	36–103
Farnesol	ND		ND		ND		ND	
Citral	ND		ND		ND		25	48–1,088
Limonene	ND		ND		ND		78	6–9,443
Linalool	90[b]	47,000 (mean)	ND		97	9–1,927	61	3–439
Chloroatranol[d]	87[c]	0.004–53	ND		ND		ND	
Atranol[d]	77[c]	0.012–190	ND		ND		ND	

ND not done; *NQ* not quantified; *NG* not given; *PPM* μg/mL (10,000 ppm = 1%)

[a] Consecutively tested patients

[b,c] Selected patients with fragrance sensitivity

[d] Allergens in oak moss absolute

33

Table 33.4 Fragrance allergens from FM I and FM II found on the label of 300 consumer products in Britain [37]

Fragrance ingredients, INCI name (chemical name)	Found in number (%) of consumer products
Fragrance mix I	
α-Amyl cinnamal	22 (7)
Cinnamal	17 (6)
Eugenol	80 (27)
Geraniol	126 (42)
Hydroxycitronellal	52 (17)
Isoeugenol	27 (9)
Evernia prunastri (oak moss absolute)	13 (4)
Fragrance mix II	
HICC	88 (29)
Citral	74 (25)
Farnesol	23 (8)
Citronellol	145 (48)
α-Hexyl cinnamal	125 (42)
Coumarin	90 (30)

All substances were most frequently found in women's perfumes except for α-Amyl cinnamal, which was seen most often on the label of other make-up, and α-Hexyl cinnamal in personal care products. HICC=hydroxyisohexyl 3-cyclohexene carboxaldehyde

Core Messages

> Fragrance allergens are widespread in consumer products and often several allergens occur in the same product.
> Topical pharmaceutical products are also a source of contact allergy to fragrance ingredients.

33.8.2 Occupational Exposure

There are a number of occupations where fragrance exposure may occur from cosmetic or domestic products, e.g., in hairdressers, beauticians, aromatherapists, masseurs, and cleaners. Chefs and bakers are exposed to spices and flavors, which may contain fragrance allergens, e.g., cinnamal from cinnamon. Eugenol is used for dental fillings and is a rare cause of contact allergy in dentists [121]. Multivariate analysis of associations between occupation and contact allergy to the fragrance mix showed that the highest occupational risk of fragrance contact allergy was associated with work as a masseur, physiotherapist, metal furnace operator, potter or glass marker, or geriatric nurse, when using data on 57,779 patients from the German surveillance system (IVDK) [122]. In an English investigation, health care worker (medicine, dentistry, nursing, veterinary) was also the occupation with the highest overall prevalence of sensitization to FM I [92]. Metalworkers exposed to metalworking fluids and with occupational skin diseases were found to have an increased risk of sensitization to fragrances in terms of a positive patch test to FM I and MP, when compared to metalworkers with occupational disease, but not exposed to metalworking fluids; [123] this could not be explained by the use of skin care and protecting creams. According to recent information from the lubricants-producing industry, fragrances are no longer usually added to metalworking fluid concentrate. However, it may be that masking fragrances are added during usage [123]. It is recommended that cases of fragrance allergy in metal workers should be thoroughly investigated for a causal relationship [124]. Another association to fragrance allergy was found in workers producing rotor blades for wind turbines with an epoxy-based technology [125]. A significant relationship between contact allergy to epoxy resins and FM I was found, and the

investigated by the ingredient labeling of 300 product bought on the retail market [37]. Ingredients from the FM I and FM II were frequently found (Table 33.4). The two top scorer were linalool and limonene, each found in 63% of the products. The mean number of labeled fragrance allergens was between 1.1 (dental products) and 12 (women perfumes) [37]. An investigation of more than 3,820 topical pharmaceutical products in Belgium showed that 10% contained fragrance ingredients and cases of iatrogenic fragrance contact allergy were identified [120].

The exposure to naturals extracts, which may have a significant allergenic potential, is virtually unknown, as it is only possible to quantify the exposure to identified chemicals. The demonstration of the main allergens in the extract oak moss absolute and their presence in almost all investigated perfumes/aftershaves is an example of a hidden exposure to important allergens in naturals [3, 65].

same association was found among male eczema patients undergoing patch testing, possibly due to concommitant sensitization. Cross-reactivity has been suggested but never proven [125].

33.9 Diagnosis of Fragrance Contact Allergy

The basic investigation of suspected fragrance contact allergy is made by patch testing with the standard patch test series, which currently entail four potential indicators of fragrance contact allergy: FM I, FM II, MP, hydroxyisohexyl 3-cyclohexene carboxaldehyde. Further, a positive reaction to colophony may in some cases indicate fragrance allergy. FM I has been used as an indicator of fragrance contact allergy since the late 1970s. The ingredients of the mix have remained unchanged since, while the test concentration of the mix was lowered from 16% originally to 8% in 1984, as data suggested that the higher concentration gave irritant reactions [126]. Thus, the individual ingredients were lowered from 2 to 1%, which may give rise to false-negative results when testing the ingredients separately [127]. The emulsifier sorbitan sesquioleate was later added to the individual ingredients, as it was shown to improve the positive rate [128]. FM I is a heterogeneous mix, which means that it contains molecules that differ widely in size and reactivity [8]. In this way, it is a realistic imitation of perfumes. Further, its composition has been shown to be a relevant reflection of exposure [129]. It has been assessed that FM I detects 50–80% of eczema patients with reactions to perfumes in cosmetics [40, 130, 131]. The same applies if individual fragrance allergens are tested [21, 23, 24, 27–29]. However, the developments in the fragrance industry, changing fashion, and regulatory interventions mean that the exposure pattern is constantly changing and fragrance ingredients other than FM I are relevant to test [20, 22–24, 27–29, 112, 130, 132].

An EU-funded research program was aimed at designing an additional screening test for fragrance allergy, fragrance mix II (FM II) [25, 26]. Based on previous investigations [20–22, 27–29, 46], published information in general, and the IFRA guidelines, a selection of candidates for testing was made, chemicals [23] and naturals [24]. Fourteen chemical were tested in 1,855 patients; the six chemicals with the highest reactivity following FM I were hydroxyisohexyl 3-cyclohexene carboxaldehyde (2.7%), citral (1.1%), farnesol (0.5%), citronellol (0.4%), α-hexylcinnamal (0.3%), and coumarin (0.3%) [23]. These six chemicals were further tested as a mixture in three different concentrations, and with the corresponding individual ingredients in 1,701 consecutive patients [25]. Positive reactions to the FM II were dose-dependent and 2.9% reacted to the FM II in a test concentration of 14%, which was recommended as an additional diagnostic screening tool [25]. About one-third of those reacting to FM II, 14% were negative at testing with FM I. In breakdown testing of the single ingredients, 74% gave a response, if doubtful reactions were included [26], and the rank order of the ingredients was as in the first study [23], except that no unequivocal positive reaction to coumarin was observed. Hydroxyisohexyl 3-cyclohexene carboxaldehyde was the dominant single constituent, with positive reactions in 36% of patients reacting to 14% FM II and was recommended for inclusion in the baseline series in Germany [133]. Assessments made of clinical relevance by different methods showed that FM II detects additional relevant cases of contact allergy to fragrances [25, 26] (Fig. 33.3).

Both the FM II 14% pet. and hydroxyisohexyl 3-cyclohexene carboxaldehyde 5% pet., as a fragrance ingredient of special importance, are in the most recent edition of the European baseline series [77]. The allergens present in FM I and II also cover the most frequent fragrance allergens detected in patients with hand eczema: citral, hydroxycitronellal, hydroxyisohexyl 3-cyclohexene, and eugenol [54], though oxidized limonene, which gave positive patch tests in 0.9% of chronic hand eczema patients [54], is not commercially available.

The function of MP as an indicator of fragrance contact allergy is more complex and heterogeneous than FM and may vary in different parts of the world due to local habits. MP contains ingredients also present in FM I, such as cinnamates, which comprise more than 35% of the MP constituents and isoeugenol/eugenol [71]. Hausen has hypothesized that the pattern of reactions may indicate sources of exposure, so that contact allergy to MP and isoeugenol/eugenol can be traced back to fragrances, especially if the reaction to FM I is moderate or strong, while reactions to cinnamal/cinnamates can be traced to essential oils and possible sunscreens [71].

A statistically significant relationship between reactions to FM I and MP was seen in a study covering several countries [26]. This may be explained by the contents of mutual allergens, while only a weak

33

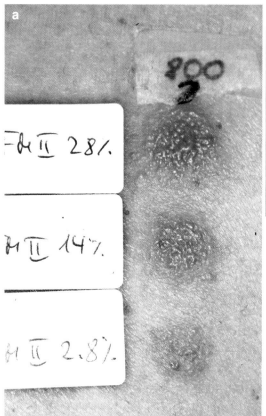

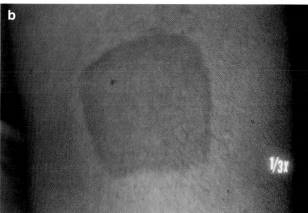

Fig. 33.3 Patch test reaction to the new fragrance mix (FM II) in dose-dependent intensity (day 3) (**a**). Breakdown testing revealed high sensitivity to HICC (Lyral). The repeated open application test (ROAT) with HICC (Lyral) was strongly positive already on day 4 (**b**) (courtesy of P.J. Frosch)

association was seen with FM II, the ingredients of which are not in MP, except for farnesol in trace amounts [71]. MP functions as an indicator of fragrance allergy, but has not in its crude form been used in perfumery since 1982 [72]. Only extracts, Peru Balsam oil and Peru Balsam absolute, are used. Their main ingredient is benzyl benzoate, which accounts for at least half of the composition, in addition a number of cinnamate-derivatives are present, but not cinnamal itself, neither any other ingredient of the FM I, according to fragrance industry [72]. Still, a majority of patients with MP contact allergy react to the MP-derivatives at patch testing (personel communication M Bruze) and may, thus, have a relevant fragrance allergy.

In 2005 an ingredient labeling of 26 fragrance ingredients identified as allergens in the consumer came into force, and concerns cosmetic products as well as detergents. The selection was done in 1998 and based on the comprehensive work of de Groot and Frosch [75]. The list entails the eight ingredients of the FM I and the six of the FM II and additional 12 substances (Table 33.5). These extra 12 substances are commercially available for patch testing in cases suspected of fragrance allergy. A screen with the 26 substances done in Germany showed that some of the substances seldom gave reactions, while others were frequent causes of positve patch test reactions [33]. A revision of the list is ongoing. Recently, the optimal patch test concentrations for the 12 ingredients not part of the FM I or FM II have been identified [134]. The recommended patch test concentration for 10 of the 12 ingredients are higher than those being used currently, identical for evernia furfurcea (1%), and lower for one substance, methyl 2-octynate (chemical name: methyl heptine carbonate). Methyl 2-octynate has caused

Table 33.5 Fragrance ingredients to be labeled as ingredients if present in cosmetics or detergents

INCI name	CAS no. concentration	Recommended test of individual ingredients in w/w % [77, 134]
Ingredients of FM I[a]		
Amyl cinnamal	122–40–7	1
Cinnamal	104–55–2	1
Cinnamyl alcohol	104–54–1	1
Eugenol	97–53–0	1
Evernia prunastri (oak moss) extract	90028–68–5	1
Geraniol	106–24–1	1
Hydroxycitronellal	107–75–5	1
Isoeugenol	97–54–1	1
Ingredients of FM II[b]		
Citral	5392–40–5	2
Citronellol	106–22–9	1
Coumarin	91–64–5	5
Farnesol	4602–84–0	5
Hexyl cinnamal	101–86–0	10
Hydroxyisohexyl 3-cyclohexene carboxaldehyde	31906–04–4	5
Additional substances		
Alpha-Isomethyl ionone	127–51–5	10
Amylcinnamyl alcohol	101–85–9	5
Anisyl alcohol	105–13–5	10
Benzyl alcohol	100–51–6	10
Benzyl benzoate	120–51–4	10
Benzyl cinnamate	103–41–3	10
Benzyl salicylate	118–58–1	10
Butylphenyl methylpropional (Lillial)	80–54–6	10
Evernia furfuracea (tree moss) extract	90028–67–4	1
d-Limonene	5889–27–5	10[c]
Linalool	78–70–6	10[c]
Methyl 2-octynoate	111–12–6	0.2[d]

The presence of the substance must be indicated in the list of ingredients when its concentration exceeds 0.001% in leave-on products and 0.01% in rinse-off products (http://ec.europa.eu/enterprise/cosmetics/cosing)

[a]FM I: fragrance mix I 8% in pet; [b]FM II: fragrance mix II 14% in pet; [c]Test concentration for unoxidised d-limonene, linalool; [d]Methyl 2-octynate have caused active sensitization when tested in 1% in pet and 2% in pet.; 0.2% has been tested without any problems was noted [134]

33

active sensitization when tested at 1 and 2% in pet., the concentration recommended for future testing is 0.2% in pet [134, 135].

In addition, benzenpropanol (Majantol®) 5% has recently been recommended for screening of fragrance-allergic individuals and is commercially available [99].

Some advances in the diagnostics of contact allergy to natural fragrance ingredients have also been attempted [24, 27–29]. Larsen tested a natural mix consisting of jasmine absolute, ylang ylang oil, narcissus absolute, sandalwood oil, and spearmint oil, and found that it identified 84% of perfume-allergic patients [30]. Natural extracts, such as ylang ylang oil, narcissus oil, sandalwood oil, and jasmine absolute, were identified as frequent sensitizers by Frosch [24], and relevant cases are missed by only testing with FM I. Still, a screening series of naturals awaits development and it is not known to which extent MP and oil of turpentine are good indicators of fragrance allergy to natural extracts in general, as has been suggested previously [64].

The role of colophony in detecting fragrance contact allergy is minor compared to MP, FM I, and FM II. Colophony has many different applications and it is uncertain if it is used in fragrances; however, ingredients of colophony may be present in fragrances or cross-reactivity may occur. No relationship between reactions to FM I or FM II and colophony was found in consecutive eczema patients tested in a European multicenter study [26]. While a significant relationship between colophony and FM I, as well as colophony and MP, was found in 747 patients suspected of fragrance contact allergy [102], it was also shown that the probability of a reaction to an extended fragrances series increased with the number of positive reactions to the fragrance indicators of the standard series [102]. In a recent investigation entailing a datamaterial of 10,128 patients, significant realtionships were found between FM I and colophony, FM I and MP, FM I and hydroxyisohexyl 3-cyclohexene carboxaldehyde, and between colophony and MP, all associations with an odds ratio over 5 [48].

As none of the current diagnostic tools is perfect, it is important to test with the cosmetic products, fine fragrances, essential oils, etc. used by the patient. It should generally be confined to stay-on products, as wash-off products, due to their irritant nature, make the interpretation of patch test reactions difficult. Further investigations of reactions to commercial products can be made based on the ingredient labeling of

sensitizing fragrance substances introduced for cosmetics and detergents in the EU region in 2005 (Table 33.5), by obtaining information/ingredients from the manufacturer [136] or by chemical fractionation in special cases [49] see Chap. 5.

> ### Core Message
>
> › A new fragrance mixture called FM II has been developed, which detects additional relevant cases of fragrance contact allergy. A validated screening agent or screening series for contact allergy to natural fragrance extracts is needed.

33.10 Clinical Relevance and Patient Advice

Clinical relevance can be assessed based on the patient's history of rashes to perfumes/perfumes products. A significant relationship between such a history and positive patch test to FM I has been shown previously [100, 128]. Currently, a higher proportion of patients giving a positive history is found among those reacting to the newly developed FM II than those reacting to FM I [25]. Assessment of exposure is an important component of clinical relevance. In a case study, all patients with a positive patch test to FM I ingredients were shown to be exposed to these allergens in cosmetic products causing eczema [129]. Similar findings exist for hydroxyisohexyl 3-cyclohexene carboxaldehyde [31, 129] and other FM II ingredients [29]. Simulations of exposure by repeated open application tests (ROAT) with commercial products containing FM I allergens have been shown to cause eczema in 60% of exposed patients who patch tested positive to FM I [40, 105]. Dummy products spiked with a single fragrance allergen in realistic concentrations have also been tested. In a series of deodorant exposure studies with cinnamal and hydroxycitronellal, 94–100% of eczema patients sensitized to the ingredient in question reacted, while all controls were negative [106, 107]. ROAT with realistic concentrations of hydroxyisohexyl 3-cyclohexene carboxaldehyde applied in ethanol caused reactions in 16 of 18 (89%) sensitized patients [116] and in 14/14 (100%) using a deodorant spiked with hydroxyisohexyl 3-cyclohexene carboxaldehyde [49].

Another indicator of clinical relevance is the strength of the patch reaction. Patients with strong reactions to the standard patch test FM I are more likely to react to the individual ingredients of the mix, to a low level of allergen [137], and to give a positive ROAT with the allergen in question [138]. Further, they are more likely to have a positive history of adverse reactions to fragranced products [128].

Thus, the advice given to the patient depends on the clinical presentation and the degree of allergy. Some patients have a weak degree of allergy and no chronic or recurrent eczema problem; they can usually tolerate (some) scented products on the skin. Others are more sensitive and have to abstain from stay-on products, while some cannot use any scented products at all, including wash-off products, such as shampoos. Patients with a chronic or relapsing eczema disease should be advised to use unscented emollients, regardless of whether they are allergic to fragrances or not, due to the risk of becoming sensitized and aggravation of their disease. In this context, it is important for the patient to know that the labeling "fragrance-free" may be misleading [139, 140]. Such products may contain fragrance ingredients, which are often various flower or plant extracts or chemicals acting as preservatives, e.g., geraniol and farnesol.

The mandatory labeling of 26 fragrance ingredients will enable the fragrance-allergic patient, who may wish to use fragranced cosmetics, to make a preselection of products based on the ingredient information. Further, it will provide the dermatologists with a tool for improving diagnostics and assessing clinical relevance. In a recent investigation of 147 fragrance-allergic patients, 45.3 % had found some kind of scented product they could tolerate, 31.6 % had not tried to find any scented products and 22 % had tried, but could not find any .The methods most often used were trying different products and reading the ingredient label [141].

The limits for labeling of the individual 26 ingredients are 10 ppm in stay-on products and 100 ppm in wash-off products. These limits are administrative and decided, as, otherwise, a labeling of all perfumed cosmetics was expected due to the presence of chemical allergens in trace amounts in essential oils. Information about presence of other fragrance ingredients in cosmetics can be obtained on a case basis by contact to the fragrance industry [136]. Clinical relevance is not a static phenomenon, especially not in the area of fragrance allergy. It is a question of interaction between individual predisposition/susceptibility and environmental exposures. Changes in general exposure to the allergens by interventions, e.g., legislation or just changes of fashion, will affect the clinical consequences of being contact allergic, defined by a positive patch test. These dynamics mean that assessment of the value of a diagnostic test such as FM I or FM II at a given time is only a snapshot. The focus, which has been on the ingredients of FM I and FM II by research programs on an EU-commission-level and by consumer organizations, means that exposure may decrease [98], as actually intended by these initiatives. The consequence is that fewer individuals will become sensitized to the allergens in question, as already indicated for FM I [73], and that fewer of those already sensitized will have clinical problems.

This should not lead to the confusion that the lack of clinical relevance is a sign of false-positive patch tests. It is a consequence of changing exposures and may be different in other geographical regions or may change again with time and exposure.

> **Core Message**
>
> › Twenty six fragrance ingredients with a sensitization potential has been mandated on the label of cosmetics and detergents from 2005 as information to the consumer. An administrative limit for the labeling has been set to 10 ppm. for stay-on products and 100 ppm. for wash-off products.

33.11 Other Skin Effects

33.11.1 Immediate Reactions

Fragrances have been reported to cause contact urticaria of the nonimmunological type. This is a high-dose effect, and cinnamal, cinnamic alcohol, and MP are known causes of contact urticaria, but others have been reported also [142–144]. The reactions to MP may be due to its containing cinnamates [71]. A relationship to delayed contact hypersensitivity has been suggested [145], but in a recent study no significant difference was found between a fragrance-allergic group and a control group in the frequency of immediate reactions to fragrance ingredients [144]. This is in keeping with a nonimmunological basis for the reactions seen [144]. A case of contact uricaria leading to anaphylaxis following an open patch test with cinnamal has been reported [146].

33.11.2 Photoallergy/Phototoxic Reactions

Musk ambrette produced a considerable number of photocontact allergic reactions in the 1970s [147, 148] and was later banned. Today, photoallergic contact dermatitis is uncommon [149]. Psoralens in naturally occurring fragrance ingredients were previously the cause of phototoxic reactions, giving rise to erythema, followed by hyperpigmentation in its characteristic form, called Berloque dermatitis [150]. There are now limits of the amount of psoralens in fragrance products. Phototoxic reactions still occur, but are rare [151].

33.11.3 Irritant Contact Dermatitis

Irritant effects of single fragrance ingredients are well known, e.g., citral [53, 55]. Autooxidation of fragrance terpenes not only increase the allergenicity, but also the irritant potential [152]. Probably, irritant contact dermatitis is frequent; however, no investigations exist substantiating this [75]. Many more people complain about rashes to perfumes/perfumed products than are proven allergic by testing [100]. This may be due to irritant effects or insufficient diagnostic apparatus.

33.12 Case Reports

A 23-year-old-woman presented with a long history of axillary dermatitis. Symptoms improved on changing to a different deodorant spray and worsened again with reuse of the former deodorant. Patch testing with the deodorant "as is" showed a ++ reaction, no reaction was seen to FM I 8% or colophony, while a ?+ was seen to MP. The perfume of the deodorant was tested in the same concentration as in the product and showed

a + reaction. Farnesol was present in the deodorant and gave ++ reaction upon testing at 1% in pet. [153].

Comment: Many cases of perfume allergy due to farnesol in deodorants have probably been overlooked in the past. It is important to test with the relevant products used by the patient and to use this test as guidance for further investigation. Farnesol is a constituent of the new diagnostic test FM II and is entailed by the ingredient labeling of selected fragrance allergens.

A 50-year-old-woman presented with an erythematous eruption, characterized by papules, vesicles, and crusting over the neck and chest. At patch testing, initially, the only positive reaction observed was with her own eau de toilette, named Women. FM I was negative. Chemical fractionation of the Women's perfume concentrate was combined with a sequenced patch testing procedure and with SAR studies. Ingredients supplied by the manufacturer were also included in the study. Benzophenone-2, Lyral®, α-hexyl cinnamic aldehyde, and alpha-damascone were found to be responsible for the patient's contact allergy to the eau de toilette, Women [154].

Comment: It is important to test with relevant products used by the patient. Light absorbers, such as benzophenone-2, are used in perfumes to protect against degradation. These may also be the cause of contact allergy. Some patients are allergic to several fragrance ingredients. Information about the contents of fragrance ingredients can be obtained from the fragrance manufacturer [136] and for selected fragrance allergens from the label of the product.

References

1. Müller J (1992) The H&R book of perfume. Understanding fragrance. Origin, history, development. Guide to fragrance ingredients. Glöss, Hamburg
2. Poucher WA (1993) Poucher's perfumes, cosmetics and soaps. The production, manufacture and application of perfumes, vol 2, 9th edn. Chapman and Hall, London
3. Bernard G, Giménez-Arnau E, Rastogi SC, Heydorn S, Johansen JD, Menné T, Goossens A, Andersen K, Lepoittevin JP (2003) Contact allergy to oak moss: search for sensitizing molecules using combined bioassay-guided chemical fractionation, GC-MS, and structure-activity relationship analysis. Arch Dermatol Res 295:229–235
4. Bauer K, Garbe D, Surburg H (1990) Common fragrance and flavor materials, 2nd edn. VCH Verlagsgesellschaft, Weinheim
5. Johansen JD (2002) Contact allergy to fragrances: clinical and experimental investigations of the fragrance mix and its ingredients. Contact Dermat 46(Suppl 3):4–31

6. Harder U (1998) The art of creating a perfume. In: Frosch PJ, Johansen JD, White IR (eds) Fragrances – beneficial and adverse effects. Springer, Berlin, Heidelberg, New York, pp 3–5

7. Christensson JB, Johansson S, Hagvall L, Jonsson C, Börje A, Karlberg AT (2008) Limonene hydroperoxide analogues differ in allergenic activity. Contact Dermat 59(6):344–352

8. Lepoittevin JP, Mutterer V (1998) Molecular aspects of fragrance sensitisation. In: Frosch PJ, Johansen JD, White IR (eds) Fragrances – beneficial and adverse effects. Springer, Berlin, Heidelberg, New York, pp 49–56

9. Christensson JB, Matura M, Gruvberger B, Bruze M, Karlberg AT (2010) Linalool–a significant contact sensitizer after air exposure. Contact Dermat 62(1):32–41

10. Hagvall L, Bäcktorp C, Svensson S, Nyman G, Börje A, Karlberg AT (2007) Fragrance compound geraniol forms contact allergens on air exposure. identification and quantification of oxidation products and effect on skin sensitization. Chem Res Toxicol 20:807–814

11. Basketter DA (1992) Skin sensitization to cinnamic alcohol: the role of skin metabolism. Acta Derm Venereol (Stockh) 72:264–265

12. Nilsson AM, Jonsson C, Luthman K, Nilsson JL, Karlberg AT (2004) Inhibition of the sensitizing effect of carvone by the addition of non-allergenic compounds. Acta Derm Venereol (Stockh) 84:99–105

13. Karlberg AT, Nilsson AM, Luthman K, Nilsson JL (2001) Structural analogues inhibit the sensitizing capacity of carvone. Acta Derm Venereol (Stockh) 81:398–402

14. Johansen JD, Skov L, Volund A, Andersen K, Menné T (1998) Allergens in combination have a synergistic effect on the elicitation response: a study of fragrance-sensitized individuals. Br J Dermatol 139:264–270

15. Marzulli FN, Maibach HI (1980) Contact allergy: predictive testing of fragrance ingredients in humans by Draize and maximization methods. J Environ Pathol Toxicol 3: 235–245

16. Patlewicz GY, Wright ZM, Basketter DA, Pease CK, Lepoittevin JP, Arnau EG (2002) Structure-activity relationships for selected fragrance allergens. Contact Dermat 47:219–226

17. Rastogi SC, Lepoittevin JP, Johansen JD, Frosch P, Menné T, Bruze M, Dreier B, Andersen KE, White I (1998) Fragrances and other materials in deodorants – search for potentially sensitizing molecules using combined GC–MS and structure activity relationship (SAR) analysis. Contact Dermat 39:293–303

18. Patlewicz GY, Basketter DA, Pease CK, Wilson K, Roberts DW, Bernard G, Arnau EG, Lepoittevin JP (2004) Further evaluation of quantitative structure activity relationship models for the prediction of the skin sensitization potency of selected fragrance allergens. Contact Dermat 50:91–97

19. Larsen WG (1977) Perfume dermatitis. A study of 20 patients. Arch Dermatol 113:623–626

20. Malten KE, van Ketel WG, Nater JP, Liem DH (1984) Reactions in selected patients to 22 fragrance materials. Contact Dermat 11:1–10

21. de Groot AC, Liem DH, Nater JP, van Ketel WG (1985) Patch tests with fragrance materials and preservatives. Contact Dermat 12:87–92

22. Frosch PJ, Pilz B, Andersen KE, Burrows D, Camasara JG, Dooms-Goossens A, Ducombs G, Fuchs T, Hannuksela M, Lachapelle JM, Lahti A, Maibach HI, Menne T, Rycroft RJG, Shaw S, Wahlberg JE, White IR, Wilkinson JD (1995) Patch testing with fragrances: results of a multicenter study of the European Environmental and Contact Dermatitis Research Group with 48 frequently used constituents of perfumes. Contact Dermat 33:333–342

23. Frosch PJ, Johansen JD, Menné T, Pirker C, Rastogi SC, Andersen KE, Bruze M, Goossens A, Lepoittevin JP, White IR (2000) Further important sensitizers in patients sensitive to fragrances. I. Reactivity to 14 frequently used chemicals. Contact Dermat 47:78–85

24. Frosch PJ, Johansen JD, Menné T, Pirker C, Rastogi SC, Andersen KE, Bruze M, Goossens A, Lepoittevin JP, White IR (2002) Further important sensitizers in patients sensitive to fragrances. II. Reactivity to essential oils. Contact Dermat 47:279–287

25. Frosch PJ, Pirker C, Rastogi SC, Andersen KE, Bruze M, Svedman C, Goossens A, White IR, Uter W, Arnau EG, Lepoittevin JP, Menné T, Johansen JD (2005) Patch testing with a new fragrance mix detects additional patients sensitive to perfumes and missed by the current fragrance mix. Contact Dermat 52:207–215

26. Frosch PJ, Rastogi SC, Pirker C, Brinkmeier T, Andersen KE, Bruze M, Svedman C, Goossens A, White IR, Uter W, Arnau EG, Lepoittevin JP, Johansen JD, Menné T (2005) Patch testing with a new fragrance mix – reactivity to the single constituents and chemical detection in relevant cosmetic products. Contact Dermat 52:216–225

27. Larsen W, Nakayama H, Lindberg M, Fischer T, Elsner P, Burrows D, Jordan W, Shaw S, Wilkinson J, Marks J Jr, Sugawara M, Nethercott J (1996) Fragrance contact dermatitis: a worldwide multicenter investigation, part I. Am J Contact Dermat 7:77–83

28. Larsen W, Nakayama H, Fischer T, Elsner P, Frosch P, Burrows D, Jordan W, Shaw S, Wilkinson J, Marks J Jr, Sugawara M, Nethercott M, Nethercott J (2001) Fragrance contact dermatitis: a worldwide multicenter investigation, part II. Contact Dermat 44:344–346

29. Larsen W, Nakayama H, Fischer T, Elsner P, Frosch P, Burrows D, Jordan W, Shaw S, Wilkinson J, Marks J Jr, Sugawara M, Nethercott M, Nethercott J (2002) Fragrance contact dermatitis: a worldwide multicenter investigation, part III. Contact Dermat 46:141–144

30. Larsen W, Nakayama H, Fischer T, Elsner P, Frosch P, Burrows D, Jordan W, Shaw S, Wilkinson J, Marks J Jr, Sugawara M, Nethercott M, Nethercott J (1998) A study of new fragrance mixtures. Am J Contact Dermat 9:202–206

31. Frosch PJ, Johansen JD, Menné T, Rastogi SC, Bruze M, Andersen KE, Lepoittevin JP, Arnau EG, Pirker C, Goossens A, White IR (1999) Lyral is an important sensitizer in patients sensitive to fragrances. Br J Dermatol 141:1076–1083

32. Enders F, Przybilla B, Ring J (1989) Patch testing with fragrance mix 16% and 8%, and its individual constituents. Contact Dermat 20:237–238

33. Schnuch A, Uter W, Geier J, Lessmann H, Frosch PJ (2007) Sensitization to 26 fragrances to be labelled according to current European regulation. Results of the IVDK and review of the literature. Contact Dermat 57(1):1–10

34. Buckley DA, Wakelin SH, Holloway D, Rycroft RJG, White IR, McFadden JP (2000) The frequency of fragrance allergy in a patch test population over a 17-year period. Br J Dermatol 142:279–283

35. Meding B, Wrangsjo K, Brisman J, Jarvholm B (2003) Hand eczema in 45 bakers – a clinical study. Contact Dermat 48:7–11

36. Bauer A, Geier J, Elsner P (2002) Type IV allergy in the food processing industry: sensitization profiles in bakers, cooks and butchers. Contact Dermat 46:228–235

37. Buckley DA (2007) Fragrance ingredient labelling in products on sale in the UK. Br J Dermatol 157(2):295–300

38. Elahi EN, Wright Z, Hinselwood D, Hotchkiss SA, Basketter DA, Pease CK (2004) Protein binding and metabolism influence the relative skin sensitization potential of cinnamic compounds. Chem Res Toxicol 17:301–310

39. Tananka S, Royds C, Buckley D, Basketter DA, Goossens A, Bruze M, Svedman C, Menné T, Johansen JD, White IR, McFadden JP (2004) Contact allergy to isoeugenol and its derivatives: problems with allergen substitution. Contact Dermat 51:288–291

40. Johansen JD, Rastogi SC, Menné T (1996) Contact allergy to popular perfumes; assessed by patch test, use test and chemical analysis. Br J Dermatol 135:419–422

41. Barratt MD, Basketter DA (1992) Possible origin of the skin sensitization potential of isoeugenol and related compounds, (I). Preliminary studies of potential reactions mechanisms. Contact Dermat 27:98–104

42. Bertrand F, Basketter DA, Roberts DW, Lepoittevin JP (1997) Skin sensitization to eugenol and isoeugenol in mice: possible metabolic pathways involving ortho-quinone and quinone methide intermediates. Chem Res Toxicol 10:335–343

43. White JM, White IR, Glendinning A, Fleming J, Jefferies D, Basketter DA, McFadden JP, Buckley DA (2007) Frequency of allergic contact dermatitis to isoeugenol is increasing: a review of 3636 patients tested from 2001 to 2005. Br J Dermatol 157(3):580–582

44. Rastogi SC, Johansen JD (2008) Significant exposures to isoeugenol derivatives in perfumes. Contact Dermat 58(5):278–281

45. Basketter DA, Wright ZM, Warbrick EV, Dearman RJ, Kimber I, Ryan CA, Gerberick GF, White IR (2001) Human potency predictions for aldehydes using the local lymph node assay. Contact Dermat 45:89–94

46. Fenn RS (1989) Aroma chemical usage trends in modern perfumery. Perfumer Flavorist 14:1–10

47. Uter W, Geier J, Schnuch A, Frosch PJ (2007) Patch test results with patients' own perfumes, deodorants and shaving lotions: results of the IVDK 1998-2002. J Eur Acad Dermatol Venereol 21(3):374–379

48. Nardelli A, Carbonez A, Ottoy W, Drieghe J, Goossens A (2008) Frequency of and trends in fragrance allergy over a 15-year period. Contact Dermat 58(3):134–141

49. Jørgensen PH, Jensen CD, Rastogi S, Andersen KE, Johansen JD (2007) Experimental elicitation with hydroxy-isohexyl-3-cyclohexene carboxaldehyde-containing deodorants. Contact Dermat 56(3):146–150

50. Braendstrup P, Johansen JD, Danish Contact Dermatitis Group (2008) Hydroxyisohexyl 3-cyclohexene carboxaldehyde (Lyral) is still a frequent allergen. Contact Dermat 59(3):187–188

51. Goossens A, Merckx L (1997) Allergic contact dermatitis from farnesol in a deodorant. Contact Dermat 37:179–180

52. Schnuch A, Uter W, Geier J, Lessmann H, Frosch PJ (2004) Contact allergy to farnesol in 2021 consecutively patch tested patients. Results of the IVDK. Contact Dermat 50:117–121

53. Heydorn S, Menné T, Andersen KE, Bruze M, Svedman C, White IR, Basketter DA (2003) Citral a fragrance allergen and irritant. Contact Dermat 49:32–36

54. Heydorn S, Johansen JD, Andersen KE, Bruze M, Svedman C, White IR, Basketter DA, Menné T (2003) Fragrance allergy in patients with hand eczema – clinical study. Contact Dermat 48:317–323

55. Rothenborg HW, Menné T, Sjolin KE (1977) Temperature dependent primary irritant dermatitis from lemon perfume. Contact Dermat 3:37–48

56. Mutterer V, Gimenez Arnau E, Lepoittevin JP, Johansen JD, Frosch PJ, Menné T, Andersen KE, Bruze M, Rastogi SC, White IR (1999) Identification of coumarin as the sensitizer in a patient sensitive to her own perfume but negative to the fragrance mix. Contact Dermat 40:196–199

57. Kunkeler AC, Weijland JW, Bruynzeel DP (1998) The role of coumarin in patch testing. Contact Dermat 39:327–328

58. Johansen JD, Andersen KE, Svedman C, Bruze M, Bernard G, Gimenez-Arnau E, Rastogi SC, Lepoittevin JP, Menné T (2003) Chloroatranol, an extremely potent allergen hidden in perfumes: a dose-response elicitation study. Contact Dermat 49:180–184

59. Vocanson M, Valeyrie M, Rozières A, Hennino A, Floc'h F, Gard A, Nicolas JF (2007) Lack of evidence for allergenic properties of coumarin in a fragrance allergy mouse model. Contact Dermat 57(6):361–364

60. Matura M, Goossens A, Bordalo O, Garcia-Bravo B, Magnusson K, Wrangsjo K, Karlberg AT (2003) Patch testing with oxidized R-(+)-limonene and its hydroperoxide fraction. Contact Dermat 49:15–21

61. Matura M, Goossens A, Bordalo O, Garcia-Bravo B, Magnusson K, Wrangsjo K, Karlberg AT (2002) Oxidized citrus oil (R-limonene): a frequent skin sensitizer in Europe. J Am Acad Dermatol 47:709–714

62. Skold M, Borje A, Matura M, Karlberg AT (2002) Studies on the autoxidation and sensitizing capacity of the fragrance chemical linalool, identifying a linalool hydroperoxide. Contact Dermat 46:267–272

63. Skold M, Borje A, Harambasic E, Karlberg AT (2004) Contact allergens formed on air exposure of linalool. Identification and quantification of primary and secondary oxidization products and effects on skin sensitization. Chem Res Toxicol 17:1697–1705

64. Schnuch A, Lessmann H, Geier J, Frosch PJ, Uter W, IDVK (2004) Contact allergy to fragrances: frequencies of sensitization from 1996 to 2002. Results of the IVDK. Contact Dermat 50:65–76

65. Rastogi SC, Bossi R, Johansen JD, Menné T, Bernard G, Giménez-Arnau E, Lepoittevin JP (2004) Content of oak moss allergens atranol and chloroatranol in perfumes and similar products. Contact Dermat 50:367–370

66. Nardelli A, Giménez-Arnau E, Bernard G, Lepoittevin JP, Goossens A (2009) Is a low content in atranol/chloroatranol safe in oak moss-sensitized individuals? Contact Dermat 60(2):91–95

67. Nakayama H (1998) Fragrance hypersensitivity and its control. In: Frosch PJ, Johansen JD, White IR (eds) Fragrances – beneficial and adverse effects. Springer, Berlin, Heidelberg, New York, pp 83–91

68. Hagvall L, Sköld M, Bråred-Christensson J, Börje A, Karlberg AT (2008) Lavender oil lacks natural protection against autoxidation, forming strong contact allergens on air exposure. Contact Dermat 59(3):143–150

69. Hausen BM, Simatupang T, Bruhn G, Evers P, Koenig WA (1995) Identification of new allergens constituents and proof of evidence for coniferyl benzoate in balsam of Peru. Am J Contact Dermat 6:199–208

70. Hjorth N (1961) Eczematous allergy to balsams. Allied perfumes and flavoring agents – with special reference to balsam of Peru. Thesis, University of Copenhagen, Denmark

71. Hausen BM (2001) Contact allergy to balsam of Peru. II. Patch test results in 102 patients with selected balsam of Peru constituents. Am J Contact Dermat 12:93–102

72. Api AM (2006) Only Peru Balsam extracts or distillates are used in perfumery. Contact Dermat 54(3):179

73. Thyssen JP, Linneberg A, Menné T, Nielsen NH, Johansen JD (2009) The prevalence and morbidity of sensitization to fragrance mix I in the general population. Br J Dermatol 161:95–101

74. Karlberg AT (2000) Colophony. In: Kanerva L, Elsner P, Wahlberg J, Maibach H (eds) Handbook of occupational dermatology, vol 64. Springer, Berlin, Heidelberg, New York, pp 509–516

75. de Groot AC, Frosch PJ (1997) Adverse reactions to fragrances. A clinical review. Contact Dermat 36:57–87

76. Cronin E (1980) Perfumes: contact dermatitis. Churchill Livingstone, Edinburgh, pp 158–170

77. Bruze M, Andersen KE, Goossens A (2008) Recommendation to include fragrance mix 2 and hydroxyisohexyl 3-cyclohexene carboxaldehyde (Lyral®) in the European Baseline patch test series. Contact Dermat 58:129–133

78. Maouad M, Fleischer AB, Sherertz EF, Feldman SR (1999) Significance-prevalence index number: a reinterpretation and enhancement of data from the North American Contact Dermatitis group. J Am Acad Dermatol 41:573–576

79. Li LF, Guo J, Wang J (2004) Environmental contact factors in eczema and the results of patch testing Chinese patients with a modified European standard series of allergens. Contact Dermat 51:22–25

80. Greig JE, Carson CF, Stuckey MS, Riley TV (2000) Prevalence of delayed hypersensitivity to the European standard series in a self-selected population. Australas J Dermatol 41:86–89

81. Mortz CG, Lauritsen JM, Bindslev-Jensen C, Andersen KE (2002) Contact allergy and allergic contact dermatitis in adolescents: prevalence measures and associations. The Odense Adolescence Cohort Study on Atopic Diseases and Dermatitis (TOACS). Acta Derm Venereol (Stockh) 82:352–358

82. Nielsen NH, Menné T (1992) Allergic contact sensitization in an unselected Danish population. The Glostrup Allergy Study. Acta Derm Venereol (Stockh) 72:456–460

83. Nielsen NH, Linneberg A, Menné T, Madsen F, Frolund L, Dirksen A, Jorgensen T (2001) Allergic contact sensitization in an adult Danish population: two cross-sectional surveys eight years apart (the Copenhagen Allergy Study). Acta Derm Venereol (Stockh) 81:31–34

84. Dotterud LK (2007) The prevalence of allergic contact sensitization in a general population in Tromsø, Norway. Int J Circumpolar Health 66(4):328–334

85. Schnuch A, Uter W, Geier J, Gefeller O, IDVK study group (2002) Epidemiology of contact allergy: an estimation of morbidity employing the clinical epidemiology and drug-utilization research (CE-DUR) approach. Contact Dermat 47:32–39

86. Thyssen JP, Carlsen BC, Menné T, Johansen JD (2008) Trends of contact allergy to fragrance mix I and Myroxylon pereirae among Danish eczema patients tested between 1985 and 2007. Contact Dermat 59(4):238–244

87. Bruynzeel DP, Diepgen TL, Andersen KE, Brandão FM, Bruze M, Frosch PJ, Goossens A, Lahti A, Mahler V, Maibach HI, Menné T, Wilkinson JD, European Environmental and Contact Dermatitis Research Group (2005) Monitoring the European standard series in 10 centres 1996-2000. Contact Dermat 53(3):146–149

88. Uter W, Hegewald J, Aberer W, Ayala F, Bircher AJ, Brasch J, Coenraads PJ, Schuttelaar ML, Elsner P, Fartasch M, Mahler V, Belloni Fortina A, Frosch PJ, Fuchs T, Johansen JD, Menné T, Jolanki R, Krêcisz B, Kiec-Swierczynska M, Larese F, Orton D, Peserico A, Rantanen T, Schnuch A (2005) The European standard series in 9 European countries, 2002/2003 – first results of the European Surveillance System on Contact Allergies. Contact Dermat 53(3):136–145

89. Zug KA, Warshaw EM, Fowler JF Jr, Maibach HI, Belsito DL, Pratt MD, Sasseville D, Storrs FJ, Taylor JS, Mathias CG, Deleo VA, Rietschel RL (2009) Patch-test results of the North American Contact Dermatitis Group 2005-2006. Dermatitis 20:149–160

90. Boonchai W, Lamtharachai P, Sunthonpalin P (2008) Prevalence of allergic contact dermatitis in Thailand. Dermatitis 19:142–145

91. Geier J, Lessmann H, Uter W, Schnuch A (2006) experiences with fragrance mix II – the German perspective. Contact Dermat 55:12

92. Buckley DA, Rycroft RJG, White IR, McFadden JP (2003) The frequency of fragrance allergy in patch-tested patients increases with their age. Br J Dermatol 149:986–989

93. Uter W, Schnuch A (2004) Fragrance allergy increases with age. Br J Dermatol 150:1212–1234

94. Mortz C, Andersen KE (1999) Allergic contact dermatitis in children and adolescents. Contact Dermat 41:121–130

95. Heine G, Schnuch A, Uter W, Worm M (2004) Frequency of contact allergy in German children and adolescents patch tested between 1995 and 2002: results from the Information Network of Departments of Dermatology and the German Contact Dermatitis Group. Contact Dermat 51:111–117

96. Johansen JD, Menné T, Christophersen J, Kaaber K, Veien N (2000) Changes in the sensitization pattern to common allergens in Denmark between 1985–1986 and 1997–1998, with a special view to the effect of preventive strategies. Br J Dermatol 142:490–495

97. White JML, White IR, Kimber I, Basketter DA, Buckley DA, McFadden JP (2009) Atopic dermatitis and allergic reactions to individual fragrance chemicals. Allergy 64:312–316

98. Rastogi SC, Menné T, Johansen JD (2003) The composition of fine fragrances is changing. Contact Dermat 48: 130–132

33

99. Schnuch A, Geier J, Uter W, Frosch PJ (2007) Majantol® a new inportant fragrance allergen. Contact Dermat 57:48–50

100. Johansen JD, Andersen TF, Veien N, Avnstorp C, Andersen KE, Menné T (1997) Patch testing with markers of fragrance contact allergy. Do clinical tests correspond to patients' self-reported problems? Acta Derm Venereol (Stockh) 77:149–153

101. Katz AS, Sheretz F (1999) Facial dermatitis: patch test results and final diagnosis. Am J Contact Dermat 10:153–156

102. Wöhrl S, Hemmer W, Focke M, Görtz M, Jarisch R (2001) The significance of fragrance mix, balsam of Peru, colophony and propolis as screening tools in the detection of fragrance allergy. Br J Dermatol 145:268–273

103. Edman B (1994) The influence of shaving method on perfume allergy. Contact Dermat 31:291–292

104. Johansen JD, Andersen TF, Kjøller M, Veien N, Avnstorp C, Andersen KE, Menné T (1998) Identification of risk products for fragrance contact allergy: a case-referent study based on patients' histories. Am J Contact Dermat 2:80–87

105. Johansen JD, Rastogi SC, Bruze M, Andersen KE, Frosch PJ, Dreier B, Lepoittevin JP, White IR, Menné T (1998) Deodorants: a clinical provocation study in fragrance-sensitive individuals. Contact Dermat 39:161–165

106. Svedman C, Bruze M, Johansen JD, Andersen KE, Goossens A, Frosch PJ, Lepoittevin JP, Rastogi S, White IR, Menne T (2003) Deodorants: an experimental provocation study with hydroxycitronellal. Contact Dermat 48:217–223

107. Bruze M, Johansen JD, Andersen KE, Frosch P, Lepoittevin JP, Rastogi S, Wakelin S, White I, Menne T (2003) Deodorants: an experimental provocation study with cinnamic aldehyde. J Am Acad Dermatol 48:194–200

108. von Peter C, Hoting E (1993) Anwendungstest mit parfümierten Kosmetika bei Patienten mit positivem Epikutantest auf Duftsstoff-Mischung. Dermatosen 41:237–241

109. Heydorn S, Menné T, Johansen JD (2003) Fragrance allergy and hand eczema – a review. Contact Dermat 48:59–66

110. Buckley DA, Rycroft RJG, White IR, McFadden JP (2000) Contact allergy to individual fragrance mix constituents in relation to primary site of dermatitis. Contact Dermat 43:304–305

111. Christophersen J, Menne T, Tanghoj P, Andersen KE, Brandrup F, Kaaber K, Osmundsen PE, Thestrup-Pedersen K, Veien NK (1989) Clinical patch test data evaluated by multivariate analysis. Danish Contact Dermatitis Group. Contact Dermat 21:291–299

112. Katsarma G, Gawkrodger DJ (1999) Suspected fragrance contact allergy requires extended patch testing to individual fragrance allergens. Contact Dermat 41:193–197

113. Veien NK (1989) Systemically induced eczema in adults. Acta Derm Venereol Suppl (Stockh) 147:1–58

114. Niinimaki A (1995) Double-blind placebo-controlled peroral challenges in patients with delayed-type allergy to balsam of Peru. Contact Dermat 33:78–83

115. Veien NK, Hattel T, Laurberg G (1996) Can oral challenge with balsam of Peru predict possible benefit from a low-balsam diet? Am J Contact Dermat 7:84–87

116. Johansen JD, Frosch PJ, Svedman C, Andersen KE, Bruze M, Pirker C, Menné T (2003) Hydroxyisohexyl 3-cyclohexene carboxaldehyde – known as Lyral: quantitative aspects and risk assessment of an important fragrance allergen. Contact Dermat 48:310–316

117. Rastogi SC, Johansen JD, Menné T (1996) Natural ingredient based cosmetics. Content of selected fragrance sensitizers. Contact Dermat 34:423–426

118. Rastogi SC, Johansen JD, Menné T, Frosch PJ, Bruze M, Andersen KE, Lepoittevin JP, Wakelin S, White IR (1999) Contents of fragrance allergens in children's cosmetics and cosmetic-toys. Contact Dermat 41:84–88

119. Rastogi SC, Heydorn S, Johansen JD, Basketter D (2001) Fragrance chemicals in domestic and occupational products. Contact Dermat 45:221–225

120. Nardelli A, D'Hooghe E, Drieghe J, Dooms M, Goossens A (2009) Allergic contact dermatitis from fragrance components in specific topical pharmaceutical products in Belgium. Contact Dermat 60(6):303–313

121. Wallenhammar LM, Ortengren U, Andreasson H, Barregard L, Bjorkner B, Karlsson S, Wrangsjo K, Meding B (2000) Contact allergy and hand eczema in Swedish dentists. Contact Dermat 43:192–199

122. Uter W, Schnuch A, Geier J, Pfahlberg A, Gefeller O, IVDK study group. Information Network of Departments of Dermatology (2001) Association between occupation and contact allergy to the fragrance mix: a multifactorial analysis of national surveillance data. Occup Environ Med 58:392–398

123. Geier J, Lessmann SA, Uter W (2004) Contact sensitization in metalworkers with occupational dermatitis exposed to water-based metalworking fluids: results of the research project "FaSt". Int Arch Occup Environ Health 77:543–551

124. Owen CM, August PJ, Beck MH (2000) Contact allergy to oak moss resin in a soluble oil. Contact Dermat 43:112

125. Pontén A, Björk J, Carstensen O, Gruvberger B, Isaksson M, Rasmussen K, Bruze M (2004) Associations between contact allergy to epoxy resin and fragrance mix. Acta Derm Venereol (Stockh) 84:151–175

126. Larsen WG (1987) Detection of allergic dermatitis to fragrances. Acta Derm Venereol (Stockh) 134:83–86

127. de Groot AC, van der Kley AM, Bruynzeel DP, Meinardi MM, Smeenk G, van Joost T, Pavel S (1993) Frequency of false-negative reactions to the fragrance mix. Contact Dermat 28:139–140

128. Frosch PJ, Pilz B, Burrows D, Camarasa JG, Lachapelle J-M, Lahti A, Menné T, Wilkinson JD (1995) Testing with fragrance mix. Is the addition of sorbitan sesquioleate to the constituents useful? Contact Dermat 32:266–272

129. Johansen JD, Rastogi SC, Menné T (1996) Exposure to selected fragrance materials. A case study of fragrance-mix-positive eczema patients. Contact Dermat 34:106–110

130. Trattner A, David M (2003) Patch testing with fine fragrances: comparison with fragrance mix, balsam of Peru and a fragrance series. Contact Dermat 49:287–289

131. Johansen JD, Rastogi SC, Andersen KE, Menné T (1997) Content and reactivity to product perfumes in fragrance mix positive and negative eczema patients. A study of perfumes used in toiletries and skin-care products. Contact Dermat 36:291–296

132. de Groot AC, Coenraads PJ, Bruynzeel DP, Jagtman BA, van Ginkel CJ, Noz K, van der Valk PG, Pavel S, Vink J, Weyland JW (2000) Routine patch testing with fragrance chemicals in the Netherlands. Contact Dermat 42:184–185

133. Geier J, Brasch J, Schnuch A, Lessmann H, Pirker C, Frosch PJ, For the Information Network of Departments of Dermatology (IVDK) and the German Contact Dermatitis

Research Group (DKG) (2002) Lyral has been included in the patch test standard series in Germany. Contact Dermat 46:295–297

134. Bruze M, Svedman C, Andersen KE, Bruynzeel D, Goossens A, Duus Johansen J, Matura M, Orton D, Vigan M, On Behalf Of The ESCD (2009) Patch test concentrations for the 12 non-mix fragrance substances regulated by European legislation. Contact Dermatitis under submission

135. Heisterberg MV, Vigan M, Johansen JD (2010) Active sensitization and allergic contact dermatitis caused by methyl heptine carbonate. Contact Dermat 62(2):97–101

136. Roberts G (2002) Procedures for supplying fragrance information to dermatologists. Letter to the editor. Am J Contact Dermat 13:206–207

137. Johansen JD, Andersen KE, Rastogi SC, Menné T (1996) Threshold responses in cinnamic-aldehyde-sensitive subjects: results and methodological aspects. Contact Dermat 34:165–171

138. Johansen JD, Andersen KE, Menné T (1996) Quantitative aspects of isoeugenol contact allergy assessed by use and patch tests. Contact Dermat 34:414–418

139. Scheinman PL (2001) Exposing covert fragrance chemicals. Am J Contact Dermat 12:225–228

140. Scheinman PL (1999) The foul side of fragrance-free products: what every clinician should know about managing patients with fragrance allergy. J Am Acad Dermatol 41:1020–1024

141. Lysdal SH, Johansen JD (2009) Fragrance allergic patients-strategies for use of cosmetic products and perceived impact on life situation. Contact Dermat 61(6): 320–324

142. Safford RJ, Basketter DA, Allenby CF, Goodwin BF (1990) Immediate contact reactions to chemicals in the fragrance mix and a study of the quenching action of eugenol. Br J Dermatol 123:595–606

143. Temesvari E, Nemeth I, Balo-Banga MJ, Husz S, Kohanka V, Somos Z, Judak R, Remenyik EVA, Szegedi A, Nebenführer L, Meszaros C, Horvath A (2002) Multicentre study of fragrance allergy in Hungary. Immediate and late type reactions. Contact Dermat 46:325–330

144. Tanaka S, Matsumoto Y, Dlova N, Ostlere LS, Goldsmith PC, Rycroft RJG, Basketter DA, White IR, Banerjee P, McFadden JP (2004) Immediate contact reactions to fragrance mix constituents and Myroxylon pereirae resin. Contact Dermat 51:20–21

145. Katsarou A, Armenaka M, Ale I, Koufou V, Kalogeromitros D (1999) Frequency of immediate reactions to the European standard series. Contact Dermat 41:276–279

146. Diba VC, Statham BN (2003) Contact urticaria from cinnamal leading to anafylaxis. Contact Dermat 48:119

147. Kroon S (1979) Musk Ambrette, a new cosmetic sensitizer and photo sensitizer. Contact Dermat 5:337–338

148. Cronin E (1984) Photosensitivity to musk ambrette. Contact Dermat 11:88–92

149. Darvay A, White IR, Rycroft RJ, Jones AB, Hawk JL, McFadden JP (2001) Photoallergic contact dermatitis is uncommon. Br J Dermatol 145:597–601

150. Cronin E (1980) Phototoxic reactions. Contact dermatitis. Churchill Livingstone, Edinburgh, pp 417–432

151. Wang L, Sterling B, Don P (2002) Berloque dermatitis induced by "Florida water". Cutis 70:29–30

152. Bråred Christensson J, Forsström P, Wennberg AM, Karlberg AT, Matura M (2009) Air oxidation increases skin irritation from fragrance terpenes. Contact Dermat 60:32–40

153. Hemmer W, Focke M, Leitner B, Görtz M, Jarisch R (2000) Axillary dermatitis from farnesol in a deodorant. Contact Dermat 42:168

154. Gimenez-Arnau A, Giminez-Arnau E, Serra-Bladrich E, Lepoittevin JP, Camarasa JG (2002) Principels and methodology for identification of fragrance allergens in consumer products. Contact Dermat 47:345–352

155. Rastogi SC, Johansen JD, Frosch PJ, Menné T, Bruze M, Lepoittevin JP, Dreier B, Andersen KE, White IR (1998) Deodorants on the European market: quantitative chemical analysis of 21 fragrances. Contact Dermat 38:29–35

156. Czarnobilska E, Obtulowicz K, Dyga W, Wsolek-Wnek K, Spiewak R (2009) Contact hypersensitivity and allergic contact dermatitis among school children and teenagers with eczema. Contact Dermat 60:264–269

Hair Dyes

34

David Basketter, Jeanne Duus Johansen,
John McFadden, and Heidi Søsted

Contents

D. Basketter (✉)
DABMEB Consultancy Ltd, Incorporated in England and Wales,
2 Normans Road, Sharnbrook, Bedfordshire MK44 1PR, UK
e-mail: david.basketter@ukonline.co.uk

J.D. Johansen (✉)
Copenhagen University Hospital Gentofte, National Allergy
Research Centre, Department of Dermato-allergology,
Niels Andersens Vej 65, 2900 Hellerup, Denmark
e-mail: jedu@geh.regionh.dk

J. McFadden
Department of Cutaneous Allergy, St John's Institute of
Dermatology, St Thomas' Hospital, London SE1 7EH, UK

H. Søsted
Research Center for Hairdressers and Beauticians,
Gentofte Hospital, University of Copenhagen, 2900 Hellerup,
Denmark

34.1 Introduction

Henna was originally used in ancient Egypt to stain the fingers and toes of the Pharaohs prior to mummification. This goes back 4,000 years, and today, in the twenty first century, people still color their body and hair. The oxidative hair dye process had been invented by the end of the nineteenth century. Reactions with aromatic amines, such as *p*-phenylenediamine (PPD), toluene-2,5-diamine and *m*-aminophenols, resorcinol, and hydrogen peroxide made it possible to make a permanent coloring of hair [1]. Contact dermatitis to synthetic hair dyes has been known for many years, and in 1939, Bonnevie suggested resorcinol, PPD, and aminophenol as part of a patch test standard series for identifying patients sensitized to PPD by furs, hair dyes, or occupational exposure [2]. Even today, PPD is allowed for the coloring of human hair and the sales of hair dyes containing aromatic amines are very substantial. A Danish population-based study showed that almost 75% of women and 18% of men had dyed their hair at some point in their lives [3]. In a UK study, 47% reported having used hair dye [4]. It was found that the median age for the first hair dyeing was 16 years [3]. This means that hair coloring is not just used for covering gray hair, but is also a fashion among teenagers [5]. Hair dyes are found in three common classes and allergic contact dermatitis has been observed for all kinds of hair dyes. *Oxidative dyes* produce a permanent dyeing

J.D. Johansen et al. (eds.), *Contact Dermatitis*,
DOI: 10.1007/978-3-642-03827-3_34, © Springer-Verlag Berlin Heidelberg 2011

of the hair that cannot be washed out. They consist of two components that are mixed before use. They contain a precursor/primary intermediates; these substances could be, for example, PPD, toluene-2,5-diamine or *p*-aminophenol, and a coupler, typically, *m*-aminophenol, resorcinol, or others, all of which have been described as contact sensitizers [6–8]. Couplers determine the final shade by reaction with the oxidized form of primary intermediates, followed by further oxidative coupling reactions. Oxidants could be hydrogen peroxide, urea peroxide, or sodium percarbonate or perborate. Some oxidative dyes contain alkalinizing agents, such as ammonia, monoethanolamine, or aminomethylpropanol. *Semipermanent hair dyes* are nitrophenylenediamine, nitro-aminophenol, or azo dyes [9], which, because of their low molecular weight, enter the hair follicle. *Temporary dyes* contain larger molecules and the dye does not enter the hair follicle, but remain as a layer around each follicle.

A questionnaire study in Denmark showed that 5.3% of the people who have dyed their hair reported an adverse skin reaction compatible with allergic origin, and only about one in six of these people contacted the health care services [3]. A questionnaire study in United Kingdom showed that 14% reported eczematous reactions after clouring their hair while 3% reported features of angio-oedema and only 15% sought professional help [4]. Other studies confirm that only a minority of patients with hair dye reactions are investigated by a dermatologist [10].

> **Core Message**
>
> › Allergic contact dermatitis has been seen to occur from all kinds of hair dyes (permanent oxidative, semipermanent, and temporary dyes), but is believed to be the most common with permanent dyes.

34.2 Clinical Picture

34.2.1 Allergic Contact Dermatitis

The severity of clinical symptoms from hair dyeing may vary considerably. There may be intense edema of the face, particularly of the eyes, with exudation of the scalp. Erythema and swelling may extend down the

neck, on to the upper chest and arms, and can even become generalized. The swelling of the face may be so striking that a mistaken diagnosis of angioneurotic edema is made (see Fig. 34.1) [10, 11]. Less dramatic symptoms are periodic swelling of the eyes related to hair dyeing or acute eczema at the scalp margins, sometimes extending to the neck or face (see Fig. 34.2) [2, 11]. Men dyeing their beard may have similar symptoms, although with varying severity [12]. In hairdressers, the most common regions affected are the hands and arms; [13] however, even though patients who apply the dye themselves wear gloves, their hands and arms occasionally may be affected [11]. The onset of symptoms may be from a few hours to the following day(s). The symptoms can be long lasting, even if hair dyeing is avoided. In a study concerning 55 cases of hair dye allergy, 23 had symptoms for more than 3 weeks [10], and hair loss has been reported following severe scalp reactions [10, 14]. A number of morphological variants of disease expression occur, including leukoderma, lichenoid, and erythema multiforme-like rash [15–17].

> **Core Message**
>
> › Hair dye allergy may cause severe clinical reactions, with edema of the face, eyelids, and scalp. More moderate reactions such as erythema, suppuration, and ulceration, typically at the scalp margin, on the ears, and sometimes with evidence of eczema where the dye has run down the neck are seen.

34.3 Temporary Black Tattoos

Temporary black henna tattoos may contain PPD and give rise to the induction of PPD allergy. The level of PPD in tattoo paint has been measured to be 0.25–2.35% [18, 19]. Since PPD is allowed only in oxidizing coloring agents for hair dyeing it is not allowed to add PPD in skin painting [20]. Typically, an eczematous reaction occurs in the original tattoo days to weeks after the tattoo has been made, as a sign of primary sensitization. Individuals sensitized to PPD by semipermanent tattoos cannot tolerate hair dyes or permanent dyes for eye lashes and eye brows [21, 22] and may experience very severe clinical reactions [23]. A questionnaire study in United Kingdom ($n = 4,000$)

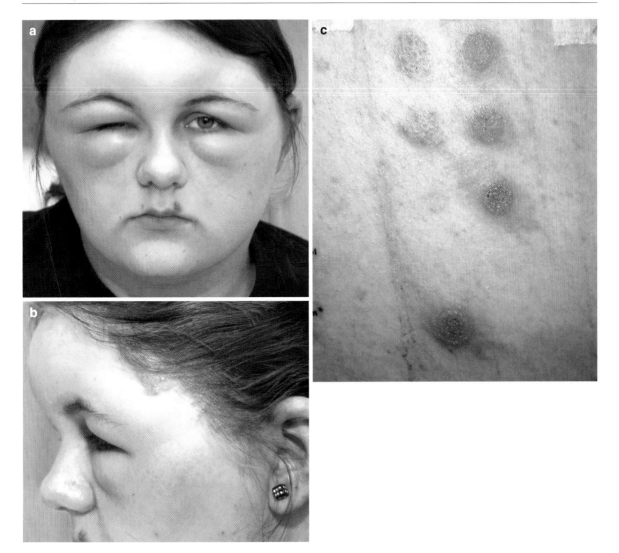

Fig. 34.1 Severe edema of the face 2 days after dyeing the hair at home (**a**). The patient was referred by the emergency physician as erysipelas because she had slight fever, nausea, and lymphadenopathy. Close inspection revealed eczematous lesions at the hairline and on the scalp (**b**). Patch testing revealed a high degree of sensitization to *p*-phenylenediamine, toluene-2.5-diamine, hydroquinone, resorcinol, benzocaine, Disperse Orange three, and to the hair dye used (2% aqueous) (**c**) (courtesy of P.J. Frosch)

showed that 7% of adults and 14% of children (age not defined) had had a temporary tattoo [4]. In Denmark 6.3% of the adult general population ($n=3,471$) reported temporary black tattoos; among those, 2.3% reported eczema where the tattoo was drawn [24].

Core Message

> Temporary black henna tattoos may contain PPD and cause primary sensitization.

34.4 Diagnosis

A key step in the diagnosis of hair dye allergy involves patch testing with commercially available screening series of hair dye ingredients for routine investigations or by workup of the individual case by obtaining the exact components in the hair dye from the producer [25, 26]. PPD is a part of the standard patch test, and screening trays with PPD-related substances are commercially available.

Based on retrospectively collected data on PPD allergy, it nevertheless represents a fairly good screen

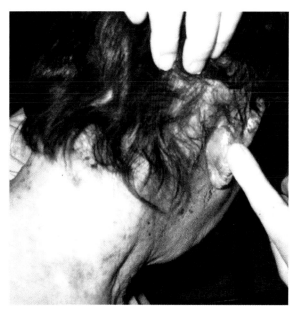

Fig. 34.2 Hair dye dermatitis with eczema at the scalp margins, extending to the neck and suppuration on the ears. The symptoms were caused by a permanent oxidative hair dye on a hairdresser's client

Table 34.1 List of commonly used hair dye ingredients, which are considered for clinical validation as an additional screening tray for hair dye allergy

INCI name	INCI name
1-Hydroxyethyl-4,5-diaminopyrazole sulfate	4-Hydroxypropylamino-3-nitrophenol
1-Naphthol	Acid violet 43
2,4,5,6-Tetraaminopyrinidine	Disperse violet 1
2,4-Diaminophenoxyethanol HCl	HC red no. 3
2,7-Naphthalenediol[a]	HC blue no. 2
2-Amino-3-hydroxypyridine	*m*-Aminophenol[a–c]
2-Amino-6-chloro-4-nitrophenol	*N*, *N*-bis(2-hydroxyethyl)-*p*-phenylenediamine
2-Methyl-5-hydroxyethylaminophenol	*o*-Aminophenol[a]
2-Methylresorcinol	*p*-Aminophenol[a–c]
3-Nitro-*p*-hydroxyethylaminophenol[a]	*p*-Methylaminophenol
4-Amino-3-nitrophenol[a]	*p*-Phenylenediamine[a–c]
4-Amino-2-hydroxytoluene	Picramic acid
4-Amino-*m*-cresol	Resorcinol[a, c]
4-Chlororesorcinol	Toluene-2,5-diamine[a–c]

[a]Reported as clinical contact allergens [6, 25]
[b]Available from Trolab Hermal, Reinbek, Germany
[c]Available from Chemotechnique Diagnostics, Malmö, Sweden

for clinical hair dye dermatitis [27, 28]. However, the existing patch test trays for diagnosing hair dye allergy may have been focused to too great an extent on PPD and PPD-related substances. About 100 ingredients are in use currently and, by a chemical structure activity analysis based on results from predictive testing in animals, many of these substances are predicted to be strong/moderate sensitizers [6–8]. In Table 34.1, a list of the substances that, based on predicted potency and volume of use, are currently being considered for clinical validation as an additional screening tray for hair dye allergy is given.

Toluene-2,5-diamine, *p*-aminophenol, and *m*-aminophenol are all available as patch test preparations, while the commonly used 4-amino-3-nitrophenol and 3-nitro-*p*-hydroxyethylamino-phenol, which have been reported as positive in PPD-negative patients, are not routinely used for the investigation of hair dye allergy [6]. If the ingredients in a hair dye are not available commercially, they may be requested from the producers. Even though the diagnostic workup of individual cases may be valuable, the complicated procedure for acquiring substances for testing probably means that patients with contact allergy to hair dyes

not reacting to PPD or only giving weak allergic reactions to PPD are overlooked [25, 26, 29].

PPD may give very strong patch test reactions, bullous or erosive, at the standard concentration of 1%. This has been observed especially in patients with PPD allergy following skin painting with temporary black henna tattoos. It has been proposed to test PPD at lower concentrations for the investigation of such patients (or patients with a history of severe clinical reactions) starting with 0.01% PPD; if the result is negative at the first reading, the concentration is stepped up to 0.1%, or even 1% [30].

Patch testing may be supplemented with the dyed hair of the patient [11] and/or the hair dye itself. In case severe reactions to the hair dye are anticipated from the original clinical presentation, a stepwise procedure can be applied as for PPD [30] by just adjusting the exposure time instead of the concentration, e.g., starting with a 30-min open exposure, followed by normal occluded exposure, if negative at the first reading. A patch test study with PPD applied on the back, the upper arm, and behind.the ears showed no differences in the sensitivity of the three anatomical regions [31]. Care should be taken in testing the hair dye itself as it may contain high levels of PPD and related substances carrying a risk of not only strong patch test reactions, but also active sensitization. Testing with the individual ingredients of the dye should be preferred.

> **Core Message**
>
> › Hair dye allergy cannot always be detected by patch testing with PPD alone.

34.5 Immediate Reactions

By far, the most common allergic reactions to hair dyes are allergic contact dermatitis. However, immediate hypersensitivity reactions, including asthma, contact urticaria, and anaphylactic shock, attributed to hair dyes have been reported [27, 32–35], and even with the very rare possibility of a fatal outcome [36]. In these cases, it appears that the reactions often tend to involve a combination of immediate and delayed effects. The presence of the immediate component can be revealed by a 20-min patch test with 1% PPD assessed within a few minutes of patch removal [32].

34.6 PPD: The Archetype

As PPD is really the "classic" hair dye allergen, it is reviewed here in greater detail than other dyes. In the EU, the current maximum use level is 6% (=3% when mixed in use), although in practice, the typical maximum level is closer to 4% [20].

34.6.1 Chemistry

p-phenylenediamine (PPD) belongs to the family of aromatic amines (see Fig. 34.3). While many haptens

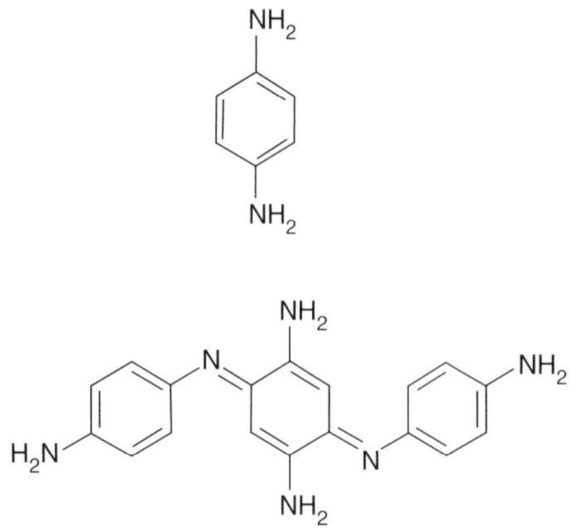

Fig. 34.3 Chemical structures of PPD and the related substance Bandrowski's base (*BB*)

contain chemically reactive groups that react directly with skin protein, PPD is a member of the class of contact allergens referred to as prohaptens, where an apparently unreactive chemical is converted to a more reactive agent [37]. PPD can be metabolized in the skin to different compounds. Mayer [38] proposed that the formation of *p*-benzoquinone in vivo is a possible explanation for both the allergenicity and cross-reactivity of aromatic amines, including PPD. However, a number of groups have tried to confirm this theory, both in predictive animal models and in clinical studies, without any success [39, 40]. Of particular note is the failure of the key putative hapten, 1,4-benzoquinone, to give positive patch test reactions in more than a small minority of PPD-allergic individuals. An alternative explanation for the allergenic effect associated with PPD was sought via the formation of Bandrowski's base (BB), which is, essentially, a trimmer of PPD that forms readily when PPD is exposed to air. Evidence for this possibility came from in vitro lymphocyte proliferation assays using cells taken from PPD-allergic subjects. Positive in vitro results were obtained with most of the subjects, whereas none of the lymphocyte populations would react to PPD itself [41]. Unfortunately, when PPD-allergic subjects are actually patch tested with BB, the large majority fails to react, and those that do react do so only weakly [42]. In reality, it seems likely that metabolic processes in skin, which, as yet, are not well understood, will play a key role in the induction of PPD allergy [43, 44]. A potential consequence of this is the possibility that it may be feasible to determine genetic markers that will

34

identify individuals likely to develop allergy to PPD [45]. The most recent chemical evidence investigates the potential role of benzoquinone diimine intermediates [46]. Nevertheless, despite the various pieces of work mentioned above, the true nature of the in vivo hapten(s) associated with PPD remains unproven.

34.6.2 Immunology

Although the real in vivo hapten(s) arising from PPD may not be known, a number of other aspects of PPD immunology have been examined. A key factor in the induction of contact allergy is the release of danger signals. Picardo (1996) found that PPD induced oxidative stress in normal human keratinocytes in culture [47, 96]. Exposure to noncytotoxic concentrations of PPD produced lipoperoxidative damage. With the overwhelming free radicals generated, an event cascade with recruitment and activation of the immune system occurs. Other authors also showed activation of multiple dermal enzymes following the application of both PPD and PPD in the presence of hydrogen peroxide [48].

Yokozeki et al. looked at the profile of T-cells involved in PPD allergy. Using a mouse model, they showed early (6 h) and late (12–24 h) swellings in adoptive transfer experiments with elicitation challenge [49]. Sieben et al. have characterized the elements of the antigen presentation pathways used during the elicitation of PPD responses [50].

In predictive allergy tests using humans, PPD has been shown to be strongly positive. Ten percent PPD sensitized all 24 subjects who were exposed to it in a human maximization test [51]. In the human repeated insult patch test, 1% PPD in petrolatum sensitized 54% of the volunteers, 0.1% sensitized 11%, and 0.01% sensitized 7% [52]. Similarly, in predictive animal tests, PPD is also strongly positive, yielding a 100% reaction rate in the guinea pig maximization test [53] and 90% in the Buehler test [54]. Currently, the murine local lymph node assay (LLNA) is the preferred standard for the establishment of the relative allergenic potencies of different haptens [55]. Potency is expressed as an EC_3 value, this being the estimated concentration of the chemical necessary to cause a threefold increase in proliferation activity. PPD is one of the most potent allergens on this basis, with an EC value of 0.1% [56]. This potency at induction also translates to a strong

ability to elicit reactions. A study on 15 PPD sensitive persons showed that the threshold value for 10% of the tested persons (ED_{10}) based on + or stronger reactions for PPD on the back was 38 ppm [31].

Given the overwhelming evidence that PPD is, indeed, one of the most powerful of contact allergens, it is not surprising that its use at levels of 1–4% in hair dyes is associated with a degree of allergic contact dermatitis.

34.6.3 Epidemiology

Since p-phenylenediame (PPD) is the most common patch test screening allergen for hair dye dermatitis, it will form the base for our understanding of the epidemiology on hair dye dermatitis. Results from a literature study showed that the weighted average positive patch test reactions to PPD among dermatitis patients was 4.4% in Asia, 4.1% in Europe, and 6.0% in North America [57]. In India, a rate of 11.5% was reported [58]. The Spanish Group for Research Into Dermatitis and Skin Allergies reported a rate of 15.2% of positive patch test reactions to PPD in 2000–2007 [59]. PPD sensitization occurred more often in south and central European patch test centers compared to scandinavian patch test centers (Denmark, Sweden) [60]. This is in line with the expectations regarding higher use levels of PPD in predominantly dark-haired populations [61]. The weighted average of PPD sensitization in the general population is estimated to be 1.0%. The highest estimate was identified in a Thai population (2.7%) [61]. In this location, the gender ratio was approximately 2:1 female:male, which is similar to the situation in Europe. No doubt, the gender bias in use will vary in different countries: in one location in India, the ratio was 2:1 male: female [58]. In countries where dyeing of facial hair is prevalent, an increase in sensitized males may be expected as beard facial hair is usually dyed weekly whereas scalp hair is usually dyed every 1–6 months.

34.6.4 Cross Reactions

For many years, the concept of "*para* group" cross sensitization has persisted, often despite real evidence. PPD belongs to the group of 1,4-substituted benzenes, along with, e.g., *p*-aminobenzoic acid, benzocaine, procaine, some sulfonamides, sunscreens, anthraquinones, and certain rubber chemicals. The reality is that the majority of 1,4-substituted benzenes most commonly do not cross react; however, there are clear exceptions: individuals sensitized to PPD may react to some other hair dyes, e.g., toluene-2,5-diamine [60, 61], *p*-aminophenol [62, 63], 2-nitro-PPD [62], and to disperse orange 3 [64]. This pattern of cross reactivity is confirmed by the evidence from predictive models [65]. PPD is not generally a good screen for azo dyes; however, cross or simultaneous reactions have been described to varying degrees [66]. Cross reactions also occur with the black rubber chemical family, including IPPD [67]. As regards local anesthetics, little evidence of cross-sensitization is published; however, this seems to occur especially in patients highly sensitized to PPD, e.g., from a temporary tattoo. Such patients may have simultaneous reactions to both local anesthetics and IPPD, without any history of prior exposure to these chemicals (Fig. 34.4). Nevertheless, it should be borne in mind that patch-test-proven reactions to *p*-aminobenzoic acid (PABA), benzocaine, and IPPD in PPD-positive subjects with hair dye allergy were less than 10% [68].

34.6.5 Occupational Allergy to PPD

This topic is discussed in Chap. 45 in this book and it is appropriate to mention here that hairdressers are at particular risk of PPD sensitization. While the prevalence

of PPD sensitization in hairdressers is not always high [13], it has been reported as a positive patch test from 15 to 45% of those tested, with relevance to ACD being high [69–71]. However, the majority of patients seen with PPD allergy are from consumer use and not occupational.

34.7 Substances Other than PPD

Hair dye substances that have caused cosmetic allergic contact dermatitis in humans are listed in Table 34.2.

Table 34.2 INCI names of hair coloring agents that have caused cosmetic allergy in humans

INCI name
2.4-Diaminophenol
2.7-Naphthalenediol
2-Aminomethyl-*p*-aminophenol HCL
2-Chloro-*p*-phenylenediamine
2-Nitro-*p*-phenylenediamine
3-Nitro-*p*-hydroxyethylaminophenol
4-Amino-3-nitrophenol
3-Amino-*m*-cresol
6-Methoxy-2-methylamino-3-aminopyridine HCL
Basic blue 99
Basic red 22
Disperse brown 1
Disperse orange 3
Henna
Hydroquinone
Lead acetate
m-Aminophenol
N-Phenyl-*p*-phenylenediamine
o-Aminophenol
p-Aminophenol
p-Phenylenediamine
Resorcinol
Solvent red 1
Toluene-2,5-diamine
Based on [5, 6, 25, 26, 79]

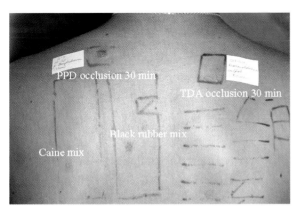

Fig. 34.4 Strong patch test reaction to PPD, day 3. Exposure time to PPD only 30 min. Cross-reactivity to caine mix (local anesthetics), *black rubber* mix, and toluene-2,5-diamine (TDA) in a patient sensitized by a temporary *black henna* tattoo (courtesy of K.E. Andersen)

34.7.1 Toluene-2,5-Diamine

Many reports on contact allergic reaction to toluene-2,5-diamine from hair dyes exist either from patients dyeing their own hair or by their occupation as hairdressers. It was the most used hair dye substance in 2002 (100 tonnage TDA vs. 80 tonnage PPD per year in Europe). Toluene-2,5-diamine is commercially available as patch test preparation in petrolatum and it often cross-reacts with PPD, but seems to give weaker reactions in PPD-positive patients at patch testing than PPD itself [62]. It can however give isolated reactions [72] and late (D7) reactions [73]. In a QSAR model, toluene-2,5-diamine was predicted to be a strong/moderate sensitizer [6] which has been confirmed in the LLNA [7]. Toluene-2,5-diamine is allowed at a concentration of 10% in hair dyes in the EU [20]. Products containing a 0.18% concentration have been reported to cause elicitation [22]. German studies showed that contact allergy to toluene-2,5-diamine is still an increasing problem among patch-tested hairdressers' clients as 8.7% had a positive patch test reaction in 1995/1996 [70] and 21.6% had a positive patch test reaction to toluene-2,5-diamine in 2005/2006 [74]. In Finland, an increase in positive patch test reactions to toluene-2,5-diamine (sulfate) from 1.4% in 1995 to 5.2% in 2002 was detected [75].

34.7.2 Resorcinol

Resorcinol is known from pharmaceuticals and has been used in hair dyes for more than 100 years. It was the second most used hair dye substance in 2002, but, taking its use into account, it is not a frequent sensitizer when used in hair dyes, an observation consistent with experimental evidence indicating that it is only of weakly sensitizing potency [76]. However, a few cases of contact allergy to resorcinol have been reported [77, 78].

34.7.3 Aminophenol

Aminophenols are frequently used hair dye substances. Aminophenols are allowed at a concentration of up to 2% in hair dyes within the EU [20] and allergic contact dermatitis has been elicited in products containing 0.067% m-aminophenol [22]. There is no restriction on the maximum use of p-aminophenol. The number of patients sensitized to p-aminophenol, in whom hair cosmetics have been considered as being causative of their contact dermatitis, increased from 3.6% in 1995 [70] to 14.2% in 2006 [74], while the frequency of m-aminophenol in sensitive consumers tested with a hairdresser series was 9.1% in 2006 [74].

34.7.4 Henna

Allergic contact dermatitis to henna from hair dyes is seen, although it is very rare [79]. Allergic contact dermatitis from henna painted on a toe has been described [80]. Immediate-type hypersensitivity with urticaria, rhinitis, and bronchial asthma on exposure to henna has been reported [81, 82].

34.7.5 Bleaching Agents

Ammonium persulfate is used to bleach hair and has been identified as the cause of occupational asthma and contact allergy in hairdressers [83]. Consumers have also been found to be sensitized [70]. A positive patch test to hydrogen peroxide was seen in a housewife who had used a dyeing cream mixed with an aqueous solution of 20–40% hydrogen peroxide. Contact dermatitis from handling hairdressers' products that contains hydrogen peroxide is frequently seen [14]. Severe chemical burns resulting in necrotic reactions that needs surgery has been reported after the use of hair lightning products. Persulfates and hydrogen peroxide were suggested to be the causative agents [84–89].

34.7.5.1 Monoethanolamine (MEA)

Monoethanolamine is used in hair cosmetics to regulate pH, and the sensitization prevalence has increased from 0.7%(2003/2004) to 3.1% (2005/2006) [74]. A case report described allergic contact dermatitis due to the cream developer trideceth-2-carboxamide MEA from a permanent hair dye product [90].

34.7.6 New Generation of Hair Dyes

A new generation of hair dyes (acid black 1, acid violet 43, acid orange 7, and acid red 33) seems to have different chemical properties to PPD and toluene-2,5-diamine [6], and a lack of cross-reaction between the two groups is described [62]. All these substances are predicted as potent contact allergens in a QSAR analysis [6].

34.8 Pretesting and Advising Patients

34.8.1 Pretesting

Hair dye allergy may result in very severe reactions and therefore any individual who has been diagnosed as allergic to hair dye chemicals such as PPD should avoid further contact. However, the reality is that many who are sensitized either have not been formally diagnosed as allergic or, even if diagnosed, will persist with the hair dyeing process. It is, therefore, desirable to predict whether such an individual has already become sensitized and should not proceed to the full hair dyeing procedure. An open test has been recommended by the hair dye producers, both in the case of home coloring and at the hairdressers [91, 92]. Another approach uses a transfer containing a lower dose of PPD [93]. The safety and benefit of these kinds of tests have been addressed by the European Commission Scientific Committee concerning cosmetics who were of the opinion that there is a risk of misleading and false-negative results by using the tests and a potential risk of inducting skin sensitization to hair dye substances [94]. This risk may be particularly high among those, who regularly dye their hair every 4–6 weeks with permanent hair dye and follow the recommendations of leading manufacturers to perform the pretest. Another important criticism has been that the peformance of these tests has not been adequately demonstrated.

34.8.2 Advising Patients

Patients with hair dye allergy are advised to stop dyeing their hair. Some hair dye ingredients are used in both permanent and temporary hair dyes [6] and,

therefore, it is not possible to give general advice that one type of hair dye can be tolerated if a reaction has occurred to the other. In addition cross-reactivities may occur. Henna may be used, but it is not always cosmetically acceptable. Some patients weakly sensitized to PPD are known to be able to continue dyeing their hair with PPD with impunity. Chan et al. found that 20 out of 33 patients with PPD allergy had a clinically relevant reaction attributed to the use of hair dyes. Follow-up showed that 3 of the 20 continued dyeing their hair using PPD hair dyes, two had recurrent dermatitis and lived with it, one had no problems, and two appeared to be clinically tolerant, as they were using PPD hair dyes at the time of patch testing but did not experience hair dye dermatitis [95].

A new generation of hair dyes has been developed, Food and Drug and Cosmetic hair dyes (FD and C) [62], but their practical value remains to be fully demonstrated. Forty hairdressers with PPD and PPD-related allergies were patch tested with ingredients and finished formulations of the FD and C dyes. Two had a positive patch test to one or more of the finished formulations. None reacted to the individual ingredients [62]. Time will show whether these hair dyes are a safe alternative to permanent hair dyes based on PPD and PPD-related substances.

Patients sensitized to PPD or PPD-related substances by hair dyeing may have cross or simultaneous sensitivity to textile dyes [64, 66]; however, it rarely causes clinical problems.

34.9 Case Reports

Presented below are two case reports whose purpose is to provide a practical illustration of the presentation of hair-dye-related allergic contact dermatitis.

> **Core Message**
>
> › A 50-year-old previously healthy woman had her hair dyed for the first time in her life at a hairdresser. No side-effects occurred. A year later, she dyed her hair with a nonpermanent hair dye at home and made the recommended preexposure test without any reaction. The following day, she developed scalp dermatitis

with severe itching, spreading to her face, neck, and upper part of the thorax. As a further complication, the patient developed vesicular hand eczema for the first time in her life. Treatment with systemic and topical steroids was given for several months, leading to the gradual clearing of the dermatitis. Patch testing was performed in several sequences with the European Standard Series supplemented with selected cosmetic allergens and a hairdressers' series. At the initial patch testing, there was a +? result to PPD at days 3 and 7. Further, she reacted with a +? to her own hair collected at day 3 after the hair dye dermatitis had erupted. An open exposure to the product, which had initiated the dermatitis, was negative both before (arm exposure at home) and after (back exposure at dermatological clinic) the allergic reaction to the product. None of the screening chemicals in the hairdressers' series gave a definite positive reaction. Only by patch testing with the individual hair dye ingredients (provided for individual patch testing by the producer) was the patient's reactions explained. The patient gave a positive patch test to 4-amino-3-nitrophenol and 3-nitro-*p*-hydroxyethylaminophenol at readings on days 3–4. These substances are not commercially available and the severe clinical reaction would have remained unexplained if patch testing had been performed only with PPD and PPD-related substances. The two substances are on the list of substances that, based on chemical considerations, have a moderate/strong allergenic potential (Table 34.1) and is considered for validation as a new screening tray [6].

> A 39-year-old women with no previous skin disease had dyed her hair tips regularly once a year at the hairdressers. Following dyeing with a permanent hair color of a reasonably fair shade, she developed facial edema and oozing scalp dermatitis 3 days later. She received medical treatment from emergency service doctors and, later, her general practitioner, who, at first, suspected mumps due to the severe edema of her face. She received treatment with antihistamines only and the symptoms subsided after 1–2 weeks. Testing with

the standard series and a hairdressers' series showed positive patch tests to PPD and PPD-related substances (toluene-2,5-diamine, nitro-*p*-toluenediamine) and 4-aminoazobenzene (probably cross-reactivity to textile azo dyes). Chemical analyzes of the hair dye showed that it contained 0.27% PPD.

> The case shows that the severe angioedema-like symptoms may be mistaken for other diseases and falsely treated as a type I reaction with only antihistamines. Furthermore, fair colors may also cause severe reactions; in this case, only 0.27% PPD was present in the hair dye, while up to 6% is permitted [20].

References

1. Balzer W, Braun HJ, Chassot L, Clausen T (2001) Diaminopyrazoles: novel primary intermediates for hair dyeing formulations. SÖFW J 127:12–16
2. Bonnevie P (1939) Aetiologie und pathogenese der Ekzemkrankheiten. Klinische Studien über die Ursachen der Ekzeme unter besonderer Berücksichtigung des Diagnostischen Wertes der Ekzemproben. Busch, Copenhagen/Barth, Leipzig
3. Sosted H, Hesse U, Menne T, Andersen KE, Johansen JD (2005) Contact dermatitis to hair dyes in an adult Danish population – an interview based study. Br J Dermatol 153:132–135
4. Orton D (2008) A UK study on the use and reported adverse reactions to hair dye. Contact Dermat 58:27–28
5. Sosted H, Johansen JD, Andersen KE, Menne T (2006) Severe allergic hair dye reactions in 8 children. Contact Dermat 54:87–91
6. Sosted H, Basketter DA, Estrada E, Johansen JD, Patlewicz GY (2004) Ranking of hair dye substances according to predicted sensitization potenzy – quantitative structure-activity relationships. Contact Dermat 51:241–254
7. Kern PS, Gerberick GF, Ryan CA, Kimber I, Aptula A, Basketter DA (2010) Historical local lymph node data for the evaluation of skin sensitization alternatives: a second compilation. Dermatitis 21:8–32.
8. Gerberick GF, Ryan CA, Kern PS, Schlatter H, Dearman RJ, Kimber I, Patlewicz GY, Basketter DA (2005) Compilation of historical local lymph node data for evaluation of skin sensitization alternative methods. Dermatitis 16:157–202
9. Nohynek GJ, Fautz R, Benech-Kieffer F, Toutain H (2004) Toxicity and human health risk of hair dyes. Food Chem Toxicol 42:517–543
10. Sosted H, Agner T, Andersen KE, Menne T (2002) 55 cases of allergic reactions to hair dye: a descriptive, consumer complaint-based study. Contact Dermat 47:299–303
11. Cronin E (1980) Hair preparations. Contact dermatitis. Churchill Livingstone, Edingburg, London, New York, pp 115–126

12. Hsu TS, Davis MD, el Azhary R, Corbett JF, Gibson LE (2002) Beard dermatitis due to para-phenylenediamine use in Arabic men. J Am Acad Dermatol 44:867–869

13. Frosch PJ, Burrows D, Camarasa JG, Dooms-Goossens A, Ducombs G, Lahti A, Menne T, Rycroft RJ, Shaw S, White IR (1993) Allergic reactions to a hairdressers' series: results from 9 European centres. The European Environmental and Contact Dermatitis Research Group (EECDRG). Contact Dermat 28:180–183

14. Aguirre A, Zabala R, Sanz de Galdeano C, Landa N, Diaz-Perez JL (1994) Positive patch tests to hydrogen peroxide in 2 cases. Contact Dermat 30:113

15. Brancaccio RR, Brown LH, Chang YT, Fogelman JP, Mafong EA, Cohen DE (2002) Identification and quantification of para-phenylenediamine in a temporary black henna tattoo. Am J Contact Dermat 13:15–18

16. Sharma VK, Mandal SK, Sethuraman G, Bakshi NA (1999) Para-phenylenediamine-induced lichenoid eruptions. Contact Dermat 41:40–41

17. Tosti A, Bardazzi F, Valeri F, Toni F (1987) Erythema multiforme with contact dermatitis to hair dyes. Contact Dermat 17:321–322

18. Avnstorp C, Rastogi SC, Menne T (2002) Acute fingertip dermatitis from temporary tattoo and quantitative chemical analysis of the product. Contact Dermat 47:119–120

19. Kang IJ, Lee MH (2006) Quantification of para-phenylenediamine and heavy metals in henna dye. Contact Dermat 55:26–29

20. European Communities. Council directive 76/768/EEC of 27 July 1976 on the approximation of the laws of the member states relating to cosmetic products, annex III amended. L262. 2004. European Communities Official Journal

21. Teixeira M, de WL, Ronsyn E, Goossens A (2006) Contact allergy to para-phenylenediamine in a permanent eyelash dye. Contact Dermat 55:92–94

22. Sosted H, Rastogi SC, Andersen KE, Johansen JD, Menne T (2004) Hair dye contact allergy: quantitative exposure assessment of selected products and clinical cases. Contact Dermat 50:344–348

23. Marcoux D, Couture-Trudel PM, Riboulet-Delmas G, Sasseville D (2002) Sensitization to para-phenylenediamine from a streetside temporary tattoo. Pediatr Dermatol 19: 498–502

24. Hansen HS, Johansen JD, Thyssen JP, Linneberg A, Sosted H (2009) Private use of hair dyes and temporary black tattoos in Copenhagen hairdressers. Ann Occup Hyg. 2010 Jan 15. [Epub ahead of print] Submitted

25. Sosted H, Menne T (2005) Allergy to 3-nitro-p-hydroxyethylaminophenol and 4-amino-3-nitrophenol in a hair dye. Contact Dermat 52:317–319

26. Sosted H, Nielsen NH, Menné T (2009) Allergic contact dermatitis to the hair dye 6-methoxy-2-methylamino-3-aminopyridine HCl (INCI HC Blue no. 7) without cross-sensitivity to PPD. Contact Dermat 60:236–237

27. Koopmans AK, Bruynzeel DP (2003) Is PPD a useful screening agent? Contact Dermat 48:89–92

28. Diepgen TL, Coenraads PJ, Wilkinson M, Basketter DA, Lepoittevin JP (2005) Para-phenylendiamine (PPD) 1% pet. is an important allergen in the standard series. Contact Dermat 53:185

29. Blanco R, de la HB, Sanchez-Fernandez C, Sanchez-Cano M (1998) Allergy to 4-amino-3-nitrophenol in a hair dye. Contact Dermat 39:136

30. Ho SG, White IR, Rycroft RJ, McFadden JP (2004) A new approach to patch testing patients with para-phenylenediamine allergy secondary to temporary black henna tattoos. Contact Dermat 51:213–214

31. Sosted H, Menne T, Johansen JD (2006) Patch test dose-response study of p-phenylenediamine: thresholds and anatomical regional differences. Contact Dermat 54:145–146

32. Wong GA, King CM (2003) Immediate-type hypersensitivity and allergic contact dermatitis due to para-phenylenediamine in hair dye. Contact Dermat 48:166

33. Pasche-Koo F, French L, Piletta-Zanin PA, Hauser C (1998) Contact urticaria and shock to hair dye. Allergy 53:904–905

34. Mavroleon G, Begishvili B, Frew AJ (1998) Anaphylaxis to hair dye: a case report. Clin Exp Allergy 28:121–122

35. Fukunaga T, Kawagoe R, Hozumi H, Kanzaki T (1996) Contact anaphylaxis due to para-phenylenediamine. Contact Dermat 35:185–186

36. Belton AL, Chira T (1997) Fatal anaphylactic reaction to hair dye. Am J Forensic Med Pathol 18:290–292

37. Landsteiner J, Jacobs JL (1936) Studies on the sensitization of animals with simple chemical compounds. II. J Exp Med 64:625–629

38. Mayer RL (1954) Group-sensitization to compounds of quinone structure and its biochemical basis role of these substances in cancer. Prog Allergy 4:79–172

39. Basketter DA, Liden C (1992) Further investigation of the prohapten concept: reactions to benzene derivatives in man. Contact Dermat 27:90–97

40. Lisi P, Hansel K (1998) Is benzoquinone the prohapten in cross-sensitivity among aminobenzene compounds? Contact Dermat 39:304–306

41. Krasteva M, Nicolas JF, Chabeau G, Garrigue JL, Bour H, Thivolet J, Schmitt D (1993) Dissociation of allergenic and immunogenic functions in contact sensitivity to para-phenylenediamine. Int Arch Allergy Immunol 102:200–204

42. White JM, Kullavanijaya P, Duangdeeden I, Zazzeroni R, Gilmour NJ, Basketter DA, McFadden JP (2006) p-Phenylenediamine allergy: the role of Bandrowski's base. Clin Exp Allergy 36:1289–1293

43. Kawakubo Y, Merk HF, Masaoudi TA, Sieben S, Blomeke B (2000) N-Acetylation of paraphenylenediamine in human skin and keratinocytes. J Pharmacol Exp Ther 292:150–155

44. Aeby P, Sieber T, Beck H, Gerberick GF, Goebel C (2009) Skin sensitization to p-phenylenediamine: the diverging roles of oxidation and N-acetylation for dendritic cell activation and the immune response. J Invest Dermatol 129: 99–109

45. Schnuch A, Westphal GA, Muller MM, Schulz TG, Geier J, Brasch J, Merk HF, Kawakubo Y, Richter G, Koch P, Fuchs T, Gutgesell T, Reich K, Gebhardt M, Becker D, Grabbe J, Szliska C, Aberer W, Hallier E (1998) Genotype and phenotype of N-acetyltransferase 2 (NAT2) polymorphism in patients with contact allergy. Contact Dermat 38:209–211

46. Eilstein J, Gimenez-Arnau E, Duche D, Rousset F, Lepoittevin JP (2007) Mechanistic studies on the lysine-induced N-formylation of 2, 5-dimethyl-p-benzoquinonediimine. Chem Res Toxicol 20:1155–1161

34

47. Picardo M, Cannistraci C, Cristaudo A, De Luca C, Santucci B (1990) Study on cross-reactivity to the para group. Dermatologica 181:104–108

48. Mathur AK, Gupta BN, Singh S, Singh A, Narang S (1992) Dermal toxicity of paraphenylenediamine. Biomed Environ Sci 5:321–324

49. Yokozeki H, Watanabe K, Igawa K, Miyazaki Y, Katayama I, Nishioka K (2001) Gammadelta T cells assist alphabeta T cells in the adoptive transfer of contact hypersensitivity to para-phenylenediamine. Clin Exp Immunol 125:351–359

50. Sieben S, Kawakubo Y, Al Masaoudi T, Merk HF, Blomeke B (2002) Delayed-type hypersensitivity reaction to paraphenylenediamine is mediated by 2 different pathways of antigen recognition by specific alphabeta human T-cell clones. J Allergy Clin Immunol 109:1005–1011

51. Kligman AM (1966) The identification of contact allergens by human assay. 3. The maximization test: a procedure for screening and rating contact sensitizers. J Invest Dermatol 47:393–409

52. Marzulli FN, Maibach HI (1974) The use of graded concentrations in studying skin sensitizers: experimental contact sensitization in man. Food Cosmet Toxicol 12:219–227

53. Basketter DA, Scholes EW (1992) Comparison of the local lymph node assay with the guinea-pig maximization test for the detection of a range of contact allergens. Food Chem Toxicol 30:65–69

54. Basketter DA, Gerberick GF (1996) An interlaboratory evaluation of the Buehler test for the identification and classification of skin sensitizers. Contact Dermat 35:146–151

55. Kimber I, Basketter DA, Berthold K, Butler M, Garrigue JL, Lea L, Newsome C, Roggeband R, Steiling W, Stropp G, Waterman S, Wiemann C (2001) Skin sensitization testing in potency and risk assessment. Toxicol Sci 59:198–208

56. Gerberick GF, Ryan CA, Kern PS, Dearman RJ, Kimber I, Patlewicz GY, Basketter DA (2004) A chemical dataset for evaluation of alternative approaches to skin-sensitization testing. Contact Dermat 50:274–288

57. Thyssen JP, White JM (2008) Epidemiological data on consumer allergy to p-phenylenediamine. Contact Dermat 59: 327–343

58. Sharma VK, Chakrabarti A (1998) Common contact sensitizers in Chandigarh, India. A study of 200 patients with the European standard series. Contact Dermat 38:127–131

59. Laguna C, de la CJ, Martin-Gonzalez B, Zaragoza V, Martinez-Casimiro L, Alegre V (2009) Allergic contact dermatitis to cosmetics. Actas Dermosifiliogr 100:53–60

60. Thyssen JP, Andersen KE, Bruze M, Diepgen T, Gimenez-Arnau AM, Goncalo M, Goossens A, Le Coz CJ, McFadden J, Rustemeyer T, White IR, White JM, Johansen JD (2009) p-Phenylenediamine sensitization is more prevalent in central and southern European patch test centres than in Scandinavian: results from a multicentre study. Contact Dermat 60:314–319

61. Basketter DA, Duangdeeden I, Gilmour NJ, Kullavanijaya P, McFadden JP (2004) Prevalence of contact allergy in an adult Thai population. Contact Dermat 50(3):128–129

62. Fautz R, Fuchs A, van der Walle HB, Henny V, Smits L (2002) Hair dye-sensitized hairdressers: the cross-reaction pattern with new generation hair dyes. Contact Dermat 46:319–324

63. Basketter DA, English J (2009) Cross-reactions among hair dye allergens. Cutan Ocul Toxicol 28:104–106

64. Goon AT, Gilmour NJ, Basketter DA, White IR, Rycroft RJ, McFadden JP (2003) High frequency of simultaneous sensitivity to Disperse Orange 3 in patients with positive patch tests to para-phenylenediamine. Contact Dermat 48: 248–250

65. Xie Z, Hayakawa R, Sugiura M, Kojima H, Konishi H, Ichihara G, Takeuchi Y (2000) Experimental study on skin sensitization potencies and cross-reactivities of hair-dye-related chemicals in guinea pigs. Contact Dermat 42:270–275

66. Seidenari S, Mantovani L, Manzini BM, Pignatti M (1997) Cross-sensitizations between azo dyes and para-amino compound. A study of 236 azo-dye-sensitive subjects. Contact Dermat 36:91–96

67. Herve-Bazin B, Gradiski D, Duprat P, Marignac B, Foussereau J, Cavelier C, Bieber P (1977) Occupational eczema from N-isopropyl-N'-phenylparaphenylenediamine (IPPD) and N-dimethy-1, 3 butyl-N'-phenylparaphenylenediamine (DMPPD) in tyres. Contact Dermat 3:1–15

68. Ho SG, Basketter DA, Jefferies D, Rycroft RJ, White IR, McFadden JP (2005) Analysis of para-phenylenediamine allergic patients in relation to strength of patch test reaction. Br J Dermatol 153:364–367

69. Guerra L, Tosti A, Bardazzi F, Pigatto P, Lisi P, Santucci B, Valsecchi R, Schena D, Angelini G, Sertoli A (1992) Contact dermatitis in hairdressers: the Italian experience. Gruppo Italiano Ricerca Dermatiti da Contatto e Ambientali. Contact Dermat 26:101–107

70. Uter W, Lessmann H, Geier J, Schnuch A (2003) Contact allergy to ingredients of hair cosmetics in female hairdressers and clients – an 8-year analysis of IVDK data. Contact Dermat 49:236–240

71. Nettis E, Marcandrea M, Colanardi MC, Paradiso MT, Ferrannini A, Tursi A (2003) Results of standard series patch testing in patients with occupational allergic contact dermatitis. Allergy 58:1304–1307

72. Winhoven SM, Rutter KJ, Beck MH (2007) Toluene-2, 5-diamine may be an isolated allergy in individuals sensitized by permanent hair dye. Contact Dermat 57:193

73. Bregnhoj A, Menne T (2008) Primary sensitization to toluene-2, 5-diamine giving rise to early positive patch reaction to p-phenylenediamine and late to toluene-2, 5-diamine. Contact Dermat 59:189–190

74. Uter W, Lessmann H, Geier J, Schnuch A (2007) Contact allergy to hairdressing allergens in female hairdressers and clients–current data from the IVDK, 2003–2006. J Dtsch Dermatol Ges 5:993–1001

75. Hasan T, Rantanen T, Alanko K, Harvima RJ, Jolanki R, Kalimo K, Lahti A, Lammintausta K, Lauerma AI, Laukkanen A, Luukkaala T, Riekki R, Turjanmaa K, Varjonen E, Vuorela AM (2005) Patch test reactions to cosmetic allergens in 1995-1997 and 2000-2002 in Finland – a multicentre study. Contact Dermat 53:40–45

76. Basketter DA, Sanders D, Jowsey IR (2007) The skin sensitization potential of resorcinol: experience with the local lymph node assay. Contact Dermat 56:196–200

77. Guerra L, Bardazzi F, Tosti A (1992) Contact dermatitis in hairdressers' clients. Contact Dermat 26:108–111

78. Vilaplana J, Romaguera C, Grimalt F (1991) Contact dermatitis from resorcinol in a hair dye. Contact Dermat 24: 151–152

79. Belhadjali H, Ghannouchi N, Amri C, Youssef M, Amri M, Zili J (2008) Contact dermatitis to henna used as a hair dye. Contact Dermat 58:182

80. Nigam PK, Saxena AK (1988) Allergic contact dermatitis from henna. Contact Dermat 18:55–56

81. Majoie IM, Bruynzeel DP (1996) Occupational immediate-type hypersensitivity to henna in a hairdresser. Am J Contact Dermat 7:38–40

82. Bolhaar ST, Mulder M, van Ginkel CJ (2001) IgE-mediated allergy to henna. Allergy 56:248

83. Fisher AA, Dooms-Goossens A (1976) Persulfate hair bleach reactions. Cutaneous and respiratory manifestations. Arch Dermatol 112:1407–1409

84. Boucher J, Raglon B, Valdez S, Haffajee M (1990) Possible role of chemical hair care products in 10 patients with face, scalp, ear, back, neck and extremity burns. Burns 16:146–147

85. Goon P, Misra A (2005) A possible chemical burn to the scalp following hair highlights. Burns 31:530–531

86. Jensen CD, Sosted H (2006) Chemical burns to the scalp from hair bleach and dye. Acta Derm Venereol 86:461–462

87. Maguina P, Shah-Khan M, An G, Hanumadass M (2007) Chemical scalp burns after hair highlights. J Burn Care Res 28:361–363

88. Peters W (2000) The hair color-highlighting burn: a unique burn injury. J Burn Care Rehabil 21:96–98

89. Schroder CM, Holler OD, Merk HF, Abuzahra F (2008) Necrotizing toxic contact dermatitis of the scalp from hydrogen peroxide. Hautarzt 59:148–150

90. Bowling JC, Scarisbrick J, Warin AP, Downs AM (2002) Allergic contact dermatitis from trideceth-2-carboxamide monoethanolamine (MEA) in a hair dye. Contact Dermat 47:116–117

91. Krasteva M, Cristaudo A, Hall B, Orton D, Rudzki E, Santucci B, Toutain H, Wilkinson J (2002) Contact sensitivity to hair dyes can be detected by the consumer open test. Eur J Dermatol 12:322–326

92. Krasteva M, Cottin M, Cristaudo A, Laine G, Nohynek G, Orton D, Toutain H, Severino V, Wilkinson J (2005) Sensitivity and specificity of the consumer open skin allergy test as a method of prediction of contact dermatitis to hair dyes. Eur J Dermatol 15:18–25

93. Basketter DA, English J (2009) in hair dye users: an assessment of the Colourstart system. Eur J Dermatol 19:232–237

94. European Commission (2007) DG Health and Consumer Protection, Scientific Committee on Consumer Products. Opinion on Sensitivity to Hair Dyes – Consumer Self Testing. SCCP/1104/07. pp 1–15

95. Chan YC, Ng SK, Goh CL (2001) Positive patch-test reactions to para-phenylenediamine, their clinical relevance and the concept of clinical tolerance. Contact Dermat 45:217–220

96. Picardo M, Zompetta C, Grandinetti M, Ameglio F, Santucci B, Faggioni A, Passi S (1996) Paraphenylene diamine, a contact allergen, induces oxidative stress in normal human keratinocytes in culture. Br J Dermatol Apr;134(4):681–685

Metals

35

Carola Lidén, Magnus Bruze, Jacob Pontoppidan Thyssen, and Torkil Menné

Contents

C. Lidén (✉)
Unit of Occupational and Environmental Dermatology,
Institute of Environmental Medicine, Karolinska Institutet,
Box 210, SE-171 77 Stockholm, Sweden
e-mail: carola.liden@ki.se

M. Bruze
Department of Occupational and Environmental Dermatology,
Malmö University Hospital, Lund University,
SE-205 02 Malmö, Sweden

J.P. Thyssen
Department of Dermato-Allergology, National Allergy
Research Centre, Gentofte Hospital, University of Copenhagen,
DK-2900 Hellerup, Denmark

T. Menné
Department of Dermato-Allergology, Gentofte Hospital,
University of Copenhagen, DK-2900 Hellerup, Denmark

J.D. Johansen et al. (eds.), *Contact Dermatitis*,
DOI: 10.1007/978-3-642-03827-3_35, © Springer-Verlag Berlin Heidelberg 2011

35.1 Introduction

There exist more than 50 metals and an enormous number of naturally occurring and manmade alloys and metal compounds. A few metals – foremost, ions and compounds of nickel, chromium, and cobalt – belong to the most important contact allergens, causing allergic contact dermatitis in a large proportion of the general population, as well as in large occupational groups.

Metals are present in the Earth's crust, usually as oxides, sulfides, and silicates, and only the precious metals in metallic form. Metallic compounds occur naturally in drinking water and food, and some are probably essential nutrients for humans. Many metallic metals and metal compounds are toxic to the environment, and some belong to the most important environmental hazards. The industrial use of many metals, their alloys, and their compounds is extremely important in modern society, as they possess valuable mechanical, electrical, and chemical properties. The most often used metals are iron, chromium, lead, nickel, cobalt, aluminum, and copper. Mining, refining, production, and trading of metals represent enormous economic values. Skin problems related to metals are caused not primarily by metals in the natural environment, but are related to human activity – by metallic metals and metal compounds in consumer products and industrial processes.

Metals are elements with a metallic luster and are good conductors of electricity and heat. The metals are divided into different overlapping groups, depending on their chemical and physical properties and their use. There are 50 metals and a few metalloids, the latter including arsenic. The expression heavy metals, which include most metals, is often used. Toxic and nonessential heavy metals (TNEM) are cadmium, mercury, and lead, which are often termed heavy metals. The toxicity of metal is, however, quite unrelated to density. Precious metals are gold, silver, rhodium, palladium, platinum, and some other platinum metals.

Metallic items are generally made of alloys, which may be combined, soldered, plated, etc. Common examples of nickel-containing alloys are stainless steels (iron/nickel/chromium), copper–nickel, and nickel–silver (nickel/copper/zinc). Brass (copper/zinc) and red gold (gold/silver/copper) are examples of nickel-free alloys. Alloys are compounds or solid solutions of more than one element in metallic form, but cannot be considered as mixtures of metals. Resistance to corrosion on skin contact varies widely between different alloys, depending on their composition. This is of great importance for the probability of alloys inducing and eliciting allergic contact dermatitis. Metal compounds are often referred to by toxicologists as soluble or insoluble. Their solubility in sweat, however, is generally not mentioned.

Why some metals act as potent or clinically important contact allergens and others do not is not fully understood. The question of multiple metal reactivity, cross-reactivity, and multiple sensitizations also remains under discussion. The clinical relevance of some metallic metals and metal compounds as contact allergens is still controversial. Some metal compounds are potent contact allergens in experiment animals, but not all of them present clinically relevant problems.

Several metallic metals and their compounds present important occupational health hazards, and several have been recognized by the International Agency for Research on Cancer (IARC) as human carcinogens. Arsenic and arsenic compounds are unique in the formation of skin cancer, related to oral medical therapy and inhalation exposure. The respiratory system is the most frequent target site of metal-induced cancers in humans, and metal-induced respiratory tumors have occurred only from inhalation exposure. Compounds of arsenic, beryllium, cadmium, chromium, and nickel have been associated with pulmonary carcinomas, and hexavalent chromium compounds and certain nickel compounds have been associated with nasosinal cavity tumors.

> **Core Message**
>
> › Nickel, chromium, and cobalt, their ions and compounds, belong to the most important skin sensitizers.
> › Consumer products and occupational skin exposure are the main sources of sensitization and elicitation.
> › The pure metals, their alloys, platings, and compounds have different abilities to cause allergic contact dermatitis.

35.2 Nickel

Nickel (Ni) was isolated in 1751 by the Swedish Baron and mineralogist, Axel Fredrik Cronstedt, as he attempted to extract copper from niccolite (kupfernickel). Since the late nineteenth century, nickel has been widely used in various alloys, particularly in stainless steel. In 1889, occupational nickel dermatitis was recognized for the first time among workers in the plating industry [1]. In 1925, nickel allergy was verified by patch testing in Kiel, Germany [2]. In 1931, consumer nickel dermatitis was reported following skin contact with spectacle frames [3]. Nickel has since been established as the most important ubiquitous contact allergen and affects 17% of women and 3% of men in Europe and North America [4].

Primary nickel sensitization is often associated with prolonged and direct skin contact with nickel-releasing consumer products such as inexpensive jewelry and clothing fasteners. Of note, new sources of nickel exposure have recently been detected, e.g., mobile phones and headsets [5]. Primary nickel sensitization and elicitation may also occur on the hands following occupational exposure. Thus, repeated and continuous occupational exposure to tools, keys, coins, and sewing needles may be of relevance in some cases. Besides contact allergy, nickel compounds may have other toxicological properties such as carcinogenicity, pulmonary effects, and general toxicity. These toxicological effects are not related to contact allergy, as they are caused by different nickel compounds and different exposures. Milestones in our understanding of nickel dermatitis are summarized in Table 35.1.

Core Message

> Occupational and, later, consumer nickel contact allergy have been frequent for the last 100 years.

35.2.1 Nickel Use and Exposure

In nature, nickel is present as oxides and sulfides bound in the ore, together with cobalt, copper, and small amounts of platinum, palladium, and gold. Global nickel deposits and reserves are large and are mainly present in

Table 35.1 Milestones in the history of nickel dermatitis

1889	Description of nickel dermatitis in plating workers
1925	Patch testing with nickel sulfate in plating workers
1935	Large-scale consumer nickel dermatitis
1950s	Suspender dermatitis with secondary spread
1970s	Jean button and zipper dermatitis
	Nickel allergy and hand eczema
	Systemic contact dermatitis
1980s	Jewelry and piercing dermatitis
	Epidemiological studies identify high prevalences of nickel allergy
	Hazard identification – risk assessment
1990s	Strategy for risk management – prevention – legislation
2000	Implementation of the EU Nickel Directive
2009	An effect of the nickel regulation is suggested in the Danish general population
	Mobile phones covered by the EU Nickel Directive

Canada, Australia, and Siberia. The main primary and end uses of nickel are shown in Table 35.2 [6]. Nickel is first and foremost used in stainless steel, together with iron and chromium. Stainless steel is one of the backbones in modern society and is widely used in industry, constructions, cars, shipbuilding, and private homes. Only a minor part of nickel is used in items designed to be in prolonged skin contact. The nickel sulfides and oxides found in nature are not allergenic. Only free nickel ions may act as haptens. The concomitant presence of nickel and cobalt in nature may explain the frequent occurrence of simultaneous contact allergy to these metals. The amount of cobalt mixed with nickel in alloys is likely to decrease as cobalt is more costly than nickel. However, it is currently unknown whether the frequency of concomitant nickel and cobalt allergy is also decreasing among patients. Nickel and chromium do not occur together in nature and combined contact allergy to these metals is therefore uncommon and mainly related to certain occupational exposures.

The most important factor for the induction and elicitation of cutaneous nickel allergy is the amount of nickel per unit area present in the epidermis. Exposure to free nickel ions may either occur in an occupational setting or as a result of skin contact to nickel-plated surfaces or nickel alloys as these are easily corroded by human sweat [7]. The unit for the quantification of

Table 35.2 Distribution and the end uses of primary nickel, 1996 [4]

Distribution of primary nickel	%	End uses of primary nickel	%
Stainless steel	65	Consumer products	19
Nonferrous alloys	13	Building and construction materials	17
Plating	9	Automobile production	11
Alloy steels	8	Process equipment	10
Foundry	3	Chemical industry	8
Other	2	Electronics	8
		General engineering	6
		Other	4
		Railway/transportation equipment	3
		Aerospace materials	3
		Petroleum industry	3
		Electric power generation	2
		Marine equipment	2
		Nickel chemicals	1

exposure to contact allergens is $\mu g/cm^2$. When it comes to nickel exposure from metal items designed to be in prolonged skin contact, the $\mu g/cm^2$ per unit time currently used as nickel release may vary over time depending on the item investigated [8].

Bang-Pedersen et al. introduced the idea that the amount of nickel released from an alloy in synthetic sweat was a significant risk factor for nickel allergy, whereas the total concentration of nickel in the alloy was not important [9]. Later studies showed that metallic items such as buttons and earrings known to induce and elicit allergic nickel dermatitis released large amounts of nickel in synthetic sweat [10, 11]. Menné et al. [8] conceptualized the idea and determined an operational limit that theoretically could prevent nickel allergy in healthy subjects and nickel dermatitis in nickel-sensitized individuals. They collected and investigated a wide range of well-defined nickel alloys and coatings, which were known to either induce nickel allergy or not to represent a nickel allergy hazard. The amount of nickel release in synthetic sweat was determined and later correlated with the alloy's ability to elicit nickel dermatitis in nickel-allergic patients. Based on this research, a nickel release limit of 0.5 $\mu g/cm^2$/week was suggested as a reasonably

safe practical compromise. Alloys releasing less than this amount, typically stainless steel or white gold, will therefore only rarely elicit dermatitis in nickel-allergic individuals, whereas alloys releasing more than 0.5 $\mu g/cm^2$/week, typically nickel-coated items, are likely to result in allergic reactions in already sensitized individuals [8, 12–14]. A recent metaanalysis reviewing past dose–response studies revealed that approximately 5% of a nickel-sensitized population will react to an occluded (e.g., wrist watch and buttons) dose of 0.44 μg nickel/ cm^2/week and also that the induction and elicitation thresholds for skin penetrating exposures (e.g., earrings) are lower [15]. Whether subjects with null-mutations in the filaggrin gene complex may develop nickel allergy when exposed to nickel concentrations below 0.5 $\mu g/cm^2$/week remains to be determined, but it seems that this gene deficiency is associated with nickel allergy [16, 17]. Roughly, the colorimetric dimethylglyoxime (DMG) spot test is able to identify items that release an excessive amount of nickel (>0.5 $\mu g/cm^2$/week) and the test may therefore work well for screening purposes [8]. However, the specificity and sensitivity are not perfect [18, 19].

Nickel has previously been used frequently as an interliner for thin (on the order of μm) gold platings. However, as they are highly porous and do not protect against nickel allergy [7, 14], their use has been more or less abandoned in Europe. If such alloys are used for ear piercing, both gold and nickel may be left in the tissue, probably explaining the high risk of induction of primary sensitization by this procedure [20].

Occupational nickel exposure on the hands is often difficult to quantify. Recently, two new methods to detect nickel on the hands were developed [21, 22]. The finger immersion method and the acid wipe sampling technique are two fairly easy ways to quantify the amount of nickel deposited on the epidermis during work and can be performed in most departments if the techniques become routine. Undoubtedly, industrial nickel exposure, particularly in the plating industry, was previously significant [1, 2], although nickel allergy seems to be a rare problem in nickel refineries. The development of tolerance in workers to inhaled nickel may possibly explain this finding [23]. Quantification of nickel exposure in different industries has previously been documented [24–26]. Many work tools release large amounts of nickel in synthetic sweat, and elicitation of nickel hand eczema is likely to occur [27]. The amount of nickel released from coins during normal handling is generally insufficient to elicit a reaction in nickel-sensitized individuals [28, 29], but a recent study showed that a significant amount of nickel is deposited on the fingers and hands when handling 1 and 2 euro coins which theoretically may lead to dermatitis [30]. Nickel exposure today is not only defined as exposures in specific industries, but is also more related to the individual job. It is therefore important in the case of a positive patch test reaction to nickel to trace the source of primary sensitization (typically, inexpensive jewelry or clothing fasteners), evaluate previous and current exposure to metal items in direct skin contact, and in the case of hand eczema, evaluate personal and occupational exposure (e.g., tools, sewing needles, CD's, and keys) using the DMG test, the acid wipe sampling methods [21, 31], the finger immersion test [22], and other exposure measurements (see Chap. 27).

Nickel is frequently found as an impurity in consumer products, including washing liquids and powders, and other household products, at a concentration of 1–5 ppm. Such concentrations will only exceptionally result in clinical disease among nickel-allergic individuals [32].

> **Core Message**
>
> › The risk of nickel sensitization depends upon nickel release from metal items designed to be in direct and prolonged contact with the skin expressed as $\mu g/cm^2$ over time.

35.2.2 Quantification of Nickel Exposure

The relevant nickel exposure parameter is the free nickel ion in the environment or the nickel skin concentration. Chemical methods have been developed to assess exposure based on atomic absorption and standardized as outlined in Chap. 27. It is particularly important to investigate nickel release from metal surfaces designed to be in direct and prolonged skin contact. The DMG test represents a rapid and easy colorimetric spot test, although both false-positive and false-negative reactions occur (See also Chap. 27). These methods are not ideal for obtaining an overall impression of nickel exposure as an individual may be exposed to many different nickel-releasing alloys and

to nickel in solutions, e.g., oils [25] and water [24]. To quantify nickel exposure, nickel in nails and in skin may be a relevant parameter. Nickel binds and accumulates in the stratum corneum and in the nail plate. A single patch test with nickel sulfate generates a deposit of nickel in the epidermis, with a high concentration in the upper part of the stratum corneum and a declining concentration gradient though the epidermis. Fullerton et al. [33, 34] and Hostynek [35] have illustrated that repeated skin tape stripping may be a powerful tool to quantify nickel exposure.

Nickel in nails may be used to quantify nickel exposure. Peters et al. [36] found a significant difference in the nail concentrations in different occupational groups (Table 35.3). Allenby and Basketter [37] observed that repeated thumb immersion in a 1-ppm nickel solution in sodium lauryl sulfate (SLS) led to the accumulation of nickel in thumbnails at up to 22.2 ppm. Nielsen et al. [38], in a blinded controlled exposure study including nickel-allergic patients with hand eczema, showed that repeated skin exposure to 10–100 ppm nickel provoked a flare-up reaction of their eczema. The corresponding nickel nail concentrations are shown in Table 35.3, together with other experimental provocation studies and occupational field studies. It appears that moderate nickel exposure, as probably present in many workplaces, gives a nickel nail

Table 35.3 Nickel in nails reflecting exposure

Type of exposure		Nickel µg/g (mean)	Reference
Occupational	None (controls)	1.19	[29]
Occupational	Moderate	29.20	[29]
Occupational	Heavy	123.00	[29]
Experimental [a]	Immersion of finger in nickel 1 ppm for 23 days, twice a day	7.80	[30]
Experimental	Immersion of finger in 10 ppm nickel once a day for 1 week	5.50	[32]
Experimental	Immersion of finger in 100 ppm nickel once a day for 1 week	12.00	[32]
Experimental	Baseline	1.58	[32]

[a]Four observations

concentration comparable with those concentrations obtained in experimental exposure studies where a significant flare-up of dermatitis was achieved. Such methods may serve as a more objective evaluation of suspected occupational nickel hand eczema. Similarly, the nickel skin concentration seems to be a useful parameter in experimental exposure studies [39]. Such methods need to be standardized and made generally available for the evaluation of the patients with nickel allergy and hand eczema.

Recently, two new methods to quantify the amount of nickel on the skin were developed [22, 31]. The Lidén method suggests that a patient or a test person is examined for nickel deposition using acid wipe sampling by cellulose wipes with 1% nitric acid. Chemical analysis is then performed by inductively coupled plasma mass spectrometry (ICP-MS) and the test result is expressed in terms of mass per unit area ($\mu g/cm^2$). This method may be useful in patients suspected with occupational nickel dermatitis on the hands [31] (see also Chap. 27, Sect. 27.2). The Staton method is also a procedure for the assessment of nickel levels in occupationally exposed individuals [22]. Briefly, the nickel content on the fingers is measured by immersing the exposed thumbs and index fingers directly into graduated sample tubes containing ultrapure water and aqueous nickel extracts. The solutions are then analyzed by inductively coupled plasma optical emission spectrometry after stabilization with nitric acid.

Core Message

> Nickel exposure can be quantified by nickel skin and nickel nail measurements.

35.2.3 Patch Testing with Nickel

The fact that nickel sulfate, and not nickel chloride, is used for patch testing is probably accidental as Schittenhelm and Stockinger [2] made the first patch test with nickel sulfate from the nickel bath to which the workers were exposed. In the 1930s, Bonnevie included nickel sulfate in the first baseline patch test series. Based on this, nickel sulfate 2.5% and nickel sulfate 5% in petrolatum are now used for the baseline series in North

America and Europe, respectively. The TRUE Test® also uses nickel sulfate and tends to elicit stronger reactions. False-positive reactions may occur in atopics, in whom follicular irritant reactions are particularly seen. The later reactions may possibly be explained by the high prevalence of null-mutations in the filaggrin gene complex among atopics [17, 40]. Filaggrin is a histidine-rich epidermal protein that is likely to chelate nickel. Thus, it is possible that the immune system in patients with filaggrin deficiency is more readily exposed to nickel, as filaggrin does not bind nickel in the epidermis, and instead, allows it to pass into the dermal compartments and meet the immune system. Weak true-positive reactions can also show a follicular pattern. False-negative reactions undoubtedly occur. In such cases, reactions can be obtained with nickel chloride 5% (actually increasing the Ni++ concentration) or by adding penetration enhancers to the patch test, such as DMSO (See also Chap. 24). None of these approaches are suitable for routine testing, as irritant reactions are common. Active patch test sensitization from nickel sulfate 5% in petrolatum has never been documented. This is in agreement with the experiences of Kligman [41] and Vandenberg and Epstein [42], who could only obtain experimental nickel sensitization by repeated exposures to high nickel concentrations in combination with irritants. When a dermatologist-obtained detailed history of nickel exposure is compared with the outcome of patch testing, there is a high degree of correspondence [43]. If the medical history is obtained via a short questionnaire, both false-positive and false-negative reports of nickel allergy are common. Typically, the nickel-sensitized patients have a history of previous inflammation, related to ear piercing or from exposure to inexpensive jewelry, and later, repeated instances of eczema related to skin contact with such metal items. False-positive histories typically include only one such incident and typically on hot summer days. The positive nickel patch test is reproducible [44], but its strength varies in the individual patients over time [45].

Skin hyperreactivity at the site of exposure tends to persist following nickel dermatitis [46]. This phenomenon is specific both with respect to allergic and irritant contact dermatitis [47]. The association between atopy and nickel allergy is controversial. In patch test studies performed in the general population, nickel allergy is equally common among those with and without a positive prick test [48]. However, hospital-based material is more difficult to interpret as both a decreased and an increased frequency of positive nickel patch test reactions have been reported among atopic patients. One explanation may be that active atopic dermatitis tends to downregulate the type IV response and, thereby, the nickel patch test. However, it is possible that the diverging study results may rather be explained by various proportions of atopic patients with filaggrin deficiency in the study materials.

Dose–response studies have been performed with nickel sulfate and nickel chloride using both occluded and nonoccluded exposure methods. The concentration threshold for reactivity to a single exposure has been established to be 1.5 $\mu g/cm^2$ in open testing [49] and 0.5 $\mu g/cm^2$ in closed applications [12, 50, 51]. For the weakest positive reactions, a papular or follicular morphology is typically observed. This is not well described in the literature and both the hair follicle and the sweat duct may be important routes for nickel absorption (see also Chap. 12). Recently, Fischer et al. showed that the elicitation threshold for the patch test was higher than the elicitation threshold (per application) for the repeated open application test (ROAT), but also that it was nearly similar to the accumulated elicitation threshold for the ROAT [52]. Also, the authors showed that for the elicitation of nickel dermatitis, the size of the exposed area (and therefore the total amount of applied nickel) influenced the elicitation reaction at some concentrations, even though the same dose per unit area was applied [53].

In vitro testing with haptens is dealt with in Chap. 2. There is comprehensive literature on the diagnosis of nickel allergy by the lymphocyte transformation test (LTT). Individuals with a positive history of metal dermatitis, but negative patch test, may have an elevated LTT. Furthermore, it has been observed that the LTT to nickel is elevated in nonallergic controls, compared to cord blood. The implication of this finding is uncertain, and the consequences for clinical disease have not been investigated [54].

Core Message

> The standard nickel patch test is safe and reproducible.

35.2.4 Clinical Picture

Historically, nickel dermatitis was most often observed as occupational hand and forearm eczema in workers in the plating industry [1, 2]. The combined effect of irritancy and contact allergy from exposure to high nickel concentrations, combined with low hygiene standards and the unavailability of treatment, led to the severe itchy dermatitis in these workers. The first cases of consumer nickel dermatitis were seen following long-term skin contact with spectacle frames and wristwatches [3]. Bonnevie [55] was the first to patch test a large group of eczema patients with a baseline series containing nickel sulfate. This led to the recognition of suspender dermatitis as a consequence of primary nickel sensitization. In the 1950s and 1960s, Calnan [56] and Marcussen [57] published a large number of nickel dermatitis cases. The separation of nickel dermatitis into a primary and a secondary eruption was introduced. "Primary eruption" means the anatomical location of primary sensitization, typically related to the suspender area or other metal contact sites. "Secondary eruption" typically means symmetrical eruptions with vesicular hand eczema, eczema in the flexural areas, and on the eyelids. It was speculated that the tendency of nickel dermatitis to spread was caused by cutaneous nickel dissemination or by a hematogenous spread caused following nickel absorption through the area of suspender dermatitis. Research on systemic allergic contact dermatitis from nickel (see later in this chapter) in the 1970s and 1980s indicated that the secondary eruptions in females with persistent metal object dermatitis (e.g., earrings) were equivalent to systemic allergic contact dermatitis and were caused by systemic nickel exposure from nickel skin absorption. The causes of primary nickel eruptions (sensitization) have changed with fashion, from suspenders to buttons in blue jeans and, more recently, to ear piercing [20, 58–60] and perhaps mobile phones [5]. The primary eruption of nickel allergy differs around the world, depending on local fashion and regulation of nickel skin exposure (see later in this chapter). The severity of nickel dermatitis depends upon how early the condition is recognized and, furthermore, whether nickel exposure from metal items in direct and prolonged skin contact is avoided, and finally whether occupational nickel contact can be minimized.

35

35.2.5 Systemic Allergic Contact Dermatitis

Systemic allergic contact dermatitis in general and systemic allergic contact dermatitis elicited by drugs are dealt with in Chaps. 17 and 38, respectively. Systemic allergic contact dermatitis may lead to various clinical patterns, including vesicular hand eczema, flexural eczema, flare-up reactions at earlier sites of contact dermatitis, and the "baboon syndrome" [61] that is observed in individuals with contact allergy in case they are exposed systemically (e.g., orally, by inhalation, or transcutaneously) to the specific hapten. The early reports of nickel dermatitis described a tendency to more widespread dermatitis reactions [2]. Christensen and Möller [62] were the first to provoke systemic allergic contact dermatitis experimentally in patients with nickel allergy. A number of later studies have confirmed their observations. There is a clear tendency toward a dose–response relationship, with few reacting at a dose below 0.5 mg elemental nickel and the majority reacting at 5.6 mg [63]. Flare-up reactions depend upon the degree of previous exposure and the time period since the last eruption [57]. Experimental provocation doses have traditionally been higher than the daily nickel intake in food, which ranges between 100 and 300 µg/day. Under normal circumstances, a number of factors interfere with the amount of nickel absorbed; among them are alcohol intake, atopy [64], drugs, and the composition of food. Release of nickel from infusion cannulae, dialysis equipment, internal prostheses, and dental braces is a rare cause of systemic nickel contact dermatitis.

35.2.6 Tolerance to Nickel

Though nickel is ubiquitous in the environment, only a subset of nickel-exposed individuals become allergic. This may be explained by uneven environmental nickel exposure, null-mutations in the filaggrin gene complex, and finally the development of tolerance in some individuals. Retrospective epidemiological studies have demonstrated tolerance to nickel following oral exposure [65, 66]. Among 1501 Danish adolescents from the general population and among 2,176 patients from patch test clinics, application of dental braces prior to ear piercing was associated with a significantly reduced prevalence of nickel allergy. Along the Norwegian–Russian border, the prevalence of nickel allergy was significantly lower among Russian women than among Norwegian women, although the prevalence of ear piercing was equally high [67]. This finding was explained by a long period of high nickel concentrations in the drinking water on the Russian side of the border caused by pollution from two nickel factories. Several clinical studies have also looked into the exacerbation of dermatitis following high oral nickel intake, as well as the reduction of hand dermatitis in nickel-allergic individuals following low-nickel diets [68, 69]. Finally, oral administration of nickel in animals prevented sensitization upon experimental cutaneous exposure [70]. The immunological background for the development of tolerance has been increasingly elucidated. In a simplified model, nickel allergy and dermatitis result from the concomitant intervention of antigen-specific effector CD8+ T-cells that cause tissue damage and from the amplification caused by T helper 1 (Th1) CD4+ cells. In subjects without nickel allergy, nickel reactive CD4+ T-cells can be isolated from peripheral blood, which suggests a tolerance reaction in these individuals [71]. Furthermore, a subset of CD4+ T-cells, named T regulatory 1 (Tr1), isolated from non-allergic individuals secrete IL-10 that may effectively block the maturation of dendritic cells. Nickel-specific Tr1 cells can also be isolated from nickel-allergic individuals, but in much lower concentrations [72]. Another subtype of CD4+ T-cells expresses CD25 antigens and also has a regulatory function in nonallergic subjects [73]. These cells mainly work through cell-to-cell interaction and are found in high numbers in the skin of non-allergic subjects following patch testing. Also, the depletion of CD4+ CD25 T-cells resulted in reduced oral tolerance in already tolerant animals [74] and in increased nickel specific responsiveness in T-cells isolated from nonallergic individuals [75]. Finally, Wu et al. showed that there was an inverse dose–response relationship between the amount of oral nickel uptake and nickel sensitization in mice [76]. Taken together, the immunological mechanisms in tolerance are several and seem to have lasting reactions.

> **Core Message**
>
> ❯ Tolerance to nickel may follow oral exposure to nickel from, e.g., drinking water or dental braces. The immunological background remains to be completely elucidated.

35.2.7 Epidemiology

It was previously believed that the number of patients receiving medical treatment reflected the number of individuals with a contact allergy to nickel. Based upon this assumption, Marcussen [77] estimated that the prevalence of nickel allergy was 1 in 10,000 women. In the 1970s, this belief was questioned and it was rather believed that contact allergy to nickel, and also to other haptens, was common and that those cases seen by dermatologists only represented the most severe and complicated cases. The latter ideas were confirmed by patch test studies in Scandinavia and the US [78–80] as they estimated that the prevalence of nickel allergy in the general population was approximately 10% in women and 1–2% in men. Later, more comprehensive studies confirmed these findings as they found a high prevalence of nickel allergy in the youngest age groups [81]. A recent review including patch test studies performed in the general population mainly in Europe and North America showed that up to 17% of women and 3% of men are nickel-allergic and that the proportion of nickel allergy out of contact allergy in general increased significantly between the 1960s and 1990s from 5 to 65% [4]. Risk factors of nickel allergy in the general population include female gender, ear piercing, and also tobacco smoking [4, 82]. Recently, general population studies have suggested a decrease of nickel allergy among Danish women, which is likely to be an effect of the regulation on nickel exposure [83, 84]. The majority of nickel-allergic subjects in the general population have a healthy skin at the time of examination, but they report previous ear piercing, jewelry dermatitis, and/or hand eczema. The nickel problem in the general population seems to be a global phenomenon [4].

Clinical patch test data published over the last 50 years have invariably put nickel as the most common contact allergen among female dermatitis patients worldwide. While the prevalence of contact allergy to most other allergens from the baseline series is between 2 and 4%, the prevalence of nickel allergy is usually between 15 and 25%. The marked difference in prevalence is mainly explained by an unrestricted exposure to nickel in women from consumer items such as inexpensive jewelry, suspenders, clothing fasteners, and ear piercing. Thus, the difference is not explained by the potency of nickel as the human maximization test [41] has classified nickel as a medium–strong sensitizer. Whether the recognition of nickel ions by human T-cells may influence the high prevalence is currently unknown. Gamerdinger et al. recently suggested that the high prevalence of nickel allergy could be explained by the fact that nickel may directly link the T cell receptor (TCR) and the major histocompatibility complex (MHC) in a peptide independent manner [85]. Such a connection between the TCR and the MHC mimics that of superantigens, but could not be found for other metals. The different prevalences of nickel allergy observed among patients from patch test centers in different countries may not necessarily reflect major differences in the pattern and burden of nickel exposure, but rather

35

differences regarding referral in the medical systems, the availability of patch testing, and their interpretation.

Data, overtime, from the same patch test center may be more interesting to study as major variables can be controlled. In Malmö, Sweden [45], the prevalence of nickel allergy increased from 7% in 1962 to 29% in 1997 among women, and from 1 to 6% among men during the same time period. In recent years, several studies have found a change in the epidemiology of nickel allergy in Europe. Three Danish patch test centers, using similar patch test methods with unchanged staff and unchanged referral patterns, compared patch data from 1986 to 1998, standardized with respect to sex, age, atopy, leg ulcers, and occupation (MOAHL index). The prevalence of nickel allergy in children (0–18 years of age) decreased significantly from 25.8% in 1986 to 9.2% in 1998 [86]. Present or past jewelry dermatitis was identified in most patients with a positive patch test reaction. 33.2% of nickel-allergic patients seen in 1998 were judged to have a current nonoccupational exposure to nickel, as compared to 73.5% in 1986. Patch test studies from Germany and Denmark (both in University hospitals and in private dermatology practice) have demonstrated similar trends, i.e., a decrease of nickel allergy in younger age groups and increasing prevalences of nickel allergy in middle-aged and older age groups, probably as a result of cohort effects [87–90]. However, the strongest evidence of an effect of the EU Nickel Directive comes from two repeated cross-sectional general population studies performed in Copenhagen, Denmark in 1990 and 2006 [84]. The studies showed that around 6.9% of 18–69-year-old Danish women who ear-pierced after the Danish nickel regulation was passed in 1990 were nickel-allergic in comparison to 15.6% of those who ear-pierced before 1990 and 3.0% of those never pierced. It is likely that these changes are a consequence of the regulation on nickel skin exposure as the prevalence of nickel allergy has increased during the same period in countries without regulations, e.g., the US [91].

> **Core Message**
>
> › Nickel is the most common contact allergen in females, affecting 17% of all women worldwide. Frequencies between 20 and 30% are observed among patch tested patients.

35.2.8 Hand Eczema and Nickel Allergy

Nickel may cause or aggravate hand eczema by four different pathogenic mechanisms (Table 35.4). Hand eczema is frequently a multifactorial disease and the different types of pathogenesis may operate together. Atopy is known to be an aggravating factor for the prognosis of nickel hand eczema, although it is unknown whether it is an independent risk factor [51]. It has been demonstrated that the concentration threshold that leads to skin reactivity is lower in anatomical regions with previous nickel dermatitis than in regions without previous nickel dermatitis [46]. This mechanism and its combination with irritants might also enact together with the four main etiologies [92].

There is solid historical evidence to support that high concentrations of nickel sulfate or nickel chloride in the plating industry could induce and elicit hand eczema [1, 2]. However, there is less clinical evidence to support that moderate nickel exposure (point two in Table 35.4) may aggravate hand eczema. Wall and Calnan [26] described seven workers in the electronic industry, in whom allergic nickel eczema was primarily induced on the hands by an exposure concentration of 40 ppm. A controlled hand exposure study in nickel-allergic subjects using a 1 ppm concentration did not provoke any aggravation [37]. In a double-blind placebo controlled exposure study over 2 weeks, a statistically significant aggravation was observed when patients with nickel allergy and low-grade hand eczema were exposed to 10–100 ppm nickel [38]. This exposure level is probably not uncommon in many industries, as indicated by nickel nail measurements. Also, Lidén et al. showed that locksmiths and carpenters have relatively high deposits of nickel on especially

Table 35.4 Mechanisms which can cause and aggravate hand eczema in the nickel-sensitive population

Occupational exposure to high (not further defined) concentration of nickel. Where nickel acts both as an allergen and an irritant, e.g., in electroplating
Exposure (occupational) to moderate nickel salt concentrations in the region of 10–100 ppm, probably in combination with irritants. Many different jobs in industry
Transcutaneous absorption of nickel released from metal items worn in prolonged skin contact, e.g., costume jewelry, suspenders, buttons, etc.
Systemic nickel exposure from food or nickel released from, e.g., dental braces

the fingers due to their work routines [21] (see also Chap. 27, Sect. 27.2 "Skin Exposure Assessment").

Vesicular hand eczema caused by transcutaneous absorption of nickel following jewelry dermatitis is probably still common today [93]. The vesicular eruption appears on the hands as a systemic allergic contact dermatitis reaction because of transcutaneous absorption of nickel. It has been demonstrated that elimination of metal items causing contact dermatitis may lead to enhanced prognosis in a significant number of patients with hand eczema [93].

Finally, nickel hand eczema may be a part of systemic allergic contact dermatitis, with vesicular hand eczema provoked by nickel in food or nickel released from dental braces or metal prostheses (see also Chap. 17).

The frequency of occupational nickel hand eczema will vary from one country to another, depending upon the perception of the disease entity, regional industries, and local laws [94]. In the period 1984–1991, a total number of 1,486 cases of occupational nickel dermatitis were notified to the Danish authorities in a background population of five million people [95]. Most cases were reported by dermatologists based on patch test results, occupational history, and assessment of exposure to nickel at a workplace by using the DMG test. Developments of objective methods such as the acid wipe sampling test may improve the quality of the medico-legal process (see also Chap. 27, Sect. 27.2).

General population studies have shown that nickel-allergic individuals have an increased risk of developing hand eczema [4]. However, the strength of this association seems to diminish as nickel exposure has been reduced in the general population in Europe [96, 97].

> **Core Message**
>
> › Nickel allergy can cause hand eczema, either as a consequence of occupational or domestic exposure or as a part of systemic allergic contact dermatitis.

35.2.9 Specific Treatment

Besides general treatment recommendations (see Chap. 49), specific treatment modalities partly experimentally exist for nickel dermatitis. Nickel hand eczema as described in the literature is known to have a notoriously bad prognosis, but, undoubtedly, many mild cases exist unnoticed in the population. Contributing to the bad prognosis are secondary bacterial infection, atopy, multiple contact allergies, and frequent nickel exposure, either transcutaneously or systemically. In the evaluation of the patients with nickel hand eczema, all these factors need consideration. If standard evaluation and treatment fail to help patients, a diet with low-nickel content may help [69]. The diet is recommended to be evaluated over 1–2 months. Chelating drugs have an effect on nickel dermatitis, when used both topically and systemically [98]. Statistically significant effects of systemic diethyldithiocarbamate (Antabuse) have been found in a controlled study [99], but the treatment has not found general acceptances because of possible side effects, such as flare-up of nickel dermatitis and, in some patients, liver toxicity.

35.2.10 Prevention and Legislation

The Danish nickel regulation was passed in 1990 [100]. It dictated that certain consumer products such as jewelry, buttons, spectacle frames, and wristwatches should not release more than 0.5 µg nickel/cm^2/week, an exposure limit identified in the nickel alloy study performed by Menné et al. [8]. Nickel contact dermatitis has since decreased among dermatitis patients in Denmark and epidemiological studies indicate that the frequency of nickel allergy has also decreased significantly among young subjects in the general population [86]. A European Nickel Directive primarily based on the Danish regulation was passed in 1994.

The original requirement (before 2005) dictated that nickel was prohibited in postassemblies used during epithelialization after piercing, unless they were homogenous and the nickel concentration was less than 0.05%. However, a new requirement from 2005 replaced the original requirement and dictates that nickel release from all items inserted into pierced parts of the body (not only during epithelialization after piercing) should be less than 0.2 µg/cm^2/week. Finally, the Nickel Directive dictates that coated products covered by the directive should not release more nickel than 0.5 µg nickel/cm^2/week within their first 2 years of use (Table 35.5).

A group led by Lidén, within the European Committee for Standardization (CEN), developed analytical methods

35

Table 35.5 The EU Nickel Directive (94/27/EC, adopted 1994, in force 2000, part of REACH 2009) and analytical methods by European Committee for Standardization (CEN)

Part	Nickel may not be used	CEN standard for control of limit
1	*To September 2005*: In postassemblies used during epithelization, unless they are homogeneous and the concentration of nickel is less than 0.05%	EN 1810 (nickel content by atomic absorption spectrometry)
1 rev.	*From September 2005*: In all postassemblies which are inserted into pierced ears and other pierced parts (not only during epithelization), unless the nickel release is less than 0.2 µg/cm² per week	EN 1811 (nickel release in artificial sweat)
2	In products intended to come into direct and prolonged contact with the skin, such as earrings, necklaces, wristwatch cases, watch straps, buttons, tighteners, zips, and mobile phones, if nickel release is greater than 0.5 µg/cm² per week	EN 1811 (nickel release in artificial sweat) CR 12471 (screening test by dimethylglyoxime)
3	In coated products, unless the coating is sufficient to ensure that the nickel release will not exceed 0.5 µg/cm² per week after 2 years of normal use	EN 12472 (wear and corrosion test)

for the control of compliance with the requirements of the Directive (Table 35.5). This European regulation developed by collaboration between the industry and dermatologists has come into effect from 2000. Based on the Danish experience and the outcome of other allergen exposure limitations, e.g., the European cosmetics directive and limitation of exposure to hexavalent chromate in cement in Scandinavian countries, a major impact can be expected [83, 87, 88]. The frequency on the market of items under part 2 of the Nickel Directive that release nickel has been investigated. A baseline study before (1999) and a follow-up study 2 years after the Directive came into force (2002/2003) revealed a significant adaptation to the requirements [101, 102]. These findings should be regarded in a global setting as a recent DMG test study performed in San Francisco showed that the prevalence of DMG positive earrings is high in an American city [103]. It is important to realize that the present EU regulation concerns well-defined nickel-containing metallic consumer items designed to be in direct and prolonged skin contact, e.g., costume jewelry, buttons, and spectacles. Recently, it was decided that mobile phones should also be covered by the EU Nickel Directive as these are often in prolonged and direct skin contact. Thus, occupational exposure to tools and, e.g., coins and other materials is not included. Whether such items need any kind of regulation may depend upon future risk assessment.

> **Core Message**
>
> › Regulating nickel release from consumer items designed to be in direct and prolonged skin contact effectively prevents nickel dermatitis.

35.2.11 Suggested Reading

In 1956, Calnan [56] published clinical data from a large group of patients with nickel dermatitis. He described the primary eruption from metal consumer items and the tendency to secondary eruptions, particularly vesicular hand eczema. Christensen and Möller in 1975 [62] provoked nickel-allergic individuals with an oral nickel dose and observed lesions similar to the secondary eruptions described earlier by Calnan. The studies led to the general understanding that a limited allergic contact dermatitis may lead to a widespread eruption through a systemic exposure based on a transcutaneous absorption. By repeating the oral nickel provocation studies by Christensen and Möller, we observed skin changes that led to description of the "baboon syndrome" [61] as a part of systemic allergic contact dermatitis.

35.3 Chromium

Crocoite – a lead-containing chromium (Cr) ore – was found in Russia by Pallas in 1765. Chromium metal was isolated in 1797 in France by Vauqelin [104]. Since the nineteenth century, chromium has found many industrial uses including leather tanning, production of alloys, and chrome plating. In 1925, Parkhurst was the first to report chromium contact allergy based on skin testing in a blue print processor [105]. Open testing with a 0.5% aqueous solution of potassium dichromate produced a papulovesicular reaction in 24 h. Thereafter, chromium compounds have been established as important ubiquitous contact allergens.

Historically, the most common cause of chromium sensitization has derived from skin contact with hexavalent chromium in wet cement. Thus, allergic contact dermatitis from chromate was a significant occupational skin disease among construction workers. Although this is still the case in many parts of the world, the epidemiological pattern is now changing in Europe following the regulation on chromium content in cement. Today, chromium exposure from skin contact with, namely, leather gloves and shoes is considered the most common cause of chromium allergy among dermatitis patients [106]. Besides contact allergy, chromium compounds have other toxicological properties, such as carcinogenicity, caustic capacity, and general toxicity [107, 108]. A chemical burn from chromic acid can be life-threatening (see also Chap. 16 "Clinical aspects of irritant contact dermatitis"). The same type of chromium compounds may induce both contact allergy and cancer, while the other toxicological effects are unrelated to contact allergy. Finally, revival of metal-on-metal total hip arthroplasties [109], which typically consist of a forged, high-carbon, cobalt-chromium-molybdenum material [110], may pose a problem in chromium-allergic individuals as it has been suggested that the prevalence of metal allergy may be higher among patients with implant failure [109, 111]. Further studies are needed to confirm or reject such an association.

Milestones in our understanding of chromium dermatitis are summarized in Table 35.6.

Table 35.6 Milestones in the history of chromium dermatitis

1900s	"Cement itch" in construction workers
1925	Chromium contact allergy in a blue print processor
1931	Patch testing with potassium dichromate, ammonium chromate, and sodium dichromate
1950	Detection of hexavalent chromium in cement
1970s	Detection of new sources of chromium exposure Chemical studies on iron sulfate and cement
1980s	Legislation in Nordic countries – iron sulfate added to cement
1990s	Epidemiological studies – general population and construction workers
2005	EU legislation on hexavalent chromium in cement
2009	Consumer dermatitis from leather exposure is the dominant cause in Europe – the possibility of a regulatory intervention is raised

> **Core Message**
>
> › Occupational and, later, consumer product chromium allergy have been frequent for the last 100 years.

35.3.1 Physicochemical Aspects and Sensitizing Potential

Chromium is one of the most widely distributed metals. Chromite ($FeOCr_2O_3$) is the principal ore of chromium. Chromium exists in every oxidation state from 0 to +6, but only the ground states 0, +2, +3, and +6 are common. Many chromium compounds have the capacity to induce sensitization and elicit chromium contact allergy. However, in contrast to other sensitizing metals, metallic chromium (ground state 0) is not sensitizing, due to its capacity to form a poorly soluble layer of oxide on the surface [7]. Therefore, it is probably more accurate to use the term "chromate allergy." The question whether there is one or more chromium haptens is not firmly resolved. Most hexavalent chromium compounds are freely water-soluble and pass through the epidermis more readily than most trivalent chromium compounds, which are insoluble [112]. It is thought that hexavalent chromium penetrates the skin and is then reduced enzymatically to trivalent chromium, which combines with protein as the hapten [113]. It has previously been demonstrated using a baseline patch test technique that if the concentration of trivalent chromium is high enough and the exposure time sufficiently prolonged, positive tests will also result [114]. More recent data indicate that patch testing with serial dilutions of hexavalent and trivalent chromium may result in positive reactions down to low concentrations [115]. Principally, the capacity to induce and elicit chromium contact allergy depends on the concentration of the chromium compound, oxidation state, and solubility, the latter often being dependent on the pH [116].

Hexavalent chromium exists as chromates and dichromates of potassium, sodium, calcium, and ammonium, which are highly water-soluble, while barium, lead, and zirconium chromates and dichromates are poorly soluble. Zinc dichromate is soluble, while zinc chromate is less soluble.

Trivalent chromium exists as salts of inorganic and organic acids, for example, chlorides, nitrates, sulfates,

35

and oxalates. Most of these salts are water-soluble, but penetrate the skin to a lesser degree than water-soluble hexavalent chromium compounds. In an alkaline environment, poorly soluble chromium hydroxide is precipitated from trivalent chromium salts. On the other hand, basic chromium (III) sulfate used for leather tanning is also water-soluble in an alkaline environment. Chromium (III) oxide and chromium hydroxide are virtually water-insoluble.

Tetravalent chromium compounds, such as chromium dioxide, can be partly transformed to hexavalent and trivalent chromium in the presence of water.

35.3.2 Chromium Use and Exposure

Chromium as a metal is present in various alloys, for example, in stainless steel, together with nickel and iron and on chrome-plated surfaces.

Chromium compounds are present in the raw materials used for the production of cement. Cement is produced at a high temperature in an alkaline environment and with an excess of oxygen, by which trivalent chromium compounds are partly oxidized to hexavalent chromium. The content of water-soluble hexavalent chromium in cement varies widely in different countries, mainly due to the variation in chromium content of the raw materials used [117, 118], but it is also due to the amount of alkali sulfate in the cement [119]. However, there is no correlation between the total content of chromium compounds in cement and its content of water-soluble hexavalent chromium [116].

Primer paints, usually yellow, red, and orange, often contain poorly water-soluble zinc, lead, and barium chromates (VI). Also, freely soluble and, thus, sensitizing alkali chromates (VI) can be present. When iron treated with such anticorrosion paints is tooled, hexavalent chromium can be extracted by the cutting fluids. Chromates in paints for wood do not contain the sensitizing alkali chromates.

Zinc-galvanized sheet metal is often coated (chromated) with both trivalent and hexavalent chromium compounds to prevent the metal dulling. When such chromated metal is handled, chromates can leach out and be transferred to volar parts of the hands. The Directive in the Restriction of the use of certain Hazardous Substances (RoHS) in the EU has recently banned the use of hexavalent chromium more or less

for the passivation of zinc and coating on aluminum for the electronic and automotive industry. A lot of these conventional coatings have now been replaced by trivalent chromium doped with different type of cobalt oxides.

On welding of stainless steel and nonstainless steel, hexavalent chromium can be released and generated, respectively, and distributed to the face via the welding fume.

Hexavalent chromium compounds are used in special tanks for chrome plating, a process consisting of applying a layer of metallic chromium to the surface. To avoid chrome ulcers from skin contact with such caustic chromium compounds, the process is automated, which not only prevents chrome ulcers, but also reduces the risk of chromate sensitization.

It is estimated that 90% of the global leather production is tanned using chromium sulfates [120]. Though only trivalent chromium is used for the tanning process, hexavalent chromium is often detected in leather, probably as a result of high heat and pH [121–123]. The Federal Institute for Risk Assessment in Germany recently recommended that the levels of chromium in leather goods should be strictly limited as the regulatory authorities of the federal states found that more than half of 850 leather goods contained hexavalent chromium, and that in one sixth, the levels were higher than 10 mg/kg leather (http://www.bfr. bund.de/cd/9575). Also, in a recent Danish study, 35% of 43 leather products on the Danish market contained hexavalent chromium above the detection limit of 3 ppm (range 4–15 ppm) [124]. Tannery workers may become sensitized following exposure to trivalent chromium [125], but the vast majority of patients are sensitized and develop allergic contact dermatitis from chromium in finished leather products, such as gloves and shoes [121, 126–130].

Besides the above-mentioned causes of chromate sensitization, there are many other possibilities, including the wood pulp industry, ash either from burnt wood or matches with chromate in the match head, coolants and machine oils, defatting solvents, brine added to yeast residues, the dye industry (due to either a dye, a reducing agent, or a mordant), printing, glues, foundry sand, boiler linings, television work (ammonium dichromate to produce cross-linking of light-sensitive polyvinyl alcohol magnetic tape (chromium dioxide)), solutions used to facilitate tire fitting, and preservatives used in milk testing.

Table 35.7 Occupational exposure to chromium is possible during contact with the following chemicals and work procedures

Analytic standards reagents

Anticorrosion agents

Batteries

Catalysts (for hydrogenation, oxidation, polymerization)

Ceramics

Drilling muds

Chromium lignosulfonates (from sodium dichromate using lignosulfate waste)

Electroplating and anodizing agents

Engraving

Explosives

Fire retardant

Magnetic tapes

Metallic chromium

Milk preservatives

Paints and varnishes

Paper

"Chrome cake" (containing sodium sulfate and small amounts of sodium dichromate)

Photography

Roofing

Sutures

Tanning leather

Textile mordants and dyes

Television screens

Wood preservatives

Traditionally, exposure to chromium compounds is most likely to occur occupationally and, above all, in jobs where men traditionally predominate. Examples of occupational exposure to chromium chemicals and work procedures are given in Table 35.7. A recent study showed that occupational skin contact with chromated metal products is a hazard in chromium-allergic patients as nearly half reacted to patch testing with chromated metal rings [131]. However, chromate allergy is increasingly caused by leather exposure in female and male dermatitis patients [106], which may result in foot dermatitis [132] or hand dermatitis [106]. High levels of chromium in detergents and bleaches have been suggested as a possible cause of chromate allergy in women in Spain, France, Belgium, and Israel [133–135], while bleaches had only trace levels of chromate in the USA [136]. When the presence of chromate in detergents and bleaches was investigated chemically, chromium above 1 ppm was detected in most of the products and with a top value at 546 ppm for one detergent [134]. The clinical relevance of chromate in household products was investigated in a study including 17 dermatitis patients with contact allergy to hexavalent chromium [137]. The patients were patch tested with serial dilutions of potassium dichromate and ROAT was performed with aqueous solutions containing 1% SLS and potassium dichromate in the concentration range 5–50 ppm. The respective solution was applied to the antecubital fossa twice daily for 1 week and 57% failed to react to 50 ppm, while 20% tested positively to 5 ppm.

In certain areas of the USA, Scotland, Mexico, and Japan, large volumes of chromite ore-processing residue (COPR) containing hexavalent chromium have been used to fill low-lying areas [138]. Because of concern about the potential risk of chromate allergy, sensitization, and particularly, elicitation in already sensitized individuals, several studies have been conducted to elucidate the problem in the 1990s [138–144]. Based on the results of a patch test study in which the threshold dose (g/cm^2) (MET) for allergic contact dermatitis was measured among those who had previously been sensitized [141] and estimations and assumptions on exposure assessment regarding soil-on-skin adherence and the bioavailability of hexavalent chromium in COPR, it was concluded that direct contact with soil concentrations at least as high as 1,240 ppm should not elicit allergic contact dermatitis in sensitized individuals [140]. In a recent study, the potential for the elicitation of allergic contact dermatitis from skin contact with chromium in standing water in the environment was investigated [138]. Twenty six people known to be allergic to hexavalent chromium were exposed to 25–29 ppm chromium by immersion of one arm for 30 min/day for three consecutive days in a potassium dichromate bath [138]. Ten of the volunteers developed a few papules or vesicles, mild redness, and pruritus on the chromate-challenged arm. Histopathologically, there was perieccrine and perivascular inflammation with spongiosis, consistent with an allergic mechanism, but in some specimens, epidermal necrosis spoke more in favor of an irritant mechanism. Generally, participants with the lowest MET to hexavalent chromium were more likely to react [138]. Due to the lack of a control group of nonsensitized individuals, it was impossible to tell whether the reactions were allergic or irritant in nature. In spite of the development of inflammatory reactions in 10 out of 26 (38%) volunteers, the authors state: "Based on these data, concentrations of 25–29 mg/L Cr (VI) in water can be considered the no-effect levels for allergic contact dermatitis and irritant contact dermatitis for Cr-sensitized persons for nearly all plausible environmental exposures to standing water" [138]. However, our interpretation is that these inflammatory reactions in the ten volunteers were allergic in nature, as the concentration of aqueous potassium dichromate needed to cause irritant reactions on patch testing is around 1,000 ppm and allergic patch test reactions can be elicited by concentrations lower than 25 ppm [145, 146].

Sometimes, chemical investigations are required to demonstrate present exposure to chromium in a chromate-sensitive person. Most often, atomic absorption spectroscopy is used, but it is important to stress that this method measures the total chromium level, while it is only the chromate level that is of interest from a contact allergic standpoint. Atomic absorption spectroscopy has been used [147] to demonstrate the accumulation of chromium in the fingernails of chromate-sensitive patients with hand dermatitis, after the fingers had been immersed in aqueous chromate solutions for 10 min/day for a period of 2 weeks. In Chap. 27, a method to evaluate hexavalent chromium content is described. Finally, Lidén et al. recently developed a new technique to sample chromium deposition on the hands by using cellulose wipes with 1% nitric acid [31]. Following the sampling procedure, chemical analysis is performed by inductively coupled plasma mass spectrometry (ICP-MS) and the test result is expressed in terms of mass per unit area (μg/cm^2). In a study including 18 participants (carpenters, locksmiths, secretaries, and cashiers), chromium was sampled in all subjects. It turned out that locksmiths had the largest amount of chromium on their hands as shown by the mean values of all samples (chromium 0.045 μg/cm^2/h) [21].

> **Core Message**
>
> › Particularly hexavalent chromium compounds are significant for chromium allergy. Cement and leather are important sources of hexavalent chromium.

35.3.3 Patch Testing with Chromate

In 1931, there were three publications on allergic contact dermatitis from chromate. Hexavalent chromium compounds, ammonium chromate 1% [148], potassium dichromate 0.5% [149], and sodium dichromate 0.1% [150], respectively, were used for patch testing. Also in the 1930s, Bonnevie included potassium dichromate in the first baseline patch test series [151]. Today, potassium dichromate 0.5% in petrolatum is still present in the baseline series for Europe, while the same salt at 0.25% is recommended in North America. The TRUE Test also uses potassium dichromate. There is a major problem with these baseline test preparations, as irritant reactions can be elicited – reactions that morphologically resemble allergic reactions may incorrectly be interpreted as allergic reactions. Retesting, both epicutaneously and intracutaneously, has been done at some centers when test reaction have been considered possibly irritant [152, 153]. When lower concentrations of potassium dichromate, 0.375% and 0.25%, are used, there will be fewer irritant reactions, but these preparations will also miss some true chromate allergies [154]. Patch testing with trivalent salts such as chromium trichloride and chromium sulfate produces a high percentage of false-negatives [141, 155]. Compared to hexavalent chromium, the patch test activity of trivalent compounds has previously been reported to be in the order of 1/10 for oxalate, 1/100 for chloride, and 1/1,000 for the acetate [114], which is in contrast with the results of a recent study in which patients hypersensitive to hexavalent chromium were patch tested with dilutions of both hexavalent chromium (potassium dichromate) and trivalent chromium (chromium trichloride hexahydrate) [115]. Both compounds were capable of eliciting dermatitis at low concentrations.

There are several reports of patch test studies performed to determine the threshold concentration of hexavalent chromium to elicit erythema or dermatitis [115, 137, 141, 144–146, 156]. Expectedly, the results vary with the population studied, patch test technique and vehicles used, and the definition of end point. In the presence of SLS, the threshold was lowered almost ten times [137]. Based on the literature, the threshold for elicitation of allergic contact dermatitis from hexavalent chromium is 1–10 ppm (corresponding to 0.03–0.3 μg/cm^2 for a Finn Chamber with a diameter of 0.8 cm and application of 15 μL to the patch unit)

[145, 146]. With the TRUE Test technique, the concentration threshold for a single exposure has been established at 0.089 g/cm^2 [141].

Leucocyte migration inhibition and lymphocyte blast transformations tests have been used to examine contact sensitivity to chromium. These tests can supplement patch testing. Equivalent results for trivalent and hexavalent chromium compounds have been reported [157, 158]. Recently, a study showed that the sensitivity of the lymphocyte proliferation test (LPT) is still moderate [159]. However, in a different study, the LTT revealed that chromium-allergic individuals with dermatitis displayed significantly higher LTT responses than sensitized volunteers without dermatitis and controls ($p<0.05$ and $p<0.01$, respectively) [160].

> **Core Message**
>
> › Patch testing with 0.5% potassium dichromate is needed to not miss chromium allergy, but this concentration may elicit irritant reactions.

35.3.4 Clinical Picture

Allergic contact dermatitis from chromate is eczematous, sometimes widespread and very persistent [161, 162]. Although the reasons for the persistence of chrome dermatitis are unknown, a common explanation is the presence of unrecognized chromium in the environment. A pattern resembling nummular eczema may be seen. Frequent and marked dryness and lichenification make it resemble atopic dermatitis. Cement eczema caused by hexavalent chromium is initially localized to the dorsal aspect of the hands and often has a nummular pattern. Later, the cement eczema can also involve the volar parts of the hands. Foot dermatitis is also a frequent clinical manifestation following contact with leather shoes, boots, or sandals [163, 164].

> **Core Message**
>
> › Allergic contact dermatitis from chromate may present as a widespread persistent dermatitis, resembling nummular eczema.

35.3.5 Systemic Contact Dermatitis

Chromium, trivalent or hexavalent, is an essential element required for normal carbohydrate and lipid metabolism. Studies on patients under total parenteral nutrition have indicated that a lack of chromium may cause disturbances in glucose metabolism [165]. The chromium intake of healthy subjects consuming normal diets is suboptimal [165]. There is a great difference in chromium intake depending more on the menu than on cooking in stainless steel utensils [166]. Yet, the fact that minute chromium compounds are present in food and water have made some authors speculate that oral ingestion may cause or contribute to the persistence of allergic contact dermatitis from chromium [167]. This has been questioned by others [143], since in vivo data have demonstrated that hexavalent chromium is readily reduced to trivalent chromium in the gastric fluid of the stomach before being systemically absorbed [168, 169]. However, in provocation studies with oral hexavalent chromium [167, 170], this reduction in the gastric fluid does not seem to affect the capacity of oral hexavalent chromium to elicit a systemic contact dermatitis. In patients with nickel or chromium allergy and dyshidrotic hand eczema, elbow eruptions have been reported to be characteristic of systemic allergic contact dermatitis from these metals [107, 170].

35.3.6 Epidemiology

Expectedly, the prevalence of chromium allergy varies widely in different countries due to many factors related not only to the degree and type of exposure, but also to factors related to diagnostic testing. Proctor et al. [143] have summarized the prevalence rates of chromium (VI) contact allergy in more than 30 studies published since 1950. These studies consist mostly of persons who have attended dermatological clinics in Europe and North America. The prevalence rates for specific cohorts range from 19.5% in workers with cement eczema in Switzerland in 1950 [171] to 1% for a clinical population tested from 1992 to 1996 in North America [158]. Although the prevalence of chromium allergy in dermatitis patients has been steadily decreasing over the past 25 years, several reports demonstrate that chromium allergy still is significant [126, 127, 172–176] and even increasing [106]. Several investigators have suggested that the decline in chromium allergy is most likely due to improved workplace hygiene, decreased contact with construction materials [177], and the addition of iron sulfate to cement to reduce most of the hexavalent chromium to an insoluble trivalent salt, which has negligible potential for sensitization and elicitation [86, 106, 178–180]. In countries where iron sulfate is not added to cement, chromate allergy may still be common in construction workers. Irvine et al. reported a high prevalence (17%) of chromate allergy among underground workers during the construction of the Channel Tunnel [181]. Sixty five percent of grouters patch tested had chromate allergy. The suggested causes for the decline in chromium allergy refer mainly to men. The frequency has also decreased in women, which has been attributed to the replacement of dichromate-containing bleaches with other detergents [179]. Still, there are countries where this has not been implemented, probably contributing to a high frequency of chromium allergy in housewives [134].

There are some investigations on the prevalence of chromium allergy in the European general population. In Finland, Peltonen and Fräki [182] have evaluated the prevalence of chromium (VI) sensitivity among 822 human volunteers. An overall prevalence of 1.7% was found. Seidenari et al. conducted a study in which 593 Italian cadets were patch tested with 0.5% potassium dichromate [183]. None tested positively. Lantinga et al. assessed the prevalence of allergic contact dermatitis for the general adult population in one defined area in the Netherlands [184]. Of the 1,992 individuals examined, 141 were identified as having episodes of eczema within the past 3 years. These individuals were patch tested and 9 (0.5%) of 1,992 cases tested positively to hexavalent chromium. Nielsen and Menné assessed the distribution of allergic contact dermatitis in an unselected population living in western Copenhagen, Denmark [81]. In 567 adults patch tested, a prevalence of 0.5% was observed, 0.7% in men and 0.3% in women. A higher frequency of chromium allergy was noted in a western Australasian community, where 9.1% of 219 adult volunteers were contact allergic [185]. White et al. patch tested 1,397 adult Thais with chromium and found that 2.3% were allergic. According to a recent review on allergic contact dermatitis in children and adolescents, the prevalence of chromate allergy in these groups has been reported to be between 0.2 and 7.6%, the latter

frequencies seeming, according to our experience, highly unlikely [186]. Finally, a review on contact allergy among adults in the general population showed that chromium allergy was more prevalent in the 1960s in comparison to recent years [4].

> **Core Message**
>
> › In construction workers exposed to hexavalent chromium, contact allergy rates exceeding 10% are seen, while the contact allergy rate in the European general population is around 1%.

35.3.7 Prevention and Legislation

Wass and Wahlberg have adopted a simple extraction procedure for the determination of leachable hexavalent chromium that could be used in industrial applications to check the quality of chromated products and establish a "threshold limit value" for such products [187]. Based on the results of occlusive tests with chromated discs in chromate-sensitive individuals, it was proposed that the mean release of hexavalent chromium from chromated parts should not exceed $0.3\ \mu g/cm^2$. Release above this value was found in approximately one out of four yellow chromated parts collected from a chromating plant and a car assembly plant. Wass and Wahlberg suggested that their method should be added to the tests performed to evaluate the technical quality of the chromate layers to reduce the risk of causing chromate allergy.

Basketter et al. reviewed the literature on published and unpublished industry data on transition metal contamination of consumer products and assessed the hazard in man [179]. Based on information on sensitization potential, including dose–response data, the levels of chromium found in consumer products and in relation to the known epidemiology of allergic contact dermatitis from chromium and in the context of the nature and extent of consumer exposure, Basketter et al. stated that good manufacturing practice in 1993 ensured that the chromium concentration in consumer products was less than 5 ppm. It was recommended that this was accepted as a standard for maximum concentration and that the target should be to achieve a concentration as low as 1 ppm. With these concentrations, it was thought that there will be no induction of chromate sensitization and that it is very unlikely that dermatitis will be elicited in already-sensitized individuals [179]. However, the maximum concentration should be lower than 5 ppm, as a ROAT study showed that 20% of the chromium-allergic patients reacted to an aqueous solution containing 5 ppm potassium dichromate, as well as 1% SLS [137].

In men, Portland cement has been, and still is in many countries, one of the most common causes of occupational skin conditions. In the beginning of the previous century, there were severe outbreaks of "cement itch" during the building of the Underground in London and of "la gâle du ciment" when the Mêtro in Paris was constructed. Although several investigators in the 1930s and 1940s reported that cement eczema was frequently combined with positive patch test reactions to chromate, it was not until 1950 that Jaeger and Pelloni first demonstrated the presence of hexavalent chromium in cement [171]. The content of hexavalent chromium in cement and concrete varies widely due to the source of the cement and additives used [117, 118]. It was previously demonstrated by Burckhardt that iron sulfate has the capacity to reduce hexavalent chromium to a trivalent form [188], and chemical analysis showed no demonstrable water-soluble chromium in cement to which iron sulfate had been added [189]. It is known that trivalent chromium will precipitate as chromium hydroxide in an alkaline solution. As cement has high alkalinity, this chemical process is most likely the reason that it is impossible to demonstrate water-soluble chromium in cement to which iron sulfate has been added [145]. Chromic hydroxide is also virtually insoluble in human sweat [145]. Because of this, iron sulfate has been added to all cement in connection with the manufacturing process in Scandinavian countries since 1981 in Denmark and 1983 in Sweden.

Denmark passed a legislation requiring the use of cement with lower levels of hexavalent chromium (<2 ppm) in 1983. Finland followed in 1987 and Sweden in 1989. Cement eczema is steadily decreasing in prevalence and had been doing so before the introduction of iron sulfate, and a decline is also occurring in countries where iron sulfate has not been added [190, 191]. Therefore, it had been questioned whether the decrease of hexavalent chromium in cement was a major cause of the decline in chromate allergy. However, some recent studies strongly indicate that the decrease of hexavalent chromium in cement is a significant and major factor in explaining the decreasing chromate allergy. In Singapore, a change in the manufacturing process of cement giving a lower content of hexavalent chromium has accompanied a decline in the prevalence of chromate allergy among construction workers [192]. In Denmark and Finland, where the content of hexavalent chromium in cement is below 2 ppm, the results of epidemiological investigations in construction workers concerning irritant and allergic contact dermatitis from cement strongly indicate that the decrease in chromate allergy has, to a large extent, been caused by the addition of iron sulfate [86, 178, 180, 193]. Furthermore, during the Channel Tunnel project, 332 out of 1,138 construction workers exposed to cement/concrete to which iron sulfate had not been added were diagnosed as having an occupational dermatitis [181]. Of these, 180 were patch tested and 96 (53%) were allergic to chromate. In similar building projects in Denmark and Sweden, during the construction of the combined tunnel and bridge of the Great Belt in Denmark and of the combined tunnel and bridge over Öresund, the strait between Denmark and Sweden, occupational dermatitis and chromate allergy have not been a problem ([180], [Nielsen, Sundlink Contractors HB, Malmö, Sweden, 1999, personal communication]). Based on this, it was decided in the EU that cement which human skin may be exposed to must not contain more than 2 ppm hexavalent chromium from 2005 [194].

Thus, it is highly unlikely that cement with iron sulfate added will sensitize and it is likely that such cement will be of minor significance for elicitation in already-chromate-sensitized persons [145]. However, chromate sensitization from cement may still occur in countries without legislation demanding the addition of iron sulfate, due to reluctance in the addition of iron sulfate to imported cement [180] or due to storage conditions leading to oxidation of trivalent chromium to hexavalent [195].

Core Message

> Regulating the content of hexavalent chromium in cement effectively prevents chromium dermatitis.

35.4 Cobalt

Cobalt (Co) is a silvery metal that belongs, together with nickel and chromium, to the transition elements. Cobalt is a skin and respiratory allergen. Occupational exposure to cobalt occurs mainly through the respiratory tract. Pulmonary effects, particularly in the hard-metal industry, are hard-metal pneumoconiosis and occupational asthma. Inhalation of hard-metal dust induces asthma, in some cases, by a type I immunological mechanism. Cardiomyopathy has been described among heavy consumers of cobalt-contaminated beer. Cobalt is genotoxic. It is controversial whether cobalt can give rise to human cancer. Cobalt is an essential trace element, as it occurs in vitamin B12.

35.4.1 Cobalt Use and Exposure

Since the 1930s, there has been a large increase in cobalt production, which reached 53,700 tons in 2007. Cobalt is now mainly a byproduct of nickel and copper mining; 50% of world production today has its origin in Africa. Cobalt has been used for thousands of years [196] (Table 35.8). The oxidation states of cobalt are 0, +1, +2, and +3.

Some of the main uses of cobalt are in the production of superalloys (Ni/Co/Fe; 22%), hard materials, carbides and diamond tooling (18%), colors (10%), and magnets (6%) [196] (Table 35.9). Hard metal is manufactured by combining tungsten and carbon with cobalt as a binder. The product has 90–95% of the hardness of diamond and is used for the cutting edges of tools and drills. Cobalt is used in electroplatings to produce hard, wear-resistant, and bright coatings.

The use of cobalt in objects intended for direct and prolonged contact with the skin may increase, as a substitute for nickel, which is limited by the Nickel Directive.

Based on risk assessment addressing allergic contact dermatitis, it was recommended that consumer products such as household products and cosmetics should not contain more than 5 ppm of each of nickel, chromium, or cobalt, and that the ultimate target level should be 1 ppm [32].

Table 35.8 Timetable for cobalt (based on [196])

2600 BC	Cobalt coloring of pottery and glass
1735	Metallic cobalt was isolated by Brandt
1780	Cobalt was proved as an element
1842	Cobalt electroplating
1901	Use as paint dryer
1933	Alnico magnets
1936	Dental alloy
1953	Extensive use as catalyst
1980	Co–Cr alloys in prosthetics
1991	Growth of catalyst chemical market
1994	Cobalt use in Ni/Cd, Ni/MH, Li/Co batteries
2001	Growth of catalysts, gas to liquid technology

Table 35.9 Main uses of cobalt (based on [196])

Metallurgical	Superalloys
	Wear-resistant coatings
	High-speed steels
	Prosthetic alloys
	Low-expansion alloys
	Steels
	Corrosion-resistant alloys
	Spring alloys
Magnetic alloys	Hard and soft magnets
Chemicals	Batteries
	Catalysts
	Adhesives, cobalt soaps
	Driers, pigments, colors
	Electroplating
	Agriculture and medicine
	Electromagnetic recording
Cemented carbides	
Cobalt-bonded diamonds	
Electronics	Recording material
	Matched-expansion alloys
	Leads
	Batteries
Ceramics and enamels	Colors in glass, enamels, pottery, china

Knowledge about skin exposure to cobalt is limited and is often associated with simultaneous exposure to nickel or chromate. Nickel-containing alloys, formerly, often contained traces of cobalt, but it is less likely now when the price of cobalt is much higher than nickel. Cement may contain cobalt and nickel as well as chromate [197]. Exposure to cobalt and its compounds alone is generally thought to occur mainly in hard-metal manufacturing and ceramics industries, which likely has to be modified. To increase knowledge about cobalt in relation to skin exposure, a broad selection of cobalt-containing hard-metal and dental alloys was stored in synthetic sweat for 1 week. The release of cobalt from different materials varied significantly. The highest amount released from the hard-metal alloys was 290 $\mu g/cm^2/week$ [198]. Cobalt was deposited at high levels (up to 4.5 $\mu g/cm^2/h$) when sharpening hard-metal tools [199]. Skin exposure was also described as an important route of cobalt uptake in workers sharpening hard-metal blades [200]. (see also Chap. 27, Sect. 27.2).

> ### Core Message
>
> › Cobalt is used in the production of alloys, magnets, batteries, dental and surgical implants, and in hard metals. Cobalt compounds are used as catalysts and as drying agents in paints, etc. Cobalt may also be present at a low level in consumer products and cement.

35.4.2 Allergic Contact Dermatitis

Contact allergy to cobalt chloride is common and is often associated with concomitant contact allergy to nickel or chromate. Based on patch test studies of samples of the general population in several countries, it is estimated that 1–3% of adults, and probably larger proportion of younger females, are sensitive to cobalt [4]. Contact allergy to cobalt chloride has been reported at approximately 5–8% of patch-tested dermatitis patients in Europe and North America, and generally at a higher rate in women than in men [201–205].

Far too little is known about cobalt allergy, although cobalt is one of the major contact allergens. Until now,

we have often had difficulty in explaining to patients induction, elicitation, and possible cross-reactivity. Solitary cobalt allergy is seen mainly among hard-metal workers and in the glass and pottery industries, but it is often difficult to identify the source of isolated positive cobalt patch tests.

Occupational allergic contact dermatitis caused by metallic cobalt dust in a factory producing tungsten carbide alloys was first described in 1945 [206], and in a pottery factory from exposure to wet, alkaline clay containing cobalt in 1953 [207]. Five percent of 853 hard-metal workers in another factory producing hard-metal items were allergic to cobalt [208, 209]. Individuals with concomitant nickel and cobalt allergy had more severe hand eczema than those with isolated cobalt or nickel sensitivity, or irritant contact dermatitis.

Cobalt is an important occupational contact allergen in construction workers, and it has often been associated with allergy to chromate [173, 210–212]. The high cobalt release from hard-metal tools and deposition of cobalt onto skin at tools sharpening [198, 199], and cobalt content of cement [197] may contribute to cobalt allergy in construction workers.

Metal workers with occupational contact dermatitis who are exposed to water-based metal working fluids had increased risk of cobalt allergy compared to other men with occupational contact dermatitis [213].

Case reports on dermatitis related to occupational exposure to cobalt-containing materials, such as black ink, animal feeds, and cement, have been published, and stomatitis related to cobalt-containing dentures and dermatitis related to orthopedic prostheses have also been reported [214]. Cases of dermatitis or granuloma related to cobalt in tattoos and of photocontact dermatitis have been reported.

The simultaneous reactivity to cobalt chloride and nickel sulfate or chromate is not believed to be due to cross-reactivity, but rather due to combined exposure. This is based partly on the knowledge of use and exposure and partly on the results from animal studies.

Cobalt chloride was used in a human maximization test and it sensitized 10 out of 25 volunteers [41]. It was reported to be a grade 3 allergen (highest grade being 5). Cobalt chloride is a potent sensitizer in the guinea pig. In guinea pig maximization tests, all animals were sensitized and cobalt chloride was reported to be a grade 5 allergen. Animals induced with cobalt chloride did not react to nickel sulfate or chromate – the results speaking in favor of multiple sensitization rather than

35

cross-reactivity [215, 216]. Cross-sensitization experiments in guinea pigs with cobalt chloride and rhodium chloride, however, indicate cross-reactivity [217].

> ### Core Message
>
> > The contact allergy rate to cobalt in the general population is around 1–3% and in patch-tested dermatitis patients 5–8%. Cobalt is an important contact allergen in construction workers and hard-metal workers. Allergy to cobalt is often seen together with allergy to nickel or to chromate. Solitary cobalt allergy is rare.

35.4.3 Patch Testing with Cobalt

The diagnostic patch test concentration used in the European baseline series is cobalt chloride 1% in petrolatum. However, 0.5% in petrolatum has often been used in the Swedish baseline series, due to the fact that 1% may produce porous reactions [218]. The TRUE Test also uses cobalt chloride.

A study was carried out to establish the minimum levels of cobalt chloride required to elicit a positive patch test response. On normal skin, the minimum eliciting concentration was 2,260 ppm. When the skin was pretreated for 24 h with sodium dodecyl sulfate (SDS), the minimum eliciting level was 2.3–226 ppm cobalt chloride [219].

Patch testing was carried out with a metallic cobalt disc containing 100% cobalt, supplementary to the 1% cobalt chloride in petrolatum [220]. In all, 458 consecutive dermatitis patients were patch tested and 23 were positive to cobalt chloride, of whom 11 were positive to the cobalt disc.

Patch testing was performed with discs of different cobalt-containing hard-metal alloys in 19 cobalt-sensitive subjects and in controls [198]. The alloys elicited positive test reactions, and the release of cobalt in artificial sweat was very high for several of the alloys.

> ### Core Message
>
> > Patch testing with 1% cobalt chloride is recommended. This concentration may, however, elicit nonallergic porous reactions.

35.4.4 Prevention and Legislation

There is no regulatory limitation in the use of cobalt for the prevention of contact dermatitis, such as for nickel and chromium in cement. These regulations may, however, affect exposure and sensitization to cobalt. If the use of cobalt increases, as a substitute for nickel in the items covered by the Nickel Directive, this may result in severe increase in allergic contact dermatitis due to cobalt. The risk is obvious, as cobalt is a potent skin sensitizer. An indication of such a scenario was found in a Danish retrospective patch test study. The prevalence of cobalt allergy in young female dermatitis patients was stable, while a decrease was expected as the prevalence of nickel allergy in this age group decreased [90]. It has been speculated that the limitation of chromium in cement may also decrease the risk of cobalt allergy in construction workers, secondary to the reduction of chromate dermatitis [175, 212].

> ### Core Message
>
> > To avoid an increase in cobalt allergy, it is essential that cobalt is not used instead of nickel in items in contact with the skin.

35.5 Aluminum

Aluminum (Al) is widely used and contact with aluminum in its elemental form or its salts is unavoidable.

35.5.1 Allergic Contact Dermatitis

Aluminum is a weak contact allergen. Until recently, only few case reports of contact allergy to aluminum existed. In a recent Swedish article, it was stated that among thousands of dermatitis patients patch tested with aluminum, only very few had positive reactions [221]. Patch testing is usually performed with aluminum chloride hexahydrate in pet. at 2% and an empty Finn Chamber, which is made of elemental aluminum [222]. However, if contact allergy is suspected, one may increase the dose to 10%.

Occupational contact dermatitis due to aluminum exposure has been reported in aluminum production

[223], in aircraft manufacture [224], and in a machine construction plant [225]. A rather new method for aluminum production, cold sealing, with nickel floride constitutes a new risk of dermatitis from working with aluminum. The risk is not from the aluminum itself, however, but from nickel sulfate on the surface of cold-sealed aluminum objects [226]. Water-soluble aluminum salts are used as antiperspirants and are found in most deodorants. This may sometimes cause axillary dermatitis [227], although reactions are usually irritant. Reactions to aluminum from the Finn Chambers used for patch testing have rarely been observed [228]. Systemic aluminum contact dermatitis from toothpaste has been reported [229].

Reactions to aluminum-absorbed vaccines may induce allergic contact dermatitis [230–235]. Recently, a Swedish study showed a statistically significant association between contact allergy to aluminum and persistent subcutaneous nodules in children who had had hyposensitization therapy [221]. The subcutaneous nodules were considered to be cutaneous manifestations of contact allergy. Netterlid et al. concluded that prospective, randomized, and controlled studies should be performed in patients undergoing hyposensitization therapy to explore and establish the sensitization rate to aluminum and the association between contact allergy to aluminum and clinical manifestations [221].

35.6 Beryllium

Beryllium (Be) is a ubiquitous metal present in soil and as soluble and insoluble salts in waste and salt water. Most beryllium is used as an alloy or in specialty ceramics for electrical and electronic applications, while pure beryllium finds use in the nuclear industry, aircraft, and medical devices, including dental alloys.

Beryllium has been clearly established as a human carcinogen [107]. Beryllium is extremely toxic, resulting in acute and chronic respiratory disease [236]. Chronic beryllium disease is characterized by noncaseating granulomas and interstitial pulmonary infiltrates, where the diagnosis is based on the demonstration of a cell-mediated immune response to beryllium salts, either in vitro with the beryllium LPT or in vivo with a patch test to beryllium sulfate [237].

Chemical burns, contact dermatitis, and granulomatous lesions may result from skin exposure to beryllium compounds. Soluble beryllium salts, such as beryllium chloride and beryllium fluoride, are caustic at high concentrations. Cutaneous findings were emphasized in a recent paper on occupational chronic beryllium disease [238].

35.6.1 Allergic Contact Dermatitis

In 1951, Curtis was the first to diagnose beryllium contact allergy in workers at two beryllium plants by patch testing with various beryllium salts [239]. Beryllium present in dental alloys has been reported to cause contact allergic reactions of the oral mucosa [240–242]. In Spain, three patients tested positively to beryllium chloride 1% in petrolatum [240]. One patient suffered from a stomatitis adjacent to a beryllium-containing prosthesis. When the prosthesis was replaced with one not containing beryllium, the symptoms disappeared. A dental mechanic making beryllium-containing prostheses presented with a hand dermatitis that was diagnosed as an occupational allergic contact dermatitis from beryllium [240]. Haberman et al. reported two patients who developed gingivitis adjacent to a beryllium-containing alloy in their dental prostheses [241]. Patch testing demonstrated positive reactions to beryllium sulfate 1% in petrolatum in the two patients.

The same test substance resulted in 5.4% positive reactors when 186 patients were tested because of oral disease [242].

35.7 Cadmium

Cadmium (Cd) is one of the most toxic metals and environmental poisons. Cadmium is used in pigments for plastics, paints, glass, and ceramics, in alloys, solders and platings, and nickel–cadmium batteries. The main industrial exposure is to fumes and dust by inhalation, and environmental exposure is via food and smoking. Acute toxicity causes nausea, vomiting, and pneumonitis and may be fatal, and chronic toxicity affects many organs (kidney, lung, bones, hematopoietic system). The itai-itai disease affected mainly women, probably due to higher gastro-intestinal absorption at low iron stores [243].

35

35.7.1 Allergic Contact Dermatitis

When cadmium chloride (2% in water) was included in the baseline patch test used in 1,502 dermatitis patients, 25 were patch test positive [244]. Further testing with serial dilutions was not interpreted in favor of contact allergy, as only 1 of 6 patients was positive to 1% cadmium chloride. The reactions were regarded as nonrelevant and probably irritant in nature. Cadmium chloride 0.5% in petrolatum was, based on testing in 662 dermatitis patients, recommended for patch testing [245]. In total, 791 patients, among them 59 dental technicians, were patch tested with a dental materials series including cadmium chloride (1% in petrolatum) [246]. Of the patients, 9% were patch test positive to cadmium chloride. The reactions were judged nonrelevant, as the rates were equal among dental technicians (possibly exposed) and other patients (probably not exposed). Cadmium red (cadmium selenide) has previously been used for the coloration of dentures and it was not evaluated as an allergen [247].

Yellow cadmium sulfide is used as a pigment for yellow and red tattoos, and it may cause phototoxic reactions and sarcoid-like granulomas [248]. It is not know how frequently this occurs.

The sensitizing potential of cadmium chloride was evaluated in a guinea pig maximization test, and cadmium chloride caused no statistically significant reactivity in induced animals compared to control animals [249].

35.8 Copper

Copper (Cu) is an important metal in industry. The primary use of copper, approximately half its production, is in electrical equipment. Copper is widely used in alloys together with tin, zinc, silver, and cadmium. Copper/tin alloys are called bronzes and may also contain other metals. Copper-containing alloys are used for coins, jewelry, pipes, roofs, etc. and may be used in some dental materials. Copper sulfate and organic copper salts are used in agriculture as fungicides and algicides. Copper is an essential trace element that is crucial in hemoglobin synthesis and in other enzyme functions.

35.8.1 Allergic Contact Dermatitis

Copper has been considered a rare skin sensitizer [250, 251]. Single cases of dermatitis related to the use of copper-containing intrauterine contraceptive devices (IUCD) [252, 253], contact stomatitis [254], oral pain [255], and oral lichen planus [256] have been described. When copper sulfate (2% in petrolatum) was included in the patch test series used in 1,190 dermatitis patients in Sweden, 1% positive reactions were recorded, but they were considered nonrelevant [250]. When copper sulfate (2% in petrolatum) was included in the patch test series in Austria, 3.5% were positive [257]. The authors suggested 5% copper sulfate for patch testing, but stated that positive reactions are usually of low clinical relevance, and that the reproducibility of test reactions was considered modest.

The sensitizing potential of copper sulfate was evaluated in a series of guinea pig maximization tests, and it was classified as a weak sensitizer or a grade I allergen [250]. Local lymph node assay (LLNA) in mice was positive [258].

35.8.2 Irritant Contact Dermatitis

Concentrated solutions of copper sulfate are corrosive and cause primary irritation on skin contact.

35.9 Gold

Many persons are or may be exposed to metallic gold (Au) as it is present in jewelry and dental materials. Currently, gold is a controversial sensitizer [259]. The reason for this is understandable. Until recently, gold allergy was considered to be extremely rare, so it was remarkable when a contact allergy rate to gold of around 10% was reported in consecutively patch-tested dermatitis patients [260]. Gold, maybe the most beloved and precious metal, has been used and worshipped for thousands of years without any obvious complaints of skin problems, either in those participating in mining and other ways of prospecting, or in those wearing jewelry.

35.9.1 Gold Use and Exposure

Gold is the only metal except copper that is markedly colored. It is abundant in low concentrations over almost all the Earth's crust and in seawater, above all in metallic form and also as gold telluride. Gold is found as grains in the bottom of rivers, above all in California, Australia, Alaska, and Russia, while gold ore in South Africa is harvested from mines with auriferous leaders. Gold is also produced as a byproduct from the production of copper, nickel, and lead. The world's yearly production of gold is 1,000 tons, of which 150 tons are used in the electronics industry [261].

Pure gold is very soft but malleable and ductile. To increase its strength, alloys with other metals, such as silver, copper, nickel, palladium, and zinc are common. The color of gold is influenced by the alloy addition, where silver gives a greenish yellow, copper a reddish, and nickel a light yellow to whitish gold.

Gold is resistant to corrosion as it does not combine with oxygen or other substances in the atmosphere, not even at elevated temperatures. Gold occurs in oxidation states 0, +I, and +III, the latter being most stable, and the equilibrium between these states can be altered easily [262]. All halogens attack gold, and so do halogen acids mixed with nitric acid or other oxidizers. Aqua regia, a mixture of hydrochloric and nitric acids, as well as cyanide solutions attack gold. To be a hapten, gold has to be ionized. When subjecting gold-containing jewelry alloys to artificial sweat for 1 and 3 weeks, no release of gold was detected [263]. However, this does not mean that metallic gold cannot be of significance for gold sensitization, as the absence of amino acids in the synthetic sweat used [263] could affect the release rate of gold ions [7]. It has been demonstrated that gold can dissolve in water solutions that contain thiol-substituted amino acids (cysteine, glutathione) and be absorbed through animal skin [7, 262]. Furthermore, the blood level of gold is higher in dermatitis patients with dental gold compared to those without dental gold and with a correlation between the gold blood level and the number of dental gold restorations, strongly suggesting that gold is released from dental gold [264]. Studies have also demonstrated the significance of dental gold and gold-plated stents for sensitization [265–268].

Gold is found in jewelry, either as an alloy, as gold plating, or as rolled gold. In plating, a base metal such as copper is electrolytically covered with nickel and then gold of varying thickness is added. Gold is also present in alloys in dentistry to make crowns, bridges, etc. Gold hydroxide, gold oxide, and various gold salts, such as potassium and sodium gold trichloride, sodium tetrachloroaurate dihydrate, potassium dicyanoaurate, and gold sodium sulfite, find their uses to make ruby glass and to color enamel and porcelain, as well as for other decorative applications in photography, in printed circuit boards, and in electronics manufacture. In the medical profession, both elemental gold and various gold compounds are used for various purposes, for example, to treat rheumatoid arthritis [269], intracoronary stents [268], and eyelid implant [270].

Core Message

> Dental gold and intracoronary gold-plated stents are significant for gold sensitization.

35.9.2 Patch Testing with Gold and Gold Compounds

Elemental gold has been used for patch testing, but it has only occasionally elicited a positive patch test. Various gold salts/compounds, both monovalent and trivalent, such as potassium dicyanoaurate, gold sodium thiosulfate, gold sodium thiomalate, and gold chloride, have been used for patch testing. Gold (III) chloride has often been used. However, it is important to stress that a test solution of gold chloride is a solution of gold chloride in hydrochloric acid, since it is insoluble in water, and hence, a strong irritant with a risk of false-positive reactions. Nevertheless, gold chloride is a sensitizer, which has been demonstrated by Kligman in a human maximization test in the 1960s [41]. In the late 1980s, Fowler reported that gold sodium thiosulfate at 0.5% in petrolatum was a good screening preparation for tracing contact allergy to gold [271]. At the Jadassohn Congress in London in 1996, gold sodium thiosulfate in petrolatum at 2% was reported to elicit higher numbers of positive patch test reactions without giving more irritant reactions or patch test sensitization [272]. Whenever patch testing with gold sodium thiosulfate, keep in mind that a test reading should also be performed after 1 week [273]. In fact, even readings on days 14–21 may be indicated. Positive test reactions to gold sodium thiosulfate and gold sodium thiomalate have also been obtained when tested intracutaneously [260, 273, 274], as well as with in vitro tests [274–276].

> **Core Message**
>
> › Gold sodium thiosulfate is not recommended for the baseline series. It should be applied for scientific purposes and when allergic contact dermatitis from gold is suspected. Positive test reactions to gold sodium thiosulfate may appear late, which is why readings should also be performed after 1 week.

35.9.3 Clinical Picture

In patients hypersensitive to gold sodium thiosulfate, dermatitis has been reported to be overrepresented in certain locations, such as the fingers, earlobes, and the eye area [265, 270, 277, 278]. Gold dermatitis has also been reported to resemble seborrheic dermatitis [279]. In patients with gold allergy and pierced ears, persistent papular elements and nodules on the earlobes have developed [280–282]. The combination of dental gold and contact allergy to gold has manifested orally with ulcerations, erosions, and erythematous lesions [274, 283, 284], as well as with erythema and swelling of the upper lips and cheek in a patient with orofacial granulomatosis [285].

Recently, allergic contact dermatitis as a complication of lip loading in four hypersensitive patients was reported [270]. A statistically significant association was also found between contact allergy to stent material and restenosis of the coronary arteries [286]. The risk for restenosis was threefold increased when the patient was gold-allergic and stented with a gold-plated stent.

35.9.4 Systemic Contact Dermatitis

Experimentally, the drug Myocrisin (gold sodium thiomalate) has been demonstrated to elicit systemic contact dermatitis in gold sodium thiosulfate-hypersensitive individuals [287–289]. Besides flare-up reactions of previous positive patch tests to gold compounds and of previous sites of gold dermatitis, the patients have experienced "fever" reactions and, biochemically, a significant rise in inflammatory mediators has been demonstrated [288, 289]. However, there are currently no data indicating that systemic administration of gold, except for gold drug administration and the consumption of a gold-containing liquor [290, 291], has any clinical significance for the elicitation or deterioration of contact dermatitis.

35.9.5 Epidemiology

When gold sodium thiosulfate was introduced in the baseline test series in Malmö, Sweden, in the early 1990s, a contact allergy rate of 9% was noted [260]. Thereafter, contact allergy rates to gold sodium thiosulfate in the range 1–23% were reported from various countries, and in most studies with a female predominance. Similar figures have been obtained while patch-testing subgroups of the general population [292–294], and even a higher contact allergy rate of 37% in patients with a gold-plated stent [268].

There are several case reports, both occupational and nonoccupational, on allergic contact dermatitis and allergic contact stomatitis from gold. Elemental gold found in jewelry such as earrings, rings, and necklaces seems to make up the majority of cases. Sporadic cases of occupational contact dermatitis from gold salts have been reported in electroplaters, guilders, and those manufacturing and selling jewelry. Irritant contact dermatitis from gold salts, particularly potassium dicyanoaurate, has been reported. Allergic contact stomatitis and glossitis from gold have been caused by gold-containing alloys in dental appliances, such as crowns, bridges, and dentures. More information on contact allergy rates and allergic as well as irritant manifestations from gold compounds are given in [259, 261, 286, 295].

Core Message

> Contact allergy to gold sodium thiosulfate in the range 1–23% was seen in dermatitis patients and most often with a female predominance. Similar and higher rates have been noted in groups of the general population. Cases of occupational contact dermatitis from gold salts have been reported.

35.10 Mercury

Mercury (Hg) exists in three chemical forms, elemental, organic, and inorganic. Currently, the main sources of mercury exposure are: [296] dental amalgam restorations; [297] in various industries, including the manufacture of insecticides, fungicides, paper, paint, jewelry, chlorine, caustic soda, and in dentistry; and [298] mercury-containing vaccines, eye and ear drops, contact lens cleaning and storage solutions, skin-lightening creams, emulsion paints, and fungicides and herbicides used in the home [296–298].

Chronic exposure to either inorganic or organic mercury can permanently damage the brain, kidneys, and the developing fetus. The most sensitive target of low-level exposures to metallic and organic mercury, following short- or long-term exposure, appears to be the nervous system, whereas the most sensitive target of low-level exposure to inorganic mercury appears to be the kidney [298]. Mercury poisoning can result in different clinical conditions with assorted cutaneous findings [299].

35.10.1 Allergic Contact Dermatitis

All three chemical forms of mercury can sensitize. Clinically, mercury allergy can manifest as allergic contact dermatitis, allergic gingivostomatitis, and systemic contact dermatitis [298, 299] with malaise and fever [300]. There is no general consensus regarding which mercury compounds to use for patch testing patients with suspected mercury hypersensitivity. Mercury compounds may be highly irritant to the skin and aqueous solutions of mercury salts may react with aluminum in Finn Chambers to produce irritant compounds [297]. In a report on mercury allergy, both metallic mercury and ammoniated mercury were recommended for patch testing when mercury allergy is suspected [297]. More information on mercury allergy is given in the chapter on skin disease from dental materials (Chap. 39).

35.11 Palladium

Palladium (Pd) belongs to the platinum group of metals. Palladium is an inexpensive precious metal, which is less resistant to corrosion than platinum. The main uses are for electrical components alloyed with copper and silver, and as a catalyst. Smaller amounts are used in jewelry, where it is used as a whitener in white gold. Palladium is increasingly used in cast dental alloys and dental prostheses.

35.11.1 Allergic Contact Dermatitis

A case of contact dermatitis from palladium was reported in 1969 in a chemist working on precious metals analysis. He was patch test positive to nickel chloride and palladium chloride [301]. Since the beginning of the 1990s, palladium chloride has been included in the baseline series of many patch test clinics. Few reports on work-related dermatitis have been published, but several reports on positive patch test reactions to palladium chloride have been released. The frequency of contact allergy to palladium chloride among dermatitis patients has in different studies been reported to be approximately 3–10% [302]. Of nickel-sensitive individuals, 30–40% are also patch test positive to palladium chloride [303–305]. In almost every case of reactivity to palladium chloride, simultaneous reactivity to nickel is shown. Patch testing with palladium chloride is generally performed at 1% in petrolatum.

Some authors have related palladium allergy to dental alloys. Few cases of contact stomatitis or oral lichen planus related to palladium [284, 306] and of granuloma related to palladium and piercing [307] have been reported.

Patch testing with elemental palladium has been carried out, but the results do not support clinical reports of allergy to elemental palladium. None of the 12 patients who were patch test positive to palladium chloride reacted to pure palladium metal foil [308]. Metal discs made of palladium were tested in 103 nickel-sensitive patients [309]. Only one reaction was recorded in a patient who did not react to palladium chloride.

The clinical relevance of palladium chloride or elemental palladium as sensitizers is not fully understood. Cross-reactivity to palladium chloride in nickel-sensitive people seems to be the most likely, but concomitant sensitivity or contamination of palladium chloride by nickel sulfate has also been discussed [303, 308, 310].

Palladium chloride has been shown to be a potent sensitizer in the guinea pig. Animals induced with palladium chloride also reacted to nickel sulfate, and many animals induced with nickel sulfate respond at challenge with palladium chloride [311, 312]. The results speak in favor of cross-reactivity.

35.12 Platinum

Platinum (Pt) salts can induce allergic responses of the immediate hypersensitivity type, including rhinitis and asthma [313]. On the other hand, platinum as a cause of contact allergic sensitization has been questioned. Koch and Baum reported a patient with contact stomatitis due to combined sensitization to palladium and platinum, both metals being present in dental alloys in the patient's mouth [306]. Recently, occupational contact allergy to platinum traced by patch testing with platinum salts was reported in refinery workers [314], in a chemical process worker [315], and in an analytical chemist [316].

The recommended patch test preparation is ammonium tetrachloroplatinate 0.25% in petrolatum.

35.13 Rhodium

Rhodium (Rh) is one of the platinum-group metals. Little is known about the toxicology of rhodium. It is used in alloys and platings for jewelry and in some dental materials. Rhodium is also used in catalysts, high-temperature furnaces, electrical contacts, high-reflective mirrors and other optical surfaces, and in nozzles for glass-fiber spinning.

35.13.1 Allergic Contact Dermatitis

Elemental rhodium has not been described as a sensitizer. Single reports on contact allergy to rhodium salts, in platers and silversmiths, have been published. A goldsmith was patch test positive to rhodium sulfate 0.05% in water and to cobalt chloride, while 40 controls were negative to rhodium sulfate at a higher concentration [317]. Contact dermatitis, contact urticaria, and asthma among 17 out of 50 workers in a precious metals factory were reported [318]. Seven hundred and twenty consecutive dermatitis patients were patch tested with rhodium chloride in Italy. Two were tested positive to rhodium chloride, the significance of which was, however, unknown [319].

Rhodium chloride has been shown to be a potent sensitizer in guinea pigs [320]. Challenge was carried out with rhodium chloride and also with cobalt chloride, nickel sulfate, and palladium chloride. Animals induced with rhodium chloride also reacted to cobalt chloride, the clinical relevance of which is not known.

35.14 Silver

Silver (Ag) is increasingly used as biocide for surface treatment of many type of products in contact with skin (see also Chap. 47). This is highly controversial due to the environmental toxicity of silver and also due to known and suspected health risks.

The increasing use of silver in health care, particularly in wound care dressings, is controversial [321]. The effectiveness has not been proven and the risks have not been thoroughly assessed. Silver-treated textiles are sometimes used in the treatment of atopic dermatitis. Silver resistance of antibiotic-resistant bacteria and penetration of silver nanoparticles through wounded skin have been described. Argyria (grayish discoloration of skin) has been described from the exposure to soluble silver, and in the photographic industry and silver solders [322], and also from wound dressings.

Silver is not a skin sensitizer. It is, however, often used in combination with nickel that may cause dermatitis [14]. Nickel–silver (also called German silver, new silver, or alpacca) is a whitish alloy of Cu/Ni/Zn, which often is silver coated. Silver jewelry may be nickel coated to prevent oxidation. These applications are not allowed in item covered by the EU Nickel Directive (see Sect. 35.2).

Silver nitrate is widely used for cauterizing bleeding and healing wounds and to mark patch test sites. Silver nitrate might, however, be a skin sensitizer and may cause local toxic reactions when used as a patch test marker [323].

35.15 Tin

Tin (Sn) is widely used in metal alloys and most humans are exposed intraorally to the tin present in amalgam.

Nielsen and Skov [324] described a case of a worker with an airborne pattern contact dermatitis caused by exposure to dust from a tin containing metal alloy. A positive patch test with $SnCl_2$ $2H_2O$ 1% in petrolatum was present. A dilution series supports an allergic reaction. Allergy could not be supported by the attempted lymphocytic transformation test.

Earlier, nonrelevant cutaneous reactivity has been seen in consecutive patients, tested with metallic, tin, and tin chloride [325]. The recommended patch test concentration is 1% tin chloride in petrolatum, but it is only based on a single case with a relevant positive patch test.

References

1. Blascho A (1889) Die Berufsdermatosen der Arbeiter. Das Galvanisierekzem. Dtsch Med Wschr 15:925–927
2. Schittenhelm A, Stockinger W (1925) Über die Idiosynkrasie gegen Nickel (Nickel krätze) und ihre Beziehung zur Anaphylaxie. Z Ges Exp Med 45:58–74
3. McAlester AW Jr, McAlester AW III (1931) Nickel sensitization from white gold spectacle frames. Am J Ophth 14:925–926
4. Thyssen JP, Linneberg A, Menné T et al (2007) The epidemiology of contact allergy in the general population–prevalence and main findings. Contact Dermatitis 57:287–299
5. Thyssen JP, Johansen JD, Zachariae C et al (2008) The outcome of dimethylglyoxime testing in a sample of cell phones in Denmark. Contact Dermatitis 59:38–42
6. Nickel Development Institute (1997) Safe use of nickel in the workplace. Toronto pp 1–78
7. Flint GN (1998) A metallurgical approach to metal contact dermatitis. Contact Dermatitis 39:213–221
8. Menné T, Brandup F, Thestrup-Pedersen K et al (1987) Patch test reactivity to nickel alloys. Contact Dermatitis 16:255–259
9. Pedersen NB, Fregert S, Brodelius P et al (1974) Release of nickel from silver coins. Acta Derm Venereol 54:231–234
10. Fischer T, Fregert S, Gruvberger B et al (1984) Nickel release from ear piercing kits and earrings. Contact Dermatitis 10:39–41
11. Menné T, Solgaard P (1979) Temperature-dependent nickel release from nickel alloys. Contact Dermatitis 5:82–84
12. Emmett EA, Risby TH, Jiang L et al (1988) Allergic contact dermatitis to nickel: bioavailability from consumer products and provocation threshold. J Am Acad Dermatol 19:314–322
13. Haudrechy P, Mantout B, Frappaz A et al (1997) Nickel release from stainless steels. Contact Dermatitis 37:113–117
14. Lidén C, Menné T, Burrows D (1996) Nickel-containing alloys and platings and their ability to cause dermatitis. Br J Dermatol 134:193–198
15. Fischer LA, Menné T, Johansen JD (2005) Experimental nickel elicitation thresholds–a review focusing on occluded nickel exposure. Contact Dermatitis 52:57–64
16. Novak N, Baurecht H, Schäfer T et al (2008) Loss-of-function mutations in the filaggrin gene and allergic contact sensitization to nickel. J Invest Dermatol 128:1430–1435
17. Thyssen JP, Carlsen BC, Menné T (2008) Nickel sensitization, hand eczema, and loss-of-function mutations in the filaggrin gene. Dermatitis 19:303–307
18. Cavelier C, Foussereau J, Massin M (1985) Nickel allergy: analysis of metal clothing objects and patch testing to metal samples. Contact Dermatitis 12:65–75
19. Heim KE, McKean BA (2009) Children's clothing fasteners as a potential source of exposure to releasable nickel ions. Contact Dermatitis 60:100–105
20. Suzuki H (1998) Nickel and gold in skin lesions of pierced earlobes with contact dermatitis. A study using scanning electron microscopy and x-ray microanalysis. Arch Dermatol Res 290:523–527
21. Lidén C, Skare L, Nise G et al (2008) Deposition of nickel, chromium, and cobalt on the skin in some occupations - assessment by acid wipe sampling. Contact Dermatitis 58:347–354
22. Staton I, Ma R, Evans N et al (2006) Dermal nickel exposure associated with coin handling and in various occupational settings: assessment using a newly developed finger immersion method. Br J Dermatol 154:658–664
23. Morgan LG, Usher V (1994) Health problems associated with nickel refining and use. Ann Occup Hyg 38:189–198
24. Clemmensen OJ, Menné T, Kaaber K et al (1981) Exposure of nickel and the relevance of nickel sensitivity among hospital cleaners. Contact Dermatitis 7:14–18
25. Wahlberg JE, Lindstedt G, Einarsson O (1977) Chromium, cobalt and nickel in Swedish cement, detergents, mould and cutting oils. Berufsdermatosen 25:220–228
26. Wall LM, Calnan CD (1980) Occupational nickel dermatitis in the electroforming industry. Contact Dermatitis 6:414–420
27. Lidén C, Röndell E, Skare L et al (1998) Nickel release from tools on the Swedish market. Contact Dermatitis 39:127–131

28. Fournier PG, Govers TR (2003) Contamination by nickel, copper and zinc during the handling of euro coins. Contact Dermatitis 48:181–188

29. Zhai H, Chew AL, Bashir SJ et al (2003) Provocative use test of nickel coins in nickel-sensitized subjects and controls. Br J Dermatol 149:311–317

30. Lidén C, Skare L, Vahter M (2008) Release of nickel from coins and deposition onto skin from coin handling–comparing euro coins and SEK. Contact Dermatitis 59:31–37

31. Lidén C, Skare L, Lind B et al (2006) Assessment of skin exposure to nickel, chromium and cobalt by acid wipe sampling and ICP-MS. Contact Dermatitis 54:233–238

32. Basketter DA, Angelini G, Ingber A et al (2003) Nickel, chromium and cobalt in consumer products: revisiting safe levels in the new millennium. Contact Dermatitis 49:1–7

33. Fullerton A, Hoelgaard A (1988) Binding of nickel to human epidermis in vitro. Br J Dermatol 119:675–682

34. Fullerton A, Andersen JR, Hoelgaard A (1988) Permeation of nickel through human skin in vitro–effect of vehicles. Br J Dermatol 118:509–516

35. Hostynek JJ (2003) Factors determining percutaneous metal absorption. Food Chem Toxicol 41:327–345

36. Peters K, Gammelgaard B, Menné T (1991) Nickel concentrations in fingernails as a measure of occupational exposure to nickel. Contact Dermatitis 25:237–241

37. Allenby CF, Basketter DA (1994) The effect of repeated open exposure to low levels of nickel on compromised hand skin of nickel-allergic subjects. Contact Dermatitis 30:135–138

38. Nielsen NH, Menné T, Kristiansen J et al (1999) Effects of repeated skin exposure to low nickel concentrations: a model for allergic contact dermatitis to nickel on the hands. Br J Dermatol 141:676–682

39. Kristiansen J, Christensen JM, Henriksen T et al (2000) Determination of nickel in fingernails and forearm skin (stratum corneum). Anal Chim Acta 403:265–272

40. Novak N, Bieber T (2003) Allergic and nonallergic forms of atopic diseases. J Allergy Clin Immunol 112:252–262

41. Kligman AM (1966) The identification of contact allergens by human assay. 3. The maximization test: a procedure for screening and rating contact sensitizers. J Invest Dermatol 47:393–409

42. Vandenberg JJ, Epstein WL (1963) Experimental nickel contact sensitization in man. J Invest Dermatol 41:413–418

43. Cronin E (1972) Clinical prediction of patch test results. Trans St Johns Hosp Dermatol Soc 58:153–162

44. Nielsen NH, Linneberg A, Menné T et al (2001) Persistence of contact allergy among Danish adults: an 8-year follow-up study. Contact Dermatitis 45:350–353

45. Hindsén M, Bruze M, Christensen OB (1999) Individual variation in nickel patch test reactivity. Am J Contact Dermat 10:62–67

46. Hindsén M, Bruze M, Christensen OB (1997) The significance of previous allergic contact dermatitis for elicitation of delayed hypersensitivity to nickel. Contact Dermatitis 37:101–106

47. Hindsén M, Christensen OB (1992) Delayed hypersensitivity reactions following allergic and irritant inflammation. Acta Derm Venereol 72:220–221

48. Nielsen NH, Menné T (1996) The relationship between IgE-mediated and cell-mediated hypersensitivities in an unselected Danish population: the Glostrup Allergy Study, Denmark. Br J Dermatol 134:669–672

49. Menné T, Calvin G (1993) Concentration threshold of non-occluded nickel exposure in nickel-sensitive individuals and controls with and without surfactant. Contact Dermatitis 29:180–184

50. Andersen KE, Lidén C, Hansen J et al (1993) Dose-response testing with nickel sulphate using the TRUE test in nickel-sensitive individuals. Multiple nickel sulphate patch-test reactions do not cause an 'angry back'. Br J Dermatol 129:50–56

51. Hindsén M, Bruze M (1998) The significance of previous contact dermatitis for elicitation of contact allergy to nickel. Acta Derm Venereol 78:367–370

52. Fischer LA, Johansen JD, Menné T (2007) Nickel allergy: relationship between patch test and repeated open application test thresholds. Br J Dermatol 157:723–729

53. Fischer LA, Menné T, Johansen JD (2007) Dose per unit area – a study of elicitation of nickel allergy. Contact Dermatitis 56:255–261

54. Lisby S, Hansen LH, Menné T (1999) Nickel-induced proliferation of both memory and naive T cells in patch test-negative individuals. Clin Exp Immunol 117:217–222

55. Bonnevie P (1936) Der klinische Wert der ekzempropen, an der nickeldiosynkrasie erläutert. Acta Dermatovener 17:376–388

56. Calnan CD (1956) Nickel dermatitis. Br J Dermatol 68:229–236

57. Marcussen PV (1957) Spread of nickel dermatitis. Dermatologica 115:596–607

58. Boss A, Menné T (1982) Nickel sensitization from ear piercing. Contact Dermatitis 8:211–213

59. Brandrup F, Larsen SF (1979) Nickel dermatitis provoked by buttons in blue jeans. Contact Dermatitis 5:148–150

60. Larsson-Stymne B, Widström L (1985) Ear piercing–a cause of nickel allergy in schoolgirls? Contact Dermatitis 13:289–293

61. Andersen KE, Hjorth N, Menné T (1984) The baboon syndrome: systemically-induced allergic contact dermatitis. Contact Dermatitis 10:97–100

62. Christensen OB, Möller H (1975) External and internal exposure to the antigen in the hand eczema of nickel allergy. Contact Dermatitis 1:136–141

63. Jensen CS, Menné T, Johansen JD (2006) Systemic contact dermatitis after oral exposure to nickel: a review with a modified meta-analysis. Contact Dermatitis 54:79–86

64. Hindsén M, Christensen OB, Möller H (1994) Nickel levels in serum and urine in five different groups of eczema patients following oral ingestion of nickel. Acta Derm Venereol 74:176–178

65. Mørtz CG, Lauritsen JM, Bindslev-Jensen C et al (2002) Nickel sensitization in adolescents and association with ear piercing, use of dental braces and hand eczema. The Odense Adolescence Cohort Study on Atopic Diseases and Dermatitis (TOACS). Acta Derm Venereol 82:359–364

66. Van H, I, Andersen KE, Von Blomberg BM et al (1991) Reduced frequency of nickel allergy upon oral nickel contact at an early age. Clin Exp Immunol 85:441–445

67. Smith-Sivertsen T, Dotterud LK, Lund E (1999) Nickel allergy and its relationship with local nickel pollution, ear piercing, and atopic dermatitis: a population-based study from Norway. J Am Acad Dermatol 40:726–735

35

68. Santucci B, Cristaudo A, Cannistraci C et al (1988) Nickel sensitivity: effects of prolonged oral intake of the element. Contact Dermatitis 19:202–205

69. Veien NK, Hattel T, Laurberg G (1993) Low nickel diet: an open, prospective trial. J Am Acad Dermatol 29:1002–1007

70. Van Hoogstraten IM, Von Blomberg BM, Boden D et al (1994) Non-sensitizing epicutaneous skin tests prevent subsequent induction of immune tolerance. J Invest Dermatol 102:80–83

71. Cavani A, Mei D, Guerra E et al (1998) Patients with allergic contact dermatitis to nickel and nonallergic individuals display different nickel-specific T cell responses. Evidence for the presence of effector CD8+ and regulatory CD4+ T cells. J Invest Dermatol 111:621–628

72. Cavani A, Nasorri F, Prezzi C et al (2000) Human CD4+ T lymphocytes with remarkable regulatory functions on dendritic cells and nickel-specific Th1 immune responses. J Invest Dermatol 114:295–302

73. Cavani A, Nasorri F, Ottaviani C et al (2003) Human CD25+ regulatory T cells maintain immune tolerance to nickel in healthy, nonallergic individuals. J Immunol 171:5760–5768

74. Dubois B, Chapat L, Goubier A et al (2003) Innate CD4+CD25+ regulatory T cells are required for oral tolerance and inhibition of CD8+ T cells mediating skin inflammation. Blood 102:3295–3301

75. Moed H, Von Blomberg BM, Bruynzeel DP et al (2005) Regulation of nickel-induced T-cell responsiveness by CD4+CD25+ cells in contact allergic patients and healthy individuals. Contact Dermatitis 53:71–74

76. Wu X, Roelofs-Haarhuis K, Zhang J et al (2007) Dose dependence of oral tolerance to nickel. Int Immunol 19: 965–975

77. Marcussen PV (1959) Nickel eczema. Survey based on 621 cases. Ugeskr Laeger 121:1349–1353

78. Menné T, Holm NV (1983) Nickel allergy in a female twin population. Int J Dermatol 22:22–28

79. Peltonen L (1979) Nickel sensitivity in the general population. Contact Dermatitis 5:27–32

80. Prystowsky SD, Allen AM, Smith RW et al (1979) Allergic contact hypersensitivity to nickel, neomycin, ethylenediamine, and benzocaine. Relationships between age, sex, history of exposure, and reactivity to standard patch tests and use tests in a general population. Arch Dermatol 115:959–962

81. Nielsen NH, Menné T (1992) Allergic contact sensitization in an unselected Danish population. The Glostrup Allergy Study, Denmark. Acta Derm Venereol 72:456–460

82. Linneberg A, Nielsen NH, Menné T et al (2003) Smoking might be a risk factor for contact allergy. J Allergy Clin Immunol 111:980–984

83. Jensen CS, Lisby S, Baadsgaard O et al (2002) Decrease in nickel sensitization in a Danish schoolgirl population with ears pierced after implementation of a nickel-exposure regulation. Br J Dermatol 146:636–642

84. Thyssen JP, Johansen JD, Menné T et al (2009) Nickel allergy in Danish women before and after nickel regulation. N Engl J Med 360:2259–2260

85. Gamerdinger K, Moulon C, Karp DR et al (2003) A new type of metal recognition by human T cells: contact residues for peptide-independent bridging of T cell receptor and major histocompatibility complex by nickel. J Exp Med 197: 1345–1353

86. Johansen J, Menné T, Christophersen J et al (2000) Changes in the pattern of sensitization to common contact allergens in Denmark between 1985-86 and 1997-98, with a special view to the effect of preventive strategies. Br J Dermatol 142:490–495

87. Schnuch A, Uter W (2003) Decrease in nickel allergy in Germany and regulatory interventions. Contact Dermatitis 49:107–108

88. Veien NK, Hattel T, Laurberg G (2001) Reduced nickel sensitivity in young Danish women following regulation of nickel exposure. Contact Dermatitis 45:104–106

89. Thyssen JP, Hald M, Avnstorp C et al (2009) Characteristics of nickel allergic dermatitis patients seen in private dermatology clinics in Denmark: a questionnaire study. Acta Derm Venereol 89:384–388

90. Thyssen JP, Johansen JD, Carlsen BC et al (2009) Prevalence of nickel and cobalt allergy among female dermatitis patients before and after Danish government regulation: a 23-year retrospective study. J Am Acad Dermatol 61(5):799–805

91. Rietschel RL, Fowler JF, Warshaw EM et al (2008) Detection of nickel sensitivity has increased in North American patch-test patients. Dermatitis 19:16–19

92. Agner T, Johansen JD, Overgaard L et al (2002) Combined effects of irritants and allergens. Synergistic effects of nickel and sodium lauryl sulfate in nickel- sensitized individuals. Contact Dermatitis 47:21–26

93. Kalimo K, Lammintausta K, Jalava J et al (1997) Is it possible to improve the prognosis in nickel contact dermatitis? Contact Dermatitis 37:121–124

94. Shah M, Lewis FM, Gawkrodger DJ (1998) Nickel as an occupational allergen. A survey of 368 nickel-sensitive subjects. Arch Dermatol 134:1231–1236

95. Halkier-Sørensen L (1996) Occupational skin diseases. Contact Dermatitis 35:1–120

96. Josefson A, Färm G, Magnuson A et al (2009) Nickel allergy as risk factor for hand eczema: a population-based study. Br J Dermatol 160(4):828–834

97. Nielsen NH, Linneberg A, Menné T et al (2002) The association between contact allergy and hand eczema in 2 cross-sectional surveys 8 years apart. Contact Dermatitis 47: 71–77

98. Gawkrodger DJ, Healy J, Howe AM (1995) The prevention of nickel contact dermatitis. A review of the use of binding agents and barrier creams. Contact Dermatitis 32: 257–265

99. Kaaber K, Menné T, Tjell JC et al (1979) Antabuse treatment of nickel dermatitis. Chelation–a new principle in the treatment of nickel dermatitis. Contact Dermatitis 5:221–228

100. Menné T, Rasmussen K (1990) Regulation of nickel exposure in Denmark. Contact Dermatitis 23:57–58

101. Lidén C, Johnsson S (2001) Nickel on the Swedish market before the Nickel Directive. Contact Dermatitis 44:7–12

102. Lidén C, Norberg K (2005) Nickel on the Swedish market. Follow-up after implementation of the Nickel Directive. Contact Dermatitis 52:29–35

103. Thyssen JP, Maibach HI (2008) Nickel release from earrings purchased in the United States: the San Francisco earring study. J Am Acad Dermatol 58:1000–1005

104. Burrows D, Adams R (1990) Metals, 2nd edn. WB Saunders, Philadelphia, pp 349–386

105. Parkhurst HJ (1925) Dermatosis industrialis in a blue print worker due to chromium compounds. Arch Dermatol 12:253–256

106. Thyssen JP, Jensen P, Carlsen BC et al (2009) The prevalence of chromium allergy in Denmark is currently increasing as a result of leather exposure. Br J Dermatol 161(6):1288–1293

107. Costa M (1998) Carcinogenic metals. Sci Prog 81(Pt 4): 329–339

108. Hayes RB (1997) The carcinogenicity of metals in humans. Cancer Causes Control 8:371–385

109. Jacobs JJ, Urban RM, Hallab NJ et al (2009) Metal-on-metal bearing surfaces. J Am Acad Orthop Surg 17:69–76

110. Kim RH, Dennis DA, Carothers JT (2008) Metal-on-metal total hip arthroplasty. J Arthroplasty 23:44–46

111. Hallab N, Merritt K, Jacobs JJ (2001) Metal sensitivity in patients with orthopaedic implants. J Bone Joint Surg Am 83-A:428–436

112. Gammelgaard B, Fullerton A, Avnstorp C et al (1992) Permeation of chromium salts through human skin in vitro. Contact Dermatitis 27:302–310

113. Burrows D (1984) The dichromate problem. Int J Dermatol 23:215–220

114. Fregert S, Rorsman H (1966) Allergic reactions to trivalent chromium compounds. Arch Dermatol 93:711–713

115. Hansen MB, Johansen JD, Menné T (2003) Chromium allergy: significance of both Cr(III) and Cr(VI). Contact Dermatitis 49:206–212

116. Fregert S (1981) Chromium valencies and cement dermatitis. Br J Dermatol 105(suppl 21):7–9

117. Fregert S, Gruvberger B (1972) Chemical properties of cement. Berufsdermatosen 20:238–248

118. Turk K, Rietschel RL (1993) Effect of processing cement to concrete on hexavalent chromium levels. Contact Dermatitis 28:209–211

119. Fregert S, Gruvberger B (1973) Correlation between alkali sulphate and water-soluble chromate in cement. Acta Derm Venereol 53:225–228

120. Aslan A (2009) Determination of heavy metal toxicity of finished leather solid waste. Bull Environ Contam Toxicol 82(5):633–638

121. Hansen MB, Menné T, Johansen JD (2006) Cr(III) and Cr(VI) in leather and elicitation of eczema. Contact Dermatitis 54:278–282

122. Nygren O, Wahlberg JE (1998) Speciation of chromium in tanned leather gloves and relapse of chromium allergy from tanned leather samples. Analyst 123:935–937

123. Graf D (2009) Formation of Cr(VI) traces in chrometanned leather: causes, prevention and latest findings. J Am Leather Chem Assoc 96:169–179

124. Rydin S (2002) Investigation of the content of CrVI and CrIII in leather products on the Danish market. Danish Environmental Protection Agency, Copenhagen, Denmark

125. Estlander T, Jolanki R, Kanerva L (2000) Occupational allergic contact dermatitis from trivalent chromium in leather tanning. Contact Dermatitis 43:114

126. Freeman S (1997) Shoe dermatitis. Contact Dermatitis 36: 247–251

127. Geier J, Schnuch A, Frosch PJ (2000) Contact allergy to dichromate in women. Dermatol Beruf Umwelt 48:4–10

128. Oumeish OY, Rushaidat QM (1980) Contact dermatitis to military boots in Jordan. Contact Dermatitis 6:498

129. Rudzki E, Kozlowska A (1980) Causes of chromate dermatitis in Poland. Contact Dermatitis 6:191–196

130. Shackelford KE, Belsito DV (2002) The etiology of allergic-appearing foot dermatitis: a 5-year retrospective study. J Am Acad Dermatol 47:715–721

131. Geier J, Lessmann H, Hellweg B et al (2009) Chromated metal products may be hazardous to patients with chromate allergy. Contact Dermatitis 60:199–202

132. Hansen MB, Rydin S, Menné T et al (2002) Quantitative aspects of contact allergy to chromium and exposure to chrome-tanned leather. Contact Dermatitis 47:127–134

133. Garcia-Perez A, Martin-Pascual A, Sanchez-Misiego A (1973) Chrome content in bleaches and detergents. Its relationship to hand dermatitis in women. Acta Derm Venereol 53:353–358

134. Ingber A, Gammelgaard B, David M (1998) Detergents and bleaches are sources of chromium contact dermatitis in Israel. Contact Dermatitis 38:101–104

135. Lachapelle JM, Lauwerys R, Tennstedt D et al (1980) Eau de Javel and prevention of chromate allergy in France. Contact Dermatitis 6:107–110

136. Hostynek JJ, Maibach HI (1988) Chromium in US household bleach. Contact Dermatitis 18:206–209

137. Basketter D, Horev L, Slodovnik D et al (2001) Investigation of the threshold for allergic reactivity to chromium. Contact Dermatitis 44:70–74

138. Fowler JF Jr, Kauffman CL, Marks JG et al (1999) An environmental hazard assessment of low-level dermal exposure to hexavalent chromium in solution among chromium-sensitized volunteers. J Occup Environ Med 41:150–160

139. Fagliano JA, Savrin J, Udasin I et al (1997) Community exposure and medical screening near chromium waste sites in New Jersey. Regul Toxicol Pharmacol 26:S13–S22

140. Horowitz SB, Finley BL (1994) Setting health-protective soil concentrations for dermal contact allergens: a proposed methodology. Regul Toxicol Pharmacol 19:31–47

141. Nethercott J, Paustenbach D, Adams R et al (1994) A study of chromium induced allergic contact dermatitis with 54 volunteers: implications for environmental risk assessment. Occup Environ Med 51:371–380

142. Paustenbach DJ, Sheehan PJ, Paull JM et al (1992) Review of the allergic contact dermatitis hazard posed by chromium-contaminated soil: identifying a "safe" concentration. J Toxicol Environ Health 37:177–207

143. Proctor DM, Fredrick MM, Scott PK et al (1998) The prevalence of chromium allergy in the United States and its implications for setting soil cleanup: a cost-effectiveness case study. Regul Toxicol Pharmacol 28:27–37

144. Stern AH, Bagdon RE, Hazen RE et al (1993) Risk assessment of the allergic dermatitis potential of environmental exposure to hexavalent chromium. J Toxicol Environ Health 40:613–641

145. Bruze M, Fregert S, Gruvberger B (1990) Patch testing with cement containing iron sulfate. Dermatol Clin 8: 173–176

146. Eun HC, Marks R (1990) Dose-response relationships for topically applied antigens. Br J Dermatol 122:491–499

147. Nielsen NH, Kristiansen J, Borg L et al (2000) Repeated exposures to cobalt or chromate on the hands of patients with hand eczema and contact allergy to that metal. Contact Dermatitis 43:212–215

148. Smith AR (1931) Chrome poisoning with manifestations of sensitization. J Am Med Assoc 97:95–98
149. Englehardt WE, Mayer RL (1931) Über Chromekzeme im Graphischen Gewerbe. Arch Gewerbepath Hyg 2: 140–168
150. Kesten B, Laszlo E (1931) Dermatitis due to sensitization to contact substances: Dermatitis venenata occupational dermatitis. Arch Dermatol 23:221–237
151. Bonnevie P (1939) Ätiologie und Pathogenese der Eczemkrankheiten. Barth, Leipzig
152. Bruze M, Conde-Salazar L et al (1999) Thoughts on sensitizers in a standard patch test series. The European Society of Contact Dermatitis. Contact Dermatitis 41:241–250
153. Möller H (1989) Intradermal testing in doubtful cases of contact allergy to metals. Contact Dermatitis 20:120–123
154. Burrows D, Andersen KE, Camarasa JG et al (1989) Trial of 0.5% versus 0.375% potassium dichromate. European Environmental and Contact Dermatitis Research Group (EECDRG). Contact Dermatitis 21:351
155. Frosch PJ, Aberer W (1988) Chrom-Allergie. Dermatosen 36:168–169
156. Allenby CF, Goodwin BF (1983) Influence of detergent washing powders on minimal eliciting patch test concentrations of nickel and chromium. Contact Dermatitis 9: 491–499
157. Al-Tawil NG, Marcusson JA, Möller E (1983) Lymphocyte stimulation by trivalent and hexavalent chromium compounds in patients with chromium sensitivity. An aid to diagnosis. Acta Derm Venereol 63:296–303
158. Räsänen L, Sainio H, Lehto M et al (1991) Lymphocyte proliferation test as a diagnostic aid in chromium contact sensitivity. Contact Dermatitis 25:25–29
159. Martins LE, Duarte AJ, Aoki V et al (2008) Lymphocyte proliferation testing in chromium allergic contact dermatitis. Clin Exp Dermatol 33:472–477
160. Lindemann M, Rietschel F, Zabel M et al (2008) Detection of chromium allergy by cellular in vitro methods. Clin Exp Allergy 38:1468–1475
161. Thormann J, Jespersen NB, Joensen HD (1979) Persistence of contact allergy to chromium. Contact Dermatitis 5:261–264
162. Wall LM, Gebauer KA (1991) A follow-up study of occupational skin disease in Western Australia. Contact Dermatitis 24:241–243
163. Hansen MB, Menné T, Johansen JD (2006) Cr(III) reactivity and foot dermatitis in Cr(VI) positive patients. Contact Dermatitis 54:140–144
164. Olumide YM (1985) Contact dermatitis in Nigeria. Contact Dermatitis 12:241–246
165. Anderson RA (1995) Chromium and parenteral nutrition. Nutrition 11:83–86
166. Accominotti M, Bost M, Haudrechy P et al (1998) Contribution to chromium and nickel enrichment during cooking of foods in stainless steel utensils. Contact Dermatitis 38:305–310
167. Kaaber K, Veien NK (1977) The significance of chromate ingestion in patients allergic to chromate. Acta Derm Venereol 57:321–323
168. Kerger BD, Paustenbach DJ, Corbett GE et al (1996) Absorption and elimination of trivalent and hexavalent chromium in humans following ingestion of a bolus dose in drinking water. Toxicol Appl Pharmacol 141:145–158
169. Kerger BD, Finley BL, Corbett GE et al (1997) Ingestion of chromium(VI) in drinking water by human volunteers: absorption, distribution, and excretion of single and repeated doses. J Toxicol Environ Health 50:67–95
170. Kaaber K, Sjölin KE, Menné T (1983) Elbow eruptions in nickel and chromate dermatitis. Contact Dermatitis 9: 213–216
171. Jaeger H, Pelloni E (1950) Test épicutanés aux bichromates, positifs dans l'eczema au ciment. Dermatologica 100:207–215
172. Balasubramaniam P, Gawkrodger DJ (2003) Chromate: still an important occupational allergen for men in the UK. Contact Dermatitis 49:162–163
173. Bock M, Schmidt A, Bruckner T et al (2003) Occupational skin disease in the construction industry. Br J Dermatol 149:1165–1171
174. Goon AT, Goh CL (2000) Epidemiology of occupational skin disease in Singapore 1989-1998. Contact Dermatitis 43:133–136
175. Kanerva L, Jolanki R, Estlander T et al (2000) Incidence rates of occupational allergic contact dermatitis caused by metals. Am J Contact Dermat 11:155–160
176. Uter W, Ruhl R, Pfahlberg A et al (2004) Contact allergy in construction workers: results of a multifactorial analysis. Ann Occup Hyg 48:21–27
177. Estlander T (1990) Occupational skin disease in Finland. Observations made during 1974-1988 at the Institute of Occupational Health, Helsinki. Acta Derm Venereol Suppl (Stockh) 155:1–85
178. Avnstorp C (1991) Risk factors for cement eczema. Contact Dermatitis 25:81–88
179. Basketter DA, Briatico-Vangosa G, Kaestner W et al (1993) Nickel, cobalt and chromium in consumer products: a role in allergic contact dermatitis? Contact Dermatitis 28: 15–25
180. Zachariae CO, Agner T, Menné T (1996) Chromium allergy in consecutive patients in a country where ferrous sulfate has been added to cement since 1981. Contact Dermatitis 35:83–85
181. Irvine C, Pugh CE, Hansen EJ et al (1994) Cement dermatitis in underground workers during construction of the Channel Tunnel. Occup Med (Lond) 44:17–23
182. Peltonen L, Fräki J (1983) Prevalence of dichromate sensitivity. Contact Dermatitis 9:190–194
183. Seidenari S, Manzini BM, Danese P, Motolese A (1990) Patch and prick test study of 593 healthy subjects. Contact Dermatitis 23:162–167
184. Lantinga H, Nater JP, Coenraads PJ (1984) Prevalence, incidence and course of eczema on the hands and forearms in a sample of the general population. Contact Dermatitis 10:135–139
185. Greig JE, Carson CF, Stuckey MS et al (2000) Prevalence of delayed hypersensitivity to the European standard series in a self-selected population. Australas J Dermatol 41: 86–89
186. Mørtz CG, Andersen KE (1999) Allergic contact dermatitis in children and adolescents. Contact Dermatitis 41:121–130
187. Wass U, Wahlberg JE (1991) Chromated steel and contact allergy. Recommendation concerning a "threshold limit value" for the release of hexavalent chromium. Contact Dermatitis 24:114–118

188. Burckhardt W, Frenk E, de SD et al (1971) Decrease of the eczematous effect of cement by ferrous sulphate. Dermatologica 142:271–273

189. Fregert S, Gruvberger B, Sandahl E (1979) Reduction of chromate in cement by iron sulfate. Contact Dermatitis 5:39–42

190. Färm G (1986) Changing patients in chromate allergy. Contact Dermatitis 15:298–299

191. Gailhofer G, Ludvan M (1987) Change in the allergen spectrum in contact eczema 1975-1984. Derm Beruf Umwelt 35:12–16

192. Goh CL, Gan SL (1996) Change in cement manufacturing process, a cause for decline in chromate allergy? Contact Dermatitis 34:51–54

193. Roto P, Sainio H, Reunala T et al (1996) Addition of ferrous sulfate to cement and risk of chromium dermatitis among construction workers. Contact Dermatitis 34:43–50

194. Thyssen JP, Johansen JD, Menné T (2007) Contact allergy epidemics and their controls. Contact Dermatitis 56:185–195

195. Bruze M, Gruvberger B, Hradil E (1990) Chromate sensitization and elicitation from cement with iron sulfate. Acta Derm Venereol 70:160–162

196. Cobalt Development Institute (CDI). Cobalt facts. www.thecdi.com/cobaltfacts.php

197. Tandon R, Aarts B (1993) Chromium, nickel and cobalt contents of some Australian cements. Contact Dermatitis 28:201–205

198. Julander A, Hindsén M, Skare L et al (2009) Cobalt-containing alloys and their ability to release cobalt and cause dermatitis. Contact Dermatitis 60:165–170

199. Julander A, Skare L, Mulder M et al (2010) Skin deposition of nickel, cobalt and chromium in production of gas turbines and space propulsion components. Ann Occup Hyg 54:340–350

200. Linnainmaa M, Kiilunen M (1997) Urinary cobalt as a measure of exposure in the wet sharpening of hard metal and stellite blades. Int Arch Occup Environ Health 69:193–200

201. ESSCA Writing Group (2008) The European Surveillance System of Contact Allergies (ESSCA): results of patch testing the standard series, 2004. J Eur Acad Dermatol Venereol 22:174–181

202. Fowler JF Jr (1990) Allergic contact dermatitis to metals. Am J Contact Dermat 1:212–223

203. Fregert S, Rorsman H (1966) Allergy to chromium, nickel and cobalt. Acta Derm Venereol (Stockh) 46:144–148

204. Hegewald J, Uter W, Pfahlberg A et al (2005) A multifactorial analysis of concurrent patch-test reactions to nickel, cobalt, and chromate. Allergy 60:372–378

205. Lindberg M, Edman B, Fischer T et al (2007) Time trends in Swedish patch test data from 1992 to 2000. A multicentre study based on age- and sex-adjusted results of the Swedish standard series. Contact Dermatitis 56:205–210

206. Schwartz L, Peck SM, Blair KE et al (1945) Allergic dermatitis due to metallic cobalt. J Allergy Clin Immunol 16:51–53

207. Pirilä V (1953) Sensitivity to cobalt in pottery workers. Acta Derm Venereol (Stockh) 33:193–198

208. Fischer T, Rystedt I (1983) Cobalt allergy in hard metal workers. Contact Dermatitis 9:115–121

209. Rystedt I, Fischer T (1983) Relationship between nickel and cobalt sensitization in hard metal workers. Contact Dermatitis 9:195–200

210. Condé-Salazar L, Guimaraens D, Villegas C et al (1995) Occupational allergic contact dermatitis in construction workers. Contact Dermatitis 33:226–230

211. Geier J, Schnuch A (1995) A comparison of contact allergies among construction and nonconstruction workers attending contact dermatitis clinics in Germany: results of the Information Network of Departments of Dermatology from November 1989 to July 1993. Am J Contact Dermat 6:86–94

212. Uter W, Rühl R, Pfahlberg A et al (2004) Contact allergy in construction workers: results of a multifactorial analysis. Ann Occup Hyg 48:21–27

213. Geier J, Lessmann H, Schnuch A et al (2004) Contact sensitizations in metalworkers with occupational dermatitis exposed to water-based metalworking fluids: results of the research project "FaSt". Int Arch Occup Environ Health 77:543–551

214. Burrows D, Adams RM, Flint GN (1999) Metals. In: Adams RM (ed) Occupational skin disease, 3rd edn. Saunders, Philadelphia, pp 395–433

215. Lidén C, Wahlberg JE (1994) Cross-reactivity to metal compounds studied in guinea pigs induced with chromate or cobalt. Acta Derm Venereol (Stockh) 74:341–343

216. Wahlberg JE, Lidén C (2000) Cross-reactivity patterns of cobalt and nickel studied with repeated open applications (ROATs) to the skin of guinea pigs. Am J Contact Dermat 11:42–48

217. Lidén C, Wahlberg JE, Maibach HI (1995) Skin. In: Goyer RA, Klaassen CD, Waalkes MP (eds) Metal toxicology. Academic Press, New York, pp 447–464

218. Fischer T, Rystedt I (1985) False-positive, follicular and irritant patch test reactions to metal salts. Contact Dermatitis 12:93–98

219. Allenby CF, Basketter DA (1989) Minimum eliciting patch test concentrations of cobalt. Contact Dermatitis 20:185–190

220. de Fine OF, Menné T (1992) Skin reactivity to metallic cobalt in patients with a positive patch test to cobalt chloride. Contact Dermatitis 27:241–243

221. Netterlid E, Hindsén M, Björk J et al (2009) There is an association between contact allergy to aluminium and persistent subcutaneous nodules in children undergoing hyposensitization therapy. Contact Dermatitis 60:41–49

222. Bruze M, Lundh K, Gruvberger B et al (2008) Aluminium chloride hexahydrate at 2% is insufficient to trace contact allergy to aluminium. Contact Dermatitis 59:183–184

223. Johannessen H, Bergan-Skar B (1980) Itching problems among potroom workers in factories using recycled alumina. Contact Dermatitis 6:42–43

224. Hall AF (1944) Occupational contact dermatitis among aircraft workers. J Am Med Assoc 125:179–185

225. Peters T, Hani N, Kirchberg K et al (1998) Occupational contact sensitivity to aluminium in a machine construction plant worker. Contact Dermatitis 39:322–323

226. Lidén C (1994) Cold-impregnated aluminium. A new source of nickel exposure. Contact Dermatitis 31:22–24

227. Williams S, Freemont AJ (1984) Aerosol antiperspirants and axillary granulomata. Br Med J (Clin Res Ed) 288:1651–1652

228. Dwyer CM, Kerr RE (1993) Contact allergy to aluminium in 2 brothers. Contact Dermatitis 29:36–38

229. Veien NK, Hattel T, Laurberg G (1993) Systemically aggravated contact dermatitis caused by aluminium in toothpaste. Contact Dermatitis 28:199–200

230. Frost L, Johansen P, Pedersen S et al (1985) Persistent subcutaneous nodules in children hyposensitized with aluminium-containing allergen extracts. Allergy 40:368–372

231. Veien NK, Hattel T, Justesen O et al (1986) Aluminium allergy. Contact Dermatitis 15:295–297

232. Clemmensen O, Knudsen HE (1980) Contact sensitivity to aluminium in a patient hyposensitized with aluminium precipitated grass pollen. Contact Dermatitis 6:305–308

233. Bøhler-Sommeregger K, Lindemayr H (1986) Contact sensitivity to aluminium. Contact Dermatitis 15:278–281

234. Fawcett HA, McGibbon D, Cronin E (1985) Persistent vaccination granuloma due to aluminum sensitivity. Br J Dermatol 113(suppl 29):101–102

235. Nielsen AO, Kaaber K, Veien NK (1992) Aluminum allergy caused by DTP vaccine. Ugeskr Laeger 154:1900–1901

236. Kriebel D, Sprince NL, Eisen EA et al (1988) Beryllium exposure and pulmonary function: a cross-sectional study of beryllium workers. Br J Ind Med 45:167–173

237. Bobka CA, Stewart LA, Engelken GJ et al (1997) Comparison of in vivo and in vitro measures of beryllium sensitization. J Occup Environ Med 39:540–547

238. Berlin JM, Taylor JS, Sigel JE et al (2003) Beryllium dermatitis. J Am Acad Dermatol 49:939–941

239. Curtis CH (1951) Cutaneous hypersensitivity to beryllium: a study of 13 cases. Arch Dermatol Syphilol 64:470–482

240. Vilaplana J, Romaguera C, Grimalt F (1992) Occupational and non-occupational allergic contact dermatitis from beryllium. Contact Dermatitis 26:295–298

241. Haberman AL, Pratt M, Storrs FJ (1993) Contact dermatitis from beryllium in dental alloys. Contact Dermatitis 28:157–162

242. Torgersson RR, Davis MDP, Bruce AJ et al (2007) Contact allergy in oral disease. J Am Acad Dermatol 57:315–321

243. Vahter M, Åkesson A, Lidén C et al (2007) Gender differences in the disposition and toxicity of metals. Environ Res 104:85–95

244. Wahlberg JE (1977) Routine patch testing with cadmium chloride. Contact Dermatitis 3:293–296

245. Geier J, Vieluf D, Fuchs T (1996) Patch testing with cadmium chloride. Contact Dermatitis 34:73–74

246. Gebhart M, Geier J (1996) Evaluation of patch test results with denture material series. Contact Dermatitis 34:191–195

247. Kaaber S, Cramers M, Jepsen FL (1982) The role of cadmium as a skin sensitizing agent in denture and non-denture wearers. Contact Dermatitis 8:308–313

248. Björnberg A (1963) Reaction to light in yellow tattoos from cadmium sulfide. Arch Dermatol 88:267–271

249. Wahlberg JE, Boman A (1979) Guinea pig maximization test method – cadmium chloride. Contact Dermatitis 5:405

250. Karlberg A-T, Boman A, Wahlberg JE (1983) Copper – a rare sensitizer. Contact Dermatitis 9:134–139

251. Hostynek JJ, Maibach HI (2003) Copper hypersensitivity: dermatologic aspects – an overview. Rev Environ Health 18:153–183

252. Barranco VP (1972) Eczematous dermatitis caused by internal exposure to copper. Arch Dermatol 106:386–387

253. Romaguera C, Grimalt F (1981) Contact dermatitis from a copper-containing intrauterine contraceptive device. Contact Dermatitis 7:163–164

254. Nordlind K, Lidén S (1992) Patch test reactions to metal salts in patients with oral mucosal lesions associated with amalgam restorations. Contact Dermatitis 27:157–160

255. Santosh V, Ranjith K, Shenoi SD et al (1999) Results of patch testing with dental materials. Contact Dermatitis 40:50–51

256. Frykholm KO, Frithiof F, Fernström AI et al (1969) Allergy to copper derived from dental alloys as a possible cause of oral lesions of lichen planus. Acta Derm Venereol (Stockh) 49:268–281

257. Wöhrl S, Hemmer W, Focke M et al (2001) Copper allergy revisited. J Am Acad Dermatol 45:863–870

258. Basketter DA, Gerberick GF, Kimber I et al (1996) The local lymph node assay: a viable alternative to currently accepted skin sensitization tests. Food Chem Toxicol 34:985–997

259. Bruze M, Andersen KE (1999) Gold – a controversial sensitizer. European Environmental and Contact Dermatitis Research Group. Contact Dermatitis 40:1–5

260. Björkner B, Bruze M, Möller H (1994) High frequency of contact allergy to gold sodium thiosulfate. An indication of gold allergy? Contact Dermatitis 30:144–151

261. Isaksson M, Bruze M (2000) Gold. In: Kanerva L, Elsner P, Wahlberg JE, Maibach HI (eds) Handbook of occupational dermatology. Springer, Berlin

262. Brown DH, Smith WE, Fox P et al (1982) The reactions of gold (0) with amino acids and the significance of these reactions in the biochemistry of gold. Inorg Chim Acta 67:27–30

263. Lidén C, Nordenadler M, Skare L (1998) Metal release from gold-containing jewelry materials: no gold release detected. Contact Dermatitis 39:281–285

264. Ahnlide I, Ahlgren C, Björkner B et al (2002) Gold concentration in blood in relation to the number of gold restorations and contact allergy to gold. Acta Odontol Scand 60:301–305

265. Bruze M, Edman B, Björkner B et al (1994) Clinical relevance of contact allergy to gold sodium thiosulfate. J Am Acad Dermatol 31:579–583

266. Schaffran RM, Storrs FJ, Schalock P (1999) Prevalence of gold sensitivity in asymptomatic individuals with gold dental restorations. Am J Contact Dermat 10:201–206

267. Ahlgren C, Ahnlide I, Björkner B et al (2002) Contact allergy to gold is correlated to dental gold. Acta Derm Venereol (Stockh) 82:41–44

268. Ekqvist S, Svedman C, Möller H et al (2007) High frequency of contact allergy to gold in patients with endovascular coronary stents. Br J Dermatol 157:730–738

269. Eisler R (2003) Chrysotherapy: a synoptic review. Inflamm Res 52:487–501

270. Björkner B, Bruze M, Möller H et al (2008) Allergic contact dermatitis as a complication of lip loading with gold implants. Dermatitis 19:148–153

271. Fowler JF Jr (1987) Selection of patch test materials for gold allergy. Contact Dermatitis 17:23–25

272. Bruze B, Björkner B, Möller H (1999) Patch testing with gold sodium thiosulfate. Jadassohn Centenary Congress, London, UK (abstract book 14)

273. Bruze M, Hedman H, Björkner B et al (1995) The development and course of test reactions to gold sodium thiosulfate. Contact Dermatitis 33:386–391

274. Räsänen L, Kalimo K, Laine J et al (1996) Contact allergy to gold in dental patients. Br J Dermatol 134:673–677

275. Räsänen L, Kaipiainen-Seppänen O, Myllykangas-Luosujärvi R et al (1999) Hypersensitivity to gold in gold sodium thiomalate-induced dermatosis. Br J Dermatol 141:683–688

276. Vamnes JS, Gjerdet NR, Morken T et al (1999) In vitro lymphocyte reactivity to gold compounds in the diagnosis of contact hypersensitivity. Contact Dermatitis 41:156–160

277. Rietschel RL, Warshaw EM, Sasseville D et al (2007) Common contact allergens associated with eyelid dermatitis: Data from the North American Contact Dermatitis Group 2003-2004 study period. Dermatitis 18:78–81

278. Fowler JF Jr, Taylor J, Storrs F et al (2001) Gold allergy in North America. Am J Contact Dermat 12:3–5

279. McKenna KE, Dolan O, Walsh MY et al (1995) Contact allergy to gold sodium thiosulfate. Contact Dermatitis 32:143–146

280. Kobayashi Y, Nanko H, Nakamura J et al (1992) Lymphocytoma cutis induced by gold pierced earrings. J Am Acad Dermatol 27:457–458

281. Armstrong DKB, Walsh MY, Dawson JF (1997) Granulomatous contact dermatitis due to gold earrings. Br J Dermatol 136:776–778

282. Park YM, Kang H, Kim HO, Cho BK (1999) Lymphomatoid eosinophilic reaction to gold earrings. Contact Dermatitis 40:216–217

283. Möller H (2002) Dental gold alloys and contact allergy. Contact Dermatitis 47:63–66

284. Raap U, Stiesch M, Reh H et al (2009) Investigation of contact allergy to dental metals in 206 patients. Contact Dermatitis 60:339–343

285. Lazarov A, Kidron D, Tulchinsky Z et al (2003) Contact orofacial granulomatosis caused by delayed hypersensitivity to gold and mercury. J Am Acad Dermatol 49:1117–1120

286. Svedman C, Ekqvist S, Möller H et al (2009) A correlation found between contact allergy to stent material and restenosis of the coronary arteries. Contact Dermatitis 60:158–164

287. Möller H, Björkner B, Bruze M (1996) Clinical reactions to systemic provocation with gold sodium thiomalate in patients with contact allergy to gold. Br J Dermatol 135:423–427

288. Möller H, Ohlsson K, Linder C et al (1998) Cytokines and acute phase reactants during flare-up of contact allergy to gold. Am J Contact Dermat 9:15–22

289. Möller H, Ohlsson K, Linder C et al (1999) The flare-up reactions after systemic provocation in contact allergy to nickel and gold. Contact Dermatitis 40:200–204

290. Möller H, Björkner B, Bruze M et al (1996) Flare-up at contact allergy sites in a gold-treated rheumatic patient. Acta Derm Venereol (Stockh) 76:55–58

291. Russell MA, Langley M, Truett AP 3rd et al (1997) Lichenoid dermatitis after consumption of gold-containing liquor. J Am Acad Dermatol 36:841–844

292. Gruvberger B, Bruze M, Almgren G (1998) Occupational dermatoses in a plant producing binders for paints and glues. Contact Dermatitis 38:71–77

293. Fleming C, Lucke T, Forsyth A et al (1998) A controlled study of gold contact hypersensitivity. Contact Dermatitis 38:137–139

294. Isaksson M, Zimerson E, Bruze M (1999) Occupational dermatoses in composite production. J Occup Environ Med 41:261–266

295. Fowler JF Jr (2001) Gold. Am J Contact Dermatitis 12:1–2

296. Langan DC, Fan PL, Hoos AA (1987) The use of mercury in dentistry: a critical review of the recent literature. J Am Dent Assoc 115:867–880

297. Handley J, Todd D, Burrows D (1993) Mercury allergy in a contact dermatitis clinic in Northern Ireland. Contact Dermatitis 29:258–261

298. Öskaya E, Mirzojeva L, Ötkur B (2009) Systemic allergic dermatitis caused by "white precipitate" in a skin lightening cream. Contact Dermatitis 60:61–63

299. Boyd AS, Seger D, Vannucci S et al (2000) Mercury exposure and cutaneous disease. J Am Acad Dermatol 43:81–90

300. Lerch M, Bircher AJ (2004) Systemically induced allergic exanthem from mercury. Contact Dermatitis 50:349–353

301. Munro-Ashman D, Munro DD, Hughes TH (1969) Contact dermatitis from palladium. Trans St Johns Hosp Dermatol Soc 55:196–197

302. Larese Filon L, Uderzo D, Bagnato E (2003) Sensitization to palladium chloride: a ten-year evaluation. Am J Contact Dermat 14:78–81

303. Kanerva L, Kerosuo H, Kullaa A et al (1996) Allergic patch test reactions to palladium chloride in schoolchildren. Contact Dermatitis 34:39–42

304. Brasch J, Geier J (1997) Patch test results in schoolchildren. Results from the Information Network of Departments of Dermatology (IVDK) and the German Contact Dermatitis Research Group (DKG). Contact Dermatitis 37:286–293

305. Bordel-Gómez MT, Miranda-Romero A, Castrodeza-Sanz J (2008) Isolated and concurrent prevalence of sensitization to transition metals in a Spanish population. J Eur Acad Dermatol Venereol 22:1452–1457

306. Koch P, Baum H-P (1996) Contact stomatitis due to palladium and platinum in dental alloys. Contact Dermatitis 34:253–257

307. Goossens A, De Swerdt A, De Coninck K et al (2006) Allergic contact granuloma due to palladium following ear piercing. Contact Dermatitis 55:338–341

308. Todd DJ, Burrows D (1992) Patch testing with pure palladium metal in patients with sensitivity to palladium chloride. Contact Dermatitis 26:327–331

309. Uter W, Fuchs T, Häusser M et al (1995) Patch test results with serial dilutions of nickel sulfate (with and without detergent), palladium chloride, and nickel and palladium metal plates. Contact Dermatitis 32:135–142

310. Hindsén M, Spirén A, Bruze M (2005) Cross-reactivity between nickel and palladium demonstrated by systemic administration of nickel. Contact Dermatitis 53:2–8

311. Wahlberg JE, Boman AS (1992) Cross-reactivity to palladium and nickel studied in the guinea pig. Acta Derm Venereol (Stockh) 72:95–97

312. Wahlberg JE, Lidén C (1999) Cross-reactivity patterns of palladium and nickel studied by repeated open applications (ROATs) to the skin of guinea pigs. Contact Dermatitis 41:145–149

313. Baker DB, Gann PH, Brooks SM et al (1990) Cross-sectional study of platinum salts sensitization among precious metals refinery workers. Am J Ind Med 18:653–664

314. Santucci B, Valenzano C, de Rocco M et al (2000) Platinum in the environment: frequency of reactions to platinum-group elements in patients with dermatitis and urticaria. Contact Dermatitis 43:333–338

315. Dastychová E, Semrádová V (2000) A case of contact hypersensitivity to platinum salts. Contact Dermatitis 43:226

316. Watsky KL (2007) Occupational allergic contact dermatitis to platinum, palladium and gold. Contact Dermatitis 57: 382–383

317. de la Cuadra J, Grau-Massanés M (1991) Occupational contact dermatitis from rhodium and cobalt. Contact Dermatitis 25:182–184

318. Nakayama H, Imai T (1982) Occupational contact urticaria, contact dermatitis and asthma caused by rhodium hypersensitivity. In: Proceedings of the 6th international symposium on contact dermatitis and joint meeting between ICDRG and JCDRG, Tokyo, Japan

319. Stingeni L, Brunelli L, Lisi P (2004) Contact sensitivity to rhodium and iridium in consecutively patch tested subjects. Contact Dermatitis 51:316–317

320. Lidén C, Maibach HI, Wahlberg JE (1995) Skin. In: Goyer RA, Klaassen CD, Waalkes MP (eds) Metal toxicology. Academic Press, New York, pp 447–464

321. Lansdown AB (2006) Silver in health care: antimicrobial effects and safety in use. Curr Probl Dermatol 33:17–34

322. Drake PL, Hazelwood KJ (2005) Exposure-related health effects of silver and silver compounds: a review. Ann Occup Hyg 49:575–585

323. Iliev D, Elsner P (1998) Unusual edge effect in patch testing with silver nitrate. Am J Contact Dermat 9:57–59

324. Nielsen NH, Skov L (1998) Occupational allergic contact dermatitis in a patient with a positive patch test to tin. Contact Dermatitis 39:99–100

325. Menné T, Andersen KE, Kaaber K et al (1987) Tin: an overlooked contact sensitizer? Contact Dermatitis 16:9–10

Metalworking Fluids

36

Johannes Geier and Holger Lessmann

Contents

J. Geier (✉) and H. Lessmann
Information Network of Departments of Dermatology (IVDK),
University of Göttingen, von-Siebold-Straße 3,
37075 Göttingen, Germany
e-mail: jgeier@ivdk.org

36.1 Metalworking Fluids: Usage and Ingredients

Metalworking fluids (MWF) are used in metal processing for cooling and lubricating purposes, corrosion inhibition and for flushing away of metal chips. Two groups of MWF can be distinguished: water-based MWF (wb MWF), usually emulsions, which are prepared at the metalworking company by aqueous dilution of a concentrate delivered by the lubricant producer; and neat oils, which are non-water-miscible oily preparations used as obtained from the manufacturer. Wb MWF are used in drilling, cutting, turning and grinding of metal parts, and neat oils in cutting, grinding and honing. Their complex composition is commonly based on mineral oils or (semi-)synthetic hydrocarbon compounds. Various admixtures such as emulsifiers, buffers, stabilisers, anti-fog-additives, foam inhibitors, tensides, solubility enhancers, lubricants, corrosion inhibitors, extreme-pressure-additives and biocides (bactericides and fungicides) are usually added, according to the respective needs [1–5]. In the comments on the German occupational exposure threshold limit values ("MAK-Werte") published in 2000, more than 200 components used in MWF are listed [2]. During the working process, wb MWF are subject to change: the concentration may rise due to vaporisation of water, the emulsion might break and the pH may shift due to heating at the workpiece or bacterial contamination. Biocides other than those contained in the original MWF may be added to prevent microbial growth during the long time of use, and slideway oils or hydraulic oils from the processing machines may contaminate the MWF by leakage [4–7] (Fig. 36.1).

J.D. Johansen et al. (eds.), _Contact Dermatitis_,
DOI: 10.1007/978-3-642-03827-3_36, © Springer-Verlag Berlin Heidelberg 2011

36

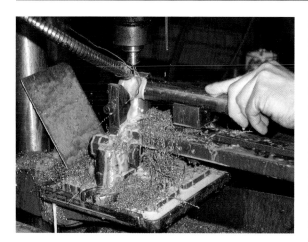

Fig. 36.1 Drilling with wb MWF. The worker's hand is permanently wetted with MWF. No gloves are allowed at this workplace because of the risk of injury from rotating tools (courtesy of H.-G. Englitz)

Core Message

> Two types of MWF can be distinguished: water-based MWF (wb MWF) and neat oils. Their composition is complex. Many components and additives are in use. Wb MWF are subject to change during the working process.

36.2 Occupational Skin Disease Due to Metalworking Fluids

Occupational contact dermatitis (OCD) is common in metal workers exposed to MWF [8–19]. In an epidemiological study on 286 metalworkers exposed to MWF, de Boer et al. found hand dermatitis in 26% of the employees [10, 11]. Forty-seven of two hundred and one trainees (23%) had had hand dermatitis at least 1 time during the study period of 2.5 years in the Swiss Prospective Metal Worker Eczema Study (PROMETES) [9]. The 3-year-incidence of hand eczema was 15.3% among metalworker apprentices in a German prospective cohort study in the car industry (PACO-study) [12]. In a Swedish cross-sectional study on 163 MWF exposed metalworkers with skin complaints, OCD was diagnosed in 14.1% [14]. Of 726 Finnish metalworkers, 20% reported recurring or prolonged dermatitis on their hands or forearms during the past 12 months in structured telephone interviews [19]. In a pooled data analysis from two prospective cohort studies in Europe, the European Community Respiratory Health Survey II (ECRHS II)

and the Swiss Cohort Study on Air Pollution and Lung and Heart Disease in Adults 2 (SAPALDIA 2), current skin symptoms were reported by 10% of metalworkers and were associated with frequent use of oil-based MWF and organic solvent/degreasing agents [15]. In most of these and other studies on OCD in metalworkers [8, 13], irritant contact dermatitis (ICD) was more frequently observed than allergic contact dermatitis (ACD). However, as in any other comparable occupational situation, ICD promotes and often precedes sensitization [20]. Hence, the frequency of ACD in a given study population depends on the average duration of exposure and skin disease. Moreover, a simple dichotomization in ICD and ACD does not reflect reality, because other factors such as atopy are also important, and in most cases, the occupational skin disease is a mixture of constitutional, and irritant and/or ACD [4, 13, 16, 17, 19, 21]. It is likely that contact allergy due to MWF is under-diagnosed because not every possible allergenic substance is being tested in the patients concerned [7, 22, 23].

Clinically, OCD due to MWF usually presents as vesicular or rhagadiform eczema of the web spaces, the lateral aspects of the fingers and the backs of the hands. Often, the dermatitis spreads to the palms and the wrists up to the forearms. Bacterial super-infections are possible [3, 8, 16, 17]. MWF dermatitis may have an unsatisfactory prognosis. Pryce et al. performed a follow-up study on 121 metalworkers concerned, and found skin symptoms in more than 70% of the patients still present after 2 years, partly in spite of job discontinuation [16]. Shah et al. made similar findings [24]. However, the authors admit that the outcome depends very much on the individuals concerned, particularly on the patients' understanding of the cause of the disease and on their willingness to change their behaviour at the workplace. A recent study on 1,355 metalworkers in Germany showed that the acceptance of skin protective measures, in particular barrier creams, was very low, which certainly contributed to recalcitrant dermatitis [25].

Core Message

> MWF are a frequent cause of OCD, with ICD being diagnosed more often than ACD. However, in most cases, the occupational skin disease is a mixture of constitutional dermatitis, ICD and/or ACD. Contact allergy due to MWF may be under-diagnosed.

36.3 Irritant Contact Dermatitis Due to Metalworking Fluids

MWF, in particular wb MWF, exhibit irritant effects to the skin. Due to the risk of injury from rotating tools, it is prohibited to wear protective gloves at most MWF workplaces. Skin irritation by wb MWF is not only caused by wet work, but also by the alkaline pH, usually ranging from 8.5 to 9.6 [5]. Additionally, emulsifiers damage the epidermal barrier and biocides have irritant properties [16, 17]. In many workplaces, there is no continuous exposure to wb MWF, but the skin is contaminated at some repetitive operations, e.g., when changing the workpiece. Mostly, the wb MWF splashes are not removed for other operations such as control measurements or burr removing. They dry up on the skin within few minutes, and as a consequence, the wb MWF is concentrated due to vaporisation and irritancy increases [26]. Additionally, it could be shown in the PROMETES study that not only chemical irritation but also mechanical factors play a role in the damage of the epidermal barrier in metalworkers [9]. Moreover, in metal processing, like in any other comparable occupational setting, a too short recovery time after repetitive minor irritant exposures eventually leads to clinically visible irritant skin damage, following the model described by Malten [9, 27].

Core Message

> In most MWF workplaces, no gloves are allowed. Irritant effects of wb MWF are due to wet work, alkalinity, emulsifiers and biocides. In wb MWF splashes that dry up on the skin, concentration of the components increases within minutes, thus enhancing irritancy.

36.4 Contact Allergy Due to Metalworking Fluids

In 1985, Alomar et al. found an increased number of contact allergies to p-phenylenediamine (PPD), dichromate and cobalt in the standard series, and to benzisothiazolinone (BIT), 1,3,5-tris(2-hydroxyethyl)-hexahydrotriazine (Grotan BK) and triethanloamine (TEA) in a MWF test series in their study on 230 MWF exposed metalworkers with OCD [8]. However, the clinical relevance of the positive reactions to the standard series allergens

could not be stated definitely in most cases [8]. In a study performed in 1986/1987 on 174 patients with suspected MWF dermatitis, Grattan et al. saw an increase of sensitizations to nickel, colophonium, formaldehyde, the formaldehyde releaser Dowicil 200 (Quaternium 15) and other biocides [13]. In 1989, de Boer et al. published an investigation on 286 metalworkers exposed to MWF, of which 75 had had hand eczema. A patch test was performed in 40 of these 75 patients, and 8 of them had a contact allergy [11]. Occupational sensitizations in these cases were due to formaldehyde and (chloro-)methylisothiazolinone (MCI/MI) [11]. Nethercott et al. investigated 27 metalworkers exposed to MWF with hand dermatitis in 1990. Thirteen of these patients had had ACD, and 11 of them were sensitised to MCI/MI, which was used in the MWF [28]. In the beginning of the 1990s, two retrospective studies on contact allergies in metalworkers were published by the Information Network of Departments of Dermatology (IVDK). However, these data analyses were focussed neither on patients exposed to MWF nor on those with OCD. In both analyses, a surprisingly high frequency of sensitization to p-aminoazobenzene (PAAB) was found [29, 30]. Brinkmeier et al. performed an investigation on 408 metalworkers and found positive patch test reactions to Biobans P 1,487, CS 1246, and CS 1135 in 13 patients (3.4%). Most of the test reactions were weak positive and could be reproduced on re-testing in only two out of ten patients [31]. In the course of a large German study on contact allergies among patients with OCD (FaSt study), 160 metalworkers were investigated from 1999 to 2001 [32]. Most frequently, sensitizations to monoethanolamine (MEA), colophonium/abietic acid, and fragrance mix were observed. Additionally, cobalt, diethanolamine (DEA), formaldehyde, formaldehyde releasers and other biocides were important allergens in these patients. Metalworkers exposed to wb MWF with OCD had a significantly increased risk of sensitization to colophonium, formaldehyde and fragrance mix, when compared to metalworkers with OCD who were *not* exposed to wb MWF, or men not working in the metal industry [32]. In 2003, a Swedish study on OCD among the employees of a metalworking plant was published by Gruvberger et al. [14]. Of 164 metalworkers with skin complaints, ten were found to have occupationally induced ACD, and four of them were sensitised to BIT, while three patients had a contact allergy due to the extreme-pressure-additive ethylhexylzinc dithiophosphate (EHZDTP) [14]. Madan and Beck recently reported contact allergy to the formaldehyde releaser N,N-methylene-bis-5-methyl-oxazolidine in 15 out of 318

(4.7%) metalworkers with suspected occupational dermatitis exposed to MWF. Of these, 11 (73%) also reacted to formaldehyde [33]. MWF were the most common source of sensitization to formaldehyde or formaldehyde releasers in patients patch tested at the Finnish Institute of Occupational Health [34]. In two recent multi-centre patch test studies including components of wb MWF, which are not part of the commercially available MWF patch test series, sensitization to diglycolamine and 4,4'-methylenebis morpholine could be detected in 2.2 and 4.9% of the patients, respectively [35, 36].

During the last decade, sensitizations to the following MWF components have been reported in case reports of metalworkers with OCD: diglycolamine [37], ethylenediamine [38], also possibly as an indicator of sensitization to other amines [39], MEA [40, 41], alkanolamineborates [42], a condensate of boric acid, MEA and fatty acids [43], fatty acid polydiethanolamide [44], oleyl alcohol [40], tertiary-butylhydroquinone [45], imazalil [46], iodopropynyl butylcarbamate (IPBC) [47], sodium pyrithione [48, 49], EHZDTP [44, 50], oak moss resin [41], glyoxal [51], 2,5-dimercapto-1,3,4-thiadiazole [6] and phenyl-alpha-naphtylamine [6].

Core Message

> In several studies, formaldehyde and other biocides, particularly formaldehyde releasers, were frequent MWF allergens. Additionally, sensitizations to colophonium/abietic acid, PPD, PAAB, dichromate and cobalt have been described, but the clinical relevance of these findings could not always be established. In case reports, a variety of other allergens in MWF have been described.

36.5 Important Allergens in Metalworking Fluids

36.5.1 Monoethanolamine (MEA), Diethanolamine (DEA), Triethanolamine (TEA) and Diglycolamine

In wb MWF, MEA, DEA and TEA are used as rust preventive agents with emulsifying properties, while diglycolamine serves as an emulsifier [36, 52]. MEA ranked first among the allergens in wb MWF in two German studies [32, 53]. MEA may be present in the MWF as reaction products of MEA with boric acid or other MWF components, and probably only a certain fraction of MEA is present as such. Cases of contact allergy due to such reaction products have been reported, partly without reaction to MEA [42, 43]. Due to a potential formation of carcinogenic N-nitrosamines, the concentration of DEA is limited to 0.2% in the MWF concentrate in Germany by law since 1993 [54]. Due to this limitation, the use of DEA in wb MWF has declined in the following years. This is probably reflected by the far lower frequency of sensitizations to DEA compared to MEA in the two above-mentioned studies [32, 52, 53]. TEA, which is also frequently used in other industrial products and as an emulsifier in creams and cosmetics, was found to be a rare MWF allergen [52]. Although used widely, no exposure associated with an increased risk of TEA sensitization could be identified in an analysis of data from the IVDK. Of the patients tested with TEA 2.5% pet., only 0.4% showed a positive reaction. The profile of patch test reactions indicated a slightly irritant potential rather than a true allergic response in many cases. Therefore, the risk of sensitization to TEA seems to be very low [52]. Diglycolamine was first described as MWF allergen in 2002 [37], and was not included in a MWF test series before 2003 [53]. Hence, experience with this substance is still limited, but it seems to be an important MWF allergen, though.

36.5.2 Colophonium/Abietic Acid

A positive patch test reaction to colophonium indicates a sensitization to oxidation products of abietic acid and other resin acids which are contained in colophonium [55]. The concentrate of a wb MWF may contain 4–8% (in some cases up to 10%) distilled tall oil (DTO). Usually, this concentrate is diluted with water down to 5%. In this case, the concentration of DTO in the final wb MWF (to which the metalworker is exposed), is in a range of 0.2–0.4%. According to the information from the industry, about 30% of the DTO are resin acids, and of these, about one third is abietic acid. In other words: the content of resin acids in the wb MWF is 0.06–0.12%, the content of abietic acid is 0.02–0.04%. Recently, a Finnish study on allergens in MWF was published. The authors could detect resin acids at a concentration of

0.41–3.8% in MWF concentrates [22]. At a commonly used dilution of 5%, the resin acid concentration in the wb MWF would be 0.02–0.2%. On exposure to air, which occurs during normal use of wb MWF, the resin acids oxidise rather quickly [56–58]. The fact that resin acids form alkanolamine salts in the wb MWF probably has no influence on the oxidation because different parts of the resin acid molecules are involved in the formation of salts and the oxidation process, respectively [56]. The concentration of resin acids in the wb MWF may seem rather low. However, in most workplaces, the wb MWF dries up on the contaminated skin, and the concentration rises within minutes [26]. Furthermore, if the irritant damage to the epidermal barrier of the exposed skin is taken into account, occupational exposure to wb MWF carries a high risk of sensitization. This is illustrated by epidemiological data. In the above-mentioned FaSt study (1999–2001), metalworkers with OCD and exposure to wb MWF had an eightfold increased risk of sensitization to colophonium (odds ratio (OR) 8.0; 95%-confidence interval (CI) 1.7–73.5) when compared to metal workers with OCD who were *not* exposed to wb MWF [32].

36.5.3 Fragrances

In the same study, metalworkers exposed to wb MWF with OCD had an increased risk of sensitization to fragrances in terms of positive patch test reactions to fragrance mix and myroxylon pereirae (MPR; Balsam of Peru), when compared with metalworkers with OCD who were *not* exposed to wb MWF [32]. If the use of barrier creams or emollients was taken into account in an adjusted logistic regression analysis, the risk estimate was even higher. This strongly indicated that the exposure to wb MWF itself was the relevant risk factor. Until about 1990, fragrances or odour masks, even MPR, were mentioned as common components of wb MWF [11, 17, 59]. According to recent information from the lubricant producing industry, normally no fragrances are added to the MWF concentrate nowadays. However, it cannot be excluded that odour masks are added by the metalworking companies during the usage of the wb MWF. Corresponding products are being offered on the market. Of course, this does not imply that every fragrance allergy in exposed metalworkers is acquired by wb MWF. In every individual

case, a complete history has to be taken carefully, particularly with respect to other allergen sources (after shave, deodorant etc.). Sometimes, however, this investigation will reveal occupational causation of fragrance allergy induced by wb MWF [41].

36.5.4 Cobalt, Nickel and Dichromate

Six comprehensive studies about cobalt, nickel and dichromate in MWF have been published as yet [60–65]. In most of these studies, analyses were done by atomic absorption spectrometry (AAS), and mostly, it was not stated if the contents of metal particles (abrasion of tools or workpieces) or of metal ions were determined. The valence state of the metal ions was not investigated. The "bio-availability" was not fully undeceived; hence it cannot be excluded that in some cases, hardly soluble metal oxides or metal sulphides were described, which are not so important from the allergological point of view. Results of these studies can be summarised as follows: cobalt, nickel and chromium are not present in fresh, unused MWF (concentration <1 ppm). The presence of cobalt in used MWF mainly depends on the metals or alloys processed. If no cobalt containing hard metals were processed, the cobalt concentration was usually below 3 ppm. When processing hard metals containing cobalt, the cobalt concentration was up to 300 ppm, in single cases even up to 550 ppm. The elicitation threshold in patients allergic to cobalt is regarded to be about 100–1,000 ppm cobalt ions [66, 67]. In pre-damaged skin, reactions could even be elicited with 10 ppm cobalt [68]. Hence, if cobalt is present as dissolved ions, concentrations found in MWF which are used in hard metal processing could be sufficient to elicit an allergic reaction, possibly even to induce sensitization. In the above-mentioned studies, concentrations of nickel and chromium in used MWF usually were below 1 ppm. However, there were some exceptions with concentrations of nickel up to 130 ppm and chromium up to 280 ppm, which might be sufficient for elicitation in high-grade sensitised individuals, provided the metals are present in a suitable, ionised form. If chromium is present in the hexavalent state, an induction of contact allergy seems possible with the exceptionally high concentrations mentioned, whereas the induction of nickel allergy seems unlikely this way.

In two studies, an increased frequency of cobalt allergies among metalworkers with OCD exposed to MWF was found [8, 32], and in one study each, an increase of sensitizations to nickel [13] and dichromate [8], respectively, was described. However, the clinical relevance of these findings could not be established clearly. In a multi-factorial analysis of data from the IVDK in more than 80,000 patients, Uter et al. could not find an increased risk of sensitization to cobalt, nickel or dichromate in metalworkers [69]. Hence, in each case of contact allergy to these metals in metalworkers exposed to MWF, it is mandatory to elucidate the source of exposure and establish the clinical relevance of the positive test reaction. Occupational exposure other than MWF (e.g. work-pieces, tools, handles) or private exposure (e.g. jeans button, costume jewellery, piercing) has to be considered.

36.5.5 Formaldehyde and Formaldehyde Releasers

Several years ago, it was common to use formaldehyde solution for additional preservation of wb MWF during usage, but this seems to be obsolete today. Nowadays, usually formaldehyde releasers, mainly *O*-formals (acetals, semiacetals) and *N*-formals (aminals, semiaminals), are used for the preservation of wb MWF and in system cleansers [7, 22, 34, 70]. The amount of formaldehyde released varies, depending on various factors such as pH, temperature, microbial contamination, etc. [71]. Peak formaldehyde concentrations may result from additional preservation during the usage. An increased frequency of sensitizations to formaldehyde among metalworkers with OCD exposed to wb MWF has been known from the studies of the 1980s [11, 13]. In the FaSt study (1999–2001), it could be shown that the risk of formaldehyde allergy was significantly increased in these patients when compared to men not working in the metal industry (OR 4.1; 95%-CI 1.5–9.2) [32]. In the above-mentioned multi-factorial IVDK data analysis of 80,000 patients, the metalworkers' risk of formaldehyde allergy ranked second after health care workers, who are exposed to it by disinfectants [69]. Sensitizations to formaldehyde releasers may be directed against the whole molecule or the formaldehyde released [33, 34, 71]. In conclusion, formaldehyde as well as formaldehyde releasers has to be considered important MWF allergens [18, 33–35, 53]. There is only a limited correlation between the ability to release formaldehyde and concomitant patch test reactions to formaldehyde and the releaser [71]. Studies on this subject are hampered by the fact that patch test reactions to formaldehyde releasers are often weak and poorly reproducible [31, 71].

36.5.6 Methyldibromo Glutaronitrile (MDBGN) and 2-Phenoxyethanol (PE)

MDBGN has been used for the preservation of wb MWF some years ago. According to the information from the lubricant industry, it is currently not in use for this purpose [7]. This is confirmed by the recently published chemical analyses of MWF, where no MDBGN could be detected [22]. However, MDBGN had been widely used as a preservative in creams, cosmetics and skin care products in the last 20 years, causing contact sensitization in numerous cases [72]. Eventually, this led to the prohibition of its use in cosmetics and skin care products [73]. Hence, in metalworkers, sensitization to MDBGN diagnosed at present may be due to former MDBGN exposure in protective creams or emollients, private skin care products, or wb MWF. MDBGN had been patch tested in a fixed combination with PE because this mixture had frequently been used as a preservative. However, PE, which, in contrast to MDBGN, is still in use as a preservative in wb MWF, plays no role as a sensitizer. So, in the vast majority of the cases, MDBGN was the relevant allergen in positive test reactions to MDBGN/PE [74].

36.5.7 Methylchloroisothiazolinone/ Methylisothiazolinone (MCI/MI)

Due to its chemical properties, MCI/MI is not used as a preservative in the MWF concentrate, but it may be added to the wb MWF at the workplace as additional biocide (top up biocide) [7, 18]. Particularly in the beginning of the 1990s, MCI/MI was very frequently found as a preservative in skin care products, but in the following years, its use declined dramatically due to the "epidemic" of sensitization in these years [75]. Recently, MCI/MI has come back into this field, albeit with lower concentrations, which will probably not induce new sensitizations

[76, 77]. Hence, the particular exposure to MCI/MI has to be established in every metalworker sensitised with special regard to additional preservation of the wb MWF during its use. BIT and Octylisothiazolinone (OIT), which are also currently used for the preservation of wb MWF [22], do not cross react with MCI/MI [78]. We have no reliable information about the usage of methylisothiazolinone (MI) in MWFs, but it should be kept in mind that MI, too, is a sensitizer, albeit weaker than MCI.

36.5.8 Other Biocides

As mentioned above, various other biocides, particularly formaldehyde releasers, isothiazolinones such as BIT and OIT and IPBC are being, or have been, used as preservatives in wb MWF, and cases of sensitization have been observed. Corresponding test substances are part of the respective MWF test series (see below). In every case of a metalworker with OCD, a detailed history including additional preservation of the MWF during its use has to be taken, and in case of weak or doubtful patch test reactions to biocides, a repeated open application test (ROAT) or provocative use test (PUT) can be recommended.

36.5.9 p-Aminoazobenzene (PAAB)

PAAB is tested as a supposed marker for contact allergy to para di-substituted aromatic amines or azo dyes [79] and was a part of MWF patch test series. Until the beginning of the 1990s, it was common to dye MWF [17, 59], partly with azo dyes. Nowadays, MWF are produced without the dye, but occasionally, some metalworking companies add colours to their MWF systems. In contrast, most technical oils such as hydraulic oils or slideway oils are coloured, but azo dyes should not be used for this purpose [4]. MWF often become contaminated with these technical oils by leakage and thus, they might be a source of exposure to dyes for the metalworker. However, while concomitant reactions to PAAB and PPD are frequent and probably indicate a contact allergy to para-amino compounds [79], we know from the analysis of data concerning allergic reactions to textile dyes that PAAB is not a reliable marker for contact allergy to azo dyes [80]. An increased risk of active sensitization has been described

when PAAB and PPD are patch tested in parallel [81]. In view of these circumstances, PAAB should be deleted from the MWF test series, although it was one of the frequent allergens in a recent IVDK data analysis [53]. In cases concerned, which may, however, not be easily suspected, the actual dyes in technical oils from the patients' workplace should instead be tested.

36.6 MWF Patch Test Series

Patch test series for diagnostics in metalworkers are commercially available. However, regarding the wide variety of substances and components used in MWF [2], it seems likely that relevant contact allergies may be overlooked, because far from all potentially allergenic MWF components are available as standardised patch test preparations. Additionally, the composition of MWF changes with time, due to technological progress. Hence, for a valid allergy diagnostic in this field, it is important to continuously adapt the MWF test series to the current spectrum of occupational exposure. In 2000, the interdisciplinary working party on allergy diagnostics in the metal branch compiled two lists of MWF allergens commercially available as patch test substances [7]. The first list contains substances currently used in MWF, and the second list substances which have only been used previously, mostly before 1994 [7]. Based on this information, at the end of 2001, the DKG established two corresponding MWF series. These series are to be tested in patients with suspected ACD and exposure to MWF in addition to the standard, the ointment base and the preservative series. This design was chosen, because it usually makes sense also to test the latter two series, as skin care products are another possible allergen source in metalworkers with suspected OCD. To avoid duplicate patch tests, the DKG omitted from the MWF series those potential MWF allergens that are contained in the standard, ointment base, or preservative series. Based on the results obtained with these test series [53], current and former MWF allergens which should be tested in metalworkers with suspected MWF dermatitis are compiled in Tables 36.1 and 36.2.

However, as patch testing with these series does not cover all potentially allergenic MWF components, MWF from the patient's workplace and their components should be tested in every case concerned.

36

Table 36.1 MWF allergens to be tested in metalworkers with suspected MWF dermatitis (modified from [4, 7, 53])

Substance	Occurrence in MWF	Function in MWF	Patch test concentration
MWF series (current allergens)			
Benzylhemiformal	wb MWF	Biocide, formaldehyde releaser	1% pet.
4,4-Dimethyl-1,3-oxazolidine/ 3,4,4-trimethyl-1,3-oxazolidine (Bioban CS 1135®)	wb MWF	Biocide, formaldehyde releaser	1% pet.
7-Ethylbicyclooxazolidine (Bioban CS 1246®)	wb MWF	Biocide, formaldehyde releaser	1% pet.
Iodopropynyl butylcarbamate (IPBC)	wb MWF	Biocide	0.2% pet.
N,N'-Methylene-bis-5-methyl-oxazolidine	wb MWF	Biocide, formaldehyde releaser	1% pet.
1,2-Benzisothiazolin-3-one, sodium salt	wb MWF	Biocide	0.1% pet.
Octylisothiazolinone	wb MWF	Biocide	0.025% pet.
2-Phenoxyethanol	wb MWF	Biocide	1% pet.
Sodium-2-pyridinethiol-1-oxide (sodium omadine)	wb MWF	Biocide	0.1% aq.
1,3,5-Tris(2-hydroxyethyl)-hexahydrotriazine (Grotan BK®)	wb MWF	Biocide, formaldehyde releaser	1% pet.
Benzotriazole	wb MWF and neat oils	Rust preventive	1% pet.
Diethanolamine (DEA)[a]	wb MWF	Rust preventive	2% pet.
Monoethanolamine (MEA)	wb MWF	Rust preventive	2% pet.
p-Tert-butylphenol	Neat oils	Antioxidant	1% pet.
Abietic acid	wb MWF	Emulsifier/surfactant	10% pet.
Diglycolamine (2-(2-aminoethoxy)ethanol)	wb MWF	Emulsifier	1% pet.
German standard series			
Formaldehyde[b]	wb MWF	Top up biocide	1% aq.
(Chloro-)methylisothiazolinone (MCI/MI)	wb MWF	Top up biocide	0.01% aq.
Lanolin alcohol	wb MWF	Anti-wear additive	30% pet.
Zinc diethyldithiocarbamate (ZDEC)[c]	Neat oils	Anti-wear additive	1% pet.
Cetearyl alcohol	wb MWF	Stabiliser/anti-wear additive	20% pet.
Colophonium[d]	wb MWF	Emulsifier/surfactant	20% pet.
Mercaptobenzothiazole	wb MWF	Rust preventive	2% pet.
Ointment base series			
Propylene glycol	wb MWF	Stabiliser	5% pet.
Polyethylene glycol (tested as polyethylene glycol ointment base)	–	Stabiliser/anti-wear additive	100%

Table 36.1 (continued)

Substance	Occurrence in MWF	Function in MWF	Patch test concentration
Triethanolamine (TEA)	wb MWF	Rust preventive	2.5% pet.
Butylhydroxy toluol (BHT)	Neat oils	Antioxidant	2% pet.
Preservative series			
Triclosan	Neat oils	Biocide	2% pet.

[a]Use in MWF limited by law in Germany since 1993

[b]Released from formaldehyde releasers

[c]Tested as a marker for sodium diethyldithiocarbamate

[d]Allergic reaction indicates contact allergy to oxidation products of resin acids

Table 36.2 Former MWF allergens to be tested in metalworkers with suspected MWF dermatitis (modified from [4, 7, 53])

Substance	Occurrence in MWF	Function in MWF	Patch test concentration (% pet.)
MWF series (former allergens)			
Chlorocresol	Neat oils	Biocide	1
Chloroxylenol	wb MWF	Biocide	1
4-(2-Nitrobutyl) morpholine/4,4'-(2-ethyl-2-nitro-trimethylene) dimorpholine (Bioban P 1487®)[a]	wb MWF	Biocide, formaldehyde releaser	1
Morpholinyl mercaptobenzothiazole (MOR)	wb MWF	Rust preventive	0.5
Standard series			
Paraben mix	wb MWF	Biocide	16
Methyldibromo glutaronitrile (MDBGN)	wb MWF	Biocide	0.2
Myroxylon pereirae resin (MPR, balsam of Peru)	wb MWF	Odour mask	25
Fragrance mix[b]	wb MWF	?	8
Ointment base series			
Coconut diethanolamide[a]	wb MWF	Emulsifier	0.5
Preservative series			
Bronopol® (2-bromo-2-nitropropane-1,3-diol)[c]	wb MWF	Biocide	0.5
Chloroacetamide	wb MWF	Biocide	0.2

[a]Prohibited in MWF by law in Germany since 1993

[b]It is unclear which fragrances are used, if at all, in MWF

[c]No longer used in MWF, but in skin care products

36.7 Patch Testing with MWF from the Patient's Workplace

Patch testing with MWF from the patient's workplace is an important additional diagnostic tool in patients with suspected MWF dermatitis, which has been employed in several studies on occupational dermatitis in metalworkers [8, 11, 13, 14]. However, in these studies, as in published recommendations for patch testing with MWF, test concentrations and vehicles have varied much [3, 8, 11, 13, 14, 82, 83]. A retrospective study on MWF patch tests in 141 metalworkers showed that wb MWF can be tested at workplace concentration and neat oils at 50% in olive oil without undue risk of irritant test reactions [84]. With lower concentrations, relevant allergic reactions might be missed.

The interdisciplinary working party on allergy diagnostics in the metal branch has published recommendations on how to patch test MWF from the patient's workplace in 2002 [5]. The essential points of these recommendations, which are as yet published in German only, are: of every MWF used by the patient, two samples should be taken, i.e. one fresh, and one used sample. In the case of wb MWF, a sample of the fresh, undiluted MWF concentrate should be obtained. The used samples are to be taken from the inflows of the machines (and not from the so-called sumps) to avoid contamination with metal chips which might cause irritant patch test reactions. Samples of used wb MWF must be stored in a refrigerator, and be tested within 3–5 days because otherwise microbial contamination will change or even destroy the emulsion. Fresh concentrate of the wb MWF should be tested 5% aq., which is an average workplace concentration. Used wb MWF can be patch tested as is, provided the concentration at the workplace is ≤8%. In the case of higher workplace concentrations, further dilution to an end concentration of 4–8%, as required, is recommended. As a rule of thumb, this can be achieved by a 1:1 aqueous dilution of the wb MWF. Usually, wb MWF are alkaline (pH 8.6–9.5), but experience shows that this is tolerated by patients on patch testing. Neat oils should be tested 50% in olive oil. Used wb MWF samples must be accompanied by information about concentration and pH at the time of sampling, date of the last change of the MWF, system cleaner used, date of last preservation, name of bactericide and fungicide used, name of other additives and date of addition, material processed in the machine and possible influx of hydraulic oils, slideway oils or other oils by leakage. For neat oils, only data on the last change of the MWF, additives, material processed in the machine, and possible influx of other oils needs to be documented. Drafts of information sheets and test protocols as well as instructions for patch testing can be downloaded in German language at www.ivdk.org (section "downloads") or at www.hautstadt.de as part of a training course for patch testing with material brought in by the patient.

The interdisciplinary working party emphasises that false-negative test reactions to MWF may occur even under the recommended conditions [5]. Allergenic components in the MWF may be diluted too much and thus may not elicit any reaction on patch testing in the intact skin of the upper back although they may cause ACD on the pre-damaged skin of the hands under workplace conditions. Hence, patch testing with the single components

of the MWF should not only be performed in case of a positive patch test reaction to the MWF from the workplace, but also in clinically suspected cases, in whom no test reaction to the individual MWF could be seen (cp. [85, 86]). However, to get the maximum benefit from a breakdown test with single components of the MWF, complete information on the ingredients and additives of the MWF must be at hand. Obtaining detailed, allergologically useful information about the ingredients and additives of the MWF is a very time-consuming business. First, the patient and his or her employer have to cooperate in providing information about the workplace exposure, in particular, correct identification of the products and batches used and their manufacturers. In the material safety data sheets of the MWF, far from every component which might be responsible for the individual patient's disease is listed [22]. Usually, only those chemicals that are known sensitizers and are present above a threshold concentration, which requires labelling with the risk phrase R 43, are named. If at all mentioned, chemicals may be denoted using synonyms not known to the clinician. Some lubricant producers are very co-operative and readily supply additional information, while others are not. As time is limited in the hospital routine, these difficulties are presumably one reason why additional diagnostics are rarely performed, and why the clinical relevance of positive reactions to standardised MWF allergens often remains unclear in the individual case. The adequate concentration for the patch testing of many MWF components does not necessarily correspond to their use concentration. Thus, performing a breakdown test with the single MWF components is hampered by uncertainty concerning correct patch test concentrations (on the producer's as well as on the physician's part), and consequently that concerning the interpretation of test reactions with these preparations. Additionally, often, the producers cannot deliver chemically defined components, because reaction products may be formed in the production process of the MWF which are not completely characterised. In this connection, reaction products of boric acid and alkanolamines may serve as an example: usually, more than one alkanolamine such as MEA, diglycolamine etc. is added to the MWF base which contains boric acid, and the reaction products are not analysed. Hence, contact allergy to these reaction products – although well known from several case reports [42, 43] – is not easy to diagnose.

Against this background, the "occupational contact allergy network" (OCA Network) has been established in Germany in 2008, funded by the German Social Accident Insurance (DGUV). The centre of the OCA Network, located at the IVDK headquarters, provides support in obtaining information on and samples of single constituents of the occupational material (workplace MWF) and helps in finding adequate patch test preparations and central documentation of patch test results, thus allowing quality control of patch testing by continuous adaptation of test recommendations, and lastly, detection of new allergens.

> **Core Message**
>
> > Patch testing with MWF from the patients' workplace is a time-consuming, but very useful additional diagnostic step, which is not easy to perform correctly. Recommendations for the adequate performance are available in German at www.ivdk.org (section "downloads") or at www.hautstadt.de as part of a training course for patch testing with material brought in by the patient.

36.8 Preventive Measures

Working with wb MWF is connected with wet work, and corresponding preventive measures have to be taken. Additionally, some peculiarities should be considered. If the skin is wetted with MWF only intermittently, the MWF should not dry up on the skin but should be removed, in order to avoid a rise in concentration by vaporisation of water and the resulting increase of irritancy. Cleaning clothes used for tools or workpieces should easily be distinguishable from those for wiping off the hands. Skin contact with MWF should be minimised by automation, encapsulation of machines etc. For degreasing of workpieces, hooks, sieves or similar devices should be used for immersing, thus reducing the alternating skin irritation by MWF and solvent.

Pollution of the MWF by dirt, food etc. has to be avoided. Workplaces have to be kept clean. Concentration and pH of the MWF have to be controlled weekly in order to recognise and eliminate any increase of concentration or pH in time. Bacterial contamination itself does not affect skin irritancy of the MWF. However, there is an indirect effect because in case of a too high microbial colonisation, additional preservation is necessary due to

technical reasons. Every additional preservation has to be documented exactly (date, amount, product used). Most suitable, additional preservation is performed after the last shift on Friday, so that the biocide is almost completely dispensed at the beginning of work on Monday morning. In companies without weekend break, as few metalworkers as possible should be exposed to the maximum biocide concentration, and all workers must be informed about the additional preservation. System cleansers should not be used during operation hours as they contain high concentrations of biocides. The same precautions as with additional preservation have to be taken.

At most MWF workplaces, it is prohibited to wear protective gloves because of the risk of injury from rotating tools. If gloves are allowed, a denseness guaranty should be demanded from the glove manufacturer. A skin protection plan has to be set up. For protection against wb MWF, water-in-oil emulsion is recommended. Creams containing tannins may be helpful under gloves. Usually, mild tensides are sufficient for skin cleaning. Regular skin care after work is as important as skin protection before work.

References

1. Anon (1991) DIN 51385 Schmierstoffe; Kühlschmierstoffe; Begriffe. Beuth, Berlin
2. Anon (2000) Kühlschmierstoffe. In: Greim H (ed) Gesundheitsschädliche Arbeitsstoffe. Toxikologisch-arbeitsmedizinische Begründungen von MAK-Werten. 31. Lieferung. VCH, Weinheim
3. Foulds IS (2000) Cutting fluids. In: Kanerva L, Elsner P, Wahlberg JE, Maibach HI (eds) Handbook of occupational dermatology. Chapter 86. Springer, Berlin, pp 691–700
4. Geier J, Lessmann H, Schmidt A, Englitz H-G, Schnuch A (2003) Kontaktekzeme durch Kühlschmierstoffe in der Metallindustrie. Akt Dermatol 29:185–194
5. Tiedemann K-H, Zoellner G, Adam M, Becker D, Boveleth W, Eck E, Eckert Ch, Englitz H-G, Geier J, Koch P, Lessmann H, Müller J, Nöring R, Rocker M, Rothe A, Schmidt A, Schumacher Th, Uter W, Warfolomeow I, Wirtz C (2002) Empfehlungen für die Epikutantestung bei Verdacht auf Kontaktallergie durch Kühlschmierstoffe. 2. Hinweise zur Arbeitsstofftestung. Dermatol Beruf Umwelt 50:180–189
6. Aalto-Korte K, Suuronen K, Kuuliala O, Jolanki R (2008) Contact allergy to 2, 5-dimercapto-1, 3, 4-thiadiazole and phenyl-alpha-naphtylamine, allergens in industrial greases and lubricant oils – contact allergy to water-insoluble greases is uncommon but needs to be considered in some workers. Contact Dermatitis 58:93–96
7. Geier J, Lessmann H, Schumacher Th, Eckert Ch, Becker D, Boveleth W, Buß M, Eck E, Englitz H-G, Koch P, Müller J, Nöring R, Rocker M, Rothe A, Schmidt A, Uter W,

36

Warfolomeow I, Zoellner G (2000) Vorschlag für die Epikutantestung bei Verdacht auf Kontaktallergie durch Kühlschmierstoffe. 1. Kommerziell erhältliche Testsubstanzen Dermatol Beruf Umwelt 48:232–236

8. Alomar A, Conde-Salazar L, Romaguera C (1985) Occupational dermatoses from cutting oils. Contact Dermatitis 12:129–138

9. Berndt U, Hinnen U, Iliev D, Elsener P (2000) Hand eczema in metalworker trainees – an analysis of risk factors. Contact Dermatitis 43:327–332

10. de Boer EM, van Ketel WG, Bruynzeel DP (1989) Dermatoses in metal workers. (I). Irritant contact dermatitis. Contact Dermatitis 20:212–218

11. de Boer EM, van Ketel WG, Bruynzeel DP (1989) Dermatoses in metal workers. (II). Allergic contact dermatitis. Contact Dermatitis 20:280–286

12. Funke U, Fartasch M, Diepgen TL (2001) Incidence of work-related hand eczema during apprenticeship: first results of a prospective cohort study in the car industry. Contact Dermatitis 44:166–172

13. Grattan CEH, English JSC, Foulds IS, Rycroft RJG (1989) Cutting fluid dermatitis. Contact Dermatitis 20:372–376

14. Gruvberger B, Isaksson M, Frick M, Pontén A, Bruze M (2003) Occupational dermatoses in a metalworking plant. Contact Dermatitis 48:80–86

15. Mirabelli MC, Zock J-P, Bircher AJ, Jarvis D, Keidel D, Kromhout H, Norbäck D, Olivieri M, Plana E, Radon K, Schindler C, Schmid-Grendelmeier P, Torén K, Villani S, Kogevinas M (2009) Metalworking exposures and persistent skin symptoms in the ECRHS II and SAPALDIA 2 cohorts. Contact Dermatitis 60:256–263

16. Pryce DW, Irvine D, English JSC, Rycroft RJG (1989) Soluble oil dermatitis: a follow-up study. Contact Dermatitis 21:28–35

17. Pryce DW, White I, English JSC, Rycroft RJG (1989) Soluble oil dermatitis: a review. J Soc Occup Med 39:93–98

18. Suuronen K, Aalto-Korte K, Piipari R, Tuomi T, Jolanki R (2007) Occupational dermatitis and allergic respiratory diseases in Finnish metalworking machinists. Occup Med 57:277–283

19. Suuronen K, Jolanki R, Luukkonen R, Alanko K, Susitaival P (2007) Self-reported skin symptoms in metal workers. Contact Dermatitis 57:259–264

20. Hornstein OP (1984) Ekzemkrankheiten. Therapiewoche 34:400–409

21. Skudlik C, Schwanitz H-J (2003) Berufsbedingte Handekzeme – Ätiologie und Prävention. Allergo J 12:513–520

22. Henriks-Eckerman M-L, Suuronen K, Jolanki R (2008) Analysis of allergens in metalworking fluids. Contact Dermatitis 59:261–267

23. Scheinman PL (1996) Multiple sensitizations in a machinist using a new cooling fluid. Am J Contact Dermat 7:61

24. Shah M, Lewis FM, Gawkrodger DJ (1996) Prognosis of occupational hand dermatitis in metalworkers. Contact Dermatitis 34:27–30

25. Kütting B, Weistenhöfer W, Baumeister T, Uter W, Drexler H (2009) Current acceptance and implementation of preventive strategies for occupational hand eczema in 1355 metalworkers in Germany. British Journal of Dermatology, e-pub ahead of print, DOI 10.1111/j.1365-2133.2009.09085.x

26. Krbek F, Schäfer Th (1991) Untersuchungen an Tropfen und Rückständen von wassermischbaren Kühlschmierstoffen. Arbeitsmed Sozialmed Präventivmed 26:411–416

27. Malten KE (1981) Thoughts on irritant contact dermatitis. Contact Dermatitis 7:238–247

28. Nethercott JR, Rothman N, Holness DL, O'Toole T (1990) Health problems in metal workers exposed to a coolant oil containing Kathon 886 MW. Am J Contact Dermat 1:94–99

29. Uter W, Geier J, Ippen H (1996) Nachrichten aus dem IVDK: Aktuelle Sensibilisierungshäufigkeiten bei der DKG-Testreihe "Metallverarbeitung". Derm Beruf Umwelt 44:34–36

30. Uter W, Schaller S, Bahmer FA, Brasch J et al (1993) Contact allergy in metal workers – a one-year analysis based on data collected by the "Information Network of Dermatological Clinics" (IVDK) in Germany. Derm Beruf Umwelt 41:220–227

31. Brinkmeier T, Geier J, Lepoittevin J-P, Frosch PJ (2002) Patch test reactions to Biobans in metal workers are often weak and not reproducible. Contact Dermatitis 47:27–31

32. Geier J, Lessmann H, Schnuch A, Uter W (2004) Contact sensitizations in metalworkers with occupational dermatitis exposed to water-based metalworking fluids. Results of the research project "FaSt". Int Arch Occup Environ Health 77:543–551

33. Madan V, Beck MB (2006) Occupational allergic contact dermatitis from N, N-methylene-bis-5-methyl-oxazolidine in coolant oils. Contact Dermatitis 55:39–41

34. Aalto-Korte K, Kuuliala O, Suuronen K, Alanko K (2008) Occupational contact allergy to formaldehyde and formaldehyde releasers. Contact Dermatitis 59:280–289

35. Geier J, Lessmann H, Becker D, Bruze M, Frosch PJ, Fuchs T, Jappe U, Koch P, Pföhler C, Skudlik C (2006) Patch testing with components of water-based metalworking fluids: results of a multicentre study with a second series. Contact Dermatitis 55:322–329

36. Geier J, Lessmann H, Frosch PJ, Pirker C, Koch P, Aschoff R, Richter G, Becker D, Eckert C, Uter W, Schnuch A, Fuchs Th (2003) Patch testing with components of water-based metalworking fluids. Contact Dermatitis 49:85–90

37. Geier J, Lessmann H, Graefe A, Fuchs Th (2002) Contact allergy to diglycolamine in a water-based metalworking fluid. Contact Dermatitis 46:121

38. Crow KD, Peachey RDG, Adams JE (1978) Coolant oil dermatitis due to ethylenediamine. Contact Dermatitis 4:359–361

39. Fisher AA (1998) Ethylenediamine hydrochloride versus amines in cutting oils. Am J Contact Dermat 9:139

40. Koch P (1995) Occupational allergic contact dermatitis from oleyl alcohol and monoethanolamine in a metalworking fluid. Contact Dermatitis 33:273

41. Owen CM, August PJ, Beck MH (2000) Contact allergy to oak moss resin in a soluble oil. Contact Dermatitis 43:112

42. Bruze M, Hradil E, Eriksohn I-L, Gruvberger B, Widström L (1995) Occupational allergic contact dermatitis from alkanolamineborates in metalworking fluids. Contact Dermatitis 32:24–27

43. Jensen CD, Andersen KE (2003) Allergic contact dermatitis from a condensate of boric acid, monoethanolamine and fatty acids in a metalworking fluid. Contact Dermatitis 49:45–46

44. Kanerva L, Tupasela O, Jolanki R (2001) Occupational allergic contact dermatitis from ethylhexylzinc dithiophosphate and fatty acid polydiethanolamide in cutting fluids. Contact Dermatitis 44:193–194

45. Meding B (1996) Occupational contact dermatitis from tertiary-butylhydroquinone (TBHQ) in a cutting fluid. Contact Dermatitis 34:224

46. Piebenga WP, van der Walle HB (2003) Allergic contact dermatitis from 1-[2-(2, 4-dichlorophenyl)-2-(2-propenyloxy) ethyl]-1H-imidazole in a water-based metalworking fluid. Contact Dermatitis 48:285–286

47. Majoie IML, van Ginkel CJW (2000) The biocide iodopropynyl butylcarbamate (IPBC) as an allergen in cutting oils. Contact Dermatitis 43:238–240

48. Isaksson M (2002) Delayed diagnosis of occupational contact dermatitis from sodium pyrithione in a metalworking fluid. Contact Dermatitis 47:248–249

49. Le Coz C-J (2001) Allergic contact dermatitis from sodium pyrithione in metalworking fluid. Contact Dermatitis 45: 58–59

50. Isaksson M, Frick M, Gruvberger B, Pontén A, Bruze M (2002) Occupational allergic contact dermatitis from the extreme pressure (EP) additive, zinc, bis ((O, O'-di-2-ethylhexyl)dithiophosphate) in neat oils. Contact Dermatitis 46:248–249

51. Aalto-Korte K, Mäkelä EA, Huttunen M, Suuronen K, Jolanki R (2005) Occupational contact allergy to glyoxal. Contact Dermatitis 52:276–281

52. Lessmann H, Uter W, Schnuch A, Geier J (2009) Skin sensitizing properties of the ethanolamines mono-, di-, and triethanolamine. Data analysis of a multicentre surveillance network (IVDK) and review of the literature. Contact Dermatitis 60:243–255

53. Geier J, Lessmann H, Dickel H, Frosch PJ, Koch P, Becker D, Jappe U, Aberer W, Schnuch A, Uter W (2004) Patch test results with the metalworking fluid series of the German Contact Dermatitis Research Group (DKG). Contact Dermatitis 51:118–130

54. Anon (1993) Technische Regeln für Gefahrstoffe (TRGS) 611, Verwendungsbeschränkungen für wassermischbare bzw. wassergemischte Kühlschmierstoffe, bei deren Einsatz N-Nitrosamine auftreten können. Carl Heymanns, Cologne

55. Hausen BM, Brinkmann J, Dohn W (1998) Lexikon der Kontaktallergene, 6. Ergänzungs-Lieferung, Kolophonium, K 4. Ecomed, Landsberg, pp 1–15

56. Hausen BM, Börries M, Budianto E, Krohn K (1993) Contact allergy due to colophonium. (IX). Sensitization studies with further products isolated after oxidative degradation of resin acids and colophonium. Contact Dermatitis 29:234–240

57. Hausen BM, Krohn K, Budianto E (1990) Contact allergy due to colophonium. (VII). Sensitizing studies with oxidation products of abietic and related acids. Contact Dermatitis 23:352–358

58. Karlberg A-T (1991) Air oxidation increases the allergenic potential of tall-oil rosin. Colophonium contact allergens also identified in tal-oil rosin. Am J Contact Dermat 2:43–49

59. Ippen H (1979) Allergische Hautschäden bei der Metallbearbeitung. Derm Beruf Umwelt 27:71–74

60. Einarsson Ö, Eriksson E, Lindstedt G, Wahlberg JE (1979) Dissolution of cobalt from hard metal alloys by cutting fluids. Contact Dermatitis 5:129–132

61. Einarsson Ö, Kylin B, Lindstedt G, Wahlberg JE (1975) Chromium, cobalt and nickel in used cutting fluids. Contact Dermatitis 1:182–183

62. Lehmann E, Fröhlich N (1993) Kühlschmierstoffe – Zusätzliche Belastungen durch Metallionen? Amtliche Mitteilungen der Bundesanstalt für Arbeitsschutz, Januar, pp 1–7

63. Minkwitz R, Fröhlich N, Lehmann E (1983) Untersuchungen von Schadstoffbelastungen an Arbeitsplätzen bei der Herstellung und Verarbeitung von Metallen – Beryllium, Cobalt und deren Legierungen. Schriftenreihe der Bundesanstalt für Arbeitsschutz, Fb. 367, Dortmund

64. Pfeiffer W, Breuer D, Blome H, Deninger C et al (1996) BIA-Report 7/96 Kühlschmierstoffe. Herausgegeben vom Hauptverband der gewerblichen Berufsgenossenschaften (HVBG), Sankt Augustin

65. Wahlberg JE, Lindstedt G, Einarsson Ö (1977) Chromium, cobalt and nickel in Swedish cement, detergents, mould and cutting oils. Berufsdermatosen 25:220–228

66. Rystedt I (1979) Evaluation and relevance of isolated test reactions to cobalt. Contact Dermatitis 5:233–238

67. Wahlberg JE (1973) Thresholds of sensitivity in metal contact allergy. 1. Isolated and simultaneous allergy to chromium, cobalt, mercury and-or nickel. Berufsdermatosen 21: 22–33

68. Allenby CF, Basketter DA (1989) Minimum eliciting patch test concentrations of cobalt. Contact Dermatitis 20:185–190

69. Uter W, Gefeller O, Geier J, Lessmann H, Pfahlberg A, Schnuch A (2002) Untersuchungen zur Abhängigkeit der Sensibilisierung gegen wichtige Allergene von arbeitsbedingten sowie individuellen Faktoren. Schriftenreihe der Bundesanstalt für Arbeitsschutz und Arbeitsmedizin, Forschung, Fb 949. Wissenschaftsverlag NW, Bremerhaven

70. Thamm H (1997) Formaldehyd und Formaldehydabspalter in Kühlschmierstoffen: Aktueller Stand. Allergologie 20: 232–238

71. Geier J, Lessmann H, Schnuch A, Fuchs Th (1997) Kontaktallergien durch formaldehydabspaltende Biozide. Eine Analyse der Daten des IVDK aus den Jahren 1992 bis 1995. Allergologie 20:215–224

72. Wilkinson JD, Shaw S, Andersen KE, Brandao FM et al (2002) Monitoring levels of preservative sensitivity in Europe. A 10-year overview (1991-2000). Contact Dermatitis 46:207–210

73. Commission Directive 2007/17/EC of 22 March 2007. http://eur-lex.europa.eu/LexUriServ/LexUriServ.do?uri=OJ:L:20 07:082:0027:0030:EN:PDF. Accessed May 2009

74. Geier J, Schnuch A, Brasch J, Gefeller O (2000) Patch testing with Methyldibromoglutaronitrile. Am J Contact Dermat 11:207–212

75. Mowad CM (2000) Methylchloroisothiazolinone revisited. Am J Contact Dermat 11:114–118

76. Fewings J, Menné T (1999) An update of the risk assessment for methylchloroisothiazolinone/methylisothiazolinone (MCI/MI) with focus on rinse-off products. Contact Dermatitis 41:1–11

77. Robinson MK, Gerberick GF, Ryan CA, McNamee P, White IR, Basketter DA (2000) The importance of exposure estimation in the assessment of skin sensitization risk. Contact Dermatitis 42:251–259

78. Geier J, Schnuch A (1996) No cross sensitization between MCI/MI, benzisothiazolinone, and octylisothiazolinone. Contact Dermatitis 34:148–149

79. Uter W, Lessmann H, Geier J, Becker D, Fuchs Th, Richter G (2002) The spectrum of allergic (cross-)sensitivity in clinical

36

patch testing with 'para amino' compounds. Allergy 7: 319–322

80. Bauer A, Geier J, Lessmann H, Elsner P (2004) Kontaktallergien gegen Textilfarbstoffe. Ergebnisse des Informationsverbundes Dermatologischer Kliniken (IVDK). Aktuelle Dermatol 30:23–27

81. Arnold WP, van Joost T, van der Valk PGM (1995) Adding *p*-aminoazobenzene may increase the sensitivity of the European standard series in detecting contact allergy to dyes, but carries the risk of active sensitization. Contact Dermatitis 33:444

82. Frosch PJ, Pilz B, Peiler D, Dreier B, Rabenhorst S (1997) Die Epikutantestung mit patienteneigenen Produkten. In: Plewig G, Przybilla B (eds) Fortschritte der praktischen Dermatologie und Venerologie 15. Springer, Berlin, pp 166–181

83. Jolanki R, Estlander T, Alanko K, Kanerva L (2000) Patch testing with a patient's own materials handled at work. In: Kanerva L, Elsner P, Wahlberg JE, Maibach HI (eds) Handbook of occupational dermatology. Chapter 47. Springer, Berlin, pp 375–383

84. Geier J, Uter W, Lessmann H, Frosch PJ (2004) Patch testing with metalworking fluids from the patient's workplace. Contact Dermatitis 51:172–179

85. Malten KE (1987) Old and new, mainly occupational dermatological problems in the production and processing of plastics. In: Maibach HI (ed) Occupational and industrial dermatology, 2nd edn. Yearbook Medical, Chicago, p 310

86. Rycroft RJG (1987) Cutting fluids, oil, and lubricants. In: Maibach HI (ed) Occupational and industrial dermatology, 2nd edn. Yearbook Medical, Chicago, p 289

Plastic Materials

37

Bert Björkner, Malin Frick-Engfeldt, Ann Pontén, and Erik Zimerson

Contents

Plastics generally consist of large molecules called polymers as well as additives that are used to modify the properties of the material. Polymers are formed by the stepwise reaction between monomers by which larger molecules are formed. In this polymerization process, primarily dimers, trimers, and higher molecular weight (MW) molecules (i.e., oligomers) are formed until finally the polymer is completed. If only one type of monomer is involved in forming the polymer, it is called a homopolymer, e.g., polyethylene. If two or more different monomers are used, it is called a copolymer, e.g., propylene ethylene copolymer. This type of polymerization is usually controlled by the addition of a small amount of catalyst or initiator. Another terminology is used for the production of, for example, epoxy and polyurethane plastics. These are two-component systems in which mixing of the two components, generally in equal amounts (same number of functional groups), starts the polymerization. In some of these resins, the two components are already mixed but so unreactive that heat is required to bring

B. Björkner, M. Frick-Engfeldt, A. Pontén (✉)
and E. Zimerson
Department of Occupational and Environmental
Dermatology, Ing 73 pl 5, Skane University Hospital,
205 02 Malmö, Sweden
e-mail: ann.ponten@skane.se

J.D. Johansen et al. (eds.), *Contact Dermatitis*,
DOI: 10.1007/978-3-642-03827-3_37, © Springer-Verlag Berlin Heidelberg 2011

37

about polymerization. One of the components is called the hardener (curing agent), and the other is called the resin. The hardener and/or the resin may consist of relatively pure substances, but may also constitute a mixture of low-, medium-, and high MW molecules, i.e., a mixture of monomers, dimers, and oligomers. In the formation of plastics, several auxiliary compounds are added to modify the final product. Examples of groups or classes of additives are plasticizers, fillers, antioxidants, UV-stabilizers, antiozonants, antistatic agents, biostabilizers, heat stabilizers, blowing agents, flame retardants, dyes, fragrances, etc.

Polymers and plastics can be classified as thermoplastic or thermosetting. Thermoplastics are linear polymers that soften or melt upon heating and can thus be reshaped. Thermosetting polymers, on the other hand, are rigid cross-linked networks that gain their final form when cured (Fig. 37.1).

The final plastic products, when completely cured or hardened, are generally considered to be inert and non-hazardous to the skin. However, the chemicals that take part in the production of the plastic are often reactive, which implies that they might also be contact allergens. Sensitizers in plastic systems might be the monomers or oligomers of the resin, hardeners, modifiers, or additives.

In the following chapters, plastics of different types are described with respect to their applications, chemistry, skin exposure, contact allergy, irritancy, patch testing, and prevention.

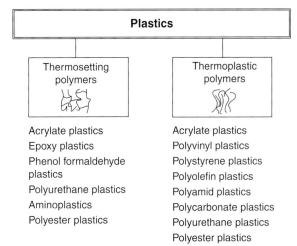

Fig. 37.1 Polymers and plastics can be classified as thermoplastic or thermosetting. Many of the plastics described in this chapter can, depending on the number of functional groups in the monomers, serve as both thermoplastic and thermosetting

37.1 Acrylic Plastics

The term acrylates can have different meanings, which sometimes is confusing. Acrylates can mean esters of acrylic acid exclusively, but sometimes, its use includes esters of acrylic acid and methacrylic acid as well as some other derivatives of these acids. To avoid confusion, we use the term acrylates in the narrower meaning, esters of acrylic acid. The terms acrylic plastics and acrylate plastics are usually used for plastics based on polymers both of acrylates and methcrylates as well as of copolymers of these. It can also include plastics made from other acrylate derivatives, e.g., acrylic fibers for textiles made from the monomer acrylonitrile

37.1.1 Applications

Acrylic plastics are used in an extremely wide range of applications (Table 37.1). As for most other plastics, it is when skin contact with the uncured plastic material that the risk of sensitization is greatest. Common applications of acrylic plastics in which contact with the uncured plastic material is encountered are printing inks, coatings, paints, varnishes, and adhesives, and furthermore, within dentistry and when doing artificial nails. Hearing aids, noise protectors, and bone cement in orthopedic surgery are other common applications. Acrylic plastics can be part of composite materials.

37.1.2 Chemistry

The acrylates belong to a group of chemicals often referred to as α,β-unsaturated carbonyl compounds (Fig. 37.2). The carbon in the carbonyl group is electron-deficient and can act electron-withdrawing on the double bond, but the carbonyl group can also act electron-releasing. In both cases, the double bond becomes activated, and as a result, the acrylates react readily with electrophils, nucleophils, and free radicals.

Methacrylates differ from the corresponding acrylates by having an extra methyl group bound in the α-position of the double bond. The extra methyl group donates electrons to the double bond in the methacrylate group, making the activation of it less pronounced. The methyl group also constitutes steric hindrance and

Table 37.1 Examples of acrylates and methacrylates used in different applications

Application	Substances
Bone cement, two component (also dentures, hearing aids, noise protectors)	*Part A* Prepolymer of methyl methacrylate Benzoyl peroxide (initiator) *Part B* Methyl metacrylate N,N-dimethyl-p-toluidine (accelerator)
Spectacle frames	Butyl acrylate
Pressure-sensitive adhesives	2-Ethylhexyl acrylate
UV-curable inks and coatings	2-Hydroxyethyl acrylate
	2-Hydroxypropyl acrylate
	2-Hydroxypropyl methacrylate
	2-Hydroxyethyl methacrylate
	2-Ethylhexyl acrylate
	Di-, tri- or tetra- acrylates and methacrylates
	1,6-Hexanediol diacrylate
	Pentaerythritol triacrylate
	Trimethylolpropane triacrylate
Water-based acrylic latex paints	Various monoacrylates and monomethacrylates
Artificial nail preparations	Metacrylic acid
	Monoacrylates
	Monomethacrylates
	Dimethacrylates
	Tripropylene glycol acrylate
Dental materials	1,6-Hexanediol diacrylate
	1,3-Butyleneglycol diacrylate
	Glycerol phosphate dimethacrylate
	Most of the methacrylates in Table 37.2
Anaerobic sealants	Diethylene glycol dimethacrylate
	Urethane dimethacrylate
	Dimethacrylates
Synthetic fibers	Acrylonitrile
Synthetic rubber	
Plastics (ABS-plastics)	
Electroforesis gel	Acrylamide
Grouting agents	Bis-acrylamide
	Methylol-acrylamide

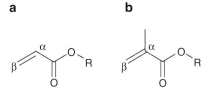

Fig. 37.2 Schematic structure of (**a**) acrylates and (**b**) methacrylates

both these factors contribute to a lower reactivity of the methacrylates as compared to the corresponding acrylates. The different reactivities of acrylates and methacrylates are reflected in their sensitizing capacities.

Acrylic acid and methyl, ethyl, butyl, and 2-ethylhexyl acrylate are examples of important monofunctional acrylates. There are many available acrylates, but there is probably a larger number of methacrylates available, among which the simplest one, methyl metacrylate, is still most important. Special functional groups can be introduced into the monomers to provide adhesion, cross-linking capability, or changed solubility. Some acrylates and metacrylates are difunctional or tri-functional, and some can have even more functional groups. Acrylates and metacrylates that have three or more acrylate or methacrylate groups in the molecule are often referred to as polyfunctional. To prevent spontaneous polymerization of the acrylic and methacrylic monomers, an inhibitor is added. This is often monomethyl ether of hydroquinone (10–15 ppm for esters and 100–200 ppm for the acids), hydroquinone, or alkylphenols. Some monomers that are closely related to the mentioned acrylic monomers are acrylonitrile, cyanoacrylates, and acrylamides. Examples of common acrylates and methacrylates are shown in Tables 37.2 and 37.3, respectively.

The acrylates and methacrylates with low MW have relatively high vapor pressure, which means that they easily evaporate and can reach high air concentrations at normal temperatures. Generally, most acrylates and methacrylates are fat soluble compounds. However, acrylic acid and metacrylic acid 2-hydroxyethyl methacrylate are some examples of acrylic compounds that are water soluble.

Acrylate or methacrylate groups can be introduced into epoxy, urethane, polyether, and polyester compounds giving acrylic or methacrylic prepolymers called acrylated epoxy resins, acrylated polyurethanes, acrylated polyethers, and acrylated polyesters.

The majority of polymers are produced by the addition of free-radical initiators such as peroxides, hydroperoxides,

37

Table 37.2 Examples of acrylates

Substance (acrylates)	Abbreviation	CAS
Alkyl-acrylates		
Methyl acrylate		96-33-3
Ethyl acrylate		140-88-5
Propyl acrylate		925-60-0
Isopropyl acrylate		689-12-3
Butyl acrylate		141-32-2
Isobutyl acrylate		106-62-8
2-Ethylhexyl acrylate	2-EHA	103-11-7
Acrylic acid esters of ethylene glycol and other glycols		
2-Hydroxyethyl acrylate	2-HEA	818-61-1
2-Hydroxypropyl acrylate	2-HPA	999-61-1
Ethylene glycol monoacrylate	EGA	818-61-1
Ethylene glycol diacrylate	EGDA	2274-11-5
Diethylene glycol diacrylate	DEGDA	4074-88-8
Triethylene glycol diacrylate	TREGDA	109-16-0
Propylene glycol diacrylate	PGDA	999-61-1
1,3-Propanediol diacrylate		25151-33-1
1,4-Butanediol diacrylate		31442-13-4
1,6-Hexanediol diacrylate	HDDA	
Multifunctional acrylates		
Pentaerythritol triacrylate	PETA	3524-68-3
Trimethylolpropane triacrylate	TMPTA	15625-89-5

The most common abbreviations are included in the table

Table 37.3 Examples of methacrylates

Substance (methacrylates)	Abbreviation	CAS
Alkyl-methacrylates		
Methyl methacrylate	MMA	80-62-6
Ethyl methacrylate	EMA	97-63-2
Propyl methacrylate		2210-28-8
Isopropyl methacrylate		4655-43-9
n-Butyl methacrylate		97-88-1
2-Ethylhexyl methacrylate		688-84-6
n-Octyl methacrylate		2157-01-9
Hydroxyalkyl methacrylates		
2-Hydroxyethyl methacrylate	2-HEMA	868-77-9
2-Hydroxypropyl methacrylate	2-HPMA	923-26-2
3-Hydroxypropyl methacrylate		2761-09-3
2,3-Dihydroxypropyl methacrylate		5919-74-4
Metacrylic acid esters of glycols		
Ethylene glycol dimethacrylate	EGDMA	97-90-5
1,2-Propanediol dimethacrylate		7559-82-2
1,4-Butanediol dimethacrylate	BUDMA	2082-81-7
Diethylene glycol dimethacrylate	DEGDMA	2358-84-1
Triethylene glycol dimethacrylate	TREGDMA	109-16-0
Tetraethylene glycol dimethacrylate	TEGDMA	109-17-1
1,6-Hexanediol dimethacrylate		6606-59-3
Multifunctional methacrylates		
Trimethylolpropane trimethacrylate	TMPTMA	3290-92-4
Pentaerythritol tetramethacrylate		3253-41-6
Metacrylic acid esters of resins and prepolymers		
2,2-Bis[4-(2-hydroxy-3-methacryloxypropoxy) phenyl]propane	BIS-GMA Bis-GMA	1565-94-2
2,2-Bis[4-(methacryloxy) phenyl]-propane	BIS-MA	
2,2-Bis[4-(2-methacryloxyethoxy) phenyl]-propane	BIS-EMA	24448-20-2
2,2-Bis[4-(3-methacryloxypropoxy) phenyl]-propane	BIS-PMA	

The most common abbreviations are included in the table

and azo compounds (e.g., 2,2'-azobisisobutyronitrile), but photochemical and radiation-initiated polymerization is also used. Initiators, accelerators, and catalysts can be added to speed up the process. The free radicals start a chain reaction between the double bonds of the monomers, which then become connected in a long carbon-chain backbone. Some monomers or formulated products with monomers polymerize in contact with water (moist surfaces), while contact with metal in the absense of air (oxygen) brings about polymerization of others.

Acrylic acid, methacrylic acid, simple alkyl-acrylates, and alkyl-methacrylates are often used in commercial polymers. Polymers from methacrylates are relatively stable, hard, and stiff compared to polymers from acrylates. Methacrylates can be copolymerized with other methacrylates or with acrylates, and this gives a great variety of polymers with applications from extremely tacky adhesives over flexible but hard materials to hard sheets. When the polymer is made from a monofunctional monomer, the result will be a thermoplastic polymer. When difunctional monomers are present in the polymerization process, more branched polymer chains will form, and if the presence of difunctional and/or polyfunctional monomers is high enough, a thermosetting acrylic polymer is formed. In the polymerization process, the monomers are consumed, but there is always a small but varying amount of unreacted monomer left in the polymer.

Acrylic plastics can contain plasticizer, antistatic agents, dyes, etc. There is, however, very little information on additives to acrylic polymers, which might indicate that not very much additives are used in acrylic plastics.

37.1.3 Skin Exposure

As for other plastics, it is the skin contact with the uncured monomers and prepolymers that most often cause sensitization. A case of a chemical burn from dipropylene glycol diacrylate (DPGDA) spilt on working shoes followed by active sensitization has been described [1]. Airborne exposure may occur when the contact allergen in question has a relatively high vapor pressure, and therefore, volatile, e.g., methyl methacrylate. In a furniture factory, nine out of nine workers with dermatitis and exposed to an aerosol of acrylate monomers developed contact allergy to pentaerythritoltriacrylate (PETA-3) [2]. Airborne exposure may also occur when dust is produced, e.g., when grinding plastic material that is not completely cured (Fig. 37.3). Examples of applications where uncured acrylic plastics are encountered are mentioned above, under applications (Table 37.1).

37.1.4 Skin Hazards

37.1.4.1 Contact Allergy

There are many reports of contact allergy to monoacrylates and monomethacrylates in humans. Contact dermatitis due to 2-HPMA in printers exposed to printing plates, as well as to UV-curing inks, has been reported [3, 4] (Fig. 37.4). Contact allergy to 2-HEMA, one of the ingredients in a photoprepolymer mixture,

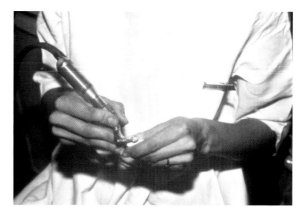

Fig. 37.3 When grinding prosthesis, uncured acrylates can cause dermatitis in sensitized dental personal

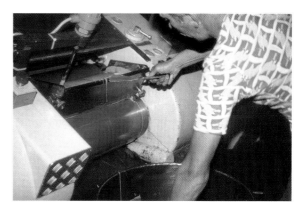

Fig. 37.4 UV-curable acrylic inks mixed with color pigments. Protected gloves are highly recommended

has been described [5]. Orthopedic surgeons, surgical technicians, nurses, and dental technicians are exposed to methyl methacrylate monomer while preparing bone cement and dentures. 2-HEMA is a water-soluble methacrylate and is, therefore, commonly used as a dentine-bonding compound. 2-HEMA is a common allergen in dental personnel. Fingertip dermatitis has been common in dentists and dental nurses allergic to dentine-bonding acrylates [6–10], but seems to have diminished with the awareness of the risk of sensitization and as the manufacturers have changed the design of the application utensils.

In recent decades, many reports of contact allergy caused by various di and triacrylates and the corresponding methacrylates have been published [10–16]. At risk of developing contact allergy to di and triacrylates are those working with UV-curable inks or coatings, while contact allergy to dimethacrylates is more commonly

37

seen in dentistry, in those working with anaerobic acrylic sealants and those exposed to the application of acrylic nails [6–11, 14, 15, 17–24]. Epoxy acrylates are strong sensitizers in animal studies [11], but allergic contact dermatitis caused by epoxy dimethacrylates seems to be rare in workers exposed to ultraviolet-cured inks [25, 26] There are some reports of allergic contact dermatitis from dimethacrylates based on bisphenol A in dental composite materials. At risk of developing contact dermatitis are dentists and dental technicians, as well as dental patients [6–10, 15, 18, 21, 24]. Methacrylates have also caused asthma and rhinoconjunctivitis in dental personnel [19, 22, 23]. Patients allergic to BIS-GMA may also react to diglycidyl ether of bisphenol A (DGEBA) [18, 27, 28]. It is uncertain whether any residual epoxy resin monomer is left unreacted [27, 29], or whether there is cross-reactivity between these relatively similar compounds. In a retrospective survey, contact allergies to bis-GMA, bis-GA, GMA, and bis-EMA were usually found in patients with simultaneous contact allergy to DGEBA and with a history of exposure to epoxy resin [30]. Methyl methacrylate and 2-HEMA can cause paresthesia of the fingertips for months after discontinuation of contact with the monomer [31–33]. The prevalence of acrylate/methacrylate allergy among two populations of dermatitis patients patch tested with the baseline series has been found to be 1 and 1.4%, respectively [34].

There are a few reports of contact allergy to the acrylonitrile monomer [35, 36]. Polyacrylamide products are generally considered nonhazardous. The monomer can be irritating and cause contact allergy. Skin problems are seen among printers exposed to photopolymerizing printing plates. Acrylamide and their acrylamide compounds N, N-methylene-bis-acrylamide, N-methylol acrylamide, and N-[2-(diethylamino) ethyl] acrylamide have been described as allergens [37, 38]. Allergic contact dermatitis from piperazine diacrylamide, used as a reagent and a cross-linker for acrylamide gels in electrophoreses and column chromatography, has been described by Wang et al. [39]. Contact sensitization to cyanoacrylates has been considered extremely rare, due to the immediate bonding of the cyanoacrylate to the surface keratin [40]. The adhesive was, therefore, believed to have never come into contact with immunocompetent cells deeper in the epidermis. For instance, Parker and Turk [41] were unable to sensitize guinea pigs with methyl or butyl 2-cyanoacrylate. However, in the last decade,

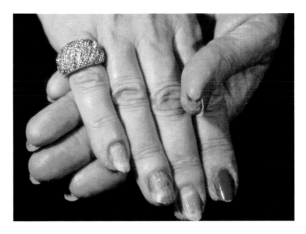

Fig. 37.5 Onychodystrophy in a patient allergic to give for artificial nails based on cyanoacrylate

some case reports have been published that strongly indicate that cyanoacrylates are able to induce contact allergy [42–55] (Fig. 37.5).

37.1.4.2 Animal Studies

The sensitizing potential and cross-reactivity of many acrylates, methacrylates, and acrylated prepolymers in guinea pigs have been thoroughly studied by numerous authors [11, 27, 41, 56–62]. Tests have shown that monoacrylates are strong sensitizers, while monomethacrylates have weak to moderate sensitizing potential [11, 41, 59, 62]. Of the multifunctional acrylates, the di and triacrylic compounds should be regarded as potent sensitizers [11, 27, 56]. The multifunctional methacrylates are weak sensitizers [11, 27]. Cross-reactions of multifunctional methacrylates and acrylates have been reviewed by Kanerva [63]. In a local lymph node assay (LLNA) methyl acrylate, ethyl acrylate, butyl acrylate, and 2-ethylhexyl acrylate were found to be relatively weak sensitizers [64]. Although there are few reports on contact allergy in humans, acrylonitrile has shown strong allergenic potential in the guinea pig maximization test (GPMT) [35]. Acrylamide, N-hydroxymethyl acrylamide, and N, N-methylene-bis-acrylamide are moderate sensitizers when tested in guinea pigs [61].

Evaluation of the irritant potential of various acrylic monomers has shown that the diacrylates are strong irritants, monoacrylates weak to moderate irritants, and monomethacrylates and dimethacrylates nonirritant or weak irritants to guinea-pig skin [11, 27, 41, 56–59, 61,

62]. Di and multifunctional acrylates as well as acrylated prepolymers seem to be more irritating than the corresponding methacrylates. These effects have been seen while patch testing both humans and guinea pigs [11].

37.1.4.3 Irritancy

Bullous irritant skin reactions in workers exposed to tetramethylene glycol diacrylate have been reported [65]. The irritant effect of various acrylate compounds has been reviewed by Kanerva et al. [66, 67]. Vaporized cyanoacrylates are known to irritate the eyes and respiratory tract. Irritation and discomfort of the face and eyes may occur in workers due to associated low humidity [40, 68].

37.1.5 Prevention

Gloves are recommended to protect the hands against the various acrylic compounds. Methyl methacrylate, as well as other acrylic monomers, such as butylacrylate and acrylamide, easily penetrates natural rubber latex gloves, and vinyl gloves are even worse in this respect [61, 69–75]. Polyethylene gloves give the best protection against methyl methacrylate diffusion [61]. Nitrile gloves give better protection than neoprene gloves against UV-curable acrylate resins [75]. New multilayer glove material of the folio type, with ethylene-vinyl-alcohol copolymer laminated with polyethylene on both sides, has especially good chemical resistance [76]. The protective effect of gloves against acrylates in dentine-bonding systems was tested on acrylate-sensitized patients and showed clear differences in the protective efficacy between types of gloves [69, 70]. Because acrylics used in dentine-bonding systems are strong sensitizers and quickly penetrate most gloves, dentists and dental personnel should use no-touch techniques [10, 76].

As most of the acrylic compounds used in UV-curable acrylic resins are regarded as irritants and relatively potent sensitizers, care should be taken accordingly to minimize their contact with the skin.

Measures that seem effective in preventing the occurrence of dermatitis include the use of impermeable protective gloves and protective clothing. Face shields and goggles are recommended whenever there is a risk of splattering. The contaminated skin should be washed with soap and water and contaminated clothing should be removed promptly. It is essential to separate clean from contaminated clothing. Thorough education of employees regarding skin hazards is also recommended.

> **Core Message**
>
> › Because acrylics used in dentine-bonding systems are strong sensitizers and quickly penetrate most gloves, dentists and dental personnel should use no-touch techniques and adequate gloves.

37.1.6 Patch Testing

In general, a patch test concentration of 2% in petrolatum is recommended for methacrylates and 0.1% in petrolatum for acrylates to avoid patch test sensitization [77]. A marked decrease in the number of positive test responses, including to cyanoacrylates, has been noticed when acetone and alcohol, instead of petrolatum, have been used as the test vehicle for various acrylic compounds [43] The petrolatum vehicle probably prevents the acrylic monomers from polymerizing. A rapid polymerization of acrylic monomers was also seen when an aluminum test chamber was used instead of a plastic test chamber. Aluminum oxide probably enhances the polymerization process [43]. When acrylic compounds are patch tested, it is recommended to use petrolatum as the test vehicle in a plastic test chamber. Patch test substances suitable for screening for acrylate/methacrylate contact allergy have been investigated [78–80].

> **Core Message**
>
> › When acrylic compounds are patch tested, it is recommended to use petrolatum as test vehicle in a plastic test chamber.

37.2 Epoxy Plastics

The term epoxy plastics will be used for the cured plastic material and epoxy resin system (ERS) for the uncured plastic material.

37.2.1 Applications

Epoxy plastics are used in a wide range of applications in which strong, flexible, and light-weight construction materials are required. They are also used when chemical, thermal, and mechanical resistance or electrically insulating capacity is needed. Products in which epoxy plastics are used are adhesives, paints, powder paints, insulating materials for electric, and electronic devices. Glass fibers and carbon fibers can be impregnated with epoxy plastics on location, but may also be preimpregnated (prepreg) and sold in rolls or sheets and used in the aircraft industry, in the manufacture of electronic circuit boards, and in the construction of wind turbine rotor blades, among many other applications [81–84]. Epoxy plastics can be used in cement and stone work. The insides of food-cans can be coated with epoxy plastics.

37.2.2 Chemistry

The term epoxy resin system(s) (ERS(s)) is used for uncured epoxy plastics and is a combination of epoxy resins, curing agents, modifiers, and additives. Epoxy resins and curing agents (hardeners) are the two mandatory components of ERSs. The term "epoxy resin" will be used for uncured epoxy resins containing epoxy groups (see below). When epoxy resins are used in two-component products, the hardeners are added to the resins immediately preceding the application, and the subsequent polymerization occurs at either ambient or at elevated temperatures. One-component products contain latent curing agents that are inactive at normal storage temperatures, but initiate polymerization when heated. Modifiers and additives are diluents, fillers, resinous modifiers, plasticizers, and pigments. The majority of the epoxy plastics are thermosetting.

37.2.2.1 Epoxy Resins

Epoxy (or ethoxylin) resins contain at least two epoxy groups, also called oxirane or epoxide groups, in their molecules. The epoxy group is formed when two carbon atoms and one oxygen atom bind chemically to form a ring. The commercially most important epoxy resins are produced by polymerization of reacting compounds with at least two hydroxy groups and epichlorohydrin [85, 86]. The majority of epoxy resins are based on DGEBA, formed by combining epichlorohydrin and bisphenol A [synonyms: 4,4'-(1-methylethylidene)bisphenol; 4,4'-isopropylidene-diphenol; 2,2'-bis(4-hydroxyphenyl)propane] [85, 86]. When the proportions of epichlorohydrin and bisphenol A are varied during the manufacturing process, epoxy resins with varying average MW are formed. The general chemical structure of DGEBA resin is shown in (Fig. 37.7). The repeating part of the resin molecule has MW 284. When $n=0$ (Fig. 37.7), an epoxy resin containing only the monomer DGEBA with MW 340 is obtained. Low-MW epoxy resins are semisolid or liquid and have an average MW of less than 900, and a large amount of the monomer DGEBA. Resins with an average MW of more than 900 are solids, but may contain more than 15% DGEBA [87, 88]. Commercial epoxy resins are, thus, mixtures of oligomers of different MWs, 340 ($n=0$), 624 ($n=1$), 908 ($n=2$), 1.192 ($n=3$), etc. When needed, diglycidyl ether of tetra-bromo-bisphenol A (4Br-DGEBA) can be used for production of a flame retardant polymer. In composite materials difficulties are encountered with adherence to carbon fibers with DGEBA resins. Epoxy resins based on other epoxy compounds than DGEBA have been developed; among them are tetraglycidyl-4,4'-methylene dianiline (TGMDA), triglycidyl p-aminophenol (TGPAP), and o-diglycidyl phthalate [84]. Instead of bisphenol A, bisphenol F or phenolic novolak resins can be used for the manufacture of epoxy resins. The monomers of these resins are the three isomers of diglycidyl ether of bisphenol F (DGEBF). The DGEBF resins can be mixed with DGEBA resins and have improved chemical and physical resistance. Further examples of polyhydroxy compounds that can be used for the production of epoxy resins are resorcinol, glycerol, ethylene glycol, pentaerythritol, and trimethylolpropane. Aliphatic epoxy resins are constituents of paints. Cycloaliphatic epoxy resin can occur in neat oils and jet aviation hydraulic fluid [89, 90]. Triglycidyl isocyanate (TGIC) and terephthalic acid diglycidylester are epoxy compounds that may be present in polyester powder paints (see Sect. 37.5.2) [91–93].

Fregert and Trulsson have described methods used for detecting the presence of epoxy resins of the bisphenol A type [94, 95]. The thin-layer chromatography method described for DGEBA has 150–200 times lower sensitivity for DGEBF [88].

Core Message

› ERSs contain epoxy resins and hardeners and may contain modifiers and additives.

37.2.2.2 Curing Agents

A large group of curing agents comprises derivatives of ethylenediamine. Generally, aromatic amines, such as 4,4'-diaminodiphenylmethane, require higher curing temperatures than aliphatic amines, such as the ethylene-diamine derivatives, which cure the epoxy resin at room temperature. Among cycloaliphatic amines, isophorone-diamine is the most widely used [96]. The hardeners used in cold-curing are mostly polyamines, polyamides, or isocyanates, and those used for thermal curing are car-boxylic acids and anhydrides or aldehyde condensation products, e.g., phenol-formaldehyde resins, melamine-formaldehyde resins, and urea-formaldehyde resins. Ideally, all epoxy groups of the epoxy resin have reacted when it is cured. Accelerators, e.g., tertiary amines, can be added to speed up the polymerization of epoxy resins. An example is 2,4,6-tris-(dimethylaminomethyl)phenol [96, 97]. Hexavalent chromate may be present in accelerators of ERS [97]. Examples of hardeners for composite epoxy resins are methyl nadic anhydride, *N,N*-dimethylbenzylamine, 4,4-diaminodiphenyl sulfone (DDS), and dicyandiamide (DICY) [96]. A list of hard-eners and catalysts is given in Table 37.4.

37.2.2.3 Reactive Diluents

Reactive diluents are used to modify epoxy resins, princi-pally by reducing their viscosity. They are epoxy com-pounds and thus contain one or more epoxide groups that react with the hardener at approximately the same rate as the resin. Most of the reactive diluents on the market are used in the cold-curing process. They are blended in with commercial epoxy resin at a concentration of 10–30% [98, 99]. The epoxy-reactive diluents are generally glyci-dyl ethers, but sometimes glycidyl esters of aliphatic or aromatic structure. Aliphatic reactive diluents include compounds as 1,4-butanediol diglycidyl ether, *n*-butyl glycidyl ether (BGE), allyl glycidyl ether, or other alkyl glycidyl ethers with longer carbon chains (C_8–C_{14}), e.g., epoxide 7 and epoxide 8. Examples of aromatic reactive diluents are phenyl glycidyl ether (PGE) and cresyl gly-cidyl ether (CGE) [98, 99].

Core Message

> Epoxy resin systems are important occupational contact allergens.

Table 37.4 Commonly used hardeners and catalysts (compiled using [96, 97])

Aliphatic amines and derivatives
Ethylenediamine (EDA)
Diethylenetriamine (DETA)
Triethylenetetramine (TETA)
Tetraethylenepentamine (TEPA)
Dipropylenetriamine (DPTA)
Diethylaminopropylamine (DEAPA)
3-Dimethylaminopropylamine (DMAPA)
Trimethylhexamethylenediamine (TMDA)
Cycloaliphatic polyamines
Isophoronediamine (IPDA)
N-Aminoethylpiperazine
3,3'- Dimethyl-4,4'-diaminodicyclohexylmethane
Menthanediamine
4,4'-Diaminodicyclohexyl methane
Aromatic amines
N,N-dimethylbenzylamine
4,4'-Diaminodiphenylmethane (DDM)=4,4'-Methylene dianiline (MDA)
m-Phenylenediamine (MPDA)
4,4'-Diaminodiphenylsulphone (DDS)=bis (4-aminophenylsulphone); (Dapsone)
3,3'-Diaminodiphenyl sulfone
2,4,6-Tris-(dimethylaminomethyl)phenol
m-Xylylenediamine
Polyaminoamides
Condensation products of ethyleneamines and carboxylic acids.
Adducts
Based on the reaction between aliphatic or aromatic amines and epoxy resin, epoxy-reactive diluents, ethylene oxide etc.
Acid anhydrides
Phthalic anhydride (PA)
Maleic anhydride (MA)
Hexahydrophthalic anhydride (HHPA)
Methyl nadic anhydride
Tetrahydrophthalic anhydride (THPA)
Methyltetrahydrophthalic anhydride (MTHPA)
Methylhexahydrophthalic anhydride (MHHPA)
Trimellitic anhydride (TMA)
Miscellaneous
Cyanoguanidine (DICY)
Di and polyisocyanates
Polymercaptans
Polyphenols
Phenolic novolacs
Cresol novolacs
Urea-formaldehyde resins
Melamine-formaldehyde resins
1,3,5-Triglycidyl isocyanurate[a]
Terephthalic acid diglycidylester[a]
Trimellitic acid triglycidylester[a]

[a]Epoxy compounds in polyester resin systems

37.2.3 Skin Exposure

In several occupations, such as within the construction industry, there is a high risk of direct contamination of the skin. When the resin and hardener are mixed, the skin might be contaminated by the epoxy resin, which can be both sticky and transparent and does not irritate the skin and therefore might go unnoticed. Airborne exposure to the skin can be due to both the relatively high vapor pressure of some components of the ERS and the grinding dust containing uncured epoxy resin. It has been experimentally shown that elevated curing temperature was more effective in reducing the DGEBA concentration than simply waiting until the next day [100].

37.2.4 Skin Hazards

37.2.4.1 Contact Allergy

ERSs have been found to be one of the most frequent causes of occupational allergic contact dermatitis [98, 101–104]. In a study performed in an epoxy-based construction industry, it was found that 16.4% of the workers had acquired occupational contact allergy to ERSs within 1 year of employment [105]. Most cases were sensitized to DGEBA resin. Among hardeners, *m*-xylylene diamine has been reported to be most common contact allergen.[102].

Epoxy Resins

It was initially suspected that the hardeners were responsible for the majority of cases with dermatitis due to ERS, but in 1977, Fregert and Thorgeirsson [106, 107] showed that the main sensitizer was the DGEBA monomer with a MW of 340. In the GPMT, the oligomer with a MW of 624 was also a sensitizer, but was considerably weaker than the monomer DGEBA. The sensitizing capacity of epoxy resin decreases as the average MW increases [106, 107]. In many cases, allergic epoxy dermatitis develops after accidental contact with epoxy resin, and frequent causative agents for epoxy dermatitis are paints and the raw material for paint [103, 108]. High MW epoxy resin in solvents for painting or epoxy resin powder for electrostatic coating of metals is thought to rarely cause sensitization because of the low content of

MW 340 oligomer. However, chemical analyses have shown that a solid epoxy resin, which was not declared as a sensitizer, contained 18% DGEBA [88]. An epidemic of occupational contact allergy was caused by DGEBA resin in an immersion oil for microscopy [109]. It is not unusual to find a positive patch test reaction to DGEBA resin where the cause of the sensitization is unknown. Dermatitis caused by ERSs is localized mostly to the hands and forearms, but the face and genital area may also be involved. When the face and eyelids are involved, the dermatitis may be caused by airborne exposure [110]. When DGEBA resins are cured by polyamine hardeners at room temperature, the amounts of unreacted DGEBA or polyamine decrease rapidly within 1 or 2 days, but, thereafter, the decrease is slow. Nevertheless, after 1-week's cure, 0.02–12% of free DGEBA and 0.01–1% of free diethylenetriamine (DETA) were found when six different epoxy resin products were experimentally cured by DETA [98]. Allergic contact dermatitis may, thus, be elicited in previously sensitized individuals. Traces of nonhardened epoxy resin have been found in twist-off caps, film cassettes, furniture, metal pieces, signboards, textile labels, stoma pouches, polyvinylchloride plastic, nasal cannulas, hemodialysis sets, cardiac pacemakers, fiberglass, brass door knobs, tool handles, and in bowling ball and golf clup repair [94, 111–113].

Non-DGEBA epoxy resins are also potential causes of allergic contact dermatitis. The monomers of epoxy resins of the DGEBF type are strong sensitizers and cross-react to a high degree with DGEBA in animal studies [114], and many patients simultaneously react to both DGEBA and DGEBF resins [102, 115, 116]. Epoxy resins based on *o*-diglycidyl phthalate, tetraglycidyl-4,4-methylenedianiline (TGMDA), TGPAP, and 4Br-DGEBA are used in composite materals and all are sensitizers in humans [82, 84]. Testing with DGEBA resin may not reveal contact allergy to these. Bisphenol A has been identified as a contact allergen in vinyl gloves [117, 118]. Photosensitivity has been reported in relation to the heating of DGEBA resin [119] and the use of epoxy powder paints [120]. The photosensitivity has been suspected to be due to bisphenol A contained in the resin [119]. Persistent light reactivity has been found in mice photosensitized by bisphenol A [121].

Reactive diluents contain epoxy groups and are strong sensitizers that may or may not cross-react with epoxy resins [122, 123]. Several cases with contact allergy to reactive diluents have been described [124, 125]. Reactive diluents may cause airborne allergic contact dermatitis and also depigmentation [124, 126]. Contact allergy to PGE may occur with or without simultaneous contact allergy to epoxy resin. Results from a GPMT have shown that PGE is a strong sensitizer. With respect to cross-reactivity, induction with DGEBA resulted in a statistically significant number of animals reacting to PGE, but when induced with PGE, the animals did not react significantly to DGEBA. The results imply that the exposure primarily either to PGE or DGEBA might be of importance for the pattern of contact allergy to these allergens [122]. A rather high risk of sensitization to epichlorohydrin has been reported for workers in plants manufacturing epoxy resin [127–129].

Occupational contact allergies can occur to epoxy compounds in products other than ERSs, such as cycloaliphatic epoxy resin in neat oil and jet aviation hydraulic fluid and 2,3-epoxypropyl trimethyl ammonium chloride (EPTMAC) used in a starch modification factory [89, 90, 130]. Contact allergy to epoxy compounds in polyester paints has been reported [91–93].

A statistically significant association between contact allergy to DGEBA resin and fragrance mix has been found [131]. This association has been confirmed and shown to be traced to contact allergy to α-cinnamal and isoeugenol [132].

Polyamine hardeners can be both sensitizers and irritants (Table 37.4) [67, 97, 125]. In patients with allergic contact dermatitis, isolated contact allergy to the hardeners of the ERSs may occur [97]. In an industrial investigation among workers exposed to epoxy resins systems, 30% of the workers had contact allergy exclusively to at least one hardener [105]. The aliphatic polyamines, cycloaliphatic polyamines, 2,4,6-tris-(dimethylaminomethyl)phenol, and *m*-xylylenediamine are all sensitizers (Table 37.4) [83, 97, 123, 133–137]. Hardeners of the polyaminoamide type are nonsensitizers, but may contain aliphatic amines. Amine-epoxy adducts can contain free amines, but no free DGEBA [87, 98]. Contact allergy to methylhexahydrophthalic anhydride present in ERSs has been described [138].

Contact urticaria can be caused by DGEBA resin, the hardeners methylhexahydrophthalic anhydride and methyltetrahydrophthalic anhydride, as well as by aliphatic polyamine hardeners [103, 139–142].

37.2.4.2 Irritancy

In workers handling fiberglass or carbon fibers, irritant dermatitis can be induced by fiber fragments [81, 143]. DGEBA is considered nonirritant, but other epoxy resin monomers as well as reactive diluents might be irritants. Amine hardeners are alkaline and might cause irritant dermatitis.

37.2.5 Patch Testing

Approximately 60–80% of the cases with contact allergy to ERSs are sensitized to DGEBA resin [131, 144]. A patch test with the low-molecular-weight epoxy resin containing a high amount of oligomer MW 340 is, thus, adequate in the majority of cases. It is recommended to patch test with the epoxy resin 1% in petrolatum and this allergen is included in most standard series. When the tests are read only once and not after 1 week, approximately 15% of contact allergies might be missed. For other types of epoxy resins, a patch test concentration of 0.25–1% is recommended [84, 116, 145]. There are too many hardeners and reactive diluents on the market to be used in routine testing. However, if contact allergy to hardeners or reactive diluents is suspected, it is necessary to obtain information and samples from the manufacturer and to test the components of the ERSs separately. The recommended test concentration for hardeners and reactive diluents is 0.1–1% in petrolatum, acetone, or ethanol [97, 98]. Studies have shown that 17–43% of cases with occupational contact allergy to ERSs were diagnosed only by specialized patch test series developed for the investigated work place [105, 146]. These results show the importance of patch testing with the patients' own work materials in an adequate concentrations.

> **Core Message**
>
> › Epoxy resin in the standard patch test series does not detect all contact allergies to ERSs.

37.2.6 Prevention

Studies have shown that 50–100% of workers sensitized to ERSs acquired their contact allergy within their first year of employment, making early preventive measures very important [105, 135].

Workers handling ERSs should be informed of the risk of skin sensitization. The simultaneous use of irritant chemicals, e.g., organic solvents and amine hardeners, increases the risk of sensitization. The highly alkaline amine hardeners can be replaced by

37

Fig. 37.6 (**a–c**) Contamination at epoxy industry

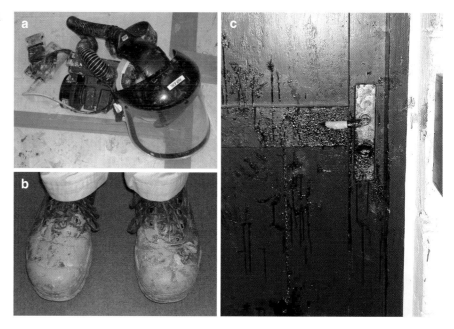

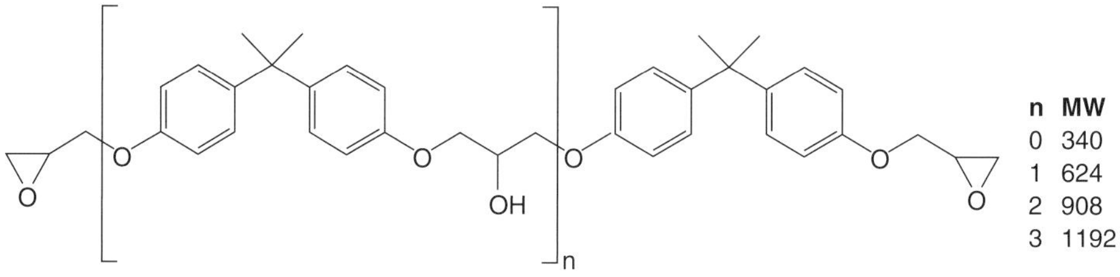

Fig. 37.7 Diglycidylether of bisphenol A (DGEBA) epoxy resin

n	MW
0	340
1	624
2	908
3	1192

polyaminoamides or amine-epoxy adducts; this reduces the irritability of the ERSs. Management personnel as well as the workers who come into contact with ERSs should be advised to refrain from skin contact. Approximately 95% of exposed workers report wearing the gloves as recommended; still, the frequency of occupational contact allergy is high [105]. A study among Taiwanese tunnel workers indicates that the recommendation to wash the hands immediately after contamination of the skin is an important preventive measure [147]. The use of proper personal protective measures, especially careful hand protection and regular cleaning and maintenance of all contaminated equipment, should be imperative (Fig. 37.6a–c). Epoxy resins are able to penetrate plastic and rubber gloves. Only heavy-duty vinyl gloves provide sufficient protection [148]. Multilayered glove material of folio type (4H gloves) has been shown to give even better protection against epoxy resins and the auxiliary compounds used with them [149].

Barrier creams have been reported to protect against epoxy resins from minutes to some hours [76, 150, 151]. To reduce the allergenic properties of DGEBA resins, the use of the MW 340 oligomer at the lowest possible concentration and the use of high MW reactive diluents is recommended. However, all epoxy resins should be regarded as potential sensitizers, and preferably, they should be marked with labels specifying the concentrations of epoxy compounds with low MW.

37.3 Phenol-Formaldehyde Plastics

Phenol-formaldehyde resins were used to make one of the first syntetic plastic materials, phenol-formaldehyde plastics or bakelite. Since then, the field of phenol-formaldehyde resins has developed and includes resins and plastics made from different phenols and aldehydes with varying applications.

37.3.1 Applications

Phenol-formaldehyde and *p-tert*-butylphenol-formaldehyde resins have many industrial applications, although other polymers/plastics have replaced the use of these resins in many fields. Glues and glue films based on phenol-formaldehyde resins are used in the plywood industry. Because of their moisture resistance, the glues and laminates are used in the building industry and in boat and aircraft construction. The resins are also good insulators against electricity; they are thus used in electronic and electric appliances. In addition, they can be used for the production of decorative laminates and coatings, and to coat rigid constructions, e.g., pipelines and reaction vessels, because of their high chemical resistance. They are also used as binders for glass and mineral fibers in the production of heat-, noise-, and fire-insulating materials, as well as in foundry molding sand and abrasives, such as sandpaper, abrasive cloth, and flexible sanding disks. Novolak resins can be used in the production of grinding wheels, brake linings, and clutch facings. They are also used as raw materials for polyfunctional epoxy resins [152–154].

p-tert-Butylphenol-formaldehyde resin is used in adhesives based on neoprene and other rubbers. These adhesives can be used in shoes, leather products, automobile interior upholstery, furniture, adhesive tapes and labels, and in the gluing of certain floor coverings [152, 153]. *p-tert*-Butylphenol-formaldehyde resin is also used as adhesives for leather, artificial fingernails, and labels.

The third largest group is phenolic resins modified by natural resins. Rosin-modified phenolic resins are used as binders for book offset-printing inks [152].

37.3.2 Chemistry

Phenol-formaldehyde resins (phenolic resins) are reaction products of phenols and aldehydes, in particular, phenol and formaldehyde. They are divided into resols and novolaks. When phenol reacts with an excess of formaldehyde under alkaline conditions, a resol resin is produced. When formaldehyde reacts with a phenol, a methylol group (hydroxymethyl group) is formed on the phenol molecule, resulting in the creation of a methylol phenol. This methylol phenol can become reactive and react with other phenol or methylol phenol molecules. As formaldehyde is in excess in the process, various methylolphenol compounds

are formed, such as monomers, dimers, and molecules of higher MW. The base-catalyzed polymerization of the products is stopped deliberately before complete curing. During processing, the polymerization can be restarted by heating to achieve complete curing of the resin. The resols can be considered as prepolymers [153].

Novolak resins are formed when formaldehyde reacts with an excess of phenols under acidic conditions. Mainly, dimers such as dihydroxydiphenylmethanes (bisphenol F isomers) are formed, but also molecules of higher MW. However, the formed molecules in this case have no or few methylol groups. The novolaks can only be cured by the addition of curing agents, such as formaldehyde, paraformaldehyde, or hexamethylenetetramine, in addition to heating. The cured polymer for both novolaks and resols constitutes the phenol-formaldehyde plastic, which also can be called resite or C-stage resin [152, 153]. *p-tert*-Butylphenol-formaldehyde resin is mainly used as the resol prepolymer due to its sticky quality which makes it functions as a binder in different chemico-technical products.

Commercially available phenol-formaldehyde resins are most commonly based on phenol itself, but other phenols such as cresols, xylenols, resorcinol (1,3-dihydroxybenzene), bisphenol A (4,4'-isopropylidenediphenol), *p-tert*-butylphenol, 4-isooctylphenol, and 4-nonylphenol can be used. Besides formaldehyde, other aldehydes, e.g., acetaldehyde, glyoxal, and furfural (2-furancarboxaldehyde), can also be used [152, 153]. Phenolic resins are available as solids (fragments, flakes, pastilles, or granules), or as solutions and liquids [153].

37.3.3 Skin Hazards

The adverse effects in workers handling phenol-formaldehyde resins are mostly skin problems. Contact dermatitis is common and is usually caused by the development of contact allergy. Most of the reported cases of contact dermatitis are due to sensitization to *p-tert*-butylphenol-formaldehyde resin. Reviews on *p-tert*-butylphenol-formaldehyde resin-induced occupational eczema have been published [152, 155–157]. In general, population allergy frequencies of 0.5–2.1% are reported from different European countries [158–160].

Many of the substances found in *p-tert*-butylphenol-formaldehyde resin are allergens. However, patch testing with dilution series of components from the resin in sensitized patients and sensitization studies in animals have shown that the methylol-substituted dimers, 4-*tert*-butyl-2-(5-*tert*-butyl-2-hydroxy-3-hydroxymethyl-benzyloxymethyl)-6-hydroxymethyl-phenol (Fig. 37.8a), and 4-*tert*-butyl-2-(5-*tert*-butyl-2-hydroxy-3-benzyloxymethyl)-6-hydroxymethyl-phenol (Fig. 37.8b) are major sensitizers in this type of resin [161, 162]. Among the monomers, 2,6-dimethylol-*p*-*tert*-butylphenol (Fig. 37.8c) and 5-*tert*-butyl-2-hydroxy-3-hydroxymethyl-benzaldehyde (Fig. 37.8d) are considered to be the most important allergens [163–166]. The strong sensitizer *p*-*tert*-butylcatechol (Fig. 37.8e) has been shown to be present in *p*-*tert*-butylphenol-

formaldehyde resin and to be of relevance considering allergic reactions to this resin. *p*-*tert*-Butylcatechol is also an antioxidant used as a stabilizer for a number of other monomers used in the production of plastics. The raw materials for the production of *p*-*tert*-butylphenol-formaldehyde resin are formaldehyde and *p*-*tert*-butylphenol (Fig. 37.8f, PTBP). Few patients allergic to *p*-*tert*-butylphenol-formaldehyde resin are reported to react positively to the raw materials, indicating that these substances are not important allergens in the resin [165, 167]. However, guinea pigs sensitized to *p*-*tert*-butylcatechol showed cross-reactions when tested with PTBP [168].

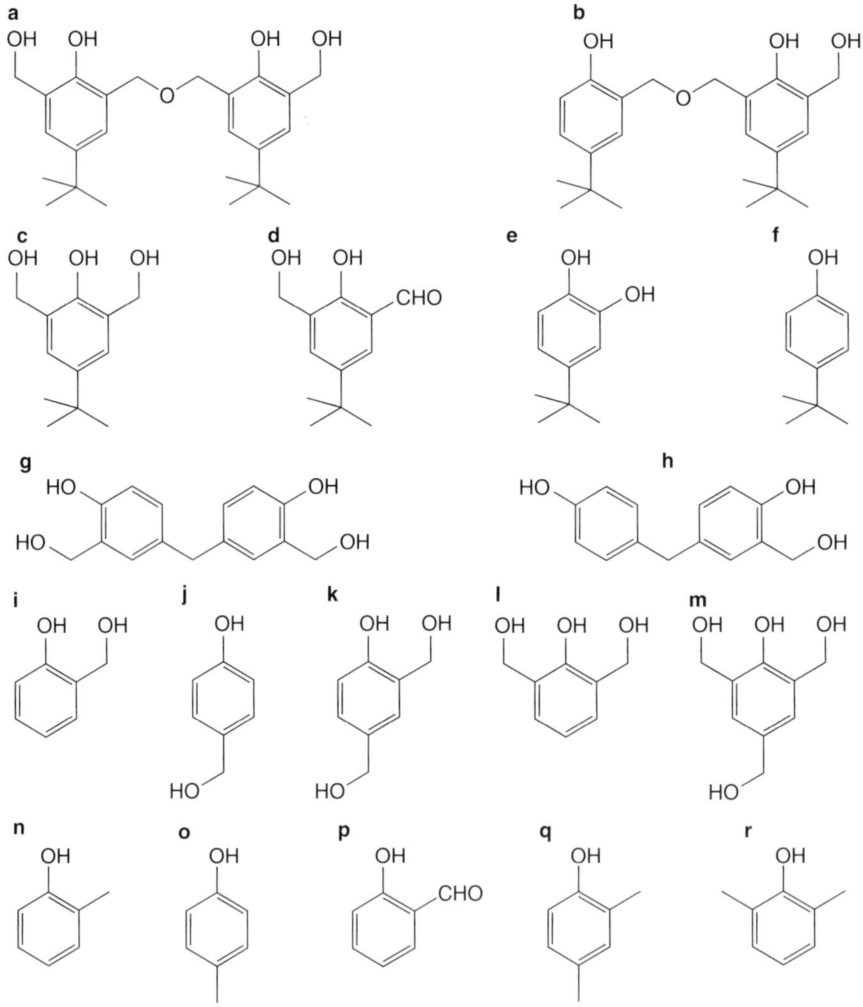

Fig. 37.8 Chemical structures of allergens in *p*-*tert*-butylphenol-formaldehyde resin (**a–f**), phenol-formaldehyde resin (**g–n**), and substances that are cross-reactors in patients allergic to phenol-formaldehyde resin (**o–r**). (**a**) 4-*tert*-butyl-2-(5-*tert*-butyl-2-hydroxy-3-hydroxymethyl-benzyloxymethyl)-6-hydroxymethyl-phenol; (**b**) 4-*tert*-butyl-2-(5-*tert*-butyl-2-hydroxy-3-benzyloxymethyl)-6-hydroxymethyl-phenol; (**c**) 2,6-dimethylol-*p*-*tert*-butylphenol; (**d**) 5-*tert*-butyl-2-hydroxy-3-hydroxymethyl-benzaldehyde; (**e**) *p*-*tert*-butylcatechol; (**f**) *p*-*tert*-butylphenol; (**g**) 4,4'-dihydroxy-3,3'-dihydroxymethyl-diphenylmethane; (**h**) 4,4'-dihydroxy-3-hydroxymethyl-diphenylmethane; (**i**) 2-methylolphenol; (**j**) 4-methylolphenol; (**k**) 2,4-dimethylolphenol; (**l**) 2,6-dimethylolphenol; (**m**) 2,4,6-trimethylolphenol; (**n**) *o*-cresol; (**o**) *p*-cresol; (**p**) salicylaldehyde; (**q**) 2,4-dimethylphenol; (**r**) 2,6-dimethylphenol

The allergens in resins based on phenol and formaldehyde have also been investigated, and several substances among the monomers and the dimers have been shown to be allergens. Methylol-substituted dimers were found to be major allergens in these resins, such as 4,4-dihydroxy-3,3-dihydroxymethyl-diphenylmethane (Fig. 37.8g) and 4,4-dihydroxy-3-hydroxymethyl-diphenylmethane (Fig. 37.8h). Examples of allergens among the monomers are 2-methylolphenol (Fig. 37.8i), 4-methylolphenol (Fig. 37.8j), 2,4-dimethylolphenol (Fig. 37.8k), 2,6-dimethylolphenol (Fig. 37.8l), 2,4,6-trimethylolphenol (Fig. 37.8m), and o-cresol (Fig. 37.8n). The monomers were, however, weaker allergens than the dimers [152, 169–176]. A patch test study in patients with contact allergy to phenol-formaldehyde resin indicates that p-cresol (Fig. 37.8o), salicylaldehyde (Fig. 37.8p), 2,4-dimethylphenol (Fig. 37.8q), and 2,6-dimethylphenol (Fig. 37.8r) are cross-reacting substances, possibly after metabolic conversion into the corresponding methylolphenols in the skin. The observed cross-reactions can indicate a connection between allergy to phenol-formaldehyde resin and tar as the methylphenols (Fig. 37.8n–r) can be found in tar [177]. Formaldehyde is not the main sensitizer in phenol-formaldehyde resins [167]. Simultaneous reactions to phenol-formaldehyde resins, colophony/hydroxyabietyl alcohol, and balsam of Peru/fragrance mix may occur [178].

Phenol-formaldehyde resins may also irritate the skin and cause chemical burns and depigmentation. Phenols and aldehydes are primary skin irritants and concentrated phenol may even cause corrosive chemical burns. Besides being a sensitizer, formaldehyde is also a skin irritant.

Irritant contact dermatitis has been reported in the manufacture of an electric insulation material (Bakelite), which is phenol-formaldehyde resin made of incompletely condensed resin powder in molds [179]. Irritant contact dermatitis was also common among workers in the manufacture of decorative laminates made of paper sheets impregnated with phenol-formaldehyde resins [167, 180].

Immediate contact reactions to p-tert-butylphenol-formaldehyde resin have also been reported [181, 182].

> **Core Message**
>
> › The raw materials (formaldehyde and phenol) are not the main sensitizers in phenol-formaldehyde resins.

37.3.4 Patch Testing

In addition to p-tert-butylphenol-formaldehyde resin, it is also necessary to patch test with the actual resin to which the worker is exposed, as there is no single reliable test substance to detect allergy to the wide variety of phenolic resin types. Bruze found 2.5 times more patients with contact allergy to phenol-formaldehyde resins when routinely patch testing with a resin based on phenol and formaldehyde (P-F-R-2), in addition to p-tert-butylphenol-formaldehyde resin [183].

While detecting contact allergy to p-tert-butylphenol-formaldehyde resin in patients for whom no clinically relevant contact with the resin can be found, the possibility of p-tert-butylcatechol as the eliciting factor should be considered, and patch testing with this substance should be performed when indicated. However, due to observed active sensitization when using a patch test concentration of 1% p-tert-butylcatechol in pet., Estlander et al. recommend a lower concentration of 0.25% pet. [184].

> **Core Message**
>
> › There is no single reliable test preparation to detect allergy to phenolic resins and patch testing with the patients own phenol-formaldehyde resin should be considered in the investigation.

> **Core Message**
>
> › Phenol-formaldehyde resin allergy could indicate sensitivity to tar and simultaneous reactions to colophony/hydroxyabietyl alcohol, balsam of Peru, and fragrance mix may occur.

> **Core Message**
>
> › When no clinically relevant contact with p-tert-butylphenol-formaldehyde resin can be found, p-tert-butylcatechol should be considered as the eliciting factor and patch tested.

37.4 Isocyanates and Polyurethane Plastics

37.4.1 Applications

Isocyanates, compounds containing the functional group –NCO, are used mainly as raw material in the production of polyurethane plastics such as paints, glues, castings, surface coatings, adhesives, and soft and rigid foam. Flexible polyurethane foams are used for mattresses, cushions, dashboards, and packages [185].

37.4.2 Chemistry

Isocyanates can be classified based on the number of –NCO groups in the molecule (i.e., monoisocyanates contain one –NCO, diisocyanate contains two –NCO, and polyisocyanates contain multiple –NCO groups). The chemical structures of the most common diisocyanate monomers and their technical grade counterparts are shown in Fig. 37.9. Di and polyisocyanates are widely used in the plastics industry since they form polyurethane upon addition reaction with multifunctional alcohols (polyols). Generally, the polyols are polyesters or polyethers with terminal hydroxyl groups, or castor oil or tall oil with secondary hydroxyl groups [185], but other compounds containing active hydrogen atoms such as water and amines can also serve as polyols. Isocyanates can also be classified as either aromatic (containing one or more aromatic rings) or aliphatic. The aromatic isocyanates dominate the market. The most commonly used aromatic diisocyanate is diphenylmethane diisocyanate (MDI) followed by toluene diisocyanate (TDI). They are frequently used in the production of rigid and flexible foam, but also in coatings, adhesives, binders, and elastomers. Aliphatic isocyanates such as isophorone diisocyanate (IPDI) and hexamethylene diisocyanate (HDI) are generally more expensive to produce, but they are used when the performance of aromatic isocyanates is inadequate, mainly because of their tendency to undergo oxidative discoloration upon exposure to light and moisture [186]. Due to their light and weather resistance, the aliphatic isocyanates are commonly used in lacquers, coatings, and paints. The production of both aromatic and aliphatic diisocyanates is mainly based on synthesizing the corresponding molecular structure with primary amine groups. The amino groups are then transformed into isocyanate groups by treatment with phosgene [187].

Most isocyanate systems used in the manufacturing of polyurethane plastics are supplied as reactive liquids or powder coatings, which after blending with polyols form thermosetting polyurethane plastics. However, there are also thermoplastic polyurethanes, which are supplied as fully-reacted products in the form of granulate and pellets that can be reshaped by conventional thermoplastic processing techniques into the required final form. The thermoplastic properties are obtained by incorporating soft segments formed by the reaction of diisocyanate and substantially linear long-chain diols with hard segments formed by the reaction of diisocyanate and short-chain diols [188]. The majority of thermoplastic polyurethanes are based on MDI, but all the other diisocyanates mentioned above are also utilized for specialist niche products [188].

In industry, technical grade isocyanate products are mainly used. They often consist of a mixture of isomers of monomers (i.e., diisocyanates) and oligomers (i.e., higher MW molecules with more than two –NCO groups), and they are often referred to as polyisocyanates of the diisocyanate monomer. TDI is industrially available as mixtures of the 2,4- and 2,6-TDI isomers at ratios of 80:20 or 65:35 (2,4:2,6) or as pure 2,4-TDI (Fig. 37.9). Commercial MDI products generally contain a complex mixture of 25–80% monomeric 4,4'-MDI as well as oligomers containing predominately three to six aromatic rings, but also smaller amounts of oligomers containing a higher number of rings (Fig. 37.9). They also contain low amounts of the monomeric isomers 2,2'-MDI and 2,4'-MDI [189]. These MDI mixtures are usually referred to as polymeric MDI (PMDI), but the synonyms crude MDI and polymethylene polyphenyl isocyanate (PAPI or PMPPI) are sometimes also used. Technical products of HDI and IPDI are often produced by reacting the monomeric isocyanates either with themselves (di- or trimerization) to form uretdiones, biurets, and isocyanurates, or with urea or urethane compounds to form higher MW polyisocyanates [187] (Fig. 37.9). The monomer content in the technical products of IPDI and HDI is generally low [190].

Several auxiliary substances are also used in the manufacturer of PU products. The hardening process can be modified by heat or with a catalyst, usually tertiary amines and/or organometallics (primarily tin compounds) [191]. Other additives, e.g., fire retardants, fillers, coloring

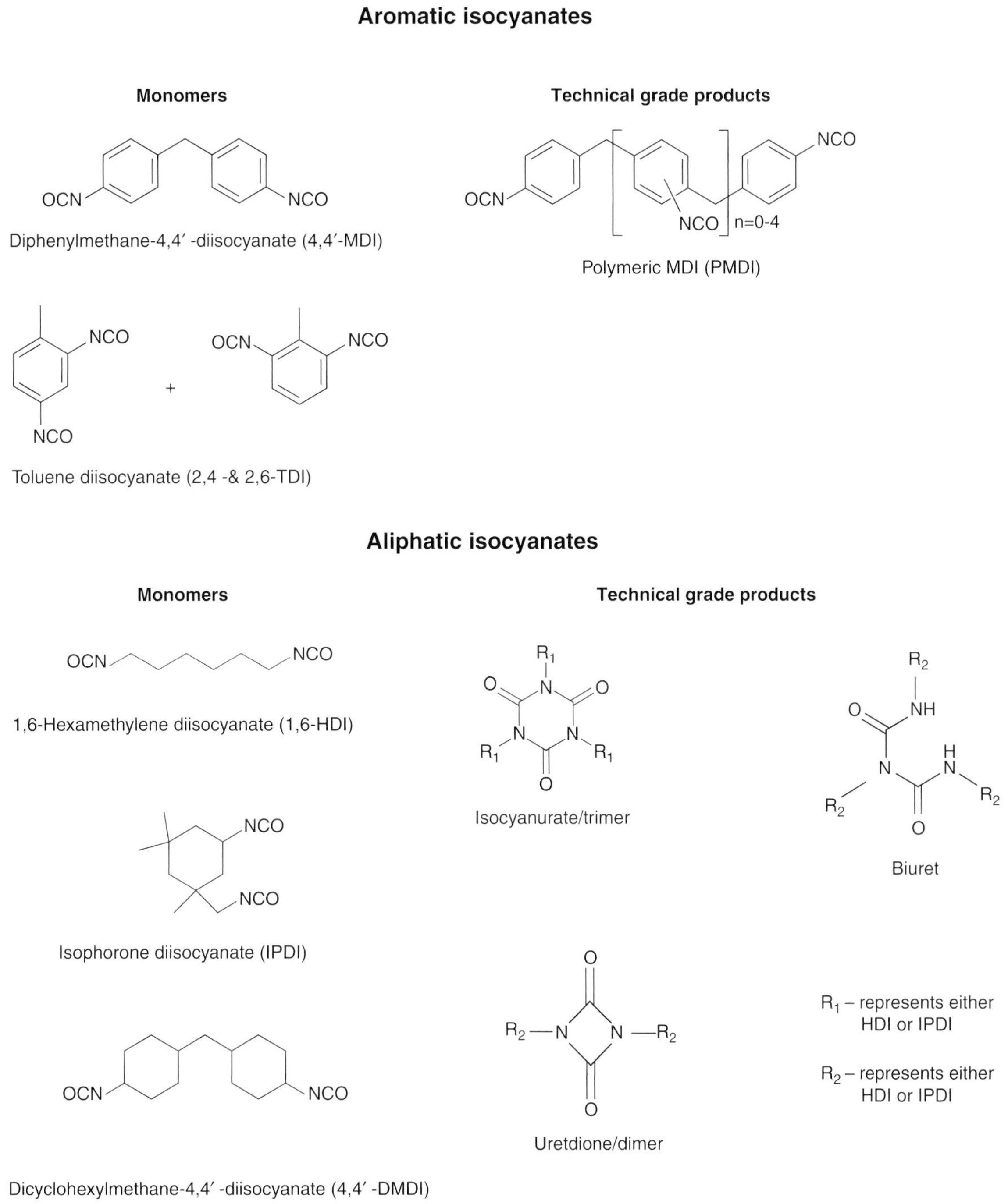
Aromatic isocyanates
Monomers
OCN
NCO
Diphenylmethane-4,4′ -diisocyanate (4,4′-MDI)
Technical grade products
OCN
NCO
NCO
n=0-4
Polymeric MDI (PMDI)
NCO
NCO
OCN
NCO
+
Toluene diisocyanate (2,4 -& 2,6-TDI)
Aliphatic isocyanates
Monomers
OCN
NCO
1,6-Hexamethylene diisocyanate (1,6-HDI)
NCO
NCO
Isophorone diisocyanate (IPDI)
OCN
NCO
Dicyclohexylmethane-4,4′ -diisocyanate (4,4′ -DMDI)
Technical grade products
R1
O
N
O
R1
N
N
R1
O
Isocyanurate/trimer
R2
O
NH
H
N
N
R2
R2
O
Biuret
O
R2—N
N —R2
O
Uretdione/dimer
R1 – represents either HDI or IPDI
R2 – represents either HDI or IPDI

Fig. 37.9 Chemical formulae of various isocyanates used in the production of polyurethane plastics

agents and cross-linking agents, can be added to modify the polyurethane reaction as well as the properties of the final product. In the production of foamed plastics, blowing agents, e.g., pentane, carbon dioxide, or water, are also added [192]. When used as activators or hardeners, diisocyanates are often dissolved in aliphatic or aromatic hydrocarbon solvents or a mixture of different organic solvents, e.g., aliphatic hydrocarbon solvents, petroleum, and butyl acetate. Adhesives, varnishes, and paints may also contain solvents.

> **Core Message**
>
> › Polyurethane plastics are formed by reacting a
>   di or polyfunctional isocyanate with a polyol in
>   the presence of suitable catalysts and additives.

37.4.3 Skin Exposure

Exposure to isocyanates is mainly an occupational problem that occurs in work places where isocyanates or PUR are manufactured and processed. However, there have recently been reports describing isocyanate exposure in domestic settings [193, 194]. Occupational exposure has been considered to occur mainly through inhalation, which has led to strict regulations regarding occupational exposure limits for airborne isocyanates in order to avoid adverse health effects on the respiratory tract. Monomeric diisocyanates with high vapor pressures, such as TDI, IPDI, and HDI, cause airborne exposure already at room temperature. MDI and most prepolymers, on the other hand, have low vapor pressures and are only volatile at elevated temperatures. Isocyanate exposure has also been reported in spraying applications, in which exposure to isocyanates with low vapor pressures becomes significant even at room temperature [195]. Completely hardened polyurethane products usually do not cause skin problems. Unreacted isocyanate monomer may, however, remain in excess inside polyurethane foams even after curing. This can create a health hazard due to isocyanate exposure when polyurethane dust is produced during machining or cutting [9, 196]. Additionally, processing of PUR materials at temperatures above 150°C causes thermal degradation, which leads to dissociation of the PUR into a complex mixture of isocyanates, amines, and aminoisocyanates [197].

Recently, concerns have been raised about the role of skin exposure from isocyanates in the development of occupational asthma [198], and animal studies have shown that animals sensitized by dermal contact alone exhibit respiratory response upon inhalation of isocyanates [199].

37.4.4 Skin Hazards

Exposure to isocyanates may result in both allergic and irritant contact dermatitis, as well as urticaria [200–203], and the typical localization is hands and face.

According to Liippo et al., facial dermatitis seems more common in patients with positive patch test reactions to TDI and/or IPDI than in patients with positive reactions to MDI [204], which is in accordance with the fact that TDI and IPDI are more volatile than MDI. However, the most well-known health risk of isocyanate exposure is the adverse effect on the respiratory tract, including both airway irritation and immunologically mediated outcomes, which include for example hypersensitive pneumonitis and diisocyanate-induced asthma [205]. Compared to respiratory symptoms, reports on skin hazards from isocyanates are few in number.

37.4.4.1 Contact Allergy

Diisocyanates are strong contact sensitizers, judged by the results of animal studies [206, 207]. Animal experiments have also shown that polyisocyanate prepolymers are capable of causing skin sensitization in guinea pigs [208]. However, in spite of this, reports on allergic contact dermatitis are relatively few in number considering the extensive use of these chemicals in manufacturing processes and other applications. The low contact allergy frequency has been explained by the fact that (1) contamination of the skin is minimized by the application of strict regulations to the handling of isocyanates in order to avoid respiratory problems; (2) that the reactive isocyanates react before penetrating the skin; [209] and (3) that the patch test diagnostics of isocyanates is inadequate due to instability of patch test allergens and lack of late readings (i.e., reading after day 7) [210, 211].

Heavy exposure to diisocyanates may result in a rapid sensitization within a week to some months after exposure [212, 213]. It has been proposed that aromatic diisocyanates are strong respiratory sensitizers but weak cutaneous sensitizers [196], and that the opposite could be true for aliphatic diisocyanates [214]. Contact allergy to MDI, TDI, IPDI, HDI, dicyclohexylmethane diisocyanate (DMDI), and trimethyl hexamethylene diisocyanate (TMDI) has been reported [68, 194, 200, 204, 212, 213, 215–221]. Most recorded cases were sensitized to MDI or DMDI.

DMDI has been reported as a very potent dermal sensitizer [196, 216, 222]. In a company manufacturing medical equipment, 13 out of 100 workers were sensitized to DMDI, which was used in a glue [216]. At a factory making car badges, two out of seven workers showed positive patch test reactions to DMDI. It was also believed that irritant contact dermatitis from DMDI was the cause of three of the workers' skin problems [222]. Recently, a case describing allergic contact dermatitis to DMDI in an office environment where DMDI-charged cartridges were used was described [223]. DMDI-exposed patients have been reported to show positive reactions to TDI, HDI, and IPDI without any previously known contact with the substances in question [193, 216]. Militello et al. [193] attributed this to cross-sensitivity, referring to Thorne et al. who investigated MDI, TDI, HDI, and DMDI and showed cross-reactions between all isocyanates, regardless of whether they were aromatic or aliphatic, in animal experiments based on the mouse-ear swelling test [207]. In the same study, it was postulated that HDI was the most potent sensitizer, followed by DMDI, MDI, and TDI in declining the order of potency [207].

MDI-positive patients may also react to the corresponding amine diaminodiphenylmethane (MDA) [200, 204, 212, 213, 219, 224]. In 1967, Fregert [224] was the first to report these simultaneous reactions. He attributed this to cross-reactivity. In 1976, Rothe [219] suggested that MDA might be the actual allergen and that it is formed from hydrolysis of MDI when MDI comes into contact with the skin. Several reports describe workers exposed to MDI with positive patch test reactions to MDA, but negative reactions to MDI [200, 212, 213, 225, 226], and it has been proposed that MDA might be an important marker for MDI hypersensitivity [200, 212, 213]. MDA may also represent cross-allergy to *p*-phenylenediamine [219, 227].

37.4.4.2 Irritancy

Isocyanates are described as mild to strong irritants and irritant contact dermatitis seems to have been more common than allergic contact dermatitis [67]. Amine accelerators, e.g., MDA, triethylenediamine, and triethylamine, used in the polyurethane production can also cause skin irritation.

37.4.5 Patch Testing

Commercially available patch test preparations of TDI and MDI only contain one isomer of the respective monomers. Therefore, patients are generally tested with the isomers 4,4'-MDI and 2,4-TDI. Patch test preparations of DMDI are not commercially available, but are normally tested as the 4,4'-DMDI isomer. Most reports found in literature refer to contact allergy to these specific isomers. However, when previously described, the general abbreviations MDI, TDI, and DMDI have often been used.

Isocyanates are highly reactive, and their stability in patch test preparations has been discussed. In 1992, Estlander et al. [212] suggested that preparations of TDI and 4,4-MDI could be used for over a year since preparations that were 5.5 and 15.5 months old had elicited positive reactions in two patients. No chemical analyses were done. In 2004 and 2005, Frick et al. and Frick-Engfeldt et al. [228, 229] performed chemical analysis on commercially available patch test preparations from isocyanate series obtained from four American and nine European patch testing departments showing that patch test preparations of 2,4-TDI, 1,6-HDI, and IPDI contained the declared concentrations, but the concentration of 4,4'-MDI was generally so low that patch testing with the same could not be considered reliable. It was concluded that there is a high risk of false-negative reactions when using these preparations of 4,4'-MDI, and therefore, additional patch testing with the patients' own fresh work material was recommended [229]. The same recommendation was given by Gossens et al. [200] when reporting 13 patients with positive patch test reactions to isocyanate-based products and where only one of these patients reacted to any commercially available patch test preparation of diisocyanates. In the case of MDI, it has been suggested that patch test preparations of PMDI with a monomer content of at least 35% are used instead of preparations of 4,4'-MDI. The recommended patch test concentration was 2% in petrolatum [211]. Additionally, preparations should be stored in a freezer, for no longer than 1 year in order to ensure stability [211].

Patch testing workers exposed to polyurethane chemicals should include relatively fresh preparations of the most common diisocyanates MDI, TDI, HDI, and IPDI, as well as MDA, and the actual chemicals to which the workers have been exposed. It has been proposed that positive reactions to isocyanates appear late, and therefore it is advisable that isocyanate patch tests are also read on day 7 and that patients should be advised to make contact with the clinic, if any reactions appear after day 7 [211].

One case of a possible active patch test sensitization with TDI 1% in pet. has been reported [230].

37

> ## Core Message
>
> > When patch testing workers are exposed to polyurethane chemicals, it is advisable to test with their own work material, in addition to the commercially available patch test preparations of diisocyanates. A second reading on day 7 is advisable since positive reactions may appear late. Positive reactions to MDA should be taken into account as it may be an important marker for MDI sensitivity.

37.4.6 Prevention

The hazardous effect of isocyanates on the respiratory tract can be reduced by making the diisocyanates less volatile. There are three main ways of doing this, either by prepolymerising or prereacting the diisocyanates, or by blocking them. In all cases, a larger molecule is brought about. There are, however, always residues of free diisocyanate in prepolymerized or blocked products. Prepolymers are produced by mixing small amounts of di or polyfunctional alcohols with an excess of isocyanate. Blocked, i.e., temporarily inactivated isocyanates are used in heat-setting applications. When heated, the blocking groups escape, thereby releasing the isocyanate groups and enabling them to react [192].

To avoid skin exposure, general precautions such as using gloves and protective clothing should be imperative. Data on the workplace performance of protective gloves and clothing are limited, and although nitrile gloves have been suggested as preferable to latex, studies have shown that isocyanates can be detected underneath both types of gloves [231].

37.5 Other Plastics

37.5.1 Amino Plastics

Amino plastics is the common name for plastics formed by the reaction between an aldehyde and a compound with one or more amino groups. The most common aldehyde is formaldehyde, but sometimes, hexamethylenetetramine, which is a formaldehyde releaser, can be used.

The most common amino-containing compounds are urea (carbamide) and melamine, 2,4,6-triamino-1,3,5-triazine. The reaction with formaldehyde produces thermosetting urea-formaldehyde and melamine-formaldehyde resins, respectively. The amino resins are cured by heat, commonly with an acid as catalyst, e.g., *p*-toluenesulfonic acid. Both amino plastics can be utilized to improve the wet strength of paper and the crease-resistance of textiles. Nowadays, the amino plastics used in textiles release lower levels of free formaldehyde than previously [232]. Amino plastics are widely used as laminating and bonding materials in the wood and furniture industry and in conjunction with fillers and reinforcements, such as glass mat and cloth, silica, cotton fabrics, and certain synthetic fibers. Urea-formaldehyde resins can be used for the manufacture of containers for cosmetics, electric fittings, bottle caps, lavatory seats, and buttons, and furthermore, for insulation of refrigerators and walls of houses. Melamine-formaldehyde resin powders filled with cellulose are used for tableware. High-quality decorative laminates are made of melamine-formaldehyde resins.

37.5.1.1 Skin Hazards from Amino Plastics

Urea and melamine do not cause contact allergy. Sensitization to amino plastics has developed from urea-formaldehyde resin used in fiberboard [233], from melamine-formaldehyde resin in orthopedic casts [234], and gypsum molds [232]. Contact allergy to different types of amino plastics used as textile finish has been found in patients with suspected textile dermatitis [232, 235]. Contact allergy to amino resins may or may not be combined with contact allergy to formaldehyde [232, 235, 236]. However, to establish the frequency of simultaneous contact allergies, the patch test technique of both the formaldehyde test preparation and the amino resin test preparations should be optimized.

Patch testing with freshly prepared test preparations of the urea-formaldehyde and melamine-formaldehyde resins might be needed to establish the contact allergy (pers. communication Magnus Bruze, June 2009).

37.5.2 Polyester Plastics

Polyester resins are classified as saturated or unsaturated. Unsaturated polyesters have double bounds in their backbone that enables them to crosslink with unsaturated monomers, and thereby form thermosetting plastics with applications such as reinforced fiber glass, coatings, finishes, lacquers, cements, and glues. Saturated polyesters do not contain double bounds and instead form thermoplastics with applications such as synthetic fibers, PET beverage bottles, and plastic film.

The saturated polyesters, also termed unmodified alkyd resins, are produced from dicarboxylic acids, usually phthalic acid or maleic acid, mainly used in their anhydride forms, and polyalcohols, usually glycerol, pentaerythritol, or trimethylolpropane.

The saturated polyesters synthesized in this way are macromolecules commonly used as plasticizers for other plastic materials. Saturated polyesters can also be modified with oils containing fatty acids leading to the incorporation of unsaturated groups into the polyester polymer enabling it to crosslink. Such modified resins are called alkyd resins and are used in modern water-based paints and surface coatings.

Unsaturated polyesters are produced through esterification of organic acids or their anhydrides, e.g., maleic anhydride, phthalic anhydride, or fumaric acid, and diols, e.g., diethylene glycol or 1,2-propylene glycol. Unsaturated monomers, e.g., styrene, are used as solvents and for copolymerization with unsaturated groups along the polyester chain. Vinyl toluene and methyl methacrylate may also be used for cross-linking. An initiator or catalyst is required to start the cross-linking process. The catalyst is usually a peroxide, such as benzoyl peroxide or methyl ethyl ketone peroxide. Accelerators, e.g., cobalt naphthenate, or tertiary amines such as dimethyl aniline, diethyl aniline, and dimethyl-*p*-toluidine, are necessary for the curing of plastics at room temperature. In styrene, there are usually inhibitors, e.g., *p-tert*-butylcatechol or hydroquinone. The peroxide-cured unsaturated polyesters have been used commercially for many years, but unsaturated polyesters cured by UV-light have equivalent properties. The UV-curable polyester system is used in the furniture industry as topcoats and for orthopedic casts. Casts cured by UV-light usually consist of unsaturated polyester with vinyl toluene as the cross-linking agent and a benzoin-ether molecule as photo-initiator. The resin is impregnated into woven glass fiber. Reactive acrylate or methacrylate groups can be attached to the molecular backbone of the unsaturated polyesters through functional groups such as hydroxyl and anhydride, forming acrylated polyesters used in UV-curable inks or coatings for wood and paper.

37.5.2.1 Skin Hazards from Polyester Plastics

Contact dermatitis from saturated polyesters and alkyd resins appears to be rare. Allergic contact dermatitis has, however, been caused by a tri-functional epoxy compound, triglycidyl isocyanurate (TGIC), used as cross-linker in heat-cured polyester paints [91, 237, 238] and to terephtalic acid diglycidylester in a powder coating [92].

Phthalic anhydrides used in the manufacturing of saturated polyesters and alkyd resins have been reported to cause irritation [239], immediate IgE-mediated hypersensitivity, asthma, allergic rhinitis, and urticaria [138, 142, 240, 241].

Unsaturated polyester resins are also rare sensitizers. Those at risk are mainly workers employed in the manufacturing industry [67, 242–245]. According to Malten, unsaturated polyester no longer appears to have sensitizing capacity, presumably because the formation of sensitizing, free maleic acid esters is prevented by the avoidance of monoalcoholic impurities [217]. Should the diols contain monoalcohols such as ethanol and butanol, then ethyl maleate and dibutyl maleate can be formed, which are strong contact sensitizers. Diethyl maleate was reported to be a sensitizer in four men working with unsaturated polyester resins [244]. Allergic contact dermatitis from unsaturated polyester resins has more frequently been reported to be due to the auxiliary ingredients, such as cobalt salt of carboxylic acids and tertiary amines used as accelerators, peroxides used as catalysts, and cross-linking agents such as styrene [246–253]. Unsaturated polyester dust from reinforced-plastic products [254] or unsaturated polyester in automobile-repair putty [245, 255] has also been reported to cause allergic contact dermatitis.

The main irritants in unsaturated polyester resin systems are styrene and organic peroxides. Unsaturated polyester resin may contain 30–60 wt% styrene. Styrene is classified as a mild skin irritant [67, 256]. Repeated skin contact with liquid styrene, however, causes drying of the skin and may also cause irritant contact dermatitis [257–259]. In addition, workers in the reinforced plastics industry are exposed to numerous other skin irritants, such as glass fiber, organic solvents, and other additives. Peroxides are used at 3–10 wt% to catalyze the hardening process of unsaturated polyester resins. These reactive organic peroxides are weak sensitizers but strong irritants [260] and have also been reported to cause stinging on uncovered skin areas during spray lamination [256].

37.5.3 Polyvinyl Chloride Plastics

Polyvinyl chloride (PVC) is used in applications such as wallpapers, toys, garden hoses, wire coatings for electric cables, shower curtains, foils, bandages, casts, and protective gloves, while rigid PVC gives rise to application in sewage systems, agricultural products, drinking water pipes, furniture, window frames, dishes, and packages of various shapes.

PVC usually contains approximately 10–70% plasticizers and other additives. The plasticizers can be phthalic acid esters, e.g., diethylhexyl phthalate (DEHP) or esters of adipic acid or other di or multifunctional acids. There are various other additives in PVC plastics, such as antioxidants, light stabilizers, initiators, flame-retardants heat stabilizers, and pigments. PVC liberates hydrogen chloride when exposed to high temperatures and the heat stabilizers are added to prevent damage by the hydrochloric acid. Sometimes, uncured epoxy resin is added as a plasticizer and a heat stabilizer to PVC.

37.5.3.1 Skin Hazards from Polyvinyl Chloride Plastics

Workers processing PVC plastics can develop contact dermatitis [261]. In the final PVC product, there are always molecules of the monomer as well as a number of additives, which may, although it is rare, cause allergic contact dermatitis [262–266], irritant contact dermatitis [267], and contact urticaria [268, 269]. A recent study indicates that delayed patch test reactions might be as common to PVC reusable gloves as to natural latex rubber gloves when tested as *as is* [270]. Bisphenol A has been identified as a contact allergen in vinyl gloves [117, 118]. Contact allergies to 1,2-benzisothiazolin-3-one (BIT) in disposable PVC gloves have recently been reported [271]. Allergic contact reactions to epoxy resin in PVC plastic film and to phenylthiourea and phenyliso-thiocyanate in PVC adhesive tape have also been reported [263, 272]. Diphenylthiourea is a heat stabilizer in PVC and is partly decomposed to phenyl isothiocyanate.

The irritancy of polyvinyl resins has been proposed to be due to the plasticizers and stabilizers, dibutyl thiomaleate, dibutyl sebacate, or dioctyl phthalate (DOP) [67, 267]. PVC powder may irritate in a particular environment: an outbreak of acneiform eruptions that

occurred in a PVC manufacturing factory has been described [273]. The cause was probably the combination of heat, high humidity, and irritation from the PVC powder. Toxic PVC disease, from the manufacturing of PVC, consisting of Raynaud's phenomenon, lytic disease of bone, and scleroderma, has been reported [274].

37.5.4 Polystyrene Plastics

Polystyrene (PS) is a hard and transparent plastic. It is manufactured by polymerization of styrene, using peroxide as an initiator. PS resin is one of the thermoplastics. As a foam, PS plastic is an important packaging and insulation material. Modified PS plastics with a co or ter-polymer structure, e.g., styrene-butadiene (SB), styrene-acrylonitrile (SAN), acrylonitrile-butadiene-styrene (ABS), are used in household utensils, toys, electrical appliances, handles, bags, and pipes. PS products are also widely used in food packaging and disposable tableware. PS products can usually be identified by their metallic sound when dropped on a hard surface. To increase the light stability of styrene-based plastics, stabilizers such as benzophenones, benzotriazoles, and organic nickel compounds are usually added.

37.5.4.1 Skin Hazards from Polystyrene Plastics

Contact allergy to styrene is extremely rare. One patient, sensitive to styrene, cross-reacted on patch testing to 2-, 3-, and 4-vinyltoluene (2-, 3-, and 4-methylstyrene) and to the metabolites styrene epoxide and 4-vinylphenol (4-hydroxy-styrene). It is assumed that styrene is a pro-hapten metabolized in the skin by arylhydrocarbon hydroxylase to styrene epoxide, which acts as a true hapten. Styrene occurs both in nature and as a synthetic product and vinyltoluenes (methylstyrenes) occur as synthetic products in plastics [253]. A case of occupational contact dermatitis has been reported [258]. Cases of immediate allergy to styrene have also been reported [259]. Though styrene is generally classified as a mild irritant [67, 256], it has, on occasions, been reported to cause chemical burns [257]. Phenols like p-tert-butyl-catechol are added to styrene to prevent spontanous polymerization and this type of additives should be consedered in cases of suspected allergy to styrene monomer or PS plastics.

37.5.5 Polyolefin Plastics

The most important polyolefins are polyethylene produced from ethene and polypropylene produced from propene. Polyethylene is the most widely used plastic with primary application in films and sheets for packaging use and shopping bags [275]. Polymerization is produced at high or low pressures, aided by catalysts and initiators. According to their density, polyethylenes are grouped into three main categories: low-density polyethylenes, linear low-density polyethylenes, and high-density polyethylenes. Because low-density polyethylene is soft, flexible, and transparent, it is used for food packaging. Low-density polyethylene has outstanding chemical and frost resistance and is therefore used for hoses, sleeves of electric cables and wires, and many kinds of household utensils such as jars, containers, and deep-freeze boxes and cases. High-density polyethylenes are used mainly for bottles and containers, but also for shopping bags and pipes.

Polypropylene is similar to high-density polyethylene, but slightly harder and tougher. In addition to filament applications, such as home furnishings, nonwoven products, and carpets, polypropylene is generally used for pipes and films.

Polyethene and polypropene usually contain low amounts (1–5%) of additives compared to several other plastics.

37.5.5.1 Skin Hazards from Polyolefin Plastics

Irritant and allergic contact dermatitis from polyethylene and polypropylene are rare. Contact allergy to a surgical suture composed of polypropylene [276] and contact urticaria due to polyethylene gloves [277] has been reported. When sawing and grinding polyolefins, the frictional heat may decompose the plastic material and release volatile chemicals, e.g., aldehydes, ketones, and acids, which might cause airborne contact dermatitis and itching [278]. Airborne irritant contact dermatitis caused by mechanical strain from synthetic fibers of polypropene and polyethylene released from an air-conditioning filter has been reported [279].

37.5.6 Polyamide Plastics

The transparency of polyamide films makes them very useful for packaging purposes. Hospital wares made of polyamide plastics have good stability at sterilization temperatures, and combined films of laminates are used, for example, in vacuum packaging of meat.

The polyamides are thermoplastics manufactured by reacting diamines with dicarboxylic acids. One type of the most well-known polyamide, nylon, is produced by polymerization of adipic acid and hexamethylene diamine. Other ways to produce polyamides is through polymerization of the cyclic amide caprolactam.

37.5.6.1 Skin Hazards from Polyamide Plastics

Irritant and allergic contact dermatitis from polyamides are rare. Contact dermatitis caused by polyamide trousers pockets has been described [280]. Contact dermatitis in the nylon production is usually caused by various additives [281–284]. Contact urticaria due to nylon has been reported [285].

37.5.7 Polycarbonate Plastics

The -O-CO-O- group characterizes a polycarbonate plastic. It can be made from phosgene ($COCl_2$) and bisphenol A (4,4-dihydroxydiphenyl-2,2-propane). Bisphenols other than bisphenol A can also be used. Polycarbonate plastic is a very transparent, tough, and inert material that is extremely resistant to sunlight and weather. It is used, among other things, in safety helmets, bullet-proof windows, shields, doors, bottles, and lamp globes. However, the plastic is relatively expensive and, therefore, has limited applications.

37.5.7.1 Skin Hazards from Polycarbonate Plastics

Irritant and allergic contact dermatitis from polycarbonates are rare.

37.5.8 Rare Plastics

Plastics of less dermatological importance are couma-
rone-indene polymers, cellulose polymers, and cyclohexanone resins. Cyclohexanone is used as an
intermediate in the production of nylon. It can be used as
a PVC solvent to facilitate the gluing of materials to plastic [286]. Only very few cases with contact allergy to
cyclohexanone have been reported [286]. It is not fully
known if the monomers, additives, or impurities are the
cause of the dermatitis in the few reported cases of contact allergy to the cyclohexanone resins [287, 288].

37.6 Plasticizers and Other Additives

Additives are used to modify the properties of the plastic material. The major classes of additives to plastics
are plasticizers, fillers and reinforcements, biocides,
flame retardants, heat stabilizers, antioxidants, ultraviolet-light absorbers, blowing agents, initiators, lubricants and flow-control agents, antistatic agents, curing
agents, colorants, solvents, and optical brighteners.

There are nearly 2,500 individual chemicals or mixtures that are utilized in the above major classes of
additives. In the plastics industry, the word compound
is used for a chemical product of plastic resin mixed
with additives. Compounds are delivered to the plastic
industry as powders or pellets. Masterbatch is a concentrated mixture of additives in the plastics.

37.6.1 Plasticizers

Plasticizers constitute a broad range of chemically and
thermally stable products of a variety of chemical classes
that are added to improve the flexibility, softness, and processing of plastics. Their principal use is in thermoplastic
resins, and 80–85% of the world's production of plasticizers is used in PVC manufacturing. Approximately 450
plasticizers are commercially available. Many are esters
of carboxylic acids (e.g., phthalic, isophthalic, adipic,
benzoic, abietic, trimellitic, oleic, sebacic acids) or phosphoric acid. Other plasticizers are chlorinated parafines,
epoxidized vegetable oils, and adipate polymers.

Although there are about 100 phthalates that have
been employed as plasticizers, around 14–15 phthalates
account for over 90% of commercial phthalate production. The commonly used phthalate, diethylhexyl phthalate (DEHP) is also called dioctyl phthalate (DOP) but
DOP can also mean di-n-octyl phthalate which is another
member in the phthalate group. Other plasticizers used
are butyl benzyl phthalate (BBP), diisononyl phthalate
(DINP), diisodecyl phthalate (DIDP), methyl-, ethyl-,
butyl phthalate, dialkyl (C_6C_{11}) phthalate, and diethylhexyl adipate. Adipates and other aliphatic diesters are
used in low-temperature applications, while trimelitates
are used for high-temperature applications. Methyl-,
ethyl-, and butyl phthalates are more often used as solvents than plasticizers in the plastics industry.

37.6.2 Flame Retardants

Flame retardants are required for high-performance
thermoplastic resins because of their use in electrical
and high-temperature applications. Numerous chemicals are used as flame retardants. Chlorine- and bro-
mine-containing aliphatic, cycloaliphatic, and aromatic
compounds are the most widely used. Others are antimony trioxide, aluminum hydrate, and chlorparaffins.
A more fire-resistant epoxy resin can be produced by
brominating bisphenol A in epoxy resins to tetrabro-
mobisphenol A.

37.6.3 Heat Stabilizers

Plastics, particularly chlorine-containing polymers,
are susceptible to thermal decomposition when exposed
to high temperatures or prolonged heating. There are
several kinds of stabilizers on the market. The most
important contain lead, tin, calcium and zinc or barium
and zinc. Epoxidized oils and esters are also used.
Diphenylthiourea is used as heat stabilizer in PVC.

37.6.4 Antioxidants

Oxidative degradation of polymers during the manufacturing process or during their useful lifetime is a
major industrial concern. Examples of antioxidants are

alkylated phenols and polyphenols (e.g., butylated hydroxytoluenes (BHT) and 4-tertiary-butylcatechol), epoxidized soyabean oil, propylphenol phosphite, thiobisphenol, organic phosphates, bisphenol A, benzophenone, hydroquinones, and triazoles.

37.6.5 Ultraviolet-Light Absorbers

Radiation from the sun or fluorescent light rapidly degrades most plastics. The most widely used UV absorbers belong to six distinct chemical classes:

Benzophenones
Benzotriazoles
Salicylates
Acrylates
Organo-nickel derivatives
Hindered amines
Metal complexes with dialkyldithiocarbamate

The most widely used UV absorbers are 2-hydroxy-benzophenones, 2-hydroxy-phenyl-benzotriazoles, and 2-cyanodiphenyl-acrylate

37.6.6 Initiators

A chain-reaction polymerization process produces most commercial synthetic polymers. Some of the many initiators used are various peroxides (e.g., benzoyl peroxide, di-tertiary-butyl peroxide, cyclohexanone peroxide, and methyl ethyl ketone peroxide). There are more than 65 commercially available organic peroxides in over 100 formulations.

37.6.7 Biocides

Biostabilizers will prevent the growth of microorganisms on the surface and in the pores of plastics. Plastic materials easily attacked by microorganisms are PVC, polyurethane, silicon products, and fiber products based on polypropene and polyamide. Microorganisms usually cause discoloration but can also cause cracks in plastic materials. Biocides are usually added to plastic products used in environments of high temperature

and humidity, e.g., saunas, showers, pools, and boats. The most widely used biocides are methyl and octyl isothiazolinones and oxybisphenoxarsine (OBPA).

37.6.8 Colorants (Dyes and Pigments)

Pigments are inert and, unlike dyes, insoluble in the medium in which they are incorporated. Both inorganic and organic pigments are used in plastics. Most colorants are inorganic pigments.

37.6.9 Metals and Metal Salts

Many metals, metal salts, and metallic compounds are used as additives in plastics. They act as stabilizers, pigments, fillers, flame retardants, and antistatics. The most commonly used metals are aluminum, titanium, lead, zinc, antimony, tin, chromium, and molybdenum. Nickel, copper, and zirconium compounds are used to a lesser degree.

37.6.10 Skin Hazards from Additives

Allergic and irritant contact dermatitis from various additives were briefly mentioned in connection with the various plastics. In spite of phthalates being widely used additives in plastics, there are only a few reports in the literature of skin problems caused by them. Allergic contact dermatitis from dibutyl phthalate has been reported when used in a plastic watchstrap, an antiperspirant spray, and a corticosteroid cream [289–292]. Contact dermatitis from diethyl phthalate has been reported from spectacle frames and a hearing aid of cellulose ester plastics [293, 294]. Two cases of contact allergy to dimethyl phthalate in computer "mice" have been reported [295].

An outbreak of dermatitis occurring in an aircraft factory was caused by the epoxy compound o-diglycidyl phthalate, among other chemicals [82]. Burrows and Rycroft have reported contact allergy to tricresyl ethylphthalate in a plastic nail adhesive [296], and Hills and Ive allergic contact dermatitis from di-isodecylphtalate in a PVC identity band [264].

Phthalates can also appear in deodorant formulations, perfumes, emollients, and insect repellents

37

[297]. A case of contact urticaria syndrome due to di(2-ethylhexyl)phtalate in work clothes has been described [269]. Triphenylphosphate allergy from spectacle frames has been reported [298, 299].

In 1976, the International Contact Dermatitis Research Group (ICDRG) examined the incidence of sensitization to the flame retardant tris(2,3-dibromopropyl)phosphate and found two positives among 1,103 patients. One of these two cases has been reported in detail by Andersen [300].

Contact allergy to ultraviolet-light absorbers such as 2-hydroxybenzophenone, resocinol monobenzoate, 2-(2-hydroxy-5-methylphenyl)benzotriazole (Tinuvin P), and *bis*-(2,2,6,6)-tetramethyl-4-piperidyl-sebacate has been encountered [301, 302].

Organic pigments, mostly of the azo type, are potentially sensitizing additives in plastics [303, 304]. Allergic contact dermatitis from perinone-type plastic dyes, C.I. Solvent Orange 60 and C.I. Solvent Red 179, used in spectacle frames has been described [305, 306]. C.I. Solvent Orange 60 has also been found to cause contact allergy in workers exposed to polyamide plastics (Zimerson, personal communication).

Cobalt, nickel, and mercury used in plastic shoes, personal computer (PC) mouse, and polyester resins have been reported [307–309].

References

1. Isaksson M, Zimerson E (2007) Risks and possibilities in patch testing with contaminated personal objects: usefulness of thin-layer chromatograms in a patient with acrylate contact allergy from a chemical burn. Contact Dermatitis 57:84–88
2. Saval P, Kristiansen E, Cramers M et al (2007) Occupational allergic contact dermatitis caused by aerosols of acrylate monomers. Contact Dermatitis 57:276
3. Björkner B (1984) Contact allergy to 2-hydroxypropyl methacrylate (2-HPMA) in an ultraviolet curable ink. Acta Derm Venereol 64:264–267
4. Pedersen NB, Senning A, Nielsen AO (1983) Different sensitising acrylic monomers in Napp printing plate. Contact Dermatitis 9:459–464
5. Malten KE, Bende WJ (1979) 2-Hydroxy- ethyl-methacrylate and di- and tetraethylene glycol dimethacrylate: contact sensitizers in a photoprepolymer printing plate procedure. Contact Dermatitis 5:214–220
6. Kanerva L, Estlander T, Jolanki R (1994) Occupational skin allergy in dental profession. In: Taylor S (ed) Dermatologic clinics vol 12, Saunders, Philadelphia
7. Kanerva L, Henriks-Eckerman M, Estlander T (1994) Occupational allergic contact dermatitis and composition of acrylates in dental bonding systems. J Eur Acad Derm Venereol 3:157–168
8. Kanerva L, Estlander T, Jolanki R (1995) Dental problems. In: Giun JD (ed) Practical contact dermatitis. McGraw-Hill, New York
9. Kanerva L, Jolanki R, Estlander T (1997) 10 years of patch testing with the (meth)acrylate series. Contact Dermatitis 37:255–258
10. Kanerva L, Estlander T, Jolanki R et al (1994) Dermatitis from acrylates in dental personnel. In: Menne T, Maibach HI (eds) Hand eczema. CRC, Boca Raton
11. Björkner B (1984) Sensitizing capacity of ultraviolet curable acrylic compounds. Thesis, University of Lund, Lund
12. Estlander T, Jolanki R, Kanerva L (1998) Occupational allergic contact dermatitis from UV-cured lacquer containing dipropylene glycol diacrylate. Contact Dermatitis 39:36
13. Geukens S, Goossens A (2001) Occupational contact allergy to (meth)acrylates. Contact Dermatitis 44:153–159
14. Goon AT, Rycroft RJ, McFadden JP (2002) Allergic contact dermatitis from trimethylolpropane triacrylate and pentaerythritol triacrylate. Contact Dermatitis 47:249
15. Kanerva L, Estlander T, Jolanki R (1989) Occupational allergic contact dermatitis from acrylates: observations concering anaerobic acrylic sealants and dental composite resins. In: Frosch PJ, Dooms-Goossens A, Lachapelle JM et al (eds) Current topics in contact dermatitis. Springer, Berlin
16. Moffitt DL, Sansom JE (2001) Occupational allergic contact dermatitis from tetrahydrofurfuryl acrylate in a medical-device adhesive. Contact Dermatitis 45:54
17. Henriks-Eckerman ML, Alanko K, Jolanki R et al (2001) Exposure to airborne methacrylates and natural rubber latex allergens in dental clinics. J Environ Monit 3:302–305
18. Kanerva L, Alanko K, Estlander T (1999) Allergic contact gingivostomatitis from a temporary crown made of methacrylates and epoxy diacrylates. Allergy 54:1316–1321
19. Kanerva L, Estlander T, Jolanki R et al (1992) Occupational pharyngitis associated with allergic patch test reactions from acrylics. Allergy 47:571–573
20. Kanerva L, Rantanen T, Aalto-Korte K et al (2001) A multicenter study of patch test reactions with dental screening series. Am J Contact Dermat 12:83–87
21. Koch P (2003) Allergic contact stomatitis from BIS-GMA and epoxy resins in dental bonding agents. Contact Dermatitis 49:104–105
22. Lindström M, Alanko K, Keskinen H et al (2002) Dentist's occupational asthma, rhinoconjunctivitis, and allergic contact dermatitis from methacrylates. Allergy 57:543–545
23. Piirila P, Hodgson U, Estlander T et al (2002) Occupational respiratory hypersensitivity in dental personnel. Int Arch Occup Environ Health 75:209–216
24. Wrangsjö K, Swartling C, Meding B (2001) Occupational dermatitis in dental personnel: contact dermatitis with special reference to (meth)acrylates in 174 patients. Contact Dermatitis 45:158–163
25. Carmichael AJ, Gibson JJ, Walls AW (1997) Allergic contact dermatitis to bisphenol-A-glycidyldimethacrylate (BIS-GMA) dental resin associated with sensitivity to epoxy resin. Br Dent J 183:297–298

26. Jolanki R, Kanerva L, Estlander T (1995) Occupational allergic contact dermatitis caused by epoxy diacrylate in ultraviolet-light-cured paint, and bisphenol A in dental composite resin. Contact Dermatitis 33:94–99

27. Björkner B, Niklasson B, Persson K (1984) The sensitizing potential of di-(meth)acrylates based on bisphenol A or epoxy resin in the guinea pig. Contact Dermatitis 10: 286–304

28. Kanerva L, Estlander T, Jolanki R (1989) Allergic contact dermatitis from dental composite resins due to aromatic epoxy acrylates and aliphatic acrylates. Contact Dermatitis 20:201–211

29. Niinimaki A, Rosberg J, Saari S (1983) Traces of epoxy resin in acrylic dental filling materials. Contact Dermatitis 9:532

30. Aalto-Korte K, Jungewelter S, Henriks-Eckerman ML et al (2009) Contact allergy to epoxy (meth)acrylates. Contact Dermatitis 61:9–21

31. Bohling HG, Borchard U, Drouin H (1977) Monomeric methylmethacrylate (MMA) acts on the desheathed myelinated nerve and on the node of Ranvier. Arch Toxicol 38:307–314

32. Kanerva L, Verkkala E (1986) Electron microscopy and immunohistochemistry of toxic and allergic effects of methylmethacrylate on the skin. Arch Toxicol Suppl 9:456–459

33. Mathias CG, Caldwell TM, Maibach HI (1979) Contact dermatitis and gastrointestinal symptoms from hydroxyethylmethacrylate. Br J Dermatol 100:447–449

34. Goon AT, Bruze M, Zimerson E et al (2008) Screening for acrylate/methacrylate allergy in the baseline series: our experience in Sweden and Singapore. Contact Dermatitis 59:307–313

35. Bakker JG, Jongen SM, Van Neer FC et al (1991) Occupational contact dermatitis due to acrylonitrile. Contact Dermatitis 24:50–53

36. Chu CY, Sun CC (2001) Allergic contact dermatitis from acrylonitrile. Am J Contact Dermat 12:113–114

37. Garnier R, Levy-Amon L, Malingrey L (2003) Occupational contact dermatitis from N-(2-(diethylamino)-ethyl) acrylamide. Contact Dermatitis 48:343–344

38. Pedersen NB, Chevallier MA, Senning A (1982) Secondary acrylamides in Nyloprint printing plate as a source of contact dermatitis. Contact Dermatitis 8:256–262

39. Wang MT, Wenger K, Maibach HI (1997) Piperazine diacrylamide allergic contact dermatitis. Contact Dermatitis 37:300

40. Calnan CD (1979) Cyanoacrylate dermatitis. Contact Dermatitis 5:165–167

41. Parker D, Turk JL (1983) Contact sensitivity to acrylate compounds in guinea pigs. Contact Dermatitis 9:55–60

42. Belsito DV (1987) Contact dermatitis to ethyl-cyanoacrylate-containing glue. Contact Dermatitis 17:234–236

43. Björkner B, Niklasson B (1984) Influence of the vehicle on elicitation of contact allergic reactions to acrylic compounds in the guinea pig. Contact Dermatitis 11:268–278

44. Bruze M, Björkner B, Lepoittevin JP (1995) Occupational allergic contact dermatitis from ethyl cyanoacrylate. Contact Dermatitis 32:156–159

45. Conde-Salazar L, Rojo S, Guimaraens D (1998) Occupational allergic contact dermatitis from cyanoacrylate. Am J Contact Dermat 9:188–189

46. Fisher AA (1985) Reactions to cyanoacrylate adhesives: "instant glue". Cutis 35:18

47. Fitzgerald DA, Bhaggoe R, English JS (1995) Contact sensitivity to cyanoacrylate nail-adhesive with dermatitis at remote sites. Contact Dermatitis 32:175–176

48. Foti C, Cassano N, Conserva A et al (2003) Irritant paronychia with onychodystrophy caused by cyanoacrylate nail glue. Contact Dermatitis 48:274–275

49. Guin JD, Wilson P (1999) Onycholysis from nail lacquer: a complication of nail enhancement? Am J Contact Dermat 10:34–36

50. Guin JD, Baas K, Nelson-Adesokan P (1998) Contact sensitization to cyanoacrylate adhesive as a cause of severe onychodystrophy. Int J Dermatol 37:31–36

51. Isaksson M, Siemund I, Bruze M (2007) Allergic contact dermatitis from ethylcyanoacrylate in an office worker with artificial nails led to months of sick leave. Contact Dermatitis 57:346–347

52. Jacobs MC, Rycroft RJ (1995) Allergic contact dermatitis from cyanoacrylate? Contact Dermatitis 33:71

53. Kanerva L, Estlander T (2000) Allergic onycholysis and paronychia caused by cyanoacrylate nail glue, but not by photobonded methacrylate nails. Eur J Dermatol 10:223–225

54. Pigatto PD, Giacchetti A, Altomare GF (1986) Unusual sensitization to cyanoacrylate ester. Contact Dermatitis 14:193

55. Tomb RR, Lepoittevin JP, Durepaire F et al (1993) Ectopic contact dermatitis from ethyl cyanoacrylate instant adhesives. Contact Dermatitis 28:206–208

56. Björkner B (1981) Sensitization capacity of acrylated prepolymers in ultraviolet curing inks tested in the guinea pig. Acta Derm Venereol 61:7–10

57. Björkner B (1982) Sensitization capacity of polyester methacrylate in ultraviolet curing inks tested in the guinea pig. Acta Derm Venereol 62:153–154

58. Björkner B (1984) Sensitizing potential of urethane (meth) acrylates in the guinea pig. Contact Dermatitis 11:115–119

59. Cavelier C, Jelen G, Herve-Bazin B et al (1981) Irritation et allergie aux acrylates et methacrylates. Premiere partie. Monoacrylates et monomethacrylates simples. Ann Dermatol Venereol 108:549–556

60. Rustemeyer T, de Groot J, von Blomberg BM et al (1998) Cross-reactivity patterns of contact-sensitizing methacrylates. Toxicol Appl Pharmacol 148:83–90

61. Waegemaekers T (1985) Some toxicological aspects of acrylic monomers, notably with reference to the skin. Thesis, Katholieke Universiteit te Nijmegen

62. van der Walle HB (1982) Sensitizing potential of acrylic monomers in guinea pig. Thesis, Katholieke Universiteit te Nijmegen, Holland, Kripps Repro Meppel

63. Kanerva L (2001) Cross-reactions of multifunctional methacrylates and acrylates. Acta Odontol Scand 59:320–329

64. Dearman RJ, Betts CJ, Farr C et al (2007) Comparative analysis of skin sensitization potency of acrylates (methyl acrylate, ethyl acrylate, butyl acrylate, and ethylhexyl acrylate) using the local lymph node assay. Contact Dermatitis 57:242–247

65. Beurey J, Mougeolle JM, Weber M (1976) Accidents cutanes des resines acryliques dans l'imprimerie. Ann Dermatol Syphiligr (Paris) 103:423–430

66. Anon (1992) Acrylate compounds, uses and evaluation of health effects. Finnish Advisory Board of Chemicals, Government Printing Office, Helsinki

37

67. Kanerva L, Björkner B, Estlander T (1996) Plastic materials: occupational exposure, skin irritancy and its prevention. In: van der Valk PGM, Maibach HI (eds) The irritant contact dermatitis syndrome. CRC, Boca Baton

68. Malten KE (1982) Old and new, mainly occupational dermatological problems in the production and processing of plastics. In: Maibach HI, Gellin GA (eds) Occupational and industrial dermatology. Year Book Medical, Chicago

69. Andersson T, Bruze M, Björkner B (1999) In vivo testing of the protection of gloves against acrylates in dentin-bonding systems on patients with known contact allergy to acrylates. Contact Dermatitis 41:254–259

70. Andersson T, Bruze M, Gruvberger B et al (2000) In vivo testing of the protection provided by non-latex gloves against a 2-hydroxyethyl methacrylate-containing acetone-based dentin-bonding product. Acta Derm Venereol 80:435–437

71. Andreasson H, Boman A, Johnsson S et al (2003) On permeability of methyl methacrylate, 2-hydroxyethyl methacrylate and triethyleneglycol dimethacrylate through protective gloves in dentistry. Eur J Oral Sci 111:529–535

72. Munksgaard EC (1992) Permeability of protective gloves to (di)methacrylates in resinous dental materials. Scand J Dent Res 100:189–192

73. Nakamura M, Oshima H, Hashimoto Y (2003) Monomer permeability of disposable dental gloves. J Prosthet Dent 90:81–85

74. Pegum JS, Medhurst FA (1971) Contact dermatitis from penetration of rubber gloves by acrylic monomer. Br Med J 2:141–143

75. Rietschel RL, Huggins R, Levy N et al (1984) In vivo and in vitro testing of gloves for protection against UV-curable acrylate resin systems. Contact Dermatitis 11:279–282

76. Estlander T, Jolanki R (1988) How to protect the hands. In: Taylor JS (ed) Occupational dermatoses. Saunders, Philadelphia

77. Kanerva L, Estlander T, Jolanki R (1988) Sensitization to patch test acrylates. Contact Dermatitis 18:10–15

78. Aalto-Korte K, Alanko K, Kuuliala O et al (2008) Occupational methacrylate and acrylate allergy from glues. Contact Dermatitis 58:340–346

79. Goon AT, Isaksson M, Zimerson E et al (2006) Contact allergy to (meth)acrylates in the dental series in southern Sweden: simultaneous positive patch test reaction patterns and possible screening allergens. Contact Dermatitis 55:219–226

80. Teik-Jin Goon A, Bruze M, Zimerson E et al (2007) Contact allergy to acrylates/methacrylates in the acrylate and nail acrylics series in southern Sweden: simultaneous positive patch test reaction patterns and possible screening allergens. Contact Dermatitis 57:21–27

81. Bruze M, Edenholm M, Engström K et al (1996) Occupational dermatoses in a Swedish aircraft plant. Contact Dermatitis 34:336–340

82. Burrows D, Fregert S, Campbell H et al (1984) Contact dermatitis from the epoxy resins tetraglycidyl-4, 4'-methylene dianiline and o-diglycidyl phthalate in composite material. Contact Dermatitis 11:80–82

83. Fregert S (1981) Manual of contact dermatitis, 2nd edn. Munksgaard, Copenhagen

84. Kanerva L, Jolanki R, Estlander T et al (2000) Airborne occupational allergic contact dermatitis from triglycidyl-p-aminophenol and tetraglycidyl-4, 4'-methylene dianiline in

preimpregnated epoxy products in the aircraft industry. Dermatology 201:29–33

85. Ellis B (1993) The synthesis and manufacture of epoxy resins. In: Ellis B (ed) Chemistry and technology of epoxy resins, 1st edn. Blackie Academic, Glasgow

86. Muskopf JW, McCollister SB (1987) Epoxy resins. In: Gerhartz W, Yamamoto YS, Kaudy L et al (eds) Ullmann's encyclopedia of industrial chemistry, vol A9, 5th edn. VCH Verlagsgesellschaft, Weinheim

87. Henriks-Eckerman M-L, Laijoki T (1986) Glycidyl ethers in epoxy resin products (in Finnish with English summary). Työterveyslaitoksen tutkimuksa 41–46 (summary p 70)

88. Ponten A, Zimerson E, Sörensen O et al (2004) Chemical analysis of monomers in epoxy resins based on bisphenols F and A. Contact Dermatitis 50:289–297

89. Jensen CD, Andersen KE (2003) Two cases of occupational allergic contact dermatitis from a cycloaliphatic epoxy resin in a neat oil: case report. Environ Health 2:3

90. Maibach HI, Mathias CT (2001) Allergic contact dermatitis from cycloaliphatic epoxide in jet aviation hydraulic fluid. Contact Dermatitis 45:56

91. Allmaras S (2003) Worker exposure to 1, 3, 5-triglycidyl isocyanurate (TGIC) in powder paint coating operations. Appl Occup Environ Hyg 18:151–153

92. Geier J, Oestmann E, Lessmann H et al (2001) Contact allergy to terephthalic acid diglycidylester in a powder coating. Contact Dermatitis 44:43–44

93. Mathias CG (1988) Allergic contact dermatitis from triglycidyl isocyanurate in polyester paint pigments. Contact Dermatitis 19:67–68

94. Fregert S (1988) Physiochemicals methods for detection of contact allergens. In: Taylor JS (ed) Occupational dermatoses, dermatological clinics, vol 6. Saunders, Philadelphia

95. Fregert S, Trulsson L (1978) Simple methods for demonstration of epoxy resins of bisphenol A type. Contact Dermatitis 4:69–72

96. Ashcroft WR (1993) Curing agents for epoxy resins. In: Ellis B (ed) Chemistry and technology of epoxy resins. Blackie Academic, Glasgow

97. Kanerva L, Estlander T, Jolanki R (1996) Occupational allergic contact dermatitis caused by 2, 4, 6-tris-(dimethylaminomethyl)phenol, and review of sensitizing epoxy resin hardeners. Int J Dermatol 35:852–856

98. Jolanki R (1991) Occupational skin diseases from epoxy compounds. Epoxy resin compounds, epoxy acrylates and 2, 3-epoxypropyl trimethyl ammonium chloride. Acta Derm Venereol Suppl (Stockh) 159:1–80

99. Shaw SJ (1993) Additives and modifiers for epoxy resins. In: Ellis B (ed) Chemistry and technology of epoxy resins, 1st edn. Blackie Academic, Glasgow

100. Hansson C (1994) Determination of monomers in epoxy resin hardened at elevated temperature. Contact Dermatitis 31:333–334

101. Dickel H, Kuss O, Schmidt A et al (2002) Occupational relevance of positive standard patch-test results in employed persons with an initial report of an occupational skin disease. Int Arch Occup Environ Health 75:423–434

102. Geier J, Lessmann H, Hillen U et al (2004) An attempt to improve diagnostics of contact allergy due to epoxy resin systems. First results of the multicentre study EPOX 2002. Contact Dermatitis 51:263–272

103. Jolanki R, Estlander T, Kanerva L (1987) Occupational contact dermatitis and contact urticaria caused by epoxy resins. Acta Derm Venereol Suppl (Stockh) 134:90–94

104. Uter W, Ruhl R, Pfahlberg A et al (2004) Contact allergy in construction workers: results of a multifactorial analysis. Ann Occup Hyg 48:21–27

105. Ponten A, Carstensen O, Rasmussen K et al (2004) Epoxy-based production of wind turbine rotor blades: occupational dermatoses. Contact Dermatitis 50:329–338

106. Fregert S, Thorgeirsson A (1977) Patch testing with low molecular oligomers of epoxy resins in humans. Contact Dermatitis 3:301–303

107. Thorgeirsson A, Fregert S (1977) Allergenicity of epoxy resins in the guinea pig. Acta Derm Venereol 57:253–256

108. Kanerva L, Tarvainen K, Pinola A et al (1994) A single accidental exposure may result in a chemical burn, primary sensitization and allergic contact dermatitis. Contact Dermatitis 31:229–235

109. Le Coz CJ, Coninx D, Van Rengen A et al (1999) An epidemic of occupational contact dermatitis from an immersion oil for microscopy in laboratory personnel. Contact Dermatitis 40:77–83

110. Dahlquist I, Fregert S (1979) Allergic contact dermatitis from volatile epoxy hardeners and reactive diluents. Contact Dermatitis 5:406–407

111. Amado A, Taylor JS (2008) Contact dermatitis in the bowling pro shop. Dermatitis 19:334–338

112. Isaksson M, Möller H, Ponten A (2008) Occupational allergic contact dermatitis from epoxy resin in a golf club repairman. Dermatitis 19:E30–E32

113. Lyon CC, O'Driscoll J, Erikstam U et al (1998) Bowlers' grip. Contact Dermatitis 38:223

114. Ponten A, Zimerson E, Sörensen O et al (2002) Sensitizing capacity and cross-reaction pattern of the isomers of diglycidyl ether of bisphenol F in the guinea pig. Contact Dermatitis 47:293–298

115. Lee HN, Pokorny CD, Law S et al (2002) Cross-reactivity among epoxy acrylates and bisphenol F epoxy resins in patients with bisphenol A epoxy resin sensitivity. Am J Contact Dermat 13:108–115

116. Ponten A, Bruze M (2001) Contact allergy to epoxy resin based on diglycidyl ether of bisphenol F. Contact Dermatitis 44:98–99

117. Aalto-Korte K, Alanko K, Henriks-Eckerman ML et al (2003) Allergic contact dermatitis from bisphenol A in PVC gloves. Contact Dermatitis 49:202–205

118. Matthieu L, Godoi AF, Lambert J et al (2003) Occupational allergic contact dermatitis from bisphenol A in vinyl gloves. Contact Dermatitis 49:281–283

119. Allen H, Kaidbey K (1979) Persistent photosensitivity following occupational exposure to epoxy resin. Arch Dermatol 115:1307–1310

120. Göransson K, Andersson R, Andersson G (1984) An outbreak of occupational photodermatosis of the face in a factory in northern Sweden. In: Berglund B, Lindvall T, Sundell J (eds) Indoor air, vol 3. Swedish Council for Building Research, Stockholm

121. Maguire HC Jr (1988) Experimental photoallergic contact dermatitis to bisphenol A. Acta Derm Venereol 68:408–412

122. Ponten A, Zimerson E, Bruze M (2009) Sensitizing capacity and cross-reactivity of phenyl glycidyl ether studied in the guinea-pig maximization test. Contact Dermatitis 60:79–84

123. Thorgeirsson A (1978) Sensitization capacity of epoxy resin hardeners in the guinea pig. Acta Derm Venereol 58:323–326

124. Angelini G, Rigano L, Foti C et al (1996) Occupational sensitization to epoxy resin and reactive diluents in marble workers. Contact Dermatitis 35:11–16

125. Jolanki R, Tarvainen K, Tatar T et al (1996) Occupational dermatoses from exposure to epoxy resin compounds in a ski factory. Contact Dermatitis 34:390–396

126. Silvestre JF, Albares MP, Escutia B et al (2003) Contact vitiligo appearing after allergic contact dermatitis from aromatic reactive diluents in an epoxy resin system. Contact Dermatitis 49:113–114

127. Prens EP, de Jong G, van Joost T (1986) Sensitization to epichlorohydrin and epoxy system components. Contact Dermatitis 15:85–90

128. van Joost T (1988) Occupational sensitization to epichlorohydrin and epoxy resin. Contact Dermatitis 19:278–280

129. van Joost T, Roesyanto ID, Satyawan I (1990) Occupational sensitization to epichlorohydrin (ECH) and bisphenol-A during the manufacture of epoxy resin. Contact Dermatitis 22:125–126

130. Estlander T, Jolanki R, Kanerva L (1997) Occupational allergic contact dermatitis from 2, 3-epoxypropyl trimethyl ammonium chloride (EPTMAC) and Kathon LX in a starch modification factory. Contact Dermatitis 36:191–194

131. Ponten A, Björk J, Carstensen O et al (2004) Associations between contact allergy to epoxy resin and fragrance mix. Acta Derm Venereol 84:151–152

132. Andersen KE, Christensen LP, Volund A et al (2009) Association between positive patch tests to epoxy resin and fragrance mix I ingredients. Contact Dermatitis 60:155–157

133. Dahlquist I, Fregert S (1979) Contact allergy to the epoxy hardener isophoronediamine (IPD). Contact Dermatitis 5:120–121

134. Jolanki R, Estlander T, Kanerva L (1987) Contact allergy to an epoxy reactive diluent: 1, 4-butanediol diglycidyl ether. Contact Dermatitis 16:87–92

135. Jolanki R, Kanerva L, Estlander T et al (1990) Occupational dermatoses from epoxy resin compounds. Contact Dermatitis 23:172–183

136. Lachapelle JM, Tennstedt D, Dumont-Fruytier M (1978) Occupational allergic contact dermatitis to isophorone diamine (IPD) used as an epoxy resin hardener. Contact Dermatitis 4:109–112

137. Mathias CG (1987) Allergic contact dermatitis from a non-bisphenol A epoxy in a graphite fiber reinforced epoxy laminate. J Occup Med 29:754–755

138. Kanerva L, Hyry H, Jolanki R et al (1997) Delayed and immediate allergy caused by methylhexahydrophthalic anhydride. Contact Dermatitis 36:34–38

139. Kanerva L, Pelttari M, Jolanki R et al (2002) Occupational contact urticaria from diglycidyl ether of bisphenol A epoxy resin. Allergy 57:1205–1207

140. Kanerva L, Jolanki R, Tupasela O et al (1991) Immediate and delayed allergy from epoxy resins based on diglycidyl ether of bisphenol A. Scand J Work Environ Health 17:208–215

141. Stutz N, Hertl M, Loffler H (2008) Anaphylaxis caused by contact urticaria because of epoxy resins: an extraordinary emergency. Contact Dermatitis 58:307–309

142. Tarvainen K, Jolanki R, Estlander T et al (1995) Immunologic contact urticaria due to airborne methylhexahydrophthalic and methyltetrahydrophthalic anhydrides. Contact Dermatitis 32:204–209

143. Eedy DJ (1996) Carbon-fibre-induced airborne irritant contact dermatitis. Contact Dermatitis 35:362–363

144. Jolanki R, Estlander T, Kanerva L (2001) 182 patients with occupational allergic epoxy contact dermatitis over 22 years. Contact Dermatitis 44:121–123

145. Jolanki R, Sysilampi ML, Kanerva L et al (1989) Contact allergy to cycloaliphatic epoxy resins. In: Frosch PJ, Dooms-Goossens A, Lachapelle JM et al (eds) Current topics in contact dermatitis. Springer, Berlin

146. Romyhr O, Nyfors A, Leira HL et al (2006) Allergic contact dermatitis caused by epoxy resin systems in industrial painters. Contact Dermatitis 55:167–172

147. Chu CY, Ponten A, Sun CC et al (2006) Concomitant contact allergy to the resins, reactive diluents and hardener of a bisphenol A/F-based epoxy resin in subway construction workers. Contact Dermatitis 54:131–139

148. Pegum JS (1979) Penetration of protective gloves by epoxy resin. Contact Dermatitis 5:281–283

149. Roed-Petersen J (1989) A new glove material protective against epoxy and acrylate monomer. In: Frosch PJ, Dooms-Goossens A, Lachapelle JM et al (eds) Current topics in contact dermatitis. Springer, Berlin

150. Blanken R, Nater JP, Veenhoff E (1987) Protective effect of barrier creams and spray coatings against epoxy resins. Contact Dermatitis 16:79–83

151. Blanken R, Nater JP, Veenhoff E (1987) Protection against epoxy resins with glove materials. Contact Dermatitis 16:46–47

152. Bruze M (1985) Contact sensitizers in resins based on phenol and formaldehyde. Acta Derm Venereol Suppl (Stockh) 119:1–83

153. Elvers B, Hawkins S, Schulz G (1991) Ullman's Encyclopedia of Industrial Chemistry, vol A19, 5th edn. VCH Verlagsgesellschaft, Weinheim

154. Estlander T, Tarvainen K, Jolanki R et al (1993) Occupational sensitization to a resin binder used in rock wool. In Books of abstracts, 3rd congress of the European Academy of Dermatology and Venereology, 26–30 Sept. Copenhagen, Denmark

155. Foussereau J, Cavelier C, Selig D (1976) Occupational eczema from para-tertiary-butylphenol formaldehyde resins: a review of the sensitizing resins. Contact Dermatitis 2:254–258

156. Schubert H, Agatha G (1979) Zur Allergennatur der para-tert. Butylphenolformaldehydharze. Derm Beruf Umwelt 27:49–52

157. White IR (1990) Adhesives. In: Adams RM (ed) Occupational skin disease. Saunders, Philadelphia

158. Barros MA, Baptista A, Correia TM et al (1991) Patch testing in children: a study of 562 schoolchildren. Contact Dermatitis 25:156–159

159. Dotterud LK, Falk ES (1995) Contact allergy in relation to hand eczema and atopic diseases in north Norwegian schoolchildren. Acta Paediatr 84:402–406

160. Nielsen NH, Menné T (1992) Allergic contact sensitization in an unselected Danish population. The Glostrup Allergy Study, Denmark. Acta Derm Venereol 72:456–460

161. Zimerson E, Bruze M (2000) Sensitizing capacity of 5, 5'-di-tert-butyl-2, 2'-dihydorxy-(hydroxymethyl)-dibenzyl ethers in the guinea pig. Contact Dermatitis 43:72–78

162. Zimerson E, Bruze M (2000) Contact allergy to 5, 5'-di-tert-butyl-2, 2'-dihydroxy-(hydroxymethyl)-dibenzyl ethers, sensitizers, in p-tert-butylphenol-formaldehyde resin. Contact Dermatitis 43:20–26

163. Zimerson E, Bruze M (1998) Contact allergy to the monomers of p-tert-butylphenol-formaldehyde resin in the guinea pig. Contact Dermatitis 39:222–226

164. Zimerson E, Bruze M (2002) Low-molecular-weight contact allergens in p-tert-butylphenol-formaldehyde resin. Am J Contact Dermat 13:190–197

165. Zimerson E, Bruze M (2002) Contact allergy to the monomers in p-tert-butylphenol-formaldehyde resin. Contact Dermatitis 47:147–153

166. Zimerson E, Bruze M (2002) Sensitizing capacity of two monomeric aldehyde components in p-tert-butylphenol-formaldehyde resin. Acta Derm Venereol 82:418–422

167. Bruze M, Fregert S, Zimerson E (1985) Contact allergy to phenol-formaldehyde resins. Contact Dermatitis 12:81–86

168. Zimerson E, Bruze M, Goossens A (1999) Simultaneous p-tert-butylphenol-formaldehyde resin and p-tert-butylcatechol contact allergies in man and sensitizing capacities of p-tert-butylphenol and p-tert-butylcatechol in guinea pigs. J Occup Environ Med 41:23–28

169. Bruze M (1986) Sensitizing capacity of 2-methylol phenol, 4-methylol phenol and 2, 4, 6-trimethylol phenol in the guinea pig. Contact Dermatitis 14:32–38

170. Bruze M (1986) Sensitizing capacity of 4, 4(1)-dihydroxy-(hydroxymethyl)-diphenyl methanes in the guinea pig. Acta Derm Venereol 66:110–116

171. Bruze M (1986) Sensitizing capacity of dihydroxydiphenyl methane (bisphenol F) in the guinea pig. Contact Dermatitis 14:228–232

172. Bruze M, Zimerson E (1985) Contact allergy to 3-methylol phenol, 2, 4-dimethylol phenol and 2, 6-dimethylol phenol. Acta Derm Venereol 65:548–551

173. Bruze M, Zimerson E (1985) Contact allergy to dihydroxydiphenyl methanes (bisphenol F). Derm Beruf Umwelt 33:216–220

174. Bruze M, Zimerson E (2002) Contact allergy to o-cresol–a sensitizer in phenol-formaldehyde resin. Am J Contact Dermat 13:198–200

175. Bruze M, Fregert S, Persson L et al (1986) Contact allergy to 4,4'-dihydroxy-(hydroxymethyl)-diphenyl methanes: sensitizers in a phenol-formaldehyde resin. J Invest Dermatol 87:617–623

176. Bruze M, Fregert S, Persson L et al (1987) Contact allergy to 2, 4'-dihydroxy-(hydroxymethyl)-diphenyl methanes. Sensitizers in a phenol-formaldehyde resin. Derm Beruf Umwelt 35:52–55

177. Bruze M, Zimerson E (1997) Cross-reaction patterns in patients with contact allergy to simple methylol phenols. Contact Dermatitis 37:82–86

178. Bruze M (1986) Simultaneous reactions to phenol-formaldehyde resins colophony/hydroabietyl alcohol and balsam of Peru/perfume mixture. Contact Dermatitis 14:119–120

179. Fregert S (1980) Irritant dermatitis from phenol-formaldehyde resin powder. Contact Dermatitis 6:493

180. Bruze M, Almgren G (1988) Occupational dermatoses in workers exposed to resins based on phenol and formaldehyde. Contact Dermatitis 19:272–277

181. Kalimo K, Saarni H, Kytta J (1980) Immediate and delayed type reactions to formaldehyde resin in glass wool. Contact Dermatitis 6:496

182. Katsarou A, Armenaka M, Ale I et al (1999) Frequency of immediate reactions to the European standard series. Contact Dermatitis 41:276–279

183. Bruze M (1988) Patch testing with a mixture of 2 phenol-formaldehyde resins. Contact Dermatitis 19:116–119

184. Estlander T, Kostiainen M, Jolanki R et al (1998) Active sensitization and occupational allergic contact dermatitis caused by para-tertiary-butylcatechol. Contact Dermatitis 38:96–100

185. Estlander T, Kanerva L, Jolanki R (2000) Polyurethane resins. In: Kanerva L, Elsner P, WJ E et al (eds) Handbook of occupational dermatology. Springer, Berlin

186. Ulrich H (2002) Diisocyanates. In: Ulrich H (ed) Chemistry and technology of isocyanates. Wiley, Chichester

187. Thorpe D (2002) Isocyanates. In: Lee S (ed) The Huntsman polyurethanes book, 1st edn. Wiley, Chichester

188. Kapasi V (2002) Thermoplastic polyurethanes. In: Lee S (ed) The Huntsman polyurethanes book. Wiley, Chichester

189. Anon TA: Concise International Chemical Assessment Document (CICAD) PG:25 p YR:2001 IP:VI:27

190. Marand A, Dahlin J, Karlsson D et al (2004) Determination of technical grade isocyanates used in the production of polyurethane plastics. J Environ Monit 6:606–614

191. Zimmerman R (2002) Catalysts. In: Lee S (ed) The Huntsman polyurethanes book, 1st edn. Wiley, UK

192. Anon (1996) Thermosetting plastics. Statue Book of the Swedish National Board of Occupational Safety and Health. AFS 1996:4

193. Militello G, Sasseville D, Ditre C et al (2004) Allergic contact dermatitis from isocyanates among sculptors. Dermatitis 15:150–153

194. Morgan CJ, Haworth AE (2003) Allergic contact dermatitis from 1, 6-hexamethylene diisocyanate in a domestic setting. Contact Dermatitis 48:224

195. Crespo J, Galan J (1999) Exposure to MDI during the process of insulating buildings with sprayed polyurethane foam. Ann Occup Hyg 43:415–419

196. Emmett EA (1976) Allergic contact dermatitis in polyurethane plastic moulders. J Occup Med 18:802–804

197. Karlsson D, Dalene M, Skarping G et al (2001) Determination of isocyanic acid in air. J Environ Monit 3:432–436

198. Bello D, Redlich CA, Stowe MH et al (2008) Skin exposure to aliphatic polyisocyanates in the auto body repair and refinishing industry: II. A quantitative assessment. Ann Occup Hyg 52:117–124

199. Rattray NJ, Botham PA, Hext PM et al (1994) Induction of respiratory hypersensitivity to diphenylmethane-4, 4'-diisocyanate (MDI) in guinea pigs. Influence of route of exposure. Toxicology 88:15–30

200. Goossens A, Detienne T, Bruze M (2002) Occupational allergic contact dermatitis caused by isocyanates. Contact Dermatitis 47:304–308

201. Larsen TH, Gregersen P, Jemec GB (2001) Skin irritation and exposure to diisocyanates in orthopedic nurses working with soft casts. Am J Contact Dermat 12:211–214

202. Stingeni L, Bellini V, Lisi P (2008) Occupational airborne contact urticaria and asthma: simultaneous immediate and delayed allergy to diphenylmethane-4, 4'-diisocyanate. Contact Dermatitis 58:112–113

203. Valks R, Conde-Salazar L, Barrantes OL (2003) Occupational allergic contact urticaria and asthma from diphenylmethane-4, 4'-diisocyanatae. Contact Dermatitis 49:166–167

204. Liippo J, Lammintausta K (2008) Contact sensitization to 4, 4'-diaminodiphenylmethane and to isocyanates among general dermatology patients. Contact Dermatitis 59:109–114

205. Klees JE, Ott MG (1999) Diisocyanates in polyurethane plastics applications. Occup Med 14:759–776

206. Tanaka K, Takeoka A, Nishimura F et al (1987) Contact sensitivity induced in mice by methylene bisphenyl diisocyanate. Contact Dermatitis 17:199–204

207. Thorne PS, Hillebrand JA, Lewis GR et al (1987) Contact sensitivity by diisocyanates: potencies and cross-reactivities. Toxicol Appl Pharmacol 87:155–165

208. Zissu D, Binet S, Limasset JC (1998) Cutaneous sensitization to some polyisocyanate prepolymers in guinea pigs. Contact Dermatitis 39:248–251

209. Malten KE (1984) Dermatological problems with synthetic resins and plastics in glues. Part II. Derm Beruf Umwelt 32:118–125

210. Frick-Engfeldt M, Isaksson M, Zimerson E et al (2007) How to optimize patch testing with diphenylmethane diisocyanate. Contact Dermatitis 57:138–151

211. Frick-Engfeldt M, Zimerson E, Karlsson D et al (2007) Is it possible to improve the patch-test diagnostics for isocyanates? A stability study of petrolatum preparations of diphenylmethane-4, 4'-diisocyanate and polymeric diphenylmethane diisocyanate. Contact Dermatitis 56:27–34

212. Estlander T, Keskinen H, Jolanki R et al (1992) Occupational dermatitis from exposure to polyurethane chemicals. Contact Dermatitis 27:161–165

213. Frick M, Isaksson M, Björkner B et al (2003) Occupational allergic contact dermatitis in a company manufacturing boards coated with isocyanate lacquer. Contact Dermatitis 48:255–260

214. Rietschel RL, Fowler JF (2001) Fisher's contact dermatitis, 5th edn. Lipingcott, Williams & Wilkins, Philadelphia

215. Belsito DV (2003) Common shoe allergens undetected by commercial patch-testing kits: dithiodimorpholine and isocyanates. Am J Contact Dermat 14:95–96

216. Frick M, Björkner B, Hamnerius N et al (2003) Allergic contact dermatitis from dicyclohexylmethane-4, 4'-diisocyanate. Contact Dermatitis 48:305–309

217. Malten KE (1984) Dermatological problems with synthetic resins and plastics in glues. Part I. Derm Beruf Umwelt 32:81–86

218. Mancuso G, Reggiani M, Berdondini RM (1996) Occupational dermatitis in shoemakers. Contact Dermatitis 34:17–22

219. Rothe A (1976) Zur Frage arbeitsbedingter Hautschadigungen durch Polyurethanchemikalien. Berufsdermatosen 24:7–24

220. Schröder C, Uter W, Schwanitz HJ (1999) Occupational allergic contact dermatitis, partly airborne, due to isocyanates and epoxy resin. Contact Dermatitis 41:117–118

221. Thompson T, Belsito DV (1997) Allergic contact dermatitis from a diisocyanate in wool processing. Contact Dermatitis 37:239

222. White IR, Stewart JR, Rycroft RJ (1983) Allergic contact dermatitis from an organic di-isocyanate. Contact Dermatitis 9:300–333

223. Kerre S (2008) Allergic contact dermatitis to DMDI in an office application. Contact Dermatitis 58:313–314

224. Fregert S (1967) Allergic contact reaction to diphenyl-4, 4'-diisocyanate. Contact Dermat Newslett 2:17

225. Alomar A (1986) Contact dermatitis from a fashion watch. Contact Dermatitis 15:44–45

226. Tait CP, Delaney TA (1999) Reactions causing reactions: allergic contact dermatitis to an isocyanate metabolite but not to the parent compound. Australas J Dermatol 40:116–117

227. Uter W, Lessmann H, Geier J et al (2002) The spectrum of allergic (cross-)sensitivity in clinical patch testing with 'para amino' compounds. Allergy 57:319–322

228. Frick-Engfeldt M, Zimerson E, Karlsson D et al (2005) Chemical analysis of 2, 4-toluene diisocyanate, 1, 6-hexamethylene diisocyanate and isophorone diisocyanate in petrolatum patch-test preparations. Dermatitis 16:130–135

229. Frick M, Zimerson E, Karlsson D et al (2004) Poor correlation between stated and found concentrations of diphenylmethane-4, 4'-diisocyanate (4, 4'-MDI) in petrolatum patch-test preparations. Contact Dermatitis 51:73–78

230. Le Coz CJ, El Aboubi S, Ball C (1999) Active sensitization to toluene di-isocyanate. Contact Dermatitis 41:104–105

231. Bello D, Herrick CA, Smith TJ et al (2007) Skin exposure to isocyanates: reasons for concern. Environ Health Perspect 115:328–335

232. Belsito DV (1993) Textile dermatitis. Am J Contact Dermat 4:249

233. Bell HK, King CM (2002) Allergic contact dermatitis from urea-formaldehyde resin in medium-density fibreboard (MDF). Contact Dermatitis 46:247

234. Ross JS, Rycroft RJ, Cronin E (1992) Melamine-formaldehyde contact dermatitis in orthopaedic practice. Contact Dermatitis 26:203–204

235. Metzler-Brenckle L, Rietschel RL (2002) Patch testing for permanent-press allergic contact dermatitis. Contact Dermatitis 46:33–37

236. Aalto-Korte K, Jolanki R, Estlander T (2003) Formaldehyde-negative allergic contact dermatitis from melamine-formaldehyde resin. Contact Dermatitis 49:194–196

237. Dooms-Goossens A, Bedert R, Vandaele M et al (1989) Airborne contact dermatitis due to triglycidylisocyanurate. Contact Dermatitis 21:202–203

238. McFadden JP, Rycroft RJ (1993) Occupational contact dermatitis from triglycidyl isocyanurate in a powder paint sprayer. Contact Dermatitis 28:251

239. Tarvainen K (1996) Occupational dermatoses from plasic composites based on polyester resins, epoxy resins and vinyl ester resins. People Work 11:1–66

240. Jolanki R, Kanerva L, Estlander T (1997) Skin allergy caused by organic acid anhydrides. In: Amin S, Lahti A, Maibach HI (eds) Contact urticaria syndrome. CRC, Boca Raton

241. Venables KM (1989) Low molecular weight chemicals, hypersensitivity, and direct toxicity: the acid anhydrides. Br J Ind Med 46:222–232

242. Dooms-Goossens A, De Jong G (1985) Letter to the editor. Contact Derm 12:238

243. MacFarlane AW, Curley RK, King CM (1986) Contact sensitivity to unsaturated polyester resin in a limb prosthesis. Contact Dermatitis 15:301–303

244. Malten KE (1964) Occupational dermatoses in the processing of plastics. Trans St John's Hosp Dermatol Soc 59:78–119

245. Tarvainen K, Jolanki R, Estlander T (1993) Occupational contact allergy to unsaturated polyester resin cements. Contact Dermatitis 28:220–224

246. Anavekar NS, Nixon R (2006) Occupational allergic contact dermatitis to cobalt octoate included as an accelerator in a polyester resin. Australas J Dermatol 47:143–144

247. Bhushan M, Craven NM, Beck MH (1998) Contact allergy to methyl ethyl ketone peroxide and cobalt in the manufacture of fibreglass-reinforced plastics. Contact Dermatitis 39:203

248. Guin JD (2001) Sensitivity to adipic acid used in polyester synthesis. Contact Dermatitis 44:256–257

249. Kanerva L, Tarvainen K, Estlander T (2000) Polyester resins. In: Kanerva L, Elsner P, Wahlberg JE et al (eds) Handbook of occupational dermatology. Springer, Berlin

250. Minamoto K, Nagano M, Inaoka T et al (2002) Allergic contact dermatitis due to methyl ethyl ketone peroxide, cobalt naphthenate and acrylates in the manufacture of fibreglass-reinforced plastics. Contact Dermatitis 46:58–59

251. Minamoto K, Nagano M, Yonemitsu K et al (2002) Allergic contact dermatitis from unsaturated polyester resin consisting of maleic anhydride, phthalic anhydride, ethylene glycol and dicyclopentadiene. Contact Dermatitis 46: 62–63

252. Pfaffli P, Jolanki R, Estlander T et al (2002) Identification of sensitizing diethyleneglycol maleate in a two-component polyester cement. Contact Dermatitis 46:170–173

253. Sjöborg S, Fregert S, Trulsson L (1984) Contact allergy to styrene and related chemicals. Contact Dermatitis 10:94–96

254. Tarvainen K, Kanerva L, Jolanki R (1995) Occupational dermatoses from the manufacture of plastic composite products. Am J Contact Dermat 6:95–104

255. Kanerva L, Estlander T, Alanko K et al (1999) Occupational allergic contact dermatitis from unsaturated polyester resin in a car repair putty. Int J Dermatol 38:447–452

256. Schmunes E (1990) Solvents and plasticizers. In: Adams RM (ed) Occupational skin diseases, 2nd edn. Saunders, Philadelphia

257. Bruze M, Fregert S, Gruvberger B (2000) Chemical skin burns. In: Menne T, Maibach HI (eds) Hand eczema. CRC, Boca Raton

258. Conde-Salazar L, Gonzalez MA, Guimaraens D et al (1989) Occupational allergic contact dermatitis from styrene. Contact Dermatitis 21:112

259. Moscato G, Biscaldi G, Cottica D et al (1987) Occupational asthma due to styrene: two case reports. J Occup Med 29:957–960

260. Haustein UF, Tegetmeyer L, Ziegler V (1985) Allergic and irritant potential of benzoyl peroxide. Contact Dermatitis 13:252–257

261. Park SG, Lee EC, Hong WK et al (2008) A case of occupational allergic contact dermatitis due to PVC hose. J Occup Health 50:197–200

262. Fregert S, Rorsman H (1963) Hypersensitivity to epoxy resins used as plasticizers and stabilizers in polyvinyl chloride (PVC) resins. Acta Derm Venereol 43:10–13

263. Fregert S, Trulson L, Zimerson E (1982) Contact allergic reactions to diphenylthiourea and phenylisothiocyanate in PVC adhesive tape. Contact Dermatitis 8:38–42

264. Hills RJ, Ive FA (1993) Allergic contact dermatitis from di-isodecyl phthalate in a polyvinyl chloride identity band. Contact Dermatitis 29:94–95

265. Huh WK, Masuji Y, Tada J et al (2001) Allergic contact dermatitis from a pyridine derivative in polyvinyl chloride leather. Am J Contact Dermat 12:35–37

266. Ito A, Imura T, Sasaki K et al (2009) Allergic contact dermatitis due to mono(2-ethylhexyl) maleate in di-(n-octyl) tin-bis(2-ethylhexyl maleate) in polyvinyl chloride gloves. Contact Dermatitis 60:59–61

267. Di Lernia V, Cameli N, Patrizi A (1989) Irritant contact dermatitis in a child caused by the plastic tube of an infusion system. Contact Dermatitis 21:339–340

268. Osmundsen PE (1980) Contact urticaria from nickel and plastic additives (butylhydroxytoluene, oleylamide). Contact Dermatitis 6:452–454

269. Sugiura K, Sugiura M, Hayakawa R et al (2002) A case of contact urticaria syndrome due to di(2-ethylhexyl) phthalate (DOP) in work clothes. Contact Dermatitis 46:13–16

270. Ponten A, Dubnika I (2009) Delayed reactions to reusable protective gloves. Contact Dermatitis 60:227–229

271. Aalto-Korte K, Ackermann L, Henriks-Eckerman ML et al (2007) 1, 2-benzisothiazolin-3-one in disposable polyvinyl chloride gloves for medical use. Contact Dermatitis 57: 365–370

272. Fregert S, Meding B, Trulsson L (1984) Demonstration of epoxy resin in stoma pouch plastic. Contact Dermatitis 10:106

273. Goh CL, Ho SF (1988) An outbreak of acneiform eruption in a polyvinyl chloride manufacturing factory. Derm Beruf Umwelt 36:53–57

274. Veltman G, Lange CE, Stein G (1978) The vinyl-chloride disease. Hautarzt 29:177–182

275. Piringer OG, Baner AL (2008) Plastic packaging: interactions with food and pharmaceuticals. Wiley-VCH, Weinheim

276. Sanchez-Morillas L, Reano Martos M, Rodriguez Mosquera M et al (2003) Delayed sensitivity to Prolene. Contact Dermatitis 48:338–339

277. Sugiura K, Sugiura M, Shiraki R et al (2002) Contact urticaria due to polyethylene gloves. Contact Dermatitis 46:262–266

278. Thestrup-Pedersen K, Madsen JB, Rasmussen K (1989) Cumulative skin irritance from heat-decomposed polyethylene plastic. In: Frosch PJ, Dooms-Goossens A, Lachapelle JM et al (eds) Current topics in contact dermatitis. Springer, Berlin

279. Patiwael JA, Wintzen M, Rustemeyer T et al (2005) Airborne irritant contact dermatitis due to synthetic fibres from an air-conditioning filter. Contact Dermatitis 52:126–129

280. Grimalt F, Romaguera C (1981) Contact dermatitis caused by polyamide trouser pockets. Derm Beruf Umwelt 29: 35–39

281. Batta K, McVittie S, Foulds IS (1999) Occupational allergic contact dermatitis from N, N-methylene-bis-5-methyl-oxazolidine in a nylon spin finish. Contact Dermatitis 41:165

282. Savage J (1978) Chloracetamide in nylon spin finish. Contact Dermatitis 4:179

283. Tanaka M, Kobayashi S, Miyakawa S (1993) Contact dermatitis from nylon 6 in Japan. Contact Dermatitis 28:250

284. Valsecchi R, Leghissa P, Piazzolla S et al (1993) Occupational dermatitis from isothiazolinones in the nylon production. Dermatology 187:109–111

285. Dooms-Goossens A, Duron C, Loncke J et al (1986) Contact urticaria due to nylon. Contact Dermatitis 14:63

286. Pazzaglia M, Tullo S, Voudouris S et al (2003) Contact dermatitis due to cyclohexanone: a further case. Contact Dermatitis 49:313

287. Bruze M, Boman A, Bergqvist-Karlsson A et al (1988) Contact allergy to a cyclohexanone resin in humans and guinea pigs. Contact Dermatitis 18:46–49

288. Heine A, Laubstein B (1990) Contact dermatitis from cyclohexanone-formaldehyde resin (L2 resin) in a hair lacquer spray. Contact Dermatitis 22:108

289. Calnan CD (1975) Dibutyl phthalate. Contact Dermatitis 1:388

290. Husain SL (1975) Dibutyl phthalate sensitivity. Contact Dermatitis 1:395

291. Sneddon IB (1972) Dermatitis from dibutylphthalate in an aerosol anti-perspirant and deodorant. Contact Dermat Newslett 12:308

292. Wilkinson SM, Beck MH (1992) Allergic contact dermatitis from dibutyl phthalate, propyl gallate and hydrocortisone in Timodine. Contact Dermatitis 27:197

293. Oliwiecki S, Beck MH, Chalmers RJ (1991) Contact dermatitis from spectacle frames and hearing aid containing diethyl phthalate. Contact Dermatitis 25:264–265

294. Smith EL, Calnan CD (1966) Studies in contact dermatitis. XVII. Spectacle frames. Trans St Johns Hosp Dermatol Soc 52:10–34

295. Capon F, Cambie MP, Clinard F et al (1996) Occupational contact dermatitis caused by computer mice. Contact Dermatitis 35:57–58

296. Burrows D, Rycroft RJ (1981) Contact dermatitis from PTBP resin and tricresyl ethyl phthalate in a plastic nail adhesive. Contact Dermatitis 7:336–337

297. Hamanaka S, Hamanaka Y, Otsuka F (1992) Phthalic acid dermatitis caused by an organostannic compound, tributyl tin phthalate. Dermatology 184:210–212

298. Camarasa JG, Serra-Baldrich E (1992) Allergic contact dermatitis from triphenyl phosphate. Contact Dermatitis 26:264–265

299. Carlsen L, Andersen KE, Egsgaard H (1986) Triphenyl phosphate allergy from spectacle frames. Contact Dermatitis 15:274–277

300. Andersen KE (1977) Sensitivity to a flame retardant, tris(2, 3-dibromopropyl)phosphate (Firemaster LVT 23 P). Contact Dermatitis 3:297–300

301. Ikarashi Y, Tsuchiya T, Nakamura A (1994) Contact sensitivity to Tinuvin P in mice. Contact Dermatitis 30: 226–230

302. Niklasson B, Björkner B (1989) Contact allergy to the UV-absorber Tinuvin P in plastics. Contact Dermatitis 21:330–334

303. Jolanki R, Kanerva L, Estlander T (1987) Organic pigments in plastics can cause allergic contact dermatitis. Acta Derm Venereol Suppl (Stockh) 134:95–97

304. Kanerva L, Jolanki R, Estlander T (1985) Organic pigment as a cause of plastic glove dermatitis. Contact Dermatitis 13:41–43

305. Shono M, Kaniwa MA (1999) Allergic contact dermatitis from a perinone-type dye C.I. Solvent Orange 60 in spectacle frames. Contact Dermatitis 41:181–184

306. Tsunoda T, Kaniwa MA, Shono M (2001) Allergic contact dermatitis from a perinone-type dye C.I. Solvent Red 179 in spectacle frames. Contact Dermatitis 45:166–167

307. Goossens A, Bedert R, Zimerson E (2001) Allergic contact dermatitis caused by nickel and cobalt in green plastic shoes. Contact Dermatitis 45:172

308. Kanerva L, Kanervo K, Jolanki R et al (2001) Cobalt–a possible sensitizer in personal computer (PC) mouse and polyester resins. Contact Dermatitis 45:126–127

309. Koch P, Nickolaus G (1996) Allergic contact dermatitis and mercury exanthem due to mercury chloride in plastic boots. Contact Dermatitis 34:405–409

Topical Drugs

38

Francisco M. Brandão and An Goossens

Contents

F.M. Brandão (✉)
Department of Dermatology, Hospital Garcia de Orta, Avenue
Torrado da Silva, 2800, Almada, Portugal
e-mail: fmbrandao@sapo.pt

A. Goossens
Department of Dermatology, University Hospital KU Leuven,
Kapucijnenvoer 33, 3000, Leuven, Belgium

38.1 Incidence and Prevalence

38.1.1 Incidence

Cutaneous adverse drug reactions are usually an iatrogenic disease induced in patients. More rarely, they are an occupational disease, either in health personnel or in pharmaceutical industry employees.

The incidence of topical reactions to drugs varies from one area to another and from one country to another, depending on local prescribing and self-medication habits. Prescribing habits are changing, and some medicaments that were common allergens 30–40 years ago, such as sulphonamides, penicillin and anti-histamines, have now been replaced by other allergenic drugs, such as non-steroidal anti-inflammatory drugs (NSAID), corticosteroids (CSs) and transdermal delivering systems.

The real incidence of adverse reactions to topical medicaments is not known and most of the data about prevalence are quite old. Bandmann et al. [20] found that 14% of 4,000 patients, tested in several European countries, were allergic to medicaments. In Belgium [61], 17% of 2,025 patients were allergic to ingredients of pharmaceutical products, while in Italy, in the 1980s [10, 255], about 20.5% of 8,230 patients were allergic to topical drugs. In Sweden, 40% of all recorded allergic reactions were due to medicaments [69], which was equivalent to an annual incidence of 43/100,000. In Singapore [107], 22.5% of patients tested had medicament sensitivity, while in India 10% of patch-tested patients were allergic to topical medicaments [18]. In Portugal, over a 6-year period (2002–2007), 17.2% of all patch-tested patients were sensitized to medicaments (Table 38.1).

These differences are not only due to geographic differences, but also to the type of patient selection – leg

J.D. Johansen et al. (eds.), *Contact Dermatitis*,
DOI: 10.1007/978-3-642-03827-3_38, © Springer-Verlag Berlin Heidelberg 2011

38

Table 38.1 Incidence of medicament contact allergy in Portugal, 2002–2007 (data from the Portuguese Contact Dermatitis Group)

Year	Total patients patch tested	Patch tests positive to medicaments (%)
2002	2,681	490 (18.3)
2003	2,849	426 (14.9)
2004	2,806	513 (18.3)
2005	2,932	417 (14.2)
2006	2,844	535 (18.8)
2007	2,799	523 (18.7)
Total	16,911	2,904 (17.2)

ulcer patients, anogenital dermatitis, etc. to specific interests of some investigators and age of the patients. Some reports support that as age increases, the prevalence of contact allergy to topical medicaments increases, and that it is independent of leg ulcer patients [116, 281]. A prevalence of allergic reactions to medicaments of about 15%, excluding leg ulcers or other high-risk patients, seems a realistic figure to be expected in a contact dermatitis clinic. However, this figure does not include other clinical entities such as irritant contact dermatitis or contact urticaria, among others.

> **Core Message**
>
> › A prevalence of up to 15% of allergic contact dermatitis to topical medicaments is, probably, a realistic figure in most contact clinics.

38.2 Factors Predisposing to Medicament Contact Dermatitis

Many factors may contribute, in various ways, to cutaneous drug sensitization. The environment, on the whole, must be considered the more important contributing factor, although there is some individual predisposition, which mainly depends on genetic factors. The intrinsic sensitizing potential of each drug is by far the most important factor (see Chap. 4), although sometimes impurities, contaminants and degradation products may be the allergenic material [10]. Moreover, compound allergy [259] and quenching phenomena [83] may interfere with this intrinsic capacity. However,

many of the more potent allergens, such as sulphonamides and penicillin, have now been banished from our prescribing habits and from the market; on the other hand, some weak sensitizers, such as neomycin, are so widely used that several new cases are seen every year.

The use of medicaments in high concentrations or in vehicles that increase skin penetration favours their irritant and sensitizing capacities. The same applies when medications are used in folds, under occlusive dressings or in transdermal devices, which lead to a much greater skin absorption, and thus, increase the probability of developing contact allergy.

Damage to the skin barrier is another very important factor favouring sensitization. Leg ulcer and stasis dermatitis patients are known to have a very high incidence of medicament allergy [10, 61]. In addition, patients with otitis externa, eye problems, perianal and vulval dermatoses, chronic hand and foot dermatitis are known to frequently develop secondary medicament allergy.

In other chronic dermatological conditions, however, such as atopic dermatitis and psoriasis, this possibly increased contact allergy seems to be an open question. In atopic patients, the defective T-cell population and the difficulty in sensitizing patients to DNCB would suggest that these patients would not develop allergic contact dermatitis as often as non-atopic individuals [28]. However, nowadays, most authors tend to consider that atopic patients, namely children, become sensitized to topical medicaments at least as often as non-atopics [101, 165, 176, 196].

It has also been suggested that psoriatic patients are not easily sensitized [76, 128], and that sensitization could be associated with certain localizations (palmoplantar and flexural [91]), although this could not be confirmed by other authors [84, 263]. Sensitization was found to be equal in other patients, especially to antipsoriatic medicaments [23, 133, 197, 232], although seemingly less to CSs [36, 84].

> **Core Message**
>
> › The use of medicaments under occlusion or in folds increases its absorption and allergenic potential. It is not unanimous if atopic and psoriatic patients do sensitize more or less to topical medicaments.

38.3 Clinical Patterns of Contact Reactions

Allergic contact dermatitis is by far the more common and more important clinical entity caused by topical drugs. However, other pathological clinical entities, either through direct cutaneous aggression, by immunoallergic mechanisms or by local or systemic pharmacological effects, may be caused by medicaments (Table 38.2) [60, 113, 240].

38.3.1 Irritant Contact Dermatitis

There are several medicaments that can irritate the skin [60, 94] (Table 38.3). Most are well-known mildly irritant drugs, and their irritancy is usually expected and sometimes desired as part of their therapeutic action – tretinoin, benzoyl peroxide, 5-fluorouracil, dithranol, sulphur compounds and others. The first contact usually does not produce any visual alteration or abnormal subjective symptoms. However, after repeated contact the skin becomes dry, erythematous and scaly, with pruritus or burning sensation, usually confined to the application area. If applied for a longer time, in higher concentrations, or in occluded areas, they may cause acute irritant contact dermatitis with oedema, erythema, vesicles or bullae that may sometimes be difficult to differentiate from allergic contact dermatitis (Fig. 38.1).

Airborne irritant contact dermatitis predominates in exposed areas but, as opposed to photosensitive dermatitis, it does not spare areas such as the upper eyelids, retroauricular folds or sub-mental area.

The subjective irritant sensation of "stinging" may be immediate or delayed and be caused by several drugs.

38.3.2 Contact Urticaria

Since the first reports [194], the contact urticaria syndrome (CUS) has been frequently studied. It includes

Table 38.2 Clinical patterns of eruptions caused by topical medicaments [60, 113, 240]

Allergic contact dermatitis
Irritant contact dermatitis
Photoallergic contact dermatitis
Phototoxic contact dermatitis
Contact urticaria
Photocontact urticaria
Dermographism
Airborne allergic contact dermatitis
Airborne irritant contact dermatitis
Airborne photoallergic contact dermatitis
Airborne phototoxic contact dermatitis
Erythema multiforme-like eruptions
Lichenoid contact dermatitis
Purpuric contact dermatitis
Skin necrosis
Dyschromia
Pustular contact dermatitis
Lymphomatoid contact dermatitis
Acne/folliculitis/rosacea
Granulomatous eruption
Interactions with cutaneous microbial flora
Pharmacological local effects
Systemic side effects

Table 38.3 Topical drugs that can induce irritant contact dermatitis. (Courtesy of [60, 94])

Oxidizing agents	Hydrogen peroxide, benzoyl peroxide, cantharidin, sodium hypochlorite, potassium permanganate, bromine, iodine, povidone iodine
Denaturing agents	Formaldehyde, mercuric chloride
Keratolytic drugs	Salicylic acid, sulphur compounds, resorcinol, pyrogallol
Organic solvents	Alcohols, propylene glycol, ethyl ether, chloroform, acetone
Anti-neoplastic drugs	Carmustine, mechlorethamine, 5-fluorouracil
Other compounds	Quaternary ammonium compounds, tar, dithranol, thimerosal, gentian violet, brilliant green, hexachlorophene, mercurial compounds, chlorhexidine, capsaicin, non-steroidal anti-inflammatory drugs, tretinoin, calcipotriol, urea, lactic acid and other α-hydroxy acids, dimethylsulfoxide, phenol, monobenzone, podophyllotoxin, selenium sulphide, methyl nicotinate

38

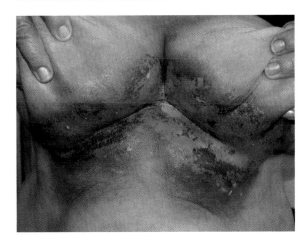

Fig. 38.1 Acute irritant contact dermatitis due to dithranol

the localized cutaneous forms (immunological and non-immunological), as well as a broad spectrum of non-cutaneous involvement (generalized urticaria, asthma and anaphylaxis). The list of medicaments causing immunological contact urticaria (ICU) or non-immunological contact urticaria (NICU) is very long (Table 38.4) [7, 152, 297] (see also Chap. 7). Chlorpromazine has been reported as causing photo-contact urticaria [193].

38.3.3 Other Important Clinical Patterns

Topical medicaments may cause other non-eczematous contact reactions (see Chap. 22). Erythema multiforme-like eruptions or urticarial papular and plaque eruption may be caused by several drugs [60, 62, 106, 113, 240] (Table 38.5). This eruption is usually preceded by an eczematous allergic reaction, which becomes urticarial, disseminates after a few days and persists longer than the initial reaction.

Skin necrosis induced by medicaments is a rare event. Gentian violet and brilliant green may cause necrosis, especially when applied in the genital area [30]. Quaternary ammonium compounds in high concentration, dichlorhexidine, 5-fluorouracil, phenol and povidone iodine have also been incriminated as causing skin necrosis [60].

Purpuric reactions may be due to proflavine [106] and benzoyl peroxide [288]. Aminoglycoside antibiotics

Table 38.4 Topical drugs that can induce ICU and NICU [7, 152, 297]

NICU	ICU
Alcohols	Alcohols
Benzoic acid/sodium benzoate	*Antibiotics*
Benzocaine	Ampicillin
Camphor	Bacitracin
Capsaicin	Cephalosporins
DMSO	Chloramphenicol
Formaldehyde	Clioquinol
Nicotinic acid esters	Gentamicin
Sorbic acid/sorbates	Mezlocillin
Tar extracts	Neomycin
Tincture of benzoin	Penicillin
	Rifamycin
	Streptomycin
	Virginiamycin
	Aescin
	Benzocaine
	Lidocaine
	Carboxymethyl cellulose
	Benzophenone
	Phenothiazines
	Promethazine
	Chlorpromazine
	Levomeprazine
	Non-steroidal anti-inflammatory drugs
	Aminophenazone
	Diclofenac
	Etofenamate
	Ketoprofen
	Loxoprofen
	Propyphenbutazone
	Salicylic acid
	Mechlorethamine
	Ketoconazole
	Clobetasol propionate
	Polyethylene glycol

Table 38.4 (continued)

NICU	ICU
	Polysorbate 60
	Parabens
	Cetyl alcohol
	Nicotine
	Pentamidine
	Pilocarpine
	Polyvinyl pyrrolidone

Table 38.5 Topical drugs inducing erythema multiforme-like eruptions [60, 113, 161, 162, 168, 240]

Ethylenediamine	Phenylbutazone
Pyrrolnitrin	Econazole
Sulphonamides	IDU
Promethazine	Furazolidone
Mephenesin	Nifuroxime
Mafenide	Scopolamine hydrobromide
Proflavine	Mechlorethamine
Clioquinol	Povidone iodine
Chloramphenicol	DNCB
Neomycin	Diphenylcyclopropenone
Lincomycin	Ketoprofen
Vitamin E	Bufexamac
Tea tree oil	

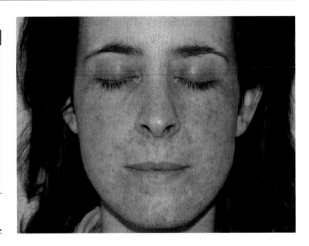

Fig. 38.2 Rosacea-like dermatitis due to long-standing application of a corticosteroid cream on the face

Long-term application of potent CSs to the whole skin promotes skin absorption of large amounts of the drug, which may induce Cushing's syndrome.

The percutaneous absorption of other drugs can rarely provoke toxic systemic effects. The degree of absorption depends on the physicochemical properties of the substance, the use of occlusive dressings, the vehicle in which the substance is incorporated, the drug concentration, the site of application, age, temperature, and the integrity of the skin barrier. Boric acid, carmustine, clindamycin, gentamicin, hexachlophene, lindane, malathion, mercurial compounds, phenol, salicylic acid, and selenium sulphide [60] represent some of the drugs that have been noted to cause systemic toxicity.

can cause lichenoid reactions [186]. Mercury salts may cause either hyper- or hypo-pigmentation [99].

The effects of application of topical CSs, mainly potent fluorinated steroids, over long periods are well known. Women with a seborrhoeic diathesis, using steroids on the face, may develop acneiform or rosaceiform eruptions, perioral dermatitis or hypertrichosis, leading to the so-called "topical drug addiction" [37] (Fig. 38.2). On the face, as well as in other areas, they induce cutaneous atrophy, telangiectasia, purpura, ecchymoses (which evolve into pseudostellate scars), susceptibility to minor trauma, striae distensae and vellus hair growth. When applied on skin infections, mainly tinea, but also other fungal, viral or parasitic diseases, they can mask and aggravate the pre-existing disease, leading, for example, to "tinea incognito" or converting common scabies into the "Norwegian" type.

> **Core Message**
>
> ❯ Beyond allergic contact dermatitis, topical drugs may induce several other clinical patterns, like irritant dermatitis, contact urticaria, erythema multiforme, skin necrosis, purpuric and lichenoid reactions, hyper- and hypo-pigmentation and others.

38.3.4 Allergic Contact Dermatitis

Most contact reactions to medicaments are of the allergic type, whether by direct contact or an airborne

38.4.2 Antibiotics and Antimicrobials

Antibiotics and other antimicrobials and antiseptics
that are used on the skin may cause contact allergy.
Their sensitizing capacity is quite variable, depending
not only on their intrinsic potential, but also on percutaneous penetration, site of application, basic cutaneous state (e.g. chronic venous insufficiency and otitis
externa) and frequency of prescription and use [100].

Aminoglycoside antibiotics, especially neomycin,
form the most important group of topical antibiotics.
Neomycin, which is included in the baseline series, has
a wide use and is rarely used systemically. It is often
combined with topical CSs, not only for use on the skin,
but also in many eye and ear preparations (Fig. 38.3a,
b). This association may mask the neomycin sensitization, due to the corticosteroid anti-inflammatory activity. In most statistics, neomycin appears as the leading
allergenic medicament [10, 17, 20, 61, 213]. Gentamicin,
though is a potent sensitizer [191], is less used and
seems to be less allergenic than neomycin [17, 290],
with which it may cross-react [245]. Occupational sensitization through the contact with bone cements [191]
has been reported. Other less frequently used aminoglycosides are mainly found in ophthalmic and ear
preparations, or sensitize through occupational medical
or veterinary contact – streptomycin, tobramycin, kanamycin, paromomycin, butirosin, ribostamycin, amikacin, sisomicin, framycetin (neomycin B, soframycin).
With the exception of streptomycin, aminoglycosides
often cross-react [17, 100, 164, 191, 243, 245].

Tylosin tartrate, virginiamycin and spiramycin are
mainly of veterinary use. Veterinary surgeons and farmers are those usually affected [135, 292]. Virginiamycin
can cross-react with pristinamycin.

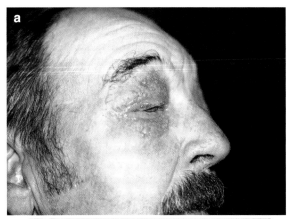
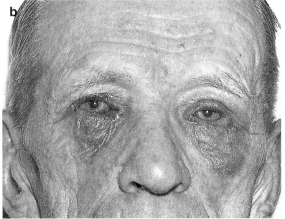

Fig. 38.3 (**a**, **b**) Allergic contact dermatitis from neomycin in eyedrops (**a**) and associated with severe conjunctivitis (**b**) (courtesy of
P.J. Frosch)

Bacitracin causes contact urticaria [74] and contact allergy, especially in leg ulcers/stasis dermatitis
patients [100, 153, 261, 309]. The concomitance of
reactions to both neomycin and polymyxin B is not
due to cross-reaction, but to their frequent association
in topical medicaments [115]. Contact allergy to
chloramphenicol is uncommon and usually due to the
use of eye preparations [267]. As with other antimicrobials, allergy to sodium fusidate seems to occur
especially in leg ulcer patients [213]. Tetracyclines
[244], clindamycin [100] (which may cross-react with
lincomycin), rifamycin [100] and mupirocin [310] are
generally rare sensitizers. Erythromycin base is a
weak sensitizer [81], but its salts (sulphate, stearate
and ethylsuccinate) may more readily induce contact
allergy [204].

38

In the past, penicillin became a frequent sensitizer in some countries, but it is hardly used nowadays topically. Semi-synthetic penicillins and derivatives – ampicillin, amoxycillin, pivampicillin, cloxacillin and cephalosporins (first, second or third generation) – can cause either allergic contact dermatitis [46, 86, 124, 212] or contact urticaria [45] in health care personnel, pharmaceutical industry workers, veterinary surgeons or farmers.

Having been one of the major sensitizers some decades ago [10, 20], topical sulphonamides are now used very little in skin products. They are still present in ophthalmic preparations (sulphathiazol and sulphacetamide) and vaginal creams (sulphathiazol), but reports of sensitization are scarce. Sulphanilamide-containing powders and creams may, however, be a problem in leg ulcer patients. Silver sulphadiazine, marketed in some countries for use on burns, seems to be almost non-allergenic and does not cross-react with other sulphonamides [59].

Nitrofurazone is a local antiseptic used in ointment or lubricated dressings for wounds and burns. It is a well-known sensitizer that can induce very severe reactions in some patients. Clioquinol (Vioform) and chlorquinaldol (Sterosan) are usually combined with CSs in topical preparations. They are weak sensitizers and may cross-react, clioquinol being the more important of the two allergens [5].

One of the most extensively used local antiseptics in the present days is povidone iodine. Besides skin irritation and necrosis, there have been a few reports of contact allergy [201], but in suspected cases investigation must be complete in order to rule out irritant reactions [175]. Thimerosal (thiomersal) contains two sensitizing moieties, mercury and thiosalicylic acid [112]. It is used in merthiolate tincture, and as a preservative in vaccines, toxoids, contact lens solutions and other eye preparations. The relevance of a positive patch test to thimerosal is usually very difficult to establish. Most cases seem to be due either to vaccines or to ophthalmic products [85, 211, 274]. Patients sensitized to the thiosalicylic moiety of thimerosal are at risk of developing photosensitization to piroxicam [44, 112]. Other mercury compounds include merbromin and phenylmercury salts. Merbromin (mercurochrome) had wide use in some countries, but its use has now almost been abandoned; it may cause anaphylaxis [39]. Quaternary ammonium compounds are largely used antiseptics and disinfectants and can cause irritation and necrosis, as well as contact sensitization [3].

Triphenylmethane dyes include gentian violet (pyoctanin), brilliant green, malachite green, methyl green, rosaniline, chrysoidine and eosin. They are rare sensitizers [169, 253].

> ### Core Message
>
> › Neomycin is still a frequent allergen and may cross-react with most aminoglycosides, with the exception of streptomycin. Penicillin and sulphonamides are, currently, rare sensitizers. Bacitracin can cause immediate and delayed reactions and, often, reacts simultaneously with neomycin and polimyxin B.

38.4.3 Antivirals

Tromantadine hydrochloride and acyclovir are the two most widely prescribed antiviral drugs. Tromantadine is a potent sensitizer, with several cases of contact allergy reported [11]. It usually causes a very severe acute exudative eczema around the lips, characteristically in patients who have already used tromantadine several times for the treatment of recurrent herpes simplex (Fig. 38.4). Acyclovir, though much more extensively used, is a weak sensitizer. Some of the cases of contact dermatitis from Zovirax cream are probably due to compound allergy [167]. Due to seemingly poor penetration of acyclovir through the skin, patch tests may be negative or doubtful; scratch-patch tests may

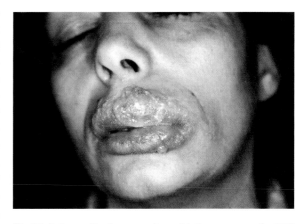

Fig. 38.4 Acute allergic contact dermatitis from tromantadine HCl

be necessary to obtain a positive reaction [222]. Patients with allergic contact dermatitis to acyclovir may develop systemic contact dermatitis to valaciclovir, ganciclovir and famciclovir [26, 177, 293], the only valid alternative being foscarnet and cidofovir [293]. Idoxuridine (IDU) [11] and trifluridine [209] are mainly used in ophthalmologic preparations.

Core Message

> Acyclovir is a weak allergen. Patients sensitized to this antiviral may develop systemic contact dermatitis if administered valaciclovir, ganciclovir or famciclovir.

38.4.4 Antimycotics

Most antimycotics can cause contact allergy; these include hydroxyquinoline, undecylenic acid [12] and its derivatives, pyrrolnitrin, nystatin [49], tolnaftate [111], naftifine [307], amorolfine [78, 172], as well as several imidazole derivatives, for which contact and cross-allergic reactions have been missed because of problems with the correct choice of vehicle for patch testing [66]. An extensive study on the sensitizing capacity (in guinea pigs) of imidazoles [121, 122], triazoles – mostly used in agriculture – [121], and azoles [123] was performed by Hausen et al. and they could demonstrate that imidazoles, the most commonly used antimycotics, have only very weak sensitization properties compared to, for example, naftifine [122]. The most frequently reported imidazoles that caused allergic contact dermatitis [66, 121, 122] are the substances most commonly used, i.e. miconazole, econazole, isoconazole – that may provoke pustular contact dermatitis [179] – and tioconazole [126] (probably due to its use in a 28% concentration in a nail solution) (Fig. 38.5). Croconazole, which is only marketed in the Far East, seems to be a strong allergen, both clinically and experimentally [121]. Clotrimazole considered to be an unusual allergen [51] but reported as an occupational allergen in a nurse [223], sulconazole, ketoconazole, oxiconazole, bifonazole (that showed a moderate sensitizing capacity [121]), enilconazole and fenticonazole [66, 117] have been less frequently reported as causes of contact allergy.

Cross-sensitivity has been reported mainly within the group of the phenylethylimidazoles, for example, between miconazole, econazole and isoconazole as well as sulconazole, and also between isoconazole and tioconazole [66, 73], but not ketoconazole. They do not seem to cross-react with the phenylmethylimidazoles, i.e. clotrimazole, bifonazole and croconazole, for which cross-reactions between them may [71], but not necessarily [262], occur. The more recent reports

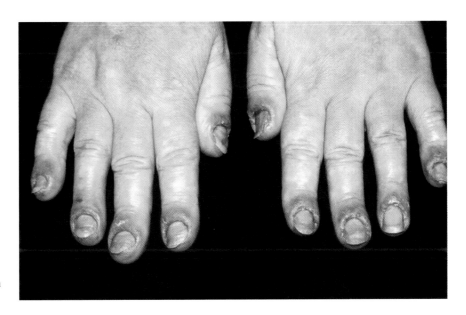

Fig. 38.5 Paronichia due to allergic contact dermatitis from tioconazole nail solution (courtesy of O. Bordalo)

deal with neticonazole [156, 257, 279] (with possible cross-reactivity with econazole and sulconazole [156]), lanoconazole [218, 260, 278, 279], sertaconazole (cross-reactivity to miconazole and econazole) [105] and luliconazole [258, 268]. Patch testing suggested in both cases that luliconazole sensitivity might have been attributable to its dithioacetal structure and revealed that lanoconazole-sensitive individuals have a high risk of reacting to luliconazole as well.

In a recently performed German study [207], 1,254 patients were tested with antifungal allergens, i.e. ciclopiroxolamine, nystatin (only active against yeasts), clotrimazole, croconazole and ketoconazole. Positive reactions were altogether rare, with ciclopiroxolamine yielding the highest number of clearly positive reactions ($n=4$), followed by nystatin and clotrimazole ($n=3$) and croconazole ($n=2$). The results obtained with commercialized products that were tested are more difficult to interpret since other ingredients may also be responsible.

Finally, drug eruptions after systemic administration have been described for example, immediate reactions to ketoconazole [287, 289], systemic reactions due to nystatin – also in lozenges [50] and a generalized exanthematous pustulosis (confirmed by a positive patch test result) to terbinafine [159].

Core Message

> The imidazoles are not strong sensitizers, but as they are very extensively used, several cases have been described. Cross-reaction between them has been reported mainly within the group of phenylethylimidazoles (miconazole, econazole, isoconazole, sulconazole and tioconazole). Systemic contact dermatitis may occur with antimycotics.

38.4.5 Corticosteroids

CSs, which are potent anti-inflammatory and immuno-modulator agents used in the treatment of various inflammatory diseases including allergic diseases, can in some cases produce immediate or delayed hypersensitivity reactions. The first documented allergic

reactions to CSs, following local application and injections of hydrocortisone, were described towards the end of 1950s [14].

Diagnosing an allergic reaction to CSs remains a challenge for clinicians. Its clinical presentation is frequently atypical and tests may be difficult to interpret. Moreover, its frequency is undoubtedly under-estimated. While knowledge of delayed hypersensitivity as a secondary effect of topical CSs (allergic contact eczema) is improving, little is known about immediate and delayed reactions to systemic CSs. It is critical to address such reactions, since appropriate diagnostic work-up should determine potential replacement agents(s) that can still be tolerated by the patient.

The most common sensitization route is through cutaneous use. Locoregional routes, including respiratory (nasal or mouth inhalation), digestive and intra-articular administration, have been less frequently implicated. Sensitization related to systemic administration of a CS, of which the intravenous route is the most common, occurs less frequently [178].

Patients who suffer from a long-term disease are at a higher risk of sensitization when treated with topical CSs: these include chronic eczema, stasis dermatitis, chronic ulceration, chronic actinic dermatitis, facial, anogenital, and hand and foot dermatitis. Changes to the skin barrier and/or a local pro-inflammatory environmental (favouring and priming antigen-presenting cells such as Langerhans cells) are the most likely determining factors.

It is not clear whether atopy represents a risk factor for the development of a CS allergy. Those patients who are allergic to a CS often exhibit co-sensitization to multiple allergens (e.g. preservatives, excipients and antibiotics) [145]. Not unexpectedly, contact allergy to CSs is only rarely occupationally induced.

According to the literature, the prevalence of allergic reactions to CSs is extremely variable. Several factors such as regional differences in prescribing habits (i.e. the types of CSs commonly prescribed and the number of prescriptions given out), awareness of topical CS allergy among medical professionals, patient selection and referral and diagnostic procedures may have an influence.

The literature reports that the frequency of CS allergy following topical application ranges from 0.2 to 0.5% or more. Despite the wide use of inhaled CSs, very few cases of asthmatic patients experiencing allergic reactions have been reported. Isaksson and colleagues [147], who examined patients with asthma or allergic rhinitis who were treated with tixocortol pivalate, observed a CS sensitization rate of 1.4%. Among non-asthmatic patients, however, the rate of sensitization was 0.9% and the difference was not statistically significant. Malik et al [198] were the first to evaluate the incidence of CS allergies in patients with digestive tract inflammation who were treated with steroid enemas. Of 44 patients, 9% tested positive for one or more CS.

Allergic reactions following systemic administration of CSs have rarely been reported in the literature and most often concern isolated cases. The prevalence of such reactions has been estimated to be between 0.1 and 0.3% [92]. About a hundred publications have reported immediate reactions after oral or parenteral administration of CSs, the allergic nature of which was not always proven, while the prevalence of systemic contact dermatitis or systemic allergic dermatitis [270] to CSs has not been examined.

Recognizing CS allergy can be difficult, as its clinical presentation tends to be neither specific nor spectacular (Fig. 38.6): the clinical signs are usually minor or display a completely atypical chronology, which is due to the anti-inflammatory properties of the CS. Indeed, the clinical manifestation of such reaction depends on two competing effects that are of variable intensity and offset in time: the immunological allergic response and the pharmacological "anti-allergic" effect. The lesions may manifest themselves as eczema, exanthema, purpura, urticaria and so on, with type IV or delayed hypersensitivity being much more common than type I or immediate hypersensitivity [14].

Type IV hypersensitivity can be identified by skin tests, mainly patch tests. The principal markers for Cs contact allergy are tixoxortol pivalate (although not for skin use), budesonide and hydrocortisone 17-butyrate, the first two having been introduced to the European baseline series in the early 2000s [143]. A slight difference between the sensitization rate to tixocortol pivalate (2–5%) and to budesonide (1–2%) is reported, but taken together, these two allegens are said to detect nearly 90% of CS allergic patients [13, 14]. However, all CS preparations used by the patient should also be tested, along with their ingredients.

While petrolatum works well for tixocortol pivalate and budesonide, for most CSs, ethanol is the first choice of vehicle [142]. Due to the anti-inflammatory activity of CSs, weakly sensitized patients exhibit an inverse

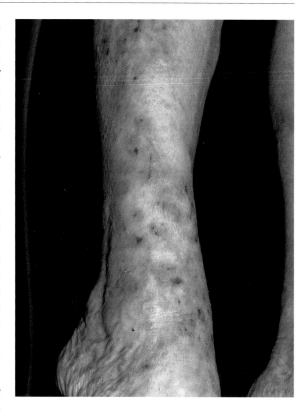

Fig. 38.6 Allergic contact dermatitis to hydrocortisone with minor inflammatory symptoms (courtesy of A. Goossens)

relation between the concentration of the test solution and the rate of positive responses. If the concentration is too low, false negative tests can result, unless the test is applied to eczematous skin. If the concentration is too high, the anti-inflammatory effect dominates and again a false negative result is possible. Comparative studies have shown that the 0.01% budesonide and 0.1% tixocortol pivalate tests will detect most patients being allergic to CSs [146]. According to studies carried out by Isaksson and colleagues [141, 148], however, in some cases even weaker solutions (between 0.02 and 0.002%) are necessary to diagnose patients with contact allergy to budesonide, which has more potent anti-inflammatory properties. Most other CSs are tested at a concentration of 0.1–1% [13]. The anti-inflammatory effect of a CS also influences the reading time. For this reason, numerous authors have proposed readings on day 6 or day 7, or even later [140].

In 1989, based on structural and clinical characteristics, Coopman et al have classified CSs into four reacting groups, namely group A, B, C and D. In 1995

Lepoittevin et al carried out conformational analysis of the observed cross-reactions, which supported this classification and the central role of constituents of the D-ring (Fig. 38.7). Further clinical data led Matura and Goossens to further subdivide group D into two subgroups, i.e. D1 and D2 (Table 38.6). Beside the recognition site of the D-ring influenced by C16, C17 substitutions, Wilkinson et al. considered the A-ring to be a second immune recognition site and halogenation of the CS structure (C6 and/or C9) to be of utmost importance as to the cross-sensitivity patterns observed with CSs [13]. The allergen does not seem to be the CS itself, but a byproduct from its skin metabolism; assuming that all CSs interact with proteins in the same manner, steroid glyoxals or 21-dehydrocorticosteroids (aldehydes), being the principal metabolites, are the most probably haptens that bind to nucleophilic protein residues. It has been shown that steroid glyoxals can bind to any aminoacid except to proline and hydroxyproline. The arginine reaction, however, is clearly predominant and also irreversible: Wilkinson et al. [305] showed that CSs with a greater capacity to bind to arginine do have stronger allergenic properties and, recently, Berl et al. [29] confirmed that steroids were indeed selectively reacting with arginine to form important adducts.

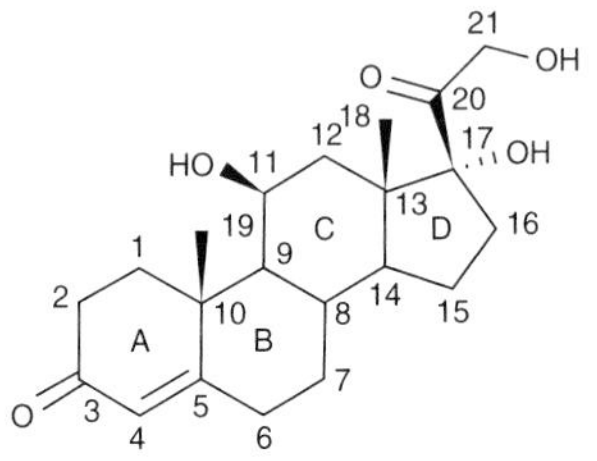

The CSs in groups C and D1 have provoked very few allergic reactions and usually do not interact with CSs from the other groups. In mometasone furoate, for example, the specific configuration of the C17 lateral chain explains the low number of positive skin reactions observed. Fluticasone propionate possesses not only a fluorine atom at C9, but also a methyl substitution at C16 and a unique structure at C17 that prevents the hapten-protein bond from forming. The risk of primary sensitization to this CS is extremely low and its cross-reactions with other CSs are weak. The CSs in group D2, on the other hand, along with those in group A and also budesonide, produce allergy more frequently. These agents often cross-react, both within the same group and with agents belonging to other groups.

The CSs of group D2 are rapidly transformed in the skin, becoming analogs with free C21 and/or C17 hydroxyls. Thus, while the agent applied to the skin

Fig. 38.7 Chemical structure of hydrocortisone with the conventional numbering of atoms

Table 38.6 Classification of corticosteroids based on cross-reaction patterns

	Characteristics of the group	Typical members	Possible cross-reactions with corticosteroids outside the group
Group A	No methyl substitution on C16, no side chain on C17, possibly short side chain on C21	Cloprednol, fludrocortisone acetate, hydrocortisone acetate, hydrocortisone, methylprednisolone, prednisolone, tixocortol pivalate	D2 group labile steroids: hydrocortisone aceponate, hydrocortisone-17-butyrate, methyl-prednisolone aceponate, prednicarbate
Group B	Cis diol or ketal function on C16 and C17, possibly a side chain on C21	Budesonide (R-isomer), amcinonide, desonide, fluocinolone acetonide, triamcinolone acetonide	–
Group C	Methyl substitution on C16, no side chain on C17, possibly a side chain on C21	Betamethasone, dexamethasone, flumethasone pivalate, halomethasone	–
Group D1	Methyl substitution on C16 (so far halogenation on the basic structure), side chain ester on C17 and often also on C21	Betamethasone dipropionate, betamethasone-17-valerate, clobetasol propionate, fluticasone propionate, mometasone furoate	–
Group D2	No methyl substitution on C16 (up to now no halogenation of the four-ring structure), side chain ester on C17, possibly a side chain on C21	Hydrocortisone aceponate, hydrocortisone buteprate, hydrocortisone-17-butyrate, methyl-prednisolone aceponate, prednicarbate	Budesonide S-isomer, Group A corticosteroids

is one of the "labile ester" CSs (D2), its metabolite corresponds more closely to group A. One example of intracutaneous biometabolization is the conversion of hydrocortisone 17-butyrate (group D2) to hydrocortisone 21-butyrate, followed by an enzymatic transformation into hydrocortisone (group A). This illustrates the typical cross-reaction observed between group A and group D2. Budesonide can be considered a unique case in the following sense: its acetal function is actually an equal mixture of the R and S diastereoisomers. Both R and S diastereoisomers can develop cross-reactions with group B CSs, but only the S diastereoisomer can cross-react with group D2 CSs. An analysis of their configuration shows that while the R isomer exhibits symmetry that is characteristic of the B group, the S isomer can take on an asymmetric aspect. The result is a large hydrophobic "cavity" at the C17 ester function, similar to group D2 agents. Some patients sensitized to CSs respond positively to skin tests with other steroids, such as the sex-hormonal steroids, which is in most cases an expression of cross-reactivity. However, CS allergy can induce an allergy to, for example, endogenous progesterone, for which the clinical presentation is a generalized eczematous eruption that gets worse during the pre-menstrual period, the so-called autoimmune progesterone dermatitis (AIPD). On the other hand, any patient presenting symptoms compatible with AIPD should also be tested for CS allergy.

The ABCD classification, however, cannot explain all observed cross-reactions and possible adjustments need to be considered. For example, according to the purely structural analysis of CSs and, recently, also by the analysis of patch tests results obtained in a large series of patients tested with many different CSs [13], the existence of a separate group C cannot be justified.

Contact allergy to CSs is an important problem in patients suffering from (chronic) dermatitis, and certain molecules such as those belonging to A, B and D2 (the labile) esters are more apt to induce sensitization than others (e.g. group D1). Moreover, testing with the CSs allergy markers in the baseline, as well with the CSs used by the patient, is necessary.

38.4.6 Antihistamines

Topical antihistamines are mainly used for their antipruritic properties. However, their sensitizing capacity greatly exceeds their beneficial effects. Beyond that, oral antihistamines or chemically related substances may induce systemic contact dermatitis in patients topically sensitized. Thus, they are now becoming less frequently used. Diphenhydramine (which belongs to the ethanolamine group) can cause allergic [127] and photoallergic contact dermatitis [308]; chorpheniramine is a sensitizer, either in topical application [125] or in eye drops [228] and promethazine and chlorpromazine (which are phenothiazines) are well-known sensitizers and photosensitizers (Fig. 38.8). Promethazine cream still exists in some European countries and several cases of allergy and photoallergy are seen every year. Chlorpromazine, which is now much less employed, previously sensitized mainly health care personnel handling this medicament and pharmaceutical industry workers [38].

> **Core Message**
>
> › Allergic contact dermatitis to CSs is more common than previously judged and should be suspected whenever a chronic dermatitis is exacerbated by or does not respond to local corticosteroid therapy. Four groups of cross-reacting molecules have been proposed. It has been recommended that budesonide and tixocortol pivalate should be added to the baseline series as screening agents for corticosteroid allergy.

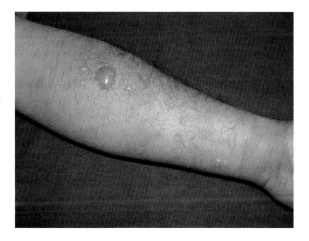

Fig. 38.8 Photoallergic contact dermatitis from prometazine

38

Doxepin, a tricyclic antidepressive drug with antihistamine activity, has been widely used for pruritus relief. Several cases of allergic and systemic contact dermatitis have been reported [32, 33].

38.4.7 Non-steroidal Anti-Inflammatory Drugs

Topical NSAIDs have been introduced onto the market in the past few decades for the treatment of soft tissue trauma, inflammatory and musculoskeletal disorders and some inflammatory skin diseases, as an alternative to topical CSs. They have the advantage of being simple to apply, of having low systemic absorption and of avoiding the well-known systemic side effects [1, 227]. However, they do cause frequent local side effects, which led to the withdrawal of some of these substances from the market – benoxaprofen, suprofen, and in some countries, phenylbutazone and oxyphenbutazone.

They belong to eight different groups [227]: salicylates, pyrazolone derivatives, p-aminophenol derivatives, indomethacin and sulindac, arylacanoic acid, tolmetins, arylpropionic acid derivatives and oxicans.

Cutaneous side effects include skin irritation, phototoxicity, contact urticaria, erythema multiforme-like eruptions and, mainly, allergic and photoallergic contact dermatitis. Since many of these compounds may also be used systemically, the possibility of the development of systemic contact dermatitis, in patients topically sensitized, must always be born in mind [15, 174, 235].

With the exception of pyrazolones and bufexamac, which are used in northern European countries, most of the former reports in the literature were coming from the Mediterranean area. This could partially be explained by the earlier extensive use of these drugs in these countries and also by the higher UV radiance in southern Europe, contributing to the development of photosensitization [138]. However, they are currently used in many other countries and recent reports from the northern Europe can be found [134, 205].

Arylpropionic acid derivatives, mainly ketoprofen, are responsible for the majority of cases of allergy and photoallergy being reported to date (Fig. 38.9a, b). Since the first reports [6, 284] to the present day [2, 68, 134, 180], several dozen cases have been published. Cross-reactivity of ketoprofen with other drugs of the same

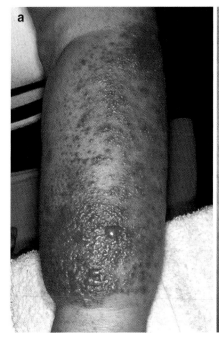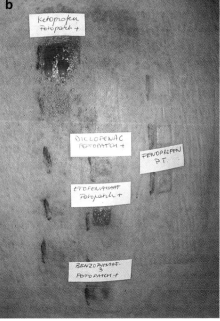

Fig. 38.9 (**a**, **b**) Photoallergic contact dermatitis from ketoprofen (**a**). Positive photopatch test to ketoprofen and related materials (**b**) (courtesy of A. Goossens)

group is controversial. Although cross-reactivities have been reported for ibuproxam [55], flubiprofen [155, 215] and suprofen [174, 264], they were not found by Le Coz et al. [180], who regarded them as concomitant reactions. These authors suggested that benzophenone is the sensitizing moiety of ketoprofen, which could explain the almost constant cross-reaction with tiaprofenic acid [15, 233] and with unsubstituted benzophenone, and the frequent cross-reaction with fenofibrate [15, 134, 254] and other monosubstituted benzophenones, such as oxybenzone [15, 134, 138, 151, 154].

Ibuproxam is another arylpropionic acid derivative, which sensitizes mainly by contact [233, 234]. Isolated reports of allergy or photoallergy to other NSAIDs of this group include ibuprofen [283], suprofen [174], piketoprofen [104, 221] and tiaprofenic acid [180]. Dexketoprofen is also an arylpropionic acid derivative NSAID that induces photoallergic contact dermatitis and cross-reacts with ketoprofen [54, 102, 282], but not with piketoprofen [134].

From the other groups, some emphasis should be given to etofenamate, which can cause contact dermatitis [132, 295], contact urticaria [236] and photocontact allergy [248]. It can cross-react with flufenamic acid and other anthranilic derivatives [295]. Bufexamac, which is widely used in some northern countries as an alternative to topical CSs, seems to have a high sensitizing capacity [1, 173] and may cause erythema multiforme-like eruptions [168]. Some years ago, it has been suggested that it should be added to the standard series in some countries [173] because of the high rate of sensitization and the serious clinical pictures of bufexamac allergy, but the use of this drug should be critically reassessed [238]. Diclofenac, which is now being used for the treatment of actinic keratoses, and aceclofenac have also been reported as sensitizers and photosensitizers [103, 160, 171, 237].

Benzydamine hydrochloride is mainly a photoallergen [40]. Piroxicam is usually a systemic photosensitizer in patients allergic to the thiosalicylic acid moiety of thimerosal [44, 79], but can also sensitize and photosensitize topically [234].

Indomethacin [27] and the pyrazolone derivatives are now less used, but can cause allergic contact dermatitis [235, 300] and erythema multiforme-like reactions [161]. Thiocolchicoside, not exactly an NSAID, is a muscle relaxant that was reported as a contact allergen [88] and photoallergen [89].

Core Message

> Non-steroidal anti-inflammatory drugs are very widely used and are frequent sensitizers. Ketoprofen induces allergic and photoallergic contact dermatitis and cross-reacts with arylpropionic acid derivatives, tiaprofenic acid, as well as with benzophenone, oxybenzone and fenofibrate. Bufexamac is strongly allergenic and its use should, probably, be discontinued.

38.4.8 Ingredients of the Vehicles

Active products are incorporated in vehicles, which may contain several different substances, with different purposes – preservatives, emollients, emulsifiers, humectants, antioxidants, fragrances – which may also induce contact allergy.

Sensitization to white and yellow petrolatum is rare [48, 63], but white petrolatum, which is purer than yellow petrolatum, seems to be less allergenic [10]. Lanolin is a natural product from sheep fleece and consists of a complex mixture of sterols (wool wax alcohols), fatty alcohols and fatty acids, whose composition varies from time to time and from place to place [8]. It is an important sensitizer in patients with long-standing eczemas, especially in leg ulcer patients, in whom it is usually one of the main allergens (Fig. 38.10). However, it seems to be a very weak allergen when used on non-eczematous skin or in cosmetics [8, 166, 299]. The allergen fraction resides mainly in the wool wax alcohols. Therefore, 30% wool wax alcohols in petrolatum is the recommended concentration for patch testing. Acetylated lanolin [252], dewaxed lanolin, hydrogenated lanolin [224] and purified anhydrous lanolin [709] have been claimed to cause less sensitization, although they may reduce the effectiveness of lanolin as an excipient.

Propylene glycol (PPG) is a viscous hygroscopic liquid. It may cause irritant and allergic contact dermatitis, as well as NICU and subjective or sensory irritation [96]. PPG patch test reactions are often difficult to evaluate and reports of contact allergy in the literature must, therefore, be interpreted with caution. Cases of allergy to PPG in corticosteroid creams, EEC electrodes and gel and other creams have been reported

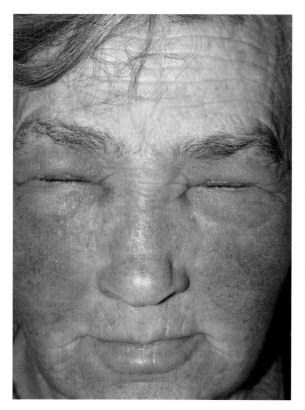

Fig. 38.10 Ectopic allergic contact dermatitis to lanolin contained in an emolient cream applied to stasis dermatitis

[114, 304]. Patients sensitized topically through medicaments usually can tolerate cosmetics preserved with parabens – the paraben paradox [80].

Sorbic acid, which induces NICU and contact allergy [239], chlorocresol [225] and non-oxynols [65] are other preservatives reported as causes of contact allergy.

Formaldehyde and formaldehyde-releasers, isothiazolinones and methyldibromoglutaronitrile, as well as a few other preservatives are mainly used in cosmetics (see Chap. 32). Finally, many topical medicaments may contain unnecessary fragrances, which may induce iatrogenic allergic contact dermatitis. In a recent report from Belgium, 10% of all topical pharmaceutical products were found to contain a total of 66 different fragrance substances [220].

> **Core Message**
>
> › Lanolin is an important allergen in patients with stasis dermatitis and leg ulcers, but it rarely induces allergy when used in non-eczematous skin or in cosmetics. Similarly, parabens may be safely used in cosmetics, but can induce sensitization in patients with long-standing eczemas.

[47, 75, 90]. Polyethylene glycols (PEG) are the condensation products of glycols with ethylene oxide, with variable molecular weight (200–6,000 Da), depending on the condensation degree. Their sensitizing capacity is higher for lower molecular weights [16]. Emulsifiers and emollients like long-chain aliphatic fatty alcohols – lauryl, myristyl, oleyl, cetyl and stearyl alcohols – may sensitize, especially in leg ulcer patients [157, 230]. Oleyl alcohol seems to be the stronger sensitizer [275]. Contact sensitivity to other emulsifiers, like sorbitan sesquioleate (Arlacel 83) [200], sorbitan stearate and oleate (Span 60 and 80) and polysorbates (Tween 40 and 80), has also been reported [119, 273].

Parabens are the most widely used preservatives, either in cosmetics or in topical medicaments. There are four esters (methyl, ethyl, propyl and butyl), which are used in combination, mainly methyl and propyl esters, in concentrations up to 0.1–0.3%. Some decades ago, they were used in much higher concentrations (up to 5%), but in the currently used concentrations, the benefits largely exceed the risks of sensitization, which remains at about 0.5–1% of all patch-tested patients

38.4.9 Other Allergens

Several other topical drugs, either in therapeutic or occupational use, may sensitize. Psoriatic patients may become topically sensitized, which can aggravate and possibly be, in some cases, a trigger factor for their skin disease [133]. Although extensively used, CSs seem rarely to sensitize these patients [84, 197]; however two such cases have been reported by Heule et al. [133]. More often, tars [36, 133], dithranol [36, 41, 197], calcipotriol [95, 229, 311] and tacalcitol [163] are the main offenders. Patients sensitive to calcipotriol can tolerate calcitriol and tacalcitol [87].

A case of allergic contact dermatitis to pimecrolimus has been reported [247] as well as another to tacrolimus [256], with cross-reaction to pimecrolimus.

Anti-neoplastic drugs may induce contact urticaria (cysplatine [250] and mechlorethamine [57]) and allergic contact dermatitis (5-fluorouracil [9] (Fig. 38.11), mitomycin C [285], mechlorethamine [298] and azathioprine [35]).

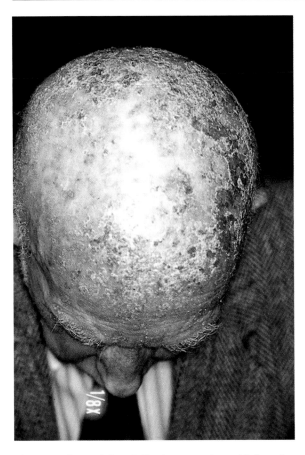

Fig. 38.11 Severe infected allergic contact dermatitis from flu-orouracil ointment used for the treatment of actinic keratoses (courtesy of P.J. Frosch)

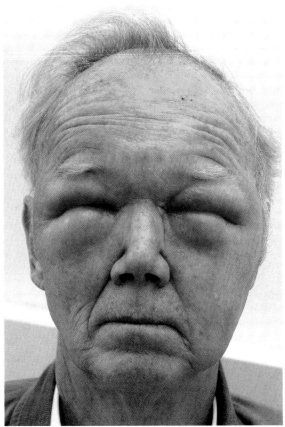

Fig. 38.12 Severe allergic facial dermatitis after 2nd treatment with Metvix photodynamic therapy for actinic keratoses of the scalp (courtesy of K.E. Andersen)

Other possible allergenic topical drugs include pro-flavine [108], minoxidil [266, 272] (which can also photosensitize [272] and cause pigmentation [276]), metronidazole [294], retinoic acid [19], zinc pyrithione [231], salicylic acid [109], acaricides like crotamiton [24], benzyl benzoate and mesulfen [206], resorcinol [82], ethanol [226], benzoyl peroxide, mainly when used for leg ulcer treatment [4] and methyl aminolevulinate (Metvix®) (Fig. 38.12) [120].

Topical traditional Chinese medicaments are largely sold as OTC products, not only in the Far East, but also in Asian communities in some European countries and in the USA. The components usually include terpenes, salicylates and essential oil extracts [187]. They may irritate [183] and sensitize [22, 184, 187]. Colophony, fragrance and myrrh seem to be rather frequent aller-gens in these preparations [22, 170, 185, 190]. Four patients who reacted to five Chinese medicaments were also allergic to fragrance mix, and three to *Myroxylon pereirae* (balsam of Peru), which strongly

suggests cross-sensitization with the plant extracts contained in these medicaments [187]. In a study con-ducted in Taiwan, thirty patients were tested with 27 traditional Chinese crude drugs and other selected material. Fifteen out of the 30 patients reacted to, at least, one of 23 crude drugs; seven were positive to *M. pereirae* resin and six to colophony, which was a much higher incidence than in the patients without contact dermatitis to Chinese medicaments [43].

> **Core Message**
>
> › Traditional Chinese medicaments can induce sensitization. They contain several different chemical products, colophony, fragrances and myrrh being the main sensitizers.

38

38.4.10 Transdermal Therapeutic Systems

These therapeutic devices were introduced to the market more than two decades ago, and an increasing number of drugs are being used this way. They have made possible effective rate-controlled transcutaneous administration of the drugs. In addition, gastro-intestinal absorption and first-pass hepatic metabolism are avoided and an improved compliance, with decreased administration cycle, is obtained. However, they also have some disadvantages. The effect of occlusion for 1–7 days may induce miliaria and irritant contact dermatitis [216], and these conditions predispose to inducing hypersensitivity to one or more components [136, 137, 216].

There are now reports of allergy to seven different transdermal therapeutic systems. Contact allergy may be due to a component of the adhesive layer – ethanol, hydroxypropyl cellulose, polyisobutylene, methacrylates – or, more commonly, to the drug itself (Fig. 38.13) – scopolamine, clonidine, nitroglycerin, estradiol and norethisterone, nicotine, testosterone [216] and buprenorphine [139].

Core Message

> The occlusion these systems provoke predisposes to inducing hypersensitivity. Several different drugs have been reported to cause allergy – scopolamine, clonidine, nitroglycerin, estradiol, norethisterone, nicotine, testosterone and buprenorphine.

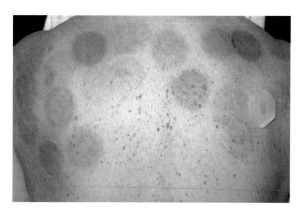

Fig. 38.13 Allergic contact dermatitis to a transdermal device containing rivastigmin (courtesy of M. Goncalo)

38.5 Sites at Risk

Several skin sites, for one reason or another, may be at special risk of developing contact sensitization. They are usually sites where skin conditions are prone to be chronic and, for that reason, many topical medicaments are applied over the course of time. Besides that, particular anatomical and pathological conditions, or special application methods, can increase skin penetration, which also increases the sensitizing capacity of pharmaceutical products. In this short review, we will consider special sites and pathological conditions – ophthalmic and ear, nose and throat (ENT) preparations, anogenital dermatoses and stasis dermatitis and leg ulcers.

38.5.1 Ophthalmic and ENT Preparations

Such medicaments are quite a common cause of contact sensitization [42, 129–131, 267]. Patients with glaucoma who are chronically treated with several ophthalmic drugs are likely to become sensitized. Symptoms may be limited to the eye (allergic contact conjunctivitis) or may involve the periocular skin and the eyelids. Allergic contact conjunctivitis often goes undiagnosed, since it usually occurs in patients who are already affected by ocular inflammation due to other causes and its clinical features are not specific. Clinical examination reveals pronounced vasodilatation and chemosis of the conjunctiva. Watery discharge and papillary response can be present. Possible complications include punctate keratitis and corneal opacities.

Patch tests should be carried out with the eye preparations used by the patient and their individual ingredients (Table 38.7). Patch testing only the preparations may give false-negative results, especially when the responsible allergen is a preservative. To increase patch test sensitivity, pre-treatment with sodium lauryl sulphate may be useful [52]. The diagnosis of allergic contact conjunctivitis may be confirmed by a provocative test with the responsible eye preparation.

Both preservatives and active ingredients may produce contact sensitization. Preservatives are certainly the most important sensitizers in eye drops, and since each preservative is contained in a large number of ophthalmic preparations, not only does allergic

Table 38.7 Substances reported to have caused contact allergy in ophthalmics (modified from [42, 93, 129–131, 267])

Preservatives

Benzalkonium chloride
Benzethonium chloride
Chlorhexidine gluconate
Cetalkonium chloride
Parabens
Phenylmercuric nitrate
Sorbic acid
Thimerosal

β-blockers

Befunolol
Betaxolol
Carteolol
Levobunolol
Metipranol
Metoprolol
1-Pentbutol
Timolol

Mydriatics

Apraclonidine
Atropine
Brimonidine
Cyclopentolate
Dipivalyl-epinefrine
Homatropine
Phenylephrine
Scopolamine
Tropicamide

Antibiotics

Bacitracin
Cefradine
Chloramphenicol
Gentamicin
Kanamycin
Neomycin
Oxytetracycline
Penicillin
Polymyxin B
Sodium colistimethate
Sulphathiazole
Tobramycin
Vancomycin

Antiviral drugs

Idoxiuridine
Trifluridine
β-interferon

Antihistaminics

N-acyl-aspartyl glutamic acid (NAAGA-DCI)
Amlexanox
Chlorpheniramine
Ketotifen
Pheniramine maleate
Sodium cromoglycate

Anaesthetics

Benzocaine
Procaine
Oxybuprocaine
Proxymetacaine
Proparacaine
Tetracaine

Enzymatic cleaners

Papaine
Tegobetaine L7

Antioxidants

Pirenoxone
Sodium bisulphite

Carbonic anhydrase inhibitors

Dorzolamide

Prostaglandins

Latanoprost

Mucolytics

N-acetylcysteine

Others

Apraclonidine
Bismuth oxide
Boric acid
Brominidine
D-Penicillamine
Diclofenac
Dorzolamide
Echothiopate iodine
ε-aminocaproic acid
Pilocarpine
Prednisolone
Resorcinol
Rubidium iodide
Tolazoline
Trometanol

conjunctivitis due to these compounds frequently go undetected, but it can actually be prolonged by the very eye drops that are prescribed to relieve the patient's ocular discomfort. Thimerosal sensitization is probably the main allergological problem in eye drop users, as it is also in contact lens wearers [274]. Preservative-free monodose eye drops are now available for the most important ophthalmic ingredients.

Active ingredients of the ophthalmic products that may cause sensitization include β-adrenergic blocking agents [150], mydriatics, antibiotics, antiviral drugs, antihistamines, anti-inflammatory

38

drugs, CSs, anaesthetics, carbonic anhydrase inhibitors, mucolytics and prostaglandins [42, 93, 129–131, 267].

ENT patients, namely those suffering from otitis externa, do also sensitize quite often. The use of medicaments on inflamed skin plus an occlusive effect probably account for this high rate of sensitization. Aminoglycoside antibiotics (neomycin, framycetin and gentamycin) are responsible for most of the reactions, other allergens being less important – preservatives, antiseptics and CSs [158, 210]. Several cases of allergic contact dermatitis to Cerumenex®, a preparation used to dissolve earwax, have been reported. The allergen – triethanolamine polypeptide oleate condensate – can also be present in shampoos [62, 249].

38.5.2 Anogenital Dermatoses

Patients with chronic vulval dermatoses, mainly pruritus vulvae, lichen sclerosus and lichen simplex chronicus, frequently apply several topical preparations that may contribute to maintain, prolong and aggravate the local symptomatology. Vulval skin is hyper-reactive to local irritants [34], which in conjunction with the local conditions – occlusion, friction, high temperature and moisture – and an increased permeability of vulvovaginal mucosae compared to that of keratinized skin [72] are factors that predispose to inducing sensitization. Contact allergy incidence in these patients is high (29–58%) [188, 189, 203, 296, 301] and is higher in patients with simultaneous anogenital dermatoses [25, 110].

Fragrances and topical medicaments are the main relevant allergens. Among topical drugs, antibiotics – particularly neomycin, LA, CSs, antiseptics and preservatives should be highlighted. In a few cases contact urticaria to latex (from condoms) and protein contact dermatitis from seminal fluid must be suspected [219].

Patients with pruritus ani and haemorrhoids are submitted to the same local and general conditions, as well as to the application of multiple topical drugs. Therefore, allergic contact eczema is frequently seen in these patients [25, 110]. LA are, by far, the more common allergens [25, 182, 192, 280], but several other topical drugs or components of medicaments have been reported as contact allergens in this area – CSs, nifuratel, sodium metabisulphite, glyceryl trinitrate, enoxolone, trimebutine and bufexamac [238]. This induced a generalized

eruption, "baboon syndrome", similar to the one induced by 5-aminosalicylic acid enemas [98].

> **Core Message**
>
> › A hyper-reactive skin mucosa, in conjunction with local conditions like occlusion and high temperature, and an increased permeability are factors that predispose to sensitization in these patients. LA are the more common allergens, but antibiotics, CSs, antiseptics and preservatives should not be forgotten.

38.5.3 Stasis Dermatitis and Leg Ulcer Patients

Stasis dermatitis and leg ulcer patients have a well-known increased risk of becoming sensitized. The long course of these pathological conditions, the damage to the skin barrier and the use of occlusive bandages promoting skin penetration are all factors that favour polysensitization. There is usually a very high incidence of medicament contact allergy in these patients, varying in different series from 58 to 86% [21, 61, 97, 149, 195, 246, 269, 306, 309].

The more important allergen groups are the following:

- Myroxylon pereirae and fragrances
- Lanolin – despite all the polemics about its sensitizing capacity, lanolin remains a constant finding as one of the main sensitizers in these patients
- Antibiotics and other chemotherapeutic agents – neomycin, bacitracin, polymyxin B, chloramphenicol, nitrofurazone, clioquinol, sodium fusidate
- Corticosteroids (Fig. 38.14)
- Preservatives and antiseptics – parabens, benzalkonium chloride, cetrimide, povidone iodine, benzoyl peroxide
- Emollients and emulsifiers – cetearyl alcohol (Lanette O), Lanette N and Lanette E, sorbitan sesquioleate and others
- Topical traditional Chinese medicaments

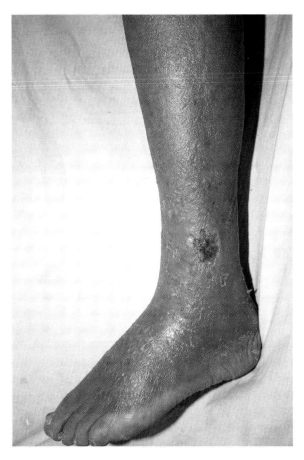

Fig. 38.14 Allergic contact dermatitis from methylprednisolone aceponate in a patient with leg ulcer (courtesy of O. Bordalo)

In the last two decades, new wound dressings, such as hydrocolloids, hydrogels, alginates and polyurethane foams, are being used with increasing frequency. They are generally well tolerated, but can occasionally cause irritant contact dermatitis. Some publications report allergic contact dermatitis from components of these dressings, mainly from hydrocolloids. Pentalin (pentaerythritol ester of hydrogenated rosin), a tackifying agent that usually cross-reacts with colophony, and Vistanex (polyisobutylene), another tackifier, are the main allergens reported [67, 199, 251]. PPG proved to be the sensitizer in patients allergic to hydrogels [97, 214]. Carboxymethyl cellulose in a hydrocolloid dressing induced a generalized urticarial rash [152]. Other possible allergens are rubber additives (thiurams and carbamates) in rubber-containing bandages [53, 149, 246].

Core Message

> A high percentage of stasis dermatitis and leg ulcer patients are contact allergic to several topical drugs – fragrances, lanolin, topical antibiotics, CSs and emulsifiers are the main allergens. Some components of recent wound dressings may rarely sensitize.

38.6 Systemic Contact Dermatitis

Systemic contact dermatitis or systemic allergic dermatitis, as recently has been proposed [270], is a very important matter which is dealt with much more detail elsewhere in this textbook (Chap. 17). It is an inflammatory skin disease that may develop from the systemic administration of a substance in patients topically sensitized to it or to a chemically related substance [208]. The route of administration may be oral, rectal, vaginal, parenteral, intra-articular, by inhalation or through percutaneous penetration.

Drugs are, by far, the most frequent causes of systemic contact dermatitis and, because of the possibility of severe generalized reactions, one should always bear this clinical entity in mind. The more important drugs and chemically related substances that may cause systemic contact dermatitis are listed in Table 38.8.

Systemic contact dermatitis may assume several different clinical cutaneous manifestations, which in some severe cases may be accompanied by general symptomatology, like fever, malaise, headache, arthralgia, nausea, vomiting, diarrhoea or even syncope [60, 208, 241, 270]:

- Flare-up of previous eczema or patch-test reaction sites
- Vesicular hand eczema, with or without erythema, localized to the palms, volar aspects and sides of the fingers
- Generalized maculopapular rash – this is the commonest eruption, which may become more severe and lead to erythroderma (Fig 38.15)
- Erythema multiforme, purpura, vasculitis
- Generalized acute exanthematic pustulosis
- Urticaria and anaphylaxis

38

- The "baboon syndrome" – this well-recognized syndrome has a characteristic distribution pattern, with diffuse pink or dark violet erythema of the buttocks and inner thighs, like an inverted triangle or V-shaped; sometimes the axillae are also involved. Several drugs may cause the baboon syndrome, particularly ampicillin, erythromycin, other antibiotics and mercury

Table 38.8 Drugs and chemically related substances that may cause systemic contact dermatitis [60, 208, 241, 270]

Topical drugs	Substances (groups) that can induce systemic contact dermatitis
Benzocaine	Para-amino compounds
Cinchocaine	Cinchocaine
Clindamycin	Clindamycin
Chloramphenicol	Chloramphenicol
Erythromycin	Erythromycin and other macrolides
Gentamicin	Neomycin and other aminiglycoside antibiotics
Neomycin	Aminoglycoside antibiotics, except streptomycin
Norfloxacin	Clioquinol
Pristinamycin	Neomycin and other aminoglycoside antibiotics
Penicillin/semi-synthetic penicillins	Penicillin/semi-synthetic penicillins and synthetic penicillins
Sodium fusidate	Fusidic acid
Sulphonamides	Sulphonamides, sulphonylureas, para-amino compounds
Acyclovir	Acyclovir
Valaciclovir	Acyclovir
Famciclovir	Acyclovir
Mercury compounds	Mercury compounds (organic and inorganic)
Thimerosal	Thimerosal, piroxicam
Halogenated hydroxyquinolines	Vioform, chlorquinaldol
Iodine	Iodides, iodinated organic compounds
Antimycotic imidazoles	Antimycotic imidazoles, metronidazole
Nystatin	Nystatin
Terbinafine	Terbinafine
Corticosteroids	Corticosteroids
Phenothiazines	Phenothiazines (antihistamines and other)
Diphenhydramine	Diphenhydramine
Ethylenediamine	Ethylenediamine anti-histamines (hydroxyzine), aminophylline
Doxepin	Doxepin
Non-steroidal anti-inflammatory drugs	Non-steroidal anti-inflammatory drugs
Propylene glycol	Propylene glycol (in foods)
Parabens	Parabens
Sorbic acid	Sorbic acid, sorbates
Mitomycin C	Mitomycin C
5-Fluorouracil	5-Fluorouracil
Ephedrine	Pseudoephedrine
Pseudoephedrine	Ephedrine, phenylephrine
Clonidine	Clonidine
Nitroglycerin	Nitroglycerin
Captopril	Captopril
Estradiol	Estradiol
Ethyl alcohol	Alcohol-containing medicaments and beverages
Methyl salicylate	Acetyl salicylic acid
Vitamins B1/C	Vitamins B1/C
Vitamin B6	Vitamin B6

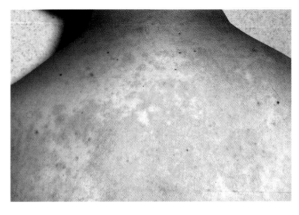

Fig. 38.15 Systemic reaction to an injection of methylprednisolone in a patient previously sensitized by a topical preparation containing the same corticosteroid (courtesy of A. Goossens)

> ### Core Message
>
> > Several topical medicaments can induce systemic contact dermatitis in sensitized patients, if administered by other route. Multiple different clinical patterns may be seen, "Baboon" syndrome being a well-recognized manifestation that can be provoked by several medicaments.

Mercury may induce other exanthematic reactions, such as mercury exanthema – a diffuse symmetrical erythema predominantly of major flexures – and even acute generalized exanthematic pustulosis. These eruptions are currently much less common than some years ago.

38.7 Diagnosis and Prognosis

Correct diagnosis of the many cutaneous drug reactions is not always an easy task. Non-allergic reactions are in most cases diagnosed on a presumptive basis, according to the clinical history and course, with reference to the available literature. The evaluation of immediate reactions (ICU/NICU) should follow the test procedures suggested by Amin et al. [7]. Other allergic non-eczematous patterns, like erythema multiforme, purpura or lymphomatoid reactions, may be diagnosed by patch tests, although patch test reactions are usually eczematous, not reproducing the clinical features.

In cases of suspected allergic contact dermatitis, besides the history and the whole clinical picture, patch tests are of utmost importance. The patient must be tested with all and every medicament he has applied, as well as all the active principles and other suspected substances. This may prove rather difficult in many instances, because patients often use many different medicaments and, in cases of ectopic dermatitis, the offending drugs may be disregarded.

Several difficulties arise in testing these patients:

- Some allergenic drugs are also irritants or, at least, marginal irritants – PPG, dithranol, calcipotriol, 5-fluorouracil, some counterirritants and others. Patch test interpretation may be quite difficult and false-positive reactions may be misinterpreted
- Most commercial medicaments have a complex composition. False-negative reactions may be expected to the whole medicament, if the allergenic substance is used at a low concentration in the final product
- The possibility of testing all the components of a commercial product depends largely on the manufacturer's goodwill. This may make the identification of individual allergens impossible
- Contact allergy to some medicaments may be due to compound allergy. Here again, the identification of the allergenic substance may prove a hard task
- Correct concentrations and vehicles for patch testing have not yet been determined for many drugs, which can lead to false-positive/negative reactions. In the case of a positive reaction to an uncommon allergen, the use of serial dilutions and patch tests in controls is mandatory
- In polysensitized patients, the occurrence of an excited skin syndrome must not be overlooked

Patients with medicament contact allergy usually have a good prognosis. However, in some circumstances, there is a high propensity for relapse – in patients with long-standing eczemas this is a rather common phenomenon due to possible cross-reactions with other drugs, the difficulty in completely avoiding some allergens like lanolin or the possibility of systemic contact dermatitis.

38.8 Appendix: Allergens in Medicaments

(*pet.* petrolatum, *aq.* aqueous, *eth.* ethanol, *o.o.* olive oil)

Anaesthetics
Amethocaine (tetracaine) – 1% pet.
Amylocaine – 5% pet.
Benzamine lactate – 1% pet.
Benzocaine – 5% pet.
Bupivacaine – 1% pet.
Butacaine – 5% pet.
Butethamine – 5% pet.

Butyl aminobenzoate – 5% pet.
Cyclomethycaine – 1% pet.
Dibucaine (cinchocaine) – 5% pet.
Diperocaine – 1% pet.
Lidocaine – 5% pet.
Mepivacaine – 1% pet.
Orthocaine – 1% pet.
Oxybuprocaine – 1% pet.
Polidocanol – 3% pet.
Pramocaine – 1% pet.
Prilocaine – 5% pet.
Procaine – 1% pet.
Propanidid – 5% pet.
Proparacaine (proxymetacaine) – 2% pet.
Propipocaine – 1% pet.

Antibiotics
Ampicillin – 5% pet.
Amikacin – 20% pet.
Azidamphenicol – 2% pet.
Bacitracin – 20% pet.
Cephalosporins – 5–20% aq. or pet.
Chloramphenicol – 5% pet.
Clindamycin – 1% aq.
Erythromycin base – 1% pet.
Erythromycin salts – 1% pet.
Framycetin – 20% pet.
Gentamicin – 20% pet.
Kanamycin – 10% pet.
Lincomycin – 1% aq.
Mupirocin – 10% pet.
Neomycin – 20% pet.
Paramomycin – 10% pet.
Penicillin (benzyl) – 10,000 U/g pet.
Polymyxin B – 3% pet.
Pristinamycin – 5% pet.
Ribostamycin – 20% pet.
Rifamycin – 2.5% pet.
Sisomicin – 20% pet.
Sodium colistimethate – 1% pet.
Sodium fusidate – 2% pet.
Spiramycin – 10% pet.
Streptomycin – 2.5% pet.
Sulphonamides – 5% pet.
Tetracyclines – 3% pet.
Thiamphenicol – 5% pet.
Tobramycin – 20% pet.
Tylosin tartrate – 5% pet.

Vancomycin – 5% aq.
Virginiamycin – 5% pet.

Antivirals
Acyclovir – 5% pet.
Famciclovir – 10% aq.
Ganciclovir – 20% aq.
Idoxuridine – 1% pet.
Trifluridine – 5% pet.
Tromantadine – 1% pet.
Valaciclovir – 10% aq.

Antiseptics/antibacterials
Ammoniated mercury – 1% pet.
Chlorquinaldol – 5% pet.
Clioquinol – 5% pet.
Cycloheximide – 1% pet.
Merbromin – 2% aq. or pet.
Mercuric chloride – 0.1% pet.
Nitrofurazone – 1% pet.
Phenylmercuric salts – 0.05% pet.
(acetate, borate, nitrate)
Povidone iodine – 0.4% aq.
Proflavine HCl – 1% pet.
Ethacridine – 2% pet.
Triphenylmethane dyes – 2% aq.
Thimerosal – 0.1% pet.

Antimycotics
Amorolfine – 1% pet.
Chlorphenesin – 1% pet.
Dibenzthione – 3% pet.
Haloprogin – 1% pet.
Bifonazole – 1% eth.
Clotrimazole – 1% eth.
Croconazole – 1% eth.
Econazole – 1% eth.
Enilconazole – 1% eth.
Fenticonazole – 1% eth.
Isoconazole – 1% eth.
Ketoconazole – 1% eth.
Lanoconazole – 1% eth.
Luliconazole – 1% eth.
Miconazole – 1% eth.
Neticonazole – 1% eth.
Oxiconazole – 1% eth.
Sertaconazole – 1% eth.
Sulconazole – 1% eth.

Tioconazole – 1% eth.
Naftifine – 5% eth.
Nystatin – 2% pet.
Pecilocin – 1% pet.
Pyrrolnitrin – 1% pet.
Tolnaftate – 1% pet.
Undecylenic acid – 2% pet.

Antihistamines
Amlexanox – 1% pet.
Antazoline – 1% pet.
Chlorpheniramine – 5% pet.
Chlorpromazine – 0.1% pet.
Diphenhydramine – 1% pet.
Doxepin – 5% pet.
Ketotifen – 0.7% aq.
Pheniramine maleate – 1% aq.
Promethazine – 1% pet.
Pyrilamine – 2% pet.
Sodium cromoglycate – 2% aq.
Tripelennamine – 1% pet.

Anti-neoplastic drugs
Azathioprine – 1% pet.
Chlorambucil – 2% pet.
Fluorouracil – 1% pet.
Mechlorethamine – 0.02% aq
Mitomycin C – 0.1% pet.

Antiparasitic
Benzyl benzoate – 5% pet.
Crotamiton – 3% pet.
Mesulfen – 5% pet.
Metronidazol – 1% pet.

NSAID
Aceclofenac – 1% pet.
Benzydamine – 5% pet.
Bufexamac – 5% pet.
Carprofen – 5% pet.
Cinnoxicam – 1% pet.
Desketoprofen – 1% pet.
Diclofenac – 1% pet.
Etofenamate – 2% pet.
Fenoprofen – 5% pet.
Feprazone – 5% pet.
Flufenamic acid – 1% pet.
Flurbiprofen – 5% pet.

Ibuprofen – 5% pet.
Ibuproxam – 2.5% pet.
Indomethacin – 5% pet.
Ketoprofen – 2.5% pet.
Mefenamic acid – 1% pet.
Mofebutazone – 1% pet.
Naproxen – 5% pet.
Oxyphenbutazone – 1% pet.
Phenylbutazone – 1% pet.
Piketoprofen – 2.5% pet.
Piroxicam – 1% pet.
Sulindac – 1% pet.
Suprofen – 0.1% pet.
Tenoxicam – 1% pet.
Thiocolchicoside – 1% pet.
Tiaprofenic acid – 1% pet.
Trometamol – 1% aq.

Antipsoriatic drugs
Calcipotriol – 2 µg/mL eth.
Calcitriol – 2 µg/mL eth.
Dithranol – 0.02% pet.
Tacalcitol – 2 µg/mL eth.
Tars (coal tar) – 5% pet.

Corticosteroids
Alclometasone dipropionate – 1% eth.
Amcinonide – 0.1% eth.
Betamethasone dipropionate – 1% eth.
Betamethasone-17-valerate – 1% eth.
Budesonide – 0.1% pet.
Clobetasol propionate – 1% eth.
Clobetasone butyrate – 1% eth.
Cloprednol – 1% eth.
Desonide – 1% eth.
Desoxymethasone – 1% eth.
Dexamethasone acetate – 1% eth.
Dexamethasone phosphate – 1% eth.
Diflorasone diacetate – 1% eth.
Diflucortolone pivalate – 1% eth.
Fludrocortisone acetate – 1% eth.
Flumethasone acetate – 1% eth.
Fluocinolone acetonide – 1% eth.
Fluocinonide – 1% eth.
Fluocortolone – 1% eth.
Fluticasone propionate – 1% eth.
Halcinonide – 1% eth.
Halomethasone – 1% eth.

Hydrocortisone – 1% eth.
Hydrocortisone aceponate – 1% eth.
Hydrocortisone acetate – 1% eth.
Hydrocortisone buteprate – 1% eth.
Hydrocortisone-17-butyrate – 1% eth.
Methyl-prednisolone aceponate – 1% eth.
Methyl-prednisolone acetate – 1% eth.
Mometasone furoate – 1% eth.
Prednicarbate – 1% eth.
Prednisolone – 1% eth.
Tixocortol pivalate – 1% pet.
Triamcinolone acetonide – 1% eth.

β-Blockers
Befulenol – 1% aq.
Betaxolol – 1% aq.
Carteolol – 1% aq.
Levobunolol – 1% aq.
Metipranolol – 2% aq.
Metopronolol – 3% aq.
1-Pentbutolol – 2% aq.
Timolol – 0.5% aq.

Mydriatics
Apraclonidine – 1% aq.
Atropine – 1% pet.
Brimonidine – 0.2% aq.
Cyclopentolate – 0.5% aq.
Dipivalyl-epinephrine – 1% aq.
Homatropine – 1% aq.
Phenylephrine –10% aq.
Scopolamine – 0.25% aq.
Tropicamide – 1% pet.

Preservatives/antioxidants
Benzyl alcohol – 1% pet.
Bithionol – 1% pet.
Butylated hydroxyanisol – 2% pet.
Butylated hydroxytoluene – 2% pet.
Chloroacetamide – 0.2% pet.
Chlorhexidine gluconate – 0.5% aq.
Chlorocresol – 1% pet.
Chloroxylenol – 1% pet.
Dichlorophene – 1% pet.
Ethyl alcohol – 10% aq.
Nonoxynols – 5% aq.
Nordihydroguaiaretic acid – 2% pet.
Quaternary ammonium compounds – 0.1% aq.
Propyl gallate – 1% pet.

Sorbic acid – 2% pet.
α-Tocopherol – 10% pet.
Triclocarban – 1% pet.
Triclosan – 1% pet.
Zinc pyrithione – 1% pet.

Vehicle ingredients
Amerchol L-101 – 50% pet.
Carbowaxes – as is
Castor oil – as is
Cetyl alcohol – 5% pet.
Cetearyl alcohol – 20% pet.
Ethyl sebacate – 2% eth.
Ethylenediamine – 1% pet.
Eucerin – as is
Lanette E – 20% pet.
Lanette N – 20% pet.
Lanolin – as is
Myristyl alcohol – 5% pet.
Oleyl alcohol – 30% pet.
Petrolatum – as is
Polyethylene glycols – pure
Polysorbate [20, 40, 80] – 5% pet.
Propylene glycol – 5% aq.
Sesame oil – as is
Sodium bisulphite – 1% pet.
Sodium lauryl sulphate – 0.1% aq.
Sorbitan laureate – 5% aq.
Sorbitan oleate – 5% aq.
Sorbitan palmitate – 5% aq.
Sorbitan sesquioleate – 20% pet.
Stearyl alcohol – 30% pet.
Triethanolamine – 2.5% pet.
Wool wax alcohols – 30% pet.

Miscellaneous
N-acetylcysteine – 10% aq.
Allantoin – 0.5% aq.
e-Aminocaproic acid – 1% aq.
5-Aminolaevulinic acid – 20% pet.
Benzoyl peroxide – 1% pet.
Bismuth oxide – 5% pet.
Boric acid – 10% pet.
Clonidine – 1% pet.
Cocamidopropyl betaine – 1% aq.
Dexpanthenol – 50% aq.
Dorzolamide – 5% aq.
Echothiopate iodine – 1% aq.
Ephedrine – 1% pet.

Epinephrine – 1% aq.

Estradiol – 2% eth.

Ichthammol – 10% pet.

Methyl salicylate – 2% pet.

Metvix® cream – as is

Minoxidil – 5%: 20% PPG/aq.

Monobenzylether hydroquinone – 1% pet.

Nicotine – 10% pet.

Nitroglycerin – 1% pet.

Norethisterone acetate – 1% eth.

Papain – 1% pet.

D-Penicillamine – 1% aq.

Pilocarpine – 1% pet.

Pimecrolimus – 1% pet.

Pirenoxone – 1% aq.

Resorcinol – 1% pet.

Retinoic acid – 0.005% pet.

Rubidium iodide – 1% pet.

Salicylic acid – 1% pet.

Scopolamine hydrobromide – 0.25% aq.

Tacrolimus – 2.5% eth.

Testosterone propionate – 1% eth.

Thioxolone – 0.5% eth.

Tolazoline – 10% aq.

Triethanolamine polypeptide oleate condensate – 25% o.o.

Rubidium iodide – 0.1%

References

1. Achten B, Bourlond A, Haven E et al (1973) Étude du bufexamac crème et du bufexamac onguent dans le traitement de diverses dermatoses. Dermatologica 146:1–7
2. Adamski H, Benkalfate L, Delavai Y et al (1998) Photodermatitis from nonsteroidal anti-inflammatory drugs. Contact Dermatitis 38:171
3. Afzelius H, Thulin H (1979) Allergic reactions to benzalkonium chloride. Contact Dermatitis 5:60
4. Agathos M, Bandmann HJ (1984) Benzoyl peroxide contact allergy in leg ulcer patients. Contact Dermatitis 11:316–317
5. Agner T, Menné T (1993) Sensitivity to clioquinol and chlorquinaldol in the quinoline mix. Contact Dermatitis 29:163
6. Alomar A (1985) Ketoprofen photodermatitis. Contact Dermatitis 12:112–113
7. Amin S, Tanglertsampan C, Maibach HI (1997) Contact urticaria syndrome: 1997. Am J Contact Dermat 8:15–19
8. Andersen KE, Maibach HI (1983) Drugs used topically. In: de AL Weck, Bundgaard H (eds) Allergic reactions to drugs. Springer, Berlin
9. Anderson LL, Welch ML, Grabski WJ (1997) Allergic contact dermatitis and reactivation phenomenon from iontophoresis of 5-fluorouracil. J Am Acad Dermatol 36:478–479
10. Angelini G, Vena GA, Meneghini CL (1985) Allergic contact dermatitis to some medicaments. Contact Dermatitis 12:263–269
11. Angelini G, Vena GA, Meneghini CL (1986) Contact allergy to antiviral agents. Contact Dermatitis 15:114–115
12. Anguita JL, Escutia B, Mari JI et al (2002) Allergic contact dermatitis from undecylenic acid in a common antifungal nail solution. Contact Dermatitis 46:109
13. Baeck M, Chemelle JA, Terreux R et al (2009) Delayed hypersensitivity to corticosteroids in a series of 315 patients: clinical data and patch test results. Contact Dermatitis 61:163–175
14. Baeck M, Marot L, Nicolas J-F et al (2009) Allergic hypersensitivity to topical and systemic corticosteroids: a review. Allergy 64:978–994
15. Bagheri H, Lhiaubet V, Montrastuc JL et al (2000) Photosensitivity to ketoprofen: mechanisms and pharmacoepidemiological data. Drug Saf 22:339–349
16. Bajaj AK (1990) Contact sensitivity to polyethyleneglycols. Contact Dermatitis 22:291–292
17. Bajaj AK, Gupta SC, Chatterjee AK (1992) Contact sensitivity to topical aminoglycosides in India. Contact Dermatitis 27:204–205
18. Bajaj AK, Saraswat A, Mukhija G et al (2007) Patch testing experience with 1000 patients. Ind J Dermatol Venereol Lepr 73:313–318
19. Balato N, Patruno C, Lembo G et al (1995) Allergic contact dermatitis from retinoic acid. Contact Dermatitis 332:51
20. Bandmann HJ, Calnan CD, Cronin E et al (1972) Dermatitis from applied medicaments. Arch Dermatol 106:335–337
21. Barbaud A, Collet E, Le Coz CJ et al (2009) Contact allergy in chronic leg ulcers: results of a multicentre study carried out in 423 patients and proposal for an updated series of patch tests. Contact Dermatitis 60:279–287
22. Barbaud A, Mougeole JM, Tang JQ et al (1991) Contact allergy to colophony in Chinese Musk and Tiger-Bone Plaster. Contact Dermatitis 25:324–325
23. Barile M, Cozzani E, Anonide A et al (1996) Is contact allergy rare in psoriatics? Contact Dermatitis 35:111–114
24. Batista A, Barros MA (1992) Contact dermatitis to crotamiton. Contact Dermatitis 27:59
25. Bauer A, Geier J, Elsner P (2000) Allergic contact dermatitis in patients with anogenital complaints. J Reprod Med 45:649–654
26. Bayrou O, Gaouar H, Leynadier F (2000) Famciclovir as a possible alternative treatment in some case of allergy to acyclovir. Contact Dermatitis 42:42
27. Beller V, Kaufmann R (1987) Contact dermatitis to indomethacin. Contact Dermatitis 17:121
28. Beltrani V (1996) Clinical manifestations of atopic dermatitis. In: Leung DYM (ed) Atopic dermatitis: from pathogenesis to treatment. Springer, Berlin
29. Berl V, Claudel E, Gerberick G et al (2008) Allergic contact dermatitis to corticosteroids: a mechanistic study. Contact Dermatitis 58:10
30. Bjornberg A, Mobacken H (1976) Necrotic skin reactions caused by 1% gentian violet and brilliant green. Acta Derm Venereol 52:55–60
31. Blaschke V, Fuchs T (2001) Periorbital allergic contact dermatitis from oxybuprocaine. Contact Dermatitis 44:198

38

32. Bonnel RA, La Grenade L, Karwoski CB et al (2003) Allergic contact dermatitis from topical doxepin: Food and Drug Administration's post marketing surveillance experience. J Am Acad Dermatol 48:294–296

33. Brancaccio RR, Weinstein S (2003) Systemic contact dermatitis to doxepin. J Drugs Dermatol 2:409–410

34. Britz MB, Maibach HI (1979) Human cutaneous vulvar reactivity to irritants. Contact Dermatitis 5:375–377

35. Burden A, Beck MH (1992) Contact hypersensitivity to azathioprine. Contact Dermatitis 27:329–330

36. Burden AD, Muston H, Beck MH (1994) Intolerance and contact allergy to tar and dithranol in psoriasis. Contact Dermatitis 31:185–186

37. Burry JN (1973) Topical drug addiction: adverse effects of fluorinated corticosteroid creams and ointments. Med J Aust 1:393–396

38. Calnan CD, Frain-Bell W, Cuthbert JW (1962) Occupational dermatitis from chlorpromazine. Trans St John Derm Soc 48:49

39. Camarasa JMG (1976) Contact dermatitis from mercurochrome. Contact Dermatitis 2:120

40. Canelas MM, Gonçalo M, Figueiredo A (2008) Photocontact dermatitis from benzydamine in eight patients. Contact Dermatitis 58(suppl 1):22–23

41. Chadha V, Shenoi SD (1999) Allergic contact dermatitis from dithranol. Contact Dermatitis 41:166

42. Chaudhari PR, Maibach HI (2007) Allergic contact dermatitis from ophtalmics: 2007. Contact Dermatitis 57:11–13

43. Chen HH, Sun CC, Tseng MP et al (2003) A patch test study of 27 crude drugs commonly used in Chinese topical medicaments. Contact Dermatitis 49:8–14

44. Cirne de Castro JL, Freitas JP, Brandao FM et al (1991) Sensitivity to thimerosal and photosensitivity to piroxicam. Contact Dermatitis 24:187–192

45. Conde-Salazar L, Guimaraens D, Gonzalez MA et al (2001) Occupational allergic contact urticaria from amoxicillin. Contact Dermatitis 45:109

46. Conde Salazar L, Guimaraens D, Romero LV et al (1986) Occupational dermatitis from cephalosporins. Contact Dermatitis 14:70–71

47. Connolly M, Buckley DA (2004) Contact dermatitis from propyleneglycol in ECG electrodes, complicated by medicament allergy. Contact Dermatitis 50:42

48. Conti A, Manzini BM, Schiavi ME et al (1995) Sensitization to white petrolatum used as vehicle for patch testing. Contact Dermatitis 33:201–202

49. Cooper SM, Reed J, Shaw S (1999) Systemic reaction to nystatin. Contact Dermatitis 41:345–346

50. Cooper SM, Shaw S (1999) Contact allergy to nystatin: an unusual allergen. Contact Dermatitis 41:120

51. Cooper SM, Shaw S (1999) Contact allergy to clotrimazole: an unusual allergen. Contact Dermatitis 41:168

52. Corazza M, Virgili A (2005) Allergic contact dermatitis from ophthalmic products: can pre-treatment with sodium lauryl sulfate increase patch test sensitivity. Contact Dermatitis 52:239–241

53. Cravo M, Gonçalo M, Figueiredo A (2008) Allergic contact dermatitis to rubber-containing bandages in patients with leg ulcers. Contact Dermatitis 58:371–372

54. Cuerda E, Goday JJ, Del Pozo JDP et al (2003) Photocontact dermatitis due to dexketoprofen. Contact Dermatitis 48:283–284

55. Cusano F, Capozzi M (1992) Photocontact dermatitis from ketoprofen and cross reactivity to ibuproxam. Contact Dermatitis 27:50–51

56. Dannaker CJ, Maibach HI, Austin E (2001) Allergic contact dermatitis to proparacaine with subsequent cross-sensitization to tetracaine from ophthalmic preparations. Am J Contact Dermat 12:177–179

57. Daughters D, Zacheim H, Maibach HI (1973) Urticaria and anaphylactoid reactions after topical applications of mechloretamine. Arch Dermatol 107:429

58. Dawe RS, Watt D, O'Neill S et al (2002) A laser-clinic nurse with allergic contact dermatitis from tetracaine. Contact Dermatitis 46:306

59. Degreef H, Dooms-Goossens A (1985) Patch testing with silver sulfadiazine cream. Contact Dermatitis 12:33–37

60. De Groot AC, Weyland JW, Nater JP (1994) Unwanted effects of cosmetics and drugs used in dermatology, 3rd edn. Elsevier, Amsterdam

61. Dooms-Goossens A (1982) Allergic contact dermatitis to ingredients used in topically applied pharmaceutical products and cosmetics. Katholieke Universitat Leuven, Leuven

62. Dooms-Goossens A, Debusschère K, Dupré K et al (1988) Can eardrops induce a shampoo dermatitis? A case study. Contact Dermatitis 19:143–145

63. Dooms-Goossens A, Degreef H (1980) Sensitization to yellow petrolatum used as a vehicle for patch testing. Contact Dermatitis 6:146–147

64. Dooms-Goossens A, Degreef H (1991) Airborne contact dermatitis: an update. Contact Dermatitis 25:211–217

65. Dooms-Goossens A, Deveylder H, Alam AG et al (1989) Contact sensitivity to nonoxynols as a cause of intolerance to antiseptic preparations. J Am Acad Dermatol 21:723–727

66. Dooms-Goossens A, Matura M, Drieghe J et al (1995) Contact allergy to imidazoles used as antimycotic agents. Contact Dermatitis 33:73–77

67. Downs AMR, Sharp LA, Sansom JE (1999) Pentaerythritol-esterified gum rosin as a sensitizer in Granuflex® hydrocolloid dressing. Contact Dermatitis 41:162–163

68. Durieu C, Marguery MC, Giornado-Labadie F et al (2001) Allergies de contact photoaggravées et photoallergies de contact au ketoprofène: 19 cas. Ann Dermatol Venereol 128:1020–1024

69. Edman B, Moller H (1986) Medicament contact allergy. Dermat Beruf Umwelt 34:139–143

70. Edman B, Moller H (1989) Testing a purified lanolin preparation by a randomized procedure. Contact Dermatitis 20:287–290

71. Erdmann S, Hertl M, Merk HF (1999) Contact dermatitis from clotrimazole with positive patch-test reactions also to croconazole and itraconazole. Contact Dermatitis 40:47

72. Farage MF (2005) Vulvar susceptibility to contact irritants and allergens: a review. Arch Gynecol Obstet 272:167–172

73. Faria A, Gonçalo S, Gonçalo M et al (1996) Allergic contact dermatitis from tioconazole. Contact Dermatitis 35:250–252

74. Farley M, Pak H, Carregal V et al (1995) Anaphylaxis to topical applied bacitracin. Am J Contact Dermat 6:28–31

75. Farrar CW, Bell HK, King CM (2003) Allergic contact dermatitis from propyleneglycol in Efudix cream. Contact Dermatitis 48:35

76. Fedler R, Stromer K (1993) Nickel sensitivity in atopic, psoriatics and healthy subjects. Contact Dermatitis 29:65–69

77. Fernandez-Redondo V, Léon A, Santiago T et al (2001) Allergic contact dermatitis from local anaesthetic on peristomal skin. Contact Dermatitis 45:238

78. Fidalgo A, Lobo L (2004) Allergic contact dermatitis due to amorolfine nail lacquer. Am J Contact Dermat 15:54

79. Figueiredo A, Ribeiro CF, Gonçalo S et al (1987) Piroxicam induced photosensitivity. Contact Dermatitis 17:73–79

80. Fisher AA (1973) The paraben paradox. Cutis 12:830–832

81. Fisher AA (1976) The safety of topical erythromycin. Contact Dermatitis 2:43–44

82. Fisher AA (1982) Resorcinol – a rare sensitizer. Cutis 29:331

83. Fisher AA, Dooms-Goossens A (1976) The effect of perfume "ageing" on the allergenicity of individual perfume ingredients. Contact Dermatitis 2:155–159

84. Fleming CJ, Burden AD (1997) Contact allergy in psoriasis. Contact Dermatitis 36:274–276

85. Forstrom L, Hannuksella M, Kousa M et al (1980) Merthiolate hypersensitivity and vaccination. Contact Dermatitis 6:241–245

86. Foti C, Bonamonte D, Trenti R et al (1997) Occupational contact allergy to cephalosporins. Contact Dermatitis 36:104–105

87. Foti C, Carnimeo L, Bonamonte D et al (2005) Tolerance to calcitriol and tacalcitol in three patients with allergic contact dermatitis to calcipotriol. J Drugs Dermatol 4:756–759

88. Foti C, Cassano N, Mazzarella F et al (1997) Contact allergy to thiocolchicoside. Contact Dermatitis 37:134

89. Foti C, Veña GA, Angelini G (1992) Photocontact allergy due to thiocolchicoside. Contact Dermatitis 27:201–202

90. Fowler JF (1993) Contact allergy to propyleneglycol in topical corticosteroids. Am J Contact Dermat 4:37

91. Fransson J, Storgards A, Hammer H (1985) Palmoplantar lesions in psoriatic patients and their relation to inverse psoriasis, tinea infection and contact allergy. Acta Derm Venereol 65:218–223

92. Freymond N, Catelain A, Queille E et al (2003) Allergic reaction to methylprednisolone. Rev Med Int 24:698–700

93. Friedlander MH (1995) A review of the causes and treatment of bacterial and allergic conjunctivitis. Clin Ther 17:800–810

94. Frosch PJ, John SM (2006) Clinical aspects of irritant contact dermatitis. In: Frosch PJ, Menné T, Lepoittevin J-P (eds) Textbook of contact dermatitis, 4th edn. Springer, Berlin

95. Frosch PJ, Rustemeyer T (1999) Contact allergy to calcipotriol does exist. Report of an unequivocal case and review of the literature. Contact Dermatitis 40:66–71

96. Funk JO, Maibach HI (1994) Propyleneglycol dermatitis: re-evaluation of an old problem. Contact Dermatitis 31:236–241

97. Gallenkemper G, Rabe E, Bauer R (1998) Contact sensitization in chronic venous insufficiency: modern wound dressings. Contact Dermatitis 38:274–278

98. Gallo R, Parodi A (2002) Baboon syndrome from 5-aminosalicylic acid. Contact Dermatitis 46:110

99. Garcia-Bravo B, Martinez Falero AA (1998) Reacciones por mercuriales. Mapfre Med 9(suppl 1):16–20

100. Gehrig KA, Warshaw EM (2008) Allergic contact dermatitis to topical antibiotics: Epidemiology, responsible allergens, and management. J Am Acad Dermatol 58:1–21

101. Giordano-Labadie F, Rancé F, Pellegrin F et al (1999) Frequency of contact allergy in children with atopic dermatitis: results of a prospective study of 137 cases. Contact Dermatitis 40:192–195

102. Goday-Bujan JJ, Rodriguez-Lozano J, Martinez-Gonzalez MC et al (2006) Photoallergic contact dermatitis from dexketoprofen: study of 6 cases. Contact Dermatitis 55:59–61

103. Goday JJ, Garcia GM, Martinez W et al (2001) Photoallergic contact dermatitis from aceclofenac. Contact Dermatitis 45:170

104. Goday JJ, Oleaga M, Gonzalez M et al (2000) Photoallergic contact dermatitis from piketoprofen. Contact Dermatitis 43:115

105. Goday JJ, Yanguas I, Aguirre A et al (1995) Allergic contact dermatitis from sertaconazole with cross sensitivity to miconazole and econazole. Contact Dermatitis 32:370–371

106. Goh CL (1987) Erythema multiforme-like and purpuric eruption due to contact allergy to proflavine. Contact Dermatitis 17:53–54

107. Goh CL (1989) Contact sensitivity to topical medicaments. Int J Dermatol 28:25–28

108. Goh CL (1989) Contact sensitivity to topical antimicrobials. I. Epidemiology in Singapore. Contact Dermatitis 21:46–48

109. Goh CL, Ng SK (1986) Contact sensitivity to salicylic acid. Contact Dermatitis 14:114

110. Goldsmith PC, Rycroft RJG, White IR et al (1997) Contact sensitivity in women with anogenital dermatoses. Contact Dermatitis 36:174–175

111. Gonzalez Perez R, Aguirre A, Oleaga JM et al (1995) Allergic contact dermatitis from tolnaftate. Contact Dermatitis 32:173

112. Gonçalo M, Figueiredo A, Gonçalo S (1996) Hypersensitivity to thimerosal: the sensitizing moiety. Contact Dermatitis 34:201–203

113. Goon A, Goh CL (2006) Noneczematous contact reactions. In: Frosch PJ, Menné T, Lepoittevin J-P (eds) Textbook of contact dermatitis, 4th edn. Springer, Berlin

114. Goossens A, Claes L, Drieghe J (1998) Antimicrobials: preservatives, antiseptics and desinfectants. Contact Dermatitis 39:133–134

115. Grandinetti PJ, Fowler JF (1990) Simultaneous contact allergy to neomycin, bacitracin and polymyxin. J Am Acad Dermatol 23:646–647

116. Green CM, Holden CR, Gawkrodger DJ (2007) Contact allergy to topical medicaments becomes more common with advancing age: an age-stratified study. Contact Dermatitis 56:229–231

117. Guidetti HS, Vicenzi C, Guerra L et al (1995) Contact dermatitis due to imidazole antimycotics. Contact Dermatitis 33:282

118. Gunson TH, Greig DE (2008) Allergic contact dermatitis to all three classes of local anaesthetics. Contact Dermatitis 59:126–127

119. Hannuksella M, Kousa M, Pirilä V (1976) Contact sensitivity to emulsifiers. Contact Dermatitis 2:201–204

120. Korshoj S, Solvsten H, Erlandsen M et al (2009) Frequency of sensitization to methyl aminolevulinate after photodynamic therapy. Contact Dermatitis 60:320–324

121. Hausen BM, Angel M (1992) Studies on the sensitizing capacity of imidazole and triazole derivatives. Part II. Am J Contact Dermat 3:95–101

122. Hausen BM, Heesch B, Kiel U (1990) Studies on the sensitizing capacity of imidazole derivatives. Part I. Am J Contact Dermat 1:25–33

123. Hausen BM, Lücke R, Rothe E et al (2000) Sensitizing capacity of azole derivatives. Part III. Investigations with antihelmintics, antimycotics, fungicides, antithyroid compounds and proton pump inhibitors. Am J Contact Dermat 11:80–88

124. Häuserman P, Bircher AJ (2002) Immediate and delayed hypersensitivity to ceftriaxone, and anaphylaxis due to intradermal testing with other β-lactam antibiotics, in a previously amoxicillin-sensitized patient. Contact Dermatitis 47:311–312

125. Hayachi K, Kawachi S, Saida T (2001) Allergic contact dermatitis due to both chlorpheniramine maleate and dibucaine hydrochloride in an over-the-counter medicament. Contact Dermatitis 44:38–39

126. Heikkila H, Stubb S, Reitamo S (1996) A study of 72 patients with contact allergy to tioconazole. Br J Dermatol 134:678–680

127. Heine A (1996) Diphenhydramine: a forgotten allergen? Contact Dermatitis 35:311–312

128. Henseler T, Christophers E (1995) Disease concomitance in psoriasis. J Am Acad Dermatol 32:982–986

129. Herbst RA, Maibach HI (1991) Contact dermatitis caused by allergy to ophtalmic drugs and contact lens solutions. Contact Dermatitis 25:305–312

130. Herbst RA, Maibach HI (1992) Contact dermatitis caused by allergy to ophtalmics: an update. Contact Dermatitis 27:335–336

131. Herbst RA, Maibach HI (1997) Allergic contact dermatitis from ophtalmics: update 1997. Contact Dermatitis 37:252–253

132. Hergueta JP, Ortis FJ, Iglesias L (1994) Allergic contact dermatitis from etofenamate: report of 9 cases. Contact Dermatitis 31:60–62

133. Heule F, Tahapary GJM, Bello CR et al (1998) Delayed-type hypersensitivity to contact allergens in psoriasis. A clinical evaluation. Contact Dermatitis 38:78–82

134. Hindsén M, Zimerson E, Bruze M (2006) Photoallergic contact dermatitis from ketoprofene in Southern Sweden. Contact Dermatitis 54:150–157

135. Hjorth N, Weissmann K (1973) Occupational dermatitis among veterinary surgeons caused by spiramycin, tylosin and penethamate. Acta Derm Venereol 5:229–232

136. Hogan DJ, Maibach HI (1990) Adverse dermatologic reactions to transdermal drug delivery systems. J Am Acad Dermatol 22:811–814

137. Holdiness MR (1989) A review of contact dermatitis associated with transdermal therapeutic systems. Contact Dermatitis 20:3–9

138. Horn HM, Humphreys F, Aldridge RD (1998) Contact dermatitis and prolonged photosensitivity induced by ketoprofen and associated with sensitivity to benzophenone-3. Contact Dermatitis 38:353–354

139. Hulst KV, Amer EP, Jacobs C et al (2008) Allergic contact dermatitis from transdermal buprenorphine. Contact Dermatitis 59:366–369

140. Isaksson M (2007) Corticosteroid contact allergy–the importance of late readings and testing with corticosteroids used by the patients. Contact Dermatitis 56:56–57

141. Isaksson M, Andersen KE, Brandao FM et al (2000) Patch testing with budesonide in serial dilutions. A multicentre study of EECDRG. Contact Dermatitis 42:352–354

142. Isaksson M, Beck MH, Wilkinson SM (2002) Comparative testing with budesonide in petrolatum and ethanol in a standard series. Contact Dermatitis 47:123–124

143. Isaksson M, Brandao FM, Bruze M et al (2000) Recommendation to include budesonide and tixocortol pivalate in the European standard series. Contact Dermatitis 43:41–42

144. Isaksson M, Bruze M (2003) Corticosteroid cross-reactivity. Contact Dermatitis 49:53–54

145. Isaksson M, Bruze M (2005) Corticosteroids. Dermatitis 16:3–5

146. Isaksson M, Bruze M, Björkner B et al (1999) The benefit of patch testing with a corticosteroid at a low patch test concentration. Am J Contact Dermat 10:31–33

147. Isaksson M, Bruze M, Hörnblad Y et al (1999) Contact allergy to corticosteroids in asthma/rhinitis patients. Contact Dermatitis 40:327–328

148. Isaksson M, Bruze M, Matura M et al (1997) Patch testing with low concentrations of budesonide detects contact allergy. Contact Dermatitis 37:241–242

149. Jankicevic J, Vesic S, Vukisevic J et al (2008) Contact sensitivity in patients with venous leg ulcers in Serbia: comparison with contact dermatitis patients and relationship to ulcer duration. Contact Dermatitis 58:32–36

150. Jappe U, Uter W, Menezes de Pádua CA et al (2006) Allergic contact dermatitis due to β-blockers in eye drops: a retrospective analysis of multicentre surveillance data 1993–2004. Acta Derm Venereol 86:509–514

151. Jeanmougin M, Petit A, Manciet JR et al (1996) Eczema photoallergique de contact au ketoprofène. Ann Dermatol Venereol 123:251–255

152. Johnson M, Fiskerstrand EJ (1999) Contact urticaria syndrome due to carboxymethylcellulose in a hydrocolloid dressing. Contact Dermatitis 41:344–345

153. Katz BE, Fisher AA (1987) Bacitracin: a unique topical antibiotic sensitizer. J Am Acad Dermatol 17:1016–1027

154. Kawada A, Aragane Y, Asai M et al (2001) Simultaneous photocontact sensitivity to ketoprofen and oxybenzone. Contact Dermatitis 44:370

155. Kawada A, Aragane Y, Maeda A et al (2000) Contact dermatitis due to flurbiprofen. Contact Dermatitis 42:167–168

156. Kawada A, Hiruma M, Fujioka A et al (1997) Contact dermatitis from neticonazole. Contact Dermatitis 36:106–107

157. Keilig W (1983) Kontaktallergie auf Cetylstearylalkohol (Lanette O) als therapeutisches Problem bei Stauungsdermatitis und Ulcus cruris. Derm Beruf Umwelt 31: 50–54

158. Keir J, English J, Fergie N (2009) Patch testing in allergic contact dermatitis. J Laryngol Otol 123:558–559

159. Kempinaire A, De Raeve L, Merckx M et al (1997) Terbinafine induced acute generalized exanthematous pustulosis confirmed by a positive patch test result. J Am Acad Dermatol 37:653–655

160. Kerr OA, Kavanagh G, Horn H (2002) Allergic contact dermatitis from topical diclofenac in Solaraze® gel. Contact Dermatitis 47:175

161. Kerre S, Busschotts A, Dooms-Goossens A (1995) Erythema-multiforme-like contact dermatitis due to phenylbutazone. Contact Dermatitis 33:213–214

162. Khanna M, Qasem K, Sasseville D (2000) Allergic contact dermatitis to tea tree oil with erythema multiforme-like id reaction. Am J Contact Dermat 11:238–242

163. Kimma K, Katayama I, Nishioka K (1995) Allergic contact dermatitis from tacalcitol. Contact Dermatitis 33:441

164. Kimura M, Kawada A (1998) Contact sensitivity induced by neomycin with cross sensitivity to other aminoglycoside antibiotics. Contact Dermatitis 39:148–150

165. Klas PA, Corey G, Storrs FJ et al (1996) Allergic and irritant patch test reactions in atopics. Contact Dermatitis 34:121–124

166. Kligman AM (1998) The myth of lanolin allergy. Contact Dermatitis 39:103–107

167. Koch P (1995) No evidence of contact sensitization to acyclovir in acute dermatitis of the lips following application of Zovirax® cream. Contact Dermatitis 33:255–257

168. Koch P, Bahmer FA (1994) Erythema-multiforme-like, urticarial papular and plaque eruptions from bufexamac: report of 4 cases. Contact Dermatitis 31:97–101

169. Koch P, Bahmer FA, Hausen BM (1995) Allergic contact dermatitis from purified eosin. Contact Dermatitis 32:92–95

170. Koh D, Lee BL, Ong HY et al (1997) Colophony in topical traditional Chinese medicaments. Contact Dermatitis 37:243

171. Kowalzick L, Ziegler H (2006) Photoallergic contact dermatitis from topical diclofenac in Solaraze® gel. Contact Dermatitis 54:348–349

172. Kramer K, Paul E (1996) Contact dermatitis from amorolfine-containing cream and nail lacquer. Contact Dermatitis 34:145

173. Kranke B, Szolar-Platzer C, Komericki P et al (1997) Epidemiological significance of bufexamac as a frequent and relevant contact sensitizer. Contact Dermatitis 36:212–215

174. Kurumaji Y, Ohshiro Y, Miyamoto C et al (1991) Allergic photocontact dermatitis due to suprofen. Contact Dermatitis 25:218–223

175. Lachapelle J-M (2005) Allergic contact dermatitis from povidone-iodine: a re-evaluation study. Contact Dermatitis 52:9–10

176. Lammintausta K, Kalimo K, Fagerlund VL (1992) Patch test reactions in atopic patients. Contact Dermatitis 26:234–240

177. Lammintausta K, Mäkelä L, Kalimo K (2001) Rapid systemic valaciclovir reaction subsequent to acyclovir contact allergy. Contact Dermatitis 45:181

178. Lauerma AI, Reitamo S (1994) Allergic reactions to topical and systemic corticosteroids. Eur J Dermatol 5:354–358

179. Lazarov A, Ingber A (1997) Pustular allergic contact dermatitis to isoconazole nitrate. Am J Contact Dermat 8:229–230

180. Le Coz CJ, Bottlaender A, Scrivener JN et al (1998) Photocontact dermatitis from ketoprofen and tiaprofenic acid: cross reactivity study in 12 consecutive patients. Contact Dermatitis 38:245–252

181. Le Coz CJ, Cribier BJ, Heid E (1996) Patch testing in suspected allergic contact dermatitis due to EMLA cream in haemodialysed patients. Contact Dermatitis 35:316–317

182. Lee TY (1998) Allergic contact dermatitis from dibucaine in Proctosedyl ointment without cross-reaction. Contact Dermatitis 39:261

183. Lee TY, Lam TH (1988) Irritant contact dermatitis due to a Chinese herbal medicine Lu-Shen-Wan. Contact Dermatitis 18:213–218

184. Lee TY, Lam TH (1991) Contact dermatitis due to Chinese orthopaedic tincture, Zheng Gu Shui. Contact Dermatitis 24:64–65

185. Lee TY, Lam TH (1993) Myrrh is the putative allergen in bone setter's herbs dermatitis. Contact Dermatitis 29:279

186. Lembo G, Balato N, Patruno C et al (1987) Lichenoid contact dermatitis due to aminoglycoside antibiotics. Contact Dermatitis 17:122–123

187. Leow YH, Ng SK, Wong WK et al (1995) Contact allergic potential of topical traditional Chinese medicaments in Singapore. Am J Contact Dermat 6:4–8

188. Lewis FM, Harrington CD, Gawkrodger DJ (1994) Contact sensitivity in pruritus vulvae: a common and manageable problem. Contact Dermatitis 31:264–265

189. Lewis FM, Shah M, Gawkrodger DJ (1997) Contact sensitivity in pruritus vulvae: patch test results and clinical outcome. Am J Contact Dermat 8:137–140

190. Li L-F, Wang J (2002) Patch testing in allergic contact dermatitis caused by topical Chinese herbal medicine. Contact Dermatitis 47:166–168

191. Lippo J, Lammintausta K (2008) Positive patch test reactions to gentamicin show sensitization to aminoglycosides from topical therapies, bone cements, and from systemic medications. Contact Dermatitis 59:268–272

192. Lodi A, Ambonati M, Coassini A et al (1999) Contact allergy to "caines" caused by anti-hemorrhoidal ointments. Contact Dermatitis 41:221–222

193. Lovell CR, Cronin E, Rhodes EL (1986) Photocontact urticaria from chlorpromazine. Contact Dermatitis 14:290–291

194. Maibach HI, Johnson HL (1975) Contact urticaria syndrome: contact urticaria to diethyltoluamide (immediate type hypersensitivity). Arch Dermatol 111:726–730

195. Machet L, Couhe C, Perrinaud A et al (2004) A high prevalence of sensitization still persists in leg ulcer patients: a retrospective series of 106 patients tested between 2001 and 2002 and a meta-analysis of 1975-2003 data. Br J Dermatol 150:929–935

196. Mailhol C, Lawuers-Cances V, Rancé F et al (2009) Prevalence and risk factors for allergic contact dermatitis to topical treatment in atopic dermatitis: a study in 641 children. Allergy 64:801–806

197. Malhotra V, Kaur I, Saraswat A et al (2002) Frequency of patch-test positivity in patients with psoriasis: a prospective controlled study. Acta Derm Venereol 82:432–435

198. Malik M, Tobin AM, Shanahan F et al (2007) Steroid allergy in patients with inflammatory bowel disease. Br J Dermatol 157:967–969

199. Mallon E, Powell SM (1994) Allergic contact dermatitis from Granuflex hydrocolloid dressing. Contact Dermatitis 30:110–111

200. Mallon E, Powell SM (1994) Sorbitan sesquioleate: a potential allergen in leg ulcer patients. Contact Dermatitis 30:180–181

201. Marks JG (1982) Allergic contact dermatitis to povidone iodine. J Am Acad Dermatol 6:473–475

202. Marques C, Faria E, Machado A et al (1995) Allergic contact dermatitis and systemic contact dermatitis from cinchocaine. Contact Dermatitis 33:443

203. Marren P, Wojnarowska F, Powell SM (1982) Allergic contact dermatitis and vulvar dermatoses. Br J Dermatol 126:52–56

204. Martins C, Freitas JD, Gonçalo M et al (1995) Allergic contact dermatitis from erythromycin. Contact Dermatitis 33:360

205. Matthieu L, Meuleman L, Van Ecke E et al (2004) Contact and photocontact allergy to ketoprofen. The Belgian experience. Contact Dermatitis 50:238–241

206. Meneghini CL, Veña GA, Angelini G (1982) Contact dermatitis to scabicides. Contact Dermatitis 8:285–286

38

207. Menezes de Pádua, CA, Uter W, Geier J et al (2008) Contact allergy to topical antifungals. Allergy 63:946–947

208. Menné T, Veien N, Sjolin K-E et al (1994) Systemic contact-type dermatitis. Am J Contact Dermat 5:1–12

209. Millan-Parrilla F, De la Cuadra J (1990) Allergic contact dermatitis from trifluridine in eye drops. Contact Dermatitis 22:289

210. Millard TP, Orton DI (2004) Changing patterns of contact allergy in chronic inflammatory ear disease. Contact Dermatitis 50:83–86

211. Moller H (1980) Why thimerosal allergy? Int J Dermatol 19:29

212. Moller NE, Nielsen B, Von Wurden K (1986) Contact dermatitis to semi-synthetic penicillins in factory workers. Contact Dermatitis 14:307–311

213. Morris SD, Rycroft RJ, White IR et al (2002) Comparative frequency of patch test reactions to topical antibiotics. Br J Dermatol 146:1047–1051

214. Motolese A, Capriata S, Simonelli M (2009) Contact sensitivity to advanced wound dressings in 116 patients with leg ulcers. Contact Dermatitis 60:107

215. Mozzanica N, Pigatto PD (1990) Contact and photocontact allergy to ketoprofen: clinical and experimental study. Contact Dermatitis 23:336–340

216. Musel AL, Warshaw EM (2006) Cutaneous reactions to transdermal therapeutic systems. Dermatitis 17:109–122

217. Nakada T, Iijima M (2000) Allergic contact dermatitis from dibucaine hydrochloride. Contact Dermatitis 42:283

218. Nakano R, Miyoshi H, Kanzaki T (1996) Allergic contact dermatitis from lanoconazole. Contact Dermatitis 35:63

219. Nardelli A, Degreef H, Goossens A (2004) Contact allergic reactions of the vulva: a 14-year review. Dermatitis 15:131–136

220. Nardelli A, D'Hogghe E, Drieghe J et al (2009) Allergic contact dermatitis from fragrance components in specific topical pharmaceutical products in Belgium. Contact Dermatitis 60:303–313

221. Navarro LA, Jorro G, Morales LC et al (1995) Allergic contact dermatitis due to piketoprofen. Contact Dermatitis 32:181

222. Nino M, Balato N, Constanzo LD et al (2009) Scratch-patch test for the diagnosis of allergic contact dermatitis to acyclovir. Contact Dermatitis 60:56–57

223. Nöhle M, Straube M, Czliska C et al (1997) Beruflich erworbene Sensibilisierungen gegen Clotrimazole. Dermat Beruf Umwelt 45:232–234

224. Oleffe JA, Blondeel A, Boschmans S (1978) Patch testing with lanolin. Contact Dermatitis 4:233–234

225. Oleffe JA, Blondeel A, Connick A (1979) Allergy to chlorocresol and propyleneglycol in a steroid cream. Contact Dermatitis 5:53

226. Okazawa H, Aihara M, Nagatani T et al (1998) Allergic contact dermatitis due to ethyl alcohol. Contact Dermatitis 38:233

227. Ophaswongse S, Maibach HI (1993) Topical nonsteroidal anti-inflammatory drugs: allergic and photoallergic contact dermatitis and phototoxicity. Contact Dermatitis 29:57–64

228. Parente G, Pazzaglia M, Vincenzi C et al (1999) Contact dermatitis from pheniramine maleate in eye drops. Contact Dermatitis 40:338

229. Park YK, Lee JH, Chung WJ (2002) Allergic contact dermatitis from calcipotriol. Acta Derm Venereol 82:71–72

230. Pasche-Koo F, Piletta PA, Hunziker N et al (1994) High sensitization rate to emulsifiers in patients with chronic leg ulcers. Contact Dermatitis 31:226–228

231. Pereira F, Fernandes C, Dias M et al (1995) Allergic contact dermatitis from zinc pyrithione. Contact Dermatitis 33:131

232. Pigatto P (2000) Atopy and contact sensitization in psoriasis. Acta Derm Venereol Suppl 211:19–20

233. Pigatto PD, Bigardi A, Legori A et al (1996) Cross reaction in patch testing and photopatch testing with ketoprofen, tiaprofenic acid and cinnamic aldehyde. Am J Contact Dermat 7:220–223

234. Pigatto PD, Mozzanica N, Bigardi AS et al (1993) Topical NSAID allergic contact dermatitis. Italian experience. Contact Dermatitis 29:39–40

235. Pigatto PD, Riboldi A, Morelli M et al (1985) Allergic contact dermatitis from oxyphenbutazone. Contact Dermatitis 12:236–237

236. Piñol J, Carapeto FJ (1984) Contact urticaria to etofenamate. Contact Dermatitis 11:132–133

237. Pitarch Bort G, de la Cuadra OJ, Torrijos Aguilar A et al (2006) Allergic contact dermatitis due to aceclofenac. Contact Dermatitis 55:365–366

238. Proske S, Uter W, Schnuch A et al (2003) Severe allergic contact dermatitis with generalized spread due to bufexamac presenting as the "baboon"syndrome. Dtsch Med Wochenschr 128:545–547

239. Ramsing DW, Menné T (1993) Contact sensitivity to sorbic acid. Contact Dermatitis 28:124

240. Rietschel RL, Fowler JF (2001) Noneczematous contact dermatitis. In: Rietschel RL, Fowler JF (eds) Fisher's contact dermatitis, 5th edn. Lippincott Williams & Wilkins, Philadelphia

241. Rietschel RL, Fowler JF (2001) Systemic contact-type dermatitis. In: Rietschel RL, Fowler JF (eds) Fisher's contact dermatitis, 5th edn. Lippincott Williams & Wilkins, Philadelphia

242. Rietschel RL, Fowler JF (2001) Local anesthetics. In: Rietschel RL, Fowler JF (eds) Fisher's contact dermatitis, 5th edn. Lippincott Williams & Wilkins, Philadelphia

243. Rudzki E, Rebandel P (1996) Cross reactions with 4 aminoglycoside antibiotics at various concentrations. Contact Dermatitis 35:62

244. Rudzki E, Rebandel P (1997) Sensitivity to oxytetracycline. Contact Dermatitis 37:136

245. Rudzki E, Zakrzewski Z, Rebandel PW et al (1988) Cross reactions between aminoglycoside antibiotics. Contact Dermatitis 18:314–316

246. Saap L, Fahim S, Arsenault E et al (2004) Contact sensitivity in patients with leg ulcers. A North American study. Arch Dermatol 140:1241–1246

247. Saitta P, Brancaccio R (2007) Allergic contact dermatitis to pimecrolimus. Contact Dermatitis 56:43–44

248. Sanchez-Perez J, Sanchez TS, Garcia-Diez A (2001) Combined contact and photocontact allergic dermatitis to etofenamate in flogoprofen gel. Am J Contact Dermat 12:215–216

249. Sasseville D, Moreau L (2005) Allergic contact dermatitis from triethanolamine polypeptide oleate condensate in eardrops and shampoo. Contact Dermatitis 52:233

250. Schena D, Barba A, Costa G (1996) Occupational contact urticaria to cisplatin. Contact Dermatitis 34:220–221

251. Schliz M, Rauterberg A, Weiss J (1996) Allergic contact dermatitis from hydrocolloid dressings. Contact Dermatitis 34:146–147

252. Schlossman ML, McCarthy JP (1979) Lanolin and derivatives chemistry. Relationship to allergic contact dermatitis. Contact Dermatitis 5:65–72

253. Schoppelrey HP, Mily H, Agathos M et al (1997) Allergic contact dermatitis from pyoctanin. Contact Dermatitis 36:221–224

254. Serrano G, Fortea JM, Latasa JM et al (1992) Photosensitivity induced by fibric acid derivatives and its relation to photocontact dermatitis to ketoprofen. J Am Acad Dermatol 27:204–208

255. Sertoli A, Francalanci S, Acciai MC et al (1999) Epidemiological survey of contact dermatitis in Italy (1984-1993) by GIRDCA (Gruppo Italiano Ricerca Dermatiti da Contatto e Ambientali). Am J Contact Dermat 10:18–30

256. Shaw DW, Maibach HI, Eichenfield LF (2007) Allergic contact dermatitis from pimecrolimus in a patient with tacrolimus allergy. J Am Acad Dermatol 56:342–345

257. Shono M (1997) Allergic contact dermatitis from neticonazole hydrochloride. Contact Dermatitis 37:136–137

258. Shono M (2007) Allergic contact dermatitis from luliconazole. Contact Dermatitis 56:296–297

259. Smeenk G, Kerckoffs HP, Schreurs PH (1987) Contact allergy to a reaction product in Hirudoid cream: an example of compound allergy. Br J Dermatol 116:223–231

260. Soga F, Katoh N, Kishimoto S (2004) Contact dermatitis due to lanoconazole, cetylalcohol and diethyl sebacate in lanoconazole cream. Contact Dermatitis 50:49–50

261. Sood A, Taylor JS (2003) Bacitracin: allergen of the year. Am J Contact Dermat 14:3–4

262. Steinmann A, Mayer G, Breit R et al (1996) Allergic contact dermatitis from croconazole without cross sensitivity to clotrimazole and bifonazole. Contact Dermatitis 35: 255–256

263. Stinco G, Frattasio A, De Francesco V et al (1999) Frequency of delayed-type hypersensitivity to contact allergens in psoriatic patients. Contact Dermatitis 40:323–324

264. Sugyiama M, Nakada T, Hosaka H et al (2001) Photocontact dermatitis to ketoprofen. Am J Contact Dermat 12:180–181

265. Suhonen R, Kanerva L (1997) Contact allergy and cross reactions caused by prilocaine. Am J Contact Dermat 8:231–235

266. Suzuki K, Suzuki M, Akamatsu H et al (2002) Allergic contact dermatitis from minoxidil: study of the cross-reaction to minoxidil. Am J Contact Dermat 13:45–46

267. Tabar I, Garcia BE, Rodriguez E et al (1990) Etiologic agents in allergic contact dermatitis by eyedrops. Contact Dermatitis 23:50–51

268. Tanaka T, Satoh T, Yokozeki H (2007) Allergic contact dermatitis from luliconazole: implication of the dithioacetal structure. Acta Derm Venereol 87:271–272

269. Tavadia S, Bianchi J, Dawe RS et al (2003) Allergic contact dermatitis in venous leg ulcer patients. Contact Dermatitis 48:261–265

270. Thyssen JP, Maibach HI (2008) Drug-elicited systemic allergic (contact) dermatitis – update and possible pathomechanisms. Contact Dermatitis 59:195–202

271. Thyssen JP, Menné T, Elberling J et al (2008) Hypersensitivity to local anaesthetics – update and proposal of evaluation algorithm. Contact Dermatitis 59:69–78

272. Tosti A, Bardazzi F, Padova MP et al (1985) Contact dermatitis to minoxidil. Contact Dermatitis 13:275–276

273. Tosti A, Guerra L, Morelli R et al (1990) Prevalence and source of sensitization to emulsifiers: a clinical study. Contact Dermatitis 23:68–72

274. Tosti A, Tosti G (1988) Thimerosal: a hidden allergen in ophthalmology. Contact Dermatitis 18:268–272

275. Tosti A, Vicenzi C, Guerra L et al (1996) Contact dermatitis from fatty alcohols. Contact Dermatitis 35:287–289

276. Trattner A, David M (2002) Pigmented contact dermatitis from topical minoxidil 5%. Contact Dermatitis 46:246

277. Turner TW (1977) Contact dermatitis to lignocaine. Contact Dermatitis 3:210–211

278. Umebayashi Y (1999) Three cases of contact dermatitis due to lanoconazole. Environ Dermatol (Japan) 6:122

279. Umebayashi Y, Ito S (2001) Allergic contact dermatitis due to lanoconazole and neticonazole. Contact Dermatitis 44:48–49

280. Urrutia I, Jauregui I, Gamboa P et al (1998) Photocontact dermatitis from cinchocaine (dibucaine). Contact Dermatitis 39:139–140

281. Uter W, Geier J, Pfahlberg A et al (2002) The spectrum of contact allergy in elderly patients with and without leg dermatitis. Dermatology 204:266–272

282. Valenzuela N, Puig L, Barnadas MA et al (2002) Photocontact dermatitis due to dexketoprofen. Contact Dermatitis 47:237

283. Valsecchi R, Cainelli T (1985) Contact dermatitis from ibuprofen. Contact Dermatitis 12:286–287

284. Valsecchi R, Falghieri G, Cainelli T (1983) Contact dermatitis from ketoprofen. Contact Dermatitis 9:163–164

285. Valsecchi R, Imberti G, Cainelli T (1991) Mitomycin C contact dermatitis. Contact Dermatitis 24:70–71

286. Van der Hove J, Decroix J, Tennstedt D et al (1994) Allergic contact dermatitis from prilocaine, one of the local anaesthetics in EMLA cream. Contact Dermatitis 30:239

287. Van Dijke CPH, Veerman FR, Haverkamp HC (1983) Anaphylatic reactions to ketoconazole. BMJ 287:1673

288. Van Joost T, Van Ulsen J, Vuzevski VD et al (1990) Purpura contact dermatitis to benzoyl peroxide. J Am Acad Dermatol 22:359–361

289. Van Ketel WG (1983) An allergic eruption probably caused by ketoconazole. Contact Dermatitis 9:113

290. Van Ketel WG, Bruynzeel DP (1989) Sensitization to gentamycin alone. Contact Dermatitis 20:303

291. Van Ketel WG, Bruynzeel DP (1991) A forgotten topical anaesthetic sensitizer – butylaminobenzoate. Contact Dermatitis 25:131–132

292. Veien NK, Hattel T, Justesen O et al (1980) Occupational contact dermatitis due to spiramycin and/or tylosin among farmers. Contact Dermatitis 6:410–413

293. Vernassiere C, Barbaud A, Trechot PH et al (2003) Systemic acyclovir reaction subsequent to acyclovir contact allergy: which systemic antiviral drug should then be used? Contact Dermatitis 49:155–157

294. Vicenzi C, Lucente P, Ricci C et al (1997) Facial contact dermatitis to metronidazole. Contact Dermatitis 36:116–117

295. Villar MA, Pagan JA, Palacios L et al (2008) Allergic contact dermatitis to etofenamate. Cross-reaction to other nonsteroidal anti-inflamatory drugs. Contact Dermatitis 58:118–119

296. Virgili A, Corazza M, Bacilieri S et al (1997) Contact sensitivity in vulvar lichen simplex chronicus. Contact Dermatitis 37:296–297

38

297. Von Krogh G, Maibach HI (1981) The contact urticaria syndrome: an update review. J Am Acad Dermatol 5:328–342

298. Vonderheid EC, Van Scott EJ, Johnson WC et al (1977) Topical chemotherapy and immunotherapy of mycosis fungoides: intermediate term results. Arch Dermatol 113:454–462

299. Wakelin SH, Smith H, White IR et al (2001) A retrospective analysis of contact allergy to lanolin. Br J Dermatol 145:28–31

300. Walchner M, Rueff F, Przybilla B (1997) Delayed-type hypersensitivity to mofebutazone underlying a severe drug reaction. Contact Dermatitis 36:54–55

301. Warshaw EM, Furda LM, Maibach HI et al (2008) Anogenital dermatitis in patients referred for patch testing. Arch Dermatol 144:749–755

302. Warshaw EM, Schram SE, Belsito DV et al (2008) Patch-test reactions to topical anesthetics: retrospective analysis of cross-sectional data, 2001 to 2004. Dermatitis 19:81–85

303. Weightman W, Turner T (1998) Allergic contact dermatitis from lignocaine: report of 29 cases and review of the literature. Contact Dermatitis 39:265–266

304. Wilkinson JD, Shaw S, Andersen KA et al (2002) Monitoring levels of preservative sensitivity in Europe. A 10-year overview (1991-2000). Contact Dermatitis 46:207–210

305. Wilkinson SM, Jones MF (1996) Corticosteroid usage and binding to arginine. Determinants of corticosteroid hypersensitivity. Br J Dermatol 135:225–230

306. Wilson CL, Cameron J, Powell SM et al (1991) High incidence of contact dermatitis in leg ulcer patients – implications for management. Clin Exp Dermatol 16:250–253

307. Willa-Craps C, Wyss M, Elsner P (1995) Allergic contact dermatitis from naftifine. Contact Dermatitis 32:369–370

308. Yamada S, Tanaka K, Kawahara Y et al (1998) Photoallergic contact dermatitis due to diphenhydramine hydrochloride. Contact Dermatitis 38:282

309. Zaki I, Shall L, Dalziel KL (1994) Bacitracin: a significant sensitizer in leg ulcer patients? Contact Dermatitis 31:92–94

310. Zappi EG, Brancaccio RR (1997) Allergic contact dermatitis from mupirocin ointment. J Am Acad Dermatol 36:266

311. Zollner TM, Ochsendorf FR, Hensel O et al (1997) Delayed-type reactivity to calcipotriol without cross sensitivity to tacalcitol. Contact Dermatitis 37:250

Dental Materials

39

Marléne Isaksson

Contents

M. Isaksson
Department of Occupational and Environmental Dermatology, Malmö University Hospital, 205 02 Malmö, Sweden
e-mail: marlene.isaksson@skane.se

39.1 Introduction

Dental professionals and dental patients are exposed to virtually the same contactants, but the clinical outcome is very different. Dentists, dental nurses and assistants, and dental laboratory technicians suffer predominantly from irritant contact dermatitis. While in the last 25–30 years, allergic contact dermatitis to acrylates and rubber products was seen to be more frequent but to a lesser degree, the equivalent of this in the mouth, allergic contact stomatitis, was a rare phenomenon.

39.2 Dental Personnel

The prevalence of skin problems is high compared to other groups. The frequency of occupational contact dermatitis in dental personnel was considered to be about 40% in the early 1990s [1], and according to the Finnish Register of Occupational Diseases (FROD), the occurrence of occupational diseases among dental personnel increased threefold in the 1990s due to the increased usage of acrylics [2, 3]. Most of these diseases are hand dermatitis, but respiratory diseases such as asthma have also increased.

Two-thirds of dental personnel with acrylate contact allergy gave a history of having had hand eczema some time or the other [4]. In another study, the 1-year prevalence of hand eczema was 14% in 527 dental personnel [5]. Of 72, 41 were patch tested and four were allergic to acrylics. In another study from Sweden comprising 700 dental personnel, a frequency of 8% occupational skin allergy was reported [4, 6]. In a survey of Swedish dentists, dental nurses, and dental technicians, overall, 3% had dermatitis due to allergy to acrylics [6]. Among

J.D. Johansen et al. (eds.), *Contact Dermatitis*,
DOI: 10.1007/978-3-642-03827-3_39, © Springer-Verlag Berlin Heidelberg 2011

174 Swedish dental personnel referred for screening for occupational skin disease, hand eczema was diagnosed in 63%. Of these, 67% were classified as irritant contact dermatitis and 33% as allergic. Seventy seven of the one thirty one patch tested (59%) presented at least one positive test reaction to substances in the baseline series and 44/109 (40%) to substances exclusive to a dental series. The most common sensitizers in the baseline series were nickel (37%), cobalt (17%), fragrance mix (12%), colophony (8%), and thiuram mix (8%). Of the 109 tested to the dental series, 24 (22%) had positive reactions to methacrylates, the majority reacting to several preparations. Reactions to 2-hydroxyethyl methacrylate (2-HEMA), ethyleneglycol dimethacrylate (EGDMA), and methyl methacrylate (MMA) were the most frequent. Almost 2/3 of the dental personnel with occupational hand eczema who were hypersensitive to an acrylic, were also positive to one of the allergens in the baseline, mainly nickel. Immediate-type, IgE-mediated allergy to natural rubber latex (NRL) was diagnosed in 10% of patients [4]. In Northern Sweden, a significantly higher prevalence of conjunctivitis and atopic dermatitis was found among dentists, both male and female. Hypersensitivity to dental materials was reported by significantly more dental personnel than by referents [7].

A questionnaire study in Danish dentists revealed a 1-year prevalence of 21.4% of skin reactions related to occupation. The main causes reported were hand washing and soaps, latex gloves and (di)methacrylate-containing materials occurring at point prevalences of 7.1, 1.3, and 1.7%, respectively [8]. In a Swedish survey of dentists, the 1-year prevalence of self-reported hand eczema was 15%. The hand eczema diagnosis was confirmed in 94% of the dentists examined, yielding a minimum 1-year prevalence of 11.6%. Four percent of those with hand eczema had been on sick leave, mainly due to side effects from protective gloves. Fifty percent of those who were patch tested reacted to at least one allergen. The most frequent allergens were nickel sulfate, fragrance mix, gold sodium thiosulfate (GSTS), and thiuram mix. Five percent of the dentists with hand eczema during the previous 12 months had positive reactions to acrylics and all those to 2-HEMA and six also to EGDMA. The prevalence of contact allergy to acrylics was below 1% in the population of responding dentists and did not have serious medical, social, or occupational consequences. Irritant contact dermatitis was seen in 67% of those with hand eczema and in 28% with allergic contact dermatitis. The most frequent combination of diagnoses was irritant contact dermatitis and atopic hand eczema [9]. Eczema was confirmed in 94% of those 158 dentists who attended a consultation. Irritant contact dermatitis was diagnosed in 2/3 and allergic contact dermatitis in 1/3 [10].

Out of 923 Finnish female dental nurses, 799 answered a questionnaire, and of the 328 (almost one third) who reported work-related dermatitis on hands, forearms, or face, 245 participated in an interview. Hundred and seven were chosen for further examination and both patch tests and prick tests were performed in 86. The prevalence of occupational skin disease was 6.5% in the surveyed dental nurse population. Allergic contact dermatitis was the most common diagnosis (3.6%), methacrylates (1.3%) and rubber chemicals (1.3%) being the most common causes. Contact urticaria (1.9%) was, in all cases but one, caused by NRL (1.8%). Frequent hand washing was the main cause to irritant contact dermatitis (1.5%) [11]. In a report from Poland on 46 dental nurses with suspected occupational dermatitis, 26% were allergic to glutaraldehyde, 12% to formaldehyde, and 11% to thimerosal. All the three or related chemicals are used as disinfectants in Poland [12]. Also, colophony has sensitized dental nurses [13].

A Danish questionnaire study among dental technicians reported the 1-year prevalence of skin problems on the hands to be 43%. There were no statistical differences in skin problems on the hands in relation to seniority [14]. In a questionnaire study in the early 1990s comprising 1,132 German dental technicians, 36% reported skin lesions attributed to work and 1/3 suspected plastic materials as the primary cause. Among the 55 dental technicians who were examined and patch tested, 64% had allergic contact dermatitis and 24% irritant contact dermatitis. 74% of the allergens were found in plastic materials. Contact allergy to MMA, 2-HEMA, and EGDMA was seen in 16, 33, and 27%, respectively [15]. In dental technician trainees, a 23% increase in the prevalence of skin problems occurred during their first 8 months of school [16]. A retrospective cohort study among former dental technician students in Sweden showed the risk of hand eczema to be more than doubled compared to controls and that the work involves frequent and unprotected exposure to acrylates and wet work [17]. Dental technicians can get allergic to colophony present at 7.5% in dental base plate molding materials and have occupational hand eczema and forearm dermatitis [18].

39.2.1 Irritant Contact Dermatitis

Dental personnel are exposed to a variety of irritants. The following are examples of such exposure: soaps and detergents, disinfectants used for personal hygiene or to clean surfaces or instruments, wearing of protective gloves due to the hydrating effect, water, frequent hand washing, seasonal influences that worsened the dermatitis during the cold and dry winter period, contact with plasters and polish dusts, metals, ceramics and plastics, mechanical friction, thermal changes, tissue fixatives, and (meth)acrylates [15]. In dental technicians wet work, grinding, working with plaster, and physical irritation when polishing metal and plastic materials were the major causes of irritant contact dermatitis in several surveys [15, 19]. Washing of hands up to 100 times a day also contributed [19]. In one case, a floor cleaner was being used as a liquid soap [15].

Latex gloves have caused skin irritation [20], and the finger webs were significantly more affected in latex glove wearers [14]. In Denmark, a study on dental technicians showed acrylates to be the major culprit; of 69 with hand eczema, 64 used MMA and cyanoacrylate glues on a regular basis, most often daily [14]. Therefore, working in dental practice poses a risk for contracting irritant contact dermatitis [15]. About 50% of the personnel in public dentistry reported occupation-related health problems, the majority of which was probably irritative dermatoses of exposed hands [21]. A German study showed 24% of dental technicians with suspected occupational skin disease to have irritant contact dermatitis [15]. In a questionnaire study among dentists, latex gloves were responsible for irritant contact dermatitis in 30.1%, [8], hand washing/soaps in 67.2%, and disinfectants/tissue fixatives in 2.8%. The latter can release or contain aldehydes and essential oils such as eugenol [8, 22]. In a Swedish study on dental personnel referred for screening for occupational skin disease, 67% of all hand eczema was classified as irritant [4].

Core Message

> Dental personnel are exposed to a variety of irritants such as frequent hand washing, soaps and detergents, disinfectants, and protective gloves.

39.2.2 Clinical Picture of Irritant Contact Dermatitis in Dental Personnel

The dorsum of fingers, especially on the dominant hand, the finger webs, and the lateral aspects of fingers are the most common sites of irritant dermatitis in dental personnel. Eighty percent of the dermatitis was present on the dorsum of fingers and around 70% on the lateral aspects of fingers in a study investigating dental technicians. Nine patients showed lesions on the face, neck, and forearms [15]. Symptoms and signs range from pain and stinging to scaling, erythema, dry skin with fissures, vesicles, and hyperkeratosis, respectively.

39.3 Dental Patients

39.3.1 Irritant Contact Stomatitis

Contact stomatitis is the inflammation and pain of the oral mucosa due to irritant substances. Irritants include heat, frictional trauma, or chemicals [23]. A chronic irritant lesion may develop due to contact with irritants of low concentration for prolonged periods of time. Such reactions can be seen in the oral mucosa when this is in close contact with amalgam or other filling materials. Mechanical effects may explain the reactions. It may be very difficult to distinguish these lesions from contact allergic lesions. Therefore, it is necessary to perform patch tests with relevant allergens. A negative patch test to dental materials is then needed to rule out an allergic origin.

39.3.2 Clinical Picture of Irritant Contact Stomatitis in Dental Patients

The mucosa is considered to be more resistant to irritating substances than the skin, and the saliva and buffer capacity can modify the appearance of stomatitis. Inflammation with erythema and ulcers or lichenoid lesions may however be present.

39

39.4 Allergic Contact Dermatitis

Dental personnel are exposed to a variety of contact allergens, the most important being acrylics, rubber additives, fragrances, formaldehyde, and metals. In the case of occupational contact dermatitis, dental professionals present with hand or facial eczema or respiratory symptoms [12]. Overall, the frequency of occupational contact allergy was estimated to be 1% in dental occupations [20]. Specifically, dentists were seriously affected (4%) [8], while dental technicians had lower figures, i.e., 2% methacrylate allergy. However, in a group of dental technicians with suspected contact dermatitis, allergic contact dermatitis was diagnosed in 64% [15]. The prevalence of contact allergy to (meth)acrylates was below 1% in a study on Swedish dentists with hand eczema. Results showed that all allergic dentists reacted to 2-HEMA [9]. In another Swedish study where referred dental personnel were patch tested, contact allergy to methacrylates was diagnosed in 22%. Reactions to 2-HEMA, EGDMA, and MMA were most frequent [4]. Figures from the FROD from the 1990s showed more than two-thirds of reported contact dermatitis in dentists and dental nurses to be allergic in origin, the most common sensitizers being methacrylates, disinfectants and antimicrobials, rubber chemicals, and mercury [2, 3]. A 10-year retrospective study on patch test results from dental personnel and dental patients tested with dental series containing acrylics showed 2.3% of dental patients and 5.8% of dental personnel to react to methacrylates. The most common allergen for both groups was 2-HEMA followed by EGDMA and triethyleneglycol dimethacrylate (TREGDMA) [24]. Methacrylate and acrylate allergy (36 acrylic monomers) in dental personnel was summarized from 12 years of patch testing at the Finnish Institute of Occupational Health (FIOH). 2-HEMA was the most important allergen in dentists and dental nurses, whereas MMA and EGDMA dominated among dental technicians [25].

> **Core Message**
>
> › Dental personnel are exposed to a variety of contact allergens, the most important being acrylics, rubber additives, fragrances, formaldehyde, and metals.

39.4.1 Clinical Picture of Allergic Contact Dermatitis in Dental Personnel

In occupational acrylic contact allergy, in 93% of cases, the fingertips were most often affected [15]. Pulpitis usually affects the first three fingers. Also, in over 80% of cases, the lateral aspects of the fingers were affected, while the dorsal aspects of the fingers and back of hands were affected in 68 and 46%, respectively [15]. Even occupational conjunctivitis has been described [19]. Signs and symptoms range from very dry skin, scaling, fissures, rhagades, vesicles, bullae, hyperkeratosis, and erythema to itching, smarting, pain, stinging, burning, tingling, slight numbness of the fingertips, and reduced sensitivity, respectively. Mild paresthesia may persist for weeks or months after the dermatitis has subsided. Paresthesia may also develop without contact allergy. Paresthesia is caused by a local effect of acrylics on the peripheral nerves without systemic neural effects [26]. Nail folds may become swollen and red [27]; ectopic allergic dermatitis may present in the face, on eyelids, or on other exposed areas, by means of spread from contaminated hands or via airborne exposure [28].

39.5 Allergic Contact Stomatitis and Cheilitis

The main allergic reactions found in dental patients include delayed hypersensitivity to metals, cosmetics, food additives, flavors, and acrylates [12]. In patients with clinical symptoms, the frequency of contact allergy to denture base materials was 28% [29, 30], but only rarely is contact allergy to acrylics in dental patients reported.

39.5.1 Clinical Picture of Allergic Contact Stomatitis and Cheilitis in Dental Patients

Contact stomatitis is the inflammation and pain of the oral mucosa due to allergic substances. Oral flavorings, preservatives, and dental materials are common allergens [23]. Clinical manifestations of gingivostomatitis are variable and include painful burning sensations in the mouth, local irritation, erythema, erosions, ulcerations, mucosal swelling, sore mouth, and tingling in the mouth. Clinical signs are frequently less pronounced than subjective symptoms. Allergic stomatitis is also rare [31]. Acrylics and metals such as mercury, gold, palladium, and manganese have caused stomatitis. Facial eruptions, systemic reactions, and even anaphylaxis can be seen. Diffuse erythema-like prosthesis stomatitis with stinging is seldom due to contact allergy, but most often caused by *Candida Albicans* in combination with an ill-fitting denture.

Cheilitis is a dermatitis of the lips. A study from Australia, in which 75 cheilitis patients were patch tested, revealed an irritant cause in 36% of cases, 25% was due to contact allergy and 19% to atopic dermatitis [32]. Sensitizers reported to have caused cheilitis are medicaments, toothpaste ingredients, potassium persulphate (in denture cleanser), colophony in dental floss, nail varnish, cosmetics, and nickel [12, 32–34]. A recent compilation of patch test results from 129 patients with chronic eczematous cheilitis revealed the most frequent causes of allergic cheilitis to be nickel, fragrances, *Myroxylon Pereirae*, and chromium and manganese salts present primarily in cosmetics, dental materials and oral hygiene products [35]. An acute lip swelling can imply an immediate-type allergy to latex and must be ruled out. Allergens in toothpastes such as eugenol, mint, or cinnamaldehyde can cause lip swelling [32, 36].

Granulomatous cheilitis is a condition where there may be a coexisting contact allergy to foodstuffs like chocolate [12].

39.6 Lichen and Lichenoid Lesions

Oral manifestations of lichen are subdivided into two entities, oral lichen planus (OLP) and oral lichenoid lesions (OLL). The etiology to OLP is not known, but explanations such as drug exposure, hepatitis C or chronic liver disease, systemic diseases such as diabetes, and psychosocial factors such as stress have been postulated [37], while OLL is thought to be a reaction to dental materials. The clinical and histological picture is the same. The only difference is the localization of the lesions; while OLL is found in areas in direct contact with a specific dental restorative material, OLP is mainly present on the buccal mucosa, gingiva, and on the lateral edges of the tongue [37]. Intraoral lichen is present in a red and a white form [38] with patterns such as lacelike reticular or papular lesions with white striae and white plaques, or erosive lesions in the buccosal mucosa, on the gingiva, or on the lateral edges of the tongue. Sometimes atrophic or bullous lesions are present. More than one form can be seen simultaneously and in the same location [37]. The diagnosis is based on the patient's history, clinical investigation, and eventually a biopsy. In general, the whitish lesions are most often symptomless, while the reddish lesions can give irritation and a varying degree of stinging.

When symptomless lesions of OLP are present, there is no need to investigate them except for regular check-ups at the dentist. When the diagnosis is OLL, a patch test aimed at dental restorative materials should be carried out. If a positive reaction is seen to an allergen, the dental material should be changed to a material that the patient is expected to tolerate, based on the results of the patch test. Even if no contact allergy is detected, a change of materials should be contemplated. OLP is treated with local antifungals and often followed by topical corticosteroids; both are prescribed in the form of an oral paste or an oral gel. OLP is a premalignant condition, although the risk for malignant transformation is considered to be very small [38].

A case-control study examining the association of dental materials with OLP showed apparent associations between OLP, the corrosion status of amalgams, the presence of a galvanic effect from dissimilar dental metals in continuous contact (bimetallism), and the presence of gold in the mouth [37].

In OLL, amalgam is the major cause, without or with contact allergy, as the material as such causes irritation. According to some reports, 2% of the adult population in Sweden has OLL. Lingua geographica-like lesions and stomatitis geographica lesions can also be seen. An Australian study showed that in 13 of 19 patients with OLL in close contact with amalgam fillings and who showed positive patch test reactions to mercury, replacement of their amalgam fillings led to complete recovery, and one patient had marked improvement [39]. In a Finnish study, it was shown that of 118 patients with OLL, 80 had metal allergy, 78 were allergic to mercury, and 11 to gold [40]. Fifty-one patients with OLL and/or OLP were patch tested and 74.5% had at least one positive reaction to a metal allergen. The positive patch test reactions were significantly more common for chromate, gold, and thimerosal compared to dermatitis patients. Forty-nine percent showed sensitivity to one or more mercury-containing compounds [41]. In contrast, another study showed 41% metal allergy in patients with OLP [42]. Of 55 OLL-patients tested to dental metals, 45% showed allergic patch tests to 1 or more dental metals. Seventy-six percent of the allergic patients were positive to mercury alone, 20% to mercury and gold, and 4% to gold alone. It was considered that all reactions to mercury were potentially relevant to the OLL. Thirteen of twenty five had the dental metal to which they had reacted removed, and in eight of nine available for follow-up after 1 year, the OLL had improved and was asymptomatic. The authors concluded that contact allergy to mercury and to a lesser extent to gold seems to be relevant to the causation of OLL in a proportion of subjects, but not all [43]. Another study showed 1/12 to be hypersensitive to mercury [12]. Removal of the amalgam restoration next to the area of OLL gave healing or much improvement in 102 of 105 cases [44] and in 86.7% of patients with OLL adjacent to amalgam fillings with sensitization to inorganic mercury [45]. OLL may in certain cases be caused by irritancy and the removal of the amalgam may then also be beneficial, even if patients are patch test negative to mercury [44, 46]. Other metals in dental prostheses, e.g., chromium and cobalt, have occasionally been responsible for OLL [47]. In patients with silver amalgam fillings and OLL adjacent to this restorative material, a high frequency of contact allergy to mercury and other base metals in dental amalgam has been noticed [48].

39.7 Causative Agents in Allergic Contact Dermatitis and Stomatitis/Cheilitis

39.7.1 Acrylics and Other Plastic Chemicals

Since the 1990s, acrylics (acrylates and methacrylates) have taken the place of amalgam in dental restorations. In particular, methacrylates have been identified as major occupational contact sensitizers. Three groups of acrylics are important in dentistry: (a) monofunctional methacrylates such as MMA and 2-HEMA, the latter being common in bonding products, and both being semivolatile; (b) multifunctional methacrylates such as EGDMA, TREGDMA, triethyleneglycol diacrylate (TREGDA); and (c) acrylated and methacrylated prepolymers such as 2,2-bis[4-(2-hydroxy-3-methacryloxypropoxy)phenyl]-propane (bis-GMA) (Bowen resin) and urethane dimethacrylate (UEDMA), the former in dentin bonding products and both present in dental filling materials [49]. Hypersensitivity to MMA in prostheses was already reported in the 1940s [50–52], and in 1954, Fisher reported on two dentists and two dental mechanics with hand eczema and allergic contact dermatitis from MMA. In those patients MMA was patch tested at 100% [53]! Dental prostheses, dental composite resins (DCR), and dentin bonding agents all have caused occupational allergic contact dermatitis from acrylics. Contact allergy frequencies to methacrylates are lower in dental patients than personnel, because patients are exposed to uncured acrylics for a shorter time than dental personnel and the sensitization capacity in the oral mucosa may be lower [54, 55], and salivary flow prevents adequate contact [56].

39.7.1.1 Dental Composite Resins

DCR based on bisphenol A and glycidyl (meth)acrylates have been used since 1962 [57]. The most commonly used is bis-GMA. It can also be manufactured by an addition-reaction between diglycidyl ether of bisphenol A (DGEBA) resin and methacrylic acid. Therefore, bis-GMA can be classified as a dimethacrylated epoxy, even if it does not contain a reactive epoxy group [49]. DCR may, as a result, contain DGEBA resin as an impurity. Hence, a person sensitized to DGEBA resin may react to bis-GMA or vice versa, especially if that person has a strong hypersensitivity to DGEBA resin and/or bis-GMA, i.e., reacts to low concentrations of the allergen when it is patch tested in a serial dilution [28]. We have seen one patient who was previously sensitized to DGEBA resin and had severe stomatitis adjacent to a newly made DCR restoration (containing bis-GMA) in the mouth and, in addition, an eczema on the cheek just overlying the DCR filling. Another patient had a systemic contact dermatitis with vesicular hand eczema for many weeks after she had a DCR restoration containing bis-GMA. She was occupationally sensitized to DGEBA resin several years preceding this occasion. Some authors have discussed cross-reactivity between DGEBA resin and epoxy acrylates but a lack of cross-reactivity between these two compounds was also reported [58].

(Meth)acrylated urethanes are also used in DCR but to a lesser extent. The aliphatic urethane methacrylates such as UEDMA are the most common, but aromatic urethanes are also used. Contact allergy to methacrylated urethanes and bis-GMA is rare. Both have a high molecular weight and a relatively high viscosity. To dilute these monomers, other methacrylates or dimethacrylates of lower viscosity are added, e.g., MMA, TREGDMA, and EGDMA [59].

Dental personnel: bis-GMA and epoxy diacrylate sensitized four dental nurses with occupational allergic contact dermatitis in the 1980s at FIOH [56], and since then, a few new cases from dental practice have been reported [4, 60].

Dental patients: Few patients have been reported to have been sensitized to DCR. Allergic stomatitis from a DCR filling material containing TREGDMA and bis-GMA was reported in 1983. The dental patient reacted to DGEBA resin in the baseline series and the filling materials used, parts A and B, both tested at 1% petrolatum (pet). The authors suspected that the reaction to DGEBA resin was due to cross-reactivity to the bisphenol A derivatives in DCR [61]. Allergic contact stomatitis and perioral allergic contact dermatitis from bis-GMA in DCR was reported for the first time in 1998. The same patient also reacted to DGEBA resin [62]. Acute gingivostomatitis due to contact allergy to methacrylate in a dental restorative material was also reported [63]. Aphthous ulcerations from TEGDMA have also been reported [64]. Other acrylics have been described as being present in DCR: monomers of low viscosity such as MMA, 2-HEMA, EGDMA, diethyleneglycol dimethacrylate (DEGDMA), TREGDMA, and tetraethyleneglycol dimethacrylate (TEGDMA) [65]; dimethacrylate derivatives of bisphenol A such as 2,2-bis[4-(methacryloxy)phenyl]propane (bis-MA), 2,2-bis[4-(2-methacryloxyethoxy)phenyl]propane (bis-EMA), and 2,2-bis[4-(3-methacryloxy-propoxy)phenyl]propane (bis-PMA); and dimethacrylate monomers containing urethane groups such as UEDMA and tetraurethane dimethacrylate (TUDMA) [56].

Polymerization may be accomplished by the peroxide/amine method, UV radiation, and, today, most often by visible light [56]. Residual monomers are present even after curing, but the effect of leaking residual monomers is not known.

In addition, additives such as initiators and inhibitors and also substances not usually allergenic such as pigments, inorganic fillers (glass, zirconium ceramics, quartz powder, amorphous silica), and polymerized waxes are present in DCR [56].

39.7.1.2 Dentin Bonding Agents are Plastics Without Fillers and are Called Resins

The first dentin bonding agent was *N*-phenyl glycine glycidyl methacrylate, Bowen's resin. Bonding systems formerly contained a primer and an adhesive, but nowadays, it is usually a one-step procedure. After etching the surface to be treated with 37% phosphoric acid, the dentin is covered by the bonding agent (adhesive) which is pressed out into the cavity with pressurized air. Polymerization is then accomplished by blue visible light, and subsequently, the DCR is applied to the cavity of the tooth in layers and cured either with chemicals or with the same visible light as above. 2-HEMA is most often present in bonding systems as it is water soluble and does not damage the pulp, but bis-GMA, TREGDMA, and UEDMA can also be present. Because bis-GMA may be used in dentin bonding agents, DGEBA resin may also be present as an impurity in these resins.

Dental personnel: A female dentist repeatedly developed pharyngitis at work. A chamber provocation test indicated that her symptoms were caused by acrylics. Prick tests with acrylics were negative, while patch tests were strongly positive without the patient having any skin lesions [66]. A dental laboratory worker developed symptoms of conjunctivitis. He was exposed to chemically curable and light-curable methacrylates and was sensitized to multiple methacrylates including MMA, 2-HEMA, EGDMA, and TREGDMA. Conjunctivitis may be caused by type IV allergy to methacrylates [67]. Acrylate compounds are reported to also cause occupational laryngitis [68].

Dental patients: A woman presented with edema, erythema, and ulceration of the mucosa of the upper lip after dental work on her front teeth. The dentist had used a primer containing maleic acid and 2-HEMA and an adhesive containing 2-HEMA and bis-GMA. Contact allergy to 2-HEMA and TEGDMA was noted, even though the adhesive system declared only 2-HEMA to be present. The reaction to TEGDMA was thought to be due to cross-sensitivity between the two methacrylates [69].

or photoallergic mechanism. They usually arise as a complication of a pre-existing, possibly eczematous, dermatosis.

The clinical picture is usually an acute dermatitis – erythema, oedema, papules and vesicles, sometimes with exudation and scaling, and always accompanied by intense pruritus. When a previous dermatosis is being treated, aggravation of the picture may suggest superimposed sensitization. However, if the sensitization is particularly due to a corticosteroid or an ingredient of a corticosteroid cream, this acute picture is usually mild or absent due to the anti-inflammatory properties of the steroid. In these circumstances, if the dermatosis does not improve, despite correct treatment, a secondary contact allergy should be suspected.

In patients with stasis dermatitis and/or leg ulcers, or other chronic eczemas, it is not rare to see dissemination of the eczema (haematogenous route – systemic contact dermatitis) to the other leg at first, then to the entire integument, leading sometimes to erythroderma; this is mainly seen in older patients with long-standing eczemas. Sometimes there is scant local symptomatology, and the first acute symptoms are seen at a distance, usually by ectopic dissemination (on the face, for example). In our experience, elderly patients with eyelid dermatitis should arouse the suspicion of allergy to topical drugs applied on the lower limbs, i.e. NSAID and venotropic drugs.

Airborne [64] and photoallergic contact dermatitis have a similar clinical expression – acute or sub-acute dermatitis on exposed areas. They differ from toxic dermatitis because they have a more polymorphic clinical picture, not precisely limited to exposed areas. However, as stated with the irritant type, there are some locations spared in photodermatitis, which may be affected in the airborne type, such as the upper eyelids, under the chin, behind the ears, the back of the neck or even the scalp.

38.4 Allergens

Topical medicaments include active principles and ingredients of the vehicles, many of which are found in cosmetics. Most substances in a medicament may, at some point, induce cutaneous sensitization.

38.4.1 Local Anaesthetics

Local anaesthetics (LA) can induce allergic contact dermatitis and, more rarely, IGE-mediated type 1 reactions [271].

They can be divided into two main groups – esters and amides – based on their structural similarities. Ester anaesthetics are derived from p-aminobenzoic acid and include benzocaine, procaine (novocaine), amethocaine (or tetracaine), cocaine and proxymetacaine (or proparacaine) [242, 271, 302]. They are used to treat pruritus ani, haemorrhoids [192] or pruritus vulvae [188], but occupational cases have been reported [58]. Benzocaine is still the principal allergen in this group [302] and may cross-react with other components of the para-group, especially with p-phenylenediamine. Nowadays, they have largely been replaced by anaesthetics of the amide group.

The amide LA comprises two subgroups, aminoacylamides (lidocaine, bupivacaine, articaine, mepivacaine and prilocaine) and aminoalkylamides (procainamide and dibucaine or cinchocaine).

Dibucaine is currently more frequently used in the same topical medicaments. It can cause allergic [25, 217, 302] and systemic contact dermatitis [202].

Other amides, like lidocaine (lignocaine, xylocaine), bupivacaine (marcaine), mepivacaine (carbocaine) and prilocaine (citanest), are less potent sensitizers. However, as they are now more often used than p-aminobenzoic esters, there have been several cases of sensitization reported. Since the first descriptions [277], many other cases of allergy to lidocaine have been reported [302, 303]. It may cross-react with mepivacaine and less often with bupivacainwwe and prilocaine [303]. Contact sensitization to prilocaine is rare [265] and it has been primarily induced by EMLA® cream [181, 286]; in none of these cases there was cross-reaction with lidocaine.

Concomitant reactions to LA of both groups are not common, but have been reported [118, 302].

Several other LA, including butacaine, proxymetacaine (proparacaine) [56], oxybuprocaine (in ophthalmic preparations) [31], propipocaine, pramocaine (pramoxine), amylocaine, cyclomethycaine, propanidid (intravenous anaesthetic), diclonine hydrochloride [60] and butylaminobenzoate [291], have been reported as sensitizers.

39.7.1.3 Prosthetic Materials: Prostheses

One of the most important groups of materials used in the prosthetic area is plastics or polymers used in dentures or prostheses, fixed bridges and crowns, facades, orthodontic devices, models, trays, and occlusal splints. Dental technicians previously handled methacrylates with bare hands [70], but nowadays they use protective gloves when possible, even if it is less common than among dentists and dental nurses. The methylmethacrylate and polymethylmethacrylate system is the most important system for removable prosthesis or dentures. Polymethyl methacrylate (PMMA) denture base has dominated the market for over 50 years [71]. The basement sheets are made from MMA liquid, which is mixed with PMMA powder resulting in a mass that is molded, manually or mechanically. The powder may contain copolymers of other acrylates such as polyisobutyl acrylate or polystyrene [72]. In the powder, there may also be organic peroxide initiators, X-ray contrast substances, pigments for color, cadmium and ferric salts, iron oxides, titanium dioxide to control translucency, and dyed synthetic fibers for esthetics [70]. Potential allergens are pigments, dyes, nylon fibers, and titanium or zinc oxides.

The liquid may contain other monomers such as *n*-butyl methacrylate, isobutyl methacrylate, or lauryl methacrylate, hydroquinone inhibitor, dimethacrylates or cross-linking agents like EGDMA, an organic amine accelerator if cold-curing or self-curing, and UV-absorbers [70, 72]. The polymerization starts after the molding process by means of heat, chemicals, or UV radiation or visible light. In the heat-polymerization process, the monomer solution may contain cross-linking bifunctional (meth)acrylates such as 1,4-butanediol dimethacrylate, 1,4-butanediol diacrylate, ethyleneglycol methacrylate, or EGDMA [70]. Cross-linking helps the dilution of high-viscosity monomers and makes the 3-dimensional structure more rigid [70]. The monomer solution which is polymerized chemically may contain *N,N*-dimethyl-*p*-toluidine as an accelerator. Another amine accelerator is 4-tolyldiethanolamine [70]. Hypoallergenic denture base materials exist, and significantly lower residual MMA monomer content was found when comparing these denture base materials to PMMA [71]. Other alternatives for prosthetic materials are polymers such as phenol formaldehyde resins, polyamides, polyurethanes, polyvinyl chloride (PVC), polyvinyl acetate, polystyrene, and polystyrene copolymers. Polycarbonates can also have this function.

Dental technicians nowadays use more complex light-cured acrylics similar to DCR in composition and hence are exposed to methacrylates with a higher sensitizing potential than MMA and thus pose a higher risk of contracting occupational contact dermatitis [73].

Dental personnel: An orthodontist developed pulpitis because of exposure to MMA liquid when remodeling children's dental devices with cold-curing acrylics without protective gloves. She was allergic to MMA, which was her only exposure, but also reacted to butyl acrylate, ethyl acrylate, and 2-hydroxypropyl methacrylate, possibly due to cross-reactivity with MMA [70]. Animal studies showed that animals sensitized to methacrylates may show cross-reactivity to acrylates but not vice versa [74]. A dental technician with hand eczema was allergic to MMA when patch tested and also to MMA liquid in 1% pet and 100% PMMA powder, which is very uncommon as this is a polymerized material and should not contain more than minute amounts of monomers [70].

Dental patients: The first report of cheilitis from acrylates in prosthesis was a male patient who had cheilitis on both lips with dermatitis extending beyond the vermilion border with additional involvement of the oral mucosa. He was allergic to MMA and the test reaction was still evident on the back 7 weeks after the testing [75]. When dentures made from MMA and PMMA are incompletely polymerized, residual monomers can dissolve into the mouth. A woman developed contact stomatitis from residual MMA. She was MMA-allergic and MMA was extracted from the denture even after 15 years of use (showed by chromatography). She was patch tested to the extract of the denture, made in 100% methanol, and was positive [76]. Another case was allergic to MMA and PMMA thought to be present in her denture base material [77]. In another case of allergic contact stomatitis from MMA in a dental prosthesis, MMA was tested in 25 and 2% pet and the patch test reactions lasted for 30 days [78]. An acrylic-metal prosthesis gave dermatitis around the mouth and swelling of eyelids and lips. Contact allergy to MMA and PMMA tested at 25% pet was positive [79]. A woman had labial edema due to an acrylic dental prosthesis made from MMA and PMMA and EGDMA as the cross-linker. She was found to be allergic to MMA and EGDMA [80]. An unusual case is the 12-year-old boy who was allergic to bis-GMA and the bonding paste in his orthodontic prosthesis and who had worn his appliance for over 1 year without any oral changes [81]. He had however extraoral eczema due to bis-GMA-allergy.

Atypical forms of contact allergic reactions to acrylic dental prostheses are chronic urticaria without mucosal or perioral lesions [82], and stomatitis and edema of the tongue, lips, eyelids, and hands [83].

Crowns and bridges or facades are made from PMMA powder and MMA liquid or paste. The liquid contains monomers of MMA and tetrahydrofurfuryl methacrylate, the crosslinkers and dimethacrylate monomers EGDMA, TREGDMA, and 1,4-butanediol dimethacrylate and the prepolymer uretan dimethacrylate. The inhibitor hydroquinone stabilizes the monomers, and the activator *N,N*-dimethyl-*p*-toluidine acts as an initiator. The powder is usually PMMA with inorganic fillers.

The light- and heat polymerizing dental materials can contain dimethacrylates, diacrylates, trimethacrylic monomers, and oligomers containing several urethane and dimethacrylate groups in the molecule.

39.7.1.4 Additives in Dental Acrylics-Initiators, Activators, Stabilizers

Benzoyl peroxide is an initiator and a catalyst for acrylic and polyester resins. Few cases of contact allergy have been reported in the dental profession. Two cases of allergic contact dermatitis in the manufacture of dental prostheses [84] as well as one dentist being allergic to benzoyl peroxide and mercury [85] have been published . Airborne allergic contact dermatitis from benzoyl peroxide has also been reported from molten candle wax and when sawing plastic materials into particles that became airborne [86, 87]. When patch testing with this substance, false-positive reactions may be seen as benzoyl peroxide is also an irritant.

At room temperature, cold-cured or self-cured acrylics need an accelerator or activator for the polymerization reaction. The activator most used is the tertiary aromatic amine *N,N-dimethyl-p-toluidine* which is a rare sensitizer.

Dental patients: Among 52 denture wearers, only one case of contact allergy to this substance was found [29]. A case of contact stomatitis from the accelerator was reported in a woman wearing a new dental prosthesis. When she discontinued wearing her denture she recovered completely [88]. Another lady allergic to her denture material containing *N,N*-dimethyl-4-toluidine was free of symptoms when she stopped wearing them [89].

A further activator is the amine accelerator *4-tolyl diethanolamine*, which induces polymerization of acrylic resins at room temperature. Contact allergy is rare.

Dental personnel: A dentist with occupational allergic contact dermatitis was allergic to 4-tolyl diethanolamine [90].

Camphoroquinone is an initiator for visible-light-cured dental acrylic composite materials and primers. So far, no dental contact allergy has been reported even if a case of patch test sensitization has been reported [91].

The inhibitors *hydroquinone* and methyl hydroquinone are used to prevent unintended spontaneous polymerization. *p*-methoxyphenol and butylated cresols are also inhibitors. 2,6-di-(*tert*-butyl)-4-methylphenol (BHT) is another rare sensitizer and inhibitor [19].

Dental patients Hydroquinone released from acrylic dentures caused allergic contact cheilitis and stomatitis in a woman [92].

39.7.1.5 UV-Absorbers

To improve color stability of the plastic, and to prevent it from yellowish discoloration and darkening with age, *UV stabilizers* are added [59]. These may be benzophenones such as 2,2-dihydroxy-4-methoxybenzophenone (UV9, Eusolex 4360), 2-hydroxy-4-methoxybenzophenone, and 2,4-dihydroxybenzophenone or 2(2-hydroxy-5-methylphenyl)benzotriazole (Tinuvin P), phenyl salicylate, methyl salicylate, resorcinol monobenzoate, or stilbene [70]. 2,2-dihydroxy-4-methoxybenzophenone (Eusolex 4360) may be present in DCR. Allergic contact dermatitis and photocontact dermatitis from sunscreens has been reported.

Dental professionals: There are no reports on occupational allergic contact dermatitis in dental personnel.

Dental patients: A dental patient had allergic gingivitis from Tinuvin P present in a restorative material as shown by high performance liquid chromatography [93].

Plasticizers are added to plastics to improve the flexibility and pliability. Dibutyl phthalate may be added to the solution in prosthetic and rebasing materials [70]. There are no reports of contact allergy in dental practice.

39.7.1.6 Bisphenol A and DGEBA Resin

Bisphenol A is used in the production of epoxy resins and polycarbonates, but is also used as an additive in the manufacture of PVC plastics. Bisphenol A has been found in PVC gloves. It is a rare sensitizer in dental care. Sixteen brands of disposable PVC gloves for medical use covering at least 80% of the Finnish market were analyzed for the presence of bisphenol A, and only one brand contained a small amount of it [94].

Dental professionals: A dental assistant with hand eczema was allergic to bisphenol A which was found in the DCR she handled by means of chemical analysis. She became free of symptoms after avoiding exposure to DCR [95]. An oral hygienist apprentice and a dentist were sensitized to bisphenol A from disposable PVC gloves of the same make. Bisphenol A was detected in the dentist's glove [94].

Dental patients: A dental patient with the burning mouth syndrome had a denture of unknown composition and was found to be hypersensitive to DGEBA resin and bisphenol A thought to have been used in a glue to mend the denture [77]. DGEBA resin may be present in a concentration of 30% in root canal sealant materials.

Dental patients: A woman had painful swelling of the oral mucosa for half a day following root canal treatment with a product containing DGEBA resin [96]. She was hypersensitive to both DGEBA resin and bisphenol F resin and also to bis-GMA. The origin of sensitization to bis-GMA was unclear.

39.7.1.7 Ethyl Cyanoacrylate Glue

Cyanoacrylates are widely used as instant contact adhesives for metal, glass, rubber, and plastics, in surgery to bind tissues and seal wounds, and in nail wrapping to create an artificial nail or to glue premade artificial fingernails on to the natural nail. Dental technicians use this type of glue regularly [14]. Cyanoacrylates polymerize almost instantaneously in air at room temperature and bond immediately and strongly to surface keratin. Due to this, many authors have considered allergic reactions to be virtually impossible. However, there are a few cases published even if not from the dental field. A hairstylist presented with acute periorbital eczema and marked edema of the eyelids and dry eczema of her fingertips. The dermatitis was due to hypersensitivity to cyanoacrylate glue used when attaching pieces of false hair to bald scalps. She had to leave her job to get well. Three women used cyanoacrylate glue in nail wrapping processes to create an artificial nail and were sensitized [97]. An office worker glued prefabricated plastic fingernails on to her natural nail to cover them which caused allergic contact dermatitis and nail dystrophy and led to months of sick leave [98].

39.7.1.8 Plastic and Fillers Composite

Fillers are inorganic materials such as finely ground glass, zirconium ceramics, quartz powder, and amorphous silica (SiO_2).

Glass ionomers are used as dental filling materials, for cementing and as fissure sealants and contain polyacrylic acid or polymaleic acid and glass powder.

An example of a *resin-modified glass ionomer* cement is triple-cured hybrid-glass ionomers which were introduced in the 1990s and contain the same sensitizing methacrylates as DCR and bonding agents. Conventional glass ionomer cements are mixed with acrylate monomers, which should be water soluble and hence 2-HEMA is used and initiators. The mixture thus contains 2-HEMA and often modified polyacrylic acid linked to methacrylate units. They are polymerized by light, when 2-HEMA and methacrylate units link together. The principle gives better strength and better esthetic properties. If they are mixed manually, there is a risk of becoming occupationally sensitized, which is why no-touch techniques should be applied. A potential hazard is the fact that 2-HEMA is released from the ionomer to the oral cavity, which makes it not biocompatible [99].

Dental personnel: A dental nurse suffered from pulpitis from acrylic tri-cure glass ionomer she worked with. The light-cured hybrid-glass ionomer system was composed of a powder, a primer, and a liquid, the latter two containing 2-HEMA, which she reacted to at patch testing. She also reacted to the hybrid-glass ionomer primer and liquid tested at 1% pet. [100]. *Compomers* are composite plastics where the acrylate monomer is modified with carboxylic acid groups and the filler is glass – much the same as in ionomers. Compomers are used as a filling material and cement. When used, it should be preceded by a bonding plastic.

39.7.1.9 Two Materials for Short-term Use

1. *Temporary fillings*
   Temporary fillings may contain zinc oxide and eugenol from cements.
   Eugenol is the main component of IRM liquid (>99%), used in temporary fillings.

Dental personnel: two dental nurses were occupationally sensitized to IRM, and eugenol was suspected to be the primary sensitizer [11].

2. *Dental or surgical packings*
   After periodontal surgery a dental packing or dressing may be used to protect the operated area. A liquid and powder is mixed, where the liquid can contain 60% eugenol with *Myroxylon Pereirae* and the powder zinc oxide and 40% colophony.

39.7.1.10 Impression Materials and Resin Carriers

Impression materials are used when inlays, bridges, and crowns are to be made. These materials may be silicon-based, alginate, beeswax or Scutan, based on etylenimine derivatives and containing bisphenol A. There are no reports of reactions to silicon-based materials in dental personnel, but two cases of contact allergy have been reported, caused by a catalyst in a silicon-based material [101]. Alginate has been implicated in oral vesicular reactions in dental students following multiple alginate impressions. Patch testing was negative and the mechanism unclear [102]. Occupational dermatitis has been reported to be from beeswax, which makes up at least 17% of dental modeling wax [103]. Contact allergy from the catalyst in Scutan, methyl-*p*-toluene sulphonate, has been reported both in dental personnel and dental patients [50, 104].

39.7.1.11 Resin Carrier

N-ethyl-p-toluene-sulfonamide functions as a resin carrier in materials used for isolating cavities below restorations [59].

Dental personnel: A dentist occupationally sensitized to several chemicals at work also reacted to this chemical [90].

39.7.1.12 Product Analysis of Acrylic Resins

Acrylic products often contain undeclared acrylates/methacrylates which makes it hard to know what patients/workers are exposed to. A few attempts have been made to compare the material safety data sheets to the actual composition of the product. DCR and bonding materials were analyzed by gas chromatography and mass spectrometric methods. Analyzed acrylate products contained undeclared acrylics, most of which had been reported to be contact sensitizers [105]. A recent chemical investigation of commercial dental restorative materials showed 2-HEMA and bis-GMA to be the most frequently occurring methacrylates in the bonding materials, and bis-GMA and TREGDMA in composite resins. The main methacrylate of two glass ionomers was 2-HEMA or trimethylolpropane trimethacrylate. In about half of the material safety data sheets, the methacrylates were declared to be present [65]. Better material safety data sheets are required from the industry before products are put on the market.

> **Core Message**
>
> › Acrylic products often contain undeclared acrylates/methacrylates. The material safety data sheets are often inadequate.

39.7.2 Rubber and Plastics in Gloves

Protective gloves are the most common cause of occupational allergy to rubber products [70]. Since the 1980s, protective gloves have been a mainstay in the dental professionals to protect the dentists and nurses from contracting HIV and hepatitis from infected patients. Natural rubber gloves were most prominent in the 1980s, whereas synthetic rubber and plastic gloves are more common nowadays. Contact allergy to additives in the natural rubber gloves is mostly directed to the accelerators thiuram, dithiocarbamate, and mercaptobenzothiazole. The same additives may also be present in synthetic rubber gloves. These allergens are present in most baseline series. A special rubber series may sometimes be helpful. Hexamethylenetetramine and 1,3-diphenylguanidine gave allergic patch test reactions in a Finnish patient working in rubber gloves [70]. It may be difficult to get information on the actual additives used in the production of gloves, and new sensitizers may also be formed during the manufacture. A test with the glove "as is" may sometimes be sufficient, but if it is negative, an extract made from the glove may have to be tested [106]. The eluent should be chosen on the basis of which sort of glove is being investigated and which potential substance(s) should be eluted. The clinical picture of an allergic contact dermatitis to glove components may be a patchy eczema on the dorsal aspects of the hands or an eczema covering the whole hand from the dorsal fingers up to the end of the glove. When a patient is rubber allergic, the best advice would be to make him/her refrain from using rubber gloves and use plastic gloves if possible. Using inner gloves from cotton or wool may also be an option. If inner gloves are worn, it is important that they do not extend beyond the outer glove, because then there is a risk of contaminating the inner glove. Contaminants may be substances that are harmless when present on open skin but may be harmful under occlusion.

Contact allergy to chemicals in plastic gloves is uncommon. 1,2-benzisothiazolin-3-one (BIT) is used as a biocide in the manufacture of PVC. In Finland, BIT in powder-free PVC gloves has caused a small epidemic of allergic contact dermatitis in dental personnel. Thirty one disposable PVC glove brands were investigated for the presence of BIT and 30% contained the preservative. A concentration of 20 ppm BIT seems to suffice for sensitization [107]. Accordingly, patients with hand eczema using PVC gloves should be tested to BIT. Other vinyl gloves contained biphenol A that sensitized dental personnel [94, 95].

> **Core Message**
>
> › Protective gloves are the most common cause of occupational allergy to rubber products.
> › A test with the glove "as is" may be sufficient, but if negative, an extract made from the glove should be tested. The eluent should be chosen on the basis of which sort of glove is being investigated and which potential substance(s) should be eluted.

39.7.2.1 Protective Effect of Medical Gloves

Medical gloves for single use are not impermeable to various acrylate monomers. The breakthrough times for typical gloves made from NRL and PVC are normally less than 10 min [4, 108]. The protective effect from gloves worn by dental professionals has been investigated. Double gloves increased the breakthrough times in an experimental setting [108]. A thin copolymer glove under a medical glove for single use offered the best protection in one study [109]. A study from Malmö showed that a commonly used ethanol-based dental adhesive containing the potent sensitizers 2-HEMA and TREGDMA penetrated all the gloves except one, the 4H glove, Safety four A/S, Lyngby, Denmark. The second best glove was a nitrile glove followed by a latex glove [110]. The same authors also showed that a glove giving a poor protection might be as bad as or even worse than no glove at all. The best protection against 2-HEMA was neoprene gloves [111]. A thin inner glove made of polythene may be of protective value as a complement to a more resilient outer glove, such as neoprene or nitrile. An in vitro study showed this [108] and the better protective capacity of a neoprene glove vs. a nitrile glove against a mixture of 2-HEMA (50%) and TREGDMA (50%). The laminated multilayered disposable glove, the 4H-glove, protects against acrylics, but is an industrial glove with poor anatomical fit. However, a fingertip piece of the 4H-glove under a disposable latex or PVC glove can been recommended [49, 50]. The best way not to get sensitized is to work with a "no touch" technique, which dentists nowadays learn early in their training. If their hands get contaminated by an acrylic material they should remove their gloves at once, wash their hands with soap and water and don new gloves [110]. Nobecutan contains thiurams. One dental nurse was sensitized to thiurams after using Nobecutan for small cuts [56].

39.7.3 Metals

On the European market, some 1,000 different odontological alloys are present. Most of the casting alloys are based on the precious metals gold, platinum, palladium, and titanium. Gold and the platinum group metals are used for inlays, crowns, and bridges.

Metal ceramic materials are made from porcelain placed on an alloy. Stainless steel prostheses, previously widely used, have in the 1990s been replaced by alloys containing chromium (30%), cobalt (60%), and manganese (5%) [112]. In Sweden, there has, since decades, been a recommendation not to use nickel-containing casting alloys for permanent prosthetic replacements, even if these type of alloys have been used in other countries without prominent side effects [113]. In Sweden, casting alloys for permanent metal ceramic materials did not previously contain chromium-cobalt, but this type of alloy is nowadays used there; for removable dentures, casting alloys are based on chromium-cobalt 25–30 and 60%, respectively. As one of the main allergens used by dentists, metals are present in amalgams, inlays, crowns, bridges, posts, cores, and braces. Mercury unites with other metals to form amalgams. Dental amalgams are therefore a mixture of metallic mercury (50%) with tin (6–13%), silver (22–36%), zinc (<1%), or copper (1–15%) that are allowed to solidify at room temperature in the patient's mouth [114]. Since almost 100 years, amalgams have been used for the permanent filling of cavities in the inner part of the mouth. Dental cements may contain amalgams composed of zinc (1%), tin (12%), and mercury, while amalgams of mercury with gold, silver (34%), or copper (3%) are used as fillings for teeth [50]. Systemic contact dermatitis induced by metals in orthodontic appliances such as from nickel, cobalt, and chromium has been reported [115].

Corrective orthodontic appliances such as wires may be made from steel containing 17–19% chromium and 10–13% nickel. Other steel alloys may contain 10–27% chromium and 12–34% nickel [115]. Nickel-titanium thread containing 54% nickel and 46% titanium may also be used. In nickel-allergic individuals, the use of nickel-free materials, such as plastic brackets or nickel-free orthodontic thread made of beta-titanium should be adopted [116]. An extraoral orthodontic apparatus such as a facial bow can be coated with a plastic layer if the material contains nickel. Other metals used in dental products are cobalt, chromium, molybdenum, beryllium, gallium, rhodium, and iridium [12]. The most frequent contact allergies among dental materials are caused by metals such as gold, nickel, and mercury [117, 118], whereas methacrylates are the most common plastic sensitizers [12]. Occupational skin disease from metals used in the dental profession has seldom been reported.

39.7.3.1 Aluminum

Aluminum is used as a pure metal or as an alloy in dental materials and as salts in dental ceramics. Contact allergy is rare. There are no reports in dental care [119].

39.7.3.2 Beryllium

This metal may be added to some nickel-chromium alloys for technical reasons. It tends to migrate to the surface because of its small atomic radius [114]. Because it increases the corrosion of other metals, alloys containing beryllium should not be used.

Dental personnel: A dental technician was thought to have developed berylliosis from occupational exposure to beryllium. Testing with beryllium sulfate was positive [120].

Dental patients: Beryllium sensitized two patients having allergic gingivitis from a beryllium-containing alloy in dental prostheses. Beryllium was present in a concentration of 1.8% [114].

39.7.3.3 Chromium

In Sweden, cast alloys for permanent metal ceramic materials did not previously contain chromium-cobalt, but this type of alloy is nowadays used there and is an alternative to the more expensive gold alloys. Chromium-cobalt alloys have been used in other countries for a long time. In Sweden, cast alloys for removable dentures are based on chromium-cobalt 25–30 and 60%, respectively. Chromium allergy seldom arises from dental metals [121].

Dental patients: A dental prosthesis containing chromium and cobalt led to OLL in a patient hypersensitive to chromium [47]. A woman previously sensitized to chromium, cobalt, and nickel had systemic contact dermatitis from dental crowns containing chromium, cobalt, and nickel [122]. Another case is a patient sensitized to chromium from a chromium dental plate which led to a reactive intraoral erythema and a generalized eczematous dermatitis [123]. A girl wearing an orthodontic appliance with wires made of steel containing 17–19% chromium had a vesicular dermatitis on her hands shortly after the fitting of the wires. She had no stomatitis. Hypersensitivity to potassium dichromate

39

was detected. A placebo-controlled oral challenge with 2.5 mg chromium resulted in a flare of vesicular dermatitis on the fingers after challenge with the chromate tablet. The dermatitis faded completely 2 months after the appliance was removed and did not recur [115].

39.7.3.4 Cobalt

Cast alloys for removable dentures based on chromium-cobalt contain about 60% cobalt. Cobalt sensitization seldom originates from dental products.

Dental patients: A dental prosthesis containing cobalt and chromium led to OLL in a patient hypersensitive to cobalt [47]. A woman previously sensitized to chromium, cobalt, and nickel had systemic contact dermatitis from dental crowns containing chromium, cobalt, and nickel [122]. A patient who was allergic to cobalt, present in a metal denture, developed hand eczema [124].

39.7.3.5 Copper

Dental amalgams may contain copper. Contact allergy has been considered very rare by some [119, 125], but others claim that positive patch tests to copper do not seem to be a rare finding and that they originate in a cross-reactivity to nickel. However, patch tests to copper are of low clinical relevance [126]. Nickel may be present as an impurity in the patch test substance of copper. Hence, the allergic reactions seen when patch testing the copper preparation may have been attributed to nickel allergy instead of copper allergy [127].

Dental patients: Acute urticaria has been described in a case having a tooth temporarily filled with black copper cement [128]. Copper allergy was noted in three patients with orodynia, except for one who also had OLP adjacent to a restoration [129]. A woman was thought to have been sensitized to copper through long-term exposure to copper-rich amalgam fillings, previously used in childhood dentistry in Sweden (before the 1960s), and had diffuse symptoms from the oral cavity without any clinical signs. Her plastic dental splint to prevent teeth grinding during sleep was discolored green on the surface due to deposition of copper compounds from the saliva caused by increased copper intake from drinking water [130].

39.7.3.6 Gold

Gold alloys contain varying amounts of gold mixed with silver, copper, smaller amounts of platinum, palladium, and zinc [12]. Gold has been used in casting alloys for inlays, in crowns, bridges, and in gold posts (gold pin in a root canal). Gold salts can be strong sensitizers but reactions to metallic gold have been considered rare. GSTS is the gold salt of choice for patch testing, e.g., 2.0 and 5.0% in petrolatum [131]. Gold chloride is not recommended due to a lower pick-up rate and risk of primary toxic reactions [132].

Dental patients: In a questionnaire study and in several clinical studies from the Department of Occupational and Environmental Dermatology in Malmö, Sweden, it has been shown that there is a statistically significant connection between dental gold and gold allergy. There is also a quantitative relationship between contact allergy to gold and the amount of gold areas in the oral cavity. A frequency of 30.4% gold allergy was recorded in dermatitis patients having been patch tested to GSTS present in a baseline series. There was no statistical relationship between oral lesions and contact allergy to gold [133]. In other studies on dermatitis, patient frequencies of 4.6, 8.6, and 10.0% were found [134–136], and gold allergy was second only to nickel in frequency of occurrence among dermatitis patients at the Department of Occupational and Environmental Dermatology in Malmö, Sweden [134]. Today, gold still is second only to nickel in frequency of occurrence among dermatitis patients and is the number one sensitizer in dental patients in the Malmö clinic (Table 39.3).

In a study of 134 patch tested dental patients, gold allergy was noted in 14% [118]. A multicenter study of patch test reactions with dental screening series from Finland revealed a contact allergy frequency of 7.7% for gold and 10.3% for mercury [117]. It is estimated that two million Swedes have dental gold. A patient allergic to gold should not have new gold restorations fitted in their mouth, but removal of gold restorations in an allergic patient without apparent signs of contact allergy should probably not be done.

Dental patients: Metallic gold in crowns and other restorations has caused allergic contact stomatitis and gingivitis [137] (Fig. 39.1a, b).

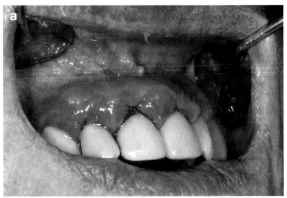

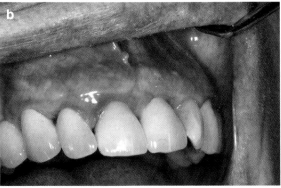

Fig. 39.1 (**a**) A patient with gingivitis due to gold allergy. Metal ceramic crowns containing gold in his front teeth. (**b**) The same patient after replacement of the gold crowns with another material he tolerated

39.7.3.7 Indium

Indium was reported to be present in dental alloys (in 0.5–6%) and in white gold (in 0.4–4.5%) in the 1990s [114, 138]. The metal was patch tested in a series of dental patients, most of whom lacked oral mucosal reactions but had subjective systemic symptoms, and 3.9% reacted with positive reactions. No clinical relevance was discussed [138].

39.7.3.8 Iridium

Iridium is one of the platinum group metals in the periodic table of the elements. Iridium was reported to be present in dental alloys and in white gold (in 0.1–0.2%) in the 1990s. The metal was patch tested in a series of dental patients, most of whom lacked oral mucosal reactions but had subjective systemic symptoms, and 1% reacted with positive reactions. No clinical relevance was discussed [138].

39.7.3.9 Manganese

Manganese is a transitional metal increasingly used in dental prostheses as nickel has been replaced. Isolated cases of positivity to manganese have been observed in prosthesis-wearers and with past or unknown relevance [139]. In Malmö at the Department of Occupational and Environmental Dermatology, we have patch tested manganese chloride 2.0% pet in 486 consecutively patch tested dental patients in Finn Chambers and recorded four positive reactions. The four patients reacted only on day 4 and not on day 7. Two were retested and did not react at all. Six reactions were regarded as toxic and 54 as doubtful. We suspect manganese chloride 2.0% pet to give false-positive reactions and have therefore ceased to test with this substance in our dental screening series.

Dental patients: A woman had allergic contact stomatitis due to manganese present in her removable partial denture (content was 0.5%). She was patch-test positive to manganese chloride 5% petrolatum. Fifteen controls were negative [139].

39.7.3.10 Mercury

Hypersensitivity to mercury is seldom reported. In Sweden, mercury in amalgams has been replaced by acrylics because of the environmental risks and the public´s opinion on worry of toxic effects. Since 2009, mercury is also prohibited to be used in dental practice.

In Malmö, we have retrospectively collected data on the 1,364 dental patients who were patch tested during a period of 11 years. Mercury 0.5% pet from Chemotechnique Diagnostics, Vellinge, Sweden and mercury 1.6% softisan made at our department were used throughout the study period. Reaction to mercury was shown by 9.3%. Thirty-four percent of the mercury contact allergies would have been missed had not a day 7 reading been performed. The most common reasons for referral from the dentists were OLL (39%) and inflammation in the oral mucosa (16%), whereas the most common subjective symptoms were burning sensation in the oral mucosa (13%) [140]. In a recent study of 134 patch tested dental patients, mercury allergy was noted in 9.9%. Mercury was not a significant factor for OLL. There was a strong association between orofacial granulomatosis and contact allergy to mercury from dental fillings in two patients [118].

Dental personnel: Occupational contact allergy to mercury is extremely rare. One dentist and two dental nurses, all three with hand eczema due to uncured amalgam contact with bare hands, have been described. They reacted positively when patch tested to metallic mercury [141–143].

Dental patients: Amalgam fillings may cause OLP or OLL on the buccal mucosa as a contact reaction with or without contact allergy.

39.7.3.11 Nickel

In Sweden, casting alloys for permanent metal ceramic materials do not contain nickel.

There has been a recommendation in Sweden for several decades not to use casting alloys containing nickel in permanent prosthetic appliances. However, in other countries, nickel has been used in casting alloys without any major problems even in nickel-allergic individuals.

Nickel and cobalt are often present in the same alloy, and in the process, it is difficult to separate the two. Therefore, nickel alloys often contain small amounts of cobalt (less than 1%) and vice versa. If more than 0.1% nickel is present in an alloy, it must be declared, but alloys containing less than 0.1% nickel are considered nickel-free.

In orthodontic alloys, such as those used in wires and brackets, stainless steel containing 18% chromium and 8% nickel is mostly used, but one may also use nickel- titanium thread, containing 54% nickel and 46% titanium. Orthodontic treatment with nickel-containing material in the mouth prior to ear piercing (nickel-sensitization) does not seem to sensitize but rather give tolerance, and adverse reactions in nickel-allergic patients with orthodontic appliances containing nickel are uncommon [144].

Dental patients: The use of 66% nickel in crowns and bridges in nickel-allergic patients did not give any adverse reactions in 16 patients followed for 3 years [113]. Nickel in a dental prosthesis has been thought to cause a dermatitis or to exacerbate a dermatitis around the mouth or in a more widespread distribution, e.g., on the hands and feet [12]. Concerning nickel reactivity and orthodontic appliances, a suggested prevalence of 0.03% adverse reactions was put forward in a survey of

orthodontists. Intra- and extraoral reactions were mild, and one case of urticaria was presented [145]. Facial eczema from a fixed retainer wire made of stainless steel in a patient with nickel allergy and without oral signs has been published recently. The patient's eczema disappeared within weeks after the retainer was taken out [146]. Systemic contact dermatitis caused by nickel in a stainless steel orthodontic appliance was presented in 1997 [147], but it was considered extremely rare. A woman previously sensitized to chromium, cobalt, and nickel had systemic contact dermatitis from dental crowns containing chromium, cobalt, and nickel [122].

39.7.3.12 Palladium

Palladium is one of the platinum group metals in the periodic table of the elements. It is resistant to corrosion. Palladium is a very common component of dental casting alloys of all types, e.g., together with dental gold, silver, zinc, and copper [12], in dental plates, and as a catalyst in white gold. The risk of using palladium in dental casting alloys appears to be extremely low because of the low dissolution rate of the palladium ions from these alloys [148], that even allergic patients tolerate them. Thirty percent of those allergic to nickel react to palladium when patch tested, especially those with a strong contact allergy to nickel. Cross-reactivity between the two metals has been proposed and also shown in a scientific study by systemic administration of nickel [149]. The clinical significance of allergic reactions caused by palladium remains unclear. However, there are a few cases published on contact allergy and allergic symptoms from palladium.

Dental patients: A patient with mouth irritation and systemic symptoms was cleared when a dental bridge containing palladium was taken out. An allergic reaction to both palladium and nickel was noted. A patient with chronic facial swelling was allergic to palladium and removal of the crowns containing palladium produced a cure [12].

39.7.3.13 Platinum

Metallic platinum is used in dentistry. It rarely causes allergic contact dermatitis [119]. Occupational contact urticaria, asthma, and allergic rhinoconjunctivitis have been described more often than contact dermatitis [50].

39.7.3.14 Silver

Silver is used together with palladium ,zinc, and copper in alloys.[12]. Dental amalgams containing metallic silver do not cause allergic contact dermatitis [128].

39.7.3.15 Tin

Tin is used in dental metal preparations such as amalgams. Contact allergy to tin is rare [150] and was first described in 1987 [151].

39.7.3.16 Titanium

Dental implants based on titanium have been used since decades. Titanium allergy among dental patients is considered rare or nonexisting, even if some reports indicate that titanium may act as an allergen [152, 153]. A retrospective study on dental patients tested to three titanium preparations (elemental titanium as powder 50% pet, calcium titanate 10.0% pet, titanium nitride 5.0% pet) during a period of 11 years and titanium oxalate 5.0% pet for 1 year revealed one patient out of 1,373 to react to calcium titanate on day 7. There were 31 doubtful reactions in total. The authors concluded that titanium does not seem to sensitize dental patients and that it can be recommended for dental implants and frameworks for removable partial dentures [154].

39.7.3.17 Zinc

Allergic patch test reactions have also been described to rare metals such as zinc and rhodium [112]. A correlation between palmoplantar pustulosis (PPP) and metal allergy has been reported in the Japanese population, and recently, a new case report discussed the relationship between PPP and zinc allergy. A woman had new dental metal restorations containing gold, indium, silver, palladium, copper, and zinc since 1 year, and after 6 months, inflammatory skin lesions resembling PPP covered her palms and soles. She was patch test positive to zinc chloride 2% pet and her skin lesions healed within 4 weeks of removing the zinc fillings [155]. At the Department of Occupational and Environmental Dermatology in Malmö, we have patch tested 483 dental patients with zinc chloride 1.0% pet

and have seen four reactions judged as positive. In none of the cases was there any suspicion of clinical relevance. Ten reactions were regarded as toxic and 50 as doubtful. We suspect the preparation to give false-positive reactions, and therefore we have omitted it from the dental screening series.

39.7.4 Disinfectants

Formaldehyde is present in the baseline series and is a common sensitizer [156] and a common cause of occupational allergic contact dermatitis among dental personnel [56, 157]. The source of formaldehyde allergy in dental work can be from hand creams, hand wash products, or instrument care [11].

Glutaraldehyde is used as a germicidal agent in the cold sterilization of surgical instruments and is a moderate irritant and a sensitizer. It is also a common cause of occupational allergic contact dermatitis among dental personnel [56, 157]. Formaldehyde and glutaraldehyde do not cross-react.

Dental personnel: Contact allergy to glutaraldehyde has been reported in dental nurses [158, 159] and contact dermatitis has been reported in dental assistants.

Tego is the commercial name for certain disinfectants where the active ingredient is dodecyl-di-(aminoethyl)glycine. It is used as an antiseptic for instruments in dental practice. It is sold under various trade names e.g., Tego, Tego 103G, Tego 51, Ampholyte G, and Ampholyte 103G. Recommended patch test concentration is 0.5% aqua [13].

Dental personnel: Tego was found to be the number one antimicrobial to cause allergic occupational eczema in dental personnel in Finland during the 1970s to the 1990s [56].

39.7.4.1 Povidone-Iodine

Polyvinylpyrrolidone-iodine (povidone-iodine 10%, Betadine) is a compound of iodine and povidone with additives such as glycerine and nonoxynol-9. It is used as an antiseptic and antibacterial agent with low irritating and toxic potential. Povidone itself may be present in toothpastes [160]. Those allergic to povidone-iodine are most often not reacting to iodine [161].

Dental personnel: Occupational allergic contact dermatitis is rare but has been described in a dentist and operating room nurse [162].

Potassium persulfate is used in antiseptics, toothpastes, and other bleaching agents of teeth. It can be used in products for disinfection of surfaces and instruments. The agent may irritate the skin and cause immediate, e.g., asthma, and delayed allergic reactions. No allergic contact dermatitis has been reported in dental care, but a laboratory assistant in a water laboratory was occupationally sensitized [163].

39.7.5 Eugenol, Colophony, Carvone

Eugenol (4-allyl-2-methoxy phenol) is the essential component of clove oil (85%) and is also present in the oil of cinnamon (10%), oil of bay (60%), perfumes, soaps, oil of carnation (80%), pimento oil (80%), flower oils, food spices, and flavors. Eugenol is also used in toothache drops, mouthwash, and antiseptics. In dentistry, eugenol is mixed with zinc oxide to form zinc-eugenol cement (ZOE), which is used as a provisional restorative material, base material, root canal filling material, in impression pastes, as sealers and periodontal packs. Cements and liners have antiseptic and anesthetic properties with a palliative action on the dental pulp. These sealers may also be used as lubricants and fillers in teeth [164]. As eugenol is highly soluble, it is continuously released from ZOE. Eugenol is also used as an intermediate two-component restorative material with PMMA powder, and a dental nurse was sensitized to eugenol from working with this intermediate restorative liquid material containing >99% eugenol [165].

Eugenol is present as one of the eight components of fragrance mix in the baseline series. *Myroxylon Pereirae* contains eugenol, and eugenol-hypersensitive individuals may react to *Myroxylon Pereirae*. Therefore, a dental worker who reacts to *Myroxylon Pereirae* in the baseline series should be investigated for occupational allergic contact dermatitis from eugenol. Eugenol in dental preparations has been reported to cause contact urticaria, gingivitis, stomatitis venenata, and allergic hand eczema in dental personnel [165]. Eugenol is considered to be a less common sensitizer than isoeugenol, cinnamic aldehyde, or cinnamic alcohol.

Dental personnel: In two patients an allergic eczematous reaction followed handling eugenol [165].

Dental patients: A eugenol impression paste gave allergic cheilitis and stomatitis in one patient [165]. Type I allergy to eugenol impression paste can present as urticaria.

39.7.5.1 Colophony

Colophony is ubiquitous and present in several dental materials such as periodontal dressings, impression materials (often with eugenol), and cavity varnishes (e.g., Hartskloroform in Sweden) and caries prophylactic varnish (fluoride dental coatings) (Duraphat). Zinc oxide-eugenol (ZOE) cements may contain colophony. The temporary filling material Nobetec in Sweden contains both colophony, eugenol, Canada balsam, and *Myroxylon Pereirae*.

Dental personnel: Occupational allergic contact dermatitis from colophony present in Duraphat fluoride varnish has been reported in dental personnel with hand eczema, one Swedish dental nurse [166] and two Finnish dental nurses [13]. Hartskloroform can give urticaria due to immediate allergy.

39.7.5.2 Carvone

The terpene l-carvone is a constituent of spearmint oil and may be present in toothpastes and chewing gums [33, 167]. Testing with toothpastes "as is" may be done, but it can lead to false-negative reactions because of a too low concentration of the sensitizer or false-positive reactions because of the content of soaps, detergents, and abrasives, which may irritate the skin [33]. Toothpaste reactions are rare.

Dental patients: Carvone has caused contact allergy in users of spearmint toothpaste and chewing gums [33, 167]. We inform our patients to buy carvone-free toothpaste, which may be difficult to obtain. Menthol is an important sensitizer in peppermint and l-carvone in spearmint. Both have been reported as causes of erosive cheilitis and should be tested in patients with oral ulcerations, OLL, and glossodynia, and in perioral eczema and cheilitis [168].

39.7.6 Local Anesthetics

The anesthetic compounds can be divided into two main, but chemically different groups, namely the ester type and the "amides." The ester type anesthetics are all derivatives of *p*-aminobenzoic acid, while the "amides" include aminoacrylamides such as lidocaine, prilocaine, and mepivacaine, and aminoalcylamides such as procainamide and the quinoline derivative dibucaine. Since their introduction in the 1940s, the amide-type anesthetics have been used most frequently for local anesthesia because of longer half-life in tissues and infrequent observations of true allergies [169]. Benzocaine is present in most baseline series because it is a common and potent sensitizer. It is a *p*-aminobenzoic acid derivative and cross-reacts with procaine and tetracaine, hair dyes, drugs such as para-aminobenzoic acid, para-salicylic acid, antidiabetic medications and is said to cross-react with sulfonamides [128]. Benzocaine and tetracaine are used in products such as analgesics, astringents, oral antibacterial preparations, preparations for toothache, teething, and denture irritation [128].

Dental personnel: Earlier dentists were often allergic to local anesthetics because they came into contact with the agents when rubbing a preparation containing a "caine" on to the surface of the gum or when gauze packs were made for postextraction sockets, or by injecting a "caine" compound into the buccal area and spilling on to the fingers when retracting or holding the syringe [128]. Fisher described four dentists who were sensitized to tetracaine, with cracking and scaling of finger pulps, especially the first three fingers [128]. Lidocaine, the amide-type anesthetic, is a rare allergen with only a few reports on contact allergy [50, 128, 170] and does not cross-react with benzocaine or tetracaine. Procaine, another local anesthetic, cross-reacts with benzocaine or tetracaine. Contact allergy to procaine used to be common among dentists [50, 128] but is not seen today.

39.8 Patch Testing

A dental series of 21 chemicals was composed in Sweden in the early 1980s and has since been modified [59]. The Swedish Contact Dermatitis Research Group has suggested two different dental series, based on previous patch test data from 15 clinics, one for the investigation of dental patients and one for the dental personnel (Tables 39.1 and 39.2). Dental personnel with suspected contact dermatitis from dental materials should be patch

Table 39.1 Dental screening series for dental personnel recommended by the Swedish Contact Dermatitis Research Group

Test substance	Concentration % w/w
Methyl methacrylate	2.0
Triethyleneglycol dimethacrylate	2.0
Ethyleneglycol dimethacrylate	2.0
Bis-GMA	2.0
2-hydroxyethyl methacrylate	2.0
Tetrahydrofurfuryl methacrylate	2.0
1,4-butanediol methacrylate	2.0
Mercury	0.5
Eugenol	2.0
Glutaraldehyde	0.2

Vehicle is petrolatum

tested with a dental plus a baseline series, whereas in dental patients, a dental series is sufficient. Sometimes, it may be difficult to judge the clinical relevance between a positive test and the patient's signs and symptoms. The connection is best judged by the patient's dentist in cooperation with the dermatologist.

Patch test preparations containing sensitizers that are used in dental practice are sold by Chemotechnique Diagnostics, Vellinge, Sweden and Trolab Hermal, Hamburg, Germany.

Patch test readings should be carried out on day 3 or 4 and also on day 7 (late reading), as allergic reactions to acrylics [171], gold [172], and mercury [12, 140] have a tendency to appear late. Concerning mercury, if a day 7 reading had not taken place, 30% of the contact allergy would have been missed [140], and for 2-HEMA, our figures would have been 25% missed reactions.[24]. In most studies looking at contact allergy frequencies a day 7 reading has not been performed consistently.

> ## Core Message
>
> › When patch testing with a dental series, patch test readings should be carried out on day 3 or 4 and also on day 7 (late reading), as allergic reactions to acrylics, gold, and mercury have a tendency to appear late.

Table 39.2 Dental screening series for dental patients recommended by the Swedish Contact Dermatitis Research Group

Test substance	Concentration % w/w
Methyl methacrylate	2.0
Triethyleneglycol dimethacrylate	2.0
Ethyleneglycol dimethacrylate	2.0
Bis-GMA	2.0
Bis-EMA	2.0
2-hydroxyethyl methacrylate	2.0
N,N-Dimethylaminoethyl methacrylate	0.2
Tetrahydrofurfuryl methacrylate	2.0
1,4-Butanediol methacrylate	2.0
1,6-Hexanediol diacrylate	0.1
Potassium dichromate	0.5
Mercury	0.5
Cobalt chloride	0.5
Gold sodium thiosulfate	2.0
Nickel sulfate	5.0
Eugenol	2.0
Colophony	20.0
N-Ethyl-4-toluenesulfonamide	0.1
Palladium chloride	2.0
R-Carvone	5.0
2-(2'-Hydroxy-5'-methylfenyl)-benzotriazole	1.0
Myroxylon Pereirae	25.0
Epoxy resin of bisphenol A	1.0

Vehicle is petrolatum

39.8.1 Indications for Patch Testing

Among dental professionals, those with evident or suspected occupational contact dermatitis or worsening of an endogenous dermatitis in dental work should at least be patch tested with the baseline series and a dental series to find contact allergies or to rule them out.

For dental patients, we have three major indications for patch testing:

1. when a patient has objective signs in the oral mucosa localized next to a dental restorative material and when the clinical picture is a lichenoid reaction or when there is a strong suspicion of contact allergy to a dental restorative material.

2. presence of dermatitis in the face or elsewhere on the body and with a temporal relation to some dental treatment.

3. when a patient has planned to go through a major dental restorative treatment and there is a history of intolerance to dental materials that will be used, and to rule out contact allergy.

4. a relative indication is the burning mouth syndrome.

In the burning mouth syndrome physical signs of mucosal disease are missing. Most patients are denture wearers and some have infection with *Candida Albicans*. In others, "psychological factors" are considered most important [12]. Patch testing is usually negative [173, 174], but 6 of 22 had contact allergy to acrylics [175]. In another study, 28% of the investigated patients had contact allergy to dental base materials including MMA and additives [29]. Also, contact urticaria and pressure urticaria was ruled out in eight denture-wearing patients with normal-appearing mucosa [173]. In denture wearers with previous allergic diseases and burning mouth syndrome, a high incidence of allergic skin reactions to denture allergens, especially methacrylates and formaldehyde, has been reported [48]. In Table 39.3, the outcome for positive patch test reactions to dental allergens from the dental patient series 2008 in Malmö is given.

39.8.2 Patch Test Sensitization

Active sensitization is an iatrogenic sensitization to a chemical induced by the application of a patch test. Some acrylics have been incriminated in active sensitization. Ethylacrylate, 2-hydroxypropyl acrylate, and 2-hydroxyethyl acrylate sensitized patients in Finland and the patch test concentration was lowered and some substances were even removed from the test series [176]. Acrylics are strong allergens and should never be applied undiluted to the skin, because a single such exposure can induce sensitization [177]. Therefore, patch testing patients with undiluted acrylic products may be hazardous and requires knowledge on the sensitizing potential of the tested substance. Acrylate products can usually be tested in 0.1% and methacrylate products in 2.0%. If the vehicle is petrolatum,

Table 39.3 Statistics for the dental patients' series 2008 in Malmö – top 10

Substance	Concentration in %/vehicle	Positive/tested	Frequency in %
Gold sodium thiosulfate	2.0% pet	14/57	24.1
Nickel sulfate	5.0% pet	13/57	22.4
Palladium chloride	2.0% pet	4/58	6.9
Cobalt chloride	1.0% pet	4/58	6.9
Thimerosal	0.1% pet	3/58	5.2
Sodium metabisulfite	2.0% pet	3/58	5.2
Colophony	20.0% pet	3/58	5.2
Benzoyl peroxide	1.0% pet	3/58	5.2
Mercury	0.5% pet	2/58	3.4
Potassium dichromate	0.5% pet	2/57	3.4
Triethyleneglycol dimethacrylate	2.0% pet	1/58	1.7
Mercury	1.6% softisan	1/58	1.7
Carvone	5.0% pet	1/58	1.7
Myroxylon Pereirae	25.0% pet	1/58	1.7
Zinc chloride	1.0% pet	1/58	1.7
For the rest of the allergens, there were no reactions	–	–	–

a metal chamber works fine, e.g., the Finn Chamber, but if the acrylic is diluted in acetone or some other solvent, a plastic chamber should be used so as not to risk polymerization of the acrylic monomers and a false-negative patch test reaction [178]. A dental patient was actively sensitized to acrylics by her dentist who performed a "use test" on intact skin with undiluted glass ionomer containing sensitizing acrylics, e.g., 2-HEMA. According to some authors, dentists should be warned against performing use tests with dental acrylics [177].

Core Message

> Acrylics are strong allergens and should never be tested undiluted. Acrylate products can usually be tested in 0.1% and methacrylate products in 2.0%. If the vehicle is petrolatum, a metal chamber works fine, but if the acrylic is diluted in acetone or some other solvent, a plastic chamber should be used so as not to risk polymerization of the acrylic monomers and a false-negative patch test reaction.

39.8.3 Screening for Contact Allergy to Acrylics

MMA was previously a standard allergen for screening for acrylate allergy. However, it is a weak sensitizer and not a very good screening substance for such allergy. The newer (meth)acrylates are much more potent sensitizers than MMA. In Malmö we have seen that 2-HEMA would have picked up all our dental personnel looking at figures 10 years back, and 2-HEMA in addition to bis-GMA would have picked up all of our dental patients [24]. A study in Malmö and Singapore has screened for contact allergy to acrylics in the baseline series during more than 2 years of testing. The tested acrylics were 2-HEMA, MMA, EGDMA, TREGDA, and 2-hydroxypropyl acrylate (2-HPA). The prevalence of acrylate allergy was 1.4% in Malmö and 1.0% in Singapore. The positive reactions in the baseline series in Malmö, in order of frequency, were: 2-HEMA, TREGDA, 2-HPA, EGDMA, and MMA. In Singapore, the substances in order of frequency were: TREGDA, EGDMA, and 2-HEMA [179]. When comparing these figures with older

39

figures from Singapore, we saw that only two allergens were in common in both centers, (unpublished data) and that over time, the frequencies for the various allergens change [180]. Hence, no single abbreviated series could be recommended for different centers.

Core Message

> ❯ No single abbreviated acrylate test series could be recommended for different centers because over time, the frequencies for the various allergens change.

39.9 Immediate Reactions

Immediate reactions may be allergic or nonallergic. Allergic reactions are IgE-mediated reactions usually caused by proteins. However, certain low-molecular-weight chemicals may also elicit similar immediate hypersensitivity reactions caused by both allergic and unknown mechanisms.

39.9.1 Clinical Picture

The first sign of type I allergy on the skin is typically contact urticaria, which usually develops in minutes but most often less than 30 min, after the skin has come into contact with the offending allergen. There is erythema on the contact areas, wheals appear and the skin may get swollen with smarting or itching. Contact urticaria may also disappear within hours if the offending allergen no longer is in contact with the skin, leaving the skin totally blank and symptomless. Other symptoms of immediate allergy are also common, e.g., itching of the eyes, conjunctivitis, and rhinitis, and there may be coughing, dyspnea, or even asthma. A life-threatening anaphylactic shock may develop in the worst scenario.

Type I allergy on the skin may also develop into the so-called protein contact dermatitis, which is seen in people who mostly have or have had an irritant eczema prior to the protein contact dermatitis. The phenomenon is confined to atopics and the dermatitis cannot be distinguished from other forms of hand eczema, irritant or allergic.

39.9.2 Causative Agents

39.9.2.1 Proteins in Natural Rubber Latex and Corn Starch

Natural rubber is derived from the milky sap of the rubber tree, *Hevea Brasiliensis*. The monomer is cis-1,4-polyisoprene intermingled with a variety of other rubber plant proteins [181]. NRL gloves are the most common cause of immediate-type allergy to latex in dental personnel [182]. To prevent NRL allergy, PVC gloves or NRL gloves with a low-protein content is recommended. Immediate-type allergy to latex is also the most common type I allergic reaction in dental patients [12]. If a patient is latex allergic, he can get symptoms ranging from contact urticaria from latex gloves and rubber dams to anaphylactic reactions from dams and latex gloves. Hundred and forty-six workers at Swedish dental care centers were examined for latex allergy with skin prick tests with different latex extracts. Blood samples from 144 were RAST-analyzed using the CAP system. Sensitization to latex diagnosed by a positive skin prick test and/or by demonstration of specific antibodies in serum analyses was found in 2.1% of the subjectsinvestigated. Latex sensitivity was one explanation to reported glove intolerance. The authors diagnosed latex allergy in less than 10% of the cases of glove-related skin complaints reported in an interview investigation and concluded that the majority of skin complaints from gloves are caused by skin irritation rather than by allergy [183]. In a study from 2000, immediate-type latex allergy was reported in 10% of dentists, 6% of dental nurses, and 4% of dental hygienists [5]. From Australia, a self-reporting questionnaire study on dentists showed that 1/3 had experienced hand dermatoses during the last year, 15% during the previous 3 weeks. Eleven percent reported dermatitis after the use of latex gloves [184]. One important cause of respiratory hypersensitivity is NRL. Based on the statistics from the FROD between 1975 and 1998, the following was reported on dental personnel: one case of asthma, seven cases of rhinitis, and two cases of combined rhinitis and conjunctivitis caused by NRL [185].

Corn Starch Powder

A study on skin prick tests to a commercial corn extract (ALK Laboratories, Denmark) in 146 individuals from dental care centers in Sweden showed negative results in all but one case, supporting earlier findings that intolerance reactions to glove powder are often not provoked by the corn starch itself. Latex allergens are absorbed by the starch powder and contact with the powder from gloves may provoke latex-allergic reactions [183].

39.9.2.2 Gutta-Percha

A transpolyisoprene, is a rubber-like gum used in dentistry and obtained from the viscous milky latex of the *Palaquium* tree from Southeast Asia. Compared with the manufacture of rubber, no preservatives or vulcanizing agents are added, but synthetic plasticizers, zinc oxide, barium sulfate, and pigment are added to the final product. Because gutta-percha is derived from trees of the same botanical family as natural rubber a potential for cross-reactivity exists.

Dental patients: A dental hygienist with known immediate latex allergy went through root canal surgery, when gutta-percha points were inserted into a maxillary molar. This resulted in immediate oral discomfort, lip and gum swelling, a throbbing sensation around the tooth, and diffuse urticaria. Not until the gutta-percha was removed 1 month later did her urticaria and oral discomfort disappear. The authors were not able to demonstrate a positive prick test or IgE antibodies to gutta-percha [181].

39.9.2.3 Low-Molecular-Weight Chemicals

Haptens may cause IgE-mediated reactions. The hapten binds to proteins in the skin or to other macromolecules, and the hapten-carrier complex acts as an allergen [186].

Eugenol, a *para*-substituted phenolic compound, is used in dental impression materials, in periodontal packs, and various sealers. It is known to cause contact urticaria and chronic urticaria [187], and recently acute urticaria was described in a patient fitted with a PMMA temporary dental bridge fixed with a zinc oxide-eugenol sealer. A skin prick test was positive for eugenol [164].

Colophony: A case of occupational rhinitis caused by Nobetec containing colophony was diagnosed at the FIOH [185].

Formaldehyde is commonly used as a disinfectant for root-canal treatment. Formaldehyde frequently provokes contact dermatitis but IgE-mediated response to formaldehyde is rare.

Dental patients: Most cases of Type I allergy have been reported in patients receiving dental treatment using (para)formaldehyde-containing tooth fillings. A common characteristic feature is the delay in time of 2–12 h between the dental treatment with (para)-formaldehyde and the allergic symptoms. This is probably due to formaldehyde being gradually released from (para) formaldehyde, then penetrating through the dentin, and gradually increasing in concentration in the circulating blood after root-canal treatment until reaching the threshold to trigger symptoms [10]. A case of anaphylaxis within minutes of exposure in a patient with immediate-type allergy to formaldehyde was described [12]. *Chlorhexidine*, a synthetic cationic bis-biguanide antiseptic and disinfectant, was introduced in 1954. It has a wide range of usages. It is used for topical application on skin or mucous membranes, wounds, burns, surgical instruments, and surfaces. It is found in toothpaste, gargles, and mouthwashes. Discoloration of teeth and tongue, distorted taste, and desquamative gingivitis are rare side effects. In spite of its common usage the sensitization rate seems low. Hypersensitivity reactions comprise delayed hypersensitivity reactions such as contact dermatitis, fixed drug reactions, and photosensitivity reactions and immediate-type hypersensitivity reactions such as contact urticaria, occupational asthma, and anaphylactic shock [188]. Contact sensitivity was first reported in 1962 [189]. Some larger studies showed a sensitization rate of 2%. Immediate anaphylactic reactions are even rarer. The first cases were published in the 1980s. Its application to mucous membranes can cause severe anaphylactic reactions, and in Japan, the Ministry of Health in 1984 recommended avoiding the use on mucous membranes. However, the use of 0.05% chlorhexidine on wounds and intact skin was considered safe, as no severe anaphylactic reactions had been reported. Recently, the second case of severe anaphylaxis due to topical skin application was reported. The author's caution its use even at a low concentration of 0.05%. The risk is higher when used on mucous membranes [188].

Chloramine-T is used as a disinfectant for instruments and surfaces in dental work. It can cause occupational contact urticaria similar to persulfates, also used for disinfection. Chloramine-T is an important cause of respiratory hypersensitivity. Based on the statistics from the FROD, three cases of asthma and one case of rhinitis caused by chloramine-T was diagnosed in 1990–1998 [185].

Phenylmercuric acetate gave an immediate hypersensitivity reaction with facial edema, rhinoconjunctivitis, and asthma in a farmer's wife exposed to this agent present in pesticides and herbicides [190].

39.9.2.4 Local Anesthetics

Immediate-type allergy to local anesthetics is rare even though adverse reactions following the administration of such substances are seen in approximately 0.5% of cases [12].

39.9.2.5 Fibrin Tissue

Bovine fibrin tissue caused an immediate-type allergic reaction in a woman who had a tooth extracted and where the extraction socket was filled with fibrin tissue to stop the bleeding [191]. A similar case has been published [192].

39.9.2.6 Metals

Nickel has caused both immediate and delayed allergy with contact urticaria, rhinitis, asthma, and contact dermatitis [193]. A case of chronic urticaria from nickel-containing dental prostheses was also reported [194]. Platinum itself is a strong type I allergen [195], and several other metals of the platinum group such as iridium, which caused respiratory allergy and contact urticaria [196], palladium, rhodium, and ruthenium, have caused immediate allergy [197, 198]. Mercury salts [190] and sodium fluoride [199], present in 31% of the toothpastes sold in Finland [200] were reported to give contact urticaria.

39.9.2.7 Methacrylates

Methacrylates are important causes of respiratory hypersensitivity. Based on the statistics from the FROD between 1975–1998, the following was reported on dental personnel: sixty four cases of occupational respiratory diseases, of which two were from the period

between 1975 and 1989 and the rest from 1990. Twenty-eight were occupational asthma, 18 of which were caused by methacrylates; 28 occupational rhinitis, six caused by methacrylates; seven allergic alveolit; and one organic dust toxic syndrome [185]. Most of the cases of asthma are from the 1990s by when the usage of plastic fillings had increased significantly [65]. Cyanoacrylates have also been implicated in causing asthma [201]. Five patients had asthma provoked by cyanoacrylates and one dental assistant got asthma from MMA when mixing MMA with PMMA to make a paste used in the manufacture of dental prosthetic trays [202]. The mechanism of respiratory hypersensitivity is still not known and there is doubt that it is IgE-mediated [203].

References

1. Rustemeyer T, Frosch PJ (2000) Occupational contact dermatitis in dental personnel. In: Kanerva L, Elsner P, Wahlberg JE, Maibach HI (eds) Handbook of occupational dermatology. Springer, Berlin
2. Kanerva L, Lahtinen A, Toikkanen J et al (1999) Increase in occupational skin diseases of dental personnel. Contact Dermatitis 40:104–108
3. Kanerva L, Alanko K, Estlander T et al (2000) Statistics on occupational dermatitis from (meth)acrylates in dental personnel. Contact Dermatitis 42:175–176
4. Wrangsjö K, Swartling C, Meding B (2001) Occupational dermatitis in dental personnel: contact dermatitis with special reference to (meth)acrylates in 174 patients. Contact Dermatitis 45:158–163
5. Lindberg M, Silverdahl M (2000) The use of protective gloves and the prevalence of hand eczema, skin complaints and allergy to natural rubber latex among dental personnel in the county of Uppsala, Sweden. Contact Dermatitis 43:4–8
6. Ohlson C-G, Svensson L, Mossberg B et al (2001) Prevalence of contact dermatitis among dental personnel in a Swedish rural county. Swed Dent J 25:13–20
7. Lönnroth EC, Shahnavaz H (1998) Adverse health reactions in skin, eyes, and respiratory tract among dental personnel in Sweden. Swed Dent J 22:33–45
8. Munksgaard EC, Hansen EK, Engen T et al (1996) Self reported occupational dermatological reactions among Danish dentists. Eur J Oral Sci 104:396–402
9. Wallenhammar L-M, Örtengren U, Andreasson H et al (2000) Contact allergy and hand eczema in Swedish dentists. Contact Dermatitis 43:192–199
10. Kunisada M, Adachi A, Asano H et al (2002) Anaphylaxis due to formaldehyde released from root canal disinfectant. Contact Dermatitis 47:215–218
11. Alanko K, Susitaival P, Jolanki R et al (2004) Occupational skin diseases among dental nurses. Contact Dermatitis 50:77–82
12. Gawkrodger DJ (2005) Investigation of reactions to dental materials. Br J Dermatol 153:479–485

13. Kanerva L, Estlander T (1999) Occupational allergic contact dermatitis from colophony in 2 dental nurses. Contact Dermatitis 41:342–343

14. Mürer AJL, Poulsen OM, Roed-Petersen J et al (1995) Skin problems among Danish dental technicians. A cross-sectional study. Contact Dermatitis 33:42–47

15. Rustemeyer T, Frosch PJ (1996) Occupational skin disease in dental laboratory workers. (I) Clinical picture and causative factors. Contact Dermatitis 34:123–133

16. Mürer AJL, Poulsen OM, Tüchsen F et al (1995) Rapid increase in skin problems among dental technicians trainees working with acrylates. Contact Dermatitis 33: 106–111

17. Meding B, Hosseiny S, Wrangsjö K et al (2004) Hand eczema, skin exposure and glove use in dental technicians. Contact Dermatitis 50:203

18. Cockayne SE, Murphy R, Gawkrodger DJ (2001) Occupational contact dermatitis from colophonium in a dental technician. Contact Dermatitis 44:42–43

19. Estlander T, Rajaniemi R, Jolanki R (1984) Hand dermatitis in dental technicians. Contact Dermatitis 10:201–205

20. Uveges RE, Grimwood RE, Slawsky LD et al (1995) Epidemiology of hand dermatitis in dental personnel. Mil Med 160:335–338

21. Jacobsen N, Aasenden R, Hensten-Pettersen A (1991) Occupational health complaints and adverse patient reactions as perceived by personnel in public dentistry. Community Dent Oral Epidemiol 19:155–159

22. Camarasa JG (1995) Health personnel. In: Rycroft RJG, Menné T, Frosch PJ (eds) Textbook of contact dermatitis. Springer, Berlin

23. LeSueur BW, Yiannias JA (2003) Contact stomatitis. Dermatol Clin 21:105–114

24. Goon ATJ, Isaksson M, Zimerson E et al (2006) Contact allergy to (meth)acrylates in the dental series in southern Sweden: simultaneous positive patch test reaction patterns and possible screening allergens. Contact Dermatitis 55: 219–226

25. Aalto-Korte K, Alanko K, Kuuliala O et al (2007) Methacrylate and acrylate allergy in dental personnel. Contact Dermatitis 57:324–330

26. Kanerva L, Mikola H-E (1998) Fingertip paresthesia and occupational allergic contact dermatitis caused by acrylics in a dental nurse. Contact Dermatitis 38:114–116

27. Kanerva L, Henriks-Eckerman M-L, Estlander T et al (1997) Dentist's occupational allergic paronychia and contact dermatitis caused by acrylics. Eur J Dermatol 7: 177–180

28. Isaksson M, Zimerson E, Svedman C (2007) Occupational airborne allergic contact dermatitis from methacrylates in a dental nurse. Contact Dermatitis 57:371–375

29. Kaaber S, Thulin H, Nielsen E (1979) Skin sensitivity to denture base materials in the burning mouth syndrome. Contact Dermatitis 5:90–96

30. Waakker-Garritsen BG, Timmer LH, Nater JP (1975) Etiological factors in the denture sore mouth syndrome. Contact Dermatitis 1:337–343

31. Tosti A, Piraccini BM, Peluso AM (1997) Contact and irritant stomatitis. Semin Cutan Med Surg 16:314–319

32. Freeman S, Stephens R (1999) Cheilitis: analysis of 75 cases referred to a contact dermatitis clinic. Am J Contact Dermat 10:198–200

33. Andersen KE (1978) Contact allergy to toothpaste flavors. Contact Dermatitis 4:195–198

34. Le Coz C-J, Bezard M (1999) Allergic contact cheilitis due to effervescent dental cleanser: combined responsibilities of the allergen persulfate and prosthesis porosity. Contact Dermatitis 41:268–271

35. Schena D, Fantuzzi F, Girolomoni G (2008) Contact allergy in chronic eczematous lip dermatitis. Eur J Dermatol 18: 688–692

36. Holmes G, Freeman S (2001) Cheilitis caused by contact urticaria to mint flavoured toothpaste. Australas J Dermatol 42:43–45

37. Martin MD, Broughton S, Drangsholt M (2003) Oral lichen planus and dental materials: a case-control study. Contact Dermatitis 48:331–336

38. Götrick B (2009) Lichen i munhålan. (in Swedish) Läkemedelsbulletinen 3:3

39. Pang BK, Freeman S (1995) Oral lichenoid lesions caused by allergy to mercury in amalgam fillings. Contact Dermatitis 33:423–427

40. Laine J, Kalimo K, Happonen R-P (1997) Contact allergy to dental restorative materials in patients with oral lichenoid lesions. Contact Dermatitis 36:141–146

41. Scalf LA, Fowler JF Jr, Morgan KW (2001) Dental metal allergy in patients with oral, cutaneous, and genital lichenoid reactions. Am J Contact Dermat 12:146–150

42. Yiannias JA, el-Azhary RA, Hand JH et al (2000) Relevant contact sensitivities in patients with the diagnosis of oral lichen planus. J Am Acad Dermatol 42:177–182

43. AthavalePN SKW, Yeoman CM et al (2003) Oral lichenoid lesions and contact allergy to dental mercury and gold. Contact Dermatitis 49:264–265

44. Dunsche A, Kastel I, Terheyden H et al (2003) Oral lichenoid reactions associated with amalgam: improvement after amalgam removal. Br J Dermatol 148:70–76

45. Koch P, Bahmer FA (1999) Oral lesions and symptoms related to metals used in dental restorations: a clinical, allergological and histologic study. J Am Acad Dermatol 41:422–430

46. Wong L, Freeman S (2003) Oral lichenoid lesions and mercury in amalgam fillings. Contact Dermatitis 48:74–79

47. Sockanathan S, Setterfield J, Wakelin S (2003) Oral lichenoid reaction due to chromate/cobalt in dental prosthesis. Contact Dermatitis 48:342–343

48. Kaaber S (1990) Allergy to dental materials with special reference to the use of amalgam and polymethylmethacrylate. Int Dent J 40:359–365

49. Kanerva L, Estlander T, Jolanki R (1994) Occupational skin allergy in the dental profession. Dermatol Clin 12: 517–532

50. Kanerva L, Estlander T, Jolanki R (1995) Dental problems. In: Guin JD (ed) Practical contact dermatitis. A handbook for the practitioner. McGraw-Hill, New York, St. Louis

51. Moody WL (1941) Severe reaction from acrylic liquid. Dent Digest 47:305

52. Stevenson WJ (1941) Methyl-methacrylate dermatitis. Contact Point 18:171–173

53. Fisher AA (1954) Allergic sensitization of skin and oral mucosa to acrylic denture materials. J Am Med Assoc 156: 238–242

54. Fisher AA (1975) Contact dermatitis, 2nd edn. Lea and Febiger, Philadelphia

55. Lowney ED (1968) Tolerance of a control sensitizer in man. Lancet 11:1137

39

56. Kanerva L, Estlander T, Jolanki R (1989) Allergic contact dermatitis from dental composite resins due to aromatic epoxy acrylates and aliphatic acrylates. Contact Dermatitis 20:201–211

57. Bowen RL (1962) Dental filling material comprising vinyl silane treated fused silica and a binder consisting of the reaction product of bisphenol A and glycidyl acrylate. US Patent 3,066,112

58. Nethercott JR (1981) Allergic contact dermatitis due to an epoxy acrylate. Br J Dermatol 104:697–703

59. Axell T, Björkner B, Fregert S et al (1983) Standard patch test series for screening of contact allergy to dental materials. Contact Dermatitis 9:82

60. Geukens S, Goossens A (2001) Occupational contact allergy to (meth)acrylates. Contact Dermatitis 44:153–159

61. Niinimäki A, Rosberg J, Saari S (1983) Allergic stomatitis from acrylic compounds. Contact Dermatitis 9:148

62. Kanerva L, Alanko K (1998) Stomatitis and perioral dermatitis caused by epoxy diacrylates in dental composite resins. J Am Acad Dermatol 38:116–120

63. Martin N, Bell HK, Longman LP et al (2003) Orofacial reactions to methacrylates in dental materials: a clinical report. J Prosthet Dent 90:225–227

64. Guerra L, Vincenzi C, Peluso AM et al (1993) Role of contact sensitizer in the burning mouth syndrome. Am J Contact Dermat 4:154–157

65. Henriks-Eckerman M-L, Suuronen K, Jolanki R et al (2004) Methacrylates in dental restorative materials. Contact Dermatitis 50:233–237

66. Kanerva L, Estlander T, Jolanki R et al (1992) Occupational pharyngitis associated with allergic patch test reactions from acrylics. Allergy 47:571–573

67. Estlander T, Kanerva L, Kari O et al (1996) Occupational conjunctivitis associated with type IV allergy to methacrylates. Allergy 51:56–59

68. Sala E, Hytönen M, Tupasela O et al (1996) Occupational laryngitis with immediate allergic or immediate type specific chemical hypersensitivity. Clin Otolaryngol Allied Sci 21:42–48

69. Agner T, Menné T (1994) Sensitization to acrylates in a dental patient. Contact Dermatitis 30:249–250

70. Kanerva L, Estlander T, Jolanki R et al (1993) Occupational allergic contact dermatitis caused by exposure to acrylates during work with dental prostheses. Contact Dermatitis 28:268–275

71. Pfeiffer P, Rosenbauer E-U (2004) Residual methyl methacrylate monomers, water sorption, and water solubility of hypoallergenic denture base materials. J Prosthet Dent 92:72–78

72. Finnish Advisory Board of Chemicals (1992) Acrylate Compounds: Uses and Evaluation of Health Effects. Government printing Centre, Helsinki, Finland, pp 1–60

73. Kanerva L, Estlander T, Jolanki R et al (1994) Dermatitis from acrylates in dental personnel. In: Menné T, Maibach HI (eds) Hand eczema. CRC, Boca Raton

74. Van der Walle HB (1982) Sensitizing potential of acrylic monomers in guinea pig. Thesis, Katholieke Universiteit te Nijmegen, Krips Repro Meppel 1–112

75. Kobayashi T, Sakuraoka K, Hasegawa Y et al (1996) Contact dermatitis to an acrylic dental prosthesis. Contact Dermatitis 35:370–371

76. Kanzaki T, Kabasawa Y, Jinno T et al (1989) Contact stomatitis due to methyl methacrylate monomer. Contact Dermatitis 20:146–148

77. van Joost TH, van Ulsen J, van Loon LAJ (1988) Contact allergy to denture materials in the burning mouth syndrome. Contact Dermatitis 18:97–99

78. Corazza M, Virgili A, Martina S (1992) Allergic contact stomatitis from methyl methacrylate in a dental prosthesis, with persistent patch test reaction. Contact Dermatitis 26:210–211

79. Ölveti É (1991) Contact dermatitis from an acrylic-metal dental prosthesis. Contact Dermatitis 24:57

80. Ruiz-Genao DP, Moreno de Vega MJ, Sánchez Pérez J et al (2003) Labial edema due to an acrylic dental prosthesis. Contact Dermatitis 48:273–274

81. Menni S, Lodi A, Coassini A et al (2003) Unusual widespread vesicular eruption related to dental composite resin sensitization. Contact Dermatitis 48:174

82. Lunder T, Rogi-Butina M (2000) Chronic urticaria from acrylic dental prosthesis. Contact Dermatitis 43:232–233

83. Bauer A, Wollina U (1998) Denture-induced local and systemic reactions to acrylate. Allergy 53:722–723

84. Calnan CD, Stevenson CJ (1963) Studies in contact dermatitis. XV. Dental materials. Trans St John's Hosp Dermatol 49:9–26

85. Kanerva L, Tarvainen K, Estlander T et al (1994) Occupational allergic contact dermatitis caused by mercury and benzoyl peroxide. Eur J Dermatol 4:359–361

86. Cronin E (1980) Contact dermatitis. Churchill Livingstone, Edinburgh

87. Quirce S, Olaguibel JM, Garcia BE et al (1993) Occupational airborne contact dermatitis due to benzoylperoxide. Contact Dermatitis 29:165

88. Tosti A, Bardazzi F, Piancastelli E et al (1990) Contact stomatitis due to N,N-dimethyl-paratoluidine. Contact Dermatitis 22:113

89. Verschueren GLA, Bryunzeel DP (1991) Allergy to N,N-dimethyl-p-toluidine in dental materials. Contact Dermatitis 24:149

90. Kanerva L, Jolanki R, Estlander T (1993) Dentist's occupational allergic contact dermatitis caused by coconut diethanolamide, N-ethyl-4-toluene sulphonamide and 4-tolyldiethanolamine. Acta Derm Venereol (Stockh) 73:126–129

91. Malanin K (1993) Active sensitization to camphoroquinone and bouble active sensitization to acrylics with long-lasting patch test reactions. Contact Dermatitis 29:284–285

92. Torres V, Mano-Azul AC, Correia T et al (1993) Allergic contact cheilitis and stomatitis from hydroquinone in an acrylic dental prosthesis. Contact Dermatitis 29:102–103

93. Björkner B, Niklasson B (1997) Contact allergy to the UV absorber Tinuvin P in a dental restorative material. Am J Contact Dermat 8:6–7

94. Aalto-Korte K, Alanko K, Henriks-Eckerman M-L et al (2003) Allergic contact dermatitis from bisphenol A in PVC gloves. Contact Dermatitis 49:202–205

95. Jolanki R, Kanerva L, Estlander T (1995) Occupational allergic contact dermatitis caused by epoxy diacrylate in ultraviolet-light-cured paint, and bisphenol A in dental composite resin. Contact Dermatitis 33:94–99

96. Koch P (2003) Allergic contact stomatitis from BIS-GMA and epoxy resins in dental bonding agents. Contact Dermatitis 49:104–105

97. Tomb RR, Lepoittevin J-P, Durepaire F et al (1993) Ectopic contact dermatitis from ethyl cyanoacrylate instant adhesices. Contact Dermatitis 28:206–208

98. Isaksson M, Siemund I, Bruze M (2007) Allergic contact dermatitis from ethylcyanoacrylate in an office worker with artificial nails led to months of sick leave. Contact Dermatitis 57:346–347

99. Nicholson JW, Czarnacka B (2008) The biocompatibility of resin-modified glass-ionomer cements for dentistry. Dent Mater 24:1702–1708

100. Kanerva L, Estlander T, Jolanki R (1997) Occupational allergic contact dermatitis caused by acrylic tri-cure glass ionomer. Contact Dermatitis 37:49–50

101. Ölveti É, Hegedus C (1994) Contact allergy reactions to Silodent impression material (in Hungarian). Fogorv Sz 87:115–119

102. Rice CD, Barker BF, Kestenbaum T et al (1992) Intraoral vesicles occurring after alginate impressions. Oral Surg Oral Med Oral Pathol 74:698–704

103. Camarasa G (1975) Occupational dermatitis from beeswax. Contact Dermatitis 1:124

104. Van Ketel WG (1977) Reactions to dental impression materials. Contact Dermatitis 3:55

105. Henriks-Eckerman M-L, Kanerva L (1997) Product analysis of acrylic resins compared to information given in material safety data sheets. Contact Dermatitis 36:164–165

106. Bruze M, Trulsson L, Bendsoe N (1992) Patch testing with ultrasonic bath extracts. Am J Contact Dermat 3:133–137

107. Aalto-Korte K, Ackermann L, Henriks-Eckerman ML et al (2007) 1, 2-benzisothiazolin-3-one in disposable polyvinyl chloride gloves for medical use. Contact Dermatitis 57: 365–370

108. Mäkelä EA, Väänänen V, Alanko K et al (1999) Resistance of disposable gloves to permeation by 2-hydroxyethyl methacrylate and triethyleneglycol dimethacrylate. Occup Hyg 5:121–129

109. Boman A, Röndell E, Sandborgh-Englund G et al (1999) Contamination and protection during dental work. 12th International Contact Dermatitis Symposium, San Francisco

110. Andersson T, Bruze M, Björkner B (1999) In vivo testing of the protection of gloves against acrylates in dentin-bonding systems on patients with known contact allergy to acrylates. Contact Dermatitis 41:254–259

111. Andersson T, Bruze M, Gruvberger B et al (2000) In vivo testing of the protection provided by non-latex gloves against a 2-hydroxyethyl methacrylate-containing acetone-based dentin-bonding product. Acta Derm Venereol 80:435–437

112. Vilaplana J, Romaguera C, Cornellana F (1994) Contact dermatitis and adverse oral mucous membrane reactions related to the use of dental prostheses. Contact Dermatitis 30:80–84

113. Spiechowicz E, Glantz PO, Axell T et al (1999) A long-term follow-up of allergy to nickel among fixed prostheses wearers. Eur J Prosthodont Restor Dent 7:41–44

114. Haberman AL, Pratt M, Storrs FJ (1993) Contact dermatitis from beryllium in dental alloys. Contact Dermatitis 28:157–162

115. Veien NK, Borchorst E, Hattel T et al (1994) Stomatitis or systemically-induced contact dermatitis from metal wire in orthodontic materials. Contact Dermatitis 30:210–213

116. Hensten-Pettersen A, Gjerdet NR, Kvam E et al (1984) Nikkelallergi og kjeveortopedisk behandling. Nor Tannlegeforen Tid (in Norwegian) 94:567–572

117. Kanerva L, Rantanen T, Aalto-Korte K et al (2001) A multicenter study of patch test reactions with dental screening series. Am J Contact Dermat 12:83–87

118. Khamaysi Z, Bergman R, Weltfriend S (2006) Positive patch test reactions to allergens of the dental series and the relation to the clinical presentations. Contact Dermatitis 55:216–218

119. Wahlberg JE (2000) Other metals. In: Kanerva L, Elsner P, Wahlberg JE, Maibach HI (eds) Handbook of occupational dermatology. Springer, Berlin

120. Müller-Quernheim J, Zissel G, Schopf R et al (1996) Differential diagnosis of berylliosis/sarcoidosis in a dental technician (in German). Dtsch Med Wochenschr 121: 1462–1466

121. Burrows D (1986) Hypersensitivity to mercury, nickel and chromium in relation to dental materials. Int Dent J 36:30–34

122. Guimaraens D, Gonzalez MA, Condé-Salazar L (1994) Systemic contact dermatitis from dental crowns. Contact Dermatitis 30:124–125

123. Hubler WR Jr, Hubler WR Sr (1983) Dermatitis from chromium dental plate. Contact Dermatitis 9:377–383

124. Glendenning WE (1971) Allergy to cobalt in metal denture as a cause of hand dermatitis. Contact Dermat Newslett 10:225–226

125. Morris A, English J (1998) Copper is unlikely to cause contact allergy. BMJ 316:1902–1903

126. Wöhrl S, Hemmer W, Focke M et al (2001) Copper allergy revisited. J Am Acad Dermatol 45:863–870

127. Karlberg A, Boman A, Wahlberg JE (1983) Copper – a rare sensitizer. Contact Dermatitis 9:134–139

128. Fisher AA (1986) Contact dermatitis, 3rd edn. Lea and Febiger, Philadelphia

129. Santosh V, Ranjith K, Shenoi SD et al (1999) Results of patch testing with dental materials. Contact Dermatitis 40:50–51

130. Gerhardsson L, Björkner B, Karlsteen M et al (2002) Copper allergy from dental copper amalgam? Sci Total Environ 290:41–46

131. Bruze M, Björkner B (1996) Patch testing with gold sodium thio-sulfate. Abstract 49, Jadassohn Centenary Congress, London

132. Möller H, Ahnlide I, Gruvberger B et al (2004) Gold trichloride as a marker of contact allergy to gold. Contact Dermatitis 50:176

133. Ahlgren C, Ahnlide I, Björkner B et al (2002) Contact allergy to gold is correlated to dental gold. Acta Derm Venereol (Stockh) 82:41–44

134. Björkner B, Bruze M, Möller H (1994) High frequency of contact allergy to gold sodium thiosulfate. An indication of gold allergy? Contact Dermatitis 30:144–151

135. Bruze M, Edman B, Björkner B et al (1994) Clinical relevance of contact allergy to gold sodium thiosulfate. J Am Acad Dermatol 31:579–583

136. McKenna KE, Dolan O, Walsh MY (1995) Contact allergy to gold sodium thiosulfate. Contact Dermatitis 32:143–146

137. Laeijendecker R, van Joost T (1994) Oral manifestations of gold allergy. J Am Acad Dermatol 30:205–209

39

138. Marcusson JA, Cederbrant K, Heilborn J (1998) Indium and iridium allergy in patients exposed to dental alloys. Contact Dermatitis 38:297–298

139. Pardo J, Rodriguez-Serna M, de la Cuadra J et al (2004) Allergic contact stomatitis due to manganese in a dental prosthesis. Contact Dermatitis 50:41

140. Jalili S, Bruze M, Isaksson M (2008) Contact allergy to mercury in dental amalgam. Elective study, Faculty of Medicine, Lund University, Malmö

141. Ancona A, Ramos M, Suarez R et al (1982) Mercury sensitivity in a dentist. Contact Dermatitis 8:218

142. Goh CL, Ng SK (1988) Occupational allergic contact dermatitis from metallic mercury. Contact Dermatitis 19:232–233

143. Kanerva L, Komulainen M, Estlander T et al (1993) Occupational allergic contact dermatitis from mercury. Contact Dermatitis 28:26–28

144. Kerosuo H, Kullaa A, Kerosuo E et al (1996) Nickel allergy in adolescents in relation to orthodontic treatment and piercing of ears. Am J Orthod Dentofacial Orthop 109:148–154

145. Volkmann KK, Inda MJ, Reichl PG et al (2007) Adverse reactions to orthodontic appliances in nickel-allergic patients. Allergy Asthma Proc 28:480–484

146. Feilzer AJ, Laeijendecker R, Kleverlaan CJ (2008) Facial eczema because of orthodontic fixed retainer wires. Contact Dermatitis 59:118–120

147. Kerosuo H, Kanerva L (1997) Systemic contact dermatitis caused by nickel in a stainless steel orthodontic appliance. Contact Dermatitis 36:112–113

148. Wataha JC, Hanks CT (1996) Biological effects of palladium and risk of using palladium in dental casting alloys. J Oral Rehabil 23:309–320

149. Hindsén M, Spirén A, Bruze M (2005) Cross-reactivity between nickel and palladium demonstrated by systemic administration of nickel. Contact Dermatitis 53:2–8

150. De Fine OF, Balslev E, Menné T (1993) Skin reactivity to tin chloride and metallic tin. Contact Dermatitis 29:110–111

151. Menné T, Andersen KE, Kaaber K et al (1987) Tin: an overlooked contact sensitizer? Contact Dermatitis 16:9–10

152. Dunlapp CL, Vincent SK, Barker BF (1989) Allergic reaction to orthodontic wire. JAMA 118:449–450

153. Schweitzer A (1997) Erstfeststellung einer Titan-Allergie. Dermatosen 45:190

154. Jalili S, Bruze M, Isaksson M (2008) 11 years of patch testing with titanium in the dental series. Abstract European Society of Contact Dermatitis meeting, Estoril, Portugal

155. Yanagi T, Shimizu T, Abe R et al (2005) Zinc dental fillings and palmoplantar pustulosis. Lancet 366:1050

156. Flyvholm M-A (2000) Formaldehyde and formaldehyde releasers. In: Kanerva L, Elsner P, Wahlberg JE, Maibach HI (eds) Handbook of occupational dermatology. Springer, Berlin

157. Nethercott JR, Holness DL, Page E (1988) Occupational contact dermatitis due to glutaraldehyde in health care workers. Contact Dermatitis 18:193–196

158. Cusano F, Luciano S (1993) Contact allergy to benzalkonium chloride and glutaraldehyde in a dental nurse. Contact Dermatitis 28:127

159. Kanerva L, Miettinen P, Alanko K et al (2000) Occupational allergic contact dermatitis from glyoxal, glutaraldehyde and neomycin sulphate ina dental nurse. Contact Dermatitis 42:116–117

160. Velázques D, Zamberk P, Suárez R et al (2009) Allergic contact dermatitis to povidone-iodine. Contact Dermatitis 60:348–349

161. Ancona A, de la Torre RS, Macotela E (1985) Allergic contact dermatitis from povidone-iodine. Contact Dermatitis 13:66–68

162. Kanerva L, Estlander T (1999) Occupational allergic contact dermatitis caused by povidone-iodine (Betadine). Environ Dermatol 6:101–104

163. Kanerva L, Alanko K, Jolanki R et al (1999) Occupational allergic contact dermatitis from potassium persulfate. Contact Dermatitis 40:116–117

164. Bhalla M, Thami GP (2003) Acute urticaria due to dental eugenol. Allergy 58:158; 137

165. Kanerva L, Estlander T, Jolanki R (1998) Dental nurse's occupational allergic contact dermatitis from eugenol used as a restorative dental material with polymethylmethacrylate. Contact Dermatitis 38:339–340

166. Isaksson M, Bruze M, Björkner B et al (1993) Contact allergy to Duraphat. Scand J Dent Res 101:49–51

167. Hausen BM (1984) Zahnpasta-Allergie. Dtsch Med Wschr 109:300–302

168. Morton CA, Garioch J, Todd P et al (1995) Contact sensitivity to menthol and peppermint in patients with intra-oral symptoms. Contact Dermatitis 32:281–284

169. Klein CE, Gall H (1991) Type IV allergy to amide-type local anesthetics. Contact Dermatitis 25:45–48

170. Fregert S, Tegner E, Thelin I (1979) Contact allergy to lidocaine. Contact Dermatitis 5:185

171. Isaksson M, Lindberg M, Sundberg K et al (2005) The development and course of patch-test reactions to 2-hydroxyethyl methacrylate and ethyleneglycol dimethacrylate. Contact Dermatitis 53:292–297

172. Bruze M, Hedman H, Björkner B et al (1995) The development and course of test reactions to gold sodium thiosulfate. Contact Dermatitis 33:386–391

173. Helton J, Storrs F (1994) The burning mouth syndrome: lack of a role for contact urticaria and contact dermatitis. J Am Acad Dermatol 31:201–205

174. Virgili A, Corazza M, Trombelli L et al (1996) Burning mouth syndrome: the role of contact hypersensitivity. Acta Derm Venereol (Stockh) 76:488–490

175. Dutree Meulenberg RO, Kozel MM, van Joost T (1992) Burning mouth syndrome: a possible etiological role for local contact hypersensitivity. J Am Acad Dermatol 26:935–940

176. Kanerva L, Estlander T, Jolanki R (1988) Sensitization to patch test acrylates. Contact Dermatitis 18:10–15

177. Kanerva L, Lauerma AI (1988) Iatrogenic acrylate allergy complicating amalgam allergy. Contact Dermatitis 38:58–59

178. Bruze M, Björkner B, Lepoittevin JP (1995) Occupational allergic contact dermatitis from ethyl cyanoacrylate. Contact Dermatitis 32:156–159

179. Goon AT, Bruze M, Zimerson E et al (2008) Screening for acrylate/methacrylate allergy in the baseline series: our experience in Sweden and Singapore. Contact Dermatitis 59:307–313

180. Goon ATJ, Bruze M, Zimerson E et al (2007) Contact allergy to acrylates/methacrylates in the acrylate and nail acrylics series in southern Sweden: simultaneous positive

patch test reaction patterns and possible screening allergens. Contact Dermatitis 57:21–27

181. Boxer MB, Grammer LC, Orfan N (1994) Gutta-percha allergy in a health care worker with latex allergy. J Allergy Clin Immunol 93:943–944

182. Jolanki R, Estlander T, Alanko K et al (1999) Incidence rates of occupational contact urticaria caused by natural rubber latex. Contact Dermatitis 40:329–331

183. Wrangsjö K, Osterman K, Hage-Hamsten M (1994) Glove-related skin symptoms among operating theatre and dental unit personnel. (II). Clinical examination, tests and laboratory findings indicating latex allergy. Contact Dermatitis 30:139–143

184. Leggat PA, Smith DR (2006) Prevalence of hand dermatoses related to latex exposure amongst dentists in Queensland, Australia. Int Dent J 56:154–158

185. Piirilä P, Hodgson U, Estlander T et al (2002) Occupational respiratory hypersensitivity in dental personnel. Int Arch Occup Environ Health 75:209–216

186. Kanerva L (1997) Contact urticaria from dental products. In: Amin S, Lahti A, Maibach HI (eds) Contact urticaria syndrome. CRC/LLC, Boca Raton, FL

187. Grade AC, Martens BPM (1989) Chronic urticaria due to dental eugenol. Dermatologica 178:217–220

188. Krautheim AB, Jermann THM, Bircher AJ (2004) Chlorhexidine anaphylaxis: case report and review of the literature. Contact Dermatitis 50:113–116

189. Calnan CD (1962) Contact dermatitis from drugs. Proc R Soc Med 55:39–42

190. Torresani C, Caprari E, Manara GC (1993) Contact urticaria syndrome due to phenylmercuric acetate. Contact Dermatitis 29:282–283

191. Ockenfels HM, Seemann U, Goos M et al (1995) Allergy to fibrin tissue in dental medicine. Contact Dermatitis 32:363–364

192. Wüthrich B, Bianchi-Kusch E, Johansson SG (1996) Allergic urticaria and angioedema caused by a hemostatic sponge of bovine fibrin used in tooth extraction. Allergy 51:49–51

193. Estlander T, Kanerva L, Tupasela O et al (1993) Immediate and delayed allergy to nickel with contact urticaria, rhinitis, asthma and contact dermatitis. Clin Exp Allergy 23:306–310

194. Espana A, Alonso ML, Soria C et al (1989) Chronic urticaria after implantation of 2 nickel-containing dental prostheses in a nickel-allergic patient. Contact Dermatitis 21:204–205

195. Schena D, Barba A, Costa G (1996) Occupational contact urticaria to cisplatin. Contact Dermatitis 34:220–221

196. Bergman A, Svedberg U, Nilsson E (1995) Contact urticaria and anaphylactic reactions caused by occupational exposure to iridium salt. Contact Dermatitis 32:14–17

197. Murdoch RD, Pepys J (1987) Platinum group metal sensitivity: reactivity to platinum group metal salts in platinum halide salt-sensitive workers. Ann Allergy 59:464–469

198. Murdoch RD, Pepys J, Hughes EG (1986) IgE-antibody response to platinum group metals: a large scale refinery survey. Br J Ind Med 43:37–43

199. Camarasa JG, Serra-Baldrich E, Lluch M et al (1993) Contact urticaria from sodium fluoride. Contact Dermatitis 28:294

200. Sainio E-L, Kanerva L (1995) Contact allergens in toothpastes and a review of their hypersensitivity. Contact Dermatitis 33:100–105

201. Savonius B, Keskinen H, Tuppurainen M et al (1993) Occupational respiratory disease caused by acrylates. Clin Exp Allergy 23:416–424

202. Davison LS, AG HA et al (1985) Occupational asthma due to methyl methacrylate and cyanoacrylates. Thorax 40:836–839

203. Piirilä P, Kanerva L, Keskinen H et al (1998) Occupational respiratory hypersensitivity caused by preparations containing acrylates in dental personnel. Clin Exp Allergy 28:1404–1411

Clothing

40

Christophe-J. Le Coz

Contents

40.1 Introduction

Clothes help to regulate skin temperature and moisture and protect from environmental injuries. They should be safe, with no toxicity, carcinogenicity, or allergenicity. Reports of clothing dermatitis are frequently individual, except rare epidemics [1, 2] occurring from furs dyed by *p*-phenylenediamine (PPD) and its derivatives in the 1920s [3], dyed nylon stockings in the 1940s [3, 4], or black "velvet" clothing and blouses in the 1980s [5, 6]. Epidemiological studies regarding this topic are most often not controlled and habitually report a frequency of positive patch tests to textile additives, mainly dyes or finishes [7–17]. Thus, the prevalence of sensitization to substances potentially implicated in textile dermatitis is difficult to establish [18], being around 1–5% of tested patients, although the interest and the clinical relevance of such tests are frequently questionable. For example, a recent study in 1,012 tested patients, indicated that 31 patients (3%) reacted to at least one clothing dye, but only ten reactions were relevant [16]. It is difficult to determine its exact incidence for these reasons, but many data suggest that clothing dermatitis is not exceptional [4, 7, 14, 17, 18].

Variations in fashion, styling, new leisure activities, and technological progress explain the variations of clinical patterns and allergens in clothing dermatitis. For instance, sock-suspenders, hats, or corsets are out of fashion in most countries. Conversely, many people wear sports clothing daily, and most clothing are treated against shrinkage, creasing, or development of odors. Concerning allergens, ester gum (abietic acid and alcohol) used as an adhesive was responsible for the epidemics of dermatitis in the 1940s [19]; allergy to formaldehyde in garments is rarer than it was previously, since more recent textile finish resins (TFR) release little or no formaldehyde, as new dyestuffs are regularly synthesized before coming into

C.-J. Le Coz
Cabinet de Dermatologie & Laboratoire de Dermatochimie,
4 rue Blaise Pascal, 67070 Strasbourg, France
e-mail: christophe.lecoz@wanadoo.fr

J.D. Johansen et al. (eds.), *Contact Dermatitis*,
DOI: 10.1007/978-3-642-03827-3_40, © Springer-Verlag Berlin Heidelberg 2011

the market. It is arduous to detect the newer allergens and ascertain the disappearance of the older ones, because the chemicals used in textiles are not declared, contrary to the case with cosmetics. The manufacturing and legislation modifications in developed countries permit a dramatic reduction of formaldehyde release [20] and the interdiction of textile dyes that are carcinogenic or that can release carcinogenic aromatic amines [21]. Some industrial labels such as Oeko-Tex Standard 100 want to promote "safe textiles" as well [22]. However, such resolutions risk to be counterbalanced by the level of imported clothing from Far East or underdeveloped countries, which contain various textile additives.

The diagnosis of clothing dermatitis requires cautious examination of both the patient and the suspected article. A poor history, lack of clinical information, or no examination of the clothing often lead to a missed diagnosis [3, 10]. We have principally considered dermatitis due to clothing itself and excluded damage from accessories such as jewels or belts, or those provoked by gloves and shoes.

40.2 Clinical Examination

Contact dermatitis from clothing generally has the clinical feature of a typical eczema [3, 10, 23], though dry rather than vesicular. The lesions can progress and be severe, generalized, or even erythrodermic, as long as contact with the allergen is not avoided. Follicular or nummular eczema is possible with finish resins [14, 23]. Pigmented contact dermatitis arises mainly in patients with a phototype IV or V, and has been described from Naphthol AS [1] as well. In some instances, the lesions can be monomorphic and infiltrated [7]. They may simulate an atopic dermatitis in popliteal areas [3], demonstrate a persistent erythematous or urticarial-type dermatitis, or even present solely as diffuse itching [10]. Purpuric clothing dermatitis, described during the Second World War, was due to textile finishes in British soldiers' uniforms. This rare instance occurred with rubber compounds such as isopropyl-phenyl p-phenylenediamine (IPPD), with the azo dyes Disperse Blue 85 [24], Disperse Blue 106/124 [25], or Disperse Yellow 27 [26]. It is not clear if purpuric reactions are of allergic and/or toxic mechanism. Cocarde lesions are rarely described [10].

The dermatitis generally occurs on the sites of intimate contact with the garment [3, 13–15], and the

lesions are sometimes symmetrical (Figs. 40.1 and 40.2). Friction or perspiration sites are preferentially involved, particularly in hypersensitivity from TFR [3, 4, 23, 27], and a clinical pattern of textile dermatitis is generally described: neck, major skin folds, and inner thighs. The areas protected by underclothing or the lining of the skirt are often free of symptoms [28, 29]. The face can be involved from handling of the

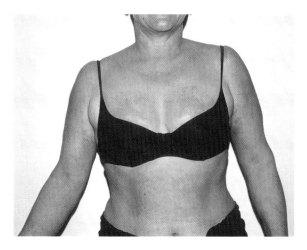

Fig. 40.1 Allergic contact dermatitis from clothing dye in black dress containing Disperse Blue 106/124

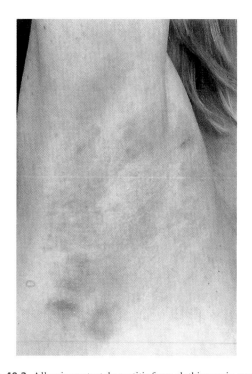

Fig. 40.2 Allergic contact dermatitis from clothing resin around axillary borders

Table 40.1 Localization of dermatitis according to garment type

Type of garment	Localization of the lesions
Socks	Feet, legs
Stockings	Lower legs, feet, toes, popliteal fossa
Blouses	Back, chest, axillary borders
Dresses	Back, neck, elbows, axillary borders, forearms, wrists
Jackets	Dorsum of hands, wrists and forearms
Trousers	Thighs, lower legs, dorsum of hands

dyes. Some peculiar localizations, in accordance with the form of the garment, are reported in Table 40.1.

Dermatitis from *socks* will be distributed on the feet and lower legs [3]. Hypersensitivity to *stockings* or tights (panty hose) will start on the lower legs, dorsum of feet and toes, and then spread to the popliteal fossa [3]. In the case of dermatitis from *blouses and dresses*, the back is typically involved.

In addition, dress dermatitis affects the neck, elbows, and axillae, predominates around the axillary borders [4], and can involve the forearms and wrists [3].

Allergy from *jackets* involves the back of the hands or wrists [4]. Dermatitis from *trousers* occurs on the thighs and lower legs and in the popliteal fossa. The dorsum of the hands is affected in patients who often put them in their pockets [3, 4].

Examination of the garment is indispensable. The labeling indicates the fiber composition (if the ratio >5%) and can guide to specific dyes or textile finishes. The practitioner should examine the different parts of the fabric and take some of them, of different colors or textures, for patch testing or for further chemical analysis.

Core Message

> Allergy from textiles frequently offers a typical pattern, mainly located in body areas in contact with the garment. Sweating and friction promote dermatitis.

40.3 The Inducers of Dermatitis

Irritant dermatitis is more frequent than allergic, either of delayed or immediate type. In addition, obtaining the final diagnosis by the way of the exact composition

of a garment is often a challenge, which necessitates tenacity and cooperation between the practitioner, the patient, and the manufacturer.

40.3.1 Textile Fibers

The exact fiber composition of a garment is generally designated on the label when ≥5% amount of fibers are present. Textile fibers are numerous and industrial developments are extensive. Natural fibers are cellulose (cotton, linen) or protein based (wool, silk). Synthetic fibers mainly consist of cellulose derivatives (rayon, acetate, and triacetate), polyamides such as nylon (Perlon®, Antron®, Quiana®), polyesters (Dacron®, Tergal®, Terylene®), acrylics (Acrylan®, Acribel®, Dralon®, Courtelle®), elastomers (Lycra®, Vyrene®), or new fibers derived from nylon such as aramids (Kevlar®, Nomex®). Fibers are frequently blended, sometimes even with metal. Cosmetics like deodorants, perfumes, and even moisturizing agents can be added during manufacture: their concentration generally fades away with wearing or after a few washing.

Textile fibers themselves, except rubber, are usually not implicated in allergic contact dermatitis [3, 30]. Observations of allergy from *wool* are often ancient and questionable [30, 31]. *Silk* can seldom provoke immediate or delayed hypersensitivity. Allergens are controversial and could be the fibers, sericin in raw silk, or silkworm protein [32]. Allergic contact dermatitis from *nylon* itself is exceptional [30] but can be due to the monomer of nylon six, epsilon-aminocaproic acid [33]. *Spandex*, a poly(urethane-urea) elastomer used in brassieres and girdles formerly contained mercaptobenzothiazole [30]. *Neoprene rubber* is a synthetic rubber based on polychloroprene polymerized with sulfur and 2,3-dichloro-1,3-butadiene. It is used to make wet suits, swimming gear, slimming suits, and clothing for fire fighters and contains especially thiourea derivatives such as ethylene-thiourea, and diethyl-, dibutyl-, and diphenyl-thiourea that have been described as allergens [34–36].

Textile fibers are mainly responsible for irritant contact dermatitis, and patients suffering from atopic dermatitis or dry skin often complain of intolerance to garments. The irritant potential of wool and that of synthetic fibers is significantly higher in such patients, while cotton garments are best tolerated [37]. This is

40

due to the structure of wool and many synthetic fibers that have a thorny surface. Irritation can be diffuse or much localized, occurring, for example, at the site of cutaneous contact with clothing tags, frequently made of synthetic coarse fibers. This has been described as "label dermatitis" [38].

Nylon, because of poor sweat absorption, can promote miliaria-like eruptions [31]. Other synthetic fibers such as rayon, polyester, and acrylics can be irritant and provoke pruritus and maceration [31, 37].

With the exception of rubber derivatives, textile fibers mostly induce irritant dermatitis.

40.3.2 Textile Resins and Formaldehyde

TFR, also named durable-press resins or permanent press clothing finishes, are especially and widely used for cotton, cotton/polyester, or wrinkle-resistant linen. TFR can facilitate bleaching and dyeing, and ameliorate nylon and make it electrically antistatic. They give textile body, improve their quality, touch, and appearance. Fabrics are crease-resistant, waterproof, nonshrinkable, mothproof, and noniron [3, 23, 39]. It is hard, if ever possible, to know the exact composition of the TFR used today by the manufacturers (personal communications). Two major types of TFR have been developed for textile industry: the older ones are formaldehyde-based resins (urea-formaldehyde resins and melamine formaldehyde resins), whereas the more recent ones are cyclized urea derivatives, which are preponderant in Europe. Most TFR release more or less high amounts of formaldehyde

due to the necessity of the formaldehyde to synthesize the resin, due to subsequent degradation of the resin during storage, during wearing because of sweat, during an acid washing [3] or by the use of chlorine during laundry [19]. Industrial washing, although expensive, decreases the presence of unreacted formaldehyde and resins at the surface of the garment. Glyoxal, another aldehyde, is sometimes used as a substitute of formaldehyde in systems which subsequently release no formaldehyde.

Urea formaldehyde (methylol urea) resins derive from the polymerization of urea and formaldehyde with a curing agent. The intermediate products are monomethylolurea CAS [1000-82-4], dimethylolurea (also named carbamol or oxymethurea) CAS [140-95-4], and methyleneurea CAS [13547-17-6]. The second stage consists of condensation of the methylolureas to low molecular polymers by methylene and methylene-ether linkages that secondarily polymerize within the interstices of the textile fibers [3, 27]. These resins release large amounts of free formaldehyde, particularly under moist and hot conditions, but are no more used for clothing in most countries (Fig. 40.3).

Melamine formaldehyde resins result from the condensation of formaldehyde and melamine CAS [108-78-1], which is obtained by the dehydratation of urea. Trimethylolmelamine CAS [1017-56-7] and hexamethylolmelamine CAS [531-18-0] are the main compounds, resulting from the condensation of melamine with three and six formaldehyde molecules, respectively. They polymerize into resins in the interstices of the fibers. Some unpolymerized methylol residues (R-CH$_2$-OH) contained in such resins can subsequently be degraded into free formaldehyde (CH$_2$=O). These TFR release large amounts of formaldehyde [27], but are out of fashion in Europe for clothing (Fig. 40.4).

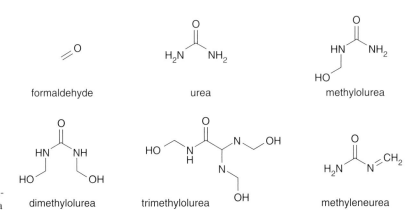

Fig. 40.3 Structures of formaldehyde, urea, (mono)methylolurea, dimethylolurea, trimethylolurea, and methyleneurea

Fig. 40.4 Structures of melamine, trimethylol-melamine, and hexamethylolmelamine

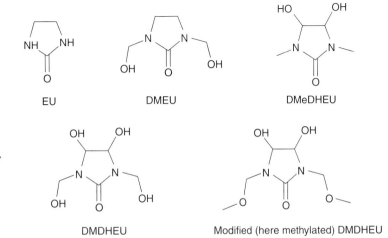

Fig. 40.5 Simplified scheme of the ether reaction between cyclized urea and cellulosic fibers

Fig. 40.6 Structures of ethylene urea (EU), dimethylol ethylene urea (DMEU), dimethyl-dihydroxy ethylene urea (DMeDHEU), dimethylol-dihydroxy ethylene urea (DMDHEU), and modified DMDHEU (here methylated dimethylol-dihydroxy ethylene urea)

Cyclized urea derivatives, the current TFR, are reticulating agents based on *N*-alkoxymethylated cyclized urea. With magnesium chloride to initiate the reaction, their *N*-methylol (N–CH$_2$–OH) groups crosslink with the hydroxyl (OH) groups of the cellulosic textile fibers to form stable ether bonds (Fig. 40.5).

These numerous molecules mainly consist of substituted ethylene ureas, such as dimethylol ethylene urea (DMEU) CAS [136-84-5], dimethyl-dihydroxy ethylene urea (DMeDHEU) CAS [3923-79-3], and dimethylol-dihydroxy ethylene urea (DMDHEU, CAS [1854-26-8]), and substituted propylene ureas such as dimethylol propylene urea (DMPU), CAS [3270-74-4], dimethylol-dihydroxy propylene urea (DMDHPU), dimethylol-5-hydroxy propylene urea, and dimethylol-4-methoxy-5,5-dimethylol propylene urea. Other molecules are dimethylol-hexahydrotriazone and urons

(uron-formaldehyde) such as dimethoxymethyl uron CAS [7388-44-5]. All of them are marketed with tenths of names (>30 for DMDHEU e.g.,) (Figs. 40.6, 40.7 and 40.8).

DMDHEU and its derivatives are now the main TFR used in Europe. During polymerization free formaldehyde is released. Inadequate curing also leads to the liberation of formaldehyde at high temperature. A number of approaches have been developed to limit the amount of formaldehyde released, such as after washing of cured fabrics, the addition of formaldehyde scavengers such as carbohydrazide to the bath, the use of urea in the pad-bath or application through a spray, and the modification of DMDHEU. Such substitutions of the molecule are expected to decrease the release of formaldehyde, and DMDHEU can be modified to etherized, glycolated, or methylated DMDHEU – so as to give

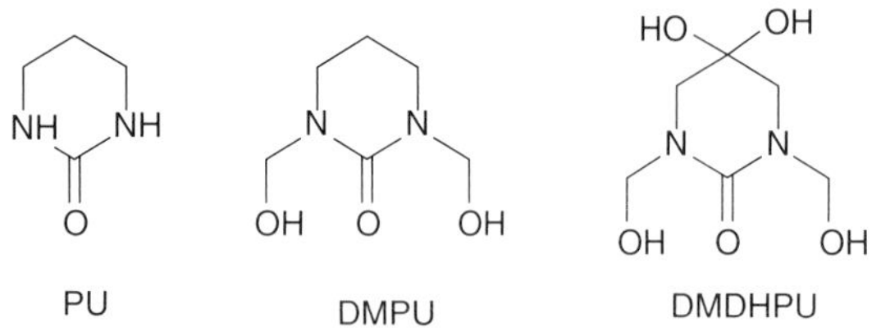

40

Fig. 40.7 Structures of propylene urea (PU), dimethylol propylene urea (DMPU), and dimethylol-dihydroxy propylene urea (DMDHPU)

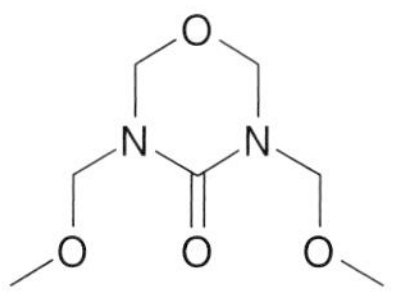

Fig. 40.8 Dimethoxy-methyl uron

dimethoxymethyl dihydroxyethylene urea – known as modified DMDHEU. Commercially, it is the modified DMDHEU (glycolated or methylated) that is much used today. The product is prebuffered to prevent premature curing and also preblended with a catalyst, magnesium-based catalysts being the most popular in use today. Such resins release various amounts of free formaldehyde: a moderate rate (100–1,000 ppm) for DMPU, DMEU, and urons, a low rate (<100 ppm) for DMDHEU and DMMDHEU, and a very low rate (<30 ppm) for blended or substituted DMDHEU [27, 31, 39].

Alternatives to DMDHEU are also being researched, but *other durable-press resins are of less importance in industry and in allergic contact dermatitis.*

Carbamate derivatives are particularly used in the USA for mixed cotton-polyester. For example, (di) methylolcarbamates are usually used in white shirts [31]. They release moderate amounts of formaldehyde [27, 31, 39] (Fig. 40.9).

Polycarboxylic acid systems such as butane 1,2,3,4-tetracarboxylic acid (BTCA), citric acid, or

modified polycarboxylic acids have been more recently developed. However, BTCA is expensive to use and citric acid causes yellowing. Although they could be "safe" TFR, they are not of interest in allergologic routine [27, 31, 39]. Another approach has been to use polymers of maleic acid to form ester cross-links, and yet another to fix a quaternary group through an epoxidation reaction to the cellulose chain to form cross-links. Research on all these alternatives continues.

The incidence of TFR-related contact dermatitis seems to be lower than 0.5% in patch tested patients [40] and higher in women than in men [23, 27], probably because of the frequency of wearing treated garments [19]. Patients positive to TFR are generally allergic to formaldehyde released by TFR [3, 23, 27]. Such people can be sensitive to formaldehyde released by preservatives used in cosmetics and have an associated facial dermatitis [27], which is a source of error in diagnosis. Previous studies have demonstrated the presence of free formaldehyde (1–3,500 ppm) in synthetic and natural fibers, particularly in 100% rayon, or in cotton-blended fabrics [3, 41]. The threshold rate for allergic contact dermatitis is 500 or 750 ppm free formaldehyde in the garment [27, 41]. During recent years, a 10–30-fold decrease in free formaldehyde has been noted in fabrics [19, 27]. First regulation was observed in Japan and Finland. European norms EN ISO 14184 part 1 and 2 [20] are based on three principles: no detectable formaldehyde in infant garments (in fact <20 ppm, which is the threshold of detection associated to Japanese regulation Law 112), level <75 ppm for garments with direct skin contact, and level <300 ppm for clothing that are not in contact with the skin. This decrease to 10–100 ppm is due to the use of DMDHEU and its derivatives, or nonformaldehyde-based resins. So, the former estimation that 8.6% of patients sensitized to formaldehyde were sensitive to textiles [40], is currently overestimated. In some instances, patients seem to be allergic to the resin itself, without formaldehyde sensitivity [8, 14, 19, 27, 42].

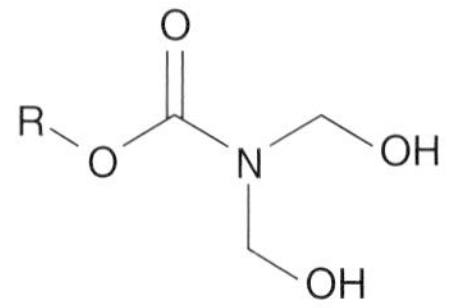

Fig. 40.9 Dimethylol carbamates. R = alkyl, hydroxyalkyl, or alkoxyalkyl chain

Textile resins are used to enhance the touch and quality of clothing (nonshrinkable and noniron). Some of them (urea-formaldehyde and melamine formaldehyde) significantly release formaldehyde. Current cyclized urea resins derived from DMDHEU release fewer or no formaldehyde.

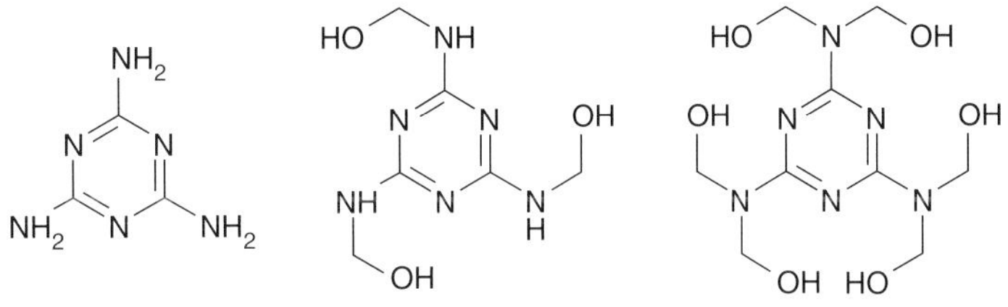

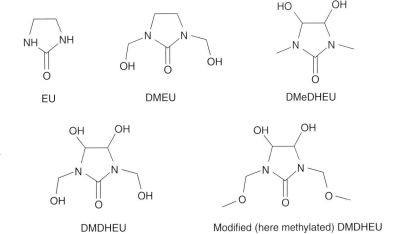

Fig. 40.4 Structures of melamine, trimethylol-melamine, and hexamethylolmelamine

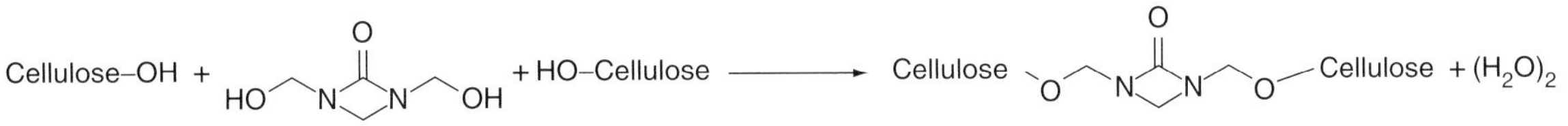

Fig. 40.5 Simplified scheme of the ether reaction between cyclized urea and cellulosic fibers

Fig. 40.6 Structures of ethylene urea (EU), dimethylol ethylene urea (DMEU), dimethyl-dihydroxy ethylene urea (DMeDHEU), dimethylol-dihydroxy ethylene urea (DMDHEU), and modified DMDHEU (here methylated dimethylol-dihydroxy ethylene urea)

Cyclized urea derivatives, the current TFR, are reticulating agents based on *N*-alkoxymethylated cyclized urea. With magnesium chloride to initiate the reaction, their *N*-methylol (N–CH$_2$–OH) groups cross-link with the hydroxyl (OH) groups of the cellulosic textile fibers to form stable ether bonds (Fig. 40.5).

These numerous molecules mainly consist of substituted ethylene ureas, such as dimethylol ethylene urea (DMEU) CAS [136-84-5], dimethyl-dihydroxy ethylene urea (DMeDHEU) CAS [3923-79-3], and dimethylol-dihydroxy ethylene urea (DMDHEU, CAS [1854-26-8]), and substituted propylene ureas such as dimethylol propylene urea (DMPU), CAS [3270-74-4], dimethylol-dihydroxy propylene urea (DMDHPU), dimethylol-5-hydroxy propylene urea, and dimethylol-4-methoxy-5,5-dimethylol propylene urea. Other molecules are dimethylol-hexahydrotriazone and urons

(uron-formaldehyde) such as dimethoxymethyl uron CAS [7388-44-5]. All of them are marketed with tenths of names (>30 for DMDHEU e.g.,) (Figs. 40.6, 40.7 and 40.8).

DMDHEU and its derivatives are now the main TFR used in Europe. During polymerization free formaldehyde is released. Inadequate curing also leads to the liberation of formaldehyde at high temperature. A number of approaches have been developed to limit the amount of formaldehyde released, such as after washing of cured fabrics, the addition of formaldehyde scavengers such as carbohydrazide to the bath, the use of urea in the pad-bath or application through a spray, and the modification of DMDHEU. Such substitutions of the molecule are expected to decrease the release of formaldehyde, and DMDHEU can be modified to etherized, glycolated, or methylated DMDHEU – so as to give

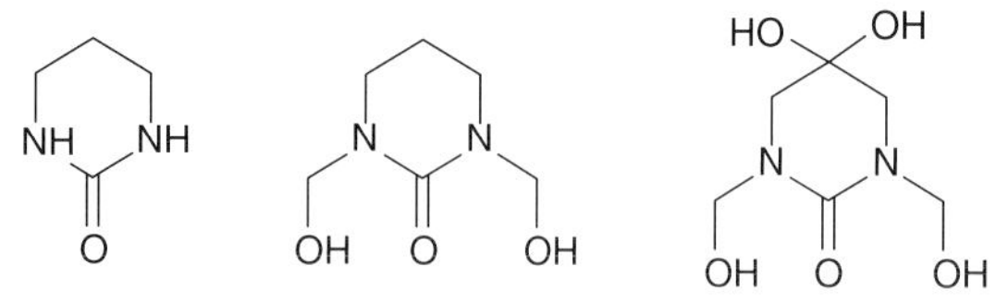

Fig. 40.7 Structures of propylene urea (PU), dimethylol propylene urea (DMPU), and dimethylol-dihydroxy propylene urea (DMDHPU)

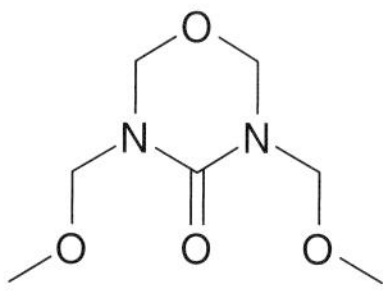

Fig. 40.8 Dimethoxy-methyl uron

dimethoxymethyl dihydroxyethylene urea – known as modified DMDHEU. Commercially, it is the modified DMDHEU (glycolated or methylated) that is much used today. The product is prebuffered to prevent premature curing and also preblended with a catalyst, magnesium-based catalysts being the most popular in use today. Such resins release various amounts of free formaldehyde: a moderate rate (100–1,000 ppm) for DMPU, DMEU, and urons, a low rate (<100 ppm) for DMDHEU and DMMDHEU, and a very low rate (<30 ppm) for blended or substituted DMDHEU [27, 31, 39].

Alternatives to DMDHEU are also being researched, but *other durable-press resins are of less importance in industry and in allergic contact dermatitis.*

Carbamate derivatives are particularly used in the USA for mixed cotton-polyester. For example, (di) methylolcarbamates are usually used in white shirts [31]. They release moderate amounts of formaldehyde [27, 31, 39] (Fig. 40.9).

Polycarboxylic acid systems such as butane 1,2,3,4-tetracarboxylic acid (BTCA), citric acid, or modified polycarboxylic acids have been more recently developed. However, BTCA is expensive to use and citric acid causes yellowing. Although they could be "safe" TFR, they are not of interest in allergologic routine [27, 31, 39]. Another approach has been to use polymers of maleic acid to form ester cross-links, and yet another to fix a quaternary group through an epoxidation reaction to the cellulose chain to form cross-links. Research on all these alternatives continues.

The incidence of TFR-related contact dermatitis seems to be lower than 0.5% in patch tested patients [40] and higher in women than in men [23, 27], probably because of the frequency of wearing treated garments [19]. Patients positive to TFR are generally allergic to formaldehyde released by TFR [3, 23, 27]. Such people can be sensitive to formaldehyde released by preservatives used in cosmetics and have an associated facial dermatitis [27], which is a source of error in diagnosis. Previous studies have demonstrated the presence of free formaldehyde (1–3,500 ppm) in synthetic and natural fibers, particularly in 100% rayon, or in cotton-blended fabrics [3, 41]. The threshold rate for allergic contact dermatitis is 500 or 750 ppm free formaldehyde in the garment [27, 41]. During recent years, a 10–30-fold decrease in free formaldehyde has been noted in fabrics [19, 27]. First regulation was observed in Japan and Finland. European norms EN ISO 14184 part 1 and 2 [20] are based on three principles: no detectable formaldehyde in infant garments (in fact <20 ppm, which is the threshold of detection associated to Japanese regulation Law 112), level <75 ppm for garments with direct skin contact, and level <300 ppm for clothing that are not in contact with the skin. This decrease to 10–100 ppm is due to the use of DMDHEU and its derivatives, or nonformaldehyde-based resins. So, the former estimation that 8.6% of patients sensitized to formaldehyde were sensitive to textiles [40], is currently overestimated. In some instances, patients seem to be allergic to the resin itself, without formaldehyde sensitivity [8, 14, 19, 27, 42].

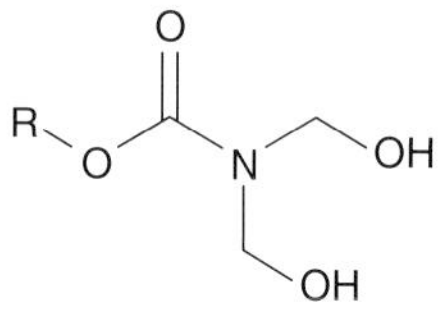

Fig. 40.9 Dimethylol carbamates. R=alkyl, hydroxyalkyl, or alkoxyalkyl chain

Textile resins are used to enhance the touch and quality of clothing (nonshrinkable and noniron). Some of them (urea-formaldehyde and melamine formaldehyde) significantly release formaldehyde. Current cyclized urea resins derived from DMDHEU release fewer or no formaldehyde.

40.3.3 Textile Dyes

Sensitization to textile dyes in clothing necessitates a transfer of the dye from the garment to the skin. However, "bleeding" of textile dyes, which induces skin discoloration, is a nonallergic phenomenon unnecessary for sensitization [4]. Sensitization occurs from the dye itself, intermediate products during the dyeing process or after-treatments, orfrom metabolites arising in the skin. Attributing an allergy to a textile dye is a hard process, and even if a textile dye is found to be positive on patch testing, the precise identification of the sensitizer in the garment is extremely difficult. There are thousands of textile dyes, marketed under different names (up to 30 for some of them) and the Color Index (CI) does not contain all information about them. A final textile color often results from a subtle mixture of several dyes. Because of this, a priori unexpected dyes can be employed as yellow, red, or orange dyes, for black or blue garments, respectively. For example, Serisol Black L 1944, used to dye black "velvet" clothes, contained five disperse dyes, namely Blue 124 and 106, Red 1, Yellow 3, and Blue 1 [5]. Moreover, a commercial dye often comprises one or two major components, and even impurities [43]. While Disperse Yellow 3 is generally pure, Disperse Red 153 or Disperse Blue 35 contains two major fractions, and Disperse Red 1 comprises one major compound and at least two other minor substances [28, 43]. Disperse Blue 124 also contains several dyes and traces of Disperse Blue 106, and "nonazo" impurities as ascertained by comparative thin layer chromatography (personal observation). These impurities can also be responsible for sensitization [3, 44]. The manufacturing processes are complex and additional procedures such as bleaching can also lead to allergenic products [2]. Skin metabolism may be responsible for the transformation of dyes. For example, Disperse Orange 3 is degraded to PPD and nitroaniline in the skin [3, 45] (Fig. 40.10).

According to their chemical structures and the Color Index system, dyes can be classified into 17 groups: nitro dyes, triphenylmethane derivatives, xanthenes, acridine derivatives, quinoline derivatives, azines,

anthraquinones, indigoid dyes, phthalocyanines dyes, oxydation bases, insoluble azo dye precursors, and azo dyes (classes XII to XVII) [46]. In practice, textile dyes are classified into different application classes: disperse, acid, basic, direct, vat, fiber-reactive, sulfur, premetallic, solvent dyes, and naphthols [11, 31, 46]. The principal allergenic textile dyes are reported in Table 40.2.

40.3.3.1 Disperse Dyes

Disperse dyes are partially soluble in water [47] and are used to color synthetic fibers such as polyester, acrylic, and acetate, and sometimes nylon, particularly in stockings. They are not employed for natural fibers. *These molecules are the main sensitizers.* Women seem to be more prone than men to become sensitized [9, 48] but these data are not constant [47].

> Disperse dyes (azo or anthraquinone type) are the most employed dyes, and the most frequent inducers of textile allergy, due to synthetic fibers.

Anthraquinone Dyes

These dyes consist of substituted anthraquinones [3, 46]. They are plastosoluble and used to stain synthetic fibers such as polyester, acetate, or nylon [47].

Disperse Blue 1, also used in coloring fabrics and plastics or for semipermanent hair colorations such as anthraquinone dyes Disperse Blue 3 and 7 , Disperse Red 11 and 15, Disperse Violet 1, 4, and 15 [49], induced urinary bladder carcinomas and sarcomas in rats. It is anticipated to be a reasonable human carcinogen [50], like Disperse Orange 11 (CI 60700).

Among these disperse anthraquinone dyes, *Disperse Red 11*, *Disperse Blue 3*, and *Disperse Blue 35* have been reported as causes of contact dermatitis from dresses, trousers, or nylon stockings [13, 15, 46, 51, 52]. Disperse Blue 35 is also a phototoxic compound

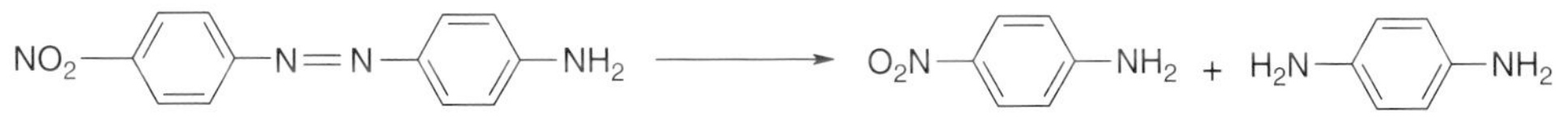

Fig. 40.10 Degradation of Disperse Orange 3 into nitroaniline and PPD

40

Table 40.2 Main textile dyes reported as allergens

Names of the dyes	CI number	CAS number	Application class	Chemical class	Test concentration (% pet.)	Suppliers
Acid Black 48	65005	1328-24-1	Acid	Anthraquinone	1	F
Acid Red 118	26410	12217-35-5	Acid	Azoic	5	C
Acid Red 359	–	–	Premetallic	Azoic (chrome)	5	C
Acid Violet 17	42650	4129-84-4	Acid	Triphenylmethane	1	
Acid Yellow 36	13065	587-98-4	Acid	Azoic	1	T
Acid Yellow 61	18968	12217-38-8	Acid	Azoic	5	C
Basic Black 1	50431	–	Basic	Azine		
Basic Brown 1 (Bismarck Brown R)	21000	1052-38-6	Basic	(Di)azoic	0.5	F, T
Basic Red 46	–	12221-69-1	Basic	Azoic	1	C
Direct Black 38[a]	30235	1937-37-7	Direct	(Tri)azoic	1	
Direct Orange 34	40215	12222-37-6	Direct	Azo (stilbene)	5	C
Direct Orange 39	40215	1325-54-8	Direct	Azoic		
Direct Yellow 169	–	–	Direct	Azoic		
Disperse Black 1	11365	60-11-7	Disperse	Azoic	1	F
Disperse Black 2	11255	6232-57-1	Disperse	Azoic	1	
Disperse Blue 1[a,b]	64500	2475-45-8	Disperse	Anthraquinone	1	
Disperse Blue 3[c]	61505	2475-46-9	Disperse	Anthraquinone	1	C, F, T
Disperse Blue 7[c]	62500	3179-90-6	Disperse	Anthraquinone	1	
Disperse Blue 26[c]	63305	3860-63-7	Disperse	Anthraquinone	1	
Disperse Blue 35[c]	–	12222-75-2	Disperse	Anthraquinone	1	C
Disperse Blue 85	11370	3177-13-7	Disperse	Azoic	1	C
Disperse Blue 102[c]	–	12222-97-8	Disperse	Azoic	1	
Disperse Blue 106[c] (formerly 357)	111935	12223-01-7 104573-53-7	Disperse	Azoic (cf. DB 124)	1	C, C[d], T[d]
Disperse Blue 124[c]	–	15141-18-1 61951-51-7	Disperse	Azoic (cf. DB 106)	1	C, C[d], F, T[d]
Disperse Blue 153	–	–	Disperse	Anthraquinone	1	C
Disperse Brown 1[c]	11152	23355-64-8	Disperse	Azoic	1	C
Disperse Orange 1[c]	11080	2581-69-3	Disperse	Azoic	1	C
Disperse Orange 3[c]	11005	730-40-5	Disperse	Azoic	1	C, F, T
Disperse Orange 13	26080	6253-10-7	Disperse	Azoic	1	

Disperse Orange 76[c] (formerly 37)	11132	51811-42-8	Disperse	Azoic	1	
Disperse Red 1[c]	11110	2872-52-8	Disperse	Azoic	1	C, F, T
Disperse Red 11[c]	62015	2872-48-2	Disperse	Anthraquinone	1	T
Disperse Red 17[c]	11210	3179-89-3	Disperse	Azoic	1	C, F, T
Disperse Red 153	–	78564-87-1	Disperse	Azoic	1	
Disperse Yellow 1[c]	10345	119-15-3	Disperse	Nitro	1	
Disperse Yellow 3[a,c]	11855	2832-40-8	Disperse	Azoic	1	C, F, T
Disperse Yellow 9[c]	10375	6373-73-5	Disperse	Nitro	1	C, F, T
Disperse Yellow 27	–	73299-30-6	Disperse	Azoic	1	
Disperse Yellow 39[c]	–	12236-29-2	Disperse	Methine	1	
Disperse Yellow 49[c]	–	54824-37-2	Disperse	Methine	1	
Disperse Yellow 54	47020	7576-65-0 12223-85-7	Disperse	Quinoline	1	
Disperse Yellow 64	47023	10319-14-9 12223-86-8	Disperse	Quinoline	1	
Naphthol AS	37505	92-77-3	Coupling agent	Naphthol	1	T
p-Aminophenol	76550	123-30-8		Related to some azo dyes	1	C, F, T
p-Aminoazobenzene (solvent yellow 1)	11000	60-09-3		Related to some azo dyes	0.251	C, F, T
p-Phenylenedi-amine	76060	106-50-3		Related to some azo dyes	1	C, F, T
Reactive Black 5[b]	20505	17095-24-8	Reactive	Azoic	1	C
Reactive Blue 21[b]	18097	12236-86-1 73049-92-0	Reactive	Phthalocyanine (copper)	1	C
Reactive Blue 238[b]	–	149315-83-3	Reactive	(Di)azoic	1	C
Reactive Orange 107[b]	–	90597-79-8	Reactive	Azoic	1	C
Reactive Red 123[b]	–	61969-31-1	Reactive	Azoic	1	C
Reactive Red 228[b]	–	–	Reactive	Azoic	1	C
Reactive Red 238[b]	–	–	Reactive	Azoic	1	C
Reactive Violet 5[b]	18097	12226-38-9	Reactive	Azoic	1	C
Vat Green 1	59825	128-58-5	Vat dye	Anthraquinone	1	

C Chemotechnique® (Malmö, Sweden); *T* Trolab® (Hermal, Reinbeck, Germany); *F* F.I.R.M.A (Firenze, Italia)
[a]Also considered as carcinogenic
[b]Not considered a allergenic for consumers, only if occupational exposure
[c]Dye banned as allergenic by the label Oeko-Tex®
[d]In Disperse Blue mix 106–124

[46, 53]. *Disperse Blue 3* has a structure close to that of Disperse Blue 7 and was positive in several patients tested with a dye series [15, 46, 48]. With Disperse Orange 76 (an azo dye), Disperse Red 11 was thought to be one of the most common causes of dye allergy in men [48]. Disperse Blue 26, one of the most used dyes in the world, is forbidden in garments with label Oeko-Tex® because of its allergenicity [22] (Fig. 40.11).

Azo Dyes

Azo dyes are characterized by an R1-N=N-R2 chemical structure. They represent the majority of commercial colorants, enabling a broad spectrum of shades and fastness properties. They are suitable for coloring various substrates, including both synthetic and natural fibers. These molecules are trapped within the fibers in which they are formed during the dyeing process. Azo dyes, disperse type, are used in synthetic fibers. They are the molecules most often implicated in textile dye dermatitis, mainly in nylon stocking, socks, trousers, dresses, and underwear. Disperse Yellow 3, Disperse Orange 3, and Disperse Red 1 were the principal sensitizers in a retrospective 1940–1984 study [54]. Today, Disperse Blue 124 and/or 106, Disperse Orange 3, Red 1 or Yellow 3 are frequently encountered [7, 10, 15]. A recent classification divided them into four chemical subgroups [28].

The monoazoic compound *Disperse Blue 124* is the most frequent positive dye on patch testing with textile series [9, 10, 15, 16, 55], particularly in women [9, 48]. It is probably the main cause of textile contact dermatitis today [5, 56–58]. It is closely related to another azo dye *Disperse Blue 106*, marketed since 1985 and formerly known as Disperse Blue 357. Both are frequently used together, and Disperse Blue 124 contains traces of Disperse Blue 106 as ascertained by comparative thin layer chromatography (Fig. 40.12). The latter seems to have a stronger sensitizing potential [5, 6, 13, 56] and can provoke infiltrated lesions [7, 57]. Concomitant positive reactions to both Disperse Blue 106 and 124 are almost constant [5, 7].

The delay necessary for the diagnosis may be long [57].

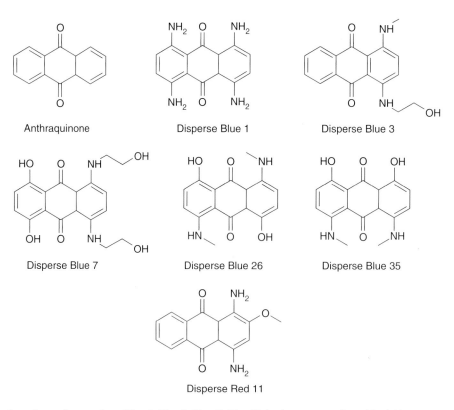

Fig. 40.11 Anthraquinone disperse dyes: Blue 1, Blue 3, Blue 7, Blue 35 (major compound), and Red 11

Disperse Blue 102 was detected in the suspect fabric of four patients with allergic contact dermatitis. It was always associated to Disperse Yellow 3 in the fabric. The four patients were all sensitized to Disperse Blue 106/124 [59].

Disperse Orange 1 was the most common allergen in a study with a disperse dye mix, with a sensitization rate of 0.5% [17]. Among the 17 positive patients, 14 were also sensitive to the Black rubber mix. Actually, it is interesting to see that Disperse Orange 1 is closely related to the components of the Black rubber mix, namely *N,N'*-diphenyl-1, 4 phenylenediamine (DPPD),

N-cyclohexyl-*N'*-phenyl-1,4-phenylenediamine (CPPD), and *N*-isopropyl-*N'*-1,4-phenylenediamine (IPPD).

Disperse Orange 3 was cited in reports of stocking dermatitis [3, 48], and remains a frequent allergen [12, 15]. Patients are sensitized to PPD at an average of 2/3, and primary sensitization to Disperse Orange 3 seems to have been acquired from hair dyes [9, 15]. *p*-aminoazobenzene (PAAB, Solvent Yellow 1) and *p*-dimethylaminoazobenzene (PDMAAB) are positive in about 2/3 patients sensitized to Disperse Orange 3 [15] (Fig. 40.13).

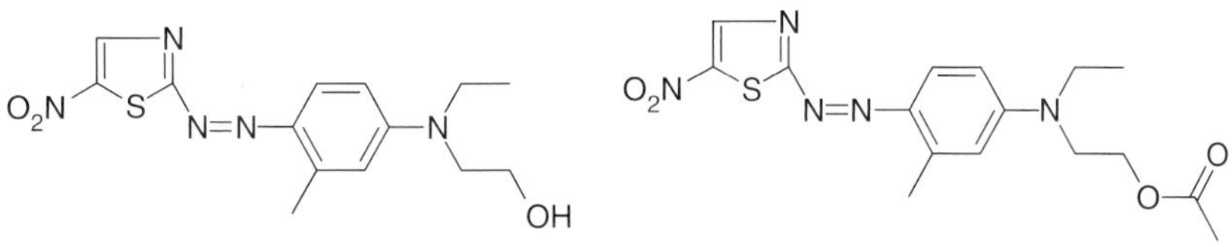

Fig. 40.12 Azo disperse dyes Disperse Blue 106 and Disperse Blue 124

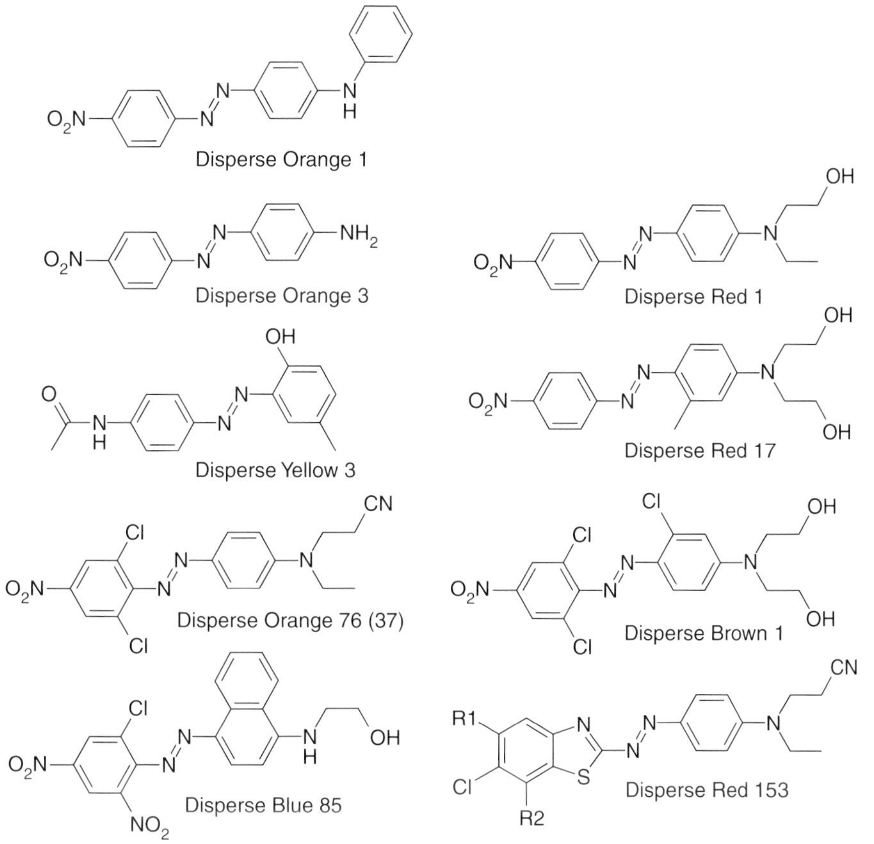

Fig. 40.13 Azo disperse dyes Orange 1, Orange 3, Red 1, Yellow 3, Red 17, Orange 76 (37), Brown 1, Blue 85, and Red 153 (R1 = Cl or H and R2 = H or Cl, respectively)

40

Disperse Red 1 was implicated in dermatitis from stocking [48], and it is frequently observed on patch testing [10, 16], especially in subjects under 12 years of age [15].

Disperse Red 17 gave positive patch test reactions in patients sensitized to other azo dyes [10, 15, 28], and was cited as a stocking dye [3, 23].

Disperse Brown 1 is less frequently positive, as is Disperse Brown 2 [28].

Disperse Orange 76 also formerly named *Disperse Orange 37*, is often positive and was thought to be one of the main causes of dye allergy in men, together with Disperse Blue 3 (an anthraquinone dye) [3, 15, 48].

Reactions to *Disperse Yellow 3* are frequent [3, 7, 9, 10, 16]. The first cases reported concerned nylon stocking dermatitis, and this azo dye is still used to dye such garments ([3, 4, 23], personal observation). This dye is regarded as a carcinogen.

Disperse Red 153 is based on two structurally close compounds [28].

Disperse Black 1 and 2 are rarely positive [13, 15].

Among disperse azo dyes, Disperse Blue 106/124 are currently the main sensitizers, found in synthetic fibers like cellulose acetate or polyamide.

Methine, Nitro, and Quinoline Dyes

Disperse Yellow 39, a methine dye, was implicated in trouser dermatitis [4, 45]. Disperse Yellow 54 and its brominated derivative Disperse Yellow 64 (quinoline), Disperse Yellow 1, and Disperse Yellow 9 (nitro) were cited in some reports [4, 46, 48] (Fig. 40.14).

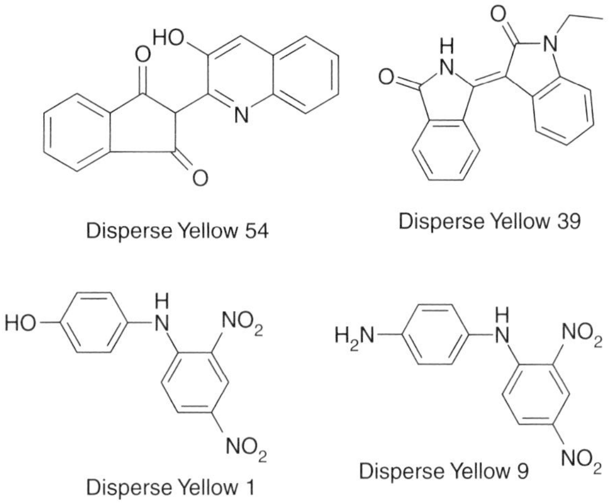

40.3.3.2 Acid Dyes

These are used to color silk, wool, and other animal protein fibers, or nylon (polyamide) when high wet-fastness is needed [31, 47]. Such dyes include monoazoic, diazoic, triphenylmethane, and anthraquinone compounds. Acid Yellow 23, Acid Black 48, Acid Black 63 [3], and Acid Violet 17 (triphenylmethane derived) were reported in the literature, mainly before 1985 [4, 46]. Acid Yellow 61, Acid Red 359, and Acid Red 118 each tested 5% pet., and removed at 3 days (sic) were positive in 5, 2, and 1 out of 1,814 consecutive patients,

Fig. 40.14 Disperse Yellow 54 (quinoleine), Disperse Yellow 39 (quinoleine), Disperse Yellow 1, and Disperse Yellow 9 (nitro)

respectively. Relevance was considered possible in four patients [11]. Acid Red 26 (CI 16150) is regarded as a carcinogen and is forbidden in the EU (Fig. 40.15).

Acid dyes used for protein or nylon fibers are rare allergens.

40.3.3.3 Basic Dyes

These are mainly used to dye wool and silk, acrylic, modacrylic, nylon, polyester, and blends of these fibers with cotton. They can be applied to cotton with a mordant [47]. Basic dyes comprise monoazoic, diazoic, and azine compounds. Basic Red 46, a monoazoic dye was implicated in occupational [60], and in clothing dermatitis sweater [61]. It seems to be an important cause of foot dermatitis, being a frequent allergen in acrylic socks [62]. Basic Brown 1, Basic Black 1, Brilliant Green (CI 42040), Turquoise Reactive, and Neutrichrome Red have also been reported as allergens [3, 13, 47].

Basic Red 9 (Magenta, CI 42500) and Basic Violet 14 (CI 42510) are regarded as carcinogens (Fig. 40.16).

Among basic dyes, Basic Red 46 seems to be an important allergen in acrylic socks.

Fig. 40.15 Acid Yellow 36 (monazoic), Acid Violet 17 (triphenyl-methane), and Acid Black 38 (anthraquinone)

Acid Yellow 36

Acid Violet 17

Acid Black 48

Fig. 40.16 Basic Brown 1 and Basic Red 46

Basic Brown 1

Basic Red 46

Fig. 40.17 Direct Black 38

40.3.3.4 Direct Dyes

These dyes are directly applied on fibers, most often cotton, wool, flax, or leather in a neutral or alkaline bath. They have low wet-fastness, and frequently need after-treatments [47]. Direct Black 38, a triazoic compound dye used for cotton, wool, and silk [45], has been implicated in patients wearing black clothes, with concomitant immediate-type reactions in some cases [63] (Fig. 40.17).

The azo dye Direct Orange 34 (CI 40230) was positive during systematic testing in 8/1,814 patients [11].

Direct Black 38 (CI 30235), Direct Blue 6 (CI 22610), and Direct Red 28 (CI 22120) are regarded as carcinogens.

40.3.3.5 Vat Dyes

Such water-insoluble dyes are applied in a reduced soluble form and then reoxidized to the original insoluble form once absorbed into the fiber. They have high wet-fastness and are used to dye cotton, flax, wool, and rayon fibers. They mostly comprise Vat Blue 6, formerly responsible for cosmetic dermatitis [46] and Vat Green 1. Vat Blue 1 (indigoid dye) is used to dye Levi Strauss 501 "shrink to fit" blue jeans [31]. Vat Green 1, an anthraquinone derivative, has only been reported as a cause of clothing contact dermatitis, from navy-blue uniforms in nurses [64] (Fig. 40.18).

Vat dyes are exceptional allergens.

40.3.3.6 Fiber Reactive Dyes

Reactive dyes consist of a two-part, direct coloring agent. The first moiety is a chromophore with an azo, anthraquinone, or phthalocyanine derivative structure. This moiety is connected to a second reactive group, which is able to form covalent bonds with the amine or sulfhydryl groups of proteins in the textile fibers. Such dyes are used for coloring cellulosic fibers (cotton, silk), wool, or polyamides and are widely used for the production of clothes, most sources of sensitization being occupational. In a study of 1,813 consecutive patients tested with an additional textile series of 12 reactive dyes, 18 (0.99%) were found to be sensitized to reactive dyes [8]. However, only five patients had a history of intolerance to garments, and two of four patch tests performed with pieces of garment were positive. In practice, reactive dyes in clothing should not be sensitizers. If they can be extracted from fibers, they are in a hydrolyzed, nonsensitizing form [45]. Exceptionally, if the garment has not been correctly washed during the industrial process, residues of native reactive dyes can induce dermatitis [65]. With the exception of occupational exposure, we feel that reactive dyes should not be tested in patients, although the risk of active sensitization [66] is theoretically of little consequence (Fig. 40.19).

Reactive dyes cause dermatitis only under their native form, i.e., in occupational circumstances, but not in consumers if the garments are correctly washed.

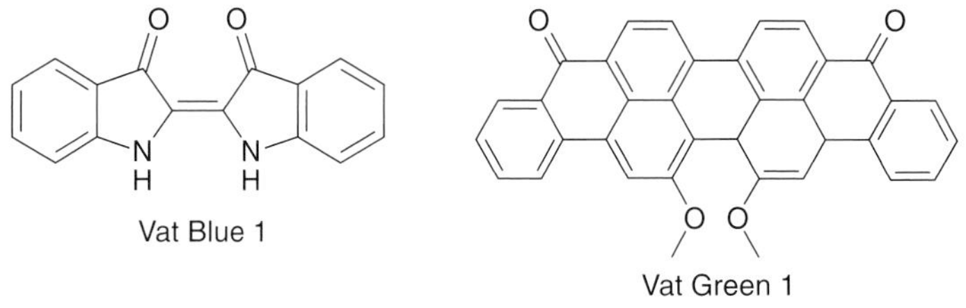

Fig. 40.18 Vat Blue 1 (synthetic indigo) and Vat Green 1

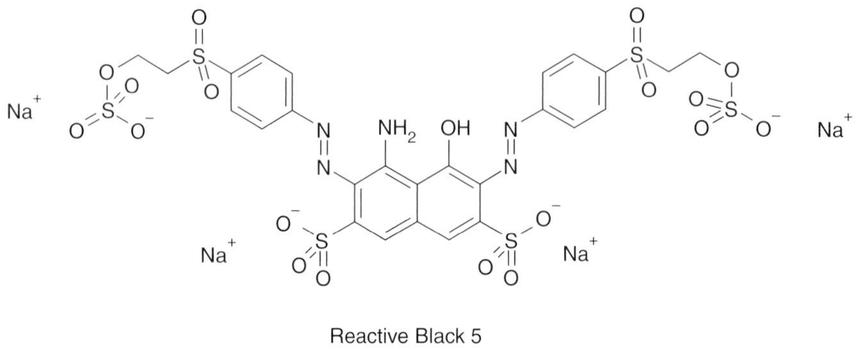

Fig. 40.19 Structure of Reactive Black 5

40.3.3.7 Sulfur, Solvent, and Nondisperse Azoic Dyes

Sulfur dyes are used for cotton in work clothes [31]. Solvent dyes are mono- or diazoic compounds used to dye oils, greases, varnishes, solvents, and cosmetics [45]. Solvent Yellow 1 (PAAB), a monoazoic compound, was positive in patients sensitized to stockings [4].

40.3.3.8 Dye-Fixing and Dye-Coupling Agents

Naphthols are coupling agents, used for staining and dyeing. *β-Naphthol* (2-naphthol, Azoic coupling component 1, CAS [135-19-3]) is no longer used in textile industry.

Naphthol AS (3-hydroxy-2-naphthoic acid anilide, Azoic Coupling Component 2), a coupling agent used for cotton dyeing, has replaced beta-naphthol because of a stronger affinity for cellulose. Naphthol AS first caused pigmented contact dermatitis in workers at a textile factory in Mexico in the 70s, where it was widely used. It was reported as an agent of -sometimes-pigmented contact dermatitis in several patients [1, 47]. We observed a similar case due to a colored foulard imported from India. Patch tests were bullous (+++) to a piece of textile and strongly positive to Naphthol AS 1% pet. The presence of this agent in the foulard was ascertained by a comparative thin-layer chromatography (TLC) [67] (Fig. 40.20).

Several other naphthols are used for textile dyeing, such as Naphthol ASD (3-hydroxy-2naphthoic acid *o*-toluidine), Naphthol AS-E (2-naphtalenecarboxamide, 3-(acetyloxy)-*N*-(4-chloro-phenyl)-, and azoic Coupling Component 10), but they have not been reported as contact allergens.

> Naphthol AS is a classical cause of allergic contact dermatitis due to colored cotton clothing.

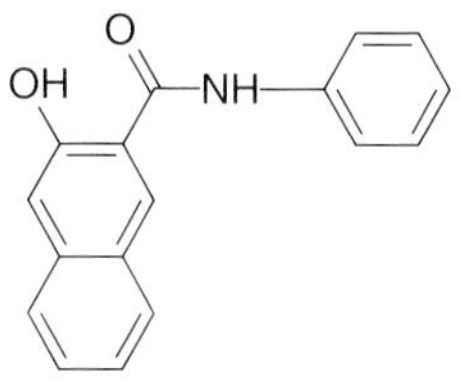

Fig. 40.20 *Naphthol AS*

40.3.4 Rubber

Latex, extracted from *Hevea brasiliensis*, is rarely (and doubtfully) a type IV sensitizer. The main allergens in rubber are vulcanization inhibitors and accelerators, dyes, and antioxidants. Sources are various such as gloves, boots, or garter-belts. They mainly include mercaptobenzothiazole and the components of the mercaptomix (dibenzothiazyl disulfide, *N*-cyclohexylbenzothiazyl sulfenamide, morpholinylmercaptobenzothiazole), thiurams (tetramethylthiuram monosulfide and disulfide, tetraethylthiuram disulfide and dipentamethylenethiuram disulfide), cyclohexylthiophthalimide, and N,N'-isopropyl-phenyl-paraphenylenediamine (IPPD). This last agent, usually present in gray or black rubber, was formerly implicated in purpuric dermatitis from rubber in the elastic of undergarments [3, 31]. Carbamates (diethyl-, dibutyl- and dibenzyldithiocarbamates) can be degraded into carbamyl compounds by chlorine used as a bleaching agent and provoke allergic contact dermatitis [3, 31, 68]. The presumed allergen is *N,N*-dibenzyl carbamyl chloride: patch tests are negative with the standard rubber allergens, but they are positive to the bleached clothing [69].

Neoprene rubber, used to make wet suits, swimming gear, and clothing for fire fighters, contains thiourea derivatives. Diethyl-, dimethyl-, dibutyl-, diphenyl-, and ethylbutyl-thiourea can be responsible for allergic contact dermatitis [34, 35].

40.3.4.1 Other Components of Garments

Trivalent *chromium salts* used to tan leather, are sometimes utilized as a mordant in wool dyeing. They caused allergic contact dermatitis from military textiles [4, 31, 64].

Colophony may be present in some garments, particularly in paper-based clothing such as surgical growns [70].

p-tert-butylphenol-formaldehyde resin (PTBPFR), the allergen of many neoprene glues, caused contact dermatitis from the adhesive of the pad of a derotation brace in a recently operated patient. The dermatitis relapsed after he wore a raincoat fabric which contained PTBPFR used as a finishing agent [71].

40

40.3.4.2 Cleaners, Softeners, and Other Auxiliaries

Waterproofing and *mothproofing agents* are not sensitizers [19, 31].

Biocides are used for several purposes. Antifungal (antimildew) properties of tributyltin oxide (a strong irritant), mercurial compounds, phenols such as pentachlorophenol, carbamates, or mercaptobenzothiazoles can be contained in outdoor materials but are no more authorized in garments, as previously described [20, 48]. Newer molecules and processes have been developed. Triclosan is largely for its antifungal and antibacterial properties, particularly to prevent odor forming in undergarments like socks or underpants. It can be applied on the textile, or incorporated in a specific thread used during weaving. Only one observation concerned clothing allergy [31]. Dimethylfumarate, used as an industrial wide-spectrum biocide in Asia and mainly in China , provoked a worldwide epidemic of severe contact dermatitis due, initially, to Chinese sofas [72, 73]. It also induced severe dermatitis and burning due to shoes [74], and to contaminated clothing as well [75]. This chemical, CAS registry number [624-49-7], is present as a white powder or tablets contained in little bags disposed around the materials for protection. It progressively evaporates and therefore contaminates the textiles, although direct contamination is possible. It is forbidden in the European Union.

The *ultraviolet light absorber* 2-(2-Hydroxy-5-methylphenyl) benzotriazole (Tinuvin® P), used as a photoprotector in plastics and textile fibers, provoked an allergic contact dermatitis from a spandex tape sewn into underwear [76] and from a plastic watch strap [77].

Flame retardants, used to treat cotton, rayon, and polyester, to retard the different phases of combustion such as the presently withdrawn tris (2,3-dibromopropyl) phosphate CAS [126-72-7] or diammonium dihydrogen phosphate, are rare allergens [19, 78]. They are now replaced by fibers that have inherent fireproof properties like blends of Kevlar® and Nomex®.

Cleaners remaining on the fabric, like 1,1,1-trichloroethane [3], are able to cause irritant contact dermatitis. Contact urticaria was reported from the marking nut *Semecarpus anacardium*, used by the launderer to identify the clothing in his shop [79].

Washing detergents are generally not reported as allergens, except rare cases of hypersensitivity to whitening agents. Enzymes, frequently added to enhance the efficacy at lower temperature, can induce dermatitis

by direct contact but are not harmful for the consumers [80]. Surfactants, especially anionic, can induce irritant dermatitis if they persist on the textile after laundry. High doses of detergent, insufficient rinsing, and use of cold tap water for washing and rinsing clothes are promoting factors for dermatitis [81]. Interest of patch testing with detergents [82] is questionable, since they are irritant, even at low concentrations.

Softeners are frequently suspected by patients and even practitioners. Such products diminish the fiber's coefficient of friction and enhance the pleasant and silky touch of garments. Numerous molecules consisting of fatty acids, polyethylens, polymers based on silicon, urethane, or acrylic are used in industry or in consumer goods. Many of them contain preservatives such as formaldehyde, glutaraldehyde, or fragrances. As the amount of residues on clothing is very low , they seem to be safe [14, 20, 83], and we usually recommend the use of softeners, slightly or not perfumed, in our patients with dermatitis.

Cosmetics can be included in garments, generally underwear. Allergens can be preservatives, perfumes, etc.

Accidental contamination is possible, and clothing may contain various articles or be contaminated by many chemical agents, mainly of occupational origin. They include metalworking fluids, resins and paints, pesticides, insecticides and repellents, plants and plant extracts, metallic particles, and fiberglass [3, 19, 84, 85]. A topical drug applied by the patient can also persist for a long time in a glove, a bandage, a shoe, a slipper, or a garment, and induce a further relapse of allergic contact dermatitis: cases have been observed with ketoprofen or salicylamide [86], personal observations.

> Washing detergents and textile softeners are not allergenic.

40.4 Patch Testing

Standard screening patch test series are inadequate for reliable detection of textile sensitivity [7, 12, 14, 47, 48].

The most essential ones are the *clothing patch tests*, which remain the gold standard for diagnosis of clothing allergic contact dermatitis. They are performed with pieces cut from suspected garments (1×1–3×3 cm), according to the pattern of eczema. This material may be moistened with a drop of water. In some cases, an extract from clothing (in water, ethanol, or acetone) can be more sensitive than clothing itself [3, 14]. For "velvet" fabrics, however, testing with pieces may induce active sensitization because of the high level of dyes [5]. Coarse fabrics may irritate the skin and cause a mild erythema or a slight edema at the 2 day reading, but it generally fades in 4 days [48]. Negativity of patch tests with the fabric is frequent, particularly in cases of textile resin sensitivity [3, 14, 31, 48] and does not invalidate the diagnosis of clothing dermatitis [19, 87]. Leaving the fabric patch test on for more than 2 days or winding a piece of garment around the arm may be helpful. However, negative patch test with the suspected garment makes its responsibility for an allergic phenomenon questionable: other garments or an irritant dermatitis (on atopic skin or, for example, pilar keratosis) have to be suspected. In such cases, a challenge test (stop and wear again) seems to be more practical to confirm or contradict allergy ([10, 48], personal observations).

However, many studies on clothing dermatitis, and even reports which focus on one allergen, do not affirm the responsibility of allergens, since they are generally not identified in garments [62, 87]. In a recent study on 20 patients with proved clothing allergic dermatitis, on 32 garments suspected by the patient, 22 actually contained an allergenic dye, and nine contained a dye the patient had reacted to [59].

Formaldehyde (1% aq.) is of importance since it can be a marker of sensitivity to textile finishes which release high or medium amounts of free formaldehyde. The cost-benefit ratio of the use of more complete textile finish series seems to be very poor [40]. Urea-formaldehyde resin (dimethylol urea) 10% pet. [40] and the mixture ethylene urea+melamine formaldehyde resin 5% pet. [2, 42] have been good screening agents. Such data are currently doubtful, since formaldehyde resins, ethylene urea, and melamine formaldehyde are no more used for clothing in our countries. DMDHEU [88] or modified DMDHEU could be better screening agents at present. However, all textile resins available for patch testing (Table 40.3) have a free, nonfixed form. They can be degraded and release formaldehyde (personal observation, Fig. 40.21). Actually, most tests positive to TFR are associated and due to sensitization to formaldehyde. So,

Table 40.3 Textile finish resin allergens available

Allergen	CAS number	Concentration	Type	Formaldehyde release	Suppliers
Formaldehyde (methylal)	50-00-0	1% aq.			C, F, T
Urea formaldehyde (dimethylol urea, carbamol, oxymethurea) (UF) (Kaurit® S)	140-95-4	10% pet.	UF	High	C, F
Melamine formaldehyde (MF) (Kaurit® M70)		7% pet.	MF	High	C
Dimethyl dihydroxy ethylene urea (DMeDHEU) (Fixapret® NF)		4.5% aq.	CU	Low	C
Dimethylol dihydroxy ethylene urea (DMDHEU) (Fixapret® CPN)	1854-26-8	4.5% aq., 10% pet.	CU	Low	C, F
Dimethylol dihydroxy ethylene urea, modified (modified DMDHEU) (Fixapret® ECO)		5% aq.	CU	Low	C
Dimethylol propylene urea (DMPU)	3270-74-4	10% pet.	CU	Medium	F
Ethylene urea *and* MF		5% pet.[a]	CU+MF	Medium and high	C

UF urea formaldehyde resin; *MF* melamine formaldehyde resin; *CU* cyclized urea derivatives

Allergens are available from Chemotechnique (Malmö, Sweden), F.I.R.M.A. (Firenze, Italia), and Trolab (Hermal, Reinbeck, Germany)

[a]Emulsified with sorbitan sesquioleate 5%

40

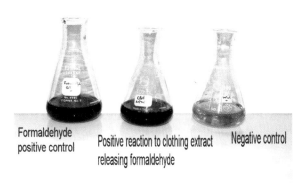

Fig. 40.21 Positive reaction with chromotropic acid method, showing liberation of formaldehyde by textile resins (formaldehyde solution on the *left* as a positive control, negative control on the *right*)

positive reactions to TFR in patients sensitive to formaldehyde have to be carefully interpreted.

PPD is an unreliable screening agent for hypersensitivity to textile dyes [5, 7, 13] and should theoretically be a detector of some azo dyes only, such as Disperse Orange 3, Disperse Red 1, and Red 17. Patients positive to PPD are frequently sensitized to Disperse Orange 3 [3, 9], but the contrary is not so [7]. PPD is hardly ever positive in patients sensitized to the frequently positive Disperse Blue 106 or Disperse Blue 124 [5, 6, 13, 28, 29, 55], *p*-aminophenol [7, 29], or Disperse Yellow 3 [3, 7, 29]. Positive reactions to both diaminodiphenylmethane and Disperse Orange 3 are observed, because of their close chemical structures and probably a similar metabolite [56]. Cross-reactions are possible among other azo dyes such as Disperse Orange 3 and Disperse Red 1 [10, 56]. Reactivity is constant to both Disperse Blue 124 and Disperse Blue 106 [5]. Therefore, some authors suggest routine patch testing with a specific textile series containing disperse dyes [8, 10, 47]. Disperse Blue 106 seems to have a good sensitivity [7]. Supplementation of the standard series with four disperse dyes (Disperse Blue 124, Disperse Red 1, Disperse Yellow 3, Disperse Orange 3) has been useful for some authors [10], but systematic addition of a more complete 16 textile dyes series [12] is of questionable value, although being scientifically interesting in patients with dye sensitivity [7]. A disperse dyes mix has been recommended, but further studies are needed to determine ideal substances and concentrations [13, 16, 89–91]. This mixture was positive in 26 out of 31 patients positive with individual dyes [16]. A recent study with a mix composed of eight disperse dyes (Disperse

Blue 35, 106 and 124, D Yellow 3, D Orange 1 and 3, and D Red 1 and 17) gave a sensitization rate of 1.5% [17], but 17 of the 47 positive patients were negative or had only a doubtful (8/17) reaction to the individual dyes.

The practitioner has to be vigilant about the purity of allergens. We could observe on a 2002–2004 period that several batches of Disperse Orange 3 provided by Chemotechnique, although prepared with both disperse and orange dye, contained no Disperse Orange 3. The mistake was discovered because successive patients sensitive to PPD and tested with textile series, reacted to Disperse Red 1, and Disperse Red 17, but not to the orange dye, as generally observed. Comparative thin layer chromatographies, nuclear magnetic resonance, and high-performance liquid chromatography detected Disperse Orange 31 that had been wrongly substituted for Disperse Orange 3 [92]. This situation also explained that a relatively low percentage of patients positive to PPD were positive to Disperse Orange 3, although a coreaction is explained to be very frequent because of skin transformation of Disperse Orange 3 into PPD [92, 93].

Caution is also needed regarding patch testing with dyes series for several reasons. A positive patch test, as a result of sensitivity to a dye, is not always relevant and can be the result either of a primary sensitization, or of a co- or cross-reaction. For example, a positive reaction to Disperse Orange 3, expected at least in 2/3 of people sensitized to PPD is almost constant in our experience. Therefore, even if a textile dye is found to be positive, this is no guarantee of its presence in the garment. Purity of some dyes in commercial patch test series is doubtful and only some dyes seem to be pure [45] (Fig. 40.22). This

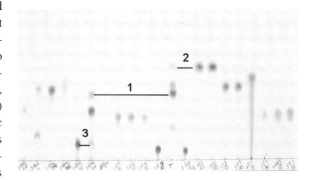

Fig. 40.22 Thin layer chromatography performed with acetone extract of a black-textile (T) and with several disperse dyes. See the different dyed fractions of T, corresponding to a component of Disperse Blue 124 (*1*) and to Disperse Orange 1 (*2*). See components of "pure" dyes, particularly Disperse Blue 124, which contains Disperse Blue 106 (*3*)

can lead to false-positive reactions when an impurity is the cause of a positive reaction. In some cases of multiple reactions [13, 55, 56], an "angry back" or excited skin syndrome should also be taken into consideration. Such a situation or nonallergic papular reactions could account for the strong differences observed between the frequencies of positive reactions to such close allergens in some observations (12.5 and 20% to Disperse Blue 106 and Disperse Blue 124, respectively in one study) [94, 95].

Regarding allergens other than textile resins and dyes, rubber compounds are mainly included in the standard series. Thiourea derivatives like diethyl-, dimethyl-, dibutyl-, diphenyl-, and ethylbutyl-thiourea can also be tested [34, 35].

The gold standard is patch testing with patient's clothing. Tests are sometimes irritant, inducing slight erythema and oedema fading at the second reading.

DMDHEU and modified DMDHEU should be good screeners for sensitivity to TFR. Patch test reactions to TFR are frequently associated to formaldehyde sensitivity, and it is sometimes difficult to establish relevance of routinely performed tests.

Standards series are unable to detect textile dyes allergy. Systematic addition of textile dye(s) like Disperse Blue 106 can be recommended.

Patch tests with textile dye series have to be cautiously interpreted, according to clinical presentation, particularly + (weakly positive, sometimes irritant) and diffuse (+++ and/or angry-back) reactions.

40.5 Chemical Analyses

40.5.1 Identification of Formaldehyde

In industry and toxicological studies, the most widely used methods for the detection of formaldehyde are based on spectrophotometry, but other methods, such as colorimetry, fluorimetry, high-performance liquid chromatography, polarography, gas chromatography, infrared detection, and gas detector tubes, are also used. The most sensitive of these methods is flow injection, which has a detection limit of 9 ppt (0.011 µg/m3). Another commonly used method is high-performance liquid chromatography, which offers a detection limit of 0.0017 ppm (0.002 mg/m^3). For the practitioner, identification of formaldehyde in garments can be useful for patients suspected of clothing dermatitis and sensitized to formaldehyde, since it may prevent relapses of their dermatitis. Several methods are available [3, 23, 31].

40.5.1.1 Chromotropic Acid Method

The reaction is exothermic and necessitates caution. Put 2 g of the garment into 100 mL water for 24 h. Filter the solution. Put 1 mL in an Erlenmeyer flask. Add 5 mL of distilled water and 1 mL of 5% fresh solution of chromotropic acid (powder stored in dark and in fridge) plus 5 mL of concentrated sulfuric acid. A violet discoloration, due to formation of 3,4,5,6-dibenzoxanthylium, is specific and indicates the presence of formaldehyde at >0.005% (50 ppm) concentration. Other aldehydes or ketones can give a yellowish, orange, reddish, or brownish, but not violet coloration.

40.5.1.2 Schiff's Reagent Method

Cut a small strip of material (8 cm²). Immerse it in about 5 mL of 0.1 N hydrochloric acid (HCl). Heat in water bath for 10 min and remove fabric. Add five drops of Schiff's aldehyde reagent (stored in fridge). A violet color indicates the presence of an aldehyde.

40.5.1.3 Acetylacetone Method

Cut a small trip of material (0.5 g), and put it into a glass jar. Add 2.5 mL of Nash reagent (15 g of ammonium acetate, 0.3 mL of glacial acetic acid, 0.2 mL of Acetylacetone, and distilled water to 1 L), stick and heat (for low concentration of formaldehyde) at 60°C for 10 min. Formaldehyde reacting with two molecules of acetylacetone and with one molecule of ammonia, will form a yellow compound 3,5-diacetyl-1,4-dihydrolutidine. Its concentration can be more exactly determined spectrophotometrically at 412 nm. Positive

40

(10, 5, and 2.5 µg/mL formaldehyde solutions) and negative (distilled water) controls are needed. This method sensitive down to 4 ppm, is contraindicated with dyed clothing [96–98].

> Identification of formaldehyde in textile is possible for the practitioner by chromotropic acid, Schiff's, or acetylacetone methods.

40.5.2 Identification of Dyes

TLC can be carried out with the dye extracted from the textile. It necessitates comparison with one or several dyes whose chemical composition is known, [3, 5, 43].

In some cases, TLC permits patch testing with different fractions of the dye mixture used in the garment. Pieces of textiles are cut into shreds and extracted with an eluent like chloroform. TLC is done with the solution put on TLC plates, using chloroform and methanol as eluents. Combination of TLC, magnetic resonance spectroscopy, and infrared spectrometry is sometimes useful to identify some dyes [3].

We have developed a method which we named EpiCAT [44], consisting of Epicutaneously Chromatogram Applied Test. A variant has been developed [99]. This method clearly indicates the dyes and/or the impurities the patients are allergic to [44, 100]. Patch testing with thin-layer chromatograms in 21 patients allergic to Disperse Blue 106 or/and 124 demonstrates that around 25% of the patients do not react to the dye itself, but to impurities [100].

Our procedure is the following:

– Cut a piece of garment (e.g.,1 g), and put it in a weigh-filter
– Add acetone in order to have a 5% solution (here add 19 g acetone)
– Leave it until apparition of a colored solution (30 min to 7 days)
– Perform a TLC with a spot of colored solution on a TLC aluminum sheet with silica gel (Merck, Darmstadt, Germany), then put in a blend of 60% ethyl acetate and 40% hexane as eluents
– Vary the eluent proportions, in order to separate the dye spots well, if necessary

– Repeat the procedure with a band of dye solution, to obtain bands of separated dyes
– Put the round-shaped TLC plate on the patient's upper back covered with an adhesive tape for 48 h
– Read at D2 and D3 or D4. Linear positive reaction(s) will occur in front of allergenic dye (Fig. 40.23)
– Repeat comparative TLC or further analysis to identify the offending dye.

Extraction of dyes from clothing is useful to ascertain the diagnosis of allergy and to identify the offending dye(s) in textiles. Patch tests can be directly realized with the TLC (EpiCAT).

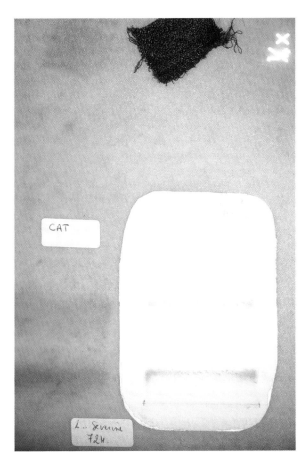

Fig. 40.23 Patch testing with a piece of garment, and EpiCAT (performed with TLC). Linear allergic reactions occur regarding 2 components of Disperse Blue 124 present in the textile

40.6 Patient Advice

Patients sensitized to textile resins (a rare situation in fact) have to replace their garments by untreated fabrics, and avoid "dry-drip," "crease resistant," "durable-press," "permanent-press," "easy care," "easy to iron," "no iron," "wash and go" or "wash and wear" textiles, particularly rayon, 100% cotton, or blends of those fibers. Most blended textiles are treated and are consequently to be avoided, such as permanent press or wrinkle resistant garments. Wool, linen, denim, nylon, or silk are unlikely to be treated and should be preferred. New textiles can be submitted for chemical analysis in hypersensitive patients (see above). Washing all new textiles at least twice before using is useful, because formaldehyde

transfer is possible from treated to untreated fabrics [19]. However, free formaldehyde will be washed out in water, but the resin will persist in the garment [23]. Wearing a protective undergarment is sometimes useful [19].

Concerning textile dye hypersensitivity, it is generally of little importance to the patient to know whether he is allergic to one or several textile dyes. Because of cross-reactions, it is frequent to observe that the patients are sensitized to dyes which are not present in a garment, even after TLC [13, 48]. However, cross-reactions occur among same, but not between different, chemical classes. Strongly colored synthetic textiles should be avoided. Lightly colored garments can be permitted, like pure (100%) natural fibers (cotton, linen, silk, wool), even dark colored [7].

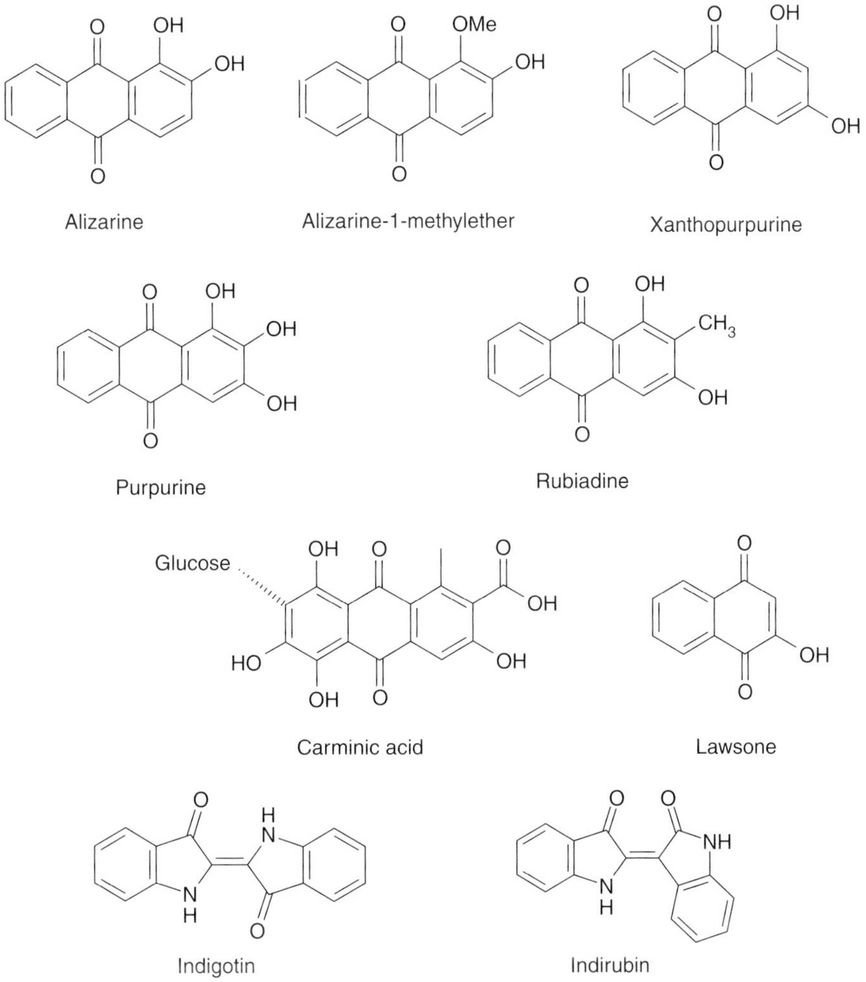

Fig. 40.24 Natural dyes alizarine, alizarine-1-methylether, xanthopurpurine, purpurine, rubiadine (Rubiaceae), carminic acid (cochineal), lawsone (henna), idigotin, and indirubin (indigo)

40

Natural clothing dyes of vegetable origin such as henna -containing lawsone- or indigo -containing indirubine and indigotin (natural indigo or Vat Blue 1)- or of animal source such as cochineal -containing the anthraquinone compounds carminic and kermesic acids that give the carmine color- can be used to color wool, cotton, and silk fabrics. Among frequent natural dyes, we can cite alizarine and its derivative alizarine-1-methylether, purpurine, xanthopurpurine, and rubiadine contained in the Rubiaceae family to which belongs madder (*Rubia tinctorum* L.) [101]. Natural dyes are generally not mentioned as a cause of clothing dermatitis, although lawsone and carminic acid can be allergenic [46, 102] (Fig. 40.24).

We generally propose to our patients who are sensitive to disperse dyes to perform a spot test with a cotton bud impregnated with acetone. If rubbing on the garment, and particularly on synthetic lining, does not produce any color transfer, it is unlikely that the garment will be allergenic. This was observed and confirmed in our disperse dye(s) allergic patients.

Patients with textile dermatitis and sensitized to finish resins or formaldehyde should avoid "no-iron" clothing.

Patients sensitized to textile dyes have to avoid synthetic fibers (if sensitized to disperse dyes), strongly colored or dark synthetic garments (if sensitized only to disperse dyes Blue 106 and 124) or cotton colored dyes (if positive to Naphthol AS).

Clothing treated with natural dyes are well tolerated by patients sensitized to synthetic dyes.

When negative, a spot-test performed with acetone is generally a good indicator of nonallergenicity of dyes in a textile.

References

1. Roed-Petersen J, Batsberg W, Larsen E (1990) Contact dermatitis from Naphthol AS. Contact Dermatitis 22:161–163
2. Kojima S, Momma J, Kaniwa MA, Ikarashi Y, Sato M, Nakaji Y, Kurokawa Y, Nakamura A (1990) Phosgene (chlorophenyl)hydrazones, strong sensitizers found in yellow sweaters bleached with sodium hypochlorite, defined as causative allergens for contact dermatitis by an experimental screening method in animals. Contact Dermatitis 23:129–141
3. Foussereau J (1987) Les eczémas allergiques cosmétologiques, thérapeutiques et vestimentaires. Masson, Paris
4. Hatch KL, Maibach HI (1985) Textile dye dermatitis. A review. J Am Acad Dermatol 12:1079–1092
5. Hausen BM (1993) Contact allergy to Disperse Blue 106 and Blue 124 in black "velvet" clothes. Contact Dermatitis 28:169–173
6. Menezes-Brandao F, Altermatt C, Pecegueiro M, Bordalo O, Foussereau J (1985) Contact dermatitis to Disperse Blue 106. Contact Dermatitis 13:80–84
7. Dooms-Goossens A (1992) Textile dye dermatitis. Contact Dermatitis 27:321–323
8. Manzini BM, Motoles A, Conti A, Ferdani G, Seidenari S (1996) Sensitization to reactive textile dyes in patients with contact dermatitis. Contact Dermatitis 34:172–175
9. Balato N, Lembo G, Patruno C, Ayala F (1990) Prevalence of textile dye contact sensitization. Contact Dermatitis 23:111–126
10. Seidenari S, Manzini BM, Danese P (1991) Contact sensitization to textile dyes: description of 100 subjects. Contact Dermatitis 24:253–258
11. Seidenari S, Manzini BM, Schiavi ME, Motolese A (1995) Prevalence of contact allergy to non-disperse azo dyes for natural fibers: a study in 1814 consecutive patients. Contact Dermatitis 33:118–122
12. Borrego L, Ortiz-Frutos J (1996) Textile dye dermatitis: Spanish experience. J Am Acad Dermatol 34:715–716
13. Lisboa C, Barros MA, Azenha A (1994) Contact dermatitis from textile dyes. Contact Dermatitis 31:9–10
14. Sherertz EF (1992) Clothing dermatitis: practical aspects for the clinician. Am J Contact Dermat 3:55–64
15. Seidenari S, Mantovani L, Manzini BM, Pignatti M (1997) Cross-sensitizations between azo dyes and para-amino compound. A study of 236 azo-dye-sensitive subjects. Contact Dermatitis 36:91–96
16. Lodi A, Ambonati M, Coassini A, Chiarelli G, Mancini LL, Crosti C (1998) Textile dye contact dermatitis in an allergic population. Contact Dermatitis 39:314
17. Ryberg K, Isaksson M, Gruvberger B, Hindsén M, Zimerson E, Bruze M (2006) Contact allergy to textile dyes in southern Sweden. Contact Dermatitis 54:313–321
18. Hatch KL, Maibach HI (2000) Textile dye allergic contact dermatitis prevalence. Contact Dermatitis 42:187–195
19. Hatch KL, Maibach HI (1986) Textile chemical finish dermatitis. Contact Dermatitis 14:1–13
20. Le Coz C (1999) Dermites de contact aux apprêts et ennoblisseurs textiles. Progrès en dermato-allergologie, Lyon. John Libbey Eurotext, Paris

21. Official Journal of the European Communities. N° L 243/15. Directive 2002/61/EC of the European Parliament and of the Council of 19 July 2002 amending for the nineteenth time Council Directive 76/769/EEC relating to restrictions on the marketing and use of certain dangerous substances and preparations (azocolourants)

22. http://www.oeko-tex.com

23. Cronin E (1963) Formalin textile dermatitis. Br J Dermatol 75:267–273

24. Van der Veen JPW, Neering H, de Haan P, Bruynzeel DP (1988) Pigmented purpuric clothing dermatitis due to Disperse Blue 85. Contact Dermatitis 19:222–223

25. Komericki P, Aberer W, Arbab E, Kovacevic Z, Kränke B (2001) Pigmented purpuric contact dermatitis from Disperse Blue 106 and 124 dyes. J Am Acad Dermatol 45:456–458

26. Foti C, Elia G, Filotico R, Angelini G (1998) Purpuric clothing dermatitis due to Disperse Yellow 27. Contact Dermatitis 39:273

27. Fowler JF, Skinner SM, Belsito DV (1992) Allergic contact dermatitis from formaldehyde resins in permanent press clothing: an underdiagnosed cause of generalized dermatitis. J Am Acad Dermatol 27:962–968

28. Nakagawa M, Kawai K, Kawai K (1996) Multiple azo disperse dye sensitization mainly due to group sensitizations to azo dyes. Contact Dermatitis 34:6–11

29. Mathelier-Fusade P, Aïssaoui M, Chabane MH, Mounedji N, Leynadier F (1996) Chronic generalized eczema caused by multiple dye sensitization. Am J Contact Dermat 7:224–225

30. Hatch KL, Maibach HI (1985) Textile fiber dermatitis. Contact Dermatitis 12:1–11

31. Rietschel RL, Fowler JF (1994) Fisher's contact dermatitis, 4th edn. Wiliams & Wilkins, Baltimore, pp 358–392

32. Inoue A, Ishido I, Shoji A, Yamada H (1997) Textile dermatitis from silk. Contact Dermatitis 37:185

33. Tanaka M, Kobayashi S, Miyakawa S-I (1993) Contact dermatitis from nylon 6 in Japan. Contact Dermatitis 28: 250

34. Kerre S, Devos L, Verhoeve L, Bruze M, Gruvberger B, Dooms-Goossens A (1996) Contact allergy to diethylthiourea in a wet suit. Contact Dermatitis 35:176–178

35. Reynaers A, Goossens A (1998) La diéthylthiourée: allergène de contact dans divers objets en néoprène. La lettre du GERDA 15:60–61

36. Alcántara M, Martínez-Escribano J, Frías J, García-Sellés FJ (2000) Allergic contact dermatitis due to diphenylthiourea in a neoprene slimming suit. Contact Dermatitis 43: 224–225

37. Diepgen TL, Stäbler A, Hornstein OP (1990) Textilunverträglichkeit beim atopischen Ekzem. Eine kontrollierte klinische Studie. Zeitschrift für Hautkrankheiten 65: 907–910

38. Veien NK, Hattel T, Laurberg G (1991) Can "label dermatitis" become "creeping neurotic excoriations"? Contact Dermatitis 27:272–273

39. Hatch KL, Maibach HI (1995) Textile dermatitis: an update (I). Resins, additives and fibers. Contact Dermatitis 32: 319–326

40. Andersen KE, Hamann K (1982) Cost benefit of patch testing with textile finish resins. Contact Dermatitis 8:64–67

41. Schorr WF, Keran E, Plotka E (1974) Formaldehyde allergy. The quantitative analysis of american clothing for free formaldehyde and its relevance in clinical practice. Arch Dermatol 110:73–76

42. Marks JG, Belsito DV, DeLeo VA, Fowler JF, Fransway AF, Maibach HI et al (1998) North American Contact Dermatitis Group patch test results for the detection of delayed-type hypersensitivity to topical allergens. J Am Acad Dermatol 38:911–918

43. Foussereau J, Dallara JM (1986) Purity of standardized textile dye allergens: a thin layer chromatography study. Contact Dermatitis 14:303–306

44. Le Coz CJ, Lefebvre C, Haberkorn L (2002) Epicutaneous chromatogram applied test (EpiCAT): an original test method for allergic contact dermatitis (ACD) from clothing dyes. Contact Dermatitis 46(suppl 4):34

45. Cavelier C, Foussereau J, Tomb R (1988) Allergie de contact et colorants (2e partie). Cahiers de notes documentaires de l'INRS 133:615–647

46. Cavelier C, Foussereau J, Tomb R (1988) Allergie de contact et colorants (1e partie). Cahiers de notes documentaires de l'INRS 132:421–443

47. Hatch KL, Maibach HI (1995) Textile dye dermatitis. J Am Acad Dermatol 32:631–639

48. Cronin E (1980) Contact dermatitis. Edinburgh, Churchill Livingstone, pp 36–92

49. Wenninger JA, Canterbery RC, McEwen Jr GN (eds) (2000) International cosmetic ingredient dictionary and handbook, 8th edn. The Cosmetic, Toiletry, and Fragrance Association, Washington DC

50. Report on Carcinogens, 10th edn (2002) US Department of Health and Human Services, Public Health Service, National Toxicology Program, December 2002

51. Cronin E (1968) Studies in contact dermatitis, dyes in clothing. Trans St John's Hosp Derm Soc 54:156–164

52. Cronin E (1968) Studies in contact dermatitis, nylon stocking dyes. Trans St John's Hosp Derm Soc 54:165–169

53. Dabestani R, Reszka KJ, Davis DG, Sik RH, Chignell CF (1991) Spectroscopic studies of cutaneous photosensitizing agents-XVI. Disperse blue 35. Photochem Photobiol 54: 37–42

54. Hausen BM, Sawall EM (1989) Sensitization experiments with textile dyes in guinea pigs. Contact Dermatitis 20:27–31

55. Dejobert Y, Martin P, Thomas P, Bergoend H (1995) Multiple azo dye sensitization revealed by the wearing of a black "velvet" body. Contact Dermatitis 33:276–277

56. Massone L, Anonide A, Isola V, Borghi S (1991) 2 cases of multiple azo dye sensitization. Contact Dermatitis 24:60–63

57. Pecquet C, Assier-Bonnet H, Artigou C, Verne-Fourment L, Saïag P (1999) Atypical presentation of textile dye densitization. Contact Dermatitis 40:51

58. Guin JD, Dwyer G, Sterba K (1999) Clothing dye dermatitis masquerading as (coexisting) mimosa allergy. Contact Dermatitis 40:45

59. Hatch K, Motschi H, Maibach HI (2003) Disperse dyes in fabrics of patients patch-test-positive to disperse dyes. Am J Contact Dermat 14:205–212

60. Chave TA, Nicolaou N, Johnston GA (2003) Hand dermatitis in a student caused by Basic Red 46. Contact Dermatitis 49:161–162

61. Foussereau J (1986) Contact dermatitis to Basic Red 46. Contact Dermatitis 15:106

62. Opie J, Lee A, Frowen K, Fewings J, Nixon R (2003) Foot dermatitis caused by the textile dye Basic Red 46 in acrylic blend socks. Contact Dermatitis 49:297–303

63. Noferi A, Ferrante E, Testa A (1966) Dermatosi allergiche da nero diretto colorante azoico solubile. Folia Allerg 13: 478–480

64. Wilson HTH, Cronin E (1971) Dermatitis from dyed uniforms. Br J Dermatol 85:67–69

65. Moreau L, Goossens A (2005) Allergic contact dermatitis associated with reactive dyes in a dark garment: a case report. Contact Dermatitis 53:150–154

66. Sommer S, Wilkinson SM (2000) A series of 3 patients sensitized to reactive dyes during patch testing. Contact Dermatitis 43:227–228

67. Le Coz CJ, Lepoittevin JP (2001) Clothing dermatitis from Naphthol AS. Contact Dermatitis 44:366–367

68. Jordan WP, Bourlas M (1975) Allergic contact dermatitis to underwear elastic. Arch Dermatol 111:593–595

69. Blancas-Espinosa R, Ancona-Alayón A, Arévalo-López A (2000) Allergic contact dermatitis to socks presenting as bleached rubber syndrome. Am J Contact Dermat 11:97–98

70. Bergh M, Menné T, Karlberg AT (1994) Colophony in paper-based surgical clothing. Contact Dermatitis 31: 332–333

71. Hayakawa R, Ogino Y, Suzuki M, Kaniwa M (1994) Allergic contact dermatitis from para-tertiary-butylphenol-formaldehyde resin (PTBP-F-R). Contact Dermatitis 30:187–188

72. Rantanen T (2008) The cause of the Chinese sofa/chair dermatitis epidemic is likely to be contact allergy to dimethylfumarate, a novel potent contact sensitizer. Br J Dermatol 159:218–221

73. Imbert E, Chamaillard M, Kostrzewa E, Doutre MS, Milpied B, Beylot-Barry M, Le Coz CJ, Fritsch C, Chantecler ML, Vigan M (2008) Allergie au fauteuil chinois: une nouvelle dermite de contact. Ann Dermatol Venereol 135:777–779

74. Vigan M, Biver C, Bourrain JL, Pelletier F, Girardin P, Aubin F, Humbert P (2009) Eczéma aigu d'un pied au diméthylfumarate. Ann Dermatol Venereol 136:281–283

75. Foti C, Zambonin CG, Cassano N, Aresta A, Damascelli A, Ferrara F, Vena GA (2009) Occupational allergic contact dermatitis associated with dimethyl fumarate in clothing. Contact Dermatitis 61:122–124

76. Arisu K, Hayakawa R, Ogino Y, Matsunaga K, Kaniwa M-A (1992) Tinuvin® P in a spandex tape as a cause of clothing dermatitis. Contact Dermatitis 26:311–316

77. Niklasson B, Björkner B (1989) Contact allergy to the UV-absorber Tinuvin® P in plastics. Contact Dermatitis 21: 330–334

78. Moreau A, Dompmartin A, Castel B, Remond B, Michel M, Leroy D (1994) Contact dermatitis from a textile flame retardant. Contact Dermatitis 31:86–88

79. Shankar DS (1992) contact urticaria induced by Semecarpus anacardium. Contact Dermatitis 26:200

80. Andersen PH, Bindslev-Jensen C, Mosbech H, Zachariae H, Andersen KE (1998) Skin symptoms in patients with atopic dermatitis using enzyme-containing detergents. Acta Derm Venereol (Stockh) 78:60–62

81. Kiriyama T, Sugiura H, Uehara M (2003) Residual washing detergent in cotton clothes: a factor of winter deterioration of dry skin in atopic dermatitis. J Dermatol 30:708–712

82. Belsito DV, Fransway AF, Fowler JF Jr, Sherertz EF, Maibach HI, Marks JG Jr et al (2002) Allergic contact dermatitis to detergents: a multicenter study to assess prevalence. J Am Acad Dermatol 46:200–206

83. Kofoed ML (1984) Contact dermatitis to formaldehyde in fabric softeners. Contact Dermatitis 11:254

84. Hafner J, Ruegger M, Kralicek P, Elsner P (1995) Airborne irritant contact dermatitis from metal dust adhering to semisynthetic working suits. Contact Dermatitis 32: 285–288

85. Le Coz CJ, Lepoittevin JP (2001) Occupational erythema-multiforme-like dermatitis from sensitization to costus resinoid, followed by flare-up and systemic contact dermatitis from beta-cyclocostunolide in a chemistry student. Contact Dermatitis 44:310–311

86. Hindsén M, Isaksson M, Persson L, Zimersson E, Bruze M (2004) Photoallergic contact dermatitis from ketoprofen induced by drug-contaminated personal objects. J Am Acad Dermatol 50:215–219

87. Khanna M, Sasseville D (2001) Occupational contact dermatitis to textile dyes in airline personnel. Am J Contact Dermat 12:208–210

88. Metzler-Brenckle L, Rietschel RL (2002) Patch testing for permanent-press allergic contact dermatitis. Contact Dermatitis 46:33–37

89. Francalanci S, Angelini G, Balato N, Berardesca E, Cusano F, Gaddoni G, Lisi P, Lodi A, Schena D, Sertoli A (1995) Effectiveness of disperse dyes mix in detection of contact allergy to textile dyes: an Italian multicentre study. Contact Dermatitis 33:351

90. Sousa-Basto A, Azenha A (1994) Textile dye mixes: useful screening tests for textile dye allergy. Contact Dermatitis 30:89–190

91. Sertoli A, Francalanci S, Giorgini S (1994) Sensitization to textile disperse dyes: validity of reduced-concentration patch tests and a new mix. Contact Dermatitis 31:47–48

92. Le Coz CJ, Jelen G, Goossens A, Vigan M, Ducombs G, Bircher A et al (2004) Disperse (yes), Orange (yes), 3 (no): what do we test in textile dye dermatitis? Contact Dermatitis 50:126–127

93. Goon AT, Gilmour NJ, Basketter DA, White IR, Rycroft RJ, McFadden JP (2003) High frequency of simultaneous sensitivity to Disperse Orange 3 in patients with positive patch tests to para-phenylenediamine. Contact Dermatitis 48: 248–250

94. Lazarov A, Trattner A, David M, Ingber A (2001) Textile dermatitis in Israel: a retrospective study. Am J Contact Dermat 11:26–29

95. Uter W, Geier J, Lessmann H, Hausen BM (2001) Contact allergy to Disperse Blue 106 and Disperse Blue 124 in German and Austrian patients, 1995 to 1999. Contact Dermatitis 44:173–177

96. Fregert S, Dahlquist I, Gruvberger B (1984) A simple method for the detection of formaldehyde. Contact Dermatitis 10:132–134

97. Gryllaki-Berger M, Mugny C, Perrenoud D, Pannatier A, Frenk E (1992) A comparative study of formaldehyde detection using chromotropic acid, acetylacetone and HPLC in cosmetics and household cleaning products. Contact Dermatitis 26:149–154

98. Le Coz CJ (2002) Allergie de contact au formaldéhyde. Ann Dermatol Venereol 129:68–69

99. Bruze M, Frick M, Persson L (2003) Patch testing with thin-layer chromatograms. Contact Dermatitis 48: 278–279

100. Ryberg K, Goossens A, Isaksson M, Gruvberger B, Zimerson E, Persson L, Bruze M (2009) Patch testing of patients allergic to Disperse Blue 106 and Disperse Blue 124 with thin-layer chromatograms and purified dyes. Contact Dermatitis 60:270–278

101. Cardon D (2003) Le monde des teintures naturelles. Belin, Paris

102. Lepoittevin JP, Le Coz C (2007) Dictionary of contact allergens. Springer, Berlin

Shoes

41

An Goossens and James S. Taylor

Contents

41.1 Introduction

Allergic contact dermatitis (ACD) of the feet caused by shoe allergens is fairly common [1, 2] and should be considered in all patients with chronic foot eczema. Shoe allergy may be acute, subacute, intermittent, or chronic and may appear superimposed on endogenous eczema [3–8]. Thus, the patient may have more than one diagnosis, e.g., both atopic and contact dermatitis, and more than one allergen, e.g., shoe component plus a topical medicament.

41.2 Epidemiology

Data on the prevalence of shoe allergy are available from patch test clinics and range from 1.5 to 11% [3, 4, 7, 9–17]. The highest prevalence rates have been recorded in warm climates [2, 12, 14], and shoes have even become the most common source of ACD in India [18]. The disorder may affect both sexes and all age groups, including children [3, 6, 7, 12, 19–22].

41.3 Risk Factors

Major risk factors for shoe dermatitis include heat, friction, occlusion, hyperhidrosis, and atopy [1–3, 7, 8, 12]. A hot, humid environment within the shoes is ideal for the development of ACD to shoe ingredients [23, 24]. The allergens leach by sweating in heavy, occlusive footwear and traverse the socks to contact skin [25]. Hence, sportsmen and [26, 27] military personnel [25] have a high risk of developing ACD to shoe ingredients since

A. Goossens (✉)
Department of Dermatology, University Hospital,
Katholieke Universiteit Leuven, Leuven, Belgium
e-mail: an.goossens@uz.kuleuven.ac.be

J.S. Taylor
Department of Dermatology, Cleveland Clinic, Cleveland,
OH, USA

J.D. Johansen et al. (eds.), *Contact Dermatitis*,
DOI: 10.1007/978-3-642-03827-3_41, © Springer-Verlag Berlin Heidelberg 2011

41

the probability of skin exposure to allergens, particularly to rubber [7, 28] and chromium [29, 30], is increased.

Core Message

> Patients with intermittent or chronic foot dermatitis should be considered as having ACD to shoes, until proven otherwise.

41.4 Clinical Presentation and Clues Pointing to Allergens

The onset of shoe dermatitis is often sudden with a history of a reaction to a new pair of shoes. Clinical signs such as erythema, papules, vesicles or blisters, oozing, scaling, and crusting at the sites of contact are presumptive of shoe allergy [8, 31]. There may be lichenification and hyperpigmentation in chronic cases [25].

Pruritus and pain may be devastating [8, 12, 31]. Other potential foot reactions from shoes include contact urticaria and other immediate contact reactions from natural rubber latex and dermatitis as a result of the bleached rubber syndrome [1].

Although any part of the foot may be affected by shoe dermatitis [6], the typical and most frequent localization is the dorsa of feet and toes, sparing the interdigital spaces [7, 12, 25, 30, 31] (Fig. 41.1); its large surface area and thin stratum corneum, along with intimate and prolonged contact with shoe upper [12], make this part of the feet vulnerable to shoe allergy. The lesions are accentuated around the metatarsophalangeal joints and/or over the central dorsal aspect of the foot, and/or over the plantar aspect of the foot [7]. Calves and shins of military personnel may be affected with ACD from boots [25]. Bilateral symmetrical dermatitis is the norm, although it may be patchy and unilateral [7, 11, 24]. The instep and flexural creases of the toes and thicker-skinned heel area are also usually spared [7, 8, 13, 25, 30] (Fig. 41.2).

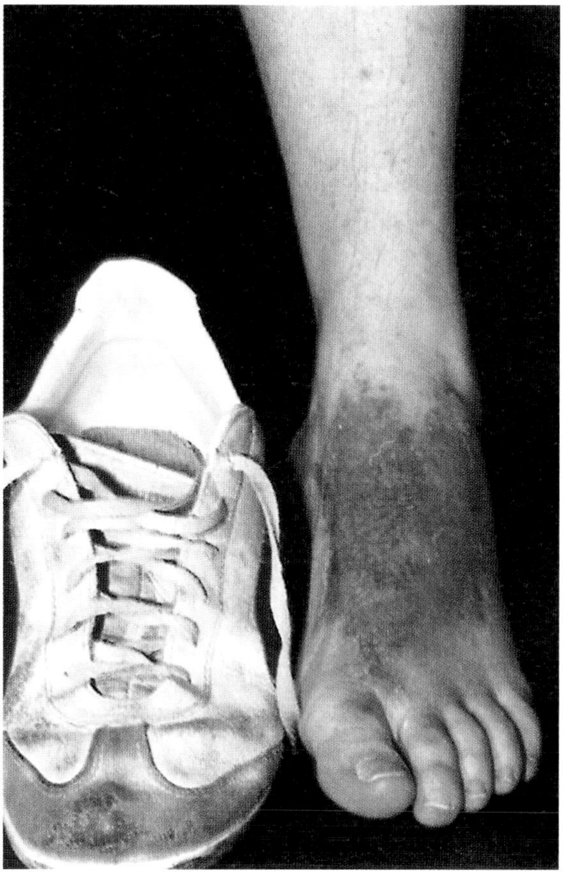

Fig. 41.1 Dorsal foot allergic contact dermatitis (ACD) (courtesy of P. Frosch)

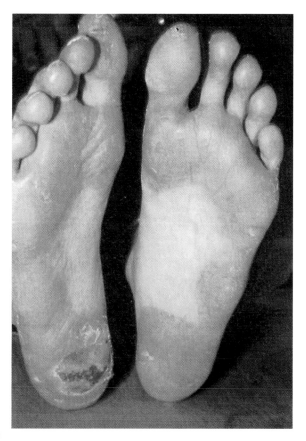

Fig. 41.2 Plantar foot ACD

Shoe allergy is typical of many other instances of ACD in that the pattern of presentation suggests the diagnosis, but the causative allergen is elusive. The initial pattern of presentation may hold the clue for the causative allergen and allow aimed patch testing with specific groups of chemicals. Dorsal foot dermatitis points to an allergen in the shoe upper or tongue of shoe. In a study comparing the localization of foot dermatitis with causative allergens [32], potassium dichromate and cobalt chloride (in leather) were most often found in association with dermatitis of the entire foot with a small predominance on the dorsum; this is in agreement with another report [24]. This was also the case for para-phenylenediamine (PPDA), colophonium, and PTBP-F resin.

With plantar dermatitis (Fig. 41.2) sparring the instep and toe creases, allergens present in the insole or shoe lining or the adhesive, which holds these two layers in place, should be suspected. The anterior portion of the sole may be involved exclusively [11]. The most important allergens were found to be rubber chemicals, MBT, and mercapto mix, and to a lesser extent thiuram mix. Instep involvement may suggest athletic shoe dermatitis or endogenous eczema. Eczema across the dorsal toes and around the heels suggests allergy to the heel and toe stiffeners or counters, which are parts of shoes that contain a wide variety of chemicals.

Interdigital dermatitis is more likely to be a microbial infection [1].

In chronic or severe cases, the presenting pattern may be obscured, making diagnosis more difficult. Shoe allergens can migrate to other parts of the shoe or even to socks or stockings, disguising the presenting pattern [33–35]. ACD to medicaments [7, 16, 36–38] and compounds present or retained in the socks [11, 39–41], for example mercaptobenzothiazoles [33], may also confound the clinical presentation. ACD can subsequently spread beyond the initial site of contact by inadvertent exposure or autosensitization, and the dermatitis may be widely and bizarrely distributed [7]. Finally, hand eczema may be present concomitantly [42–44], which often clears upon resolution of the foot eruption. Some allergens are common to both locations [45].

Shoe allergy can mimic other dermatoses of the feet. ACD to MBT is reported to simulate palmoplantar psoriasis or pustular psoriasis [7]. Purpuric eruptions from shoes [46] and black rubber boots [47] have been reported. Leukoderma can also be associated with shoe dermatitis [48–51] and is more commonly seen in developing countries as, for example, in India [49–51], where monobenzyl ether of hydroquinone in bathroom clogs and rain shoes was identified among the causes of dorsal foot depigmentation [50]. Figure 41.3 illustrates hypopigmentation in a patient reacting to PTBP-F resin.

Sites of common allergens in shoes are shown in Table 41.1 [1].

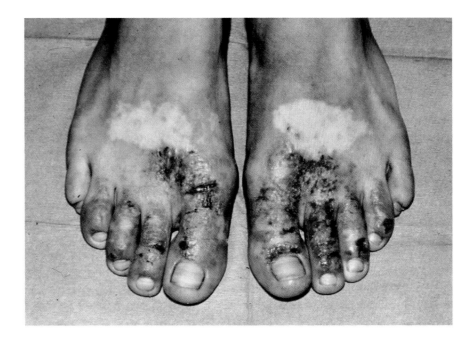

Fig. 41.3 Illustration of hypopigmentation in a patient reacting to PTBP-F resin

Table 41.1 Sites of common allergens in shoes[a]

Allergen	Location	Avoid
Mercaptobenzothiazole Tetramethylthiuram disulfide	Rubber Neoprene adhesives Adhesive + leather treatment biocides Leather finish coats	Rubber foam uppers + insoles Solid rubber shoe soles + heels Sock lining adhesives Fiberboard insoles Highly finished leathers
Dibenzothiazyl disulfide (MBT mix)	Solid or adhesive neoprene Rubber	Sock lining adhesive Rubber soles or heels Rubber insole sponge
Thiourea	Solid or foam neoprene	EVA-neoprene-nylon combination insole
Diaminodiphenyl methane	Polyurethane	Shiny upper foam Comination shoe soles
Colophony	Tackifying resins	Natural rubber latex cement (sock lining adhesive) Heel and toe counters
Paratertiary butyl phenol formaldehyde resin	Tackifying resins	Neoprene adhesives (sock lining adhesive) Heel and toe counters
Nickel	Metal trim	Dimethylglyoxime positive eyelets
Formaldehyde	Leather tanning Biocides in natural rubber latex adhesives	Lutidine positive leather or soft perspiration proof leather
Chromate	Leather tanning	Leather Athletic shoe uppers

[a]Modified from Patricia Podmore MD, Londonderry, Northern Ireland and Frances J Storrs, MD, Portland, OR.

Core Message

› Shoe allergy may mimic other chronic dermatoses and may be accompanied by hyperhidrosis.

41.5 Allergens in Shoes

Having detailed information about shoe construction and all component chemicals is a helpful and ideal approach in diagnosing shoe allergy [1]. However, this information is often hard to obtain from the manufacturers, and identification of all the constituents of a shoe may practically be impossible [1, 7, 52]. The allergens in shoes are gradually changing as a consequence of modifications in footwear manufacture technologies and constant flux in material selection and style design. Leather and shoe dyes were the most common allergens in shoe dermatitis during the 1930s and 1940s [7, 28]. However, chromium compounds, which are not only used as tanning agents for leather but also as dyes for both leather and nonleather synthetic uppers

of the shoes [32], are still the most important shoe allergens in many European countries [16, 32] and, according to a recent study, also in India [53].

This is in contrast to other parts of the world such as USA, Canada [7, 17, 28, 32], Brazil [15], and Asia [14], where rubber allergens that became more important since the 1950s are more predominant. This probably reflects a dramatic change in footwear style with much greater use of rubber components [7, 28]. In rubber or adhesives, mercaptobenzothiazoles are the most important allergens [7, 14, 24, 25] followed by thiurams, carbamates, and PPDA derivatives. Besides thiurams, thiourea compounds are allergens in neoprene rubber and adhesives [54–57]. Heel and toe counters, fibreboard lasting boards, and leather finish coats all contain rubber resins, which may include MBT or thiurams [52, 58]. Recently, the popular shoes Crocs® [59] caused dermatitis in a 14-year-old boy who is allergic to rubber additives, but the specific allergen was not identified.

Among the adhesive components, para-tert-butylphenolformaldehyde resin (PTBPF-R), another important sensitization source [32], although less so in the UK [16], was found to be the most common individual shoe allergen in a recent study in the USA [17]. PTBP-F resin is the main tackifier used in neoprene adhesives and is found mainly in shoe-lining and shoe-insole glues. It is also encountered in heel and toe counters [3, 12]. Together with chromate, it is also an important allergen in orthopedic shoes and orthopedic prostheses [60].

Colophonium and modified colophonium are also tackifiers occasionally found in heel and toe stiffeners, as well as in rubber latex or neoprene adhesives used to glue shoe insoles and linings in place [3, 13, 52, 61]. Patients sensitive to colophonium and PTBP-F resin should be advised to wear either unlined shoes or leather-lined shoes with the lining stitched, not glued, in place and shoes with no heel or toe supports.

Other shoe allergens include formaldehyde in leather tanning and nickel in decoration and trim, eyelets, or buckles [12]. Metal salts such as nickel and cobalt may also be used as dyes or pigments in plastic footware worn by medical personnel [23].

Allergies to dyes are rarely encountered, with the exception of redyed leather or fabric shoes [1, 13, 41]. The most commonly used dyes are azo-aniline group dyes related to PPDA and para-aminoazobenzene [1].

41.6 Hidden Sources of Shoe Allergens

Despite our knowledge of shoe components, it may be difficult to cure patients completely, perhaps because not all shoe allergens have been identified and/or patients may react to less-known allergens. Even lanolin may be a shoe allergen due to its presence in shoe polish [1].

Styrenated phenol has been identified as an allergen in athletic shoes, in addition to thioureas [62–64]. Diaminodiphenylmethane is a polyurethane precursor and potential allergen in polyurethane upper foam [65], and dodecylmercaptan is a polymerization inhibitor present in polyurethane resins [12, 56].

Not all cases of PTBP-F resin sensitivity are detected by testing with the standard series. PTBP itself should be tested, as well as the actual PTBP-F resin used in the shoes [66]; some of the monomers and/or contaminants are the actual allergens [67]. In this regard, a nonrelevant positive test to balsam of Peru in the baseline series may be an indication of a relevant contact allergy to phenol-formaldehyde resin, such as e.g. PFR-2 due to cross-reactivity between phenolic compounds [68].

Also, biocides and fungicides may be responsible for shoe dermatitis, such as 2-*n*-octyl-4-isothiazolin-3-one, a biocide used during leather finishing [12, 56], and 2-(thiocyanomethylthio)-benzothiazole (TCMTB), a fungicide in leather tanning [1]. Recently, several cases have been reported from France [69] and Spain [70] in particular, concerning severe contact dermatitis cases due to dimethylfumarate present as an antifungal agent in sachets in the footware itself or in the boxes used for packing them, the same substance having been responsible for a widespread epidemic of Chinese armchair dermatitis all over Europe.

Cyclohexylthiophtalimide is the most widely used vulcanization retarder in the rubber industry. ACD to this substance may develop following exposure to rubber shoes [71].

A vesicular dermatitis of the soles due to ACD to cinnamon powder that is used as an odor-neutralizing agent in insoles has been reported as well [72].

41.7 Occupational Dermatitis

Reports of occupational dermatitis in shoe production or shoe repair may also point to other shoe allergens [73–80]. These include 1,2-benzisothiazolin-3-one (another biocide) (BIT) [75], ethyl cyanoacrylate [74], propolis [77], epichlorohydrin (a volatile component of epoxy resin) [78] in shoe adhesives, PTBP-F resin [80], and phthalates in PVC shoes [76]. A study of an Italian shoe factory provided a long list of chemicals; the major occupational allergens, however, were PTBP-F resin and MBT [73].

Last but not the least, chemicals contacted at work may remain on footwear causing sensitization and/or contact dermatitis, for example, acrylates [81].

41.8 Patch Testing for Shoe Allergy

Testing for shoe allergy is performed with (a) chemicals from the baseline series, (b) other shoe chemicals present in an expanded shoe series, and (c) pieces of shoes worn by the patient. Many cases of shoe allergy can be diagnosed by patch testing with the baseline series or the T.R.U.E. Test panel [7, 11]. Allergens that are not covered by standard screening series may be identified by additional patch testing with a series of other shoe constituents [1, 2, 6, 11, 28, 55, 82-84], and selected shoe chemicals are available from standard patch test suppliers.

Podmore [55] assembled a series of chemicals by breaking down all the constituents of shoes and identifying all possible culprits. These and other lists [6, 11] include resins, rubber accelerators, dyes, plasticizers, tanning agents, antioxidants, and UV stabilizers. Other authors have included p-aminoazobenzene and other dyes; the biocides such as thimerosal, chloroacetamide, and phenyl mercuric nitrate; hydroquinone in rubber; vegetable tannins; glutaraldehyde, a rare sensitizer as a leather tannin; polyurethane chemicals (Desmodur, Desmocoll 400, Desmodur R and RF and dodecyl mercaptan); urethane adhesives; and other adhesive components [1, 8, 11, 85, 86]. A specific shoe series has recently been suggested in the UK [87] and includes urea formaldehyde (heat setting resin), gum rosin (colophonium derivative not picked up by testing with colophonium in the baseline series), acid yellow 36 and several disperse dyes, glutaraldehyde (leather tanning), octyl- and methyl-and methylchloro-isothiazolinones (boicides), benzotriazole (UV stabilizer), and some additional rubber allergens.

However, patients who are suspected of having ACD to shoes may be patch test negative to the baseline and additional shoe allergens, but positive to shoe pieces [1, 3]. Thus, careful testing with properly selected pieces of material from the shoe itself, from an area in contact with the affected skin, is an important adjunct in the diagnosis of shoe allergy [1].

The pieces should be wafer-thin to avoid false-positive, irritant pressure effects. Since the standard Finn chamber holds portions not larger than 5 mm², many prefer to patch test either with the larger Finn chamber or vander Bend chambers. Tests may also be performed without a chamber, utilizing only occlusive tape (Fig. 41.4). With the latter technique, 1 cm² or larger shoe pieces should be used [11, 55]. It may be helpful to leave the shoe pieces in place for 4 or 5 days [11] or even for a prolonged 14-day exposure [88], rather than the usual 48-h. To help replicate the conditions of shoe wearing, Jordan [89] suggests soaking the shoe pieces (each in a separate container) in water for 15 min before testing. However, patch testing with ultrasonic bath extracts (or extracts after soaking for 24 h) of shoe pieces might be the best method to identify contact allergy, which would otherwise go unrecognized [90].

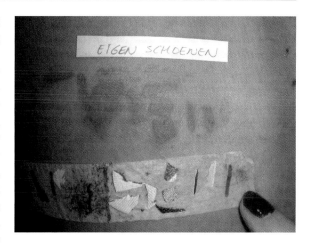

Fig. 41.4 Positive tests to pieces of shoes, utilizing only occlusive tape. The only allergen identified was thiuram mix

Finally, it must be emphasized that topical medications may be absorbed by the shoes, in which case shoe pieces may cause false-positive patch test reactions from the medication, rather than the shoe itself.

Core Message

> Patch testing for shoe allergy should ideally include the baseline series, a shoe chemical series, pieces from shoes worn by the patient as well as topical medications, foot powders, and shoe inserts used by the patient.
> Chemical analysis.

Detailed chemical analysis of shoe extracts by various types of chromatography and mass spectroscopy and the subsequent patch testing of the fractions have identified undetected allergens in several studies. These include dibenzothiazyl disulphide – a dimer of MBT, styrenated phenol, and 6-ethoxy-2, 2,4-trimethyl-1,2-dihydroquinoline (ETMDQ). Using this method, unknown shoe allergens were isolated, identified, and added to a shoe test series [61, 91, 92].

Mercury chloride, an unexpected allergen, was identified by atomic absorption spectrometry and polarography in new polyvinylchloride boots. The boots were worn by a 5-year-old child with a history of skin intolerance to Mercurochrome (merbromin), who developed ACD and a mercury exanthem after wearing them [93].

A related study found that the amounts of thioureas and MBT leached from rubber articles were greater than the patch test elicitation threshold for these chemicals. Such studies may be helpful to manufacturers in designing products that do not release allergens in sufficient amounts to cause reactions in consumers [94].

Core Message

> Differential diagnosis of shoe allergy includes dye allergy in stockings, topical medications used, juvenile plantar dermatosis, other eczematous skin disease, and tinea pedis.

41.9 Differential Diagnosis

Allergy to various textile dyes has been reported to constitute up to 10% of foot ACD. The risk correlates with the ease of leaching of the dye from the fabric [95]. Shoe dermatitis may be imitated by sock or stocking allergy from disperse [11, 40] and nondisperse azo dyes [39, 41], such as the cationic azo dye that has caused lots of shoe dermatitis in Australia [95]. Although PPD is traditionally used as an indicator of textile dye dermatitis, it may be negative in azo dye-sensitive patients and is not always accepted as a reliable marker [41].

Nylon stocking allergy may spare the toe webs, while involving the rest of the feet and legs.

ACD of the feet may be an iatrogenic complication of topical medications being used for a preexisting nonallergic foot dermatosis [7, 12]. Topical antibiotics such as neomycin, bacitracin, and gentamycin, topical corticosteroids and nonsteroidal anti-inflammatory drugs, antimycotics, and in fact, any topical pharmaceutical (or cosmetic) component may lead to a primary allergic foot dermatitis [7, 36–38, 96].

Juvenile plantar dermatosis is a condition with distinctive, symmetrical glazed, cracked skin of weight-bearing areas, sparing the web spaces. It presents with erythema and pain, is rarely itching, and is found in children usually between 3 and 14 years of age, and rarely in infants and adults. The dermatitis is thought to result from excessive sweating and overdrying of the feet due to modern occlusive footwear in children with atopic background. Patch tests and fungal scrapings are consistently negative in this disorder [8, 97].

Other differential diagnoses include irritant contact dermatitis, atopic eczema, especially involving the ankle and dorsal first toe, tinea pedis, psoriasis, lichen planus, dyshidrotic eczema, and id reactions [1, 80].

41.10 Prognosis and Outcome

Shoe allergy may become chronic and recalcitrant to therapy, disabling with painful fissuring, and may be complicated by secondary infection – cellulitis and lymphangitis [3, 30]. Despite these possibilities, the outcome is generally good. In Freeman's study [3] involving adults, 87.5% of patients afflicted with shoe dermatitis had improved or resolved completely. In a prospective study on children, 72% of patients with foot dermatitis showed improvement or resolution of symptoms at the end of 6 months. However, atopy was a poor prognostic factor [6].

41.11 Allergen Substitution

The only effective treatment that will resolve shoe dermatitis is the avoidance of the shoes likely to contain the allergen(s) [7, 8], as patients often present with multiple positive patch tests. Patch testing with pieces from the patient's shoes may identify patch-test negative shoes (although false-negative reactions are often obtained), which the patient can continue to wear, discarding those which are patch-test positive [4].

Patients with ACD to shoe components are usually advised to use hypoallergenic substitute shoes [1]. Recommendations should be on the basis of the information about shoe manufactures in individual countries. In USA, valuable information on footwear alternatives for patients with rubber, chrome, and other shoe chemical allergies and on custom shoemakers for patients with contact allergies is available [98].

Dermatitis confined to the soles may be treated by replacing the insoles with composition, cork, or felt, which is glued in with a nonrubber cement. Commercially available insole inserts may be very useful, but one needs to know their composition (e.g., urethane, neoprene, latex, etc.) including additives (fragrance, deodorizers, etc.). Shoe substitution for contact dermatitis of other foot areas may include all-leather shoes such as moccasins with no insole and no attached outer sole, injection-molded plastic shoes, or wooden shoes for rubber allergy. Vinyl shoes may be an acceptable alternative in patients with allergy to rubber or leather [8, 98, 99].

For patients with chromium allergy and clinically relevant shoe dermatitis, wearing good quality, new, leather shoes and discarding them after a few months (thus preventing the allergens from leaching out), and wearing extra pairs of large cotton socks in shoes (thus preventing contact with the allergens) may help in clearing foot dermatitis [1, 3]. Although not always successful, hypoallergenic shoe leather (present in shoes from Trippen, Loint's, Think, Miss Clair, Brako, etc. in the EU and for which information can be found on their websites) can also be recommended for such patients, however, preferably after having patch tested with extracts from such leathers since some patients may still present with (severe) positive patch tests to them (Fig. 41.5). It is not known whether this is due to unidentified allergens or to very low amounts of chromium that are still present (according to information from the manufacturers, primary chrome-tanning is not excluded). Indeed, the presence of low amounts of chromium or relevant leather-related allergens (e.g., other tanning agents) and dyes has been documented in hypoallergenic shoe leather [1]. Alternatives in such cases are the use of all-plastic or all-fabric (canvas) shoes. If leather insoles are chrome-tanned, they should be

removed. Wooden clogs with vegetable-tanned leather, if tolerated, may also be helpful for chrome allergy [1, 11], and if there is concomitant adhesive allergy, the vegetable-tanned leather uppers can be stapled rather than glued in place.

Pedorthists or orthotists who are knowledgeable about shoe composition may also be helpful in suggesting temporary shoe substitutes or inserts. Some manufacturers will make custom shoes, but these are often expensive [3, 98], and it is important to know as much about the composition of the shoe as possible, especially dyes and adhesives [11, 100]. Again, patch testing with extracts of the substitute shoe in advance is useful. However, there is no guarantee about the success of substitute shoes, especially in the case of hybrid eczema in which the patient has both exogenous and endogenous dermatitis. Moreover, concomitant topical therapy is very important: absorbent powders may control hyperhidrosis and topical steroids may help to clear the dermatitis [8].

41.12 Conclusion

Shoe contact dermatitis is a frequent phenomenon, both in men and women, according to our experience, particularly in women who are liable to develop shoe dermatitis since they wear shoes without stockings in summer, thereby being in direct contact with the potential allergens [32]. It still remains a difficult condition to manage. It is important to give patients appropriate and detailed advice on avoidance, because with proper evaluation, the prognosis of shoe dermatitis remains very good in most patients who are successful in finding alternative footwear through a number of different strategies [3, 6]. Even then, some cases remain insoluble and must be managed empirically with hypoallergenic footwear, such as plastic or wooden shoes with vegetable-tanned uppers sewn or stapled rather than glued in place.

41.13 Case Report

History: A 48-year-old consultant developed foot dermatitis with erythematous scaly patches and plaques on her doral feet and soles with linear patches

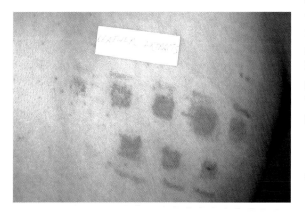

Fig. 41.5 Positive patch test reactions to several "hypoallergenic" leather extracts obtained from different companies in a patient allergic to potassium dichromate

corresponding to the sites of shoe contact. The eruption began 14 months earlier while she was on vacation and has persisted chronically since then. She was initially treated by her family physician with topical antifungals and topical and systemic corticosteroids with some improvement. A dermatologist diagnosed shoe dermatitis and suggested referral to a center for patch testing. She has a history of allergic rhinitis, but no personal or family history of eczema.

Patch testing: The patient was patch tested with the standard tray and pieces of her shoes and had positive reactions to thiuram mix (1+), *p*-tertbutylphenol formaldehyde resin (2+), mixed di-alkylthioureas (2+), ethyl acrylate (1+), and methyl methacrylate (1+); additionally, she had 1+ to 2+ reactions to pieces of insole and inner foam and other materials from five different pairs of her everyday shoes. She was patch test negative only to pieces of *Think* shoes

Diagnosis: ACD to neoprene, neoprene adhesives, and rubber. The reactions to the shoe components were relevant to the three main allergen groups; she had previously reacted to leather watch bands, foam rubber, foam rubber ear phones, as well as her shoes.

Treatment and course: She was given information on alternative special order shoes without the allergens; Follow-up information 4 months later revealed that she had remained clear by wearing the patch test negative *Think* shoes; she also sent her patch test results to several other shoe manufacturers that she identified from the internet and successfully wears these alternative shoes.

Comment: Prior to patch testing, the patient thought that she was allergic to chrome tanned leather. Trial and error changes in shoes along with topical and systemic therapy did not clear her dermatitis. Patch testing allowed her to identify the specific chemicals and shoes to which she was allergic and remain clear of the eruption.

41.14 Classic Articles

1. Calnan CD, Sarkany L (1959) Studies in contact dermatitis: IX. Shoe dermatitis. Tran St John Hosp Derm Soc 43:8–26 [70].
   This classic article reviews the shoe dermatitis literature upto 1959 and reports the demographics,

clinical findings, and patch test results from 102 cases of shoe dermatitis seen at the St Johns Hospital for Skin Diseases in London. Shoe allergy occurred in all age groups was three times more common in women, and primarily affected the dorsal feet and toes and anterior soles. Rubber allergy occurred in one-third of cases and leather allergy in two-thirds, with specific allergens often unknown; chromate allergy was uncommon. In addition to patch testing with a small shoe chemical series, the necessity of patch testing with pieces of every shoe worn by the patient is emphasized. Many leather-sensitive patients were able to remain clear of dermatitis by wearing the patch-test negative shoes.
   This report emphasizes the need to patch test with shoe pieces in order to adequately diagnose and manage shoe allergy, and it still holds true today and is also emphasized in other "classic" articles on shoe contact allergy. [3, 69]

2. Freeman S (1997) Shoe dermatitis. Contact Dermatitis 36:247–251 [3]
   Follow-up study of 55 cases of shoe allergy published 36 years after the Calnan article (70) emphasizes the chronic disabling nature of shoe allergy, the frequent delay before patch testing is performed, the value of testing standard tray allergens in identifying cases, and the absolute necessity of testing with shoe pieces. Follow-up showed that 87.5% of cases improved or resolved completely and most patients were able to find alternative shoes.
   This follow-up study shows that shoe allergy has a good prognosis with careful history and patch testing with the standard screening tray and shoe pieces, as well as success in obtaining shoe substitutes.

3. Jung JH, McLaughlin JL, Stannard J, Guin JD (1988) Isolation, via activity-directed fractionation, of mercaptobenzothiazole and dibenzothiazyl disulfide as 2 allergens responsible for tennis shoe dermatitis. Contact Dermatitis 19:254–259.

This article emphasizes the fact that the causative allergen is frequently not known in shoe allergy cases. Reliance cannot always be placed on results of the standard screening tray because such testing may be negative. Even when positive, the relevance of the positive screening tests is often unknown since the allergen is almost never extracted from the patient's shoes. Testing with shoe pieces is often positive, but the

41

specific allergen is usually never identified. Industrial-grade chemicals may contain contaminants and new allergens may be created via oxidation or other chemical reactions. A case of dermatitis to a tennis shoe insole was studied further by isolating and identifying the causative allergens by step-by-step patch test monitoring of the active fractions obtained by chromatographic separation.

This is one of the first articles to identify and clarify the allergens in a case of shoe allergy by chemical analysis of the incriminated shoe piece. Since the chemical composition of many shoes is essentially unknown, studies of this type may be the only way to identify shoe allergens in the future.

References

1. Taylor JS, Erkek E, Podmore P (2006) Shoes. In: Frosch PJ et al (eds) Contact dermatitis, 4th edn, Chap 38. Springer, Berlin, pp 703–716
2. Trattner A, Farchi Y, David M (2003) Shoe contact dermatitis in Israel. Am J Contact Dermat 14:12–14
3. Freeman S (1997) Shoe dermatitis. Contact Dermatitis 36:247–251
4. Roul S, Ducombs G, Leaute-Labrege C (1996) Footwear contact dermatitis in children. Contact Dermatitis 34:334–336
5. Cronin E (1966) Shoe dermatitis. Br J Dermatol 78:617–625
6. Cockayne SE, Shok M, Messinger AG (1998) Foot dermatitis in children: causative allergens and followup. Contact Dermatitis 38:203–206
7. Shackelford KE, Belsito DV (2002) The etiology of allergic-appearing foot dermatitis: a 5-year retrospective study. J Am Acad Dermatol 47:715–721
8. Guenst BJ (1999) Common pediatric foot dermatoses. J Pediatr Health Care 13:68–71
9. Lynde CW, Warshawski L, Mitchell JC (1982) Patch test results with a shoe wear screening tray in 119 patients (1977–1980). Contact Dermatitis 8:423–425
10. Saha M, Srinivas CR, Shenoy SD (1993) Footwear dermatitis. Contact Dermatitis 28:260–264
11. Storrs FJ (1986) Dermatitis from clothing and shoes. In: Fisher AA (ed) Contact dermatitis. Lea and Febiger, Philadelphia, pp 283–337
12. Rani Z, Hussain I, Haroon TS (2003) Common allergens in shoe dermatitis: our experience in Lahore, Pakistan. Int J Dermatol 42:605–607
13. Strauss RM, Wilkinson SM (2002) Shoe dermatitis due to colophonium used as leather tanning or finishing agent in Portuguese shoes. Contact Dermatitis 47:59
14. Chen HH, Sun CC, Tseng MP (2004) Type IV hypersensitivity from rubber chemicals: a 15-year experience in Taiwan. Dermatology 208:319–325
15. Lazzarini R, Duarte I, Marzagao C (2004) Contact dermatitis of the feet: a study of 53 cases. Dermatitis 15:125–130
16. Holden CR, Gawkrodger DJ (2005) 10 years' experience of patch testing with a shoe series in 230 patients: which allergens are important? Contact Dermatitis 53:37–39
17. Warshaw EM, Schram SE, Belsito DV, DeLeo VA, Fowler JF Jr, Maibach HI, Marks JG Jr, Mathias CGT, Pratt MD, Rietschel RL, Sasseville D, Storrs FJ, Taylor JS, Zug KA (2007) Shoe allergens: retrospective analysis of cross-sectional data from the north American contact dermatitis group. Dermatitis 18:191–202
18. Bajaj AK, Saraswat A, Mikhija G, Rastogi S, Yadav S (2007) Patch testing experience with 1000 patients. Indian J Dermatol, Venereol Leprol 73:313–318
19. Belsito DV (2004) Patch testing with a standard allergen ("screening") tray: rewards and risks. Derm Ther 17: 231–239
20. Teixeira M, Machado S, Teixeira A, Silva E (2005) Severe contact allergy to footwear in a young child. Contact Dermatitis 52:159–160
21. Beattie PE, Green C, Lowe G, Lewis-Jones MS (2007) Which children should we patch test? Clin Experimental Dermatol 32:6–11
22. Romaguera C, Vilaplana J (1998) Contact dermatitis in children: 6 years experience (1992-1997). Contact Dermatitis 39:277–280
23. Goossens A, Bedert R, Zimerson E (2001) Allergic contact dermatitis caused by nickel and cobalt in green plastic shoes. Contact Dermatitis 45:172
24. Rietschel RL, Fowler JF Jr (eds) (2001) Shoe contact dermatitis In: Fisher's contact dermatitis. Lippincott Williams & Wilkins, Philadelphia, pp 305–319
25. Oumeish OY, Parish LC (2002) Marching in the army: common cutaneous disorders of the feet. Clin Dermatol 20:445–451
26. Brooks C, Kujawska A, Patel D (2003) Cutaneous allergic reactions induced by sporting activities. Sports Med 33: 699–708
27. Metelitsa A, Barankin B, Lin AN (2004) Diagnosis of sports-related dermatoses. Int J Dermatol 43:113–119
28. Belsito DV (2003) Common shoe allergens undetected by commercial patch-testing kits: dithiodimorpholine and isocyanates. Am J Contact Dermat 14:95–96
29. Hansen MB, Johansen JD, Menne T (2003) Chromium allergy: significance of both Cr(III) and Cr(VI). Contact Dermatitis 49:206–212
30. Wolf R, Orion E, Matz H (2002) Contact dermatitis in military personnel. Clin Dermatol 20:439–444
31. Fishman TD (2000) Wound assessment and evaluation. Dermatol Nurs 12:194–195
32. Nardelli A, Taveirne M, Drieghe J, Degreef H, Goossens A (2005) The relation between the localisation of foot dermatitis and the causative allergens in shoes: a 13-year retrospective study. Contact Dermatitis 53:201–206
33. Rietschel RL (1984) Role of socks in shoe dermatitis. Arch Dermatol 120:398
34. Maibach H (1984) Panty hose dermatitis resembling and complicating tinea pedis. Contact Dermatitis 1:329
35. Bugnet LD, Sanchez-Politta S, Sorg O, Piletta P (2008) Allergic contact dermatitis to colophonium-contaminated socks. Contact Dermatitis 59:127–128
36. Saha M, Srinivas CR, Shenoy SD (1993) Sensitivity to topical medicaments among suspected cases of footwear dermatitis. Contact Dermatitis 28:44–45

37. Hindsén M, Isaksson M, Persson L, Zimersson E, Bruze M (2004) Photoallergic contact dermatitis from ketoprofen induced by drug-contaminated personal objects. J Am Acad Dermatol 50:215–219

38. Zirwas MJ (2009) Allergy to imidazole antifungals retained in shoes. Dermatitis 20:172–173

39. Saha M, Srinivas CR (1993) Footwear dermatitis possibly due to para-phenylenediamine in socks. Contact Dermatitis 28:295

40. Giusti F, Massone F, Bertoni L, Pellacani G, Seidenari S (2000) Contact sensitization to disperse dyes in children. Pediatr Dermatol 20:393–397

41. Wilkinson SM, Thomson KF (2000) Foot dermatitis due to non-disperse azo dyes. Contact Dermatitis 42:162–163

42. Lear JT, English JS (1996) Hand involvement in allergic contact dermatitis from mercaptobenzothiazole in shoes. Contact Dermatitis 34:432

43. Li LF, Wang J (2002) Contact hypersensitivity in hand dermatitis. Contact Dermatitis 47:206–209

44. Warshaw EM (2004) Therapeutic options for chronic hand dermatitis. Derm Ther 17:240–250

45. Vani G et al (2005) Allergic contact dermatitis of the hands and/or feet- common sensitizers. Contact Dermatitis 52:50

46. Verma GK, Sharma NL, Mahajan VK, Tegta GR, Shanker V (2007) Purpuric contact dermatitis from footwear. Contact Dermatitis 56:362–364

47. Calnan CD, Peachey RDG (1972) Allergic contact purpura. Clin Allergy 1:287

48. Zaitz ID, Proenca NG, Broste D (1987) Achromatizing contact dermatitis caused by rubber sandals (Portuguese). Medicina Cutanea Ibero-Latino-Americana 15:1–7

49. Pandhi KK, Kumar AS (1985) Contact leukoderma due to "Bindi" and footwear. Dermatologica 170:260–262

50. Bajaj AK, Supta SC, Challerjee AK (1996) Footwear depigmentation. Contact Dermatitis 35:117–118

51. Ghosh S, Mukhopadhyay S (2009) Chemical leucoderma: a clinico-aetiological study of 864 cases in the perspective of a developing country. Br J Dermatol 160:40–47

52. Koch P (2001) Occupational contact dermatitis. Recognition and management. Am J Clin Dermatol 2:353–365

53. Chowdhuri S, Ghosh S (2007) Epidemio-allergological study in 155 cases of footwear dermatitis. Indian J Dermatol Venereol Leprol 73:319–322

54. Warshaw EM, Cook JW, Belsito DV, DeLeo VA, Fowler JF Jr, Maibach HI, Marks JG Jr, Mathias CGT, Pratt MD, Rietschel RL, Sasseville D, Storrs FJ, Taylor JS, Zug KA (2008) Positive patch-test reactions to mixed dialkyl thioureas: cross-sectional data from the North American Contact Dermatitis Group, 1994-2004. Dermatitis 19:190–201

55. Podmore P (1995) Shoes. In: Guin JD (ed) Practical contact dermatitis. McGraw-Hill, New York, pp 325–332

56. Aye M, Masson EA (2002) Dermatological care of the diabetic foot. Am J Clin Dermatol 3:463–474

57. Lammintausta K, Kalimi K (1995) Sensitivity to rubber. Study with rubber mixes and individual rubber chemicals Dermatosen 33:204–208

58. Fogh A, Pock-Steen B (1992) Contact sensitivity to thiuram in wooden shoes. Contact Dermatitis 27:348

59. Castanedo-Tardan MP, Gelpi C, Jacob SE (2008) Allergic contact dermatits to Crocs®. Contact Dermatitis 58: 248–249

60. Corazza M, Lauriola MM, Mantovani L, Virgili A (2006) Allergic contact dermatitis due to orthopedic shoes and a prosthesis for an amputated foot. Contact Dermatitis 55:115–117

61. Lyon CC, Tucker SC, Gafvert E, Karlberg AT, Beck MH (1999) Contact dermatitis from modified rosin in footwear. Contact Dermatitis 41:102–103

62. Kaniwa MA, Jsoma K, Nakomura O et al (1994) Identification of causative chemicals of allergic contact dermatitis using a combination of patch testing in patients and chemical analysis. Application to cases from rubber footwear. Contact Dermatitis 30:26–34

63. Roberts JL, Hanifin JM (1979) Athletic shoe dermatitis, contact allergy to ethylbutylthiourea. JAMA 241:275–276

64. Roberts JL, Hanifin JM (1980) Contact allergy and cross-reactivity to substituted thiourea compounds. Contact Dermatitis 6:138–139

65. Cronin E (1980) Contact dermatitis. Churchill Livingstone, Edinburgh, p 738

66. Malten K, Seutter E (1985) Allergic degradation products of paratertiary butyl phenol for formaldehyde plastic. Contact Dermatitis 12:222–224

67. Zimerson E, Bruze M (2002) Contact allergy to the monomers in p-tert-butylphenol-formaldehyde resin. Contact Dermatitis 47:147–153

68. Bruze M (1994) A nonrelevant contact allergy to balsam of Peru as an indication of a relevant contact allergy to phenol-formaldehyde resin. Am J Contact Dermat 3:162–168

69. Vigan M, Biver C, Bourrain JL, Pelletier F, Girardin P, Aubin F, Humbert P (2009) Acute dimethylfumarate-induced eczema on the foot. Ann Dermatol Venereol 136: 281–283

70. Giménez-Arnau A, Silvestre JF, Mercader P, De La Cuadra J et al (2009) Shoe contact dermatitis from dimethyl fumarate: clinical manifestations, patch test results, chemical analysis, and source of exposure. Contact Dermatitis 61:249–260

71. Huygens S, Barbaud A, Goossens A (2001) Frequency and relevance of positive patch tests to cyclohexylthiophthalimide, a new rubber allergen. Eur J Dermatol 11:443–445

72. Hartmann K, Hunzelmann N (2004) Allergic contact dermatitis from cinnamon as an odour-neutralizing agent in shoe insoles. Contact Dermatitis 50:253–254

73. Mancuso G, Reggiani M, Berdonidini RM (1996) Occupational contact dermatitis in shoemakers. Contact Dermatitis 34:17–22

74. Bruze M, Bjoskner B, Lepoittevin JP (1995) Occupational allergic contact dermatitis from ethyl cyanoacrylate. Contact Dermatitis 32:156–159

75. Ayadi M, Martin P (1999) Pulpitis of the fingers from a shoe glue containing 1, 2-benzisothiazolin-3-one (BIT). Contact Dermatitis 40:115–116

76. Vidovic R, Kansky A (1985) Contact dermatitis in workers processing polyvinyl chloride. Derm Beruf Umwelt 33: 104–105

77. Henschel R, Agathos M, Breit R (2002) Occupational contact dermatitis from propolis. Contact Dermatitis 47:52

78. Machado S, Silva E, Sanches M, Massa A (2003) Occupational airborne contact dermatitis. Am J Contact Dermat 14:31–32

79. Adams RM (1990) Shoe repairers. In: Adams RM (ed) Occupational skin disease. W. B. Saunders Company, Philadelphia, pp 662–663

80. White IR (1990) PTBP resins. In: Adams RM (ed) Occupational skin disease. W. B. Saunders Company, Philadelphia, pp 402–403

81. Isaksson M, Zimerson E (2007) Risks and possibilities in patch testing with contaminated personal objects: usefulness of thin-layer chromatograms in a patient with acrylate contact allergy from a chemical burn. Contact Dermatitis 57:84–88

82. Taylor JS (1986) Rubber. In: Fisher AA (ed) Contact dermatitis. Lea and Febiger, Philadelphia, pp 603–643

83. Dooms-Goossens A et al (1987) Shoe dermatitis. Boll Dermatol Allergol Profess 2:120–126

84. Grimalt F, Romaguera C (1975) New resin allergens in shoe contact dermatitis. Contact Dermatitis 1:169–174

85. Jelen G, Cavelier C, Protois JP (1989) A new allergen responsible for shoe allergy: chloracetamide. Contact Dermatitis 21:110–111

86. Lynch PJ (1969) Indian sandal strap dermatitis JAMA 209:1906

87. Katugampola RP, Statham BN, English JSC, Wilkinson MM, Foulds IS, Green CM, Ormerod AD, Stone NM, Horne HL, Chowdhury MMU (2005) A multicentre review of the footwear allergens tested in the UK. Contact Dermatitis 53:133–135

88. Hansen M, Menne T, Johansen JD (2006) Cr(III) and Cr(VI) in leather and elicitation of eczema. Contact Dermatitis 54:278–282

89. Jordan WP (1972) Clothing and shoe dermatitis. Postgrad Med 52:143

90. Bruze M et al (1992) Patch testing with ultrasonic bath extracts. Am J Contact Dermat 3:133–137

91. Jung JH, McLaughlin JL, Stannard J, Guin JD (1988) Isolation, via activity-directed fractionation, of mercapto-benzothiazole and dibenzothiazyl disulfide as 2 allergens responsible for tennis shoe dermatitis. Contact Dermatitis 19:254–259

92. Nishioka K et al (1996) Contact dermatitis due to rubber boots worn by Japanese farmers, with special attention to 6-ethoxy-2, 2, 4-trimethyl-1, 2-dihydroquinoline (ETMDQ) sensitivity. Contact Dermatitis 35:241–245

93. Koch P, Nickolaus G (1996) Allergic contact dermatitis and mercury exanthem due to mercury chloride in plastic boots. Contact Dermatitis 34:405–409

94. Emmett EA, Risby TH, Taylor JS (1994) Skin elicitation threshold of ethylbutylthiourea and mercaptobenzothiazole with relative leaching from sensitizing products (published erratum in Contact Dermatitis 1994, 31:208). Contact Dermatitis 30:85–90

95. Opie J, Lee A, Frowen K, Fewings J, Nixon R (2003) Foot dermatitis caused by the textile dye Basic Red 46 in acrylic blend socks. Contact Dermatitis 49:297–303

96. Baeck M, Marot L, Nicolas J-F, Pilette C, Tennstedt D, Goossens A (2009) Allergic hypersensitivity to topical and systemic corticosteroids: a review. Allergy 64:978–994.

97. Steck WD (1983) Juvenile plantar dermatosis: the "wet and dry foot syndrome". Cleve Clin Q 50:145–149

98. Scheman A, Jacob S, Zirwas M, Warshaw E, Nedorost S, Katta R, Cook J, Castanedo-Tardan MP (2008) Contact allergy: alternatives for the 2007 North American Contact Dermatitis Group (NACDG) Standard Screening Tray. Dis Mon 54:96–98

99. Brar KJ, Shenoi SD, Balachandran C, Mehta VR (2005) Clinical profile of forefoot eczema: a study of 42 cases. Indian J Dermatol Venereol Leprol 71:179–181

100. Downs AM, Sansom JE (1999) Severe contact allergy to footwear responding to handmade shoes. Contact Dermatitis 40:218

Occupational Contact Dermatitis

42

Peter J. Frosch and Katrin Kügler

Contents

P.J. Frosch (✉) and K. Kügler
Hautklinik, Klinikum Dortmund gGmbH,
Beurhausstr. 40, 44137 Dortmund, Germany
e-mail: peter.frosch@klinikumdo.de

42.1 Introduction

Contact dermatitis of the hands is primarily caused by occupational factors. The huge variety of occupations requires detailed information about the patient by an experienced dermatologist and/or occupational physician. Many cases are complex and result from endogenous (primarily atopic) and exogenous factors (wet work, irritants, allergens, heat, cold, friction). After establishing the diagnosis, a strategy for treatment and prevention is often successful. In recalcitrant cases a reevaluation is necessary – in rare instances, this may lead to retraining for a different occupation.

42.2 Definition

Occupational contact dermatitis is the most frequent type of occupational skin diseases, but followed by a long list of other conditions: calluses resulting from pressure and friction, folliculitis due to oil, miliaria from excessive sweating, chronic actinic damage and white skin cancer following extensive sun light exposure, vitiligo from chemicals toxic to melanocytes, etc. – for further details see Table 42.1. Several textbooks on occupational dermatology cover this subspeciality including asthma, urticaria, and systemic toxicity by skin absorption of occupational chemicals [1–5]. The reader will also benefit from studying a series of original papers published recently [6–13]. Furthermore, in nearly every chapter of this book, occupational aspects as the principal factor or cofactor are discussed. The focus of this chapter is on describing the often difficult

J.D. Johansen et al. (eds.), *Contact Dermatitis*,
DOI: 10.1007/978-3-642-03827-3_42, © Springer-Verlag Berlin Heidelberg 2011

Table 42.1 Occupational skin manifestations other than contact dermatitis (further details [1–4])

Clinical findings	Causative factors
Hyperkeratosis, callus	Pressure, friction
Xerosis, dry skin	Low humidity, increased air flow, low temperature
Pruritus, papular eruptions	Fiberglass and other types of fibers, dust of various nature
Granulomas	Beryllium, Zirconium (production of fluorescent lamps and steel alloys), cut hairs (hairdresser; "barber's sinus"), sheep wool, microorganisms (mycobacteria)
Hemorrhages, "black heel"	Pressure, friction, pounding (athletes, various sporting activities)
Green hair	Copper in swimming pool water
Tattoos	Coal dust, dirt trapped in injuries
Nail dystrophy, paronychia	Mechanical damage, mycotic or bacterial infections
Erythema ab igne, miliaria, intertrigo	Excessive heat
Frost bites, acrocyanosis, cold panniculitis, chilblains (perniosis)	Excessive cold
Raynaud's phenomenon	Cold, Hand-held vibrating tools
Urticaria	Pressure, cold, heat, UV-light, local contact with various chemicals and biological agents
Various entities, partially with a pathognomonic morphology	Biologic causes: orf virus, human papilloma viruses, herpes simplex virus, various bacteria, fungi and aquatic organisms
Acne	Pressure, friction, chemicals (polychlorbiphenyls, dioxins)
Folliculitis	Oils, greases
Skin cancer	UV-light – association with squamous cell carcinoma is well established, less with basal cell carcinoma and malignant melanoma, various chemicals (arsenic, polycyclic aromatic hydrocarbons, tar)
Oral mucosa (gingivitis, pharyngitis, discolorations, leukoplakia), tooth damage	Various chemicals (acids, arsenic, pesticides, enzymes, nickel, cadmium, silver)
Solar elastosis, comedones, epidermal cysts	UV-light
Hyperpigmentation	Postinflammatory (burns, injury), after phototoxic reactions, arsenic, polychlorinated biphenyl, dioxins, azo dyes, various metals (silver, mercury, bismuth)
Hypopigmentation, leukoderma	Postinflammatory, various chemicals (monobenzylether of hydroquinone, alkylphenols and catechols)
Systemic sclerosis, scleroderma – like disease	Vinylchloride, organic solvents (perchlorethylene, trichlorethylene)
Systemic lupus erythematosus and silicosis	Silica (high exposure in miners of ore and uranium, stone cutting)

diagnostic pathway in a case of eczema that is suspected to be occupational.

The first author has based the approach on his 30 years of experience in Germany at three Dermatology centers with a long tradition of occupational dermatology. The guidelines given in this chapter may, therefore, be different in other countries with other medical infrastructures and insurance systems (see also Chap. 53).

After careful diagnostic workup, a dermatitis has to be regarded as occupational, if occupational factors are considered to be key in causing or aggravating the disease. A close time relationship between flares of the dermatitis and occupational activity should be present. This medical definition may deviate from legal definitions with regard to compensation claims in different countries.

42.3 Clinical Aspects

The dermatitis in occupational cases is usually localized on the hands and most prominent on those parts that have the highest frequency of contact with the occupational irritant(s) and/or allergen(s). Most cases of the dermatitis do not always correspond to the preferred hand of the worker – usually the right hand. In certain occupations, the dermatitis is most pronounced on the opposite nondominant (left) hand if a certain object is held there and comes in contact with occupational materials, e.g., dental technicians working on prosthetic parts using methacrylates or metal workers (grinders, lathe operator) operating CNC machines who have to measure the objects regularly and thus have intensive contact with the cutting fluids primarily with thumb, index, and middle finger of the left hand (Figs. 42.1 and 42.2). If a contact allergy is present, the dermatitis may be strictly confined to the areas of contact, e.g., in case of the so-called "tulip fingers" on the tips of the grasping fingers (see Chaps. 15 and 46). The recently abandoned acid permanent wave caused an epidemic in hairdressers by sensitization to glyceryl monothioglycolate – the dermatitis usually started on the pulps of those fingers which had most contact with the hair (Fig. 42.3). Another example could be the facial dermatitis confined to the rubber mask of a pilot or diver. In many occupations eczematous lesions are present on the worker's lower arms, neck, and face. This may be due to dusts (wood, stone) or vapors of fluids and gases. Mild forms are usually caused by irritants, severe types with lichenification, and vesicles are mostly allergic to, e.g., acrylates or plants. Further instructive clinical pictures are shown in Fig. 42.4 and in Chap. 15. If the degree of sensitization is high, a

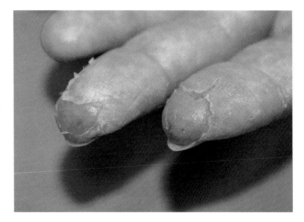

Fig. 42.2 Allergic contact dermatitis in a dentist practicing for 30 years. She had her own laboratory and performed final fittings of prosthetic parts by shaping and abrading. The freshly hardened polymer objects were held primarily in the left nondominant hand where the dermatitis was most pronounced. Patch testing revealed multiple sensitizations (methyl methacrylate, ethylenegylcol-dimethacrylate, HEMA, TEGDMA, HPMA)

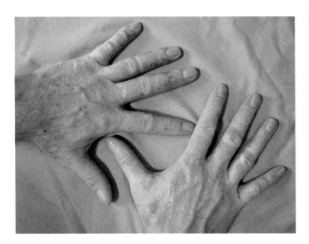

Fig. 42.1 Moderate chronic irritant dermatitis in a metal CNC (computer numerical control) machine operator. Extensive patch testing including the patient's own cutting fluids was negative. The dermatitis was more pronounced on the left hand due to holding the produced small metal objects (still contaminated with the cutting fluids) for periodical measurements

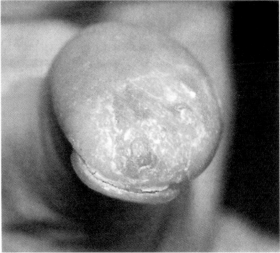

Fig. 42.3 Allergic contact dermatitis of the pulps of a hairdresser's hands from glyceryl monothioglycolate. The strength of the wave was checked with the unprotected finger tips before applying the fixative

Fig. 42.4 Occupational allergic contact dermatitis from gloves in a female surgeon (**a**). She was patch test positive to thiuram mix and the glove's manufacturer confirmed the presence of a thiuram derivative. Note that the dermatitis is the most severe on the back of the hands and least so on the palms (**b**)

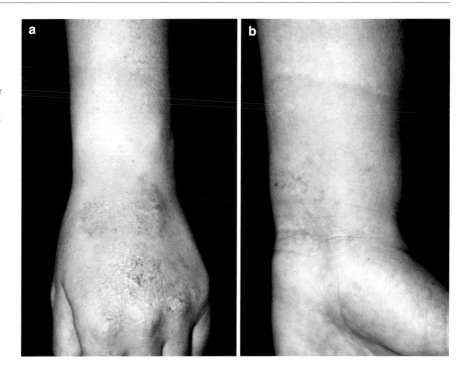

dermatitis may develop in "ectopic areas" by the transfer of small amounts from the fingers to the periorbital or genital region (e.g., as observed with the immersion oil dermatitis by epoxy resin (see Chap. 42)).

42.4 Causative Factors

Tables 42.2–42.5 list major irritants and allergens and the corresponding work field where an occupational contact dermatitis is seen at a relatively high frequency. Some of the original publications read like detective stories – first an irritant cause was suspected, then after careful testing of many possible culprits and their constituents a new allergen has been identified [5, 14–19]. The same holds true for the opposite – what may look like an epidemic of an occupational allergen turns out to be an unusual type of delayed irritation [20–22]. Further reports are of high didactic value in regard to the methodology of resolving difficult cases of occupational contact dermatitis and are recommended particularly to the less experienced "novice" in this field [23–35].

It has taken a long time until water, by itself, has been recognized as an irritant. Wet work over several hours each day is an important factor or cofactor for the

Table 42.2 Common high-risk occupations for irritant contact dermatitis

Baker
Butcher
Cooks
Cleaner
Construction worker
Dental technician
Florist
Food handler
Hairdresser
Healthcare worker
Homemaker
Horticulturist
Masseur/masseuse
Metalworker
Motor mechanic
Nurse
Painter
Printer
Tiler

Table 42.3 Principal occupational contact irritants

Water
Soaps and detergents
Alkalis
Acids
Metalworking fluids
Organic solvents
Other petroleum products
Oxidizing agents
Reducing agents
Animal products
Physical factors

Table 42.4 Common high-risk occupations for allergic contact dermatitis

Adhesives/sealants/resins/plastics worker
Agriculturalist/farmer
Cement caster
Construction worker
Dental technician
Florist
Glass worker
Graphics worker
Hairdresser and barber
Horticulturist/Gardener
Leather tanner
Painter
Pharmaceutical/chemical worker
Rubber worker
Textile worker
Tiler and terrazzo-maker
Woodworker

Table 42.5 Principal occupational contact allergens

Biocides (including isothiazolinones)
Chromate (cobalt)
Dyes
Essences and fragrances
Formaldehyde
Formaldehyde resins
(Meth)acrylates
Plants and woods
Rubber-processing chemicals

events of vesiculation on the fingers ("dyshidrotic eczema"). Friction is often neglected as a contributing factor for skin damage. Paper, strings, rough surfaces on various objects, sharp edges on wires, etc. may break the valuable stratum corneum barrier. Heat and cold are further hazards. Patients with rosacea or seborrhoic dermatitis often experience an exacerbation in hot humid working environments. Physical types of urticaria may develop or be aggravated by extreme climatic conditions. Low temperatures (starting already at 10°C) may cause Raynaud's phenomenon, worsen acrocyanosis in young females, or rarely induce cold panniculitis and acquired cold urticaria. These cases are often a subject of controversy among experts because endogenous factors may be evident to the physician but difficult to accept by the patient and lawyer.

42.5 Diagnostic Workup

42.5.1 History

Taking a detailed occupational history is nearly an art and reflects the knowledge and experience of the physician. Nevertheless, it can be learned and success in individual cases is stimulating and rewarding. The description of the work place by the patient is only a starting point. The worker can usually not provide names and manufacturers of all materials he or she have contact with. Inquiries about the safety engineer or owner of the company beforehand are useful. We are using a questionnaire sent out with the appointment

development of an irritant dermatitis (e.g., hairdresser apprentices, food handlers). Occlusion under nonpermeable gloves is a major problem in many occupations. The worker complains of discomfort and itching; patients with an atopic background frequently develop

42

date. It contains questions regarding the products for skin cleansing, the use of barrier creams at work, skin care after work, and protective gloves. Cooling fluids and all other materials the skin comes in contact with are to be listed in detail with the exact name, manufacturer, use concentration at work, etc. If present, safety data sheets are to be provided. In Germany, the insurance institutions now frequently visit the work place and ask detailed questions regarding the working procedure and all skin contactants. A detailed report is written including a photo of the work environment. This is very helpful for the examining physician. In some countries (e.g., Sweden), this task is performed by an occupational dermatologist or state licensed occupational physician. A most important question is the time relationship of the dermatitis to the working activities. In most cases the dermatitis has clearly developed at work after some time. Depending on the occupation, this can be few months (e.g., irritant hand eczema in a hairdresser apprentice) or even several years (e.g., dermatitis in a tiler due to chromate containing cement). In other cases, an atopic dermatitis turns out, upon detailed questioning, to have been present in a mild form during childhood on typical locations, but never on the hands before. In our experience, mild cases of psoriasis have often been missed by the previous examining physicians – atypical forms of "eczema" recalcitrant to various therapeutic approaches may turn out to be psoriasis of the hands, aggravated by the working conditions. The diagnosis can often be made only after all treatment is discontinued for a minimum of 10 days, a biopsy is taken, and the clinical pattern is followed for some time after an antipsoriatic treatment has been started. Another not rare example is tinea incognita – under the wrong diagnosis, "eczema," a mycotic infection of the hand, is treated for months/years with corticosteroids.

In clear-cut cases the worker will describe a close relationship between the acuity of the dermatitis and the work activities. However, in chronic cases this relationship becomes more diffuse and the dermatitis, if severe in particular, does not completely heal even during a long vacation of 2 or 3 weeks. An important diagnostic clue in our experience is the question of relapse after resuming work. If the first symptoms with itching and redness develop within few hours or 1–2 days, a contact allergy is often present. If the flare is slight and takes several days to develop, it is an irritant dermatitis in all likelihood. We also may deal with a

"hybrid," a combination of irritant and allergic factors. To elucidate this is a real challenge in occupational dermatology.

42.5.2 Information on Workplace Materials

The above-mentioned questionnaire is helpful in obtaining information on the materials the patient has contact with at work. However, the manufacturing procedures today are often very complex and change rapidly due to increased cost efficiency and quality assurance. The number of materials with potential skin contact sometimes exceeds one hundred or more. Individual materials may be used only for a short period and be substituted by another one after few weeks, not always recognized by the workers in the production line. Metal workers often report that a certain cutting fluid had caused "problems" in many workers and was replaced by a new one. Careful patch testing may reveal a sensitization to one of the ingredients of the old cutting fluid after some time has passed when the company has kept good records, e.g., to one of the Biobans as preservatives [36]. But this is often not the case and the examining physician is provided only with information on the currently used materials. Safety data sheets are often incomplete in regard to all constituents [37]; depending on the legislation, the constituents have to be declared only if they are known sensitizers or irritants and exceed concentrations considered to be "safe." The nomenclature is sometimes confusing and requires further inquiries with chemists. Manufactures sometimes deny the presence of a certain material because they use it under a different name or they are not aware of the possible links to sensitizers. For example, as pointed out by Geier and Lessmann in the chapter on metal workers, the high prevalence of sensitization to colophony in this profession is due to the addition of distilled tall oils (DTO) to cutting fluids. DTO contain resin acids and even abietic acid, the main sensitizer in colophony. The manufacturers deny the presence of colophony and usually do not know about the sensitizing properties of DTO. There are numerous reports in the literature demonstrating that only the chemical analysis of the patch test positive material of the patient could reveal the sensitizer (see Chap. 27).

Therefore, in recalcitrant cases or "mini-epidemics" in a factory, the close cooperation with analytical chemists is necessary and rewarding [38].

42.5.3 Diagnostic Testing

Patch testing is indispensable in dealing with occupational skin disease. The standard series has to be supplemented by the series as recommended by international study groups (EECDRG, GERDA, German Contact Dermatitis Research Group) for certain professions and working areas (see Chap. 24). Hairdresser, health workers, and food handlers are at special risk and require a high degree of attention and expertise in their diagnostic workup; an in-depth discussion of these professions therefore follows this chapter. Patch testing of the patient's own materials is of particular interest in this respect. Before testing, detailed information on the local and systemic toxicity must be obtained in order to avoid caustic reactions with the risk of claims for legal compensation. The semi-open patch test is very practical, safe, and often provides the clue for the diagnosis. For further details, see Chap. 57.

Screening tests for atopy are also mandatory in our experience. Many cases of occupational hand eczema have an endogenous atopic disposition of variable degree. Next to a detailed history ("Erlangen score for atopy" [39]), prick testing with the typical allergens is performed. We also measure the total IgE in serum.

The diagnosis has to be based on (1) detailed history, (2) in-depth information on the workplace, (3) results of careful patch testing, and (4) observation of the course of the disease. Complex cases can often only be resolved after evaluation while following the patient and giving advice after the first "working diagnosis."

42.6 Therapy and Prevention

The principles of therapy and prevention, as described in detail in other chapters (49 and 50), hold true also for cases of occupational contact dermatitis. Based on our experience, we would like to emphasize the following points. Clear-cut cases of contact allergy to a certain material are often the easiest to treat, and the prognosis is excellent if the sensitizing material can be substituted by another one without this risk. Common examples would be dichromate containing leather gloves, rubber gloves with a frequently sensitizing thiuram as accelerator, face masks with black neoprene, a cutting fluid with a well-known sensitizer as preservative, a barrier cream used at work with a sensitizing fragrance or preservative, etc. However, in practice, most cases are more complicated and resistant to a simple solution. Often the employer is reluctant to change to a different product because of economic reasons. Cooling fluids in the metal industry have to meet special requirements for the type of metal and cutting procedure; they are therefore not easily replaceable by others. The employer will often only act if several workers have skin problems clearly associated with this material. A therapeutic challenge are the cases of chronic irritant contact dermatitis, particularly with an atopic background. Avoidance of irritant factors at work is often not possible. Gloves can be helpful particularly if well designed for a specific task, allowing a fine grip and being not too occlusive. In "eczema schools" the workers can be trained to minimize skin damage and get used to work with gloves whenever possible and allowed by general safety instructions. The use of barrier cream is of very limited benefit in our experience, confirmed by recent reports [41, 40]; the number of irritants is often large and very different in chemical nature, the effect is not long-lasting, and many workers do not like it on their skin and complain of various

> **Core Message**
>
> › Occupational contact dermatitis is the most frequent cause of occupational skin diseases. It has a major socioeconomic impact. Affected people often experience severe impairment in the quality of life. The ratio of irritant to allergic contact dermatitis varies considerably among occupations and depends on the experience and diagnostic thoroughness of the examining dermatologist.

42

disadvantages (increased sweating, loss of grip capacity, itching under gloves, etc.). The increased motivation of skin care after work is of great benefit in our experience. If a skin care product with good acceptance for the individual patient can be found – and there is a wide array available – the skin condition will always improve. Acute events of the eczema must be treated by a dermatologist the patient has frequent access to. Corticosteroids of medium to strong potency should be used intermittently rather than weak ones continuously. Some workers, particularly older ones not eligible for retraining or in danger of losing the job, can only be managed by treating them with all options available today: local and systemic corticosteroids, tacrolimus ointment, ciclosporin, acitretin, alitretinoin, and last but not the least, phototherapy.

If all measures fail, the case should be carefully reevaluated, preferably in a specialized center on occupational dermatology. There may be a missed allergen at work or at home, the endogenous part of the disease may be overwhelming in the meantime, the patient's compliance may have decreased, or – in rare cases – the patient produces artifacts in order to obtain legal compensation [40, 42–45]. The persistence of skin symptoms after all occupational exposures have been discontinued is now classified as "persistent postoccupational dermatitis" (PPOD) and may be more common than previously thought [46, 47]. The impairment in quality of life by chronic hand dermatitis is substantial and has been underestimated for a long time as recent studies have shown [48–51].

Core Message

> The main goal in the treatment and prevention is avoiding chronicity of the contact dermatitis. After a working diagnosis has been established, this goal can only be achieved by intensive cooperation with the patient and the employer. All contact irritants (chemical, thermal, mechanical) and contact allergens (workplace, skin care products, protective garments, etc.) must be evaluated as the cause or as contributory factors. Together with the employer and safety engineer, these factors must be scrutinized and, if possible, reduced or eliminated.

References

1. Adams R (1999) Occupational skin disease. Saunders, Philadelphia
2. Kanerva L, Elsner P, Wahlberg JE, Maibach HI (2000) Handbook of occupational dermatology. Springer, Heidelberg
3. Marks JG, de Leo VA (1997) Contact and occupational dermatology. Mosby, St. Louis
4. Lachapelle JM, Frimat P, Tennstedt D, Ducombs G (1992) Précis de dermatologie professionnelle et de l'environment. Masson, Paris
5. Aalto-Korte K, Suuronen K, Kuuliala O, Jolanki R (2008) Contact allergy to 2, 5-dimercapto-1, 3, 4-thiadiazole and phenyl-alpha-naphtylamine, allergens in industrial greases and lubricant oils-contact allergy to water-insoluble greases is uncommon but needs to be considered in some workers. Contact Dermatitis 58:93–96
6. McCall BP, Horwitz IB, Feldmann SR, Balkrishnan R (2005) Incidence rates, costs, severity, and work-related factors of occupational dermatitis: a workers' compensation analysis of Oregon, 1990-1997. Arch Dermatol 14:713–718
7. Warshaw EM, Schram SE, Maibach HI, Belsito DV, Marks JG Jr, Fowler JF Jr, Rietschel RL, Taylor JS, Mathias CG, DeLeo VA, Zug KA, Sasseville D, Storrs FJ, Pratt MD (2008) Occupation-related contact dermatitis in North American health care workers referred for patch testing: crosssectional data, 1998 to 2004. Dermatitis 19:261–274
8. Keegel T, Erbas B, Cahill J, Noonan A, Dharmage S, Nixon R (2007) Occupational contact dermatitis in Australia: diagnostic and management practices, and severity of worker impairment. Contact Dermatitis 56:318–324
9. Carstensen O, Rasmussen K, Pontén A, Gruvberger B, Isaksson M, Bruze M (2006) The validity of a questionnaire-based epidemiologica study of occupational dermatosis. Contact Dermatitis 55:295–300
10. Curr N, Dharmage S, Keegel T, Lee A, Saunders H, Nixon R (2008) The validity and reliability of the occupational contact dermatitis disease severity index. Contact Dermatitis 59:157–164
11. Dhir H (2006) Hand dermatitis and nail disorders of the workplace. Clin Occup Environ Med 5:381–396
12. Meding B, Lantto R, Lindahl G, Wrangsjö K, Bengtsson B (2005) Occupational skin disease in Sweden – a 12-year follow up. Contact Dermatitis 53:308–313
13. Skoet R, Olsen J, Mathiesen B, Iversen L, Johansen JD, Agner T (2004) A survey of occupational hand eczema in Denmark. Contact Dermatitis 51:159–166
14. Aalto-Korte K, Ackermann L, Henriks-Eckerman ML, Välimaa J, Reinikka-Railo H, Leppänen E, Jolanki R (2007) 1, 2-benzisothiazolin-3-one in disposable polyvinyl chloride gloves for medical use. Contact Dermatitis 57:365–370
15. Isaksson M, Zimerson E (2007) Risks and possibilities in patch testing with contaminated personal objects: usefulness of thin-layer chromatograms in pathient with acrylate contact allergy from a chemical burn. Contact Dermatitis 57:84–88
16. Milkovic-Kraus S, Macan J, Kanceljak-Macan B (2007) Occupational allergic contact dermatitis from azithromycin in pharmaceutical workers: a case series. Contact Dermatitis 56:99–102

17. Romyhr O, Nyfors A, Leira HL, Smedbold HT (2006) Allergic contact dermatitis caused by epoxy resin systems in industrial painters. Contact Dermatitis 55:167–172

18. Aalto-Korte K, Mäkelä EA, Huttunen M, Suurone K, Jolanki R (2005) Occupational contact allergy to glyoxal. Contact Dermatitis 52:276–281

19. Corazza M, Borghi A, Virgili A (2004) A medicolegal controversy due to a hidden allergen in cutting oils. Contact Dermatitis 50:254–255

20. Malten KE, den Arend JACJ, Wiggers RE (1979) Delayed irritation: hexanediol diacrylate and butanediol diacrylate. Contact Dermatitis 5:178–184

21. Heras-Mendaza F, Casado-Farinas I, Paredes-Gascon M, Conde-Salazar L (2008) Erythema multiforme-like eruption due to an irritant contact dermatitis from a glyphosate pesticide. Contact Dermatitis 59:54–56

22. Lensen G, Jungbauer F, Goncalo M, Coenraads PJ (2007) Airborne irritant contact dermatitis and conjunctivitis after occupational exposure to chlorothalonil in textiles. Contact Dermatitis 57:181–186

23. Paulsen E, Larsen FS, Christensen LP, Andersen KE (2008) Airborne contact dermatitis from Eucalyptus pulverulenta "Baby Blue" in a florist. Contact Dermatitis 59:171–193

24. Inoue T, Yagami A, Sano A, Nakagawa M, Abe M, Mori A, Sasaki K, Matsunaga K (2008) Contact dermatitis because of antimicrobial coating desk mat. Contact Dermatitis 58:123–124

25. Aalto-Korte K, Alanko K, Henriks-Eckerman ML, Kuuliala O, Jolanki R (2007) Occupational allergic contact dermatitis from 2-N-octyl-4-isothiazolin-3-one. Contact Dermatitis 56:160–163

26. Piskin G, Meijs MM, van der Ham R, Bos JD (2006) Glove allergy due to 1, 3-diphenylguanidine. Contact Dermatitis 54:61–62

27. Peramiquel L, Serra E, Dalmau J, VilaAT MJM, Alomar A (2005) Occupational contact dermatitis from simvastatin. Contact Dermatitis 52:286–287

28. Zemtsov A, Fett D (2005) Occupational allergic contact dermatitis to sodium lauroyl sarcosinate in the liquid soap. Contact Dermatitis 52:166–167

29. Kwon S, Campbell LS, Zirwas MJ (2006) Role of protective gloves in the causation and treatment of occupational irritant contact dermatitis. J Am Acad Dermatol 55:891–896

30. Geier J, Lessmann H, Uter W, Schnuch A (2003) Occupational rubber glove allergy: results of the Information Network of Departments of Dermatology (IVDK), 1995-2001. Contact Dermatitis 48:39–44

31. Sato K, Kusaka Y, Suganuma N, Nagasawa S, Deguchi Y (2004) Occupational allergy in medical doctors. J Occup Health 46:165–170

32. McDonald JC, Beck MH, Chen Y, Cherry NM (2006) Incidence by occupation and industry of work-related skin diseases in the United Kingdom, 1996-2001. Occup Med (Lond) 56:398–405

33. Pal TM, de Wilde NX, van Beurden MM, Coenraads PJ, Bruynzeel DP (2009) Notificatioin of occupational skin diseses by dermatologists in The Netherlands. Occup Med (Lond) 59:38–43

34. Turner S, Carder M, van Tongeren M, McNamee R, Lines S, Hussey L, Bolton A, Beck MH, Wilkinson M, Agius R (2007) The incidence of occupational skin disease as reported to The Health and Occupation Reportin (THOR) network between 2002 and 2005. Br J Dermatol 157:713–722

35. Tanko Z, Diepgen TL, Weisshaar E (2008) Is nickel allergy an occupational disease? Discussion of the occupational relevance of a type IV allergy to nickel (II) sulfate using case reports. J Dtsch Dermatol Ges 6:346–349

36. Brinkmeier T, Geier J, Lepoittevin JP, Frosch PJ (2002) Patch test reactions to Biobans in metalworkers are often weak and not reproducible. Contact Dermatitis 47:27–31

37. Keegel T, Saunders H, LaMontagne AD, Nixon R (2007) Are material safety data sheets MSDS useful in the diagnosis and management of occupational contact dermatitis? Contact Dermatitis 57:331–336

38. Henriks-Eckermann ML, Suuronen K, Jolanki R (2008) Analysis of allergens in metalworking fluids. Contact Dermatitis 59:261–267

39. Diepgen TL, Sauerbrei W, Fartasch M (1996) Development and validation of diagnostic scores for atopic dermatitis incorporating criteria of data quality and practical usefulness. J Clin Epidemiol 49:1031–1038

40. Cahill J, Keegel T, Nixon R (2004) The prognosis of occupational contact dermatitis in 2004. Contact Dermatitis 51:219–226

41. Winker R, Salameh B, Stokovich S, Nikl M, Barth A, Ponocny E, Drexler H, Tappeiner G (2009) Effectiveness of skin protection creams in the prevention of occupational dermatitis: results of a randomized, controlled trial. Int Arch Occup Environ Health 82:653–667

42. Cohen AD, Vady DA (2006) Dermatitis artevacta in soldiers. Mil Med 171:497–499

43. Shab A, Matterne U, Diepgen TL, Weisshaar E (2008) Are obsessive-compulsive disorders and personality disorders sufficiently considered in occupational dermatoses? A discussion based on three case reports. J Dtsch Dermatol Ges 11:947–951

44. Isaksson M, Siemund I, Bruze M (2007) Allergic contact dermatitis from ethylcyanoacrylate in an office worker with artificial nails led to months of sick leave. Contact Dermatitis 57:346–347

45. Cvetkovski RS, Zachariae R, Jensen H, Olsen J, Johansen JD, Agner T (2006) Quality of life and depression in a population of occupational hand eczema patients. Contact Dermatitis 54:106–111

46. Sajjachareonpong P, Cahill J, Keegel T, Saunders H, Nixon R (2004) Persistent post-occupational dermatitis. Contact Dermatitis 51:278–283

47. Keogh SJ, Gawkrodger DJ (2006) Persistent post-occupational dermatitis: report of five cases. Acta Derm Venereol 86:248–249

48. Cvetkovski RS, Zachariae R, Jensen H, Olsen J, Johansen JD, Agner T (2006) Prognosis of occupational hand eczema: a follow-up study. Arch Dermatol 142:305–311

49. Belsito DV (2005) Occupational contact dermatitis: etiology, prevalence, and resultant impairment/disability. J Am Acad Dermatol 53:303–313

50. Agner T, Andersen KE, Brandao FM, Bruynzeel DP, Bruze M, Frosch P, Goncalo M, Goossens A, Le Coz CJ, Rustemeyer T, White I, Diepgen T (2009) Contact sensitisation in hand eczema patients – relation to sub diagnosis, severity and QoL. Contact Dermatitis 61:291–296

51. Kütting B, Weistenhöfer W, Baumeister T, Uter W, Drexler H (2009) Current acceptance and implementation of preventive strategies for occupational hand eczema in 1355 metalworkers in Germany. Br J Dermatol 161(2):390–396. doi: 10.1111/j.1365-2133.2009.09085

Occupational Contact Dermatitis: Health Personnel

43

Ana M. Giménez-Arnau

Contents

A.M. Giménez-Arnau
Department of Dermatology, Hospital del Mar, IMAS,
Universitat Autònoma, Barcelona, Spain
e-mail: agimenez@imas.imim.es
e-mail: 22505aga@comb.cat

43.1 Introduction

Health personnel carry out a wide spectrum of jobs. All of them are susceptible to different forms of contact dermatitis. A hospital is like a large factory. Many facts and substances can be dangerous to the health workers skin. This group of workers belong to the fifth high-risk occupational category [1]. Mahler [2] reported an average annual incidence of 7.3 occupational skin diseases per 10,000 workers. Highest incidence affects younger people. Biological and physical causes are not considered in this chapter. Radiation and viral, fungal, bacterial or animal factors may all cause occupational dermatoses in health personnel, but rarely of the contact dermatitis type. Protective measures and general prevention must be organized at the health services as in the big enterprises [3].

> **Core Message**
>
> › Health workers have high occupational risk, mainly in younger people.

43.2 Range of Occupations

Health personnel can be divided into three main groups. The first of these includes physicians, surgeons, medical specialists, radiologists, laboratory specialists and dental personnel. The second group includes nurses, clinical assistants, laboratory and radiology technicians, biologists, pharmacists, physiotherapists and dialysis workers. The third group includes office personnel, technical service workers, kitchen and laundry

J.D. Johansen et al. (eds.), *Contact Dermatitis*,
DOI: 10.1007/978-3-642-03827-3_43, © Springer-Verlag Berlin Heidelberg 2011

workers, cleaners and disinfection and sterilization area workers. Veterinarians deserve special attention because of their wide spectrum of work.

43.3 Type of Cutaneous Disease

Health care workers mainly suffer from irritant and/or allergic contact dermatitis and contact urticaria. The prevalence of such diseases, using patch and prick test, in health care workers ($n=55$) was found to be 61% of irritant contact dermatitis, 31% of allergic contact dermatitis and 27% of contact urticaria to latex [4]. Eleven percent of them showed both allergic contact dermatitis related to thiuram and contact urticaria to latex [4]. Ninety five percent of them were deemed to be work-related [4]. Nettis et al. [5] found work-related irritant and allergic contact dermatitis in 44.4% and 16.5% of diagnosis, respectively. Mahler et al. [2] observed 54% of irritant and 51% of allergic contact dermatitis. Health care workers with occupational disease are more likely to be females, who suffer hand dermatitis and a history of atopy [6].

> **Core Message**
>
> › Health workers mainly suffer from irritant and/or allergic contact dermatitis and less frequently contact urticaria.

43.4 Irritant Contact Dermatitis

Health care personnel have exposure to a variety of cutaneous irritants. The most common type of contact dermatitis in health workers is irritant contact dermatitis. The frequent use of disinfectant solutions, detergents and soaps for hand washing can induce stratum corneum lipid disturbances and consequently a skin barrier defect [7]. Trans-epidermal water loss with brush washing is increased compared to the simple hand washing [8]. Cumulative irritant contact dermatitis readily favours sensitization to a broad number of commonly employed substances. Recently, we have learned from different studies that disinfection with alcohol-based solutions containing emollients or alternate use of a disinfectant/

detergent causes less skin irritation than that with only a detergent [9, 10]. The nurses' perceptions of the benefits of alcohol hand rubs vs hygienic hand washing were no longer demonstrated in a multi-centre questionnaire-based study [11]. Educational programmes should promote alcoholic disinfection as a procedure with good efficiency and skin tolerability to reduce the prevalence of hand eczema in nurses and enhance compliance with hand hygiene standards. This type of prevention cannot substitute primary preventive measures.

43.5 Atopy as a Risk Factor

Atopy is a risk factor. Personal or family background of atopy favours the development of hand dermatitis and contact urticaria [12]. Hand dermatitis occurred in 65% of persons with atopic symptoms and in 75% of those who had unusually dry skin and atopic relatives. Among the remaining workers, only 33% had had eczema elsewhere on the skin or on the hands [13, 14].

43.6 Wet Work

Hospital wet work also increases the risk of hand eczema. Previous irritant contact dermatitis produced by wet working predisposes to allergic reactions, mostly to nickel, fragrances or rubber chemicals. Of persons with allergic contact dermatitis, 55% had suffered irritant hand dermatitis previously, compared to 44% of those without positive patch test reactions. Of those with sensitivity to fragrance, 70% had suffered from hand dermatitis [15].

> **Core Message**
>
> › Atopy condition and wet work increases the risk of hand eczema in healthy workers.

43.7 Hand Dermatitis

Self-reported hand eczema in a hospital population is around 23% [16] or 22% [17]. The frequencies were significantly higher among assistant nurses (32%), nurses (30%) and nursing aids (27%). Health care professionals have a higher prevalence of skin irritation than that seen in general population, because of the necessity for frequent hand hygiene during patient care. As many as 75% of the occupational skin diseases in hospital cleaners were hand irritant contact dermatitis, 21% were allergic contact dermatitis and 4% were candidosis of the finger webs. The causes of irritant contact dermatitis were detergents, alkaline soaps, acids, sodium perborate and hypochlorite and also hypobromide compounds [18–20]. The ways to minimize the adverse effects of hand hygiene include selecting less irritating products, using skin moisturizers and modifying certain hand hygiene practices such as unnecessary washing. Among the allergic causes, the frequency of type IV thiuram allergy hand dermatitis has been showing statistically significant increase (odds ratio 2.55, 95% confidence interval 1.25–5.20, $P=0.01$) since 1983 [21]. Euxyl K-400 is a preservative that is well recognized as a sensitizer, but only occasionally involved in occupational cases. It has been described in a liquid detergent named Prilan® causing allergic contact dermatitis of the fingers in a female hospital cleaner [22]. Local and general prophylactic measures must be extended in order to reduce occupational hand dermatitis among hospital workers, including surgeons, nurses, cleaning personnel, kitchen workers and clinical assistants, among many others. Prevention of occupational hand eczema in health care workers also requires specific educational programmes [23].

43.8 Nurses, Clinical Assistants and Cleaners

Nurses, clinical assistants and cleaners commonly have their hands exposed to irritants, and so, often suffer irritant contact dermatitis of the hands and forearms. This is significantly more frequent in women under 30 years of age, mostly workers in training grades and surgical fields. In the majority of cases (90%), the lesions are irritant, and mainly related to disinfectants. A decreased prevalence of the well-established natural rubber latex allergy has been observed due to different preventive measures, for example, its substitution by other materials such as neoprene or nitrile rubber [24]. Some pharmaceutical products have special relevance in nurses (Table 43.1).

Table 43.1 Special allergens for nurses [1]

	Test
Cetrimide	0.25% pet.
Chlorhexidine digluconate	0.5% aq.
Chlorpromazine	0.1% pet.
Chloroxylenol	1% pet.
Formaldehyde	1% aq [46].
Glutaraldehyde	1% aq. or pet.
Penicillin	10,000 IU/g pet.[a]
Povidone-iodine	10% pet.

[a]See table, "Medicaments"

Special cases of individual allergic contact reactions are due to the direct contact with drugs (Table 43.2) Of 14,689 patients (1978–2001) suspected of contact allergy, 33 health care workers showed occupational allergic contact dermatitis from drugs [25].

1,5-Pentanedial (glutaraldehyde) at 2% is employed as a cold sterilizer for many instruments in hospitals (in bronchoscopy, cytoscopy, anaesthetics, renal dialysis, etc.) [26]. It causes brown discolouration, irritant and allergic contact dermatitis mainly in nurses, clinical assistants and cleaning workers in hospitals because of different sources of exposure [27, 28]. Clinical symptoms often show some chronicity (Fig. 43.1). Although glutaraldehyde and formaldehyde do not seem to cross-react [29, 30], some patients show positive allergic reactions to both substances [31, 32] (test 1% aq. or pet., but beware of false-positive reactions [33]). Waters et al. [34] investigated work practices and glutaraldehyde exposure in relation to cutaneous symptoms and lung function. Skin symptoms were 3.6 times more likely to be reported by exposed workers. Although in USA, the National Institute of Occupational Safety and Health has published guidelines for safe handling of glutaraldehyde, allergy appears to continue to rise. In Australia, the occupational exposure standard expressed as permissible exposure limit ceiling value was reduced from 0.20 to 0.10 ppm (1995). In the USA (American Conference of Government Industrial Hygienists, 1998) it is of 0.05 ppm. Natural rubber latex glove material is more permeable to glutaraldehyde than styrene-ethylene-butadiene-styrene thermoplastic elastomer material [35]. Ortho-phtalaldehyde, a mixture of hydrogen peroxide and paracetic acid, has been proposed as a substitute of glutaraldehyde.

Table 43.2 Occupational drug-induced contact dermatitis in nurses

Antibiotics

Aminoglycosides
  Streptomycin
  Amika cin
  Gentamicin

Penicillin
  Ampicillin
  Amoxycillin
  Cloxacillin
  Oxacillin
  Flucoxacillin

Cephalosporins
  Ceftizoxime
  Cefotaxime
  Cefodizime
  Ceftazidime
  Cefuronide
  Cephazolin
  Cefuroxime
  Ceftriaxome

Pentamidine isothionate
  Meropenem

Analgesics
  Propacetamol hydrochloride
  Dipyridamole
  Caffeine and diacetylmorphine (heroin)

Chlorpromazine

Maclofenoxate

Cyanamide (carbodiimide), tetraethylthiuram disulphide (Antabuse)

Potassium chloride

Ranitidine hydrochloride

Ethylenediamine which is used to make theophylline soluble

Mesna (sodium 2-mercapto-ethane sulphonate)

Anti-neoplastic drugs
  Cisplatin
  Ammonium tetrachloroplatinate
  Ammonium hexachloroplatinate

Vitamin B_6

Meglumine diatrizoate (Angiografine®, Urografine®, contrast media)

Papain

Tylosin

Boldo (diuretic herbal medicine),

Cascara (anthraquinone stimulant laxative)

Methylprednisolone

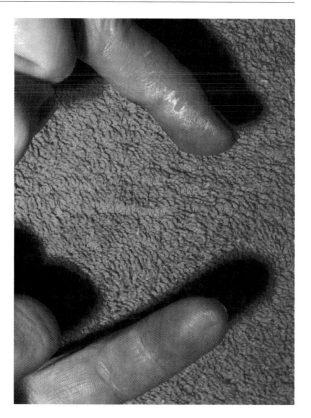

Fig. 43.1 Allergic contact dermatitis in a laboratory technician caused by immersion oil (Leica®). She was positive in an open patch test with the immersion oil and also patch test positive to the constituent epoxy resin [46] (courtesy of A. Goossen)

Ampholytics have been used as disinfectants by hospital personnel. Desimex®, Ampholyt G® and Tego 103 G® are dodecyldiaminoethylglycine hydrochloride. Ampholyt G® does not contain benzyl alcohol or formaldehyde. Tego 103 G® contains the active ingredients: 9-lauryl-3,6,9-triazanonanoic acid and 7-dilauryl-1,4,7-triazaheptane, benzyl alcohol and a small quantity of formaldehyde. Cases of allergic contact dermatitis have been described. Because of the chemical nature of these substances, some patients may also be reactive to ethylenediamine, but this special cross-reaction is rare [36, 37]. Diodecyldimethylammonium chloride and bis(aminopropyl)-laurylamine are detergents, disinfectants and amphoteric tensioactives sometimes used to clean operating rooms and other areas. They are bactericidal, virucidal and active against HIV_1. Their concentration for use is 0.25%. Both may cause allergic contact dermatitis in hospital workers. Patch tests must be from 0.01% aq. to 0.1 and 1% aq. [38]. The use of protective gloves and systematic prevention of contact is recommended. Dimethyldidecylammonium chloride 0.1%, *N,N*-bis (3-aminopropyl) dodecylamine 1.0% and *N,N*-bis (3-aminopropyl)dodecylamine included in Gigasept AF®, a detergent-disinfectant for surgical instruments, can induce eyes burns and coughing fits after direct exposure to its vapour. Despite protective measures (gloves and masks), skin lesions and other symptoms persisted [39].

The antiseptics that commonly cause contact dermatitis in nurses, clinical assistants and cleaners are widely used in different hospital wards. Chloramine-T (sodium *p*-toluenesulphonchloramine) has been described as a sensitizer for nurses (test 0.05% aq.) [40]. Allergic contact dermatitis from undecylenamide diethanolamide in a liquid soap has been described in a hospital worker [41]. Methyldibromo glutaronitrile (1,2-dibromo-2,4-dicyanobutane) used as preservative in soaps and many other products induced occupational allergic contact dermatitis in two nurses [42].

Diisocyanates are found in hospitals as a constituent of soft casts. They are a cause of occupational asthma and have been described as causing cutaneous problems, both as irritants and sensitizers. When using soft casts, the extremity is covered by layer gauze. The cast is dipped into water and applied while wearing rubber gloves and, sometimes, a barrier cream. Because of the potential for asthma, the ventilation is often switched on during the casting. When dipping the cast, the forearms above the level of the gloves often get into contact with the water. After having applied the cast, the extremity of the patient is rubbed in light circular motions so that the cast fits perfectly. The dipping water is reused several times, accumulating diisocyanates from each use. Larsen et al. [43] conducted a study among the nursing staff of an orthopaedic outpatient clinic patch testing five types of diisocyanates and concluded that diisocyanates are primarily irritants rather than sensitizers in the professional setting studied.

Thiomersal originally caused allergy when a nurse was vaccinated against viral hepatitis. As a result of further contact with this preservative during the vaccination of schoolchildren, she showed allergic contact dermatitis on the hands. The vaccines from Biomed, that she had been exposed to, contained 0.01% thiomersal [44]. Two cases (an ophthalmologist and a nurse) of occupational dermatitis due to mercury vapour from broken sphygmomanometer have been described. Patients suffered from itchy erythema with high fever followed by generalized exanthem. The air concentration of mercury vapour was higher than permissible levels (0.05 mg/m³ and a concentration of 9.9 mg/m³) [45].

> ### Core Message
>
> ❭ Nurses suffer mainly from irritant contact dermatitis. Although a decreased prevalence of natural rubber latex allergy has been observed, contact allergic reactions with drugs are common, the *risk of sensitization being high.*

43.9 Surgeons

Chemical components of rubber gloves commonly cause allergic contact dermatitis of the hands and forearms in surgeons. Although many different substances can sensitize, the most frequent ones are those that are tested in the thiuram mix of the standard series. Less frequent ones are mercaptobenzothiazole and others tested in the mercapto mix. Release of thiurams and carbamates from rubber gloves varies between brands. Glove powder contributes to enhance contact dermatitis and urticaria. The knowledge about cutaneous reactions from gloves has increased enormously in recent years. The main reason is the broad knowledge in type I allergy to natural rubber latex and recognition of the relatively large number of patients and health care personnel who suffer from this hypersensitivity.

Orthopaedic surgeons use acrylic bone cement, for fixation of prostheses to the bone of the hip joint. Bone cement contains methyl methacrylate monomer and polymethyl methacrylate. The monomer is a strong lipid solvent. The hand dermatitis caused by allergy to methacrylate is usually a dry, pruriginous, fissured, chronic eczema of the fingertips, sometimes with paresthesia and tingling or burning sensations. Gloves usually do not protect the hands from acrylic bone cement. Indeed, even if two pairs of rubber gloves worn, the sensitized surgeon may still suffer from contact with the acrylic cement, because enough acrylic penetrates both the pairs if the surgeon has contact for a sufficient time [46–48]. Colophony has also been identified as a causative agent of allergic contact dermatitis in an orthopaedic surgeon who suspected paper-based surgical clothing as the cause [49].

43

Antiseptics are present in surgical scrubbing agents in the pre-operating room. Some surgeons contract chronic, dry, pruritic, irritant contact dermatitis of the dorsum of the hands from such agents. It is not infrequent for superimposed allergic contact dermatitis to appear, because these substances also have allergic capacity. The most commonly involved substances are: hexachlorophene G 11 (test 1% pet.), dichlorophene G 4 (test 1% aq.), tribromosalicylanilide (test 1% pet.), dibromosalicylanilide (test 1% pet.), triclosan (Irgasan DP 300) (test 2% pet.), Fentichlor (test 1% pet.), chlorhexidine (test both acetate and gluconate 0.5% aq.) [50], *p*-cresol (test 1% aq.), Dowicides (phenolic substances) (test 1% pet.), imidazolidinyl urea (test 2% pet.), sodium hypochlorite (test 0.5% aq.), sodium hyposulphite (test 1% aq.) and benzydamine hydrochloride (test 5% aq. or pet.) [51].

Some quaternary ammonium compounds are of special interest. The most common and widely used one is benzalkonium chloride (alkylbenzyldimethylammonium chloride), a cationic detergent used as a pre-operative skin disinfectant, and also for surgical instruments. Some people allergic to benzalkonium chloride may need to avoid other quaternary ammonium compounds because of cross-reaction. Patch testing with 0.1% aq. can also provoke irritant reactions. True allergic responses may be obtained by testing with 0.01% aq., but a dilution series plus ROAT is recommended.

Table 43.3 Occupational contact sensitizers involved in laboratory personnel

2-Aminophenyl disulphide
3-4-Dicarbethoxy hexane-2,5-dione
Alcohols
Azathioprine
Aephalosporins
Cephalosporine
Codeine
Cytosine arabinoside
d-Limonene
Dicyclohexyl carbodiimide
Diisopropyl carbodiimide
Diglycidyl ether of bisphenol A
Dimethylaminopropylethyl carbodiimide
Ethyl-2-bromo-*p*-methoxyphenylacetate
Ethyl chloro oximido acetate
Isothiazolinone
n-Acetyl-cysteine
Propylene oxide
Pyridine
Simvastatin
Sodium bisulphite
Vitamin A acetate
Vitamin K

> **Core Message**
>
> › Chemical components of rubber gloves commonly cause allergic contact dermatitis of the hands and forearms in surgeons. Antiseptics present in surgical scrubbing agents in the pre-operating room induce irritant contact dermatitis of the dorsum of the hands.

43.10 Laboratory Personnel

Laboratories use many other different substances capable of producing dermatitis in their personnel. As the working environments are so diverse, aimed patch testing needs to be performed, guided by a careful history. In pharmaceutical laboratories, mainly in product synthesis areas, contact dermatitis may arise in the pharmacologists who synthesize such products. Very often the sensitizers are not the final compounds. Sensitizations have been published as individual case reports, and substances mentioned are reported in Table 43.3

Contact dermatitis caused by alcohols is of special interest. Amyl, butyl, ethyl, methyl and isopropyl alcohols can all cause allergic contact dermatitis, though rarely. Contact allergy to alcohols may cause a generalized allergic reaction when alcohol is ingested. Nevertheless, contact reactions to alcohol do not necessarily signify that a systemic reaction will develop after drinking alcoholic liquor. Alcohol can be an allergen for nurses, physicians and laboratory technicians. It can produce irritant contact dermatitis and non-immunological contact urticaria. Its effects can be produced by external or internal exposure. Contaminants are common in alcohol. Pure ethanol should be used for patch testing. Because of its volatility, the interpretation of the results can be difficult. In occlusive patch testing, immediate fading of the reaction suggests irritancy. If the reaction remains clearly visible after 4 days, it may be allergic. Repeated testing with lower dilutions may confirm this. Alcohols can be tested undiluted, although many different concentrations have been used, the lowest being 1% [52].

Propylene oxide used for preparing tissue specimens in a histopathological laboratory (test in ethanol at 0.1–11%) [53] or *dl*-Limonene (dipentene) (Figs. 43.1 and 2) that has been used as a non-toxic substitute for xylene as a wax solvent and cleaning agent for use by laboratory technicians [54] is among the substances that have been described as causing allergic contact dermatitis in laboratory technicians. Allergic contact dermatitis to diglycidyl ether of bisphenol A (MW 340 Da), a low molecular weight monomer constituent of Leica immersion oil (Leica Microsystems, Wetzler, Germany) was described during the nineties. It was initially described by Sommer et al. [55] and by Le Coz and Goossens [56]. Technicians and physicians working in cytogenetic, bacteriology and haematology laboratories were the main target. Contact dermatitis or airborne allergy mainly involved forearms and hands and also face and neck. Irritant reactions must also be considered. According to the material safety data sheet, the contents of this ecological oil are as follows: modified cyclohexyl epoxy resin (45%), modified bisphenolic epoxy resins (35%), 1,4 butanediol diglycidylether (10%) and phthalates (4%). A breakdown performed with the oil's ingredients confirmed sensitization to liquid modified epoxy resin components contained at >80% concentration. Positive reactions have been described also to cycloaliphatic epoxy resin and to the diluents such as phenyl glycidyl ether and cresyl glycidyl ether [57]. In the meantime, the manufacturer has withdrawn this product (the epoxy resin was added for improvement of optical qualities). This "epidemic" could have been avoided by obtaining advice from experts on contact allergy beforehand.

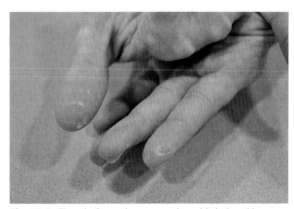

Fig. 43.2 Chronic finger tips contact dematitis induced by occupational exposure to pure *dl*-Limonene in a technician from a neuropharmacology laboratory in spite of the use of nitril gloves

43.11 Other Therapists

Some substances have been reported as being responsible for occupational contact dermatitis in other personnel involved in special therapeutic procedures. A physiotherapist suffered allergic contact dermatitis from benzydamine hydrochloride and lavender fragrance, contained in Difflam® gel, a topical no steroidal anti-inflammatory agent [58]. Isothiazolinone derivatives contained in Parmetol® caused allergic contact dermatitis in a radiology technician. Parmetol is used in radiographic developing solutions [59]. Metaproterenol produced airborne contact dermatitis in a respiratory therapist who routinely administered Alupent® (metaproterenol sulphate), Mucomyst® (acetylcysteine) and Bronkosol® (isoetharine) in aerosolized forms [60]. Benzoyl peroxide included in a hardener substance, Lucidol® hardening gel, has been demonstrated to induce recurrent eczema of the face, neck and arms for 2 years in an orthopaedic technician [61].

43.12 Veterinarians

Veterinarians are exposed to many organic, biological and chemical substances that may produce allergic contact dermatitis. Occupational dermatoses have been reported in 48–77% of veterinarians. Sensitized veterinarians can suffer asthma, rhinitis and contact dermatitis from dander, hair, bristles or saliva from cows, horses, cats or dogs [62, 63]. Specific IgE and prick/scratch tests are diagnostic. Clinically, allergic contact

> **Core Message**
>
> › Epoxy resin is a strong contact allergen. Their incorporation to microscopic immersion oil was an unnecessary and avoidable oversight.

urticaria, allergic contact dermatitis or both reactions can be observed. Bovine amniotic fluid (BAF) caused a severe and extensive eruption in a 30-year-old non-atopic veterinarian. Patch test and prick test proved negative, though a weak reaction to the patch was visible by the fourth day. Only an intra-dermal test was positive to BAF pure and at 1/10. In other similar patients, RAST has been useful to confirm the allergic nature of the relatively common protein contact dermatitis.

Certain antibiotics are more often used in veterinary than in human medicine. Spiramycin, tylosin and benzyl penicillin diethylaminoethylester (penethamate) are the most important ones. Spiramycin and tylosin are used to treat enteritis in pigs, mastitis in cows and respiratory infections in household pets. Penethamate hydriodide is used for local or intra-lesional treatment of mastitis in cows. It cross-reacts with penicillin [64, 65].

Hormones, vitamins, minerals, antibiotics, growth stimulants, preservatives, metals, antioxidants and certain other substances are present in animal feeds (Table 43.4). Health personnel who handle these additives may experience allergic contact dermatitis. For example, vitamin A and vitamin D_3 contain 5% ethoxyquin as an antioxidant preservative. Ethoxyquin (6-ethyl-1,2-dihydro-2,2,4-trimethylquinoline) is a contact sensitizer. Quindoxin, a growth promoting factor, is a common sensitizer and also induces photodermatitis. Quindoxin is an antibiotic of the quinoxaline group, a growth promoter. It has been reported to induce contact and photocontact dermatitis. Its derivatives olaquindox and carbadox have been used as feed additives for growth promotion in pigs, rabbits and other animals. It is extremely difficult for breeders to avoid exposure to dust containing relatively highly concentrations of olaquindox. A very low dose of olaquindox produces contact dermatitis mainly by phototoxic or photoallergic mechanisms. In some cases, persistent light reactors are developed. Olaquindox has an absorption spectrum between 256 and 373 nm [66–68].

The patients suffer eczema of the hands, wrists, forearms, face and neck with severe itching and light intolerance. In some cases, farmers have a history of other photoallergy, for example, to chlorpromazine, sunscreens, cosmetics and others. Halquinol, a chlorinated derivative of 8-hydroxyquinoline, is added to animal feeds for the prevention of *Escherichia coli* and

Table 43.4 Animal feed additives

	Function	Test
Amprolium	Growth promoter	10% aq.
Arsanilic acid	Growth promoter	10% pet.
Bacitracin zinc	Growth promoter	20% pet.
Chlortetracycline hydrochloride	Growth promoter	5% pet.
Sulphacetamide	Growth promoter (prevents enteral infections)	5% pet.
Tylosin tartrate	Growth promoter (prevents Gram-negative infections)	5% pet.
Diethylstilboestrol	Fattening cattle	1% pet.
Ethoxyquin	Antioxidant preservative	1% pet.
Ethylenediamine	Antiseptic	1% pet.
Medroxyprogesterone acetate	Abortions	1% pet.
Neomycin sulphate	Prevention of dysentery	20% pet.
Nitrofurazone	Prevention of *Salmonella* infection	1% pet.
Penicillin	Prevention of mastitis	10,000 IU
Thiabendazole	Worm control	1% pet.
Piperazine	Worm control	1% pet.
Phenothiazines	Worm control	1% pet.

Salmonella infections. Halquinol causes irritant, allergic and photoallergic dermatitis, and sometimes allergic contact urticaria and airborne dermatitis [69].

Dinitolmide, which is used to control coccidiosis in chicken factories, and nitrofurazone, used for the treatment of salmonellosis in pigs and as a growth promoting factor for cattle and swine, can also cause allergic contact dermatitis in veterinarians. Chlorpromazine and other phenothiazine derivatives are used by veterinarians and farmers for the sedation of animals. Contact and photodermatitis in a farmer due to chlorpromazine used for sedation of pigs suggest that this type of medicament should be included in a patch test series for veterinarians (Table 43.5). Occupational contact allergy to lincomycin and spectinomycin in chicken vaccinators has been documented [70].

Table 43.5 Contact allergens reported in veterinarians

Penicillin	10,000 IU (g pet.ª)	Formaldehyde	1% aq.
Streptomycin	1% pet.	Mercaptobenzothiazole	2% pet.
Dihydrostreptomycin	0.1% pet.	Merthiolate	0.1% pet.
Erythromycin base	1% pet.	Piperazine	1% aq.
Oxytetracycline	3% pet.	Tuberculin	10% aq.
Penethamate	1% pet.	Bovine tuberculin	10% aq.
Spiramycin (Rovamycin)	10% pet.	Ethoxyquin	1% pet.
Tylosin (tartrate)	5% pet.	Quindoxin	0.1% pet.
Procaine HCl	1% pet.	Chlorpromazine	0.1% pet.
Benzocaine	5% pet.		

43.13 Laboratory Animal Handlers

Allergic disease is a serious occupational health concern for individuals who have contact with laboratory animals. Urticaria is the most common skin manifestation, although contact dermatitis may also occur. The overall prevalence of allergic disease among laboratory animal handlers is about 23% and respiratory allergy is much more common than skin allergy. There are only sparse data on the incidence or prevalence of skin conditions. A study performed in Sweden by Agrup and Sjöstedt [71] revealed a prevalence of 14% of contact urticaria to rats, but this appears to be an unusually high rate. Another study of pharmaceutical industry and university laboratory workers found no increase in urticaria [72]. Evidence from the study of Aoyama et al. indicates that skin allergy tends to be accompanied by respiratory allergy symptoms [73].

43.14 Conclusion

Health care workers are exposed to many agents capable of inducing irritant or allergic contact dermatitis and also contact urticaria. Skin complaints should be assessed with both prick and patch testing. It is necessary the identification of the responsible agents in order to learn how to avoid them. There is a need, to develop effective prophylactic and preventive measures.

Acknowledgements With gratitude, I dedicate this review chapter to Professor Jose G. Camarasa, who made us understand and love immunodermatology.

References

1. Stingeni L, Lapomarda V, Lisi P (1995) Occupational hand dermatitis in hospital environments. Contact Dermatitis 33:172–176
2. Mahler V (2007) Skin protection in health care setting. Curr Probl Dermatol 34:120–132
3. Camarasa JG, Conde Salazar L (1988) Occupational dermatoses in sanitary workers. In: Orfanos CE, Stadler R, Gollnick H (eds) Dermatology in five continents. Proceedings of the XVIIth world congress of dermatology, Berlin, 24–29 May 1987. Springer, Berlin, pp 1045–1048
4. Holness DL, Mace SR (2001) Results of evaluating health care workers with Prick and Patch testing. Am J Contact Dermatitis 12:88–92
5. Nettis E, Colanardi MC, Soccio AL, Ferrannini A, Tursi A (2002) Occupational irritant and allergic contact dermatitis among healthcare workers. Contact Dermatitis 46:101–107
6. Suneja T, Belsito DV (2008) Occupational dermatosis in health care workers evaluated for suspected allergic contact dermatitis. Contact Dermatitis 58:285–290
7. Kikuchi-Numagami K, Saishu T, Fukaya M, Kanazawa E, Tagami H (1999) Irritancy of scrubbing up for surgery with or without a brush. Acta Derm Venereol 79:230–232
8. Hachem JP, De Paepe K, Sterckx G, Kaufman L, Rogiers V, Roseeuw D (2002) Evaluation of biophysical and clinical parameters of skin barrier function among hospital workers. Contact Derm 46:220–223
9. Pedersen LK, Held E, Johansen JD, Agner T (2005) Short-term effects of alcohol-based disinfectant and detergent on skin irritation. Contact Derm 52:82–87

43

10. Slotosch CM, Kampf G, Löffler H (2007) Effects of disinfectants and detergents on skin irritation. Contact Derm 57: 235–241

11. Stutz N, Becker D, Jappe U, John SM, Ladwig A, Spornraft-Ragaller P, Uter W, Löffler H (2009) Nurses' perceptions of the benefits and adverse effects of hand disinfection: alcohol-based hand rubs vs. hygienic handwashing: a multicentre questionnaire study with additional patch testing by the German Contact Dermatitis Research Group. Br J Dermatol 160:565–572

12. Valsecchi R, Leghissa P, Cortinovis R, Cologni L, Pomesano A (2000) Contact urticaria from latex in healthcare workers. Dermatology 201:127–131

13. Lammintausta K, Kalimo K (1981) Atopy and hand dermatitis in hospital wet work. Contact Derm 7:301–308

14. Nilson E, Mikaelsson B, Andersson S (1985) Atopy, occupation and domestic work as risk factors for hand eczema in hospital workers. Contact Derm 13:216–223

15. Lammintausta K, Kalimo K, Havu VK (1982) Occurrence of contact allergy and hand eczemas in hospital wet work. Contact Derm 8:84–90

16. Flyvholm M-A, Bach B, Rose M, Frydendall Jepsen K (2007) Self-reported hand eczema in hospital population. Contact Derm 57:110–115

17. Lan C-C E, Feng W-W, Lu Y-W, Wu C-S, Hung S-T, Hsu H-Y, Hsin-Su Y, Ko Y-C, Lee C-H, Yang Y-H, Chen G-S (2008) Hand eczema among university hospital nursing staff: identification of high-risk sector and impact in quality of life. Contact Derm 59:301–306

18. Hansen KS (1983) Occupational dermatoses in hospital cleaning women. Contact Derm 9:343–351

19. Singgih SIR, Lantinga H, Nater JP, Woest Kruyt-Gaspersz JA (1986) Occupational hand dermatoses in hospital cleaning personnel. Contact Derm 14:14–19

20. Gawkrodger DJ, Lloyd MH, Hunter JAA (1986) Occupational skin disease in hospital cleaning and kitchen workers. Contact Derm 15:132–135

21. Gibbon KL, McFadden JPM, Rycroft RJG, Ross JS, Chinn S, White IR (2001) Changing frequency of thiuram allergy in healthcare workers with hand dermatitis. Br J Dermatol 144:347–350

22. Aalto-Korte K, Jolanki R, Estlander T, Alanko K, Kanerva L (1996) Occupational allergic contact dermatitis caused by Euxyl K 400. Contact Derm 35:193–194

23. Weisshaar E, Radulescu M, Bock M, Albrecht U, Diepgen TL (2006) Educational and dermatological aspects of secondary individual prevention in healthcare workers. Contact Derm 54:254–260

24. Crippa M, Balbiani L, Baruffini A, Belleri L, Draicchio F, Feltrin G, Larese F, MAaggio GM, Marcer G, Micheloni GP, Montomoli L, Moscato G, Previdi M, Sartorelli P, Sossai D, Spatari G, Zanetti C (2008) Consensus document. Update on latex exposure and use of gloves in Italian health care settings. Med Lav 99:387–399

25. Gielen K, Goossens A (2001) Occupational allergic contact dermatitis from drugs in healthcare workers. Contact Derm 45:273–279

26. Lyon TC (1971) Allergic contact dermatitis due to Cidex. Oral Surg 32:895

27. Schnuch A, Geier J UW, Frosch PJ (1998) Patch testing with preservatives, antimicrobials and industrial biocides. Results from a multicentric study. Br J Dermatol 138:467–476

28. Shaffer MP, Belsito DV (2000) Allergic contact dermatitis from glutaraldehyde in health-care workers. Contact Derm 43:150–156

29. Neering H, van Ketel WG (1974) Glutaraldehyde and formaldehyde allergy. Contact Dermatitis Newslett 16:518

30. Maibach HI (1975) Glutaraldehyde: cross reaction to formaldehyde. Contact Derm 1:326

31. Nethercott JR, Holness DL, Page E (1988) Occupational contact dermatitis due to glutaraldehyde in health care workers. Contact Derm 18:193–197

32. Hansen KS (1983) Glutaraldehyde occupational dermatitis. Contact Derm 9:81–82

33. Hansen EM, Menné T (1990) Glutaraldehyde: patch test, vehicle and concentration. Contact Derm 23:369–370

34. Waters A, Beach J, Abramson M (2003) Symptoms and lung function in health care personnel exposed to glutaraldehyde. Am J Ind Med 43:196–203

35. Lehman PA, Franz TJ, Guin JD (1994) Penetration of glutaraldehyde through glove material: Tactylon™ versus natural rubber latex. Contact Derm 30:176–177

36. Foussereau J, Samsoen M, Hecht MT (1983) Occupational dermatitis to Ampholyt G in hospital personnel. Contact Derm 9:233–234

37. Suhonen R (1980) Contact allergy to dodecyldi (aminoethyl) glycine (Desimex i). Contact Derm 6:290–291

38. Dejobert Y, Martin P, Piette F, Thomas P, Bergoend H (1997) Contact dermatitis from didecyldimethylammonium chloride and bis-(aminopropyl)-laurylamine in a detergent-disinfectant used in hospital. Contact Derm 37:95–96

39. Dibo M, Brasch J (2001) Occupational allergic contact dermatitis from N,N-bis(3-aminopropyl)dodecylamine and dimethyldidecylammonium chloride in 2 hospital staff. Contact Derm 45:40

40. Lombardi P, Gola M, Acciai MC, Sertoli A (1984) Unusual occupational allergic contact dermatitis in a nurse. Contact Derm 20:302

41. Cristersson S, Wrangsjö K (1991) Contact allergy to undecylenamide diethanolamide in a liquid soap. Contact Derm 27:191–192

42. Diba VC, Chowdhury MMU, Adisesh A, Statham BN (2003) Occupational allergic contact dermatitis in hospital workers caused by methyldibromoglutaronitrile in a work soap. Contact Derm 48:118–119

43. Larsen TH, Gregersen P, Jemec GBE (2001) Skin irritation and exposure to diisocyanates in orthopedic nurses working with soft casts. Am J Contact Dermat 12:211–214

44. Kiec-Swierczynska M, Krecisz B, Swierczynska-Machura D (2003) Occupational allergic contact dermatitis due to thiomerosal. Contact Derm 48:337–338

45. Suzuki K, Matsunaga K, Umemura Y, Ueda H, Sasaki K (2000) 2 cases of occupational dermatitiis due to mercury vapor from a broken sphygmomanometer. Contact Derm 43:175–177

46. Pegum J, Medhurst FA (1971) Contact dermatitis from penetration of rubber gloves by acrylic monomer. Br Med J 2:141

47. Fries JB, Fisher AA, Salvati EA (1975) Contact dermatitis in surgeons from methylmethacrylate bone cement. J Bone Joint Surg Am 57:547

48. Fisher AA (1979) Paresthesia of the fingers accompanying dermatitis due to methylmethacrylate bone cement. Contact Derm 5:56

49. Bergh M, Menné T, Karlberg AT (1994) Colophony in paper-based surgical clothing. Contact Derm 31:332–333
50. Knudsen BB, Avnstorp C (1991) Chlorhexidine gluconate and acetate in patch testing. Contact Derm 24:45–49
51. Foti C, Vena GA, Angelini G (1992) Occupational contact allergy to benzydamine hydrochloride. Contact Derm 27:328–329
52. Ophaswongse S, Maibach HI (1994) Alcohol dermatitis: allergic contact dermatitis and contact urticaria syndrome, a review. Contact Derm 30:1–6
53. Steinkraus V, Hansen BM (1994) Contact allergy to propylene oxide. Contact Derm 31:120
54. Wakelin SH, McFadden JP, Leonard JN, Rycroft RJG (1998) Allergic contact dermatitis from d-limonene in a laboratory technician. Contact Derm 38:164–165
55. Sommer S, Wilkinson SM, Wilson CL (1998) Airborne contact dermatitis caused by microcopy immersion fluid containing epoxy resin. Contact Derm 39:141–142
56. Le Coz C, Goossens A (1998) Contact dermatitis from an immersion oil for microscopy. N Engl J Med 339:406–407
57. Hughes R, Taylor JS (2002) Surveillance of allergic contact dermatitis: Epoxy resin and microscopic immersion oil. J Am Acad Dermatol 47:965–966
58. Rademaker M (1994) Allergic contact dermatitis from lavender fragrance in Difflam® gel. Contact Derm 31:58–59
59. Pazzaglia M, Vincenzi C, Gasparri F, Tosti A (1996) Occupational hypersensitivity to isothiazolinone derivatives in a radiology technician. Contact Derm 34:143
60. Fung MA, Geisse JK, Maibach HI (1996) Airborne contact dermatitis from metaproterenol in a respiratory therapist. Contact Derm 35:317–318
61. Forschner K, Zuberbier T, Worm M (2002) Benzoyl peroxide as a cause of airborne contact dermatitis in an orthopaedic technician. Contact Derm 47:241
62. Camarasa JG (1986) Contact eczema from cow saliva. Contact Derm 2:117
63. Prahl P, Roed-Petersen J (1979) Type I allergy from cows in veterinary surgeons. Contact Derm 5:33–36
64. Hjorth N (1967) Occupational dermatitis among veterinary surgeons caused by penethamate. Berufsdermatosen 15:163
65. Melhorn HC, Beetz D (1971) Das Antioxydant Aethoxyquin als berufliches Ebenzatogen bei einem Futtermitteldosierer. Berufsdermatosen 19:84
66. Burrows D (1975) Contact dermatitis in animal feed mill workers. Br J Dermatol 92:167
67. Caplan RM (1973) Contact dermatitis from animal feed additives (letter to editor). Arch Dermatol 107:918
68. Shander S, Schröder W, Geier J (1996) Olaquindox-induced airborne photoallergic contact dermatitis followed by transient or persistent light reactors in 15 pig breeders. Contact Derm 35:344–354
69. Bleumink E, Nater JP (1973) Allergic contact dermatitis to dinitolmide (letter to editor). Arch Dermatol 108:423–424
70. Nelder KM (1972) Contact dermatitis from animal feed additives. Arch Dermatol 106:722–723
71. Agrup G, Sjöstedt L (1985) Contact urticaria in laboratory technicians working with animal. Acta Derm Venereol 65:111–115
72. Davies GE, McArdle LA (1981) Allergy to laboratory animals: a survey by questionnaire. Int Arch Allergy Appl Immunol 64:302–307
73. Aoyama K, Ueda A, Manda F, Matsushita T, Ueda T (1992) Allergy to laboratory animals: an epidemiological study. Br J Ind Med 49:41–47

Occupational Contact Dermatitis: Chefs and Food Handlers

44

Vera Mahler

Contents

44.1 Epidemiology and Risk Factors of Occupational Skin Diseases in Chefs and Food Handlers

Chefs and food handlers are at high risk of developing an occupational skin disease (OSD) (mainly irritant (ICD) or allergic contact dermatitis (ACD)). In a population-based study from Germany [1], the overall incidence rates of OSD per 10,000 workers per year were 33.2 for bakers, 23.9 for pastry cooks, 6.6 for cooks and 2.9 for butchers and food processing industries [1]. An occupation with an incidence rate of more than seven cases per 10,000 workers per year is considered an "exceedingly high risk occupation" for an OSD, and those with three to seven cases are considered "high risk occupations" [1]. Only the occupational group of hairdressers exhibited an even higher overall incidence rate (97.4) than bakers. In this register, overall, the male gender was predominant with regard to OSD in bakers, butchers and the food processing industry, whereas in pastry cooks and cooks, the female gender was more frequent [1]. In a previous analysis from the same register, it could be demonstrated that incidence rates were sex- and age-related [2]: Females developed OSD at higher incidence rates compared to males. OSD occurred mostly at young age (between 15 and 24 years) after a median occupational exposure of 26 months in bakers and confectioners compared to 43 months in cooks [2].

Of the different dermatological conditions caused by contact with food (ICD, ACD, protein contact dermatitis (PCD), occupational contact urticaria (OCU), phototoxic and photoallergic contact dermatitis), ICD is the most frequent OSD in chefs and food handlers [2–6]. However, the ratio of irritant vs. ACD varies between the different occupational fields [5]: ICD was

V. Mahler
Department of Dermatology, University Hospital Erlangen,
Hartmannstr.14, 91052 Erlangen, Germany
e-mail: vera.mahler@uk-erlangen.de

J.D. Johansen et al. (eds.), *Contact Dermatitis*,
DOI: 10.1007/978-3-642-03827-3_44, © Springer-Verlag Berlin Heidelberg 2011

44

observed most frequently in pastry cooks (76% ICD vs. 11% ACD and 7% combined ICD and ACD). In cooks, ICD was present in 69% of patients, ACD in 7% and a "hybrid" contact dermatitis (a combination of ACD and ICD) in 13%. Sixty three percent of food handlers and butchers suffered from ICD, 13% from ACD and 9% from a hybrid contact dermatitis. Compared to these occupational fields, a higher rate of ACD was found in bakers: With a share of 53%, ICD was still the most frequent OSD among bakers; however, 23% had ACD and 17% combined ICD and ACD [5]. These ratios between ICD and ACD in the respective food occupations were confirmed by a population-based survey of occupational hand eczema in Denmark [6].

Less frequently, due to protein contact with the skin, two IgE-mediated (sometimes overlapping) clinical conditions can be observed in chefs and food handlers: occupational contact urticaria (OCU) and protein contact dermatitis (PCD) [6, 7]. The frequency of OCU varies significantly with the group of patients examined: While Bauer et al. detected 1.5% of patients with OCU in a retrospective data analysis of patch test data of $n = 873$ employees in the food processing industry [8], up to 18.2% of butchers with OSD displayed OCU in a population-based survey of occupational hand eczema in Denmark [6]. In the same survey, 11.8% of bakers were diagnosed with OCU, and an additional 5.9% developed OCU based on ICD. In cooks and kitchen workers, OCU was present in 5.7%, and in an additional 10%, OCU and ICD were diagnosed [6]. While PCD is relatively rare in the general population, it is regularly seen in chefs and food handlers [9, 10]. PCD was diagnosed in 2.7% of $n = 873$ employees from the food handling industries [4]. A recent analysis of the database of the Information Network of Departments of Dermatology (IVDK) of $n = 140,840$ patients patch tested from 1994 to 2008 in the German-speaking countries revealed an overall frequency of PCD of 0.2%. In contrast, the frequency of PCD was 4% in bakers and pastry cooks, 1.9% in meat and fish processing industries and 1.5% in cooks and caterers (unpublished results of the PCD working group of the German contact dermatitis research group). Atopic eczema and irritant skin damage are predisposing factors for PCD [10].

The percentage of atopic dermatitis (based on the information about past flexural eczema or currently diagnosed atopic dermatitis by a dermatologist) in the examined group of food occupations was 14–18%, which was not higher than the percentage in the general population in a recent survey from Denmark [6].

Assuming an atopic skin diathesis (ASD) of 20% in the general population, the relative risk (RR) of an employee with an ASD developing OSD in one of the three occupations (baker, confectioner, cook) has been calculated to be increased in average by 3.6× [2].

The potential impact of an ASD on OSD could be confirmed in food preparation workers (pastry cooks, bakers, cooks) in the context of preventive strategies: Assuming a prevalence of 20% ASD in the total population, ASD accounts for about 50% (attributable risk (AR)) of the overall annual OSD incidence of 20.6 cases per 10,000 workers in pastry cooks. In consequence, at least half of this OSD rate could be prevented if ASD among the working population was surveyed [11]. Similarly, the AR of an ASD to OSD was found to be 47.3% in bakers, 34.9 in cooks, and 24% in butchers and the food processing industry [11]. However, it cannot be concluded from these data that applicants with an ASD need to be discouraged from entering risk occupations generally, because of the large number of applicants with this risk factor [11]. In contrast, effective preventive strategies can be implemented including educational programmes where individuals with an ASD are specially advised on skin protection and skin care measures [11]. An ASD (>10 points, "atopy score"), flexural dermatitis or previous hand dermatitis (as the strongest factor) proved to be predictive factors for the development of hand dermatitis in food industry apprentices; however, no association was found to respiratory atopy, metal sensitization or gender [8].

The need for and benefit of effective secondary preventive measures (exposure-analysis-based individual and group training in preventive measures, protective gloves and use of skin care and protection products), combined with medical treatment, could be demonstrated in bakers and confectioners with occupational hand dermatitis [12].

> Young bakers and pastry cooks are at exceedingly high risk to develop an OSD, mainly ICD.

> PCD is rare in the general population, but commonly seen in chefs and food handlers. Atopic eczema and irritant skin damage are predisposing factors for PCD.

An ASD (>10 points, "atopy score"), flexural dermatitis or previous hand dermatitis (as the strongest factor) are predictive factors for the development of hand dermatitis in the food industry.

44.2 Specific Exposures to Irritants, Contact and Protein Allergens in Chefs and Food Handlers

Chefs and food handlers have skin contact not only with foods and their innate ingredients (e.g. proteins and flavours) but also with added food additives and colours. Besides, working standards for food handler hygiene, hand washing and use of protective equipment [13] implicate frequent contact to water, cleaning agents, disinfectants and rubber gloves, which may cause irritant and ACD as well.

44.2.1 Irritants in Food Handling Occupations

Wet work (water and soap), food (e.g. flour, vegetables, fruits, essential oils from spices, meat, fish) and disinfectants have been identified as relevant occupational exposures inducing ICD [6, 14].

The foods that most commonly induce ICD are garlic, onion, citrus fruit, potatoes, sweetcorn, carrots, spices (e.g. cayenne pepper and jalapenos due to the irritancy of capsaicin), mustard, horseradish, radish, hot radish (syn. daikon radish), cabbage, cauliflower, broccoli (all due to the irritancy of allyl isothiocyanate) and pineapple (due to the irritant properties of bromelain) [3]. Bromelain, the proteolytic enzyme found in pineapple juice, causes a separation in the epidermis along with an increase in capillary permeability. The resulting histamine release causes pruritis and a wheal reaction [14]. Bromelain is also used as a food additive functional as flavour enhancer, flour treatment agent, stabilizer and thickener (e.g. in dairy products, cheeses, spreads, processed meat and poultry, soy and dietetic products) [15].

Some of the many food additives, which may irritate the skin, are acetic acid (E260), ascorbic acid (E 300), citric acid (E 330), calcium acetate (E263), calcium sulphate, lactic acid (E 270), sodium and potassium nitrate and nitrite (E 249–252 used as curing salts, antimicrobial preservative, colour fixative in salted meats and fish, charcuterie, corned beef, hard cheese), potassium bicarbonate, potassium iodide, potassium bromate and yeast [3, 14, 15].

Especially hand washing more than 20× per day constitutes a relevant risk factor for ICD [8].

Wet work and skin contact to disinfectants, food and food additives are of irritant potency in the food handling occupations.

44.2.2 Contact Allergens in Food Handling Occupations

As relevant food-derived contact allergens, spices, flour and other non-specified allergens could be identified [6]. Spice allergy usually presents as a contact dermatitis on the palmar sides of the fingers or hands [14]. Of the approximately 60 spices and their essential oils used in cooking, over 20 are reported to be the causes of ACD [14]. Contact dermatitis has been most frequently described to be due to the following spices (*from different plant species*): bay leaves (*Laurus nobilis*), cardamom (*Elettaria cardamomum*), cinnamon (*Cinnamomum zeylanicum*), cloves (*Syzygium aromaticum*), coriander (*Coriandrum sativum*), curry (a mixture of spices), mace (*Myristica fragans*), nutmeg (*Myristica fragans*), paprika (*Capsicum annuum*), turmeric (*Curcuma longa*) and vanilla (*Vanilla planifolia*) [16].

A number of fragrance materials contained in herbs, spices and vegetables have been identified to be causing contact allergy in food occupations: Anethole (synonyms: 1-methoxy-4-(1-propenyl)benzene, *p*-propenylanisole; a flavouring ingredient in anise, star anise, licorice and fennel), carvone (from spearmint), cinnamic acid (in cinnamon and tomato), cinnamic aldehyde (from cinnamon), citral (ginger), eugenol (in cloves, cinnamon, bay leave, Jamaican pepper), geraniol (from spearmint), limonene (from the peel of citrus fruits, dill, peppermint, spearmint, cardamon, caraway, celery seed oil, parsley, parsnips and carrots), linalool (in basil and coriander), phellandrene (from ginger), pinene (from Bay leaf, peppermint, spearmint, parsley, parsnips, celery and carrots), vanillin (from vanilla) [3, 14, 17]. Since contact dermatitis to spices is often based on contact

44

sensitivity to a contained fragrant component, the patch test reactions to fragrance mix, balsam of Peru and colophony may be positive and have been suggested as screening agents [18].

Carnosol (a phenolic antioxidant and tumour-suppressant in extracts from rosemary) has been identified as contact allergen from rosemary. Urushiol (an oleoresin also present in poison ivy and poison oak) is the responsible contact allergen for mango dermatitis following the skin contact with the sap, fruit skin, leaf or stem of the mango tree [14]. Cardol, a phenol similar to urushiol, is contained in ginko seed and cashew nut oil [14].

Allyl isothiocyanate (mustard oil) is responsible for the pungent taste in mustard and horseradish. It is, at the same time, a sensitizer and irritant found in horseradish, cabbage, cauliflower, broccoli, brussel sprouts, kale, turnip and radish [14, 17]. Sesquiterpene lactones are relevant contact allergens contained in artichoke, lettuce, endive, chicory and chamomile [14].

Due to the characteristic pattern of skin involvement (fingers DI to DIII of the non-dominant hand), contact allergy to garlic (and therein contained contact allergens diallyl disulfide and, to a lesser extent, allyl-propyldisulfide and allicin) remains the best known and recognizable of all forms of contact dermatitis in chefs [14].

In addition to the food's natural ingredients, numerous food additives and colours added to food for various purposes may be relevant inducers of skin symptoms in the individual chef or food handler. The "Codex General Standard for Food Additives" (GSFA, Codex STAN 192-1995) contained in the *Codex Alimentarius*, a collection of internationally adopted food standards, guidelines and codes of practice, sets forth the conditions under which permitted food additives may be used in foods [15]. Codex standards are voluntary and non-binding recommendations. Although their implementation is not controlled, many governments implement them because they see the benefit for their consumers and trade. The use of food additives may vary in concordance with national legal authorities, e.g. ammonium persulfate had formerly been used in a number of European countries (but not in the United States) as a "flour improver" to render the flower white. After

persulfate sensitivity had become a major problem among bakers, in the second half of the twentieth century, ammonium persulfate had been banned as a food additive in many European countries. In contrast, the FDA recently reviewed the safety of ammonium persulfate, and in 2008, approved its use as a multi-purpose food additive (<0.075%) for direct addition to food and as an indirect food additive in industrial starch (<0.3 or <0.6% in alkaline starch) in U.S. [19, 20].

Therefore, concerning specific food additives, national differences in legislation and subsequent use and exposure at the workplace have to be regarded in the allergological evaluation.

In the United States, more than 3,000 additives are on file with the Food and Drug Administration, of which more than half are regulated [19]. In Europe, where in 2002 the EFSA (European Food Safety Authority) succeeded the Scientific Committee on Foods as the keystone of European Union (EU) risk assessment regarding food and feed safety, the European Parliament and Council Directives (94/36/EC) and (95/2/EC) and subsequent amendments determine the legal grounds for colours and additives in foods. Table 44.1 gives an overview of food additives and contaminants that may cause contact allergic skin reactions upon skin contact in the individual chef or food handler. Contaminants of food of exogenous or endogenous/natural origin can complicate the process of identifying the offending agent [17]. Difficulties in identifying these agents (which may not be listed on the food label (e.g. contaminants)) and obstacles in obtaining such substances for the allergological examination may occur. Furthermore, except for patch testing for ACD, the diagnostic reliability of skin testing and in vitro tests with food additives is limited [17].

In spite of this ample variety of possible contact allergens in the occupational field of chefs and food handlers, which may be relevant in the individual case [14, 17], a limited number of contact allergens contribute to the majority of contact allergies [4, 21, 22]. Significantly higher rates of sensitization were found in employees of the food processing industry compared to the total test population for the following:

Table 44.1 Among the numerous food additives, several are known for having induced allergic contact dermatitis

I	Food additives	E-number	Predominant current uses in foods	Predominant type(s) of reaction
1.	*Preservatives*			
	Benzoic acid	E 210	Acidic foods/beverages, candied/dried fruits, fruit and vegetable preparations, fermented foods, salads, vinegar, dairy and egg-based deserts	NICU; ACD
	Benzoates	E 211–213	Acidic foods/beverages, candied/dried fruits, fruit and vegetable preparations, fermented foods, salads, vinegar, dairy and egg-based deserts	ACD; NICU
	Parabens	E 214–219	Fruit/vegetable purees, jams, juices, soft drinks, candy, milk, packaged meat/poultry/fish	ACD
	Sorbic acid	E 200	Baked goods, cheese, meat/fish products, fruits/vegetables, pickles, juices, wine	NICU; ACD
	Sorbates	E 201–203	Baked goods, cheese, meat/fish products, fruits/vegetables, pickles, juices, wine	ACD; NICU
2.	*Antioxidants*			
	Butylated hydroxyanisole	E 320	Breakfast cereals, baked goods, beverages, butter oil, vegetable oil/fat, ghee, fat emulsions, lard, tallow, fish oil other animal fats, spreads, confectionery, cocoa and chocolate products, decorations, toppings, ice cream, sherbet, desserts, milk powder, cream powder, frozen/canned/ fermented/dried/semi-preserved/smoked/salted fish and seafood, processed meats/poultry/game, dried vegetables, herbs, spices, seasonings, condiments, sauces, soups and broths, precooked pasta, chewing gum, processed nuts, potato snacks, yeast	ACD
	Butylated hydroxytoluene	E 321	As butylated hydroxyanisole	ACD
	Ethylenediamine		Indirect food additive: antimicrobial in cane sugar/beet sugar mills; food packaging adhesive and coating	ACD
	Dodecyl gallate (=lauryl gallat)	E 312	Margarine	ACD
	Octyl gallate	E 311	Margarine	ACD
	Propyl gallate	E 310	Breakfast cereals, baked goods, mixes for bakery products and soups, sauces, butter oil, ghee, vegetable oil/fat, fat emulsions, spreads, confectionary, decorations, cocoa and chocolate products, herbs, spices, seasonings, condiments, precooked pasta, desserts, milk powder, cream powder, processed meats/poultry/game, fermented/dried/smoked/salted fish and seafood, chewing gum, processed nuts, snacks (potato/cereal/flour/starch-based, whole/broken/flaked grains), rice, water-based flavoured and energy drinks-based and energy drinks	ACD

(*continued*)

Table 44.1 (continued)

I	Food additives	E-number	Predominant current uses in foods	Predominant type(s) of reaction
	Citrus red 2		Surface of oranges from Florida	ACD
	Ponceau (=cochineal Red A)	E 124	Alcoholic beverages, water-based flavoured drinks and energy drinks, dairy products, surface of cheese, canned fruits, fruit fillings/puree/spreads jams, jelly, marmalade, chewing gum, fine bakery ware, confectionary, surface decoration of chocolate, decorations, toppings, sweet sauces, ice cream, sherbet, syrups, desserts, surimi and fish roe, seafood, preserved/canned/fermented fish and seafood, edible casings, mustard, salads, sauces, seasonings, condiment, soups, broths, processed nuts, dietetic foods, surface labelling of eggs	ACD
	Tartrazine	E 102	Bakery products, bakery mixes, confectionary, water-based flavoured drinks and energy drinks, ice cream, sauces, desserts, snacks, soups and broth, cereals, rice and pasta products, candy, chewing gum, jams, jelly, marmalade, gelatins, mustards, horseradish, yogurt, pickled products, fruit squash[b]	NICU
	Sunset yellow	E 110	Alcoholic beverages, water-based flavoured drinks and energy drinks, dairy-based drinks, surface of cheese, breakfast cereals, fruit fillings/puree/spreads jams, jelly, marmalade, chewing gum, fine bakery ware, confection-ary, surface decoration of chocolate, further decorations, toppings, sweet sauces, ice cream, sherbet, syrups, desserts, surimi and fish roe, fish, seafood, fish and seafood, edible casings, instant noodles, snacks, mustard, fermented vegetables, animal derived fats/oils, sauces, seasonings, condiment, soups, broths, dietetic food	NICU
	Natural dyes			
	Carmine		Alcoholic beverages, water-based flavoured drinks and energy drinks, dairy products, bread products, batters, breakfast cereals, fruit fillings/puree/spreads jams, jelly, marmalade, surface of cheese, desserts, chewing gum, cocoa production, confectionary, decorations, toppings, sweet sauces, ice cream, sherbet, frozen/cooked/smoked fish and seafood, caviar, fish roe, mustard, sauces, soups, broths, snacks, Surface labelling of eggs and further fresh food	ACD; (spec. IgE, urticaria upon ingestion)
6.	*Bleaches*			
	Ammonium persulfate		Multi-purpose food additive (<0.075%) for direct addition to food, indirect food additive in industrial starch[c]	ACD, CU
	Potassium persulfate		Coating on fresh citrus fruits	ACD
	Benzoyl peroxide		Flour, wheat products	ACD
7.	Natural and synthetic flavours			
	Anethole		Anise-like scent and taste in alcoholic drinks, seasoning and confectionery applications, natural berry extracts	ACD
	Balsam of Peru		Contains about 200 components, which may be used in candy, chocolate, marzipan, bakery products, ice cream, desserts, water-based flavoured drinks, liquors, aromatised tea	ACD; NICU

(continued)

Table 44.1 (continued)

44

I	Food additives	E-number	Predominant current uses in foods	Predominant type(s) of reaction
	Carvone		L-carvone (=$R(-)$-carvone): scent and taste of spearmint, D-carvone (=$S(+)$-carvone): scent and taste of caraway	ACD
	Cinnamic acid		Scent and taste of cinnamon (e.g. in ice cream, candy, beverages, chewing gum)	ACD; NICU
	Cinnamic aldehyde		Scent and taste of cinnamon (e.g. in ice cream, candy, beverages, chewing gum)	ACD; NICU
	Citral		Citral A (=geranial): strong scent and taste of lemon. Citral B (=neral): less intense, but sweeter scent and taste of lemon	ACD
	Eugenol		Spicy, clove-like aroma	ACD
	Geraniol		Rose-like scent used in flavours such as peach, raspberry, grapefruit, red apple, plum, lime, orange, lemon, watermelon, pineapple and blueberry	ACD
	Limonene		D-limonene (=$R(+)$-limonen) strong scent of orange	ACD
	Linalool		Floral scent with a touch of spiciness: D-Linalool (=$S(+)$-linalool=coriandrol) is perceived as sweet and floral, whereas L-linalool (=$R(-)$-linalool=licareol) more woody and lavender-like	ACD
	Vanillin		Vanilla-taste. Used in ice cream, chocolate, confectionery and baked goods	ACD
II	*Exogenous contaminants*			
	Fertilizers, fungicides, herbicides, insecticides, lead, mercury		Plant foods	ACD, ICD
III	*Endogenous/natural contaminants*			
	Histamine		Eggplant, spinach, fermented foods, cheeses, alcoholic beverages, vinegars, microbial contamination of foods, histamine-releasing preservatives (e.g. benzoates)	NICU
	Serotonine		Mushrooms, walnut, plantain, pineapple, banana, kiwifruit, plums, tomatoes, chocolate	Itch may occur after ingestion or as cofactor when skin barrier function is impaired (however, of lesser potency than histamine)
	Nickel		Cocoa, chocolate, soy beans, oatmeal, hazelnuts and almonds, fresh and dried legumes	Flares of ACD may occur after ingestion[d]
	Cobalt		Fish, crustaceans, milk, dairy products, offal, dried fruits, nuts, condiment, oils, sugar, cereals (such as oats), broccoli and spinach	Flares of ACD may occur after ingestion[d]

Food additives and contaminants of reported potency to elicit allergic contact dermatitis upon skin contact (modified from [15, 19, 32–34])

[a]Banned in the US

[b]Banned in Norway

[c]In the US

[d]Skin contact with metal containing food has not been reported to initiate primary induction of contact sensitization [17]

- Compositae mix (food-related, since direct skin contact to compositae like lettuce, chicory, endive, iceberg lettuce, artichoke, mugwort etc. exists in food handling occupations)
- Thiuram mix (linked with preventive measures such as gloves)
- Formaldehyde (contained in disinfectants and cleaning agents)
- Nickel sulphate (which could be released from stainless steel cooking instruments) [4]
- A broad sensitization to flavouring agents or spices in food processing occupations could not be confirmed in this retrospective analysis [4].
- Sensitizations to gallates, sulfites and persulfates were only occasionally found [4].

For patch testing in food workers, patch testing of the standard, rubber and compositae series, as well as patients' own products according to the individual history and exposure, is recommended [4]. To rule out false-positive/irritant results obtained with non-standardized patient-specific natural food materials should be evaluated in the context of patch tests performed in (at least three) control individuals [14].

> For patch testing in food workers, patch testing of the standard, rubber and compositae series, as well as patients' own products according to the individual history and exposure, is recommended.

44.2.3 Elicitors of Phototoxic and Photoallergic Reactions in Food Handling Occupations

Phototoxic reactions ("phytophotodermatitis") may rarely occur in chefs and food handlers after skin contact with psoralen-containing plant material (e.g. fig, peel of lime, lemon, grapefruit, bitter and bergamot orange, carrot, celery, fennel, parsley and parsnip, dill, clove) and concomitant intense light exposure primarily in the UVA range (320–400 nm) [14].

Photoallergic reactions in which the allergen is photo-activated by either sunlight or artificial light in the UVA range as a prerequisite to incite a delayed hypersensitivity reaction (mostly including the dorsa of the hands, extensor forearms, face, posterior neck, ears, "V area" of the chest, superior aspects of the back and shoulders) may rarely occur in chefs and

food handlers after skin contact with food and spices (e.g. garlic) (see also Chap. 18 and 29).

44.2.4 Elicitors of Protein Contact Dermatitis, Immunological Contact Urticaria and Non-immunological Contact Urticaria in Food Handling Occupations

Chefs and food handlers belong to the occupations that are also at risk for PCD and OCU (see also Chaps. 7 and 21) [9, 23]. OCU can be subdivided into two categories: Immunological (IgE-mediated, e.g. due to foods) or, more frequently, non-immunological (NICU) due to a variety of low-molecular weight substances such as preservatives, fragrances and foodstuff [24, 25].

Most potent and best-studied food preservatives and flavouring triggering a NICU are benzoic acid, sodium benzoate, sorbic acid, abietic acid, nicotinic acid esters, cinnamic acid, cinnamic aldehyde and balsam of Peru [3, 9, 14]. Furthermore, foodstuff that contain a high genuine content of histamine (sauerkraut, pineapple, yeast, red wine, mature cheeses, pickled herring) and contaminated tuna, as well as those that cause direct release of histamine (strawberries, tomatoes and alcohol), are often associated with NICU [3].

NICU (with few exceptions) remains restricted to the site of skin contact and rarely causes systemic reactions [9].

In contrast, IgE-mediated OCU may not be limited to the contact site but may present as a multi-systemic disease (including generalized urticaria with or without angioedema, symptoms of the respiratory and gastrointestinal tracts, and as worst case, scenario anaphylactic shock) [26]. A great number of relevant protein allergens causing IgE-mediated allergic reactions to foods have been identified on molecular grounds [27]. For the current list of characterized food allergens, see "The Official List of Allergens" (http://www.allergen.org/Allergen.aspx) regularly updated by the Allergen Nomenclature Sub-committee that operates under the auspices of the International Union of Immunological Societies (IUIS). During food processing (e.g. cooking), conformational epitopes of the protein-allergen may be destroyed in many foods, leading to a reduced allergenicity and reduced skin test reactivity of the cooked product in some patients. However, this cannot be generalized for

44

all allergens and patients, as some allergens are heat resistant (e.g. lipid transfer proteins, LTP), and patients may be sensitized to linear epitopes as well, which are less prone to modification during the cooking process. Scientific approaches to reduce the allergen content of tedious highly cross-reactive panallergens present in various plant foods (e.g. profilin; LTP) have been successfully addressed and resulted in profilin-reduced and LTP-reduced tomatoes; however, these are far from being marketed [28].

The same protein sources causing OCU may induce PCD [7]. PCD in the food handling occupations most frequently presents as a chronic or recurrent eczema which usually affects the hands and forearms. However, sometimes the fingertips or proximal nail folds (i.e. chronic paronychia) may be involved exclusively [7, 10, 23]. In distinguishing PCD from hand eczema of other origin, associated immediate symptoms of burning, itching or stinging few minutes after skin contact may be relevant [23]. A reduced stratum corneum barrier integrity (e.g. due to atopic dermatitis or ICD) may facilitate penetration of high molecular weight proteins and induction of PCD [7, 10].

The ever-expanding list of occupational protein sources inducing PCD has been divided into four groups: group 1: fruits, vegetables, spices, plants, woods; group 2: animal proteins (e.g. epithelia, meat and body organs, various body fluids, dairy products, seafood etc); group 3: grains (e.g. rye, wheat, barley, oat, cornstarch); group 4: enzymes (e.g. α-amylase, glucoamylase, cellulase, xylanase, protease, papain) [7, 14, 23]. PCD (with or without accompanying respiratory symptoms) due to high molecular flour proteins (predominantly from wheat and rye) and enzymes used as dough enhancers (predominantly from α-amylase, less frequently due to Aspergillus niger-derived cellulase, hemicellulase and xylanase) are primarily reported among bakers [10, 29] (Fig. 44.1).

Diagnostic tests for IgE-mediated OSDs (OCU and PCD) include skin prick or scratch tests with the fresh and commercial material as well as *in vitro tests* for specific IgE (see also Chaps. 25 and 28). Scratch and scratch-patch (scratch chamber) tests may be helpful in the individual case, but bear a higher risk of irritant and false-positive reactions [7, 30]. Serially diluted allergens applied in prick and scratch tests are generally

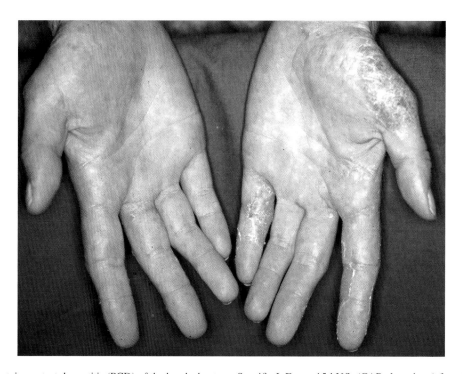

Fig. 44.1 Protein contact dermatitis (PCD) of the hands due to IgE-mediated reaction against wheat and rye flour and α-amylase in a 33-year-old female baker. The patient had an insignificant atopy score of five points. After having worked as a baker for 3 years, work-related rhino conjunctivitis first occurred (at age 31), and 2 years later, PCD of the hands, forearms and face. Specific IgE was 15 kU/L (CAP class three) for wheat and rye flour, skin prick tests were highly positive for wheat and rye flour (mean wheal diameter 6 mm) and α-amylase (mean wheal diameter 3 mm), whereas patch tests were negative. The respiratory symptoms as well as the skin lesions cleared entirely after contact to flour was stopped

regarded as safe, but since systemic reactions may occur rarely, a setting where trained personnel and resuscitation equipment are available is required for precautious reasons. Some authors have recommended open skin application testing prior to the performance of prick and scratch tests since it is thought to be less hazardous than these more invasive methods [9, 10]. Placing or rubbing the food on intact skin usually is negative. Therefore, the importance of applying this test on damaged or eczematous skin has been emphasized [9, 10, 30]. The test substances are applied for 15–30 min to the skin and readings are taken immediately after their removal, as well as 30 and 60 min later [9]. Suspected foods often give positive test results only with the native substances since commercial food extracts are often unreliable [9]. For example, wheat and rye flour skin prick test (SPT) solutions from three companies for diagnosis of type I-allergy in bakers differed extremely in protein concentrations and composition with the consequence of widely differing SPT results: Sensitivity of SPTs in comparison with allergen-specific bronchial challenge as a gold standard for respiratory symptoms was between 40 and 67% (i.e. 33–60% of SPTs were false-negative) [31]. Due to

Food allergens causing IgE-mediated immediate type reactions identified on molecular grounds are listed in the "The Official List of Allergens" provided by the IUIS (http://www.allergen.org/Allergen.aspx).

Protein sources inducing PCD belong to four groups: group 1: fruits, vegetables, spices, plants, woods; group 2: animal proteins; group 3: grains; group 4: enzymes.

these limitations, testing with several commercial SPT solutions at the time, as well as fresh food materials applied in a prick to prick test, is recommended. Patch tests (performed on intact skin) with food are usually negative in PCD [7, 10].

44.3 Conclusion for the Treatment of OSD in Chefs and Food Handlers

Chefs and food handlers belong to the group of occupations that are at (exceedingly) high risk for OSDs.

A complex variety of occupational exposures to irritants, contact and protein allergens is linked with the food handling occupations (as outlined above) and may result in seven different disease entities (ICD, ACD, immunological OCU, NICU, PCD, and rarely, phototoxic or photoallergic reactions). It should be kept in mind that the same substance can trigger several distinct mechanisms and may originate different clinical pictures in the affected individual.

The prerequisite for a successful treatment is the individual identification and exclusion of the disease eliciting factors. Diagnostic procedures include, according to the patient's history, patch testing of commercially available test series and individual foodstuff, rub and/or prick tests, in vitro tests, avoidance and/or provocation tests with the culprit substances/allergen(s), as well as an enduring implementation of a skin protection concept at the workplace.

References

1. Dickel H, Kuss O, Blesius CR, Schmidt A, Diepgen TL (2001) Occupational skin diseases in Northern Bavaria between 1990 and 1999: a population based study. Br J Dermatol 145:453–462
2. Tacke J, Schmidt A, Fartasch M, Diepgen TLD (1995) Occupational contact dermatitis in bakers, confectioners and cooks. A population-based study. Contact Dermatitis 33:112–117
3. Amado A, Jacob SE (2007) Contact dermatitis to foods. Actas Dermosifiliogr 98:452–458
4. Bauer A, Geier J, Elsner P (2002) Type IV allergy in the food processing industry: sensitization profiles in bakers, cooks and butchers. Contact Dermatitis 46:228–235
5. Dickel H, Kuss O, Schmidt A, Kretz J, Diepgen TL (2002) Importance of irritant contact dermatitis in occupational skin disease. Am J Clin Dermatol 3:283–289
6. Skoet R, Olsen J, Mathiesen B, Johansen JD, Agner T (2004) A survey of occupational hand eczema in Denmark. Contact Dermatitis 51:159–166
7. Amaro C, Goossens A (2008) Immunological occupational contact urticaria and contact dermatitis from proteins: a review. Contact Dermatitis 58:67–75
8. Bauer A, Bartsch R, Hersmann C, Stadeler M, Kelterer D, Schneider W, Seidel A, Schiele R, Elsner P (2001) Occupational hand dermatitis in food industry appretices: results of a 3-year follow-up cohort study. Int Arch Occup Environ Health 74:437–442
9. Doutre MS (2005) Occupational contact urticaria and protein contact dermatitis. Eur J Dermatol 15:419–424
10. Levin C, Warshaw E (2008) Protein contact dermatitis: allergens, pathogenesis, and management. Dermatitis 19:241–251
11. Dickel H, Bruckner TM, Schmidt A, Diepgen TL (2003) Impact of atopic skin diathesis on occupational skin disease. J Invest Dermatol 121:37–40

44

12. Bauer A, Kelterer D, Stadeler M, Schneider W, Kleesz P, Wollina U, Elsner P (2001) The prevention of occupational hand dermatitis in bakers, confectioners and employees in the catering trades. Preliminary results of a skin prevention program. Contact Dermatitis 44:85–88

13. Smith TA, Kanas RP, McCoubrey IA, Belton ME (2005) Code of practice for food handler activities. Occup Med 55:369–370

14. Brancaccio RB, Alvarez MS (2004) Contact allergy to food. Derm Ther 17:302–313

15. Codex Alimentarius (2008) "General Standard for Food Additives" (GSFA, Codex STAN 192-1995), 9th revision. http://www.codexalimentarius.net/gsfaonline/additives/index.html

16. Dooms-Goossens A, Dubelloy R, Degreef H (1990) Contact and systemic contact type dermatitis to spices. Dermatol Clin 8:89–93

17. Bahna SL (2004) Adverse food reactions by skin contact. Allergy 59(suppl 78):66–70

18. Van den Akker TW, Roesyanto Mahadi ID, Van Toorenenbergen AW, Van Joost T (1990) Contact allergy to spices. Contact Dermatitis 22:267–272

19. U.S. Food and Drug Administration. Center for Food Safety and Applied Nutrition: "Everything" Added to Food in the United States (EAFUS): A Food Additive Database of 17 Oct 2008. http://vm.cfsan.fda.gov/~dms/eafus.html

20. U.S. Food and Drug Administration (2008) Code of Federal Regulations, Title 21, Volume 3 (21CFR172.892): Subchapter B – Food for human consumption, Part 172 – Food additives permitted for direct addition to food for human consumption, Subpart I–Multipurpose Additives revised as of 1 Apr 2008

21. Dickel H, Kuss O, Schmidt A, Diepgen TL (2002) Occupational relevance of positive standard patch-test results in employed persons with an initial report of an occupational skin disease. Int Arch Occup Environ Health 75:423–434

22. Nethercott JR, Holness DL (1989) Occupational dermatitis in food handlers and bakers. J Am Acad Dermatol 21:485–490

23. Hjorth N, Roed-Petersen J (1976) Occupational protein contact dermatitis in food handlers. Contact Dermatitis 2:28–42

24. Wakelin SH (2001) Contact urticaria. Clin Exp Dermatol 26:132–136

25. Warner MR, Taylor JS, Leow YH (1997) Agents causing contact urticaria. Clin Dermatol 15:623–635

26. Von Krogh C, Maibach HI (1981) The contact urticaria syndrome. An update review. J Am Acad Dermatol 5:328–342

27. Chapman MD, Pomés A, Breiteneder H, Ferreira F (2007) Nomenclature and structural biology of allergens. J Allergy Clin Immunol 119:414–420

28. Le LQ, Mahler V, Lorenz Y, Scheurer S, Biemelt S, Vieths S, Sonnewald U (2006) Reduced allergenicity of tomato fruits harvested from Lyc e 1-silenced transgenic tomato plants. J Allergy Clin Immunol 118:1176–1183

29. Harris-Roberts J, Robinson E, Waterhouse JC, Billings CG, Proctor AR, Stocks-Greaves M, Rahman S, Evans G, Garrod A, Curran AD, Fishwick D (2009) Sensitization to wheat flour and enzymes and associated respiratory symptoms in British bakers. Am J Ind Med 52:133–140

30. Niinimäki A (1987) Scratch-chamber tests in food handler dermatitis. Contact Dermatitis 16:11–20

31. Sander I, Merget R, Degens PO, Goldscheid N, Brüning T, Raulf-Heimsoth M (2004) Comparison of wheat and rye flour skin prick test solutions for diagnosis of baker's asthma. Allergy 59:95–98

32. Bend J, Bolger M, Knaap AG, Kuznesof PM, Larsen JC, Mattia A, Meylan I, Pitt JI, Resnik S, Schlatter J,Vavasour E, Rao MV, Verger P, Walker R, Wallin H, Whitehouse B, Abbott PJ, Adegoke G, Baan R, Baines J, Barlow S, Benford D, Bruno A, Charrondiere R, Chen J, Choi M, DiNovi M, Fisher CE, Iseki N, Kawamura Y, Konishi Y, Lawrie S, Leblanc JC, Leclercq C, Lee HM, Moy G, Munro IC, Nishikawa A, Olempska-Beer Z, de Peuter G, Pronk ME, Renwick AG, Sheffer M, Sipes IG, Tritscher A, Soares LV, Wennberg A, Williams GM, Joint FAO/WHO Expert Committee on Food Additives (2007) Evaluation of certain food additives and contaminants. World Health Organ Tech Rep Ser 947:1–225

33. European Parliament and Council Directive (94/36/EC) of 30 June 1994 on colours for use in foodstuffs. http://ec.europa.eu/food/fs/sfp/addit_flavor/flav08_en.pdf

34. European Parliament and Council Directive (95/2/EC) of 20 Feb 1995 on food additives other than colours and sweeteners, as amended by Directives 96/85/EC, 98/72/EC and 2001/5/EC

Occupational Contact Dermatitis: Hairdressers

45

Heidi Søsted

Contents

H. Søsted
Research Centre for Hairdressers and Beauticians
Department of Dermato-Allergology
Copenhagen University Hospital Gentofte
Niels Andersens Vej 65, 2900 Hellerup-Denmark
e-mail: hesos@geh.regionh.dk

45.1 Epidemiology of Hand Eczema

Hairdressing is one of the occupations with the highest incidence of Occupational Contact Dermatitis in Europe [1, 2]. In United Kingdom, hairdressers had the highest incidence rate with 23.9/100,000 workers [3]. The annual prevalence of hand eczema is estimated to be 6–11% in the general population in Northern Europe [4–6], while it is around 13–18% among hairdressers [6].

The average incidence rate of hand dermatitis reported in a study on Dutch hairdressers was 32.8 cases per 100 person-years [7]. The risk of hairdressers having to leave the profession is most often because of asthma or hand eczema [8], and change of job due to hand eczema was reported almost 3 times more often by hairdressers than by a matched control group [6].

Hairdresser apprentices seem to be at high risk for developing occupational hand eczema compared to other occupations, though the debut age for hand eczema is 19–21 years [4, 9]. A German study shows that younger hairdressers have higher risk for developing hand eczema compared to older hairdressers [10], but this trend is probably seen because many hairdressers change career because of their skin problems. In many cases, the hand eczema is a combination of an irritant and allergic variety. A hairdresser can acquire a dry irritant dermatitis to the wet work while shampooing a client's hair or allergic contact dermatitis due to p-phenylenediamine (PPD) or toluene-2,5-diamine in the hair dye, see Fig. 45.1.

In an Irish study it was shown that up to 54.8% of the hairdressers with ACD or ICD left the occupation because of skin problems [11]. A similar investigation in Germany among hairdresser apprentices showed that 30.1% of those students that dropped out reported skin problems as the reason [12, 13]. Early intervention is, therefore, important.

J.D. Johansen et al. (eds.), *Contact Dermatitis*,
DOI: 10.1007/978-3-642-03827-3_45, © Springer-Verlag Berlin Heidelberg 2011

45

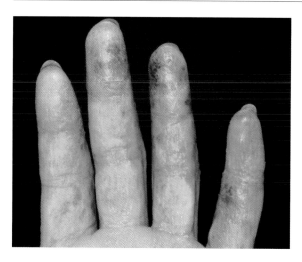

Fig. 45.1 Hand dermatitis and discolouration of the fingers in a 16-year-old female. She used to wash newly dyed hair in a hair dresser salon after school. Patch test was positive to PPD

45.1.1 Smoking

Tobacco smoking is known to influence various inflammatory skin diseases. Smoking among hairdressers, more than ten cigarettes per day, may result in a slightly increased risk of hand eczema [14].

45.1.2 Atopic Dermatitis

Diagnosed atopic dermatitis increases the risk of occupational skin or respiratory diseases threefold among hairdressers [15].

> **Core Message**
>
> › Hairdressing is a high-risk occupation for hand eczema.

45.1.3 Exposure to Allergens

Four basic chemical ingredients are responsible for the majority of contact allergies among hairdressers: Glyceryl monothioglycolate (GMT), PPD, toluene-2,5-diamine and ammonium persulfate. Among the preservatives, methylchloroisothiazolinone is an important

allergen [10, 16]. In a study where hairdressers worked with radiolabelled PPD, PPD was detected in the hairdressers' urine during working conditions, while PPD was under the limit of detection in blood samples [17].

45.1.3.1 Hair Dye

Hair dyes and precursors are some of the major allergens in hairdressers' dermatitis. Hair dyes as PPD, toluene-2,5-diamine, m-aminophenol, 2-methylresorcinol and the coupler resorcinol have been detected on hairdressers' hands during the working day in the salon. The dyes come from the products, newly dyed hair and also from the contaminated salon [18]. Hair dyes have especially been found on the hairdressers' hand after cutting and drying customers' hair [17].

45.1.3.2 Persulfates

Persulfates are used in (almost) every bleaching and highlighting product in a hairdresser's salon. Some companies have changed the formulation of the products from dust to granulate in order to decrease the number of bronchial reactions. However, still many hairdressers suffer from airway symptoms. In a Finnish study ammonium persulfate caused 90% of the respiratory diseases and 27% of hand dermatoses [15]. If hairdressers suffer from occupational rhinitis or asthma, they could be prick tested with ammonium persulfate [19]. Bronchial provocations with persulfates are possible, but a standardized method is needed [19].

45.1.3.3 Hydrogen Peroxide

Hydrogen peroxide is a part of oxidative hair dyes (see Table 34.1). It serves as an oxidizer, but is also able to bleach hair and used as a neutralizing agent in permanent waving. The usual patch test concentration is 3% aq. The substance is an irritant and can rarely cause contact dermatitis.

45.1.3.4 Glyceryl Monothioglycolate

GMT is an important ingredient in permanent wave products. GMT causes very severe cases of contact dermatitis, and many sensitized hairdressers are subject to disabling flare-ups, even when they are no longer working with GMT. This is caused by contamination of the hairdressing salons and persistence of the substance on clients' hair [10, 16]. A paper from European Environmental Contact Dermatitis Research Group showed great regional differences in Europe due to differences in the used products – highest figures for GMT in Germany, lowest in Finland and France; at that time, GMT perms were rarely used in these two latter countries [20]. GMT was removed from the German market by an agreement between the hairdressers' insurance agencies and manufacturers. Furthermore, a national legislation came into effect in 1995. This contributed to a significant decline of the incidence of occupational skin diseases among hairdressers between 1990 and 1999 [21]. Other European countries also saw a decrease in the use of GMT in their salons. Nowadays, German hairdressers are obliged to use gloves according to safety regulations of the insurance institutes. In Germany the frequency of positive patch test to GMT decreased from 31.2% in 1995/1996 to 7.5% in 2005/2006 [10, 22].

45.1.3.5 Cysteamine Hydrochloride

Due to the decrease of the use of GMT in permanent wave solutions in several European countries, suppliers of permanent wave solutions have started to market cysteamine hydrochloride. Cysteamine hydrochloride functions as a reducing agent and is found typically at concentrations between 5 and 12% in permanent solutions. Cross-reactions between cysteamine hydrochloride and thioglycolates are unlikely because they are structurally distinct from each other. But a Swedish hairdresser and 16 Dutch hairdressers were found to be sensitized to cysteamine hydrochloride, when tested 0.5% in pet, all of which were clinically relevant for their dermatitis (year 1994–2004). In all cases, there was an evident occupational exposure to cysteamine hydrochloride [23]. No cases have been reported since 2004 when searched on PubMed on the internet (28 May 2009 www.ncbi.nlm.nih.gov/sites/entrez).

45.1.3.6 Nickel

Nickel allergy is prevalent among hairdressers and it is an often raised question whether work tools can sensitize and elicit eczema in hairdressers. The prevalence of nickel allergy was found to be lower among young female hairdressers (11.3%) in comparison to older hairdressers (42.1%) in a Danish study. This may possibly be a result of the EU Nickel Directive or a consequence of a decreased use of nickel releasing work tools in salons. In hairdressers' salons in Copenhagen, Denmark, 200 scissors were dimethylglyoxime tested and only one scissor released nickel, while 7 out of 13 crochet hooks released nickel. Other areas of the world may have more inexpensive scissors that might release nickel. When nickel allergic hairdressers present with hand eczema, their work tools should be investigated for nickel release, when possible [24].

45.1.3.7 Fragrance Ingredients

An important group of allergens among hairdressers is fragrances. Among hairdressers seen at departments of dermatology in Germany, 10.2% had a positive patch test reaction to fragrance mix I, but fragrance mix II is also important since 6.3% had a positive reaction. Sensitization prevalences did not differ significantly between hairdressers and clients. The formulation of fragrance mixtures used in (hair) cosmetics undergoes continuous change, which results in a need for updating the hairdressing series. While the sensitization prevalence for fragrance mix I in hairdressers as well as in clients did not exceed 8.7% for all female patients in the period 2001–2004, a higher prevalence of sensitization towards hydroxyisohexyl 3-cyclohexenecarboxaldehyde in hairdressers was notable (4.7 vs. 2.7%) in the same period. It cannot be concluded from the data if this higher rate is due to occupational exposure or the high degree of personal use of decorative cosmetics or perfume among hairdressers. This limitation – the inability to definitely incriminate exposure to hair cosmetics as the source of sensitization – also applies to all other allergens not exclusively found in hair cosmetics [10].

45.1.3.8 Pyrogallol

Pyrogallol was forbidden in the European Union in 1992 and it is not likely to be a part of any legal cosmetic product any more [10]. Pyrogallol is normally not important in patch testing young European hairdressers.

45.1.3.9 Methyldibromo Glutaronitrile

The preservative methyldibromo glutaronitrile has been forbidden in cosmetic products in the European Union since 2007 [25].

45.2 Gloves

To prevent hand dermatitis, it is important that the hairdressers do not get in touch with hair dyes, bleaching agents or permanent wave products without wearing gloves. This includes a clean salon and very strict use of suitable gloves. Disposable nitrile rubber gloves have been tested for penetration of PPD, toluene-2,5-diamine sulphate and resorcinol, and no breakthrough was detected [26]. Disposable poly vinyl chloride (PVC) gloves cannot be used repeatedly when in contact with hair dyes. Furthermore, PVC can result in environmental problems. Natural latex gloves provide adequate protection against the chemicals, but induce the risk of sensitization to latex. Hydrogen peroxide (which is the oxidative agent in most oxidative hair dye products) did not accelerate chemical breakthrough [27]. Since nitrile gloves are suitable for the hairdresser work, these gloves are recommendable, but one should be aware of possible sensitizing thiuram and carbamate compounds. Research Centre for Hairdresser and Beauticians (Denmark) recommends disposable nitrile accelerator free gloves. They can be distributed by Abena A/S phone+45 74 31 17 00, but there could be several other companies selling gloves without thiuram and carbamates that are suitable for hairdressers.

> **Core Message**
>
> › Protective gloves that can reduce contact with the hairdressing chemicals are essential for preventing hand eczema. Disposable nitrile gloves are suitable to restrain chemicals in the hairdressers' work.

45.3 Nail Disorders

The human fingernail plate is highly keratinized. The keratin structure is held together by disulfide bonds. The organic elements – sulphur and nitrogen – occur almost exclusively in amino acids of the nail plate. Hairdressers who do not use gloves while working with dyes display in their fingernails significantly lower percentages of sulphur, but higher percentages of carbon than unexposed controls. The occupational use of chemical agents leads to decreased sulphur levels in the exposed persons, probably due to diminution of sulphur-rich proteins in the nails, resulting from destruction of disulfide bonds by alkaline and acid groups. Thus, the carbon/sulphur ratio seems to be a useful indicator for the amount of damage of nail protein by harmful agents. The observed changes in the hairdressers' fingernails were changes in colour and structure, changes in strength and pigmentation of the nails [28]. Some of the nail disorders in hairdressers' nails are caused by the chemicals they work with.

45.4 Contact Urticaria

Contact urticaria is not unusual among hairdressers because of their exposure to protein allergens in latex gloves, plants and certain low molecular weight substances. Contact urticaria gives a wheal-and-flare response within 30–60 min after exposure to certain agents, which disappears within 24 h and usually within a few hours. Sometimes the symptoms are itching, burning or tingling, alone or accompanied by erythema.

The whealing reactions can be strictly confined to the area of contact, but they can appear as generalized urticaria, sometimes associated with extra-cutaneous symptoms (bronchospasms, rhino-conjunctivitis, swelling of the upper airways, gastro-intestinal manifestations) and anaphylactic reactions. When urticaria has been induced by airborne contact (e.g. ammonium persulfate), the parts of the body most often affected are the uncovered areas [29].

> **Core Message**
>
> › To prevent hand eczema in hairdressers, reduction of skin-damaging exposures is essential.

Table 45.1 Allergens frequently reported in the hairdressers

Compound	Concentration/Vehicle % (w/w)
Bleaching	
Ammonium persulfate	2.5 pet
Fragrance	
Fragrance mix I	8.0% pet
Fragrance mix II	14% pet
Balsam Peru	25.0 pet
Hydroxyisohexyl-3-cyclohexene carboxaldehyde (Lyral)	5.0% pet
Gloves	
Thiuram mix	1.0% pet
Hair dyes	
p-Phenylenediamine[a]	1.0 pet
Toluene-2,5-diamine	1.0 pet
2-Nitro-4-phenylenediamine	1.0 pet
Resorcinol	1.0 pet
3-Aminophenol	1.0 pet
4-Aminophenol	1.0 pet
Hydroquinone	1.0 pet
Metals	
Nickel sulphate	5.0 pet
Cobalt chloride	1.0 pet
Permanent waving	
Ammonium thioglycolate	2.5 aq
Glyceryl Monothioglycolate	1.0 pet
Preservatives	
Chloroacetamide	0.2% pet
Formaldehyde	1.0 aq
Chlorocresol	1.0 pet
Chloroxylenol	1.0 pet
2-Bromo-2-nitropropane-1,3-diol	0.5 pet
Methylchloroisothiazolinone/methylisothiazolinone 3:1	0.01 aq
Imidazolidinyl urea	2.0 aq
Diazolidinyl urea	2.0 pet
Paraben mix	16 % pet
Others	
Cocamidopropylbetaine[b]	1.0 aq
Zink pyrithione	1.0 pet
Monoethanolamine (MEA)	2.0 pet

The table is based on different reports in the literature [9, 10, 32, 35]

In patch testing, especially of elderly hairdressers, the forbidden substances pyrogallol and captan (0.5% pet) can give positive reactions. Furthermore, it can still be relevant to patch test with the hair dye 4-Aminobenzenesulfonic acid (CAS No 121-57-3) that should not be sold to consumers in Europe after 18/6/2008 and methyldibromo glutaronitrile that has been forbidden recently [25]. If hairdressers suffer from occupational rhinitis or asthma, they should be prick tested with persulfates [36]

[a]In Standard tray

[b]Cocamidopropylbetaine often produces irritative reactions

45.5 Suggestions for a Patch Test Series for Hairdressers

Since hairdressers have a potential exposure to many different cosmetic products, it might be relevant to test hairdressers with different series. Table 45.1 is a suggestion for a "series for hairdressers", but optimally it can be relevant, furthermore, to test with allergens from the following series (available from Trolab®Hermal, Germany and Chemotechnique Diagnostics, Sweden):

- Cosmetic series (Trolab, Chemotechnique)
- Fragrance, essential oils (Trolab, Chemotechnique)
- Hairdressing (Trolab, Chemotechnique)
- Plant series, relevant in products containing herbal ingredients (Trolab, Chemotechnique)
- Preservatives (Trolab)
- Rubber additive series (gloves) (Trolab, Chemotechnique)
- Vehicles, emulsifiers (Trolab)

If it seems relevant in view of the clinical manifestations, it is recommended to test the hairdresser with the specific ingredients in products [30, 31]. Besides, it can be recommended to test hairdressers with an extended hair dye series (see Table 34.1). Many of these ingredients are currently not available from commercial patch test suppliers [32], but ingredients from the hair dyes in use in the saloon can be obtained from the producers.

Table 45.2 Prick testing with persulphates in hairdressers

If hairdressers suffer from occupational rhinitis or asthma, they should be prick tested with persulfate [36], in addition to standard prick testing with inhalant proteins and latex

Test solutions should be freshly prepared

Ammonium persulfate, 2% solutions [15] prepared by adding 0.7 mL sterile water to 14 mg ammonium persulfate [36]

Potassium persulfate, 2% solutions [15] prepared by adding 0.7 mL sterile water to 14 mg potassium persulfate [36]

This recommendation is based on a Finnish study where 138 patients were prick tested as above, seven patients who are all hairdressers had a positive prick test reaction to one of the persulfates and 20 controls were negative [36]. One should be aware that some of the hypersensitivity reactions to persulfates may be IgE-mediated [36]. Skin prick test results have showed that allergy to human dandruff and pityrosporum ovale was common among Finnish hairdressers [15]

45

Table 45.3 Protection of hands in hairdressers

Use disposable gloves when washing, colouring, styling newly coloured hair, bleaching and perming
Mix the hair dyes and bleaching in separate cupboard to prevent contamination of the salon
Cut the client's hair before colouring
Disposable gloves have to be new, clean and dry
Use a cotton glove inside the protection glove
Use gloves as long as needed, but as short as possible
Use a moisturizing cream without fragrances and with high lipid content before starting work and during the day
Apply moisturizing cream on your entire hands, particularly after work
Avoid wearing fingerrings on the job
Use protective gloves during wet work in your spare time
Use warm gloves when you are outside in the cold month
Never reuse disposable gloves

Recommendation to reduce contact with irritants and allergens. Based on Lind et al. [18]

45.6 Cancer

The occupational exposures of a hairdresser were classified by the International Agency for Research on cancer (IARC) as probably being carcinogenic (Group 2A) [33]. This classification has recently been supported by Italian researchers who suggest that hairdressers' occupational exposure can induce DNA damage in hairdressers with irritative contact dermatitis and increase the TNFa levels, particularly in hairdressers with allergic contact dermatitis [34].

References

1. Pal TM, de Wilde NS, van Beurden MM, Coenraads PJ, Bruynzeel DP (2009) Notification of occupational skin diseases by dermatologists in The Netherlands. Occup Med (Lond) 59:38–43
2. Skoet R, Olsen J, Mathiesen B, Iversen L, Johansen JD, Agner T (2004) A survey of occupational hand eczema in Denmark. Contact Derm 51:159–166
3. Shum KW, Meyer JD, Chen Y, Cherry N, Gawkrodger DJ (2003) Occupational contact dermatitis to nickel: experience of the British dermatologists (EPIDERM) and occupational physicians (OPRA) surveillance schemes. Occup Environ Med 60:954–957
4. Diepgen TL, Coenraads PJ (1999) The epidemiology of occupational contact dermatitis. Int Arch Occup Environ Health 72:496–506
5. Meding B, Jarvholm B (2002) Hand eczema in Swedish adults – changes in prevalence between 1983 and 1996. J Invest Dermatol 118:719–723
6. Lind ML, Albin M, Brisman J, Kronholm DK, Lillienberg L, Mikoczy Z, Nielsen J, Rylander L, Toren K, Meding B (2007) Incidence of hand eczema in female Swedish hairdressers. Occup Environ Med 64:191–195
7. Smit HA, van RA, Vandenbroucke JP, Coenraads PJ (1994) Susceptibility to and incidence of hand dermatitis in a cohort of apprentice hairdressers and nurses. Scand J Work Environ Health 20:113–121
8. Leino T, Tuomi K, Paakkulainen H, Klockars M (1999) Health reasons for leaving the profession as determined among Finnish hairdressers in 1980–1995. Int Arch Occup Environ Health 72:56–59
9. Valks R, Conde-Salazar L, Malfeito J, Ledo S (2005) Contact dermatitis in hairdressers, 10 years later: patch-test results in 300 hairdressers (1994 to 2003) and comparison with previous study. Dermatitis 16(1):28–31
10. Uter W, Lessmann H, Geier J, Schnuch A (2007) Contact allergy to hairdressing allergens in female hairdressers and clients–current data from the IVDK, 2003–2006. J Dtsch Dermatol Ges 5:993–1001
11. Laing ME, Powell FC, O'Sullivan D, Nagle CM, Keane FM (2006) The influence of contact dermatitis on career change in hairdressers. Contact Derm 54:218–219
12. Uter W, Pfahlberg A, Gefeller O, Schwanitz HJ (1998) Prevalence and incidence of hand dermatitis in hairdressing apprentices: results of the POSH study. Prevention of occupational skin disease in hairdressers. Int Arch Occup Environ Health 71:487–492
13. Uter W, Pfahlberg A, Gefeller O, Schwanitz HJ (1999) Hand dermatitis in a prospectively-followed cohort of hairdressing apprentices: final results of the POSH study. Prevention of occupational skin disease in hairdressers. Contact Derm 41:280–286
14. Meding B, Alderling M, Albin M, Brisman J, Wrangsjo K (2009) Does tobacco smoking influence the occurrence of hand eczema? Br J Dermatol 160:514–518. Ref Type: Journal
15. Leino T, Tammilehto L, Hytonen M, Sala E, Paakkulainen H, Kanerva L (1998) Occupational skin and respiratory diseases among hairdressers. Scand J Work Environ Health 24:398–406
16. van der Walle HB (1994) Dermatitis in hairdressers (II). Management and prevention. Contact Derm 30:265–270
17. Hueber-Becker F, Nohynek GJ, Dufour EK, Meuling WJ, De Bie AT, Toutain H, Bolt HM (2007) Occupational exposure of hairdressers to [14C]-para-phenylenediamine-containing oxidative hair dyes: a mass balance study. Food Chem Toxicol 45:160–169
18. Lind ML, Boman A, Sollenberg J, Johnsson S, Hagelthorn G, Meding B (2005) Occupational dermal exposure to permanent hair dyes among hairdressers. Ann Occup Hyg 49: 473–480
19. Moscato G, Pignatti P, Yacoub MR, Romano C, Spezia S, Perfetti L (2005) Occupational asthma and occupational rhinitis in hairdressers. Chest 128:3590–3598
20. Frosch PJ, Burrows D, Camarasa JG, Dooms-Goossens A, Ducombs G, Lahti A, Menne T, Rycroft RJ, Shaw S, White IR (1993) Allergic reactions to a hairdressers' series: results from

9 European centres. The European Environmental and Contact Dermatitis Research Group (EECDRG). Contact Derm 28: 180–183

21. Dickel H, Kuss O, Schmidt A, Diepgen TL (2002) Impact of preventive strategies on trend of occupational skin disease in hairdressers: population based register study. BMJ 324: 1422–1423

22. Uter W, Lessmann H, Geier J, Schnuch A (2003) Contact allergy to ingredients of hair cosmetics in female hairdressers and clients – an 8-year analysis of IVDK data. Contact Derm 49:236–240

23. Isaksson M, van der WH (2007) Occupational contact allergy to cysteamine hydrochloride in permanent-wave solutions. Contact Derm 56:295–296

24. Thyssen JP, Milting K, Bregnhøj A, Søsted H, Johansen JD, Menné T (2009) Nickel allergy in patch tested female hairdressers and assessment of nickel release from hairdressers work tools. Contact Derm 61(5):281–286

25. Council directive 76/768/EEC of 27 July 1976 on the approximation of the laws of the member states relating to cosmetic products, amended. European Communities off. Journal L262 27.9.1976

26. Lind ML, Johnsson S, Meding B, Boman A (2007) Permeability of hair dye compounds p-phenylenediamine, toluene-2, 5-diaminesulfate and resorcinol through protective gloves in hairdressing. Ann Occup Hyg 51:479–485

27. Lee HS, Lin YW (2009) Permeation of hair dye ingredients, p-phenylenediamine and aminophenol isomers, through protective gloves. Ann Occup Hyg 53:289–296

28. Schumacher E, Dindorf W, Dittmar M (2009) Exposure to toxic agents alters organic elemental composition in human fingernails. Sci Total Environ 407:2151–2157

29. Doutre MS (2005) Occupational contact urticaria and protein contact dermatitis. Eur J Dermatol 15:419–424

30. Sosted H, Menné T (2005) Allergy to 3-nitro-p-hydroxyethylaminophenol and 4-amino-3-nitrophenol in a hair dye. Contact Derm 52:317–319

31. Sosted H, Nielsen NH, Menné T (2009) Allergic contact dermatitis to the hair dye 6-methoxy-2-methylamino-3-aminopyridine HCl (INCI HC Blue no. 7) without cross-sensitivity to PPD. Contact Derm 60:236–237

32. Sosted H, Basketter DA, Estrada E, Johansen JD, Patlewicz GY (2004) Ranking of hair dye substances according to predicted sensitization potenzy – quantitative structure-activity relationships. Contact Derm 51:241–254

33. Anon (1993) Occupational exposures of hairdressers and barbers and personal use of hair colourants. IARC Monogr Eval Carcinog Risks Hum 57:43–118

34. Cavallo D, Ursini CL, Setini A, Chianese C, Cristaudo A, Iavicoli S (2005) DNA damage and TNFalpha cytokine production in hairdressers with contact dermatitis. Contact Derm 53:125–129

35. Test advice for Hairdressers (2009) http://www.hermal.de/her_en/gfx/trolab/trolab_downloads/Hairdressers_05_08.pdf

36. Aalto-Korte K, Makinen-Kiljunen S (2003) Specific immunoglobulin E in patients with immediate persulfate hypersensitivity. Contact Derm 49:22–25

Plants and Plant Products

46

Christophe J. Le Coz, Georges Ducombs, and Evy Paulsen

Contents

C.J. Le Coz (✉)
Cabinet de Dermatologie, Laboratoire de Dermatochimie,
4 rue Blaise Pascal, 67070 Strasbourg, France
e-mail: christophe.lecoz@wanadoo.fr

G. Ducombs
Cabinet de Dermatologie, 50 Avenue Thiers, 33100 Bordeaux,
France

E. Paulsen
Department of Dermatology, Odense University Hospital,
5000 Odense, Denmark

46.1 Introduction

Contact dermatitis from plants or plant products, *phytodermatitis*, is frequently observed in clinical practice. It is likely that the most frequent reactions of this type, which occur due to occasional and irritant contacts such as those encountered during leisure activities, are not seen by dermatologists. Practitioners usually come across more severe dermatitis cases, with irritant or allergic mechanisms, of immediate or delayed type and sometimes photoworsened or even photoinduced dermatitis.

The exact incidence of dermatitis from plants and plant products is not known, but this problem is not rare. Many patients likely self-medicate following self-diagnosis or diagnosis by a pharmacist or attend their family doctor who prescribes palliative treatment without necessarily ascertaining the cause of the skin reaction. In other instances, cases do reach the dermatologist. For example, among 1,752 patients

J.D. Johansen et al. (eds.), *Contact Dermatitis*,
DOI: 10.1007/978-3-642-03827-3_46, © Springer-Verlag Berlin Heidelberg 2011

considered to have occupational dermatitis, Fregert found that 8% of women and 6% of men were reacting to plant-derived products [1]. We can, therefore, estimate that among patients attending dermatologic clinics for dermatitis, an average of 5–10% suffer from dermatitis caused by plants or plant products. It is, however, evident that geographical variations in flora considerably influence the epidemiology of plant dermatitis.

In Europe, many phytodermatitis cases are occupationally acquired. Florists, gardeners, horticulturists, foresters, woodworkers, farmers, cookers, and people in contact with food preparation are at risk, as described by Paulsen [2–4]. Hobby gardeners, housewives, and those who handle or come into contact with plant materials nonoccupationally are also at risk. Indeed, any people enjoying leisure pursuits in the garden or countryside (children playing, campers, walkers, and so on) are likely to come into contact with plant material with the potential to cause contact dermatitis.

For plants and plant products, reactions of mixed etiology are frequent, like allergic reactions superimposed on irritant reactions due to Asteraceae, or mechanical plus chemical irritations evoked by stinging nettles. It is frequently hard to distinguish between allergic and irritant mechanisms in clinical examination and during patch test procedure, and the reader will have to bear this in mind constantly. We will limit this chapter to plant contact and will not consider the effect of systemic administration of plants or plant extracts.

It is clearly impossible to provide an exhaustive catalog of cutaneous side effects of plants in this chapter and the reader will sometimes be invited to examine the question in more detail using other sources. Some books are prominent in botanical dermatology, like those written by Mitchell and Rook [5], Lovell [6], Sell [7], or Benezra, Ducombs, Sell and Foussereau [8]. Others focus on, are devoted to, or are restricted to geographical areas [9]. Many (but not all) important medical articles and reviews are indexed in international databases like the United States National Library of Medicine (see http://www.nlm.nih.gov/). We also warmly recommend the website BoDD (Botanical Dermatology Database, owner Richard J. Schmitt, see http://bodd.cf.ac.uk/) for its interesting content [10] and the website Botaderma (owners Jean-Claude Rzeznik & Yves Sell, see http://botaderma.com) that proposes a very interesting and practical system to identify the offending plant [11].

46.2 Clinical Pictures

46.2.1 Immediate-Type Reactions

The types of reaction reviewed in this section belong to the class of immediate responses that have immunological or nonimmunological mechanisms.

46.2.1.1 Contact Urticaria

Contact urticaria appears within minutes following contact with the plant. It has been described for various species [12, 13].

Nonimmunological Contact Urticaria

Probably, the best-known urticant plants are the nettles belonging to family Urticaceae, like *Urtica dioica* L., *U. urens* L., and *U. pilulifera* L. The stinging hairs are disposed on the ventral faces of the leaves, permitting skin penetration of histamine, acetylcholine and 5-hydroxytryptamine after only a very slight touch. Nettles are used for rheumatic disorders in folk medicine [7, 14].

Among other nonprotein substances, plant-derived pharmacological elicitors of urticaria are numerous and include *Myroxylon pereirae* (balsam of Peru) and the cinnamic acid derivatives contained therein (Fig. 46.1), thapsigargin from *Thapsia garganica* L. (family Apiaceae) [12, 15, 16], and capsaicin from different species of capsicum, such as paprika and cayenne (*Capsicum* spp., family Solanaceae). The mechanism by which nonimmunologic urticant agents elicit their effect (at least for those agents listed above) appears to involve the release of histamine from mast cells.

> **Core Message**
>
> › Contact urticaria from nonprotein chemicals is most often due to a nonimmunological mechanism.

Immunological (IgE-mediated) Contact Urticaria

Fruits and vegetables may induce allergic contact urticaria, mainly in people with previous dermatitis,

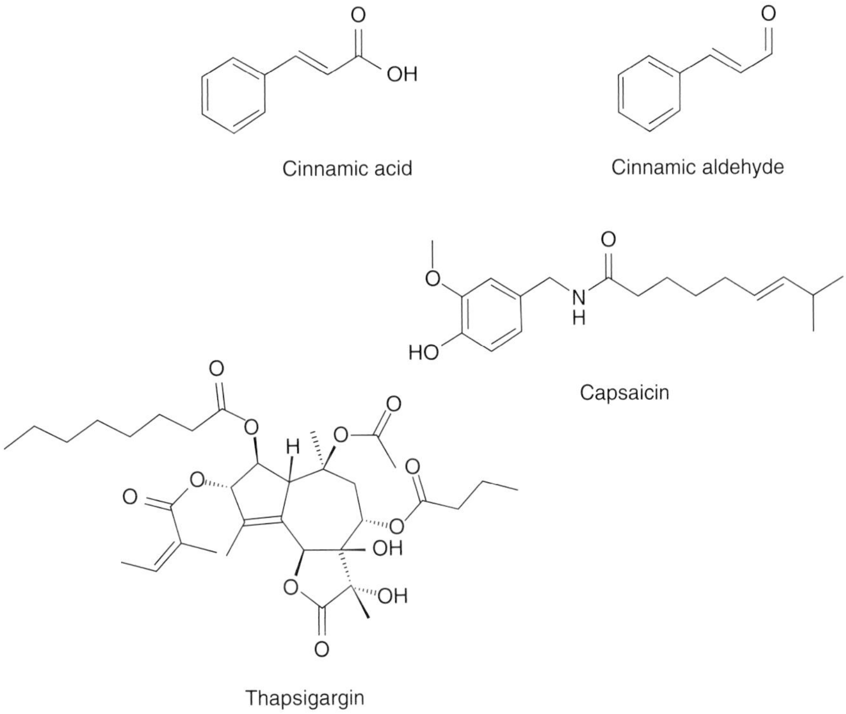

Fig. 46.1 Cinnamic acid, CAS
621–82–9, cinnamic aldehyde,
CAS 104–55–2, thapsigargin,
CAS 67526–95–8 and
capsaicin CAS 404–86–4

Cinnamic acid   Cinnamic aldehyde

Capsaicin

Thapsigargin

like atopic dermatitis (see Sect. 46.2.1.2). For example, sensitization from birch pollen (*Betula alba* L.,
family Betulaceae) may be complicated by immediate symptoms occurring after ingestion (mouth
swelling) or skin contact (contact urticaria) due to
apples, hazelnuts, almonds, plums, apricot, peach,
cherries, or celery and carrot. This is due to strong
homologies with the birch pollen allergens Bet v 1
and/or Bet v 2.

A case report of occupational contact urticaria and
type I sensitization attributable to a gerbera (probably
Gerbera jamesonii Bolus, family Asteraceae) has been
reported. Conjunctivitis and respiratory symptoms are
possible [17].

Airborne contact urticaria can be associated with
rhinitis, conjunctivitis, or asthma. This has been
largely reported as an occupational problem in health
workers with hypersensitivity to latex proteins from
rubber gloves made with natural latex (usually derived
from *Hevea brasiliensis* Muell.Arg., family
Euphorbiaceae). Airborne transmission of the latex
allergens is enhanced by their adsorption onto the
cornstarch (derived from *Zea mays* L., family
Gramineae) used as glove powder [18]. Airborne contact urticaria reported in a warehouseman resulted
from exposure to dust derived from cinchona bark
(*Cinchona* spp., family Rubiaceae) [19].

Allergic urticaria may spread from the initial site of
contact, become generalized, or be associated with
systemic symptoms of anaphylaxis.

> **Core Message**
>
> › Immunologic-type contact urticaria is due to spe-
>   cific IgE synthesis, mainly to proteins, and can be
>   severe, with generalized or systemic symptoms.

46.2.1.2 Protein Contact Dermatitis

Protein contact dermatitis is mostly seen in people
(with atopy in 50% of cases) who handle food, meat,
or vegetables and has been described with frequent
food like onion, lettuce, potato, carrot, or more rarely,
with asparagus (personal observation). It generally
consists of a chronic dermatitis, mainly located on
hands and forearms, with acute urticaria appearing
within minutes of contact with food proteins, which
rapidly disappears. It is followed by the worsening of
the dermatitis within hours or days [20–24]. Protein
contact dermatitis can be of irritant (nonspecific) or
allergic (IgE-mediated) type. In such cases, atopy with
immediate-type sensitizations to pollens is frequent.

46

> **Core Message**

> › Protein contact dermatitis due to plant or plant
> products consists of contact urticaria followed
> by the worsening of a previous dermatitis,
> mainly occurring in food handlers.

46.2.2 Irritant Contact Dermatitis

46.2.2.1 Mechanical Irritation

A number of plants can provoke "macrotraumatic"
injury by mechanical means due to their armament of
prickles, spines, or thorns. Others, because of the knife-
like morphologies of their leaf edges, may lacerate the
skin. Although typically a trivial and self-limiting event,
such mechanical damage may lead to the development
of sores, secondary infections such as pyodermitis or
tetanus, and granulomatous lesions that may develop
insidiously some time after the initial trauma, after it
has been forgotten. For instance, in arid regions of the
Americas, cacti (family Cactaceae) are responsible for
injuries that may become granulomatous, after dermal
embedding of plant material [25, 26] (Fig. 46.2).

Certain plants are injurious because their bristles or
barbs (named *trichomes* or *glochids*, respectively) can
cause "microtrauma." These structures can penetrate
the outer layer of the skin and cause papular dermatitis, prurigo, and even symptoms of urticaria. In 1956,
Shanon and Sagher [27] described "Sabra dermatitis"
due to occupational contact with the prickly pear, also
named the Indian or Barbary fig (*Opuntia ficus-indica*
Miller, family Cactaceae) (Fig. 46.3). Dermatitis is
caused by penetration of glochids from the spine cushions of the plants and their fruits through the skin, and
it simulates chronic eczema or scabies.

Microtrauma (and chemical irritant action) from calcium oxalate needle crystals (named *raphides*) also
causes a characteristic dermatitis resembling that from
glass fiber [28]. Irritant contact dermatitis occur almost
systematically in people who handle plants that contain
crystals such as blue agave (*Agave tequilana* Weber)
[29]. Penetration of such raphides into the skin may be
accompanied by intracutaneous injection of plant sap.
This can result in an irritant or allergic skin reaction to
one or more of the sap constituents. Thus, preparation of
the tubers of various aroids (plants of Araceae family)

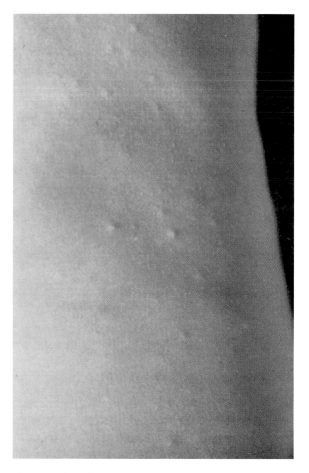

Fig. 46.2 Granulomatous lesions on a child's arm from cactus
(courtesy of F. Vakilzadeh)

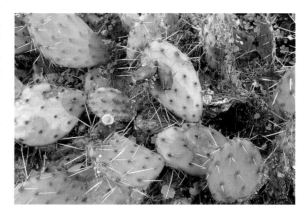

Fig. 46.3 Indian or Barbary fig (*Opuntia ficus-indica* Miller,
family Cactaceae)

for food use (for example the malanga or cocoyam,
Xanthosoma sagittifolium L.) carries with it the risk of
dermatitis from the calcium oxalate needle crystals and
the saponins it contains [30]. Similarly, calcium oxalate

raphides in dumbcanes (*Dieffenbachia* spp., family Araceae), which are commonly grown as decorative house plants, are responsible for an edematous urticaria-like dermatitis, and/or an edematous and bullous stomatitis in people who have handled damaged plant material or accidentally chewed the leaves. The reaction in the mouth renders the victim speechless (hence the common name of the plant, dumbcanes) and may even be life-threatening if the airway becomes obstructed. The severity of the reaction has been ascribed to the presence of a protease named dumbcain in the plant sap, which contributes to the irritant reaction [31].

> ### Core Message
>
> › Trauma due to plants may be due to several mechanisms. Prickles, spines, or thorns provoke macrotraumas, and leaves may act like knifes. Microtrauma may be due to dermo-epidermic penetration of trichomes (bristles), glochids (barbs), or raphides (calcium oxalate needle crystals).

46.2.2.2 Chemical Irritation

Many plants contain irritant substances (Table 46.1) that vary from weakly irritant compounds, requiring repeated exposure or a damaged skin barrier to exert their effects, to some of the most irritant compounds known to Man, which can elicit inflammation in microgram quantities, like those contained in Euphorbiaceae. Such potent skin irritants are also mucous membrane irritants and can cause violent purgation after ingestion and intense ocular irritation that may lead to blindness when there is contact with the eyes. The mechanical role of calcium oxalate needles has been described above; they, moreover, enhance the action of toxic chemicals such as the proteloytic enzyme bromelain (of pineapple), or the toxic glucosides contained herein, the so-called saponins.

Acute irritant dermatitis can arise after some minutes or hours. Chronic dermatitis develops after repeated contact with the irritant agent or on the background of previous contact with weakened skin. The clinical presentation of irritant contact dermatitis is various, but lesions are generally monomorphous in a patient (as with burns) and are limited to sites of contact, such as the hands, forearms, mucous membranes, perioral regions, buttocks, and so on. They consist of simple dryness of the skin, cracking and hyperkeratosis, inflammatory reactions with edema, erythema, papules, and vesicles. Pain, rather than itching, is also a feature. Strong irritant plants like spurges (*Euphorbia* spp., family Euphorbiaceae) may induce blisters, ulceration, or necrosis by the way of their acrid milky juice. Ranunculaceae, such as *Ranunculus bulbosus* L. or *R. repens* L., are sometimes used in traditional medicine and have been reported to be strong irritants, inducing bullous or even necrotizing dermatitis by the way of ranunculin [7, 14, 32].

> ### Core Message
>
> › Chemical irritation from plants (such as Euphorbiaceae) may induce severe chemical burns.

46.2.3 Allergic Contact Dermatitis

Allergic contact dermatitis (ACD) from plants can present in many forms, depending upon both the allergen and the method of exposure. Typical forms are represented by acute ACD, fingertips or periungueal chronic ACD, airborne ACD, contact urticaria, and erythema multiforme-like eruptions.

46.2.3.1 Acute ACD: Acute Eczema

The normal presentation is that of a typical ACD, involving exposed parts such as the hands, forearms, eyelids, and sometimes the genitals if the allergen is transported by the hands or clothing. Lesions' onset at the site of contact is frequently diffuse, spreading on unexposed areas. The initial maculopapular or vesicular eruption may provoke blisters or develop into a full-blown erythroderma, for example, with *Frullania* (Jubulaceae family) dermatitis.

46.2.3.2 Chronic ACD and the Example of "Tulip Fingers"

A number of examples of usually occupationally acquired finger dermatitis have been described, with some typical features. This takes the form of fingertip dermatitis, painful rather than pruritic, fissured and hyperkeratotic, of which the best-known example is "tulip fingers," seen in tulip pickers (*Tulipa* spp. and cultivars, family Liliaceae).

Table 46.1 Main plants responsible for chemical irritant contact dermatitis

Family	Botanical name	English name	French name	German name	Offending chemicals
Agavaceae	*Agave americana* Linné	Agave	Agave d'Amérique	Amerikanische Agave	Calcium oxalate Sapogenins
Amaryllidaceae	*Narcissus pseudo-narcissus*	Daffodil	Jonquille	Gelbe Narzisse	Calcium oxalate
	Narcissus poeticus L.	Poet's narcissus	Narcisse des poètes	Dichternarzisse	Calcium oxalate
Araceae	*Dieffenbachia picta* Schott	Dumb cane	Dieffenbachia	Dieffenbachie	Calcium oxalate
	Philodendron spp.	Philodendron	Philodendron	Baumlieb	
Bromeliaceae	*Ananas cosmosus*	Pineapple Bromel(a)in	Ananas	Ananas	Calcium oxalate
Brassicaceae	*Armoracia rusticana*	Horse radish	Raifort	Meerrettich	Isothiocyanates
	Brassica oleracea var. *italica*	Broccoli	Brocoli	Brokkoli	
	Brassica nigra L.	True mustard	Moutarde noire	Schwarzer Senf	
	Raphanus sativus L. var. *sativus*	Small radish	Radis	Radieschen	
	Sinapis alba L.	White mustard	Moutarde blanche	Weisser Senf	
Euphorbiaceae	*Euphorbia* spp.	Spurge	Euphorbe	Wolfsmilch	Latex
	Euphorbia pulcherrima Willdenow	Poinsettia	Poinsettia	Weinachtsstern	Esters of phorbol
	Codiaeum variegatum	Croton	Croton	Wunderstrauch	Esters of ingenol
	Hippomane mancinella	Manchineel tree	Mancellinier	Manzanillbaum	
	Ricinus communis L.	Castor bean	Ricin	Rizinus, Wunderbaum	
Liliaceae	*Hyacinthus orientalis* L.	Hyacinth	Jacinthe	Gartenhyazinthe	Calcium oxalate
Polygonaceae	*Rheum rhaponticum* L.	Rhubarb	Rhubarbe	Rhabarber	Calcium oxalate
Ranunculaceae	*Anemone pavonina* Lam.	Anemone	Anémone	Anemone	Protoanemonin
	Ranunculus acer L.	Meadow butter-cup	Bouton d'or	Butterblume	
	Aquilegia vulgaris L.	Columbine	Ancolie des jardins	Gemeine Akelei	
	Caltha palustris L.	Yellow marsh marigold	Souci d'eau	Sumpfdotterblume	
Solanaceae	*Capsicum frutescens* L.	Chillies	Piment de Cayenne, langue d'oiseau	Cayennepfeffer	Capsaicin
	Capsicum annuum L.	Sweet pepper, capsicum	Poivron, piment doux and piment fort	Tachepfeffer, paprika	

Fig. 46.4 (**a**) *Alstroemeria* spp. family Alstroemeriaceae. (**b**) Allergic contact dermatitis in a nursery gardener from Alstroemeria (courtesy of P.J. Frosch)

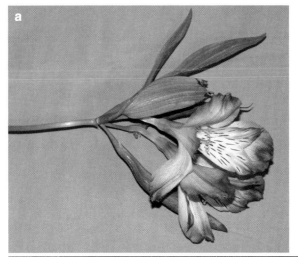

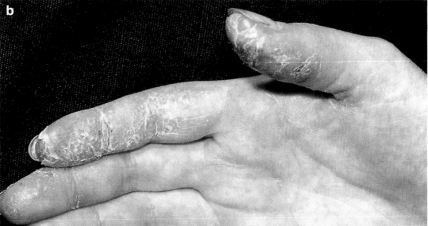

Lesions frequently spread on periungueal sites, inducing onychosis. Similar reactions may arise in people handling daffodil and narcissus bulbs (*Narcissus* spp. and cultivars, family Amaryllidaceae), Alstroemeria flowers (*Alstroemeria* spp. and cultivars, family Alstroemeriaceae) (Fig. 46.4a, b), garlic (*Allium sativum* L., family Alliaceae), and so on. The most frequently involved fingers are those that are in direct and prolonged contact with the bulb. For garlic dermatitis in cooks, the nondominant hand is generally involved, since it is the one used to maintain the bulb. Although nominally an immunological delayed-type reaction, tulip fingers and related eruptions such as "daffodil itch" or "lily rash" in daffodil bulb or flower handlers [33] may arise in part from mechanical and/or chemical irritation.

46.2.3.3 Erythema Multiforme-like and Atypical Dermatitis

Bonnevie first described an erythema multiforme-like rash that developed after contact with leaves of *Primula obconica* Hance (family Primulaceae) [34]. The clinical picture resembles that of a drug eruption, with confluent pseudo-cockades arising on the contact area. Histopathological features are those of ACD with severe edema and keratinocyte necrosis. Several authors have reported similar features following contact with poison ivy [35] or tropical woods such as Rio rosewood (*Dalbergia nigra* Allemão; pao ferro, *Machaerium scleroxylon* Tul., family Leguminosae) [36–39] (Fig. 46.5). Further nonoccupational cases

46

Fig. 46.5 Erythema multiforme-like reaction in a carpenter caused by wood dust (pao ferro) (courtesy of P.J. Frosch)

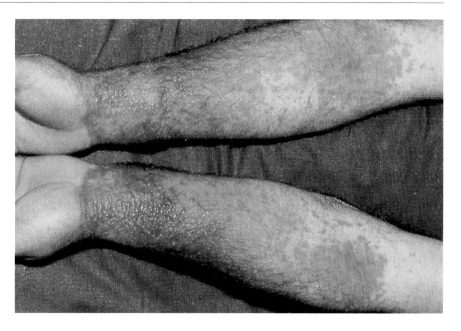

have been reported in the literature. An occupationally acquired airborne erythema multiforme-like eruption was due to pyrethrum (*Tanacetum* spp., family Compositae) used as a pesticide [40].

Erythema multiforme-like dermatitis can be the expression of an active sensitization for several days following initial contact [41].

Intense blistering can evoke pemphigoid, as was observed in the wife of a woodworker who had been helping her husband work with bois d'Olon, a kind of satinwood (*Fagara heitzii* Aubrév. and Pellegrin, family Rutaceae) [42].

46.2.3.4 Airborne Contact Dermatitis

Hjorth et al [43] described an airborne ACD of plant origin, due to air-conveyed oleoresins of Compositae, mimicking and often misdiagnosed as a photodermatitis. However, some features may differentiate it from photodermatitis, since airborne contact dermatitis involves the upper eyelids, the triangle of skin behind the earlobe, and the backs of facial folds without involving the the triangle under the chin (Fig. 46.6). Although pollens were formerly incriminated as the causative agents of airborne phytodermatitis, it is likely that finely pulverized materials derived from dead plants are the more likely etiological agents in the case of ragweeds (*Ambrosia* spp.) and related members of the Compositae family. The final proof that airborne plant material may carry allergens was obtained in the case of feverfew (*Tanacetum parthenium* (L) Schultz-Bip.) when the nonvolatile sesquiterpene lactone parthenolide was isolated from plant particles trapped in a high volume air sampler [44]. Vaporized allergens may be responsible for airborne contact dermatitis in florists exposed to chrysanthemums (*Dendranthema* cultivars, family Compositae) ([45] or to *Alstroemeria* L. [46]). It was also noted that simply walking in a forest may bring on an attack of eczema in patients who are sensitized to liverworts of the genus Frullania (*Frullania dilatata Dum.*, family Jubulaceae for example), suggesting that either particles of liverwort or vaporized allergens are the causative agents [47]. Other reports describe airborne contact dermatitis from lichen particles [48, 49] or pine dust (unidentified species of the family Pinaceae) [50]. The last cases exhibited positive patch test reactions to colophony.

In North America and elsewhere, it is recognized that the smoke from burning poison ivy (*Toxicodendron* spp.) and related plants in the Anacardiaceae family may sensitize if the allergenic oleoresin is vaporized rather than pyrolyzed [51]. Airborne contact dermatitis to feverfew or congress grass (*Parthenium hysterophorus* L., Asteraceae family) is a major dermatological problem, particularly in northern India. The classical form involves exposed areas, but seborrheic-like dermatitis, widespread dermatitis, photosensitive lichenoid

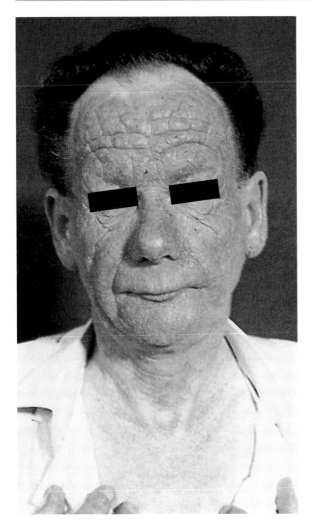

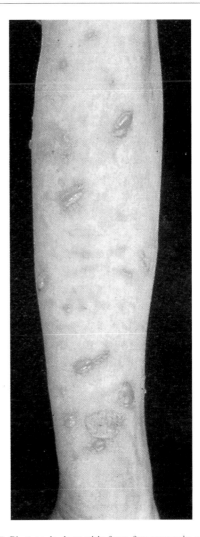

Fig. 46.6 Airborne contact dermatitis from Compositae in a farmer. Note the marked infiltration on the forehead and the sharp upper border from wearing a hat (courtesy of N. Hjorth)

Fig. 46.7 Phototoxic dermatitis from furocoumarin-containing plants (courtesy of P.J. Frosch)

reactions, and prurigo nodularis-like eruptions have been reported [9, 52]. Patients suffer seasonal relapses, but sensitivity is lifelong and sometimes complicated by the development of photosensitivity [52].

46.2.4 Photodermatitis (Phytophotodermatitis)

46.2.4.1 Phytophototoxicity

Oppenheim first described dermatitis bullosa striata pratensis, or "meadow dermatitis," in 1926 [53, 54].

The condition only develops under particular circumstances. The individual, having been out in the sun for some time with areas of bare skin and having been sunbathing on damp grassy vegetation, notices the appearance, over several hours, of a pruritic erythematous and bullous rash in a distribution pattern mimicking the shape of the grass or the veins of leaves (Fig. 46.7). Damp vegetation may be replaced by atmospheric humidity or perspiration. The linear, figurate, and vesiculobullous nature of the lesions on sun-exposed skin leads one to suspect the phototoxic nature of the dermatitis. Dermatitis generally peaks around 72 h, and healing is accompanied by postinflammatory hyperpigmentation. Currently, Oppenheim dermatitis occurs frequently after gardening, and the so-called strimmer rash appears to be a variant of this condition, having a diffuse rather than striated or figurate presentation; a "strimmer" (string trimmer) is an ingenious handheld device for cutting vegetation with a mechanically whirled string (nylon filament) [55, 56]. Oppenheim dermatitis can easily be reproduced in individuals exposed to the same conditions [57], rapidly suggesting a nonallergic mechanism. Some peculiar situations have been reported, such as the epidemic of Oppenheim dermatitis in 58 soldiers on an exercise in open country [58], or the phytophototoxicity with extensive linear and blistering skin lesions on the back of an 8-year-old-girl that was mistaken for signs of whipping by her father [59].

Meadow dermatitis and associated conditions are commonly ascribed to contact with members of the Apiacea/Umbelliferae plant family that grow in grassy meadows. In Europe, in late summer, these plants are in fact a common cause of bullous dermatitis, which may present in a wide variety of circumstances. Such dermatitis is caused by furocoumarins (also known as furanocoumarins or psoralens) (Fig. 46.8), which are present in the implicated plants and cause exaggeration of the burning potential of sunlight or artificial ultraviolet light, generally UVA. Numerous plants contain psoralens, although they have a limited distribution in the plant kingdom, the most important sources being the families Apiaceae/Umbelliferae, Fabaceae/Leguminosae, Moraceae, and Rutaceae [5, 8, 60].

Coumarin derivatives such as isopimpinellin and limettin also possess photosensitizing properties, and large amounts have been isolated from citrus peels [61].

Another category of photosensitizers are the furoquinolines, and among them, dictamnine is isolated from the roots of Rutaceae such as *Dictamnus albus* L., *Skimmia repens* Nakai, *Aegle marmelos* Correa, *Zanthoxylum alatum* Roxb., and *Ruta graveolens* L. [62–64] (Fig. 46.9). Important examples of phototoxic plants are reported in Table 46.2.

Phototoxic contact dermatitis may present as the so-called berloque dermatitis, induced by perfumes or perfumed cosmetics containing high amounts of psoralens, in particular oil of bergamot. Berloque dermatitis normally begins in the neck or décolleté, with erythema at the site where perfume runs down the skin and is irradiated by the sun. Again, this is normally followed by postinflammatory hyperpigmentation, which may last months or years. This dermatitis is currently rare due to the avoidance of fragrances containing psoralens, but can be observed with artisan or traditional fragrances [65].

46.2.4.2 Phytophotoallergic Contact Dermatitis

Plant or plant-product-induced photoallergic dermatitis occurs only very rarely. Perhaps, the only well-authenticated cases are a reaction to *Parthenium hysterophorus* L. (family Asteraceae) [66] and a photoallergy to psoralens [67]. However, experimentally induced photoallergies to psoralens and to other coumarins that are known to occur naturally have been described [68]. It is difficult to differentiate between a photoworsened ACD and a true photoallergy. Photoworsening of an ACD is the more likely diagnosis than true photoallergy when plant material is implicated as the cause of a photosensitivity reaction of

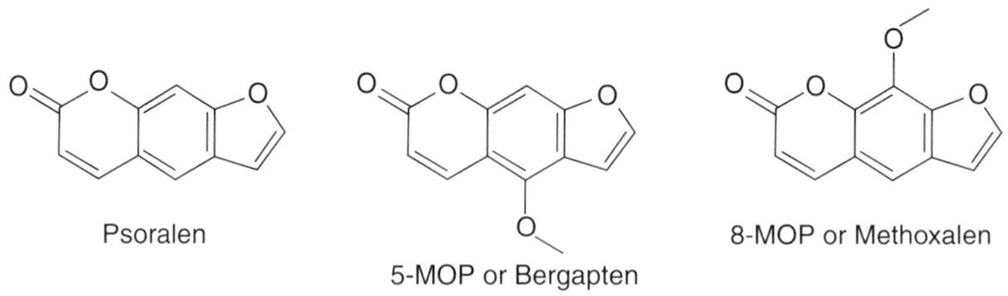

Fig. 46.8 Structures of psoralens. Psoralen (ficusin) CAS 66–97–7, 5-methoxypsoralen (bergapten) CAS 484–20–8, and 8-methoxypsoralen (xanthotoxin or methoxalen) CAS 298–81–7

Psoralen

5-MOP or Bergapten

8-MOP or Methoxalen

Fig. 46.9 Structures of limettin CAS 487–06–9, isopimpinellin CAS 482–27–9, and dictamnine, CAS 482–27–9

Limettin

Isopimpinellin

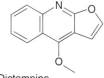

Dictamnine

Table 46.2 Main phototoxic plants

Family	Botanical name	English name	French name	German name
Apiaceae or Umbelliferae	*Ammi majus* L.	Bullwort, Bishop's weed	Ammi élevé	Grosse Knorpelmöhre
	Angelica archangelica L.	Garden angelica	Angélique	Engelwurz, Garten Angelik
	Angelica sylvestris L.	Wild angelica	Angélique des bois	Wilde Engelwurz
	Anthriscus sylvestris Hoffmann sauvage	Cow parsley	Chérophylle sauvage, cerfeuil	Wiesen-Kerbel
	Apium graveolens L.	Wild celery	Céleri sauvage, ache puante	Echte Sellerie, Epf
	Apium graveolens var. *dulce* Persoon	Celery	Céleri à côtes	Stielsellerie
	Daucus carota L. ssp *sativus* Hayek	Common garden carrot	Carotte	Karotte, Möhre
	Foeniculum vulgare Miller	Fennel	Fenouil	Gemeiner Fenchel
	Heracleum lanatum Michaux.	Cow parsnip, masterwort	Grande berce laineuse	Herkulesstaude, Bärenklau
	Heracleum mantegaz-zianum Somm and Lev.	Giant hogweed, parsnip tree	Berce du Caucase	Kaukasicher Bärenklau
	Heracleum sphondylium L.	Hogweed	Grance berce	Wiesen-Bärenklau
	Heracleum stevenii Manden	Palm of Tromsø	–	–
	Pastinaca sativa L.	Parsnip, madnep queenweed	Panais, pastenade	Pastinak, Hammelmöhre
	Petroselinum crispum	Parsley	Persil	Petersilie
Fabaceae or Leguminosae	*Psoralea corylifolia* L.	Babchi, bakuci	Psoralier	Harzklee
	Myroxylon peirerae Klotzsch	Balsam tree	Baume du Pérou	Balsam Baum
Moraceae	*Ficus carica* L.	Fig tree	Figuier	Feigenbaum
Rutaceae	*Citrus aurantifolia* Swingle	Lime	Citron vert	Limone
	Citrus aurantium L.	Bitter orange	Bigaradier, orange amère	Bittere orange, Pomeranze
	Citrus bergamia Risso and Poit.	Bergamot orange	Bergamote	Bergamottzitronen, Bergamotte
	Citrus limetta Riss.	Sweet lemon	Citron doux	Süsse Zitrone
	Citrus limon (L.) Burm.	Lemon	Citron	Zitrone
	Citrus paradisi Macfad.	Grapefruit	Pamplemousse	Pumpelmuss
	Citrus sinensis Osbeck	Sweet orange	Orange douce	Apfelzine
	Cneoridium dumosum	Bushrue, berryrue	–	–
	Dictamnus albus L.	Gasplant, fraxinella, burning bush	Fraxinelle, buisson ardent	Weisser Diptam
	Pelea anisata H. Mann	Mokihana fruits	Mokihana	Mokihana
	Ruta chalepensis L.	Fringed rue	Rue à feuilles étroites, rue d'Alep	Aleppo-Raute
	Ruta graveolens L.	Rue, Herb of grace	Rue fétide, rue des jardins	Weinraute, Garten-Raute

the skin [48, 49] in lichen pickers with a history of photosensitivity.

A rather different relationship between contact allergy and photosensitivity is seen in chronic actinic dermatitis (persistent light reaction, photosensitive eczema, or actinic reticuloid). In such patients, generally men over 50 years, dermatitis occurs in photoexposed areas during the sunny season, which then worsens with a chronic course, including itching, lichenified, and extensive lesions or even erythroderma. Patients have a marked broad spectrum photosensitivity to UVB, UVA, or even visible radiations. It is frequent to observe contact sensitivity (but not photoallergic reactions) to oleoresins from members of the plant family Asteraceae and sesquiterpene lactones contained herein, or photosensitivity to photoallergens such as musk ambrette or sunscreens, but the disease expresses itself even in the absence of exposure to the plant material. It appears that an initial contact sensitization progresses to a generalized photosensitivity state with a relationship between plants of the family Compositae, the sesquiterpene lactones they contain, and chronic actinic dermatitis [69–72].

46.3 Inducers of Dermatitis

It is not possible to consider the whole panorama of plants liable to elicit contact dermatitis here, but the plants most often incriminated are described below. Occupational contacts [13, 73] are usually the most frequent inducers of plant contact dermatitis.

46.3.1 Alliaceae (Onion Family)

Members of the family Alliaceae are widely grown and used for culinary purposes. In addition, garlic (*Allium sativum* L.) has both a contemporary and a folkloric history of use as a medicinal agent. While the lachrymatory properties of onions (*Allium cepa* L.) are widely appreciated, they are rarely discussed in the medical literature. Most commonly reported is occupational dermatitis from garlic, and to a lesser extent, from onion; this includes both immediate and delayed reactions [20, 74–79]. A typical presentation is a circumscribed irritant hyperkeratotic eczema on the fingers of one or both hands; sometimes the thumb, index, and middle fingers of the nondominant (usually left) hand

may be used to grasp the garlic bulb, while the knife is held in the right hand [80]. Less distinct patterns of eczema are likely more frequent than the presentation described above, but remarkable situations can occur, such as haemorrhagic and blistering contact dermatitis [81], cheiropompholyx associated with the ingestion of garlic extract [82], dermatitis of the elbow flexures, lower back and periorbital regions with cheilitis [83], or airborne dermatitis due to garlic powder, which was also reported as a cause of immediate-type reactions such as conjunctivitis, rhinitis, and asthma [84].

Garlic and other *Allium* species have often been reported to have both irritant and allergenic properties, due to phytochemicals not present in undamaged plant material, but released as a response to damage. They are derived from a variety of sulfur-containing amino acids present in the intact plants. A minor structural difference between the principal precursor compounds, namely S-(1-propenyl)-L-cysteine sulfoxide and S-(2-propenyl)-L-cysteine sulfoxide or alliin for garlic, results in an enzymatic transformation by the thermolabile alliinase: the lachrymatory thiopropanal-S-oxide from onion, but allicin and diallyldisulfide from garlic, as illustrated in Fig. 46.10 [85]. Diallyldisulfide, allylpropyldisulfide, and allicin have been identified as the principal low-molecular-weight allergens of garlic [86]. Commercial diallyldisulfide seems to be a suitable preparation for the investigation of garlic dermatitis, although 1% pet. may carry a lower risk of irritancy or can be negative. Irritant reactions with plants are expected with fresh garlic concentrations higher than 10%, but concentrations up to 50% for garlic and onion in arachnid oil were considered to be safe [79]. It is likely that each different extraction procedure affects the manner in which the irritants/allergens are released, making it virtually impossible to produce a standard extract. So, patch tests with plant extracts or plant material used as is must be interpreted with some caution [87]. Delayed-type cross-reactions between garlic and onion, although occasionally described, are unlikely.

46.3.2 Alstroemeriaceae (Alstroemer Family) and Liliaceae (Lily Family)

These two families are considered together because members of the genera *Alstroemeria* L. (Peruvian lily, Inca lily) and *Bomarea* Mirb. (family Alstroemeriaceae), and the genus *Tulipa* L. (family Liliaceae) produce the

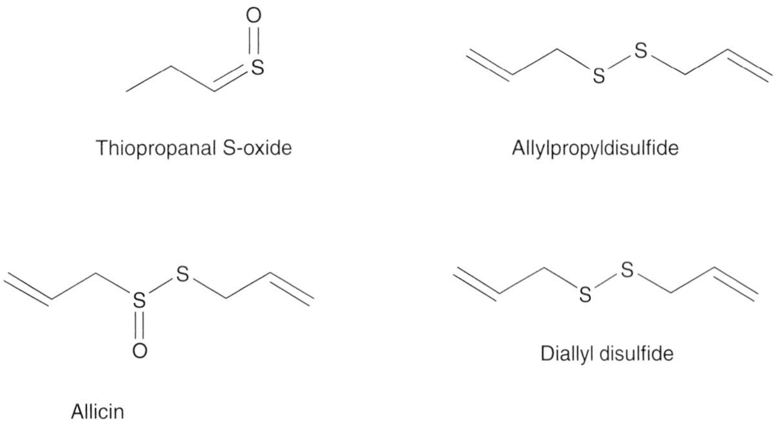

Fig. 46.10 Structures of thipropanal S-oxide CAS 32157–29–2, allicin CAS 539–86–6, diallyl disulfide CAS 2179–57–9, and allypropyl disulfide CAS 2179–59–1

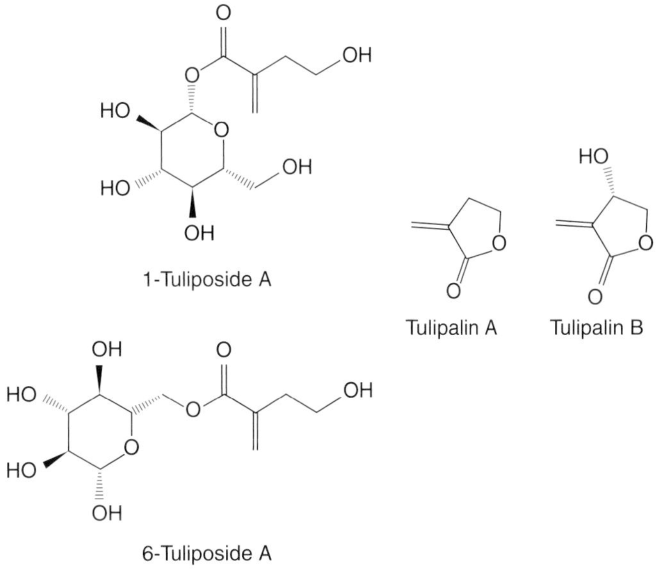

Thiopropanal S-oxide

Allylpropyldisulfide

Allicin

Diallyl disulfide

Fig. 46.11 Structures of 1- and 6-tuliposides A (glycosidic precursors of tulipalin A) CAS 19870–30–5 and CAS 19870–31–6, respectively, tulipalin A (α-methylene-γ-butyrolactone) CAS 547–65–9 and tulipalin B (β-hydroxy-α-methylene-γ-butyrolactone) CAS 38965–80–9

1-Tuliposide A

Tulipalin A   Tulipalin B

6-Tuliposide A

same allergen, tulipalin A (Fig. 46.11). The substance is released when the plant material (flowers, stems and leaves) is damaged [88–91]. Tulipalin A, otherwise known as α-methylene-γ-butyrolactone, is obtained from a glucoside precursor known as tuliposide A. This one can be present as 1-tuliposide A [92] or more frequently identified as 6-tuliposide A [93–95].

Tulips contain a second glucoside, 6-tuliposide B [90], which is classically considered to be a nonsensitizer and has antibiotic properties, protecting the plant against bacteria [96]. Patients sensitive to tulips reportedly do not react to either tuliposide B or tulipalin B. However, it was demonstrated that tulipalin B (β-hydroxy-α-methylene-γ-butyrolactone) is a sensitizer in guinea pigs, and that cross-reactivity between tulipalins A and B does occur [97]. Other tuliposides

have been detected in *Alstroemeria* species, e.g., tuliposide D [95]. There is evidence that the tuliposides themselves can elicit ACD [89, 93], but this may be the outcome of some spontaneous degradation to tulipalin A on the skin [98].

Garden tulips are available both as "species tulips" and cultivars of hybrid origin. Dermatitis among bulb handlers and florists is a frequent but unpleasant occupational hazard. Bulb collectors, sorters, and packers develop a characteristic dermatitis called "tulip fingers," a painful dry fissured hyperkeratotic eczema, at first underneath the true margin of the nails, spreading to the periungueal regions, fingers, and hands [99]. Sometimes the dermatitis spreads to the face, forearms, and genital region. It seems certain that both irritant and ACD occurs. "Tulip fingers" is common in the Netherlands and other parts of Europe. The allergen is found mainly in the epidermis of the bulb, but dermatitis may also occur in those who handle the cut flowers [100].

Alstroemeria hybrids have been popular in the cut-flower trade since the 1980s due to their long-lasting and colored flowers (Fig. 46.4a, b). Horticulturists and florists are at high risk of both irritant and ACD, and the rate of sensitization for tulipalin A can exceed 50% in workers of *Alstroemeria* cultivation [101]. Handling of cut flowers provokes a dermatitis affecting mainly the fingertips, which is similar to "tulip fingers" [102–104]. Depigmentation may follow the resolution of *Alstroemeria* dermatitis or a positive patch test to plant [105]. Contact urticaria and rhinoconjunctivitis, with positive prick tests, were described for *Alstroemeria* [106].

In the preparation of plant material for patch testing, it should be remembered that the various cultivars of *Alstroemeria* and *Tulipa* do not necessarily contain similar levels of tuliposide A or associated contact allergens. For example, the cultivar Rose Copeland is a notorious sensitizer [107], whereas *Tulipa fosteriana* Hoog cv Red Emperor has been found to contain very much less tuliposide than other cultivars [99]. Nonsystematic concomitant patch test reactions between tulips and *Alstroemeria* [102, 105] may be due to differences in the amount of allergens. Different ways of performing patch testing have been recommended, since the so-called short ether extracts of *Alstroemeria* are too rich in tulipalin A and carry the risk of active sensitization [92]: a filtered 96% ethanol extract of the reference bulb of *Tulipa* cv Apeldoorn or an 80% acetone extract of the bulbs diluted with 70% ethanol immediately prior to use [99], a tuliposide-rich methanolic extract incorporated into petrolatum [92], a 50-μL application of 6-tuliposide A at 0.01% or an α-methylene-γ-butyrolactone at 0.001% in ethanol [93]. Currently, the 0.01% concentration in petrolatum seems to be effective and safe for detecting sensitive people [92, 108].

Core Message

> Tulipalin A (α-methylene-γ-butyrolactone) is the main contact allergen in *Alstroemeria* and *Tulipa* species. It frequently induces a fingertip allergy known as "tulip fingers," mostly in people who have occupational contact with flowers and bulbs.

Common hyacinth (*Hyacinthus orientalis* L.) has been described above as inducers of irritant contact dermatitis, due to calcium oxalate present in their bulbs. It is noteworthy that bulbs evoke pruritus in almost all workers who manipulate them, but dermatitis is less frequent [109]. We observed an unusual exposure in two schoolteachers who decided to describe the structure of bulbs and explained in detail the way to cultivate hyacinth bulbs to their pupils (personal observations). Hyacinths likely contain as-yet unidentified allergens [107].

46.3.3 Amaryllidaceae (Daffodil Family)

The Amaryllidaceae family comprises some 1,100 species of plant in 85 genera, many of which are cultivated for their showy flowers. Among these, daffodils (*Narcissus* spp. and cultivars) are the most common, involving several species such as trumpet narcissi (*Narcissus pseudonarcissus* L.), narcissi (other species, e.g., *N. poeticus*), and jonquils (*Narcissus jonquilla* L.), which constitute a significant dermatological hazard because of their irritant and allergenic properties. An important bulb and cut-flower industry exists in the Netherlands and the Isles of Scilly in the United Kingdom, and with it exists the occupational disease known as "daffodil itch" or "lily rash" [99, 107], sometimes clinically close to "tulip fingers."

The rash has long been ascribed in part to the calcium oxalate needle crystals present in both the dry outer scales of the bulbs and in the sap exuding from cut flower stems [99]. Observation in the field related the method of picking and then gathering the flowers to the development of the daffodil pickers' rash, at the points of contact of plant sap with the skin like the finger webs, the dorsum of the hand, and the anterior aspect of the wrist [110]. Dermatitis may involve the neck, face, and the genitals [8]. It is likely that the "lily rash" is mainly caused by an irritant mechanism [109], but that an allergic reaction is possible [111]. Among many irritant alkaloids, two allergenic ones were identified from *N. pseudonarcissus* L., namely masonin and homolycorine (Fig. 46.12) [33]. Patch tests may be performed with leaves, stems, and flowers, or with ethanol, acetone, or water [8].

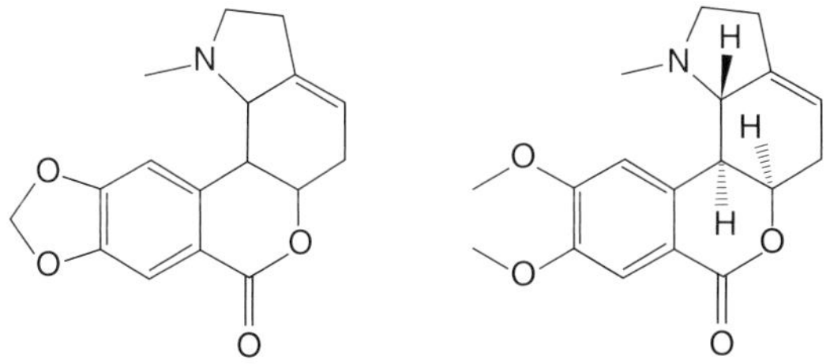

Fig. 46.12 Structures of masonin CAS 568–40–1 and homolycorine, CAS 477–20–3

46.3.3.1 Anacardiaceae, Ginkgoaceae, and Proteaceae

These plant families are considered together because they contain similar contact allergens, and hence, cause similar dermatitis. Nevertheless, the clinical picture may vary depending upon the precise mode of contact.

Anacardiaceae (Cashew Family)

The Anacardiaceae family includes 60 genera comprising some 600 species of trees and shrubs, distributed throughout the tropics, and also found in warm temperate regions of Europe, eastern Asia, and the Americas. They are considered to cause more dermatitis than all other plant families combined [5]. Some tropical species are of economic importance, such as *Mangifera indica* L. that provides mango fruits, *Anacardium occidentale* L. that yields cashew nuts, cashew nut shell oil that is used in the manufacture of brake linings, *Semecarpus anacardium* L.f. that is known as the Indian marking nut tree that provides black juice used as an indelible ink when labeling clothing, the Japanese lacquer tree *Toxicodendron verniciuum* F. Barkley, or several other species used for dying or tanning. The main dermatologically important plants are reported in Table 46.3.

Although these and many other species in the family Anacardiaceae are dermatologically hazardous [112–121], perhaps the most important genus is *Toxicodendron*. This genus includes the poison ivy complex (*Toxicodendron radicans* Kuntze and subspecies such as *T. radicans* Kuntze *var. rydbergii* Erskine), the poison oak complex with *Toxicodendron diversilobum* Greene (in western North America) and *Toxicodendron toxicarium* Gillis (in eastern North America), and the poison sumac (*Toxicodendron striatum* Kuntze, *T.*

vernix Kuntze) of North America and elsewhere [122–126]. Over half of the population of the United States is sensitive to poison ivy and its relatives [127], and as the plants are not a part of the natural flora, poison ivy dermatitis is generally unknown in Europe [128]. Clinical aspects vary with exposure. Dermatitis initially appears on the fingers, forearms, arms, legs, and sometimes genitalia [8, 127]. Lesions consist of papules, vesicles, and/or blisters. Erythema multiforme-like eruption is sometimes observed. Systemic contact dermatitis may occur after accidental, medicinal, or alimentary ingestion of plant materials. It may present as eczema, as a generalized maculopapular eruption or as erythroderma occurring generally within 48 h following administration. When generalized rash occurs, leukocytosis and neutrophilia are frequent and liver dysfunction is possible [129, 130]. The same features with eczematous eruption of flexural regions, mouth, and anal itching may occur after ingestion of cashew nuts in people previously sensitized to poison ivy [131]. The "black spot poison ivy dermatitis" is a rarer condition, consisting of black enamel spots, due to colored and dried plant sap, secondarily surrounding patch dermatitis, mainly of allergic origin [132].

Early literature refers to poison ivy and its relatives as species of *Rhus*. On the basis of morphological grounds and phytochemical distinction, it appears that *Toxicodendron* is more suited and that the genus *Rhus* must be distinguished from the genus *Toxicodendron* [10, 133], although other authors argue for using the term *Rhus* [7]. There is consequently a frequent nomenclatural confusion in the dermatological literature, especially with the numerous synonyms. Individual subspecies of *Toxicodendron* rarely appear in the dermatological literature, largely because case reports of poison ivy dermatitis hardly warrant publication, partly because of the difficulty in precisely identifying the subspecies of the plants. The distributions of the various *Toxicodendron* species and subspecies have been described for the United States [133–135]. The "black spot test" consists of carefully crushing sap from the leaves of the plant onto white paper: the test is positive with *Toxicodendron*, the stain darkening on exposure to the air [136]. The same phenomenon occurs with wood sap (Fig. 46.13). Poison ivy, poison oak, and poison sumac are native to North America, but can be exported. The dermatitis can present after an individual has been in contact with the plant while visiting an endemic area. As the plant has the potential to grow in

Table 46.3 Dermatologically important Anacardiaceae plants

Botanical name	Synonyms	English name	French name	German name
Anacardium occidentale L.		Cashew nut tree	Anacardier, noix de cajou, pomme cajou	Kaschu, Elefantenlaus Baum, westindischer Nierenbaum
Comocladia dodonaea Urban	*Comocladia ilicifolia* Sw., *Ilex dodonaea* L.	Christmas bush, poison ash	Bois de houx	
Gluta laccifera Ding Hou	*Melanorrhoea laccifera* Pierre	Camboge lacquer	Arbre à laque du Cambodge	
Gluta renghas L.		East coast rengas, ape-nut		
Gluta usitata Ding Hou	*Melanorrhoea usitata* Wallich. theetsee	Burmese lacquer tree, de Birmanie	Arbre à laque	
Holigarna ferruginea March.				
Lithraea caustica Hook. and Arn.	*Lithraea venenosa* Miers.	Litre, aroeira		
Mangifera indica L.		Mango tree	Manguier	Mangobaum
Metopium toxiferum Krug and Urban	*Rhus metopium* L.	Poisonwood, coral sumac, Florida poison tree, Honduras walnut		
Semecarpus anacardium L.	*Anacardium orientale* Auct.	Indian marking nut tree, bhilawa tree	Anacarde d'Orient	Tintenbaum
Smodingium argutum E. Mey.		African poison ivy, um-tovane, tovana, rainbow leaf	Smodingie, lierre toxique d'Afrique	Afrikanischer Giftefeu
Toxicodendron diversilobum Greene	*Rhus diversiloba* Torr. and Gray. *R. toxicodendron* L. ssp. *diversiloba* Engl.	Western poison oak, Pacific poison oak	Sumac irrégu-lièrement lobé, sumac de l'ouest	Sumach, verschieden-lappiger Sumach
Toxicodendron radicans L. ssp. *barkleyi* Gillis	*Rhus villosum* Sessé and Moçino	Western poison oak		
Toxicodendron radicans L. ssp. *divaricatum* Gillis	*T. divaricatum* Greene, *Rhus divaricata* Greene	Western poison oak		
Toxicodendron radicans L. ssp. *eximium* Gillis	*T. eximium* Greene, *Rhus eximia* Stanley	Western poison oak		
Toxicodendron radicans L. ssp. *hispidum* Gillis	*Rhus toxicodendron* L. var. *hispida* Engl.. *R. intermedia* Hayata	Taiwan tsuta-urushi		
Toxicodendron radicans L. ssp. *negundo* Gillis	*T. negundo* Greene, *T. arborigunum* Greene	Taiwan tsuta-urushi	Herbe à puce grimpante	

Toxicodendron radicans L. ssp. *orientale* Gillis	*T. orientale* Greene, *Rhus orientalis* Schneider	Tsuta-urushi		Sumach, Kletter-Giftsumach, Rankender Sumach, Giftefeu
Toxicodendron radicans L. ssp. *pubens* Gillis	*R. toxicodendron* L. var. *pubens* Engelm.	Tsuta-urushi		
Toxicodendron radicans L. ssp. *radicans* Gillis	*T. radicans* Kuntze, *Rhus radicans* L., *Rhus toxicodendron* L.	Poison ivy, three-leaved ivy, eastern poison ivy, poison vine, black vine, markweed	Sumac radicant, lierre toxique, herbe à puce de l'est	
T. radicans L. ssp. *verrucosum* Gillis	*T. verrucosum* Greene, *Rhus verrucosa* Scheele	Poison ivy, three-leaved ivy, poison vine, black vine, markweed		
Toxicodendron rydbergii Greene poison ivy	*T. radicans* Kuntze var. *rydbergii* Erskine, *Rhus rydbergii* Small, *R. toxicodendron* L. var. *rydbergii* Garnett	Rydberg's poison ivy, western poison ivy	Herbe à puce de Rydberg	
Toxicodendron striatum	*Rhus striata* Ruiz and Pavón, *R. juglandifolia* Willd	Manzanillo, hinchador Kuntze		
Toxicodendron succedaneum Kuntze	*Rhus succedanea* L.	Japanese wax tree		
Toxicodendron toxicarium Gillis	*T. quercifolium* Greene, *T. toxico-dendron* L. Britten, *Rhus querci-folia* Steudel, *R. toxicodendron* L. var. *quercifolium* Michx., *R. toxicarium* Salisb.	Eastern poison oak, oak leaf ivy	Sumac véné-neux à feuilles de chêne	Echter Giftsumac
Toxicodendron vernicifluum Barkley	*Rhus verniciflua* Stokes, *R. vernicifera* DC	Japanese lacquer tree, varnish tree	Sumac à laque, vernis vrai	Lacksumach
Toxicodendron vernix Kuntze	*Rhus vernix* L., *R. venenata* DC	Poison sumac, poison dogwood, swamp sumac, poison elder	Sumac à vernis, bois chandelle	Giftsumach

46

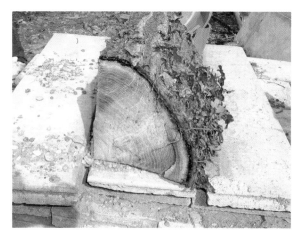

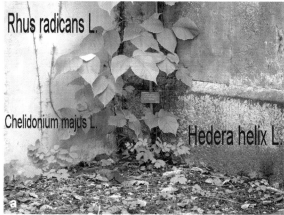

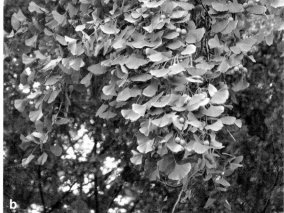

Fig. 46.13 Stain darkening of the sap of *Toxicodendron* species is the basis of the "black spot test," here demonstrated with sap of a recently cut down Japanese lacquer tree (*Toxicodendron vernicifluum* Barkley)

Fig. 46.14 (**a**) *Toxicodendron radicans* growing in the botanical garden of Strasbourg, France. (**b**) Female Ginkgo tree (*Ginkgo biloba* L.) bearing ovules (Jardin botanique, Strasbourg, France)

Europe too (Fig. 46.14a), it is possible for an individual to be sensitized and subsequently develop the rash without leaving their country [137], particularly in the case of workers at botanical gardens (personal observations).

Cross-reactivity between Anacardiaceae has been reported for a long time. Similarities between urushiols from poison ivy and cashew nut shell oil are well known. In South America, species of *Lithraea*, and especially *L. caustica* Hook. and Arn. [10], are a frequent cause of a poison ivy-like dermatitis. In 17 *Lithraea*-sensitized subjects, reactions to poison oak urushiol were constant, and reactions to extracts prepared from *Lithraea molleoides* Engl. and *Lithraea brasiliensis* Marchand occurred in 13/17. The responses to poison oak urushiol were stronger and occurred at lower concentrations than those to *Lithraea* extracts [138]. Similar studies of cross-reactivity between *Lithraea* and other members of the Anacardiaceae were reported [139, 140]. Concomitant reactions have been observed, but without systematic cross-reactivity, as in a patient sensitized to poison ivy or poison oak (*Toxicodendron* spp.) while in the United States and who subsequently showed apparent cross-reactions to *Rhus copallina* L., *R. semialata* Murray (syn. *R. javanica* L.), and *R. trichocarpa* Miq. [128].

Ginkgoaceae (Maidenhair Family)

Ginkgo biloba L., the ginkgo tree, is the solitary representative of the family Ginkgoaceae and is regarded as one of the world's oldest surviving tree species. Contact dermatitis from the ginkgo tree is not due to its leaves, but to its malodorous fruits [141], in fact to the ovules exclusively borne by female trees (Fig. 46.14b). Contact occurs through inadvertent contamination of the skin with the fruit pulp [142], collecting and using the nut within the fruit in an Asian cooking style [142, 143], or in children through playing marbles with the fallen fruits. The lesions consist of erythematous papules and vesicles, with severe swelling in severe cases. They usually affect the face, the forearms, and the thighs, and sometimes the genitalia [143, 144]. Stomatitis, cheilitis, and proctitis following ingestion of ginkgo fruit were described [145].

Cross-reactions between ginkgo fruit pulp, poison ivy, or ginkgo and cashew nut have been discussed [146]. They were, however, not supported by a recent study of the ginkgolic acids found in *Ginkgo* fruits and urushiol from *Toxicodendron* [147]. Patch testing can be performed with fruit pulp in 1% acetone [145].

Proteaceae

The Proteaceae family comprises 1,050 species in 62 genera found in tropical areas. In Australia, members of the family Proteaceae are the cause of a poison ivy-like dermatitis. The best known are probably the so-called silky oak or silver oak (*Grevillea robusta* Cunn.) and related *Grevillea* species and cultivars. Contact with the wild and cultivated tree [148–150], as well as with objects made from the wood [151], has been recorded as being allergenic. "Grevillea poisoning" was described as a severe contact dermatitis on exposed areas in people cutting trees or maintaining electric power lines in the Los Angeles area [152]. Allergic

dermatitis following contact with flowers of Kahili or Bank's Grevillea (*Grevillea banksii* R. Br.) was described in Hawaii [153].

Allergens

The allergenic agents in all these members of the Anacardiaceae, Ginkgoaceae, and Proteaceae are derivatives of catechol, phenol, resorcinol, or salicylic acid with a side chain (-R) (Fig. 46.15). This side chain is mostly a C_{15} (sometimes a C_{17}) alkyl (saturated) or alkenyl (one, two, or three double bonds C=C) chain [4, 8]. The alk(en)yl catechols are also known as *urushiol*, a generic name that in fact refers to the blend of several close molecules (urushiols) naturally contained in the plant. An urushiol with a C_{15} side chain is named pentadecylcatechol (a term sometimes employed in medical literature for poison ivy

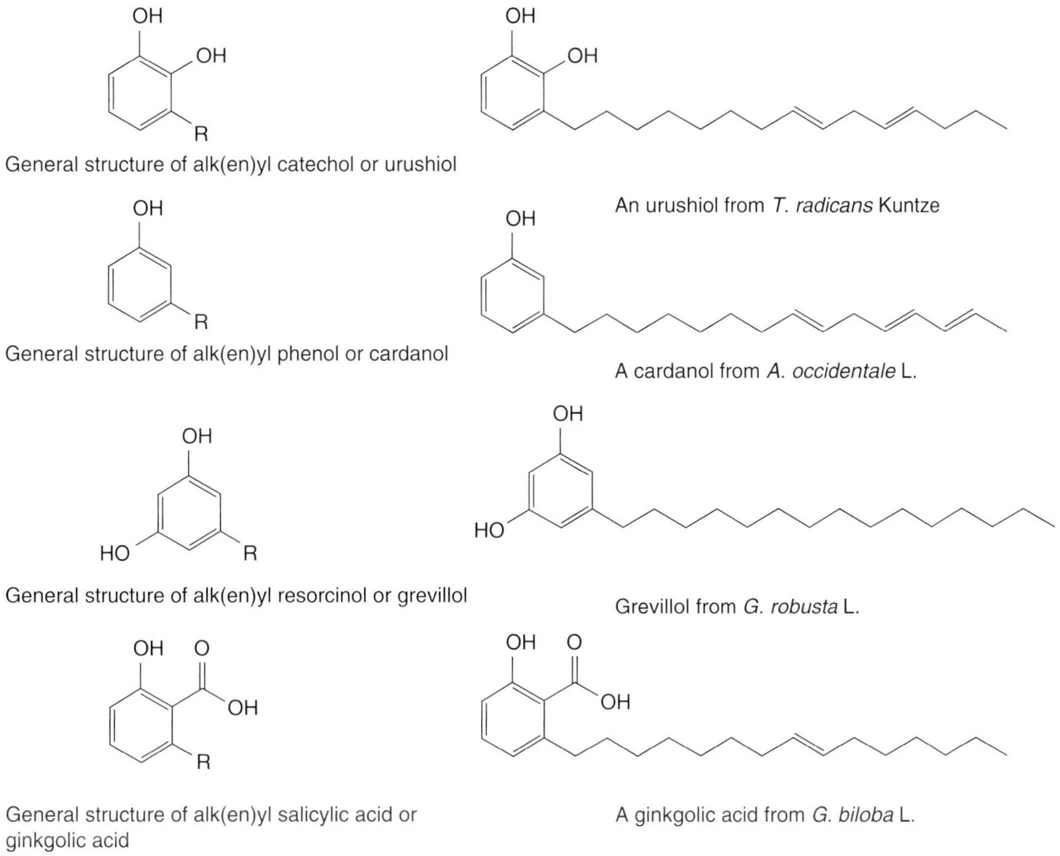

General structure of alk(en)yl catechol or urushiol

An urushiol from *T. radicans* Kuntze

General structure of alk(en)yl phenol or cardanol

A cardanol from *A. occidentale* L.

General structure of alk(en)yl resorcinol or grevillol

Grevillol from *G. robusta* L.

General structure of alk(en)yl salicylic acid or ginkgolic acid

A ginkgolic acid from *G. biloba* L.

Fig. 46.15 Structures of urushiol and related allergens from Anacardiaceae (*T. radicans* Kuntze, *A. occidentale* L.), Proteaceae (*G. robusta* L.), and Ginkgoaceae (*G. biloba* L.) families

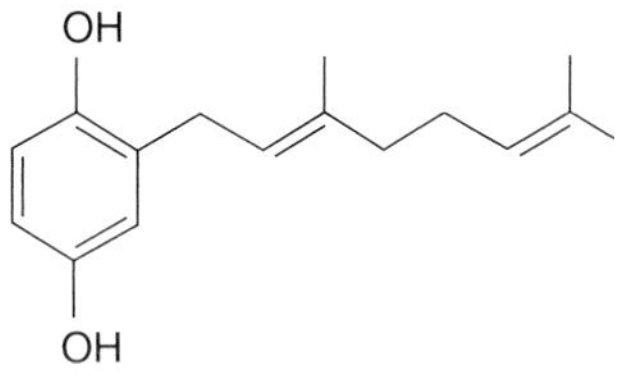

Fig. 46.16 Structure of geranylhydroquinone CAS 10457–66–6, from *Phacelia crenulata* Torrey

urushiol), and an urushiol with a C_{17} side chain is a heptadecylcatechol (mostly encountered in poison oak urushiol). Phenol, resorcinol, and salicylic acid compounds substituted with an alk(en)yl chain have traditionally been called *cardanol, grevillol,* and *ginkgolic acid,* respectively. Because the allergenic natural plant material is a mixture of closely related compounds, and because of the close similarity between individual compounds from a variety of botanical sources, there is the possibility of cross-sensitization between different species throughout the world [154].

The risk of cross-sensitization extends to families other than those described in this section. The genus *Philodendron* (family Araceae) yields sensitizing alkyl resorcinols [155]. The genera *Phacelia* and *Wigandia* belonging to the Hydrophyllaceae family yield alkenyl hydroquinones. Prenylated quinones and prenylated phenols were identified in *W. caracasana* Kunth [156], and geranylhydroquinone in *P. crenulata* Torrey (Fig. 46.16); this molecule does not cross-react with poison oak or ivy [157].

Core Message

> Plants of the family Anacardiaceae are frequent causes of contact dermatitis. The skin reaction occurs following sensitization to various alkyl or alkenyl catechols (urushiol), phenols, resorcinols, or salicylic acid derivatives. These compounds are also primary irritants.

46.3.4 Compositae (Asteraceae) and Liverworts

The two families are considered together because they contain sesquiterpene lactones as allergens.

46.3.4.1 Asteraceae/Compositae (Daisy Family)

The family Asteraceae/Compositae comprises some 25,000 species in over 1,500 genera. Representatives are found throughout the world, and examples may be found living in almost every situation, the majority being herbaceous plants. The family provides a number of food plants, for example, lettuce, endive, chicory, dandelion, salsify, scorzonera, and artichoke. Many more are grown for their decorative flowers, such as chrysanthemums, dahlias, and heleniums. Others are widespread and common weeds [158]. Additionally, some species such as arnica, chamomile, or feverfew are used medicinally, by skin application or systemic administration. It is, therefore, difficult to avoid contact with these plants. Plants of dermatological interest are indicated in Table 46.4.

ACD from Asteraceae has several clinical presentations (Fig. 46.6). Accidentally exposed subjects can develop an acute and single episode of dermatitis. Chronic exposure, e.g., of occupational origin, can induce acute dermatitis that can often relapse, or a primary chronic and secondarily lichenified dermatitis. When the lesions are localized to the elbow or knee flexures, they can simulate atopic dermatitis. The eczema, which may be localized initially on the face, hands, and genitals, can become generalized as an erythroderma and can even be, in rare instances, fatal [159].

Exposure to the sesquiterpene lactones by the way of airborne plant material produces an airborne contact dermatitis (sometimes mistaken for a photodermatitis). In the United States, this is known as "ragweed dermatitis" because it is largely caused by ragweeds, which are species of *Ambrosia* [160, 161] or "weed dermatitis" in regions where other composite weeds predominate [162], such as , *Artemisia, Helenium,* and *Iva* [163–172] species. For example, cases of severe airborne ACD from triangle-leaf bursage (*Ambrosia deltoidea*) were reported in the USA, with positive reactions, in one case, to both ether extracts of the plant and a filter from an outdoor air sampler placed near the plants [173].

In Australia, the same condition is described as "bush dermatitis" due to genera such as *Arctotheca, Cassinia, Conyza, Cynara,* and *Dittrichia* [168, 174–177]. In India, another variant has been called "parthenium dermatitis" [9, 178, 179] after the offending plant (*Parthenium hysterophorus* L.).

Table 46.4 Dermatologically important Asteraceae/Compositae plants

Correct name	Synonyms	English name	French name	German name
Achillea millefolium L.	*Achillea lanulosa* Nuttall	Yarrow, nosebleed, milfoil, thousand leaf	Achilée mille-feuille, herbe àla coupure	Gemeine Schafgarbe
Ambrosia acanthicarpa Hook.	*Franseria acanthicarpa* Cov.	Bur-ragweed, sandbur	Franserie lampourde	Falsche Ambrosie
Ambrosia artemisiifolia L.	*Ambrosia elatior* L.	Short ragweed, common ragweed	Ambroisie à feuille d'armoise, ambroisie élevée	Beifussblättrige Ambrosie, hohes Tauben-kraut, Wermutblätt-rige Ambrosie
Ambrosia psilostachya DeCambolle		Western ragweed, perennial ragweed, common ragweed	Herbe à poux vivace	Ausdauernde Ambrosie
Ambrosia trifida L.	*Ambrosia aptera* DC.	Giant ragweed, tall ragweed		Dreispaltige Ambrosie
Anthemis arvensis L. ssp. arvensis		Field chamomile, corn chamomile (scentless)	Fausse camomille, camomille sauvage, anthémis des champs	Acker Hundskamille
Anthemis cotula L.	*Maruta cotula* DC	Stinking chamomile, corn chamomile (scented)	Anthémis cotule, anthémis fétide	Stinkende Hundskamille
Arctotheca calendula Levyns	*Arctotis calendulacea* L., *Cryptostemma calendu- lacea* R. Br.	Capeweed	Artothèque souci	Dune Calendula
Arnica montana L.		Arnica, mountain tobacco, wolf's bane	Arnica, tabac des Vosges, quinqui- na des pauvres	Berg-Wohlverleih, Arnika
Artemisia ludoviciana Nutt.	*Artemisia ludoviciana* Nutt., *Artemisia purshiana*	Dark-leafed mugwort, prairie sage	Armoise argentée	Edelraute
Artemisia vulgaris L.		Common mugwort	Armoise vulgaire, herbe aux cent goûts	Gewöhnlicher Beifuss, Fliegenkraut
Cassinia aculeata R. Br.		Common cassinia, dogwood, cauliflower bush		
Chamaemelum nobile All	*Anthemis nobilis* L.	Roman chamomile, dog fennel	Camomille romaine	Römische Kamille
Cichorium endivia L. spp. *endivia* L.		Common endive	Endive, chicorée des jardins	Winter Endivie
Cichorium intybus L.		Chicory, wild chicory	Chicorée sauvage, barbe de capucin	Wilde Zichorie, gemeine Wegwarte, Sonnenwedel
Conyza bonariensis Cronq.	*Erigeron bonariensis* L. *Conyza ambigua* DC., *Conyza crispa* Rupr.	Fleabane	Érigéron crépu	Südamerikanisches Berufskraut

(continued)

Table 44.1 (continued)

I	Food additives	E-number	Predominant current uses in foods	Predominant type(s) of reaction
	Sulfites e.g. sodium bisulfite	E 221–228 E 222	Alcoholic beverages, vinegar, water-based flavoured and energy drinks-based and energy drinks, fruit/vegetable juices/concentrates, dried/canned/fermented/frozen fruits/vegetables, peeled/cut/shredded fresh vegetables, surface treated fresh fruit, frozen/smoked/dried/fermented/salted fish and seafood, fresh seafood, jam, jelly marmalade, sugars, syrups, herbs, spices, seasonings, condiments, sauces, mead, mustard, starch, snacks (potato/cereal/flour/starch-based)	ACD; (urticaria upon ingestion; rarely spec. IgE)
	Tocopherols	E 306–309	Butter oil, ghee, further oils and fats, dressings, desserts, chewing gum	ACD
3.	*Stabilizers*			
	Gums			
	Guaiac		Lard, tallow, fish oil, further animal oils, vegetable oils and fats, sauces, chewing gum	ACD
	Guar	E 412	Dairy-based products, egg-based products, cheeses, fat spreads/emulsions, ice cream, sherbets, processed/cooked/canned fruits/vegetables, breakfast cereals, bakery products, soybean products, confectionary, precooked pasta and rice, processed meats/poultry/game, edible casings, seasonings, condiments, vinegar, mustard, sauces, soups, broths, salads, yeast, alcoholic beverages, water-based flavoured and energy drinks-based and energy drinks, dietetic products, desserts	ACD, OCU
	Karaya (=sterculia gum)	E 416	As guar	ACD
	Acacia (=gum arabic)	E 414	As guar	ACD
	Tragacanth	E 413	As guar	ACD
	Waxes			
	Beeswax	E 901	Glaze of confectionary and fine bakery ware, decorations, toppings, sweet sauces, cocoa and chocolate products, coffee beans, surface-treated fresh fruits and nuts, chewing gum, water-based flavoured and energy drinks	ACD
	Carnauba	E 903	Glaze of confectionary, processed fruit, and as beeswax	ACD
	Carrageenan	E 407	Desserts, ice cream, milk shakes, sweetened condensed milks, sauces, pâtés and processed meat, soy products, diet drinks	ACD
4.	*Emulsifiers*			
	Propylene glycol	E 1520	Humectant, solvent for food colours and flavourings, chewing gum	ACD
5.	*Dyes*			
	Azo dyes			
	Amaranth (=FD&C Red 2)	E 123	Caviar, alcoholic beverages[a]	NICU

Botanical name	English	French	German
Saussurea lappa C.B. Clarke / *Saussurea costus* Lipsch.	Costus	Costus	Costus
Silybum marianum Gaertn.	Blessed milk-thistle, holy thistle	Chardon de Marie	Mariendistel
Tagetes minuta L. / *Tagetes glandulifera* Schrank marigold	Small-flowered stinking roger	Tagète des décombres	Tagetes
Tanacetum cinerariifolium Schultz-Bip. / *Chrysanthemum cinerariifolium* Vis., *Pyrethrum cinerariifolium* Trevir.	Pyrethrum, Dalmatian pyrethrum	Pyrèthre	Dalmatinische Insektenblume
Tanacetum parthenium Schultz-Bip. / *Chrysanthemum parthenium* Bernh., *Matricaria parthenium* L.	Feverfew	Grande camomille	Mutterkraut, Falsche Kamille
Tanacetum vulgare L. / *Chrysanthemum tanacetum* Karsch., *C. vulgare* Bernh.	Tansy, bitter buttons	Tanaisie, tanacée, herbe aux vers	Gemeiner Rainfarn, Wurmkraut
Taraxacum officinale Weber / *Leontodon taraxacum* L., *Taraxacum dens-leonis* Desf., *T. taraxacum* Karst	Dandelion, blowball	Pissenlit, laitue de chien, dent de lion	Gebräulicher Löwen-zahn, Kuhlblume
Xanthium spinosum L.	Spiny cocklebur	Lampourde épineuse, petite bardane	Dornige Spitzklette
Xanthium strumarium L.	Noogoora burr	Lampourde ordi-naire, herbe aux écrouelles	Gemeine Spitzklette, Kropfspitzklette
X. italicum Moretti / *X.-californicum* Greene, *Xanthium strumarium* L. ssp *italicum* D. Löve	Californian burr	Lampourde d'Italie	Italienische Spitzklette

The environmental conditions favoring ragweed dermatitis and its variants in hot and arid climates are not normally encountered in the temperate regions of Europe. Nevertheless, there are also European variants of ragweed dermatitis which have been described in rather specialized circumstances, with feverfew (*Tanacetum parthenium* Schultz-Bip.) [44, 180, 181], chicory (*Cichorium intybus* L.) and lettuce (*Lactuca sativa* L.) [182], liverworts of the genus *Frullania* [47], and the chrysanthemums of florists [45].

In its classical form, contact dermatitis from ragweed particularly affects male subjects and spares women and children [159], but newer reports from both the USA and Europe point to a more equal female:male ratio in Compositae dermatitis in general, depending on exposure [183, 184]. Furthermore, atopic dermatitis seems to be a risk factor for Compositae sensitization in children [185].

Many cases have been described with sensitization to Asteraceae [5, 8] like with yarrow (*Achillea millefolium* L.) [163], chamomile (*Anthemis* spp L.) [167], arnica (*Arnica montana* L.) [169], small-flowered marigold (*Tagetes minuta* L.) [186], pyrethrum (*Tanacetum cinerariifolium* Schultz-Bip) [187], dandelion (*Taraxacum officinale* Wiggers) [188], elecampane (*Inula helenium* L.) [189, 190], sunflower (*Helianthus annuus L.)* [191], guayule (*Parthenium argentatum* Gray) [192], or Noogoora Burr (*Xanthium strumarium* L.) [193]. Cultivated plants, such as dahlia or chrysanthemum cultivars, are an important source of occupational contact allergy [194–198]. Botanical and vernacular names of dermatologically important Asteraceae are reported in Table 46.4.

Phototoxicity may theoretically occur following contact with α-terthienyl, a natural phototoxic thiophene compound of many Asteraceae species [199], but no authentic clinical cases appear to have been described in the literature.

Contact urticaria has been described with this family [13, 200].

Core Message

> The large Asteraceae/Compositae family is a frequent inducer of ACD, due to the sesquiterpene lactones contained in the plants.

46.3.4.2 Liverworts (Jubulaceae)

Liverworts, together with mosses and hornworts, comprise a group of small, nonvascular plants known as bryophytes [201]. Typically, they grow as epiphytes in damp locations, although they can withstand periods of desiccation. Of the liverworts, only a few species of *Frullania* have been described as causes of ACD. These are found on trees in several regions of the world, notably in British Columbia in Canada, the Pacific Northwest of the United States (Oregon), and in the Bordeaux and Strasbourg regions of France. They are a cause of occupational contact dermatitis in forest workers and woodcutters [202, 203], and domestic allergy in people who use lobe-leaved trees as firewood. *Frullania dilatata* Dum., *F. tamarisci* Dum., and *F. tamarisci* Dum. ssp. *nisquallensis* Hatt. are the most aggressive species. Instances of cross-sensitivity reactions between *Frullania* species and members of the Compositae family are accounted for by the occurrence of structurally similar sesquiterpene lactones in the plants concerned, such as costunolide [8, 204]. More specifically, *Frullania dilatata* Dum. and *tamarisci* Dum. are sources of (+)- and (−)-frullanolide, respectively [205, 206]. There is a risk of active sensitization by patch testing [202], sometimes occult, as revealed by a new patch test session (personal observations).

Core Message

> The liverwort *Frullania* spp. induces contact allergy in foresters and people who are in contact with raw woods (firewood).

46.3.4.3 Sesquiterpene Lactone Allergens

The main allergens of Asteraceae are sesquiterpene lactones, and different ones may occur in a single species. They are characterized by the presence of a γ-butyrolactone ring bearing an exocyclic α-methylene group (Fig. 46.17). Hundreds of molecules have been (and continue to be) identified to date [207]. They are also present in other plant families such as Magnoliaceae, Winteraceae, Jubulaceae, Apiaceae, Aristolochiaceae, and Lauraceae [208].

The range of structures encountered among sesquiterpene lactones known to be allergenic is very wide, and

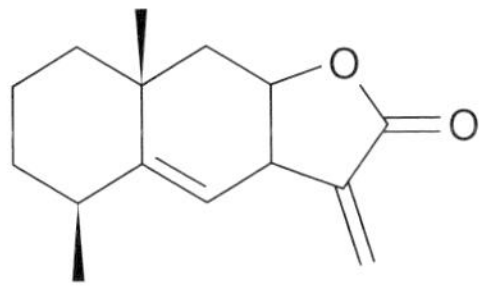

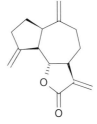
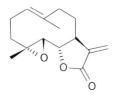

Alantolacone from
inula helenium L.

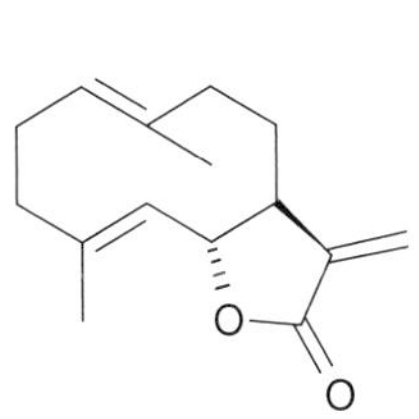

Costunolide (Costus lactone)
from *Saussurea lappa* C.B. Clarke

Dehydrocostus lactone from
Saussurea lappa C.B. Clarke

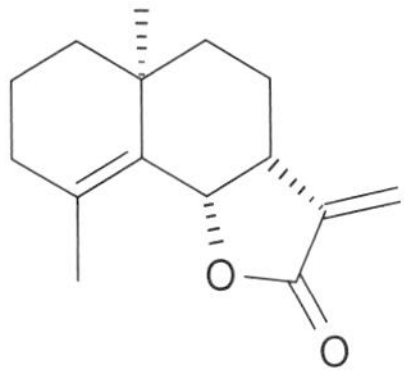

(+) D-Frullanolide
from *Frullania dilatata* Dum.

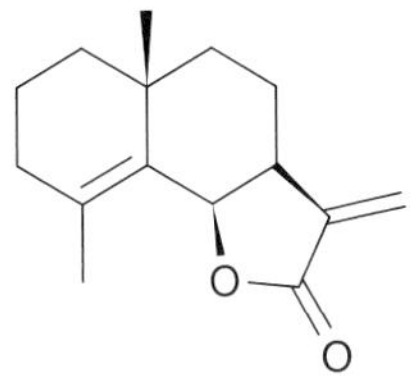

(–) L-Frullanolide
from *Frullania tamarisci* Dum.

Parthenolide from *Chrysanthemum parthenium* (L.) Bernh.

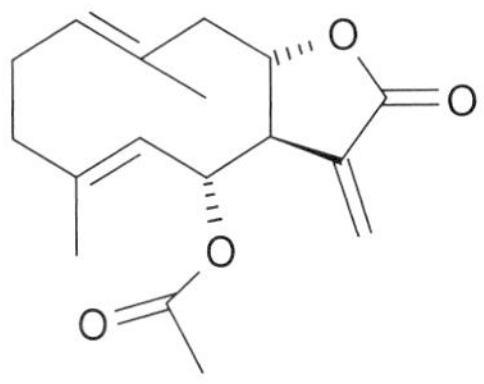

Laurenobiolide from
Laurus nobilis L.

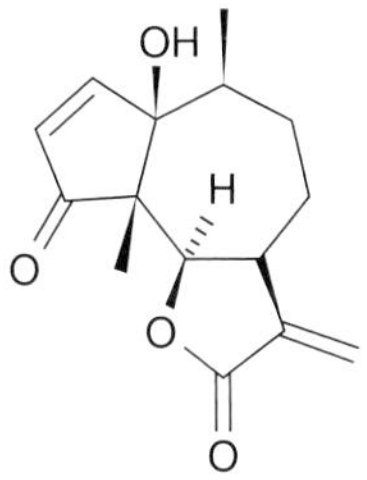

Parthenin from
Parthenium hysterophorus L.

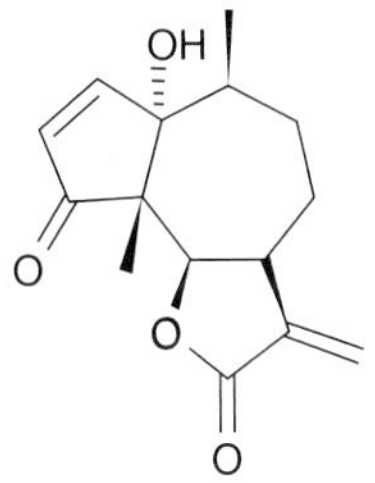

Hymenin from
Parthenium hysterophorus L.

Fig. 46.17 Structures of some allergenic sesquiterpene lactones. Alantolactone CAS 546–43–0, costunolide CAS 553–21–9, dehydrocostus lactone CAS 477–43–0, D-frullanolide CAS 40776–40–7, L-frullanolide CAS 27579–97–1, parthenin CAS 508–59–8 and its diastereoisomer hymenin, parthenolide CAS 20554–84–1, and laurenobiolide

each individual species contains a more or less complex mixture of these compounds. So, cross-sensitivity between various species in the Asteraceae is common, but neither complete nor predictable [170, 197, 209]. This unpredictability may be exemplified by the fact that individual cultivars of the autumn-flowering chrysanthemums (*Dendranthema* cultivars) do not necessarily cross-react [45, 196, 210], while cross-reactions between members of the Compositae and liverworts of the genus *Frullania* (family Jubulaceae), laurel (*Laurus nobilis* L., family Lauraceae), and various members of the family Magnoliaceae, such as *Michelia lanuginosa,* have been reported [5, 47, 211–215]. Data have been reviewed in the literature [216]. Cross-reactivity between sesquiterpene lactones largely depends on their stereochemistry.

Parthenin and hymenin are examples of diastereoisomers found in the same plant (*Parthenium hysterophorus* L.), but not produced in the same region, since parthenin is found in India and hymenin is found in South America. There is no cross-reactivity between the disatereoisomers parthenin and hymenin [217].

A vast number of species in the Compositae family have been described either as causes of contact dermatitis or as elicitors of positive patch test reactions. Many more may be regarded as potential contact allergens on the basis of their reported content of sesquiterpene lactones bearing an α-methylene-γ-butyrolactone ring.

In order to facilitate the diagnosis of sesquiterpene lactone-induced ACD, a mixture of three representative lactones from various structural classes (alantolactone, costunolide, and dehydrocostus lactone) has been made available for testing. This mixture, called *Sesquiterpene lactone mix*, has been widely tested, but detects only between 35 and 65% of cases of sensitization [218–221]; this poor sensitivity is partially explained by phytogeographic variations [222]. *Compositae mix* 6% pet., now discontinued, was an alternative preparation comprising a mixture of plant extracts (arnica, yarrow, tansy, German chamomile, and feverfew), which seemed to detect a higher proportion of cases [219, 223]. Other blends have been proposed, such as a blend of *Achillea millefolium* L., *Chamaemelum nobile* All. (syn. *Anthemis nobilis* L.), *Helianthus annuus* L., *Tagetes minuta* L., and *Tanacetum vulgare* L. [224], or the present commercially available

Compositae mix 5% pet., consisting of a mixture of short ether extracts of arnica, Roman chamomile, tansy, yarrow, and the sesquiterpene lactone parthenolide (Table 46.5). Dandelion and feverfew extracts, together or individually [225, 226], also appear to be more useful than sesquiterpene lactone mix alone.

Core Message

> Sesquiterpene lactones are potent contact allergens in Asteraceae/Compositae and liverworts. The numerous molecules generally do not cross-react.

Table 46.5 Commercially available plant allergens (*C* Chemotechnique Diagnostics, Malmö, Sweden, *F* Firma, Italy, *T* Trolab Hermal, Reinbeck, Germany)

Allergens	Concentration (%)	Sources of exposure	Providers
Achillea millefolium extract	1	Yarrow	C, T
Alantolactone	0.1		C, F
α-methylene-γ-butyrolactone[a]	0.01 (C), 0.005 (F)	*Tulipa, Alstroemeria, Bomarea, Disocorea Hispida, Erythronium, Gagea, Fritillaria*	C, F
Arnica montana extract	0.5	Mountain tobacco	C, T
Chamomilla romana (Anthemis nobilis) extract	1 (C), 2.5 (T)	Roman chamomile	C, T
Chrysanthemum cinerariifolium extract	1	Pyrethrum	C
Compositae mix	5 (C) (F)		C, F
Diallyl disulfide	1 (C), 2 (F)	Garlic	C, F
Lichen acid mix (atranorin, usnic acid, evernic acid)	0.3		C
Parthenolide	0.1	*Tanacetum parthenium* (feverfew)	C
Primin	0.01	*Primula obconica*, Primulaceae	C, F, T
Propolis	10	Beekeepers, medications	C
Sesquiterpene lactone mix (Alantolactone, costunolide, (*Frullania*) dehydrocostus lactone, each 0.033%)	0.1	Asteraceae/Compositae, Jubulaceae	C
Tanacetum parthenium extract	1	Feverfew	T
Tanacetum vulgare extract	1	Tansy	T, C
Taraxacum officinale extract	2.5	Dandelion	C
Usnic acid	0.1 (T), 1 (F)	Lichens	T, F

[a]Only 0.01% can be considered safe [92])

46.3.5 *Cruciferae (Cabbage or Mustard Family, Brassicaceae)*

The Brassicaceae family contains about 3,200 species in 375 genera, covering a large number of food plants such as cabbages (*Brassica oleracea* L.) with several varieties, for example, curly kale (*B. oleracea* var. *fimbriata* Miller), cauliflower (*B. oleracea* var. *botrytis* L.), Brussels sprouts (*B. oleracea* var. *gemmifera* DC.), kohl rabi (*B. oleracea* var. *gongyloides* L.), broccoli (*B. oleracea* var. *botrytis* ssvar. *Cymosa* Lam), turnips (Brassica *campestris* L. *var rapifera* Metz), radishes, rutabagas, mustard, and cress.

Together with the smaller Cleomaceae (which comprises the increasingly popular garden flower cleome or Spider flower, *Cleome spinosa* Jacq., syn. *C. pungens*) and Capparaceae (Capparidaceae) families, Cruciferae characteristically contains glucosidic compounds (glucosinolates), which, in many species, release mustard oils (isothiocyanates, Fig. 46.18) when the plant material is damaged. These mustard oils impart pungency to the Cruciferae that contributes to the value of many food or as irritants in traditional counterirritant remedies and rubefacient ointments. The most commonly used compound is the oil from black mustard seed (*Brassica nigra* Koch), which principally contains allyl isothiocyanate. This isothiocyanate is produced from its glucosinolate precursor sinigrin [227] by the action of an enzyme named myrosinase, activated when the plant material is damaged.

Notwithstanding the irritant properties of mustard oils and pharmaceutical preparations made from them, Coulter [228] observed no irritant reactions following rough handling of Cruciferae. Clinically, these plants are more commonly found to be responsible for ACD in food handlers [7]. Radishes induced finger dermatitis in a waitress who chopped them (*Raphanus sativus* L.) [229]. Cabbages (*Raphanus sativus* var. *capitata* Alef.) provoked occupational contact dermatitis [230], and cabbage juice produced positive patch test reactions in 5/53 patients with hand dermatitis suspected to have been caused by vegetables [76].

To avoid irritant reactions, patch test concentrations with isothiocyanates should be prepared in the range 0.1–0.05% pet. [5, 231]. Positive patch test reactions to all four of these isothiocyanates have been reported in various circumstances, but cross-reactions, if they exist, are not systematic [229, 232]. Methyl isothiocyanate [233] should be tested if plants belonging to the Capparaceae family are suspected as being the cause of dermatitis.

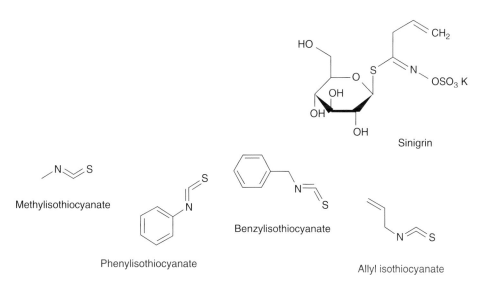

Fig. 46.18 Structures of methyl isothiocyanate CAS 556–61–6, phenyl isothiocyanate CAS 103–72–0, benzyl isothiocyanate CAS 622–78–6 and ally isothiocyanate CAS 57–06–7, and its precursor sinigrin CAS 3952–98–5

> **Core Message**
>
> › Brassicaceae are irritant and allergenic, due to the isothiocyanates they release when the plant is damaged.

46.3.6 Euphorbiaceae (Spurge Family)

The Euphorbiaceae family comprises some 5,000 species in about 300 genera, which, with the exception of the polar regions, are found throughout the world. The largest and most widely distributed genus is *Euphorbia*. In Europe, euphorbias are small weeds known as spurges; tropical species are shrubs or trees, often resembling cacti in arid parts of Africa. They contain a latex which, in many species, is a skin irritant. The irritant compounds are diterpene esters belonging to three general classes: the tiglianes, ingenanes, and daphnanes. These irritant diterpenes are also found in other genera of the Euphorbiaceae and, interestingly, in the unrelated family Thymelaeaceae (daphne family). Reviews deal with the distributions of these compounds within the two families, their irritant properties, and their tumor-promoting and other biologically hazardous properties [234–236].

Irritant contact dermatitis from Euphorbiaceae and Thymelaeaceae is rarely seen by European practitioners, but it is likely that accidental skin contact occurs quite frequently. As the irritant reaction resolves spontaneously within 1–2 days, it is unlikely to be seen in a dermatology clinic. Thus, though there is extensive anecdotal literature supported by numerous scientific studies of the irritant compounds, clinical studies and case reports are rare: 60 cases of irritant contact dermatitis from the infamous manchineel tree (*Hippomane mancinella* L.) of tropical America [237], irritant contact dermatitis from the African milk bush (*Synadenium grantii* Hook.f.) in a gardener [238], an irritant patch test reaction to the petty spurge (*Euphorbia peplus* L.), a garden weed presented by the patient as a house plant [239], and perioral dermatitis from a pencil tree (*Euphorbia tirucalli* L.) [240]. Several authors described the irritant properties of the friendship cactus (*Euphorbia hermentiana* Lemaire) following the use of this plant by a bank as an inducement to open a savings account [241], examined the irritant properties of a number of tigliane, ingenane, and daphnane polyol esters in humans [242], or described a case of an 8-year-old-girl who developed irritation and swelling of the face and eyelids as a result of a fight in which a boy beat her with snow-on-the-mountain (*Euphorbia marginata* Pursh) [243]. We have observed irritant dermatitis in a botanist who had botanized and made contact with euphorbia (Fig. 46.19).

It is frequently difficult to ascertain whether Euphorbiaceae are responsible for irritant or ACD. Allergy rather than irritation is documented for two common ornamental Euphorbiaceae, namely croton (*Codiaeum variegatum* Blume var. *pictum* Muell. Arg.) and poinsettia (*Euphorbia pulcherrima* Willd.), although the allergens have not yet been characterized [244–248].

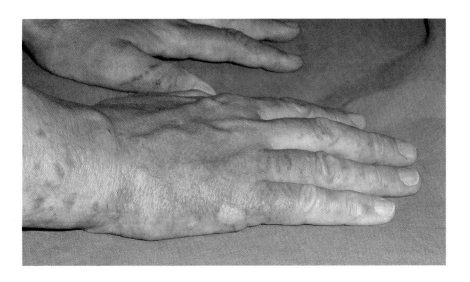

Fig. 46.19 Bullous irritant hand dermatitis due to *Euphorbia* spp

Out of 305 cases of contact dermatitis presented at the dermatology clinic on the Hawaiian island of Kauai, 61 were attributable to contact with plants. Among the most frequently blamed, Mango (*Mangifera indica* L., family Anacardiaceae) caused ACD, and mokihana (*Pelea anisata* H. Mann, family Rutaceae) induced irritant photodermatitis, but the mechanism of the reactions to the euphorbias, allergic, or irritant was not stated [249]. It should be remembered that the irritant properties of these plants are sometimes utilized in popular remedies, for treating warts and basal cell carcinomas [250]. The potential for using euphorbias to produce dermatitis artefacta should also be recognized.

Among the irritants isolated from Euphorbiaceae (Fig. 46.20), 12-Deoxyphorbol-13-phenylacetate is an example of a tigliane polyol ester, found in the common sun spurge (*Euphorbia helioscopia* L.) [251]. Resiniferatoxin, a daphnane polyol ester that is one of the most irritant compounds known to Man, is found in officinal spurge (*Euphorbia resinifera* Berg) [252, 253]. The ingenane polyol ester 3-*O*-hexadecanoyl ingenol is

found in the caper spurge (*Euphorbia lathyris* L.) [171]. Readers interested in a comprehensive survey of the occurrence of such compounds in the Euphorbiaceae and Thymelaeaceae are referred to works by Evans [254] and Schmidt [10, 255, 256].

Core Message

> Euphorbiaceae are very strong irritant and sometimes allergenic plants.

46.3.7 Lichens

Lichens are not really plants and consist of a symbiotic association of a fungus (mycosymbiont, Kingdom Fungi) and an alga (phytosymbiont, Kingdom Protoctista), the first one providing morphology and sexual reproduction via spores, the second one producing organic materials

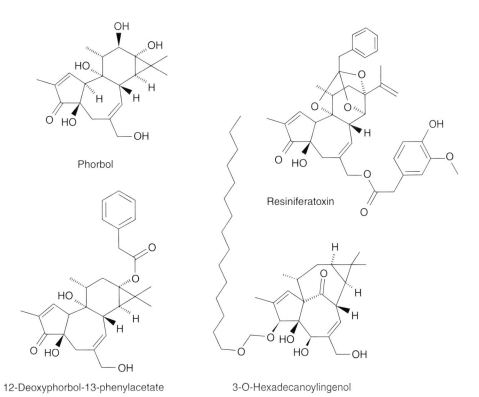

Phorbol

Resiniferatoxin

12-Deoxyphorbol-13-phenylacetate

3-O-Hexadecanoylingenol

Fig. 46.20 Structures of the irritant phorbol CAS 17673–25–5 and representative irritants from the Euphorbiaceae and Thymelaeaceae: resiniferatoxin CAS 57444–62–9, 12-deoxyphorbol-13-phenylacetate, and 3-*O*-hexadecanoylingenol

46

Fig. 46.21 Structure of some sensitizing lichen compounds. (+)-Usnic acid CAS 125–46–2, evernic acid, CAS 537–09–7, perlatolic acid, atranorin CAS 479–20–9, chloroatranorin, atranol CAS 526–37–4 and chloroatranol CAS 57074–21–2

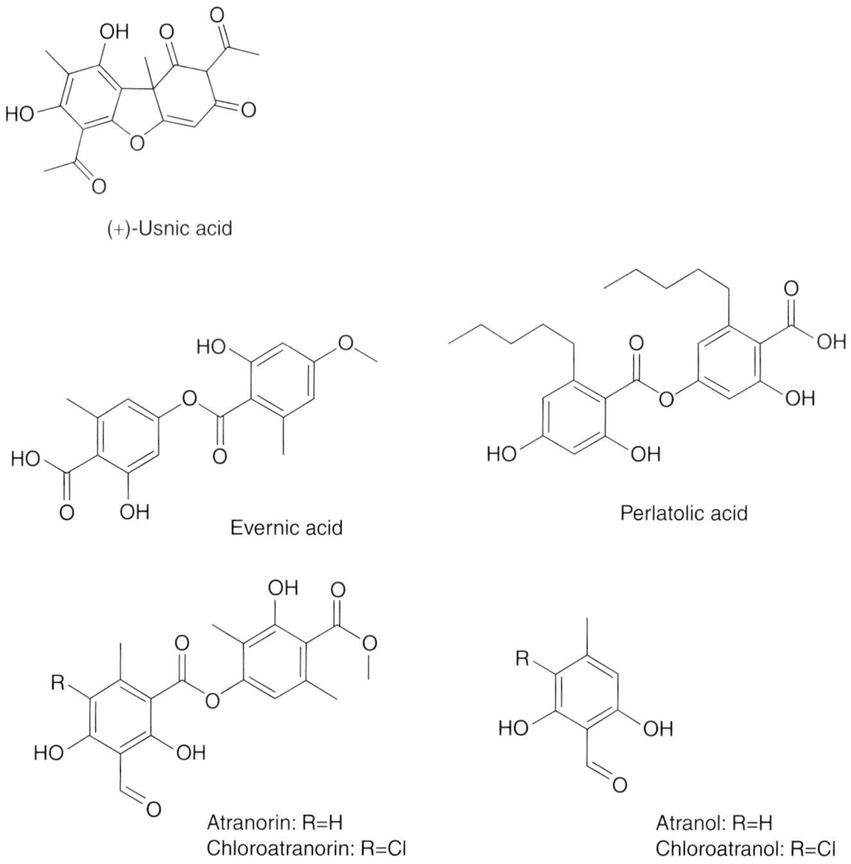

(+)-Usnic acid

Evernic acid

Perlatolic acid

Atranorin: R=H
Chloroatranorin: R=Cl

Atranol: R=H
Chloroatranol: R=Cl

by the way of photosynthesis [257]. Lichens grow on walls, roofs, trees, and rocks.

Several species are sensitizing, and those most often found to be the causes of ACD are species of *Cladonia*, *Evernia*, and *Parmelia*, although reactions have been described with other species such as *Hypogymnia*, *Platismatia*, *Physconia*, *Usnea*, and *Alectoria* (*Bryoria*) [202]. Frequent sensitizing compounds from lichens are described in Fig. 46.21. Dermatitis usually affects forestry workers and lichen pickers and appears on the hands, forearms, face, and other exposed areas [258, 259]. Allergy to lichens may also be observed following exposure to perfumes containing oak moss (which is not a moss!), which is extracted from *Evernia prunastri* (L.) Ach. and related species [260, 261]. *E. prunastri* contains atranorin and chloroatranorin, depsides that lead to the formation of atranol and chloroatranol during preparation of oak moss absolute. With methyl-β-orcinol carboxylate, they are potent allergens identified in oak moss absolute [262–264].

A history of abnormal photosensitivity is associated with lichen sensitivity and has been discussed below. Irradiation of patch tests to lichens and their extracts may elicit enhanced responses [265–268]. An airborne contact dermatitis simulating photodermatitis has also been suggested to contribute to the clinical features seen in patients with lichen allergy [48]. Immediate-type allergies with asthma and urticaria were described following inhalation of, or direct contact with, algae from lichens [269].

Lichens can be tested "as is," but irritant reactions may occur. Oak moss is present in the fragrance mix of the European standard series, as a mixture of mainly *Evernia prunastri* Ach. (oak moss stricto sensu) and *Pseudevernia furfuracea* Zopf. (syn. *Parmelia furfuracea* Ach., tree moss). As tree moss, growing on both lobe-leaved trees and conifers, is frequently automatically picked with bark, it may contain derivatives of colophony. Such resinic acids are responsible for some positive reactions to fragrance mix in colophony-sensitive patients [270]. Lichen-derived compounds such as atranorin, usnic acid, and evernic acid can be tested at 0.1 or 1% pet. Whether cross-sensitization occurs between structurally related lichen compounds is not clear. Because of the common occurrence of some of the lichen compounds in a number of species, concomitant sensitization is possible [258, 259].

> **Core Message**
>
> ➢ Lichens are responsible for some cases of contact allergy from plants or plant extracts in perfumes.

46.3.8 Primulaceae (Primrose Family)

This family of cosmopolitan distribution comprises 1,000 species in about 28 genera (among them *Cyclamen* spp), but only *Primula* (*Primula obconica* Hance) presents a common dermatological hazard. *P. obconica* is popularly grown in Europe as a house and greenhouse plant for its showy and long-lasting flowers, and the first report of contact allergy in 1888 by White has since been followed by many other reports [5, 271, 272]. Dermatitis (Fig. 46.22) generally affects the eyelids, face, neck, fingers, hands, and forearms, but *P. obconica* can also cause conjunctivitis and erythema multiforme-like eruption [273]. The most important allergen of *Primula* is a quinone named primin [274], formed by the oxidation of its biosynthetic precursor miconidin (which is also allergenic [275]) in minute glandular hairs (trichomes) present at the surface of the plant (Fig. 46.23). Dermatitis may be due to direct contact with plants, dust particles, or to primin released directly from intact *P. obconica* plants [276]. This explains flares of dermatitis in highly sensitized patients after entering a room containing *P. obconica*. The presence of other allergens has been suggested [272, 275, 277], for example, the quinhydrone formed from primin and miconidin [271], the flavone primetin present in *Primula mistassinica* Michaux, and skin oxidized into a quinone derivative [278]. These could explain ACD with positive allergic patch test reactions to fragments of the plant, but negative to primin ([279], personal observation, Fig. 46.24). Other species of *Primula* are reported to be allergenic,

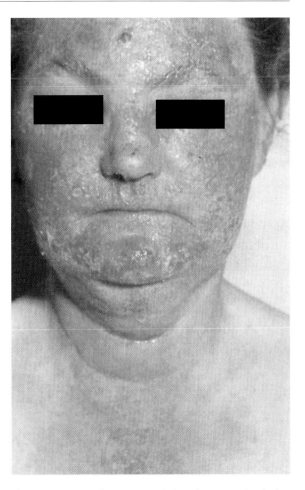

Fig. 46.22 Unusually, severe exudative edematous primula dermatitis on the face (courtesy of N. Hjorth)

such as *P. auricula* and *P. denticulata* [280, 281]. For a number of years, *P. obconica* was the most common cause of plant-induced contact dermatitis in Europe, but has become less of a problem in recent years, as its reputation has stimulated a widespread avoidance response. It is noteworthy that primin-free *Primula* have recently been developed, among them includes the "Touch Me" cultivar [282].

Because the content of primin in the leaves varies with the season, method of cultivation, and cultivar identity [283, 284], the outcome of using fresh plant material as such for patch testing varies from the occurrence of false negatives during the winter months [285] to active sensitization between the months of April to August, when primin levels are at their highest [284, 286]. It was previously recommended that an ether extract of the leaves harvested in spring (60 g fresh weight dipped in

46

Fig. 46.23 Chemical structures of primin CAS 15121–94–5, miconidin CAS 34272–58–7 and primetin CAS 548–58–3

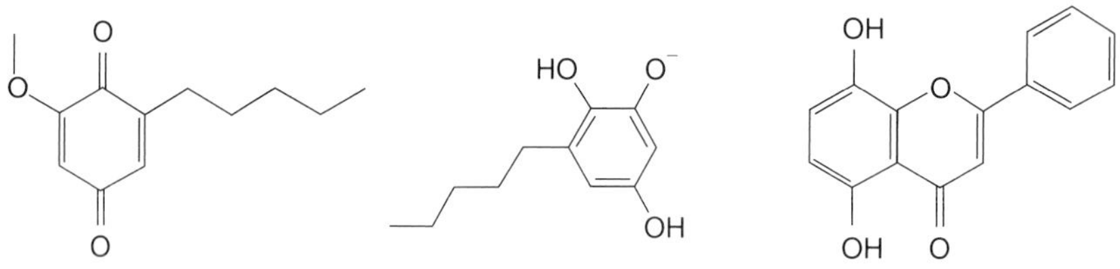

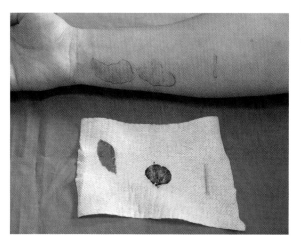

Primin   Miconidin   Primetin

Fig. 46.24 Positive patch test reactions to *Primula obconica* Hance, performed in a horticulturist negative to primin

100 mL ether before concentrating to 50 mL at room temperature) should be used [287]. Patch testing with commercially available synthetic primin carries a real risk of active sensitization if concentrations greater than the usual (0.01%) are used.

Core Message

> Primulaceae are a source of contact sensitization, mainly in florists who handle *Primula obconica* Hance.

46.3.9 Ranunculaceae (Buttercup Family)

The family contains 1,900 species in 50 genera. Mostly herbaceous with rhizomes, Ranunculaceae chiefly grow in northern temperate regions. Many members of the family are very caustic and can cause skin or mucous membrane irritation [10, 30, 32]. This has led to the use of poultices of the plants as counterirritants

in traditional medicine for the treatment of rheumatic joints, and severe adverse cutaneous reactions, with skin necrosis, may occur [288–292]. Systemic symptoms may occur after accidental ingestion of fresh plants by humans or animals, with systemic, digestive, renal, cardiorespiratory, neurologic, and possibly life-threatening symptoms.

Protoanemonin is the irritant agent in Ranunculaceae. It is released from its precursor ranunculin by an enzymatic cleavage when the plant material is damaged [293–296]. Protoanemonin rapidly loses its irritant properties by dimerization into anemonin (Fig. 46.25). Dried plants are, therefore, inoffensive.

The following genera are representative members of the Ranunculaceae that have to be regarded as possible causes of irritant contact dermatitis:

Anemone spp. with wood anemone (*Anemone nemorosa* L.)
Actaea spp. with baneberry or herb Christopher (*Actaea spicata* L.), and white baneberry (*Actaea alba* Miller)
Caltha spp. with marsh marigold or kingcup (*Caltha palustris* L.)
Clematis spp. with Traveller's Joy, called "Old Man's Beard" because of long and feathery achenes or "herbe aux gueux" because middle age mendicants scrubbed their face with sap to provoke dermatitis and pity (*Clematis vitalba* L.)
Pulsatilla spp. such as prairie crocus (*Pulsatilla patens* Miller, syn. *Anemone patens* L.), Pasque flower (*Pulsatilla vulgaris* Mill., syn. *Anemone pulsatilla* L.)
Ranunculus such as common meadow buttercup (*Ranunculus acris* L., syn. *Ranunculus acer* Auct.), corn buttercup (*Ranunculus arvensis* L.), bulbous buttercup (*Ranunculus bulbosus* L.), or creeping buttercup (*Ranunculus repens* L.)
Helleborus spp. with Christmas rose (*Helleborus niger* L.).

Fig. 46.25 Structure of ranunculin CAS 644–69–9, precursor of the strong irritant protoanemonin CAS 108–28–1, loses irritancy after dimerization into anemonin CAS 508–44–1

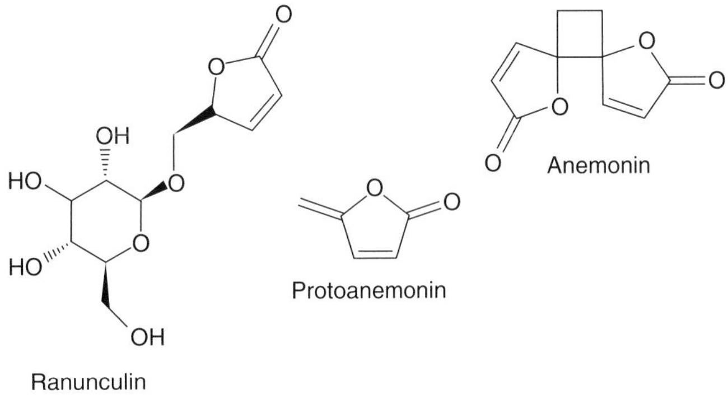

Ranunculin

Protoanemonin

Anemonin

Core Message

> Ranunculaceae are very strong irritants, containing protoanemonin. They can induce severe skin damage, as systemic intoxication after ingestion.

46.3.10 Umbelliferae/Apiaceae (Carrot Family), Rutaceae (Rue Family), and Moraceae (Mulberry Family)

Members of these families have been considered together because of their capacity to induce photodermatitis, of phototoxic origin. The phototoxicity is due to furocoumarins contained in them. The synonym psoralen is derived from the Latin name of the Indian plant babchi or bakuchi (*Psoralea corylifolia* L., Leguminosae family), a plant that was used for the treatment of vitiligo [297]. The most classical feature is Oppenheim dermatitis and its variants that are discussed below. Children using the stems of hogweeds (*Heracleum mantegazzianum* Somm. and Lev. and *H. sphondylium* L.) as toy telescopes or peashooters in late summer typically develop bullous and erythematous lesions around the eyes and mouth [298, 299]. Other exposed areas of skin may be affected if contact with the sap occurs during horseplay among these plants, which are weeds of uncultivated land along roads, railways, and streams [56]. Because several members of these families are important sources of food, phototoxic reactions may occasionally be observed following occupational or household contact and sun exposure, on areas such as hands, the upper limbs, and around the mouth.

The Apiaceae/Umbelliferae family contains 2,850 species in 275 genera with a cosmopolitan distribution, chiefly in north temperate regions. Some are food plants such as celery (*Apium graveolens* L. var. *dulce* Pers.) [300–302], parsnip (*Pastinaca sativa* L.syn. *Peucedanum sativum* Benth. and Hook.) [303, 304], carrot (Daucus carota L.) [8], angelica (*Angelica archangelica* L.) [8, 305], chervil (*Anthriscus cerefolium* Hoffm.), or parsley (*Petroselinum crispum* A.W. Hill, syns. *Apium crispum* Miller, *Petroselinum sativum* Hoffm.) [306]. Others are medicinal, wild, or cultivated plants such as Bishop's weed (*Ammi majus* L.) [307], Palm of Tromsø (*Heracleum stevenii* Manden syn. *Heracleum laciniatum* Hornem.) [308], giant hogweed (*Heracleum mantegazzianum* Somm. and Lev) [56, 298], and hogweed (*Heracleum sphondylium* L.) [309]. Several dermatologically significant plants are reported in Table 46.2.

ACD from Apiceae/Umbelliferae is possible, and has been described for carrot, celery, and parsley. Falcarinol, also contained in members of Araliaceae (see later section), is probably the delayed-type allergen present [310, 311].

The Rutaceae family comprises citrus fruits. Many of them have induced phototoxicity, such as lime [60, 61, 312], bergamot [313, 314], and orange [315, 316]. Furanocoumarins are isolated mainly from citrus rind. Pulp also contains photosensitizers, but to a lesser degree, with an average ratio of 1: 20–1: 100 [61]. Garden rue (*Ruta graveolens* L.) grows in gardens and may elicit phototoxic reactions after being picked [317, 318], as may other rue species such as *Ruta chalepensis* L. (syn. *Ruta bracteosa* DC.) [319]. Perfumes with psoralens from bergamot oil (*Citrus bergamia* Risso and Poit.) can induce phototoxicity presenting as "berloque dermatitis." Gas plant (*Dictamnus albus* L., syn. *Dictamnus fraxinella* Pers.) [60, 63, 303, 320], mokihana (*Pelea anisata* H. Mann) [321, 322], blister bush (*Phebalium anceps* DC), and Western Australian blister bush (*Phebalium argenteum* Smith) also contain psoralens [323], which largely account for the (sometimes very severe) bullous dermatitis [61].

The Moraceae family contains edible fig (*Ficus carica* L.) [324–327], breadfruit (*Artocarpus altilis*), other *Ficus* spp (naturally growing or as indoor plants in temperate countries), and the tropical wood iroko or African teak (*Chlorophora excelsa* Benth. and Hook. f.), which contains chlorophorin.

Although allergic reactions to psoralens do not seem to have been described, photoallergic reactions can occur [67, 68]. However, a number of psoralen-containing plants may also sensitize as a result of other compounds that they contain. For example, citrus oils are generally weakly allergenic, but are also irritant, and some are phototoxic [328]. Similarly, carrots (*Daucus carota* L., family Umbelliferae) have sensitized workers in the canning industry [329–331], but there is no convincing evidence that they may elicit phototoxic reactions, although weak phototoxicity has been observed experimentally [332]. Thus, if an allergic reaction is suspected, it is important to realize that irritancy and photoaggravation may occur during patch testing.

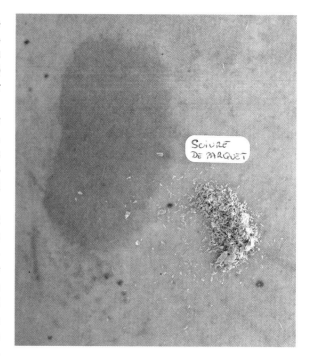

Fig. 46.26 Positive patch test reaction to woodfloor (wood dust diluted in petrolatum) in a "do it yourself" carpenter

> **Core Message**
>
> ❯ The Apiaceae/Umbelliferae family is mainly responsible for phototoxic contact dermatitis (Oppenheim dermatitis and variants) like Rutaceae (citrus family) and Moraceae (fig family) because of the furocoumarins contained in them.

46.3.11 Woods

Although woods are not derived from a botanically homogeneous source, we will consider them together for practical reasons. Most dermatoses from contact with woods are occupational and observed in carpenters, joiners, cabinet-makers, and associated tradespersons [5, 8, 13, 73, 333], as forest workers are generally affected by liverwort and lichens growing on trees. Less commonly, dermatitis is due to finished wood

products, such as violin chin-rests [334], necklaces [335], bracelets [336], and knife handles [337].

Woodworkers are highly exposed to sawdust, and contact initially occurs on exposed areas (hands and forearms, face and neck, Fig. 46.26). Standard clothing is not good protection. Airborne sawdust, however, may drift inside loosely fitting protective clothing and adhere to sweaty areas of skin like the axillae, waistband, groin, and ankles. Such areas can be prone to irritant and/or ACD.

The additional hazards of asthma and sinus ethmoidal adenocarcinoma from inhaling the sawdust of certain woods and the higher risks of Hodgkin's disease associated with woodworking, as well as of systemic symptoms if the wood contains pharmacologically active constituents, have been reviewed [338, 339]. Reviews on wood-induced dermatitis are recommended for detailed information [8, 73, 338–343], like the website (http://biodiversity.bio.uno.edu/delta/wood) [344] to which readers can refer for further information.

The most highly sensitizing woods are of tropical origin, as they commonly contain quinones as sensitizers. Because of the wide occurrence of quinones, reactivity to several woods may be expected. For example,

2,6-dimethoxy-1,4-benzoquinone is found in many woods, such as African or American mahogany (*Khaya* spp., Meliaceae family), Bubinga (*Guibourtia spp.*, family Caesalpinaceae), Capomo (*Brosimum alicastrum* Schwartz, family Moraceae), *Bowdichia* spp. (*Bowdichia nitida* Benth.) and *Diplotropis* spp. (*Diplotropis purpurea*), Doussié (*Afzelia* spp.), Afrormosia or Kokrodua (*Pericopsis elata* van Meeuwen), Makoré (*Tieghemella africana* Pierre, *T. heckelii* Pierre ex A. Chev.), Sipo (*Entandrophragma* spp., family Meliaceae), and Wengé (*Millettia* spp. *laurentii* De Wild, *Milettia stuhlmanii* Taub. family Papilionaceae) [343].

In studies with guinea pigs, cross-reactivity between primin, deoxylapachol, various dalbergiones, mansonones, and other quinones have been observed [338], but cross-sensitivity between primin and various wood quinones does not seem to occur in humans [345]. In addition to quinonoid allergens, a number of other types of low-molecular-weight allergens have been identified from woods, reflecting the variety of botanical sources from which exploitable woods are obtained. Structures of some of the best-known wood allergens are given in the following figures.

Woods provide some rather significant problems with their identification. Most are transported under a trivial rather than botanical name, and it is not unusual for these trivial names to be misapplied either inadvertently or deliberately. For example, the single milowood (*Thespesia populnea* Sol. ex Corrêa) is also named Álamo, álamo blanco, algodón de monte, beach maho, bosch-katoen, catalpa, clamor, clemón, cork-tree, cremón, emajagüilla, frescura, grós hahaut, haiti-haiti, jaqueca, John-Bull-tree, macoi, mahault de Londres, maho, mahot bord-de-mer, majagua de Florida, majagüilla, otaheita, palo de jaqueca, palu santu, portiatree, santa maría, seaside mahoe, Spanish cork, and tuliptree. It is imperative, for serious diagnosis and exploration, that a solid sample of a wood believed to be the cause of contact dermatitis (or any other pathological lesion) is sent to a wood anatomist for identification [338]. Its origin and any available trade names should also be made known to the wood anatomist.

46.3.11.1 American and Australian Woods

A variety of American and Australian woods deserve a mention in this context [10, 73, 343–347].

Australian blackwood (*Acacia melanoxylon* R. Br., Mimosaceae family) is a very important wood in Australia, inducing occupational contact dermatitis due to 2,6-dimethoxy-1,4-benzoquinone, acamelin, and melacacidin.

The Australian silky oak (*Grevillea robusta* A. Cunn., Proteaceae family) has been discussed above.

Brazilian rosewood or palissander (*Dalbergia nigra* All., Papillionaceae family) such as East India rosewood (*Dalbergia latifolia* Roxb.), cocolobo (*Dalbergia retusa* Hemsl., *Dalbergia granadilla*, and *Dalbergia hypoleuca*), or grenadil (*Dalbergia melanoxylon* Guill. and Perr.) are used for high-class furniture such as wooden jewels and musical instruments. Dalbergiones such as (*R*)-3,4-dimethoxydalbergione, (*R*)- and (*S*)-4-methoxydalbergione, (*S*)-4-methoxydalbergione, (*S*)-4,4'-dimethoxydalbergione, and (*S*)-4'-hydroxy-4-methoxydalbergione are the sensitizers (Fig. 46.27).

Grapia is a Brazilian wood (*Apuleia leiocarpa* Macbr., Caesalpinioidae family) that can induce contact dermatitis and mucous membrane symptoms. Main allergens are likely to be ayanin, oxyayanin A, and oxyayanin B, the latter also being an allergen in movingui (*Distemonanthus benthamianus* Baill., family Caesalpinioidae).

Incense cedar (*Calocedrus decurrens* Florin, Cupressaceae family) used for pencils, chests, or toys is a cause of contact dermatitis due to the allergen thymoquinone.

Pao ferro, "Santos-palissander" or caviuna vermelha (*Machaerium scleroxylon* Tul., Papilionaceae family), is frequently used as a substitute of rosewood. The sensitizers are dalbergiones, including (*R*)-3,4-dimethoxydalbergione, which is a very potent allergen.

Polynesian rosewood or milowood (*Thespesia populnea* Sol., Malvaceae family) is a wood used for small articles and wood jewels. It contains mansonones such as mansonone X.

Sucupira (*Bowdichia nitida* Spruce, Fabaceae family) is a Brazil wood, which is used for flooring and responsible for ACD in joiners and flooring workers. Among the allergens present, 2,6-dimethoxy-*p*-benzoquinone and Bowdichione are the best known.

Western cedar (*Thuja plicata* Donn., family Cupressaceae) is used as a hardwood in construction work or on boats. Its main contact allergen is

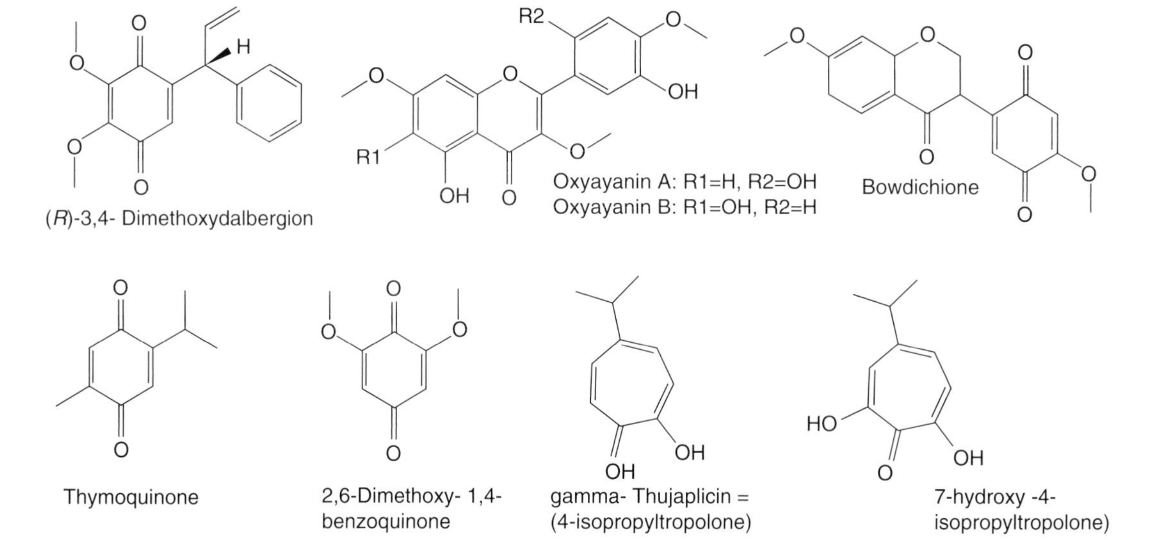

Fig. 46.27 Allergens from American and Australian woods: (*R*)-3,4-dimethoxydalbergion CAS 3755–64–4, oxyayanin A CAS and oxyayanin B CAS, bowdichione, thymoquinone CAS 490–91–5, 2,6-dimethoxy-1,4-benzoquinone CAS 530–55–2, γ-thujaplicin CAS 672–76–4, and 7-hydroxy-4-isopropyltropolone

thymoquinone. It also contains γ-thujaplicin and 7-hydroxy-4-isopropyl-tropolone.

46.3.11.2 Asian Woods

Several Asian woods are reported to be sources of allergens [10, 73, 344, 347].

Teak (*Tectona grandis* L., Verbenaceae family) is largely used for various indoor and outdoor applications (such as in doors and windows) due to its high durability. The sensitizers are naphthoquinones named deoxylapachol and lapachol, which have similar reactivities [73, 347] (Fig. 46.28).

East-Indian rosewood is similar to Brazilian rosewood in terms of use and allergens.

Macassar (*Diospyros celebica Bakh.*, family Ebenaceae) is related to coromandel and ebony.

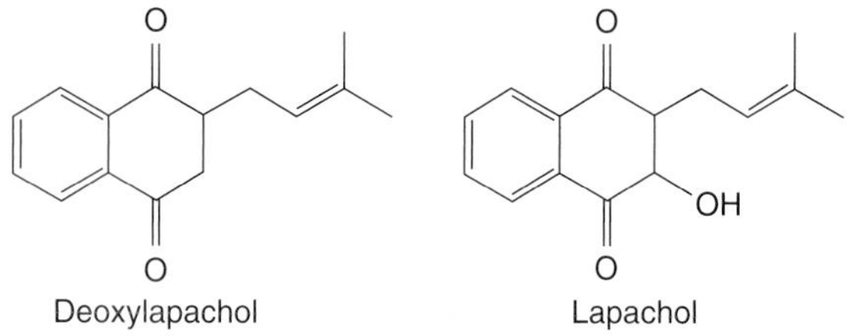

Fig. 46.28 Structure of deoxylapachol CAS 3568–90–9, and lapachol CAS 84–79–7

46.3.11.3 African Woods

The following African woods are the most relevant to this discussion [10, 73, 344, 348].

African ebony (*Diospyros crassifolia* Hiern., family Ebenaceae) and coromandel (*Diospyros melanoxylon* Roxb.) are wood species with black heartwood used for precious works.

African mahogany (*Khaya grandiflora* DC.), Khaya mahogany (*Kahya ivorensis* A. Chev.), Krala (*Khaya anthotheca* C. DC.), and Senegal mahogany (*Khaya senegalensis* A. Juss., Meliaceae family) are sensitizers by the way of allergens such as anthothecol (Fig. 46.29).

African red padauk wood (*Pterocarpus soyauxii* Taub., Papillonaceae family) is a hardwood tree used to manufacture veneer, furniture, and musical instruments.

Ayan (*Distemonanthus benthamianus* Baillon, Caesalpinaceae family) is used for flooring or windows. Its allergens are oxyayanin A and B.

Iroko, African teak or kambala (*Chlorophora excelsa* Benth and Hook. f., Moraceae family), has good strength and durability and is used for indoor and outdoor constructional work. Chlorophorin is its main allergen.

Mansonia or bete (*Mansonia altissima* A. Chev, Sterculiaceae family) is used as a substitute for walnut. It has several sensitizers called sesquiterpenoid mansonones, with the *ortho*-quinone mansonone A being the main allergen.

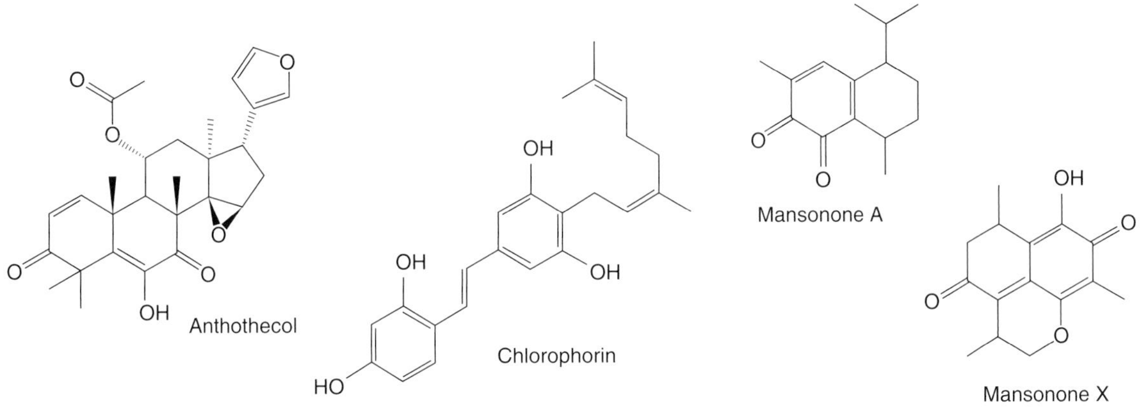

Fig. 46.29 Structures of some allergens in African woods: anthothecol CAS 10410–83–0, chlorophorin CAS 537–41–7, mansonone A CAS 7715–94–8, and mansonone X

46.3.11.4 European Woods

Woods derived from trees growing in temperate regions in Europe are also sensitizers [73, 347, 349, 350]. Dermatitis has been reported in association with alder (*Alnus* sp., Betulaceae family), ash (*Fraxinus* sp., Oleaceae family), beech (*Fagus* sp., Fagaceae family), birch (*Betula* sp. Betulaceae family), and poplar (*Populus* sp., Salicaceae family) woods.

The most extensively grown and exploited trees in temperate regions are the pines (*Pinus* spp.), spruces (*Picea* spp.), firs (*Abies* spp.), and related conifers (family Pinaceae). These are rarely implicated as causes of ACD. It is worth noting that patients with dermatitis from pine or spruce have positive reactions to colophony. Pines are sources of turpentine oil and colophony, both of which are well-known sensitizers. In both of these wood-derived products, the actual sensitizers are the hydroperoxidic autoxidation products that are formed in contact with the air, rather than the major constituents from which they are derived.

The major resinic acids in colophony are abietic and dehydroabietic acids. Abietic acid was formerly claimed to be the cause of colophony (rosin) dermatitis. However, it appears to be neither a sensitizer nor an elicitor of colophony dermatitis if rigorously purified, whereas numerous oxidation products such as 15-hydroperoxyabietic acid or products from secondary oxidation are the allergens responsible (Fig. 46.30) [351–353].

In turpentine oil, hydroperoxides of 3-carene, and not Δ3-carene itself, are sensitizers [354, 355].

> **Core Message**
>
> › Woods induce contact dermatitis, mainly in woodworkers. Irritation is frequent, and contact allergy can be severe due to potent allergens like quinones.

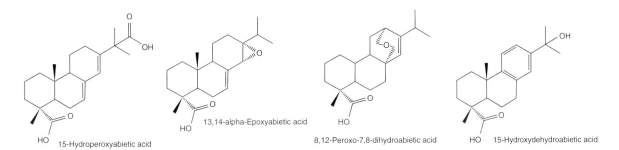

Fig. 46.30 Examples of oxidation products of colophony, responsible for sensitization

46

46.3.12 Mushrooms

Several cases of occupational ACD have been described from mushrooms, which mainly induce immediate-type symptoms. The best-known manifestation is likely shii-take dermatitis, due to contact or ingestion of raw or half-cooked black mushrooms (*Lentinula edodes* Pegler) [356]. Other mushrooms have been reported as being allergenic, such as yellow boletus (*Boletus luteus* L., syn. *Suillus luteus* Gray), cep or Polish mushroom (*Boletus* edulis Bull.Fr), meadow mushroom (*Agaricus campestris* L.), cultivated mushroom (white type: *Agaricus hortensis* Imai; brown type: *Agaricus bisporus* Pilát), orange agaric (*Lactarius deliciosus* Gray), pine yellow clavaria or fairy clubs (*Clavaria flava* Fr., syn. *Ramaria flava* Quélet), oyster (*Pleurotus ostreatus* Kummer), and yamabushitake or monkey's head mushroom (*Hericicum erinaceum* Pers.) [357–360].

46.3.13 Ferns

Ferns and related plants [361] have rarely been implicated in plant dermatitis. Leatherleaf or Baker fern (*Arachnoides adiantiformis* Tindale, Aspidiaceae, or Dryopteridaceae family) provoked ACD in a flower shop worker [362].

46.3.14 Miscellaneous Plants

Many plants have been described as inducing dermatitis. Case reports are sometimes scarce or even unique. Many are reported in dermato-botanical books, but it is interesting to cite some recent reports of dermatitis due to plants belonging to families not mentioned above.

46.3.14.1 Araliaceae (Ginseng, Aralia, Ivy Family)

Common ivy (*Hedera helix* L.) is a very common plant in Europe that may induce contact irritation and more rarely sensitization. It contains three powerful irritants and weak sensitizers, namely falcarinol, 11,12-dehydrofalcarinol and 11,12,16,17-didehydrofalcarinol (Fig. 46.31), which have moderate sensitizing potential [311, 363, 364]. These allergens or related molecules are also present in other members of this family, such as ginseng (*Panax ginseng* C. Meyer), *Schefflera arboricola* Hayata [311], or kakuremino (*Dendropanax trifidus* Makino) [365]. Falcarinone, an oxidation product of falcarinol, is commonly found in the Apiaceae/Umbelliferae family [311], and falcarinol is likely a delayed-type allergen of Apiaceae/Umbelliferae, as in carrot, celery, and parsley [310, 311].

46.3.14.2 Papaveraceae (Poppy Family)

Greater celandine, sometimes named "wart plant" (*Chelidonium majus* L., Papaveraceae family), is well known in traditional topical treatments of warts, epithelial tumors, and hyperkeratotic lesions [366]. Its orange-colored juice has irritant properties and has been reported to be a probable allergenic [367]. Systemic (liver) toxicity is possible after ingestion [368].

46.3.14.3 Guttiferae (St John's Wort or Mangosteen Family)

This family comprises herbs, lianes, shrubs, and trees that have a colored resinous juice. They are used for timbers, drugs, dyes, gums, pigments, and resins.

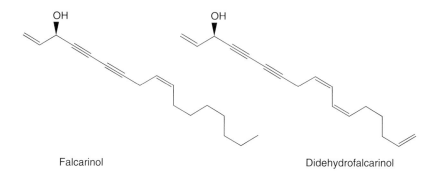

Fig. 46.31 Falcarinol, CAS 21852–80–2, and didehydrofalcarinol, CAS 110927–49–6

Falcarinol   Didehydrofalcarinol

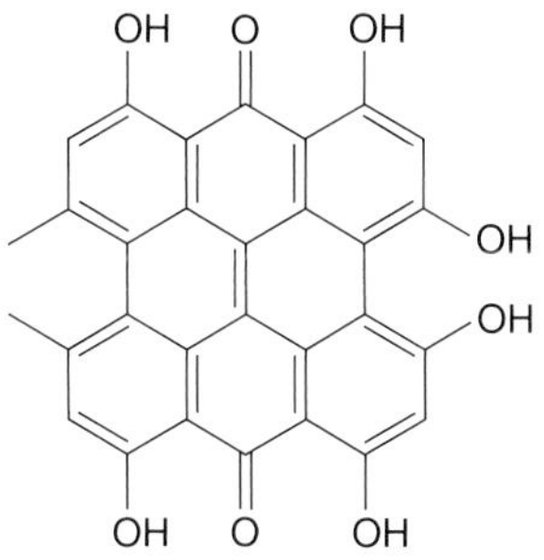

Fig. 46.32 Hypericin, CAS 548–04–9, extracted from *Hypericum perforatum* L.

St John's wort (*Hypericum perforatum* L.) has been used for centuries for wounds, burns, or dermatitis [366]. It has recently been used systemically for depression. It contains hyperforin, which has antibacterial or claimed antidepressant properties, and the phototoxic substance hypericin (Fig. 46.32), which is responsible for cutaneous side effects such as contact dermatitis and photosensitivity [369–372].

Tamanu oil (Calophyllum inophyllum), extracted from the fruits or seeds of *Calophyllum tacamahaca* L. and used as a cosmetic or traditional medicine ingredient, has been reported to be a cause of ACD, with photoworsening of patch tests [373].

46.3.14.4 Hydrangeaceae

Dermatitis due to *Hydrangea macrophylla* Thunb (Hydrangeaceae family) appears as a chronic, fissuring, and scaling dermatitis of hand and finger. Irritant dermatitis is possible, but allergy is not rare and is due to hydrangenol (Fig. 46.33). Occupational exposure is mainly found in nursery workers, florists, or gardeners. Patch tests with leaves and stems are strongly positive, as hydrangenol 0.1% pet., which gives strongly positive reactions [374].

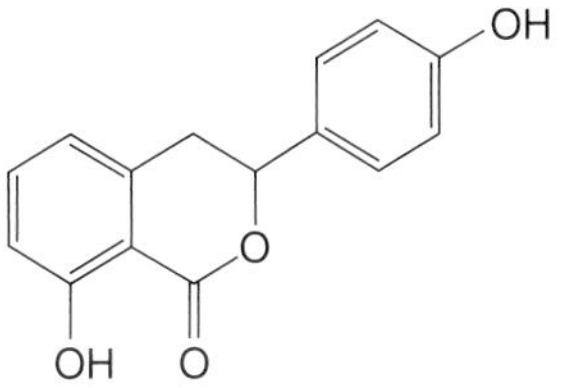

Fig. 46.33 Hydrangenol, CAS 480–87–7 the allergen of hydrangea

46.3.14.5 Iridaceae (Iris Family)

Contact dermatitis to iris (safflower) (*Iris germanica* var *florentina* Dykes) was reported, with positive reactions to petals [375], but not to leaves in one observation [376].

46.3.14.6 Labiatae (Mint Family)

This family may be named as the Labiaceae and comprises more than 5,500 species, many of them yielding essential oils. They can be used for cooking and in traditional and herbal medicine. Numerous are well known like peppermint (*Mentha piperita* L.), origanum (*Origanum vulgare* L.) and marjoram (*Origanum majorana* L.), basil (*Ocimum basilicum* L.), lavender (*Lavandula* L.), and sage (*Salvia officinalis* L.). Most of them can induce irritant and sometimes ACD. Rosemary (*Rosmarinus officinalis* L.) and thyme (*Thymus vulgaris* L.) are said to cause allergic cross-reactions [377].

46.3.14.7 Paeoniaceae (Peony Family)

The family comprises 33 species in one genus. Among them, *Paeonia officinalis* L. has been reported to cause ACD. Patient can react to all parts of the plants, both to fresh and dried materials [378].

46.3.14.8 Solanaceae (Nightshade Family)

The family contains more than 2,000 species in 90 genera, providing numerous food plants such as tomatoes (*Lycopersicon lycopersicum*), potatoes (*Solanum tuberosum* L.), paprika and pepper (*Capsicum*), and tobacco (*Nicotiana tabacum*).

Occupational hand contact dermatitis is frequent in pickers or harvesters [379], mainly irritant, but sometimes allergic. Leaves of eggplants or brinjal (*Solanum melongena* L.) were tested positive when chopped in petrolatum [380]. Fruits (aubergine) and pollens may induce immediate symptoms.

46.4 Diagnosis of Plant Dermatitis

Finding the source of a plant-induced contact dermatitis is often difficult. A provisional diagnosis may be made by asking patients about their occupation,

46

Table 46.4 (continued)

Correct name	Synonyms	English name	French name	German name
Cynara cardunculus L.	*Cynara cardunculus* L. ssp. *cardunculus*; *Cynara cardunculus* L. ssp. *flavescens*	Cardoon	Cardon, carde	Kardone, Gemüse-Artischocke
Cynara scolymus L.	*Cynara cardunculus* L. ssp. *scolymus*; *Cynara cardunculus* L. ssp. *flavescens*	Globe artichoke	Artichaut	Artischoke, Alcachofra
Dahlia variabilis Desf.	*Dahlia x hortensis*	Dahlia	Dahlia	Dahlia
Dendranthema	*Chrysanthemum x hortorum* W. Miller, *Chrysanthemum mori-folium* Ramat.	Autumn-flowering chrysanthemum	Chrysanthème de Chine, chrysanthème d'automne	Chrysanthemen, Allerseelen-Aster
Dittrichia graveolens Greuter	*Inula graveolens* Desf, *Erigeron graveolens* L.	Stinkwort	Inule fétide	Duftender Alant
Gaillardia pulchella Foug.	*Gaillardia picta* Sweet Foug.	Showy gaillardia	Gaillarde pulchella	Kurzlebige Kokardenblume
Helenium autumnale L.		Sneezeweed, swamp sunflower, false sunflower	Hélénie automnale	Sonnenbrot
Helenium amarum H. Rock	*Helenium tenuifolium* Nutt., *Gaillardia amara* Raf.	Sneezeweed, bitterweed	–	–
Helianthus annuus L.		Sunflower	Tournesol, soleil	Einjährige Sonnen-blume
Inula helenium L.		Elecampane, horseheal, scabwort	Aunée officinale, grande aunée, inule aulnée	Echter Alant, Muxiang
Iva angustifolia Nutt.		Narrow-leaf marshelder		
Iva xanthifolia Nutt.		Marshelder		
Lactuca sativa L.		Lettuce	Laitue	Lattich
Leucanthemum vulgare Lam.	*Tanacetum leucanthemum* Schultz-Bip., *Chrysanthemum leucanthemum* L.	Marguerite, ox-eye daisy	Marguerite	Gemeine Wucher-blume, Wiessen-Margerite
Matricaria chamomilla L. var *recutita* Grieson	*Matricaria chamomilla* L., *Matricaria recutita* L., *Chamomilla recutita* Rauschert	German chamomile, wild chamomile	Matricaire, camomille allemande	Echte Kamille, deutsche Kamille
Parthenium argentatum A. Gray		Guayule	Guayule	Guayule
Parthenium hysterophorus L.		Congress grass, Santa Maria, whitetop	Absinthe bâtard	Parthenium hysterophorus
Petasites albus Gaertner		White butterbur	Pétasite blanc	Weisse Pestwurz

Core Message

› Patch tests with plant or wood materials have
   to be performed cautiously, heeding recommendations, and interpreted carefully because
   of the irritant and sensitizing risk.

46.4.2 Plant Extracts

Plant allergens, which are generally low-molecular-
weight secondary plant metabolites, are likely to be
soluble in acetone, ethanol, or ether. Thus, a filtered
acetone or ethanol extract of dried plant material or a
short ether extract of fresh material usually produces a
solution suitable for patch testing. Producing water
extracts of fresh plant material is not recommended,
although this is often carried out and can produce
active substances. Water extracts seem to degrade
rapidly and lose their sensitizing power within a
month [171], due to chemical degradation and/or to
microbial contamination. For example, acetone extracts
of *Parthenium hysterophorus* have been demonstrated
to be more sensitive than water extracts, with very
good sensitivity to 1% acetone extract [52].

Extracts in organic solvents are generally more stable, but they should not be regarded as having an indef-
inite shelf life. Moreover, with time, evaporation of the
solvent may increase the concentration and sensitizing
effect of the allergen(s). Incorporating an evaporated
extract into petrolatum represents a standard means of
retaining material for patch testing, but it is questionable whether this extra manipulation of the extract
confers any benefit over the application of a known
volume of the extract onto a standard occlusive patch
chamber.

46.4.3 Allergen Identification

Identification of the phytochemical(s) responsible
requires either a supply of the purified sensitizers
known to be present in the plant, or a somewhat labori-
ous extraction, isolation, purification, and characterization procedure using, ideally, several kilograms of
fresh plant material.

46.4.4 Commercial Allergens

Relatively few plant constituents are available commercially for patch testing. Table 46.5 indicates the
main plant allergens available from Chemotechnique,
Firma, and Hermal. Some of them are natural extracts
that contain the major allergen, as well as other impurities. Volatile oil constituents, which are found in the
aromatic oils of plants, are unstable to air oxidation
and generally virtually impossible to purify (except
through derivatization and resynthesis) if liquid at
room temperature. It should be remembered that the
air oxidation products themselves may be the sensitizers. Synthetic or purified extracts contain one or a mixture of molecules.

There is an ongoing search to identify mixtures of
compounds that can be used to reliably detect particular common types of plant- or plant-product-
induced dermatitis. Thus, various authors have
recommended mixtures to detect colophony allergy,
sesquiterpene lactone allergy, lichen allergy, and so
on. It is likely that none of these mixtures will ever
be regarded as an absolutely certain means of detecting the group allergy in question. For example,
allergy to Asteraceae is difficult to screen, as discussed above. The Compositae mix gives more frequent patch test reactions than sesquiterpene lactone
mix [382, 383], but its sensitivity, ascertained by the
relevance of positive reactions, seems lower than that
of SLM [382].

46.4.5 Photopatch Testing

Airborne contact dermatitis from plants can closely
simulate photocontact dermatitis, but plant-induced
photoallergy is actually very rare. However, patients
with photosensitivity have frequent positive reactions
to plants or plant extracts. Photoworsening of patch
test reactions may be indicative of an underlying
acquired photosensitivity, a state that may or may not
be causally associated with contact with the plant
material being investigated.

Photopatch tests have to be performed in duplicate,
one series being a dark (nonirradiated) control removed
after 48 h as in usual patch tests. The series that will be
irradiated is removed after 24 or 48 h, and irradiated by
a UVA source, generally with a dose of 5 J/cm². When

a total spectrum irradiation is possible, which allows us to test both UVA and UVB sensitivity, a third series has to be applied. Two series are removed after 24 h, and then the first one is irradiated with UVA and the second one with a sunlight system, delivering 75% of the minimal erythematous dose (MED).

46.4.6 Results and Relevance

Contact urticaria appears within minutes of patch testing and disappears rapidly. Patient interrogatory, literature data, and if necessary, results from open tests, prick tests, or a search for a specific IgE will lead to the diagnosis of immunologic or nonimmunologic contact urticaria.

Contact dermatitis is much more difficult to explore. The realization of patch tests, their readings, and the validity of patch test results are often hard to determine. The relevance of positive test reactions can be difficult to establish because the patient may have handled several plants over a period of time and become sensitized to some or all. The phenomenon of cross-sensitization adds a further dimension to the problem of relevance.

False-positive reactions may be due to an irritant reaction, and it is useful to refer to guidelines before testing plants. Testing with numerous plants or extracts can cause an angry back or excited skin syndrome. Each plant part or plant extract must then be tested again separately. Sometimes, positive reactions arise from contamination of the plant material with pesticides or other agricultural/horticultural chemicals [384], or from fungal contamination. Another cause of positive reactions is the use of an extract at a concentration that is too high, whereby a subclinical sensitivity may be unmasked.

Active sensitization to the material should not be overlooked, but patch test reactions are generally delayed, occurring after 7–10 days. They are theoretically (and practically) possible with many plant materials, such as plant extracts.

False-negative reactions may arise if an inappropriate sample of plant material is tested (such as patch testing with a leaf when the allergen is contained in the stem), or if the extract contains an insufficient concentration of the allergen, perhaps as a result of using a stored extract or of seasonal variations of allergen content.

46.4.7 Multiple Plant Reactions and Cross-Sensitivity

In most cases, reactions to several plants in the same patient are not due to cross-sensitization. First, cosensitization is frequent, particularly in people who are frequently in contact with plants. Many plants contain the same hapten, and so a patient sensitized to a particular compound in one plant will react to another plant containing the same compound. Moreover, he or she will react to plants that present a different compound, but one that will be still metabolized into the same allergen. Such situations are false cross-reactions.

In rarer cases, true cross-sensitization arises when the immune surveillance process misidentifies a second compound due to its structural similarity to the primary sensitizer. Difficult and long procedures, e.g., chemical studies of spatial molecular structures, correlated to clinical reactivity patterns and clinical experimentation such as cross-retests permit us to assume a true cross-reactivity between different molecules.

Clearly, false cross-reactions and cross-reactions are almost impossible to detect with certainty in humans because the primary sensitizer cannot easily be determined. Thus, reactions may occur to plants not previously encountered by the patient, as well as to isolates that are not actually present in the sensitizing plant.

46.5 Prevention and Treatment

46.5.1 Removal of the Allergens and Irritants

As soon as the plant responsible for contact dermatitis has been identified, steps should be taken to avoid further contact. In cases of occupational phytodermatitis, work practices and occupational hygiene measures should first be reviewed because of the employer's legal responsibility to provide a safe working environment. However, the patient may have to consider a change of workplace (for example, in the case of *Primula* dermatitis), and sometimes leave his or her occupation (as in the case of foresters allergic to *Frullania*).

46.5.2 Barrier Creams

Barrier creams, used as recommended, can be helpful in the prevention of irritant dermatitis. The practitioner must carefully read their composition in relation to some allergens such as lanolin and methyldibromoglutaronitrile and other allergens.

Their use in primary and secondary prevention of ACD is discussed [385].

46.5.3 Gloves

It has been demonstrated that wearing gloves is a useful approach.

However, tuliposide A (present in *Alstroemeria* and Liliaceae) readily penetrates through vinyl gloves [104]. Nitrile gloves may prevent contact with tuliposide A [104]. A recent study shows that vinyl, polyethylene, and latex gloves are likely to be permeable to plant allergens such as α-methylene-γ-butyrolactone, primin, and diallyldisulfide. Nitrile gloves could protect from primin [386].

46.5.4 Acute Dermatitis

Acute dermatitis has to be rapidly treated with potent topical corticosteroids, such as betamethasone esters. They have to be applied once (or twice) a day, in adequate quantities (for example, an average of 20 g/day of topical 0.05% betamethasone dipropionate cream for each upper limb), every day until total healing. Pulverization, or compresses with saline (around 10 g NaCl per liter of fresh or warm water), are frequently useful. Systemic corticosteroids are used by some authors for severe cases. A high daily dose for a short period, until healing (1 mg/kg per day prednisone), is better than a lower regimen that requires a longer duration.

46.5.5 Chronic Dermatitis

Treatment is symptomatic too. We use topical corticosteroids in the same manner as described below, sometimes with emollients, until healing.

Other solutions such as UV therapy are helpful for diffuse dermatitis. Photochemotherapy with UVA and 8-MOP, or even systemic immunosuppressive chemicals such as azathioprine or ciclosporin, can be tried for severe and intractable phytophotodermatitis with or without persistent light reactions [387].

Preventive measures (wearing gloves, removal of allergens or irritants) are always indispensable.

46.5.6 Hyposensitization

Hyposensitization measures have been attempted with limited success when avoidance of contact is impractical, such as with poison ivy in certain outdoor occupations. After a note by R. Dakin in 1829, the first attempts in this direction were attributed to Schamberg in 1919 [388]. Other authors have then carried out oral or parenteral hyposensitization with varied results and sometimes severe side effects, with reports of fatal renal complications [389, 390]. Oral desensitization with daily intake of leaf extract in water has been reported as being beneficial on skin lesion and patch test results [391]. A similar approach was attempted in 24 Indian patients positive to *P. hysterophorus*, with increasing amounts of plant extracts. Of 20 patients who completed the study, six suffered worsened dermatitis and stopped treatment. In the remaining 14 patients, a progressive fall in the mean clinical severity score was noted, but no significant change in the titer of test reactivity. Long-term results are unspecified, with 3/7 patients free of symptoms after 1 year [52]. Currently, there is no scientific basis behind this practice, and the risk of toxic side effects should be considered [390, 392]. Induction of tolerance in naive subjects appears to be a more successful strategy than desensitization of those already sensitized [393].

The so-called hardening is also a procedure that has been discussed, and it has been described as an external topical hyposensitization. It consists of repeated patch test application, until the reactivity progressively fades [390].

46.6 Example of Botanical Nomenclature

The plant *kingdom*, which comprises around 350,000 species, is divided into five *divisions*: phycophytes (seaweeds or algae), bryophytes (mosses, liverworts/

46

hepatics, and hornworts), mycophytes (fungi or mycetes), pteridophytes (ferns and related), and spermatophytes (seed plants) [7, 8]. Spermatophytes are divided into two *groups*:

- Gymnosperms: conifers, cycads, ginkgos, ephedras, chlamydosperms
- Angiosperms (Magnoliophyta) group: plants with flowers, which are divided into two *classes*:
  - Dicotyledon (Magnoliopsidae) class, subdivided into nine *subclasses*
  - Monocotyledon (Liliopsidae) class, subdivided into three subclasses

Subclasses are subdivided into *orders*
Orders are divided into *families*
Each family is made up of *genera* (singular: *genus*)
Each genre is divided into *species*
Ideally, to identify a plant, we need information on its roots, stems (aerian or underground), leaves (insertion, venation, arrangement, simple or compound organization, margins), and its reproductive organs (flowers, fruits).

Following the considerable work of the Swedish naturalist Dr. Carl von Linné (1707–1778), each species is characterized by two names written in Latin: the first name is the genus, the second the species. These are often related to the name of the author who first described the species, and are frequently abbreviated.

The purple foxglove (*Digitalis purpurea* L.) belongs to the plant kingdom, the Spermatophyta division, the Angiospermae subdivision, the Dicotyledonae class, the Gamopetalae subclass, the Tubiflorales order, the Scrophulariaceae family, the Rhinanthoideae family, the genus *Digitalis*, and the species *purpurea*, as described by Linné [8]. The white dead nettle (*Lamium album* L.) belongs to the Lamiaceae family, the *Lamium* genus, and the *album* species [7].

References

1. Fregert S (1975) Occupational dermatitis in a 10-year material. Contact Derm 1:96–107
2. Paulsen E, Sogaard J, Andersen KE (1997) Occupational dermatitis in Danish gardeners and greenhouse workers. I. Prevalence and possible risk factors. Contact Derm 37: 263–270
3. Paulsen E (1998) Occupational dermatitis in Danish gardeners and greenhouse workers. II. Etiological factors. Contact Derm 38:14–29
4. Evans FJ, Schmidt RJ (1980) Plants and plant products that induce contact dermatitis. Planta Med 38:289–316
5. Mitchell J, Rook A (1979) Botanical dermatology. Plants and plant products injurious to the skin. Greengrass, Vancouver
6. Lovell CR (1993) Plants and the skin. Blackwell Scientific, Oxford
7. Sell Y, Benezra C, Guérin B (2002) Plantes et réactions cutanées. John Libbey Eurotext, Paris
8. Benezra C, Ducombs G, Sell Y, Foussereau J (1985) Plant contact dermatitis. Decker, Toronto
9. Behl PN, Captain RM (1979) Skin-irritant and sensitizing plants found in India. Chand, Ram Nagar, New Delhi
10. Schmidt RJ (2005) The botanical dermatology database: homepage. (See http://bodd.cf.ac.uk/index.html)
11. Rzeznik JC, Sell Y (2009) Botaderma database: homepage. (See http://botaderma.com/plante/index.php?page=accueil)
12. Bourrain JL (2001) Les agents étiologiques des urticaires de contact. Ann Derm Venereol (Stockh) 128:1363–1366
13. Guin JD (2000) Occupational contact dermatitis to plants. In: Kanerva L, Elsner P, Wahlberg JE, Maibach HI (eds) Handbook of occupational dermatology. Springer, Berlin, pp 730–766
14. Couplan F, Styner E (1004) Guide des plantes sauvages comestibles et toxiques. Delachaux et Niestlé, Lausanne
15. Norup E, Smitt UW, Brøgger Christensen S (1986) The potencies of thapsigargin and analogues as activators of rat peritoneal mast cells. Planta Med 52:251–255
16. Brøgger Christensen S, Norup E, Rasmussen U (1984) Chemistry and structure-activity relationship of the histamine secretagogue thapsigargin and related compounds. In: Krogsgaard-Larsen P, Brøgger Christensen S, Kofod H (eds) Natural products and drug development. Munksgaard, Copenhagen, pp 405–418 (Alfred Benzon Symposium 20)
17. Estlander T, Kanerva L, Tupasela O, Jolanki R (1988) Occupational contact urticaria and type I sensitization caused by gerbera. Contact Derm 38:118–120
18. Le Coz CJ (2001) Fiche d'éviction. Hypersensibilité au latex ou caoutchouc naturel. Ann Dermatol Venereol 128: 577–578
19. Dooms-Goossens A, Deveylder H, Duron C, Dooms M, Degreef H (1986) Airborne contact urticaria due to cinchona. Contact Derm 15:258
20. Hjorth N, Roed-Petersen J (1976) Occupational protein contact dermatitis in food handlers. Contact Derm 2:28–42
21. Hannuksela M, Lahti A (1977) Immediate reactions to fruits and vegetables. Contact Derm 3:79–84
22. Kaupinnen K, Kousa M, Reunala T (1980) Aromatic plants – a cause of severe attacks of angio-edema and urticaria. Contact Derm 6:251–254
23. Veien NK, Hattel T, Justesen O, Norholm A (1983) Causes of eczema in the food industry. Derm Beruf Umwelt 31:84–86
24. Janssens V, Morren M, Dooms-Goossens A, Degreef H (1995) Protein contact dermatitis: myth or reality? Br J Dermatol 132:1–6
25. Karpman RR, Spark RP, Fried M (1980) Cactus thorn injuries to the extremities: their management and etiology. Ariz Med 37:849–851

26. Spoerke DG, Spoerke SE (1991) Granuloma formation induced by spines of the cactus, *Opuntia acanthocarpa*. Vet Hum Toxicol 33:342–344

27. Shanon J, Sagher F (1956) Sabra dermatitis. An occupational dermatitis due to prickly pear handling simulating scabies. AMA Arch Dermatol 74:269–275

28. Snyder DS, Hatfield GM, Lampe KF (1979) Examination of the itch response from the raphides of the fishtail palm *Caryota mitis* Lour. Toxicol Appl Pharmacol 48:287–292

29. Salinas ML, Ogura T, Soffchi L (2001) Irritant contact dermatitis caused by needle-like calcium oxalate crystals, raphides, in *Agave tequilana* among workers in tequila distilleries and agave plantations. Contact Derm 44:94–96

30. Morton JF (1972) Cocoyams (*Xanthosoma caracu*, *X. atrovirens* and *X. nigrum*), ancient root- and leaf-vegetables, gaining in economic importance. Proc Fl State Hort Soc 85:85–94

31. Walter WG, Khanna PN (1972) Chemistry of the aroids. I. *Dieffenbachia seguine, amoena,* and *pitta*. Econ Bot 26:364–372

32. Metin A, Çalka O, Behçet L, Yildirim E (2001) Phytodermatitis from Ranunculus damascenus. Contact Derm 44:183

33. Gude M, Hausen BM, Heitsch H, König WA (1988) An investigation of the irritant and allergenic properties of daffodils (*Narcissus pseudonarcissus* L., Amaryllidaceae. A review of daffodil dermatitis. Contact Derm 19:1–10

34. Bonnevie P (1939) Aetiologie und Pathogenese der Ekzemkrankheiten. Nyt Nordisk Forlag, Copenhagen

35. Schwartz RS, Downham TF (1981) Erythema multiforme associated with *Rhus* contact dermatitis. Cutis 27:85–86

36. Holst R, Kirby J, Magnusson B (1976) Sensitization to tropical woods giving erythema multiforme-like eruptions. Contact Derm 2:295–296

37. Martin P, Bergoend H, Piette F (1980) Erythema multiforme-like eruption from Brasilian rosewood. 5th International Symposium on Contact Dermatitis, 28–30 March 1980, Barcelona, Spain

38. Irvine C, Reynolds A, Finlay AY (1988) Erythema multiforme-like reaction to "rosewood". Contact Derm 19:224–225

39. Athavale PN, Shum KW, Gasson P, Gawkrodger DJ (2003) Occupational hand dermatitis in a wood turner due to rosewood (*Dalbergia latifolia*. Contact Derm 48:345–346

40. García-Bravo B, Rodriguez-Pichardo A, Fernandez de Pierola S, Camacho F (1995) Airborne erythema-multiforme-like eruption due to pyrethrum. Contact Derm 33:433

41. Le Coz CJ, Lepoittevin JP (2001) Occupational erythema-multiforme-like dermatitis from sensitization to costus resinoid, followed by flare-up and systemic contact dermatitis from β-cyclocostunolide in a chemistry student. Contact Derm 44:310–311

42. Ducombs G, Félix B, Allery JP (1996) Erythème polymorphe-like dû au bois d'Olon. A propos d'un nouveau cas. Lett GERDA 13:70–71

43. Hjorth N, Roed-Petersen J, Thomsen K (1976) Airborne contact dermatitis from Compositae oleoresins simulating photodermatitis. Br J Dermatol 95:613–620

44. Paulsen E, Christensen LP, Andersen KE (2007) Compositae dermatitis from airborne parthenolide. Br J Dermatol 156:510–515

45. Schmidt RJ (1986) Compositae. Clin Dermatol 4:46–61

46. Christensen LP (1999) Direct release of the allergen tulipalin A from *Alstroemeria* cut flowers: a possible source of airborne contact dermatitis? Contact Derm 41:320–324

47. Foussereau J, Muller JC, Benezra C (1975) Contact allergy to *Frullania* and *Laurus Nobilis*: cross-sensitization and chemical structure of the allergens. Contact Derm 1:223–230

48. Thune PO, Solberg YJ (1980) Photosensitivity and allergy to aromatic lichen acids, Compositae oleoresins and other plant substances. Contact Derm 6:64–71

49. Thune PO, Solberg YJ (1980) Photosensitivity and allergy to aromatic lichen acids, Compositae oleoresins and other plant substances. Contact Derm 6:81–87

50. Watsky KL (1997) Airborne allergic contact dermatitis from pine dust. Am J Contact Dermat 8:118–120

51. Fisher AA (1965) The poison "Rhus" plants. Cutis 1:230–236

52. Sharma VK, Sethuraman G, Tejasvi T (2004) Comparison of patch test contact sensitivity to acetone and aqueous extracts of *Parthenium hysterophorus* in patients with airborne contact dermatitis. Contact Derm 50:230–232

53. Oppenheim M (1932) Dermatite bulleuse striée, consécutive aux bains de soleil dans les prés. (Dermatitis bullosa striata pratensis.). Ann Derm Venereol (Stockh) 3:1–7

54. Kissmeyer A (1933) Dermatite bulleuse striée des prés. Bull Soc Fr Dermatol Syphiligr 40:1486–1489

55. Freeman K, Hubbard HC, Warin AP (1984) Strimmer rash. Contact Derm 10:117–118

56. Ippen H (1984) Photodermatitis bullosa generalisata. Derm Beruf Umwelt 32:134–137

57. Tunget CL, Turchen SG, Manoguerra AS, Clark RF, Pudoff DE (1994) Sunlight and the plant: a toxic combination: severe phytophotodermatitis from *Cneoridium dumosum*. Cutis 54:400–402

58. Qadripur SA, Gründer K (1975) Kasuistischer Beitrag über Gruppenerkrankung mit Photodermatitis bullosa striata pratensis (Oppenheim). Hautarzt 26:495–497

59. Campbell AN, Cooper CE, Dahl MGC (1982) "Non-accidental injury" and wild parsnips. Br Med J 284:708

60. Pathak MA, Daniels F, Fitzpatrick TB (1962) The presently known distribution of furocoumarins (psoralens) in plants. J Invest Dermatol 39:225–239

61. Wagner AM, Wu JJ, Hansen RC, Nigg HN, Beiere RC (2002) Bullous phytophotodermatitis associated with high natural concentrations of furanocoumarins in limes. Am J Contact Dermat 13:10–14

62. SchempP CM, Schöpf E, Simon JC (1999) Dermatitis bullosa striata pratensis durch *Ruta graveolens* L. (Gartenraute). Hautartz 50:432–434

63. Schempp CM, Sonntag M, Schöpf E, Simon JC (1996) Dermatitis bullosa striata pratensis durch *Dictamnus albus* L. (Brennender Busch). Hautartz 47:708–710

64. El Sayed K, Al-Said MS, El-Feraly FS, Ross SA (2000) New quinoline alkaloids from *Ruta chalepensis*. J Nat Prod 63:995–997

65. Wang L, Sterling B, Don P (2002) Berloque dermatitis induced by "Florida water". Cutis 70:29–30

66. Bhutani LK, Rao DS (1978) Photocontact dermatitis caused by *Parthenium hysterophorus*. Dermatologica 157:206–209

67. Ljunggren B (1977) Psoralen photoallergy caused by plant contact. Contact Derm 3:85–90

68. Kaidbey KH, Kligman AM (1981) Photosensitization by coumarin derivatives. Arch Dermatol 117:258–263

69. Frain-Bell W, Johnson BE (1979) Contact allergic sensitivity to plants and the photosensitivity dermatitis and actinic reticuloid syndrome. Br J Dermatol 101:503–512

70. Lim HW, Cohen D, Soter NA (1998) Chronic actinic dermatitis: results of patch tests with Compositae, fragrances, and pesticides. J Am Acad Dermatol 38:108–111

71. Du P Menagé H, Ross JS, Norris PG, Breathnach SM, Hawk JLM, White IR (1995) Contact and photocontact sensitization in chronic actinic dermatitis: sesquiterpene lactone mix is an important allergen. Br J Dermatol 132:543–547

72. Du P Menagé H, Hawk JLM, White IR (1998) Sesquiterpene lactone mix contact sensitivity and its relationship to chronic actinic dermatitis: a follow-up study. Contact Derm 39: 119–122

73. Hausen BM (2000) Woods. In: Kanerva L, Elsner P, Wahlberg JE, Maibach HI (eds) Handbook of occupational dermatology. Springer, Berlin, pp 771–780

74. Bleumink E, Doeglas HMG, Klokke AH, Nater JP (1972) Allergic contact dermatitis to garlic. Br J Dermatol 87:6–9

75. Bleumink E, Nater JP (1973) Contact dermatitis to garlic: cross reactivity between garlic, onion, and tulip. Arch Dermatol Forsch 247:117–124

76. Sinha SM, Pasricha JS, Sharma RC, Kandhari KC (1977) Vegetables responsible for contact dermatitis of the hands. Arch Dermatol 113:776–779

77. Van KeteL WG, de Haan P (1978) Occupational eczema from garlic and onion. Contact Derm 4:53–54

78. Campolmi P, Lombardi P, Lotti T, Sertoli A (1982) Immediate and delayed sensitization to garlic. Contact Derm 8:352–353

79. Cronin E (1987) Dermatitis of the hands in caterers. Contact Derm 17:265–269

80. Burks JW Jr (1954) Classic aspects of onion and garlic dermatitis in housewives. Ann Allergy 12:592–596

81. Eming SA, Piontek JO, Hunzelmann RH (1999) Severe toxic contact dermatitis caused by garlic. Br J Dermatol 141: 391–392

82. Burden AD, Wilkinson SM, Beck MH, Chalmers RJ (1994) Garlic-induced systemic contact dermatitis. Contact Derm 30:299–300

83. Pereira F, Hatia M, Cardoso J (2002) Systemic contact dermatitis from diallyl disulfide. Contact Derm 46:124

84. Bassioukas K, Orton D, Cerio R (2004) Occupational airborne allergic contact dermatitis from garlic with concurrent Type I allergy. Contact Derm 50:39–41

85. Freeman GG, Whenham RJ (1976) Nature and origin of volatile flavour components of onion and related species. Int Flavours Fd Addit 7:222–227; 229

86. Papageorgiou C, Corbet JP, Menezes-Brandao F, Pecegueiro M, Benezra C (1983) Allergic contact dermatitis to Garlic (Allium sativum L.). Identification of the allergens: the role of mono-di-, and trisulfides present in garlic. A comparative study in man and animal (guinea-pig). Arch Dermatol Res 275:229–234

87. Mitchell JC (1980) Contact sensitivity to garlic (Allium). Contact Derm 6:356–357

88. Brongersma-Oosterhoff UW (1967) Structure determination of the allergenic agent isolated from tulip bulbs. Recl Trav Chim Pays Bas Belg 86:705–708

89. Verspyck Mijnssen GAW (1969) Pathogenesis and causative agent of "tulip finger". Br J Dermatol 81:737–745

90. Slob A (1973) Tulip allergens in Alstroemeria and some other Liliiflorae. Phytochemistry 12:811–815

91. Slob A, Jekel B, de Jong B, Schlatmann E (1975) On the occurrence of tuliposides in the Liliiflorae. Phytochemistry 14:1997–2005

92. Hausen BM, Prater E, Schubert H (1983) The sensitizing capacity of Alstroemeria cultivars in man and guinea pig. Remarks on the occurrence, quantity and irritant and sensitizing potency of their constituents tuliposide A and tulipalin A (α-methylene-γ-butyrolactone. Contact Derm 9:46–54

93. Santucci B, Picardo M, Iavarone C, Trogolo C (1985) Contact dermatitis to Alstroemeria. Contact Derm 12: 215–219

94. Christensen LP, Kristiansen K (1995) A simple HPLC method for the isolation and quantification of the allergens tuliposide A and tulipalin A in Alstroemeria. Contact Derm 32:199–203

95. Christensen LP, Kristiansen K (1995) Isolation and quantification of a new tuliposide (tuliposide D) by HPLC in Alstroemeria. Contact Derm 33:188–192

96. Shoji M, Kazuaki A (2003) Antimicrobial activities of anthers in tulips. Plant Biology 2003, 25–30 July 2003. Honolulu, Hawaii, USA

97. Barbier P, Benezra C (1986) Allergenic α-methylene-γ-butyrolactones. Study of the capacity of β-acetoxy- and β-hydroxy-α-methylene-γ-butyrolactones to induce allergic contact dermatitis in guinea pigs. J Med Chem 29: 868–871

98. Beijersbergen JCM (1972) A method for determination of tulipalin A and B concentrations in crude extracts of tulip tissues. Recl Trav Chim Pays Bas Belg 91:1193–1200

99. Hjorth N, Wilkinson DS (1968) Contact dermatitis. IV. Tulip fingers, hyacinth itch and lily rash. Br J Dermatol 80: 696–698

100. Guin JD, Franks H (2001) Fingertip dermatitis in a retail florist. Cutis 67:328–330

101. Van der Mei IA, de Boer EM, Bruynzeel DP (1998) Contact dermatitis in Alstroemeria workers. Occup Med (Lond) 48:397–404

102. Rycroft RJG, Calnan CD (1981) Alstroemeria dermatitis. Contact Derm 7:284

103. Rook A (1981) Dermatitis from Alstroemeria: altered clinical pattern and probable increasing incidence. Contact Derm 7:355–356

104. Marks JG (1988) Allergic contact dermatitis to Alstroemeria. Arch Dermatol 124:914–916

105. Björkner BE (1982) Contact allergy and depigmentation from alstroemeria. Contact Derm 8:178–184

106. Chan RY, Oppenheimer JJ (2002) Occupational allergy caused by Peruvian lily (Alstroemeria). Ann Allergy Asthma Immunol 88:638–639

107. Van der Werff PJ (1959) Occupational diseases among workers in the bulb industries. Acta Allergol 14:338–355

46

108. Bruze M, Björkner B, Hellstrom AC (1996) Occupational dermatoses in nursery workers. Am J Contact Dermat 7: 100–103

109. Bruynzeel DP (1997) Bulb dermatitis. Dermatological problem in the flower bulb industries. Contact Derm 37: 70–77

110. Julian CG, Bower PW (1997) The nature and distribution of daffodil picker's rash. Contact Derm 37:259–262

111. Klaschka F, Grimm WW, Beiersdorff HU (1964) Tulpen-Kontaktekzem als Berufsdermatosen. Hautarzt 15:317–321

112. Pardo-Castello V (1923) Dermatitis venenata: a study of the tropical plants producing dermatitis. Arch Dermatol Syphilol 7:81

113. Bertrand G, Brooks G (1934) Recherches sur le latex de l'arbre à laque du Cambodge (*Melanorrhoea laccifera* Pierre). Bull Soc Chim Fr 5:109–114

114. Ridley HN (1911) Rengas-poisoning. Malay Med J 9:7

115. Watt G (1906) Burmese lacquer ware and Burmese varnish. Kew Bull 5:137–147

116. Srinivas CR, Kulkarni SB, Menon SK, Krupashankar DS, Iyengar MA, Singh KK, Sequeira RP, Holla KR (1987) Allergenic agent in contact dermatitis from *Holigarna ferruginea*. Contact Derm 17:219–222

117. Sprague TA (1921) Plant dermatitis. J Bot 59:308–310

118. Kirby-Smith JL (1938) Mango dermatitis. Am J Trop Med 18:373–384

119. Jackson WPU (1946) Plant dermatitis in the Bahamas. BMJ 2:298

120. King DE, Wolfish PS, Heng MCY (1983) The much-maligned dhobie. J Am Acad Dermatol 8:258

121. Findlay GH, Whiting DA, Eggers SH, Ellis RP (1974) *Smodingium* (African "poison ivy") dermatitis. History, comparative plant chemistry and anatomy, clinical and histological features. Br J Dermatol 90:535–541

122. Corbett M, Billets S (1975) Characterization of poison oak urushiol. J Pharm Sci 64:1715–1718

123. Gross M, Baer H, Fales HM (1975) Urushiols of poisonous Anacardiaceae. Phytochemistry 14:2263–2266

124. De Hurtado I (1965) Contact dermatitis caused by the "manzanillo" (*Rhus striata*) tree. Int Arch Allergy Appl Immunol 28:321–327

125. Nakamura T (1985) Contact dermatitis to *Rhus succedanea*. Contact Derm 12:279

126. Powell SM, Barrett DK (1986) An outbreak of contact dermatitis from *Rhus verniciflua* (*Toxicodendron verniciflum*). Contact Derm 14:288–289

127. Kligman AM (1958) Poison ivy *(Rhus)* dermatitis. An experimental study. AMA Arch Dermatol 77:149

128. Ippen H (1983) Kontaktallergie gegen Anacardiaceae. Übersicht und Kasuistik zur "Poison Ivy"-Allergie in Mitteleuropa. Derm Beruf Umwelt 31:140–148

129. Oh SH, Haw CR, Lee MH (2003) Clinical and immunologic features of systemic contact dermatitis from ingestion of *Rhus* (*Toxicodendron*. Contact Derm 48:251–254

130. Cardinali C, Francalanci S, Giomi B, Caproni M, Sertoli A, Fabbri P (2004) Contact dermatitis from *Rhus toxicodendron* in a homeopathic remedy. J Am Acad Dermatol 50: 150–151

131. Marks JG Jr, DeMelfi T, McCarthy MA, Witte EJ, Castagnoli N, Epstein WL, Aber RC (1984) Dermatitis from cashew nuts. J Am Acad Dermatol 10:627–631

132. Kurlan JG, Lucky AW (2001) Black spot poison ivy: a report of 5 cases and a review of the literature. J Am Acad Dermatol 45:246–249

133. Gillis WT (1971) The systematics and ecology of poison ivy and the poison-oaks (*Toxicodendron*, Anacardiaceae). Rhodora 73:72–159; 161–237; 370–443; 465–540

134. Guin JD, Gillis WT, Beaman JH (1981) Recognizing the Toxicodendrons (poison ivy, poison oak, and poison sumac. J Am Acad Dermatol 4:99–114

135. Guin JD, Beaman JH (1986) Toxicodendrons of the United States. Clin Dermatol 4:137–148

136. Guin JD (1980) The black spot test for recognizing poison ivy and related species. J Am Acad Dermatol 2:332–333

137. Walker S William J, Lear J, Beck M (2004) Toxicodendron dermatitis in the United Kingdom. Contact Derm 50:163

138. Ale SI, Ferreira F, Gonzalez G, Epstein W (1997) Allergic contact dermatitis caused by *Lithraea molleoides* and *Lithraea brasiliensis*: identification and characterization of the responsible allergens. Am J Contact Dermat 8: 144–149

139. Lima AO (1953) Über das antigene Verhalten der Ölharze einiger Gattungen der Familie Anacardiaceae. Int Archs Allergy Appl Immun 4:169–174

140. De Hurtado I (1968) Studies on the biological activity of *Rhus striata* ("manzanillo"). 2. Skin response to patch tests in humans. Int Arch Allergy Appl Immunol 33:209

141. Mitchell JC, Maibach HI, Guin J (1981) Leaves *of Ginkgo biloba* not allergenic for Toxicodendron sensitive subjects. Contact Derm 7:47–48

142. Nakamura T (1985) Ginkgo tree dermatitis. Contact Derm 12:281–282

143. Tomb RR, Foussereau J, Sell Y (1988) Mini-epidemic of contact dermatitis from ginkgo tree fruit (*Ginkgo biloba* L.). Contact Derm 19:281–283

144. Bolus M, Raleigh NC (1939) Dermatitis venenata due to ginkgo berries. Arch Dermatol Syphilol 39:530

145. Becker LE, Skipworth GB (1975) Ginkgo-tree dermatitis, stomatitis, and proctitis. J Am Med Assoc 231:1162–1163

146. Sowers WF, Weary PE, Collins OD, Cawley EP (1965) Ginkgo-tree dermatitis. Arch Dermatol 91:452–456

147. Lepoittevin JP, Benezra C, Asakawa Y (1989) Allergic contact dermatitis to *Ginkgo biloba* L.: relationship with urushiol. Arch Dermatol Res 281:227–230

148. Occolowitz JL, Wright AS (1962) 5-(10-Pentadecenyl)resorcinol from *Grevillea pyramidalis*. Aust J Chem 15:858–861

149. Ridley DD, Ritchie E, Taylor WC (1968) Chemical studies of the Proteaceae. II. Some further constituents of *Grevillea robusta* A. Cunn.; experiments on the synthesis of 5-*n*-tridecylresorcinol (grevillol) and related substances. Aust J Chem 21:2979–2988

150. Menz J, Rossi ER, Taylor WC, Wall L (1986) Contact dermatitis from *Grevillea* "Robyn Gordon". Contact Derm 15:126–131

151. Hoffman TE, Hausen BM, Adams RM (1985) Allergic contact dermatitis to "silver oak" wooden arm bracelets. J Am Acad Dermatol 13:778–779

46

152. May SB (1960) Dermatitis due to *G. robusta* (Australian silk oak. Report of a case. Arch Dermatol 82:1006

153. Arnold HL (1942) Dermatitis to the blossom of *Grevillea banksii*. Arch Dermatol 45:1037–1051

154. Benezra C, Ducombs G (1987) Molecular aspects of allergic contact dermatitis to plants. Derm Beruf Umwelt 35:4–11

155. Knight TE (1991) Philodendron-induced dermatitis: report of cases and review of the literature. Cutis 48:375–378

156. Reynolds GW, Gafner F, Rodriguez E (1989) Contact allergens of an urban shrub *Wigandia caracasana*. Contact Derm 21:65–68

157. Reynolds G, Rodriguez E (1979) Geranylhydroquinone: a contact allergen from trichomes of *Phacelia crenulata*. Phytochemistry 18:1567–1568

158. Aeschimann D, Lauber K, Moser DM, Theurillat JP (2004) Flora alpina. Belin, Paris

159. Arlette J, Mitchell JC (1981) Compositae dermatitis. Current aspects. Contact Derm 7:129–136

160. Mitchell JC, Roy AK, Dupuis G, Towers GHN (1971) Allergic contact dermatitis from ragweeds (*Ambrosia* species). The role of sesquiterpene lactones. Arch Dermatol 104:73–76

161. Brunsting LA, Anderson CR (1934) Ragweed dermatitis. A report based on eighteen cases. J Am Med Assoc 103:1285–1290

162. Shelmire B (1939) Contact dermatitis from weeds: patch testing with their oleoresins. J Am Med Assoc 113:1085–1090

163. Mitchell JC (1975) Biochemical basis of geographic ecology, part 2. Int J Dermatol 14:301–321

164. Brunsting LA, Williams DH (1936) Ragweed (contact) dermatitis. Observations in forty-eight cases and report of unsuccessful attempts at desensitization by injection of specific oils. J Am Med Assoc 106:1533–1535

165. O'Quinn SE, Isbell KH (1969) Influence of oral prednisone on eczematous patch test reactions. Arch Dermatol 99:380–389

166. Möslein P (1963) Pflanzen als Kontakt-Allergene. Berufsdermatosen 11:24–28

167. Hausen BM, Busker E, Carle R (1984) Über das Sensibilisierungsvermögen von Compositearten VII. Experimentelle Untersuchungen mit Auszügen und Inhaltsstoffen von *Chamomilla recutita* (L.) Rauschert und *Anthemis cotula* L. Planta Med 50:229–234

168. Burry JN (1979) Dermatitis from fleabane: compositae dermatitis in South Australia. Contact Derm 5:51

169. Hausen BM (1980) Arnikaallergie. Hautarzt 31:10–17

170. Mitchell JC, Geissman TA, Dupuis G, Towers GH (1971) Allergic contact dermatitis caused by *Artemisia* and *Chrysanthemum* species. The role of sesquiterpene lactones. J Invest Dermatol 56:98–101

171. Shelmire B (1940) Contact dermatitis from vegetation; patch testing and treatment with plant oleoresins. J South Med Assoc 33:337–346

172. Mackoff S, Dahl AO (1951) A botanical consideration of the weed oleoresin problem. Minn Med 34:1169–1173

173. Schumacher MJ, Silvis NG (2003) Airborne contact dermatitis from *Ambrosia deltoidea* (triangle-leaf bursage). Contact Derm 48:212–216

174. Burry JN, Kuchel R, Reid JG, Kirk J (1973) Australian bush dermatitis: compositae dermatitis in South Australia. Med J Aust 1:110–116

175. Burry JN, Reid JG, Kirk J (1975) Australian bush dermatitis. Contact Derm 1:263–264

176. Maiden JH (1909) On some plants which cause inflammation or irritation of the skin, part II. Agric Gaz NSW 20:1073–1082

177. Burry JN, Kloot PM (1982) The spread of composite (Compositae) weeds in Australia. Contact Derm 8:410–413

178. Towers GHN, Mitchell JC, Rodriguez E, Bennett FD, Subbarrao PV (1977) Biology and chemistry of *Parthenium hysterophorus* L., a problem weed in India. J Sci Ind Res 36:672–684

179. Towers GH, Mitchell JC (1983) The current status of the weed *Parthenium hysterophorus* L. as a cause of contact dermatitis. Contact Derm 9:465–469

180. Hausen BM (1981) Berufsbedingte Kontaktallergie auf Mutterkraut (*Tanacetum parthenium* (L.) Schulz-Bip.; Asteraceae). Derm Beruf Umwelt 29:18–21

181. Mensing H, Kimmig W, Hausen BM (1985) Airborne contact dermatitis. Hautarzt 36:398–402

182. Malten KE (1983) Chicory dermatitis from September to April. Contact Derm 9:232

183. Menz J, Winkelmann RK (1987) Sensitivity to wild vegetation. Contact Derm 16:169–173

184. Paulsen E, Andersen KE, Brandão FM et al (1999) Routine patch testing with the sesquiterpene lactone mix in Europe: a 2-year experience. A multicentre study of the EECDRG. Contact Derm 40:72–76

185. Paulsen E, Otkjær A, Andersen KE (2008) Sesquiterpene lactone dermatitis in the young: is atopy a risk factor? Contact Derm 59:1–6

186. Verhagen AR, Nyaga JM (1974) Contact dermatitis from *Tagetes minuta*. A new sensitizing plant of the Compositae family. Arch Dermatol 110:441–444

187. Mitchell JC, Dupuis G, Towers GHN (1972) Allergic contact dermatitis from pyrethrum (*Chrysanthemum* spp.). The roles of pyrethrosin, a sesquiterpene lactone, and of pyrethrin II. Br J Dermatol 86:568–573

188. Hausen BM (1982) Taraxinsäure-1'-*O*-β-D-glucopyranosid, das Kontaktallergen des Löwenzahns (*Taraxacum officinale* Wiggers). Derm Beruf Umwelt 30:51–53

189. Gougerot H, Burnier B (1933) Purpura réticulé et eczéma généralisé à la suite d'application de feuille d'aunée («Inula Helenium»); sensibilisation. Bull Soc Fr Dermatol Syphiligr 40:1702–1704

190. P'iankova ZP, Nugmanova ML (1975) Dermatit ot deviasila (dermatitis due to elecampane). Vestn Dermatol Venereol 12:53–54

191. Hausen BM, Spring O (1989) Sunflower allergy. On the constituents of the trichomes of *Helianthus annuus* L. (Compositae). Contact Derm 20:326–334

192. Rodriguez E, Reynolds GW, Thompson JA (1981) Potent contact allergen in the rubber plant guayule (*Parthenium argentatum*). Science 211:1444–1445

193. Maiden JH (1918) Plants which produce inflammation or irritation of the skin. Agric Gaz NSW 29:344–345

194. Vryman LH (1933) Dahlienwurzelrinden-Dermatitis. Arch Dermatol Syphilol 168:233

195. Calnan CD (1978) Sensitivity to dahlia flowers. Contact Derm 4:168

196. Olivier J, Renkin A (1954) Eczéma par sensibilité à une seule variété de chrysanthèmes. Arch Belg Dermatol Syphiligr 10:296–297

197. Rook A (1961) Plant dermatitis. The significance of variety-specific sensitization. Br J Dermatol 73:283–287

198. Hausen BM, Schulz KH (1976) Chrysanthemum allergy. III. Identification of the allergens. Arch Dermatol Res 255:111–121

199. Towers GHN, Arnason T, Wat CK, Graham EA, Lam J, Mitchell JL (1979) Phototoxic polyacetylenes and their thiophene derivatives. (Effects on human skin.). Contact Derm 5:140–144

200. Quirce S, Tabar AI, Olaguibel JM, Cuevas M (1996) Occupational contact urticaria syndrome caused by globe artichoke (Cynara scolymus. J Allergy Clin Immunol 97:710–711

201. Douin I (1986) Nouvelle flore des mousses et des hépatiques pour la détermination facile des espèces. Belin, Paris

202. Schmidt RJ (1996) Allergic contact dermatitis to liverworts, lichens, and mosses. Semin Dermatol 15:95–102

203. Mitchell JC (1986) Frullania (liverwort) phytodermatitis (woodcutter's eczema). Clin Dermatol 4:62–64

204. Mitchell JC, Fritig B, Singh B, Towers GH (1970) Allergic contact dermatitis from Frullania and Compositae. The role of sesquiterpene lactones. J Invest Dermatol 54:233–239

205. Knoche H, Ourisson G, Perold GW, Foussereau J, Maleville J (1969) Allergenic component of a liverwort: a sesquiterpene lactone. Science 166:239–240

206. Ducombs G, Lepoittevin JP, Berl V, Andersen KE, Brandao FM, Bruynzeel DP, Bruze M, Camarasa JG, Frosch PJ, Goossens A, Lachapelle JM, Lahti A, Le Coz CJ, Maibach HI, Menné T, Seidenari S, Shaw S, Tosti A, Wilkinson JD; European Environmental and Contact Dermatitis Research Group multicentre study (2003) Routine patch testing with frullanolide mix: an European Environmental and Contact Dermatitis Research Group multicentre study. Contact Derm 48:158–161

207. Hindsen M, Christensen LP, Paulsen E (2004) Contact allergy to the sesquiterpene lactone calocephalin. Contact Derm 50:162

208. Mitchell JC, Dupuis G (1971) Allergic contact dermatitis from sesquiterpenoids of the Compositae family of plants. Br J Dermatol 84:139–150

209. Hausen BM (1979) The sensitizing capacity of Compositae plants. III. Test results and cross-reactions in Compositae-sensitive patients. Dermatologica 159:1–11

210. Schmidt RJ (1985) When is a chrysanthemum dermatitis not a chrysanthemum dermatitis? The case for describing florists' chrysanthemums as Dendranthema cultivars. Contact Derm 13:115–119

211. Asakawa Y, Benezra C, Foussereau J, Muller JC, Ourisson G (1974) Cross-sensitization between Frullania and Laurus nobilis. Arch Dermatol 110:957

212. Fernandez de Corres L, Corrales Torres JL (1978) Dermatitis from Frullania, Compositae and other plants. Contact Derm 4:175–176

213. Hausen BM, Osmundsen PE (1983) Contact allergy to parthenolide in Tanacetum parthenium (L.) Schulz-Bip. (feverfew, Asteraceae) and cross-reactions to related sesquiterpene lactone containing Compositae species. Acta Derm Venereol (Stockh) 63:308–314

214. Marzulli FN, Maibach HI (1980) Further studies of effects of vehicles and elicitation concentrations in contact dermatitis testing. Contact Derm 6:131–133

215. Cheminat A, Stampf JL, Benezra C, Farral MJ, Frechet JM (1981) Allergic contact dermatitis to costus: removal of haptens with polymers. Acta Derm Venereol (Stockh) 61:525–529

216. Warshaw EM, Zug KA (1996) Sesquiterpene lactone allergy. Am J Contact Dermat 7:1–23

217. Rao PV, Mangala A, Towers GH, Rodriguez E (1978) Immunological activity of parthenin and its diasteriomer in persons sensitized by Parthenium hysterophorus L. Contact Derm 4:199–203

218. Ducombs G, Benezra C, Talaga P, Andersen KE, Burrows D, Camarasa JG, Dooms-Goossens A, Frosch PJ, Lachapelle JM, Menné T et al (1990) Patch testing with the "sesquiterpene lactone mix": a marker for contact allergy to Compositae and other sesquiterpene-lactone-containing plants. Contact Derm 22:249–252

219. Paulsen E, Andersen KE, Hausen BM (2001) An 8-year experience with routine SL mix patch testing supplemented with Compositae mix in Denmark. Contact Derm 45:29–35

220. Green C, Ferguson J (1994) Sesquiterpene lactone mix is not an adequate screen for Compositae allergy. Contact Derm 31:151–153

221. Shum KW, English JSC (1998) Allergic contact dermatitis in food handlers, with patch tests positive to Compositae mix but negative to sesquiterpene lactone mix. Contact Derm 39:207–208

222. Lepoittevin JP, Tomb R (1995) Sesquiterpene lactone mix is not an adequate screen for Compositae allergy. Contact Derm 32:254

223. Hausen BM (1996) A 6-year experience with Compositae mix. Am J Contact Dermat 7:94–99

224. Stingeni L, Lisi P (1996) Airborne allergic contact dermatitis from Compositae. Ann Ital Dermatol Clin Sperim 50:170–173

225. Schmidt RJ, Kingston T (1985) Chrysanthemum dermatitis in South Wales; diagnosis by patch testing with feverfew (Tanacetum parthenium) extract. Contact Derm 13:120–121

226. Goulden V, Wilkinson SM (1998) Patch testing for Compositae allergy. Br J Dermatol 138:1018–1021

227. Ettlinger MG, Lundeen AJ (1956) The structures of sinigrin and sinalbin; an enzymatic rearrangement. J Ann Chem Soc 78:4172–4173

228. Coulter S (1904) The poisonous plants of Indiana. Proc Indiana Acad Sci 119:51–63

229. Mitchell JC, Jordan WP (1974) Allergic contact dermatitis from the radish, Raphanus sativus. Br J Dermatol 91:183–189

230. Leoni A, Gogo R (1964) Dermatite professionale da contatto con cavolo capuccio. Minerva Med (Roma) 39:326–327

231. Gaul LE (1964) Contact dermatitis from synthetic oil of mustard. Arch Dermatol 90:158–159

232. Fregert S, Dahlquist I, Trulsson L (1983) Sensitization capacity of diphenylthiourea and phenylisothiocvanate. Contact Derm 9:87–88

233. Richter G (1980) Allergic contact dermatitis from methyl isothiocyanate in soil disinfectants. Contact Derm 6: 183–186

234. Schmidt RJ (1986) Biosynthetic and chemosystematic aspects of the Euphorbiaceae and Thymelaeaceae. In: Evans FJ (ed) Naturally occurring phorbol esters. CRC, Boca Raton, FL, pp 87–106

235. Webster GL (1986) Irritant plants in the spurge family (Euphorbiaceae). Clin Dermatol 1:36–45

236. Evans FJ (1986) Environmental hazards of diterpene esters from plants. In: Evans FJ (ed) Naturally occurring phorbol esters. CRC, Boca Raton, FL, pp 1–31

237. Satulsky EM, Wirts CA (1943) Dermatitis venenata caused by the manzanillo tree. Further observations and report of 60 cases. Arch Dermatol Syphilol 47:797

238. Rook A (1965) An unrecorded irritant plant. Synadenium grantii. Br J Dermatol 77:284

239. Calnan CD (1975) Petty spurge (*Luphorbia peplus* L.). Contact Derm 1:128

240. Strobel M, N'Diaye B, Padonou F, Marchand JP (1978) Les dermites de contact d'origine végétale. A propos de 10 cas observés à Dakar. Bull Soc Méd Air Noire Lang Fr 23: 124–127

241. Worobec SM, Hickey TA, Kinghorn AD, Soejarto D, West D (1981) Irritant contact dermatitis from an ornamental, *Euphorbia hermentiana*. Contact Derm 7:19–22

242. Hickey TA, Worobec SM, West DP, Kinghorn AD (1981) Irritant contact dermatitis in humans from phorbol and related esters. Toxicon 19:841–850

243. Pinedo JM, Saavedra V, Gonzalez-de-Canales F, Llamas P (1985) Irritant dermatitis due to *Euphorbia marginata*. Contact Derm 13:44

244. D'Arcy WG (1974) Severe contact dermatitis from poinsettia. Arch Dermatol 109:909–910

245. Hausen BM, Schulz KH (1977) Occupational contact dermatitis due to croton (*Codiaeum variegatum* (L.) A. Juss var. *pictum* (Lodd.) Muell. Arg.). Sensitization by plants of the Euphorbiaceae. Contact Derm 3:289–292

246. Schmidt H, Ølholm-Larsen P (1977) Allergic contact dermatitis from croton (*Codiaeum*). Contact Derm 3:100

247. Cleenewerck MB, Martin P (1989) Occupational contact dermatitis due to *Codiaeum variegatum* L., *Chrysanthemum indicum* L., *Chrysanthemum* x *hortorum* and *Frullania dilatata* L. In: Frosch PJ, Dooms-Goossens A, Lachapelle JM et al (eds) Current topics in contact dermatitis. Springer, Berlin, pp 149–157

248. Santucci B, Picardo M, Cristaudo A (1985) Contact dermatitis from *Euphorbia pulcherrima*. Contact Derm 12:285–286

249. Elpern DJ (1984) The dermatology of Kauai, Hawaii, 1981–1982. Int J Dermatol 24:647–652

250. Weedon D, Chick J (1976) Home treatment of basal cell carcinoma. Med J Aust 1:928

251. Schmidt RJ, Evans FJ (1980) Skin irritants of the sun spurge (*Euphorbia helioscopia* L.). Contact Derm 6:204–210

252. Adolf W, Sorg B, Hergenhahn M, Hecker E (1982) Structure-activity relations of polyfunctional diterpenes of the daphnane type. I. Revised structure for resiniferatoxin

and structure-activity relations of resiniferonol and some of its esters. J Nat Prod 45:347–354

253. Schmidt RJ, Evans FJ (1979) Investigations into the skin-irritant properties of resiniferonol ortho esters. Inflammation 3:273–280

254. Evans FJ (1986) Phorbol: its esters and derivatives. In: Evans FJ (ed) Naturally occurring phorbol esters. CRC, Boca Raton, FL, pp 171–215

255. Schmidt RJ (1986) The daphnane polyol esters. In: Evans FJ (ed) Naturally occurring phorbol esters. CRC, Boca Raton, FL, pp 217–243

256. Schmidt RJ (1986) The ingenane polyol esters. In: Evans FJ (ed) Naturally occurring phorbol esters. CRC, Boca Raton, FL, pp 245–269

257. Tiévant P (2001) Guide des lichens. 350 espèces de lichens d'Europe. Delachaux et Niestlé, Lausanne

258. Mitchell JC (1965) Allergy to lichens. Arch Dermatol 92:142–146

259. Mitchell JC, Shibata S (1969) Immunologic activity of some substances derived from lichenized fungi. J Invest Dermatol 52:517–520

260. Dahlquist I, Fregert S (1980) Contact allergy to atranorin in lichens and perfumes. Contact Derm 6:111–119

261. Thune P, Solberg Y, Mc Fadden N, Staerfelt F, Standberg M (1982) Perfume allergy due to oak moss and other lichens. Contact Derm 8:396–400

262. Bernard G, Gimenez-Arnau E, Rastogi SC, Heydorn S, Johansen JD, Menné T, Goossens A, Andersen K, Lepoittevin JP (2003) Contact allergy to oak moss: search for sensitizing molecules using combined bioassay-guided chemical fractionation, GC-MS, and structure-activity relationship analysis. Arch Dermatol Res 295:229–235

263. Bossi R, Rastogi SC, Bernard G, Gimenez-Arnau E, Johansen JD, Lepoittevin JP, Menné T (2004) A liquid chromatography-mass spectrometric method for the determination of oak moss allergens atranol and chloroatranol in perfumes. J Sep Sci 27:537–540

264. Johansen JD, Andersen KE, Svedman C, Bruze M, Bernard G, Gimenez-Arnau E, Rastogi SC, Lepoittevin JP, Menné T (2003) Chloroatranol, an extremely potent allergen hidden in perfumes: a dose-response elicitation study. Contact Derm 49:180–184

265. Thune P (1977) Allergy to lichens with photosensitivity. Contact Derm 3:213–214

266. Tan KS, Mitchell JC (1968) Patch and photopatch tests in contact dermatitis and photodermatitis. A preliminary report of investigation of 150 patients, with special reference to "cedar-poisoning". Can Med Assoc J 98:252–255

267. Thune P (1977) Contact allergy due to lichens in patients with a history of photosensitivity. Contact Derm 3:267–272

268. Salo H, Hannuksela M, Hausen B (1981) Lichen pickers' dermatitis (*Cladonia alpestris* (L.) Rab.). Contact Derm 7:9–13

269. Champion RH (1971) Atopic sensitivity to algae and lichens. Br J Dermatol 85:551–557

270. Lepoittevin JP, Meschkat E, Huygens S, Goossens A (2000) Presence of resin acids in "Oak moss" patch test material: a source of misdiagnosis? J Invest Dermatol 115:129–130

271. Hausen BM (1979) Primelallergie. Hintergründe und Aspekte. Mat Med Nordmark 31:57–76

272. Hjorth N (1979) Primula dermatitis. In: Mitchell J, Rook A (eds) Botanical dermatology. Greengrass, Vancouver, pp 554–564

273. Virgili A, Corazza M (1991) Unusual primin dermatitis. Contact Derm 24:63–64

274. Schildknecht H (1957) Struktur des Primelgiftstoffes. Z Naturforsch 22B:36–41

275. Paulsen E, Christensen LP, Andersen KE (2006) Miconidin and miconidin methyl ether from *Primula obconica* Hance: new allergens in an old sensitizer. Contact Derm 55:203–209

276. Christensen LP, Larsen E (2000) Direct emission of the allergen primin from intact *Primula obconica* plants. Contact Derm 42:149–153

277. Cairns R (1964) Plant dermatoses: some chemical aspects and results of patch testing with extracts of *Primula obconica*. Trans St John's Hosp Dermatol Soc 50:137–143

278. Hausen BM, Schmalle HW, Marshall D, Thomson RH (1983) 5, 8-Dihydroxyflavone (primetin) the contact sensitizer of Primula mistassinica Michaux. Arch Dermatol Res 275:365–370

279. Dooms-Goossens A, Biesemans G, Vandaele M, Degreff H (1989) Primula dermatitis: more than one allergen? Contact Derm 21:122–124

280. Aplin C, Tan R, Lovell C (2000) Allergic contact dermatitis from *Primula auricula* and *Primula denticulata*. Contact Derm 42:48

281. Aplin CG, Lovell CR (2001) Hardy primula species and allergic contact dermatitis. Contact Derm 42(suppl 2):11

282. Christensen LP, Larsen E (2000) Primin-free *Primula obconica* plants available. Contact Derm 43:45–46

283. Hjorth N (1966) Primula dermatitis: sources of error in patch testing and patch test sensitization. Trans St John's Hosp Dermatol Soc 52:207–219

284. Hjorth N (1967) Seasonal variations in contact dermatitis. Acta Derm Venereol (Stockh) 47:409–418

285. Fregert S, Hjorth N, Schulz KH (1968) Patch testing with synthetic primin in persons sensitive to *Primula obconica*. Arch Dermatol 98:144–147

286. Fernández de Corres L, Leanizbarrutia I, Muñoz D (1987) Contact dermatitis from *Primula obconica* Hance. Contact Derm 16:195–197

287. Agrup G, Fregert S, Hjorth N, Övrum P (1968) Routine patch tests with ether extract of *P. obconica*. Br J Dermatol 80:497–502

288. Frenzl F (1937) Artificial dermatitis caused by *Anemone nemorosa*. Casop Lék Cesk 76:1831–1835

289. Spengler F (1946) Die therapeutische Verwendung der *Anemone nemorosa* des Buschwindröschens. Pharmazie 1:222–223

290. Rodziewicz J, Wlodarczyk S (1961) Zmiany skórne wywolane dzialaniem jaskru. Przegl Dermatol 48:429–434

291. Aaron TH, Muttitt ELC (1964) Vesicant dermatitis due to prairie crocus (*Anemone patens* L.). Arch Dermatol 90:168–171

292. Rudzki E, Dajek Z (1975) Dermatitis caused by buttercups (*Ranunculus*). Contact Derm 1:322

293. Kipping FB (1935) The lactone of γ-hydroxyvinylacrylic acid, protoanemonin. J Chem Soc 1145–1147

294. Hill R, van Heyingen R (1951) Ranunculin: the precursor of the vesicant substance of the buttercup. Biochem J 49:332–335

295. Moriarty RM, Romain CR, Karle IL, Karle J (1965) The structure of anemonin. J Am Chem Soc 87:3251–3252

296. Boll PM (1968) Naturally occurring lactones and lactames. 1. The absolute configuration of ranunculin, lichesterinic acid, and some lactones related to lichesterinic acid. Acta Chem Scand Ser B 22:3245–3250

297. Innocenti G, Dall'Acqua F, Guiotto A, Caporale G (1977) Investigation on skin-photosensitizing activity of various kinds of Psoralea. Planta Med 31:151–155

298. Camm E, Buck HWL, Mitchell JC (1976) Phytophotodermatitis from *Heracleum mantegazzianum*. Contact Derm 2:68–72

299. Dreyer JC, Hunter JAA (1970) Giant hogweed dermatitis. Scott Med J 15:315–319

300. Birmingham DJ, Key MM, Tubich GE, Prone VB (1961) Phototoxic bullae among celery harvesters. Arch Dermatol 83:73–87

301. Seligman PJ, Mathias CGT, O'Malley MA, Beier RC, Fehrs LJ, Serrill WS, Halperin WE (1987) Phytophotodermatitis from celery among grocery store workers. Arch Dermatol 123:1478–1482

302. Austad J, Kavli G (1983) Phototoxic dermatitis caused by celery infected by *Sclerotinia sclerotiorum*. Contact Derm 9:448–451

303. Sommer RG, Jillson OF (1967) Phytophotodermatitis (solar dermatitis from plants). Gas plant and the wild parsnip. N Engl J Med 276:1484–1486

304. Picardo M, Cristaudo A, de Luca C et al (1986) Contact dermatitis to *Pastinaca sativa*. Contact Derm 15:98–99

305. Coste F, Marceron L, Boyer J (1943) Dermite à l'angélique. Bull Soc Fr Dermatol Syphiligr 50:316–317

306. Arvy MP, Gallouin F (2003) Épices, aromates et condiments. Belin, Paris

307. Sidi E, Bourgeois-Gavardin J (1955) Accidents provoqués par les applications locales d' "Ammi majus". In: Tolérance et intolérance aux produits cosmétiques. Masson, Paris, pp 337–338

308. Kavli G, Midelfart K, Raa J et al (1983) Phototoxicity from furocoumarins (psoralens) of Heracleum laciniatum in a patient with vitiligo. Action spectrum studies on bergapten, pimpinellin, angelicin and sphondin. Contact Derm 9:364–366

309. Weimarck G, Nilsson E (1980) Phototoxicity in *Heracleum sphondylium*. Planta Med 38:97–100

310. Machado S, Silva E, Massa A (2002) Occupational allergic contact dermatitis from falcarinol. Contact Derm 47:109–110

311. Hausen BM, Bröhan J, König WA, Faasch H, Hahn H, Bruhn G (1987) Allergic and irritant contact dermatitis from falcarinol and didehydrofalcarinol in common ivy (*Hedera helix* L.). Contact Derm 17:1–9

312. Sams WM (1941) Photodynamic action of lime oil (*Citrus aurantifolia*). Arch Dermatol Syphilol 44:571–587

313. Opdyke DLJ (1973) Fragrance raw materials monographs. Bergamot oil expressed. Fd Cosm Toxicol 11:1031–1033

314. Girard J, Unkovic J, Delahayes J, Lafille C (1979) Étude expérimentale de la phototoxicité de l'essence de bergamote; corrélation entre l'homme et le cobaye. Dermatologica 158:229–243

315. Volden G, Krokan H, Kavli G, Midelfart K (1983) Phototoxic and contact toxic reactions of the exocarp of

46

sweet oranges: a common cause of cheilitis? Contact Derm 9:201–204

316. Fisher JF, Trama LA (1979) High-performance liquid chromatographic determination of some coumarins and psoralens found in citrus peel oils. J Agric Fd Chem 27:1334–1337

317. Gawkrodger DJ, Savin JA (1983) Phytophotodermatitis due to common rue (*Ruta graveolens*). Contact Derm 9:224

318. Zobel AM, Brown SA (1990) Dermatitis-inducing furanocoumarins on leaf surfaces of eight species of rutaceous and umbelliferous plants. J Chem Ecol 16:693–700

319. Brener S, Friedman J (1985) Phytophotodermatitis induced by *Ruta chalepensis* L. Contact Derm 12:230–232

320. Möller H (1978) Phototoxicity of *Dictamnus alba*. Contact Derm 4:264–269

321. Elpern DJ, Mitchell JC (1984) Phytophotodermatitis from mokihana fruits (*Pelea anisata* H. Mann, fam. Rutaceae) in Hawaiian lei. Contact Derm 10:224–226

322. Yoke M, Turjman M, Flynn T, Balza F, Mitchell JC, Towers GH (1985) Identification of psoralen, 8-methoxypsoralen, isopimpinellin, and 5, 7-dimethoxycoumarin in Pelea anisata H. Mann. Contact Derm 12:196–199

323. Jarvis WM (1968) The photosensitizing furanocoumarins of *Phebalium argenteum* (blister bush). Aust J Chem 21:537–538

324. Zaynoun ST, Aftimos BG, Abi Ali L, Tenekjian KK, Khalidi U, Kurban AK (1984) *Ficus carica*; isolation and quantification of the photoactive components. Contact Derm 11:21–25

325. Ippen H (1982) Phototoxische Reaktion auf Feigen. Hautarzt 33:337–339

326. Kitchevatz M (1934) Etiologie et pathogénèse de la dermite des figues. Bull Soc Fr Dermatol Syphiligr 41:1751–1759

327. Houloussi-Behdjet D (1933) Dermatite des figues et des figuiers. Bull Soc Fr Dermatol Syphiligr 40:787–796

328. Schwartz L (1938) Cutaneous hazards in the citrus fruit industry. Arch Dermatol Syphilol 37:641–649

329. Vickers HR (1941) The carrot as a cause of dermatitis. Br J Dermatol Syph 53:52–57

330. Peck SM, Spolyar LW, Mason HS (1944) Dermatitis from carrots. Arch Dermatol Syphilol 49:266

331. Klauder JV, Kimmich JM (1956) Sensitization dermatitis due to carrots. Report of cross-sensitization phenomenon and remarks on phytophotodermatitis. Arch Dermatol 74:149–158

332. Van Dijk E, Berrens L (1964) Plants as an etiological factor in phytophotodermatitis. Dermatologica 129:321–328

333. Rackett SC, Zug KA (1997) Contact dermatitis to multiple exotic woods. Am J Contact Dermat 8:114–117

334. Haustein UF (1982) Violin chin rest eczema due to East-Indian rosewood (*Dalbergia latifolia* Roxb.). Contact Derm 8:77–78

335. Hausen BM (1997) Contact dermatitis from a wooden necklace. Am J Contact Dermat 8:185–187

336. Dias M, Vale T (1992) Contact dermatitis from a *Dalbergia nigra* bracelet. Contact Derm 26:61

337. Cronin E, Calnan CD (1975) Rosewood knife handle. Contact Derm 1:121

338. Hausen BM (1981) Woods injurious to human health. A manual. De Gruyter, Berlin

339. Willis JH (1982) Nasal carcinoma in woodworkers: a review. J Occup Med 24:526–530

340. Woods B, Calnan CD (1976) Toxic woods. Br J Dermatol 95:1–97

341. Hausen BM (1986) Contact allergy to woods. Clin Dermatol 4:65–76

342. Hausen BM, Adams RM (1990) Woods. In: Adams RM (ed) Occupational skin disease. Saunders, Philadelphia, PA, pp 524–536

343. Foussereau J (1981) Bois exotiques (TA 23). Fiche d'allergologie, Dermatologie professionnell. INRS, Paris, pp 1–5

344. Richter HG, Dallwitz MJ (2005) Commercial timbers: descriptions, illustrations, identification, and information retrieval (homepage). (See http://biodiversity.bio.uno.edu/delta/wood)

345. Fernández de Corres L, Leanizbarrutia I, Muñoz D (1988) Cross-reactivity between some naturally occurring quinones. Contact Derm 18:186–187

346. Dejobert Y, Martin P, Bergoend H (1995) Airborne contact dermatitis from *Apuleia leiocarpa* wood. Contact Derm 32:242–243

347. Estlander T, Jolanki R, Alanko K, Kanerva L (2001) Occupational allergic contact dermatitis caused by wood dusts. Contact Derm 44:213–217

348. Kiec-Swierczynska M, Krecisz B, Swierczynska-Machura D, Palczynski C (2004) Occupational allergic contact dermatits caused by padauk wood (*Pterocarpus soyauxii* Taub.). Contact Derm 50:384–385

349. Weber LF (1953) Dermatitis venenata due to native woods. AMA Arch Dermatol Syphil 67:388–394

350. Majamaa H, Viljanen P (2004) Occupational facial allergic contact dermatitis caused by Finnish pine and spruce wood dusts. Contact Derm 51:157–158

351. Karlberg AT (1988) Contact allergy to colophony. Chemical identification of allergens, sensitization experiments and clinical experiences. Acta Derm Venereol (Stockh) 139:1–43

352. Karlberg AT, Bohlinder K, Boman A et al (1988) Identification of 15-hydroperoxyabietic acid as a contact allergen in Portuguese colophony. J Pharm Pharmacol 40:42–47

353. Karlberg AT (2000) Colophony. In: Kanerva L, Elsner P, Wahlberg JE, Maibach HI (eds) Handbook of occupational dermatology. Springer, Berlin, pp 509–516

354. Hellerström S, Thyresson N, Widmark G (1957) Chemical aspects of turpentine eczema. Dermatologica 115:277–286

355. Pirilä V, Kilpiö O, Olkkonen A et al (1969) On the chemical nature of the eczematogens in oil of turpentine. V. Pattern of sensitivity to different terpenes. Dermatologica 139:183–194

356. Lippert U, Martin V, Schwertfeger C, Junghans D, Ellinghaus B, Fuchs T (2003) Shiitake dermatitis. Br J Dermatol 148:178–179

357. Korstanje MJ, van de Staak WJBM (1990) A case of hand eczema due to mushrooms. Contact Derm 22:115–116

358. Kanerva L, Estlander T, Jolanki R (1998) Airborne occupational allergic contact dermatitis from champignon mushroom. Am J Contact Dermat 9:190–192

359. Maes MFJ, Van Baar HMJ, Van Ginkel CJW (1999) Occupational allergic contact dermatitis from the mushroom White Pom Pom (*Hericium eriaceum*). Contact Derm 40:289–290

360. Simeoni S, Puccetti A, Peterlana D, Tinazzi E, Lunardi C (2004) Occupational allergic contact dermatitis from champignon and Polish mushroom. Contact Derm 51:156–157

361. Prelli R (2001) Les fougères et plantes alliées de France et d'Europe ocidentale. Belin, Paris

362. Hausen BM, Schulz KH (1978) Occupational allergic contact dermatitis due to leatherleaf fern *Arachnoides adiantiformis* (Forst) Tindale. Br J Dermatol 98:325–329

363. Özdemir C, Schneider LA, Hinrichs R, Staib G, Weber L, Weiss JM, Scharffetter-Kochanek K (2003) Allergische Kontaktdermatitis auf Efeu (*Hedera helix* L.). Hautarzt 54:966–969

364. Garcia M, Fernandez E, Navarro A, del Pozo MD, Fernandez de Corres L (1995) Allergic contact dermatitis from *Hedera helix* L. Contact Derm 33:133–134

365. Oka K, Saito F (1999) Allergic contact dermatitis from *Dendropanax trifidus*. Contact Derm 41:350–351

366. Leclerc H (1927) Précis de phytothérapie. Essai de thérapeutique par les plantes françaises. Masson et Cie, Paris

367. Etxenagusia MA, Anda M, González-Mahave I, Fernández E, Fernández de Corrès L (2000) Contact dermatitis from *Chelidonium majus* (greater celandine). Contact Derm 43:47

368. Stickel F, Poschl G, Seitz HK, Waldherr R, Hahn EG, Schuppan D (2003) Acute hepatitis induced by greater celandine (*Chelidonium majus*). Scand J Gastroenterol 38:565–568

369. Holme SA, Roberts DL (2000) Erythroderma associated with St John's wort. Br J Dermatol 143:1127–1128

370. Kubin A, Wierrani F, Burner U, Alth G, Grunberger W (2005) Hypericin – the facts about a controversial agent. Curr Pharm Des 11:233–253

371. Lane-Brown MM (2000) Photosensitivity associated with herbal preparations of St John's wort (*Hypericum perforatum*). Med J Aust 172:302

372. Schempp CM, Müller KA, Winghofer B, Schöpf E, Simon JC (2002) Johanniskraut (*Hypericum perforatum* L.) – eine Pflanze mit Relevanz für die Dermatologie. Hautarzt 53:316–321

373. Le Coz CJ (2004) Allergic contact dermatitis from tamanu oil (*Calophyllum inophyllum, Calophyllum tacamahaca*). Contact Derm 51:216–217

374. Avenel-Audran M, Hausen BM, Le Sellin J, Ledieu G, Verret JL (2000) Allergic contact dermatitis from hydrangea – is it so rare? Contact Derm 43:189–191

375. Van der Willigen AH, van Joost T, Stolz E, van der Hoek JCS (1987) Contact dermatitis to safflower. Contact Derm 17:184–186

376. Dejobert Y, Arzur L, Thellart AS, Martin P, Torck M, Frimat P, Piette F, Thomas P (2004) Contact dermatitis to Iris in a florist. Contact Derm 50:163–164

377. Martínez-González MC, Goday Buján JJ, Martínez Gómez W, Fonseca Capdevila E (2007) Concomitant allergic contact dermatitis due to *Rosmarinus officinalis* (rosemary) and *Thymus vulgaris* (thyme). Contact Derm 56:49–50

378. Timmermans MWH, Pentinga SE, Rustemeyer T, Bruynzeeel DP (2009) Contact dermatitis due to Paeonia (peony): a rare sensitizer? Contact Derm 60:232–233

379. Le Coz CJ (2000) Cigarette and cigar makers and tobacco workers. In: Kanerva L, Elsner P, Wahlberg JE, Maibach HI (eds) Handbook of occupational dermatology. Springer, Berlin, pp 887–889

380. Kabashima K, Miyachi Y (2004) Contact dermatitis due to eggplant. Contact Derm 50:101–102

381. Schena D, Magnanini M, Rosina P, Chieregato C (1998) Allergic contact dermatitis due to Hygrophila salicifolia. Contact Derm 39:132

382. Assier-Bonnet H (2000) Compositae mix versus sesquiterpene lactone mix for patch testing: a French experience. Contact Derm 42(suppl 2):40

383. Bong J, English JS, Wilkinson SM (2001) Diluted Compositae mix versus sesquiterpene lactone mix as a screening agent for Compositae dermatitis: a multicentre study. Contact Derm 42(suppl 2):49

384. Bruynzeel DP, Tafelkruijer J, Wilks MF (1995) Contact dermatitis due to a new fungicide used in the tulip bulb industry. Contact Derm 33:8–11

385. Grevelink SA, Olsen EA (1991) Efficacy of barrier creams in suppression of experimentally induced Rhus dermatitis. Am J Contact Dermat 2:69

386. Gonçalo M, Mascarenhas R, Vieira R, Figueiredo A (2004) Permeability of gloves to plant allergens. Contact Derm 50:200–201

387. Wrangsjö K, Ros AM (1996) Compositae allergy. Semin Dermatol 15:87–94

388. Schamberg J (1919) Desensitization of persons against poison ivy. JAMA 73:12–13

389. Kligman AM (1958) Cashew nut shell oil for hyposensitization against Rhus dermatitis. AMA Arch Dermatol 78:359–363

390. Guin JD (1991) The case of Dr Shelmire's child's nurse: a historical look at the confusion surrounding hyposensitization to Toxicodendrons. Am J Contact Dermat 2:194–197

391. Hashimoto Y, Kawada A, Aragane Y, Tezuka T (2003) Occupational contact dermatitis from chrysanthemum in a mortician. Contact Derm 49:106–107

392. Watson ES (1986) *Toxicodendron* hyposensitization programs. Clin Dermatol 4:160–170

393. Resnick SD (1986) Poison-ivy and poison-oak dermatitis. Clin Dermatol 4:208–212

Pesticides

47

Carola Lidén

Contents

C. Lidén
Unit of Occupational and Environmental Dermatology,
Institute of Environmental Medicine, Karolinska Institutet,
Box 210, SE-171 77 Stockholm, Sweden
e-mail: carola.liden@ki.se

47.1 Introduction

Pesticides include, according to EU legislation, plant protection products and biocidal products. Most pesticides are chemicals used in agriculture to control pests, weeds, or plant diseases. Pesticides are used in horticulture, forestry, and livestock production, and some are used as vector control agents in public health programmes. Herbicides, insecticides, and fungicides are the major groups (Table 47.1). Most pesticides are synthetic products, but some such as plant extracts or microorganisms are of biological origin. The wide application of biocidal products as preservative of cosmetics, other consumer and chemical products, and for the treatment of materials results in exposure of the general population (Table 47.1).

Many pesticides are potentially very hazardous to human health (Table 47.2) and to other organisms, and they may cause damage to the ecosystem. Human exposure to plant protection and many biocidal products is generally unintentional – dermal, oral, or respiratory. Dermal exposure is often the major route through which acute and severe toxic effects are initiated, mainly by the skin's absorption of cholinesterase-inhibiting insecticides (organophosphorous compounds). Contact dermatitis and other adverse skin effects are also important (Table 47.3). Intentional ingestion during a suicide attempt is often fatal. Acute and chronic health effects of exposure to pesticides constitute a large public health problem in developing countries [1]. This chapter deals mainly with the pesticides for plant protection.

J.D. Johansen et al. (eds.), *Contact Dermatitis*,
DOI: 10.1007/978-3-642-03827-3_47, © Springer-Verlag Berlin Heidelberg 2011

47

Core Message

> Dermal exposure to pesticides may cause systemic toxic effects, dermatitis, or other adverse skin effects.

Table 47.1 Main categories of pesticides

Plant protection agents	Herbicides and desiccants
	Insecticides, acaricides, molluscicides, and nematicides
	Fungicides
	Plant growth regulators
Biocidal products	Disinfectants and general biocidal products
	Human, veterinary, private, food area applications – excluding cleaning products that are not intended to have a biocidal effect, including washing liquids, powders, and similar products
	Preservatives
	In-can preservatives, film preservatives, wood preservatives, fiber, leather, rubber, and polymerized materials preservatives, slimicides, metalworking-fluid preservatives, etc
	Pest control
	Rodenticides, insecticides, repellents, etc
	Other biocidal products
	Antifouling products, etc

Examples of groups and types

Table 47.2 Health effects of pesticides (based on [1])

Bone-marrow effects
Cancer
Developmental effects
Enzyme induction
Eye lesions
Immunological effects
Neurotoxicity
Reproductive dysfunction
Respiratory effects
Skin lesions (see Table 47.3)
Systemic poisoning

Table 47.3 Skin effects of pesticides (based mainly on [16, 19])

Absorption through the skin
Accumulation in skin
Chemical burns
Chloracne
Contact dermatitis: allergic and irritant
Hyper- and hypopigmentation
Nail dystrophy
Photosensitivity
Porphyria cutanea tarda
Sclerodermatous changes
Squamous cell carcinoma

47.2 Use of Pesticides and its Limitations

Today, about 750 active ingredients are used as pesticides for plant protection in 50,000 commercial formulations on the world market, and 25% of the world consumption of pesticides occurs in developing countries [1, 2].

Historically, the use of inorganic chemicals, sulfur, and arsenic to control insects dates back to classical Greece and Rome. Paris green, an impure copper arsenite, was introduced in 1867 for crop protection. Iron sulfate was found to be useful for weed control. The first organomercury seed dressing was introduced in 1913 in Germany. DDT was developed in 1940. Since then, a wide range of chemical compounds have been introduced as pesticides.

The use of pesticides is, in large parts of the world, surrounded by regulations concerning the substances allowed, methods, indications, and periods of application, education, and protective equipment for workers. An increasing number of pesticides have, during the last decades, been banned or severely restricted for use in large parts of Europe and in Northern America, mainly due to their unwanted effects on the environment, and in some cases due to their effects on human health. Examples are DDT and other organochlorine insecticides, many mercury compounds, some phenoxy acid herbicides, and the herbicide paraquat. Many of those pesticides are, however, widely exported to and used in developing countries [1, 3, 4]. In the EU, pesticides must be approved for sale and use under

Directive 91/414/EEC on plant protection products and Directive 98/8/EC on biocidal products.

The herbicide paraquat has its major markets in Asia, Central and South America, which use 75% of the paraquat produced. In 2003, the EC decided to authorize its use. In 2007, however, the Court of First Instance of the European Communities annulled the decision, as a result of Sweden's action. The outcome may lead to a higher level of protection of health. The substance is now banned in 13 countries.

The biocide dimethylfumarate was banned in 2009 by the EC in products placed on the market, in accordance with Directive 2001/95/EC on general product safety. This was done soon after it had been revealed that the substance had caused several cases of severe contact dermatitis in Europe, because of its use as anti-mold agent in some imported consumer goods. Dimethylfumarate is not authorized for use in the EU (see Sect. 47.5.6).

> **Core Message**
>
> › The use of pesticides in Europe and Northern America is surrounded by regulations for the protection of the environment and human health, while the use of pesticides causes severe problems in developing countries.

47.3 Terminology, Classification, and Formulations

In EC regulation, pesticides are either plant protection or biocidal products. Plant protection products are mainly used to protect plants and plant products in agriculture, forestry, and horticulture from attacks by fungi, pests, and competing plants. Biocidal products are defined as chemical or biological pesticides which do not constitute plant protection products (Table 47.1).

Pesticides are usually categorized according to what they are used against, or what they protect. The active ingredients are often mentioned by their common or trivial names, according to the International Organization for Standardization (ISO), which is the terminology used in this chapter. Many synonyms occur, and many pesticides are better known by their trade names. The WHO classification based on the degree of acute hazard to humans is widely used: class Ia is extremely

hazardous; Ib is highly hazardous; II is moderately hazardous; and III is slightly hazardous.

Pesticides are formulated in different ways – such as solid or liquid concentrates, solutions, or emulsions in water or organic solvents, aerosols, granules, powders, or mixed with sand, dusts, and fumigants. It is essential to recall that pesticide products, besides their active ingredients, also contain nonactive ingredients and possibly contaminants. Many of the nonactive ingredients and contaminants are toxic substances, and some are known skin irritants or allergens (organic solvents, formaldehyde, isocyanates). The formulants can also act as facilitators for transport into the skin and may therefore worsen a lesion. The chemical structures of some pesticides are shown in Fig. 47.1.

47.4 Skin Exposure and Absorption Through Skin

There is a broad variation in the degree of skin exposure to pesticides at work. Sprayers, mixers, loaders, packers, and mechanics perform work with high risk of direct skin contact with pesticides. Sprayers are also exposed to aerosols, during and after application. Workers may be exposed to pesticide residues on treated flowers, crops, bulbs, and wood. Some pesticides are quickly degraded while others are more or less persistent.

A number of methods of exposure assessment have been used for different pesticides [5, 6] (see also Chap. 27). Cholinesterase activity in erythrocytes or in plasma should be determined in workers using organophosphorous compounds. Paraquat and some other pesticides or their metabolites can be measured in urine. Skin exposure can be studied by hand-wash techniques, fluorescent tracer technique, and by the analysis of pesticide levels in patches on the skin. The hands are generally the part of the body with the highest exposure, but the arms and face and other unprotected or soaked parts are exposed, and with knapsack sprayers, the back and lower legs too [7].

Percutaneous absorption of pesticides varies considerably from compound to compound, as shown by experimental studies on normal skin of human volunteers, and by in vitro studies [8–12]. The regional variation in pesticide absorption through the skin is large and the highest from scrotal skin, head, and neck. Occlusion, skin damage, concentration, contact time, area, humidity, and temperature are the factors that are important for absorption.

46

hobbies, and recent excursions during which plant contact may have occurred. It is often necessary to enlist the help of a botanist to identify plants brought in by patients. If the results of an investigation of a plant-induced dermatitis are to be published, it is essential to identify the plant precisely. While photographs of plants are helpful, they are usually less helpful than accurate drawings showing features that enable similar species to be distinguished one from another. There is no substitute for a botanist who is familiar with the taxonomic literature on the plant concerned, but just as there are specialities in the medical profession, no one botanist is an expert on all plants.

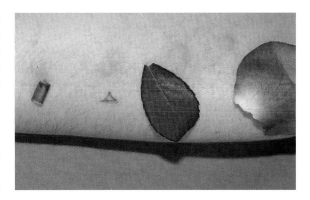

Fig. 46.34 Positive prick tests to rose (petal, stem, leave and thorn) in a florist with immediate symptoms following contact with roses

46.4.1 Raw Plants

46.4.1.1 Plant Identification

The practitioner has to consider not only the plant species itself, but also its generic and familial identity. The genetic information that groups plants into species, genera, and families actually determines to a large extent the nature of the plant's secondary metabolites. Thus, sesquiterpene lactones are a common feature of the members of the family Compositae, while mono- and dihydroxyalk(en)ylbenzenes are commonly found in the members of the family Anacardiaceae. Once a plant has been implicated and identified, reference to the literature should reveal whether or not it has been recorded as an allergenic plant.

46.4.1.2 Prick Tests

Pricks can be performed through the crude material as is or by the "prick by prick" method (prick into the plant, and then into the skin). Plant materials can be crushed and diluted with saline (for example, 1: 9 parts) in order to obtain a solution that can be easily pricked (Fig. 46.34, rose).

46.4.1.3 Patch Tests

It is often possible to carry out tests with plant material "as is," and a diagnosis of plant dermatitis can usually be established with a few grams of fresh plant

material. The practitioner has to patch test several plant pieces such as roots, stems, leaves, and reproductive organs (flowers and/or fruits). It is sometimes useful to patch test crushed leaves or slices of stem [381].

It is important to use, whenever possible, the actual plant material that is believed to be responsible for the current dermatitis. This is because distinct chemical races may exist in outwardly identical plants, where one specimen contains the allergen, while the second does not. As noted above, cultivars of plants such as tulips and chrysanthemums exhibit varying propensities to induce and elicit ACD. If an inappropriate sample of plant material is tested, the risk of a missed diagnosis clearly exists.

Woods should not be tested as is, because of the risk of irritation and active sensitization. Wood dust can be tested diluted in white petrolatum, 10–20% (weight/weight). Extracts obtained with solvents such as acetone or ethanol can be used. Controls are useful when they are negative because of the high incidence of irritancy [39, 340, 346], but they raise ethical considerations. When purified isolates from woods are available for patch testing, these may be prepared according to the recommendations of Hausen [341]. Here too, the risk of active sensitization is real ([346]; A. Goossens, personal communication).

Care should be taken with plants known to contain either irritant compounds (such as *Euphorbia* spp.) or highly allergenic compounds (such as *Primula*), where the past experiences of other dermatologists (reported in the literature, at congresses or via networks) should be heeded.

Irritant reactions are frequent with plant materials and have to be considered when doubtful or weakly positive (edema and erythema) reactions are observed.

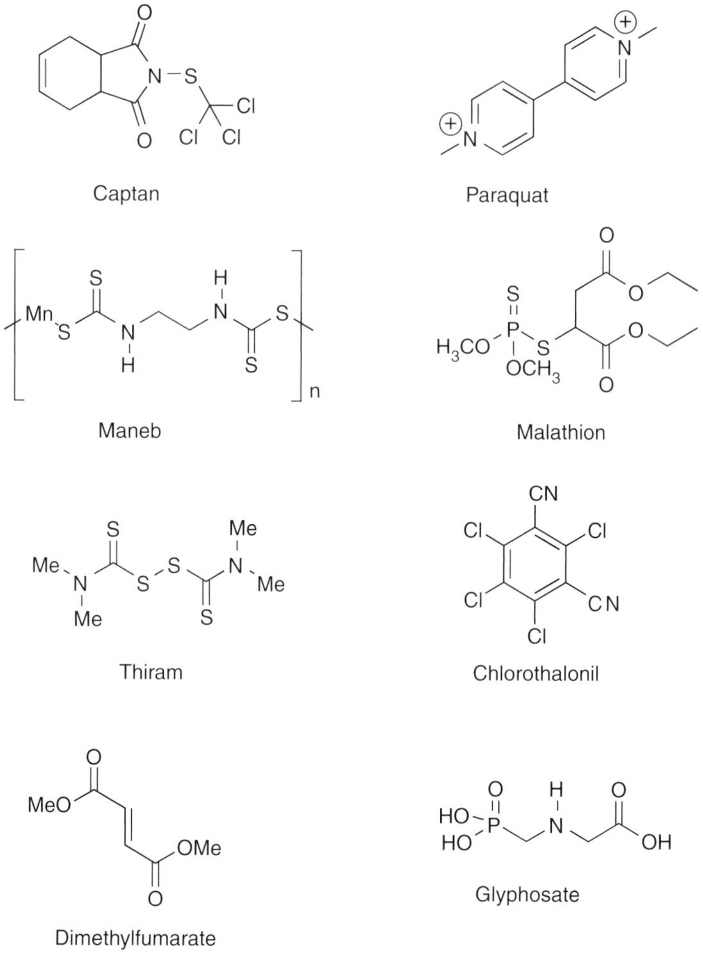

Fig. 47.1 Chemical structures of some pesticides

Captan

Paraquat

Maneb

Malathion

Thiram

Chlorothalonil

Dimethylfumarate

Glyphosate

Core Message

> Percutaneous absorption of pesticides varies between compounds. Occlusion, skin damage, concentration, contact time, and surface area are important factors for absorption. The fluorescent tracer technique and other methods may be used in exposure assessment.

47.4.1 Prevention of Skin Exposure

The most appropriate equipment for protection against exposure to hazardous pesticides depends on the type of work and the properties of the pesticide product. For the most heavily exposed groups, such as applicators, mixers, and producers, the use of coverall, apron, raincoat, gloves, hat, boots, mask, and goggles or face shields is often indicated. For protection, it is important that the equipment is used properly, is clean, and is in good shape. The gloves that generally give the best protection are nitrile/butyl rubber gloves or laminate gloves (4H or Barrier). Barrier creams have not been shown to provide effective protection.

In many parts of the world, adequate conditions are not provided for protecting pesticide workers. The reasons for insufficient protection are often a lack of resources and low level of awareness of risks due to skin exposure. It is also uncomfortable to use fully protective equipment in a hot and humid climate. In the poorest developing countries, where many of the most dangerous pesticides are used, workers may have no protection at all. Knapsack sprayers may carry out mixing and spraying dressed in just a T-shirt and shorts. Spraying by airplane is frequent and people on the ground may be unprotected. Adequate washing conditions for skin, clothes, and equipment are often not present.

Skin exposure to pesticides is heavily dependent on how the work is carried out, and on awareness of the risk caused by contamination of the skin. The use of a fluorescent tracer mixed with the pesticide has been introduced for visualization, by UV light, of skin contamination [5, 7, 13]. The method has been very useful for explaining risky techniques and occurrences to workers. Guidelines for personal protection and field surveys have been published by authorities and organizations such as WHO, US EPA (the U.S. Environmental Protection Agency), and Crop Life International (former GIFAP and GCPF).

Core Message

> Adequate protective equipment and working conditions, and awareness of risks and safe handling, are essential for the prevention of severe health effects due to skin exposure to pesticides.

47.5 Skin Effects of Some Pesticides

The true prevalence and incidence of skin disease due to pesticide exposure is not known. It is likely that many of the pesticides cause more dermatitis than that is reported. Farmers generally do not have easy access to dermatologists; many agricultural workers are temporarily employed and do not seek medical care; and in most developing countries, dermatologists are rare and patch testing is often not done.

Irritant contact dermatitis due to pesticide exposure is believed to be more frequent than allergic contact dermatitis. The most frequently reported cases of allergic contact dermatitis have been related to fungicides and insecticides. The most important fatal effects of skin exposure to pesticides are acute toxic reactions due to skin absorption of organophosphorous compounds [14, 15]. Pesticides are also known to cause other skin effects (Table 47.3).

The following examples may illustrate how the situation varies globally. In California, adverse health effects due to pesticide exposure have attracted much

attention. The agricultural sector has had the highest rate of occupational skin disease of any industry, and epidemics of contact dermatitis have been reported. One third of the illnesses and injuries due to pesticides have been reported to involve the skin [16]. In Japan, contact dermatitis was reported in 27% of 815 patients diagnosed with and treated for pesticide poisoning. The principal pesticides reported to be responsible for the dermatitis cases were fungicides and insecticides, and spraying operations were reported in 78% of cases [17]. In Denmark, clinical examination and patch testing was carried out on 253 gardeners and greenhouse workers with occupational skin symptoms identified by a questionnaire. A relatively low prevalence of contact allergy to fungicides was thought to reflect the effect of protective measures [18].

Detailed reviews on occupational skin disease related to pesticides, covering large numbers of case reports, as well as more conclusive studies, have been published [16, 19]. The results from the predictive testing of 23 pesticides in guinea pigs are presented in a review [20]. Predictive testing for sensitization and irritation are discussed [21, 22]. Some of the most relevant information on the skin effects of commonly used pesticides is summarized below.

Core Message

> Irritant and allergic contact dermatitis and other skin effects are caused by pesticide exposure. Fungicides and insecticides are the most frequently reported causes of allergic contact dermatitis. Skin absorption of organophosphorous compounds and paraquat causes severe toxic effects.

47.5.1 Herbicides and Desiccants

Glyphosate (Roundup and other trade names) is the largest selling nonselective herbicide applied in agriculture, public areas, and for home use. It has been associated with skin disease, and cases of irritant as well as allergic contact dermatitis have in recent years been reported from Japan, Panama, and Spain [4, 23–25].

Paraquat (Gramoxone and other trade names) is a nonselective contact herbicide and desiccant. It is one

47

of the most widely used pesticides for weed control. Paraquat is highly toxic when ingested, causing multiple organ failure, and there is no antidote. Irritant contact dermatitis, occupational keratoses, nail lesions with discoloration, deformity and onycholysis, necrotic ulcers, and also fatalities have been reported after skin exposure [16, 26]. Considerable amounts may be absorbed through damaged skin and under occlusion, while absorption through intact skin is limited [10, 27].

2,4-D and 2,4,5-T are phenoxy acid herbicides [6, 28]. They are selective against broad-leaved plants and used as defoliants, and are produced in enormous quantities. They may contain TCDD (dioxin), which is often formed during production. This is the explanation for several outbreaks of chloracne and porphyria cutanea tarda among workers in pesticide production, and for the disaster in Seveso, Italy, in 1976. Contact dermatitis has also been described. 2,4-D and 2,4,5-T were components of "Agent Orange," used by the United States army to defoliate jungle areas in South Vietnam.

47.5.2 Insecticides

Many insecticides are very toxic on skin contact, resulting in systemic toxicity; some are skin irritants, and others are identified as clinically relevant contact allergens. A substantial number of case reports have been published on different types of skin reaction to several insecticides. Reference is given for reviews [16, 19]. Some illustrative examples are given below.

Pyrethrins are botanical pesticides and plant extracts. They are obtained from Chrysanthemum cinerariaefolium and are moderately potent allergens. Pyrethroids are synthetic compounds with a longer duration of activity against insects than that of pyrethrum, and less toxicity to mammals than organophosphorous compounds. Paresthesias and contact urticaria following skin exposure have been described [16, 29, 30].

Malathion and parathion are examples of organophosphorous pesticides [14, 16]. Parathion is extremely toxic, and its use in Europe and Northern America is heavily restricted. Malathion, which is degraded rapidly in the body, is less dangerous. Malathion is a moderate sensitizer according to predictive testing in man and guinea pig (review by [20]). Sclerodermatous changes have occurred in workers handling malathion, parathion, DDT, and some other pesticides [31].

DDT and lindane are chlorinated hydrocarbons. Lindane is widely used and is a skin irritant [16]. Cases of irritant contact dermatitis from treatment of scabies by lindane have been described. Allergic contact dermatitis has not been convincingly reported.

47.5.3 Fungicides

Benomyl, captan, chlorothalonil, difolatan, fluazinam, mancozeb, maneb, thiram, and zineb are some of the fungicides that are most frequently, or convincingly, reported to cause allergic contact dermatitis (reviewed in [16, 19]). Several other fungicides are reported to have caused allergic contact dermatitis in single cases. Airborne contact dermatitis and photocontact dermatitis have also been reported [15, 32]. Some illustrative examples of contact allergy to fungicides are given below.

Benomyl is used for fruits, nuts, vegetables, crops, and ornamentals. Several cases of allergic contact dermatitis from exposure to benomyl have been reported. Picking plants containing residues was found to be an important source of sensitization [33].

Mancozeb, maneb, thiram, zineb, and other thiurams are members of the dithiocarbamate group. Cross-reactivity may be present in persons sensitive to these pesticides or chemically related rubber chemicals [34].

Chlorothalonil (Bravo, Daconil, and other trade names) is a broad-spectrum fungicide used on vegetables, fruits, flowers, trees, and bananas. Allergic contact dermatitis has been described in workers in floriculture and banana fields [35–37]. Chlorothalonil has been described as a possible cause of skin pigmentation (ashy dermatitis) in banana field workers, many of whom were patch test positive [38]. Chlorothalonil has also other uses (see Sect. 47.5.6).

Fluazinam caused outbreaks of contact dermatitis on the arms and face at a tulip processing company and among farmers shortly after it had been introduced. Exposed workers were patch test positive and controls patch test negative [39].

Predictive testing in animals by the guinea-pig maximization test has shown that benomyl, captan, chlorothalonil, mancozeb, maneb, and zineb are extremely potent sensitizers (reviewed in [20]). An extremely sensitizing potency of chlorothalonil was shown by the local lymph node assay (LLNA), and in guinea pigs [40].

47.5.4 Repellents

N,N-Diethyl-m-toluamide (DEET) is a much used insect repellent against mosquitoes. It has been reported to produce allergic contact dermatitis and contact urticaria, and to exacerbate seborrhea and acne. It has also been reported to cause erythema, progressing to bullae and permanent scarring [16, 41].

47.5.5 Rodenticides

Warfarin is and ANTU has been frequently used rodenticides, substances used to kill rats and mice. Only single cases of occupational contact dermatitis due to exposure to Warfarin and ANTU have been reported [16].

47.5.6 Preservatives for the Treatment of Articles and Materials

The increasing use of biocidal products as preservatives for the treatment of a wide range of articles and materials that come into contact with the skin is controversial. Many of the substances are potent skin sensitizers, and many are dangerous to the environment. Unwanted exposure is difficult to avoid. Some examples of products and applications are given.

Products used for the preservation of manufactured products in containers such as cosmetics and paints, and of metal working fluids are described in the other chapters.

The biocide dimethylfumarate caused an outbreak of allergic contact dermatitis in some European countries in 2007–2008. Many consumers developed severe dermatitis after exposure to sofas, armchairs, and shoes imported from China [42]. It was revealed that the articles were treated by dimethylfumarate in small pouches placed in the furniture or footwear boxes. Due to the alarming outbreak, the EC banned dimethylfumarate in products (see Sect. 47.2). The substance has probably not been used as pesticide by European industry.

Chlorothalonil, which has caused allergic contact dermatitis, is, besides its use as a fungicide in agriculture, used as wood preservative and in paints [40, 43, 44].

Airborne symptoms, interpreted as irritant contact dermatitis, among workers in a Portuguese trailer tent factory has also been described [45] (see Sect. 47.5.3).

Glutaraldehyde is used as a slimicide and is added to wood pulp slurry in the production of paper. Glutaraldehyde is a known contact allergen and is described in other chapters.

5-Chloro-2-methylisothiazol-3-one/2-methylisothiazol-3-one (MCI/MI) is used together with arsenic, chromium, and copper compounds in wood preservation. MCI/MI is also used as a slimicide in the production of paper, and at printing. MI is increasingly used in combination with other preservatives. Contact allergy to MCI/MI is described in other chapters.

Tributyltin oxide (TBTO) is used as a wood preservative and in antifouling paints. TBTO is a skin irritant and has caused chemical burns, but it is not known as skin sensitizer [46].

Silver and silver salts are increasingly used for the antibacterial treatment of a wide range of products including underwear, sportswear and shoes, plaster, mobile phones, and refrigerators. There is a fear that this may lead to the development of antibiotic resistant bacteria and argyria, and other negative effects on health and environment. Risks are currently under evaluation.

47.6 Patch Testing

It may be difficult to acquire adequate information concerning possible exposure to pesticide products. It is often even more difficult to obtain detailed information concerning the composition of the actual products, and to achieve access to the active ingredients for patch testing. It is also important to recall that pesticide products, in addition to the active ingredients and possible contaminants, contain other ingredients that may be toxic, irritants, or allergens, and that they are often dissolved or mixed in organic solvents or water.

At present, no commercial pesticide patch test series is available. Some patch test clinics have their own pesticides series, composed to correspond to the use of pesticides in their geographical region. As the use of pesticides changes over time and in different areas of application, it is not possible to give definite recommendations.

Patch testing should ideally be carried out with the active ingredients and other ingredients of the pesticides that the patient is exposed to. It may, however, be extremely difficult to obtain the ingredients. A practical approach is then to patch test with appropriate dilutions of the pesticide product. For many pesticide products, but not all, testing with 1% and 0.3%, and possibly 0.1% of the product in water or petrolatum is possible (Bruynzeel, personal communication). It must be stressed, however, that the active ingredient or possibly other ingredients may need further dilution. Positive

reactions should be validated by testing on control persons.

Before patch testing, previous experience of testing with the pesticide product or ingredients should be checked in recent reports and reviews. Some of the most well-documented pesticide patch test preparations are listed in Table 47.4.

Safety is important when testing such potentially hazardous compounds. The recommended amounts applied at patch testing, however, are so small that they are regarded as safe, with no risk of systemic toxicity.

Table 47.4 Recommended patch test concentrations for some pesticides (based mainly on original publications and reviews [16, 19, 47])

Active ingredient (CAS number)	Type	Patch test concentration
2,4-DNCB (97–00–7)	Alg	0.01–0.1% aq. or acet.
2-Methyl-4-isothiazolin-3-one (MI) (2682–20–4)	Slim, wood	MI: 0.05–0.1% aq.
5-Chloro-2-methyl-4-isothiazolin-3-one (MCI) (26172–55–4)	Slim, wood	MI/MCI: 0.01–0.02% aq.
Benomyl (17804–35–2)	Fung	0.1–1% pet.
Captan (133–06–2)	Fung	0.25–0.5% aq. or pet.
Chlorothalonil (1897–45–6)	Fung, wood	0.001–0.01% acet.
Dazomet (533–74–4)	Fung, herb, insect	0.1% pet. or 0.25% aq.
DDT (50–29–3)	Insect	1% pet. or acet.
Difolatan (2425–06–1)	Fung	0.1% pet. or aq.
Dimethylfumarate (624-49-7)	Fung	0.1% pet.
Fluazinam (79622–59–6)	Fung	0.5% pet.
Folpet (133–07–3)	Fung	0.1% pet.
Glutaraldehyde (111–30–8)	Slim	0.2–0.3% pet.
Glyphosate (34494–03–6; 38641–94–0; 81591–81–3)	Herb	1–10% aq.
Lindane (58–89–9)	Insect	1% pet.
Malathion (121–75–5)	Insect	0.5% pet.
Maneb (12427–38–2)	Fung	0.5–1% pet.
Paraquat (1910–42–5)	Herb	0.1% pet.
Pentachloronitrobenzene (82–68–8)	Fung	0.5–1% pet.
Pyrethrum (several CAS-numbers)	Insect	1–2% pet.
Thiram (137–26–8)	Fung	1% pet.
Warfarin (81–81–2; 129–06–6)	Rod	0.5% pet.
Zineb (12122–67–7)	Fung	1% pet.
Ziram (137–30–4)	Fung	1% pet.

(Vehicles: *acet.* acetone; *aq.* water; *pet.* petrolatum; types of pesticides: *alg* algicides; *fung* fungicides; *herb* herbicides and desiccants; *insect* insecticides; *rod* rodenticides; *slim* slimicides; *wood* wood preservatives)

> ## Core Message
>
> ❯ Patch testing may be performed with appropriate concentrations of the pesticide product or the active ingredient and other ingredients. Consult the literature for safe handling.

References

1. World Health Organization and United Nations Environmental Programme (WHO/UNEP) (1990) Public health impact of pesticides used in agriculture. WHO, Geneva
2. Wilkinson CF (1990) Introduction and overview. In: Baker SR, Wilkinson CF (eds) The effects of pesticides on human health. Princeton Scientific Publishing, Princeton, NJ, pp 5–33 (Advances in Modern Environmental Toxicology, vol XVIII)
3. Dinham B (2003) The perils of paraquat. Sales targeted at developing countries. Pesticide News 60:4–7
4. Wesseling C, Corriols M, Bravo V (2005) Acute pesticide poisoning and pesticide registration in Central America. Toxicol Appl Pharmacol 207(2 Suppl):697–705
5. Fenske RA (2005) State-of-the-art measurement of agricultural pesticide exposures. Scand J Work Environ Health 31 (suppl 1):67–73; 63–65
6. Legaspi JA, Zenz C (1994) Occupational health aspects of pesticides. Clinical and hygienic principles. In: Zenz C, Dickerson OB, Horvath EP (eds) Occupational medicine, 3rd edn, Chap 47. Mosby, St Louis, pp 617–653
7. Blanco LE, Aragón A, Lundberg I et al (2005) Determinants of dermal exposure among Nicaraguan subsistence farmers during pesticide applications with backpack sprayers. Ann Occup Hyg 49:17–24
8. Andersen KE (1999) Systemic toxicity from percutaneous absorption. In: Adams RM (ed) Occupational skin disease, 3rd edn. Saunders, Philadelphia, pp 69–85
9. Nielsen JB, Nielsen F, Sørensen JA (2004) In vitro percutaneous penetration of five pesticides – effects of molecular weight and solubility characteristics. Ann Occup Hyg 48:697–705
10. Nielsen JB, Nielsen F, Sørensen JA (2007) Defense against dermal exposures is only skin deep: significantly increased penetration through slightly damaged skin. Arch Dermatol Res 299:423–431
11. Wester RC, Maibach HI (1985) In vivo percutaneous absorption and decontamination of pesticides in humans. J Toxicol Environ Health 16:25–37
12. Wester RC, Maibach HI (1996) Percutaneous absorption: short-term exposure, lag time, multiple exposures, model variations, and absorption from clothing. In: Marzulli FN, Maibach HI (eds) Dermatotoxicology, 5th edn, Chap 4. Taylor and Francis, Washington, pp 35–48
13. Aragón A, Blanco L, López L et al (2004) Reliability of a visual scoring system with fluorescent tracers to assess dermal pesticide exposure. Ann Occup Hyg 48:601–606
14. Grandjean P (1990) Organophosphorus compounds. In: Skin penetration: hazardous chemicals at work, Ch 12. Taylor and Francis, Washington, pp 157–170
15. Mark KA, Brancaccio RR, Soter NA et al (1999) Allergic contact and photoallergic contact dermatitis to plant and pesticide allergens. Arch Dermatol 135:67–70
16. Manuskiatti W, Abrams K, Hogan DJ et al (2000) Pesticide-related dermatoses in agricultural workers. In: Kanerva L, Elsner P, Wahlberg JE, Maibach HI (eds) Handbook of occupational dermatology, Chap 92. Springer, Berlin, pp 781–802
17. Matsushita T, Nomura S, Wakatsuki T (1980) Epidemiology of contact dermatitis from pesticides in Japan. Contact Dermatitis 6:255–259
18. Paulsen E (1998) Occupational dermatitis in Danish gardeners and greenhouse workers. Contact Dermatitis 38:14–19
19. Hogan DJ, Grafton LH (1999) Pesticides and other agricultural chemicals. In: Adams RM (ed) Occupational skin disease, 3rd edn. Saunders, Philadelphia, pp 597–622
20. Wahlberg JE, Boman A (1985) Guinea pig maximization test. In: Andersen KE, Maibach HI (eds) Contact allergy predictive tests in guinea pigs. Karger, Basel, pp 59–106 (Current Problems in Dermatology, vol 14)
21. Lisi P, Caraffini S, Assalve D (1987) Irritation and sensitization potential of pesticides. Contact Dermatitis 17:212–218
22. Marzulli F, Maguire HC (1982) Usefulness and limitations of various guinea-pig test methods in detecting human skin sensitizers. Validation of guinea-pig tests for skin hypersensitivity. Food Chem Toxicol 20:67–74
23. Heras-Mendaza F, Casado-Fariñas I, Paredes-Gascón M et al (2008) Erythema multiforme-like eruption due to an irritant contact dermatitis from a glyphosate pesticide. Contact Dermatitis 59:54–56
24. Horiuchi N, Oguchi S, Nagami H et al (2008) Pesticide-related dermatitis in Saku district, Japan, 1975-2000. Int J Occup Environ Health 14:25–34
25. O'Malley MAO, Mathias CGT, Coye MJ (1989) Epidemiology of pesticide-related skin disease in California agriculture. In: Dosman JA, Cockroft DW (eds) Principles of health and safety in agriculture. CRC, Boca Raton, pp 301–304
26. Wesseling C, van Wendel de Joode B, Ruepert C et al (2001) Paraquat in developing countries. Int J Occup Environ Health 7:275–286
27. Garnier R (1995) Paraquat poisoning by inhalation or skin absorption. In: Bismuth C, Hall AH (eds) Paraquat poisoning – mechanisms, prevention and treatment. Dekker, New York, pp 211–234
28. Hayes WJ (1982) Pesticides studies in man. Williams and Wilkins, Baltimore
29. Franzosa JA, Osimitz TG, Maibach HI (2007) Cutaneous contact urticaria to pyrethrum-real? common? or not documented?: an evidence-based approach. Cutan Ocul Toxicol 26:57–72
30. Lisi P (1992) Sensitization risk of pyrethroid insecticides. Contact Dermatitis 26:349–350
31. Jablonska S (ed) (1975) Scleroderma and pseudoscleroderma. Polish Medical, Warsaw, p 603
32. Nakamura M, Arima Y, Nobuhara S et al (1999) Airborne photocontact dermatitis due to the pesticides maneb and fenitrothion. Contact Dermatitis 40:222–223
33. Guo YL, Wang BJ, Lee CC et al (1996) Prevalence of dermatoses and skin sensitization associated with use of pesticides in fruit farmers of southern Taiwan. Occup Environ Med 53:427–431

47

34. Matsushita T, Aoyama K (1981) Cross-reactions between some pesticides and the fungicide benomyl in contact allergy. Ind Health 19:77–83

35. Bruynzeel DP, van Ketel WG (1986) Contact dermatitis due to chlorothalonil in floriculture. Contact Dermatitis 14:67–68

36. Penagos HG (2002) Contact dermatitis caused by pesticides among banana plantation workers in Panama. Int J Occup Environ Health 8:14–18

37. Penagos H, Ruepert C, Partanen T et al (2005) Pesticide patch test series for the assessment of allergic contact dermatitis among banana plantation workers in Panama. Dermatitis 15:137–145

38. Penagos H, Jimenez V, Fallas V et al (1996) Chlorothalonil, a possible cause of erythema dyschromicum perstans (ashy dermatitis). Contact Dermatitis 35:214–218

39. Bruynzeel DP, Tafelkruijer J, Wilks MF (1995) Contact dermatitis due to a new fungicide used in the tulip bulb industry. Contact Dermatitis 33:8–11

40. Boman A, Montelius J, Rissanen R-L et al (2000) Sensitizing potential of chlorothalonil in the guinea pig and the mouse. Contact Dermatitis 43:273–279

41. Sudakin DL, Trevathan WR (2003) DEET: a review and update of safety and risk in the general population. J Toxicol Clin Toxicol 41:831–839

42. Rantanen T (2008) The cause of the Chinese sofa/chair dermatitis epidemic is likely to be contact allergy to dimethyl-fumarate, a novel potent contact sensitizer. Br J Dermatol 159:218–221

43. Lidén C (1990) Facial dermatitis caused by chlorothalonil in a paint. Contact Dermatitis 22:206–211

44. Spindeldreier A, Deichmann B (1980) Kontaktdermatitis auf ein Holzschutzmittel mit einer neven fungiziden Wirksubstanz. Dermatosen 28:88–90

45. Lensen G, Jungbauer F, Gonçalo M et al (2007) Airborne irritant contact dermatitis and conjunctivitis after occupational exposure to chlorothalonil in textiles. Contact Dermatitis 57:181–186

46. Lewis PG, Emmet EA (1987) Irritant dermatitis from tributyl tin oxide and contact allergy from chlorocresol. Contact Dermatitis 17:129–132

47. de Groot AC (2008) Patch testing. Test concentrations and vehicles for 4 350 chemicals, 3rd edn. Acdegroot publishing, Wapserveen

Contact Allergy in Children

48

Marie-Anne Morren and An Goossens

Contents

M.-A. Morren (✉) and A. Goossens
Department of Dermatology, University Hospital, Katholieke
Universiteit Leuven, Leuven, Belgium
e-mail: marie-anne.morren@uz.kuleuven.ac.be

J.D. Johansen et al. (eds.), *Contact Dermatitis*,
DOI: 10.1007/978-3-642-03827-3_48, © Springer-Verlag Berlin Heidelberg 2011

48.1 Introduction

Contact allergy has not been studied as extensively in children as in adults. Although there are many similarities between these two patient populations, the results obtained in adults cannot always be applied to children. A child is not simply a small version of an adult.

48.2 Prevalence and Incidence

Allergic contact dermatitis in children has always been considered rare, and their eczematous conditions have mostly been attributed to endogenous factors such as atopic or seborrheic dermatitis, sometimes in association with irritancy induced by soap, clothing, etc. [1–3]. One of the reasons for this would be their reduced exposure to environmental allergens (professional, cosmetic, pharmaceutical) for example [3, 4]. Some authors also cite a lower reactivity and sensitization capacity of children's skin [5, 6].

As allergic contact dermatitis was not often suspected in children, little patch testing was performed [7]. Since the 1980s, however, this diagnosis has been more frequently considered, for example, [8]. Photoallergic contact dermatitis seems to be rare [1, 7], although it may also be underdiagnosed.

48.2.1 Prevalence of Contact Allergy in an Unselected Population

Data on the prevalence of contact allergy in healthy children are scarce. In a population of 314 healthy children who were less than 18 years of age, Weston et al. [9] found positive patch test results in 20%; Barros et al. [10] reported a 13% incidence in 562 children aged between 5 and 14; while Dotterud and Falk [11] observed that 23% of 424 healthy children from 7 to 12 years had contact allergy. Bruckner et al. [12] found that 24.5% of 85 children between 6 months and 5 years of age, attending well-child visits and tested with a T.R.U.E. test panel, presented one [16 infants] or 2 [4 infants] positive tests. Nickel and thimerosal were the most frequent allergens identified. However, Johnke et al. [13] warn for false positive tests, especially with nickel sulfate in such young children: they found many (111/543 infants) weak transient reactions with the highest (200 µg/cm²) nickel concentration tested, of which only 8.6% could be reproduced. Hence, a single positive nickel patch test in small children should be assessed with caution! In a Danish study on adolescents between 12 and 16 years, a prevalence of 15.2% was found, the relevance of which was estimated to be 50%, for the present or the past (7.2%). Girls reacted more frequently [14]. In Poland [15], allergy screening in 7- and 16-year olds revealed that 18.7% of 3,846 six-year olds and 8.3% of 5,474 sixteen year olds reported symptoms of chronic/recurrent eczema. A representative sample of these underwent patch testing with 10 common contact allergens. In 43.8% of the 96 six-year olds tested, at least one positive test was found and a final diagnosis of allergic contact dermatitis was confirmed in 36%. Of the 133 teenagers tested, 52.6% presented with at least one positive test, and a diagnosis of allergic contact dermatitis was confirmed in 26%. This would mean that about 7% of the 6-year olds and 2% of the 16-year olds would suffer from allergic contact dermatitis. This is in accordance with the Danish study. Although this study suggests that the prevalence of contact allergy increases in the younger generations, the authors warn that this might be biased by the study design where the presence of eczema was reported by the parents in the younger and by the teenagers themselves.

48.2.2 Prevalence of Contact Allergy in a Selected Population

Several studies have been performed in children suspected of contact allergy or suffering from atopic or juvenile plantar dermatitis, orofacial granulomatosis, "dyshidrosis", psoriasis, photosensitivity, urticaria, or other dermatoses. The studies [16–46], (see Table 48.1) differ in the number and the age of the patients involved, the clinical symptoms, as well as the relevancy and the incidence of the positive reactions observed. In a study by Pambor et al. in 1991 [22], only 3.6% of the children tested showed clinically relevant positive patch tests, whereas Pevny and coworkers observed relevance rates of up to 71% [18], with the majority around 40%.

Other factors that render comparison of those studies difficult [27] include the different test populations involved (e.g., the presence or not of atopy, differences in origin and habits), the variability of the test conditions (materials, allergens, concentrations, vehicles, reading times), and the interpretation of the test results, i.e., allergic or irritant.

The question arises as to whether contact allergy in children has become more frequent in recent years. According to Björksten [47], its prevalence in 18-year-old Swedish males increased from 0.9% in 1978 to 1.5% in 1993. A polish study seems to confirm this [15].

> **Core Message**
>
> › Contact allergy in children is more frequent than previously suspected.

48.2.3 Prevalence in Relation to Genetic Factors

According to Walton et al. [48], occupational and environmental factors are essential, but the hereditary background can also be important, as could be demonstrated, for example, by the higher incidence of HLA-B35 and BW22 antigens and their correlation with an increased risk of nickel sensitization in a female population. The importance of genetic factors has also been studied in children [49–51]: these authors conclude that there is a specific genetic selection at the level of the peripheral T-lymphocyte system.

Table 48.1 Incidence of contact allergy in selected populations

Reference	Number	Age (year)	Categories	%	Relevance %	Most frequent allergens (% of children with positive test)
Veien et al. 1982 [16]	168	<14	Suspicion of ACD	46	80	Nickel > dichromate > rubber
Pevny et al. 1984 [17]	147	3–16	Suspicion of ACD	71	93	Nickel > cobalt > para-dyes > dichromate
Romaguera et al. 1985 [18]	1,023	<14	ACD and others (45% atopics)	31	69.5	Nickel/cobalt > pharmaceutical ingredients > cosmetics > shoes > clothes > professional
Rademaker and Forsyth 1989 [19]	129	<12	Atopic eczema	48	92	Metals > perfume > rubber
			Eczema			
			Atypical JPD			
			Contact dermatitis			
			Orofacial granulomatosis			
			Other			
Kuiters et al. 1989 [20]	67	<16	Dermatitis	28	84	Nickel > balsam of Peru > fragrance mix > colophony > carba-mix
Balato et al. 1989 [21]	585	<14	Eczema	14	?	Nickel > cobalt > ethylenediamine > dichromate > mercury ammonium chloride > mercaptobenzothiazole > neomycin > mercapto mix
Pambor et al. 1992 [22]	366	2–14	Atopic dermatitis (n=214)	25	5%	Nickel > chloramphenicol > parabens > turpentine
			Other dermatosis (n=142)	18	7%	
Ayala et al. 1992 [23]	323	<14	Atopic dermatitis	35.2	61.7	Metals > pharmaceutical ingredients > preservatives > fragrance > shoes
			Contact dermatitis			
			Dyshidrotic eczema			
			Foot, diaper, or perioral eczema			
			(Palmar/plantar psoriasis)			
Gonçalo et al. 1992 [24]	329	<14	ACD	51.7	65.3	Nickel, thimerosal, cobalt, mercury ammonium chloride, fragrance mix, dichromate
Sevila et al. 1994 [25]	272	2–14	ACD	37.1	54.4	Nickel, rubber, mercury chloride, cobalt, thimerosal, benzoyl peroxide, fragrance mix
Motolese et al. 1995 [26]	53	≤2	Dermatitis	60.4	62.5	Thimerosal > nickel > ammoniated mercury
Stables et al. 1996 [27]	92	3–14	Atopic dermatitis	32.6	87	Nickel, fragrance mix, balsam of Peru, thimerosal, neomycin, cobalt, lanolin, dichromate, mercapto mix
			Localized dermatitis			
			JPD			
			Orofacial granulomatosis			
			Reactions to vaccines			
			Atypical psoriasis			

(continued)

Table 48.1 (continued)

Reference	Number	Age (year)	Categories	%	Relevance %	Most frequent allergens (% of children with positive test)
Rudzki and Rebandel [28]	626	3–16	?	42.7	?	Nickel, dichromate, cobalt, mercury chloride, fragrance mix, para-phenylenediamine, neomycin, balsam of Peru
Wilkowska et al. 1996 [29]	100	5–15	Atopic dermatitis Eczema Nonallergic dermatoses	49	?	Dichromate, cobalt, neomycin
Katsarou et al. 1996 [30]	232	<16	ACD ?	43.5	?	Nickel, cobalt, fragrance mix, dichromate, para-phenylenediamine, para-tertiary-butylphenol-formaldehyde resin, mercapto mix, mercury ammonium chloride, balsam of Peru
Wantze et al. (1996) [31]	234	≤14	ACD?	49.1	?	Thimerosal > nickel > ethylmercurychloride
Brasch et al. 1997 [32]	416	6–15	ACD	41	?	Nickel, thimerosal, benzoyl peroxide, fragrance mix, cobalt, amalgam, mercury ammonium chloride, phenylmercury acetate, Amerchol L-101, cobalt chloride, dichromate, colophony
Shah et al. 1997 [33]	83	6–16	Atopic dermatitis Hand/feet dermatitis (Peri)oral dermatitis Reactions to local anesthetics Dermatoses with unusual localizations Peri-anal dermatitis Urticaria Photo reactions	49	?	Nickel, fragrance mix, cobalt, neomycin, para-phenylenediamine, colophony, para-tertiary-butylphenol-formaldehyde resin
Manzini et al. 1998 [34]	670	<12	Suspicion of ACD	42.1	?	Thimerosal > nickel > Kathon CG°
Romaguera et al. [35]	141	Up to 14	Suspicion of ACD	50	78	Nickel > cobalt > thimerosal > mercury > fragrance mix, carba mix, thiuram mix
Giordano-Labadie et al. [36]	137	<16	Sequential patients with AD	43	100	Nickel > fragrance mix, lanolin > pot. dichromate, balsam of Peru, emollient, neomycin
Roul et al. [37]	337	1–15	Suspicion of ACD	67	100	Nickel > fragrance mix > wool wax alcohols > dichromate > balsam of Peru > neomycin cobalt chloride > PTBF resin
Duarte et al. [38]	102 (91% female)	10–19	Suspicion of ACD	56	100	Nickel > tosylamide formaldehyde resin > thimerosal > cobalt > balsam of Peru, carba-mix, thiuram mix

Study	N	Age (years)	Indication	%	%	Allergens
Wohrl et al. [39]	79	1–10		49		Nickel, thimerosal, fragrance mix, cobalt, amalgam, balsam of Peru
Lewis et al. [40]	191	<16	Suspicion of ACD	41		Nickel, fragrance mix, thiuram, cobalt, p-phenylenediamine, tixocortol pivalate, balsam of Peru
Heine et al. [41]	285	6–12	Suspicion of ACD	52.6		Thimerosal, benzoyl peroxide, phenylmercuric acetate, gentamicin sulfate, nickelsulphate, ammoniated mercury, cobalt chloride, fragrance mix, bufexamac, compositae mix
	2,175	13–18	Suspicion of ACD	49.7		Nickel sulfate, thimerosal, bezoyl peroxide, phenylmercuric acetate, fragrance mix, ammoniated mercury, cobalt chloride, p-phenylenediamine, compositae mix, gentamicin sulfate
Seidenari et al. [42]	1,094	0.6–12	Suspicion of ACD	52.1		Neomycin, nickel, wool alcohols, thimerosal, propolis, Methyl(chloro)isothiazolinone, potassium dichromate, fragrance mix, p-tert-butylphenol-formaldehyde, mercaptobenzothiazole, disperse red, p-phenylenediamine, balsam of Peru
Beattie et al. [43]	114	3–15	Deterioration of AD, localized dermatitis , history of reacting to a specific allergen		54	Nickel, rubber chemicals, fragrance mix, wool alcohol and/or amerchol, cobalt, balsam of Peru, sorbitan sesquioleate, potassium dichromate
Jacob et al. [44]	65	1–18	Suspicion of ACD	83	77	Nickel sulfate, thimerosal, Balsam of Peru, cocamidopropyl betaine, neomycin, carbamates, cinnamic aldehyde, cobalt chloride, disperse blue 106, formaldehyde
Zug et al. [45]	391	0–18	Suspicion of ACD	65.7	51.2	Nickel, cobalt, thimerosal, neomycin, gold , fragrance mix
Mailhol et al. [46]	641	0–18	Atopic eczema	6.2		Own emollient, chlorhexidine, hexamedine

48

48.2.4 Prevalence Related to Sex

While some authors [9, 10, 27] detected similar incidences in both boys and girls, others, for example, [11, 31] reported a higher incidence in girls [41]. This is the case for nickel [16, 48, 52] in particular and after the age of 12 [15, 19, 28, 30] or after puberty [41]. Hormonal factors may be a contributory factor here [24, 32]. Kwangsukstith and Maibach [53] have formulated several arguments for the existence of sex-related differences in the incidence of allergic contact dermatitis: varying test results obtained depending upon the menstrual cycle; increased sensitization liability in females, in general, and enhanced reactivity to DNCB in females taking contraceptives; allergic contact dermatitis due to transdermal clonidine being more frequently observed in women than in men; and finally, a greater susceptibility of feminine skin to irritation and hence to sensitization.

48.2.5 Prevalence Related to Age

Unlike some authors [10, 15, 27, 37, 52], most report an increasing incidence of allergic contact dermatitis with age and attribute it to the increasing exposure to environmental allergens [8, 21, 25, 26, 29, 45, 54]. This also applies to the development of multiple sensitivities [24]. A reduced sensitization potential in younger children has also been suggested [5, 6]. This has been experimentally demonstrated by Uhr [55], who showed that sensitization to dinitrofluorobenzene does occur among premature infants, but less frequently than among infants carried to term, and in both of these groups, less frequently than in children aged 2–12 months. Epstein [56] obtained sensitization to pentadecylcatechol in 44% of children below 1 year of age, in about 58% between the age of 1 and 3 years, and in 87% of children between 4 and 8 years. In contrast to this, Motolese et al. [26] found contact allergy in 32 out of 53 infants (3 months to 2 years) with dermatitis. At least 20 out of the 32 were considered relevant.

Fisher reported several cases of allergic contact dermatitis in neonates and infants [57–60]: epoxy resin in a vinyl identification band in a 1-week-old neonate, three cases of ethylenediamine contact allergy (induced by Mycolog®) in children aged 6 weeks to 1 year, one case of nickel allergy due to earrings in a 4-week-old girl, neomycin as a cause of allergic contact dermatitis on the penis of a 5-week-old boy who was circumcised, and balsam of Peru in an ointment to treat diaper rash in a 8-week-old girl

(who had received this treatment for only 1 week), and finally, nickel in underwear causing a row of contact dermatitis lesions on the back of a 7-month-old boy. Seidenari [61] also described three remarkable contact allergy cases (two of them connubial) in babies: nickel present in the bars of a crib caused "dyshidrosis" of the hands and feet in a 12-month-old atopic boy; nickel in his mother's jewelry (she wore rings on all her fingers) exacerbated the atopic eczema of a 6-month-old boy; and para-phenylenediamine in the mother's dyed hair caused hand dermatitis in a 12-month-old girl. Aihara and Ikezawa [62] have reported a neonate who was allergic to a mydriatic agent used for fundoscopy (the responsible allergen was not detected).

Moreover, in infants, several cases of contact allergy due to the rubber antileaking system in their diapers have been reported [63–65] and also to disperse dyes used in the colored parts [66]. A list of the different allergens reported in allergic diaper dermatitis is given by Smith and Jacob [67]: rubber allergens (cyclohexylthiopthalimide, mercaptobenzothiazole, and iodopropinylcarbamate), glues (p-tert-butylphenol-formaldehyde), disperse dyes, and ingredients of topical products (fragrance mix and balsam of Peru, sorbitan sesquioleate, an emulsifier, and preservatives like bromonitropropanediol). We have reported the case of an atopic infant with therapy-resistant diaper dermatitis, allergic to parabens and fragrance mix present in baby toilet tissues and several baby creams, respectively [68].

We also diagnosed contact allergy to the electrodes used to monitor an infant for sudden death. An allergy to PTBP-resin was found; however, we were not able to confirm the presence of this allergen in the electrode.

48.2.6 Prevalence Related to Origin

The exposure of children to certain contact allergens varies throughout the world [8]. For example, in contrast to Europe, poison ivy (and other members of the *Rhus* family) is particularly apt to induce sensitization in certain parts of North and South America [1, 8]. In Scandinavian countries, plant dermatitis in children is rare, except for reactions to *Heracleum* spp. [3].

Exposure and subsequent sensitivity to neomycin also seems to vary geographically: for example, there is a high incidence in Portugal [10], Italy [42], and certain areas in the USA [45] such as Denver [9], as opposed to Philadelphia [69]. In Germany, bufexamac is a frequent allergen in atopic children as this topical medication is frequently used to treat mild atopic dermatitis [41]. Thimerosal and aluminum are present in vaccines in some countries and not in others [41].

In contrast to Scandinavian countries [3], shoe dermatitis seems to be particularly common in the USA [70], mainly due to rubber [69]. Regional variations in the type of clothing and living conditions clearly influence the allergen spectrum [16].

In developing countries, occupational allergy is more common in older children as compared to Western countries [38]. In 8 and 6% of adolescents in Germany, hairdressing and health care, respectively, were found to be the sources of allergic contact dermatitis [41].

48.2.7 Prevalence in Relation to the Sensitization Source

Objects or materials common to the child's environment may give rise to some unusual allergen sources. Diapers [63–67], and, for example, sucked-on objects [71], are not at all rare causes of allergic diaper dermatitis and allergic cheilitis and perioral dermatitis (e.g., also due to rubber allergens), respectively, particularly in the younger age group. This also applies to mercurials [32, 70] in vaccines and topical pharmaceuticals used to treat abrasions and infections of the skin. However, nickel [23, 32], cosmetic ingredients [8], and occupational allergens [5, 17, 38, 41] are more frequent causes of allergy in older children. With changing lifestyle, adolescents might nowadays be at risk of developing allergic problems from electronic devices, although this seems to be quite rare [72]. The incidence of the allergens found mainly depends on the exposure, which itself varies with the age of the population [31].

48.3 The Clinical Picture

The clinical characteristics of allergic contact dermatitis are, in general, the same in children as in adults. It is of utmost importance to take a detailed history, in order to specify the environment of the child and of those taking care of it, and to examine thoroughly the topography of the lesions. The localization is often an indication of the allergen or allergens involved [8]. Based on data published in the literature, we compiled a list of allergens in relation to specific body sites (see Table 48.2).

Sometimes the clinical picture is unusual:

- A hypertrophic verrucous cheilitis due to the topical application of thimerosal used to treat fissures [73].
- A bullous dermatitis induced by a neomycin-containing finger bandage; patch tests were positive to neomycin, colophony, and thiuram mix [17].
- A "baboon syndrome" [74, 75] from mercury, due to the intake of erythromycin to treat an infection of the throat [76].
- An EEM-like eruption on the thighs spreading to the trunk after an initial contact eczematous reaction induced by a plant extract containing St John's wort [77], a temporary henna tattoo [78], disperse dyes in a 2-year-old boy [79], tea tree oil [80] as well as mephenesin (own observation).
- A lichenoid contact dermatitis on the feet, hands, and buttocks of 6-year duration due to topical aminoglycosides in which lichenoid positive patch test were also obtained [81] (a papular pattern of allergic contact dermatitis does not seem to be rare, for example, with nickel [82]); this lichenoid pattern of reaction is also frequently seen in reactions to PPD in temporary tattoos [83]. Healing may be with depigmentation [78, 84].
- Itching nodules and granulomas may persist for months or even years at the injection site of vaccines due to a delayed reaction to aluminum in vaccines [85].
- A generalized nummular dermatitis in both a boy and a girl was induced by application of an ethylenediamine-containing preparation to the groins and the feet, respectively [86]; a positive reaction to thimerosal was found in five atopic children (7–28 months old) with nummular eczema on the trunk, limbs, and face [87].
- A generalized eczema occurred twice in an 18-month-old boy caused by sensitivity to phenoxyethanol used as a preservative in a DTP vaccine [88]; the third booster vaccine containing thimerosal as the preservative did not produce a reaction.
- A systemic contact dermatitis occurred in a 14-year-old boy caused by an orthodontic appliance that contained nickel [89].

48

Table 48.2 Correlation between the localization of the lesions and the nature of the allergens

Face	Ingredients of topical pharmaceutical products (e.g., benzoyl peroxide), cosmetics (e.g., methyl (chloro)isothiazolinone), and perfume components; plants; nickel or chromium in cell phones; plants (compositae)
Periorbital area	Ophthalmic preparations; nickel, cobalt; nail lacquer; plants (spices)
Perioral area	Sucked-on objects (rubber additives); nickel, cobalt, and palladium; flavoring agents (cinnamic aldehyde)
Ears	Nickel, cobalt, chromium (cell phones), eardrops
Neck	Nickel, nail lacquer, perfume components
Trunk	Clothing dyes (axillae, inner thighs), rubber additives, nickel (peri-umbilically), PTBP-resin (electrode), PPD and essential oils in temporary tattoos
Arms	Cosmetics (e.g., sunscreens), aluminum (vaccines), plants, PPD, and essential oils (temporary tattoo's)
Wrists	Nickel and cobalt, dichromate (leather watch-strap)
Hands and fingers	Preservatives (cosmetics, play gels, plasticine), nickel and cobalt, rubber and resin components, plants (compositae)
Buttocks and thighs	Aluminum (vaccines), plastic (toilet seat)
Diaper area	Topical pharmaceutical (e.g., ethylenediamine, neomycin) and cosmetic products, rubber (or glue) in antileaking system from diapers, disperse dyes in diapers
Legs	Plants orthopedic appliances (resins, such as PTBPF and epoxy)
Feet	Shoe allergens (rubber additives, glues) (PTBP), dichromate, plants, topical pharmaceutical products
Airborne distribution, especially during summer	Plants especially compositae

---

Core Message

> Certain contactants are characteristic of children (Table 48.2), and may be responsible for unusual clinical presentations.

48.4 Allergic Contact Dermatitis and Atopy

The association between atopy and contact allergy in children is a controversial subject [90].The conclusions drawn differ largely according to the allergens investigated and whether the incidence of contact allergy in atopic or the incidence of atopy in children suffering from allergic contact dermatitis is being investigated [91].

Several authors were unable to detect differences between atopic and nonatopic subjects in this regard [23, 26, 92], but others have. Some authors were able to find a higher incidence in atopic than nonatopic children [11, 29, 46, 93], and this was sometimes attributed to the greater permeability of irritated skin, for example, [11]. Others report the opposite [27, 30, 32, 55].

Nickel reactions are more often seen in atopics [26, 82, 94], and mainly in girls [95], which reflects the greater importance of sex and ear piercing than atopy as such. The latter authors (in agreement with, for example, Pambor et al. [92]), stress the irritant properties of metals and particularly nickel on atopic skin, and, indeed, papulopustular patch test reactions are a frequent finding, for example, [91]. Dotterud and Falk [95] doubt if metal sensitivity is associated with atopy. First, there is the reduced cellular immunity of atopics: positive reactions are found more often in atopic children with moderate dermatitis than in those with severe atopic eczema [96, 97]; second, there is the greater permeability of diseased skin, particularly on the hands, which facilitates the penetration of allergens [96, 98].

Besides nickel, Oranje et al. [99] also found cobalt and balsam of Peru (Myroxylon Pereirae) to be important allergens in an atopic child population; furthermore, they observed few reactions on patch testing with food.

Contact allergy to the ingredients of topical medications and emollients are also common in atopic dermatitis patients [36, 46, 90]. In a recent study, Mailhol et al. [46] found positive patch tests in 6.2% of 641 children with atopic eczema systematically patch tested with seven agents of common topical treatment. The own emollient tested was the most common allergen (47.5%); protein extracts were most frequently the responsible allergen (6 out of 9), callendula officinalis, fragrance and amerchol L 101 being the others. Chloorhexidine (in 42.5%) and hexamedine (7.5%) were also common allergens. More severe eczema, younger age at onset, and IgE-mediated sensitization were risk factors. The authors conclude that it is advisable to use emollients devoid of proteins (as was already suggested by Rancé et al. [100]) and fragrances and doubt about the need to add antiseptics to the topical treatment of these patients.

Beattie et al. [43], however, warn that a history of reactions to emollients in an atopic child is mostly suggestive of an irritant reaction. We agree on this, particularly since many emollients are reported to give immediate stinging or redness. As Mailhol et al. [46] state, it is difficult to exclude irritant reactions in some cases (many 1+ reactions; 71.8% of the patients with a positive reaction had a SCORAD of 25 or more!). In our experience, a moderate to severe eczema predisposes to irritant reactions even if the back is free of eczema at the time of the tests. These tests, particularly those with an irritant potential like metals and preservatives, frequently remain negative when retested after a prolonged period of regression of the eczema (own data).

As is the case with nonatopics, the incidence of contact allergy was found to increase with age [97, 98].

> **Core Message**
>
> › Positive reactions in atopics must be interpreted carefully, as atopic skin is readily irritated; this is especially the case for metals.

48.5 Patch Testing in Children

Patch testing is indicated not only when contact allergy is suspected, but also in cases of persistent eczema [21, 43, 44, 68] on specific localizations, such as on the hands and the feet and around the mouth [33, 43], the eyes [43], and also in the umbilical region, particularly in atopics [91]. The latter group should certainly be tested when multiple exacerbations occur, even when they are treated, or when the dermatitis is asymmetrical [33].

Most authors agree that patch testing in children is safe [9, 19, 41–46, 73, 101], the only problems being mainly technical because of the small patch-test surface [19], hypermobility (which may result in loss of patch test materials), particularly in younger children [33], and the reluctance of some parents to allow patch testing [4, 33]. Mallory [102] gives the following instructions when testing children:

- Test in different sessions if the test area is very small.
- Should the patches come off, ask the parents to report it and instruct them not to reapply them.
- It may be necessary to use a stronger adhesive than usual, though this could be irritating [9].
- The application has to be performed as quickly as possible while the child is distracted; Jacob et al. [103] suggest video distraction.
- The same authors [103] suggest demonstrating the technique on the parent in front of the child if she/he is too scared.
- Make a diagram of the tested allergens (this applies for adults too).
- Inform the parents about the test procedure and the measures that may be taken to optimize the patch test conditions.

The patch test concentrations have been discussed in detail in the literature. Some authors have recommended lower concentrations [3, 92, 104, 105]; particularly with regard to specific allergens such as nickel and formaldehyde [6, 94], mercurials [73], potassium dichromate, MBT, and thiuram mix [60]. Irritancy problems have been reported with patch testing, especially in the younger age-group [6, 9, 11, 22], while others use the same test concentrations as in adults [5, 16, 17, 26, 27, 41–45, 106, 107]. Wahlberg and Goossens [108] critically reviewed studies on the incidence of contact allergy and found that a very high prevalence is found in "healthy" children as compared with that in adults. They suspect that a lot of those reactions might be irritant and therefore conclude that all patch test concentrations used in adults are not necessarily suitable to be used in children as was already suggested for metals by Roul et al. [37]. In dubious cases, one might have to retest with a lower test concentration [91]. Moreover, as is the case with patch testing in general, false-positive as well as false-negative reactions may occur [1, 57]. It is therefore important that the relevance of the tests are further investigated, if necessary, with a serial dilution test, repeated open application test (ROAT), or a usage

48

test [7]. For marginal irritants such as dichromate, fragrance mix, formaldehyde, mercury compounds, and carba-mix in particular [108], repeated patch testing with standardized tests (e.g., T.R.U.E.-test) should be performed in order to demonstrate reproducibility, and if necessary, the concentration should be adapted. Johnke et al. [13] already demonstrated that in infants, 200 µg/cm^2 nickel sulfate produces many transient reactions (111/543), whereas reproducible tests were obtained only in 8.6% of the cases. They therefore favor a lower patch concentration for nickel in children.

Core Message

> Patch testing in children is safe, but false-positive reactions are possible. If there is a suspicion by history and clinical picture, or there is unexplained eczema at particular body sites, patch testing should be performed at all ages.

48.6 The Most Frequent Allergens in Children

48.6.1 Metals

48.6.1.1 Nickel

Nickel is the most common allergen both in children and adults in Europe, as it is in many other parts of the world. In the general population, about 10% of females react to it, the incidence being influenced by the increasing popularity of ear and other piercings [95]. Indeed, ear piercing along with atopy – the latter even in children aged between 4 and 17 months [82, 109] – have been regarded as major risk factors for the development of nickel sensitization, especially in girls [95, 110], although boys may also be affected [111]. In Poland, among 7-year-old boys, a higher rate of positive reactions was found compared with 16-year-old boys [15]; the same upward trend being reported by Vigan in France [112]. Rademaker and Forsyth [19] could not determine significant differences between boys and girls below the age of 12. Subumbilical and periumbilical, mostly papular reactions are also common and are frequently accompanied by an id-like spread [109, 113, 114].

Veien [115] attributes the high incidence of nickel allergy in young females to the common habit of wearing cheap jewelry, reduced suppressor activity correlated with their higher estrogen levels, and higher skin permeability to nickel. Permeability could be increased by decreased iron levels associated with menarche, as iron is a competitive inhibitor in the skin and on the surface of Langerhans cells.

Nickel sensitization sources in children are numerous: jewelry, even when worn by the mother [61], and particularly earrings [57, 59] (stainless steel, even though silver or gold plated is not always "safe" in this regard [116]), metal buttons, zippers and snaps, identification bracelets, safety pins, jeans and belt buckles e.g., [102, 109, 113, 114], metal accessories on shoes, coins, metal toys, magnets, medallions, keys, door handlers, school chairs, ballet balance bars [44], and so on [59, 94]. Even bed rails have caused nickel contact allergy [61, 117]. Due to restrictions on the concentration of nickel allowed in jewelry and textile accessories (<0.5 µg/cm^2/week), advised by the authorities in Europe in the beginning of the 90s, a decline in the prevalence of nickel allergy has been registered in Denmark [118] and Germany [119]. In the USA, Byer et al. [114] could only detect nickel in 10% of 74 pairs of jeans buckles, whereas the dimethylglyoxime test was positive in 25 of the 47 belts, indicating that this nickel source is more important for sensitization induction. However, even today, 6% of children's clothing fasteners out of 20 countries released more nickel than that allowed in the European Nickel Directive release limit [120]. In the UK, Beattie et al. [43] however still reported an increase during the period 1999–2002.

Orthodontic appliances may occasionally be at the origin of a nickel allergy, causing cheilitis, perioral eczema [89, 121, 122], and also stomatitis, sometimes associated with systemically induced dermatitis on the eyelids, fingers, ears, periorbital area [122], or more generalized reactions [89], even a severe deterioration of atopic dermatitis [123]. Van Hoogstraten et al. [111] were able to show that the wearing of a dental apparatus before nickel skin contact has occurred may actually induce tolerance to this metal.

A new source of nickel are cell phones; nickel has been demonstrated in case parts, headsets as well as keys in 11–33% of the phones on the market between 2004 and 2006 in Denmark [124] as well as in nearly half of popular models in the USA [125].

A low nickel diet might be useful in resistant nickel allergy cases [16].

48.6.1.2 Cobalt

Cobalt allergies are often found in association with nickel allergies in both adults and children, for example, [32]. Not only metallic objects but also certain plastic materials may release cobalt or cobalt salts and induce contact sensitivity. For example, Grimm [126] described the case of an 11-year-old boy who had suffered for 4 years from eczematous lesions at the site of his spectacle frames, on his wrist, and around his mouth. The dermatitis was attributed to cobalt present in the metallic part of his wristwatch, in the polyester resin-type plastics of the spectacle frames, and the ballpoint pen which he habitually chewed on. Kanerva [127] suggests that cobalt might also be a possible sensitizer in personal computer mice.

48.6.1.3 Potassium Dichromate

Leather seems to be the most important cause of chromium allergy; the examples published concern shoes (cf. below), a body splint [128], and a prayer strap in a 13-year-old Jewish boy [73]. Concomitant reactions to nickel have been observed [32]. More recently, allergic reactions to chromium in cell phones have been described in young adults and teenagers [129].

48.6.1.4 Mercury

Contact allergy to mercurials is very common in children, particularly in countries where they are still widely used as antiseptics (e.g., mercurochrome), such as Spain [110, 130] and Italy [42, 131]. Other sensitization sources for mercurials are other topically applied medicaments, such as eyedrops, depigmenting creams [130], pediculosis preparations [132], vaccines [41, 42, 44, 45, 133], as well as broken thermometers [75], amalgam fillings, contact lens solutions, and pesticides. Levy et al. [70] warn against the use of mercurials in medications because of their potential systemic toxicity, which may cause kidney damage, particularly when large skin surfaces are treated. As thimerosal is less frequently used in topical products including vaccines, this allergen has recently been removed from the North American and European standard screening series.

48.6.1.5 Aluminum

For aluminum, vaccines and occasionally also hyposensitization therapy in pollen allergy are reported as the most important sensitization sources [85, 134–137]. Clinically, the reactions often present as long-lasting, pruritic, excoriated, subcutaneous nodules, occasionally accompanied by hypertrichosis [85, 138]. In many cases, the contact eczema is revealed by positive reactions to Finn Chambers used in patch testing or to deodorants [134], eardrops [137], or even toothpaste [135] containing aluminum salts. Flare-ups of previous injection sites may be explained by the persistence of this metal in the skin [134]. Probably, the aluminum sensitivity is lost with time as this sensitivity is extremely rare in adults [139].

48.6.1.6 Palladium

This metal, shown to be an allergen in animals, is mainly present in orthodontic appliances and jewelry [140], which may be responsible for granulomatous reactions. As with adults, most palladium-allergic children also react to nickel [32, 141], for which cross-sensitization seems to be the most plausible explanation.

48.6.1.7 Iron

There seems to be only one case report of iron contact allergy, which was caused by an orthopedic prosthesis in a 7-year-old boy [142], so this metal seems to be an extremely rare allergen.

48.6.1.8 Copper

According to a Viennese report copper, present in dental amalgam, caused problems in children [52].

48.6.1.9 Gold

Gold is a top 10 allergen in children in the USA [45], although more than half of the reactions were not found relevant.

48

48.6.2 *Pharmaceutical Products*

Many topical pharmaceutical ingredients have been described as allergens in children and should certainly not be overlooked [143]. In a German study [41], it was the most important suspected source of relevant contact allergens in children aged between 6 and 12 years. They include antibiotics, mainly neomycin [17, 42, 45, 57], which is often used in the treatment of otitis [69]. Leyden and Kligman [69], in contrast to Weston et al. [9], suggest that neomycin allergy is less frequently seen in children than in adults. Cross-reactivity with other aminoglycosides does occur [81]. Antivirals like tromantadine (own observations) and Zovirax®, of which the responsible allergen could not be identified [144]; antihistamines like dexchlorpheniramine maleate [145]; nonsteroidal anti-inflammatory agents like fepradinol [146] and bufexamac [41] used to treat atopic dermatitis; local anesthetics, particularly benzocaine [17], which often cross-reacts with other ester-type anesthetics [102] and also with permanent hair dyes and textile dyes, which may later cause problems, because of their chemical relationship have been documented [57]. Even corticosteroid preparations may cause contact allergy in children, for example, [147], and not infrequently in atopics [148]. Tixocortol pivalate and budesonide may be used as markers in the standard series, but all topical preparations used by the child should be tested as well. Contact allergy to the new class of topical immunomodulatory drugs especially for tacrolimus has also been reported. A provocation test was positive after 1 week for lesions in the face, but only after 7 weeks when applied to the antecubital region. Patch tests were positive only after 5 days with tacrolimus 5% and 2.5% in ethanol, but neither with Protopic ointment nor with lower concentrations of tacrolimus. The authors suggest that the low percutaneous absorption through intact extrafacial skin is the reason for this delay in positive results and the need for high concentrations [149].

Other agents which have been reported include quinine present in a balsam used in the treatment of respiratory infections (the adult formulation was used and not the one for children which did not contain quinine [150]). Plant extracts may also be responsible for allergic reactions [77].

In France [46], chlorhexidine and hexamidine frequently used in infected atopic dermatitis were allergens in as much as 2.7% and 0.5%, respectively, of a cohort of systematically patch tested children with atopic dermatitis (Fig. 48.1).

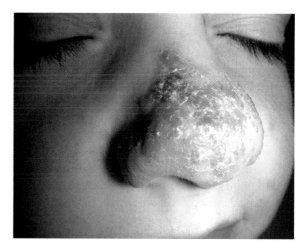

Fig. 48.1 Allergic contact dermatitis from chlorhexidine in a 6-year-old atopic boy

Allergy to certain topical medicaments specifically used in older children, are for example namely those used to treat acne such as benzoyl peroxide [1, 17].

An allergic dermatitis from the parenteral administration of vitamin K has been reported by Pigatto et al. [151].

Not only active principles but also other ingredients may be responsible for allergic reactions in children: emulsifiers and vehicle components, such as wool wax alcohols and derivatives, propyleneglycol and cetostearylalcohol, as well as a specific ingredient of eardrops – triethanolamine oleyl polypeptide – are typical examples of this [152]. Sometimes, rarer allergens such as laureth-4 [153], ethyl sebacate [147], and Tween 80 [154] are involved.

Ethylenediamine, used in Mycolog cream, has been widely used to treat various skin conditions, including diaper dermatitis [58, 86], and may cross-react with some antihistamines and aminophylline to induce severe systemic reactions [58]. This chemical is also used in ophthalmic solutions, insecticides, fungicides, epoxy hardeners, and rubber stabilizers, for example, [102].

Preservatives are not at all rare causes of allergic reactions in children, for example, [68, 155]. Goulden and Goodfield [156] reported the case of a 12-year-old boy who even reacted to a methylprednisolone injection due to his sensitivity to the preservative myristyl picolinium chloride.

Thimerosal has attracted much attention in the literature since it is frequently observed as an allergen in young children [157–159], and its inclusion in the standard series has been discussed [160, 161] and even removed from the North American and European standard screening series. It is used as an antiseptic, disinfectant, and preservative agent for contact lens solutions, eyedrops, and vaccines, the last being regarded as the main sensitization source through contamination of the tip of the needle [157, 158, 162, 163]. Many authors [45, 160, 164] state that, in most cases, an allergy to thimerosal is not relevant to the patient's skin condition. A positive reaction to thimerosal should be taken into account with hyposensitization solutions, eyedrops, eye cosmetics, or contact lens solutions, but does not seem to contraindicate future vaccinations, provided they are administered intramuscularly [163]. Furthermore, as this molecule contains two allergenic parts – mercury and thiosalicylic acid – one must consider cross-reactions with other mercurials and with the photoproduct of piroxicam, which is chemically related to the thiosalicylic acid part, for example, [133, 157, 165]. Efforts are now being made to omit thimerosal from the commonly used vaccines [80].

Also phenoxyethanol contact allergy has been described in relation with a DTP vaccine [88].

Last but not least, adhesive tape can also be a cause of allergy due to colophonium and thiuram derivatives [17]. Children may also be exposed to colophonium in preparations to treat warts [139].

48.6.3 Cosmetics

The market for cosmetic products specially formulated for children is expanding and habits common for adults such as going to "beauty farms" are adapted for this young age group. Consequently, one can expect cosmetics to become more important causes of contact allergy and indeed, recent studies confirm that it has become the most frequent cause of contact allergy in children [166], at least in the older age-group (12–18 years) [41].

Almost every ingredient may be responsible for cosmetic dermatitis. Conti [155] reviewed preservatives and found that 44% of the children reacting to chemicals such as formaldehyde and its releasers, parabens, methyl (chloro) isothiazolinone, Euxyl K400® (methyldibromo glutaronitrile and phenoxyethanol), and the antioxidant butylhydroxyanisole (BHA), were atopic. In the USA, cocamidopropyl betaine has been reported as an important allergen. It is used as nonionic surfactant in "no more tears" shampoos and baby washes [44].

The use of cosmetic products in babies and small children and particularly those containing balsam of Peru (Myroxylon Pereirae) has been described as the cause of a subsequent perfume allergy. Fisher [57, 58] has reported two such cases: one of a 4-month-old baby and another of an 11-year-old girl, both of whom became sensitized by the application of a balsam ointment in the diaper area. One developed contact eczema later from the mother's perfume and the other from a deodorant.

Fisher [71] further stated that children often become allergic to cosmetics used by the mother (or the person taking care of them). In a 7-year-old girl with allergy to cinnamic aldehyde (cinnamal), cheilitis and perioral dermatitis were caused by the mother's lipstick left after she kissed her. The localizations often involved seem to be the forehead and the cheeks, with perfume, lipstick, hairspray, or nail lacquer as the responsible agents. A PPD-allergy induced by the mother's dyed hair was observed in a 12-month-old girl [61].

However, children often use cosmetic products themselves, even though this may not always be revealed immediately! An example of "ectopic" dermatitis, localized unilaterally on the face and neck, due to repeated use of the mother's nail lacquer illustrates this [73].

Although guidelines for the maximum concentration of preservatives and fragrances in cosmetics have been provided [80], it has been demonstrated that cosmetic toys may contain much higher concentrations of fragrance [167]. There are no extrasafety requirements for those products intended for children [139].

Contact allergy to the sunscreen agents, 4-methylbenzylidene camphor, isopropyl dibenzoylmethane, and 2-ethylhexyl methoxycinnamate has been described in an 18-month-old boy [168]. Shah et al. [33] also reported on sunscreen agents as the cause of photoallergic contact dermatitis and recently, several cases due to octocrylene, a UV-B sunscreen and a stabilizer, have been observed in Belgium (own observations) and France (REVIDAL-GERDA), in children in particular. But ingredients other than the sunscreen may also be responsible, for example, triethanolamine used as an emulsifier [169], and polymers, to make the formulations more water-resistant, such as polyvinylpyrrolidone-1-triacontene copolymer [170].

More recently, hydrolyzed proteins [171], added because of their moisturizing capacities, were reported as allergens in emollients.

48

48.7 Tattoos

Temporary henna tattoos gain popularity in Western adolescents, especially during holidays. Whereas contact allergy to henna itself seems to be rare, in tourist areas, additives are added to make the process faster and to obtain a more dark pigment. PPD, coffee, oil of eucalyptus or other essential oils, mustard, clove, lemon juice, turpentine, coal tar, tea, or even fresh urine of camels or yaks are examples of such components [78, 83, 84, 172]. It has been demonstrated that the concentration of PPD in some of these tattoos is higher than those allowed for hair dyes [173], even although the use of diaminobenzene-derivatives is forbidden for dyeing skin [80].

Contact allergies to PPD, and less frequently to essential oils in temporary tattoos are increasingly reported in children [78, 83, 84, 172]. Eczematous reactions are mostly seen at the site of the tattoo and they may be long-lasting. EEM-like [78] or lichenoid reactions [83] are also described. Moreover, some patients may develop depigmentation [83, 84] or hyperpigmentation and even hypertrophic scars [174] following the acute reaction, and this may persist for several months up to more than 1 year. Moreover, these allergies may have consequences in the future of these children as certain professions become risky, for instance, hair dressing, as well as potential problems with dark tanned clothing or hair dyes may follow. These reactions may be particularly severe, needing hospitalization for systemic treatment with corticosteroids, even necessitating intensive care unit treatment in one 13-year old with severe edema of face and neck [175]. Therefore, there is an urgent need to restrict these practices world-wide as is already done in Canada [174]. As severe reactions to the patch test may be seen, a hundred fold dilution (0.01%) of PPD is advised.

48.8 Toys

Preservatives in play gels have been described as causes of acute eczema on the hands; in the two cases, parabens were found to be the responsible allergens [176, 177] (Fig. 48.2). Tosti [178], too, has described two girls who were sensitized by the preservatives methyl (chloro) isothiazolinone and 2-chloro-*N*-methyl-chloroacetamide in plasticine.

Pevny et al. [17] observed a 14-year-old boy with hand eczema from a model kit, glue, and firearm accessories: positive patch tests were found to the plastic materials he had come into contact with and to benzoyl peroxide,

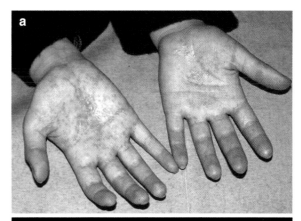

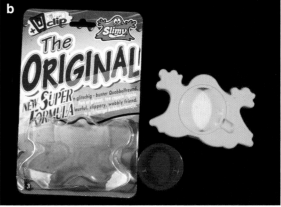

Fig. 48.2 Allergic contact dermatitis (**a**) from a play gel (**b**) containing parabens

p-tert-butyl catechol, and p-tert-butyl phenol (present in the glues), as well as to potassium dichromate in the gun oil.

Facial allergy due to contact with a cuddly toy [102] and from balloons (cf. below) has been described. An allergy to rubber from his basket ball was also the cause of persisting hand eczema in a 9-year-old boy [179].

Also music playing may provoke eczema: PPD used to stain the bow for playing cello provoked eczematous lesions of the first three fingers of the right hand in an 11-year-old girl [180]. Colophonium used as rosin for the bow or in the gripping powder used by gymnasts [181], or nickel in ballet balance bars [44] are possible allergens as well.

48.9 Electronic Devices

Electronic devices are nowadays part of the life of most teenagers, some spending hours with them. Although contact allergy is exceptional, we have to be aware of the potential hazards in these devices.

Cell phone dermatitis has been described in teenagers. Potential allergens are nickel [124], and hexavalent chromium [129]. Predilection areas are the preauricular region, the ear, and to a lesser extent, the cheek and chin, and exceptionally, more extended over the body. Lesions are often situated on one side of the face. Risk factors are prolonged use of the phone, and warm weather. As discussed before, nickel is present in many mobile phones at different sites like the keys, the encasement, and head phones [124, 125].

Prolonged use of computers may also induce contact dermatitis, although irritant or mechanically induced lesions are more frequent. Plastic components such as resorcinol monobenzoate, phtalates, or even cobalt [128] in computer mice have been described. In neoprene mouse mats and wrist rests, thiourea as well as thiurams and mercaptans can cause allergy [72].

Another potential source could be head and ear phones used in, for example, MP3 players, although no problems have yet been reported.

48.10 Rubber Items

Additives in the rubber of balloons may occasionally cause facial dermatitis [2, 181], but they may also be responsible for dermatitis due to elastic underwear, particularly when bleached [182, 183], in a ball causing persistent hand eczema [179], in rubber sponges used to apply cosmetics [183], and in gloves [180] (although a preservative in the glove, i.e., cetyl pyridinium chloride, may be an exceptional allergen as well [184]). As with balloons, for example, Type I allergic reactions may also occur, sometimes associated with a Type IV reaction, as was the case in a 6-year-old boy who had undergone multiple surgical operations and reacted to both gloves and a rubber dam used in dentistry [185]. Moreover, contact urticaria syndrome induced by natural rubber latex proteins is a frequent finding in such children, those suffering from spina bifida being particularly susceptible in this regard.

A particular type of diaper dermatitis reminiscent of a cowboy's belt and gun holsters (hence "Lucky Luke") was reported by Roul et al. [63, 64]. The reaction was provoked by the rubber parts used for the new antileaking system in these diapers. The rubber parts were positive in all children, and in some, MBT,

cyclohexyl thiophtalimide [65], and PTBP-resin, probably present in the glue (Fig. 48.3).

Thiurams, mercapto chemicals, and more seldom, carbamates are the responsible allergens for rubber allergy in children, often in shoe dermatitis (cf. below). Thiourea derivatives in neoprene may be the

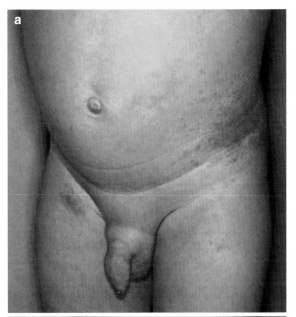

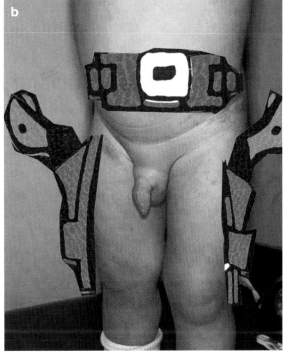

Fig. 48.3 Dermatitis from rubber derivatives in diapers (**a**) named "Lucky Luke" (**b**)

48

causal allergens in sports equipment, such as goggles [186], trainers [139], footwear [187], and diving suits (own case). Polyurethane is usually tolerated and IPPD used in industrial rubbers is unlikely to be the cause [141].

48.11 Shoes and Clothes

Shoe dermatitis generally affects the back of the feet (Fig. 48.4). Mercaptobenzothiazole and thiuram derivatives are present in rubber [43] and also in certain glues [16, 143, 188], responsible for shoe dermatitis. Other potential culprits are nickel and cobalt as well as PPD [43], which is also a possible dye allergen in socks [188], PPD-derivatives such as diaminodiphenylmethane [189], and chromates [159, 190]. Trevistan and Kokelj [159] also consider dodecylmercaptane and thimerosal, used as a preservative in leather or leather cream, to be relevant shoe allergens. Topical medication was the most frequent cause of foot dermatitis in a retrospective study by Shackelford and Belsito [191], the allergens of which persist in shoe material for a long time. On the other hand, shoe allergens may persist in cotton socks even when they are washed.

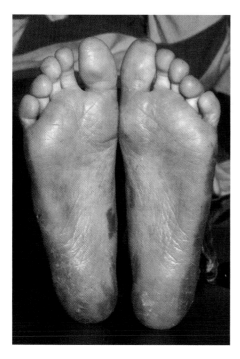

Fig. 48.4 Shoe dermatitis due to thiuram derivatives in an atopic child, complicated by corticosteroid (triamcinolone acetonide) contact allergy

When only the soles of the feet are affected, especially the first toe and fore foot, particularly in atopics, juvenile plantar dermatosis is more likely.

In Italy [192], 51 (4.6%) out of 1098 children tested positive to one or more disperse dyes used in synthetic clothes and especially to disperse yellow 3 and disperse orange 3. This is, however, much higher than what is seen in Germany [41], the UK [43], and the USA [44, 45]. As only 17% of these Italian children were also positive to PPD in the standard series, the authors suggest adding disperse dyes to the standard series [192]. We have recently observed 2 children sensitized through the application of a black henna tattoo, one reacting to disperse dyes in her black school uniform, the other to his football shirt.

In our experience, the clinical picture of clothing dermatitis may closely resemble atopic dermatitis and is difficult to diagnose especially in those children with a history of AD.

48.12 Plastic Materials and Resins

Plastic toys as well as glues have been described as typical allergen sources for children [17] (cf. above). PTBPF resin is the most frequently used phenol-formaldehyde (PF) resin and is mainly used in neoprene-type adhesives and all-purpose glues (Fig. 48.5).

Vincenzi et al. [193] reported the case of an adolescent with a linear vesicular dermatitis on the left leg caused by the glue in a knee guard. There were positive patch tests to PTBPF and PF resins. Shono et al. [194] observed four adolescents who reacted to these resins in an adhesive tape used for ankle support. One of them also reacted to sports shoes. It was also reported as the cause of contact dermatitis to a limb prosthesis in a 5-year-old boy [195] and is possibly used as glue for electrodes to monitor sudden death in infants (personal observation). PF resin and benzoyl peroxide were reported as the cause of contact allergy to swimming goggles in a 12-year-old girl; dibutylthiourea in black neoprene rubber may also be the cause [186].

Epoxy resin was the cause of dermatitis due to the glue used to fix kneepads in trousers [102] as well as an allergy to an identification band [59].

Not only the resins themselves but also preservatives, like benzalkonium chloride in plaster of Paris, may cause contact allergy [196].

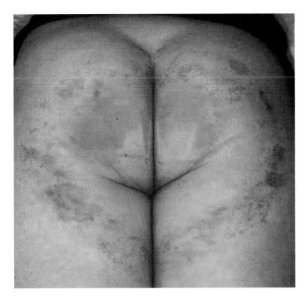

Fig. 48.5 Allergic contact dermatitis from plastic toilet seat (presence of para-tert-butylphenol-formaldehyde resin to which the child reacted upon patch testing, however, not confirmed)

48.13 Plants

Children often come into contact with plants while playing and do not know about their potential irritant, phototoxic (e.g., giant hogweed) or allergenic effects. In a review on plant dermatitis in Australia [197], children as well as gardeners are considered at risk.

48.13.1 Poison Ivy, Poison Oak, Poison Sumac

Plants belonging to the *Rhus* family are the ones most often involved in allergic contact dermatitis among children living in northern California. Exposure can be direct or indirect (e.g., transfer of the allergen via pets), the latter being more difficult to diagnose [1]. Mallory [102] reports the possible presence of black spots on the skin caused by the oleoresin in poison ivy as a clue to its diagnosis.

48.13.2 Toxicodendron succedaneum (Rhus tree)

Ten cases of phytophotodermatitis from *Toxicodendron succedaneum* in children under the age of 15 were reported in New Zealand. Generally, the face was involved [198].

48.13.3 Urtica urens

A combined contact urticarial and contact eczematous reaction on the hands and arms has been described by Edwards [199].

48.13.4 Asteraceae or Compositae

Wakelin et al. [200] reported the case of an atopic boy with exacerbations of his chronic eczema on the palmar side of his right, dominant hand. Patch tests were positive to sesquiterpene lactones, and to chrysanthemums, daisies, and dandelions, some of which he fed to his rabbits. Flohr et al. in the UK [201] suggest routine testing to compositae mix and sesquiterpene lactone mix, as well as a plant series in all children, including those with confirmed atopic eczema, when the eczema is confined to the hands or when an airborne allergen exposure is suspected. Lesions appearing in late spring and during the summer are suggestive and children living in the country side and playing outside are particularly at risk. They diagnosed a compositae allergy in three atopic children aged 3–8, one of them with a negative sesquiterpene lactone mix 0.1% in petrolatum. In Italy, 17 out of 641 consecutively patch tested children reacted to compositae mix tested routinely, 12 of them had atopic dermatitis, the youngest being 2 years old. An airborne pattern was present with, in most cases, lesions on the hands and the face [202]. The same results were found in Germany [41], where a frequency of 4.1% was found in the younger age-group. This is not surprising as the compositae family is ubiquitous and the second largest plant family comprising approximately 10% of the world's flowering plants [202].

Commens et al. [203] discussed the problem of Bindii (*Soliva pterosperma*) dermatitis, which is most often located on the palms, soles, knees, and elbows, and tends to occur in Australian children (mainly boys who play sports) in the spring and early summer. The persistence of erythematous papules for several months, and sometimes, also squamous and pustular lesions, has been ascribed to a residue of the allergenic seed in the skin. The differential diagnoses include dermatitis herpetiformis.

48.13.5 Lichens

Wood and Rademaker [204] reported a facial dermatitis in an 8-year-old atopic girl, which occurred

48

whenever she climbed trees. Patch testing was positive to lichens and usnic acid, thus indicating *Parmelia* spp as the sensitization source.

48.13.6 Gingko Fruit

Squashing the fruit of *Gingko biloba* or using it as marbles has been reported as a cause of allergic contact dermatitis in children in France [205].

48.13.7 Dioscorea Batatas Decaisne

Kubo et al. [206] described the case of a 9-year-old girl who had accidentally touched her cheek with the rasped root of this plant, which resulted in the development of both an irritant and an allergic contact dermatitis.

48.13.8 Protein Contact Dermatitis

Oat-containing moisturizers are used for maintenance therapy in atopic dermatitis. Although allergic reactions to these products are rare, protein contact dermatitis to avena extract has been reported by Pazzaglia et al. [207].

48.13.9 Various Plant Materials

Fisher [71] has reported the occurrence of allergic reactions due to the presence of various plant components or extracts in topically applied products. Moreover, as the use of herbal preparations is dramatically increasing, contact allergy to "natural" ingredients such as tea tree oil (45) causing in 14.3% of relevant reactions in 0–5 years olds!, especially when photoaged (oxidation products), *Calendula officinalis*, etc. is becoming more frequent [80].

48.14 "Occupational" Allergens

Among adolescents, certain occupational activities are likely to induce sensitization, for example, [23], particularly in hairdressers ([41], the third most frequent source of ACD in 12–18-year olds in Germany) and construction workers [18, 30] and to a lesser extent in metal workers [18].

Pre-employment patch testing is not recommended, although some authors advocate it, particularly with regard to metal allergy [208].

However, children like to help adults and this may also produce problems as in the case reported by Corazza et al. [209], who reacted to methylchloroisothiazolinone in beeswax used to polish old wooden furniture.

> **Core Message**
>
> › Metals (jewelry, mobile phones), ingredients of pharmaceutical and cosmetic products, PPD in tattoos, rubber additives (in shoes, toys, diapers, sports equipment, and so on), plastics, resins (including those used in glues, orthopedic devices, electronic devices), and plants are allergens in children. In adolescents, occupational allergens are also sometimes possible.

48.15 Is it Advisable to Test with a Shortened Standard Series for Children?

In view of the lack of chemical exposure of children compared to that of adults and the small patch test area, and especially with younger children, the risk of active sensitization, Brasch and Geier [1] as well as Roul et al. [37] proposed testing with an abbreviated standard patch test series of 16 or 17 allergens.

Vigan in 1994 proposed [210], based on four studies [18, 19, 24, 159] and a large multicenter study performed by the *Réseau de Vigilance en Dermato-Allergologie* (Revidal) created by the *Groupe d'Etudes et de Recherche en Dermato-Allergologie* (GERDA, France [211]) in 959 children below the age of 15, tested in 11 different centers from 1995 to 1997, to restrict the baseline series to 16 allergens. These are: potassium dichromate, neomycin, thiuram mix, PPD-base, cobalt chloride, formaldehyde, colophonium, balsam of Peru (Myroxylon Pereirae), wool wax alcohols (lanolin alcohol), mercapto mix, paraben mix, PTBP-FR, fragrance mix, nickel sulfate, methyl(chloro)-isothiazolinone, and mercaptobenzothiazole.

Based on a similar study conducted in Germany, an expert panel recommended in 2007 that 12 allergens

Table 48.3 Abbreviated baseline patch test series for children suggested by the German Contact Dermatitis Research Group [212]

Nickel sulfate	5% pet
Thiuram mix	1% pet
Colophony (colophonium)	20% pet
Mercaptobenzothiazole	2% pet
Fragrance mix I	8% pet
Fragrance mix II	14% pet
Mercapto mix	1% pet
Bufexamac	5% pet
Methyldibromo glutaronitrile	1% pet
Methyl (chloro) isothiazolinone	100 ppm aq
Neomycin	20% pet
Compositae mix	6% pet
P-tert.Butylphenol-formaldehyde resin*	1% pet.
Potassium dichromate*	0.5% pet
Wool alcohols (lanolin alcohol)*	30% pet
Disperse blue mix*	1% pet
Parapenylenediamine*	0.5 pet

*Only tested if the history suggests contact allergy

should be routinely tested in children, supplemented with other tests, when the history is suggestive (those with *) (Table 48.3) [212], for example, with regard to skin care products, cosmetics, clothing, or clinical findings, such as foot dermatitis. Cobalt chloride, balsam of Peru, parabens, and formaldehyde are not included in their series, although these are not rare allergens in children in other countries [15, 42–45]. Bufexamac, on the contrary, is an allergen typical for Germany (and Japan) where it is used in the treatment of atopic dermatitis; it is irrelevant for most other countries. In Italy, a screening series of 30 allergens is used, with a few markers for clothing dyes, which seems to be more of a problem there [42]. In the very young, such a restricted series seems interesting.

When corticosteroids have been used, testing with the corticosteroid allergy markers, i.e., tixocortolpivalate 0.1% pet and budesonide 0.1% pet., and the products used by the patient are indicated. Of course, according to the specific history and chemical environment of the patient, other substances should also be tested, including samples brought by the patient, for example, their emollient, pieces of shoes if lesions at the feet, plants, etc. Inclusion of compositae mix [201, 202, 212] and disperse dyes [42] in the screening series has also been suggested.

The North American Contact Dermatitis Group [45], however, proposed to test with the same screening series of 65 allergens as in adults, with the addition of other materials according to the history, and in several sessions. If only the NACDG resp. T.R.U.E. test panel screening series were used, they stated that 15%, resp. 39% of the relevant reactions would not have been found. Moreover, 4.3% of the children had only a positive reaction to non NACDG supplemental allergen [45]. It is the view of Storrs [107] that exactly the same methods as in adults can be used, sometimes requiring sequential tests. If screening series of allergens are needed, they have to be performed locally and adapted regularly as the prevalence of allergies is not the same in different countries; moreover, there are changes with time. Vigan in a more recent publication [112] came to the same conclusion.

> **Core Message**
>
> › In children, an abbreviated baseline series, supplemented with allergens suggested by the history, should be used.

48.16 Conclusions

Contact allergy in children is more frequent than previously recognized. In an unselected population, for instance, one consisting of schoolchildren, the prevalence is about 20%, while in a selected population, i.e., children suspected of contact allergy or suffering from atopic or other types of dermatitis, the prevalence is found to be variable, for example, related to geographical origin, with a mean of 40%.

Immunological differences between children (especially neonates) and adults do exist, but their impact on the clinical development of contact allergy is still unknown. Although allergic contact dermatitis has occasionally been observed in neonates, it is generally agreed that susceptibility to contact sensitization and certainly also exposure to environmental allergens increase with the child's age.

48

Whether allergic contact dermatitis is more or less frequently associated with atopy is still a matter of discussion. On the one hand, the Th1 response is reduced in acute atopic eczema, hence atopics are less likely to develop contact allergy; on the other hand, the damaged skin barrier facilitates allergen penetration. The possibility of allergic contact dermatitis in atopic children has to be considered, particularly if the distribution of the lesions is asymmetrical, when the dermatitis is located umbilically (nickel!), if an airborne pattern is found especially emerging during spring and summer (compositae), and when the dermatitis persists when being treated (disperse dyes, topical medication, or emollients).

As with adults, the history and localization of the dermatitis are crucial for the diagnosis of allergic contact dermatitis, though certain contactants and/or habits that are characteristic for the child or the adolescent may be responsible for unusual clinical presentations.

Patch testing in children is safe; most authors think that irritant reactions are not frequently observed (except in atopics, particularly with metals) and that the same patch test concentrations as in adults can be used. However, the possibility of false-positive and false-negative reactions have to be considered, and if there is doubt, lower patch test concentrations should be tested later on.

Due to reduced test surface area, diminished environmental exposure to certain allergens, and, particularly, hypermobility of young children, testing with an abbreviated standard series is recommended by some although others warn that many reactions may be missed. Anyway, it is important to take into account the history and clinical picture and to add suggestive allergens if an abbreviated series are tested.

The most important allergens observed in this population are metals such as nickel (sometimes associated with cobalt), particularly in girls, which still is attributed to the popularity of cheap jewelry, although regulations have reduced the exposure to nickel. Other sources like cell phones are however emerging. Mercury and its derivatives are still used as antiseptic agents in some countries, but the allergic reactions observed to them, even in young children, are not often clinically relevant. This is particularly true for thimerosal, for which vaccines have been regarded as the main sensitization source. However, such an allergy does not seem to be a contraindication for future vaccinations, provided the tip of the needle is not contaminated and the injection is administered intramuscularly.

Other allergens identified in children mainly concern the ingredients of pharmaceutical products and cosmetics (sometimes via another member of the household), rubber derivatives, which are often responsible for shoe or diaper dermatitis, resins, and plants. Certain occupational allergens (e.g., those associated with hairdressing, construction, and metalworking) are found in adolescents.

Last but not the least, by changing regulations concerning the presence of allergens in common products, the incidence of contact allergy might decrease in the future. This is already the case for nickel [41] in, for example, jewelry and soon, also in mobile phones [213] and will hopefully be so for p-phenylenediamine in temporary henna tattoos.

References

1. Epstein E (1971) Contact dermatitis in children. Pediatr Clin North Am 18:839–852
2. Cronin E (1980) Contact Dermatitis. Churchill Livingstone, Edinburgh, pp 20–21
3. Hjorth N (1981) Contact dermatitis in children. Acta Dermatovener 95:36–39
4. Tennstedt D, Lachapelle JM (1987) Eczéma de contact allergique chez l´enfant. Bulletin d´actualité thérapeutique 32:3223–3228
5. Pevny I, Brennenstuhl M, Razinskas G (1984) Patch testing in children (1). Contact Dermatitis 11:201–206
6. Marcussen PV (1963) Primary irritant patch-test reactions in children. Arch Dermatol 87:378–382
7. Mortz CG, Andersen KE (1999) Allergic contact dermatitis in children and adolescents. Contact Dermatitis 41:121–130
8. Weston WL, Weston JA (1984) Allergic contact dermatitis in children. Am J Dis Child 138:932–936
9. Weston WL, Weston JA, Kinoshita J, Kloepfer S, Carreon L, Toth S, Bullard D, Harper K, Martinez S (1986) Prevalence of positive epicutaneous tests among infants, children, and adolescents. Pediatrics 78:1070–1074
10. Barros MA, Baptista A, Correia TM, Azevedo F (1991) Patch testing in children: a study of 562 schoolchildren. Contact Dermatitis 25:156–159
11. Dotterud LK, Falk ES (1995) Contact allergy in relation to hand eczema and atopic diseases in north Norwegian schoolchildren. Acta Paediatr 84:402–406
12. Bruckner AL, Weston WL, Morelli JG (2000) Does sensitization to contact allergens begins in infancy? Pediatrics 105:3–9
13. Johnke H, Norberg LA, Vach W, Bindslev-Jensen C, Host A, Andersen KE (2004) Patch test reactivity to nickel sulphate and fragrance mix in unselected children. Contact Dermatitis 50:131
14. Mortz CG, Lauritsen JM, Bindslev-Jensen C, Andersen KE (2001) Prevalence of atopic dermatitis, asthma, allergic rhinitis, and hand and contact dermatitis in adolescents.

The Odense Adolescence Cohort Study on Atopic Diseases and Dermatitis. Br J Dermatol 144:523–532

15. Czarnobilska E, Obtulowicz K, Dyga W, Wsolek-Wnek K, Spiewak R (2009) Contact hypersensitivity and allergic contact dermatitis among school children and teenagers with eczema. Contact Dermatitis 60:264–269

16. Veien NK, Hattel T, Justesen O, Norholm A (1982) Contact dermatitis in children. Contact Dermatitis 8:373–375

17. Pevny I, Brennenstuhl M, Razinskas G (1984) Patch testing in children (2). Contact Dermatitis 11:302–310

18. Romaguera C, Alomar A, Camarasa JMG, Garcia Bravo B, Garcia Perez A, Grimalt F, Guerra P, Lopez Gorretcher B, Martin Pascual A, Miranda A, Moran M, Pena ML (1985) Contact dermatitis in children. Contact Dermatitis 12:283–284

19. Rademaker M, Forsyth A (1989) Contact dermatitis in children. Contact Dermatitis 20:104–107

20. Kuiters GRR, Sillevis Smitt JH, Cohen EB, Bos JD (1989) Allergic contact dermatitis in children and young adults. Arch Dermatol 125:1531–1533

21. Balato N, Lembo G, Patruno CC, Ayala F (1989) Patch testing in children. Contact Dermatitis 20:305–307

22. Pambor M, Krüger G, Winkler S (1992) Results of patch testing in children. Contact Dermatitis 27:326–328

23. Ayala F, Balato N, Lembo G, Patruno C, Tosti A, Schena D, Pigatto P, Angelini G, Lisi P, Rafanelli A (1992) A multi-centre study of contact sensitization in children. Contact Dermatitis 26:307–310

24. Gonçalo S, Gonçalo M, Azenha A, Barros MA, Sousa Bastos A, Brandao FM, Faria A, Marques MSJ, Pecegueiro M, Rodrigues JB, Salgueiro E, Torres V (1992) Allergic contact dermatitis in children. Contact Dermatitis 26:112–115

25. Sevila A, Romaguera C, Vilaplana J, Botella R (1994) Contact dermatitis in children. Contact Dermatitis 30:292–294

26. Motolese A, Manzini BM, Donini M (1995) Patch testing in infants. Am J Contact Dermatitis 6:153–156

27. Stables GI, Forsyth A, Lever RS (1996) Patch testing in children. Contact Dermatitis 34:341–344

28. Rudzki E, Rebandel P (1996) Contact dermatitis in children. Contact Dermatitis 34:66

29. Wilkowska A, Grubska-Suchanek E, Karwacka I, Szarmach H (1996) Contact allergy in children. Cutis 58:176–180

30. Katsarou A, Koufou V, Armenaka M, Kalogeromitros D, Papanayotou G, Vareltzidis A (1996) Patch tests in children: a review of 14 years experience. Contact Dermatitis 34:70–71

31. Wantke F, Hemmer W, Jarisch R, Götz M (1996) Patch test reactions in children, adults and the elderly. Contact Dermatitis 34:316–319

32. Brasch J, Geier J (1997) Patch test results in schoolchildren. Contact Dermatitis 37:286–293

33. Shah M, Lewis FM, Gawkrodger DJ (1997) Patch testing in children and adolescents: five years´ experience and follow-up. J Am Acad Dermatol 37:964–968

34. Manzini BM, Ferdani G, Simonetti V, Donini M, Seidenari S (1998) Contact sensitization in children. Pediatr Dermatol 15:12–17

35. Romaguera C, Vilaplana J (1998) Contact Dermatitis in children: 6 years experience (1992-1997). Contact Dermatitis 39:277–280

36. Giordano-Labadie F, Rancé F, Pellegrin F, Bazex J, Dutau G, Schwarze HP (1999) Incidence of contact allergy in

children with atopic dermatitis: results of a prospective study of 137 cases. Contact Dermatitis 40:192–195

37. Roul S, Ducombs G, Taïeb A (1999) Usefulness of the European standard series for patch testing in children. A 3-year single-centre study of 337 patients. Contact Dermatitis 40:232–235

38. Duarte I, Lazzarini R, Kobata CM (2003) Contact dermatitis in adolescents. Am J Contact Dermatitis 14:200–204

39. Wohrl S, Hemmer W, Focke M (2003) Patch testing in children, adults and the elderly: influence of age and sex on sensitization patterns. Pediatr Dermatol 20:119–123

40. Lewis VJ SBN, Chowdhury MMU (2004) Allergic contact dermatitis in 191 consecutively patch-tested children. Contact Dermatitis 51:155–156

41. Heine G, Schnuch A, Uter W, Worm M (2004) Frequency of contact allergy in German children and adolescents patch tested between 1995 and 2002: results from the Information Network of Departments of Dermatology and the German Contact Dermatitis Research Group. Contact Dermatitis 51:111–117

42. Seidenari S, Giusti F, Pepe P, Mantovani L (2005) Contact sensitization in 1094 children undergoing patch testing over a 7-year period. Pediatr Dermatol 22:1–5

43. Beattie PE, Green C, Lowe G (2007) Which children should we patch test? Clin Exp Dermatol 32:6–11

44. Jacob SE, Brod B, Crawford GH (2008) Clinically relevant patch test reactions in children – a United States based study. Pediatr Dermatol 25:520–527

45. Zug KA, McGinley-Smith D, Washaw EM, Taylor JS, Rietschel RL, Maibach HI, Belsito DV, Fowler JF, Storrs FJ, DeLeo VA, Marks JG, Mathias T, Pratt MD, Sasseville D (2008) Contact allergy in children referred for patch testing. North American Contact Dermatitis Group Data 2001-2004. Arch Dermatol 144:1329–1336

46. Mailhol C, Lauwers-Cances V, Rancé F, Paul C, Giordano-Labadie F (2009) Prevalence and risk factors for allergic contact dermatitis to topical treatment in atopic dermatitis : a study in 641 children. Allergy 64:801–806

47. Björkstén B (1997) The environment and sensitisation to allergens in early childhood. Pediatr Allergy Immunol 8(suppl 10):32–39

48. Walton S, Nayagam AT, Keczkes K (1986) Age and sex incidence of allergic contact dermatitis. Contact Dermatitis 15:136–139

49. Walker FB, Smith PD, Maibach HI (1967) Genetic factors in human allergic contact dermatitis. Int Arch Allergy 32:453–462

50. Hawes GE, Struyk L, van den Elsen PJ (1993) Differential usage of T-cell receptor V gene segments in CD4+ and CD8+ subsets of T lymphocytes in monozygotic twins. J Immunol 150:2033–2045

51. Thestrup-Pedersen K (1997) Contact allergy in monozygous twins. Contact Dermatitis 36:52–53

52. Wöhrl S, Hemmer W, Focke M, Götz M, Jarisch R (2003) Patch testing in children, adults and the elderly: influence of age and sex on sensitization patterns. Pediatr Dermatol 20:119–123

53. Kwangsukstith C, Maibach HI (1995) Effect of age and sex on the induction and elicitation of allergic contact dermatitis. Contact Dermatitis 33:289–298

54. Meneghini CL (1995) Contact dermatitis in children. In: Rycroft RJG, Menné T, Frosch PJ, Benezra C (eds) Textbook of contact dermatitis. Springer, Berlin, pp 403–404

55. Uhr JW (1960) Delayed-type hypersensitivity in premature neonatal humans. Nature 187:1130

56. Epstein WL (1961) Contact-type delayed hypersensitivity in infants and children: induction of Rhus sensitivity. Pediatrics 27:51–53

57. Fisher AA (1985) Allergic contact dermatitis in early infancy. Cutis 35:315–316

58. Fisher AA (1990) Perfume dermatitis in children sensitized to balsam of Peru in topical agents. Cutis 45:21–23

59. Fisher AA (1994) Allergic contact dermatitis in early infancy. Cutis 54:300–302

60. Fisher AA (1994) Patch testing in children including early infancy. Cutis 54:387–388

61. Seidenari S, Manzini BM, Motolese A (1992) Contact sensitization in infants: report of 3 cases. Contact Dermatitis 27:319–320

62. Aihara M, Ikezawa Z (1998) Neonatal allergic contact dermatitis. Contact Dermatitis 18:105

63. Roul S, Ducombs G, Léauté-Labrèze TA (1998) "Lucky Luke" contact dermatitis due to rubber components of diapers. Contact Dermatitis 38:363–364

64. Roul S, Léauté-Labrèze C, Ducombs G, Taïeb A (1998) Eczéma de contact aux changes complets type "Lucky-Luke": un marqueur de dermatite atopique ? Ann Dermatol Venereol 125 (suppl 3):3S74

65. Belhadjali H, Giordano-Labadie F, Rancé F, Bazex J (2001) "Lucky Luke" contact dermatitis from diapers: a new allergen? Contact Dermatitis 44:248

66. Alberta L, Sweeney M, Wis K (2005) Diaper dye dermatitis. Pediatrics 116:e450–e452

67. Smith WJ, Jacob SE (2009) Letter to the editor. The role of allergic contact dermatitis in diaper dermatitis. Pediatr Dermatol 26:369–370

68. Nardelli A, Morren MA, Goossens A (2009) Contact allergy to fragrances and parabens in an atopic baby. Contact Dermatitis 60:107–109

69. Leyden JJ, Kligman AM (1979) Contact dermatitis to neomycin sulfate. JAMA 242:1276–1278

70. Levy A, Hanau D, Foussereau J (1980) Contact dermatitis in children. Contact Dermatitis 6:260–262

71. Fisher AA (1995) Cosmetic dermatitis in childhood. Cutis 55:15–16

72. Wintzen M, Van Zuuren EJ (2003) Computer-related skin diseases. Contact Dermatitis 48:241–243

73. Fisher AA (1994) Allergic contact dermatitis and patch testing in childhood. Cutis 54:230–232

74. Andersen KE, Hjorth N, Menne T (1984) The baboon syndrome: systemically induced allergic contact dermatitis. Contact Dermatitis 10:97–100

75. Moreno-Ramirez D, Garcia-Bravo B, Rodriguez Pichardo A, Peral Rubio F, Camacho Martinez F (2004) Baboon syndrome in childhood: easy to avoid, easy to diagnose, but the problem continues. Pediatric Dermatol 21:250–253

76. Goossens C, Sass U, Song M (1997) Baboon syndrome. Dermatology 194:421–422

77. Torinuki W (1990) Generalized erythem-multiforme-like eruption following allergic contact dermatitis. Contact Dermatitis 23:202–203

78. Jappe U, Hausen BM, Petzoldt D (2001) Erythema-multiforme-like eruption and depigmentation following allergic contact dermatitis from a paint-on henna tattoo, due to para-phenylenediamine contact hypersensitivity. Contact Dermatitis 45:249–250

79. Baldari U, Alessandrini F, Raccagni AA (1999) Diffuse erythema multiforme-like contact dermatitis caused by disperse blue 124 in a 2 year old child. J Eur Acad Dermatol Venerol 12:180–181

80. Kütting B, Brehler R, Traupe H (2004) Allergic contact dermatitis in children – strategies of prevention and risk management. Eur J Dermatol 14:80–85

81. Lembo G, Balato N, Patruno C, Pini D, Ayala F (1987) Lichenoid contact dermatitis due to aminoglycoside antibiotics. Contact Dermatitis 17:122–123

82. Ho VC, Johnston MM (1986) Nickel dermatitis in infants. Contact Dermatitis 15:270–273

83. Schultz E, Mahler V (2002) Prolonged lichenoid reaction and cross-sensitivity to para-substituted amino-compounds due to temporary henna tattoo. Int J Dermatol 41:301–303

84. Bowling CR, Groves R (2002) Clinical picture: an unexpected tattoo. Lancet 23:649

85. Bergfors E, Trollfors B, Inerot A (2003) Unexpectedly high incidence of persistent itching nodules and delayed hypersensitivity to aluminium in children after the use of adsorbed vaccines from a single manufacturer. Vaccine 22:64–69

86. Caraffini S, Lisi P (1987) Nummular dermatitis-like eruption from ethylenediamine hydrochloride in 2 children. Contact Dermatitis 17:313–314

87. Patrizi SC, Rizzoli L, Vincenzi C, Trevisi P, Tosti A (1999) Sensitisation to thimerosal in atopic children. Contact Dermatitis 40:94–97

88. Vogt T, Landthaler M, Stolz W (1998) Generalized eczema in an 18-month-old boy due to phenoxyethanol in DPT vaccine. Contact Dermatitis 38:50–51

89. Kerosuo H, Kanerva L (1997) Systemic contact dermatitis caused by nickel in a stainless steel orthodontic appliance. Contact Dermatitis 36:112–113

90. Akhavan A, Cohen SR (2003) The relationship between atopic dermatitis and contact dermatitis. Clin Dermatol 21:158–162

91. Cohen PR, Cardullo AC, Ruszkowski AM, DeLeo VA (1990) Allergic contact dermatitis to nickel in children with atopic dermatitis. Ann Allergy 65:73–77

92. Pambor M, Winkler S, Bloch Y (1992) Allergic contact dermatitis in children. Contact Dermatitis 24:72–73

93. De La Cuadra J, Sanz J, Martorell A (1990) Prevalence of positive epicutaneous tests in atopic and non-atopic children without dermatitis. Contact Dermatitis 23:242–243

94. Fisher AA (1991) Nickel dermatitis in children. Cutis 47:19–21

95. Dotterud LK, Falk ES (1994) Metal allergy in north Norwegian schoolchildren and its relationship with ear piercing and atopy. Contact Dermatitis 31:308–313

96. Rystedt I (1985) Contact sensitivity in adults with atopic dermatitis in childhood. Contact Dermatitis 13:1–8

97. Guillet MH, Guillet G (1995) Enquête allergologique chez 251 malades atteints de dermatite atopique modérée ou sévère. Ann Dermatol Venereol 123:157–164

98. Lisi P, Simonetti S (1985) Contact sensitivity in children and adults with atopic dermatitis – a chronological study. Dermatologica 171:1–7

99. Oranje AP, Bruynzeel DP, Stenveld HJ, Dieges PH (1994) Immediate- and delayed-type contact hypersensitivity in

children older than 5 years with atopic dermatitis: a pilot study comparing different tests. Pediatr Dermatol 11: 209–215

100. Rancé F, Dargassies J, Dupuy P, Smitt AM, Guerin L, Dutau G (2001) Faut-il contre-indiquer l'utilisation des émollients à base d'avoine chez l'enfant atopique. Rev Fr Allergol Immunol Clin 41:477–483

101. Weston WL (1997) Contact dermatitis in children. Curr Opin Pediatr 9:372–376

102. Mallory SB (1995) The pediatric patient: practical contact dermatitis. In: Guin JD (ed). McGraw-Hill, New York, pp 603–616

103. Jacob SE, Steele T, Brod B, Crawford GH (2008) Dispelling the myths behind pediatric patch testing – experience from our tertiary care patch testing centres. Pediatr Dermatol 25:296–300

104. Röckl H, Müller E, Hiltermann W (1966) Zum Aussagewert positiver Epicutantests bei Säuglingen und Kindern. Archiv für klinische und experimentelle Dermatologie 226:407–419

105. Müller E, Röckl H (1975) Aussagewert von Läppchentests bei Kindern und Jugendlichen. Der Hautarzt 26:85–87

106. Rietschel RL, Rosenthal LE, North American Contact Dermatitis Group (1990) Standard patch test screening series used diagnostically in young and elderly patients. Am J Cont Derm 1:53–55

107. Storrs FJ (2008) Patch testing children – what should we change? Pediatr Dermatol 25:420–423

108. Wahlberg JE, Goossens A (2001) Use of patch test concentrations for adults in children and their influence on test reactivity. Occup Environ Dermatol 49:97–101

109. Silverberg NB, Licht J, Friedler S, Sethi S, Laude TA (2002) Nickel contact hypersensitivity in children. Pediatr Dermatol 19:110–113

110. Camarasa JMG, Aspiolea F, Alomar A (1983) Patch tests to metals in children. Contact Dermatitis 9:157–161

111. Van Hoogstraten IMW, Andersen KE, Von Blomberg BME, Boden D, Bruynzeel DP, Burrows D, Camarasa JG, Dooms-Goossens A, Kraal G, Lahti A, Menne T, Rycroft RJG, Shaw S, Todd D, Vreeburg KJJ, Wilkinson JD, Scheper RJ (1991) Reduced incidence of nickel allergy upon oral nickel contact at an early age. Clin Exp Immunol 85:441–445

112. Vigan M (2008) Usefulness of the European standard series for patch testing in children. Contact Dermatitis 58(suppl 1):24

113. Sharma V, Beyer DJ, Paruthi S, Nopper AJ (2002) Prominent pruritic periumbilical papules: allergic contact dermatitis to nickel. Pediatr Dermatol 19:106–109

114. Byer TT, Morrell DS (2004) Periumbilical allergic contact dermatitis: blue jeans or belt buckles? Pediatr Dermatol 21:223–226

115. Veien NK, Hattel T, Justesen O, Norholm A (1986) Why do young girls become nickel sensitive? Contact Dermatitis 15:306–307

116. Räsänen L, Lehto M, Mustikka-Mäki UP (1993) Sensitization to nickel from stainless steel ear-piercing kits. Contact Dermatitis 28:292–294

117. Reiffers J, Hunziker N, Brun R, Vidmar B (1974) Sensibilisations cutanées allergiques peu communes. Dermatologica 148:285–291

118. Jensen CS, Lisby S, Baadsgaard O, Volund A, Menne T (2002) Decrease in nickel sensitization in a Danish school-girl population with ears pierced after implementation of the nickel-exposure regulation. Br J Dermatol 146: 636–642

119. Schnuch A, Geier J, Lessmann H, Uter W, Kliniken ID (2003) Decrease in nickel sensitization in young patients-succesful intervention through nickel exposure regulation? Results of the IVDK, 1992-2001. Hautartz 54:626–632

120. Heim KE, McKean BA (2009) Children's clothing fasteners as a potential source of exposure to releasable nickel ions. Contact Dermatitis 60:100–105

121. Temesvári E, Rácz I (1988) Nickel sensitivity from dental prosthesis. Contact Dermatitis 18:50–51

122. Veien NK, Borckhorst E, Hattel T, Laurberg G (1994) Stomatitis or systemically-induced contact dermatitis from metal wire in orthodontic materials. Contact Dermatitis 30:210–213

123. De Silva BD, Doherty VR (2000) Nickel allergy from orthodontic appliances. Contact Dermatitis 42:102–103

124. Thyssen JP, Johansen JD, Zachariae C, Menne T (2008) The outcome of dimethylglyoxime testing in a sample of cell phones in Denmark. Contact Dermatitis 59:38–42

125. Bercovitch L, Luo J (2008) Cellphone contact dermatitis with nickel allergy. CMAJ 178:440–442

126. Grimm I (1971) Ungewöhnliche Form einer Kontaktdermatitis durch Kobalt bei einem 11 jährigen Kind. Berufsdermatosen 19:39–42

127. Kanerva L, Kanervo K, Jolanki R, Estlander T (2001) Letter to the editor. Cobalt, a possible sensitizer in personal computer (PC) mouse and polyester resins. Contact Dermatitis 45:126–127

128. Thomas SE, Tucker WFG, Bleehen SS (1986) Body splint dermatitis in childhood. Contact Dermatitis 14:320–321

129. Seishima M, Oyama Z, Yamamura M (2002) Cellular phone dermatitis. Arch Dermatol 138:272–273

130. De La Cuadra J (1993) Sensibilisation cutanée au mercure et à ses composés. Ann Dermatol Venereol 120:37–42

131. Bardazzi F, Vassilopoulos A, Valenti R, Paganini P, Morelli R (1990) Mercurochrome-induced allergic contact dermatitis. Contact Dermatitis 23:381–382

132. Anonide A, Massone L (1996) Periorbital contact dermatitis due to yellow mercuric oxide. Contact Dermatitis 35:61

133. Audicana MT, Munoz D, Dolore Del Pozo M, Fernandez E, Gastraminza G, Fernandez de Corres L (2002) Allergic contact dermatitis from mercury antiseptics and derivatives: study protocol of tolerance to intramuscular injections of thimerosal. Am J Contact Dermatitis 13:3–9

134. Veien NK, Hattel T, Justesen O, Norholm A (1986) Aluminium allergy. Contact Dermatitis 15:295–297

135. Veien NK, Hattel T, Laurberg G (1993) Systemically aggravated contact dermatitis caused by aluminium in toothpaste. Contact Dermatitis 28:199–200

136. Kaaber K, Nielsen AO, Veien NK (1990) Aluminium sensitization following vaccination. Contact Dermatitis 23:256

137. O'Driscoll JB, Beck MB, Kesseler ME, Ford G (1991) Contact sensitivity to aluminium acetate eardrops. Contact Dermatitis 24:156–157

138. Kaaber K, Kerusuo H, Kullaa A, Kerusuo E (1992) Vaccination granulomas and aluminium allergy: course and prognostic factors. Contact Dermatitis 26:304–306

139. White IR (2000) Allergic contact dermatitis. In: Harper J, Oranje A, Prose N (eds) Textbook of pediatric dermatology, vol 1. Blackwell Science Oxford, London, pp 287–294

140. Boman A, Wahlberg JE (1990) Experimental sensitization with palladium chloride in the guinea pig. Contact Dermatitis 23:256

141. Kanerva L, Kerusuo H, Kullaa A, Kerusuo E (1996) Allergic patch test reactions to palladium chloride in schoolchildren. Contact Dermatitis 34:39–42

142. Hemmer W, Focke M, Wantke F, Götz M, Jarisch R (1996) Contact hypersensitivity to iron. Contact Dermatitis 34:219–220

143. Cockayne SE, Shah M, Messenger AG, Gawkrodger DJ (1998) Foot dermatitis in children: causative allergens and follow-up. Contact Dermatitis 38:203–206

144. Vincenzi C, Peluso AM, Lameli N, Tosti A (1992) Allergic contact dermatitis caused by acyclovir. Am J Contact Dermatitis 3:105–107

145. Cusano F, Capozzi M, Errico G (1989) Contact dermatitis from dexchlorpheniramine. Contact Dermatitis 21:340

146. Gomez A, Martorell A, De La Cuadra J (1994) Allergic contact dermatitis from fepradinol in a child. Contact Dermatitis 30:44

147. Kabasawa Y, Kanzaki T (1990) Allergic contact dermatitis from ethyl sebacate. Contact Dermatitis 22:226

148. Morren MA, Dooms-Goossens A (1994) Corticosteroid allergy in children: a potential complication of atopic eczema. Eur J Dermatol 4:106–109

149. Shaw DW, Eichenfield LF, Shainhouse T, Maibach HI (2004) Allergic contact dermatitis from tacrolimus. J Am Acad Dermatol 50:962–965

150. Dias M, Conchon I, Vale T (1994) Allergic contact dermatitis from quinine. Contact Dermatitis 30:121–122

151. Pigatto PD, Bigardi A, Fumagalli M, Altomare GF, Riboldi A (1990) Allergic dermatitis from parenteral vitamin K. Contact Dermatitis 22:307–308

152. Balato N, Lembo G, Patruno C, Ayala F (1989) Allergic contact dermatitis from Cerumenex® in a child. Contact Dermatitis 21:348–349

153. Svensson A (1988) Allergic contact dermatitis to laureth-4. Contact Dermatitis 18:113–114

154. Lucente P, Iorizzo M, Pazzaglia M (2000) Contact sensitivity to Tween 80 in a child. Contact Dermatitis 43:172

155. Conti A, Motolese A, Manzini BM, Seidenari S (1997) Contact sensitization to preservatives in children. Contact Dermatitis 37:35–36

156. Goulden V, Goodfield MJD (1995) Delayed hypersensitivity reaction to the preservative myristyl picolinium chloride. Contact Dermatitis 33:209

157. Osawa J, Kitamura K, Ikezawa Z (1991) A probable role for vaccines containing thimerosal in thimerosal hypersensitivity. Contact Dermatitis 24:178–182

158. Novak M, Kuicalova E, Friedländerova B (1986) Reactions to Merthiolate in infants. Contact Dermatitis 15:309

159. Trevisan G, Kokelj F (1992) Allergic contact dermatitis due to shoes in children: a 5-year follow-up. Contact Dermatitis 26:45

160. Möller H (1994) All these positive tests to thiomersal. Contact Dermatitis 31:209–213

161. Wantke F, Hemme W, Götz M, Jarisch R (1996) Routine patch testing with thimerosal: why should it be performed? Contact Dermatitis 35:67–68

162. Cox NH, Forsyth A (1988) Thiomersal allergy and vaccination reactions. Contact Dermatitis 18:229–233

163. Aberer W (1991) Vaccination despite thiomersal sensitivity. Contact Dermatitis 24:6–10

164. Aberer W, Kränke B (1996) Reply. Contact Dermatitis 35:67–68

165. Aberer W (1997) Thiomersal-Kontaktallergie und Impfungen mit Thiomersal-konservierten Seren. Dermatosen 45:137

166. Kohl L, Blondeel A, Song M (2002) Allergic contact dermatitis from cosmetics. Dermatology 204:334–337

167. Rastogi SC, Johansen JD, Menné T, Frosch P, Bruze M, Andersen KE, Lepoittevin JP, Wakelin S, White IR (1999) Contents of fragrance allergens in children's cosmetics and cosmetic-toys. Contact Dermatitis 41:84–88

168. Helsing P, Austad J (1991) Contact dermatitis mimicking photodermatosis in a 1-year-old child. Contact Dermatitis 24:140–141

169. Chu CY, Sun CC (2001) Allergic contact dermatitis from triethanolamine in a sunscreen. Contact Dermatitis 44:41

170. Stone N, Varma S, Hughes TM, Stone NM (2002) Allergic contact dermatitis from polyvinylpyrrolidone 1-triacontene copolymer in a sunscreen. Contact Dermatitis 47:49

171. Livideanu C, Giordano-Labadie F, Carle P (2007) Contact dermatitis to hydrolized wheat protein. Contact Dermatitis 57:283–284

172. Neri I, Guareschi E, Savoia F, Patrizi A (2002) Childhood allergic contact dermatitis form Henna tattoo. Pediatr Dermatol 19:503–505

173. Brancaccio RR, Brown LH, Chang YT, Fogelman JP, Mafong EA, Cohen DE (2002) Identification and quantification of para-phenylenediamine in a temporary black henna tattoo. Am J Contact Dermatitis 13:15–18

174. Jacob S, Zapolanski T, Chayavichitsilp P, Conelly A, Eichenfield LF (2008) p-Phenylenediamine in black henna tattoos. A practice in need of policy in children. Arch Pediatri Adolesc Med 162:790–792

175. Sosted H, Johansen JD, Andersen KE (2006) Severe allergic hair dye reactions in 8 children. Contact Dermatitis 54:87–91

176. Verhaeghe I, Dooms-Goossens A (1997) Multiple sources of allergic contact dermatitis from parabens. Contact Dermatitis 36:269–270

177. Downs AMR, Sansom JE, Simmons I (1998) Let Rip! Fun Pot® dermatitis. Contact Dermatitis 38:234

178. Tosti A, Bassi R, Peluso AM (1990) Contact dermatitis due to natural plasticine. Contact Dermatitis 22:301–302

179. Rodriguez-Serna M, Molinero J, Febrer I, Aliaga A (2002) Persistent hand eczema in a child. Am J Contact Dermatitis 13:35–36

180. O'Hagan AH, Bingham EA (2001) Cellist's finger dermatitis. Contact Dermatitis 45:319

181. Rudzki E, Rebandel P (1995) 2 cases of dermatitis from rare sources of sensitization to frequent contactants. Contact Dermatitis 32:361

182. Fowler JF (1990) Case for diagnosis. Am J Contact Dermatitis 1:71

183. Fisher AA (1994) Contact allergy in children. Part 1: rubber allergy. Cutis 54:138–140

184. Castelain M, Castelain PY (1993) Allergic contact dermatitis from cetyl pyridinium chloride in latex gloves. Contact Dermatitis 28:118

185. Placucci F, Vincenzi C, Ghedini G, Piana G, Tosti A (1996) Coexistence of type 1 and type 4 allergy to rubber latex. Contact Dermatitis 34:76

186. Azurdia RM, King CM (1998) Allergic contact dermatitis due to phenol-formaldehyde resin and benzoyl peroxide in swimming goggles. Contact Dermatitis 38:234–235

187. Warshaw EM, Cook JW, Belsito DV, DeLeo VA, Fowler JF Jr, Maibach HI, Marks JG Jr, Mathias CG, Pratt MD, Rietschel RL, Sasseville D, Storrs FJ, Taylor JS, Zug KA (2008) Positive patch-test reactions to mixed thioureas: cross-sectional data from the North American Contact Dermatitis Group, 1994-2004. Dermatitis 19:190–201

188. Roul S, Ducombs G, Leaute-Labreze C, Labbe L, Taieb A (1996) Footwear contact dermatitis in children. Contact Dermatitis 35:334–336

189. Saha M, Srinivas CR (1993) Footwear dermatitis due to para-fenylenediamine in socks. Contact Dermatitis 28:295

190. Weston JA, Hawkins K, Weston WL (1983) Foot dermatitis in children. Pediatrics 72:824–827

191. Shakelford KE, Belsito DV (2002) The etiology of allergic-appearing foot dermatitis: a 5-year retrospective study. J Am Acad Dermatol 47:715–721

192. Giusti F, Massone F, Bertoni L, Pellacani G, Seidenari S (2003) Contact sensitization to disperse dyes in children. Pediatr Dermatol 20:393–397

193. Vincenzi C, Guerra L, Peluso AM, Zucchelli V (1992) Allergic contact dermatitis due to phenol-formaldehyde resins in a knee-guard. Contact Dermatitis 27:54

194. Shono M, Ezor K, Kaniwa MA, Ikarashi Y, Kojima S, Nakamura A (1991) Allergic contact dermatitis from para-tertiary-butylphenol-formaldehyde resin (PTBP-FR) in athletic tape and leather adhesive. Contact Dermatitis 24:281–288

195. Sood A, Taylor JS, Billock JN (2003) Contact dermatitis to a limb prothesis. Am J Contact Dermatitis 14:169–171

196. Stanford D, Georgouras K (1996) Allergic contact dermatitis from benzalkonium chloride in plaster of Paris. Contact Dermatitis 35:371–372

197. Southcott RV, Haegi LAR (1992) Plant hair dermatitis. Med J Aust 156:623–632

198. Rademaker M, Duffill MB (1995) Allergic contact dermatitis to Toxicodendron succedaneum (rhus tree): an autumn epidemic. N Z Med J 108:121–123

199. Edwards EK Jr, Edwards EK Sr (1992) Immediate and delayed hypersensitivity to the nettle plant. Contact Dermatitis 27:264–265

200. Wakelin SH, Marren P, Young E, Shaw S (1997) Compositae sensitivity and chronic hand dermatitis in a seven-year-old boy. Brit J Dermatol 137:289–291

201. Flohr C, Ravenscroft J, English J (2008) Compositae dermatitis in three children with hand dermatitis. Contact Dermatitis 59:370–379

202. Fortina AB, Romano I, Peserico A (2005) Contact sensitization to compositae mix in children. J Am Acad Dermatol 53:877–880

203. Commens C, McGeogh A, Bartlett B, Kossard S (1984) Bindii (Jo Jo) dermatitis (Soliva pterosperma [Compositae]). J Am Acad Dermatol 10:768–773

204. Wood B, Rademaker M (1996) Allergic contact dermatitis from lichen acids. Contact Dermatitis 34:370

205. Tomb RR, Foussereau J, Sell Y (1988) Mini-epidemic of contact dermatitis from gingko tree fruit (Ginkgo biloba L.). Contact Dermatitis 19:281–283

206. Kubo Y, Nonaka S, Yoshida H (1988) Allergic contact dermatitis from Dioscorea batatas Decaisne. Contact Dermatitis 18:111–112

207. Pazzaglia M, Jorizzo M, Parente G, Tosti A (2000) Allergic contact dermatitis due to avena extract. Contact Dermatitis 42:364

208. Kraus SM, Muselinovic NZ (1991) Pre-employment screening for contact dermatitis among the pupils of a metal industry school. Contact Dermatitis 24:342–344

209. Corazza M, Mantovani L, Bacilieri S, Virgili A (2001) A child with "occupational" allergic contact dermatitis due to MCI/MI. Contact Dermatitis 44:53

210. Vigan M, Sauvage C, Adessi B, Girardin P, Meyer JP, Vuitton DA, Laurent R (1994) Pourquoi et comment réaliser une batterie standard chez les enfants? Nouv Dermatol 13:12–15

211. Vigan M, Avenel-Audran M, Blondeel A, Bourrain JL, Castelain M, Dejobert Y, Ducombs G, Flechet ML, Goossens A, Girardin P, Jelen G, Milpied-Homsi B, Pons-Guiraud A, Roul S (1998) Interêt des allergènes de la batterie standard ICDRG pour tester les enfants: étude multicentrique REVIDAL GERDA portant sur 959 enfants. Ann Dermatol Vénéreol 125:3s76

212. Worm M, Aberer W, Agathos M, Becker D, Brasch J, Fuchs T, Hillen U, Höger P, Mahler V, Schnuch A, Szliska C (2007) Patch testing in children – recommendations of the German Contact Dermatitis Research Group (DKG). J Dtsch Dermatol Ges 5:107–109

213. Thyssen JP, Johansen D (2009) Mobile phones are now covered by the European Union Nickel Directive. Contact Dermatitis 61:56–57

Therapy and Rehabilitation of Allergic and Irritant Contact Dermatitis

49

Dimitar Antonov, Sibylle Schliemann, and Peter Elsner

Contents

The key principles for managing a patient with contact dermatitis can be summarized in the "rule of the 4 *R*s":

> *Recognize* (the causative allergic/irritant agent) – Sect. 49.1
> *Remove* (the irritant/allergen) – Sect. 49.2
> *Reduce* inflammation – Sect. 49.3
> *Restore* the skin barrier – Sect. 49.4

This chapter overviews the treatment approaches and the evidence supporting them, which are divided into categories according to the above principles.

> **Core Message**
>
> The "rule of the 4 *R* s" for managing a patient with contact dermatitis
> > *Recognize* the causative allergic/irritant agent
> > *Remove* the irritant/allergen
> > *Reduce* inflammation
> > *Restore* the skin barrier

49.1 Recognize (the Causative Allergic/Irritant Agent)

In contact dermatitis, the basis for therapy is the recognition of the causative allergen(s) and/or irritant(s). This provides the chance to avoid exposure to these causes. Therefore, a thorough history and patch testing, including patients' own substances, are necessary, as outlined in other chapters of this book. The judgement on the relevance of reactions is basically a decision whether avoidance of these substances is expected to result in the improvement or clearance of lesions.

P. Elsner (✉), D. Antonov, and S. Schliemann
Department of Dermatology, Friedrich Schiller University,
Erfurter Straße 35, 07743 Jena, Germany
e-mail: elsner@derma-jena.de

J.D. Johansen et al. (eds.), *Contact Dermatitis*,
DOI: 10.1007/978-3-642-03827-3_49, © Springer-Verlag Berlin Heidelberg 2011

However, contact dermatitis is frequently combined with endogenous disease, e.g. atopic dermatitis. In these cases, the removal of allergens/irritants may not be sufficient for healing. In other cases, no causal allergens or irritants are found, despite meticulous workup. Thus, a pragmatic symptom-oriented approach is needed for the therapeutic management.

49.2 Remove (the Irritant/Allergen)

Once the causative agent – allergen or irritant – has been identified, the key to the therapeutic success lies in its avoidance. Identifying the sources of exposure to the irritant/allergen in the home/leisure or occupational environment may be a tedious process, sometimes requiring a workplace visit or collaboration with the occupational health authorities.

> **Core Message**
>
> ❯ The key to the therapeutic success lies in the avoidance of the causative allergens/irritants.

Due to the development of hardening in ICD, decrease in the exposure frequency or intensity may be sufficient in the long-term, instead of complete avoidance of the irritant. Therefore, personal protective measures, such as barrier creams, gloves and protective clothing, are more effective in the management of irritant than allergic contact dermatitis.

The prognosis of allergic contact dermatitis depends on the avoidance of the allergen, as well as on the avoidance of intermittent irritants, and on constitutional factors (e.g. atopic predisposition). Avoiding the allergen is the most important prerequisite for long-term remission. Studies on the loss of sensitivity to contact allergens indicate that ubiquitous allergens maintain prolonged sensitivity [92]. On the other side, prolonged avoidance of the allergen may lead to the loss of hypersensitivity for avoidable and non-cross-reactive allergens, for example those used in the immunotherapy of alopecia, although they are strong allergens [87]. The prognosis for nickel or chromate allergy is poor, as they are widespread and difficult to avoid, while the prognosis is good for allergens that are easy to identify and avoid. Nevertheless, patients with established hypersensitivity should be considered at lifelong risk for developing contact dermatitis.

49.2.1 Preventive Measures

The general scheme of prevention in public health divides it into primary, secondary and tertiary prevention.

Primary prevention aims to decrease the incidence of disease by limiting the exposure to its risk factors. Its relevance to contact dermatitis translates into measures to identify potential allergens and irritants and initiate preventive actions before they can cause sensitization and/or contact dermatitis.

The purpose of secondary prevention is to decrease the prevalence of disease by prompt diagnosis and adequate treatment in order to prevent complications. In terms of contact dermatitis, this refers to the dermatologists' responsibility not to delay the diagnosis of contact dermatitis, to establish the patients' clinically relevant hypersensitivities (by means of proper testing) and initiate avoidance measures.

Tertiary prevention aims to reduce impairment and disability of established disease and promote patients' adjustment to incurable conditions. In contact dermatitis the tertiary prevention includes the treatment of chronic cases and the rehabilitation measures to help the patient return to his environment and prevent job loss.

> **Core Message**
>
> ❯ The preventive measures for contact dermatitis can be divided into primary, secondary and tertiary. The primary prevention is the most rewarding one in returning value to society for the invested efforts and resources.

In contact dermatitis, the different levels of prevention often coincide, for example primary prevention measures constitute secondary prevention in terms of preventing recurrence of dermatitis in already sensitized individuals. An example of a measure to facilitate the diagnosis of established hypersensitivity is to review and analyze the practice of patch testing. The allergens included in the patch testing series should reflect the common allergens present in consumer products and occupational environment and should not fall behind. For example, a proportion of the allergens in the fragrance mix may not be common allergens [6].

Substances intended for human use undergo extensive testing. There are legislative opportunities at this level to identify toxic and irritant substances or potential allergens. The relative potency of allergens can be quantified, and appropriate acceptable concentrations in different product types can be set (reviewed in [6]). Manufacturers' safety data sheets should contain information on the safety hazards, when a given chemical is irritant or allergen. For established allergens, protection is needed both for the consumer/user and the people involved in the manufacturing. For most allergens, there are acceptable levels of exposure, which will not lead to sensitization, while for others complete avoidance is necessary (see Chap. 51).

Understanding how people become exposed to irritants and allergens in their occupational or non-occupational environment is a cornerstone in the process of both protecting the sensitized individual and preventing new sensitizations. This can be achieved by developing programs for collective prevention in the workplace and regulatory standards for exposure levels. Changes in the processes or activities that lead to exposure are more effective than the personal protection measures. The avoidance/protection measures can be individual or collective and directed at the occupational or home/recreational environment. These include:

1. Labelling: the communication that certain chemicals can be safety hazards as irritants or allergens requires appropriate labelling. In the manufacturing process, this translates into danger signs on the chemicals and their containers. For the benefit of the consumer, the labelling of cosmetic and medicinal products should specify their constituents. Standardization of the names of ingredients and the way they are declared on the package facilitates their recognition by the user. An example of such standardization is the International Nomenclature of Cosmetic Products. Currently, the regulations for the declaration of constituents are more stringent for the cosmetics than for medicinal products, which results in the possibility of people developing allergic reactions to excipients in the medicinal products not listed on the package (unpublished observation).

2. Personal protective measures, like protective clothing, appropriate type of gloves, barrier creams and emollients, etc., need to be suited for specific exposures (see Chap. 50).

3. Appropriate use of cleaning products – soap substitutes and mild cleansers without fragrances or irritant ingredients, adequate rinse-off and drying should be recommended. Emollients should be readily available for use after washing.

4. In the occupational setting, various collective measures to limit the exposure can be implemented, if practical. These include closed production systems, chemical inactivation of allergens or substitution of allergens, ventilation, automation and change in the way materials are handled.

5. Educational measures: In many occasions, patients need to be educated how to avoid the allergen or irritant. Internet databases, such as the Contact Allergen Replacement Database (CARD) of the American Contact Dermatitis Society, are helpful to create allergen-free product lists. The CARD claims to take into account synonyms and cross-reactivity. Distributions of "allergen passports" or handouts to the patients, with general information where the allergen can be encountered, are also helpful. Additional educational measures include eczema schools (see Chap. 50), patient seminars and safety instructions at the workplace. There are examples of exposures resulting from improper handling of materials, disinfectants, etc., which would not have occurred if the manufacturer's instructions had been followed. For more information on the preventive measures in the occupational setting, see Chap. 50.

Avoidance measures need to be adapted to the needs of individual patients. Monitoring of compliance and reinforcements are frequently necessary. A qualitative study on the compliance in avoiding allergens in cosmetic products showed that patients comply with medical instructions in socially different ways. Medical instructions in clinical practice need to address the social differences, especially the limitations of the educational level [94].

> **Core Message**
>
> › Patients comply with medical instructions in socially different ways. Medical instructions need to take into account the educational and social differences.

49.2.2 Elimination Diets

Ingested allergens may induce perioral dermatitis, gingivostomatitis and other manifestations on the site of contact [51]. Pruritus ani is also reported from hyposensitization studies [140]. In addition, ingested contact allergens can provoke distant reactions, such as systemic contact dermatitis or flare-up reactions in skin-areas previously affected by contact dermatitis (see Chap. 17). It is believed that certain allergens in food may foster the high allergic sensitivity and sustain the inflammatory reactions in chronic dermatitis, especially nickel allergy in chronic hand eczema. There is evidence that a nickel elimination diet may lead to clinical improvement and even clearance of chronic contact dermatitis (reviewed in [82, 118]). Even some patients with chronic hand eczema and negative Ni-patch test are reported to have improved from low-nickel diet [82]. There are controversies, because the diet content of nickel is usually lower than the amount required to trigger a flare in most of the patients. Additionally, nickel is present in many common food and sometimes in water, which makes the diet difficult to adhere to, and the patients need to be highly motivated [82]. Other diets, such as a low cobalt and nickel diet, have also been proposed. Chelating agents, such as disulfiram and its metabolite diethyl dithiocarbamate, have been administered because of their ability to bind metal ions, but are not widely used in clinical practice. They are associated with an unexpectedly high level of hepatotoxicity, unlike when they are used for other indications. In a follow-up retrospective study of Nickel-allergic patients with hand eczema, 20% of all participants (11 out of 61) developed elevated serum transaminases and half of them showed clinical evidence of hepatitis [68].

49.3 Reduce Inflammation: Pharmacologic Therapy

Many treatment modalities are available for the treatment of contact dermatitis, most of which are traditional and few are studied extensively in quality randomized controlled trials (RCTs) [25, 130]. The choice of therapy should be based on the acuteness, severity, morphology of lesions and type of dermatitis. Additionally, the history of previous treatments may help to assess the patient's compliance and motivation and reveal anxieties towards certain treatment modalities, most commonly corticosteroids.

Acute or mild contact dermatitis should be treated thoroughly and effectively, in order to prevent it from becoming chronic. Sufficient time without contact to irritants and allergens should be planned to allow the restoration of skin barrier and normal reactivity (see Sect. 49.4). If acute contact dermatitis persists with the tendency to become sub-acute or chronic, special attention is required to rule out additional irritants or allergens, which could be present in the home/recreational or occupational environment. A change in the environment, such as hospital admission, can be helpful. A patient's compliance with the treatment and the prescribed prevention measures should also be considered. The possibility of sensitization to treatment modalities (topical corticosteroids, topical antihistamines or other ingredients of emollients and topical medicinal products) should be investigated.

In many instances, for example irritant or allergic hand eczema and persistent light reaction, the dermatitis has the tendency to persist, even when all conceivable triggering causes have been removed. The term "persistent post-occupational dermatitis", with pertinent criteria [111, 136], has been proposed for the subset of patients with occupationally related disease onset, but such cases are likely to exist also in non-occupational contact dermatitis.

49.3.1 Basic Topical Therapy

The basic topical therapy is a key component in the treatment of dermatitis. It helps to reduce inflammation and itching, has corticosteroid-sparing effects and promotes recovery. In numerous experimental studies, it has been

Table 49.1 General principles and effects of basic topical therapy in contact dermatitis, based on disease acuteness and morphology [25]

Type	Desired effect	Topical therapy
Acute	Drying, astringent, antibacterial	"Moist on moist", hand baths and soaks, moisturizing or moist dressings; wet dressings with saline, aluminium acetate (Burrow's solution), potassium permanganate (stains nails and skin), silver nitrate (0.1%, stains black); tannin-based synthetic agents; alcohol-based tinctures, lotio alba, pasta exsiccans; dyes; topical antiseptics in case of superinfection; when hand dermatitis is combined with hyperhidrosis – aluminium chloride hexahydrate, tap-water ionophoresis, botulinum toxin type A
Sub-acute	Anti-inflammatory, antipruritic, moisturizing	Tar and ichthyol preparations, Polidocanol and urea-based preparations, moisturizing water-in-oil and oil-in-water emulsions
Chronic	Keratolytic, anti-proliferative, moisturizing	Keratolytic ointments (salicylic acid up to 20%, urea 10–20%); rich ointments, including water-in-oil and oil-in-water emulsions; glycerin-based creams; Tar and ichthyol preparations, fissures: hydrocolloid dressing, argentum nitricum

shown to promote the healing of irritant and allergic contact dermatitis, without any other treatment [21, 104]. The basic topical therapy should be adjusted according to disease severity, acuteness, body area affected and stage of evolution. The general principles of dermatological therapy, such as "moist on moist", should be observed. Table 49.1 summarizes the effects and general recommendations for the use of basic topical therapy in contact dermatitis [25]. The basic topical therapy may be underestimated by patients and physicians as "bland" and without active ingredients. The result of such an attitude may be a reduced compliance, application that is inadequate or in insufficient quantity, ultimately compromising treatment [80]. Emollients should be continued even after the visible signs of dermatitis have subsided, because the functional derangements, including barrier dysfunction, take longer to heal – see below Sect. 49.4.

Core Message

> ❯ The basic topical therapy is a key component in the management of dermatitis. Its inadequate or insufficient application ultimately compromises treatment.

For an acute dermatitis, hand baths, wet dressings and soaks with solutions, which have astringent and drying effects, are recommended. Such solutions are saline, aluminium acetate (Burrow's solution, may cause irritation if used longer than 3 days [1]), potassium permanganate (e.g. 4 times a day to soak for vesiculobullous eruptions; stains the skin and nails brown, but has

excellent drying and antiseptic effects) and synthetic tannins [40]. Apart from reducing exudation, these wet dressings and soaks help soften and remove dried crusts and scales. The cooling effect is also beneficial, but the risk of hypothermia, when applied over large areas, should be considered. Bullae should be drained, without removing the roof. Topical antiseptics are used in cases of superinfection or when bacterial colonization may be an aggravating factor. Because of the risk of sensitization and bacterial resistance, preference is given to antiseptic solutions such as potassium permanganate, over topical antibiotics. Additional options include chlorhexidine, octenidine, clioquinol, etc. A variety of combined preparations with cortocosteroids are available, but the use of every particular component and especially topical antibiotic should be clearly indicated. In cases of clinical signs of infection, systemic antibiotics are indicated. In patients with atopic and non-atopic hand eczema, without clinical signs of pyodermia, corticosteroids alone reduce or eliminate colonization with *Staphylococcus aureus* [93]. When hand dermatitis is combined with hyperhidrosis, aluminium chloride hexahydrate and tap water ionophoresis are recommended, and there are reports of a beneficial effect of botulinum toxin type A (reviewed in [146]).

In sub-acute dermatitis, the topical therapy should possess anti-inflammatory, antipruritic and moisturizing effects. Urea- and polidocanol-based topical therapies are recommended. Contact allergy to polidocanol has been reported, especially in elderly patients with lower leg dermatitis [42, 126]. Ichthyol and tar preparations have additional anti-proliferative effects. However, tar preparations contain pyrenes with established animal carcinogenicity. In addition to their cutaneous

49

effects, increased systemic exposure correlates with the total amount applied and body area treated, rather than the barrier impairment [132].

In chronic dermatitis, rich moisturizing ointments are indicated. Keratolytic ointments are used in cases with hyperkeratosis, such as tylotic hand eczema. The anti-proliferative effects of the tar preparations make them useful here as well. Fissures frequently form in chronic dermatitis. They are painful, heal slowly and can be entry points for infection. Softening the epidermis and sealing the fissures improve pain and recovery.

49.3.2 Specific Therapies

The variety of specific therapies is presented in Fig. 49.1. A stepwise approach is advised, with more potent and systemic therapies reserved for more severe, more widespread, recalcitrant or chronic cases [25].

49.3.2.1 Topical Corticosteroids

Topical corticosteroids are the primary treatment and widely used for both allergic and irritant contact dermatitis. Their use is traditional and the evidence, conforming to the standards of modern-day evidence-based medicine, is insufficient. Their application in ICD has been subject to debate, with some authors reporting no benefit [78, 131] and others the opposite [75, 103]. Some consider them as providing only symptomatic relief in ICD [1]. Nevertheless, the topical steroids are well established in the clinical practice of treating both irritant and allergic contact dermatitis.

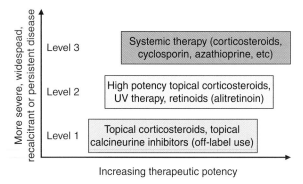

Fig. 49.1 Treatment options for contact dermatitis, in relation to disease severity

The choice of a particular product should balance the potency with the undesirable effects. To help guide such decisions, a therapeutic index (TIX) has been developed and made available online [84, 85]. Corticosteroids with higher TIX (group 2, TIX >2) have a more favourable ratio of potency to undesirable effects, while group 1 corticosteroids have a less favourable ratio (TIX <2). Usually, the group 2 preparations with the TIX >2 should be chosen. However, in acute and severe episodes it is advisable to use sufficiently potent topical corticosteroids to quickly suppress the inflammation, even though they have a lower TIX. They should be given for short periods and tapered quickly or replaced with corticosteroids with higher TIX. Additionally, in chronic dermatitis with lichenification and hyperkeratosis such as tylotic hand eczema, treatment with the most potent corticosteroids is also indicated, because of their anti-proliferative effects and presumed lower penetration [25]. On the other hand, in intertriginous and flexural areas, as well as on the face, mild-strength corticosteroids should be used. Interval and intermittent dosing regiments help to reduce the corticosteroid load and undesirable effects. For chronic hand eczema, such regimens, for example administration of potent corticosteroids only on the weekends or every other day, are shown to be safe as the long-term maintenance (up to 36 weeks) [133]. Combining topical corticosteroids with other treatment modalities may also shorten the period of application and reduce the corticosteroid load.

The topical corticosteroids are available in different vehicles, such as lotions, creams and ointments, and the choice should be guided by the acuteness and morphology of lesions, like in the basic topical therapy. It should be kept in mind that the same corticosteroid-active ingredients may have different potency in the different vehicles.

In addition to the well-known side effects of topical corticosteroids, they may induce atrophy and impair skin barrier regeneration (see below, Sect. 49.4.3). This makes them inappropriate in conditions where the contact with irritants cannot be completely excluded. Emollients may help decrease the negative effects of corticosteroids on skin barrier repair [52]. Another drawback is tachyphylaxis, where patients grow less responsive to topical steroids.

Contact sensitization to the corticosteroids or other ingredients of the topical therapy should be considered, if the condition worsens or persists (reviewed in [63]). Hypersensitivity to corticosteroids is reported to affect up to 5% of patients with dermatitis [143], but the frequency varies among countries and corticosteroids [127]. It is not easy to suspect sensitization because of the anti-inflammatory effect of the corticosteroid, but it may lead to recurrence or deterioration of dermatitis, sustained chronic inflammation, as well as other manifestations [63, 64]. Patch testing requires late readings, up to 7 days [127]. The topical corticosteroids are divided into four groups, with the cross-reactivity being low between the groups and high within [63].

49.3.2.2 Topical Calcineurin Inhibitors

The topical calcineurin inhibitors (TCIs) provide a needed alternative to corticosteroids in atopic dermatitis and other conditions [83]. Their most valuable advantage is their safety over long-term usage, without the induction of atrophy or interference with barrier repair (see below Sect. 49.4.3). TCIs are shown to be beneficial in experimental human models with Ni-induced ACD [102] and SLS-induced ICD [31, 47]. Their anti-inflammatory potency has been approximated to that of lower mid-strength corticosteroids, such as 0.1% hydrocortisone butyrate or 0.1% betamethasone-17-valerate [102, 113]. Further evidence from RCTs is needed to prove efficacy in contact dermatitis.

There are several studies in chronic hand eczema [113, 123] (reviewed in [83]) where TCI showed good therapeutic effects worthy of further study in large RCTs. As TCIs may not penetrate well through hyperkeratosis, in some of the studies they were applied under occlusion, for example twice daily with overnight occlusion [9]. In psoriasis, a TCI has been applied with 6% salicylic acid to enhance penetration and potency [83]. In addition to chronic hand eczema, there are individual case observations of good efficacy in chronic actinic dermatitis (CAD) [83].

TCIs are topical immunomodulators and should not be used when skin infections are present. Additionally, a small fraction of chronic hand eczema patients experienced burning or stinging, erythema or worsening under treatment [113]. Concerns regarding potential photocarcinogenicity have been raised, because of such established effects of systemic immunosuppressive therapy in organ transplant recipients and animal data on topical preparations. An expert review concluded that such concerns are not corroborated by the available data from animal and human studies [107]. They also concluded that combination of TCI and UV therapy is acceptable

and may be useful. Nevertheless, UV protection, such as sunscreens and appropriate clothing, is advisable in patients undergoing TCI treatment [107], and the warning against skin exposure to UV during TCI treatment, including UV and PUVA therapy, is not amended in the official prescribing information [18].

49.3.2.3 Retinoids

Alitretinoin (9-cis-retinoic acid) is a retinoid with a distinct clinical profile [12]. It has proven efficacy for the treatment of severe chronic hand eczema, unresponsive to standard therapy. With more than 2,000 patients included in different controlled trials, it is the therapy for chronic hand eczema with the highest level of evidence [25]. It is unknown why alitretinoin, in contrast to other closely related retinoids, is efficient in chronic eczema, but one suggested reason is its characteristic receptor-binding profile [12]. It binds with high affinity to all RAR and RXR receptor types [19]. Alitretinoin has anti-inflammatory and immunomodulatory effects, and similarly to other retinoids, inhibits proliferation and enhances differentiation, but in contrast to them, has minimal drying effect.

In the largest clinical trial with 1,032 patients, alitretinoin, given at 30 mg once daily after breakfast for 24 weeks, led to a "clear" or "almost clear" outcome in 48% of patients with severe hand eczema unresponsive to standard therapy [110]. Partial response was achieved by 62% of patients. The curve of patients achieving the "clear" or "almost clear" response did not reach plateau for 200 days, indicating that continued therapy may bring further benefit. The remission was sustained, with 65% being free of recurrence at 6 months. Median time to relapse was 5.5 months. The most frequent adverse effect was headache (20%), leading to 4% withdrawal. Headache was reported in the first 10 days and resolved without alitretinoin discontinuation [25]. Additional class effects were the mucocutaneous effects and dryness (noted at a lower incidence than with other retinoids), decreased TSH levels and hyperlipidemia [110].

Concerns have been raised that the degree of alitretinoin efficacy and the duration of remission might have been overstated, and that trials directly comparing alitretinoin with other treatment options are not yet available [62]. Nevertheless, and especially given the general level of evidence for the other treatment modalities in chronic hand eczema, alitretinoin stands out as

49

the best studied one so far. It is the only systemic treatment for chronic hand dermatitis, approved by the regulatory drug agencies in several European countries.

Alitretinoin is considered suitable for the long-term management of hand eczema. Patients with high blood lipids should be given 10 mg. It is teratogenic, and the necessary precautions are the same as with isotretinoin. Contraception is required up to 1 month after the therapy cessation.

Topical bexarotene, oral acitretin and etretinate [106] have also been tried in chronic hand eczema with less success. A study concluded that topical bexarotene had potential use in severe chronic hand dermatitis. A high rate of treatment-related irritation was reported (29%) [56]. Oral acitretin led to 50% average improvement in the clinical score in patients with tylotic eczema for 4 weeks, with no additional improvement with longer treatment. It might be studied in combination with other therapeutic agents [124].

Core Message

> Alitretinoin is the therapy for chronic hand eczema with the highest level of evidence.

49.3.2.4 Phototherapy

Different phototherapy modalities are well established in the treatment of eczematous diseases such as atopic dermatitis. They are also traditionally used in contact dermatitis (mainly chronic hand eczema) and photoallergic contact dermatitis, but of the many published studies, few are well-controlled and usually the number of patients is small. Broad- and narrow-band UVB, PUVA and UVA1 therapies have shown good results in chronic hand eczema. Phototherapy has a favourable effect on skin barrier function (see below Sect. 49.4.3). There is accumulated clinical experience with broad-band UVB and PUVA. UVA1 and narrow-band UVB are insufficiently studied in contact dermatitis in order to be recommended [14].

Currently, PUVA with topical psoralens is mostly used (cream-, gel-, bath- or paint-PUVA) with the advantage that only a small part of the body is subjected to psoralens and irradiation, with no systemic symptoms and systemic phototoxicity. Different protocols are employed and guidelines are available online [61]. For example, soaking of patients' hands in a psoralen solution for 15 min followed by UVA, 4 times per week, starting with 0.5 J/cm^2 and increasing with 0.5–1.0 J/cm^2 every third procedure until slight erythema [112]. Under such regimen, 93% of the patients with dyshidrotic and 86% of the patients with hyperkeratotic eczema achieved excellent or very good results [112]. Hyperkeratotic eczema was less responsive than dyshidrotic eczema, took more procedures to clear (mean 14.5, range 8–25; vs. mean 12.4, range 7–25) and needed higher cumulative UV dosage (mean 27.9 vs. 21.4 J/cm^2). In another study with three or four procedures weekly for 8 weeks, half of the patients with dyshidrosis showed complete remission [8]. Remissions have different durations; some report a mean of 6 months [112].

Both UVB and PUVA regimens may be carcinogenic, and long-term application or usage as maintenance therapy should be avoided. Topical PUVA is plausibly less carcinogenic than oral PUVA. Some patients may develop irregular patchy blistering or sunburn-reactions and consecutive hyperpigmentations in the treated areas. This is related to the method of psoralen application (bath PUVA gives a more uniform psoralen distribution than paint-PUVA). Erythema in PUVA appears later than in UVB regimens and reaches its peak 72–96 h post-exposure; thus frequent PUVA regimen, such as daily regimens, may lead to severe cumulative phototoxicity.

UVA1 is considered to be less carcinogenic than PUVA and UVB [99], but as the long-term safety is unknown, only two treatment cycles per year are recommended [97]. Good results with long remissions are reported with mid- and high-dose regimens. For example, 40 J/cm^2 5 times per week for 3 weeks (~600 J/cm^2 per treatment cycle) [99, 114], or 5 times per week for 3 weeks with increasing dosages, cumulative 1720 J/cm^2 [97].

UV-free phototherapy has been developed and is expected to be non-carcinogenic. It was reported to be effective in atopic hand and foot eczema, but further studies in efficacy and safety are needed [73].

Phototherapy can be combined with other treatments, for example topical corticosteroids or retinoids, to speed up the effect and lower the total UV dosage [120]. Combinations with systemic immunosuppressants are not recommended because of increased carcinogenicity. As a precaution against possible similar effects, combinations with TCIs are warned against in the TCIs' official prescribing information. A common drawback for phototherapies is that special facilities are required which are not always available, even more so for UVA1 therapy. Patients find it problematic to schedule regular visits within the normal working hours and to travel to the facilities. PUVA with portable home-UVA devices [129] and phototherapy with portable UBV devices [7] have been proposed, but may lead to serious safety concerns.

49.3.2.5 Ionizing Radiation Therapy

Two modalities of radiotherapy, Grenz rays and superficial X-rays, have been reported as effective treatments of refractory chronic hand eczema, less frequently for plantar eczema [32] (reviewed in [82, 91]). With the availability of other treatment options, it is considered that radiotherapy is currently justifiable only in exceptional cases and in older patients [14]. However, it is used more widely in some countries and less or not at all in others and the opinions vary. While radiation therapy for this indication is regarded as obsolete by some, according to others, the Grenz rays modality is a simple, affordable, effective, and ultimately, still a valid option [137]. A recent UK guidance [91] advises that it should be used only in the research setting in the UK. It was found that Grenz rays were not used in the UK since 1980s, as they were replaced by better therapies. While some consider the Grenz rays therapy to be an established practice, others have the opinion that if it is to be used again in the UK, it should be "regarded as novel and of uncertain safety and efficacy" [91].

Of the two radiotherapy modalities, Grenz rays were preferably used over superficial X-rays as they are safer (do not penetrate deeper than the skin). In a double-blind study with 25 patients, superficial X-rays were found to be more effective than Grenz rays, probably because of their deeper penetration (half-value layer of 13 mm in tissue vs. 0.4 mm for Grenz rays) [33]. The protocol was 1 Gy (100 rad) of superficial X-rays vs. 3 Gy (300 rad) of Grenz rays, 3 times at 21 days intervals. Superficial X-rays showed better results at 3, 6, 12 and 18 weeks after therapy initiation. Because of the carcinogenicity risks, the authors estimated that up to three courses like the above with superficial X-rays and up to five courses like the above with Grenz rays are permissible for lifetime [33]. Other protocols are also reported from different studies, with the greatest clinical improvement being most evident usually several weeks after therapy commencement. The major disadvantage of radiotherapy is the carcinogenic risk. Other adverse events are erythema and hyperpigmentation. More severe local adverse events could be induced in the event of overdosage. Additionally, radiotherapy requires specially licenced facilities and personnel.

49.3.2.6 Systemic Corticosteroids and Immunosuppressive Agents

Systemic corticosteroids may be required in extensive or severe acute contact dermatitis and exacerbations of chronic disease, usually short-term 0.5–1 mg/kg/day prednisolone equivalent with quick tapering. The long-term or frequent use is not indicated in contact dermatitis due to their well-known side effects.

There is accumulated clinical experience in dermatology with immunosuppressants such as azathioprine, methotrexate, cyclosporin and others. They are traditionally used for a variety of indications, either alone or as corticosteroid-sparing agents. There is limited evidence for their effectiveness in contact dermatitis.

Cyclosporin is reported to be beneficial in chronic hand eczema [46, 105]. In a double-blind study with 41 patients, 3 mg/kg/day of cyclosporin for 6 weeks was as effective as topical betamethasone dipropionate, leading to 57% reduction in disease severity score [46]. More experience is available with atopic dermatitis and guidelines for the use of cyclosporin in dermatology have been developed [89, 115]. Therapy with cyclosporin should be conducted for up to 6 months at the minimal effective dose, with a following 3 months tapering. In some patients, longer therapy may be required, whereas in good responders earlier discontinuation is advisable. If no clinical response is observed for 8 weeks, cyclosporin should be withdrawn. In some studies on atopic dermatitis, higher initial doses (4–5 mg/kg/day) were used to achieve faster response, but after satisfactory improvement the dosage should be reduced to the individual minimal effective dose [115]. Gastrointestinal symptoms, infections, paraesthesia and headaches are most frequently reported. These, in addition to the elevated blood pressure and the reversibly elevated serum creatinine, are dose-related, usually in doses higher than

49

3 mg/kg/day [115]. Blood pressure and serum creatinine should be monitored.

Increased cancer risk is well known for the long-term and higher dosage of cyclosporin, such as with organ transplant recipients. It is also documented for patients with previous exposure to carcinogens, such as PUVA or methotrexate [86]. Patients with psoriasis, who had undergone previous PUVA therapy above a certain threshold, had an increased skin cancer risk even with short-term use of cyclosporin [86]. Cyclosporin should not be combined with UV therapy and be used in patients who have significant cumulative life-long UV exposure (the data are insufficient to back-up specific recommendations). The cyclosporin-related risk of malignancies might be expected to be low for the dermatological patients, since they are usually treated with shorter courses and lower doses and if they have no previous significant UV or other carcinogenic exposures. However, not enough long-term data are available [128].

Azathioprine is used alone or as a corticosteroid-sparing agent. There is efficacy evidence from small RCTs in airborne contact dermatitis and CAD. Parthenium dermatitis is the commonest airborne contact dermatitis in India [135], because the Parthenium weeds are widespread and complete avoidance of the allergen is not always possible. Azathioprine 100 mg daily was as effective as a systemic corticosteroid (betamethasone 2 mg daily) over a period of 6 months in a double-blind RCT with 41 patients. The azathioprine arm had fewer side effects and fewer (but not statistically significant) relapses after 6 months post-treatment. A dose regimen of 300 mg azathioprine once weekly pulses has also been proposed for this indication [134]. A double-blind RCT of azathioprine vs. placebo with only 18 patients demonstrated the efficacy of azathioprine in CAD [90]. Of the eight patients on active therapy, five achieved full remission and the study was terminated prematurely because of the un-blinding due to the different efficacy, confirmed by the statistical analysis. In another single-group observational study, 14 CAD patients were treated with 100–200 mg daily dosage of azathioprine. There are also anecdotal reports of good results in pompholyx.

The late onset of clinical effect, after 4–8 weeks, is one of the main drawbacks of azathioprine. The bone marrow and hepatotoxicity are the most important side effects. The effectiveness and toxicity of azathioprine are related to the activity of the enzyme thyopurine methyltransferase (TPMP), one of the three inactivation pathways. The current guidelines recommend its measurement before treatment initiation [3, 145]. Due to genetic polymorphisms, 11% of the population have intermediate TPMP activity and are predisposed to toxic effects, and 1 in 300 people has low or no activity and is susceptible to life-threatening pancytopenia; other frequencies are also reported [3]. Patients with low activity should not receive azathioprine, those with intermediate can be given 1 mg/kg/day with careful monitoring and those with normal activity (88% of population) up to 2 mg/kg/day. People with higher than normal activity are likely to be non-responders and require more aggressive dosing [145]. Other dosage recommendations are also available [3]. Inhibition of the other inactivation pathways, which may be caused either by drugs such as xanthine oxidase inhibitors (allopurinol) and others, or by genetic variability, can lead to azathioprine toxicity like in the intermediate group. Therefore, dosing based on TPMP pre-treatment activity does not exclude the possibility of myelosuppression and regular monitoring is necessary, such as weekly CBC and serum liver enzymes for the first 4 weeks or until maintenance dose is achieved, then as a minimum once in 3 months [3]. The risk of malignancy in non-transplant patients is low, but may increase with longer azathioprine application, especially in patients with significant UV exposure [145].

Due to the limited data on the use of methotrexate, mycophenolate mofetil and other immunosuppressive agents in contact dermatitis, they cannot be viewed as standard therapy and should be reserved for special cases.

Methotrexate is well established in the clinical practice of dermatology. It has been reported in case series of patients with unresponsive hand dermatitis [27] and other types of recalcitrant eczema [117]. Good results were achieved with a range of initiation doses between 5 and 20 mg weekly after 1–2 months of therapy. Longer maintenance therapy with the lowest effective doses such as 2.5 or 5 mg weekly is advised in one of the reports [117]. The general safety precautions with methotrexate therapy should be observed, such as monitoring the serum liver enzymes and CBC, as well as the cumulative dosage. Mycophenolate mofetil is reported to be effective in an individual case of dyshidrotic eczema [98].

49.3.2.7 Other Treatment Approaches

For the management of cases where complete avoidance of the allergen is impossible, hyposensitization has been attempted, but the published studies have produced conflicting results, and it is not a standard therapy. A RCT on oral nickel hyposensitization with 30 patients demonstrated significant reduction of circulating lymphocytes responsive to nickel, but no effect on the clinical parameters [4]. Both beneficial effects and no effects are reported in earlier studies [82]. Successful hyposensitization in plant dermatitis, for example parthenium dermatitis [55], has also been reported.

Disodium chromoglycate and other agents have been investigated, but are not used in clinical practice. There are publications on psychological support and cognitive relaxation techniques [82].

49.4 Restore the Skin Barrier

The treatment of contact dermatitis is incomplete without measures to restore the skin barrier. The permeability barrier function of the skin is chiefly localized in the stratum corneum (SC) [30], and its functional integrity is related to SC thickness, hydration and lipid content. The barrier function of the skin is severely impaired during an episode of irritant or allergic contact dermatitis. Its recovery may take a long period of time, and this should be addressed in the treatment strategy. Additionally, when allowed to persist, the disruption of the skin barrier induces a chronic increase in inflammatory cytokines, leading to inflammation and epidermal proliferation [100] (see Chap. 6). Acceleration of barrier repair is shown to improve epidermal hyperplasia [22]. The recovery time, the effects of moisturizers, the influence on the barrier repair of the different modalities used in the treatment of dermatitis, and the additional factors affecting the recovery of the barrier function are reviewed separately below.

Core Message

> The treatment of contact dermatitis is incomplete without measures to restore the skin barrier.

49.4.1 Recovery Time

The recovery time is better studied with ICD than ACD. The complete healing of ICD has been defined as the following [76]

1. Clinically normal skin
2. Return to normal of the quantitative parameters, as measured by bioengineering instruments
3. Functional normality, including loss of irritability

Core Message

> The complete recovery of irritant contact dermatitis requires not only clinically normal skin, but also functional normality, including return to normal skin physiology and loss of irritability.

The above three objectives of the treatment of dermatitis are not achieved simultaneously. The time periods needed to quench the inflammation and restore the different bioengineering parameters are unequal and vary among individuals and dermatitis-eliciting agents. In studies with sodium-lauryl-sulphate (SLS)-induced acute irritant reactions, the times to recovery correlate with SLS exposure (in terms of time and concentration). After acute irritation with a 1% SLS patch test for 24 h in healthy volunteers, the bioengineering parameters of the skin returned to normal, without treatment, after 9 days [43]. Repeated shorter exposures to SLS model better the cumulative irritant dermatitis seen in clinical practice. In studies using such exposures, the parameters returned to normal after 14 days [20], 20–23 days [142], and up to after 4 weeks [76]. The different bioengineering parameters do not follow coincident time-courses, even more with the different irritants [39]. Some irritants, such as SLS in the chronic cumulative elicitation model, lead to erythema that persists longer than the elevation of TEWL, while other irritants, such as potassium soap, induced elevation of trans-epidermal water loss (TEWL) with no erythema [142].

Even after both the visual assessment of the skin and the bioengineering parameters are back to normal,

49

sub-clinical irritation may persist, resulting in augmented reactivity to re-challenge with irritants. Freeman and Maibach [41] reported that a re-challenge 1 week after initial acute ICD, elicited with 24 h SLS patch test, leads to higher TEWL in most patients and at most sites than the initial irritation. At the time of re-challenge, the erythematous reactions of the initial irritation had subsided and TEWL levels were close to normal. The authors concluded that although the skin may look healed, it had a functional impairment that made it more irritable than at baseline. They used the metaphor that the clinically evident dermatitis is only the tip of the iceberg of functional derangement. They also observed high variability among persons and body sites, with 5 out of 34 testings (in 11 volunteers) exhibiting a hardening phenomenon (lower TEWL on re-challenge). In later studies and with cumulative irritation, mimicking chronic ICD, both hypo- [141] and hyper- [20, 41] reactivity are reported in different time points, up to 9 and 10 weeks after the elicitation of dermatitis. The clinical relevance of these results is not straightforward, but the common conclusion is that a functional impairment of the skin persists long after the clinical and bioengineering parameters are normal, and that recovery time is longer in chronic as compared to acute contact dermatitis. It is also not clear to what extent the augmented reactivity is due to barrier-related mechanisms alone and thus whether it can be mitigated with therapies targeted at barrier repair.

The barrier dysfunction is also well documented in ACD, although it is less studied than in ICD. Usually, a 48 h nickel patch test in sensitized individuals is employed. In one such study the TEWL after ACD was still elevated 5 days after ACD, but emollient treatment significantly ameliorated it [21]. In another study with a similar dermatitis-provoking procedure, the barrier impairment after ACD was still present after 10 days in the placebo-treated areas [149]. Altered reactivity has also been observed in ACD. Increased reactivity (compared to baseline) to re-challenge with allergens has been demonstrated up to 8 months after ACD, but these late responses are attributable to immune memory rather than to the barrier dysfunction [59]. As to the barrier function, it has been shown that after irritation with a surfactant between 6 and 30 h before Ni-patch testing, ACD can be elicited with lower allergen concentrations, than in non-irritated skin [2]. It is, therefore, considered that restored

barrier function is required to diminish the exposure and penetration of allergens. Additionally, many allergens also have irritant properties and real-life situation usually involves the combined action of irritants and allergens [96].

There is accumulated evidence that after an episode of dermatitis, the permeability barrier remains disrupted for a long time. The generalization of recovery times found in experimental studies may not be straightforward, given the complexities of real-life situations, the mixed nature of action of eliciting agents and the variability of intensity, duration and body-surface area exposed. Nonetheless, the prevailing opinion is that it takes weeks to months to restore the barrier function of the skin and extended work leave may be necessary. For example, a study of tertiary individual prevention foresees a period of 6 weeks (3 weeks inpatient treatment, followed by additional 3 weeks off-work) for patients with chronic occupational contact dermatitis [119]. Further research is needed into the duration of barrier recovery after contact dermatitis in the clinical practice.

> **Core Message**
>
> › Weeks to months are necessary for the recovery of the skin barrier function after an episode of dermatitis. The recovery time is longer in chronic as compared to acute contact dermatitis.

49.4.2 The Effect of Moisturizers on Barrier Repair

The terms "moisturizers" and "emollients" are used synonymously in this chapter. They are frequently prescribed to help restore the skin barrier. There are multiple examples of moisturizers accelerating the barrier function recovery after irritant or allergic contact dermatitis.

Emollients are not always, and in all circumstances, beneficial for the skin barrier. Of note, there is no clear distinction between moisturizers that are used to restore the barrier after irritant trauma and the barrier creams used to prevent CD before the contact with the causative agents [58]. The preventive effect of barrier creams on hand eczema is reviewed in

Chap. 47. It has been shown that moisturizers and barrier creams may be harmful to the skin barrier function. Application of a moisturizer 3 times per day for 4 weeks in healthy volunteers led to increased susceptibility to SLS-induced irritation [58]. There are additional examples of moisturizers, including barrier creams intended to prevent ICD, which actually exacerbate the irritant effects [44]. In a study comparing five emollients applied for 7 weeks, four of them increased and only one decreased the susceptibility to irritation with SLS [16]. Similar effects have been observed with ACD. In a comparison between two moisturizers, the one with poorer hydrating properties (without humectants and free fatty acids) increased the skin barrier damage after 3 weeks pre-treatment in an ACD model with 48 h Ni-patch test in sensitized volunteers [53]. In another study, pre-treatment for only 7 days with a 70% lipid-rich moisturizer led to more-intense reactions to Ni-patch tests in sensitized individuals [147]. These and others examples, however, refer to pre-treatment with emollients of healthy skin, before the contact with the provoking agent. As to the recovery of the skin barrier after an episode of dermatitis, there is no doubt that moisturizers are beneficial, given that the basic principles of topical therapy are observed (see Sect. 46.3.1). It has been hypothesized that the pre-treatment with moisturizers might possibly lead to down-regulation of the lipid production in skin, and therefore, interfere with barrier recovery, but the experimental data do not corroborate this hypothesis [58].

There are multiple characteristics of the moisturizers that determine their effect on barrier repair. The mechanisms behind these effects are more or less unclear, but there are accumulated efficacy data regarding the following emollient characteristics: occlusive properties, constitution of emollients (lipid content, inclusion of humectants and other ingredients) and pH.

> **Core Message**
>
> › The emollients are key components in the therapy of contact dermatitis and the skin barrier function restoration.

49.4.2.1 Occlusive Properties

The increased TEWL after barrier disruption is a signal triggering the barrier-repair mechanisms, including lipid and DNA synthesis and keratinocyte proliferation [100]. Artificial repair of the barrier, such as occlusion with water-impermeable membranes, inhibits the increase in the lipid and DNA synthesis [35, 100] and barrier recovery. In contrast, semi-occlusive water-permeable membranes allow normal repair [49]. While keeping the epidermis moist and preventing dryness are essential for the healing process, preserving the transdermal water flux is also necessary [49]. Moisturizers exert their effects not only through the actions of their individual ingredients, but also by providing optimal occlusion.

Additionally, occlusion is studied regarding the penetration of allergens and irritants. Occlusion alone disrupts the skin barrier in healthy skin, and many studies have shown enhanced irritation and sensitization under occlusion such as under gloves (reviewed in [148]).

49.4.2.2 Lipids Content

The lipid content of the SC is a key component of the barrier function of the skin. Externally applied moisturizers may contain either physiological or non-physiological lipids, or both. The lipid composition is shown to affect the gene expression of lipid-processing enzymes in the skin [17]. The three major classes of physiologic skin lipids are cholesterol, ceramides and free fatty acids, and their relative quantities in the skin need to be in balance for the normal barrier function and recovery. For example, lower amounts of certain lipids (ceramide 1, ceramide 6I and 6II) in healthy volunteers correspond to a lowered threshold to experimental irritation [67]. The application of non-physiological lipids, such as petrolatum, occludes the skin and leads to a quick but temporary and incomplete improvement in barrier function. The non-physiologic lipids do not enter the endogenous system of lipid synthesis and secretion. In contrast, physiologic lipids and their precursors do not have an immediate effect on barrier function. However, they have a "delayed" effect indicating increased improvement of barrier repair [45]. They can enter the endogenous system of lipid synthesis and secretion, and hence, interfere with the balance of lipids. Therefore, the ratio of

49

the three lipid classes (cholesterol, ceramides and free fatty acids) in the formulation is crucial. Application of only one or two of the three components actually delays the barrier recovery [36]. The three classes need to be present in an approximately equimolar ratio (1:1:1) for the barrier repair to proceed normally [29]. The barrier recovery can be further enhanced by increasing any one of the components to a 3:1:1 ratio [29]. However, certain diseases have inherent abnormalities in the SC lipid production with a deficit in one of the lipid classes. In such cases, supplying that particular lipid by making it the dominant one in the topical formulation brings the highest benefit. For example, in ageing dry skin cholesterol synthesis is decreased and a cholesterol-dominant 3:1:1 mixture improves barrier repair, while fatty acid dominant mixture impedes it [36, 45]. Likewise, in atopic patients ceramides are insufficient and ceramide-dominant mixture is most beneficial [36, 45]. Such effects of the physiological lipids are dependent on the proper functioning of the endogenous lipid production and secretion system. In clinical conditions where this system is impaired, such as after sunburn, irritant dermatitis due to certain surfactants or retinoids and radiation dermatitis, the physiological lipids would not be able to exert their effects and non-physiological lipids should be preferred [36].

The effect of lipid content has been studied mainly in experimentally induced dermatitis. Its clinical relevance in the treatment of contact dermatitis remains to be proved. For example, a study with 30 chronic hand dermatitis patients did not observe superiority of an emollient with physiological lipids over a petrolatum-based one. In addition to the small sample size, a possible reason could be that the efficacy of physiological lipids may be related both to a specific external damage and to endogenous deficiencies [74].

49.4.2.3 Humectants and Other Ingredients

Humectants are usually added to moisturizers in order to increase the SC hydration [80]. Many topical preparations with claims to improve barrier recovery contain humectants, ingredients used in wound healing, vitamins, antioxidants, plant-derived compounds and others. The usefulness of such preparations is rarely proven in large RCTs with patients, but there are multiple reports from studies with experimentally induced irritation or barrier disruption or ACD in volunteers. Many more are studied only in experimental conditions with animals or skin organ cultures. The effects of some of the multitudinous compounds are summarized in Table 49.2. It should be noted that the effects of the below-mentioned compounds may be dependent on their concentrations and vehicles.

Table 49.2 Effects of various topically applied compounds on the barrier recovery [22, 23, 80]

Improve barrier repair	Delay barrier repair
Glycerol	–
Urea	–
Panthenol	–
Tocopheryl acetate	–
Alpha hydroxyacids	–
Niacinamide (nicotinamide, vitamin B(3))	–
Sodium salts of anionic polymers	Sodium salts of cationic polymers
Sodium-exchange resins	Chloride-exchange resin
Barium sulphate with a negative ζ potential	Barium sulphate with a positive ζ potential
Magnesium and calcium ions	Calcium ions
Magnesium ions (chloride, sulphate, lactate)	Potassium ions
Copper chloride	–
Chitin-glucan	–
–	Androgens (testosterone, androsterone), their effects are blocked by estradiol
–	Progesterone, its effects are enhanced by estradiol
Calcium channel blockers	Calcium channel agonists
H1 and H2 blockers	Histamine
nNOS inhibition, decrease of intracellular cGMP production; guanylyl cyclase inhibitors	Nitric oxide and increase in intracellular cGMP production
Caffeine (in men)	–
Trypsin-like serine protease inhibitors	–
Plasminogen activator inhibitors	–

Humectants like glycerol [37], urea, panthenol and others [80] were shown to improve barrier repair. Close to 200 compounds are used for skin hydration, but hydration and improved dryness do not always lead to better barrier function [80]. For example, 15% glycolic acid has been shown to improve xerosis on the legs, but also to increase TEWL as well as the susceptibility to externally applied irritants [80].

The topical preparations also contain emulsifiers, which may interfere with the structural organization of the cutaneous lipids, and hence, with the barrier function. SLS has been ranked as the most irritant and is used in experimental studies [5]. Although all emulsifiers can be expected to interact with the permeability barrier, non-ionic emulsifiers are considered less-irritant than ionic. Physiologic lipids, such as fatty acid and cholesterol, are also used as emulsifiers [80]. Additionally, large-molecular weight polymeric emulsifiers that cannot penetrate the skin are expected not to influence the barrier function, but may contain low molecular weight monomers [16]. Emulsifiers have been shown to have different effects on TEWL in normal vs. irritated skin [5].

49.4.2.4 pH

The acidic pH values on the skin surface (4–6 in different body sites) and the pH gradient throughout the SC regulate the activation of enzymes involved in lipids processing and desquamation. In experimentally induced barrier disruption in mice, acidic pH allowed normal barrier recovery, while neutral and alkaline pH delayed the process regardless of ions concentrations [54, 88]. In human volunteers, pre-treatment with alkaline moisturizer impaired the skin barrier function after 5 weeks of application and made the skin more susceptible to SLS irritation [70]. On the other hand, a study with experimental SLS barrier disruption in 18 healthy volunteers did not detect differences between acidic (pH 4) and neutral (pH 7) emollients in terms of both barrier repair and irritability by SLS re-challenge [15]. Further research is needed on the clinical relevance of moisturizers' effects on barrier repair in terms of their pH values.

49.4.2.5 Additional Data on Moisturizers

Barrier repair with moisturizers was extensively studied in atopic dermatitis. Different barrier therapies have proven clinical benefit in atopic dermatitis in RCTs (reviewed in [95]). Some of these topical preparations are developed on the basis of the beneficial 3:1:1 ratio of physiologic lipids, others contain humectants and ingredients such as grapevine extract, hyaluronic acid and others. Barrier therapies supplementing the lipid imbalance in atopic dermatitis not only improve the barrier function, but have shown anti-inflammatory efficacy comparable to the lower mid-potency corticosteroid fluticasone propionate 0.05% cream [30, 95].

49.4.3 The Influence on the Barrier Repair of the Different Modalities Used in the Treatment of Dermatitis

The reduction in inflammation and exudation in eczema contributes to the regeneration of the epidermis and the skin barrier, especially in ACD. Therefore, all the anti-inflammatory therapies, such as corticosteroids, calcineurin inhibitors, immunosuppressive agents and others, have the initial effect to improve the barrier function. Apart from such unspecific anti-inflammatory effects, the treatment modalities may exhibit specific effects on the rate of barrier recovery and those are reviewed here.

Additionally, the process known as skin hardening or accommodation makes the skin less sensitive to irritants and prevents further dermatitis reactions with continued exposure. The research into the hardening mechanisms and why some patients instead of hardening develop chronic dermatitis has provided little clinically relevant information so far [138].

> **Core Message**
>
> › The treatment modalities for contact dermatitis influence the barrier function repair. While both topical and systemic corticosteroids and retinoids have negative effects, the topical calcineurin inhibitors allow normal recovery and UV-phototherapy up-regulates the barrier function of the skin.

49

49.4.3.1 Corticosteroids

Both topical and systemic corticosteroids induce epidermal changes leading to impaired barrier function. In different models, the following effects of corticosteroids were demonstrated: SC thinning and reduced epidermal thickness, reduced keratinocyte size, suppression of lipid synthesis and reduction in SC lipid content, inhibition of keratinocyte proliferation, interference with keratinocyte maturation, reduction in corneodesmosomes and cohesion, etc. (reviewed in [116]). Such effects are reported even after short-term (3 days) usage of potent topical steroids [69]. These changes may not be visible, but are considered to be clinically significant [69] because they lead to both increased susceptibility to minor barrier insults and delayed recovery, as demonstrated in experiments with human volunteers [69, 71]. These negative effects can be ameliorated by reducing the corticosteroid load or with the help of emollients. Optimized dosing regiments of topical corticosteroids include intermittent use (e.g. every other day, twice a week or only at weekends), switch from short-term very potent to long-term weaker corticosteroids with better TIX, and rotational therapy (alternation of topical corticosteroid and other treatment modalities) [116]. In experiments with mice, the inhibited lipid synthesis was supplemented by physiologic lipids, applied topically in equimolar concentrations [69]. This was shown to improve or even reverse the negative corticosteroid effects on the barrier function. In experimental ACD in volunteers, a barrier-cream (without physiologic lipids) also improved the delay in barrier recovery [52]. In atopic dermatitis, emollients are shown to reduce topical corticosteroid usage [30].

49.4.3.2 Calcineurin Inhibitors

The influence of calcineurin inhibitors on barrier recovery, in comparison to corticosteroids, has been explored in studies with atopic eczema, SLS barrier disruption in healthy volunteers and in laboratory animals [31, 47, 66]. The calcineurin inhibitors are devoid of the negative effects of corticosteroids and allow the barrier function to recover normally. They lead to no skin atrophy or epidermal thinning, and the lipid formation and bi-layer structures are regular. At the same time, they have no additional benefit over the unspecific anti-inflammatory effects.

49.4.3.3 Phototherapy

The effects of UV irradiation on barrier function differ with time. The acute effect is that of a delayed barrier injury, but the following restoration makes it more resistant. In the long-term, phototherapy increases the risk of photo-ageing and this is considered to have negative effects on barrier function [34].

After a single UV irradiation, there is a delayed barrier disruption with increase in TEWL, followed by gradual restitution. The kinetics depend on factors such as UV type and dosage, skin colour, body site and others [79]. Barrier disruption can be observed not only after a single high UV dose, but also with single and repeated sub-erythematogenic doses [79], which might be dependent on the light source. The delayed barrier injury corresponds to the arrival of damaged keratinocytes at the stratum granulosum/SC junction, which do not synthesize lipids normally ("lamellar body-incompetent cells"), as demonstrated in experiments with mice [60]. Barrier recovery is associated with compensatory increase in lipid synthesis and keratinocyte proliferation [60], as well as accelerated barrier regeneration, inhibited inflammation and increased SC thickness [81]. The compensatory barrier up-regulation may be of clinical benefit for patients with impaired barrier function, such as in contact dermatitis. A study with 30 healthy volunteers demonstrated that UVA or UVB irradiation makes the skin more resistant to SLS irritation [77]. UVA and UVB did not differ in the SLS irritation, but UVB led to thickening of SC, not seen in UVA, and the increase in lipids was less pronounced in UVA. In another study with bath PUVA in patients with various diseases such as psoriasis, vitiligo, mycosis fungoides, etc., the overall effect of 20 min. bathing and PUVA was disrupted barrier and increased susceptibility to SLS irritation within a course of 15 days therapy [81]. However, the barrier function was not investigated after therapy was discontinued and the barrier allowed to recover. Further evidence is needed for the effects of UV radiation on skin barrier in patients with contact dermatitis.

Additionally, the UV radiation-induced changes are age-dependant, with attenuated UVB effects in senescent epidermis, as suggested by experiments with mice [57]. In mice models of photo-ageing, long-term UVA and UVB led to increased TEWL alongside other abnormalities [11].

49.4.3.4 Retinoids

No information is published regarding the barrier function under alitretinoin treatment of contact dermatitis and the available options to improve it. Clinical data can be derived from studies with other conditions and other retinoid compounds.

Retinoids influence proliferation and differentiation of keratinocytes and induce multiple changes, including reduced cohesion and lipid synthesis. When administered topically, they are known as irritants; oral administration induces skin xerosis, fragility and thinning of SC [28]. Both topical and oral administrations disrupt the barrier function of the skin, evident as increased TEWL [122]. However, there are variations among the different retinoids in terms of irritability, TEWL and other bioengineering parameters of barrier dysfunction [38]. The mucocutaneous side effects under oral alitretinoin therapy are reported to be less frequent than with the other retinoids [110], but no specific studies on the barrier function are published.

The negative effects of retinoids on barrier function can be ameliorated by barrier therapies. A double-blind placebo RCT with 60 patients showed that a pre- and concurrent treatment with a topical niacin-derivative can mitigate the barrier impairment and improve tolerance to topical retinoic acid in the treatment of facial photodamage [65]. Similar results are reported from another study, where niacin was combined with panthenol and tocopheryl acetate in a barrier-enhancing cosmetic facial moisturizer [26]. Irritating effects of tazarotene in psoriasis can be ameliorated with topical corticosteroids [121], but this is probably not a good approach in contact dermatitis, given the negative effects of corticosteroids on barrier function.

49.4.4 Other Factors Influencing Barrier Repair

There is an abundance of studies regarding the influence of all sorts of factors on the barrier repair and homeostasis (reviewed in [23]). Additionally, the role of environmental factors on intrinsic weaknesses of the skin barrier is reviewed in Chap. 6.

Barrier dysfunction is inherent to atopic dermatitis and there is enhanced susceptibility to irritants in atopic subjects [1]. Increased susceptibility to developing occupational contact dermatitis has been observed for people with atopic skin diathesis, indicated as a history of flexural eczema [10]. Other constitutional factors related to barrier function recovery include hormonal status [125], age, skin type (rather than race) [50] and others.

Environmental and lifestyle factors such as sauna [72], dietary supplements (with pantothenate, choline, nicotinamide, histidine and inositol, as demonstrated in dogs) [139] and water drinking [144] have a positive effects on barrier function. Alcohol consumption negatively affects barrier function [13].

Stress also interferes with barrier function [108]. It exerts its effects probably through glucocorticosteroid-related mechanisms [23]. The rate of barrier recovery is shown to have a circadian rhythm [24] and seasonal variations [109]. Visible light can also influence barrier recovery – red light accelerates, blue light delays it and white and green light have no effect [23].

There are reports of beneficial effects on skin barrier function with extracts prepared from Blue-lagoon silica mud [48] and Dead sea salts [101], indicating possible positive effects of climatotherapy.

References

1. Akhavan A, Cohen SR (2003) The relationship between atopic dermatitis and contact dermatitis. Clin Dermatol 21:158–162
2. Allenby CF, Basketter DA (1993) An arm immersion model of compromised skin (II). Influence on minimal eliciting patch test concentrations of nickel. Contact Derm 28:129–133
3. Anstey AV, Wakelin S, Reynolds NJ (2004) Guidelines for prescribing azathioprine in dermatology. Br J Dermatol 151: 1123–1132
4. Bagot M, Terki N, Bacha S et al (1999) Per os desensitization in nickel contact eczema: a double-blind placebo-controlled clinico-biological study. Ann Dermatol Venereol 126:502–504
5. Barany E, Lindberg M, Loden M (2000) Unexpected skin barrier influence from nonionic emulsifiers. Int J Pharm 195:189–195
6. Basketter DA (2008) Skin sensitization: strategies for the assessment and management of risk. Br J Dermatol 159: 267–273
7. Bayerl C, Gabea A, Peiler D et al (1999) Pilotstudie zur therapie des beruflich bedingten handekzems mit einer neuen tragbaren UVB-bestrahlungseinheit. Aktuelle Derm 25:302–305
8. Behrens S, von Kobyletzki G, Gruss C et al (1999) PUVA-bath photochemotherapy (PUVA-soak therapy) of recalcitrant dermatoses of the palms and soles. Photodermatol Photoimmunol Photomed 15:47–51

49

9. Belsito DV, Fowler JF Jr, Marks JG Jr et al (2004) Pimecrolimus cream 1%: a potential new treatment for chronic hand dermatitis. Cutis 73:31–38

10. Berndt U, Hinnen U, Iliev D et al (2000) Hand eczema in metalworker trainees–an analysis of risk factors. Contact Derm 43:327–332

11. Bissett DL, Hannon DP, Orr TV (1987) An animal model of solar-aged skin: histological, physical, and visible changes in UV-irradiated hairless mouse skin. Photochem Photobiol 46:367–378

12. Bollag W, Ott F (1999) Successful treatment of chronic hand eczema with oral 9-cis-retinoic acid. Dermatology 199: 308–312

13. Brand RM, Jendrzejewski JL, Charron AR (2007) Potential mechanisms by which a single drink of alcohol can increase transdermal absorption of topically applied chemicals. Toxicology 235:141–149

14. Brasch J, Becker D, Aberer W et al (2007) Contact dermatitis. J Dtsch Dermatol Ges 5:943–951

15. Buraczewska I, Loden M (2005) Treatment of surfactant-damaged skin in humans with creams of different pH values. Pharmacology 73:1–7

16. Buraczewska I, Berne B, Lindberg M et al (2007) Changes in skin barrier function following long-term treatment with moisturizers, a randomized controlled trial. Br J Dermatol 156:492–498

17. Buraczewska I, Berne B, Lindberg M et al (2009) Moisturizers change the mRNA expression of enzymes synthesizing skin barrier lipids. Arch Dermatol Res 301(8):587–594

18. CHCP (2009) Assessment report for protopic, p35 London: EMEA. Retrieved 10 July 2009 from http://www.emea.europa.eu/humandocs/PDFs/EPAR/protopic/Protopic-H-C-374-II-34.pdf

19. Cheng C, Michaels J, Scheinfeld N (2008) Alitretinoin: a comprehensive review. Expert Opin Investig Drugs 17: 437–443

20. Choi JM, Lee JY, Cho BK (2000) Chronic irritant contact dermatitis: recovery time in man. Contact Derm 42: 264–269

21. De Paepe K, Hachem JP, Vanpee E et al (2001) Beneficial effects of a skin tolerance-tested moisturizing cream on the barrier function in experimentally-elicited irritant and allergic contact dermatitis. Contact Derm 44:337–343

22. Denda M (2002) New strategies to improve skin barrier homeostasis. Adv Drug Deliv Rev 54(suppl 1):S123–S130

23. Denda M (2009) Methodology to improve epidermal barrier homeostasis: how to accelerate the barrier recovery? Int J Cosmet Sci 31:79–86

24. Denda M, Tsuchiya T (2000) Barrier recovery rate varies time-dependently in human skin. Br J Dermatol 142:881–884

25. Diepgen T, Elsner P, Schliemann S et al (2009) Management von handekzemen leitlinie ICD-10-ziffer: L20. L23. L24. L25. L30. J Dtsch Dermatol Ges 7:s1–s16

26. Draelos ZD, Ertel KD, Berge CA (2006) Facilitating facial retinization through barrier improvement. Cutis 78:275–281

27. Egan CA, Rallis TM, Meadows KP et al (1999) Low-dose oral methotrexate treatment for recalcitrant palmoplantar pompholyx. J Am Acad Dermatol 40:612–614

28. Elias PM (1986) Epidermal effects of retinoids: supramolecular observations and clinical implications. J Am Acad Dermatol 15:797–809

29. Elias PM (2006) Improving barrier function. In: Elias PM, Feingold KR (eds) Skin barrier. Taylor & Francis, New York

30. Elias PM (2008) Barrier repair trumps immunology in the pathogenesis and therapy of atopic dermatitis. Drug Discov Today Dis Mech 5:e33–e38

31. Engel K, Reuter J, Seiler C et al (2008) Anti-inflammatory effect of pimecrolimus in the sodium lauryl sulphate test. J Eur Acad Dermatol Venereol 22:447–450

32. Fairris GM, Jones DH, Mack DP et al (1984) Superficial X-ray therapy in the treatment of constitutional eczema of the feet. Br J Dermatol 111:500–502

33. Fairris GM, Jones DH, Mack DP et al (1985) Conventional superficial X-ray versus Grenz ray therapy in the treatment of constitutional eczema of the hands. Br J Dermatol 112:339–341

34. Farage MA, Miller KW, Elsner P et al (2007) Structural characteristics of the aging skin: a review. Cutan Ocul Toxicol 26:343–357

35. Feingold KR (1991) The regulation of epidermal lipid synthesis by permeability barrier requirements. Crit Rev Ther Drug Carrier Syst 8:193–210

36. Feingold KR (2007) Thematic review series: skin lipids. The role of epidermal lipids in cutaneous permeability barrier homeostasis. J Lipid Res 48:2531–2546

37. Fluhr JW, Darlenski R, Surber C (2008) Glycerol and the skin: holistic approach to its origin and functions. Br J Dermatol 159:23–34

38. Fluhr JW, Vienne MP, Lauze C et al (1999) Tolerance profile of retinol, retinaldehyde and retinoic acid under maximized and long-term clinical conditions. Dermatology 199(suppl 1):57–60

39. Fluhr JW, Kuss O, Diepgen T et al (2001) Testing for irritation with a multifactorial approach: comparison of eight non-invasive measuring techniques on five different irritation types. Br J Dermatol 145:696–703

40. Folster-Holst R, Latussek E (2007) Synthetic tannins in dermatology–a therapeutic option in a variety of pediatric dermatoses. Pediatr Dermatol 24:296–301

41. Freeman S, Maibach H (1988) Study of irritant contact dermatitis produced by repeat patch test with sodium lauryl sulfate and assessed by visual methods, transepidermal water loss, and laser Doppler velocimetry. J Am Acad Dermatol 19:496–502

42. Frosch PJ, Schulze-Dirks A (1989) Contact allergy caused by polidocanol. Hautarzt 40:146–149

43. Gloor M, Senger B, Langenauer M et al (2004) On the course of the irritant reaction after irritation with sodium lauryl sulphate. Skin Res Technol 10:144–148

44. Goh CL (1991) Cutting oil dermatitis on guinea pig skin (I). Cutting oil dermatitis and barrier cream. Contact Derm 24: 16–21

45. Goldstein AM, Abramovits W (2003) Ceramides and the stratum corneum: structure, function, and new methods to promote repair. Int J Dermatol 42:256–259

46. Granlund H, Erkko P, Eriksson E et al (1996) Comparison of cyclosporine and topical betamethasone-17, 21-dipropionate in the treatment of severe chronic hand eczema. Acta Derm Venereol 76:371–376

47. Grassberger M, Steinhoff M, Schneider D et al (2004) Pimecrolimus – an anti-inflammatory drug targeting the skin. Exp Dermatol 13:721–730

48. Grether-Beck S, Muhlberg K, Brenden H et al (2008) Bioactive molecules from the blue lagoon: in vitro and in vivo assessment of silica mud and microalgae extracts for their effects on skin barrier function and prevention of skin ageing. Exp Dermatol 17:771–779

49. Grubauer G, Elias PM, Feingold KR (1989) Transepidermal water loss: the signal for recovery of barrier structure and function. J Lipid Res 30:323–333

50. Gunathilake R, Schurer NY, Shoo BA et al (2009) PH-regulated mechanisms account for pigment-type differences in epidermal barrier function. J Invest Dermatol 129:1719–1729

51. Gupta G, Forsyth A (1999) Allergic contact reactions to colophony presenting as oral disease. Contact Derm 40:332–333

52. Hachem JP, De Paepe K, Vanpee E et al (2001) Combination therapy improves the recovery of the skin barrier function: an experimental model using a contact allergy patch test combined with TEWL measurements. Dermatology 202:314–319

53. Hachem JP, De Paepe K, Vanpee E et al (2002) The effect of two moisturisers on skin barrier damage in allergic contact dermatitis. Eur J Dermatol 12:136–138

54. Hachem JP, Behne M, Aronchik I et al (2005) Extracellular pH controls NHE1 expression in epidermis and keratinocytes: implications for barrier repair. J Invest Dermatol 125:790–797

55. Handa S, Sahoo B, Sharma VK (2001) Oral hyposensitization in patients with contact dermatitis from *Parthenium hysterophorus*. Contact Derm 44:279–282

56. Hanifin JM, Stevens V, Sheth P et al (2004) Novel treatment of chronic severe hand dermatitis with bexarotene gel. Br J Dermatol 150:545–553

57. Haratake A, Uchida Y, Mimura K et al (1997) Intrinsically aged epidermis displays diminished UVB-induced alterations in barrier function associated with decreased proliferation. J Investig Dermatol 108:319–323

58. Held E, Sveinsdottir S, Agner T (1999) Effect of long-term use of moisturizer on skin hydration, barrier function and susceptibility to irritants. Acta Derm Venereol 79:49–51

59. Hindsen M, Bruze M, Christensen OB (1997) The significance of previous allergic contact dermatitis for elicitation of delayed hypersensitivity to nickel. Contact Derm 37:101–106

60. Holleran WM, Uchida Y, Halkier-Sorensen L et al (1997) Structural and biochemical basis for the UVB-induced alterations in epidermal barrier function. Photodermatol Photoimmunol Photomed 13:117–128

61. Hölzle E, Gollnick H, Herzinger T et al (2002) Empfehlungen zur Phototherapie und Photochemotherapie, Leitlinien der Deutschen Dermatologischen Gesellschaft (DDG). Düsseldorf. Retrieved 13 July 2009 from http://www.uni-duesseldorf. de/AWMF/ll/013-029.htm

62. Ingram JR, Batchelor JM, Williams H (2009) Alitretinoin as a potential advance in the management of severe chronic hand eczema. Arch Dermatol 145:314–315

63. Isaksson M (2004) Corticosteroids. Dermatol Ther 17:314–320

64. Isaksson M, Bruze M (2001) Repetitive usage testing with budesonide in experimental nickel–allergic contact dermatitis in individuals hypersensitive to budesonide. Br J Dermatol 145:38–44

65. Jacobson MK, Kim H, Coyle WR et al (2007) Effect of myristyl nicotinate on retinoic acid therapy for facial photodamage. Exp Dermatol 16:927–935

66. Jensen JM, Pfeiffer S, Witt M et al (2009) Different effects of pimecrolimus and betamethasone on the skin barrier in patients with atopic dermatitis. J Allergy Clin Immunol 123:1124–1133

67. Jungersted JM, Hellgren LI, Jemec GB et al (2008) Lipids and skin barrier function–a clinical perspective. Contact Derm 58:255–262

68. Kaaber K, Menne T, Veien NK et al (1987) Some adverse effects of disulfiram in the treatment of nickel-allergic patients. Derm Beruf Umwelt 35:209–211

69. Kao JS, Fluhr JW, Man MQ et al (2003) Short-term glucocorticoid treatment compromises both permeability barrier homeostasis and stratum corneum integrity: inhibition of epidermal lipid synthesis accounts for functional abnormalities. J Invest Dermatol 120:456–464

70. Kim E, Kim S, Nam GW et al (2009) The alkaline pH-adapted skin barrier is disrupted severely by SLS-induced irritation. Int J Cosmet Sci 31(4):263–269

71. Kolbe L, Kligman AM, Schreiner V et al (2001) Corticosteroid-induced atrophy and barrier impairment measured by non-invasive methods in human skin. Skin Res Technol 7:73–77

72. Kowatzki D, Macholdt C, Krull K et al (2008) Effect of regular sauna on epidermal barrier function and stratum corneum water-holding capacity in vivo in humans: a controlled study. Dermatology 217:173–180

73. Krutmann J, Medve-Koenigs K, Ruzicka T et al (2005) Ultraviolet-free phototherapy. Photodermatol Photoimmunol Photomed 21:59–61

74. Kucharekova M, van De Kerkhof PC, van Der Valk PG (2003) A randomized comparison of an emollient containing skin-related lipids with a petrolatum-based emollient as adjunct in the treatment of chronic hand dermatitis. Contact Derm 48:293–299

75. Kucharekova M, Hornix M, Ashikaga T et al (200w3) The effect of the PDE-4 inhibitor (cipamfylline) in two human models of irritant contact dermatitis. Arch Dermatol Res 295:29–32

76. Lee JY, Effendy I, Maibach HI (1997) Acute irritant contact dermatitis: recovery time in man. Contact Derm 36:285–290

77. Lehmann P, Holzle E, Melnik B et al (1991) Effects of ultraviolet A and B on the skin barrier: a functional, electron microscopic and lipid biochemical study. Photodermatol Photoimmunol Photomed 8:129–134

78. Levin C, Zhai H, Bashir S et al (2001) Efficacy of corticosteroids in acute experimental irritant contact dermatitis? Skin Res Technol 7:214–218

79. Lim SH, Kim SM, Lee YW et al (2008) Change of biophysical properties of the skin caused by ultraviolet radiation-induced photodamage in Koreans. Skin Res Technol 14:93–102

80. Loden M (2005) The clinical benefit of moisturizers. J Eur Acad Dermatol Venereol 19:672–688; quiz 686–687

81. Löffler H, Aramaki J, Friebe K et al (2002) Changes in skin physiology during bath PUVA therapy. Br J Dermatol 147:105–109

82. Lofgren SM, Warshaw EM (2006) Dyshidrosis: epidemiology, clinical characteristics, and therapy. Dermatitis 17:165–181

83. Luger T, Paul C (2007) Potential new indications of topical calcineurin inhibitors. Dermatology 215(suppl 1):45–54

84. Luger T, Elsner P, Kerscher M et al (2009) Topische Dermatotherapie mit Glukokortikoiden – therapeutischer Index. ICD 10: L20. Leitlinien der Deutschen Dermatologischen Gesellschaft (DDG). Düsseldorf. Retrieved 9 July 2009 from http://www.uni-duesseldorf.de/AWMF/ll/013-034.htm

85. Luger T, Loske KD, Elsner P et al (2004) Topical skin therapy with glucocorticoids – therapeutic index. J Dtsch Dermatol Ges 2:629–634

86. Marcil I, Stern RS (2001) Squamous-cell cancer of the skin in patients given PUVA and ciclosporin: nested cohort crossover study. Lancet 358:1042–1045

87. Mastrolonardo M, Lopalco PL, Diaferio A (2002) Topical immunotherapy with contact sensitizers: a model to study the natural history of delayed hypersensitivity. Contact Derm 47:210–214

88. Mauro T, Holleran WM, Grayson S et al (1998) Barrier recovery is impeded at neutral pH, independent of ionic effects: implications for extracellular lipid processing. Arch Dermatol Res 290:215–222

89. Mrowietz U, Eberhard Klein C, Reich K et al (2000) Therapie mit Ciclosporin in der Dermatologie, Leitlinien der Deutschen Dermatologischen Gesellschaft (DDG). Düsseldorf. Retrieved 15 July 2009 from http://www.uni-duesseldorf.de/AWMF/ll/013-013.htm

90. Murphy GM, Maurice PD, Norris PG et al (1989) Azathioprine treatment in chronic actinic dermatitis: a double-blind controlled trial with monitoring of exposure to ultraviolet radiation. Br J Dermatol 121:639–646

91. NICE (2007) Grenz rays therapy for inflammatory skin conditions. Retrieved 03 September 2009 from http://guidance.nice.org.uk/IPG236 and attachments http://guidance.nice.org.uk/IPG236/Guidance/pdf/English and http://www.nice.org.uk/guidance/index.jsp?action=download&o=31797

92. Nielsen NH, Linneberg A, Menne T et al (2001) Persistence of contact allergy among Danish adults: an 8-year follow-up study. Contact Derm 45:350–353

93. Nilsson E, Henning C, Hjorleifsson ML (1986) Density of the microflora in hand eczema before and after topical treatment with a potent corticosteroid. J Am Acad Dermatol 15:192–197

94. Noiesen E, Larsen K, Agner T (2004) Compliance in contact allergy with focus on cosmetic labelling: a qualitative research project. Contact Derm 51:189–195

95. Ong PY (2009) Emerging drugs for atopic dermatitis. Expert Opin Emerg Drugs 14:165–179

96. Pedersen L, Johansen JD, Held E et al (2004) Augmentation of skin response by exposure to a combination of allergens and irritants – a review. Contact Derm 50:265–273

97. Petering H, Breuer C, Herbst R et al (2004) Comparison of localized high-dose UVA1 irradiation versus topical cream psoralen-UVA for treatment of chronic vesicular dyshidrotic eczema. J Am Acad Dermatol 50:68–72

98. Pickenacker A, Luger TA, Schwarz T (1998) Dyshidrotic eczema treated with mycophenolate mofetil. Arch Dermatol 134:378–379

99. Polderman MC, Govaert JC, le Cessie S et al (2003) A double-blind placebo-controlled trial of UVA-1 in the treatment of dyshidrotic eczema. Clin Exp Dermatol 28:584–587

100. Proksch E, Brandner JM, Jensen JM (2008) The skin: an indispensable barrier. Exp Dermatol 17:1063–1072

101. Proksch E, Nissen HP, Bremgartner M et al (2005) Bathing in a magnesium-rich dead sea salt solution improves skin barrier function, enhances skin hydration, and reduces inflammation in atopic dry skin. Int J Dermatol 44:151–157

102. Queille-Roussel C, Graeber M, Thurston M et al (2000) SDZ ASM 981 is the first non-steroid that suppresses established nickel contact dermatitis elicited by allergen challenge. Contact Derm 42:349–350

103. Ramsing DW, Agner T (1995) Efficacy of topical corticosteroids on irritant skin reactions. Contact Derm 32:293–297

104. Ramsing DW, Agner T (1997) Preventive and therapeutic effects of a moisturizer. An experimental study of human skin. Acta Derm Venereol 77:335–337

105. Reitamo S, Granlund H (1994) Cyclosporin A in the treatment of chronic dermatitis of the hands. Br J Dermatol 130:75–78

106. Reymann F (1982) Two years' experience with tigason treatment of pustulosis palmo-plantaris and eczema keratoticum manuum. Dermatologica 164:209–216

107. Ring J, Barker J, Behrendt H et al (2005) Review of the potential photo-cocarcinogenicity of topical calcineurin inhibitors: position statement of the European dermatology forum. J Eur Acad Dermatol Venereol 19:663–671

108. Robles TF (2007) Stress, social support, and delayed skin barrier recovery. Psychosom Med 69:807–815

109. Rogers J, Harding C, Mayo A et al (1996) Stratum corneum lipids: the effect of ageing and the seasons. Arch Dermatol Res 288:765–770

110. Ruzicka T, Lynde CW, Jemec GB et al (2008) Efficacy and safety of oral alitretinoin (9-cis retinoic acid) in patients with severe chronic hand eczema refractory to topical corticosteroids: results of a randomized, double-blind, placebo-controlled, multicentre trial. Br J Dermatol 158:808–817

111. Sajjachareonpong P, Cahill J, Keegel T et al (2004) Persistent post-occupational dermatitis. Contact Derm 51:278–283

112. Schempp CM, Muller H, Czech W et al (1997) Treatment of chronic palmoplantar eczema with local bath-PUVA therapy. J Am Acad Dermatol 36:733–737

113. Schliemann S, Kelterer D, Bauer A et al (2008) Tacrolimus ointment in the treatment of occupationally induced chronic hand dermatitis. Contact Derm 58:299–306

114. Schmidt T, Abeck D, Boeck K et al (1998) UVA1 irradiation is effective in treatment of chronic vesicular dyshidrotic hand eczema. Acta Derm Venereol 78:318–319

115. Schmitt J, Schmitt N, Meurer M (2007) Cyclosporin in the treatment of patients with atopic eczema – a systematic review and meta-analysis. J Eur Acad Dermatol Venereol 21:606–619

116. Schoepe S, Schacke H, May E et al (2006) Glucocorticoid therapy-induced skin atrophy. Exp Dermatol 15:406–420

117. Shaffrali FC, Colver GB, Messenger AG et al (2003) Experience with low-dose methotrexate for the treatment of eczema in the elderly. J Am Acad Dermatol 48:417–419

118. Sharma AD (2007) Relationship between nickel allergy and diet. Indian J Dermatol Venereol Leprol 73:307–312

119. Skudlik C, Weisshaar E, Scheidt R et al (2009) Multicenter study "Medical-occupational rehabilitation procedure skin – optimizing and quality assurance of inpatient-management (ROQ)". J Dtsch Dermatol Ges 7:122–126

120. Stege H (2008) Ultraviolet therapy in patients with chronic hand eczema. Hautarzt 59:696–702

121. Stucker M, Hoffmann M, Altmeyer P (2002) Instrumental evaluation of retinoid-induced skin irritation. Skin Res Technol 8:133–140

122. Tagami H, Tadaki T, Obata M et al (1992) Functional assessment of the stratum corneum under the influence of

oral aromatic retinoid (etretinate) in guinea-pigs and humans. Comparison with topical retinoic acid treatment. Br J Dermatol 127:470–475

123. Thelmo MC, Lang W, Brooke E et al (2003) An open-label pilot study to evaluate the safety and efficacy of topically applied tacrolimus ointment for the treatment of hand and/or foot eczema. J Dermatolog Treat 14: 136–140

124. Thestrup-Pedersen K, Andersen KE, Menne T et al (2001) Treatment of hyperkeratotic dermatitis of the palms (eczema keratoticum) with oral acitretin. A single-blind placebo-controlled study. Acta Derm Venereol 81:353–355

125. Tsutsumi M, Denda M (2007) Paradoxical effects of beta-estradiol on epidermal permeability barrier homeostasis. Br J Dermatol 157:776–779

126. Uter W, Geier J, Fuchs T (2000) Contact allergy to polidocanol, 1992 to 1999. J Allergy Clin Immunol 106: 1203–1204

127. Uter W, de Padua CM, Pfahlberg A et al (2009) Contact allergy to topical corticosteroids–results from the IVDK and epidemiological risk assessment. J Dtsch Dermatol Ges 7(34–41):34–42

128. Vakeva L, Reitamo S, Pukkala E et al (2008) Long-term follow-up of cancer risk in patients treated with short-term cyclosporine. Acta Derm Venereol 88:117–120

129. van Coevorden AM, Kamphof WG, van Sonderen E et al (2004) Comparison of oral psoralen-UV-A with a portable tanning unit at home vs hospital-administered bath psoralen-UV-A in patients with chronic hand eczema: an open-label randomized controlled trial of efficacy. Arch Dermatol 140:1463–1466

130. van Coevorden AM, Coenraads PJ, Svensson A et al (2004) Overview of studies of treatments for hand eczema-the EDEN hand eczema survey. Br J Dermatol 151:446–451

131. van der Valk PG, Maibach HI (1989) Do topical corticosteroids modulate skin irritation in human beings? Assessment by transepidermal water loss and visual scoring. J Am Acad Dermatol 21:519–522

132. Veenhuis RT, van Horssen J, Bos RP et al (2002) Highly increased urinary 1-hydroxypyrene excretion rate in patients with atopic dermatitis treated with topical coal tar. Arch Dermatol Res 294:168–171

133. Veien NK, Olholm Larsen P, Thestrup-Pedersen K et al (1999) Long-term, intermittent treatment of chronic hand eczema with mometasone furoate. Br J Dermatol 140: 882–886

134. Verma KK, Bansal A, Sethuraman G (2006) Parthenium dermatitis treated with azathioprine weekly pulse doses. Indian J Dermatol Venereol Leprol 72:24–27

135. Verma KK, Mahesh R, Srivastava P et al (2008) Azathioprine versus betamethasone for the treatment of parthenium dermatitis: a randomized controlled study. Indian J Dermatol Venereol Leprol 74:453–457

136. Wall LM, Gebauer KA (1991) A follow-up study of occupational skin disease in Western Australia. Contact Derm 24:241–243

137. Warner JA, Cruz PD Jr (2008) Grenz ray therapy in the new millennium: still a valid treatment option? Dermatitis 19: 73–80

138. Watkins SA, Maibach H (2009) The hardening phenomenon in irritant contact dermatitis: an interpretative update. Contact Derm 60:123–130

139. Watson AL, Fray TR, Bailey J et al (2006) Dietary constituents are able to play a beneficial role in canine epidermal barrier function. Exp Dermatol 15:74–81

140. Watson ES (1986) Toxicodendron hyposensitization programs. Clin Dermatol 4:160–170

141. Widmer J, Elsner P, Burg G (1994) Skin irritant reactivity following experimental cumulative irritant contact dermatitis. Contact Derm 30:35–39

142. Wilhelm K-P, Freitag G, Wolff HH (1994) Surfactant-induced skin irritation and skin repair: evaluation of a cumulative human irritation model by noninvasive techniques. J Am Acad Dermatol 31:981–987

143. Wilkinson SM, Cartwright PH, English JS (1991) Hydrocortisone: an important cutaneous allergen. Lancet 337:761–762

144. Williams S, Krueger N, Davids M et al (2007) Effect of fluid intake on skin physiology: distinct differences between drinking mineral water and tap water. Int J Cosmet Sci 29:131–138

145. Wise M, Callen JP (2007) Azathioprine: a guide for the management of dermatology patients. Dermatol Ther 20: 206–215

146. Wollina U (2008) Pompholyx: what's new? Expert Opin Investig Drugs 17:897–904

147. Zachariae C, Held E, Johansen JD et al (2003) Effect of a moisturizer on skin susceptibility to NiCl2. Acta Derm Venereol 83:93–97

148. Zhai H, Maibach HI (2002) Occlusion vs. skin barrier function. Skin Res Technol 8:1–6

149. Zhai H, Chang YC, Singh M et al (1999) In vivo nickel allergic contact dermatitis: human model for topical therapeutics. Contact Derm 40:205–208

Prevention of Hand Eczema: Gloves, Barrier Creams and Workers' Education

50

Britta Wulfhorst, Meike Bock, Christoph Skudlik, Walter Wigger-Alberti, and Swen Malte John

Contents

S.M. John (✉), B. Wulfhorst, M. Bock, C. Skudlik, and W. Wigger-Alberti
Department of Dermatology, Environmental Medicine and Health Theory, University of Osnabrueck, Sedanstraße 115, 49069 Osnabrück, Germany
e-mail: sjohn@uos.de

50.1 Introduction: Trends and Tasks in Dermatological Prevention

Hand eczema is a common, chronic disease with a high socio-economic burden and a distinctly negative impact on quality of life [1, 2]. In the general population, it is characterized by a point prevalence of 9.7% and an incidence rate of 5.5–8.8/1,000 person years [3, see Chap. 11]. Epidemiologic studies have identified risk factors for development and prognosis, and indicated the need and pivotal options for prevention, particularly in occupational settings. Occupational skin diseases – which clinically, by about 90%, impose as hand eczema – are the most frequent occupational diseases in many industrialized countries with a high socio-economic burden for society as well as for the affected individual [4, 5, see Chap. 42]. In Germany, in 2007, 18,398 new cases were officially reported to the statutory employers' liability insurance bodies (the overwhelming majority of cases being hand eczema), which is more than 25% of all reports on occupational diseases. Accordingly, the National Institute for Occupational Safety and Health (NIOSH) states that, in the USA, skin disease accounts for nearly 25% of all occupational injuries for which workers' compensation claims are filed (www.cdc.gov/niosh). NIOSH comments: "Skin diseases of occupational origin outnumber all other work-incurred illnesses. Early recognition and preventive measures can effectively reduce the incidence of occupational dermatoses in the United States".

For the above-mentioned reasons, the prevention of hand eczema has been extensively studied in occupational settings, which is why this chapter will focus on this aspect. Another reason is that in most countries, social insurance systems and law requirements allow for specific documentation and attendance to patients

J.D. Johansen et al. (eds.), *Contact Dermatitis*,
DOI: 10.1007/978-3-642-03827-3_50, © Springer-Verlag Berlin Heidelberg 2011

50

affected by occupational skin disease, thus enabling a certain epidemiological insight (however, biased by a 50–100 fold under-reporting [6–8]), and – most importantly – facilitating intervention studies.

Quite unanimously, in various high-risk professions, intervention studies have produced fair-quality evidence that prevention is effective [9–23 (for overview: see Table 50.5)]. Due to various methodological approaches, the great diversity of work place settings with largely varying exposure profiles and different outcome variables, the degree of evidence and transferability of these studies may be disputable. Thus, we certainly need further research. This should preferably take place in an international network of researchers, in order to share the gathered experiences in various countries and commonly develop robust best-practice-models for disseminating information, treatment and management of patients (compatible to various social insurance systems, professions, personal backgrounds and ethnicities), a common risk and susceptibility assessment, evidence-based standards of personal protective measures, set up of data bases and public internet information-platforms etc.

One uniform finding is common to most intervention studies: the lack of information about proper personal skin protection in affected (and unaffected) workers in all risk professions in all countries. So, there is an imminent future task of prevention to improve on workers' education. In this context, multi-disciplinary approaches seem most promising (see Sect. 50.3). Thus, further research particularly has to focus on work-related educational activities, including longitudinal studies assessing effectiveness by return to work and the course of disease as outcome variable. Furthermore, the strategies of OCD prevention need to be further clarified; however, as yet, there is already a range of some evidence-based recommendations [18, 24–26, (see Sect. 50.3)].

Paradoxically, the widely accepted effectiveness of prevention for the reduction of OCD prevalence makes it increasingly difficult – and unethical – to do controlled intervention studies, in which some affected individuals were to be exempted from preventive measures. On the other hand, the beneficial effects of prevention have started to influence relevant decision making outside of dermatology (e.g., in social insurance bodies and politics) and even in the general population. This unique consensus, for example, recently triggered off a nationwide "prevention campaign "skin" 2007–2008" in Germany. Clinicians dealing with contact dermatitis should make

use of the fact that prevention is currently favoured by public – and political – opinion. This is underlined by a recent EU-report, highlighting the problem of emerging occupational skin diseases and emphasizing the need for prevention [27]. This development may increasingly become a stronghold for future dermatology. Due to their specific knowledge and competence, dermatologists – in cooperation with other disciplines – in many cases, can save their patients' health and jobs, and thus also save expenses for tax-payers and insurance systems.

Estimated annual economic costs for occupational dermatoses exceed 1.2 billion euros per year in Germany [28], for the US at least 1 billion dollar per year was calculated [8, 29] and for England, it was well over 200 million Pounds [26]. These figures include direct costs like treatment, compensation as well as indirect costs due to absenteeism of workforce (sick leave) and lack of productivity, these indirect costs constituting the bulk of OCD economic burden (up to 90%). OCD is most frequent in small and medium-sized enterprises (SME), all too often causing unemployment and personal suffering for the affected individual. The National Institute for Occupational Safety and Health (NIOSH), Cincinnati, Ohio, USA, states that 2/3 of American workers are occupied in small plants having fewer than 500 workers. It is here that the occupational skin disease rate tends to be the highest, because they frequently lack comprehensive health care programmes. Improved prevention of OCD will therefore significantly contribute to enhanced competitiveness of SME, as costs for prolonged sick leave and loss of productivity are detrimental especially to them. This particularly holds true in times of recession. Thus, in 2010, the European Academy for Dermatology and Venereology (EADV) started a campaign ("healthy skin@work/europrevention") as a joint scientific effort for the individual and society on the whole to encourage the development of common health and safety policies to reduce OCD prevalence, stimulate further research and put science into practice. Prevention of OCD should be ascribed a higher priority in the affected industries, as every employee is entitled to a safe working environment.

Skin diseases of occupational origin outnumber all other work-incurred illnesses. Early recognition and preventive measures can effectively reduce the incidence of occupational dermatoses in the United States.

National Institute for Occupational Safety and Health
(NIOSH; www.cdc.gov/niosh)

50.1.1 Primary Prevention

Primary prevention aims at avoiding OCD in healthy individuals employed in workplaces that are hazardous to the skin. In most countries, there are detailed legal regulations providing the background for primary prevention at workplaces.

1. Primary prevention should primarily focus on workplace-related risk reduction strategies, e.g.

   - Elimination or substitution of harmful exposures (e.g. substitution of glyceryl monothioglycolate in the hairdressing trade [30] and natural rubber latex gloves from the health sector [9] or adding ferrous sulphate to cement to inhibit the formation of potentially sensitizing chromium VI; compare Chap. 52).
   - Technical measures (e.g. "no touch" techniques in cleaning by using specific leverage-systems, encapsulation of cooling fluids in the metal industry, splash-guards, dust absorbing systems, ventilation, automation, etc. [26]), changing work organization (e.g., equal distribution of wet work among all employees, introducing breaks to avoid the continuous wearing of gloves etc.).

2. Primary prevention should secondarily focus on worker-related risk reduction strategies, e.g.,

   - Identification of susceptible individuals, e.g., by dermatological pre-employment counselling: recent observations allow to define risk populations including genetic risk factors more precisely [31–33]. To such risk groups, preventive measures and education should be specifically made accessible.
   - Continuous health surveillance.
   - Optimizing personal skin protection (gloves, protective creams, after-work creams, see Sect. 50.2.1, 50.2.2).
   - Education and training, including vocational schools' curricula (see Sect. 50.3).
   - Prevention campaigns (e.g., "healthy skin@ work/europrevention").

As pointed out, primary prevention will chiefly be directed towards risk groups, particularly people in hazardous professions and only secondarily to the general population, but it will also include the dissemination of medical knowledge in terms of health promotion and health education (see Sect. 50.3). The recent nationwide skin disease prevention campaign 2007–2008 in Germany (Fig. 50.1) has shown that the awareness to the prevention of OCD can particularly be raised in people employed in risk professions but has also indicated the limits of reaching the general

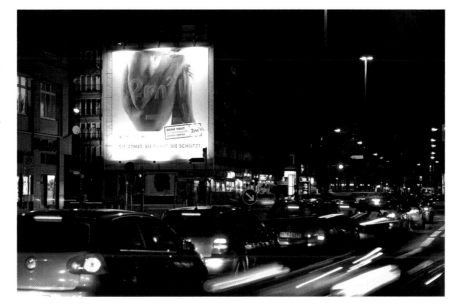

Fig. 50.1 The "Healthy Skin Campaign" in Berlin, Potsdamer Platz, 2008. Slogan: "Your skin. The two most important square meters of your life". This was postered throughout the country and accompanied by various information activities in the general public (e.g., marathon events, various outdoor activities, "skin days") and for employees in high-risk-professions at their workplaces. It was funded by the statutory health and accident insurance institutions

population, where no relevant effects of the campaign were so far detectable in randomized pre/post-telephone interviews [34]. Interestingly, the annual figure of reported occupational skin diseases has risen during the campaign, most likely due to the fact that even dermatologists became more aware of the possibilities of OCD-notification and prevention (see Sect. 50.1.2). It would not be an unwanted side-effect of the forthcoming EADV prevention campaign if the same would happen. Obviously, such campaigns, which include the general public, will reach decision makers and exert political pressure to improve preventive offers to patients and stimulate research.

50.1.2 Secondary Prevention

Target groups of secondary prevention are individuals with initial signs of OCD. Secondary prevention aims at early disease detection, thereby increasing opportunities for interventions to prevent OCD chronification or progression of symptoms. Secondary prevention requires accurate medical diagnostics and treatment, teaching offers, psychological understanding and an improvement of working conditions [35].

In Germany, due to specificities in the social insurance system, in the last decennium, specific prevention concepts aiming chiefly at early detection of OCD, but including all levels of prevention could be scientifically developed, implemented and evaluated. Meanwhile, this work has formed the basis for a nationwide systematic approach to OCD by the respective statutory employers' liability insurance bodies, the so-called multi-step intervention approach ("Stufenverfahren Haut"). This approach offers quick preventive help for all severity grades of OCD for every employee regardless of the profession, including dermatological outpatient and – if needed in severe cases – inpatient therapy, skin protection seminars and a multi-disciplinary intervention with focus on teaching and systematic follow-up [5] (Fig. 50.2). As was recently suggested, the experience gained may be helpful to further establish complex prevention strategies even in other countries with different insurance systems and work environments [36]. This is why in the following paragraphs, an overview on the German approach is given. Obviously, regardless of the social insurance systems, relevant costs to society will always have to be covered if OCD prevention is neglected – let alone the impact on the affected individual.

In the classical OCD-high-risk profession of hairdressing, the first extensive preventive experience was

Fig. 50.2 The statutory employers' liability insurances recently implemented the "multi-step intervention approach" (*Stufenverfahren Haut*) as a systematic approach to the prevention of occupational skin disease. This approach offers quick preventive help for all levels of OCD severity, including dermatological outpatient and – if needed in severe cases – inpatient therapy, skin protection seminars and a multi-disciplinary intervention with focus on teaching and systematic follow-up

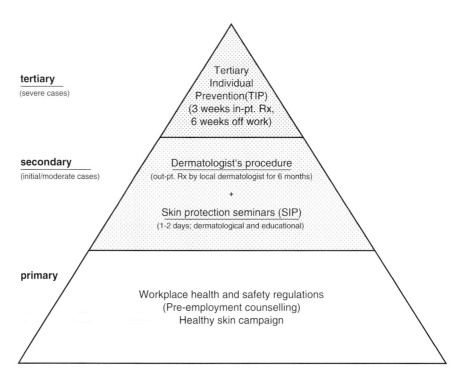

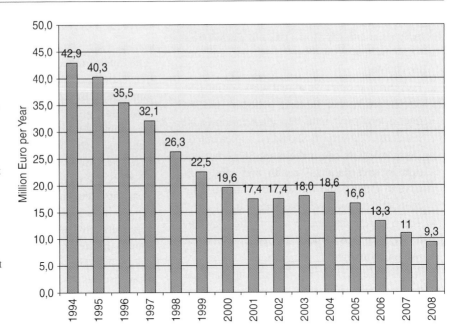

Fig. 50.3 Reduction of costs for job rehabilitation benefits/re-training due to job loss by occupational dermatitis of affected patients in hairdressing and the private health sector in Germany 1994–2008. Reduction is related to the implementation of preventive programmes. Accordingly, employers' premiums for statutory occupational accident insurance for BGW-insured businesses significantly decreased (ancillary labour costs). Source: *statutory employers' liability insurance for the health and welfare services (*Berufsgenossenschaft für Gesundheitsdienst und Wohlfahrtspflege, BGW), Hamburg, 2009

gained; an almost tenfold reduction of OCD was observed due to a systematic preventive programme [37, 38]. Similar observations were obtained in geriatric nursing and also in other parts of the health sector [19, 20, 22, 39]; this explains, as to why in the last 15 years, the expenses for OCD kept dropping in these branches. Exemplarily, the >70% cost-reduction for occupational rehabilitation after job loss due to OCD in the German health and hairdressing sector in the last decade is shown (Fig. 50.3). These data may be helpful to encourage the development of health and safety policies even in industries where OCD, in spite of its prevalence and economic burden, is not yet considered a high priority.

The question of how accident or health insurers are informed that an employee has developed an OCD is of vital importance for early intervention. In Germany, even if there is only a slight suspicion that a dermatosis may be work-related, a dermatologist's report (Hautarztbericht) is filed with the respective employers liability insurance institution [40]. This report requires the consent of the person concerned. It is based on a detailed examination, including patch tests and atopy screening. It also includes recommendations concerning therapy, personal skin protection and after-work skin care (see Chap. 53). Once the insurer has been notified, it will – if an occupational cause is likely – usually

commission the reporting dermatologist to follow up the patient with regular consultations and provide all required treatments for a consecutive 6-month-period. In an attempt to handle potential occupational dermatoses as quickly and un-bureaucratically as possible, this so-called dermatologist's procedure was recently updated and the dermatologist's fees have been raised. For the purposes of optimal early intervention, rapid medical treatment following completion of the report and documentation of progress at close intervals are now required as a rule. In doing so, rapid enforcement of an insured person's legal claim to prevention measures for purposes of preserving employment shall be guaranteed; the follow-up period of 6 months can be extended, if necessary. Additionally, multi-disciplinary skin protection seminars are offered to affected employees.

These recent initiatives show that the insurers' administrations have widely accepted that these low-threshold preventive measures eventually save money; it also demonstrates appreciation for the important role of dermatologists in the field of prevention.

For quality management, the operational effectiveness of the above-described comprehensive scheme of secondary prevention measures, which was newly introduced in 2006, is presently being analyzed in a randomized quota sample with 1 year follow-up [41].

50

Core Message

> OCD in risk professions is neither fate nor inevitable.

> Prevention is effective in real work settings.

> Recent progress in the field, including specific inter-disciplinary multi-step intervention at all levels of OCD severity should be implemented.

> Dermatologists can make a specific contribution to save patients' health and jobs, taxpayers' money, and furthermore, increase the economic competitiveness of industry.

> There is relevant public and political awareness of the role of dermatological prevention in some countries.

> At this stage, a common coordinated international approach to prevention by dermatologists seems recommendable.

50.1.3 Tertiary Prevention

The intensified comprehensive measures of tertiary prevention are indicated when, due to severe recalcitrant OCD, the cessation of the harmful occupation is threatening.

Occupational skin diseases represent a substantial expense factor for the statutory employers' liability insurance bodies in Germany. Among all occupational diseases, they result in the highest expenditures for insurants receiving job rehabilitation benefits per year. Approximately, 60% of all expenses for occupational rehabilitation are dedicated annually to this purpose. Due to the present economic situation, expenditures for occupational rehabilitation (2006: 43.1 million Euro for skin diseases) frequently do not achieve their stated objectives as re-trained claimants do not succeed in reintegrating into the employment market. On the one hand, this emphasizes the need for specific, early

Fig. 50.4 Flow chart of TIP according to the Osnabrueck Model, upon which the present multi-centre study of the German Statutory Accident Insurance (DGUV) is based: inpatient treatment and integrated consecutive outpatient care by the referring dermatologist at the patient's place of residence. Overall period of abstention from work is approximately 6 weeks, to allow for complete regeneration of the skin barrier after severe damage

Inpatient - phase

- Dermatology (Diagnostics, Treatment)
- Health education
- Health psychology
- Ergotherapy
- Case management by insurer

3 weeks

Post - inpatient - phase

- Post-inpatient sick leave. Patient stays at home. This phase is also covered by employers' liability insurer

- Outpatient care by the local (referring) dermatologist (including continuation of initiated therapy, e.g., topical PUVA, iontophoresis etc.)

3 weeks

After return to the workplace

- Realization of recommended and practised skin protection measures at the workplace
- Continuation of the outpatient dermatological counselling and stage-adapted therapy by referring dermatologist (including continuation of initiated therapy e. g., topical PUVA, iontophoresis etc.)
- Documentation of the course
- Quick intervention in case of recurrences

>3-12 months

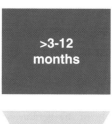

secondary prevention of OCD, and on the other hand, the need to also create options to help affected individuals, where OCD has already advanced to a recalcitrant course. Protracted phases of inability to work caused by poorly treated eczema all too frequently entail a decline into precarious employment or long-term unemployment, which is followed by a loss of income and what contributes to a person's central identity in life.

Therefore, for those cases of severe OCD, in which the above-mentioned outpatient prevention measures are not sufficiently successful, specific multi-disciplinary inpatient prevention measures have been developed (tertiary individual prevention, or TIP). TIP represents the ultima ratio within the hierarchical multi-step intervention concept (Fig. 50.2). TIP comprises 2–3 weeks of inpatient dermatological diagnostics and treatment as well as intensive health-related pedagogic and psychological counselling. Furthermore, TIP includes ergotherapeutic exercises for use tests of adequate skin protection methods in a simulation model of the workplace, counselling by the case manager of the statutory insurance institutions and – wherever possible – involvement of the employer's occupational physician. Subsequently, after discharge, the local dermatologist follows up the case at close intervals for another

3 weeks; this outpatient treatment as well as the sick leave expenses is also being covered for by the employers' liability insurance bodies ["Osnabrueck Model", 42]. Each patient remains off work for a total of 6 weeks to allow full barrier recovery (Fig. 50.4). One of the decisive factors in TIP is the seamless continuation of the initiated medical and preventive efforts when the patient re-starts working; therefore, subsequent outpatient treatment by the local dermatologist is always indicated. It may be extended up to 1 year or longer.

A total of 764 out of 1,164 (66%) TIP patients with severe OCD treated regularly by a local dermatologist for up to 1 year, were successful in remaining in their respective (risk-) professions as assessed by a questionnaire 1 year after discharge [43; Fig. 50.5]. In the past, most of these patients would have had to give up their workplaces. The continuation of employment was found to be unrelated to the type of risk occupation practiced, but was contingent upon the age of the patients at the time of receiving TIP (Fig. 50.6). Accumulation of life and professional experience in many cases act inspiringly on individual motivation to employ adequate skin protection at the workplace, and this in turn increases the probability of employment

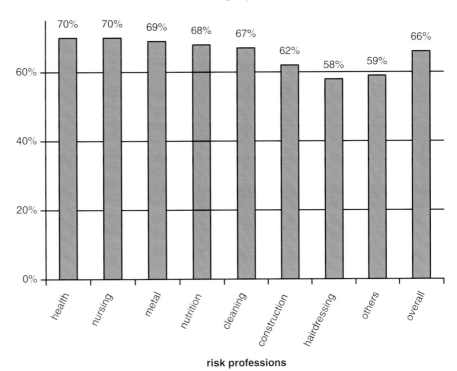

Fig. 50.5 Employment continuation of patients from various high-risk occupations 1 year after TIP (cohort 10/1994–09/2003). The comparatively low success rate in hairdressing does not result from an occupation-specific, but from an age-specific effect (i.e. a preponderance of younger age groups among this cohort of counselled hairdressers; among these age groups, the risk of career shifting is higher; cf. Fig. 50.6). N_{total} = 1,164

50

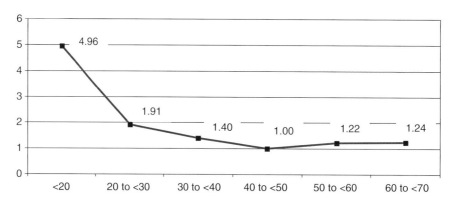

Fig. 50.6 Age-dependent risk of job loss by OCD among affected patients, 1 year after TIP (cohort 10/1994–09/2003). Logistic regression, adjusted for the implementation of advised prevention measures, supply of skin protection materials by employers, and implementation of outpatient medical treatment. 1=minimal risk of job loss. In the <20-year-old age group, the risk of job loss due to severe hand eczema is fivefold higher than in the 40- to 50-year-old age group [43]. N_{total}=1,163

continuation. Thus, TIP measures prove particularly successful in patients over 30 years of age, i.e. persons whose professional alternatives in the current employment market are limited. This observation emphasizes the socio-political dimension of such measures.

An earlier evaluation of the 2002 TIP-patient collective (n=274) showed that 91% of cases were primary OCD of the hands [44]. Clinically relevant type-IV sensitization was observed in 42% of cases, predominantly as secondarily acquired allergic contact eczema; they were most frequent in hairdressing (in 66% of cases). Now, a multi-centre study, which aims to further standardize TIP and evaluate sustainability of prevention in more depth (3-year dermatological follow-up of 1,000 OCD patients) is currently being conducted [21].

Core Message

> Recently obtained data reveal that there are scientifically sound options for multi-disciplinary prevention and patient management of OCD – dependent on disease severity – on an outpatient or a combined inpatient-outpatient basis, using a coordinated approach by a network of clinics, practices and statutory social insurance bodies.

50.2 Personal Skin Protection

50.2.1 Protective Gloves

50.2.1.1 Introduction

Gloves are probably the most common option of personal protective equipment (PPE) used to protect workers against damage to health from workplace skin exposure [45]. In the prevention of occupational contact dermatitis (OCD), gloves are important and effective against most irritants. The usage of protective gloves is one of the several possibilities to avoid developing OCD. However, current protective gloves are not perfect: depending on the glove material, some are permeable to various chemicals and do not provide the promised protection; side effects such as occlusion, latex and contact allergy are common reasons for discontinuance of their usage.

The health and safety executive (HSE) [46] states that there are four basic requirements that must be met for any suitable protective glove:

- It must be appropriate for the risks and the conditions where it is used.
- It must take into account the ergonomic requirements and state of health of the user.

- It must fit the user correctly, if necessary, after adjustments.
- It must control or prevent the risk involved without increasing the overall risk.

Table 50.1 Pictograms EN 374

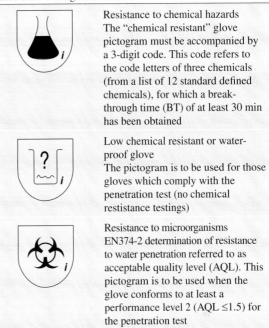

	Resistance to chemical hazards The "chemical resistant" glove pictogram must be accompanied by a 3-digit code. This code refers to the code letters of three chemicals (from a list of 12 standard defined chemicals), for which a break-through time (BT) of at least 30 min has been obtained
	Low chemical resistant or water-proof glove The pictogram is to be used for those gloves which comply with the penetration test (no chemical restistance testings)
	Resistance to microorganisms EN374-2 determination of resistance to water penetration referred to as acceptable quality level (AQL). This pictogram is to be used when the glove conforms to at least a performance level 2 (AQL ≤1.5) for the penetration test

Core Message

If protective gloves are selected or worn incorrectly, it may increase the wearers' overall risk to health, because:

> Contaminants may get inside the glove to reside permanently against the skin which could cause greater exposure than if a glove had not been worn at all.

> Wearing a glove for extended periods can lead to the development of excessive moisture (occlusion effect) on the skin which itself may act as an irritant.

> Wearing gloves can cause an allergic reaction (see Chap. 49).

50.2.1.2 Rules and Regulations

In Europe, gloves are covered by the PPE Directive 89/686/EEC "Gloves intended for protection". This Directive states the general requirements for PPE for each type of protective glove; medical gloves (MG) are dealt with separately. The PPE Directive is a part of European legislation which defines essential requirements for the product [162]. The Directive is based upon the existence of European Standards to define specifications or performance levels for the products. The Directive is passed by the European Parliament and adopted into national law, whereas the European Standard is prepared by a committee made up of various interested parties (including manufacturers, Health & Safety Specialists, Test & Certification Bodies) and represents a consensus of opinion reached by all parties.

Under European regulations, levels of risk and seriousness of the potential injury have to be determined and the protective gloves are divided into three categories:

Category I: Gloves of simple design – suitable for minimum risk.

Category II: Gloves of intermediate design – for intermediate risk.

Category III: Gloves of complex design – for protection against high risks, i.e. where skin exposure would result in irreversible damage to health or possibly death.

The different categories require different amounts of quality proofs and information. Only for category III, the number of the certified testing institute has to be marked.

According to the results of testing the penetration and permeation of chemicals, different pictograms have to be marked on each glove [47].

The EN 374 describes the pictograms and the conditions for using it (Table 50.1). The EN 374/2 indicate the level of penetration in terms of the Acceptable Quality Level. The permeation of hazardous liquids measuring the breakthrough time (BT) is defined in EN 374/3 [48].

Chemical Protective Gloves

The requirements for chemical protective gloves underline the importance of sound information about their performance. In the context of the new EC 1907/2006, the marketing of substances will depend on the description of safe exposure scenarios [49]. If an exposure scenario is safe only because gloves are used, it will be the responsibility of the person who puts a chemical on the market to investigate and document that efficient gloves are available. The best way to respond to this duty would be to provide the minimum standard of effective protective glove or product names of effective gloves in the safety data sheets [50].

All chemical protective gloves in the EU must be CE marked. Unfortunately, it is a fallacy that this enables to select the appropriate glove and can also be taken to indicate how well the glove will perform. It is not always realized that the CE marking is neither a guarantee of quality nor of the suitability of a glove for a particular purpose [45].

Medical Gloves (MGs)

In Europe, MGs which are intended to protect patients and users from cross-contamination are referred to as medical devices and are covered by the European Council Directive 93/42/EEC concerning medical devices [51].

The use of single use gloves in the health sector is being regulated by a separate European standard (EN 455) [52]. The requirements are modified to the medical workplace. It seems that these regulations are lesser than those laid down in the regulations for chemical protective gloves (EN 374-I–III) [53]. EN 455 comprises standard techniques for accessing water tightness in compliance with an acceptable Quality Level of 1.5 (penetration). Further, in Part 2, the physical properties of the MG for single use will be measured (e.g., dimension, length, wide, strength). In Part 3, the evaluation of biological safety (contents of latex protein) has to be examined. There are no regulations concerning permeation (unlike EN 374-III). The tested gloves have to be signed with the label EN455 and the pictogram for latex, if they contain this protein.

The imminent underlying hypothesis is that if a glove fulfils the criteria for penetration according to EN 374-II (meaning, particularly, that there are no holes in the glove), then this glove is also impermeable to micro organisms. It is remarkable that EN 455 does not contain any regulations as to the question of permeability of chemicals. Considering the fact that in the health sector, there is an exposure to various chemicals including allergens (like bone cement, dental acrylates, etc.),

this seems a lack. The only exception may be in the field of medication with cytostatic drugs in oncology where it is recommended to use single-use gloves, which are certified and tested by EN374, in contact with cytostatica in pharmaceutical and medical health care setting.

A recent survey of the USA rules, regulations and standards concerning protective and MG use has been presented by Henry III [54]. These regulations are highly similar to the European ones.

In 2008, in Germany, a comprehensive approach to dermal risk assessment in real work settings was published in the Technical Rule on Hazardous Substances 401 (TRGS 401) [55]. European regulations of dangerous substances do not include wet work as a skin hazard factor, whereas, the current German TRGS 401 does. Moreover, it states that it is an occupational hazard if workers are exposed to a humid environment or wear impermeable gloves for more than a total of 2 h per work shift. To our knowledge, this is the first time that wearing occlusive gloves has been legally equated to wet work and defined as occupational hazard. Recent results may advocate wet work as occupational exposure to a humid environment of a total of >2 h per work shift.

Referring to gloves, the TRGS 401 specifies that:

- The user does not have to investigate glove effectiveness if the producer of a chemical specifies the product name of the gloves.
- The effectiveness of gloves must be proven by the producer. However, as performance tests are not yet standardized, employers have to decide about the tests according to their best judgement.
- If toxicological data or other reliable information is not available for a chemical substance, it should be regarded as an R24 or R38 substance (toxic in contact to skin, irritates the skin) when selecting risk management measures.
- If only the BTs according to EN 374-III are known, it is recommended that the gloves should be worn at the most for one-third of this time.

50.2.1.3 Standard Methods for Testing the Protective Glove Barrier

Different properties have to be tested and evaluated if protective gloves are to give an adequate level of protection (EN 374).

Penetration

Penetration refers to the passage of chemicals through macroscopic holes or pores. Penetrability can result from a manufacturing process (a material defect) or from faulty or lengthy storage.

Testing of penetrability is regulated in EN 374-2 [56] and ASTM F 903 [57]. The results of an air or water leakage test determine the acceptance quality level (AQL) values as described in EN 374-2. The AQL value names the maximum share of faulty units that can be considered as satisfactory quality for sampling inspection. Table 50.2 lists the AQL values demanded for each level of performance. For MGs, an AQL of 1.5 is demanded.

Table 50.2 Penetration testing: air/water leakage test, performance levels and acceptance quality levels (AQLs)

AQL maximum number leaking gloves in percentage	4.0	1.5	0.65
Performance level	1	2	3

Permeation

Permeation refers to the migration of chemicals through the protective glove material on a molecular level (sorption, diffusion, de-sorption). There is a standard test for penetration and permeation included in EN 374-III [58] and similarly in ASTM F 739 [59] and ASTM F 1383 [60].

Key parameter for permeation measurement is the BT in minutes. BT is defined as the elapsed time between the initial application of a test chemical and the point of time at which a permeation rate (PR) of $1\ \mu g/min/cm^2$ (EN Standard) – $0.1\ \mu g/min/cm^2$ (ASTM standard) – is detected (Fig. 50.7; Table 50.3).

The standard only determines permeation under conditions of total contact, but without stretching,

Penetration

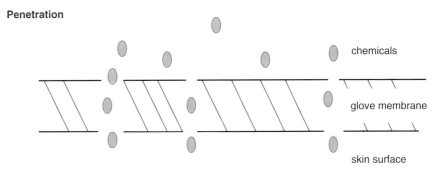

Measurements: airtight or watertight seal tested according to EN 374, part 2

Permeation

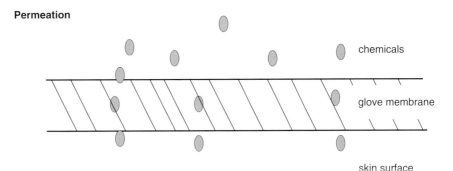

Fig. 50.7 Test parameters for barrier function of protective gloves: penetration and permeation [82]

Measurements: Two-compartment permeation cell of standard dimensions according to EN 374, part 2

Table 50.3 Permeation testing: protection Indexes and determined BTs of chemicals through glove membranes

Breakthrough time (min)	>10	>30	>60	>120	>240	>480
Class (Protection Index)	1	2	3	4	5	6

flexing or other factors that will occur when a glove is used in a real working environment. Furthermore, the standard (EN 374-III) requires that the test is conducted at a temperature of $23 \pm 1°C$. Inside an occlusive glove, the raised skin temperature will result in a higher temperature of the glove material. This can have significant effects on the permeation BT [45].

A further problem arises as most data of the manufacturers will provide information on permeation BT for individual chemicals, whereas real working environments are characterized by a mixture of chemicals. The process of permeation of mixtures is complex, depending upon several factors, in particular, concentration. Some chemicals may act as vehicles, enhancing the permeation of others.

Degradation

Degradation describes the interaction between the chemical substance and the glove material. The glove may become brittle and split, may swell and lose its mechanical strength or simply dissolve. Unfortunately, there is currently no standard, either within the European Union or the United states, for testing degradation. Different manufacturers are free to use different test methods to determine the level of degradation that will occur with their gloves in contact with different chemicals. Thus, the comparison of the degradation of gloves from different manufacturers can be misleading.

Other test methods for protective gloves and MGs like biocompatibility, in vivo testing in man or in experimental animals, have been presented by Boman and Mellström [61].

50.2.1.4 Glove Materials and Manufacturing

Mellström and Bowman [62] presented a detailed description of the materials used for gloves. Table 50.4

Table 50.4 Overview: glove materials used for PG and MG [modified from 63]

Name of material/trade names (abbreviation)	Application field
Natural rubber materials	
Natural rubber/Latex (NR)	PG, MG
Synthetic rubber materials	
Butyl rubber (BR)	PG
Chloroprene/Neoprene (CR)	PG, MG
Flour rubber/Viton (V)	PG
Polyisoprene rubber/Isolex (PIR)	PG, MG
Nitrile rubber/N-Dex, Nitrilite (NI)	PG, MG
Styrene butadiene/Elastyrene (SBR)	MG
Styrene ethylene butadien/Tactylon	MG
Styrene isoprene	MG
Plastic polymeric materials	
Ethylene methylacrylate (EMA)	PG, MG
Polyethylene (PE)	PG, MG
Polyvinylalcohol (PVA)	PG
Polyvinylchloride (PVC)	PG, MG
olyurethane (PU)	PG
E+Ethylenvinylalcohol (EVOH)+PE/Laminate, 4H-glove	PG, MG
Leather	PG
Textile	
Cotton	PG
Nylon	PG
Jersey	PG
Silk	PG
Bamboo	PG
Special fibre materials (cut resistant)	
Kevlar	PG
Lycra	
Spectra fibre	

gives a survey of glove materials used for protective gloves (PG) and MG.

The protective effect of different glove materials against hazardous substances depends on the one hand on the type and composition of the material; protective effect of the same material can differ due to manufacturing processes, variation in polymer formulation, use of additives and procedures of quality control. On the other hand, the protective effect depends on the thickness of the glove material; in a non-linear fashion, the BT increases with the thickness of glove materials [61, 63].

50.2.1.5 Unwanted Side Effects of Gloves

Selection of the Wrong Glove

Often, the employer does not know about the effective use of protective gloves. The provision of suitable protective gloves against chemical hazard is difficult because of the wide variety of gloves companies. There are companies with a high-quality level of glove production, and also low-cost producers.

The variety of available products makes it difficult for the user to select the suitable glove material. On the glove package, usually, only details of the resistance towards individual substances are declared. Only a few glove manufacturers give concrete recommendations to their glove materials for dealing with substance mixtures. In practice, in most workplaces, substance mixtures will be a relevant chemical hazard [64].

Unfortunately, all too frequently, gloves will be chosen because of the price and availability. Often, there is no understanding of glove function and the correct use of certain gloves.

Internal Contamination of Gloves

Macroscopic holes or pores or a high permeability may not be easily detected and can result in quite extensive contamination inside the glove.

Even if the correct glove has been chosen, skin contamination is common. Incorrect handling and wrong removal of gloves can result in the workers' hands becoming contaminated with the chemicals against which the glove is intended to provide protection [65]. Correct techniques for donning and removing of gloves, depending on whether the gloves are single use or will be reused are described by Packham and Packham [64].

Occlusion Effects

On the one hand, the use of impermeable gloves offers protection against occupational noxious substances. On the other hand, it is reported that long-term glove wearing may lead to irritant contact dermatitis [66, 67], also called hydration dermatitis [68, 69].

However, there is still conflicting evidence on that matter. We recently analyzed the occlusive effects of glove materials (polyvinyl chloride, natural rubber latex) on epidermal barrier function and related the findings to the definitions of wet work in the current German Technical Regulations on Hazardous Substances [55]. The study showed only very low effects by occlusion in healthy skin. A significant long-term effect after daily occlusion for 4 h during 7 days could not be demonstrated [70]. A current study by Fartasch et al. [71] concludes that repeated occlusions increase the irritability of the skin. However, differences to controls were detected only after occlusion >3 h/day and consecutive irritation.

Allergic Contact Dermatitis from Protective Gloves

Geier et al. state that at the present level of technological development, it is not possible to produce an elastic protective glove without the use of vulcanization accelerators [72]. It is known that vulcanization accelerators frequently lead to contact sensitizations (type IV-allergy). Despite a certain retrograde trend within the last few years, thiurames are by far the most frequent glove-related allergens [73, 74]. Dithiocarbamates as well as mercaptobenzothiazol and its derivatives also often appear as allergens in this area [75]. 1,3-Diphenylguanidine is seldom used in protective gloves; the test preparation often leads to wrong positive reactions [76].

Within the last few years, single cases of allergic reactions to polyvinylchloride (PVC) gloves were also described, with the bisphenol A, formaldehyde or benzisothiazolinon as the responsible allergens [77, 78].

A few years ago, the latex contact urticaria (type-I-allergy) represented a great problem in medical professions. According to evidence-based legal regulations and extensive prevention measures by the professional associations in many countries, the incidence of this occupational illness could be dramatically reduced [9].

In rare cases, type-IV-reactions to natural rubber latex (eczematous-like reactions) have also been observed [79–81].

50

50.2.1.6 Perspectives

Semi-Permeable Gloves

The principle of semi-permeable membranes is known by the application of "breathing active" functional clothing, e.g., using membranes from manufacturers like GoreTex® (W. L. Gore & Associates Inc., www.goretex.com) or Sympatex® (Sympatex Technologies Inc., www.sympatex.com). These membranes are selectively permeable; on the one hand, they prevent water penetration from the outside, while on the other hand, they allow water vapour transport from the inside medium to the outside. In an effort to transfer this working principle on to protective gloves, the benefit of prototypes of semi-permeable gloves in the prevention of occupational skin disease could be demonstrated. It was possible to avoid the negative effects of longstanding occlusion on skin barrier properties with semi-permeable gloves in healthy skin [82].

Recently, it was observed that semi-permeable membranes are also suitable in patients with pre-existing irritant skin damage (experimentally induced standardized irritation with SLS). These findings support the hypothesis that semi-permeable materials improve barrier recovery rates by providing an optimized water vapour gradient during the healing process. In conclusion, the results indicate a relevant benefit of semi-permeable protective gloves for the prevention of occupational skin diseases, particularly when considering the fact that many wet workers start using gloves only after the occurrence of initial skin damage [83]. However, as yet, the chemical resistance of these gloves is unsatisfactory. Therefore, at present, we examine the suitability of the material as a lining, worn under a chemical protective glove or in restricted work activities, where there is exposure only to humidity, but not to chemicals.

Rip Up Gloves for the Work
on Shifting Machines

A considerable problem for the protection of workers against cutting fluids in the metal industry is created by rotating machines, where for safety reasons, wearing gloves should be avoided and is legally prohibited in some countries. Particularly, if exposed workers have already developed allergies against cutting fluid

ingredients like colophony or monoethanolamine, protection with chemical-resistant gloves is essential from an allergologists' point of view. There are new developments in the creation of easy-tearing gloves in order to overcome these problems; however, so far, no published data are available.

"Hypoallergenic" Gloves

At present, industry is developing gloves which do not contain any vulcanization accelerators and have nevertheless elastic and protective properties. Some manufacturers already offer such accelerator-free gloves as "hypoallergenic". Properly designed studies assessing the technical qualities and the chemical resistance of these new developments have to show whether the "hypoallergenic" glove means progress to the prevention of the OCDs.

50.2.2 Barrier Creams

Protective creams and gels (PC) or so-called barrier creams are one of the classical measures to protect the hands against low-grade hazards at the work place. During recent years, the prevailing opinion has been for PCs that they are effective in a pure physical way, since due to their composition, a diffusion barrier against the offending irritant is built up to prevent penetration. Hazardous substances of similar physico-chemical properties are grouped (e.g., water-miscible or non-water-miscible) to simplify the product recommendation [84]. However, the theory that the product builds up only a physical barrier between the skin and the irritant, and the formulation remains unchanged after the product has been applied to the skin, is incorrect [85]. It should also be taken into consideration that in many workplaces, skin contact to both water-miscible and non-water-miscible irritants is unavoidable and a simple formulation based on only physical properties may not prevent against both types of irritants. Moreover, it has to be considered that skin protection products cannot offer protection that is comparable with gloves. Preparations marketed as "invisible glove" may feign a seeming protection that causes workers at risk to be careless of contact to irritants. On the other hand, PCs often remain the only realizable preventive measure in the case of occupations with an increased requirement for sense of touch, finger mobility or when working at rotating machines.

Basically, the concept of an integrative skin protection at the workplace consists of a three-step programme consisting of skin protection before work, skin cleansers removing aggressive substances from the skin, and skin care products to be used after work to restore the natural barrier function and to increase skin hydration and skin smoothing [84, 86, 87]. Most manufacturers offer special plans to pursue this aim. However, the benefit of the integrated skin protection based on different products still has only rarely been validated [86, 88, 89]. Not only has it been debated whether a strict distinction between skin care products used before and after work is justified, since emollients alone have been shown to treat and prevent irritant contact dermatitis [90], but also the effectiveness of PCs in general has been discussed over so many years now [91–93]. In a recent review on the evidence of each single element of that three-step programme, Kütting and Drexler [86] came to the following conclusion: In cases of impaired skin conditions, the therapeutic effect of skin protection as part of secondary prevention was undoubted. However, the benefit of PCs in primary prevention of hand eczema could not been proven according to their review. Beyond doubt was the fact that PCs facilitate the removal of sticky oils, greases and resins from the skin, thus decreasing the need to wash with potentially irritating abrasives and waterless cleansers.

50.2.2.1 Study Designs to Prove Effectiveness

Much effort has been taken to develop valid methods for the evaluation of actual protective properties of PCs. Of course, for proper assessment, intervention studies in factories are required, but double-blinded, placebo-controlled, randomized clinical tests of PCs are still missing for reasons of methodological difficulties, ethical doubts and the enormous expenditure for tests regarding the preventive benefit of PCs in practice. Publications on real intervention studies of PCs in

a workplace setting are scarce [23, 94–97]. In most studies, the interpretation is difficult because of the small sample size, short follow-up or the low incidence of hand eczema during the study period. The observed effect is always a combination of the intervention effect being measured, and a number of disturbing variables reflecting the organizational complexity of such studies [98]. Therefore, the potential effect of PCs in the prevention of work-related hand eczema has mostly been documented in a laboratory setting and on experimentally damaged skin. The extent to which experimental data from test models are generally applicable to actual occupational exposure is of course a matter of debate [89]. However, to understand the principles of skin protection preparations and to investigate their benefit at least against test irritants, a variety of models have been established and regarded as helpful. A guideline of the German Task Force for Occupational and Environmental Medicine (ABD) has recently reviewed the current literature, and gives recommendations for the selection of test models and study designs, and discusses their values and limitations [99].

Since Suskind introduced the "slide test" to evaluate PCs in the 1950s [100], various studies using penetration, diffusion and absorption models, excised human skin or reconstructed epidermis have been performed to investigate both the effects of irritants on skin barrier function and the benefit of PCs under highly experimental conditions [101–112]. However, all of these studies are not considered close enough to real work place situations.

Coming to human in vivo studies, the first standardized repeated irritation test (RIT) test in humans, with a set of four relevant irritants was presented by Frosch and Kurte in 1994 [85]. Different formulations could be simultaneously compared to the control field, which receives the irritant only, without PC-pre-treatment. Irritant cutaneous reactions were quantified by four parameters: erythema score, transepidermal water loss (TEWL), blood flow volume and stratum corneum hydration by measuring capacitance. The main conclusion was: The dogma that oil-in-water emulsions are primarily effective against lipophilic irritants, and water-in-oil emulsions against hydrophilic irritants, needs to be re-evaluated. A specific profile of PC effectiveness could be demonstrated. The interaction of the skin, the formulation and the irritant is complex and has to be evaluated in humans. These observations still hold true after many years. Most repetitive test designs used nowadays are based on the RIT [113, 114]. In a national multi-centre study, a repeated short-time occlusive irritation test (ROIT) has been evaluated in six skilled centres [115]. The skin reactions were induced by two irritants (SLS and TOL). The evaluation showed that significant results could already be achieved with a 5-day protocol. Furthermore, in spite of the expected inter-centre variations due to heterogeneity of the individual threshold of irritation, interpretation of clinical score and inter-instrumental variability, the ranking of the PCs with respect to the reduction of the irritant reaction was consistent in all centres.

In spite of promising data, it may be criticized that in all models presented, the investigation of PC effectiveness has been limited to the exposure of a single irritant only. Skin exposure in the occupational setting can be very complex. Hydrophilic and hydrophobic irritants such as the anionic surfactant SLS and the organic solvent TOL have mainly been used in studies although repetitive contact to both hydrophilic and hydrophobic substances together or, more commonly, one after the other, occurs regularly in the workplace setting. For instance, workers in the metal working industry are repetitively exposed to water-based metal working fluids, neat oils, detergents and organic solvents. Therefore, the interaction between irritant chemicals has significant practical consequences. Indeed, concurrent application of SLS and TOL was shown to induce significantly stronger reactions than those caused by twice daily application of each irritant on its own [116]. This additive effect of a mixed irritant application on skin irritation is significant for the use of PCs in practice and the way PCs should be tested. The benefit of a commercially available PC compared to non-pre-treated control sites was tested against the sequential application of two irritants in the so-called tandem repeated irritation test (TRIT) [117]. Interaction of further irritants has been investigated with attention to professions where a multitude of hazardous substances may cause irritant contact dermatitis [118].

It should not be concealed that some authors found no protection from or even aggravation of irritant contact dermatitis [114, 119–121] and the protective properties against systemic absorption of solvents were less than adequate [101, 105]. The galenic composition of a PC and their possible interaction with the offending irritant may correspond to either a protective or an irritant effect on human stratum corneum, in worse case, even a better penetration of the irritant [122]. In an experimental setting, the penetration of butoxyethanole was increased by using skin care products after artificially induced barrier disruption by tape stripping [123]. The pathomechanisms of increase or decrease of penetration of technical substances such as solvents due to skin care products is still not totally understood. Discussed to promote an enhancement are ingredients such as emulsifers [105, 124, 125].

50.2.2.2 Usage and Application

The best product cannot be of any benefit when not applied properly. PCs should be applied before contact to irritants, which includes a re-application after every break or a certain period e.g., half a work shift according to manufacturers' claim. Before the re-application of the product, the skin has to be cleaned and dried to avoid increased penetration of remaining irritants on the skin surface [84]. It is clear that the effectiveness of a PC is also influenced by the application itself. They must be applied not only frequently enough, but also in adequate amounts and to all skin areas that need protection. Studies with a fluorescent-marked PC indicated that the application was mostly incomplete in different professional groups and patients with hand eczema especially in the dorsum of the hands and the inter-digital spaces, excluding the space between the index finger and the thumb [126]. This might be an explanation why experimentally tested products fail in studies with application at the workplace. Simply, lack of protection could be

Core Message
› In vitro methods may help to discriminate between different formulations. Repetitive irritation tests in humans are more related to the workplace situation and should be performed with relevant irritants.

Core Message
› The accuracy and regularity of proper application is a basic condition for protective creams to be effective. Each interventional programme should take care of sufficient education in product application.

caused by uneven or spotty application of skin care products. Individuals should be made aware of the most commonly missed regions to ensure complete skin protection. A simple fluorescence method may be useful to quantify self-application and in worker education [127, 128].

50.2.2.3 Strategies

Though PCs are one of the common measures to prevent irritant contact dermatitis, their actual benefit at the workplace remains controversial [93]. The data of in vitro and in vivo tests underline the importance of careful selection of PCs for specific workplaces. Choosing the wrong preparation may well worsen the effect of an irritant. However, results of animal experiments may not be valid for humans, particularly when dealing with irritants, in view of their complex action mechanisms and the high inter-individual variability in susceptibility of human skin [129]. Regarding the various models to investigate the effectiveness of skin care products, the validation of a sensitive, standardized and widely accepted model proved by inter-laboratory standardization or controlled clinical studies at the workplace still seems to be necessary. Clearly, studies both under experimental conditions and in the workplace are needed before a rational recommendation can be made if a product is safe and effective for skin protection. For the evidence-based recommendation of skin protection, further studies, especially under daily working conditions evaluating the contribution of each single element of skincare programme (products, frequency of application and education programme) are needed [89]. However, repetitive studies in humans – even if they are experimental – are still the gold standard. The number of workplace substances is uncountable, and technical progress enforces the adaptation of technical substances and fluids to the new demands. For that reason, there is still is big need for experimental studies with new protection formulations which can hardly be tested in long-term randomized trials in humans at work [130].

Due to the variety of potential irritants at the workplace, mostly, standard irritants are used in order to examine the effectiveness of products in relation to groups of irritants (e.g., detergents). This may be permissible if the manufacturer refers to the fact that the examination took place in a model. Whenever protection against an individual substance, groups of working materials or other skin hazards is claimed, it has to

be proven that the skin protection was examined against these substances. If the use of PCs is recommended against a combination of irritants, models with combination of irritants should be used [117]. The same holds true for the benefit of an integrative skin protection concept and the interaction of protection, skin cleansing and regeneration [88]. The variability of results due to different formulations has been shown in a previous study on long-term treatment with moisturizers [131]. The only preparation that caused a significantly lower increase of TEWL after SLS irritation was a complex cream compared to simple formulations. The importance of specific chosen ingredients could be highlighted by a study comparing the protection of a PC and a skin care cream against irritation by SLS [104]. Both the preparations had similar basic ingredients but the PC had some specific ingredients claimed to be protective as such and the skin care formulation had ingredients which are claimed to have regeneration and barrier repair effects. In that experimental test design, only the PC demonstrated protection against irritation with SLS.

In a recent prospective, randomized, controlled trial to compare the effect of skin protection and skin care alone or in combination with cleansing against a control group, 485 workers from the building and the timber industries were examined over 1 year [23]. When evaluating the changes in TEWL values, measured at the dorsal aspects of the hands, in the building industry workers, an improvement was found for the group that used skin protection and skin care in combination and the group that used skin care alone. In the timber industry, there was an improvement for the group with skin protection and skin care in combination and even by skin protection alone. In female workers, only mild eczema increased descriptively in all groups between the first and the second visit except for the group using skin protection alone. Even the TEWL scores decreased linearly for the group using the combination and for – the right hand – the one using skin protection alone. However, the authors conclude that skin protection creams alone have a small effect on the skin barrier in workers included in the study compared with skin care alone or in combination. Nevertheless, gender effects in that study were relevant and may give an indication about the different usage habits of workers previously discussed [122]. A standardized interview in 1,355 metalworkers confirmed a poorer compliance regarding the use of PCs in men than in women [16].

Taking all these results together, it seems obvious that choosing the wrong preparation may cause aggravated irritation due to lack of effectiveness or even worse due to prolonged or increased penetration of hazardous technical substances such as solvents. But on the other hand, protective effects could be proved for some preparations in experimental test designs. Lack of effectiveness in cohort studies at the workplace has to be discussed critically as long as adequate application of products has not been investigated in these studies.

> **Core Message**
>
> › Whenever a combination of protective creams and skin care products has an advantage compared to skin protection or skin care alone (even if skin care alone was more effective than skin protection alone), the use of protection products as part of a three-step programme seems to be justified.

50.3 Workers' Education

As demonstrated above (Sect. 50.2.1), understanding the appropriate gloves for different irritants may be quite complex. In addition, Tucker stated that: "even if a glove is capable of preventing contact between a chemical and the skin, it must be worn to accomplish this preventive effect" [36, 163]. To facilitate the skin protection behaviour of workers in professions with high risks to develop OCD, educational measures have become more favourable in the last decade. Health educational measures in OCD prevention programmes are described in many papers as one part of standard measures to improve the outcome of occupational skin disease. Many authors claimed that patient educational programmes are effective, evidence based and efficient [4, 24, 26, 43, 132, 133]. Projects on primary, secondary and tertiary prevention of OCD have approached both medical and educational procedures on an inter-disciplinary and integrative level for different professions [20, 134–136]. Only a few authors are less euphoric [137], when they characterize irritant hand dermatitis as chronic in duration, despite all efforts in education [138]. Educational programmes have shown to be

effective for the reduction of the prevalence of OCD in many occupations (see Table 50.5). Health education was shown to be an effective tool in the primary, secondary and tertiary prevention of skin disorders. It has been stressed that education during apprenticeship or initial training is most important [24]. Most authors fail to reveal the reason for the effectiveness of the programmes. After the establishment of skin protection programmes including educational measures for the reduction of skin symptoms in different wet occupations in all levels of preventions (primary, secondary and tertiary), further work on evidence and refinement of the theoretical basis, the aims and outcome parameters, the methods, the structure and the implementation of skin protection programmes by different health care professionals should be initiated [24].

> **Core Message**
>
> Strategies of workers' education
>
> › Induce awareness to health hazards
> › Thus avoid complacency at the workplace
> › Identify particularly hazardous work activities
> › Develop protective strategies to avoid them
> › Dermatological pre-employment counselling should identify persons at risk, and provide them with specific instructions/teaching offers
> › Teaching should generally start before or along with job training and be repeated periodically in risk professions
> › It should stress the pathogenesis of OCD, and give practical and specific advice to best practice skin protection policy, including glove use, removal of gloves without contamination, moisture-absorbing cotton linings, protective creams, after-work creams etc.
> › It should be empowerment-based (creating motivation) and include clues to laymen's recognition of early OCD-symptoms
> › Multi-disciplinary approaches (dermatologist/educationalist) are successful
> › Include employers as on-job-multipliers (combined top-down and bottom-up strategy)
> › Include social insurance bodies and social partners in the various branches

Table 50.5 Epidemiological basis and educational aspects of intervention studies on primary, secondary and tertiary prevention of OCD

Profession(s)	Design	Aim	Outcome parameters	Results	References
Epidemiological basis					
Printers	Evaluation in two non-randomly selected companies, focus group $n=5$; direct observational studies 21	To elicit key issues that would aid the development of subsequent interventions	Skin care policy, use of gloves	Lack of skin care policy, no provision of occupational health services, less knowledge. Regular use of gloves of the correct type and size is the most practical intervention	Brown et al. [12]
Dental technicians	Retrospective Cohort Study ($n=2,139$), questionnaires, dental technicians and randomly selected population controls	To estimate occupational skin exposure, the use of skin protection and the incidence of hand eczema		Frequent and unprotected exposure to methacrylates, frequent hand washings, dental technicians have twice the risk of hand eczema than the general population. Efforts to improve skin protection and increase participation in obligatory training are important	Meding et al. [155]
Nurses	Questionnaires ($n=112$) Observation ($n=53$)	To assess the exposure levels to wet work (duration and frequency of skin irritant exposure in nursing)		Observation method showed that the actual duration of wet work was less than half the duration of subjectively estimated wet work. A questionnaire does not accurately assess the quantity of wet-work activities. The quantity of wet-work activities is different depending on the job activities, gloves were used daily for short-time periods. Prevention programmes should focus on decreasing the frequency of wet hands by encouraging the use of gloves	Jungbauer et al. [66]
Hairdressers apprentices	Total survey of hairdressers' trainees in lower Saxony, 5-year periods, standardized questionnaires: 1989: $n=4,008$, 1994: $n=2,505$, 1999: $n=2,427$, conducted by health educational specialists	To assess the incidence of hand eczema, the exposure levels, the use of skin protection, consultation of physicians		Incidence of self reported skin diseases decreased from 70 to 57% between 1989 and 1994, while during 1994 and 1999, a slight increase to 61% was observed. The use of gloves increased between 1989 and 1994. Comparison between 1994 and 1999 reveals a stagnation in the use of protective gloves. Results reason the necessity to continue preventive measures	Schlesinger et al. [156]

(continued)

50

Table 50.5 (continued)

Profession(s)	Design	Aim	Outcome parameters	Results	References
Hairdressers	Population-based study Questionnaire ($n=193$ trainees, $n=184$ practicing hairdressers)	To assess the knowledge on skin hazards, practiced skills and the use of preventive measures		70% identified chemicals as potential skin hazards, less than 15% identified the role of wet work correctly, only a small proportion recognized that chemicals could cause allergy. Use of gloves was inadequate. Recommendation of improved student education, appropriate glove use and the application of after-work emollient creams	Nixon et al. [157]
Primary prevention					
Health care trainees	RCT ($n=521$), interviews, evaluation of skin changes by examination, intervention: teaching protocol regarding all aspects of primary prevention (three times in the first, twice in the second year)	To investigate the effects of primary skin prevention employing an educational training in all aspects of occupational skin protection	Morphological changes of the hands, use of hand care creams, knowledge regarding skin care	Significantly better skin condition of the hands in the intervention group (22.6%). No difference in the amount of skin care cream used	Löffler et al. [17]
Adolescents/high school students before choice of occupation	Baseline and follow-up-questionnaire ($n=1,015$), 2 weeks after intervention (instruction by dermatologists vs. a teacher). 90-min teaching unit on occupational skin hazards and allergies, identification of risk persons, application of preventive measures, conducted by dermatologists and teachers	To inform adolescents about potentially hazardous occupations, risk groups and preventive measures before they started apprenticeships in order to minimize the risk of OCD	Knowledge, acceptance of the teaching unit	Increased knowledge after the training, acceptance of the teaching unit	Radulescu et al. [135]
Student auxiliary nurses	Intervention study ($n=107$), questionnaires, clinical evaluation of the hands, measurements of TEWL, patch testing, educational programme before starting of the practical training, follow-up 10 weeks after starting practical training	To investigate whether an educational programme was efficient in preventing work-related skin problems on the hands	Use of disinfectants, aggravation of skin problems, TEWL	Significant increase in TEWL for the control group (CG) ($p<0.005$), use of hand disinfectants was significantly lower in the intervention group ($p=0.002$), 4% of the intervention group had less problems with skin during practical training ($p>0.05$)	Held et al. [14]

Population	Study design	Aim	Outcome measures	Results	Reference
Hairdressers' apprentices	Controlled intervention study (n=185), standardized interviews and dermatological examination (four times during vocational training in year 1–3), training in skin protection measures (six seminars), training by a professional teacher, dermatological examination	Significant reduction in hand eczema	Knowledge and attitude concerning skin care management, reduction of skin lesions	At the end of the 3 years vocational training, 90% of intervention group (IG) and 75% of CG had no skin changes (p<0.05)	Riehl [158]
Bakers' apprentices	Controlled intervention study (n=94), standardized interviews, 4 monthly follow-up, training in skin protection measures	To quantify the uptake and maintenance of standard prevention techniques in first year bakers' apprentices	Point prevalence of hand dermatitis, uptake and maintenance of skin protection and skin care measures	Skin protection and skin care measures can be introduced successfully in the daily routine of a skin risk occupation and high uptake and maintenance can be achieved. Use of barrier cream in IG at follow-up: 100 vs. 3.2% in CG, use of protective gloves: 43.3% IG vs. 32.3% CG, acceptance of skin care: 88.9% IG vs. 68.1% CG	Bauer et al. [159]
Secondary prevention					
Geriatric nurses	RCT (n=209), standardized questionnaires (baseline and 3 month after intervention), severity classified clinically and by using bioengineering methods. Intervention: repeated training in skin protection measures over a period of 6 months, conducted by health educationalists and dermatologists	To evaluate the effects of an interdisciplinary prevention programme	Reduction of eczema frequencies, remain in work, use of protective measures	Significant reduction of eczema frequency in the IG (89%IG vs. 90% CG at baseline to 53% IG vs. 82% CG at follow-up, p<0.01)	Schuerer et al. [19]
Health care workers, cleaners, kitchen employees	Descriptive study (n=791) 2-day skin protection course, conducted by dermatologists, specialists in occupational medicine, hygiene specialists and staff of the insurance association	To elucidate the need for health education, advisory services, diagnostics and additional therapy in occupational dermatology	Diagnoses of participants attending a skin protection course, acceptance of the course by participants	Participants rated the course as good to excellent. 80% of the participants had skin lesions while attending the course, in 27% the dermatosis was severe	Weisshaar et al. [22]

(continued)

50

Table 50.5 (continued)

Profession(s)	Design	Aim	Outcome parameters	Results	References
Health care workers	Observational study (n=253), telephone interviews 1 year after attendance of a course in skin protection	To investigate the course of OCD and to what extent a change in health behaviour could be achieved 1 year after	Reduction of skin lesions, receiving medical care, sick leave due to skin lesions, remaining on the job, changes in skin care behaviour, impairment of QL, assessment of the course	Significant decrease of skin lesions (77% at baseline to 68% at follow up, $p=0.02$), 72% reported skin lesions had improved, 9% left their occupation due to skin disease. Skin care and skin protection had improved. Frequency of hand washing was reduced. Impairment of QL was reduced from 54% at baseline to 27% at follow-up ($p<0.001$)	Apfelbacher et al. [145]
Hairdressers	Controlled Intervention Study (n=215), Follow-up 3 months, 5 and 10 years after attendance of an educational programme, standardized questionnaires conducted by dermatologists and health educational specialists	To analyse the long-term effectiveness of a job-specific secondary programme, which was created to enable hairdressers to stay on the job despite their OCD	Frequency of job continuation, implementation of preventive measures, provision of skin protection by the employer, motivation to use it	3 month follow-up, remaining in work: 71.8% IG vs. 60% CG, give up work because of OCD: 14.7% IG vs. 22.5% CG (not significant), 5 year follow-up: remaining in work: 58.7% IG vs. 29.1% CG ($p<0.001$), give up work because of OCD: 12.8 vs. 27.3%. Ten year follow-up: stabilization of the effects shown by the 5 year follow-up results	Wulfhorst et al. [146]
Metal workers	Longitudinal Intervention study (n=90), standardized questionnaires, examination, 1-year follow-up after a 1 day skin protection course, conducted by dermatologists and health educational specialists	To improve individual skin protection, specific knowledge about the disease, decrease the severity of hand eczema	Clinical diagnoses, knowledge, acceptance of the course, skin protection behaviour	Positive tendencies of all parameters. 96.1% remained at workplace, rating of the prevention course as highly recommendable and practically relevant	Mertin et al. [160]
Health care workers, cheese dairies gut cleaners	RCT (n=1,909 health care workers, n=665 cheese dairies, n=736 gut cleaners), questionnaire surveys on baseline and 1 year follow-up – tutorial on topics (skin, how to make a skin policy for the department, training of resource-persons)	To implement evidence-based prevention programmes, significantly reduce hand eczema, use protective measures, change skin care products (to better products)	Frequency of eczema, use of protective measures	Health care workers: No significant reduction of eczema frequencies (24.2–18.5%).Cheese dairies: eczema frequencies were low (11.8 and 5.9%) in two cheese dairies, no overall changes in eczema, significant increase in the use of gloves, change in the use of skin care products. Gut cleaners: significant reduction in eczema (56–41%, $p<0.0005$),→ influence of occupational health management system in gut cleaners, significant increase in the use of gloves (39–47%), change in the use of skin care products (36%)	Flyvolm et al. [139]

Bakers and catering trade employees	Prospective controlled intervention study (n=225), development of specific recruitment strategies for an interdisciplinary Skin Disease Prevention Programme (SDPP), standard invitation vs. personalized methods	To increase the participation rate in the prevention programme	Commitment of the employees to join in the prevention programme	Commitment of employees to join the SDPP increased significantly from 30 to 54% in the group receiving the new personalized targeted invitation letter	Kaatz et al. [15]
Tertiary prevention					
Wet-work professions/ high-risk professions	Longitudinal Study (n=1,486), standardized questionnaire, 1 year follow-up after attendance of standardized interdisciplinary inpatient rehabilitation measures (2–3-weeks inpatient treatment plus intensive health-pedagogic counselling), consecutive 3-weeks outpatient treatment – (tertiary individual prevention – TIP), conducted by health educationalists, dermatologists, health psychologists	To analyse the effectiveness of intensified interdisciplinary preventive measures	Remaining in job, use of skin protection	764 (66%) of the responding 1,164 TIP patients had successfully remained in their (risk-)professions. To remain in the workplace was dependent on the individual motivation to use skin protection (p<0.001), provision of skin protection by the employer (p<0.001), (higher) age of the patient (p<0.001) and the duration of continued outpatient treatment by the local dermatologist (p<0.001) but unrelated to the kind of risk profession	Skudlik et al. [5]
Wet-work professions	Longitudinal design (n=101), questionnaire before and 3 weeks after a 3 week tertiary inpatient individual prevention programme (TIP), conducted by health psychologists and dermatologists	To evaluate whether social cognitions as embroiled by the theory of planned behaviour become more favourable during TIP and whether the modes of predictions hold in a setting to which the model has not been applied	Attitude, subjective descriptive norm, perceived behavioural control, behavioural intention	Attitude, perceived behavioural control and intention to perform skin protection significantly increased during TIP. Results emphasize the importance of health educational and psychological interventions for patients with occupational skin disease	Matterne et al. [161]

50

This chapter discusses the effectiveness of educational approaches – which actually has not been systematically reviewed. Older reviews state a lack of high-quality studies on health education in skin protective programmes [4, 137]. We will focus on the prerequisites for high-quality studies with the aim to contribute to develop standards for health educational interventional studies in the prevention of OCD.

50.3.1 Definitions

Most health professions agree on the philosophical basis of patient education and the characteristics it encompasses have been recognized, the actual process of patient education and how it should be carried out have often been interpreted more broadly. The terms patient education, patient teaching and – in the special application field of prevention of OCD – eczema schools, have been used synonymously and the term instruction used interchangeably with education. In some instances, patient education has been equated to patient information. The terms education, instruction, teaching and information each imply a focus on knowledge. Certainly, to be able to carry out treatment recommendations, patients must have knowledge about what to do. However, knowledge alone is not always a predictor to behaviour [139]. Patients' knowledge about their condition and even that of recommendations are insufficient to ensure that those recommendations will be followed. Before patient education can be effective, learning must take place. Ultimately, learning involves more than the ability to regurgitate the facts. A comprehensive definition of patient education, then, must encompass more than presenting to a passive patient [140].

50.3.1.1 Health Education

Tones [141] considers health education as a technical activity – as a set of procedures designed to achieve whatever goals have been generated by ideological preference. These often conflicting goals have one thing in common: they aim to influence decision making and behaviour. So he stated: "Health education is any intentional activity which is designed to achieve health or illness-related learning, that is,

some relatively permanent change in an individuals' capability or disposition. Effective health education may thus produce changes in knowledge and understanding or ways of thinking, it may influence or clarify values, it may bring about some shift in belief or attitude, it may facilitate the acquisition of skills, and it may even effect changes in behaviour or lifestyle".

50.3.1.2 Patient Education

In the 1960s, the term patient education was beginning to be used by health professionals to convey the idea of dissemination of information to patients who had specific disease conditions. Patient education and health education were beginning to be viewed as two separate, although related concepts. Activities were planned to encourage patients with acute or chronic conditions to participate actively and appropriately in their treatment and rehabilitations [140].

Patient education is an active, individualized process directed not only towards knowledge, but also adaptation and behaviour change that will produce positive health outcomes. To be effective, this individualized process necessitates communication between patients and health professionals in which patients' needs, experiences, attitudes, preferences and other factors that impact their health and health care are identified. Patients' perceptions themselves, their lives, and their problems can have significant impact on the effectiveness of patient education [140, p. 32].

50.3.1.3 Eczema School

The term eczema school is sometimes used with respect to health educational measures for children or adolescents with atopy [142], as in [143] the following cases: "'Eczema school' educational programmes have proved to be helpful". In relation with OCD, "eczema school" is seldom used [133].

50.3.1.4 Skin Protection Programme

The prevention of OCD, health educational measures (primary prevention) and patient education are components of skin protection programmes. A skin protection programme is defined as "a series of practical instructions about skin care aimed at a well-defined group of people. In relation to OCD the programme may be directed at a certain occupation (i.e. wet workers, mechanics, hairdressers, etc.), or at a certain workplace. It is necessary that the skin protection programme is an integrated part of an educational programme, which should provide information on healthy and diseased skin, lead to early recognition of skin symptoms, and give the employees prerequisites to understand evidence-based recommendations regarding skin protective procedures. Ideally, an educational programme should improve knowledge about skin care, followed by a change in behaviour of skin protection and a decrease in clinical symptoms. Recommendations given in a skin protection programme should be evidence-based, as far as this is available" [24, p. 254].

50.3.2   Aims and Methods of Educational Programmes

In general, educational programmes have – independent of the specific disease – been developed to improve healthcare practices, reduce morbidity and lower costs of care [144].

Specific aims of patient educational programmes are summarized as follows: To change behaviour and decrease skin symptoms in wet occupations, improve the compliance, improve the level of knowledge, inform adolescents about potentially dangerous occupations, risk groups and preventive measures before they start apprenticeships, in order to minimize the risk of occupational allergies or skin diseases, improve the health-related quality of life, acquire problem-solving skills associated with acting or participating in authentic situations [17, 24, 133, 135, 145, 146]. In recent studies, very little information about educational preventive measures is provided. Flyvholm (2005) stated that educational activities include lectures, discussions, reflection, homework and feedback [134]. Brown (2004) prefers the use of a variety of educational tools, including instructional pamphlets, videotapes and lectures [4].

50.3.3   Theoretical Approaches in Health Educational Skin Protection Programmes

"The science and art of health behaviour and health education are eclectic, rapidly evolving and reflective of an amalgamation of approaches, methods and strategies from social and health sciences. Health education is also dependent on epidemiology, statistics and medicine. They draw on the theoretical perspectives, research, and practice tools of such diverse disciplines as psychology, sociology, anthropology etc." [147, p. 4]. Therefore, it is not possible to characterize all theoretical approaches of importance and actuality, which are the basis for the conceptualization of health educational skin protection programmes. We would like to outline some often-used theories; some of their constructions were used as outcome parameters in intervention studies on the prevention of OCD (e.g., self-efficacy).

Recently, the importance of employee involvement called *participatory action research* has been emphasized. This implies that the employees and/or their representatives participate actively in all phases of the intervention process. One practical way to manage this is to first let a group of frontline employees to undergo a training programme, then let them develop written guidelines regarding skin protection and hazard management and subsequently pass on the information to their colleagues [24].

According to *Antonovsky's salutogenesis model* [148] and the Ottawa Charter of the WHO [149], health promotion endeavours to strengthen resources and skills. The WHO Ottawa Charter states that "health promotion is the process of enabling people to increase control over, and to improve, their health". Health is seen as a resource for life, not the objective of living. Aaron Antonovkys' concept of salutogenesis has become an established theoretical framework for health promotion. Within this framework, the focus is on peoples' resources rather than risk factors for disease. Another key element is the orientation towards problem solving [136].

The health action process approach (HAPA) suggests that the adoption, initiation and maintenance of health behaviours must be explicitly conceived as a process that consists of at least a motivation phase and a volition phase. The latter might be further subdivided into a planning phase, action phase and maintenance phase. It is claimed that perceived self-efficacy plays a crucial role at all stages along with other cognitions. For example, risk perceptions serve predominantly to set the stage for a contemplation process early in the motivation phase, but do not extend beyond. Similarly, outcome expectancies are chiefly important in the motivation phase when individuals balance the pros and cons of certain consequences of behaviours, but they lose their predictive power after a personal decision has been made. However, if one does not believe in one's capability to perform a desired action, one will fail to adopt, initiate and maintain it [150].

50.3.4 Professionalization of Health Education

Health education practice is strengthened by the close collaboration among professionals of different disciplines. Even though patient education may be recognized as an important aspect of quality patient care, it is often taken for granted as a skill that health professionals develop automatically [140].

Most health professionals receive no formal training for effectively conducting patient education. For the benefit of the patient and for delivery of the highest quality of patient education, it is necessary that health professionals work together in a coordinated effort. One important profession in patient education is health education [147].

Leaders in the field of health education in the USA realized the need for the standardization of practice across the profession and identification of the particular skills required of the health educator. Today, there are about 250 academic programmes provided by institutions of higher education in the US designed to prepare entry- and advanced-level health education professionals for service in schools, communities and public health venues [151]. Recently (June 2008), the International Union for Health Promotion and Education (IUHPE) addressed "the development and implementation of credentialing systems to strengthen global capacity in health promotion". Participants from Iceland, Ireland, France, Japan, Norway, Spain, United Kingdom and the US developed a consensus statement that identified eight domains required for effective practice in health promotion: (a) catalyzing change, (b) leading, (c) assessing, (d) planning, (e) implementing, (f) evaluating, (g) advocating,

and (h) developing/sustaining partnerships. This development could encourage all countries to begin the process of collaborating on the development of quality assurance mechanisms for health education practice .

In Germany, guidelines for patient education recommend the participation in a trainer workshop before starting the teaching of patients in a special patient education programme. A patient education programme for children and adolescents with atopy is recommended to be offered only by institutions with certification for the education of patients suffering atopy [152].

In OCD, workers' education is characterized by one major specificity. The cases are extremely heterogeneous: the various work place settings, wide spectra of occupational irritants and allergens, acquired work-related allergies, including sensitization against gloves/accelerators must be considered and exclude a fully standardized regimen. This is why, on the one hand, a multi-disciplinary approach is pivotal, enabling *specific* advice to the affected worker by the health educator, which must be based on a profound dermatological diagnosis. On the other hand, therefore, individual counselling (in addition to group seminars) is an indispensable element. Obviously, a sound knowledge on OCD and allergies is crucial in order to make health education in OCD effective; train-the-trainer seminars have to take this essential aspect into account.

50.3.5 Systematic Reviews on the Effectiveness of Educational Programmes in Prevention of OCD and Exemplary Studies with Educational Impact

As mentioned above (Sect. 50.1.1) in various high risk professions, intervention studies have produced fair-quality evidence that prevention is effective. OCD education programmes within skin protection programmes are complex interventions difficult to evaluate because of the problems in identifying and separately assessing the effect of the various components of the intervention. OCD patient education, to date, has demonstrated success, but most studies show limitations. To demonstrate links between outcomes and patient education programme components, there is a need for more trials which combine process and outcome evaluation. Programmes, to date, have relied too heavily on the provision of medical information to patients. Programmes which also aim to improve disease management, self-efficacy and other determinants of health behaviour should also be included. Programme components need to be clearly described and the rationale for their use justified in trial reports. This will produce an evidence base to clarify the role education programmes can play in improving outcomes, and enable the development of more effective programmes [153].

Table 50.5 summarizes recent studies on health education/patient education in the context of primary, secondary and tertiary prevention of OCD. In addition, some epidemiological studies, which focus on the legitimation of intervention studies are mentioned.

50.3.6   Further Implications in Health Educational Research in the Specific Field of OCD

The above-mentioned studies have important implications for practice and research. Incorporating educational programmes for self management into routine care of high risk professions or patients suffering from OCD may significantly improve outcomes. Although selection of a programme may depend on cost and availability, efforts should be made to incorporate models that are known to work. Future studies should focus on morbidity measurements and quality of life and directly compare strategies. Assessment of the impact of education in the prevention of OCD would be enhanced if trials were reported in a uniform way. Studies should be conducted over longer periods, and be adequately powered to determine clinically relevant effects. Future studies should test alternative components directly to determine their relative effectiveness [144].

In a recent systematic review on prevention of allergic contact dermatitis (ACD) [137], there were no studies with a good-quality rating that examined the prevention of ACD. The authors of this review recommend for future research – among other things – studies of educational interventions. Other authors [12] emphasize that many recent studies had limitations in their design and implementation including no clear theoretical basis, and too short follow-up time. An example of the ongoing process to develop standards in occupational intervention research is the development of a theoretical framework in a practical guidance by the National Institute of Occupational Safety and Health (NIOSH). Three essential phases within intervention research are defined, namely development research, implementation research and effectiveness research. Intervention development research is a necessary prerequisite to ensure success of the other phases, and aims to systematically analyse information on the current state of knowledge about the issue of concern, establish what changes are required and why, define the theoretical basis for the choice of intervention methods to implement and develop partnerships with the target population [154].

To date, there is abundant data from a number of countries, where preventive initiatives for OCD in selected settings and professions have proven significantly effective and successful; in this context, early dermatological intervention as well as specific teaching of affected individuals ("workers' education") has been demonstrated as pivotal. Of course, intervention needs to be accompanied by common regulatory efforts to limit exposure to hazardous substances. The international cooperation between researchers should be enhanced to promote integration and excellence of research in this area.

Core Message

> It is possible to verify the effectiveness of various educational programmes, for example by controlled intervention studies. The results underline the necessity of an even more pronounced implementation of health pedagogical interventions in joint multi-disciplinary initiatives for prevention of OCD. Of course, workers' education measures have to be evidence based; continuous quality-management and long-term evaluations are crucial.

References

1. Agner T, Andersen KE, Brandao FM, Bruynzeel DP, Bruze M, Frosch P, Goncalo M, Goossens A, Le Coz CJ, Rustemeyer T, White IR, Diepgen T (2008) Hand eczema severity and quality of life: a cross-sectional, multicentre study of hand eczema patients. Contact Dermatitis 59:43–47

50

2. Moberg C, Alderling M, Meding B (2009) Hand eczema and quality of life: a population-based study. Br J Dermatol 161:397–403

3. Diepgen TL, Andersen KE, Brandao FM, Bruze M, Bruynzeel DP, Frosch P, Goncalo M, Goossens A, Le Coz CJ, Rustemeyer T, White IR, Agner T (2009) Hand eczema classification: a cross-sectional, multicentre study of the aetiology and morphology of hand eczema. Br J Dermatol 160:353–358

4. Brown T (2004) Strategies for prevention: occupational contact dermatitis. Occup Med (Lond) 54(7):450–457

5. Skudlik C, Breuer K, Junger M, Allmers H, Brandenburg S, John SM (2008) Optimal care of patients with occupational hand dermatitis: considerations of German occupational health insurance. Hautarzt 59:690–695

6. Diepgen TL, Schmidt A (2002) Werden Inzidenz und Prävalenz berufsbedingter Hauterkrankungen unterschätzt? Arbeitsmed Sozialmed Umweltmed 37:477–480

7. Emmett EA (2002) Occupational contact dermatitis I: incidence and return to work pressures. Am J Contact Dermat 13:30–34

8. Mathias CGT (1985) The cost of occupational skin disease. Arch Dermatol 121:1519–1524

9. Allmers H, Schmengler J, John SM (2004) Decreasing incidence of occupational contact urticaria caused by natural rubber latex allergy in German healthcare workers. J Allergy Clin Immunol 114:347–351

10. Attwa E, el-Laithy N (2009) Contact dermatitis in car repair workers. J Eur Acad Dermatol Venereol 23:138–145

11. Bauer A, Kelterer D, Bartsch R, Stadeler M, Elsner P (2007) Skin protection in the food industry. Curr Probl Dermatol 34:138–150

12. Brown TP, Rushton L, Williams HC, English JS (2007) Intervention implementation research: an exploratory study of reduction strategies for occupational contact dermatitis in the printing industry. Contact Dermatitis 56(1):16–20

13. Held E, Agner T (2006) The Danish experience: prevention of skin problems in wet work employees. In: Frosch PJ, Menné T, Lepoittevin J-P (eds) Contact dermatitis. Springer, Berlin, pp 864–867

14. Held E, Wolff C, Gyntelberg F, Agner T (2001) Prevention of work-related skin problems in student auxiliary nurses: an intervention study. Contact Dermatitis 44:297–303

15. Kaatz M, Ladermann R, Stadeler M, Fluhr JW, Elsner P, Bauer A (2008) Recruitment strategies for a hand dermatitis prevention programme in the food industry. Contact Dermatitis 59:165–170

16. Kütting B, Weistenhöfer W, Baumeister T, Uter W, Drexler H (2009) Current acceptance and implementation of preventive strategies for occupational hand eczema in 1355 metalworkers in Germany. Br J Dermatol 161:390–396

17. Löffler H, Bruckner T, Diepgen TL, Effendy I (2006) Primary prevention in health care employees: a prospective intervention study with a 3-year training period. Contact Dermatitis 54:202–209

18. Mygind K, Borg V, Flyvholm MA, Sell L, Jepsen KF (2006) A study of the implementation process of an intervention to prevent work-related skin problems in wet-work occupations. Int Arch Occup Environ Health 79:66–74

19. Schurer NY, Klippel U, Schwanitz HJ (2005) Secondary individual prevention of hand dermatitis in geriatric nurses. Int Arch Occup Environ Health 78:149–157

20. Schwanitz HJ, Riehl U, Schlesinger T, Bock M, Skudlik C, Wulfhorst B (2003) Skin care management: educational aspects. Int Arch Occup Environ Health 76:374–381

21. Skudlik C, Weisshaar E, Scheidt R, Wulfhorst B, Diepgen TL, Elsner P, Schonfeld M, John SM (2009) Multicenter study "Medical-Occupational Rehabilitation Procedure Skin - optimizing and quality assurance of inpatient-management (ROQ)". J Dtsch Dermatol Ges 7(2):122–126

22. Weisshaar E, Radulescu M, Soder S, Apfelbacher CJ, Bock M, Grundmann JU, Albrecht U, Diepgen TL (2007) Secondary individual prevention of occupational skin diseases in health care workers, cleaners and kitchen employees: aims, experiences and descriptive results. Int Arch Occup Environ Health 80:477–484

23. Winker R, Salameh B, Stolkovich S, Nikl M, Barth A, Ponocny E, Drexler H, Tappeiner G (2009) Effectiveness of skin protection creams in the prevention of occupational dermatitis: results of a randomized, controlled trial. Int Arch Occup Environ Health 82:653–662

24. Agner T, Held E (2002) Skin protection programmes. Contact Dermatitis 47:253–256

25. Bourke J, Coulson I, English J (2009) Guidelines for the management of contact dermatitis: an update. Br J Dermatol 160:946–954

26. English JS (2004) Current concepts of irritant contact dermatitis. Occup Environ Med 61(722–726):674

27. European Agency for Safety and Health at Work (2008) European Risk Observatory report: Occupational skin diseases and dermal exposure in the EU (EU-25). http://osha.europa.eu/en/publications/reports/TE7007049ENC_skin_diseases

28. Batzdorfer L, Schwanitz HJ (2004) Direkte und indirekte Kosten berufsbedingter Hauterkrankungen. Arbeitsmed, Sozialmed, Umweltmed 11:578–582

29. National Occupational Research Agenda (o.J.) Developing dermal policy based on laboratory and field studies. A new National Institute for Occupational Safety and Health (NIOSH) research program in response to the National Occupational Research Agenda (NORA). DHHS (NIOSH) Publication No. 2000-142. www.cdc.gov/niosh/topics/skin/pdfs/NORADermal-2.pdf. Accessed 10 Aug 2009

30. Uter W, Geier J, Lessmann H, Schnuch A (2006) Is contact allergy to glyceryl monothioglycolate still a problem in Germany? Contact Dermatitis 55:54–56

31. de Jongh CM, John SM, Bruynzeel DP, Calkoen F, van Dijk FJH, Khrenova L, Rustemeyer T, Verberk MM, Kezic S (2008) Cytokine gene polymorphisms and susceptibility to chronic irritant contact dermatitis. Contact Dermatitis 58:269–277

32. de Jongh CM, Khrenova L, Verberk M, Calkoen F, van Dijk FJH, Voss H, John SM, Kezic S (2008) Loss-of-function polymorphisms in the filaggrin gene increase susceptibility to chronic irritant contact dermatitis. Br J Dermatol 159:621–627

33. Li H, Dai Y, Huang H, Li L, Leng S, Cheng J, Niu Y, Duan H, Liu Q, Zhang X, Huang X, Xie J, Feng Z, Wang J, He J, Zheng Y (2007) HLA-B*1301 as a biomarker for genetic susceptibility to hypersensitivity dermatitis induced by trichloroethylene among workers in China. Environ Health Perspect 115:1553–1556

34. Rogosky E, Zec S (2009) Präventionskampagne Haut. Deutsche Gesetzliche Unfallversicherung (DGUV), Berlin

35. John SM (2008) Occupational skin diseases: options for multidisciplinary networking in preventive medicine. GMS Ger Med Sci 6:Doc07. www.egms.de/en/gms/2008-6/000052.shtml

36. Slodownik D, Lee A, Nixon R (2008) Irritant contact dermatitis: a review. Australas J Dermatol 49(1):1–11

37. Dickel H, Kuss O, Schmidt A, Diepgen TL (2002) Impact of preventive strategies on trend of occupational skin disease in hairdressers: population based register study. BMJ 324:1422–1423

38. Nienhaus A, Rojahn K, Skudlik C, Wulfhorst B, Dulon M, Brandenburg S (2004) Secondary individual prevention and rehabilitation in female hairdressers suffering from skin diseases. Gesundheitswesen 66:759–804

39. Skudlik C, Dulon M, Wendeler D, John SM, Nienhaus A (2009) Hand eczema in geriatric nurses in Germany. Prevalence and risk factors. Contact Dermatitis 60: 136–143

40. John SM, Skudlik C, Römer W, Blome O, Brandenburg S, Diepgen TL, Harwerth A, Köllner A, Pohrt U, Rogosky E, Schindera I, Stary A, Worm M (2007) Recommendation: Dermatologist's procedure. Recommendations for quality assurance of the German Society of Dermatology (DDG) and the Task Force on Occupational and Environmental Dermatology (ABD). JDDG 5(12):1146–1148

41. Voss H, Mentzel F, Wilke A, Maier B, Gediga G, Skudlik C, John SM (2009) Optimized dermatologist's report and hierarchical multi-step invention: randomized evaluation of the cornerstones of preventive occupational dermatology. Hautarzt 60:695–701

42. Skudlik C, Junger M, Palsherm K, Breuer K, Brandenburg S, John SM (2009) Cooperation among clinics and practices: integrated medical care in occupational dermatology. Hautarzt 60:722–726

43. Skudlik C, Wulfhorst B, Gediga G, Bock M, Allmers H, John SM (2008) Tertiary individual prevention of occupational skin diseases: a decade's experience with recalcitrant occupational dermatitis. Int Arch Occup Environ Health 81:1059–1064

44. Skudlik C, Schwanitz HJ (2004) Tertiary prevention of occupational skin diseases. JDDG 2:424–434

45. Packham CL (2006) Gloves as chemical protection - can they really work? Ann Occup Hyg 50(6):545–548

46. Health & Safety Executive (2009) Choosing the right gloves to protect skin. [www.hse.gov.uk/skin/employ/gloves.htm]

47. Council Directive of 21 December 1989 on the approximation of the laws of the Member States relating to personal protective equipment: 89/686/EEC

48. CEN (2003) EN374-I -3,2003, protective gloves against chemicals and micro-organisms. Comité Européen de Normalisation, Brussels

49. EU (2006) Regulation (EC) 1907/2006. Registration, evaluation, authorisation and restriction of chemicals (REACH). Official J Eur Union (30.12.2006) L396/1-L396/849

50. Leuchtenberg-Auffahrt E, Rühl R (2007) Safety of gloves for chemical protection. Ann occup Hyg 51(8):739–740

51. Mellström GA, Carlsson B (2005) European Standards on protective gloves. In: Boman A, Estlander T, Wahlberg JE, Maibach HI (eds) Protective gloves for occupational use, 2nd edn. CRC Press, Boca Raton, pp 29–34

52. CEN (2003) EN455 I-III Medical gloves for single use. Part I: requirements and testing for freedom from holes, part II: requirements and testing for physical properties, part III: requirements and testing for biological evaluation. Comité Européen de Normalisation, Brussels

53. CEN (2003) EN374-I-III Protective gloves against chemicals and micro-organisms. Part I: terminology and performance requirements, part II: determination of resistance for penetration, part III: determination of resistance to permeation by chemicals. Comité Européen de Normalisation, Brussels

54. Henry NW III (2005) U.S. rules, regulations and standards for protective gloves for occupational use. In: Boman A, Estlander T, Wahlberg JE, Maibach HI (eds) Protective gloves for occupational use, 2nd edn. CRC, Boca Raton, pp 35–42

55. BAuA (2008) TRGS 401. Risks resulting from skin contact – determination, evaluation, measures. [www.baua.de/de/Themen-von-A-Z/Gefahrstoffe/TRGS/TRGS-401.html]

56. CEN (2003) EN374-2:2003, protective gloves against chemicals and micro-organisms. Part 2: determination of resistance to penetration. Comité Européen de Normalisation, Brussels

57. American Society of Testing and Materials ASTM (2009) F 903 standard test method for resistance of protective clothing materials to penetration by liquids. In: ASTM annual book of ASTM standards, vol 11.03. www.astm.org

58. CEN (2003) EN374-III: protective gloves against chemicals and micro-organisms. Part 3: determination of resistance to permeation by chemicals. Comité Européen de Normalisation, Brussels

59. American Society of Testing and Materials ASTM (2009) F 739 standard test method for resistance of protective clothing materials to permeation by liquids or gases under conditions of continuous contact. In: ASTM annual book of ASTM standards, vol 11.03. www.astm.org

60. American Society of Testing and Materials ASTM (2009) F 1383 standard test method for resistance of protective clothing materials to permeation by liquids or gases under conditions of intermittent contact. In: ASTM annual book of ASTM standards, vol 11.03. www.astm.org

61. Boman A, Mellström GA (2006) Protective gloves. In: Frosch PJ, Menné T, Lepoittevin JP (eds) Contact dermatitis, 4th edn. Springer, Berlin, pp 845–853

62. Mellström GA, Boman A (2005) Gloves: types, materials, and manufacturing. In: Boman A, Estlander T, Wahlberg JE, Maibach HI (eds) Protective gloves for occupational use, 2nd edn. CRC, Boca Raton, pp 15–28

63. Mellström GA, Boman A (2006) Protective gloves. In: Chew A-L, Maibach HI (eds) Irritant dermatitis. Springer, Berlin, pp 409–419

64. Packham CL, Packham HE (2005) Practical considerations when selecting and using gloves for chemical protection in a workplace. In: Boman A, Estlander T, Wahlberg JE, Maibach HI (eds) Protective gloves for occupational use, 2nd edn. CRC, Boca Raton, pp 255–285

65. Rawson BV, Cocker J, Evans PG, Wheeler JP, Akrill PM (2005) Internal contamination of gloves: routes and consequences. Ann Occup Hyg 49(6):535–541

66. Jungbauer FHW, Van der Harst JJ, Groothoff JW, Coenraads PJ (2004) Skin protection in nursing work: promoting the use of gloves and hand alcohol. Contact Dermatitis 51:135–140

67. Zhai H, Maibach HI (2001) Skin occlusion and irritant and allergic contact dermatitis: an overview. Contact Dermatitis 44:201–206

68. Kligman AM (1996) Hydration injury to human skin. In: Van der Valk PGM, Maibach HI (eds) The irritant contact dermatitis syndrome. CRC, Boca Raton, pp 187–194

69. Schäfer P, Bewick-Sonntag C, Capri MG, Berardesca E (2002) Physiological changes in skin barrier function in relation to occlusion level, exposure time and climatic conditions. Skin Pharmacol Appl Skin Physiol 15:7–19

70. Wetzky U, Bock M, Wulfhorst B, John SM (2009) Short- and long-term effects of single and repetitive glove occlusion on the epidermal barrier. Arch Dermatol Res 301(8):595–602

71. Fartasch M (2009) Veränderungen der Haut durch das feuchte Milieu versus Okklusion durch Schutzhandschuhe. JDDG (Suppl.4)7:14

72. Geier J, Krautheim A, Lessmann H (2009) Allergological diagnostics and current allergens in occupational Dermatology. Hautarzt 2009 Jul 22 Epub ahead of print, PMID: 19621203

73. Bhargava K, White IR, White JML (2009) Thiuram patch test positivity 1980-2006: incidence is now falling. Contact Dermatitis 60:222–223

74. Knudsen B, Lerbaek A, Johansen JD, Menné T (2006) Reduction in the frequency of sensitization to thiurams. A result of legislation? Contact Dermatitis 54:170–171

75. Geier J, Lessmann H, Uter W, Schnuch A (2003) Occupational rubber glove allergy: results of the Information Network of Departments of Dermatology (IVDK), 1995 to 2001. Contact Dermatitis 48:39–44

76. Geier J, Uter W, Lessmann H, Schnuch A (2003) The positivity ratio – another parameter to assess the diagnostic quality of a patch test preparation. Contact Dermatitis 48:280–282

77. Aalto-Korte K, Ackermann L, Henriks-Eckerman ML, Välimaa J, Reinikka-Railo H, Leppänen E, Jolanki R (2007) 1, 2-benzisothiazolin-3-one in disposable polyvinyl chloride gloves for medical use. Contact Dermatitis 57:365–370

78. Pontén A (2006) Formaldehyde in reusable protective gloves. Contact Dermatitis 54:268–271

79. Sommer S, Wilkinson SM, Beck MH, English JS, Gawkrodger DJ, Green C (2002) Type IV hypersensitivity reactions to natural rubber latex: results of a multicentre study. Br J Dermatol 146:114–117

80. Wilkinson SM, Beck MH (1996) Allergic contact dermatitis from latex rubber. Br J Dermatol 134:910–914

81. Wyss M, Elsner P, Wüthrich B, Burg G (1993) Allergic contact dermatitis from natural latex without contact urticaria. Contact Dermatitis 28:154–156

82. Wulfhorst B, Schwanitz HJ, Bock M (2004) Optimizing skin protection with semipermeable gloves. Dermatitis 15:184–191

83. Bock M, Wulfhorst B, John SM (2009) Semipermeable Glove Membranes – Effects on skin barrier repair following SLS-Irritation. Contact Dermatitis 61:276–280

84. Kresken J, Klotz A (2003) Occupational skin-protection products - a review. Int Arch Occup Environ Health 76:355–358

85. Frosch PJ, Kurte A (1994) Efficacy of skin barrier creams (IV). The repetitive irritation test (RIT) with a set of 4 standard irritants. Contact Dermatitis 31(3):161–168

86. Kütting B, Drexler H (2008) The three-step programme of skin protection. A useful instrument of primary prevention or more effective in secondary prevention? Dtsch Med Wochenschr 133:201–205

87. Wigger-Alberti W, Elsner P (1997) Preventive measures in contact dermatitis. Clin Dermatol 15:661–665

88. Berndt U, Gabard B, Schliemann-Willers S, Wigger-Alberti W, Zitterbart D, Elsner P (2002) Integrated skin protection from work place irritants: a new model for efficacy assessment. Exogeneous Dermatol 1:45–48

89. Kütting B, Drexler H (2003) Effectiveness of skin protection creams as a preventive measure in occupational dermatitis: a critical update according to criteria of evidence-based medicine. Int Arch Occup Environ Health 76:253–259

90. Ramsing DW, Agner T (1997) Preventive and therapeutic effects of a moisturizer. An experimental study of human skin. Acta Dermato Venereol (Stockh) 77:335–337

91. Alvarez MS, Brown LH, Brancaccio RR (2001) Are barrier creams actually effective? Curr Allergy Asthma Rep 1:337–341

92. Schliemann S (2007) Limitations of skin protection. Curr Probl Dermatol 34:171–177

93. Wigger-Alberti W, Elsner P (1998) Do barrier creams and gloves prevent or provoke contact dermatitis? Am J Contact Dermatitis 9:100–106

94. Berndt U, Wigger-Alberti W, Gabard B, Elsner P (2000) Efficacy of a barrier cream and its vehicle as protective measures against occupational irritant contact dermatitis. Contact Dermatitis 42:77–80

95. Frosch PJ, Peiler D, Grunert V, Grunenberg B (2003) Efficacy of barrier creams in comparison to skin care products in dental laboratory technicians – a controlled trial. JDDG 1(7):547–557

96. Goh CL, Gan SL (1994) Efficacies of a barrier cream and an afterwork emollient cream against cutting fluid dermatitis in metalworkers: a prospective study. Contact Dermatitis 31:176–180

97. Perrenoud D, Gallezot D, van Melle G (2001) The efficacy of a protective cream in a real-world apprentice hairdresser environment. Contact Dermatitis 45:134–138

98. Coenraads PJ, Diepgen TL (2003) Problems with trials and intervention studies on barrier creams and emollients at the workplace. Int Arch Occup Environ Health 76:362–366

99. Fartasch M, Diepgen TL, Drexler H, Elsner P, Fluhr JW, John SM, Kresken J, Wigger-Alberti W (2009) Berufliche Hautmittel (ICD-10:L23, L24) S1-Leitlinie der Arbeitsgemeinschaft für Berufs- und Umweltdermatologie (ABD) in der Deutschen Dermatologischen Gesellschaft (DDG). Arbeitsmed Sozialmed Umweltmed 44:53–67

100. Suskind RR (1955) The present status of silicone protective creams. Indust Med Surg 24:413–416

101. Boman A, Wahlberg JE, Johansson G (1982) A method for the study of the effect of barrier creams and protective gloves on the percutaneous absorption of solvents. Dermatologica 164:157–160

102. de Fraissinette A, Picarles V, Chibout S, Kolopp M, Medina J, Burtin P, Ebelin ME, Osborne S, Mayer FK, Spake A, Rosdy M, De Wever B, Ettlin RA, Cordier A (1999) Predictivity of an in vitro model for acute and chronic skin irritation (SkinEthic) applied to the testing of topical vehicles. Cell Biol Toxicol 15:121–135

103. Guillemin M, Murset JC, Lob M, Riquez J (1974) Simple method to determine the efficiency of a cream used for skin protection against solvents. Br J Ind Med 31:310–316

104. Klotz A, zur Mühlen A, Thörner B, Kietzmann M, Holtmann W, Pittermann W (2003) Testing the efficacy of skin protection products in-vivo and in-vitro. SÖFW J 129:10–16

105. Korinth G, Geh S, Schaller KH, Drexler H (2003) In vitro evaluation of the efficacy of skin barrier creams and protective gloves on percutaneous absorption of industrial solvents. Int Arch Occup Environ Health 76(5):382–386

106. Lodén M (1986) The effect of 4 barrier creams on the absorption of water, benzene, and formaldehyde into excised human skin. Contact Dermatitis 14:292–296

107. Mahmoud G, Lachapelle JM, Van Neste D (1984) Histological assessment of skin damage by irritants: its possible use in the evaluation of a 'barrier cream'. Contact Dermatitis 11:179–185

108. Marks R, Dykes PJ, Hamami I (1989) Two novel techniques for the evaluation of barrier creams. Br J Dermatol 120:655–660

109. Treffel P, Gabard B, Juch R (1994) Evaluation of barrier creams: an in vitro technique on human skin. Acta Derm Venereol (Stockh) 74:7–11

110. Zhai H, Maibach HI (1996) Percutaneous penetration (Dermatopharmacokinetics) in evaluating barrier creams. Curr Probl Dermatol 193–205

111. Zhai H, Willard P, Maibach HI (1998) Evaluating skin-protective materials against contact irritants and allergens. Contact Dermatitis 38:155–158

112. zur Mühlen A, Klotz A, Weimans S, Veeger M, Thorner B, Diener B, Hermann M (2004) Using skin models to assess the effects of a protection cream on skin barrier function. Skin Pharmacol Physiol 17:167–175

113. Wigger-Alberti W, Caduff L, Burg G, Elsner P (1999) Experimentally-induced irritant contact dermatitis to evaluate the efficacy of protective creams in vivo. J Am Acad Dermatol 40:590–596

114. Wigger-Alberti W, Rougier A, Richard A, Elsner P (1998) Efficacy of protective creams in a modified repeated irritation test (RIT): methodological aspects. Acta Derm Venereol (Stockh) 78:270–273

115. Schnetz E, Diepgen TL, Elsner P, Frosch PJ, Klotz AJ, Kresken J, Kuss O, Merk H, Schwanitz HJ, Wigger-Alberti W, Fartasch M (2000) Multicentre study for the development of an in vivo model to evaluate the influence of topical formulations on irritation. Contact Dermatitis 42:336–343

116. Wigger-Alberti W, Krebs A, Elsner P (2000) Experimental irritant contact dermatitis due to cumulative epicutaneous exposure to sodium lauryl sulphate and toluene: single and concurrent application. Br J Dermatol 143:551–556

117. Wigger-Alberti W, Spoo J, Schliemann-Willers S, Klotz A, Elsner P (2002) The tandem repeated irritation test: a new method to assess prevention of irritant combination damage to the skin. Acta Derm Venereol 82:94–97

118. Fluhr JW, Bankova L, Fuchs S, Kelterer D, Schliemann-Willers S, Norgauer J, Kleesz P, Grieshaber R, Elsner P (2004) Fruit acids and sodium hydroxide in the food industry and their combined effect with sodium lauryl sulphate: controlled in vivo tandem irritation study. Br J Dermatol 151:1039–1048

119. Boman A, Mellström GA (1989) Percutaneous absorption of 3 organic solvents in the guinea pig (III). Effect of barrier creams. Contact Dermatitis 21:134–140

120. Frosch P, Schulze-Dirks A, Hoffmann M, Axthelm I (1993) Efficacy of skin barrier creams (II). Ineffectiveness of a popular "skin protector" against various irritants in the repetitive irritation test in the guinea pig. Contact Dermatitis 29:74–77

121. Goh CL (1991) Cutting oil dermatitis on guinea pig skin (I). Cutting oil dermatitis and barrier cream. Contact Dermatitis 24:16–21

122. Xhauflaire-Uhoda E, Macarenko E, Denooz R, Charlier C, Piérard GE (2008) Skin protection creams in medical settings: successful or evil? J Occup Med Toxicol 25:3–15

123. Fartasch M, Deters A, Schnetz E, Goen T, Drexler H, Schmelz M (2006) Cutaneous penetration: its modulation by skin care products. Contact Dermatitis 55:10

124. Korinth G, Luersen L, Schaller KH, Angerer J, Drexler H (2008) Enhancement of percutaneous penetration of aniline and o-toluidine in vitro using skin barrier creams. Toxicol In Vitro 22:812–818

125. Korinth G, Weiss T, Penkert S, Schaller KH, Angerer J, Drexler H (2007) Percutaneous absorption of aromatic amines in rubber industry workers: impact of impaired skin and skin barrier creams. Occup Environ Med 64:366–372

126. Wigger-Alberti W, Maraffio B, Wernli M, Elsner P (1997) Self-application of a protective cream: pitfalls of occupational skin protection. Arch Dermatol 133:861–864

127. Kelterer D, Fluhr JW, Elsner P (2003) Application of protective creams: use of a fluorescence-based training system decreases unprotected areas on the hands. Contact Dermatitis 49:159–160

128. Wigger-Alberti W, Maraffio B, Elsner P (1997) Training workers at risk for occupational contact dermatitis in the application of protective creams: efficacy of a fluorescence technique. Dermatology 195:129–133

129. Zhai H, Maibach HI (1996) Effect of barrier creams: human skin in vivo. Contact Dermatitis 35:92–96

130. Fluhr JW, Miteva M, Elsner P (2007) Efficacy and safety testing. The clinical perspective. Curr Probl Dermatol 34:33–46

131. Buraczewska I, Berne M, Lindberg M, Törmä H, Lodén M (2007) Changes in skin barrier function following long-term treatment with moisturizers, a randomized controlle trial. Br J Dermatol Mar 156(3):492–498

132. Bikowski JB (2008) Hand eczema: diagnosis and management. Cutis Oct 82(4 suppl):9–15

133. Kalimo K, Kautiainen H, Niskanen T, Niemi L (1999) 'Eczema school' to improve compliance in an occupational dermatology clinic. Contact Dermatitis 41:315–319

134. Flyvholm MA, Mygind K, Sell L, Jensen A, Jepsen KF (2005) A randomised controlled intervention study on prevention of work related skin problems among gut cleaners in swine slaughterhouses. Occup Environ Med 62:642–649

135. Radulescu M, Bock M, Bruckner T, Ellsäßer G, Fels H, Diepgen TL (2007) Health education on occupational allergies and dermatoses for adolescents. JDDG 7:576–582

136. Wulfhorst B, Bock M, John SM (2006) Worker's education and teaching programmes: the German experience. In: Frosch PJ, Menné, Lepoittevin JP (eds) Textbook of contact dermatitis, 4th edn. Springer, Berlin

137. Saary J, Qureshi R, Palda V, DeKoven J, Pratt M, Skotnicki-Grant S, Holness L (2005) A systematic review of contact dermatitis treatment and prevention. J Am Acad Dermatol 53(5):845

138. Jungbauer FH, van der Vleuten P, Groothoff JW, Coenraads PJ (2004) Irritant hand dermatitis: severity of disease,

50

occupational exposure to skin irritants and preventive measures 5 years after initial diagnosis. Contact Dermatitis
50(4):245–251

139. Flyvolm MA, Rrydendall Jepsen K (2008) Experiences
with implementation of evidence-based prevention programmes to prevent occupational skin diseases in different
occupations. GITAL Dermatol Venereol 143(1):71–78

140. Falvo DR (2004) Effective patient education: a guide to
increased compliance. Jones & Bartlett, Sudbury

141. Tones K (2004) Health promotion, health education, and
the public health. In: Detels R, McEwen J, Beaglehole R,
Tanaka H (eds). Oxford textbooks of public health, 4th edn.
Oxford University Press, Oxford, pp 829–863

142. Ersser SJ, Latter S, Sibley A, Satherley PA, Welbourne S
(2007) Psychological and educational interventions for
atopic eczema in children. Cochrane Database Syst Rev
(Online) (3):CD004054

143. Darsow U, Lübbe J, Taïeb A, Seidenari S, Wollenberg A,
Calza AM, Giusti F, CA RJ (2005) European Task Force on
Atopic Dermatitis Titel: position paper on diagnosis and
treatment of atopic dermatitis. J Eur Acad Dermatol
Venereol 19(3):286–295

144. Guevara JP, Wolf FM, Grum CM, Clark NM (2003) Effects
of educational interventions for self management of asthma
in children and adolescents: systematic review and meta-
analysis. BMJ 326(7402):1308–1309

145. Apfelbacher CJ, Soder S, Diepgen TL, Weisshaar E
(2009) The impact of measures for secondary individual
prevention of work-related skin diseases in health care
workers: 1 year follow-Up study. Contact Dermatitis
60:144–149

146. Wulfhorst B, Bock M, Gediga G, Skudlik C, Allmers H,
John SM (2009) Sustainability of an interdisciplinary secondary prevention program for hairdressers. International
Archives of Occupational and Environmental Health 83(2):
165–171

147. Glanz K, Rimer BK, Lewis FM (eds) (2002) Health behavior and health education. Theory, Research and Practice,
3rd edn. Jossey-Bass, San Francisco, p 4

148. Lindstrom B, Eriksson M (2005) Salutogenesis. J Epidemiol
Community Health 59:440–442

149. WHO (1986) The Ottawa Charter. Who, Geneva

150. Schwarzer R (2004) Stage models of health behavior
change: advances and problems. In: Keller S, Velicer WF
(eds) Research on the transtheoretical model: where are we
now, where are we going? Pabst Science, Lengerich,
Germany, pp 110–113

151. Frauenknecht M (2005) Professional standards for health
education teacher preparation. Health Educ 37(2):24–26

152. Staab D, Diepgen TL, Fartasch M, Kupfer J, Lob-Corzilius T,
Ring J, Scheewe S, Scheidt R, Schmid-Ott G, Schnopp C,
Szepanski R, Werfel T, Wittenmeier M, Wahn U, Gieler U
(2006) Age related, structured educational programmes for
the management of atopic dermatitis in children and adolescents: muticentre, randomised controlled trial. BMJ 332:
923–940

153. Harris M, Smith BJ, Veale A (2008) Patient education programmes – can they improve outcomes in COPD? Int J
Chron Obstruct Pulmon Dis 3(1):109–112

154. Goldenhar LM, La Montagne AD, Katz T (2001) The intervention research process in occupational health: an overview from the National Occupational Research Agenda
Intervention Effectiveness Research Team. J Occup Environ
Med 43:616–622

155. Meding B, Wrangsjö K, Hosseiny S, Andersson E, Hagberg S,
Toren J, Wass K, Brisman J (2006) Occupational skin exposure and hand eczema among dental technicians – need for
improved prevention. Scand J Work Environ health 32:
219–224

156. Schlesinger T, Revermann K, Schwanitz HJ (2001)
Dermatosen bei Auszubildenden des Friseurhandwerks in
Niedersachsen. Dermatol Beruf Umwelt 49:185–192

157. Nixon R, Roberts H, Frowen K, Sim M (2006) Knowledge
of skin hazards and the use of gloves by Australian hairdressing students and practicing hairdressers. Contact
Dermatitis 54:112–116

158. Riehl U (2000) Interventionsstudie zur Prävention von
Hauterkrankungen bei Auszubildenden des Friseurhandwerks.
Rasch, Osnabrück

159. Bauer A, Kelterer D, Bartsch R, Schlegel A, Pearson J,
Stadeler M, Kleesz P, Grieshaber R, Schiele R, Elsner P,
Williams H (2002) Prevention of hand dermatitis in bakers'
apprentice: different efficacy of skin protection measures and
UVB hardening. Int Arch Occup Environ Health 75:491–499

160. Mertin M, Frosch P, Kügler K, Sieverding M, Goergens A,
Wulfhorst B, John SM (2009) Skin disease prevention
courses for secondary prevention in metal workers.
Dermatologie Beruf Umwelt 57:29–35

161. Matterne U, Diepgen TL, Weisshaar E (2009) Effects of a
health-educational and psychological intervention on socio-
cognitive determinants of skin protection behavior in individuals with occupational dermatoses. Int Arch Occup Environ
Health 83:183–189. doi 10.1007/s00420-009-0448-z

162. CEN (2003) EN 420-2003. Protective gloves – general
requirements and test methods. Comité Européen de
Normalisation, Brussels

163. Tucker SB (1988) Prevention of occupational skin disease.
Dermatol Clin 6:87–96

Prevention of Allergic Contact Dermatitis: Safe Exposure Levels of Sensitizers

51

Jacob Pontoppidan Thyssen and Torkil Menné

Contents

51.1 General Aspects of Contact Allergy Epidemics

The overall prevalence of contact allergy in the general population is high, and nickel, fragrances, and preservatives remain the most common causative allergens [1]. It is likely that the development of contact allergy in the general population replicates the development observed among patients with dermatitis. Thus, the prevalence of fragrance mix I allergy showed an increase during the 1990s, but has since decreased in both the patient population and the general population [2–5]. Thus, if a new chemical (e.g., a preservative) that is frequently used in professional as well as personal care products turns out to be a contact allergen, identical trends of contact allergy among patients and consumers are to be expected. A categorization of contact allergy epidemics was recently proposed [6]. Thus if more than 1/20, 1/100, 1/1,000, or 1/10,000 subjects in the general population are contact sensitized, one should categorize the epidemic as "outbreak," "generalized," "concentrated," and "low-level," respectively. Examples of contact allergy epidemics observed during the twentieth century were recently described (Table 51.1) [7]. It appeared that these contact allergy epidemics had several common features. Thus, allergic contact dermatitis to a given chemical was first described among workers, and later, among consumers. Once the epidemic was established, it tended to be long-lasting as allergens persisted in consumer products for decades [7]. Thus, when consumer cases are reported in the medical literature, one should suspect that many subjects in the general population are already sensitized and that morbidity may increase unless something radical is done. The control of contact allergy epidemics has traditionally been achieved

J.P. Thyssen (✉) and T. Menné
Department of Dermato-Allergology, National Allergy Research Centre, Niels Andersensvej 65, 2900 Hellerup, Denmark
e-mail: jacpth01@geh.regionh.dk

J.D. Johansen et al. (eds.), *Contact Dermatitis*,
DOI: 10.1007/978-3-642-03827-3_51, © Springer-Verlag Berlin Heidelberg 2011

Table 51.1 Characteristics of contact allergy epidemics [7]

Initial cases of allergic contact dermatitis are detected among workers
Once consumer cases are reported, the epidemic is already accelerating
The control of an epidemic is time consuming and requires that toxicologists, dermatologists and politicians communicate with each other
Industrial and public interference is usually scarce
Regulations seem mainly to be a European measure to fight epidemics

Table 51.2 Selected premarketing measures and tools to prevent contact allergy epidemics [7]

Quantitative structure-activity relationship (QSAR) [9]
Dermal sensitization threshold (DST) [45]
In vitro tests [10]
Animal testing [12, 46]
Human repeat insult patch testing (HRIPT)
Quantitative risk assessment (QRA)

through communication between toxicologists, dermatologists, and administrators. Generally, public and industrial interference is negligible and rarely affect the course of an epidemic. Finally, European governments have traditionally been more motivated to regulate contact allergy epidemics than governments on other continents.

51.2 Industrial Measures to Prevent Contact Allergy Epidemics Prior to Product Marketing

When industries choose to use a new chemical in a product or a well-known chemical in a new setting, several measures are taken to prevent skin sensitization and allergic contact dermatitis (Table 51.2). The risk assessment process generally follows a stepwise approach including hazard identification, dose–response assessment, exposure assessment, and risk characterization [8]. Quantitative structure-activity relationship (QSAR) is a process by which the chemical structure is quantitatively correlated with biological activity [9]. QSAR models are used in toxicology as well as environmental science for the purpose of risk assessment. In vitro methods generally focus on either the induction of T lymphocyte responses or the interaction of chemicals with Langerhans cells [10]. Despite substantial progress, such tests need to be further elaborated to replace animal testing. Currently, the best practice for establishing safety involves determining the sensitization potential of an ingredient using animal assays. Previously, the guinea pig maximization test (GPMT) was widely used to assess the elicitation potential of an allergen [11]. However, today, the mouse local lymph node assay (LLNA) is

more frequently used as it allows the determination of the response during sensitization rather than during elicitation [12]. Based on the LLNA, skin sensitizing chemicals are defined as chemicals that lead to a threefold increase in cell proliferation in the draining lymph node. In some cases, the absence of contact sensitization at threshold doses may be confirmed in humans by using a human repeat insult patch test (HRIPT). However, the main problems with current test methods such as the GPMT, the LLNA, and the HRIPT are the sensitivity of the test systems, the correct interpretation of test data, and their incorporation into the final risk assessment.

The No Expected Sensitization Induction Level (NESIL) estimates the sensitization threshold for a given chemical in humans. The NESIL is expressed as dose per unit area of the skin ($\mu g/cm^2$) and is based on the outcome of animal and human assays. Information about the NESIL, sensitization assessment factors (SAFs), and calculations of consumer exposure through normal product use are used to perform a quantitative risk assessment (QRA) [13]. Using these parameters, an acceptable exposure level (AEL) for humans can be calculated and compared with the expected consumer exposure level (CEL). An AEL:CEL ratio of 1 or higher is generally considered to be acceptable. The AEL:CEL ratio must be calculated for the ingredient in each product type.

51.3 Detection and Surveillance of Contact Allergy Epidemics

There are several ways to detect and monitor contact allergy epidemics [7] (Table 51.3). Health care providers and researchers are usually the first to detect and report new cases of contact allergy. A case report should always include a careful description of the clinical picture as well as the source and exposure of the contact allergen.

Table 51.3 Selected measures to detect and monitor contact allergy epidemics

Clinical case reports
Dose–response patch test studies
Repeated open application testing (ROAT) in allergic individuals
Patch test data from clinical departments
Epidemiological studies in the general population
Studies that investigate the content of consumer products
Reports with information about the amount of registered chemical products in a country

This way, other dermatologists may recognize identical or similar cases in their clinics. Recently, efficient communication between dermatologists in England and Finland revealed the etiology of a Chinese sofa/chair dermatitis epidemic caused by dimethylfumarate, a novel potent contact sensitizer [14]. Furthermore, clinicians should rapidly provide and publish dose–response patch test data to determine and suggest test concentrations that may be used for patch testing. Also, the relationship between the threshold dose of elicitation at single occluded exposure and the threshold dose of elicitation at repeated open application testing (ROAT) should be assessed for that allergen. This information is important to determine use concentration and prevent allergic contact dermatitis in sensitized individuals. In fact, it was recently proposed that a general equation should be constructed to convert patch test elicitation data into ROAT elicitation data [15]. If it becomes possible to delineate this relationship, one may use patch test data from patients with contact allergy to determine doses that will not elicit allergic contact dermatitis in real-life exposure situations. This information can be essential to industries so that they can rapidly lower the use concentrations of, for example, preservatives in personal care products. Taken together, a thorough investigation of an allergen includes determination of its potency, the dose that induces and elicits contact dermatitis, the number of repeated applications necessary to elicit contact dermatitis, time relationship, and eventually a confirmatory repeated open application test (ROAT).

Epidemiological patch test data from patients as well as subjects in the general population are essential to monitor contact allergy epidemics [1, 16–20]. Such data may be used to recognize even slight increases of contact allergy if the patch test data material is large enough.

The European Surveillance System of Contact Allergies (ESSCA) is a pan-European surveillance network with patient patch test data from departments in several countries [21]. This ongoing international surveillance system permits up-to-date comparisons of allergen sensitization frequencies across countries, which helps to monitor and detect changes in the prevalence of contact allergy. Epidemiological evaluations may, furthermore, provide evidence to support the benefits of governmental regulations on allergen exposure [22, 23] and indicate new risk factors [24–26]. Finally, dermatologists and administrators may acquire important exposure information from studies evaluating changes in the development of registered chemical products in a country [27] and from studies evaluating the allergen content or release from consumer products [28–30].

51.4 Measures to Prevent Contact Allergy Epidemics After Product Marketing

There seem to be five key players that may be involved in the solution process of a contact allergy epidemic: industries (both the producers and the users of a chemical), researchers (toxicologist, environmentalists, and dermatologists), politicians, the media, and the people. The industries may use several measures to prevent a contact allergy epidemic appearing in the first place using QRA. However, once an epidemic is established, there are a few examples of industrial willingness to limit allergen exposure in both consumer and occupational products without prior regulation. In 1981, the Danish cement producer Aalborg Portland® voluntarily added ferrous sulfate to their cement, 2 years before it became compulsory by law in Denmark. Also, in the 1990s, hair products containing acid perms with glyceryl monothioglycolate (GMT) were withdrawn from the market by German manufacturers after several cases of allergic contact dermatitis among hairdressers and consumers were reported in Germany [31, 32]. Such industrial measures are expensive for the companies as they may involve changes in several steps of the production. However, the liability of a product is vital to most companies and the money may be well spent in the long run.

Researchers and dermatologists publish their knowledge about emerging contact allergy epidemics in the scientific literature, which are often cited in public

51

media too. Media are generally interested in allergic diseases and may, therefore, publish "hot" stories about, for example, fragrances in children toys, nickel in cell phones, and severe cutaneous reactions following temporary henna tattooing. Since people in Western societies seem to have an increasing awareness of individual protection against environmental exposure, media may further enforce this tendency. Today, we agree that a significant proportion of Western consumers tend to avoid personal products that contain contact allergens when it is possible and when they find it necessary. Thus, fragrance-free personal care products such as baby nappies are popular in, for example, Denmark. However, the social use of fragrances and hair dyes seems to be unaffected by this rising "awareness culture." Taken together, people may avoid purchasing certain "risk products" and thereby indirectly change the supply of products and indirectly force companies to provide products that are safer to use.

Population health became decreasingly popular in the western world with the rise of liberalism in the late twentieth century [33]. Thus, depending on the country studied, political attention diverged more or less from population health to individual health as well as from public health to private medicine. Several reasons have been suggested to explain why population health even today may be politically underappreciated in many countries [33]: Firstly, *the rescue imperative* – modern society is often more willing to spend large resources on saving a subject or a group of subjects that are at stake (e.g., financing supplementary expensive medicine for a very small group of patients who have been widely exposed in the media) than saving statistical lives or reducing morbidity among the masses. Secondly, *the technological imperative* – public health services are less appealing than high technological solutions (e.g., scanning devices may receive more funding than little advanced information campaigns). Thirdly, *the invisibility of public health* – the people and its politicians tend to forget or neglect aspects of public health that work well (e.g., clean water and safe food). Fourthly, *the culture of individualism* – society may sometimes value individual satisfaction, responsibility, and choice over public health and safety.

The above mentioned imperatives are important to consider when one reflects on governmental initiatives to prevent allergic contact dermatitis. The political culture and climate in a country at a given time will in many cases determine how much the political system

Table 51.4 Political measures to prevent contact allergy epidemics

Prohibition
Limitation
Information campaigns
Mandatory labeling of consumer products

becomes involved in fighting contact allergy epidemics. Furthermore, the strength of industrial lobbyism should be acknowledged. Although industries may have the best intentions when they produce, test, and market a new product for occupational or personal use, the products sometimes turn out to be allergenic and lead to increasing morbidity among workers and subjects in the general population [34–36]. Thus, risk assessment failures in the past are numerous and new contact allergy epidemics are likely to come in the future as the sensitivity of the test systems remains lower than one could wish for. The political systems have several measures they can use to prevent contact allergy epidemics [7] (Table 51.4): Prohibition is the strongest political measure and has only been used for the use of methyldibromoglutaronitrile (MDBGN) in cosmetics sold in the EU. This measure is only applied when safety data prove a clear correlation between low concentration allergen exposure and clinical disease, often in conjunction with a large epidemic. Another measure is the limitation of a contact allergen. This has been used in Denmark and the EU to limit nickel release from consumer products [37, 38]. Furthermore, limitation has been used to reduce the content of methylchloroisothiazolinone/methylisothiazolinone (MCI/MI) in the EU to a concentration of 15–55 ppm in industrial products and 15 ppm in cosmetic products [39], and to reduce the content of hexavalent chromium in cement in Denmark in 1983 and in the EU in 2005 [40]. Finally, the political system may use information campaigns or make warnings or ingredient labels mandatory on consumer products to limit allergen exposure, although the effect of such measures has never been investigated. Since 2005, the Seventh Amendment to the cosmetic EU Directive 76/768/EEC required that any cosmetic product containing any of 26 raw materials above certain trigger levels should be declared. This has certainly made it easier for fragrance-allergic individuals to protect themselves from fragrance exposure, although such measures are damage controlling rather than damage eliminating.

In fact, nearly half of consumers have difficulties reading cosmetic labels [41].

The history of contact allergy prevention has several successes within the EU such as the limitation of nickel release from consumer products [16, 23, 42], the limitation of chromium in cement [22, 43], the prohibition of MDBGN in cosmetic products, etc. [44]. However, several challenges remain to be confronted, like *para*-phenylenediamine-related substance in hair dyes, hexavalent chromium in leather, and fragrances in cosmetic products.

References

1. Thyssen JP, Linneberg A, Menné T et al (2007) The epidemiology of contact allergy in the general population–prevalence and main findings. Contact Dermatitis 57:287–299
2. Nardelli A, Carbonez A, Ottoy W et al (2008) Frequency of and trends in fragrance allergy over a 15-year period. Contact Dermatitis 58:134–141
3. Schnuch A, Lessmann H, Geier J et al (2004) Contact allergy to fragrances: frequencies of sensitization from 1996 to 2002. Results of the IVDK*. Contact Dermatitis 50:65–76
4. Thyssen JP, Linneberg A, Menné T et al (2009) The prevalence and morbidity of sensitization to fragrance mix I in the general population. Br J Dermatol 161:95–101
5. Thyssen JP, Carlsen BC, Menné T et al (2008) Trends of contact allergy to fragrance mix I and Myroxylon pereirae among Danish eczema patients tested between 1985 and 2007. Contact Dermatitis 59:238–244
6. Thyssen JP, Menné T, Schnuch A et al (2009) Acceptable risk of contact allergy in the general population assessed by CE-DUR- a method to detect and categorize contact allergy epidemics based on patient data. Regul Toxicol Pharmacol 54:183–187
7. Thyssen JP, Johansen JD, Menné T (2007) Contact allergy epidemics and their controls. Contact Dermatitis 56:185–195
8. Felter SP, Ryan CA, Basketter DA et al (2003) Application of the risk assessment paradigm to the induction of allergic contact dermatitis. Regul Toxicol Pharmacol 37:1–10
9. Rodford R, Patlewicz G, Walker JD et al (2003) Quantitative structure-activity relationships for predicting skin and respiratory sensitization. Environ Toxicol Chem 22:1855–1861
10. Kimber I, Pichowski JS, Betts CJ et al (2001) Alternative approaches to the identification and characterization of chemical allergens. Toxicol In Vitro 15:307–312
11. Magnusson B, Kligman AM (1969) The identification of contact allergens by animal assay. The guinea pig maximization test. J Invest Dermatol 52:268–276
12. Kimber I, Dearman RJ, Basketter DA et al (2002) The local lymph node assay: past, present and future. Contact Dermatitis 47:315–328
13. Api AM, Basketter DA, Cadby PA et al (2008) Dermal sensitization quantitative risk assessment (QRA) for fragrance ingredients. Regul Toxicol Pharmacol 52:3–23
14. Rantanen T (2008) The cause of the Chinese sofa/chair dermatitis epidemic is likely to be contact allergy to dimethylfumarate, a novel potent contact sensitizer. Br J Dermatol 159:218–221
15. Fischer LA, Johansen JD, Menné T (2008) Methyldibromoglutaronitrile allergy: relationship between patch test and repeated open application test thresholds. Br J Dermatol 159:1138–1143
16. Johansen J, Menné T, Christophersen J et al (2000) Changes in the pattern of sensitization to common contact allergens in Denmark between 1985-86 and 1997-98, with a special view to the effect of preventive strategies. Br J Dermatol 142:490–495
17. Mortz CG, Lauritsen JM, Bindslev-Jensen C et al (2002) Contact allergy and allergic contact dermatitis in adolescents: prevalence measures and associations. The Odense Adolescence Cohort Study on Atopic Diseases and Dermatitis (TOACS). Acta Derm Venereol 82:352–358
18. Nielsen NH, Menné T (1992) Allergic contact sensitization in an unselected Danish population. The Glostrup Allergy Study, Denmark. Acta Derm Venereol 72:456–460
19. Schafer T, Bohler E, Ruhdorfer S et al (2001) Epidemiology of contact allergy in adults. Allergy 56:1192–1196
20. Wilkinson JD, Shaw S, Andersen KE et al (2002) Monitoring levels of preservative sensitivity in Europe. A 10-year overview (1991-2000). Contact Dermatitis 46:207–210
21. The ESSCA Writing Group (2008) The European Surveillance System of Contact Allergies (ESSCA): results of patch testing the standard series, 2004. J Eur Acad Dermatol Venereol 22:174–181
22. Avnstorp C (1989) Follow-up of workers from the prefabricated concrete industry after the addition of ferrous sulphate to Danish cement. Contact Dermatitis 20:365–371
23. Jensen CS, Lisby S, Baadsgaard O et al (2002) Decrease in nickel sensitization in a Danish schoolgirl population with ears pierced after implementation of a nickel-exposure regulation. Br J Dermatol 146:636–642
24. Menné T, Holm NV (1983) Nickel allergy in a female twin population. Int J Dermatol 22:22–28
25. Thyssen JP, Nielsen NH, Linneberg A (2008) The association between alcohol consumption and contact sensitization in Danish adults: the Glostrup Allergy Study. Br J Dermatol 158:306–312
26. Linneberg A, Nielsen NH, Menné T et al (2003) Smoking might be a risk factor for contact allergy. J Allergy Clin Immunol 111:980–984
27. Flyvholm MA (2005) Preservatives in registered chemical products. Contact Dermatitis 53:27–32
28. Buckley DA (2007) Fragrance ingredient labelling in products on sale in the U.K. Br J Dermatol 157:295–300
29. Rastogi SC, Johansen JD, Frosch P et al (1998) Deodorants on the European market: quantitative chemical analysis of 21 fragrances. Contact Dermatitis 38:29–35
30. Thyssen JP, Johansen JD, Zachariae C et al (2008) The outcome of dimethylglyoxime testing in a sample of cell phones in Denmark. Contact Dermatitis 59:38–42
31. Peters K-P, Frosch PJ, Uter W et al (1994) Typ-IV-Allergien auf Friseurberufsstoffe: Ergebnisse einer multizentrischen Studie in acht Kliniken der Deutschen Kontaktallergiegruppe und des 'Informationsverbundes Dermatologischer Kliniken' in Deutschland. Dermatol Beruf Umwelt 42:50–57

51

32. Schnuch A, Geier J (1995) Glycerylmonothioglykolat-Sensibilisierung bei Friseurkunden. Dermatol Beruf Umwelt 43:29

33. Gostin LO (2004) Health of the people: the highest law? J Law Med Ethics 32:509–515

34. Bjorkner B, Bruze M, Dahlquist I, Fregert S, Gruvberger B, Persson K (1986) Contact allergy to the preservative Kathon CG. Contact Dermatitis 14:85–90

35. Bruze M, Gruvberger B, Agrup G (1988) Sensitization studies in the guinea pig with the active ingredients of Euxyl K 400. Contact Dermatitis 18:37–39

36. Chan PK, Baldwin RC, Parsons RD et al (1983) Kathon biocide: manifestation of delayed contact dermatitis in guinea pigs is dependent on the concentration for induction and challenge. J Invest Dermatol 81:409–411

37. European Communities (1994). European Dir. 94/27/EC of 30 June 1994 amending for the 12th time Dir. 76/769/EEC on the approximation of the laws, regulations and administrative provisions of the Member States relating to restrictions on the marketing and use of dangerous substances. Official J Eur Communities 37:1–2

38. Menné T, Rasmussen K (1990) Regulation of nickel exposure in Denmark. Contact Dermatitis 23:57–58

39. Reinhard E, Waeber R, Niederer M et al (2001) Preservation of products with MCI/MI in Switzerland. Contact Dermatitis 45:257–264

40. Directive 2003/53/EC of the European Parliament and of the Council of 18 June 2003 amending for the 26th time Council Directive 76/769/EEC relating to restrictions on the marketing and use of certain dangerous substances and preparations (nonylphenol, nonylphenol ethoxylate and cement) Official Journal of the European Union.page L 178/24- 178/28. 17/7.-2003.

41. Noiesen E, Munk MD, Larsen K et al (2007) Difficulties in avoiding exposure to allergens in cosmetics. Contact Dermatitis 57:105–109

42. Schnuch A, Uter W (2003) Decrease in nickel allergy in Germany and regulatory interventions. Contact Dermatitis 49:107–108

43. Zachariae CO, Agner T, Menné T (1996) Chromium allergy in consecutive patients in a country where ferrous sulfate has been added to cement since 1981. Contact Dermatitis 35: 83–85

44. Johansen JD, Veien N, Laurberg G et al (2008) Decreasing trends in methyldibromo glutaronitrile contact allergy–following regulatory intervention. Contact Dermatitis 59:48–51

45. Safford RJ (2008) The Dermal Sensitisation Threshold – a TTC approach for allergic contact dermatitis. Regul Toxicol Pharmacol 51:195–200

46. Buehler EV (1965) Delayed contact hypersensitivity in the guinea pig. Arch Dermatol 91:171–177

Legislation

52

Ian R. White and David A. Basketter

Contents

52.1 Introduction

Europe has the most highly developed set of legislation regarding contact dermatitis. Rather than cataloguing the varying aspects of legislation globally, we have limited the material to a relatively brief consideration of this European perspective, since we believe that it provides a good model. Legislation and regulations regarding chemical substances, preparations, detergents and cosmetics are mentioned, together with information on legislation relating to two very important allergens, nickel and chromate.

It is important to be aware that substantial changes are planned to the Cosmetics Directive in the coming years. Intensive action on a "recast" is underway with the text having been approved at the first reading by the European Parliament in March 2009. However, at the time of writing, the new legislation is not enacted, so the material that follows focuses on the existing legislation. On the current plans, the recast of the Cosmetics Directive will come into force in 2012. At that point, it will be a Regulation, rather than a Directive, which means it automatically replaces all national legislation from its date of enactment. The Regulation will require nanomaterials to be specifically identified on product ingredient labels.

52.2 Cosmetics Directive

In Europe, cosmetic safety legislation is governed by the Cosmetics Directive (76/768/EEC), which is then

I.R. White (✉)
Department of Cutaneous Allergy,
St John's Institute of Dermatology,
St Thomas' Hospital, London SE1 7EH, UK
e-mail: ian.white@kcl.ac.uk

D.A. Basketter
DABMEB Consultancy Ltd,
Incorporated in England and Wales,
2 Normans Road, Sharnbrook,
Bedfordshire MK44 1PR, UK

European Legislation and responsibilities advance and change often. Therefore, although references to specific web pages in this chapter were accurate at the time of publication, they should be considered as pointers only.

J.D. Johansen et al. (eds.), *Contact Dermatitis*,
DOI: 10.1007/978-3-642-03827-3_52, © Springer-Verlag Berlin Heidelberg 2011

incorporated into the national legislation of the EU member states. DG Enterprise of the European Commission was responsible for this Directive but since 2010 DG Sanco has assumed responsibility. The full text is published in English on the website: http://eur-lex.europa.eu/LexUriServ/LexUriServ.do?uri=CONSLEG:1976L0768:20080424:EN:PDF.

Regular updates are published in all of the official EU languages: http://ec.europa.eu/enterprise/cosmetics/html/consolidated_dir.htm.

Annex 1 of the Cosmetics Directive provides an illustrative list of cosmetic products. Annex 2 is a list of substances that are prohibited from use in cosmetic products available in Europe. Annex 3 tabulates sub-

Annex 2
– Prohibited

Annex 3
– Restricted/conditions of use

Annex 4
– Colouring agents

Annex 6
– Preservatives

Annex 7
– UV filters

stances that may be used, but only under certain restrictions (such as for application to hair only, not for oral hygiene). Annexes 6 and 7 are positive lists of preservatives and UV filters.

As part of an exhaustive review of hair dye safety, only hair dyes listed in Annex 3 may be used.

Relatively few ingredients are included in the various annexes. However, the cosmetic industry uses several thousand substances for which there is no specific regulation. The so-called *inventory* of cosmetic ingredients (now called "CosIng") is an indicative but not exhaustive listing of these substances. Although the inventory has been the responsibility of DG Enterprise and it is published on their website (http://ec.europa.eu/enterprise/cosmetics/cosing/), it will be transferred to DG Sanco. Part 1 of the inventory lists general cosmetic ingredients; Part 2 lists fragrance ingredients. The inventory contains the INCI name (International Nomenclature for Cosmetic Ingredients) that must be used for ingredient labelling purposes in the

European Union. The INCI system is based on the CTFA nomenclature used in the USA. The important differences between the American (voluntary) system and the European one (legal) are the use of Latin scientific names for biological extracts (rather than common names in the USA), colour index numbers (FD&C in the USA) and aqua (water in USA). The prime reason for the differences was to ensure that language was "scientific" and acceptable to all nations, rather than being obviously English.

Ingredient listing was introduced in the sixth amendment of the cosmetic Directive, although a compromise was reached where fragrance compositions in cosmetics would be indicated simply by the word *parfum*. This "fragrance exception" was included because of the lobbying activities of the industry, but identification of 26 "established" fragrance allergens was done with the seventh amendment of the Directive. Since March 2005, identification has been required if one of the fragrance substances is present at levels >10 ppm for leave-on products and >100 ppm for rinse-off. This should ensure that the great majority of individuals with identified fragrance allergies can adequately avoid exposure. These levels were suggested by the European Parliament as a pragmatic solution, as the "safe" levels for most of the fragrance substances are largely unknown. The list of fragrance substances that must be labelled is under review.

Before a cosmetic ingredient is added to one of the annexes in the Cosmetics Directive, there is a requirement that a scientific evaluation of the substance is provided by the independent advisory committee of the European Commission. Until 1997, this was the Scientific Committee for Cosmetology (SCC). From 1997 until 2004, it was the Scientific Committee for Cosmetics and Non-Food Products (SCC NFP); from 2004 to 2009, the Scientific Committee for Consumer Products (SCCP); and currently, the Scientifc Committee for Consumer Safety (SCCS). All of the opinions from recent years are available on the website of DG Sanco (Directorate General for Consumer Safety and Health Protection):

Before 2004: http://ec.europa.eu/health/ph_risk/committees/sccp/sccp_opinions_en.htm
2004–2009: http://ec.europa.eu/health/ph_risk/committees/09_sccp/sccp_opinions_en.htm
and since 2009: http://ec.europa.eu/health/ph_risk/committees/04_sccs/sccs_opinions_en.htm

A request for assessment is presented to the advisory committee via the services of the European Commission. Requests are made because evaluation is required by the

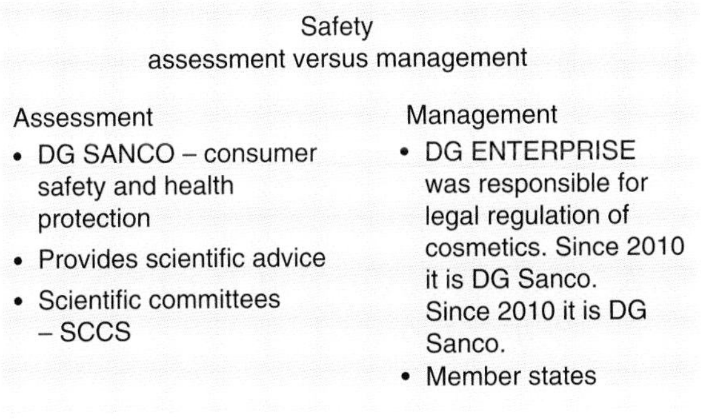

Safety
assessment versus management

Assessment
- DG SANCO – consumer safety and health protection
- Provides scientific advice
- Scientific committees – SCCS

Management
- DG ENTERPRISE was responsible for legal regulation of cosmetics. Since 2010 it is DG Sanco. Since 2010 it is DG Sanco.
- Member states

Fig. 52.1 Safety assessment vs. management

Directive; there is a concern raised by a Member State or scientific/clinical data suggest a problem that needs to be evaluated. The information evaluated by the SCCS is normally supplied in a complete dossier (containing the toxicological, chemical, epidemiological data: published, "on file" and "gray" material) of a substance provided by industry, but information may be submitted by others (which happened with methyldibromo glutaronitrile and hydroxyisohexyl 3-cyclohexene carboxaldehyde, where the dermatological community provided the data).

DG Sanco is responsible for the assessment of risk, while DG Enterprise was concerned with the management of risk; DG Sanco is now concerned with both aspects. (Fig. 52.1).

The above scientific advisory committees have produced Guidelines for the Safety Evaluation of Cosmetic Ingredients. These guidelines are regularly updated as science and technology progresses and are available from the website.

Although a cosmetic product must comply with all regulatory requirements, it is also a requirement that the safety of each cosmetic product (including that of the ingredients that have not been regulated) be independently assessed by an individual with appropriate expertise – the assessor. Every cosmetic product has an associated dossier containing technical details of the ingredients and a safety (toxicological) assessment (Fig. 52.2).

The seventh amendment also introduced a timeline for the prohibition of animal experiments used to evaluate the safety of cosmetic ingredients that must comply with the requirements of the Directive. There has been prohibition of testing of finished cosmetic products on animals since September 2004. Additionally, with exceptions, there is to be a gradual prohibition of testing of ingredients on animals as alternative validated methods are adopted. There will

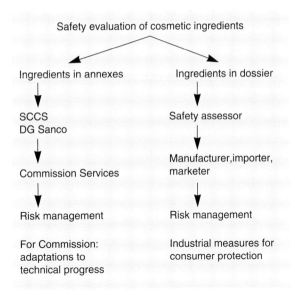

Safety evaluation of cosmetic ingredients

Ingredients in annexes

→ SCCS DG Sanco

→ Commission Services

→ Risk management

For Commission: adaptations to technical progress

Ingredients in dossier

→ Safety assessor

→ Manufacturer, importer, marketer

→ Risk management

Industrial measures for consumer protection

Fig. 52.2 Safety evaluation of cosmetic ingredients

also be a parallel prohibition of the sale of cosmetics when an ingredient has been tested on animals, within or outside of the EU, to meet the requirements of the Cosmetics Directive after March 2009. The exceptions consist of repeat dose toxicity, toxicokinetics and reprotoxicity, which will be permitted until 2013. The timeline was introduced into the seventh amendment by a process of conciliation, and was politically driven.

Hazard identification
– In vivo, in vitro tests, QSAR, epidemiology

Dose–response assessment
– NOAEL (no observed adverse effect level)

Exposure assessment
– Amount, frequency, specific groups

Risk characterization
– Margin of safety

There are several steps associated with the process of *risk assessment*:

As far as dermatological assessments are concerned, the following represents the status (2005) of the validation of and the movement towards the reduction or replacement of animal (in vivo) testing methodologies.

52

52.2.1 Skin Irritation

> Draize in vivo skin irritation test
> – OECD 404, EC B.4

Several in vitro skin irritation tests under validation

52.2.2 Skin Corrosivity

Three validated alternatives:

> TER – rat skin transcutaneous electrical resistance test (draft OECD 430, EC B.40)
> EPISKIN and EpiDerm – reconstructed human epidermal equivalent (draft OECD 431, EC B.40)

52.2.3 Eye Irritation

> No validated complete alternative to Draize in vivo test (OECD 405, EC B.5).
> ECVAM – the European Centre for Validation of Alternative Methods (http://ecvam.jrc.it/index.htm) – is currently evaluating.
> Bovine cornea opacity-permeability test
> Neutral organic chemicals
> Red blood cell; neutral red uptake
> Surfactants
> Hen's egg test – chorioallantoic membrane
> Screening finished products
> Most recently, a comprehensive summary of the strategies taken to avoid the use of animal testing has been published [1]

52.2.4 Skin Sensitization

> Magnusson Kligman Guinea Pig Maximization Test (OECD 406, EC B.6)
> Local lymph node assay (OECD draft 429)
> – Allows reduction of animal use and refinement of data obtained

Potential alternatives to animal testing are currently under review at ECVAM and included a direct peptide reactivity assay and two in vitro methods based on allergen-induced changes in dendritic like cell lines.

52.2.5 Dermal Absorption, Percutaneous Penetration

> In vivo (draft OECD Guideline 427)
> In vitro (draft OECD Guideline 428)
> – Isolated human/pig skin

52.2.6 Photoirritation

> 3T3 Neutral Red Uptake Phototoxicity Test (draft OECD 432, EC B.41)
> Expected that chemicals showing photoallergic properties may be positive

52.3 Detergent Regulations

The Detergents Regulations of the European Union came into force in October 2005: http://europa.eu.int/eur-lex/pri/en/oj/dat/2004/l_104/l_104200404.08en00010035.pdf.

This regulation requires the listing of preservatives in detergents, household and similar products when present at any concentration in a finished product, and the identification of the presence of any of the fragrance allergens itemized in the Cosmetics Directive and present at >100 ppm (such products are treated as rinse-off cosmetics). The Regulations also require that formulation details are released if needed to investigate an adverse reaction.

52.4 REACH and the Dangerous Substances Directive (DSD)

REACH (Registration, Evaluation, Authorisation and restriction of Chemicals) has replaced the older DSD [14], but for completeness, the latter is still included, as many substances have been classfied as allergens or irritants on its basis than under the newer legislation. REACH details can be found on the EU website and elsewhere [2]. It shifts much of the emphasis on the assessment of chemicals and their risk assessment to industry. Extensive guidance has been published, including for skin sensitisers and irritants [3, 4]. Toxicological evaluations also have to follow the principles set out in the GHS (globally harmonized scheme), which aim to have international harmonization of testing and assessment [5]. Currently, the GHS is being modified to allow for skin sensitizing chemicals to be classified as strong and weak, which in principle is similar to the way in which skin irritants are subdivided [6]. Read further for details of current classification categories.

The legislation embodied in the DSD deals with all new chemical substances that are being produced in the European Union [7]. Sections consider skin sensitization and skin irritation. Test methods for the identification of skin sensitizers are clearly set out [8, 9], but the legislation also admits a wide range of chemical structure and human evidence.

Where a substance is identified as a skin sensitizer, it is classified and labelled as *R43: May cause sensitization by skin contact*. Similar strategies apply to the identification of skin irritants, where the classification may be *R38: Irritant, R34: Causes burns* or *R35: Causes severe burns*, depending on the severity of the observed effects. It is unfortunate that to date, no such categorization of skin sensitizers has been adopted, despite clear proposals from a recent EU expert group [10].

The outcome of classification under the dangerous preparations directive (DPD) is reflected in the manufacturer's safety data sheet (MSDS) when that substance is supplied, for example, to a consumer product manufacturer.

52.5 Dangerous Preparations Directive (DPD)

The legislation contained in the DPD represents, in effect, the consequences of a preparation if a substance in that preparation is classified as irritating or sensitizing [5]. The key consequence is the labelling of the preparation with an appropriate warning, such as: *May cause sensitisation by skin contact*. However, all labellings are subject to largely administrative (not scientifically-based) threshold limits. Thus, for most sensitizing substances, labelling a preparation as carrying a skin sensitization risk is only required when the concentration of the sensitizing substance in the preparation is 1%. The aim here is to protect health by limiting the induction of skin sensitization. To take account of the potential failure of this legislation, such that individuals do become sensitized, additional labelling is shortly to come into force such that for a concentration between the above labelling threshold and up to a factor of ten lower, the preparation must be labelled with the name of the sensitizing substance and the words added: *May cause an allergic reaction*.

It might be considered unfortunate that even in the EU, where regulations regarding skin sensitizers and irritants are at their most developed, there is no harmonization between the legislation (for example, to protect those already sensitized, the name of the sensitizer, written in simple language, is clearly sufficient, without any additional wording). It is also most unfortunate that the relative potency of the allergen is not taken into account during labelling (except in rare cases, usually after a considerable clinical problem has arisen).

52.6 Nickel

Nickel is still the most common contact allergen in the EU (and elsewhere). However, in the EU, this is set to change because of a relatively recent Directive [11], which resulted from action originating in Denmark. The directive limits the allowed release of nickel from metal objects in prolonged contact with the skin to 0.5 mg/cm^2 per week. The impact of this limit has already paid dividends in Denmark, where a sharp reduction in nickel allergy is now evident [12]. It seems likely that the same will happen elsewhere in Europe.

52.7 Chromate

The European Union has also regulated exposure to chromate in cement. Cement and cement-containing preparations may not be used or placed on the market if they contain, when hydrated, more than 0.0002%

52

(2 ppm) of soluble chromium VI out of the total dry weight of the cement. The Member States of the European Union have been required to meet this limit since January 2005 [13].

References

1. EC (2006) Regulation No 1907/2006 of the European Parliament and of the Council of 18 December 2006 concerning the Registration, Evaluation, Authorisation and restriction of Chemicals (REACH), establishing a European Chemicals Agency, amending Directive 1999/45/EC and repealing Council Regulation (EEC) No 793/93 and Commission Regulation (EC) No 1488/94 as well as Council Directive 76/769/EEC and Commission Directives 91/155/EEC, 93/67/EEC, 93/105/EC and 2000/21/EC. Official J Eur Union L396:1–849

2. ECHA (2008) Guidance on information requirements and chemical safety assessment. Chapter R.7a: Endpoint specific guidance, European Chemicals Agency, Helsinki, pp 256–288

3. ECHA (2008) Guidance on information requirements and chemical safety assessment. Chapter R.4: Evaluation of available information 23pp. Helsinki, Finland, European Chemicals Agency. http://guidance.echa.europa.eu/docs/guidance_document/information_requirements_r4_en.pdf?vers=20_08_08. Accessed 13 Feb 2009

4. Anon (2003) Globally Harmonised System of Classification and Labelling of Chemicals (GHS). Part 3: Health and Environmental Hazards. United Nations Organisation, New York, NY, USA, and Geneva, Switzerland, pp 151–158

5. http://www.unece.org/trans/doc/2008/ac10c4/UN-SCEGHS-16-inf03e.pdf. Accessed 29 June 2009

6. Scott L, Eskes C, Hoffmann S, Adriaens E, Alepée N, Bufo M, Clothier R, Facchini D, Faller C, Guest R, Harbell J, Hartung T, Kamp H, Varlet BL, Meloni M, McNamee P, Osborne R, Pape W, Pfannenbecker U, Prinsen M, Seaman C, Spielmann H, Stokes W, Trouba K, Berghe CV, Goethem FV, Vassallo M, Vinardell P, Zuang V (2010) A proposed eye irritation testing strategy to reduce and replace in vivo studies using bottom-up and top-down approaches. Toxicol In Vitro 24(1):1–9

7. EU (1996) EU dangerous substances directive. 22nd adaptation to technical progress (96/54/EC). Official J Eur Commun L248:199

8. EU (1996) EC Test Method B6. Commission Directive 96/54/EC of 30 July 1996, adapting to technical progress for the twenty-second time Council Directive 67/548/EEC on the approximation of the laws, regulations and administrative provisions relating to the classification, packaging and labelling of dangerous substances. Methods for the determination of toxicity, B6. Acute toxicity skin sensitisation. Official J Eur Commun L248:206–212

9. OECD (2002) Guidelines for testing of chemicals. Guideline no. 429. Skin sensitisation: the local lymph node assay. Organisation for Economic Cooperation and Development, Paris

10. Basketter DA, Andersen KE, Lidén C, van Loveren H, Boman A, Kimber I, Alanko K, Berggren E (2005) Evaluation of the skin sensitising potency of chemicals using existing methods and considerations of relevance for elicitation. Contact Dermatitis 50:39–43

11. EU (1994) Nickel Directive: European Parliament and Council Directive 94/27/EC of 30 June 1994: amending for the 12th time Directive 76/769/EEC on the approximation of the laws, regulations and administrative provisions of the Member States relating to restrictions on the marketing and use of certain dangerous substances and preparations. Official J Eur Commun L188:1–2

12. Nielsen NH, Linneberg A, Menné T, Madsen F, Frolund L, Dirksen A, Jorgensen T (2002) Incidence of allergic contact sensitization in Danish adults between 1990 and 1998; the Copenhagen Allergy Study, Denmark. Br J Dermatol 147:487–492

13. EU (2003) Cement Directive: Directive 2003/53/EC of the European Parliament and of the Council of 18 June 2003 amending for the 26th time Council Directive 76/769/EEC relating to restrictions on the marketing and use of certain dangerous substances and preparations (nonylphenol, nonylphenol ethoxylate and cement). Official J Eur Commun L178:24–27

14. EU (1998) EU Council Directive 88/379/EEC of 7 June 1988 on the approximation of the laws, regulations and administrative provisions of the Member States relating to the classification, packaging and labelling of dangerous preparations. Official J Eur Commun L18:14

International Comparison of Legal Aspects of Workers' Compensation for Occupational Contact Dermatitis

53

Peter J. Frosch, Werner Aberer, Tove Agner, Paul J. August, L. Conde-Salazar, Lieve Constandt, Patricia Engasser, Felipe Heras, Swen Malte John, Antti Lauerma, Christophe J. Le Coz, Magnus Lindberg, Howard I. Maibach, Haydn L. Muston, Rosemary L. Nixon, Hanspeter Rast, W.I. van Tichelen, and Jason Williams

Contents

P.J. Frosch (✉)
Hautklinik, Klinikum Dortmund gGmbH,
Beurhausstr. 40, 44137 Dortmund, Germany
e-mail: peter.frosch@klinikumdo.de

W. Aberer
e-mail: werner.aberer@meduni-graz.at

T. Agner
e-mail: t.agner@dadlnet.dk

P.J. August, H.L. Muston, and J. Williams
e-mail: jasondlwilliams@hotmail.com

L. Conde-Salazar
e-mail: lconde@isciii.es

L. Constandt
e-mail: lieveconstandt@yahoo.com

P. Engasser and H.I. Maibach
e-mail: MaibachH@Derm.ucsf.edu

F. Heras
e-mail: fheras@isciii.es

S.M. John
e-mail: sjohn@uos.de

A.Lauerma
e-mail: antti.lauerma@ttl.fi

C.-J. Le Coz
e-mail: christophe.lecoz@wanadoo.fr

M. Lindberg
e-mail: magnus.lindberg@orebroll.se

R.L. Nixon
e-mail: rnixon@occderm.asn.au

H. Rast
e-mail: Hanspeter.rast@suva.ch

W.I. van Tichelen
e-mail: Wouter.va.tichelen@mensura.be

53.1 Introduction

In a European textbook on contact dermatitis, a chapter on legal aspects is entirely appropriate. In many cases an occupational cause is suspected and proven after careful diagnostic procedures. A number of questions then arise that are handled in different ways in different European countries. Faced with the modern enlarged European Union, with its expected labour

J.D. Johansen et al. (eds.), *Contact Dermatitis*,
DOI: 10.1007/978-3-642-03827-3_53, © Springer-Verlag Berlin Heidelberg 2011

53

migration, the occupational physician needs to know and understand the essential differences between the legislation for occupational contact dermatitis in the major countries.

This chapter is largely based on the feedback from questionnaires sent to members of the European Environmental and Contact Dermatitis Research Group (EECDRG) and other colleagues that are experienced in this field. The underlying concept of handling a case of occupational contact dermatitis in Germany and various other (mainly European) countries and the probable outcomes for three typical cases are described. Fifteen questions were asked about various aspects of such cases (including institutions involved, report forms, requirements for recognition, retraining and pension). Due to the nomenclature and country-specific legal rules, it often proved difficult for responders to answer these questions and make clear statements. Nevertheless, some major differences became apparent.

In this chapter, the authors have tried to characterize the principle legal characteristics in the various countries. Frequent comparisons are made with the German system; this is only for the ease of understanding and definitely not with any intention of suggesting that this should be regarded as the "standard". In the years to come, it will probably be necessary to create more uniform joint legislation in this area, in order to avoid socially unjust decisions.

Recent Information on occupational diseases in Europe (incidence, safety, legal aspects) can be obtained from two internet sources: http://www.euro-gip.fr/index.php?chlang=en *(EUROGIP Enquiry Report 34/E as of Jan 2009: Occupational diseases in Europe. 1990–2006 statistical data and legal news)* and the European Agency for Safety and Health at Work – European Risk Observatory report 2008: Occupational skin diseases and dermal exposure in the EU (EU-25). Policy and practice overview (http://osha.europa.eu/en/publications/reports/TE7007049ENC_skin_diseases).

53.2 Occupational Dermatitis in Germany

Peter J. Frosch, Swen M. John

In Germany, the legal basis for dealing with occupational diseases (OD) is cited in the seventh book of the State Insurance Code *Sozialgesetzbuch* (SGB 7) and the Decree on Occupational Diseases *Berufskrankheitenverordnung* ("BKV", from 31st Oct 1997; latest amendment dates from 1st July 2009). OD are defined in the official list of recognized OD; this list is included in the BKV (Anlage zur BKV) and it presently comprises 73 OD. The two skin diseases in this list are classified under:

> No. 5101: Severe or repeatedly relapsing dermatoses that have clearly necessitated the cessation of all occupational activities which were or could be responsible for causing the disease or its relapse or aggravation.
> No. 5102: Cancer or pre-cancer caused by soot, un-purified paraffins, tar, anthracene, pitch or similar substances.

The list is updated periodically. The responsibility of dealing with occupational incidents and diseases falls on non-profit Statutory Employers´ Liability Insurance Institutions, which have recently formed an umbrella organization Deutsche Gesetzliche Unfallversicherung (DGUV). These institutions cover different fields of work, such as administrative work and trade, health care (including hairdressing), construction, mechanical engineering, iron and steel industry, mining, quarrying, transport, wholesale trade and warehousing, food production, the complete school system (all pupils are insured), public administration and offices and all public services including public hospitals, etc. Agriculture, horticulture, forestry and the wood industry are also insured branches, but have a separate umbrella institution (Bundesverband der landwirtschaftlichen Berufsgenossenschaften [BLB]). All together, at the moment, there are more than 40 such statutory institutions with responsibilities for the above named branches; the number will further decrease in a concerted effort to lean management, recently implemented by law (Unfallversicherungsmodernisierungsgesetz [UVMG] from 30th Oct 2008).

Every employee must by law be insured against occupational accidents, injuries and diseases. Only employers have to pay this insurance. The system used to settle claims about occupational accidents and diseases is quite elaborate and has a very "social" feel.

Even when there is only a slight suspicion that a dermatosis case is work related, a dermatologist's report (*Hautarztbericht*) is filed with the appropriate insurance institution [1]. This report requires the consent of the person concerned. It is based on a detailed examination, including patch tests and atopy screening. It also includes recommendations concerning therapy, protection, skin care and even changing the workplace [2]. This is an attempt to handle potential occupational dermatoses as quickly and un-bureaucratically as possible. Recently, the emphasis, even more so, has been laid on the early preventative intervention (see Chap. 50 of this book). The statutory employers' liability insurances, thus, implemented the "step-wise procedure skin" (Stufenverfahren Haut) as a systematic approach to the prevention of occupational skin disease [1]. This approach offers quick preventive help for all levels of severity of contact dermatitis, including dermatological out patient, and if needed, in severe cases inpatient therapy, skin protection seminars and an interdisciplinary intervention with one's focus on teaching and systematic follow-up [3–6].

Only if the dermatosis continues and the suspicion that the disease has an occupational origin is confirmed, any doctor in contact with the person concerned is obliged *by law* to fill in a special initial report form (the medical report of an occupational disease: *Ärztliche Anzeige über eine Berufskrankheit*). This form is then sent to the relevant insurance institution or to an official government physician dealing with OD (*Staatlicher Gewerbearzt*). This does not require the consent of the person concerned.

After obtaining the report, the insurance institution investigates the case further, often by sending a specially trained adviser to inspect the workplace. The adviser gives detailed advice to the worker regarding the avoidance of irritants and potential allergens and can recommend the use of barrier creams, gloves and appropriate cleansing agents. These must be provided by the employer. If the patient continues to have skin symptoms, he or she is referred to a dermatologist or a centre specialized on occupational skin diseases, often a university hospital [1, 2, 4]. A detailed work-up is carried out, including patch testing and atopy screening, and the dermatologist's report (*Hautarztbericht*) is sent to the insurance institution. There is a moderate payment for both the initial report and the *Hautarztbericht*. The dermatologist must make a clear statement as to the origin of the disease, including occupational and non-occupational factors, and provides detailed suggestions for the avoidance of occupational risks and recommendations for preventive measures. The dermatologist will then be given the mandate (*"Behandlungsauftrag"*) to see the patient on

a regular basis for a period of initially 6 months and treat him on the expenses of the accident insurance in order to avoid job loss "by all means" [2]. If all such measures fail (as in the case of the bricklayer given below), the patient must stop working in his or her occupation, and an expert opinion from a dermatologist (usually a different one) is ordered by the insurance institution. This opinion provides the basis for rejecting or recognizing the condition as an occupational skin disease and for paying compensation and/or retraining. Recently, recommendations for standardized expert dermatological opinions in these cases have been issued by the Task Force on Occupational and Environmental Dermatology ("Bamberg Medical Bulletin"; [7]).

A copy of the initial report (*Ärztliche Anzeige*) is also sent to an official government physician (*Staatlicher Gewerbearzt*), who can then investigate the case further, order an expert opinion or decide independently whether the disease is to be classified as occupational or non-occupational. If the *Gewerbearzt* and the insurance institution disagree on a case, particularly if a monthly pension is at stake, a second or third expert's opinion is obtained. A commission (see below) then makes a decision. If the patient is dissatisfied with the decision, he or she may take the matter to court (*Sozialgericht*). After reviewing the case, the judge often orders another expert opinion from a recognized specialist in occupational dermatology.

According to German law (seventh decree on OD: 7. *Berufskrankheitenverordnung*), to be regarded as a case of occupational contact dermatitis, an eczema must be either "severe" or "repeatedly relapsing" and must have created the need for the insured person to cease all activities that are (or could be) causing the disease, aggravation or relapse of the disease (No. 5101: "*schwere oder wiederholt rückfällige Hauterkrankungen, die zur Unterlassung aller Tätigkeiten gezwungen haben, die für die Entstehung, die Verschlimmerung oder das Wiederaufleben der Krankheit ursächlich waren oder sein können*"). The severity ("*Schwere*") of the dermatitis is based on the clinical picture, the duration and the existence of a sensitization of occupational relevance. The clinical picture is considered severe if the dermatitis is highly vesicular in the acute stage or lichenified with deep fissures in the chronic stage. Further factors are pain, severe pruritus, impairment of mobility and spreading of the dermatitis beyond the original site. A duration of more than 6 months and a continuous need for medical treatment are important criteria for defining

53

the severity by the course of the disease. Sensitization to an important occupational material that cannot be avoided (e.g. by appropriate skin protection) or replaced is also part of the definition. In the case of a type I allergy, asthma, angioedema or generalized urticaria would qualify as a "severe" degree of occupational origin. Further details are given in the original German publication [8]. "Repeatedly relapsing" (*wiederholt rückfällig*) means that at least three bouts of the disease have occurred. By definition, it is also necessary that the disease has healed or at least improved considerably between two bouts.

A further specific term in the German legislation is *Minderung der Erwerbsfähigkeit* (MdE), meaning "diminution of working ability". The physician must estimate, in an abstract manner, the number of occupations in the overall labour market that the patient is unable to work in due to the occupational disease. For instance, a bricklayer who has acquired a chromate allergy and is suffering from severe hand eczema will receive an MdE of 20–30%, which means that he cannot enter about 20–30% of the occupations available in the labour market because chromate is such an ubiquitous allergen. However, these figures may change due to developments in the work environment. Chromate allergy is now slowly decreasing in Germany due to the addition of ferrous sulphate to cement. Recommendations for the MdE are therefore regularly updated by a Task Force of the German Dermatological Society [9–15]. If the estimate is below 20% (for example, 10–15% in the case of a nickel allergy with *slight* hand eczema), the case is still recognized as an occupational disease (*Anerkennung dem Grunde nach,* "basic recognition" or "admission in law"). However, 20% is a critical figure, because a patient with an MdE of 20% or more receives compensation: he or she is paid a pension equivalent to the appropriate percentage of the pension that would have been awarded if he or she were totally disabled (two-thirds of the annual earnings in the year before stopping work). This pension is paid by the insurance institution for as long as the disability lasts, often for life. Withdrawal of the compensation is difficult, but it can occur if the change in MdE is more than 5% and the new MdE is less than 20%. In every case, however, once an occupational disease has been legally acknowledged to exist, this acknowledgement can never be withdrawn. Income protection (*Übergangsgeld, Verletztengeld*) during recovery and retraining must always be covered by the insurance institution.

The *Arbeitsgemeinschaft für Berufs- und Umweltdermatologie* (Task Force on Occupational and Environmental Dermatology [ABD] of the German Dermatological Society [DDG]) has published recommendations regarding the degree of MdE based on the presence and severity of skin lesions, the intensity of allergic contact sensitization(s) and the spread (occurrence) of the allergen(s) in working life. In contrast to earlier recommendations, a severe course of a cumulative irritant dermatitis can also qualify for an MdE of 20% [16].

In the following section, three typical examples of occupational "legal cases" are given, as they were handled by the German authorities.

53.2.1 Example A

A bricklayer, aged 35 years, has to stop all occupational activities because of severe recalcitrant hand eczema, which has resulted in at least three sick leaves each of a duration of several weeks. A patch test is strongly positive for dichromate. A further attempt to work with cement of low dichromate content and the use of nitrile gloves did not improve his condition. In the expert's opinion, the dermatologist suggested that he should be retrained, that his disease should be recognized as occupational (*Berufskrankheit* 5101) and that he should be granted a pension of 20%.

The retraining is paid for by the insurance company for construction workers. The retraining programme takes 2 years and costs about 100,000€. This procedure is performed according to paragraph three of the *Berufskrankheitenverordnung* (BKV), which states that the insurer has to do everything possible to prevent the development, the aggravation or the recurrence of an occupational disease. In general, retraining procedures are not implemented for people older than 40–45 years; elder people suffering from a recognized occupational dermatosis receive partial income protection over 5 years.

53.2.2 Example B

A nurse suffers from atopic eczema, which began in childhood. She suffers from hayfever, and when she began her training as a nurse, she had slight eczema on the flexures, but not on the hands. After 2 years, she developed a hand eczema, which is considered to be irritant because patch tests with occupational allergens are negative. She has had three sick leaves and has occasionally seen a dermatologist. She has voluntarily given up her occupation and wants to be retrained for a clean, dry office job. In the expert's opinion, the physician denies the existence of an occupational skin disease because the patient is suffering from a mild atopic eczema that has been precipitated on the hands by her occupational activities. Even after stopping nursing, she has skin symptoms on the hands. This is interpreted as the expression of a primarily endogenous skin disease and not an occupational dermatitis. The physician also recommends retraining, but the costs are not covered by the insurer. In most cases like this one, the Ministry of Labour or the pension fund will cover part of the costs of retraining.

If she is to return to nursing, the employers' liability insurance will provide prophylactic skin protection seminars and also dermatological treatment, if occupationally aggravated hand eczema should recur [1, 3].

53.2.2.1 Comment

Cases like this one are often difficult to assess. Some dermatologists would recognize this case as occupational because the patient had never had symptoms on her hands before her occupational activity that triggered off the eczema at this site. Other dermatologists would recognize the occupational cause of the hand eczema, but would argue that due to the mildness of the disease, there was no objective need to cease all occupational activities. They might, however, recommend measures according to paragraph 3 BKV (therapy, protective measures) in order to prevent relapses of severe hand dermatitis if the patient returned to work as a nurse. This could, in fact, mean that the nurse would be retrained for a new job at the cost of the insurer.

If a patient appeals, the case first has to be taken to a commission at the insurance institution (*Widerspruchsausschuss*), which includes a representative of the employers and a labour union representative. Every detail of the individual case is scrutinized and the opinion of a dermatologist may be heard again.

If the commission's decision is again not accepted by the patient, he or she can appeal and take the insurer

to court (*Sozialgericht*). There are no court costs here, and lawyer costs are covered by the patient's labour union, if he or she is a member.

53.2.3 Example C

A surgeon, aged 40 years, develops a contact allergy to rubber gloves. Patch testing confirms that he is allergic to thiurams and must use more expensive, thiuram-free, latex gloves. He is free from symptoms when he uses this type of glove. In the expert's opinion, the disease is recognized as work related, but not as a fully fledged occupational disease as there are means of appropriate prevention and the surgeon can continue his work with special precautions.

He does not receive any compensation because he is not obliged to stop working (which is one of the prerequisites for the acknowledgement of occupational skin disease; see above). The costs of the more expensive allergen-free gloves must be covered by the employer. If the costs are very high, or if the surgeon is self-employed, the insurance institution may cover all or at least part of it. This is a procedure from paragraph 3 BKV used to keep the surgeon in his occupation "by all means". Medical costs are covered for by insurance institution [2].

53.3 Occupational Contact Dermatitis in Other European Countries, Australia and the USA

Table 53.1 lists the institutions primarily involved in dealing with a case of occupational dermatitis in a number of countries. In nearly all countries except the United Kingdom, where two separate systems exist (see below), such cases are initially handled outside the system of common law. Insurance institutions – private, semiprivate or governmental – deal with the first stage after the case has been reported to them. In most countries this report is filed by the family physician, by a dermatologist or by a company physician, and the suspicion (not the proof) of an occupational cause is sufficient. Further details are discussed below. Most of the institutions listed in Table 53.1 regularly compile data on occupational skin diseases: the reader may obtain these directly from them.

Table 53.1 Institutions primarily involved in the settlement of a case of occupational dermatitis

Country	Institution	Institution collecting data on occupational dermatitis
Australia	Safe Work Australia GPO Box 9880 Canberra ACT 2601 Australia http://www.safeworkaustralia.gov.au	
Austria	AUVA (*Allgemeine Unfallversicherung*), *Unfallverhütungsdienst* Webergasse 4, 1203 Vienna, Austria http://www.auva.at HAV@auva.at Court ("*Arbeits- und Sozialgericht*")	AUVA
Belgium	*Fonds voor Beroepsziekten-Fonds des Maladies Professionelles* Ave. de l'Astronomie 1, 1210 Brussels, Belgium http://www.fmp-fbz.fgov.be wouter.vantichelen@fmp-fbz.fgov.be	
Denmark	*Arbeidsskadestyrelsen* (National Board of Occupational Health) Sankt Kjelds Plads 11, Postboks 3000, 2100 Copenhagen Denmark www.ask.dk e-mail: ask@ask.dk	
Finland	Private insurance companies Finnish Institute of Occupational Health *Työsuojeluhallitus* (Government Board for Occupational Safety) http://www.ttl.fi http://www.mol.fi	Same
France	Caisse Nationale d'Assurance Maladie des Travailleurs Salariés (CNAMTS) 50, Avenue du Professeur André Lemierre 75986 PARIS CEDEX 20 Phone : (33) 01 72 60 10 00 http://www.ameli.fr/ Institut National de Recherche et de Sécurité (INRS) pour la prévention des accidents du travail et des maladies professionnelles http://www.inrs.fr/ Ministère du Travail, des Relations Sociales, de la Famille, de la Solidarité et de la Ville 127, Rue de Grenelle 75007 Paris Phone : (33) 01 44 38 38 38 http://www.travail-solidarite.gouv.fr/	
Germany	Deutsche Gesetzliche Unfallversicherung (DGUV) – Spitzenverband der Berufsgenossenschaften und Unfallkassen Mittelstraße 51, 10117 Berlin, Germany, E-Mail: info@dguv.de Internet: http://www.dguv.de *Bundesministerium für Arbeit und Soziales (BMAS)* Wilhelmstraße 49, 10117 Berlin, Germany, E-Mail: info@bmas.bund.de http://www.bmas.de	
Spain	Instituto Nacional de Seguridad e Higiene en el trabajo http://www.mtas.es	Instituto Nacional de Medicina *Seguridad del Trabajo, Corn Evaluac. de Incapacidad* Alcala 56, 28071 Madrid, Spain Private insurance companies

Table 53.1 (continued)

Country	Institution	Institution collecting data on occupational dermatitis
Sweden	*The Swedish Work Environment Authority* Lindhagensgatan 133 112 79 Stockholm arbetsmiljoverket@av.se	Occupational injury information system (ISA) *The Swedish Work Environment Authority*
Switzerland	SUVA (*Schweiz-Unfallversicherungsanstalt*) *Abteilung Arbeitsmedizin* Postfach, 6002 Luzern, Switzerland arbeitsmedizin@suva.ch http://www.suva.ch (d,f,i,e) Other insurance institutions	SUVA
UK	Department of work and pensions http://www.dwp.gov.uk Courts and lawyers (common law action) Private insurance companies	Same HSE: http://www.hse.gov.uk THOR: http://www.coeh.man.ac.uk/thor
USA	State authorities (each state's division of occupational medicine) Private insurance companies	NIOSH, Taft Highway Cincinnati, Ohio, USA

53.3.1 Australia

Rosemary L. Nixon

All states and territories have slightly different occupational health and safety and workers' compensation legislations. There are also national schemes for government workers and seafarers. Self-employed workers are not covered by workers' compensation in many circumstances.

In the state of Victoria, for example, it is the worker who must instigate a claim, except in severe injury circumstances. This requires the worker to complete a three-page claim form, to which they must attach a workers' compensation certificate from their treating doctor.

Claims are classified as standard or minor. A minor claim implies that costs have not exceeded a set dollar amount for that year (indexed annually, and was $A564 in 2008) *and/or* less than 10 days has been lost from work. Costs include medical consultations, diagnostic tests, treatments including pharmaceutical prescriptions and travel expenses. The employer must pay these costs as part of their liability. The employer must also pay the worker 95% of their wages for the lost time within their liability of less than 10 days. The employer must submit a quarterly report with details of any minor claims that do not affect the cost of their insurance premium.

A standard claim occurs when these expenses are expected to reach, or have reached, the set dollar amount for that year *and/or* the worker has lost more than 10 days from work. The employer sends the information about the claim to their workers' compensation insurance agent within 10 days of receiving it from the worker, and a decision is made by the agent as to whether to accept the claim or not. If accepted, the agent then pays all further reasonable costs and 95% of all wages while the employee is off work. Many industrial unions have negotiated workplace agreements that ensure that the employer contributes the missing 5% of pre-injury wage. If the claim is not accepted by the workers' compensation agent, the worker is referred to an independent medical examiner. If the claim is still disputed, a process of conciliation is undertaken.

If a worker remains unable to work and is assessed as having no current work capacity, he or she will be paid the following:

Ninety-five percent of pre-injury wage to a maximum of $A1,250 (2008, indexed yearly) a week for the first 13 weeks.
After 13 weeks, work capacity is re-assessed. If there is still no work capacity, he or she will be paid 75% of the pre-injury wage up to the maximum, for up to 2 years.

53

After 2 years, a review takes place and if the worker is still unable to work, he or she is paid 75% of the pre-injury wage up to the above maximum. This may continue until the retirement age, or until a degree of work capacity is shown. If a worker's condition is stable and no further change is anticipated, he or she may apply for a lump sum payment provided the worker's impairment is 30% or greater, using a formula related to the *American Medical Association's Guide to Permanent Impairment*, Fourth Edition [17].

At any time during the process, the workers' compensation insurer can review the claim and decide to terminate liability, ceasing payments. If the worker is still unable to work, he or she may apply for a disability pension. If disputation arises, especially with respect to the termination of the claim or the determination of work capacity, the claim is adjudicated by three independent medical practitioners, the "medical panel".

Self-employed sole proprietors who do not employ others are not considered "workers" under the scheme and are therefore not covered by workers' compensation. However, if they are hired as a contractor, they may be deemed to be a "worker" and therefore are covered in the contract by the employer's workers' compensation insurance. An exception is also made where sole proprietors receive a salary as the director of their own proprietary company and remuneration exceeds $A7,500 per annum.

There is considerable evidence that many Australian workers do not submit claims for occupational skin disease, especially if they do not lose appreciable time from work. As there is a subsidized national health scheme (Medicare), all patients receive a government rebate for a considerable portion of their personal medical expenses, for both general practitioner and specialist expenses. Although patients should not legally claim on Medicare for conditions caused by work, in practice, they often prefer the simplicity of this approach, rather than completing the significant amount of paperwork required for a claim and undergoing the stigma of claiming "compo". Uncertainty surrounding the clinical diagnosis and its work-relatedness often complicates the situation.

In this workers' compensation system, workers rather than medical or other practitioners instigate claims, which is different from the mode of initiating claims utilized in many other countries.

53.3.1.1 Example A

In the Australian system, the bricklayer would be compensated for his time off work. It is the responsibility of the employer to find him alternative duties at the workplace, if any work is available.

If, however, he was off work and his skin then improved, the insurance company would pay for some rehabilitation, although this would usually comprise assistance with finding a more suitable job, rather than extensive retraining for another career. Many tradespersons are disappointed that they are encouraged to take relatively unskilled and poorly paying jobs, when their previous employment involved considerable skills.

In fact, the workers' compensation authority funds an incentive scheme for alternative employers to encourage them to employ people who cannot return to their pre-injury workplace. Support is in the form of a wage subsidy on a sliding scale up to the first 24 weeks and covers training and other relevant costs. However, the worker must have the capacity to work at least 15 h a week. Unfortunately, in reality, the bricklayer may not be aware of all possible options and would probably find less-skilled work for himself, if able to do so. The insurance company would fund the costs of his medical appointments, prescriptions and any other treatments.

53.3.1.2 Example B

In the Australian system, the nurse would likely be assessed as experiencing *significant* aggravation of her dermatitis at work, so she would receive workers' compensation benefits, and if another job could not be found by her employer, she would most likely be referred to the incentive scheme mentioned above. Again, the insurance company would fund the costs of her medical appointments, prescriptions and any other treatments, such as moisturizing creams.

53.3.1.3 Example C

In the Australian system, the employing hospital would pay for appropriate gloves for the surgeon. He would not receive workers' compensation benefits, as he remains working. Although his employer could claim the costs of the more expensive gloves from the insurer, this would adversely affect the employer's workers' compensation premium payments, so the hospital may find it preferable to pay for the alternative gloves themselves.

53.3.2 Austria

Werner Aberer

In Austria, the equivalent to the German insurance institutions for OD is the *Allgemeine Unfallversicherungsanstalt* (AUVA), a non-profit, state-oriented insurance institution that is independent of other health insurers or employers. Every employer must pay a fee for each of his employees (1.4% of the total income) to be insured by the AUVA. Every physician must report a case of suspected occupational (skin) disease to the AUVA; the patient's consent is not necessary. The AUVA can then inspect the workplace and will order an expert opinion. The expert will review the case and make detailed suggestions, in a quite similar way as described for the three German examples. He will also make an estimate of the degree of disability and suggest a pension (for example, 20% for the bricklayer, example A). In general, the main cause of the disease must be occupational in order for it to be judged as a "legal case". A primarily endogenous disease (such as atopic eczema) only qualifies for compensation under special circumstances (such as the first manifestation of the disease due to occupational factors). Cumulative insult dermatitis may be recognized if it is severe, disabling and associated with frequent sick leaves.

Negligence on the part of the employer does not have to be proven. Retraining is available to patients even if they are older than 40 years and costs are met mostly by the AUVA, partly by other state authorities. Similar to the German and in contrast to the Danish system, the worker can only receive compensation if he/she stops working in the job that caused the damage.

53.3.2.1 Example A

A bricklayer, aged 35 years, has to stop all occupational activities because of severe hand eczema. There are no specific pre-defined criteria such as a certain number of sick leaves. A patch test is strongly positive for dichromate. A further attempt to work with cement

of low dichromate content and the use of nitrile gloves did not improve his condition. In the expert's opinion, the dermatologist suggested that he should be retrained, that his disease should be recognized as occupational (*Berufskrankheit* 19), and that he should be granted an MdE of about 20% (this is the minimum, less than 20% does result in no specific financial compensation).

If the skin disease is severe but controllable by protection measures under optimal conditions, the worker may be sent for rehabilitation to Opatija/Croatia for 3 weeks in order to give the skin a chance to recover. The rehabilitation measures there are not quite comparable to those taken in specialized German institutions, but the combination of vacation and abstinence from work may help to allow the patient to continue his/her work afterwards for at least some time without major problems. Such vacations are permitted and paid by the AUVA every year, if medically justified.

The retraining is paid for by the insurance company (AUVA). The retraining programme takes as long as essential, the costs are variable. In general, retraining procedures are not implemented for people older than 50 years.

53.3.2.2 Example B

A nurse suffers from atopic eczema, which began in childhood. She suffers from hayfever, and when she began her training as a nurse she had slight eczema on the flexures, but not on the hands. After 2 years, she developed a hand eczema, which is considered to be irritant because patch tests with occupational allergens are negative. She has had some sick leaves and has occasionally seen a dermatologist. She has voluntarily given up her occupation and wants to be retrained for a clean, dry office job. In the expert's opinion, the physician denies the existence of an occupational skin disease because the patient is suffering from a mild atopic eczema that has been precipitated on the hands by her occupational activities. Even after stopping nursing, she has skin symptoms on the hands. This is interpreted as the expression of a primarily endogenous skin disease and not an occupational dermatitis. The physician may recommend to stay in the job, but to intensify skin care and protection measures. If the nurse does not want to continue her job, she will find ways to make the AUVA pay her job retraining or send her into retirement.

Cases like this one are often difficult to assess. Some dermatologists would recognize this case as occupational because the patient had never had symptoms on her hands before her occupational activity that triggered off the eczema at this site. Other dermatologists would recognize the occupational cause of the hand eczema, but would argue that due to the mildness of the disease, there was no objective need to cease all occupational activities. They might, however, recommend measures in order to prevent relapses of severe hand dermatitis if the patient returned to work as a nurse. This could, in fact, mean that the nurse would be retrained for a new job at the cost of the insurer.

If a patient appeals, the case has to be taken to a commission at the Arbeits- und Sozialgericht, which includes a representative of the employers and a labour union representative. Every detail of the individual case is scrutinized and the opinion of a dermatologist may be heard again. There are no court costs here.

53.3.2.3 Example C

A surgeon, aged 40 years, develops a contact allergy to rubber gloves. Patch testing confirms that he is allergic to thiurams and must use more expensive, thiuram-free, latex gloves. He is free from symptoms when he uses this type of glove. In the expert's opinion, the disease is recognized as occupational, but the surgeon can continue his work with special precautions.

He does not receive any compensation because he is not obliged to stop working. The costs of the more expensive gloves must be covered by the employer. If the costs are very high or if the surgeon is self-employed, the insurance institution (Sozialversicherung) will cover all or at least part of it. This is a procedure used to keep the surgeon in his occupation.

More information: www.auva.at

53.3.3 Belgium

Lieve Constandt, Wouter I. van Tichelen

In Belgium, occupational skin diseases are handled primarily by the Fund for Occupational Diseases (Fund), which is a public institution with corporate capacity that falls under remit of the Ministry of Social Affairs. It is ruled by a managing committee consisting of a chairman and members nominated by federations of trade unions and employers, respectively. Both sides of the industry have equal representation on the committee.

Every employee must be insured against OD by law; the social contributions are paid by the employer. Not only employees, but also students and apprentices are covered. The law does not apply to civil servants and state railway personnel. For them, other rulings are set out. However, at the request of other governmental insurance institutions (for example the Health Insurance Service for civil servants), the Fund will carry out medical examinations of the patients who claim compensation for an occupational disease. The self-employed are not covered.

Insured people are entitled to indemnification by the Fund if they can prove that they were exposed to an agent included in the list of those causing OD and that they suffer from a disease that is related to this kind of exposure. They should be exposed to a much greater extent than the general population. However, the individual causal relationship between the disease and the exposure is legally presumed (presumption of causation). This is the so-called "list system". Practically all cases of occupational skin diseases can be recognized under this system. Compensation for a disease not mentioned in the legal list is possible, but one has to prove the causal relationship between occupation and disease (the so-called "open system").

When an occupational dermatitis is suspected, the company physician is obliged to report the case to the Ministry of Employment and Labour and to the Fund. However, any medical doctor (general practitioner, dermatologist, company physician, physician employed by the mutual sick fund) can initiate the case using a special report form that is forwarded to the Fund. The medical documents that led to the diagnosis need to be supplied. The patient's consent is required before a claim for compensation is filed.

The Fund investigates the case. A detailed work-up, including patch testing and atopy screening, is carried out by a specialist in occupational dermatology who is employed by the Fund. He or she recommends recognition or refusal. The final decision is made by the medical superintendent of the Fund, who will estimate the loss of earning capacity. A consulting engineer may inspect the workplace.

After recognition of an occupational skin disease, the worker is not bound to leave his job. Non-economic loss is generally not compensated. If the patient can continue his work eventually with special precautions, he does not receive any compensation. When he is obliged to stop working due to the occupational dermatitis, he is entitled to a monthly payment (up to 20–30% of his wages, not higher than a defined maximum) – not a lump sum – which is received together with unemployment benefits. Should he be in a position to find alternative work, and if he were to earn less in his new job, he would receive – under certain conditions – financial compensation.

Other benefits provided are the cost of medical treatment in compliance with the rules and after intervention from the sickness insurance and the cost of special gloves and shoes (up to a certain amount) that do not contain the allergen to which the patient is sensitized. Retraining is paid for by the Fund, but is rarely performed.

If the patient is dissatisfied with the decision, he or she is able to appeal to the welfare tribunal. The judge always orders another expert opinion, not necessarily from a recognized specialist in dermatology. The court costs are covered by the Fund.

An allergic contact dermatitis will be recognized providing that the triggering allergen(s) is (are) relevant to the occupation. However, the dermatitis does not have to be wholly occupational to qualify.

A chronic irritant contact dermatitis may be recognized as an occupational disease if its relationship to occupational activities is quite clear. Only medications and protective gloves are paid for by the Fund.

One exception to the rule that non-economic loss is not compensated is occupational natural rubber latex allergy. Latex-allergic health care workers, cleaning personnel and other workers using latex products will always receive financial compensation (at least 10%) because of the inconvenience and the severe allergic reactions they may experience. Thus, a nurse with latex glove-associated urticaria would receive 10% and additional financial compensation if she had to stop working in her occupation. The cost of latex-free gloves is also covered by the Fund.

53.3.4 Denmark

Tove Agner

In Denmark, occupational skin disease may be notified to the authorities either with the patient's consent, or anonymously, not mentioning the name of the patient. Cases should be reported whenever the slightest suspicion of work-related disease appears, and by law, a case should be reported within a year after the suspicion of an occupationally related disease has been raised. Cases are most often notified by dermatologists or general practitioners, but it can also be done by the employer or the patient him/herself. After the case has been notified, the authorities will in most cases call for a medical report (expert opinion) from a dermatologist. If 50% or more of the cause of the disease is due to occupational exposure, the disease can be recognized as occupational – even if the disease has disappeared. However, this does not necessarily lead to any financial compensation.

Compensation is divided into economical compensation for ongoing disease, reimbursement for medical costs, economical for supporting retraining and compensation for the loss of income. Worker's compensation for ongoing disease is only paid when symptoms are still present, or if an allergy has been achieved to a ubiquitous allergen (nickel, latex, rubber additives, chromate, formaldehyde). The degree of permanent injury is determined on the basis of the dermatological medical report. When the disease is only partially occupational, the compensation will be reduced appropriately. If the degree of injury has worsened after compensation has been paid, the case can be reviewed within 5 years. When retraining is necessary, costs are paid for by the state. In the case where an occupational disease forces a change of job, financial compensation for reduced income can be granted. A fundamental difference between the German and the Danish systems is that worker's compensation can be given to people who are continuing in the same job that caused the damage.

53.3.4.1 Example A

In the Danish system, this case would be recognized as an occupational allergic contact dermatitis to chromate, and the bricklayer would be compensated for his ongoing symptoms, according to the severity of the disease as assessed by a dermatologist in a medical report. An additional compensation will be added due to occupational sensitization to chromate, which is considered a ubiquitous allergen, and therefore, difficult to avoid. Medical costs (gloves, moisturizers, disease-related medication on prescription) will be covered by the state, as will retraining and/or compensation for reduced income. Prophylactic skin protection seminars are not available in DK.

53.3.4.2 Example B

In the Danish system, this case would be recognized as an occupational irritant contact dermatitis in a patient with previous atopic eczema. The nurse would be compensated for ongoing disease according to severity, and this compensation will be reduced by 25–33% due to previous atopic eczema (other atopic symptoms than eczema will not lead to reduction in compensation). Medical costs will be covered by the state, as will be retraining, if this is considered necessary.

53.3.4.3 Example C

In the Danish system, this case would be recognized as an occupational allergic contact dermatitis due to thiuram. Since the eczema has cleared, the surgeon will not receive compensation for ongoing disease but he will receive a minor compensation for sensitization to thiuram (rubber additive), as this is considered a ubiquitous allergen. Medical cost will be covered by the state.

More information: www.ask.dk

53.3.5 Finland

Antti Lauerma

In Finland, an employer is under the law responsible for injuries or diseases caused by work itself to the employee. However, the main economic responsibility for this is outsourced to compulsory employer's insurances provided by private insurance companies. The exception is civil servants, who get compensation from a government fund, but that follows the same practices and laws as private insurance companies, as described below.

The study of occupational disease can be started by a physician who knows the conditions of the workplace, usually an occupational health services physician. If can be also started by other physicians. Occupational skin diseases are studied mainly by dermatologists. Dermatologists involved in this include dermatologists in private practice, municipal and central hospitals. University hospitals have specialized units for patch testing and dermatological allergology and they study most patients who cannot

be diagnosed elsewhere. The most complicated cases are studied in Finnish Institute of Occupational Health (FIOH).

The study of occupational disease is usually accepted by insurance company after receiving a request document from physician to start study. The referring document can theoretically be sent also by patient, but this happens rarely. After acceptance, all costs for study and possible later costs for retraining, pension and other social costs are covered by the insurance. Insurance covers 100% of cost of study to patient and the unit doing the study.

The disease becomes an occupational disease after it fulfils two criteria, i.e. it has to be *most likely* caused by an agent that *at most part* is causative of disease, and the agent has to be of chemical, physical or biological in origin. For example psychosomatic or stress-related diseases are not covered. Irritant dermatitis is also covered if it fulfils the criteria. The clearest occupational cases are those that are caused primarily by the disease, e.g. sensitization at work. However, a disease that has started as non-occupational can also be reimbursed as occupational, if it is worsened by the work, e.g. contact to nickel in work in an individual already allergic to nickel.

When the physician studying disease makes diagnosis of occupational disease, it has to be accepted by the insurance company. The insurance company has its own physicians who review the cases. In case of doubt, they refer the patient to the university hospital or FIOH. In case of initial rejection, the patient's physician can also ask separately for such referral.

When a possible occupational disease has been studied and rejected, the patient can file a complaint to insurance company. If rejected there, the patient can file a second complaint to an independent insurance court. The final place for complaint after this is the Highest Court for Administrative Matters, whose decision is final.

If a patient is diagnosed with occupational disease, he or she contacts the employer. Usually attempts are made to change the patient's work tasks to enable continuation of work. If that is not possible, the patient continues on sick leave. Depending on the estimation of the total cost, the insurance company either retrains him or her for new work or gives disability pension. The former is the usual practice for younger people.

Disability pension is a costly choice for insurance company as the patient receives 80% of previous salary as disability pension. For this reason, studies of occupational disease have to be very precise and objective, as demands end often in the courts and may take several years to be solved. Long waiting times also usually mean that patient is out of the workforce for long times that can also increase risks of loss of work ability for other reasons than occupational disease.

The three typical examples (A, B, C) of occupational legal cases are likely to be handled in a similar way they are handled in Germany. The costs of studies and retraining are covered by the insurance companies. Retraining for persons with non-occupational disease (case B, when necessary) is covered by national welfare insurance system.

53.3.6 France

In France, the legal basis for dealing with OD is fixed in the "Code de la Sécurité Sociale" and several other statutes, one of which is the "Code Rural" for agriculture.

The French legislation is characterized by the existence of "tables of OD", which allow recognition and compensation for such conditions. According to the 25th Oct 1919 Law, an OD will be recognized only if it is listed in one of the 112 tables for the general regimen (65 for agricultural regimen). These tables are updated from time to time, and more than 45 tables concern skin disorders of allergic, irritant, cancerous or infective cause. Each table concerns a particular situation: some tables are devoted to a definite substance (e.g. Table 83 for methyl methacrylate), as other tables concern a group of substances (e.g. Table 51 for epoxy resins and their components) or a type of dermatitis (for Table 65 dermatitis of allergic mechanism). The tables are divided into three columns. The first one concerns the designation of the diseases with symptoms or lesions, like "eczematous dermatitis recurring after a new exposure or attested by patch tests" (Table 31 for aminoglycosides) or "eczema-like dermatitis" (Table 47 for woods) or dermatitis or chemical burns (Table 32 for fluorine, hydrofluoric acid and salts), or "contact urticaria" (Table 95 for latex proteins). The second column entitled "term of notice" concerns the maximal admissible delay between the last contact with the pathogenic agent and the first medical establishment of the disease: for example, the delay is 7 days in the case of cements (Table 8). The third column indicates or enumerates the occupations likely to provoke the disease. There is an indicative (non-limited) list

of works for main tables. In some cases, however, and mainly for cancerous or infective diseases or in the case of dermatitis due to epoxy resins, there is a limited list of occupations allowing recognition. The procedure is well defined. The medical certificate needed for the declaration is made in triplicate, generally by the dermatologist, sometimes by the patient's practitioner or even by the occupational physician (art. L. 461-5 of the Code de la Sécurité Sociale). The patient will fill in a declaration form and send it with the medical certificate to the Caisse Primaire d'Assurance Maladie (CPAM). The CPAM holds a medical and administrative enquiry and then notifies about acceptance or refusal. When the medical, occupational and administrative conditions indicated in the concerned table are fulfilled, a presumption of occupational origin is accorded to the worker and no additional proof is required. So, there is no need for positive tests in suspected allergic dermatitis that relapses after fresh exposure, and no need for recurrence of the dermatitis after new exposure when a patch test is positive, except for latex (Table 95). When the dermatitis is recognized as an OD, expenditures related to it are taken over. If the patient has a permanent disability, compensation can be paid. If this disability is <10%, the patient will receive a lump sum that generally does not exceed 1,500€. Exceptionally, when disability is >10%, she or he will receive a monthly pension. When the disease is not recognized as occupational, the patient can refer the Comité Régional de Reconnaissance des Maladies Professionnelles (CRRMP).

In some cases, the patient suffers dermatitis mentioned as a "dermatitis with occupational features", listed in complementary tables. For example, an occupational dermatitis due to pyridine or its derivatives is listed under n° 613. Such dermatitis, although of occupational origin, offers no compensation, but has to be declared on a special form to the Ministry of Labour (art. L. 461-6 of Code de la Sécurité Sociale). It contributes to complete, extend and bring the tables up to date.

When a patient suffers an occupational dermatitis, the occupational physician usually tries to provide him a new working area. However, in the case of repeatedly relapsing dermatitis, his occupational physician can declare the patient inapt for his job. The employer has by law to give another job in the same company, or is obliged to double the redundancy compensation, which partly depends on the age of the patient. Retraining may be carried out, but is very difficult for many patients.

53.3.6.1 Example A (Bricklayer)

Table 8 entitled "diseases due to cements" applies in this case. The OD can be officially recognized, but only if the patient himself makes the notification. A pension will be paid only if there is a residual disease, with a permanent disability that exceptionally exceeds 10%, even with severe lesions. So, occupational physicians are frequently reluctant to declare the patient inapt for his job, which means he/she will be laid off. This situation is very hard to manage, since a bricklayer frequently has many difficulties in doing another job. Many patients continue to work, despite occupational dermatitis. As unfitness is of value for a specific job in a specific work plant, many patients try to be hired in another firm, without claiming previous unfitness. For such patients, a declaration to the Commission des Droits et de l'Autonomie des Personnes Handicapées (CDAPH) that has replaced the Commission Technique d'Orientation et de Reclassement Professionnel (COTOREP) can be useful, since it can offer ways of retraining.

53.3.6.2 Example B (Nurse)

If the nurse works in a state hospital, she is considered as a civil servant and is concerned by a peculiar regimen. An administrative procedure will be carried out within the hospital. If the affection corresponds medically and administratively to one of the table, an OD will likely be recognized. In practice, the nurse will be rapidly appointed to another post in the same hospital and will not receive any compensation.

53.3.6.3 Example C (Surgeon)

The surgeon has to fill in the declaration form and send it with the medical certificate that indicates an OD corresponding to Table 65 (tetramethylthiuram sulphide). The employer will furnish adapted gloves, but the surgeon will not receive any compensatiation.

53.3.7 Spain

Luis Conde-Salazar, Felipe Heras

In Spain, any physician or worker can claim to the public commission in charge of the evaluation of occupational disabilities. This commission will then take further action, it will inspect the work place and order an expert's opinion at a specific dermatology occupational department[1]. The commission will finally make a judgment on the disability and the size of the compensation. If the worker or the employer do not agree with these conclusions, they could claim to the Labour Court.

The compensation for an occupational disease that prevents a worker from continuing with his job is granted with 55% of his salary in case he is less than 55-years-old, and with 75% of the salary if he is older. The disability is revised 2 years later, and the compensation could be removed if the skin disease does not reappear in a new occupation.

The Occupational Insurance Company of the patient ("Mutua") carries out the retraining of the worker with an occupational disease. It usually takes place during the 6–8 months of lapse time until the decision of the disability commission is made. Nevertheless, retraining is barely used for patients with occupational skin diseases.

53.3.7.1 Example A (Bricklayer)

His disease would be recognized as occupational and he would obtain a pension of 55% of his salary. His Occupational Insurance Company could carry out retraining, but it depends on the possibilities of each Insurance Company and the needs of the worker.

The worker would maintain this disability pension even if he starts working in a new occupation. Two years later, the commission for occupational disabilities will review his case to evaluate if the skin problem persists at his new work place and if the pension is still suitable.

53.3.7.2 Example B (Nurse)

Her disease would not be recognized as occupational. However, as the occupational factor worsens the dermatitis, a change of work would be recommended. The employer must then find a new workplace for the patient, with less number of irritants and less wet work. This is not always possible in small enterprises, but it could be easily achieved in a hospital. The patient would neither be granted a pension nor retraining (her salary aside), but she would not loose her work status or her income in the new workplace.

53.3.7.3 Example C (Surgeon)

As the surgeon can still work and has no disability, he would not receive any compensation. The employer will pay for the new thiuram-free gloves.

More information can be obtained from: http://www.isciii.es/htdocs/centros/medicinadeltrabajo/medicinatrabajo_presentacion.jsp

53.3.8 Sweden

Magnus Lindberg

In Sweden the Social Security Act regulates most of the social security systems including occupational injury compensation. OD and injuries are specifically covered by the Work Injury Act (LFA). Social insurance is administered by the Swedish Social Insurance Agency. For OD, there is also a complementary labour-market insurance for most employees (Labour Market No Fault Liability Insurance [TFA]). Questions regarding the working environment are handled by the Swedish Work Environment Authority, which is the administrative state authority. It was formed in 2001 by merging the Labour Inspectorate and the National Board of Occupational Safety and Health. They have the responsibility for regulation, information and also inspection of matters concerning the working environment. Among other things, they handle ISA – The Swedish Information System on Occupational Accidents and Work-related diseases. The Social insurance was revised in 2008 with a strong focus on stricter indications for sickness compensation and a more rapid rehabilitation, aiming at as rapid as possible return to a previous job or to the labour market. To provide this, a series of different programmes/activities have been introduced and are handled by the Social Insurance Agency. In addition, The Swedish National Board of Health and Welfare has launched guidelines on how to handle sick leave for different diagnosis, e.g. skin diseases such as eczema, urticaria and psoriasis are covered. The Social Insurance Agency has medical advisers employed to assist in the review of the cases. They do not see patients, but do assist in reviewing documentations from the patients' physicians to provide basis for decisions on sickness benefit, rehabilitation allowance, compensation for measures in work-oriented rehabilitation, sickness compensation and occupational injury compensation. However, it is not compulsory that a medical certificate concerning a patient with skin disease is written by a dermatologist, which might be a drawback for the patient. When a person has a reduced work capacity due to sickness, the case is initially handled in the same way whether it is an occupational disease or not. The employer pays sick pay for the first 14 days. After this period, The Swedish Social Insurance Agency has the economic responsibility. The aim is that a sick leave should not be longer than a year. Employers have the primary responsibility to rehabilitate a person on sick leave. If they cannot perform the rehabilitation within their organization, the rehabilitation will be a case for the Social Insurance. In 2002, LAF was revised. The definition of an occupational skin disease in the Social insurance is that of a disease contracted as a result of environmental conditions at work. This can be a primary disease (e.g. hand eczema due to contact allergy to a preservative in a cutting fluid) or worsening of an already present or latent skin disorder (e.g. hand psoriasis, contact eczema worsening atopic eczema). Environmental factors include chemical, physical, stress factors and also factors related to the organization of the work itself and the workplace. To define a disease as occupational, there must be a harmful stimulus (stimuli), a known mechanism, a clinical disease and a relevant association between these factors. The proof must make it probable that the harmful stimulus (stimuli) has caused the disease or worsening of a present or latent disease. In the latter case, there needs to be strong evidence speaking in favour of a connection. In case of a suspected occupational disease, the employee and employer report this together on a specific form (Notification of a work Injury). If the disease leads to an economic consequence for the employee in a longer perspective (e.g. loss of income due to a change of job or in the worse case a retirement) or to economic costs in rehabilitation and re-orientation on the labour market, the notification of work injury is reviewed by the Social Health Insurance and notified to the Swedish Work Environment Authority. For the review, a medical opinion (and in some rare cases, an inspection of the workplace) is needed. The medical examination should at best (but do mostly not) include a detailed work-up by a dermatologist including estimation of skin exposure, patch testing and an opinion on connection and relevance. A medical expert opinion does not include a decision on the degree of economic compensation, disability or

53

pension. In the decision on an occupational skin disease and the degree of compensation, the Social Insurance Agency also considers personal factors that can influence the outcome of an exposure to harmful stimulus (stimuli). In principle, a person is insured "in their current condition". An important question is if the disease is chronic or will heal with time. Today, due to economic restrictions in the Social Insurance, there are limited possibilities for economic compensation and support for, for example, change of job and rehabilitation measures such as education. Based on the above mentioned, the outcome of an occupational skin disease can differ considerably between occupations and will also depend on the size of the employer's organization. For example, in cases of hand eczema, a craftsman will probably change job or be retrained for another occupation. In some cases, this will be done with financial support from the Social Insurance and additional compensation from TFA. In the case of a healthcare worker (e.g. nurse), it will probably be possible to change the work tasks or complement the equipment used. There might be some economic compensation from Social Insurance and/or TFA for increased medical costs. Contact dermatitis, especially hand eczema, is a chronic relapsing disease which makes it difficult to be handled from an insurance point of view. There is a risk that the severity of the disease is underestimated. It would be desirable that medical opinions and clinical investigations in cases of occupational skin diseases are performed by a dermatologist, which is not obligatory in Sweden.

53.3.8.1 Example A (Bricklayer)

If a bricklayer develops an occupational skin disease, the outcome will depend on the size of the employer's organization and the quality of the medical investigation. A contact dermatitis will probably be considered as an occupational disease. The medical problem in the rehabilitation is to establish the connection between exposure and the skin disease. The medical work-up can vary considerably between individuals. When an occupational skin disease is established, it is the responsibility of the employer to adapt the working conditions by, for example, a change in working assignments or establishing protective measures. If this is not possible, there is a possibility to get some financial support from the Social

Insurance to change job or to be retrained. If the disease causes economic loss, it is possible to get some compensation from the insurance systems.

53.3.8.2 Example B (Nurse) and Example C (Surgeon)

In theory, if a nurse or a surgeon develops an occupational skin disease, they will be handled in the same way as the bricklayer in example A. There are, however, some major differences. In examples B and C, there is often a better possibility to change working positions within the organization. However, from a medical point of view, it can be more difficult to recognize the skin disease as occupational and to establish the relation between exposure and disease.

53.3.9 Switzerland

Hanspeter Rast

The basis for the insurance of accidents and OD is a law enacted in 1981 (*Unfallversicherungsgesetz*). Recognition, compensation and preventive measures are covered by it. All employees in Switzerland have to be insured. Suva (*Schweizerische Unfallversicherungsanstalt*) is the compulsory insurer for employees in industry, construction, transport and federal institutions. In addition, there are various insurers for small trades and service companies. Only Suva has a staff of technicians for local inspection of companies and medical departments for occupational medicine and rehabilitation. The patient himself and the employer are responsible for reporting the suspicion of an occupational disease. The physician treating the case is asked by the insurer for a medical report. The general rule for recognizing a disease as an occupational one is that the occupational activity must be the sole or overwhelming cause. The government has published a list of substances, exposures and occupational activities that are the basis for recognition as an occupational disease. If these factors are involved, a causal relationship of more than 50% is sufficient for an individual case to be recognized as an occupational disease. If the disease is caused by other factors not found in the official list, the causal relationship between occupational activity and disease must be at least 75% in order to suffice for recognition. In contrast to other countries, there is no official list of OD, but rather a compendium of substances and various activities and exposures that have the potential to cause certain diseases. An occupational disease, including a dermatosis, is considered to exist if medical treatment or sick leave has been required. Therefore, no special criteria for severity (as used in Germany, for example) have to be fulfilled for recognition. The insurer pays for the medical treatment and other expenses, including loss of wages. If rehabilitation fails, a pension may be paid. In a case where the employee continues on the job and suffers severe health impairment (such as for spreading contact dermatitis, many recurrences, long sick leaves), Suva is entitled to prohibit certain activities that have proven to be hazardous to the individual (declaration of "unsuitability"). This measure also provides financial security to the employee for up to 4 years. A special state insurance, the *Invalidenversicherung*, is responsible for retraining and specific rehabilitation measures.

53.3.9.1 Example A

The bricklayer's condition would be recognized as an occupational disease according to the law. Suva would notify the employee and the employer that all contacts with cement and dichromates must be discontinued. In construction, this is actually equivalent to giving up the occupation. The bricklayer would also register with the *Invalidenversicherung* and ask for retraining at his relatively low age. The employee is also entitled to a temporary financial compensation from the insurer in cases of lower wages, unemployment or retraining procedures.

   If the disease continues and the patient is considerably handicapped by it or if rehabilitation measures fail, a permanent pension will be granted. This is covered by several insurances together (*Invalidenversicherung*, accident insurance, pension fund of the former employer). If there is no loss of earnings in the new occupation after retraining, no pension will be paid (in contrast to the German system). If there is a considerable, probably lifelong dermatosis, particularly on the hands and face, an additional lump sum (*Integritätsentschädigung*) is paid once at pensionable age. Should the worker be dissatisfied with the decision of the insurer, he can appeal to the courts.

53.3.9.2 Example B

If the nurse has contact with substances in the list of occupational hazardous substances, such as formaldehyde or rubber accelerators, and these aggravate a pre-existing mild atopic dermatitis in a definite manner, the insurer will cover the case until the previous health status is re-attained. The occupational factors must be dominant, at least for some period of time. After that the regular health insurance is liable for all costs. Expert opinions often show discrepancies in such cases of endogenous disease without clear occupational sensitization. If the course of the case is severe and followed by many sick leaves, Suva might declare the "unsuitability" of the person, which usually means giving up the job. The patient can apply to the *Invalidenversicherung* for retraining with or without recognition of an occupational disease.

53.3.9.3 Example C

If the surgeon is employed in a public or a private hospital, the accident insurance under contract (usually a private one) will cover all medical costs, provided that the case is at all reported. In most cases, the hospital will cover additional costs, such as more expensive thiuram-free gloves, for a highly qualified employee. In Switzerland it is the employer's duty to provide all adequate protective measures, including gloves. If special expensive individual procedures have to be installed, the insurer may take care of a part of it.

53.3.10 *United Kingdom*

Jason D.L. Williams, Paul J. August,
Hayden L. Muston

In the UK, there are two ways of obtaining compensation for occupational dermatoses.

   Firstly, the Government administers a scheme of National Insurance through the Inland Revenue Service. Employers, the self-employed and employees must make contributions to this central fund. If an individual is unable to work from illness of any kind for longer than 4 days consecutively, he or she will be entitled to statutory sick pay from his or her employer for up to 28 weeks. On a longer term basis, Incapacity Benefit is payable by the state to those who are eligible and have been assessed as being incapable of working. Industrial Injuries Disablement Benefit is an additional payment to those suffering from what is known as prescribed industrial disease. Prescribed diseases are divided into the following:

(a) Conditions due to physical agents
(b) Conditions due to biological agents
(c) Conditions due to chemical agents
(d) Miscellaneous conditions

For dermatologists, the most relevant prescribed diseases are the following:

A11. Vibration white finger
B1.   Anthrax
B12. Orf
C21. Primary carcinoma of the skin from exposure to arsenic or tar-based products or mineral oil or soot
C25. Occupational vitiligo
C30. Chrome dermatitis and ulceration of the mucous membranes or epidermis
D5.   Non-infective dermatitis of external origin

It is left to the patient to fill in an application form. The suspicion of an occupational cause is sufficient justification for filing a report to the state. For a claim to succeed, the claimant needs to show that he/she has the prescribed disease and has been in the occupation that caused it. Initially, the assessment is made by one or two independent doctors. Definite proof and positive patch tests are not essential in cases of dermatitis. However, a report from a dermatologist will often be the basis for a further decision/opinion, and patch tests may then be undertaken. In cases of occupational dermatitis, where there have been multi-factorial contributions to the skin disorder, including constitutional and other non-occupational factors, the claim will succeed but the assessed percentage disability will be reduced proportionately. Since 1986, the claimant has to be at least 14% disabled to receive any benefit.

Establishing this is more difficult than it may sound, because the fact that the person cannot work at his or her own job is not considered disablement, which refers to impairment of everyday life. Therefore, it must be an exceptionally severe case for a skin complaint to reach 14% disablement, and only a few such cases are currently recorded each year. Disablement Benefit is usually paid as a weekly pension and may be subject to review. The claimant may ask for their case to be re-assessed in some circumstances such as ignorance of or a mistake regarding a material fact, as well as deterioration of the condition. A Medical Appeals tribunal exists which will examine claims thought to have been administered incorrectly according to the regulations. This tribunal, while set up by the state, is independent of it.

The second way of gaining compensation is for the affected individual to sue the employer for damages through the civil court. Civil actions are brought under a claim for negligence and/or a breach of statutory duty. Statutory duties are encompassed in a number of regulations with which the employer must comply. These include the Control of Substances Hazardous to Health (COSHH) and Personal Protective Equipment at Work Regulations (PPEWR). Together, these regulations provide a framework to prevent harm to the worker. Regulations ensure that knowledge of the risk, suitable training to avoid the risk, physical protection against the risk, regular review and monitoring of the harmful exposures, health surveillance and adequate information are all provided to the worker. In large claims, engineering reports will be obtained to determine whether a breach has occurred, and if it has, the extent of it. The dermatologist must establish the cause of the problem and whether negligence or a breach of the statutory regulations caused the skin disease.

Every employer in the United Kingdom has to be insured through a private insurance company for what is known as employer liability for common law action. When a claimant sues the firm, a solicitor will be consulted. Since Apr 1999, new "Woolf Rules" apply to the presentation of expert evidence. In the past, each side would instruct its own expert(s), including, where necessary, a dermatologist. The new rules mean that the court, with the agreement of all the contesting parties, is encouraged to appoint a single independent expert where possible. The expert's duty and report are addressed to the court and are independent of whoever is responsible for the fee. He or she must give an impartial and balanced assessment, and where there may be a range of opinions, this must be documented. The expert is open to questions from all sides. The contesting parties are, nevertheless, at liberty to appoint their own experts who are required to supply unbiased reports with a range of opinions that would be expected from other dermatological experts in the field. This is more likely in large or complex cases. The experts' duty is again to the court, not to one side or the other. The contesting parties have the choice of whether or not to have the court consider this evidence, in which case all of those involved must discuss the case and produce a joint report identifying any areas where there is disagreement, thereby providing the court with a condensed view of the issues in question. It is intended that this method will reduce legal expenses and the frequency of court proceedings and attendances by experts. Presently, most cases are settled without going to court.

Unless he or she is in a trade union or has legal expenses insurance, the claimant may have to fund the costs, but many solicitors work on a conditional or "no win, no fee" basis. In successful cases the defendants may be ordered to pay the claimant's expenses. In the past, if the patient did not have sufficient means, the state used to give legal aid, but this has now been withdrawn from such cases.

If the worker is suing for negligence through the courts, the claimant must prove:

> That the skin complaint was contracted at work.
> That it was avoidable and foreseeable by a reasonable employer.
> That the employer did not take adequate precautions against it.

If the claimant is suing for breach (breakdown) of statutory duty, he or she must prove:

> A breach of the statutory regulations occurred.
> This breach caused the skin complaint.

If the case is accepted as an occupational skin disease, compensation payments will take into account the following:

> Loss of earnings by the person
> Future loss of earnings (including pension)
> Loss of promotion prospects
> Loss of future employment prospects on the open job market
> Pain and suffering
> Loss of amenity in social and domestic activities (for example, if the patient has lost a hand, he or she might be unable to pursue a hobby, such as golf)
> Ongoing treatment costs (either in the private healthcare system or the National Health Service)
> Loss of congenial employment (where relevant)

Following recognition of an occupational skin disease, workers have the right to stay in the same employment, but if they are unable to fulfil their duties adequately, they may be dismissed or moved to a less well-paid post. Retraining in the UK for dermatological cases is not well organized and rarely done. Even if they are retrained, many people will find it extremely difficult to get a job because employers are reluctant to take on someone with a history of occupational skin disease, whose skin is vulnerable and who may get skin trouble in the future with the associated worry of possible litigation.

In the UK, the Health and Safety Executive (HSE) has collated statistics for occupational dermatoses from a number of sources. There is no legal requirement for employees or medical personnel to report work-related skin disorders. This means that statistics will not be altogether reliable and probably underestimate those affected.

The HSE has undertaken a study by questionnaire and interview for the years 2001/2002 entitled the self-reported work-related illness (SWI) survey. A sample of 96,000 people in England and Wales were contacted. As a result of this survey, it was concluded that there was a prevalence of 39,000 individuals with work-related skin disorders at that time (with a 95% confidence interval of 30,000–48,000). The best source of information on the incidence of occupational dermatoses in the UK comes from returns made voluntarily by occupational physicians and dermatologists to The Health and Occupation Reporting (THOR) Network based at the Centre for Occupational Health at Manchester University. These schemes are respectively known as OPRA and EPIDERM. In the last 3 years (2006–2008), the estimated number of new cases of occupational dermatosis per year has been between 9,045 and 11,479 cases. The vast majority of cases were contact dermatitis. There has been a gradual decline in the number of reported cases, but this is felt to be due to reporting bias. In contrast, an analysis of claims for Industrial Injuries Disablement Benefit for dermatitis confirmed and assessed at more than 1% disability shows the numbers to be in the region of 200 per year for the last 3 years, confirming that a low proportion of those affected make a claim. Another source of occupational skin disease statistics has been from those reported by employers under RIDDOR (reporting of injuries, diseases and dangerous occurrences regulations) to the HSE, but substantial under-reporting occurs. A more detailed account and analysis of these figures can be found on the THOR and HSE websites (http://www.manchester.ac.uk/medicine/oeh/thor/epiderm/ and http://www.hse.gov.uk/). No formal feedback of any kind is provided by the state or legal system about the outcomes of cases in which dermatologists have provided expert opinions. In the state system, this information is also not available on request; in the legal system, it will usually be granted, but the dermatologist will rarely know when to ask, since most cases are settled out of court with no further reference to him or her.

Regarding the examples (A, B and C) described earlier, there is no formal retraining programme for such cases in the UK. Any retraining must, therefore, be undertaken at the affected individual's own expense. The employer should pay statutory sick pay when there is time off work due to dermatitis for up to 28 weeks. Thereafter, incapacity benefit would have to be claimed if the affected person is still not working and eligible for the benefit. Some employers may provide income protection insurance. Otherwise, it is up to the individual to consider paying for this, but regrettably, the vast majority of workers fail to obtain insurance cover.

None of the cases is likely to achieve the 14% disablement needed to receive Disablement Benefit as a result of the prescribed disease of dermatitis. The bricklayer and the nurse would both have entered the state disability statistics had they applied for such a pension, but they are unlikely to have done this because of the growing knowledge in the community of the small probability of obtaining such benefit for skin disease. Otherwise, it is unlikely that any of these persons would have appeared in official Government statistics. Nevertheless, if they do see a dermatologist or occupational physician who is an active participant in the voluntary reporting scheme (EPIDERM and OPRA), they will be incorporated into the figures kept by HSE.

The bricklayer could take court action, but would need to prove negligence or a breach of statutory duty if he is going to succeed in a claim for damages.

As the nurse has stopped work voluntarily, he or she is unlikely to resort to a civil court action, even though it can be argued that despite the constitutional background, the condition of the hands would not have arisen if she had not been nursing. Furthermore, the employer should have recognized at the pre-employment medical that there was a foreseeable increased risk of irritant contact dermatitis, bearing in mind the long-standing history of atopic eczema. If she did make a claim and it is shown in court that her employer did not take appropriate action to prevent the dermatitis and act promptly when she did, she would succeed in a claim for damages. The ongoing nature of her hand problem is a further issue, as the concept of persistent occupational dermatitis is now well recognized.

The surgeon is unlikely to have applied for any form of compensation: if he were directly employed in the National Health Service, the additional expense of his gloves would be met by the employer; if self-employed (as are all dental surgeons, for example), he or she would have to meet the extra cost.

53.3.11 *United States*

Howard I. Maibach, Patricia Engasser

Laws establishing worker compensation in the United States were first passed in 1911. In the first decade, coverage was for accidents only. In 1920, illnesses were included, and in recent decades, coverage has been extended to disorders caused by cumulative trauma and conditions arising from emotional trauma. As is the case with the laws of most other nations, the basic tenet is *liability without fault*, eliminating the requirement that the worker proves negligence on the part of the employer. The intent was to prevent an adverse climate in the workplace. The system is operated through insurance, which may be a state-supported insurance company, a private insurance company or self-insurance in the case of large, financially sound companies. Some states permit all methods to be used. Federal employees are covered under a special federal programme. Heavy penalties exist for companies that fail to insure their workers. *Medical care* is available without restriction and may be provided not only by doctors of medicine and osteopathy, but also by dentists, podiatrists, optometrists, physical therapists and chiropractors. In some states, Christian Science practitioners and naturopaths are authorized to treat these patients, but only if the employer is notified of this choice prior to injury. While some states provide a free choice of physician, certain states require treatment under a physician designated by the employer for the first 30 days or so, unless the employee makes prior arrangements.

Income protection during recovery is a basic tenet in all states, with a maximum and minimum. The employer assumes the cost through an insurance carrier or, if self-insured, through the company, usually a subsidiary.

Although unusual in dermatology, *death benefit*, when the death is due to illness related to the workplace, is provided with automatic payments to the surviving dependents. Payments usually equal the worker's temporary disability indemnity benefit. Burial expenses are included, with a maximum cost permitted.

Disputes arise in fewer than 10% of cases, but when there is disagreement and *dispute resolution* is necessary, lawyers for the opposing sides may request depositions from the various physicians. Later, the case may be presented before a judicial hearing officer (often called a "referee"). The purpose of the hearing is to clarify the issues, with the intent to decide the case fairly and according to the law. If the hearing officer's decision is unacceptable to either party, an appeals board can be requested to hear the case. At that time, an *independent medical examiner* is usually appointed to evaluate the case. If there are still unresolved issues, the state appeals court may be petitioned to study the problem; an appellate court is next in line, and finally the state supreme court, but the majority of cases are settled in the lower courts. An important difference between workers' compensation law and ordinary civil law is that the court that has originally decided an award may alter its decision if there is reasonable cause, or if the worker's condition changes.

Rehabilitation services are available in most states, but are unequal in extent and funding. Job training is available for workers unable to return to their previous work and is especially important for patients with allergic contact dermatitis in which a workplace allergen has been positively identified.

The following three cases (examples A, B and C) show the way in which compensation would be handled in the United States:

Rehabilitation training in most states continues indefinitely, even past the normal retirement age of 65. The rating for pension indemnity is based upon the percentage of the workplace from which the worker (the bricklayer in this case) is precluded because of the skin condition. This determination involves a complicated process, requiring the recommendations of rehabilitation specialists, vocational disability experts and industrial engineers, as well as the examining/reporting physicians.

The insurance company is required to pay for that period of time in which there was clearly work aggravation of this pre-existing condition (atopic dermatitis for the nurse in this case). Furthermore, if the work appears to have brought a previously inactive condition to clinical activity, which is not uncommon in atopics, the treatment period allowed may be longer. Even if there is no work relationship, rehabilitation services are provided.

In this case, the contact allergy of the surgeon would be considered work related, and the cost of the alternative gloves would be paid for by the insurance company. Unfortunately, however, the company (in this case, the hospital) might find other reasons to discharge this surgeon because of the excessive cost of the gloves and the possible increase in insurance premiums.

53.3.11.1 Conclusions and Comment

Profound differences in legislation on occupational skin disease become apparent when the systems used in various European countries are compared. In Germany and Scandinavian countries, recognition of a dermatosis as being occupational is proposed in a relatively easy manner by initiating well-developed and frequently used governmental and insurance pathways. An irritant contact dermatitis or atopic hand eczema will be recognized in most cases if the disease is severe and causes frequent sick leave, and if its relationship to occupational activities is quite clear. A patient might receive compensation or retraining for an alternative "clean" job. In a country such as Spain, much more responsibility is placed on the

53

employer to help employees after they have acquired a skin disease in the working environment. The system seems to be less institutionalized and more "privatized".

In most countries, a bricklayer with dichromate allergy would receive financial compensation, but lump sums are preferred to monthly payments. In Germany, retraining is rarely performed after the age of 40 years, while in most other countries the patient can be older than 40. In the questionnaire, the question of the value of retraining and the course of the skin disease was answered by the overwhelming majority in the following way:

> Most patients find a job only with difficulty after retraining.
> They continue to have skin problems quite frequently.

Regarding the overall evaluation of retraining programmes, out of seven responders, three decided it was "very valuable in some cases", two "very valuable", one "of some value" and one "of little value".

These judgments of experienced occupational dermatologists should stimulate further thinking and work. Should we be more restrictive with retraining, because most patients will have problems in finding new satisfying work and will continue to have major skin problems? Are we retraining patients at too late a stage, once the disease has manifested itself and taken on a more endogenous character (see Chaps. 19, 41 and 45)? Is more cooperation necessary among physicians, social workers and specialists in occupational safety, with regard to inspecting the workplace and making far-reaching recommendations for the patient with an occupational skin disease? In every country a striking shortcoming exists: the workplace is rarely inspected by a physician! Based on many reports in the literature, we know that this is an extremely important aspect of dealing with an occupational disease (see Chaps. 41, 46 and 53). The patient inevitably and unintentionally sometimes omits important details from the history that turn out to be diagnostic clues if detected by a trained observer. On visits to dental laboratories, for example, we learned that most technicians are not aware of the risk of sensitization from acrylates and do not avoid frequent direct skin contact [18].

In most countries, the legislation seems to be rather inaccurate and unclear with regard to important aspects and to the definitions of terms such as "severity of disease", "recurrence" and "frequency of relapses". This also holds true for the degree of disability and estimates of the pensionable lump sum for compensation. In connection with the protection of personal data, it seems important to point out that the patient's consent for a report to be made to the insurer or governmental institution is not obligatory in every country. Considering the possibility that the patient may experience retaliation of various kinds in the workplace after the case for compensation has been initiated, the patient's consent to this procedure should be made mandatory.

In order to harmonize the various systems for dealing with occupational dermatoses, we recommend the formation of a committee under the auspices of the European Community.

References

1. John SM, Skudlik C (2006) New forms of management in dermatology. Integrated in-patient-out-patient prevention of severe occupational dermatoses: cornerstones for an effective integrated management in clinics and practices; PMID: 17203451. Gesundheitswesen 68(12):769–774
2. John SM, Skudlik C, Römer W, Blome O, Brandenburg S, Diepgen TL, Harwerth A, Köllner A, Pohrt U, Rogosky E, Schindera I, Stary A, Worm M (2007) Recommendation: Dermatologist's procedure. Recommendations for quality assurance of the German Society of Dermatology (DDG) and the Task Force on Occupational and Environmental Dermatology (ABD). JDDG 5:1146–1148
3. Skudlik C, Junger M, Allmers H, Brandenburg S, John SM (2008) Optimal care of patients with occupational hand dermatitis: considerations of German occupational health insurance. Hautarzt 59:690; 692–695
4. John SM (2008) Occupational skin diseases: options for multidisciplinary networking in preventive medicine. GMS Ger Med Sci 2008;6:Doc07 (Online-Publikation: http://www.egms.de/en/gms/2008-6/000052.shtml)
5. Skudlik C, Wulfhorst B, Gediga G, Bock M, Allmers H, John SM (2008) Tertiary individual prevention of occupational skin diseases – a decade's experience with recalcitrant occupational dermatitis. Int Arch Occup Environ Health 81:1045–1058
6. Skudlik C, Weisshaar E, Wulfhorst B, Scheidt R, Schönfeld M, Elsner P, Diepgen TL, John SM (2009) Multicenter study "Medical-Occupational Rehabilitation Procedure Skin – optimizing and quality assurance of inpatient-management (ROQ)". JDDG 7:122–127

7. Diepgen TL, Bernhard-Klimt C, Blome O, Brandenburg S, Dienstbach D, Drexler H, Elsner P, Fartasch M, Frank KH, John SM, Kleesz P, Köllner A, Otten H, Pappai W, Römer W, Rogosky E, Sacher J, Skudlik C, Zagrodnik F (2008) Bamberg Medical Bulletin: Recommendations for the assessment of skin diseases and skin cancers. Part I: skin diseases. Occup Environ Dermatol 56:132–150

8. Fartasch M, Schmidt A, Diepgen TL (1993) Die Schwere der Hauterkrankung nach BKVO 5101 in der gutachterlichen Beurteilung. Dermatosen 41:242–245

9. Diepgen TL Dickel H, Becker D et al (2002) Beurteilung der Auswirkung von Allergien bei der Minderung der Erwerbsfähigkeit im Rahmen der BK 5101. Dermatol Beruf Umwelt 50:139–154

10. Diepgen TL, Dickel H, Becker D et al (2005) Evidenzbasierte Beurteilung der Auswirkung von Typ-IV-Allergien bei der Minderung der Erwerbsfähigkeit. Hautarzt 56:207–223

11. Diepgen TL, Dickel H, Becker D, John SM, Geier J, Mahler V, Rogosky E, Schmidt A, Skudlik C, Wagner E, Weisshaar E (2008) für die Arbeitsgruppe "Bewertung der Allergene bei BK 5101" der Arbeitsgemeinschaft für Berufs- und Umweltdermatologie in der Deutschen Dermatologischen Gesellschaft: Beurteilung der Auswirkung von Allergien bei der Minderung der Erwerbsfähigkeit im Rahmen der BK 5101: Thiurame, Mercaptobenzothiazole, Dithiocarbamate, N-Isopropyl-N'-phenyl-p-phenylendiamin. [Evaluation of the effects of allergies on the reduction in earning capacity in the context of BK 5101: thiurams, mercaptobenzothiazoles, dithiocarbamates, N-isopropyl-N'-phenyl-p-phenylene diamine]. Dermatol Beruf Umwelt 56(1):11–24

12. Geier J, Lessmann H, Becker D, Dickel H, John SM, Mahler V, Rogosky E, Skudlik C, Wagner E, Weisshaar E, Diepgen TL (2008) für die Arbeitsgruppe "Bewertung der Allergene bei BK 5101" der Arbeitsgemeinschaft für Berufs- und Umweltdermatologie in der Deutschen Dermatologischen Gesellschaft: Formaldehydabspalter. [Formaldehyde releasers]. Dermatol Beruf Umwelt 56(1):34–36

13. Geier J, Lessmann H, Skudlik C, John SM, Becker D, Dickel H, Mahler V, Rogosky E, Wagner E, Weisshaar E, Diepgen TL (2008) für die Arbeitsgruppe "Bewertung der Allergene bei BK 5101" der Arbeitsgemeinschaft für Berufs- und Umweltdermatologie in der Deutschen Dermatologischen Gesellschaft: Auswirkungen berufsbedingter Mehrfachsensibilisierungen gegen Nickel, Chromat und/oder Kobalt bei der BK 5101. [Impact of a combined occupational contact allergy to nickel, cobalt and/or dichromate in cases of occupational skin disease]. Dermatol Beruf Umwelt 56(3):122–123

14. Mahler V, Becker D, Dickel H, Geier J, John SM, Lessmann H, Rogosky E, Skudlik C, Wagner E, Weisshaar E, Diepgen TL (2009) für die Arbeitsgruppe "Bewertung der Allergene bei BK 5101" der Arbeitsgemeinschaft für Berufs- und Umweltdermatologie in der Deutschen Dermatologischen Gesellschaft: Begründung für die Beurteilung der Auswirkung einer Allergie auf Bronopol. [Relevance and occupational consequences of Type IV-allergy to Bronopol]. Dermatol Beruf Umwelt 57(1):36–37

15. Skudlik C, John SM, Becker D, Dickel H, Geier J, Lessmann H, Mahler V, Rogosky E, Wagner E, Weisshaar E, Diepgen TL (2008) für die Arbeitsgruppe "Bewertung der Allergene bei BK 5101" der Arbeitsgemeinschaft für Berufs- und Umweltdermatologie in der Deutschen Dermatologischen Gesellschaft: Begründung für die Beurteilung einer Duftstoffallergie (Allergene des Duftstoff-Mix, Allergene des Duftstoff-Mix II, Lyral) im Rahmen der MdE-Bewertung. [Justification for the evaluation of fragrance allergies (allergens of fragrance mix, allergens of fragrance mix II, Lyral) in the context of the evaluation of the reduction in earning capacity]. Dermatol Beruf Umwelt 56(1):25–30

16. Blome O, Bernhard-Klimt C, Brandenburg S, Diepgen T, Dostal W, Drexler H, Frank K, John S, Kleesz P, Schindera I, Schmidt A, Schwanitz H (2003) Begutachtungsempfehlungen für die Berufskrankheit Nr. 5101 der Anlage zur BKV. Dermatol Beruf Umwelt/Occup Environ Dermatol 51: D2–D14

17. AMA (1995) Guides to the evaluation of permanent impairment, 4th edn. American Medical Association, Chicago, IL

18. Rustemeyer T, Frosch PJ (1996) Occupational skin diseases in dental laboratory technicians. Contact Dermatitis 34:125–133

Further Reading

1. Fabry H, Frosch PJ (2001) Probleme der ärztlichen Begutachtung aus der Dermatologie. In: Fritz E, May B (eds) Die ärztliche Begutachtung. Steinkopf, Darmstadt, pp 893–953

2. Health and Safety Commission (1999) Health and safety statistics 1998/1999. HSC (HSE), London, ISBN 0-7176-1717-5

3. Lips R, Rast H, Elsner P (1996) Outcome of job change in patients with occupational chromate dermatitis. Contact Dermatitis 34:268–271

4. Meding B (1995) Skin disease as an occupational injury. Arbeite Och Hälsa Sci Publ Ser 16:155–169

5. National Board of Occupational Safety and Health, the Swedish Work Environment Fund (ed) (1987) Occupational injuries in Sweden 1983. National Board of Occupational Safety and Health, Solna, Sweden

6. Rast H, Bircher A (2006) Begutachtung von Berufsdermatosen aus Sicht des Unfallversicherungsträgers. Gesetzliche Bestimmungen in der Schweiz. In: szliska C, Brandenburg S, John SM (eds.) Berufsdermatosen. Dustri, Deisenhofen, pp 8c.1–8c.10

7. Suva (2003) Wegleitung der Suva durch die Unfallversicherung. Schweizerische Unfallversicherung Suva, Luzern (available also in French)

8. Schwanitz HJ (2003) Präventionsmaßnahmen. In: Schwanitz HJ, Wehrmann W, Brandenburg S, John SM (eds) Gutachten Dermatologie. Steinkopff, Darmstadt, pp 17–31

Databases and Networks. The Benefit for Research and Quality Assurance in Patch Testing

54

Wolfgang Uter, Axel Schnuch, Ana Giménez-Arnau, David Orton, and Barry Statham

Contents

W. Uter (✉)
Department of Medical Informatics, Biometry and Epidemiology, University of Erlangen-Nürnberg, Waldstrasse 6, 91054 Erlangen, Germany
e-mail: wolfgang.uter@imbe.med.uni-erlangen.de

A. Schnuch
Information Network of Departments of Dermatology (IVDK), University Skin Hospital, von-Siebold-Strasse 3, 37075 Göttingen, Germany

A. Giménez-Arnau
Department of Dermatology, Hospital del Mar, IMAS. Universitat Autònoma, Barcelona, Spain

D. Orton
Amersham Hospital, Environmental and Contact Dermatitis Unit, Whielden Strasse, Amersham, Buckinghamshire HP7 0JD, UK

B. Statham
Department of Dermatology, Singleton Hospital, Abertawe Bro Morgannwg University NHS Trust, Swansea SA2 8QA, Wales, UK

54.1 Scope

The present chapter summarises several information technology (IT) applications in the research field of contact dermatitis intended to support the clinical management of patients and/or research. Today, due to the overwhelming speed of IT innovation, there seem to be few strictly technical problems. However, it seems to be an important issue to integrate IT into everyday work in such a way that it is not perceived as an intrusion, but rather as a support by its users. The starting point for a successful contact allergy research application is the implementation of user-friendly patch test software to document relevant parts of the patient's history and patch test results. After an overview of the relevant issues, this presentation focuses on the usefulness of electronically collected data for quality control purposes within a patch test network. In this context, quality control is both an outcome and also a prerequisite for further use of this data for scientific purposes, e.g., surveillance of contact allergy or other dedicated analyses. The successful use of such databases generated by different networks is illustrated by several examples. As an aid in the daily management of contact dermatitis patients, a number of auxiliary sources of information are briefly outlined in the final section.

J.D. Johansen et al. (eds.), *Contact Dermatitis*,
DOI: 10.1007/978-3-642-03827-3_54, © Springer-Verlag Berlin Heidelberg 2011

54

54.2 Patch Test Software

Electronic health records are being introduced into many areas of medical care. This process is not primarily driven by research interests, but is motivated by the intended increase in the efficiency of procedures, improved data availability and both economic and clerical reasons. Still, such data can be scientifically analysed, keeping in mind the possible limitations of both precision and validity. However, several groups have realised early on that in the special situation of contact allergy research, namely for the analysis of patch test results with the Baseline Series or other series over time, dedicated (local) databases and software, respectively, are a prerequisite [1–6]. Acceptability of data collection for research purposes by those users entering patch test data can be increased by two opposite strategies: (a) minimising the amount of data entered, thus effectively collecting only aggregated patient information ("minimal add-on", e.g., current SIDAPA system), (b) fully covering all departmental documentation needs, thus eliminating the necessity for additional routine documentation ("replacement", [3, 7]). The European Surveillance System on Contact Allergies (ESSCA, www.essca-dc.org) has elaborated a "minimal dataset", i.e., a collection of mandatory and optional anamnestic items (latest revision seen at http://www.ivdk.gwdg.de/essca/doc/minidat8_2003_06.pdf; last accessed 2009-06-29). A suggested list of occupations, based on the ISCO-88 COM classification, is found at http://www.ivdk.gwdg.de/essca/doc/occup_ESSCA_01-02.pdf; last accessed 2009-06-29. At present, both above-mentioned strategies are being followed, depending on the preferences and scope of the respective research networks. A special line of development focused on decision support by an expert system that derived rules dynamically based on an accumulating body of data [8, 9], or the inclusion of information on product ingredients – both not necessarily in the context of a network [10–12]. In a number of research networks, these approaches have proven viable in the past decades with, however, a varying degree of flexibility (and complexity) of the "patch test software" used, which will be illustrated here:

- Possibly, the most basic way to electronically document history and patch test results is to transfer this information from paper patient's records to an electronic spreadsheet, following a "minimal add-on" strategy. In this spreadsheet, the rows usually represent single patients, and the columns different attributes of these patients, such as age, gender, occupation, etc. With regard to patch test results, one reading of one allergen will usually occupy one column, rendering such a sheet fairly "broad". Furthermore, this system is highly inflexible, as (a) changes in the scope of allergens will either lead to new versions of the sheet incompatible with the previous ones or further extension of columns and (b) the reading frame is usually restricted to two readings, e.g., day 2 and day 4, possibly supplemented by a statement on clinical relevance. As an absolute minimum, only one summary reaction, possibly combined with a statement on relevance, could be documented for each allergen tested.

- A more flexible way to collect patch test data, allowing for the inclusion of (different versions of) test series applied to one patient, has been implemented by the British group. Here, a basic set of personal characteristics is recorded for each patient along with results with any number of pre-defined test series. The database system has been implemented in Microsoft Access, distributed in uniform versions across the British network, allowing for relatively easy pooling of this highly standardised, yet flatly structured data. In this system, the fixed reading frame (two readings per allergen and the evaluation of clinical relevance case of positive reactions) imposes some restriction. Moreover, centre-specific test series, reflecting local exposures or research interests, or patients' own materials are not included in the database.

Both solutions already mentioned illustrate the correlation between flexibility and complexity, that is, potential difficulties in setting up, maintaining and analysing a database. This relationship is further illustrated by those more flexible and complex systems which fully exploit the conceptual framework of data representation by either using event-based data representation or, most often in this field, a relational database system.

- A number of solutions for storing patch test data have used, and are using, a relational database format (among others, [1, 3, 7, 12] – probably a non-comprehensive list as many investigators did not publish on the methodological aspects of their patch test software). As one example, the WinAlldat software used by the German-Swiss-Austrian IVDK-network had been developed some 20 years ago [3, 7]. Continuous expansion of functionality presently includes multilingual capabilities ("WinAlldat/ESSCA" [13], used by the European Surveillance System on Contact Allergies (ESSCA)), administration of centre-specific test series and series with patients' own materials, use of prick-, scratch and similar tests, network integration, an interface to hospital information systems, and most recently, a data mining tool to examine the contents of the database with a set of freely definable filters. The aim is to both cover all departmental documentation needs ("replacement" strategy) and provide electronic data capturing of the full scope of data (except personal identifiers which are not transmitted to the data centre). However, the development and maintenance of such dedicated software for patch testing and support of users necessitates specialised personnel and appropriate resources, not to mention means for a data centre for pooling and analysis of data collected (see below). Hence, only (larger, adequately funded) networks will possibly be in a position to invest in such an undertaking. Single centres or smaller groups are advised to join the existing networks after carefully checking the evidence of previous productivity (list of publications using the system) and indicators of future viability.
- While locally distributed patch test software and databases may have advantages, especially in terms of data protection possibilities, and certainly have been justified before the advent of the World Wide Web, today, the option of one centrally hosted database, accessed by any number of registered departments via the Internet using a browser, virtual private network (VPN) and other software tools to ensure data protection is well worth considering when setting up a network from scratch. However, a whole range of measures must be employed to satisfy current (legal) standards of data protection, including server and client certificates, connection preferably via VPNs, as well as requirements for data backup and easy access to the service. The Italian SIDAPA has recently started a Web-based multi-centre documentation facility, exemplifying this interesting alternative to the multiple distributed databases used elsewhere. The scope of data includes important demographic and clinical information, the series tested, selected from a list of pre-defined batteries, and documentation of positive (and, implicitly, of non-positive) reactions without information on reading time (http://www.epidemiologiadermatiti.it/, last accessed 2009-04-27, Pigatto 2009, personal communication). At the time of writing this chapter, detailed experience and scientific publications based on this system are not yet available.

Independent of the actual system used to record patch test results and patient histories on-site, the question of data transmission (secure, anonymous) and the storage format of pooled data remain to be addressed. Regarding the latter, any proprietary structure can be used, provided it is consistent, complete and self-explanatory (or documented accordingly). One possible structure for the representation of clinical study data has been elaborated by an international consortium of stakeholders (http://www.cdisc.org/, last accessed 2009-04-14). It is called the "operational data model" which involves a set of conventions for storing information about, and actual data from any clinical study in a common format based on the XML standard.

Core Message

> The computerised registration of patch test results along with relevant clinical and demographic data can not only be used for medical letter writing, but also exploited for quality auditing and clinical epidemiology research.

54

54.3 The Centre of a Multi-Centre Network

As soon as several centres co-operate as a multi-centre network, the issue of handling data coming in from the different departments arises. While it is possible to collect data from local distributed databases *ad hoc* on demand for a study project (as in the GERDA system, Drieghe 2009, personal communication), a "permanent" data centre, while costlier, has advantages in terms of ongoing feed-back and quality control. The tasks of a data centre include:

- Checking of incoming data for completeness and formal correctness.
- Labelling of data with the respective centre identifier and adequate archiving.
- Preparation of a set of useful descriptive analyses as feed-back for the Department (see also section "quality-control").
- Coordination of requests for analyses and publication of projects coming in from the members of the network.
- Analysing pooled, quality-controlled data (see next section) for scientific projects initiated by any member of the network.

The ways these tasks are fulfilled will largely depend on the actual setting, i.e., data structure, software used and individual experience of the researchers involved, and are thus not addressed in detail here. The resources needed to maintain a data centre, possibly in addition to those devoted to development and support of patch test software, should not be underestimated.

54.4 Quality Control in Patch Test Networks

Quality control is a key part of the process of Clinical Governance embracing all aspects of patient care by assuring high standards based on the best available clinical evidence. In the field of contact allergy research (and patient care), quality control comprises a set of very different issues ranging from laboratory controls

to the elaboration of scientific guidelines regarding this diagnostic procedure. Each scientific network analysing pooled data should be aware of the variation introduced by the full range of potential methodological differences (patch test material, storage of allergens, selection of test series based on history and clinical picture – dependent upon the training of the clinician, amount of allergen applied, timeframe of readings and, possibly most crucial, visual reading of the test reactions). The latter aspect can be addressed in terms of standardisation by regular training sessions with live patients, or evaluation of (digital) images of patch test reactions [14], e.g., in the course of scientific meetings of the network (The online patch test training tool by the German Contact Dermatitis group is accessible via http://www.ivdk.gwdg.de/dkg, select "PT Reading Course", after initial registration). In this section, we primarily address the comparison of local patch test reading results with the group's average to identify possible methodological variation. Once identified, efforts should follow to eliminate the "technical" source(s) of divergence. Comparisons between local results and results from the remaining centres could address the following:

- The % positive reactions to a set of allergens, mostly the allergens from the (European) Baseline Series, and also to "difficult" allergens [15] as these may indicate diverging reading methods even better.
- The pattern of reactivity, i.e., the proportion of doubtful or irritant vs. positive reactions (operationalised as "Reaction Index" [16]) or the proportion of weak positive among all positive reactions ("Positivity Ratio" [15]).

Differences in the spectrum of allergens diagnosed in the different centres can also be due to differences in patient characteristics. This observation led to the development of the MOHL-index some decades ago, recently expanded to the MOAHLFA-index. This incorporates the most important demographic and clinical characteristics, helping to put patch test results into this perspective [17, 18]. The aim of comparing contact allergy prevalences of one department with the average is to identify those "outliers" which are not "explained" by an underlying variation of patient characteristics. Admittedly, this is a difficult process which cannot be automated, but needs careful consideration and discussion with the respective department. In contrast, other characteristics of the patch test reaction profile of allergens are probably less dependent on the underlying population of patients, such as the proportion of weak positive reactions among all positive reactions or the proportion of doubtful or irritant reactions among all reactions. Moreover, it has proven useful to analyse the proportion of reactions documented as positive to a set of "problematic" allergens which are expected to yield mostly false-positive reactions. If the reaction profile diverges from the average, or prevalences of "positive" reactions to problematic allergens are consistently higher in one department, with no indications of exceptionally frequent true-positive reactions to these allergens, the suspicion of divergent patch test reading standards arises and should be discussed bilaterally.

A further reason for variation in the frequencies of positivity between different patch test centres may be the proportion of patients in a catchment population who undergo testing. If the proportion of patients tested is too low, this may give rise to a falsely high percentage of positive results as those tested may not be representative of the population at risk of sensitisation (who should be patch tested). Such differences may arise through too restrictive use of diagnostic testing, but in many instances, it arises due to geographic dispersal of patients making it difficult for patients to travel for investigation. At the other end of the scale, a high rate of referral may not lead to a declining rate of relevant allergens. M. Beck demonstrated that patch testing up to 1 in 700 of a catchment population led to no drop off in the rate of identification of relevant allergens [19]. Quality control is important also to assure patients and healthcare providers that the individual/department performing the patient assessment and investigation is doing so in a competent manner. This can be approached from varying perspectives such as those outlined in the guidelines; detailing the training requirements for individuals providing contact dermatitis services as well as ways of demonstrating the maintenance of competency by various means including benchmarking of patch testing results with other departments in the data network. While it is unlikely that any single measure of quality will indicate a cause for concern with regard to local methodology and interpretation of results, examining variance in positivity, particularly when repeated in data pooled over 2–3 years, will lead to a careful reflection of the reasons for variance, including the standards of grading and interpretation of positive results [20].

In comparison to the "soft" criteria mentioned above, the proportion of missing data for a set of core items can be regarded as a straightforward benchmark of data quality; "acceptable" proportions of missing data can be decided by the peer group [21].

Quality control is thus not only a prerequisite for networking, but also an outcome not available otherwise. In other words, a single department never putting its data to the test misses the chance to be alerted of possible methodological difficulties. Moreover, beyond a certain start-up and consolidation period of a network, only those data fulfilling the set quality criteria should be used in pooled scientific analyses – i.e., data of "poor quality" should be excluded. This should enhance the credibility of scientific results, which are often the basis for important regulatory decisions.

54.5 Surveillance of Contact Allergy

One of the most obvious outcomes of continuously collecting patch test data in a quality-controlled network is the possibility of using this data for monitoring the frequency of contact allergy among patients. Given sufficient size, the network may be regarded as a sample of the national level. The main interest of surveillance is to identify emerging allergens (in a subgroup) and to identify persisting problems. However, the degree of success of preventative action can also be monitored by following up the time trend of the contact allergen in question. A number of examples from different networks are given in the following section.

To be valid, any comparison across time or between departments has to take the differing age distribution, gender or other factors associated with specific contact sensitisation, into account (see also Chap. 11). If, for instance, the increasing average age of patients as observed in the IVDK-network is not considered in the analysis of time trends of those specific sensitisations associated with age, confounding will occur, obscuring the true trend of sensitisation prevalence over time [18].

The primary objective of contact allergy surveillance is the monitoring of sensitisation prevalences in patients patch tested, taking relevant patient characteristics into account to arrive at valid comparisons across time or space. However, as the prevalence or incidence in the general population is also of interest – but rarely addressed by population-based epidemiological studies – a method has been developed to grossly estimate morbidity at the population level. This methodology is based on clinical surveillance data and national information on

54

sales of patch test materials, ("CE-DUR" [22]). According to the studies in Denmark and Germany, the estimates derived from this very economical method are well in line with the scant epidemiological data available [23].

54.6 Detection of New Contact Allergens

Surveillance as discussed above is largely based on patch testing with standardised series of commercial allergens often used uniformly on a national or even international level (e.g., the "European Baseline Series"). In addition to these batteries, departmental special series and in particular patients' own materials are also used clinically to improve diagnostic sensitivity. The analysis of departmental/national series can reveal new allergens that may be important beyond the local catchment area. Electronically collected (multi-centre) test results with patients' own materials, although not standardised and thus difficult to analyse on a large scale, may identify certain "problematic" products and certain allergens not yet covered by the series used ([24], see also Chap. 57). In this section, a number of ways to collect evidence on new allergens using different approaches are described.

Cosmetovigilance (CV) can be regarded as a special part of contact allergy surveillance. It does not involve continual analysis of "routine" patch test data, but *ad hoc* reporting of case series with patch test results to certain (types of) products obtained within an established CV network [25]. As such, CV is based on patch testing with patients' own materials (see Chap. 54) and with standardised breakdown test results allowing for the identification of potential new allergens. In a slightly different approach, a "service institution" for the cosmetic industry has been implemented in Germany ("IDOK" [26]). IDOK provides advice on adequate preparation of patch test allergens in case a dermatologist requests single ingredients of the product for breakdown testing. This service is especially useful for small and medium enterprises without in-house toxicological expertise in this area, increasing the quality of patient care. The results of breakdown testing are then transmitted to IDOK, accumulating an ever-increasing body of data on patch test results with cosmetic ingredients usually not present in commercial series. The potential problems encountered with this system include: (a) a low level of dermatologists

feed-back, 50% in this system (also due to a considerable drop-out rate of patients who did not appear for the second patch test), (b) the quality of patch testing seems to be more heterogeneous, compared to a closed network of experienced experts as in France and (c) the publication of results with ingredients still protected by a patent is difficult.

In contrast to these "bottom-up" approaches, targeting diagnostic efficacy and collecting data on an individual patient level, an entirely different strategy to improve diagnostics could be labelled a "top-down" approach: if all relevant stakeholders involved with a certain area of exposure, e.g., cutting fluids, could be persuaded to join an expert panel screening currently used products for potential allergens, these putative additional allergens could be compiled into a provisional test series, and the diagnostic benefits of this approach could be explored. In Germany, the employer's liability insurance of the metal industry has brought together clinical researchers, chemical scientists, major representatives of cutting fluid producers and safety engineers. This collaboration has resulted in the development of two patch test series, namely, the "historical" and "current" cutting fluid additives later on used by dermatologists [27]. As one spin-off of these activities, diglycolamine has been identified as a new important cutting fluid allergen. Moreover, valid recommendations on the handling of fresh or used cutting fluid samples intended for patch testing have been issued [28]. Applying a similar approach, epoxy resin systems were screened for potential allergens, which were then compiled into an experimental test series yielding interesting insights into the spectrum of sensitisation and cross-reactivity; respective additions to an epoxy resin test series were recommended [29].

> ### Core Message
>
> › Given sufficient quality, pooled data of a contact allergy network can be used for surveillance (time trends, subgroup analyses). Moreover, data collected beyond routine documentation in sub-systems (e.g., Cosmetovigilance) can be systematically analysed for the detection of new allergens, or new sources of exposures to known allergens.

54.7 Examples from Existing Databases/Networks

It is well-known that national or international contact dermatitis research groups (e.g., EECDRG or ICDRG) have undertaken several multi-centre studies addressing a wide range of important scientific issues. These studies have usually been performed, and are still being performed, in a prospective manner, in an effort to collect sufficient data, analyse these and publish the results within a reasonable time period. The data networks as defined here go beyond this *ad hoc* approach: complete information on all patients tested in the network is routinely collected in a standardised way and can be analysed retrospectively and in terms of regular, e.g., yearly, surveillance. At the same time, these networks obviously offer the infrastructure for special prospective studies, if necessary, supplementing anamnestic items or the scope of patch test series. Examples

from existing networks mentioned in this section pertain to published output from such existing networks – for an overview see Table 54.1.

54.7.1 Increasing Contact Allergy Frequency

Time and again, new contact allergens, or well-known allergens used in new types of products, cause epidemics, i.e., an increasing frequency of positive reactions in patch tested patients (review in [30]). While these epidemics may start small and locally, open markets and broad exposure in the population may give rise to a generalised epidemic. Biocides used in cosmetic products are particularly well-recognised for causing epidemics, followed by intervention (reduction of use concentration, regulation or withdrawal) and subsequent decrease

Table 54.1 Examples of published outcomes of currently active contact allergy networks, i.e., not including multi-centre studies of national contact dermatitis groups that are not based on a formal, pre-existing IT-based network infrastructure

Network (area covered)	Main results	References
Danish Contact Dermatitis Group	Clinical network: many international publications covering different topics	(Selected examples see text)
BCDS (UK)	Clinical network: many international publications covering different topics	Examples: [48–51]
IVDK (Germany, Austria, Switzerland)	Tri-national clinical network (www.ivdk.org): many international publications covering different topics	(Selected examples see text)
REVIDAL-GERDA (France)	Cosmetovigilance: six cases of allergic contact dermatitis after application of mascara, in five cases due to shellac (20% ethanol) according to a complete breakdown testing. Clinical network with electronic data capturing using dedicated software developed by Goossens/Drieghe	[52](Goossens 2009, personal communication)
GEIDAC (Spain)	Started in 2008	
NEICDG (North-East Italy Contact Dermatitis Group)	Regional clinical network: Example: a comparison of PT results in patients aged >65 years and those who are 20–40 years old	[53]
SIDAPA	National Internet-based network collecting clinical data along with patch test results with fixed series (positive vs. non-positive); started 2009	(Pigatto 2009, personal communication)
NACDG	Clinical network: many international publications addressing time trends, standard series allergens, special subgroups and single allergens	
ESSCA (EU), working group of the ESCD	Meta-network (www.essca-dc.org): Continual analysis of sensitisation prevalence to allergens of the European Baseline Series and selected allergens of interest	[37, 38]

The list maybe non-exhaustive; possible omissions of eligible networks are not intentional

of sensitisation prevalence [31]. Single departments may, independent of each other, note increased sensitisation prevalence in their patients, which may become significant after some time. However, only the pooling of a large amount of data from several departments renders statistical analyses sufficiently powerful allowing for an earlier identification of an epidemic, and, of course, earlier primary intervention.

54.7.2 Decreasing Contact Allergy Frequency

With surprisingly little delay, the beneficial effect of interventions reducing exposure to a certain allergen can be recognised in surveillance data [32]. Recent examples include the decline of primin contact allergy in Denmark [33], and of nickel contact allergy noted in young Danish females after national nickel regulation [34]. In Germany, a decline and eventual vanishing of contact allergy to glyceryl monothioglycolate in young German hairdressers after withdrawal of this compound from the German market has been observed [35]. These examples also illustrate that changes in morbidity may not be observed on the level of all patients, young and old, female and male, but only in certain subgroups. In fact, it is necessary to target those persons (patients) who are young enough not to have been exposed prior to intervention, but who would have most likely been exposed if the intervention had not happened for the sensitive surveillance of intervention effects. The prevalence of contact allergy in such a subgroup is the closest possible approximation of the incidence of specific contact sensitisation, which is usually not directly measurable.

54.7.3 Persisting Contact Allergy Problems

Sometimes, the frequency of contact sensitisation to a certain allergen will not reach 0% after intervention action, even if the subgroup of patients most sensitive to intervention effects (see above) is being monitored. The example of nickel contact allergy in Denmark already quoted above [34], and very similar German data [36] point to relevant persisting exposure(s) to this allergen.

In the case of other allergens such as colophony, rubber allergens or p-phenylene diamine, no particular intervention efforts have been taken so far, and sensitisation prevalence remain at a high level of several percent in consecutively tested patients (e.g., [37, 38]).

54.7.4 Subgroup or Multi-Factorial Analyses

Rare exposures, represented by job title, contactants, special test series or other patient characteristics, require a large overall clinical sample to achieve sufficient power for statistical testing or sufficient precision of estimates of morbidity or risk. Evidently, the pooling of quality-controlled data from several centres provides many more possibilities for subgroup analyses. As certain high risk exposures may emerge in a small subgroup, this is an important asset. The appearance of MCI/MI as important allergen in male patients exposed to paints in a non-occupational context (a relatively small subgroup) can be regarded as an example of a subgroup analysis. After recognition of the problem and lowering of the concentration of MCI/MI in water-based paints, the prevalence of sensitisation decreased to a "normal" level [39].

Multi-factorial analyses are used to obtain estimates of sensitisation risk associated with a number of factors of interest and potential confounders, respectively, where each risk estimate is adjusted for all other factors (see Chap. 11). The Danish contact dermatitis group has been the first to apply this standard epidemiological approach to contact allergy data, exploiting the possibilities of networking [40]. With an increasing number of factors and complexity of the model, and also with a decreasing prevalence of the outcome (specific sensitisation), the sample size needs to increase massively. Otherwise, a situation will arise, whereby, analysts will be forced to make their model more parsimonious, i.e., omit one or more factors. Consequently, detailed analyses are often only possible based on several 10,000s of patients, and, thus, only based on network data. One recent example is the multi-factorial analysis of risk factors for sensitisation to standard allergens in construction workers [41], revealing not only chromium, but also epoxy resin and thiurams as significant occupational allergens, or the identification of polysensitisation as an important characteristic of susceptibility [42].

54.7.5 Link with Other Data

"Routine" data collected electronically in a network can be linked, prospectively or in retrospect, with external data sources. These may include diverse data such as prescription data on topical drugs, to estimate a numerator of exposure for risk assessment in a recent pharmacoepidemiological project [43] or meteorological data at the time of patch testing addressing the association with irritant/doubtful, weak, and strong positive patch test reactions to standard allergens [44]. Moreover, the data collected can serve to identify cases and controls for studies involving laboratory analyses, e.g., polymorphisms potentially relevant for sensitisation (e.g., [45]).

54.8 Auxiliary Databases

While this chapter focuses on how databases and networks with (anonymous) patient data can support contact allergy research, other sources of information that support clinical and scientific work also deserve mention. The following section cannot claim to cover all relevant resources; often, specific helpful information may be available only in the national language. The websites of the national contact dermatitis groups often include useful links to (national) sources of information. The sites listed should present relevant information, be scientifically correct, updated continually and easily accessible. Moreover, the National groups' websites could host a discussion forum covering practical

problems or current issues relevant for the patch test clinic. The BCDS website, for instance, hosts a discussion forum restricted to those with password-controlled access. The forum facilitates discussion on any topic related to contact dermatitis or concerning or the BCDS contact dermatitis database. Many topics ranging from advice about unusual allergens to guidance on the interpretation of borderline positive/irritant patch test reactions have been discussed.

54.8.1 Information on Allergens

Often, well-known websites such as PubMed (http://www.ncbi.nlm.nih.gov/sites/entrez?db=pubmed, last accessed 2009-04-27), Google (Scholar) or other search engines identify information pertaining to a certain allergen. The CAS number is a particularly useful and usually unique identifier of chemical compounds. A number of internet-based resources in English language are listed in Table 54.2.

54.8.2 Product Databases

The necessity to keep information up to date is particularly acute with regard to information on the ingredients of products, as the composition of products may change more or less frequently. In the field of pharmaceutical agents, inventories such as "Rote Liste"

Table 54.2 Selected internet resources regarding information on allergens

URL	Description	Access
http://hazmap.nlm.nih.gov/	A relational database of hazardous chemicals and occupational exposures (job titles), including contact allergy	Free
http://ec.europa.eu/enterprise/cosmetics/cosing/	Inventory of cosmetic ingredients (INCI)	Free
http://www.cdeskpro.be/	Comprehensive information system available for dermatologists	Restricted
http://www.ifraorg.org	Collection of IFRA Standards	Free
http://www3.interscience.wiley.com/cgi-bin/mrwhome/104554790/HOME	List of MAK and BAT values (German regulations) for chemicals with expert statements, including contact allergy	Restricted
http://eur-lex.europa.eu	Legal decisions on R classification	Free
http://bodd.cf.ac.uk/index.html	Botanical names and further information on plants	Free

54

(http://www.rote-liste.de/, last accessed 2009-04-27) in Germany in or http://www.medicines.org.uk/ (last accessed 2009-04-27) in the United Kingdom are examples of useful resources. With regard to cosmetics, the INCI labelling system (see Table 54.2) provides useful qualitative information for diagnosis, final evaluation of relevance and prevention (if appropriately implemented by industry and sensibly used by the patient). Unfortunately, product information for industrial products is far less complete or available in most countries. In Denmark, the "PROBAS" database is a unique resource containing information on more than 75,000 (mostly industrial) products [46]; however, it is not freely accessible. Generally, databases representing exposure can potentially be used to estimate the extent of exposure in the workplace [47]. Moreover, if exposure information is combined with information on specific morbidity (sensitisation), the risk of sensitisation can be more validly estimated than based on human sensitisation data alone (one example in the field of active topical ingredients: [43]).

References

1. Bahmer FA (1989) The Homburg model for computer-based documentation in allergy. Semin Dermatol 8:99–100
2. Beck MH, Hiller V (1989) Computer analysis of patients undergoing contact dermatitis investigation. Semin Dermatol 8:105
3. Diepgen TL, Stüben O (1989) ALLDAT: an allergy data system for storage and analysis of test data with regard to epidemiological and occupational dermatology. Semin Dermatol 8:101–102
4. Gailhofer G (1989) Evaluation of patch test data using a personal computer system. Semin Dermatol 8:103–104
5. Sertoli A, Gola M, Martinelli C, Angelini G, Ayala F et al (1989) Epidemiology of contact dermatitis. Semin Dermatol 8:120–126
6. Shaw S, Wilkinson JD (1989) Desk-top, stand-alone computer system for patch test clinic. Semin Dermatol 8:106–112
7. Uter W, Diepgen TL, Arnold R, Hillebrand O, Pietrzyk PM, Stüben O, Schnuch A (1992) The informational network of departments of dermatology in Germany – a Multicenter Project for Computer-assisted Monitoring of Contact Allergy – Electronic Data Processing Aspects. Derm Beruf Umwelt 40:142–149 (published erratum: p 197)
8. Albert J, Geier J, Lehmann M, Schoof J (1997) Lernende Klassifizierungssysteme zur fallbasierten Auswertung von Allergietestdaten. Allergo J 6:408
9. Dooms-Goossens A, Drieghe J, Degreff H, Dooms M (1990) The "Codex-E": an expert system for contact dermatitis. Contact Dermatitis 22:180–181
10. Dooms Goossens A, Degreef H, Drieghe J, Dooms M (1980) Computer assisted monitoring of contact dermatitis patients. Contact Dermatitis 6:123–127
11. Edman B (1989) DALUK: The Swedish Computer System for Contact Dermatitis. Semin Dermatol 8:97–98
12. Rantanen T (1989) INFODERM – a microcomputer database system with finnish product files. Semin Dermatol 8:94–95
13. Uter W, Arnold R, Wilkinson J, Shaw S, Perrenoud D, Rili C, Vigan M, Ayala F, Krecisz B, Hegewald J, Schnuch A (2003) A multilingual European patch test software concept: Win Alldat/ESSCA. Contact Dermatitis 49:270–271
14. Uter W, Becker D, Schnuch A, Gefeller O, Frosch P.J. (2007) The validity of rating patch test reactions based on digital images. Contact Dermatitis 57:337–342
15. Geier J, Uter W, Lessmann H, Schnuch A (2003) The positivity ratio–another parameter to assess the diagnostic quality of a patch test preparation. Contact Dermatitis 48:280–2
16. Brasch J, Henseler T (1992) The reaction index: a parameter to assess the quality of patch test preparations. Contact Dermatitis 27:203–204
17. Smith HR, Wakelin SH, McFadden JP, Rycroft RJ, White IR (1999) A 15-year review of our MOAHLFA index. Contact Dermatitis 40:227–228
18. Uter W, Gefeller O, Geier J, Schnuch A (2008) Changes of the patch test population (MOAHLFA index) in long-term participants of the Information Network of Departments of Dermatology, 1999–2006. Contact Dermatitis 59:56–57
19. Bhushan M, Beck MH (1999) An audit to identify the optimum referral rate to a contact dermatitis investigation unit. Br J Dermatol 141:570–572
20. Bourke J, Coulson I, English J (2009) Guidelines for the management of contact dermatitis: an update. Br J Dermatol 160:946–954
21. Uter W, Mackiewicz M, Schnuch A, Geier J (2005) Interne Qualitätssicherung von Epikutantest-Daten des multizentrischen Projektes "Informationsverbund Dermatologischer Kliniken" (IVDK). Dermatol Beruf Umwelt 53:107–114
22. Schnuch A, Uter W, Geier J, Gefeller O (2002) Epidemiology of contact allergy: an estimation of morbidity employing the clinical epidemiology and drug-utilization research (CE-DUR) approach. Contact Dermatitis 47:32–39
23. Thyssen JP, Uter W, Schnuch A, Linneberg A, Johansen JD (2007) 10-year prevalence of contact allergy in the general population in Denmark estimated through the CE-DUR method. Contact Dermatitis 57:265–272
24. Uter W, Balzer C, Geier J, Frosch PJ, Schnuch A (2005) Patch testing with patients' own cosmetics and toiletries–results of the IVDK*, 1998–2002. Contact Dermatitis 53:226–233
25. Vigan M (1997) Les nouveaux allergenes des cosmetiques. La cosmetovigilance. Ann Dermatol Venereol 124:571–575
26. Lessmann H, Uter W, Geier J, Schnuch A (2006) Die informations- und Dokumentationsstelle für Kontaktallergien (IDOK) des Informationsverbundes Dermatologischer Kliniken (IVDK). Dermatol Beruf Umwelt 54:160–166
27. Geier J, Lessmann H, Frosch PJ, Pirker C, Koch P, Aschoff R, Richter G, Becker D, Eckert C, Uter W, Schnuch A, Fuchs T (2003) Patch testing with components of water-based metal-working fluids. Contact Dermatitis 49:85–90
28. Tiedemann K-H, Zöllner G, Adam M, Becker D, Boveleth W, Eck E, Eckert C, Englitz HG, Geier J, Koch P, Lessmann H, Müller J, Nöring R, Rocker M, Rothe A, Schmidt A,

Schumacher T, Uter W, Warfolomeow I, Wirtz C (2002) Empfehlungen für die Epikutantestung bei Verdacht auf Kontaktallergie durch Kühlschmierstoffe. 2. Hinweise zur Arbeitsstofftestung. Dermatol Beruf Umwelt 50:180–189

29. Geier J, Lessmann H, Hillen U, Jappe U, Dickel H, Koch P, Frosch PJ, Schnuch A, Uter W (2004) An attempt to improve diagnostics of contact allergy due to epoxy resin systems. First results of the multicentre study EPOX 2002. Contact Dermatitis 51:263–272

30. Thyssen JP, Johansen JD, Menné T (2007) Contact allergy epidemics and their controls. Contact Dermatitis 56:185–195

31. Dillarstone A (1997) Cosmetic preservatives. Contact Dermatitis 37:190

32. Wesley NO, Maibach HI (2003) Decreasing allergic contact dermatitis frequency through dermatotoxicologic and epidemiologic based intervention? Food Chem Toxicol 41:857–860

33. Zachariae C, Engkilde K, Johansen JD, Menné T (2007) Primin in the European standard patch test series for 20 years. Contact Dermatitis 56:344–346

34. Johansen J, Menné T, Christophersen J, Kaaber K, Veien N (2000) Changes in the pattern of sensitization to common contact allergens in denmark between 1985–86 and 1997–98, with a special view to the effect of preventive strategies. Br J Dermatol 142:490–5

35. Uter W, Geier J, Lessmann H, Schnuch A (2006) Is contact allergy to glyceryl monothioglycolate still a problem in Germany? Contact Dermatitis 55:54–56

36. Schnuch A, Uter W (2003) Decrease in nickel allergy in Germany and regulatory interventions. Contact Dermatitis 49:107–108

37. Hegewald J, Uter W, Aberer W, Ayala F, Beliauskiene A, Belloni Fortina A, Bircher A, Brasch J, Chowdhury MM, Coenraads PJ, Schuttelaer M-L, Elsner P, English J, Fartasch M, Mahler V, Frosch PJ, Fuchs T, Gawkrodger DJ, Giménez-Arnau AM, Green CM, Johansen JD, Menné T, Jolanki R, King CM, Krecisz B, Kiec-Swierczynska M, Larese F, Ormerod AD, Orton D, Peserico A, Rantanen T, Rustemeyer T, Sansom JE, Statham BN, Corradin MT, Wallnofer W, Wilkinson M, Schnuch A (2008) The European Surveillance System of Contact Allergies (ESSCA): results of patch testing the standard series, 2004. J Eur Acad Dermatol Venereol 22:174–181

38. Uter W, Rämsch C, Aberer W, Ayala F, Balato A, Beliauskiene A, Belloni Fortina A, Bircher AJ, Brasch J, Chowdhury MMU, Coenraads P-J, Schuttelaar M-LA, Cooper S, Corradin MT, Elsner P, English J, Fartasch M, Mahler V, Frosch PJ, Fuchs T, Gawkrodger DJ, Giménez-Arnau AM, Green CM, Horne HL, Jolanki R, King CM, Krêcisz B, Kiec-Swierczynska M, Ormerod AD, Orton D, Peserico A, Rantanen T, Rustemeyer T, Sansom JE, Simon D, Statham B, Wilkinson M, Schnuch A (2009) The European Baseline Series in 10 European Countries, 2005/2006 - Results of the European Surveillance System on Contact Allergies (ESSCA). Contact Dermatitis 61:31–38

39. Schnuch A, Uter W, Geier J, Lessmann H, Hillen U, Roßkamp E (2002) Kontaktallergien gegen Dispersionsfarben Epidemiologische Überwachung durch den IVDK – Intervention des Umweltbundesamtes und erfolgreiche Primärprävention? Allergo J 11:39–47

40. Christophersen J, Menné T, Tanghoj P, Andersen KE, Brandrup F, Kaaber K, Osmundsen PE, Thestrup Pedersen K, Veien NK (1989) Clinical patch test data evaluated by multivariate analysis. Danish Contact Dermatitis Group. Contact Dermatitis 21:291–299

41. Uter W, Rühl R, Pfahlberg A, Geier J, Schnuch A, Gefeller O (2004) Contact allergy in construction workers: results of a multifactorial analysis. Ann Occup Hyg 48:21–27

42. Schnuch A, Brasch J, Uter W (2008) Polysensitization and increased susceptibility in contact allergy: a review. Allergy 63:156–167

43. Menezes de Pádua CA, Schnuch A, Nink K, Pfahlberg A, Uter W (2008) Allergic contact dermatitis to topical drugs – epidemiological risk assessment. Pharmacoepidemiol Drug Saf 17:813–821

44. Uter W, Hegewald J, Kränke B, Schnuch A, Gefeller O, Pfahlberg A (2008) The impact of meteorological conditions on patch test results with 12 standard series allergens (fragrances, biocides, topical ingredients). Br J Dermatol 158:734–739

45. Reich K, Westphal G, König IR, Mossner R, Krüger U, Ziegler A, Neumann C, Schnuch A (2003) Association of allergic contact dermatitis with a promoter polymorphism in the IL16 gene. J Allergy Clin Immunol 112:1191–4

46. Flyvholm MA, Andersen P, Beck ID, Brandorff NP (1992) PROBAS: the Danish product register database. A national register of chemical substances and products. J Hazard Mater 30:59–69

47. Brandorff NP, Flyvholm MA, Beck ID, Skov T, Bach E (1995) National survey on the use of chemicals in the working environment: estimated exposure events. Occup Environ Med 52:454–463

48. Jong CT, Statham BN, Green CM, King CM, Gawkrodger DJ, Sansom JE, English JS, Wilkinson SM, Ormerod AD, Chowdhury MM (2007) Contact sensitivity to preservatives in the UK, 2004-2005: results of multicentre study. Contact Dermatitis 57:165–168

49. Kalavala M, Statham BN, Green CM, King C, Ormerod AD, Sansom J, English JS, Wilkinson MS, Horne H, Gawkrodger D (2007) Tixocortol pivalate: what is the right concentration? Contact Dermatitis 57:44–46

50. Katugampola RP, Statham BN, English JS, Wilkinson MM, Foulds IS, Green CM, Ormerod AD, Stone NM, Horne HL, Chowdhury MM (2005) A multicentre review of the footwear allergens tested in the UK. Contact Dermatitis 53:133–135

51. Katugampola RP, Statham BN, English JS, Wilkinson MM, Foulds IS, Green CM, Ormerod AD, Stone NM, Horne HL, Chowdhury MM (2005) A multicentre review of the hairdressing allergens tested in the UK. Contact Dermatitis 53:130–132

52. Le Coz CJ, Leclere JM, Arnoult E, Raison-Peyron N, Pons-Guiraud A, Vigan M (2002) Allergic contact dermatitis from shellac in mascara. Contact Dermatitis 46:149–152

53. Piaserico S, Larese F, Recchia GP, Corradin MT, Scardiglis F, Gennaro F, Carriere C, Semenzato A, Brandolisio L, Peserico A, Belloni Fortina A (2004) Allergic contact sensitivity in elderly patients. Aging Clin Exp Res 16:221–5

Contact Dermatitis Research Groups

55

Derk P. Bruynzeel

Contents

55.1 Introduction

This textbook was the initiative of the members of the European Environmental and Contact Dermatitis Research Group (EECDRG). The EECDRG, founded in 1985, had publishing a textbook and founding a society focused on contact dermatitis as their main goals. Rightly, they felt that promotion of knowledge of contact dermatitis was of immense importance. Their second goal, founding of the European Society of Contact Dermatitis (ESCD), was established in 1988 in a meeting at the end of a contact dermatitis congress organized by Peter Frosch in Heidelberg. The first official congress of the ESCD was organized by Jean-Marie Lachapelle in Brussels, in 1992 (Chap. 1). The first edition of the textbook was published in the same year. The Society has since held every second year a congress and organized meetings and courses to disseminate expertise and knowledge to make young colleagues enthusiastic about the clinical and experimental aspects of contact dermatitis. At these well-attended congresses, the opportunities for making professional contacts and friends the essential network, are great.

Today, it is easy to find information on persons and all subjects, and also contact dermatitis, via the Internet, though it can be quite time-consuming. Therefore, it can be handy to have the addresses of the chairperson and /or secretary of contact dermatitis groups and other colleagues who are interested in contact dermatitis. It is quite sure that if they can provide you with information on their group or persons you are looking for in their country, it will be a great help. A disadvantage of such a list is always that due to the delay in collecting the information and publication, addresses may have changed; but in practice, this not really a big problem.

D.P. Bruynzeel
Burg. Dedelstraat 42, NL-1391 GD Abcoude, Amsterdam, The Netherlands
e-mail: d.bruynzeel@chello.nl

J.D. Johansen et al. (eds.), *Contact Dermatitis*,
DOI: 10.1007/978-3-642-03827-3_55, © Springer-Verlag Berlin Heidelberg 2011

The information might help you form and extend your network among those who are active in the fields of occupational and contact dermatitis. Since the number of colleagues involved is not so numerous, you will easily be able to meet them on the congresses and symposia of the American Contact Dermatitis Society (ACDS) and ESCD. It is something like a big family and a group of friends.

ACDS: www.contactderm.org/

ESCD: www.escd.org/

55.2 Contact Dermatitis Groups

Australia	Australasian College of Dermatologists' Contact Dermatitis Group
Chairperson:	Rosemary Nixon Occupational Dermatology Research and Education Center, Skin and Cancer Foundation Victoria, 1/80 Drummond Street, Carlton, Vic 3053, Australia rnixon@occderm.asn.au
Austria	Arbeitsgruppe Allergologie der Österreichischen Gesellschaft für Dermatologie und Venerologie
Chairperson:	Stefan Woehrl Department of Dermatology, Medical University of Vienna, Währinger Gürtel 18–20, 1090 Vienna, Austria stefan.woehrl@meduniwien.ac.as
Secretary:	Thomas Hawranek Department of Dermatology, Paracelsus Private Medical University Salzburg, Muellner Hauptstrasse 48, 5020 Salzburg, Austria t.hawranek@salk.at
Belgium	Belgian Contact and Environmental Dermatology Group (BCEDG)
Chairperson:	Stefan Kerre Gijmelse Steenweg 16, 3200 Aarschot, Belgium
Secretary:	An Goossens Department of Dermatology – Contact Allergy Unit, University Hospital K.U. Leuven, 3000 Leuven, Belgium an.goossens@uz.kuleuven.ac.be
Brazil	Brazilian Contact Dermatitis Study Group
Chairperson:	Ida Duarte Rua Wanderley 1223/116, São Paulo, São Paolo CEP 05011-001, Brazil idaduarte@terra.com.br
Secretary:	Mario Cezar Pires Rua Caraibas 533/101, São Paulo, São Paolo CEP 05020-000, Brazil mapires@webcable.com.br
Czech Republic	Group for Dermatological Allergology and Occupational Dermatology
Chairperson:	Eliška Dastychová First Department of Dermatovenerology, Faculty Hospital St Anna, Pekařská 53, 656 91 Brno, Czech Republic eliska.dastychova@fnusa.cz
Secretary:	Dagmar Košťálová Dermatology private practice, Karlovarská 30, 301 00 Plzeň, Czech Republic
Denmark	Danish Contact Dermatitis Research Group
Chairperson:	Jeanne Duus Johansen National Allergy Research Center, Department of Dermatology-allergology, Gentofte Hospital, University of Copenhagen, 2900 Hellerup, Denmark jedu@geh.regionh.dk

Europe	European Environmental and Contact Dermatitis Research Group (EECDRG)
Chairperson:	Magnus Bruze Department of Occupational and Environmental Dermatology, University Hospital Malmo, 205 02 Malmo, Sweden magnus.bruze@derm.mas.lu.se
Secretary:	Tove Agner Department of Dermatology, Bispebjerg Hospital, Denmark t.agner@dadlnet.dk
European Society of Contact Dermatitis (ESCD)	
Chairperson:	An Goossens Deptartment of Dermatology – Contact Allergy Unit, University Hospital K.U., Leuven, 3000 Leuven, Belgium
Secretary:	Ana Giminez-Arnau Department of Dermatology, Hospital del Mar, IMAS, Universitat Autonome, Barcelona, Passeig Maritim 25–29, 08003 Barcelona, Spain 22505aga@comb.es
Finland	Finnish Contact Dermatitis Group
Chairperson:	Riita Jolanki Finnish Institute of Occupational Health (FIOH), Team of Control of Hypersensitivity Diseases, Topeliuksenkatu 41 a A, 00250 Helsinki, Finland riita.jolanka@ttl.fi
Secretary:	Arja Laukkanen Kuopio University Hospital (KUH), Department of Dermatology, P.O.Box 1777, 70211, Kuopio, Finland arja.laukkanen@kuh.fi
France	Groupe d'Etude et de Recherches en Dermato-Allergologie (GERDA)
Chairperson:	Martine Vigan Unité d'Allergologie, Dermatologie II, Center Hospitalier St Jacques, 19 Quai Vauban, 25030 Besançon cedex, France mvigan@chu-besancon.fr
Secretary:	Gilbert Jelen 92 Grande Rue, 67700 Saverne, France gilbert.jelen@wanadoo.fr
Germany	German Contact Dermatitis Research Group (DKG)
Chairperson:	Johannes Geier Information Network of Departments of Dermatology, University of Goettingen, von-Siebold-Str. 3, 37075 Goettingen, Germany jgeier@gwdg.de
Secretary:	Vera Mahler Department of Dermatology, University Hospital Erlangen, Hartmannstr. 14, 91052 Erlangen, Germany vera.mahler@uk-erlangen.de
Arbeitsgemeinschaft Berufs- und Umweltdermatologie (ABD)	
Chairperson:	Swen M. John Department of Dermatology, Environmental Medicine and Health Theory, University of Osnabrueck, Sedanstrasse 115, 49069 Osnabrück, Germany sjohn@uos.de
Secretary:	Thomas L. Diepgen Departmentof Social Medicine, Occupational and Environmental Dermatology, Thibaubstr. 3, 69115 Heidelberg, Germany thomas.diepgen@med.uni-heidelberg.de

(*continued*)

55

Hungary	Hungarian Contact Dermatitis Research Group
Chairman:	Erzsébet Temesvári Mária u 41, 1085 Budapest, Hungary temerz@bor.sote.hu
Secretary:	Valéria Kohánka OMFI. Nagyvárad tér 2, 1096 Budapest, Hungary kohankav@okk.antsz.hu

International Contact Dermatitis Research Group (ICDRG)

Chairperson:	Jean-Marie Lachapelle 26 Avenue de Vincennes, Montigny-le-Tilleul 6110, Belgium jean-marie.lachapelle@uclouvain.be
Secretary:	Peter Elsner Department of Dermatology and Allergy, Fridrich-Schiller University Jena, Erfurter Strasse 35, 07740 Jena, Germany elsner@derma-jena.de
Israel	Israeli Contact Dermatitis Society
Chairperson:	Akiva Trattner Department of Dermatology, Rabin Medical Center, Petah Tiqva 49100, Israel atrattner@clalit.org.il
Secretary:	Dani Slodownik Department of Dermatology, Hadassah University Hospital, Eim Kerem, Jerusalem, Israel gbds@netvision.net.il
Italy	Italian Society of Allergologic Occupational and Environmental Dermatology (SIDAPA)
Chairperson:	Antonella Tosti Department of Dermatology, University of Bologna, Via Massarenti 1, 40138 Bologna, Italy Antonella.tosti@unibo.it
Secretary:	Massimiliano Nino Via S Pansini 5, 80131 Napoli, Italy Massimilianonino@yahoo.it
Japan	Japanese Society for Dermatoallergology and Contact Dermatitis (JSDACD)
Chairperson:	Kayoko Matsunaga Department of Dermatology, Fujita Health University School of Medicine, 1-98 Dengakugakubo, Kutsukake-cho, Toyo-ake, Aichi 470-1192, Japan kamatsu@fujita-hu.ac.jp
Secretary:	Fukumi Furukawa Department of Dermatology, Wakayama Medical University, 8111-1 Kimiidera, Wakayama 641-0012, Japan dajs@wakayama-med.ac.jp
Korea	Korean Society for Contact Dermatitis and Skin Allergy
Chairperson:	Jun Young Lee Department of Dermatology, The Catholic University of Korea, Seoul, St Mary's Hospital, 505 Banpo-dong, Seocho-gu, Seoul 137-701, Korea jylee@catholic.ac.kr
Secretary:	Shin Jeong Hyun Department of Dermatology, Inha University Hospital, 7-206, Shinhung-dong Jung-gu, Incheon 400-711, Korea mikie2001@hanmail.net
Mexico	Mexican Group for Research on Contact Dermatitis and Professional Dermatoses

Chairperson:	Roberto Blancas-Espinosa Anaxágoras 963, Colonia del Valle, CP 03100 Mexico D.F., Mexico rblancase@hotmail.com
Secretary:	Alfredo Arévalo-López Peten 284 Colonia Narvarte, CP 03020 Mexico D.F., Mexico alfarelo@yahoo.com
The Netherlands	Dutch Eczema and Allergy Workingparty
Secretary:	Albert Wolkerstorfer, Department of Dermatology, AMC University of Amsterdam, Meibergdreef 35, 1105 AZ Amsterdam, The Netherlands a.wolkerstorfer@amc.uva.nl
North America	American Contact Dermatitis Society (ACDS)
Chairperson:	Suzanne Connolly Department of Dermatology, Mayo Clinic, Scottsdale, AZ 85259, USA
Secretary:	Glen Crawford Department of Dermatology, University of Pensylvania, Philadelphia, PA 19104, USA
Secretariat:	138 Palm Coast Parkway NE #333, Palm Coast, FL 32137, USA info@contactderm.org
North American Contact Dermatitis Group (NACDG)	
Chairperson:	Joseph F. Fowler, Jr 501 South second Street, Louisville, KY 40202, USA fowlerjoe@msn.com
Secretary:	Kathryn A. Zug Section of Dermatology, Dartmouth-Hitchcock Medical Center, Dartmouth Medical School, 1, Medical Center Drive, Lebanon, NH 03756, USA kzug@hitchcock.org
Poland	Allergology Section of the Polish Association of Dermatology
Chairperson:	Beate Krecisz Nofer Institute of Occupational Medicine, Teresy 8, 91-348 Lodz, Poland krecisz@imp.lodz.pl
Secretary:	Dorota Chomiczewska Nofer Institute of Occupational Medicine, Teresy 8, 91-348 Lodz, Poland krecisz@imp.lodz.pl
Portugal	Grupo Português de Estudo das Dermites de Contacto (GPEDC)
Chairperson:	Raquel Silva Serviço de Dermatologia, Hospital Santa Maria, Av. Prof. Egas Moniz, 1649-035 Lisboa, Portugal rpalminhas@netcabo.pt
Secretary:	Maria Raquel Santos Cerviço de Dermatologia, Hospital Curry Cabral, Rua da Beneficiênda 8, 1069-166, Lisboa, Portugal mrsantos@hccabral.min-saude.pt
Singapore	Environmental and Occupational Dermatology Society (EODS)
Chairperson:	Leow Yung Hian National Skin Center, 1 Mandalay Road, Singapore 308205, Republic of Singapore yhleow@nsc.gov.sg
Secretary:	Kenneth Choy Block C, 120 Kim Seng Road, Singapore 239436, Republic of Singapore kennethchoy@mom.gov.sg
South America	South American Contact Dermatitis Research Group (DERMOSUR)

(continued)

55

Chairperson:	Aliche Alchorne Rua Iraúna 469, Jardim Novo Mundo, SP 04518-060 Sao Paulo, Brasil
Secretary:	S. Iris Ale Arazatí 1194, PC 11300 Montevideo, Uruguay
Spain	Spanish Contact Dermatitis Group (GEIDAC)
Secretary:	Esther Serra Baldrich Department of Dermatology, Hospital de Ant Pau, Av Sant Antoni Maria Claret 167, 08025 Barcelona, Spain essera@santpau.cat
Sweden	Swedish Contact Dermatitis Research Group (SCDRG)
Chairperson:	Marléne Isaksson Department of Occupational and Environmental Dermatology, Lund University, Malmö University Hospital, Malmö 205 02, Sweden marlene.isaksson@skane.se; marlene.isaksson@med.lu.se
Secretary:	Mihaly Matura Unit of Occupational and Environmental Dermatology, Institute of Environmental Medicine, Karolinska Institute, Norrbacka, Stockholm 17176, Sweden mihaly.matura@ki.se
Switzerland	Swiss Contact Dermatitis Research Group (SCDRG)
Chairperson:	Dagmar Simon Department of Dermatology, Inselspital, Bern University Hospital, 3010 Bern, Switzerland dagmar.simon@insel.ch
Secretary:	Rita Sigg Falkenstrasse 3, 6004 Luzern, Switzerland siggrita@bluewin.ch
United Kingdom	British Contact Dermatitis Society (BCDS)
Chairperson:	Mark Wilkinson Department of Dermatology Leeds General Infirmary, Great George Street, Leeds, West Yorkshire LS1 3EX, UK mark.wilkinson@@leedsth.nhs.uk
Secretary:	David Orton Department of Dermatology and Allergy, Amersham Hospital, Whielden Street, Amersham, Buckinghamshire HP7 0JD, UK david.orton@buckshosp.nhs.uk

Patch Test Concentrations and Vehicles for Testing Contact Allergens

56

Anton C. De Groot and Peter J. Frosch

Contents

Patch testing is a safe and fairly reliable method for identifying contact allergens in patients with contact dermatitis. The technique of patch testing is described in Chap. 24. All patients are tested with the European baseline series [1], containing the most frequent contact allergens in European countries (Table 56.1). Often, standard series patch testing is not enough, and additional allergens or potential allergens need to be tested, based on the patient's history and clinical examination. Examples are products and chemicals to which the patient is exposed occupationally or in his/her home environment. Test series containing the most frequent allergens in certain products (preservatives, fragrances, dental materials, plastics and glues, medicaments) or certain occupations (hairdressing, pesticides, oil and cooling fluid) are very helpful. Approximately, 560 patch test materials are commercially available from Almirall Hermal GmbH (Scholtzstrasse 3, 21462 Reinbek, Germany, (www.almirall.de), Chemotechnique Diagnostics (Modemgatan 9, 235 39, Vellinge, Sweden, www.chemotechnique.se) and Brial Allergen GmbH (Bövemannstrasse 8, 48268 Greven, Germany, www.brial.com; for Canada and the US: www. allergeaze.com).

For other chemicals and products, the investigator must decide how to apply them as a patch test. Chemicals usually need to be diluted, and it is of utmost importance to use an appropriate patch test concentration and vehicle to avoid both false-negative and false-positive (irritant) reactions. The most useful reference source for documented test concentrations and vehicles of chemicals, groups of chemicals, and products is the book *Patch Testing* [2]. Other useful lists are provided in recent textbooks on contact dermatitis [3, 4].

Guidelines for testing the patient's own contact materials are provided in Chap. 57.

A.C. De Groot (✉)
acdegroot publishing, Schipslootweg 5,
8351 HV Wapserveen, The Netherlands
e-mail: antondegroot@planet.nl

P.J. Frosch
Hautklinik, Klinikum Dortmund gGmbH,
Beurhausstr. 40, D-44137 Dortmund, Germany
e-mail: peter.frosch@klinikumdo.de

J.D. Johansen et al. (eds.), *Contact Dermatitis*,
DOI: 10.1007/978-3-642-03827-3_56, © Springer-Verlag Berlin Heidelberg 2011

56

Table 56.2 lists alphabetically all the chemicals mentioned in this book for which test concentrations and vehicles were suggested by various authors. In addition, all commercially available allergens are also listed with their supplier(s), their test concentrations, and vehicles as supplied. It should be appreciated that for a considerable number of allergens, the concentrations vary between suppliers. Table 56.3 provides a list of test concentrations for *groups* of chemicals as suggested by various authors in this book. Table 56.4 finally is an alphabetical listing of commonly used abbreviations and their full chemical synonyms.

Table 56.1 The European baseline [1]

Chemical	Concentration % (w/w) and vehicle	Concentration in mg/cm^{2a}
Metals		
Cobalt chloride	1% pet.	0.4
Nickel sulfate	5% pet.	2.0
Potassium dichromate	0.5% pet.	0.2
Rubber chemicals		
Thiuram mix	1% pet.	0.4
Dipentamethylenethiuram disulfide (0.25%)		0.1
Tetramethylthiuram disulfide (0.25%)		0.1
Tetraethylthiuram disulfide (0.25%)		0.1
Tetramethylthiuram monosulfide (0.25%)		0.1
N-Isopropyl-*N*'-phenyl-*p*-phenylenediamine	0.1% pet.	0.04
Mercapto mix	2% pet.	0.8
N-Cyclohexylbenzothiazyl sulfenamide (0.5%)		0.2
Dibenzothiazyl disulfide (0.5%)		0.2
Mercaptobenzothiazole (0.5%)		0.2
Morpholinyl mercaptobenzothiazole (0.5%)		0.2
Mercaptobenzothiazole	2% pet.	0.8
Medicaments		
Budesonide	0.01% pet.	0.004
Benzocaine	5% pet.	2.0
Neomycin sulfate	20% pet.	8.0
Clioquinol	5% pet.	2.0
Tixocortol pivalate	0.1% pet.	0.04
Cosmetic ingredients		
Myroxylon pereirae (balsam of Peru)	25% pet.	10.0
Methylchloroisothiazolinone, methylisothiazolinone	0.01% aq.	0.003
Colophonium (rosin)	20% pet.	8.0

Table 56.1 (continued)

Chemical	Concentration % (w/w) and vehicle	Concentration in mg/cm^{2a}
Formaldehyde	1% aq.	0.3
Fragrance mix I (including 5% sorbitan sesquioleate)	8% pet.	3.2
α-Amylcinnamaldehyde (1%)		0.4
Cinnamal(dehyde) (1%)		0.4
Cinnamyl alcohol (1%)		0.4
Eugenol (1%)		0.4
Geraniol (1%)		0.4
Hydroxycitronellal (1%)		0.4
Isoeugenol (1%)		0.4
Evernia prunastri (oakmoss absolute) (1%)		0.4
Fragrance mix 2	14% pet.	5.6
Citral (1%)		0.4
Citronellol (0.5%)		0.2
Coumarin (2.5%)		1.0
Farnesol (2.5%)		1.0
α-Hexylcinnamaldehyde (5%)		2.0
Hydroxyisohexyl 3-cyclohexene carboxaldehyde (2.5%)		1.0
Methyldibromo glutaronitrile	0.5% pet.	0.2
Paraben mix	16% pet.	6.4
Butylparaben (4%)		1.6
Ethylparaben (4%)		1.6
Methylparaben (4%)		1.6
Propylparaben (4%)		1.6
p-Phenylenediamine base	1% pet.	0.4
Quaternium-15	1% pet.	0.4
Wool wax alcohols (lanolin alcohol)	30% pet.	12.0
Hydroxyisohexyl 3-cyclohexene carboxaldehyde (Lyral®)	5% pet.	2.0
Miscellaneous		
p-tert-Butylphenol formaldehyde resin	1% pet.	0.4
Epoxy resin	1% pet.	0.4
Primin	0.01% pet.	0.004
Sesquiterpene lactone mix	0.1% pet.	0.04
Alantolactone (0.033%)		0.013
Dehydrocostus lactone and Costunolide (0.067%)		0.027

[a]Calculations based on the use of the Finn chamber (diameter 0.8 cm) technique with the application of 20 mg pet. preparation or where appropriate (in water) 15 μL aqueous test solution (1)

Table 56.2 Test concentrations, vehicles, and commercial availability of contact allergens

Allergen	Test concentration and vehicle Listed in this book	Suppliers Almirall	Chemo	Brial
Abietic acid (icr)	10% pet.	+	+	+
Acebutolol hydrochloride				2% pet.
Aceclofenac	1% pet.			
Acetaminophen (paracetamol) (de)	10% pet.		+	+
Acetyl cysteine	10% aq.			
Acetylsalicylic acid (icr)	10% pet.		+	+
Achillea millefolium (yarrow extract)	1% pet.		+	
Acid black 48 (CI 65005)	1% pet.			
Acid blue 3 (CI 42051)				0.25% coca/glyc.
Acid red 14 (azorubine)				0.1% alc.
Acid red 118 (CI 26410)	5% pet.		+	
Acid red 359	5% pet.		+	
Acid violet 17 (CI 42650)	1% pet.			
Acid yellow 36 (CI 13065, metanil yellow)	1% pet.	+	+	+
Acid yellow 61 (CI 18968)			5% pet.	
Acyclovir (fde)	5–10% pet.		10% pet.	
Alantolactone (icr)	0.1% pet.		0.33% pet.	
Alclometasone-17, 21-dipropionate	1% alc.		1% pet.	
Alcohol, ethyl (icr)	10% aq.			
Algin (sodium alginate)				1% coca
Alimemazine tartrate	See trimeprazine tartrate			
Aluminium chloride hexahydrate	2–10% pet.		2% pet.	
Aluminium hydroxide				10% pet.
Allylisopropylacetylurea	See apronalide			
Amalgam		5% pet.		
Amalgam alloying metals	20% pet.	+		+
Amalgam non gamma 2				5% pet.
Amaranth				0.1% coca/glyc.
Amcinonide	1% alc.	0.1% pet.		0.1% pet.
Amerchol® L-101	See lanolin alcohol and paraffinum liquidum			
Amethocaine	see tetracaine			
Amikacin sulfate	20% pet.			
p-Aminoazobenzene (solvent yellow 1,CI 11000)	0.25–1% pet.	1% pet.	0.25% pet.	1% pet.
ε-Aminocaproic acid	1% aq.			

Table 56.2 (continued)

Allergen	Test concentration and vehicle	Suppliers		
	Listed in this book	Almirall	Chemo	Brial
Amino-4-*N*,*N*-diethylaniline sulfate (TSS Agfa®)			1% pet.	
2-2(Aminoethoxy)ethanol	See diglycolamine			
Amino-4-*N*-ethyl-*N*-(methanesulfon-aminoethyl)-*m*-toluidine (CD 3)		1% pet.	1% pet.	
δ-Aminolevulinic acid	20% pet.			
m-Aminophenol	1% pet.	+	+	+
p-Aminophenol (CI 76550) (icr)	1% pet.	+	+	+
Amlexanox (fde)	1% pet.			
Ammoniated mercury	1% pet.	+		+
Ammonium bituminosulfonate	See ichthammol			
Ammonium heptamolybdate				1% aq.
Ammonium hexachloroplatinate (icr)	0.1% aq.		+	
Ammonium persulfate (icr)	2.5% pet.	+	+	+
Ammonium tetrachloroplatinate (icr)	0.25% pet.	+		+
Ammonium thioglycolate	1% pet, fresh/2,5% aq.		2.5% aq.	1% pet.
Amorolfine	1% pet.			
Amoxicillin trihydrate (de)	10% pet.		+	
Ampicillin (icr)	5% pet.		+	+
Amprolium hydrochloride	10% aq.			
α-Amylcinnamic alcohol	5% pet.	1% pet.	+	
α-Amylcinnamaldehyde (icr)	1% pet.	+	2% pet.	+
Amylocaine hydrochloride	5% pet.		+	
Anethole			5% pet.	
Aniline				1% pet.
Anisyl alcohol	10% pet.	1% pet.	10% Softisan	
Antazoline	1% pet.			
Anthemis nobilis (*Chamomilla romana*)	1–2.5% pet.		1% pet.	
Apraclonidine	1% aq.			
Arnica montana (arnica extract)	0.5% pet.		+	
Arsanilic acid	10% pet.			
Aspartame				0.1% coca
Atranorin (ph)			0.1% pet.	
Atropine sulfate	1% pet.	1% aq.		1% aq.
Azathioprine	1% pet.			

(continued)

Table 56.2 (continued)

Allergen	Test concentration and vehicle	Suppliers		
	Listed in this book	Almirall	Chemo	Brial
Azidamfenicol	2% pet.			
Azodiisobutyrodinitrile			1% pet.	
Azorubine	See acid red 14			
Bacitracin (icr)	20% pet.	+	5% pet.	+
Bacitracin zinc	20% pet.			
Balsam of Peru	See *Myroxylon pereirae*			
Balsam of Tolu	See *Myroxylon toluiferum*			
Basic brown 1	See Bismarck brown R			
Basic red 46			1% pet.	
Beech tar	See *Fagus sylvatica*			
Befunolol	1% aq.			
Benomyl	0.1–1% pet.			
Benoxinate	See oxybuprocaine			
Benzaldehyde (icr)	5% pet.	+		+
Benzalkonium chloride (BAK)	0.01–0.1% aq.	0.1% pet.	0.1% aq.	0.1% pet.
Benzamine lactate	1% pet.			
2-Benzimidazolethiol (2-mercaptobenzimidazole)			1% pet.	
Benzisothiazolinone (BIT) (ph)	0.1% pet.	+	0.05% pet.	+
Benzocaine (icr) (ph)	5% pet.	+	+	+
Benzoic acid (icr) (ph)			5% pet.	5% pet. and 1% alc./glyc.
Benzoin resin	See *Styrax benzoin*			
Benzophenone-3 (oxybenzone) (ph)	10% pet.	+	+	+ and 3% pet.
Benzophenone-4 (sulisobenzone) (ph) (icr)	2% pet.	10% pet.	2% pet.	10% pet.
Benzophenone-10 (mexenone) (ph)	10% pet.		+	
IH-Benzotriazole	1% pet.	+	+	+
Benzoyl peroxide (icr)	1% pet.	+	+	+
Benzydamine hydrochloride (ph)	1–5% pet. or 5% aq.			
Benzyl alcohol (icr)	10% pet.	1% pet.	+	1% pet.
Benzyl benzoate	10% pet.	1% pet.	+	5% pet.
Benzyl cinnamate	10% pet.	5% pet.	+	
Benzylhemiformal	1% pet.	+		+
Benzyl salicylate	10% pet.	1% pet.	+	1% pet.
Bergamot oil	see *Citrus bergamia*			
Beryllium chloride or sulfate	1% pet.			
Betamethasone dipropionate	1% alc.			

Table 56.2 (continued)

Allergen	Test concentration and vehicle	Suppliers		
	Listed in this book	Almirall	Chemo	Brial
Betamethasone-17-valerate	1% alc.	0.12% pet.	1% pet.	0.12% pet.
Betaxolol hydrochloride	1% aq.			
Betula alba (birch tar)			3% pet.	
BHA (butylated hydroxyanisole) (icr)	2% pet.	+	+	+ and 2% alc.
BHT (butylated hydroxytoluene) (icr)	2% pet.	+	+	+ and 1% alc.
Bifonazole	1% alc.			
Bioban® CS-1135	1% pet.		+	+
Bioban® CS-1246	1% pet.	+	+	+
Bioban® P 1487	1% pet.	+	0.5% pet.	+
Bis(aminopropyl)-lauramine	0.01–0.1–1% aq.			
Bis(dibutyldithiocarbamato) zinc	See zinc dibutyldithiocarbamate			
Bis(diethyldithiocarbamato) zinc	See zinc diethyldithiocarbamate			
BIS-EMA	2% pet.		1% pet.	
BIS-GMA	2% pet.	+	+	+
BIS-MA	2% pet.		+	
Bismarck brown (vesuvine brown, basic brown 1, CI 21000)	0.5% pet.	+		+
Bismuth oxide	5% pet.			
Bisphenol A	See 4,4′-Isopropylidenediphenol			
Bisphenol A dimethacrylate				2% pet.
Bithionol (ph) (icr)	1% pet.	+	+	+
Black rubber mix (*N*-Isopropyl-*N*-phenyl-*p*-phenylenediamine, *N*-cyclohexyl-*N*-phenyl-*p*-phenylenediamine, *N,N*-diphenyl-*p*-phenylenediamine)			0.25% pet.	0.6%
Boric acid	10% pet.			
Brilliant black				0.1% coca/glyc.
Brimonidine	0.2% aq.			
5-Bromo-4′-chlorosalicylanilide (ph)		1% pet.		
2-Bromo-2-nitropropane-1,3-diol (icr)		0.5% pet.	0.25% pet.	0.25 and 0.5% pet.
Budesonide	0.1% pet.	+	0.01% pet.	+ and 0.01%
Bufexamac	5% pet.	+		+
Bupivacaine	1% pet.			
Butacaine	5% pet.			
1,4-Butanediol diacrylate (BUDA)	0.1% pet.		+	

(*continued*)

Table 56.2 (continued)

56

Allergen	Test concentration and vehicle	Suppliers		
	Listed in this book	Almirall	Chemo	Brial
1,4-Butanediol diglycidyl ether	0.25% pet.	+	+	
1,4-Butanediol dimethacrylate (BUDMA)	2% pet.		+	+
Butethamine hydrochloride	5% pet.			
Butyl acrylate (BA)	0.1% pet.		+	+
Butyl aminobenzoate	5% pet.			
Butylated hydroxyanisole	see BHA			
Butylated hydroxytoluene	see BHT			
4-*tert*-Butylbenzoic acid			1% pet.	
p-tert-Butylcatechol (PTBC)	0.25% pet.	+	+	1% pet.
Butyl glycidyl ether	0.25% pet.			
t-Butyl hydroquinone	1% pet.	+	+	+
n-Butyl methacrylate (BMA)	2% pet.		+	
Butyl methoxydibenzoylmethane (ph)	10% pet.	+	+	+
p-tert-Butyl-α-methylhydrocinnamic aldehyde (butylphenyl methyl propional, Lilial)	10% pet	+	+	
Butylparaben (icr)	3% pet.	+	+	+
p-tert-Butylphenol	1% pet.	+	+	+
p-tert-Butylphenolformaldehyde resin (PTBP)	1% pet.	+	+	+
Butylphenyl glycidyl ether	0.25% pet.			
Butylphenyl methyl propional	See *p-tert*-Butyl-α-methylhydrocinnamic aldehyde			
Cadmium chloride (ph)	0.5–1% pet.			0.5% pet.
Caine mix I (procaine hydrochloride, dibucaine hydrochoride)			3.5% pet.	
Caine mix II (dibucaine hydrochloride, lidocaine, tetracaine)			10% pet.	
Caine mix III (benzocaine, dibucaine, tetracaine)			10% pet.	7 and 10% pet.
Caine mix IV (amylocaine, lidocaine, prilocaine)			10% pet.	
Calcipotriol	2 µg/mL alc.			
Calcitriol	2 µg/mL alc.			
Camphor (icr)				1% pet.
Camphoroquinone			1% pet.	
Cananga odorata (cananga oil, ylang-ylang oil)		10% pet.	2% pet.	2% pet.

Table 56.2 (continued)

Allergen	Test concentration and vehicle	Suppliers		
	Listed in this book	Almirall	Chemo	Brial
Captan	0.25–0.5% aq. or pet.		0.5% pet.	
Captopril (de)	5% pet.		+	
˟Carbamazepine (de) (fde) (phde)	1% pet.		+	
Carba mix (N,N-diphenylguanidine, zinc dibutyl dithiocarbamate, zinc diethyldithiocarbamate)			3% pet.	3% pet.
Carmine				0.5% coca/glyc.
Carprofen	5% pet.			
Carteolol	1% aq.			
Carvone	5% pet.		+	+
Castor oil	pure			
CD 2 (color developer 2)	See methyl-3-amino-4-N, N-diethyl-aniline			
CD 3 (color developer 3)	See amino-4-N-ethyl-N(methanesulfon-aminoethyl)-m-toluidine			
CD 4 (color developer 4)	See 4-(N-Ethyl-N-2-hydroxyethyl)-2-methyl-phenylenediamine sulfate			
Cedarwood oil	See *Cedrus atlantica*			
Cedrus atlantica (cedarwood oil) (ph)	10% pet.	+		+
Cephalexin (de)			10% pet.	
Cephotaxim sodium salt (de)			10% pet.	
Cephradine (de)			10% pet.	
Cetalkonium chloride		0.1% pet.		0.1% pet.
Cetrimide	See Cetrimonium bromide			
Cetrimonium bromide (Cetrimide)	0.25% pet.			
Cetyl alcohol (icr)	5% pet.		+	
Cetyl alcohol, stearyl alcohol	20% pet.	+	+	+
Cetylpyridinium chloride	0.1% pet.	+		+
Chamomilla romana	See *Anthemis nobilis*			
Chlorambucil	2% pet.			
Chloramine-T (icr)	0.05% aq.			
Chloramphenicol (icr)		5% pet.	5% pet.	10% pet.
Chlorhexidine diacetate (ph, icr)	0.5% aq.		+	
Chlorhexidine digluconate (ph) (icr)	0.5% aq.	+	+	+
Chloroacetamide	0.2% pet.	+	+	+
p-Chloro-m-cresol (PCMX) (icr)	1% pet.	+	+	+
5-Chloro-2-methyl-4-isothiazolin-3-one	0.01–0.02% aq.			

(continued)

Table 56.2 (continued)

Allergen	Test concentration and vehicle	Suppliers		
	Listed in this book	Almirall	Chemo	Brial
Chlorothalonil (icr)	0.001–0.01% acet.			
Chloroxylenol	1% pet.	+	0.5% pet.	+
Chlorphenesin	1% pet.			
Chlorpheniramine maleate	5% pet.			+
Chlorpromazine hydrochloride (phde) (icr)	0.1% pet.		+	1% pet.
Chlorquinaldol (ph)	5% pet.	+	+	+
Chlortetracycline hydrochloride	5% pet.			1% pet.
Chromic chloride				1% pet.
Chromic potassium sulfate				2% aq.
Chromic sulfate				0.5% pet.
Cinchocaine®	See dibucaine hydrochloride			
Cinnamal (cinnamic aldehyde) (ph) (icr)	1% pet.	+	2% pet.	+
Cinnamonum cassia (cinnamon oil) (ph)(icr)				0.5% pet.
Cinnamyl alcohol	1–5% pet.	1% pet.	2% pet.	1% pet.
Cinnoxicam	1% pet.			
Ciprofloxacin (fde)			10% pet.	
Citral	2% pet.	+	+	
Citronellal				2% pet.
Citronellol	1% pet.	+	+	
Citrus aurantium dulcis (neroli oil) (ph)	2% pet.	+		+
Citrus bergamia (bergamot oil) (ph)				2% pet.
Citrus dulcis (orange oil) (ph)		2% pet.		
Citrus limonum (lemon oil) (ph)		2% pet.		2% pet.
Clioquinol (icr)	5% pet.	+	+	+
Clarithromycin (fde)			10% pet.	
Clindamycin phosphate (de)	1% aq.		10% pet.	
Clobetasol-17-propionate (icr)	1% alc.	0.25% pet.	1% pet.	0.25 and 1% pet.
Clobetasone butyrate	1% alc.			
Clonidine	1% pet.			
Cloprednol	1% alc.			
Clotrimazole	1% alc.	5% pet.		5% pet.
Clove oil	See *Eugenia caryophyllus*			
Coal tar	See Pix ex carbone			

Table 56.2 (continued)

Allergen	Test concentration and vehicle	Suppliers		
	Listed in this book	Almirall	Chemo	Brial
Cobalt chloride (ph) (icr)	1% pet.	+	+	+
Cobaltous sulfate (ph)				2.5% pet.
Cocamide DEA	0.5% pet.	+	+	+
Cocamidopropyl betaine	1% aq.	+	+	+
Cochenille red				1% coca/glyc.
Cold cream				pure
Colophonium (rosin) (ph) (icr)	20% pet.	+	+	+
Compositae mix (*Tanacetum vulgare, Arnica montana, parthenolide, Chamomilla romana, Achillea millefolium*)	5–6% pet.		5% pet.	6% pet.
Copper sulfate	See cupric sulfate			
Corticosteroid mix (budesonide, tixocortol pivalate, hydrocortisone-17-butyrate)			2.1% pet.	
Cotrimoxazole (de)			10% pet.	
Coumarin (ph)	5% pet.	+	+	1% pet.
p-Cresol	1% aq.			
Cresyl glycidyl ether (icr)	0.25% pet.	+		+
Croconazole	1% alc.			
Cromoglycate sodium	See cromolyn			
Cromolyn (cromoglycate sodium) (icr)	2% aq.			2% pet.
Crotamiton	3% pet.			
Cupric sulfate (copper sulfate) (icr)	2% pet.	1% aq.	2% pet.	1% aq. and 2% pet.
Cyclohexanone resin			1% pet.	
Cycloheximide	1% pet.			
N-Cyclohexylbenzothiazyl sulfenamide (CBS)	1% pet.	+	+	+
N-Cyclohexyl-*N*-phenyl-*p*-phenylene-diamine (CPPD)			1% pet.	
Cyclohexyl thiophthalimide	1% pet.	0.5% pet.	+	+
Cyclomethycaine hydrochloride	1% pet.			
Cyclopentolate hydrochloride	0.5% aq.			
Cymbopogon schoenanthus (lemon grass oil) (ph)		2% pet.		2% pet.
Cysteamine hydrochloride	0.5% pet.			
Dandelion	See *Taraxacum officinale*			

(continued)

Table 56.2 (continued)

Allergen	Test concentration and vehicle	Suppliers		
	Listed in this book	Almirall	Chemo	Brial
Dazomet	0.1% pet. or 0.25% aq.			
Decyl glucoside				5% pet.
Dermatophagoides mix			30% pet.	
Desketoprofen	1% pet.			
Desonide	1% alc.			
Desoxymethasone (ph)	1% alc.			1% pet.
Dexamethasone				0.5% pet.
Dexamethasone acetate	1% alc.			
Dexamethasone phosphate	1% alc.			
Dexamethasone 21-phosphate disodium salt			1% pet.	
Dexpanthenol	See panthenol			
Dialkyl thiourea mix (diethyl thiourea, dibutyl thiourea)			1% pet.	
Diallyl disulfide			1% pet.	
4,4′-Diaminodiphenylmethane (ph)	0.5% pet.	+	+	+
Diazolidinyl urea	2% pet.	+	+	+ and 1% pet. and 1% aq.
Dibenzothiazyl disulfide (MBTS)	1% pet.	+	+	+
Dibenzthione (sulbentine)	3% pet.			
1,2-Dibromo-2,4-dicyanobutane	See methyldibromo glutaronitrile			
Dibromosalicylanilide (ph)	1% pet.			
Dibucaine hydrochloride (Cinchocaine®) (ph)	5% pet.	+	+	+ and 2.5% pet.
Dibutyl phthalate		5% pet.	5% pet.	5% pet.
Dibutylthiourea	1% pet.	+	+	+
Dibutyl- and diethylthiourea mix			1% pet.	
Dichlorophene (ph)	0.5% pet./1% aq.	0.5% pet.	1% pet.	0.5% pet.
Diclofenac sodium (ph)	1–5% pet.		1% pet.	5% pet.
Dicloxacillin sodium salt hydrate (de)			10% pet.	
Diethanolamine	2% pet.	+		+
2-(4-Diethylamino-2-hydroxybenzoyl)-benzoic acid hexylester (Uvinul® A+)			10% pet.	
Diethyleneglycol diacrylate (DEGDA)	0.1% pet.		+	
Diethylenetriamine (DETA)	1% pet.	0.5% pet.	+	
Diethylhexyl butamido triazone (Uvasorb® HEB)		10% pet.		
Di-2-ethylhexyl phthalate (DEHP)	See dioctyl phthalate			
Diethyl phthalate				5% pet.

Table 56.2 (continued)

Allergen	Test concentration and vehicle	Suppliers		
	Listed in this book	Almirall	Chemo	Brial
Diethylstilbestrol	1% pet.			
Diethylthiourea	1% pet.		+	
Diflorasone diacetate	1% alc.			
Diflucortolone pivalate	1% alc.			
Diglycolamine (2-(2-aminoethoxyethanol)	1% pet.	+		
Dihydrostreptomycin	0.1% pet.			
4,4′-Dihydroxydiphenyl		0.1% pet.		0.1% pet.
Diltiazem hydrochloride (de)			10% pet.	
N,N-Dimethylaminoethyl methacrylate			0.2% pet.	
Dimethylaminopropylamine			1% aq.	1% aq. and 1% pet.
Dimethyl dihydroxyethyleneurea			4.5% aq.	4.5% aq.
Dimethyl fumarate	0.01–0.1% pet.			
Dimethylol dihydroxyethyleneurea	4.5% aq./10% pet.			5% aq.
Dimethylol dihydroxyethyleneurea, modified				5% aq.
4,4-Dimethyloxazolidine/ 3,4,4,trimethyl-oxazolidine	See Bioban® CS-1135			
Dimethyl phthalate	5% pet.	+		+
Dimethylol propylene urea	10% pet.	5% aq.		
N,N-Dimethyl-p-toluidine		2% pet.	5% pet.	2% pet.
N,N-Di-β-naphthyl-p-phenylenediamine (DBNPD)			1% pet.	
2,4-Dinitrochlorobenzene (DNCB) (icr)	0.01–0.1% aq. or acet.			
Dioctyl phthalate (di-2-ethylhexyl phthalate) (icr)		5% pet.	2% pet.	5% pet.
Dipentamethylenethiuram disulfide		0.25% pet.	1% pet.	0.25% pet.
Dipentamethylenethiuram tetrasulfide				0.25% pet.
Dipentene (d-limonene)	10% pet.	2% pet.	+	3% pet.
Diphenhydramine hydrochloride (ph)	1% pet.		+	
1,3-Diphenylguanidine (DPG) (icr)	1% pet.	+	+	+
Diphenylmethane 4,4-diisocyanate (MDI) (icr)			2% pet.	1% pet.
N,N′-Diphenyl-p-phenylenediamine (DPPD)		0.25% pet.	1% pet.	0.25% pet.
Diphenylthiourea (DPTU)	1% pet.	+	+	+
Dipivalyl epinephrine hydrochloride	1% aq.			
Dipyrone (metamizol) (fde) (icr)				1% pet.

(continued)

Table 56.2 (continued)

Allergen	Test concentration and vehicle	Suppliers		
	Listed in this book	Almirall	Chemo	Brial
Direct black 38 (CI 30235)	1% pet.			
Direct orange 34 (CI 40215)			5% pet.	
Disodium EDTA (edetic acid disodium salt)		1% pet.	1% pet.	1% pet.
Disodium phenyl dibenzimidazoletetra-sulfonate (Neoheliopan AP)			10% pet.	
Disperse black 1 (CI 11365)	1% pet.			
Disperse black 2 (CI 11255)	1% pet.			
Disperse blue 1 (CI 64500)	1% pet.			+
Disperse blue 3 (CI 61505)	1% pet.	+	+	+
Disperse blue 7 (CI 62500)	1% pet.			
Disperse blue 26 (CI 63305)	1% pet.			
Disperse blue 35 (ph)	1% pet.		+	
Disperse blue 85 (CI 11370)	1% pet.		+	
Disperse blue 102	1% pet.			
Disperse blue 106 (CI 111935)	1% pet.	0.3% pet.	+	+
Disperse blue 124	1% pet.	0.3% pet.	+	
Disperse blue 153	1% pet.		+	
Disperse blue mix (124/106)	1% pet.		+	+
Disperse brown 1 (CI 11153)	1% pet.		+	
Disperse orange 1 (CI 11080)	1% pet.		+	
Disperse orange 3 (CI 11005)	1% pet.	+	+	+
Disperse orange 13 (CI 26080)	1% pet.			
Disperse orange 76	1% pet.			
Disperse red 1 (CI 11110)	1% pet.	+	+	+
Disperse red 11 (CI 62015)	1% pet.	+		+
Disperse red 17 (CI 11210)	1% pet.	+	+	+
Disperse red 153	1% pet.			
Disperse yellow 1 (CI 10345)	1% pet.			
Disperse yellow 3 (CI 11855)	1% pet.	+	+	+
Disperse yellow 9 (CI 10375)	1% pet.	+	+	+
Disperse yellow 27	1% pet.			
Disperse yellow 39	1% pet.			
Disperse yellow 49	1% pet.			
Disperse yellow 54 (CI 47020)	1% pet.			
Disperse yellow 64 (CI 47023)	1% pet.			
Dithiocarbamate				2% pet.

56

Table 56.2 (continued)

Allergen	Test concentration and vehicle		Suppliers		
	Listed in this book	Almirall	Chemo	Brial	
4,4'-Dithiodimorpholine	1% pet.		+	+	
Dithranol	0.02% pet.				
Diurethane dimethacrylate		2% pet.		2% pet.	
DMDM hydantoin	2% aq.	+	+	+	
Dodecyl dimethyl ammonium chloride (quaternium-12)	0.01–0.1–0.5–1% aq.				
Dodecyl gallate (lauryl gallate)		0.3% pet.	0.25% pet.	0.3% pet.	
Dodecyl mercaptan	0.1% pet.		+	+	
Dorzolamide	5% aq.				
Doxepin	5% pet.				
Doxycycline (phde) (fde)	10% pet.		+ (monohy- drate)		
Drometrizole (2-(2'-hydroxy-5'-methyl-phenyl)benzotriazole)	1% pet.		+		
Drometrizole trisiloxane (ph)			10% pet.		
Echothiophate iodine	1% aq.				
Econazole nitrate	1% alc.				
Edetic acid disodium salt	See disodium EDTA				
Enilconazole	1% alc.				
Eosine (ph)			5% pet.	50% pet.	
Ephedrine hydrochloride (de)	10% pet.				
Epichlorohydrin	0.1% pet.				
Epinephrine	1% aq.				
Epoxy acrylate			0.5% pet.		
Epoxy resin (icr)	1% pet.	+	+	+	
Epoxy resin, bisphenol F	0.25% pet.		+.	+ and 1% pet.	
Epoxy resin, cycloaliphatic			0.5% pet.		
Erythromycin (base and salts) (de)	1 and 10% pet.	10% pet.	1% pet.		
Erythrosine (ph)				0.25% pet. and alc./glyc.	
Estradiol	2% alc.				
Ethacridine lactate monohydrate (Rivanol®)	2% pet.				
Ethanolamine (monoethanolamine)	2% pet.	+		+	
Ethoxyquin (ph)	1% pet.		0.5% pet.		
Ethyl acrylate (EA)	0.1% pet.		+	+	
Ethyl alcohol (icr)	10% aq.-pure				

(*continued*)

Table 56.2 (continued)

Allergen	Test concentration and vehicle	Suppliers		
	Listed in this book	Almirall	Chemo	Brial
7-Ethylbicyclooxazolidine	See Bioban® CS-1246			
Ethyl cyanoacrylate (ECA)			10% pet.	
Ethylenediamine dihydrochloride (ph) (icr)	1% pet.	+	+	+
Ethyleneglycol dimethacrylate (EGDMA)	2% pet.	+	+	+
Ethylene urea	See 2-imidazolidinone			
Ethyleneurea + melamine-formaldehyde	5% pet.		+	+
2-Ethylhexyl acrylate (EHA)	0.1% pet.		+	+
2-Ethylhexyl-*p*-dimethylaminobenzoate	See octyl dimethyl PABA			
2-Ethylhexyl-*p*-methoxycinnamate	See octyl methoxycinnamate			
bis-Ethylhexyloxyphenyl methoxyphenyl triazine (Tinosorb® S)			10% pet.	
4-(*N*-Ethyl-*N*-2-hydroxyethyl)-2-methyl-phenylenediamine sulfate (CD 4)		1% pet.	1% pet.	
Ethyl methacrylate (EMA)	2% pet.		+	
Ethylparaben (icr)	3% pet.	+	+	+
Ethyl sebacate	2% alc.			
N-Ethyl-4-toluenesulfonamide	0.1% pet.			
Etofenamate (icr) (ph)	2% pet.			
Eucalyptus globulus (eucalyptus oil)		2% pet.		2% pet.
Eucerin, anhydrous (lanolin)	pure			pure
Eugenia caryophyllus (clove oil)		2% pet.		2% pet.
Eugenol (icr) (ph)	1–2% pet.	1% pet.	2% pet.	1% pet.
Euxyl® K 400	See methyldibromoglutaronitrile and phenoxyethanol			
Evernia furfuracea (tree moss)	1% pet.	+	+	
Evernia prunastri (oak moss absolute) (ph)	1% pet.	+	+	+
Evernic acid (ph)			0.1% pet.	
Fagus sylvatica (beech tar)			3% pet.	
Famciclovir	10% aq.			
Farnesol	5% pet.	+	+	
Fenoprofen	5% pet.			
Fentichlor (ph)	1% pet.		+	
Fenticonazole	1% alc.			
Feprazone	5% pet.			
Ferrous chloride				2% alc./glyc.

Table 56.2 (continued)

Allergen	Test concentration and vehicle	Suppliers		
	Listed in this book	Almirall	Chemo	Brial
Ferrous sulfate				5% pet.
Fluazinam	0.5% pet.			
Fludrocortisone acetate	1% alc.			
Flufenamic acid	1% pet.			
Flumethasone acetate	1% alc.			
Fluocinolone acetonide	1% alc.			
Fluocinonide	1% alc.			
Fluocortolone	1% alc.			
Fluorouracil (ph)	1% pet.			
Flurbiprofen	5% pet.			
Fluticasone propionate	1% alc.			
Folpet	0.1% pet.			
Formaldehyde (ph) (icr)	1% aq.	+	+	+
Formic acid				1% aq.
Fragrance mix 1 (ph) (cinnamic alcohol, cinnamal, hydroxycitronellal, α-amyl-cinnamal, geraniol, eugenol, isoeugenol, oakmoss absolute)	8% pet.	+	+	+
Fragrance mix 2 (citral, citronellol, coumarin, farnesol, α-hexylcinnamic aldehyde, Lyral®)	14% pet.	+	+	+
Framycetin (neomycin B)	20% pet.	10% pet.		
Fusidic acid sodium salt	2% pet.	+		+
Gallium oxide				1% pet.
Ganciclovir	20% aq.			
Gentamicin sulfate (icr)	20% pet.	+	+	+
Geraniol (icr)	1% pet.	+	+	+
Geranium oil, Bourbon			2% pet.	
Glutaral	0.2–0.3% pet./1% aq. or pet.	0.3% pet.	0.2% pet.	0.3% pet.
Glyceryl thioglycolate (icr)	1% pet.	+	+	+
Glyoxal				
Glyphosate	1–10% aq.			
Gold sodium thiosulfate (icr)	2–5% pet.			
Grotan® BK	See 1,3,5-Tris(2-hydroxyethyl)-hexahydrotriazine			
Halcinonide	1% alc.			
Haloprogin	1% pet.			
Halomethasone	1% alc.			

(continued)

Table 56.2 (continued)

Allergen	Test concentration and vehicle	Suppliers		
	Listed in this book	Almirall	Chemo	Brial
Hexachlorophene (ph)	1% pet.	+	+	+ and 0.5% pet.
Hexamethylene diisocyanate (HDI)	0.1% pet.		+	
Hexamethylenetetramine	See methenamine			
Hexamethylpentylcyclohexenecarbox-aldehyde (Lyral®)	See hydroxyisohexyl 2-cyclo-hexene carboxaldehyde			
1,6-Hexanediol diacrylate (HDDA)	0.1% pet.		+	
1,6-Hexanediol diglycidyl ether	0.25% pet.	+	+	
α-Hexylcinnamaldehyde	10% pet.	+	+	
Hexylresorcinol	0.25% pet.	+		+
Homosalate (homomenthyl salicylate) (ph)	5% pet.		+	
Homatropine	1% aq.			
Hydantoin (de)			10% pet.	
Hydrangenol	0.1% pet.			
Hydrazine sulfate			1% pet.	1% pet.
Hydroabietyl alcohol	10% pet.	+	+	
Hydrochlorothiazide (phde)	1–10% pet.		10% pet.	
Hydrocortisone (ph)	1% alc.	1% pet.		1% pet.
Hydrocortisone aceponate	1% alc.			
Hydrocortisone acetate	1% alc.			
Hydrocortisone buteprate	1% alc.			
Hydrocortisone-17-butyrate	1% alc.	0.1% pet.	+	+ and 0.1% pet.
Hydrogen peroxide			3% aq.	
Hydroquinone (HQ)	1% pet.	+	+	+
Hydroquinone monobenzylether	See monobenzone			
Hydroxycitronellal (ph)	1% pet.	+	+	+
2-Hydroxyethyl acrylate (2-HEA)	0.1% pet.	+	+	
2-Hydroxyethyl methacrylate (HEMA)	2% pet.	1% pet.	+	+ and 1% pet.
Hydroxyisohexyl 3-cyclohexene carboxaldehyde (Lyral®)	5% pet.	+	+	
Hydroxylammonium chloride			0.1% aq.	
Hydroxylammonium sulfate			0.1% aq.	
2-Hydroxymethyl-2-nitro-1,3-propanediol	See tris(hydroxymethyl) nitromethane			
2-(2'-Hydroxy-5'-methyl-phenyl) benzotriazole	See drometrizole			
Hydroxymethylpentylcyclohexene-carboxaldehyde (Lyral®)	See hydroxyisohexyl 3-cyclo-hexene carboxaldehyde			

Table 56.2 (continued)

| Allergen | Test concentration and vehicle | | Suppliers | | |
	Listed in this book	Almirall	Chemo	Brial
2-Hydroxypropyl acrylate (HPA)	0.1% pet.		+	
2-Hydroxypropyl methacrylate (HPMA)	2% pet.		+	+
Hypericum perforatum (hypericum oil)				0.5% pet.
Ibuprofen (fde)	5–10% pet.		10% pet.	
Ibuproxam (ph)	2.5% pet.			
Ichthammol (ammonium bituminosulfonate)	10% pet.		+	
Idoxuridine	1% pet.			+
2-Imidazolidinone (ethylene urea)			1% pet.	
Imidazolidinyl urea	2% pet.	+	+	+ and 2% aq.
Indium (III) chloride			10% aqua	1% pet.
Indium sulfate			10% aqua	
Indomethacin	5% pet.			1% pet.
Iodoform				5% pet.
Iodopropynyl butylcarbamate	0.2% pet.	+	0.1% pet.	0.1, 0.2 and 0.5% pet.
Isoamyl-*p*-methoxycinnamate (ph)	10% pet.	+	+	+
Isoconazole nitrate	1% alc.			
Isoeugenol	1% pet.	+	2% pet.	+
α-Isomethylionone			10% pet.	
Isophoronediamine (IPD)	0.1% pet.	0.5% pet.	+	0.5% pet.
Isophorone diisocyanate (IPDI)	1% pet.		+	
Isopropyl dibenzoylmethane (ph)	10% pet.		2% pet.	
4,4′-Isopropylidenediphenol (Bisphenol A)	1% pet.	+		+
Isopropyl myristate		10% pet.	20% pet.	10% pet.
N-Isopropyl-*N*′-phenyl-*p*-phenylenediamine (IPPD)	0.1% pet.	+	+	+
Jasminum officinale (jasmine absolute, synthetic)		5% pet.	2% pet.	2% pet.
Juniperus (juniper tar)			3% pet.	
Kanamycin sulfate	10% pet.	+	+	+
Ketoconazole (icr)	1% alc.			
Ketoprofen (phde) (icr)	1–2.5% pet.		1% pet.	
Ketotifen	0.7% aq.			
Lanette E®	20% pet.			
Lanette N®	20% pet.			

(*continued*)

Table 56.2 (continued)

Allergen	Test concentration and vehicle	Suppliers		
	Listed in this book	Almirall	Chemo	Brial
Lanoconazole	1% alc.			
Lanolin	pure	+		30% pet.
Lanolin alcohol (wool wax alcohols) (icr)	30% pet.	+	+	+
Lanolin alcohol and paraffinum liquidum (Amerchol® L 101)	50% pet.	+	+	+
Laurus nobilis (laurel oil)		2% pet.		2% pet.
Lauryl gallate	See dodecyl gallate			
Lauryl glucoside			3% pet.	
Lavandula angustifolia (lavender, absolute) (ph)			2% pet.	2% pet.
Lemon grass oil	See *Cymbopogon schoenanthus*			
Lemon oil	See *Citrus limonum*			
Levobunolol hydrochloride	1% aq.			
Lichen acid mix (atranorin, evernic acid, usnic acid)	0.3% pet.		+	
Lidocaine hydrochloride (icr)	5% pet.	15% pet.	+	15% pet.
Lilial	See *p-tert*-butyl-α-methylhydro-cinnamic aldehyde			
d-Limonene	See dipentene			
Linalool		10% pet.	10% pet.	
Lincomycin hydrochloride	1% aq.			
Lindane (icr)	1% pet.			
Lomefloxacin (phde)	5–10% pet.			
Luliconazole	1% alc.			
Lyral®	See hydroxyisohexyl 3-cyclo-hexene carboxaldehyde			
Mafenide				10% pet.
Majantol	5% pet.	+		+
Malathion	0.5% pet.			
Maneb (ph)	0.5–1% pet.			
Manganese chloride	<2% pet.			
Mechlorethamine hydrochloride (icr)	0.02% aq.			
Medroxyprogesterone acetate	1% pet.			
Mefenamic acid (fde)	1% pet.			
Melaleuca alternifolia (tea tree oil)			5% pet.	5% pet.
Melamine-formaldehyde			7% pet.	
Mentha piperita (peppermint oil) (icr)		2% pet.		2% pet.
Menthol (icr)		1% pet.	2% pet.	1% pet.

Table 56.2 (continued)

Allergen	Test concentration and vehicle	Suppliers		
	Listed in this book	Almirall	Chemo	Brial
Mepivacaine hydrochloride	1% pet.			
Merbromin (mercurochrome)	2% aq. or pet.			
2-Mercaptobenzimidazole	See 2-benzimidazolethiol			
Mercaptobenzothiazole (MBT) (icr)	2% pet.			+
Mercapto mix (mercaptobenzothiazole, dibenzothiazyl disulfide, morpholinyl mercaptobenzothiazole, N-cyclohexyl-benzothiazyl sulfenamide)	1% pet.	+	+	+
Mercuric chloride	0.1% pet.			
Mercurochrome	See merbromin			
Mercury (icr)	0.5% pet.		+	+
Mesulfen	5% pet.			
Metamizol	See dipyrone			
Metanil yellow	See acid yellow 36			
Methenamine (hexamethylenetetramine)	2% pet	1% pet.	+	1% pet.
Methyl-3-amino-4-N,N-diethyl-aniline (CD 2)		1% pet.	1% pet.	
p-Methylaminophenol sulfate (Metol®)(icr)		1% pet.	1% pet.	
Methyl anthranilate			5% pet.	
4-Methylbenzylidene camphor (ph)	10% pet.	+	+	+
Methylchloroisothiazolinone, methyl-isothiazolinone (icr)	0.01% aq.	+	+ and 0.02% aq.	+
Methylcoumarin (6-MC) (ph)			1% pet.	
Methyldibromo glutaronitrile (1,2-dibromo-2,4-dicyanobutane)	0.2–0.5–1% pet.	0.2 and 0.3% pet.	0.2 and 0.5% pet.	0.1, 0.3 and 0.5% pet.
Methyldibromo glutaronitrile + phenoxyethanol (Euxyl® K 400)		1% pet.	1 and 1.5% pet.	0.1, 1 and 2% pet.
Methyl diisocyanate	2% pet.			
N,N-Methylenebisacrylamid (MBAA)			1% pet.	
Methylene-bis-benzotriazolyl tetramethyl butylphenol (Tinosorb M)			10% pet.	
Methylene-bis(methyloxazolidine)	1% pet.	+		+
α-Methylene-γ-butyrolactone (tulipaline)	0.005–0.01% pet.		0.01% pet.	
Methyl heptine carbonate		1% pet.		
Methylhydroquinone (MHQ)		1% pet.	1% pet.	
γ-Methylionone		1% pet.		
2-Methyl-4-isothiazolin-3-one	0.01–0.1% aq.	0.05% aq.		
Methyl methacrylate (MMA)	2% pet.	+	+	+

(continued)

Table 56.2 (continued)

Allergen	Test concentration and vehicle	Suppliers		
	Listed in this book	Almirall	Chemo	Brial
Methyl-2-octynoate			0.2% pet.	
N-Methylolchloroacetamide			0.1% pet.	
Methylparaben (icr)	3% pet.	+	+	+
Methylprednisolone aceponate	1% alc.			
Methylprednisolone acetate	1% alc.			
Methyl salicylate (icr)	2% pet.			+
Methyl violet				0.5% pet.
Metipranolol	2% aq.			
Metol®	See p-methylaminophenol sulfate			
Metoprolol (de)	3% aq.			
Metronidazole (fde)	1% pet.			+
Mexenone	See benzophenone-10			
Miconazole nitrate	1% alc.		+	
Minocycline hydrochloride (de)			10% pet.	
Minoxidil	5% in aq. + 20% prop.glyc.			
Mitomycin C	0.1% pet.			
Mofebutazone	1% pet.			
Mometasone furoate	1% alc.			
Monobenzone (monobenzylether of hydroquinone)	1% pet.			
Monobenzylether of hydroquinone	See monobenzone			
Monoethanolamine	See ethanolamine			
2-Monomethylol phenol			1% pet.	
Monosodium glutamate				1% coca/glyc.
Morpholinyl mercaptobenzothiazole (MOR) (icr)	0.5% pet.	+	1% pet.	+
Mupirocin	10% pet.			
Musk ambrette (ph)	5% pet.			
Musk ketone (ph)			1% pet.	
Musk mix (xylene, moskene, ketone)			3% pet.	
Musk moskene (ph)			1% pet.	
Musk xylene (ph)			1% pet.	
Myristyl alcohol	5% pet.			
Myroxylon Pereirae (balsam of Peru) (ph) (icr)	25% pet.	+	+	+
Myroxylon toluiferum (balsam of Tolu)			20% pet. 10% alc.	20% pet.

Table 56.2 (continued)

Allergen	Test concentration and vehicle	Suppliers		
	Listed in this book	Almirall	Chemo	Brial
Naftifine hydrochloride	5% alc.			
Naphthol AS (CI 37505)	1% pet.	+		+
Naphthyl mix (*N,N*-Di-β-naphthyl-*p*-phenylenediamine, *N*-phenyl-2-naphthy-lamine)			1% pet.	
Naproxen (ph)	5% pet.			
Narcissus absolute		2% pet.	2% pet.	
Neomycin sulfate (icr)	20% pet.	+	+	+
Neroli oil	See *citrus aurantium dulcis*			
Neticonazole	1% alc.			
Nickel chloride	5% pet.			
Nickel sulfate (icr)	5% pet./ 2.5% pet.	5% pet.	+	+
Nicotine (icr)	10% pet.			
Nigrosine	1% pet.		+	
(Nitrobutyl)morpholine/ (ethylnitrotri-methylen)dimorpholine	See Bioban® P 1487			
Nitrofurazone	1% pet.		+	+
Nitroglycerin (icr)	1% pet.			
2-Nitro-*p*-phenylenediamine (ONPPD)	1% pet.			
Nonoxynols	5% aq.			
Nordihydroguaiaretic acid	2% pet.			
Norethisterone acetate	1% alc.			
Norfloxacine (de)			10% pet.	
Nystatin (de)	2% pet.	+		+
Oak moss absolute	See *Evernia prunastri*			
Octocrylene (ph)			10% pet.	
Octyl dimethyl PABA (2-ethylhexyl-*p*-dimethylaminobenzoate) (ph)	10% pet.	+	+	+
Octyl gallate		0.3% pet.	0.25% pet.	0.3% pet.
Octylisothiazolinone	0.025% pet.	+	0.1% pet.	+
Octyl methoxycinnamate (2-ethylhexyl-*p*-methoxycinnamate) (ph)	10% pet.	+	+	+
Octyl phthalate				5% pet.
Octyl salicylate	10% pet.		5% pet.	
Octyl triazone (ph)			10% pet.	
Olaquindox (ph)	1% pet.		+	
Olea europeae (olive oil)			pure	
Oleamidopropyl dimethylamine			0.1% aq.	0.1% alc./aq.

(continued)

Table 56.2 (continued)

Allergen	Test concentration and vehicle	Suppliers		
	Listed in this book	Almirall	Chemo	Brial
Oleyl alcohol	30% pet.			
Oligotriacrylate 480 (OTA)			0.1% pet.	
Olive oil	See *Olea europeae*			
Orange oil	See *Citrus dulcis*			
Orthocaine	1% pet.			
Oxiconazole	1% alc.			
Oxybenzone	See benzophenone-3			
Oxybuprocaine (benoxinate)	1% pet.			
Oxyphenbutazone (de) (icr)	1% pet.			
Oxytetracycline	3% pet.	+		+
PABA (ph)	10% pet.	+	+	+
Palladium chloride (icr)	1–2% pet.	1% pet.	2% pet.	1% pet.
Panthenol (dexpanthenol) (icr)	50% aq.	5% pet.		5% pet.
Papain	1% pet.			1% pet.
Paraben mix (butyl, ethyl, methyl, propyl-paraben) (icr)	16% pet.	+	+	+
Paracetamol	See *acetaminophen*			
Paraquat	0.1% pet.			
Paromomycin	10% pet.			
Parthenolide	0.1% pet.		+	
Patchouli oil	See *Pogostemon cablin oil*			
Pecilocin	1% pet.			
Pectin				1% coca
PEG 6 (and) PEG 32 (polyethylene glycol ointment)	pure	+		+
PEG 400 (icr)				pure
Penbutolol sulfate	2% aq.			
Penethamate	1% pet.			
d-Penicillamine	1% aq.			
Penicillin G (de) (icr)	10.000 U/g pet./10% pet.		10% pet (potassium salt)	
Pentachloronitrobenzene	0.5–1% pet.			
Pentaerythritol triacrylate (PETA)			0.1% pet.	
Peppermint oil	See *Mentha piperita*			
Perfume mix (cinnamic alcohol, cinnamal, hydroxycitronellal, eugenol, isoeugenol, geraniol)			6% pet.	
Petrolatum, white (icr)	pure	+	+	+

Table 56.2 (continued)

Allergen	Test concentration and vehicle		Suppliers		
	Listed in this book		Almirall	Chemo	Brial
Phenidone®	See 1-phenyl-3-pyrazolidinone				
Pheniramine maleate	1% aq.				
Phenol-formaldehyde resin (P-F-R-2)	5% pet.		+	1% pet.	+
Phenolphthalein					0.5% pet.
Phenoxyethanol (icr)	1% pet.		+	+	+
Phenylbenzimidazol sulfonic acid (ph)	10% pet.		+	+	+
Phenylbutazone (de) (icr) (ph)	1–5% pet.				10% pet.
p-Phenylenediamine dihydrochloride				0.5% pet.	
p-Phenylenediamine free base (ph) (icr)	1% pet.		+	+	+
Phenylephrine hydrochloride	10% aq.		+		10% coca
Phenyl glycidyl ether (icr)			0.25% pet.	0.25% pet.	
α-Phenylindole				2% pet.	
Phenyl isocyanate					0.1% pet.
Phenylmercuric acetate (icr)	0.05% pet.		0.01% pet.	0.01% aq.	+
Phenylmercuric borate	0.05% pet.				
Phenylmercuric nitrate (icr)	0.05% pet.				0.01% pet.
Phenyl-β-naphthylamine (PBN)	1% pet.			+	+
o-Phenylphenol (ph) (icr)				1% pet.	
Phenyl-p-phenylenediamine					0.25% pet.
1-Phenyl-3-pyrazolidinone (Phenidone®)				1% pet.	
Phenyl salicylate	1% pet.			+	+
Phosphorus sesquisulfide (icr)				0.5% pet.	
Piketoprofen (ph)	2.5% pet.				
Pilocarpine hydrochloride (icr)	1% pet.		1% aq.		1% alc./glyc.
Pimecrolimus	1% pet.				
Pindolol					2% pet.
α-Pinene					15% pet.
Pinus (pine tar)				3% pet.	3% pet.
Piperazine (de)	1% pet.				
Pirenoxine	1% aq.				
Piroxicam (phde) (de)	1% pet.			+	
Pix ex carbone (coal tar) (ph) (icr)	5% pet.			+	+
Pogostemon cablin oil (patchouli oil)			10% pet.		
Polidocanol	3% pet.		+		+
Polyethylene glycol-400	See PEG-400				

(continued)

Table 56.2 (continued)

Allergen	Test concentration and vehicle	Suppliers		
	Listed in this book	Almirall	Chemo	Brial
Polyethylene glycol ointment	See PEG 6 (and) PEG 32			
Polymyxin B sulfate	3% pet.	+		+
Polyoxyethylene sorbitan monolaurate	See Polysorbate 20			
Polyoxyethylene sorbitan monooleate	See Polysorbate 80			
Polyoxyethylene sorbitan monopalmitate	See Polysorbate 40			
Polysorbate 20 (polyoxyethylene sorbitan monolaurate) (icr)	5% pet.			
Polysorbate 40 (polyoxyethylene sorbitan monopalmitate) (icr)	5% pet.			10% pet.
Polysorbate 80 (polyoxyethylene sorbitan monooleate) (icr)	5% pet.		+	10% pet.
Potassium dichromate (ph)	0.5% pet./0.25% pet.	+	+	+
Potassium dicyanoaurate		0.002% aq.		0.002% aq.
Povidone-iodine (icr)	10% pet./0.4% aq.			10% aq.
Pramocaine hydrochloride	1% pet.			
Prednicarbate	1% alc.			
Prednisolone	1% alc.	1% pet.		0.5% pet.
Prilocaine hydrochloride	5% pet.		+	
Primin	0.01% pet.	+	+	+
Pristinamycin (icr) (de)	5–10% pet.		10% pet.	
Procaine hydrochloride (ph) (icr)	1% pet.	2% pet.	+	2% pet.
Proflavine hydrochloride	1% pet.			
Promethazine hydrochloride (phde) (icr) (fde)	0.1–1% pet.	0.1% pet.	1% pet.	2% pet.
Propanidid	5% pet.			
Propantheline bromide				5% pet.
Propionic acid			3% pet.	
Propipocaine	1% pet.			
Propolis	10% pet.	+	+	+
Propranolol hydrochloride (de)	20% pet.			2% pet.
Propylene glycol (icr)	5% aq.	5% pet and 20% aq.	5% pet.	20 and 30% aq.
Propylene oxide	0.1–1% alc.			
Propyl gallate	1% pet.	0.5% pet.	1% pet.	0.5% pet.
Propylparaben (icr)	3% pet.	+	+	+
Propyphenazone (icr)				1% pet.

Table 56.2 (continued)

Allergen	Test concentration and vehicle		Suppliers		
	Listed in this book		Almirall	Chemo	Brial
Pyrethrum	See *Chrysanthemum cinerariaefolium*				
Pyrilamine maleate	2% pet.				
Pyrogallol			1% pet.		1% pet.
Pyrrolnitrin	1% pet.				
Quaternium-12	See dodecyl dimethyl ammonium chloride				
Quaternium-15	1% pet.		+	+2% pet.	+ and 2% pet.
Quindoxin (ph)	0.1% pet.				
Quinidine sulfate (phde)			1% pet.		1% pet.
Quinine sulfate (phde)	1% pet.			+	25% pet.
Quinoline mix (clioquinol, chlorquinaldol)				6% pet.	
Quinoline yellow					0.1% coca/glyc.
Reactive black 5 (CI 20505)	1% pet.			+	
Reactive blue 21 (CI 18097)	1% pet.			+	
Reactive blue 238	1% pet.			+	
Reactive orange 107	1% pet.			+	
Reactive red 123	1% pet.			+	
Reactive red 228	1% pet.			+	
Reactive red 238	1% pet.			+	
Reactive violet 5 (CI 18097)	1% pet.			+	
Resorcinol (icr)	1% pet.		+	+	+
Resorcinol monobenzoate				1% pet.	
Resorcinol/formaldehyde resin					5% pet.
Retinoic acid	0.005% pet.				
Rhodium chloride	1% aq.				
Ribostamycin	20% pet.				
Rifamycin (icr)	2.5% pet.				
Rivanol®	See ethacridine lactate monohydrate				
Rosa (rose oil)					0.5% pet.
Rosa centifolia (rose oil, Bulgarian)				2% pet.	
Rosemary (rosemary oil)					0.5% pet.
Rosin	See colophonium				
Rubidium iodide	1% pet.				
Ruthenium (icr)					0.1% pet.

(*continued*)

Table 56.2 (continued)

Allergen	Test concentration and vehicle	Suppliers		
	Listed in this book	Almirall	Chemo	Brial
Saccharin				0.1% coca/gly.
Salicylaldehyde		2% pet.		2% pet.
Salicylic acid (icr)	1% pet.			5% pet.
Sandalwood oil	See *Santalum album*			
Santalum album (sandalwood oil) (ph)		10% pet.	2% pet.	
Scopolamine hydrobromide	0.25% aq.			
Sertaconazole	1% alc.			
Sesamum indicum (sesame oil)		pure		
Sesquiterpene lactone mix (alantolactone, costunolide, dehydrocostus lactone)	0.1% pet.	+	+	+
Shellac				20% alc.
Silver colloidal				0.1% pet.
Silver protein				3% pet.
Sisomicin	20% pet.			
Sodium alginate	See algin			
Sodium benzoate (icr)		5% pet.	5% pet.	5% pet.
Sodium colistimethate	1% pet.			
Sodium diphosphate				1% coca/glyc.
Sodium disulfite				1% pet. and 1% coca/glyc.
Sodium formate				2% coca/glyc.
Sodium fusidate	See fusidic acid sodium salt			
Sodium glutamate	See monosodium glutamate			
Sodium hypochlorite (icr)	0.5% aq.			
Sodium hyposulfite	1% aq.			
Sodium lauryl sulfate	0.1% aq.	0.25% aq. (control irritant)		0.25% aq. (control irritant)
Sodium metabisulfite	2% pet.			
Sodium nitrite				2% aq./glyc.
Sodium omadine	See sodium pyrithione			
Sodium pyrithione (sodium omadine)	0.1% aq.		+	+
Sodium sulfite				1% coca/glyc.
Sodium thiosulfoaurate			0.25% pet.	0.25 and 0.5% pet.
Solvent red 23 (Sudan III)				1% pet.
Solvent yellow 11	See *p*-aminoazobenzene			
Sorbic acid (icr)	2% pet.	+	+	+ and 2% alc./glyc.

Table 56.2 (continued)

Allergen	Test concentration and vehicle	Suppliers		
	Listed in this book	Almirall	Chemo	Brial
Sorbitan laurate (Span® 20) (icr)	5% aq.			
Sorbitan oleate (Span® 80)	5% aq.		5% pet.	5% pet.
Sorbitan palmitate (Span® 40)	5% aq.			
Sorbitan sesquioleate (icr)	20% pet.	+	2% pet.	+
Spiramycin sulfate (de)	10% pet.		+ (base)	
Stannous chloride		0.5% pet.	1% pet.	0.5% pet.
Steraramidopropyl dimethylamine				0.1% aqua
Stearyl alcohol (icr)	30% pet.		+	+
Streptomycin (sulfate) (icr)	1–2.5% pet.			5% pet.
Styrax benzoin (benzoin resin) (icr)			2% pet.	10% alc./glyc./aq.
Sudan III	See solvent red 23			
Sulbentine	See dibenzthione			
Sulconazole nitrate	1% alc.			
Sulfamethoxazole (de)	20% pet.			
Sulfanilamide (ph)	5% pet.	+	+	+
Sulfurdioxide (icr)				2% aq.
Sulfur, pharmaceutical (precipitated)				10% pet.
Sulindac	1% pet.			
Sulisobenzone	See benzophenone-4			
Suprofen (ph)	0.1% pet.			
Tacalcitol	2 µg/mL alc.			
Tacrolimus	2.5% alc.			
Tanacetum parthenium (feverfew) extract	1% pet.			
Tanacetum vulgare (tansy extract)	1% pet.		+	
Tansy extract	See *Tanacetum vulgare*			
Tantalum				1% pet.
Taraxacum officinale (dandelion)			2.5% pet.	
Tartrazine				1% coca/glyc.
Tea tree oil	See *Melaleuca alternifolia*			
Tego® 103 G	0.05% aq.			
Tenoxicam (fde)	1% pet.			
Terephtalylidene dicamphor sulfonic acid (Mexoryl® SX)	10% aq.			
Tetracaine hydrochloride (amethocaine)	1% pet.	+	5% pet.	+
Tetrachlorosalicylanilide (TSCA) (ph)			0.1% pet.	

(continued)

Table 56.2 (continued)

Allergen	Test concentration and vehicle	Suppliers		
	Listed in this book	Almirall	Chemo	Brial
Tetracycline hydrochloride		2% pet.		2% pet.
Tetraethylene glycol dimethacrylate			2% pet.	
Tetraethylthiuram disulfide (TETD)		0.25% pet.	1% pet.	0.25% pet.
Tetrahydrofurfuryl methacrylate (THFMA)	2% pet.		+	
Tetramethylbenzidine			0.1% pet.	
Tetramethylol acetylenediurea			5% aq.	
Tetramethylthiuram disulfide (TMTD)		0.25% pet.	1% pet.	0.25% pet.
Tetramethylthiuram monosulfide (TMTM)		0.25% pet.	1% pet.	0.25% pet.
Thiabendazole	1% pet.			
Thiamphenicol	5% pet.			
Thimerosal (icr)	0.1% pet.	+		+ and 1% pet.
Thiocolchicoside	1% pet.			
Thiourea (ph)			0.1% pet.	0.1 and 1% pet.
Thioxolone	0.5% alc.			
Thiram	1% pet.			
Thiuram mix (tetramethylthiuram monosulfide, tetramethylthiuram disulfide, tetraethylthiuram disulfide, dipentamethylenethiuram disulfide)	1% pet.	+	+	+ and 1.25% pet.
Tiaprofenic acid (phde)	1% pet.			
Timolol	0.5% aq.			
Tin (icr)			50% pet.	
Tioconazole	1% alc.			
Titanium				1% pet.
Titanium-(IV)-oxide				0.1% pet.
Tixocortol pivalate	0.1–1% pet.	1% pet.	0.1% pet.	0.1 and 1% pet.
Tobramycin (de)	20% pet.			
α-Tocopherol (vitamin E) (icr)	10% pet.			pure
Tocopheryl acetate				10% pet.
Tolazoline	10% aq.			
Tolnaftate	1% pet.			
Toluene-2,5-diamine (p-toluenediamine) (PTD)	1% pet.	+	+	+
Toluene diisocyanate (TDI)	2% pet.		+	1% pet.
Toluene sulfonamide/formaldehyde resin	See tosylamine/formaldehyde resin			

Table 56.2 (continued)

Allergen	Test concentration and vehicle		Suppliers		
	Listed in this book		Almirall	Chemo	Brial
4-Tolyldiethanolamine				2% pet.	
Tosylamide/formaldehyde resin (toluene-sulfonamide/ formaldehyde resin)	10% pet.		+	+	+
Tree moss	See *Evernia furfuracea*				
Triamcinolone acetonide	1% alc.		0.1% pet.	1% pet.	0.1 and 1% pet.
Tribromsalan (TBS) (ph)	1% pet.			+	
Trichloroethylene	5% o.o.				
Triclocarban (TCC) (ph)	1% pet.				
Triclosan (ph)	1–2% pet.		2% pet.	2% pet.	2% pet.
Tricresyl phosphate	5% pet.		+	+	+
Triethanolamine	2.5% pet.		+	2% pet.	+
Triethanolamine polypeptide oleate condensate (Xerumenex®)	25% o.o				
Triethyleneglycol diacrylate (TREGDA)				0.1% pet.	
Triethyleneglycol dimethacrylate (TREGDMA)	2% pet.		+	+	+
Triethylenetetramine (TETA)	0.5% pet.		+	+	++
Trifluridine	5% pet.				
Triglycidyl isocyanurate	0.5% pet.			+	
Trimeprazine tartrate (alimemazine tartrate)					1% pet.
Trimethoprim (de) (fde)	20% pet.				
2,2,4-Trimethyl-1,2-dihydroquinoline	1% pet.			+	
Trimethylolpropane triacrylate (TMPTA)	0.1% pet.			+	
Trimethylolpropane triglycidyl ether				0.25% pet.	
Tripelennamine	1% pet.				
Triphenyl phosphate			5% pet.	5% pet.	5% pet.
Tripropyleneglycol diacrylate (TPGDA)	0.1% pet.			+	
1,3,5-Tris(2-hydroxyethyl)-hexahydrotriazine (Grotan® BK)	1% pet.		+	1% aq.	+
Tris(hydroxymethyl)nitromethane (tris nitro)				1% pet.	
Tris nitro	See tris(hydroxymethyl) nitromethane				
Trolamine	See triethanolamine				

(continued)

Table 56.2 (continued)

Allergen	Test concentration and vehicle	Suppliers		
	Listed in this book	Almirall	Chemo	Brial
Tromantadine hydrochloride	1% pet.			
Tromethamine (Trometamol)	1% aq.			
Tropicamide (icr)	1% pet.			
TSS Agfa®	See amino-4-*N*,*N*-diethylaniline sulfate			
Tuberculin (bovine)	10% aq.			
Tulipalin	See α-methylene-γ-butyrolactone			
Turpentine oil (icr)		10% pet.		
Turpentine peroxides (icr)			0.3% o.o.	0.3% pet.
Tylosin tartrate	5% pet.			
Undecylenic acid	2% pet.			
Urea formaldehyde resin	10% pet.		+	
Urethane diacrylate (aliphatic) (UDA)			0.1% pet.	
Urethane diacrylate (aromatic) (UDA)			0.05% pet.	
Urethane dimethacrylate (UDMA)	2% pet.		+	+
Usnic acid (ph)	0.1% pet.	+	+	+
Valaciclovir	10% aq.			
Vancomycin (de)	5% aq.			
Vanillin (icr)		10% pet.	10% pet.	10% pet.
Vat green 1 (CI 59825)	1% pet.			
Venice turpentine				10 and 20% pet.
Vesuvine brown	See Bismarck brown			
Virginiamycin (de) (icr)	5% pet.			
Vitamin E	See α-tocopherol			
Warfarin	0.5% pet.			
Wood mix (pine, spruce, birch, teak)			20% pet.	
Wood tar mix (pine, beech, juniper, birch) (ph)			12% pet.	12% pet.
Wool wax alcohols	See lanolin alcohol			
Xerumenex®	See triethanolamine polypeptide oleate condensate			
m-Xylylenediamine			0.1% pet.	
Yarrow	See *Achillea millefolium*			
Ylang-ylang oil	See *Cananga odorata*			
Zinc chloride (icr)			1% pet.	1% pet.
Zinc dibenzyldithiocarbamate	1% pet.	1% pet.		
Zinc dibutyldithiocarbamate (ZBC) (icr)	1% pet.	+	+	+

Table 56.2 (continued)

Allergen	Test concentration and vehicle	Suppliers		
	Listed in this book	Almirall	Chemo	Brial
Zinc diethyldithiocarbamate (ZDC) (icr)	1% pet.	+	+	+
Zinc dimethyldithiocarbamate (Ziram) (icr)	1% pet.		+	
Zinc ethylenebis(dithiocarbamate)	See Zineb			
Zinc (powder)				1% pet.
Zinc pyrithione (ph)	1% pet.		1% pet.	1% pet.
Zineb (zinc ethylenebis(dithiocarbamate)) (ph)	1% pet.		+	+
Ziram	See zinc dimethyldithiocarbamate			
Zirconium oxide				0.1% pet.

alc. alcohol; *aq.* water; *coca* isotonic sodium chloride (0.9%) and fluidized phenol (90.9%) in water; *DMSO* dimethyl sulfoxide; *glyc.* glycerin; *MEK* methyl ethyl ketone (butanone); *o.o.* olive oil; *pet.* petrolatum; *prop. glyc.* propylene glycol
+ means: available from this supplier in the concentration as mentioned in column 1
icr immediate contact reactions reported (Chaps. 7 and 28)
de drug eruption with positive patch test reported (Chap. 26)
fde fixed drug eruption with positive patch test reported (Chap. 26)
ph photosensitivity reported (Chaps. 8, 18 and 29)
phde photosensitive drug eruption with positive photopatch test reported (Chaps. 8,18, 26 and 29)

Table 56.3 Recommended test concentrations for groups of chemicals

Product	Test concentration and vehicle
Acrylates, monoacrylates	0.1% pet.
Aminoglycosides	20% pet.
Carbowaxes	Pure
Cephalosporins	5–20% aq. or pet.
Epoxy resins (DGEBA based)	1% pet.
Epoxy resins (not DGEBA based)	0.25–1% pet.
Epoxy resin hardeners	0.1–1% in pet., acet. or alc.
Epoxy resin reactive diluents	0.1–1% in pet., acet. or alc.
Imidazole antimycotics	1% alc.
Methacrylates, monomers	2% pet.
Nonoxynols	5% aq.
Phenothiazines	1% pet.
Polyethylene glycols	Pure
Quaternary ammonium compounds	0.1% aq.
Sulfonamides	5% pet.
Systemic drugs causing drug eruptions	Pure chemical 1–20% in pet., aqua, alc. or acet.
	Commercial drug: powder in pet. to obtain a concentration of 10% for the active drug. With low concentrations of active drug: powder 30% in pet.
Tetracyclines	3% pet.

acet. acetone; *alc.* alcohol; *aq.* water; *pet.* petrolatum

56

Table 56.4 List of abbreviations

BA	Butyl acrylate
BAK	Benzalkonium chloride
BIS-EMA	2,2-bis(4-(2-Methacryloxyethoxy)phenyl) propane
BIS-GA	2,2-bis(4-(2-Hydroxy-3-acryloxypropoxy) phenyl)propane (Epoxy diacrylate)
BIS-GMA	2,2-bis(4-(2-Hydroxy-3-methacryloxy-propoxy)phenylpropane
BIS-MA	2,2-bis(4-(Methacryloxy)phenyl)propane
BIT	Benzisothiazolinone
BMA	*n*-Butyl methacrylate
BUDA	1,4-Butanediol diacrylate
BUDMA	1,4-Butanediol dimethacrylate
CBS	*N*-Cyclohexylbenzothiazyl sulfenamide
CPPD	*N*-Cyclohexyl-*N*-phenyl-*p*-phenylenediamine
DBNPD	*N*,*N*-Di-β-naphthyl-*p*-phenylenediamine
DEGDA	Diethyleneglycol diacrylate
DEHP	Di-2-ethylhexyl phthalate (=dioctyl phthalate)
DETA	Diethylenetriamine
DMAEMA	*N*,*N*-Dimethylaminoethyl methacrylate
DNCB	2,4-Dinitrochlorobenzene
DOP	Dioctyl phthalate
DPG	1,3-Diphenylguanidine
DPGDA	Dipropyleneglycol diacrylate
DPPD	*N*,*N'*-Diphenyl-*p*-phenylenediamine
DPTU	Diphenylthiourea
EA	Ethyl acrylate
ECA	Ethyl cyanoacrylate
EDTA	Ethylenediaminetetraacetic acid disodium salt (see Disodium EDTA)
EGDMA	Ethyleneglycol dimethacrylate
EHA	2-Ethylhexyl acrylate
EMA	Ethyl methacrylate
HDDA	1,6-Hexanediol diacrylate
HDI	Hexamethylenediisocyanate
2-HEA	2-Hydroxyethyl acrylate

HEMA	2-Hydroxyethyl methacrylate
HPA	2-Hydroxypropyl acrylate
HPMA	2-Hydroxypropyl methacrylate
HQ	Hydroquinone
IPD	Isophorone diamine
IPDI	Isophorone diisocyanate
IPPD	*N*-Isopropyl-*N'*-phenyl-*p*-phenylenediamine
MBAA	*N*,*N*-Methylenebisacrylamid
MBT	Mercaptobenzothiazole
MBTS	Dibenzothiazyl disulfide
6-MC	Methylcoumarin
MDI	Diphenylmethane-4,4-diisocyanate
MMA	Methyl methacrylate
MOR	Morpholinyl mercaptobenzothiazole
ONPPD	2-Nitro-*p*-phenylenediamine
OTA	Oligotriacrylate
PBN	Phenyl-β-naphthylamine
PCMC	*p*-Chloro-*m*-cresol
PCMX	Chloroxylenol
PCP	Pentachlorophenol
PEA	2-Phenoxyethyl acrylate
PETA	Pentaerythritol triacrylate
P-F-R-2	Phenol-formaldehyde resin
PTBC	*p-tert*-Butylcatechol
PTBT	*p-tert*-Butylphenolformaldehyde resin
PTD	Toluene-2,5-diamine
TBS	Tribromsalan
TCC	Triclocarban
TCSA	Tetrachlorosalicylanilide
TDI	Toluene diisocyanate
TETA	Triethylenetetramine
TETD	Tetraethylthiuram disulfide
THFMA	Tetrahydrofurfuryl methacrylate
TMPTA	Trimethylolpropane triacrylate
TMTD	Tetramethylthiuram disulfide
TMTM	Tetramethylthiuram monosulfide

TPGDA	Tripropyleneglycol diacrylate
TREGDA	Triethyleneglycol diacrylate
TREGDMA	Triethyleneglycol dimethacrylate
TSS	4-Amino-*N*,*N*-dietyhylaniline sulfate

UDA	Urethane diacrylate
UDMA	Urethane dimethacrylate
ZBC	Zinc dibutyldithiocarbamate
ZDC	Zinc diethyldithiocarbamate

References

1. Bruze M, Andersen KE, Goossens A; on behalf of the ESCD and EECDRG (2008) Recommendation to include fragrance mix 2 and hydroxyisohexyl 3-cyclohexene carboxaldehyde (Lyral®) in the European baseline patch test series. Contact Dermatitis 58:129–133

2. De Groot AC (2008) Patch testing. Test concentrations and vehicles for 4350 chemicals, 3rd edn. Acdegroot publishing, Wapserveen

3. Rietschel RL, Fowler JF Jr (eds) (2008) Fisher's contact dermatitis, 6th edn. BC Decker, Hamilton

4. Kanerva L, Elsner P, Wahlberg JE, Maibach HI (eds) (2000) Handbook of occupational dermatology. Springer, Heidelberg

Patch Testing with the Patients' Own Products

57

Peter J. Frosch, Johannes Geier, Wolfgang Uter, and An Goossens

Contents

P.J. Frosch
Hautklinik, Klinikum Dortmund gGmbH,
Beurhausstr. 40, 44137 Dortmund, Germany
e-mail: peter.frosch@klinikumdo.de

J. Geier
Information Network of Departments of Dermatology (IVDK),
University of Göttingen, von-Siebold-Street 3,
37075 Göttingen, Germany
e-mail: jgeier@ivdk.org

W. Uter
Department of Medical Informatics, Biometry and
Epidemiology, Univ. Erlangen/Nürnberg, Waldstraße 6,
91054 Erlangen, Germany

A. Goossens
Department of Dermatology, University Hospital,
Katholieke Universiteit Leuven, Leuven, Belgium
e-mail: an.goossens@uz.kuleuven.ac.be

Commercially available patch test kits (standard and various supplementary series) are the basis of a diagnostic workup if an allergic contact dermatitis is to be confirmed. However, various investigators have shown that this way of testing is not sufficient. Menné et al. [1] found in a multicenter study that the European Standard Series detects only 37–73% of the responsible allergens in patients with contact dermatitis. The additional and/or separately tested allergens were positive in 5–23%; the authors emphasize the necessity of testing with the products actually used by the patient. In Italy, an analysis of 230 patients referred to a contact clinic because of suspected occupational contact dermatitis showed that the standard series alone detected 69.9% of all cases considered to be of an allergic nature [2]; 26.3% of all allergic cases were positive only to supplementary series. The agents most commonly responsible for allergic contact dermatitis were metals and *para*-phenylenediamine.

In a German study of the IVDK network, the data of 2,460 patients tested between 1989 and 1992 were evaluated [3]. In 208 patients (8.5%), type IV sensitizations were found to a total of 289 materials. In 44% of these cases, only the patients' own products were patch test positive and thought to be clinically relevant.

In a subsequent analysis of 1998–2002 data, 8.6% of 3,621 patients had a positive patch test reaction to

J.D. Johansen et al. (eds.), *Contact Dermatitis*,
DOI: 10.1007/978-3-642-03827-3_57, © Springer-Verlag Berlin Heidelberg 2011

their own skin-care products that were additionally patch tested. Of 1,333 patients, 5.3% were tested positive to their own bath and shower products. In about one-third of the patients reacting to either product category, further positive tests to commercial allergens were not observed [4, 5].

The materials most frequently tested are usually topical medications, cosmetics of various types, rubber, and leather products.

The group of Kanerva has published an impressive series of papers in which patch testing with the patients' own industrial chemicals has provided the main clue to the causative agent of allergic contact dermatitis [6]. Various constituents of plastic materials, epoxy glues and paints, reactive dyes, and industrial enzymes were identified after chemical analysis. For example, with regard to the isocyanates present in polyurethane resins, it was found that among 22 occupationally related cases, 21 reacted to the isocyanates obtained from the companies involved (13) or to diaminodiphenylmethane (marker for isocyanate allergy), but only 1 reacted to the commercially available isocyanate, diphenylmethane diisocyanate or MDI (Trolab, Chemotechnique) [7]. Indeed, Frick et al. [8], when analyzing 14 commercial preparations of MDI, found that in most cases, its concentration did not match the one stated on the label. Moreover, the isocyanates tested are not always representative of the mixtures used in industry.

Recently, reports on contact allergy to the patients' perfume where the current fragrance mix and the commercially available major allergens of perfume remained negative were published. After repeated testing with various fractions of perfumes, the causative allergens were identified: Lilial [9] and coumarin [10]. The experience with perfumes has shown that in this dynamic field, with rapid changes in trendy attractive smells, the consumer is exposed to a wide array of chemicals that may cause sensitization. This subject is reviewed in detail in Chap. 31, Sect. 31.1. Further examples documenting the high value of testing with the patients' own products are published elsewhere [11–14]. In this field and in many industrial areas, patch testing with merely the standard and supplementary series will always be inadequate until new allergens have been identified, their clinical relevance has been confirmed by several study groups, and they are eventually included in a test series.

In the following paragraphs, guidelines for testing with patients' own materials in order to harmonize this approach in daily practice will be given. Knowledge in this field is often minimal and profound mistakes are made. For example, concentrated biocides or plastic monomers are applied under occlusion in undiluted form causing bullous or ulcerative lesions and possibly active sensitization. In contrast, the material is not infrequently diluted too much or in an inappropriate vehicle resulting in a false-negative reaction.

The guidelines are presented mainly in tables in order to be used by the technicians at the work bench. They contain essential information; for more detailed information, the reader is referred to other chapters in this book (particularly Chap. 57) and the pertinent references listed at the end.

57.1 Information on the Test Material Before Patch Testing

Never apply coded material obtained from a manufacturer without knowing the details about the chemical regarding its toxicity and appropriate test concentration. Major cosmetic manufacturers now have a safety department that will supply this information and often provide the ingredients at adequate dilutions and a vehicle for patch testing. However, some tend to supply the ingredients in dilutions as used in the products, producing false-negative reactions on patch testing. Unfortunately, this cooperative attitude is rare with the manufacturers of industrial products (e.g., metalworking fluids (MWFs), glues, paints, etc.). The material safety data sheets provide only basic information and do not list all allergologically relevant ingredients. In addition, the producer selling the product is often unaware of the contaminants or materials under a different nomenclature (i.e., the manufacturer denies the presence of colophony, but admits that abietic acid, the major allergen of colophony, is present in a cooling fluid). In a recent study from Finland on dental restorative materials, a high discrepancy was found between the listing of acrylates/methacrylates in material safety data sheets and the presence of these materials as detected by chemical analytical methods. 2-Hydroxyethyl methacrylate (2-HEMA), bisphenol A glycidyl methacrylate (*bis*-GMA), ethyleneglycol dimethacrylate (EGDMA), triethylene glycol dimethacrylate (TREGDMA), and (di)urethane dimethacrylate were either omitted completely as ingredients or not listed as often as appropriate. The authors analyzed glues, composite resins, and glass isomers [15].

The German network IVDK has established a model project [16] supporting the breakdown testing of cosmetic products. In cooperation with the manufacturers, the inquiring dermatologist will receive a recommendation on how to test the product ingredients, and which constituents, not present in the standard or additional series, might be a potential allergen. These are then provided in a test kit supplied by the manufacturer (this service is limited to Germany). Ideally, the test results are fed back to the data center, and are added to the database for the identification of putative "new" allergens – a system similar to the "cosmetovigilance" established in France [17].

57.1.1 Test Method

57.1.1.1 Skin Tests

Methodological details regarding dilution, vehicle, pH measurement, open test, closed patch test, repetitive open application test (ROAT), and use test are dealt with in Chap. 22. In Dortmund, we found large Finn chambers (12 mm diameter) that are useful for testing cosmetics with low irritancy (e.g., moisturizers, lip cosmetics, sunscreens, and eye drops [18]; Fig. 57.1).

The semi-open test as described by Dooms-Goossens [19] is particularly helpful if strong irritancy under occlusion is suspected, e.g., in the case of shampoos, liquid soaps, nail varnish, and also industrial products such as glues, paints, inks, varnishes, etc. The golden rule is that when a subject comes into direct skin contact with such a product (either on purpose, e.g., cleaning products, or accidentally, e.g., soluble oils, paints), then the product may be tested in this way. Corrosive or other toxic materials (pH <3 or >10) that are normally used in closed systems only or with protection from appropriate clothing are excluded from testing. The material is applied to the skin with a cotton swab (about 15 µL) on a small area

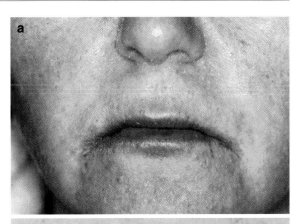

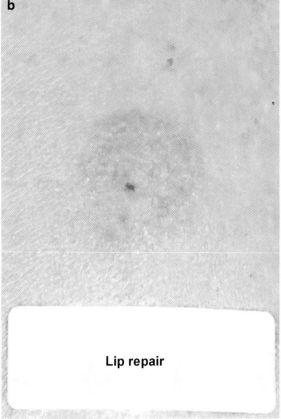

Lip repair

Fig. 57.1 Severe cheilitis with eczematous pruritic lesions in the perioral region after long-term use of a lipstick for dry lips (**a**). The patch test with the lipstick "as is" in a large Finn chamber showed a weak doubtful reaction (**b**). Breakdown testing with the ingredients provided by the manufacturer revealed contact allergy to dexpanthenol. The dermatitis cleared rapidly after discontinuance of the lipstick

(2 × 2 cm), left to dry (possibly dabbing with another Q-tip or tissue), and is then covered with acrylic tape (e.g., micropore, 3M) (Fig. 57.2)

57

Fig. 57.2 Semi-open test: after applying the test material with a cotton swab, the completely dried area is covered with acrylic tape (**a**). Comparison of positive reactions obtained with a semi-open test to the patient's own isocyanate solution and a patch test with its dilution at 2% in petrolatum (**b**); there was also a positive reaction to diaminodiphenylmethane as a marker for isocyanate contact allergy

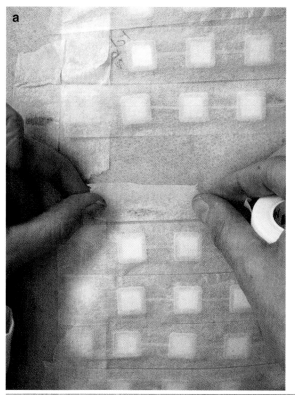

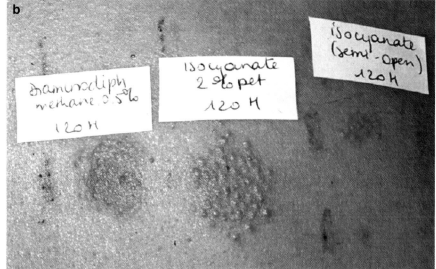

57.1.1.2 pH

At pH 4–9, very few irritant reactions are caused by the acidity or alkalinity itself [20]. The buffering solutions listed in Table 57.1 can be used to dilute water-soluble materials.

57.1.1.3 Dilution

Solid materials can be tested "as is," placing scrapings or cut pieces in the test chamber, or they can be applied on acrylic tape thus avoiding pressure effects. In this way, positive reactions to small pieces of glove, shoes,

Table 57.1 Composition of acid buffer solution, pH 4.7, and alkaline buffer solution, pH 9.9 [20]

Compound	Concentration	% of total volume
Acid buffer, pH 4.7		
Sodium acetate	0.1 N (8.2 g CH_3COONa/l aqua)	50
Acetic acid	0.1 N (6.0 g CH_3COOH/l aqua)	50
Alkaline buffer, pH 9.9		
Sodium carbonate	0.1 M (10.6 g Na_2CO_3/l aqua)	50
Sodium bicarbonate	0.1 M (8.4 g $NaHCO_3/l$ aqua)	50

rubber, or scrapings of (hard) plastic materials may be obtained (Fig. 57.3). However, the reactions often turn out to be false-negative because the concentration of the sensitizer is too low or the sensitizer is not released. Alternatively, pressure or friction effects of sharp particles may cause some sort of irritant reaction, which should, however, be clearly identifiable as such. Depending on the material, the sensitizer can be extracted with water or solvents (Table 57.2; [6]).

The correct dilution of materials for patch testing often presents a technical problem, because the calculation basis is not clear to every technician. Therefore, Table 57.3 provides a practical guideline for diluting liquid materials. For solid materials, the dilution is performed on a weight:volume basis.

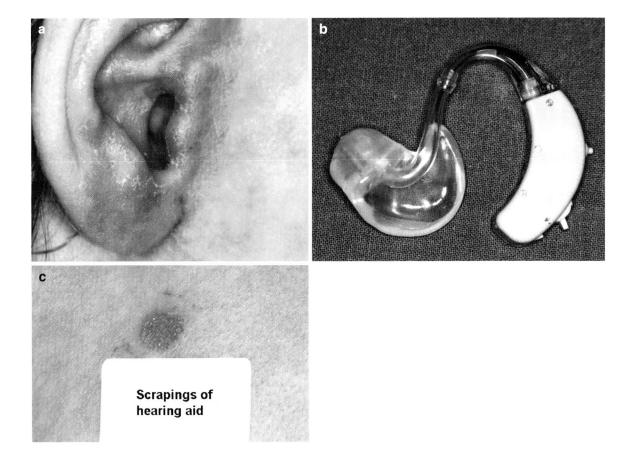

Fig. 57.3 Contact dermatitis of the ear due to a hearing aid (**a**, **b**). Patch testing with fine scrapings of the plastic material was strongly positive (**c**). In subsequent testing with the plastic series, the patient also showed a positive reaction to 2-hydroxyethyl methacrylate (*2-HEMA*) which was a component of the hearing aid as the manufacturer confirmed

Table 57.2 Materials suitable for extraction and recommended solvents [6]

Material	Solvent
Paper	Ethanol
Plants and wood dusts	Acetone, ether, ethanol, or water
Plastics, e.g., gloves	Acetone
Rubber, e.g., gloves	Acetone or water
Textiles	Ethanol

Table 57.3 Recipe for diluting materials for patch testing [31]

Desired percentage dilution (%)	Quantity (µl) to be mixed in 10 ml of vehicle
0.1	10
0.5	50
1.0	100
2.0	200
5.0	500 (0.5 ml)
10	1,000 (1.0 ml)

57.1.2 Control Tests

When a reaction to a new material which suggests a contact allergy based on morphology and development over time is observed, control tests on human volunteers should be performed. This procedure is, however, now a great problem in some countries. In most German University departments, for instance, the approval of the ethics committee has to be obtained beforehand and each volunteer has to provide informed consent.

57.2 Product Categories for Patch Testing

57.2.1 Decorative Cosmetics, Sunscreens, Toiletries (Tables 57.4 and 57.5)

Many allergens are included in the standard series, the series for vehicles, emulsifiers, and preservatives. Fine fragrances may contain ingredients that are not present in commercially available test compounds. Perfumes in alcoholic solutions can be tested as is – occasionally slight irritant reactions (erythema without infiltration) might occur; the frequency of these reactions can be

Table 57.4 Testing of decorative cosmetics and sunscreens

Cosmetic/ sunscreen	Concentration	Comment
Eye make-up		
Eye liner	As is	
Eye shadow	As is	
Mascara	As is	Semi-open test first, allow to dry (solvents)
Make-up cleanser	As is	Semi-open test first, irritation possible (amphoteric or other detergents)
Facial make-up		
Rouge	As is	
Powder	As is	
Foundation	As is	
Lip stick	As is	Photopatch test when sunscreens are incorporated
Moisturizers		
Creams, ointments, lotions	As is	Irritation possible; positive patch test reaction should be confirmed by ROAT or use test. Photopatch test when sunscreens are present
Bleaching creams	As is	
Sunscreens	As is	Photopatch test including active ingredients as commercially available
Self-tanning creams	As is	
Perfumed products		
Fine fragrances	As is	Allow to dry. Photopatch test if clinical findings suggest actinic dermatitis
Eau de Toilette	As is	
After shave	As is	
Deodorants		
Spray, roll on, stick	As is	Allow to dry. Irritation possible. Often false-negative, ROAT!
Shaving products		
Cream	1% (w)	Semi-open with product as is first. Irritation possible under occlusion
Soap	1% (w)	

ac acetone; *MEK* methyl ethyl ketone; *oo* olive oil; *pet* petrolatum; *w* water

Table 57.5 Testing of cleaning products

Product type	Concentration	Comment
Soap bar	1% (w)	Irritation possible; use test
Shampoo	1% (w)	
Shower gel	1% (w)	
Bathing foam	0.1% (w)	
Toothpaste	1% (w)	

w water

reduced by allowing the patch to dry before being applied to the skin [21].

Many moisturizing face creams now contain sunscreens as "anti-aging factors." For details on sunscreens and for photopatch testing see Chap. 27.

The detergents that are active ingredients (sodium lauryl sulfate, lauryl ether sulfates, sulfosuccinic esters, isethionates) are not important allergens. They cause irritant reactions at dilutions of 1–0.5% in most subjects, particularly in patients with sensitive skin. Perfumes and preservatives may be relevant allergens in this category of products [4, 5]. Cocamidopropyl betaine has caused allergic patch test reactions for some time. Now, the major allergen (3-dimethylaminopropylamine) has been identified and removed from this major detergent in shampoos and shower gels.

57.2.2 Hairdressing, Depilatory, and Nail Cosmetics (Table 57.6)

Major allergens are listed in the standard and supplementary series. However, as the group of Menné has recently shown, not all cases of contact dermatitis from hair dyes are identified by *para*-phenylenediamine (PPD) and its derivatives [22]. Therefore, individual testing with the patients' own hair dyes might be necessary. To reduce the risk of active sensitization, an open test must precede the closed patch test. Recently, an epidemic of allergic contact dermatitis from epilating products in France and Belgium has been elucidated [23]. By testing with the commercial products and the ingredients, it was found that modified colophonium derivatives were the main allergens (although in most patients, the colophonium of the standard series was negative); further allergens were methoxy PEG-22/dodecyl glycol copolymer and lauryl alcohol, present in the accompanying skin conditioning tissue.

Table 57.6 Testing of hair dressing products and nail cosmetics

Product	Concentration	Comment
Hair dyes	2% (w)	Active sensitization possible! Semi-open test: five drops dye and five drops oxidizing agent. If negative after 48 h, closed patch test with 2%
Hair spray	As is	Allow to dry. Irritation possible
Hair gel	As is	Semi-open test first
Depilatory	As is	Semi-open test first. Irritation possible (do not occlude)
Nail lacquer	As is	Always semi-open test only
Nail lacquer remover		Do not test (highly irritating)
Glues for artificial nails	1 and 0.1% (MEK)	Semi-open test as is. Most glues are cured with UV light

MEK methyl ethyl ketone

57.2.3 Topical Medicaments

Most topical medicaments used for dermatological conditions can be tested undiluted. Few contain irritating constituents (benzoyl peroxide, tretinoin, mustard, capsaicin, liquid antiseptic agents such as those containing PVP-iodine and nonoxynol, or quaternary ammonium, etc.) – these must be tested in a dilution series. Chapter 35 on topical drugs lists many chemicals as active ingredients that have been identified as contact allergens by patch testing the material of the patient.

57.2.4 Medical Appliances

EKG contact gel	As is
Various aids from plastic materials (prosthesis, hearing aid)	Scrapings, undiluted
Implantations, materials for osteosynthesis	
Metals in standard series	
Methylmethacrylate	2% pet
Palacos® and monomer liquids	Do not test undiluted

Do not test parts of osteosynthesis materials with sharp edges (irritant reactions).

Most patients with a metal allergy (nickel, chromium, cobalt) tolerate implanted metals. Sensitization by implanted materials after a variable latent period of weeks or months, however, has been reported; overall, it seems to be rare with modern metal alloys. Predictive testing is not indicated.

57.2.5 Dental Prosthesis and Other Dental Restorative Materials

Fine scrapings of the prosthesis can be tested in a large Finn chamber with the addition of physiological saline. An allergic contact stomatitis caused by these materials is extremely rare. Sensitizations by acrylates may occur, although these are primarily seen in dental technicians on the hands, due to daily contacts at work.

57.2.6 Disinfecting Agents

These materials are often irritating under occlusion for 48 h in a patch test. Therefore, a semi-open test should always be performed first (Table 57.7). Furthermore, it might be necessary to test with the individual constituents of the product to detect a contact allergy (e.g., to hand disinfecting agents).

57.2.7 Clothing

A piece of the suspected material – textiles, gloves, shoes – (2 × 2 cm moistened with saline solution) is applied under occlusion for 48 h on the back.

Table 57.7 Testing of disinfecting agents

Product	Concentration	Comment
Hand disinfection	As is	Semi-open test first. Closed patch test may be irritating. Use test. Test ingredients!
Disinfecting agents for instruments, floors, etc.	1, 0.1, 0.01%	Semi-open test first. Often contain strong irritants

Textile dyes, formaldehyde resins, and thioureas can be identified by further testing with the supplementary series. Acid dyes may actively sensitize if tested at high concentrations. Therefore, new dyes brought in by the patient must be initially tested at a high dilution [see also Chaps. 37 (clothing), 38 and 43 (shoes, textiles, and rubber)]. In this context, patch testing with thin-layer chromatograms can serve as an elegant adjunct to quickly identify contact allergy to a certain ingredient of a mixture, such as a textile dye, although the (variable, possibly high) detection limit may yield false-negative results [24].

57.2.8 Pesticides

Most reactions to pesticides are irritant and pose the hazard of systemic toxicity by percutaneous absorption (see Chap. 47). Therefore, we do not recommend patch testing with pesticides unless there is strong evidence for allergic contact dermatitis. Detailed information about toxicity must be obtained before sequential testing (open test, semi-open test, and closed patch test).

57.2.9 Detergents for Household Cleaning

General recommendation: 1 and 0.1% (water), semi-open test first, control for pH!

Rather than the detergents, it is usually the additives, such as perfumes, preservatives, dyes, etc., that are the sensitizers, although the frequency of contact allergy to this type of product is apparently often overestimated [25].

Harsh detergents contain quaternary ammonium compounds, which are highly irritating.

57.2.10 Food Stuff

In food handlers and bakers, a protein contact dermatitis must be excluded by prick and scratch chamber testing.

57.2.10.1 Scratch Chamber Testing [26]

After four scarifications with a fine needle, the test material is applied under a large Finn chamber for

24 h. Readings are taken after 24 and 48 h. With fruits and vegetables, irritant reactions are quite frequent.

For bakers, the flours used, the spices, and enzymes must be tested in prick and scratch chamber tests (amylase 1% in water).

In rare cases, an exposure test with the dough squeezed in the hands for 20 min might confirm a suspected protein contact dermatitis.

57.2.11 Plants

Patch testing with pieces of plants is not recommended in general, because irritant reactions are frequent and active sensitization may occur, although direct application on acrylic tape and not occluded by a chamber is less apt to do. The commercially available and standardized materials for patch testing (sesquiterpene lactone mix, primin, Compositae mix, diallyl sulfide, tulipaline, etc.) are safe and identify most cases of plant dermatitis. In professional gardeners sensitization to various plants might occur. For further details and extraction of allergens, see Chap. 41.

In cases of recalcitrant plant dermatitis and unproductive patch testing with commercially available allergens, it may be worthwhile producing an extract of the suspected plant according to Hausen [27]. The pertinent features are listed in Table 57.8.

Plant extracts may be highly irritating. Therefore, adequate control tests must be performed in every case.

Table 57.8 The production of a plant extract for patch testing according to Hausen [27]

Obtaining a concentrate of the plant juice by cutting, pressing, or smashing in a mortar; dilution with water by 1:10 and 1:100
Short extraction with diethylether (60–90 s). Working with ether is dangerous because of its explosive nature. If a suitable laboratory equipment is not available (rotation evaporation under an exhaust system), a practical alternative is the use of large open glassware filled with the solvent and the plant, left open in the air for about 1 h
Tulips, lilies, alstroemeria, and other Liliaceae are extracted more efficiently with ethanol
After evaporation of the solvent, the extract is incorporated into a suitable vehicle: water, ethanol, methanol, acetone, acidic acid ester, methylethylketone, or plant oil. The use of petrolatum is also possible. Dilution series to start with: 1:10, 1:100, 1:1,000. The material should be kept in a refrigerator

It is self evident that the exact botanical classification is necessary before starting any investigative work.

57.2.12 Woods

Fine wood dust moistened with physiological saline can be patch tested with a Finn chamber or on adhesive acrylic tape. Exotic woods can be strongly irritating and sensitizing (teak, rosewood, Macoré) – these should be diluted to at least 10% in petrolatum (sensitization might occur even at lower concentrations in rare cases).

Turpentine and colophony (peroxides) are the major allergens of conifers (pine, spruce, larch).

57.2.13 Office Work

Reactions to paper and cardboard are usually irritant in nature, particularly in atopics. In rare cases, sensitizations to colophony or formaldehyde resins may be relevant. A piece of paper (2 × 2 cm, moistened with physiological saline) is applied occlusively for 2 days. NCR (carbonless) paper can be tested in the same way after rubbing it firmly to release the encapsulated dye. Diethylendiamine and colophony have been identified as allergens in NCR paper [11]. Telefax paper may also contain contact allergens (colophony, Bisphenol A). According to Karlberg and Lidén [28], testing with paper extracts (in acetone or methanol) is more reliable than a patch test with the paper as is.

Other materials that may be relevant to chronic hand eczema in office workers are:

- Rubber articles
- Glues (colophony, various resins)
- Woods (desk tops, handles)
- Metals (nickel in metallic objects such as perforators, pens, etc.)
- Plants
- Liquid soaps, hand creams used at the work place

57.2.14 Construction Materials

- Concrete
- Cement
- Resins for various purposes
- Tile setting materials

Testing with the material as is under occlusion is absolutely contraindicated because of high irritancy. A semi-open test might be indicated in cases with a high suspicion of contact allergy, particularly when resins are involved and testing with the standard and supplementary series remains negative. The main allergen in cement is potassium dichromate, which is present in the standard series. Fast-curing cements contain epoxy resins, which are increasingly recognized as major allergens not only in the construction industry, but also in other industrial areas (painting, metal, electronics, and plastic). The epoxy resin of the standard series is insufficient to detect all cases of relevant epoxy resin allergies, as has been shown by a large German multicenter study [29]. Sometimes acrylic resins may also be present.

57.2.15 Paints, Lacquers

The chemical composition of paints and lacquers is very complex. Acrylates of various types are added for rapid curing. In the so-called biologic paints turpentine and colophony are often present. Isothiazolinones are frequently used in water-based wall paints. Before patch testing is performed with these products, detailed information from the manufacturer should be obtained. Semi-open tests can be performed. As a guideline, the concentrations as listed in Table 57.9 can be used.

57.2.16 Greases and Oils

These materials primarily used for lubrication rarely produce an allergic contact dermatitis. They are not very irritating except for hydraulic oils. Table 57.10 provides the recommended test concentrations.

Table 57.9 Testing of paints, lacquers, and solvents. Semi-open test first for all paints or lacquers

Product	Concentration	Comment
One component (water based, e.g., wall paints)	10–100% (w)	
One component (solvent- or oil-based, e.g., paints for wood, iron, etc.)	1–10% (pet)	
Diisocyanate hardeners of polyurethane paints or lacquers	2–5% (pet)	
Paints containing epoxy, polyesters, or acrylics	0.1–1.0% (pet)	Obtain detailed information on chemical composition first. Test conc. may be raised to 10% for some paints (see Chap. 34 on plastics)
Organic solvents		
Aliphatic, cycloaliphatic	1–10% (pet)	
Aromatic	1–5% (pet)	
Chlorinated	0.1–1% (pet)	
Esters	1–10% (pet)	

pet petrolatum

Table 57.10 Testing of technical greases and oils

Product	Concentration	Comment
Lubricating grease	As is and 20% (pet)	Semi-open test first
Lubricating oils	As is, 50, 10% (oo)	
Hydraulic oils	1% (oo)	

oo olive oil; *pet* petrolatum

57.2.17 Metalworking Fluids

MWFs are indispensable for the processing of metal parts. Their chemical composition varies with the purpose and the type of metal. Material safety data sheets usually do not contain all relevant allergological information. The most important allergens are rust preventives/emulsifiers, resin acids from distilled tall

Table 57.11 Testing of metalworking fluids (*MWF*) – for details see Chap. 33

Product	Concentration (%)	Comment
Water-based	5 (w)	The usual workplace concentration of fresh MWF is 4–8%. Test a freshly diluted MWF at 5%, the used one as is (provided the concentration at the workplace is less than 8% – otherwise use a dilution of at least 1:1)
Oil-based	50 (oo)	

oo olive oil; *w* water

oil, and biocides. For further details see Chaps. 33 and 39. Table 57.11 provides guidelines for testing with MWF [30].

The most common mistake when testing water-based MWF is that the concentrate brought in by the patient is patch tested without further dilution. This usually produces severe irritant, sometimes ulcerative, lesions. The concentrate is usually diluted to 4–8% by adding water in the circulatory system of the machine. Metal workers often come into contact with this dilution of the MWF and develop a chronic irritant contact dermatitis (Fig. 57.4).

Perfumes as "odor masks" are often added and may produce an allergic contact dermatitis. The same holds true for isothiazolinones and other biocides, which are also often added as "system cleaners" in excessive concentrations during the use cycle of a MWF in order to prevent degradation and bad odors. Therefore, testing of both the fresh and the used MWF is obligatory.

57.2.18 Rubber Chemicals

Rubber products can be patch tested as is. This may be particularly worthwhile with protective gloves, rubber masks, or other materials with prolonged direct skin contact. Often, the usual rubber ingredients available for patch testing remain negative. The isolation of the allergen in rubber products is extremely difficult due to the complex chemical nature and the numerous additives used for maintaining the desired technical features. As a guideline, accelerators, antioxidants, and

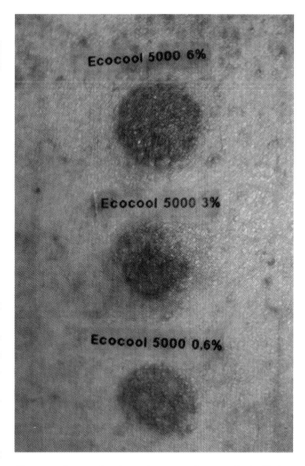

Fig. 57.4 Strong allergic patch test reactions to a fresh dilution series of a metalworking fluid (MWF) brought in by a patient with chronic occupational hand eczema (use concentration at the work place was 6% in water). He also showed positive reactions to colophony (2+), abietic acid (3+), monoethanolamine (1+), and 2-(2-aminoethoxy)ethanol (diglycolamine) (1+). These materials are often present in MWFs and may cause relevant sensitizations

other materials provided by a cooperative manufacturer can be tested at 1% in petrolatum. Positive reactions require further dilutions and testing on control persons.

57.2.19 Glues and Adhesives

This group of products is nowadays ubiquitous and frequently used at home for production and repairs in various areas. Glues are often irritating in undiluted form. Testing with acrylates in inadequate dilutions can cause active sensitization. The test concentrations

Table 57.12 Testing of glues and adhesives

Product	Concentration	Comment
Adhesive tapes	As is	
Glues (excluding epoxy, formaldehyde resin, and acrylic)		Semi-open test first. Allow to dry when patch testing
Dispersion glues	10–100% (pet or w)	
Solvent-based contact glues	1–10% (pet)	
Cyanoacrylate	2% (pet)	Strong irritant, rare allergen. Semi-open test first

pet petrolatum; *w* water

as listed in Table 57.12 provide a guideline only; before patch testing an unknown new material, detailed information from the manufacturer should be obtained. Testing should always start with a semi-open test to avoid strong irritant reactions or active sensitization.

57.2.20 Plastic Materials

With this group of chemicals, testing with the commercially available patch testing substances produced by major manufacturers is recommended. These materials have been validated on large groups of patients and the patch test concentrations can be considered as safe and nonsensitizing.

Most patients have contact only with the end product after complete curing and containing no monomers as irritating or sensitizing components. However, as described in detail in Chap. 34 on plastic materials, exceptions to this rule do occur and relevant sensitization may be detected only by patch testing fine dust particles of the plastic product or with all ingredients after time-consuming dilution series. Patch testing with a thin-layer chromatogram of a resin of unknown composition may be an interesting option to screen for the causative agent [24].

A few of these materials are carcinogenic and may cause bronchial asthma (for example, the group of

isocyanates). Therefore, these materials must be handled with great caution.

57.2.21 Do Not Test

In general, the following materials should not be tested, because they are known as strong irritants and not as contact allergens (with few exceptions).

Patch testing may be performed only if there is a high suspicion of contact allergy by history and clinical findings. In such a case, an open and semi-open test should precede closed patch testing (dilution series from 0.1 to 1%).

- Astringents (e.g., $AgNO_3$)
- Antifreeze
- Car wax
- Gasoline
- Diesel
- Floor wax
- Lime
- Organic solvents (various types)
- Kerosene
- Metal chips (coarse)
- Rust remover
- White spirit
- Toluene
- Toilet cleaners and other strong caustic cleaning agents
- Cement, concrete

All products that have a strong pungent odor and/or contain organic solvents should be tested for pH (see above). If an open and semi-open test is negative, a dilution series starting with a very high dilution can be performed under occlusion (maximum 24 h, locating on the medial aspect of the upper arm, which enables removal by the patient in case pain occurs).

If there is doubt about the nature of the patch test reaction – irritant or allergic – an expert in the field should be consulted before further testing is performed. Active sensitization of volunteers or ulcerative lesions with scar formation may be the risk factors for further investigative procedures.

References

1. Menné T, Dooms-Goossens A, Wahlberg JE, White IR, Shaw S (1992) How large a proportion of contact sensitivities are diagnosed with the European standard series? Contact Dermatitis 26:201–202
2. Nettis E, Marcandrea M, Colonardi MC, Paradiso MT, Ferrannini TA (2003) Results of standard series patch testing in patients with occupational allergic contact dermatitis. Allergy 58:1304–1307
3. Daecke CM (1994) Der Stellenwert patienteneigener Testsubstanzen bei der Epikutantestung. Hautarzt 45: 292–298
4. Balzer C, Schnuch A, Geier J, Uter W (2005) Ergebnisse der Epikutantestung mit patienteneigenen Kosmetika und Körperpflegemittel im IVDK, 1998–2002. Dermatol Beruf Umwelt 53:8–24
5. Uter W, Balzer C, Geier J, Frosch PJ, Schnuch A (2005) Patch testing with patients' own cosmetics and toiletries – results of the IVDK, 1998–2002. Contact Dermatitis 53:226–233
6. Jolanki R, Estlander T, Alanko K, Kanerva L (2000) Patch testing with a patient's own materials handled at work. In: Kanerva L, Elsner P, Wahlberg JE, Maibach HI (eds) Handbook of occupational dermatology. Springer, Berlin, pp 375–383
7. Goossens A, Detienne T, Bruze M (2002) Occupational allergic contact dermatitis caused by isocyanates. Contact Dermatitis 47:304–308
8. Frick M, Zimerson E, Karlsson D et al (2004) Poor correlation between stated and found concentration of diphenylmethane-4, 4´-diisocyanate (4, 4´-MDI) in petrolatum patch-test preparations. Contact Dermatitis 51:73–78
9. Giménez Arnau E, Andersen KE, Bruze M, Frosch PJ, Johansen JD, Menné T, Rastogie SE, White IR, Lepoittevin JP (2000) Identification of Lilial® as a fragrance sensitizer in a perfume by bioassay-guided chemical fractionation and structure-activity relationships. Contact Dermatitis 43: 351–358
10. Mutterer V, Giménez Arnau E, Lepoittevin JP, Johansen JD, Frosch PJ, Menné T, Andersen KE, Bruze M, Rastogi SC, White IR (1999) Identification of coumarin as the sensitizer in a patient sensitive to her own perfume but negative to the fragrance mix. Contact Dermatitis 40:196–199
11. Lange-Ionescu S, Bruze M, Gruvberger B, Zimerson E, Frosch PJ (2000) Kontaktallergie durch kohlefreies Durchschlagpapier. Dermat Beruf Umwelt 48:183–187
12. Magerl A, Heiss R, Frosch PJ (2001) Allergic contact dermatitis from zinc ricinoleate in a deodorant and glyceryl ricinoleate in a lipstick. Contact Dermatitis 44:119–121
13. Magerl A, Pirker C, Frosch PJ (2003) Allergisches Kontaktekzem durch Schellack und 1, 3-Butylenglykol in einem Eyliner. J Dtsch Dermatolog Ges 1:300–302
14. Uter W, Balzer C, Geier J, Schnuch A, Frosch PJ (2005) Ergebnisse der Epikutantestung mit patienteneigenen Parfüms, Deos und Rasierwässern. Ergebnisse des IVDK 1998–2002. Dermatol Beruf Umwelt 53:25–36
15. Henriks-Eckerman M, Suuronen K, Jolanki R, Alanko K (2004) Methacrylates in dental restorative materials. Contact Dermatitis 50:233–237
16. Uter W, Geier J, Lessmann H, Schnuch A (1999) Unverträglichkeitsreaktionen gegen Körperpflege- und Haushaltsprodukte: Was ist zu tun? Die Informations- und Dokumentationsstelle für Kontaktallergien (IDOK) des Informationsverbundes Dermatologischer Kliniken (IVDK). Deutsche Dermatologe 47:211–214
17. Vigan M (1997) Les nouveaux allergenes des cosmetiques. La cosmetovigilance. Ann Dermatol Venereol 124:571–575
18. Herbst RA, Uter W, Pirker C, Geier J, Frosch PJ (2004) Allergic and non-allergic periorbital dermatitis: patch test results of the Information Network of the Departments of Dermatology during a 5-year period. Contact Dermatitis 51:13–19
19. Dooms-Goossens A (1995) Patch testing without a kit. In: Guin JD (ed) Practical contact dermatitis. A handbook for the practitioner. McGraw-Hill, Philadelphia, PA, pp 63–74
20. Bruze M (1984) Use of buffer solutions for patch testing. Contact Dermatitis 10:267–269
21. Johansen JD, Frosch PJ, Rastogi SC, Menné T (2001) Testing with fine fragrances in eczema patients. Contact Dermatitis 44:304–307
22. Sosted H, Basketter DA, Estrada E, Johansen JD, Patlewicz GY (2004) Ranking of hair dye substances according to predicted sensitization potency: quantitative structure-activity relationships. Contact Dermatitis 51:241–254
23. Goossens A, Armingaud P, Avenel-Audran M et al (2002) An epidemic of allergic contact dermatitis due to epilating products. Contact Dermatitis 46:67–70
24. Bruze M, Frick M, Persson L (2003) Patch testing with thin-layer chromatograms. Contact Dermatitis 48:278–279
25. Belsito DV, Fransway AF, Fowler JF Jr, Sherertz EF, Maibach HI, Mark JG Jr, Mathias CG, Rietschel RL, Storrs FJ, Nethercott JR (2002) Allergic contact dermatitis to detergents: a multicenter study to assess prevalence. J Am Acad Dermatol 46(2):200–2006
26. Niinimäki A (1987) Scratch-chamber tests in food handler dermatitis. Contact Dermatitis 16:11–20
27. Hausen BM (1988) Allergiepflanzen, Pflanzengifte. Handbuch und Atlas der allergieinduzierenden Wild- und Kulturpflanzen. Ecomed, Landsberg Lech
28. Karlberg AT, Lidén C (1992) Colophony (rosin) in newspapers may contribute to hand eczema. Br J Dermatol 126:161–165
29. Geier J, Lessmann H, Hillen U, Jappe U, Dickel H, Koch P et al (2004) An attemt to improve diagnostics of contact allergy due to epoxy resin systems. First results of the multi-centre study EPOX 2002. Contact Dermatitis 51:263–272
30. Tiedemann KH, Zöllner G, Adam M et al (2002) Empfehlungen für die Epikutantestung bei Verdacht auf Kontaktallergie durch Kühlschmierstoffe. 2. Hinweise zur Arbeitsstofftestung. Dermatol Beruf Umwelt 50:180–189
31. Sherertz EF, Byers SV (1997) Estimating dilutions for patch testing skin care products: a practical method. Am J Contact Derm 8:181–182

Dictionary of Contact Allergens: Chemical Structures, Sources, and References

58

Christophe J. Le Coz and Jean-Pierre Lepoittevin

Contents

58.1 Introduction

This chapter has been written in order to familiarize the reader with the chemical structure of chemicals implicated in contact dermatitis, mainly as haptens responsible for allergic contact dermatitis. For each molecule, the principal name is used for classification. We have also listed the most important synonym(s), the Chemical Abstract Service (CAS) Registry Number that characterizes the substance, and its chemical structure. The reader will find one or more relevant literature references. As it was not possible to be exhaustive, some allergens have been omitted since they were obsolete, extremely rarely implicated in contact dermatitis, their case reports were too imprecise, or they are extensively treated in other chapters of the textbook. From a practical chemical point of view, acrylates, cyanoacrylates and (meth)acrylates, cephalosporins, and parabens have been grouped together.

1. Abietic acid

CAS Registry Number [514–10–3]

Abietic acid is probably the major allergen of colophony, along with dehydroabietic acid, by way of oxidation products. Its detection in a material indicates that allergenic components of colophony are present.

C.J. Le Coz (✉)
Cabinet de Dermatologie & Laboratoire de Dermatochimie,
4 rue Blaise Pascal, F-67070 Strasbourg, France
e-mail: Christophe.lecoz@wanadoo.fr

J.-P. Lepoittevin
Institut le Bel, Labo. Dermatochimie,
4, rue Blaise Pascal, 67070 Strasbourg Cedex, France
e-mail: jplepoit@unistra.fr

J.D. Johansen et al. (eds.), *Contact Dermatitis*,
DOI: 10.1007/978-3-642-03827-3_58, © Springer-Verlag Berlin Heidelberg 2011

58

Suggested Reading

Bergh M, Menné T, Karlberg AT (1994) Colophony in paper-based surgical clothing. Contact Dermatitis 31:332–333

Karlberg AT, Bergstedt E, Boman A, Bohlinder K, Lidén C, Nilsson JLG, Wahlberg JE (1985) Is abietic acid the allergenic component of colophony? Contact Dermatitis 13:209–215

Karlberg AT, Bohlinder K, Boman A, Hacksell U, Hermansson J, Jacobsson S, Nilsson JLG (1988) Identification of 15-hydroperoxyabietic acid as a contact allergen in Portuguese colophony. J Pharm Pharmacol 40:42–47

2. Acetaldehyde

Acetic Aldehyde, Ethanal, Ethylic Aldehyde

CAS Registry Number [75–07–0]

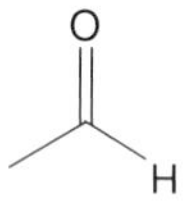

Acetaldehyde, as its metabolite, is responsible for many of the effects of ethanol, such as hepatic or neurological toxicity. A case of contact allergy was reported in the textile industry, where dimethoxane was used as a biocide agent in textiles, and its degradation led to acetaldehyde.

Suggested Reading

Eriksson CJ (2001) The role of acetaldehyde in the actions of alcohol (update 2000). Alcohol Clin Exp Res 25(suppl 5): 15S–32S

Shmunes E, Kempton RJ (1980) Allergic contact dermatitis to dimethoxane in a spin finish. Contact Dermatitis 6:421–424

3. Acid Blue 158

CAS Registry Numbers [6370-08-7], [39389-99-6], [53126-96-8]

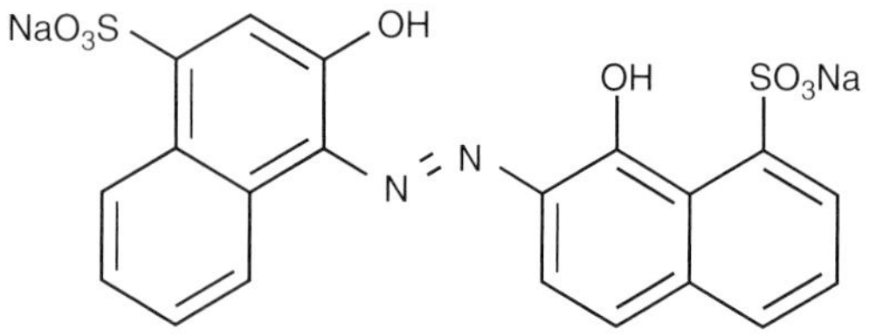

This azo dye has the Color Index nr. 14880. It is found in suture materials.

Suggested Reading

Hausen BM (2003) Allergic contact dermatitis from colored surgical suture material: contact allergy to epsilon-caprolactam and acid blue 158. Am J Contact Dermat 14:174–175

Raap U, Wieczorek D, Kapp A, Wedi B (2008) Allergic contact dermatitis to acid blue 158 in suture material. Contact Dermatitis 59:192–193

4. Acrylamide

CAS Registry Number [79–06–1]

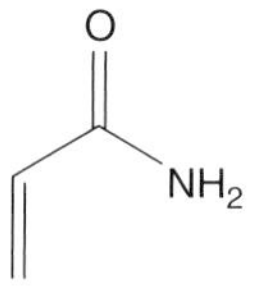

Acrylamide is used in the plastic polymers industry for water treatments and soil stabilization and to prepare polyacrylamide gels for electrophoresis. This neurotoxic, carcinogenic, and genotoxic substance is known to have caused contact dermatitis in industrial and laboratory workers.

Suggested Reading

Beyer DJ, Belsito DV (2000) Allergic contact dermatitis from acrylamide in a chemical mixer. Contact Dermatitis 42: 181–182

Dooms-Goossens A, Garmyn M, Degreef H (1991) Contact allergy to acrylamide. Contact Dermatitis 24:71–72

Lambert J, Mathieu L, Dockx P (1988) Contact dermatitis from acrylamide. Contact Dermatitis 19:65

5. Acrylates, Cyanoacrylate, and Methacrylates

Acrylic Acid and Acrylates

CAS Registry Number [79–10–7]

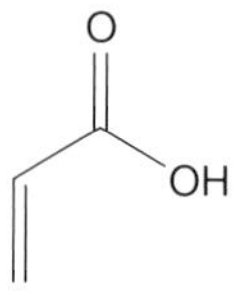

Acrylic acid 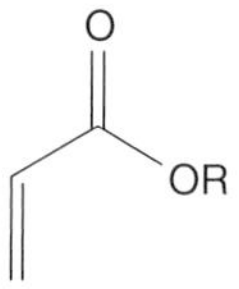   Acrylate

Acrylates are esters from acrylic acid. Occupational contact allergies from acrylates have frequently been reported and mainly concern workers exposed to the glues based on acrylic acid, as well as dental workers and beauticians.

Bisphenol A Diglycidylether Diacrylate

2,2-bis[4-(2-Hydroxy-3-Acryloxypropoxy)phenyl]-Propane (Bis-GA)

CAS Registry Number [8687–94–9]

Bis-GA is an epoxy diacrylate. It caused contact dermatitis in a process worker, being contained in ultraviolet-light-curable acrylic paints.

Suggested Reading

Aalto-Korte K, Jungewelter S, Henriks-Eckerman ML, Kuuliala O, Jolanki R (2009) Contact allergy to epoxy (meth)acrylates. Contact Dermatitis 61:9–21

Jolanki R, Kanerva L, Estlander T (1995) Occupational allergic contact dermatitis caused by epoxy diacrylate in ultraviolet-light-cured paint, and bisphenol A in dental composite resin. Contact Dermatitis 33:94–99

Bisphenol A Glycidyl Methacrylate

Bis-GMA

CAS Registry Number [1565–94–2]

Bis-GMA is an epoxy-methacrylate. Sensitization occurs in dentists, beauticians, and consumers with sculptured photopolymerizable nails.

Suggested Reading

Aalto-Korte K, Jungewelter S, Henriks-Eckerman ML, Kuuliala O, Jolanki R (2009) Contact allergy to epoxy (meth)acrylates. Contact Dermatitis 61:9–21

Kanerva L, Estlander T, Jolanki R (1989) Allergic contact dermatitis from dental composite resins due to aromatic epoxy acrylates and aliphatic acrylates. Contact Dermatitis 20:201–211

1,4-Butanediol Diacrylate

CAS Registry Number [1070–70–8]

A positive patch test was observed in a male process worker in a paint factory, sensitized to an epoxy diacrylate contained in raw materials of ultraviolet-light-curable paint. The positive reaction was probably due to a cross-reactivity.

Suggested Reading

Jolanki R, Kanerva L, Estlander T (1995) Occupational allergic contact dermatitis caused by epoxy diacrylate in ultraviolet-light-cured paint, and bisphenol A in dental composite resin. Contact Dermatitis 33:94–99

1,4-Butanediol Dimethacrylate

CAS Registry Number [2082–81–7]

Sensitization to 1,4-butanediol dimethacrylate was reported in dental technicians, with cross-reactivity to methyl methacrylate.

Suggested Reading

Rustemeyer T, Frosch PJ (1996) Occupational skin diseases in dental laboratory technicians. (I). Clinical picture and causative factors. Contact Dermatitis 34:125–133

n-Butyl Acrylate

CAS Registry Number [141–32–2]

Sensitization to n-butyl acrylate can occur in the dental profession.

58

Suggested Reading

Daecke C, Schaller J, Goos M (1994) Acrylates as potent allergens in occupational and domestic exposures. Contact Dermatitis 30:190–191

Kanerva L, Estlander T, Jolanki R, Tarvainen K (1993) Occupational allergic contact dermatitis caused by exposure to acrylates during work with dental prostheses. Contact Dermatitis 28:268–275

Rustemeyer T, Frosch PJ (1996) Occupational skin diseases in dental laboratory technicians. (I). Clinical picture and causative factors. Contact Dermatitis 34:125–133

tert-Butyl Acrylate

CAS Registry Number [1663–39–4]

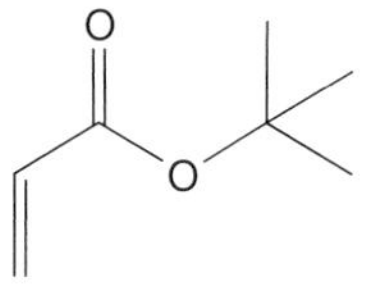

Sensitization may affect dental workers.

Suggested Reading

Kanerva L, Estlander T, Jolanki R, Tarvainen K (1993) Occupational allergic contact dermatitis caused by exposure to acrylates during work with dental prostheses. Contact Dermatitis 28:268–275

Cyanoacrylic Acid and Cyanoacrylates

2-Cyanoacrylic Acid

CAS Registry Number [15802–18–3]

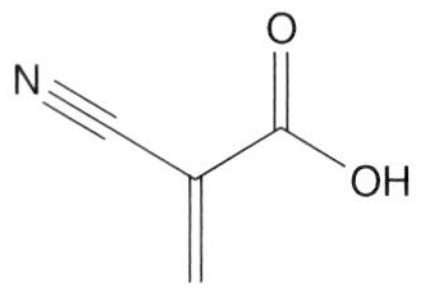

Cyanoacrylic acid 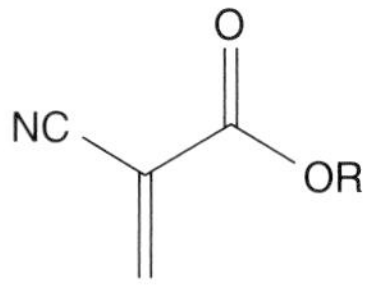   Cyanoacrylate

Cyanoacrylates, particularly 2-ethyl cyanoacrylate, are derived from cyanoacrylic acid. They are used as sealants.

Suggested Reading

Fischer AA (1985) Reactions to cyanoacrylate adhesives: "instant glue". Cutis 35:18; 20; 22

Tarvainen K (1995) Analysis of patients with allergic patch test reactions to a plastics and glue series. Contact Dermatitis 32:346–351

Diethyleneglycol Diacrylate

CAS Registry Number [4074–88–8]

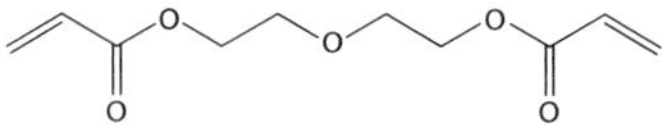

Diethyleneglycol diacrylate was positive in a painter sensitized to his own acrylate-based paint.

Suggested Reading

Nakamura M, Arima Y, Yoneda K, Nobuhara S, Miyachi Y (1999) Occupational contact dermatitis from acrylic monomer in paint. Contact Dermatitis 40:228–229

Ethyl Acrylate

CAS Registry Number [140–88–5]

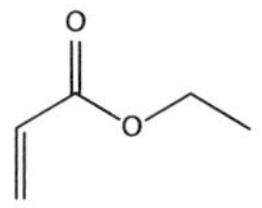

Ethyl acrylate is a sensitizer in the dental profession.

Suggested Reading

Kanerva L, Estlander T, Jolanki R, Tarvainen K (1993) Occupational allergic contact dermatitis caused by exposure to acrylates during work with dental prostheses. Contact Dermatitis 28:268–275

Rustemeyer T, Frosch PJ (1996) Occupational skin diseases in dental laboratory technicians. (I). Clinical picture and causative factors. Contact Dermatitis 34:125–133

Ethyl Cyanoacrylate

Ethyl-2-Cyanoacrylate

CAS Registry Number [7085–85–0]

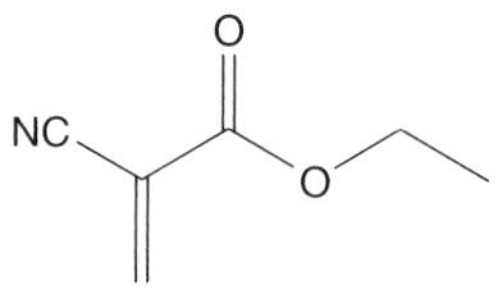

Ethyl cyanoacrylate is contained in instant glues for metal, glass, rubber, plastics, textiles, tissues, and nails. It polymerizes almost instantaneously in air at room temperature and bonds immediately and strongly to surface keratin. Beauticians are exposed to contact dermatitis from nail glues.

Suggested Reading

Bruze M, Björkner B, Lepoittevin JP (1995) Occupational allergic contact dermatitis from ethyl cyanoacrylate. Contact Dermatitis 32:156–159

Fitzgerald DA, Bhaggoe R, English JSC (1995) Contact sensitivity to cyanoacrylate nail-adhesive with dermatitis at remote sites. Contact Dermatitis 32:175–176

Jacobs MC, Rycroft RJG (1995) Allergic contact dermatitis from cyanoacrylate? Contact Dermatitis 33:71

Tomb R, Lepoittevin JP, Durepaire F, Grosshans E (1993) Ectopic contact dermatitis from ethyl cyanoacrylate instant adhesives. Contact Dermatitis 28:206–208

Ethyleneglycol Dimethacrylate

CAS Registry Number [97–90–5]

Ethyleneglycol dimethacrylate (EGDMA) is a crosslinking agent of acrylic resins and is employed to optimize the dilution of high-viscosity monomers and to link together the macromolecules constituting the polymer. It caused contact dermatitis in dental technicians and dental assistants. A case was also reported in a manufacturer of car rear-view mirrors.

Suggested Reading

Farli M, Gasperini M, Francalanci S, Gola M, Sertoli A (1990) Occupational contact dermatitis in 2 dental technicians. Contact Dermatitis 22:282–287

Kanerva L, Jolanki R, Estlander T (1995) Occupational allergic contact dermatitis from 2-hydroxyethyl methacrylate and ethylene glycol dimethacrylate in a modified acrylic structural adhesive. Contact Dermatitis 35:84–89

Rustemeyer T, Frosch PJ (1996) Occupational skin diseases in dental laboratory technicians. (I). Clinical picture and causative factors. Contact Dermatitis 34:125–133

Tosti A, Rapacchiale S, Piraccini BM, Peluso AM (1991) Occupational airborne contact dermatitis due to ethylene glycol dimethacrylate. Contact Dermatitis 24:152–153

2-Ethylhexyl Acrylate

2-EHA

CAS Registry Number [1322–13–0]

2-EHA was contained in a surgical tape and caused allergic contact dermatitis in a patient.

Suggested Reading

Daecke C, Schaller J, Goos M (1994) Acrylates as potent allergens in occupational and domestic exposures. Contact Dermatitis 30:190–191

Ethyl Methacrylate

CAS Registry Number [97–63–2]

Ethyl methacrylate is used in dental prostheses or photobonded sculptured nails.

Suggested Reading

Kanerva L, Estlander T, Jolanki R, Tarvainen K (1993) Occupational allergic contact dermatitis caused by exposure to acrylates during work with dental prostheses. Contact Dermatitis 28:268–275

Kanerva L, Lauerma A, Estlander T, Alanko K, Henriks-Eckerman ML, Jolanki R (1996) Occupational allergic contact dermatitis caused by photobonded sculptured nails and a review of (meth)acrylates in nail cosmetics. Am J Contact Dermat 7:109–115

Rustemeyer T, Frosch PJ (1996) Occupational skin diseases in dental laboratory technicians. (I). Clinical picture and causative factors. Contact Dermatitis 34:125–133

Glycidyl Methacrylate

CAS Registry Number [106–91–2]

Glycidyl methacrylate, an epoxy methacrylate, was reported as the allergenic component of the anaerobic sealant Sta-Lok.

Suggested Reading

Aalto-Korte K, Jungewelter S, Henriks-Eckerman ML, Kuuliala O, Jolanki R (2009) Contact allergy to epoxy (meth)acrylates. Contact Dermatitis 61:9–21

Dempsey KJ (1982) Hypersensitivity to Sta-Lok and Loctite anaerobic sealants. J Am Acad Dermatol 7:779–784

1,6-Hexanediol Diacrylate

Hexamethylene Diacrylate

CAS Registry Number [13048–33–4]

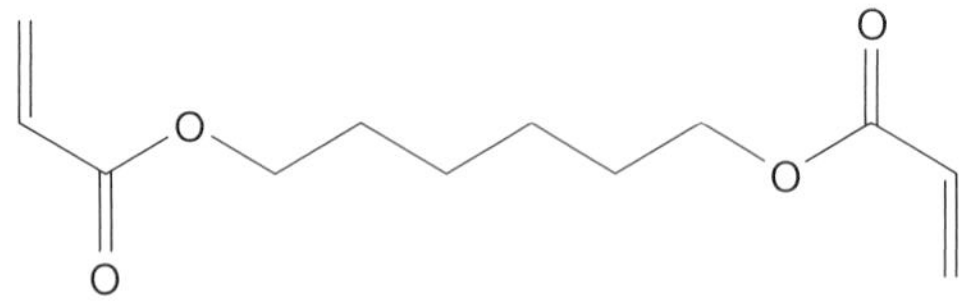

Sensitization occurred after accidental occupational exposure in an employee in the laboratory of a plastic paint factory.

Suggested Reading

Botella-Estrada R, Mora E, de La Cuadra J (1992) Hexanediol diacrylate sensitization after accidental occupational exposure. Contact Dermatitis 26:50–51

2-Hydroxyethyl Acrylate

2-HEA, Ethylene Glycol Acrylate

CAS Registry Number [818–61–1]

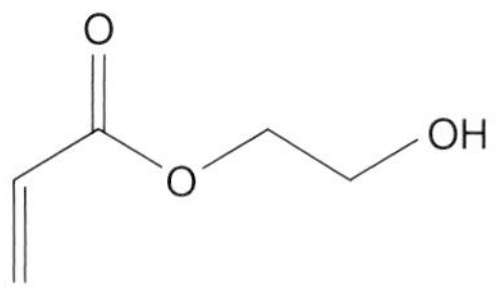

2-HEA is contained in Lowicryl 4KM and K11 M resins. It caused contact dermatitis in workers embedding media for electron microscopy. It may also be contained in UV-cured nail gel used for photobonded, sculptured nails.

Suggested Reading

Kanerva L, Lauerma A, Estlander T, Alanko K, Henriks-Eckerman ML, Jolanki R (1996) Occupational allergic contact dermatitis caused by photobonded sculptured nails and a review of (meth) acrylates in nail cosmetics. Am J Contact Dermat 7:109–115
Tobler M, Wüthrich B, Freiburghaus AU (1990) Contact dermatitis from acrylate and methacrylate compounds in Lowicryl® embedding media for electron microscopy. Contact Dermatitis 23:96–102

2-Hydroxyethyl Methacrylate

2-HEMA

CAS Registry Number [868–77–9]

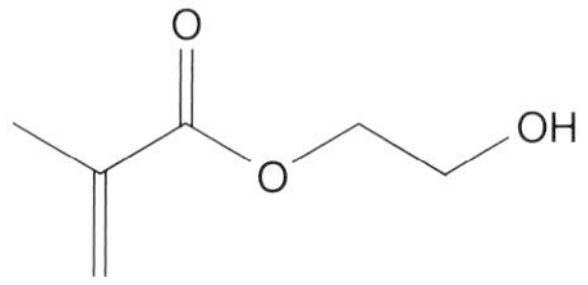

Sensitization to 2-HEMA concerns mainly dental technicians and dentists, but can also occur in other workers such as printers, beauticians, or consumers using photopolymerizable sculptured nails.

Suggested Reading

Geukens S, Goossens A (2001) Occupational contact allergy to (meth)acrylates. Contact Dermatitis 44:153–159
Jolanki R, Kanerva L, Estlander T, Tarvainen K (1994) Concomitant sensitization to triglycidyl isocyanurate, diaminodiphenyl-methane and 2-hydroxyethyl methacrylate from silk-screen printing coatings in the manufacture of circuit boards. Contact Dermatitis 30:12–15
Kanerva L, Estlander T, Jolanki R, Tarvainen K (1993) Occupational allergic contact dermatitis caused by exposure to acrylates during work with dental prostheses. Contact Dermatitis 28:268–275
Kanerva L, Jolanki R, Estlander T (1995) Occupational allergic contact dermatitis from 2-hydroxyethyl methacrylate and ethylene glycol dimethacrylate in a modified acrylic structural adhesive. Contact Dermatitis 35:84–89
Rustemeyer T, Frosch PJ (1996) Occupational skin diseases in dental laboratory technicians. (I). Clinical picture and causative factors. Contact Dermatitis 34:125–133

2-Hydroxypropyl Acrylate

CAS Registry Number [999–61–1]

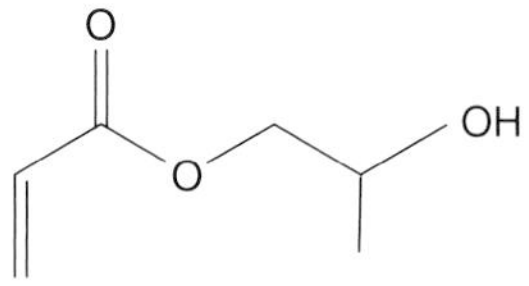

A case of occupational contact dermatitis was reported in industry.

Suggested Reading

Lovell CR, Rycroft RJG, Williams DMJ, Hamlin JW (1985) Contact dermatitis from the irritancy (immediate and delayed) and allergenicity of hydroxypropyl acrylate. Contact Dermatitis 12:117–118

2-Hydroxypropyl Methacrylate

CAS Registry Number [27813–02–1]

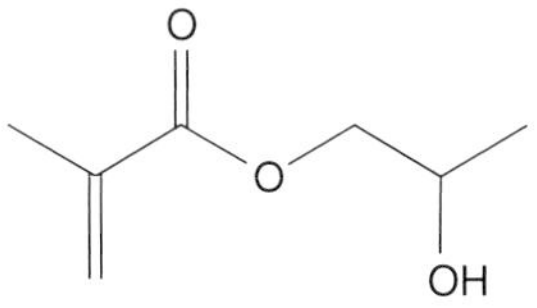

Sensitization to 2-hydroxypropyl methacrylate concerns mainly the dental profession.

Suggested Reading

Kanerva L, Estlander T, Jolanki R, Tarvainen K (1993) Occupational allergic contact dermatitis caused by exposure to acrylates during work with dental prostheses. Contact Dermatitis 28:268–275

Kanerva L, Estlander T, Jolanki R (1997) Occupational allergic contact dermatitis caused by triacrylic tri-cure glass ionomer. Contact Dermatitis 37:49

Rustemeyer T, Frosch PJ (1996) Occupational skin diseases in dental laboratory technicians. (I). Clinical picture and causative factors. Contact Dermatitis 34:125–133

Methacrylic Acid and Methacrylates

CAS Registry Number [79–41–4]

Methacrylic acid   Methacrylate

Methacrylates are derived from methacrylic acid. They are used in the production of a great variety of polymers. As they are moderate to strong sensitizers, sensitization concerns many professions. Dental technicians, assistants, and surgeons are frequently exposed. Methacrylates were reported as occupational allergens in chemically cured or photocured sculptured nails.

Methyl Acrylate

MA

CAS Registry Number [96–33–3]

MA is contained in some nail lacquers.

Suggested Reading

Kanerva L, Estlander T, Jolanki R, Tarvainen K (1993) Occupational allergic contact dermatitis caused by exposure to acrylates during work with dental prostheses. Contact Dermatitis 28:268–275

Kanerva L, Lauerma A, Estlander T, Alanko K, Henriks-Eckerman ML, Jolanki R (1996) Occupational allergic contact dermatitis caused by photobonded sculptured nails and a review of (meth) acrylates in nail cosmetics. Am J Contact Dermat 7:109–115

Methyl Methacrylate and Polymethyl Methacrylate

CAS Registry Numbers [80–62–6] and [9011–14–7]

Methyl methacrylate is one of the most common methacrylates. This acrylic monomer, the essential component of the fluid mixed with the powder, causes allergic contact dermatitis mainly in dental technicians and dentists. Cases were also reported following the use of sculptured nails and ceramic workers. Polymethyl methacrylate is the result of polymerized methyl methacrylate monomers, which are used as sheets, molding, extrusion powders, surface coating resins, emulsion polymers, fibers, inks, and films. This material is also used in tooth implants, bone cements, and hard corneal contact lenses.

Suggested Reading

Farli M, Gasperini M, Francalanci S, Gola M, Sertoli A (1990) Occupational contact dermatitis in 2 dental technicians. Contact Dermatitis 22:282–287

Gebhardt M, Geier J (1996) Evaluation of patch test results with denture material series. Contact Dermatitis 34:191–195

Kanerva L, Estlander T, Jolanki R, Tarvainen K (1993) Occupational allergic contact dermatitis caused by exposure to acrylates during work with dental prostheses. Contact Dermatitis 28:268–275

Kanerva L, Lauerma A, Estlander T, Alanko K, Henriks-Eckerman ML, Jolanki R (1996) Occupational allergic contact dermatitis caused by photobonded sculptured nails and a review of (meth) acrylates in nail cosmetics. Am J Contact Dermat 7:109–115

Kiec-Swierczynska MK (1996) Occupational allergic contact dermatitis due to acrylates in Lodz. Contact Dermatitis 34:419–422

Rustemeyer T, Frosch PJ (1996) Occupational skin diseases in dental laboratory technicians. (I). Clinical picture and causative factors. Contact Dermatitis 34:125–133

Pentaerythrityl Triacrylate

CAS Registry Numbers [3524–68–3] and others

58

Pentaerythritol triacrylate is a multifunctional acrylic monomer. It can be contained in photopolymerizable printer's ink or varnishes. Sensitization was described in dental technicians and in a textile fabric printer.

Suggested Reading

Geukens S, Goossens A (2001) Occupational contact allergy to (meth)acrylates. Contact Dermatitis 44:153–159

Kanerva L, Estlander T, Jolanki R, Tarvainen K (1995) Occupational allergic contact dermatitis and contact urticaria caused by polyfunctional aziridine hardener. Contact Dermatitis 33:304–309

Kiec-Swierczynska MK (1996) Occupational allergic contact dermatitis due to acrylates in Lodz. Contact Dermatitis 34:419–422

Rustemeyer T, Frosch PJ (1996) Occupational skin diseases in dental laboratory technicians. (I). Clinical picture and causative factors. Contact Dermatitis 34:125–133

Polyurethane Dimethacrylate

The polyurethane dimethacrylate was contained in Loctite glues of the 300 and 500 series.

Suggested Reading

Dempsey KJ (1982) Hypersensitivity to Sta-Lok and Loctite anaerobic sealants. J Am Acad Dermatol 7:779–784

Tetraethylene Glycol Dimethacrylate

CAS Registry Number [109–17–1]

Tetraethylene glycol dimethacrylate is a cross-linking agent of acrylic resins, employed to optimize the dilution of high-viscosity monomers and to link together the macromolecules constituting the polymer, to make the three-dimensional structure more rigid. Occupational dermatitis was reported in a dental technician.

Suggested Reading

Farli M, Gasperini M, Francalanci S, Gola M, Sertoli A (1990) Occupational contact dermatitis in 2 dental technicians. Contact Dermatitis 22:282–287

Triethylene Glycol Dimethacrylate

CAS Registry Number [109–16–0]

Triethylene glycol dimethacrylate (TREGDMA) is a cross-linking agent of acrylic resins, used in sealants or dental bonding resins. It is mainly used in dentistry by dental technicians and dentists.

Suggested Reading

Farli M, Gasperini M, Francalanci S, Gola M, Sertoli A (1990) Occupational contact dermatitis in 2 dental technicians. Contact Dermatitis 22:282–287

Kanerva L, Lauerma A, Estlander T, Alanko K, Henriks-Eckerman ML, Jolanki R (1996) Occupational allergic contact dermatitis caused by photobonded sculptured nails and a review of (meth) acrylates in nail cosmetics. Am J Contact Dermat 7:109–115

Kiec-Swierczynska MK (1996) Occupational allergic contact dermatitis due to acrylates in Lodz. Contact Dermatitis 34:419–422

Rustemeyer T, Frosch PJ (1996) Occupational skin diseases in dental laboratory technicians. (I). Clinical picture and causative factors. Contact Dermatitis 34:125–133

Trimethylolpropane Triacrylate

CAS Registry Number [15625–89–5]

Trimethylolpropane triacrylate (TMPTA) is a multifunctional acrylic monomer. It reacts with propyleneimine to form polyfunctional aziridine. Sensitization was observed in a textile fabric printer. Patch tests were positive with the polyfunctional aziridine hardener, but were negative to TMPTA. TMPTA caused contact dermatitis in an optic fiber manufacturing worker and was reported as a sensitizer in a floor top coat or in photopolymerizable inks.

Suggested Reading

Kanerva L, Estlander T, Jolanki R, Tarvainen K (1995) Occupational allergic contact dermatitis and contact urticaria caused by polyfunctional aziridine hardener. Contact Dermatitis 33:304–309
Kiec-Swierczynska MK (1996) Occupational allergic contact dermatitis due to acrylates in Lodz. Contact Dermatitis 34:419–422

Maurice PDL, Rycroft RJG (1986) Allergic contact dermatitis from UV curing acrylate in the manufacture of optical fibers. Contact Dermatitis 15:92–93

Tripropylene Glycol Diacrylate

CAS Registry Number [42978–66–5]

As a cause of occupational contact dermatitis, tripropylene glycol diacrylate was contained in dental resins, UV-cured inks, and nail cosmetics.

Suggested Reading

Kanerva L, Estlander T, Jolanki R, Tarvainen K (1993) Occupational allergic contact dermatitis caused by exposure to acrylates during work with dental prostheses. Contact Dermatitis 28:268–275
Kanerva L, Lauerma A, Estlander T, Alanko K, Henriks-Eckerman ML, Jolanki R (1996) Occupational allergic contact dermatitis caused by photobonded sculptured nails and a review of (meth) acrylates in nail cosmetics. Am J Contact Dermat 7:109–115

Urethane Acrylate

Urethane acrylate gave a positive reaction in a lottery-ticket-coating machine worker sensitized to epoxy acrylate oligomers contained in a UV varnish.

Suggested Reading

Guimaraens D, Gonzalez MA, del Rio E, Condé-Salazar L (1994) Occupational airborne allergic contact dermatitis in the national mint and fiscal-stamp factory. Contact Dermatitis 30:172–173

Kanerva L, Estlander T, Jolanki R, Tarvainen K (1993) Occupational allergic contact dermatitis caused by exposure to acrylates during work with dental prostheses. Contact Dermatitis 28:268–275

6. Acrylonitrile

2-Propenenitrile

CAS Registry Number [107–13–1]

Acrylonitrile is a raw material used extensively in industry, mainly for acrylic and modacrylic fibers, acrylonitrile-butadiene-styrene and styrene-acrylonitrile resins, adiponitrile used in nylon's synthesis, for nitrile rubber, and plastics. It is also used as an insecticide. This very toxic and irritant substance is also a sensitizer and caused both irritant and allergic contact dermatitis in a production manufacturer.

Suggested Reading

Bakker JG, Jongen SMJ, Van Neer FCJ, Neis JM (1991) Occupational contact dermatitis due to acrylonitrile. Contact Dermatitis 24:50–53

Chu CY, Sun CC (2001) Allergic contact dermatitis from acrylonitrile. Am J Contact Dermat 12:113–114

7. Alachlor®

2-Chloro-2,6-Diethyl-N-(Methoxymethyl)Acetanilide, 2-Chloro-N-(2,6-Diethylphenyl)-N-(Methoxymethyl) Acetamide

CAS Registry Number [15972–60–8]

Alachlor® is a herbicide. Occupational contact dermatitis was rarely observed in agricultural workers.

Suggested Reading

Won JH, Ahn SK, Kim SC (1993) Allergic contact dermatitis from the herbicide Alachlor®. Contact Dermatitis 28: 38–39

8. Alantolactone

CAS Registry Number [546–43–0]

The allergen eudesmanolide sesquiterpene lactone was isolated from elecampane (*Inula helenium* L.). With dehydrocostuslactone and costunolide, it is a component of the (sesquiterpene) lactone mix used to detect sensitization to Compositae–Asteraceae. See also Chap. 46.

Suggested Reading

Ducombs G, Benezra C, Talaga P, Andersen KE, Burrows D, Camarasa JG, Dooms-Goossens A, Frosch PJ, Lachapelle JM, Menné T, Rycroft RJG, White IR, Shaw S, Wilkinson JD (1990) Patch testing with the "sesquiterpene lactone mix": a marker for contact allergy to Compositae and other sesquiterpene-lactone-containing plants. Contact Dermatitis 22:249–252

Lamminpää A, Estlander T, Jolanki R, Kanerva L (1996) Occupational allergic contact dermatitis caused by decorative plants. Contact Dermatitis 34:330–335

9. Alkyl Glucosides

Alkyl glucosides are copolymers; based on a fatty alcohol and a glucoside polymer, they comprise decyl glucoside, coco glucoside and lauryl (dodecyl) glucoside in cosmetics, and cetearyl glucoside as a surfactant and emulsifying agent because of its higher viscosity. Due to their manufacturing processes, they are blends of several copolymers. For example, coco glucoside contains C_6, C_8, C_{10}, C_{12}, C_{14}, and C_{16} fatty alcohols. Such variations explain uncertainty when searching for the precise CAS Registry Number. Because alkyl glucosides are comparable mixtures, patients sensitive to one alkyl glucoside may also react to others. See also 127. Decyl Glucoside.

Suggested Reading

Goossens A, Decraene T, Platteaux N, Nardelli A, Rasschaert V (2003) Glucosides as unexpected allergens in cosmetics. Contact Dermatitis 48:164–166

Le Coz CJ, Meyer MT (2003) Contact allergy to decyl glucoside in antiseptic after body piercing. Contact Dermatitis 48:279–280

10. Allicin

CAS Registry Number [539–86–6]

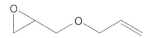

Allicin is one of the major allergens in garlic (*Allium sativum* L.). It is responsible for the characteristic flavor of the bulbs and has immunomodulating and antibacterial properties. See also Chap. 46.

Suggested Reading

Bruynzeel DP (1997) Bulb dermatitis. Dermatological problems in the flower bulb industries. Contact Dermatitis 37:70–77

Lamminpää A, Estlander T, Jolanki R, Kanerva L (1996) Occupational allergic contact dermatitis caused by decorative plants. Contact Dermatitis 34:330–335

Papageorgiou C, Corbet JP, Menezes-Brandao F, Pecegueiro M, Benezra C (1983) Allergic contact dermatitis to garlic (*Allium sativum L.*). Identification of the allergens: the role of mono-, di- and tri-sulfides present in garlic. A comparative study in man and animal (guinea pig). Arch Dermatol Res 275:229–234

11. Allyl Glycidyl Ether

CAS Registry Number [106–92–3]

Allyl glycidyl ether is a monoglycidyl derivative, used as a reactive epoxy diluent for epoxy resins. As an impurity, it was considered to be the sensitizing agent in a plastic industry worker allergic to 3-glycidyloxy-propyl trimethoxysilane, an epoxy silane compound used as a fixing additive in silicone and polyurethane.

Suggested Reading

Angelini G, Rigano L, Foti C, Grandolfo M, Vena GA, Bonamonte D, Soleo L, Scorpiniti AA (1996) Occupational sensitization to epoxy resin and reactive diluents in marble workers. Contact Dermatitis 35:11–16

Dooms-Goossens A, Bruze M, Buysse L, Fregert S, Gruvberger B, Stals H (1995) Contact allergy to allyl glycidyl ether present as an impurity in 3-glycidyloxypropyltrimethoxysilane, a fixing additive in silicone and polyurethane. Contact Dermatitis 33:17–19

Jolanki R, Kanerva L, Estlander T, Tarvainen K, Keskinen H, Henriks-Eckerman ML (1990) Occupational dermatoses from epoxy resin compounds. Contact Dermatitis 23:172–183

12. Allyl Isothiocyanate

CAS Registry Number [57–06–7]

Allyl isothiocyanate is generated by enzymatic hydrolysis of the glucoside sinigrin, present in Cruciferae–Brassicaceae, mainly the oil from black mustard seed (*Brassica nigra* Koch). It may induce irritant and sometimes allergic contact dermatitis, mimicking the "tulip finger" dermatitis. See also Chap. 46.

Suggested Reading

Ettlinger MG, Lundeen AJ (1956) The structures of sinigrin and sinalbin; an enzymatic rearrangement. J Ann Chem Soc 78:4172–4173

Lerbaek A, Chandra Rastogi S, Menné T (2004) Allergic contact dermatitis from allyl isothiocyanate in a Danish cohort of 259 selected patients. Contact Dermatitis 51:79–83

13. Allylpropyldisulfide

CAS Registry Number [2179–59–1]

With allicin and diallyl sulfide, allylpropyldisulfide is one of the allergens in garlic (*Allium sativum* L.). See also Chap. 46.

Suggested Reading

Bruynzeel DP (1997) Bulb dermatitis. Dermatological problems in the flower bulb industries. Contact Dermatitis 37: 70–77

14. Alprenolol

CAS Registry Number [13655–52–2]

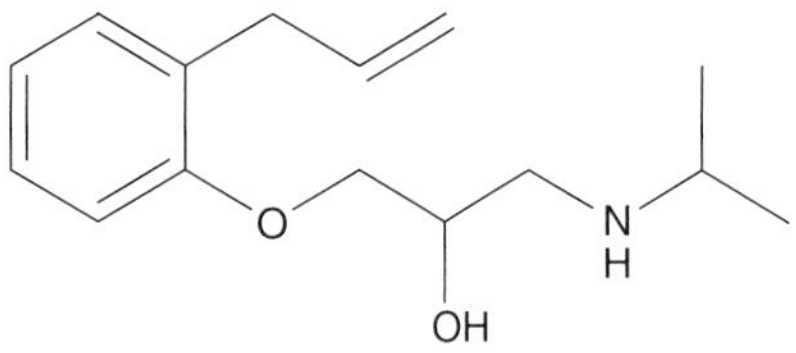

Occupational cases of contact dermatitis due to this beta-blocker were reported in the pharmaceutical industry.

Suggested Reading

Ekenvall L, Forsbeck M (1978) Contact eczema produced by α-adrenergic blocking agent (Alprenolol). Contact Dermatitis 4:190–194

15. Amethocaine

Pantocaine, Tetracaine

CAS Registry Number [136–47–0]

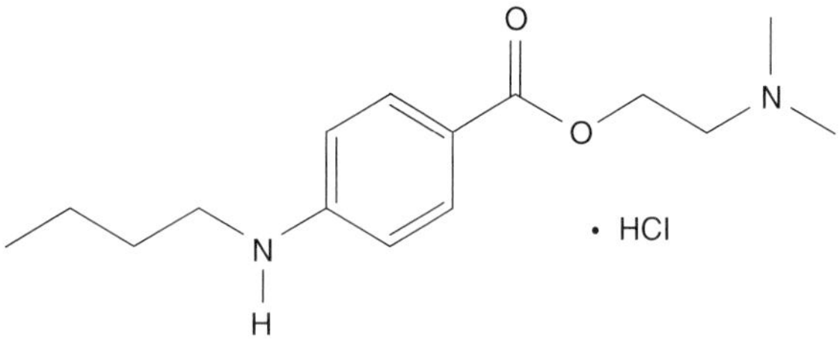

Amethocaine is a local anesthetic used in dental surgery. It was reported as an agent of contact dermatitis in dentists or dental nurses and in ophthalmologists.

Suggested Reading

Berova N, Stranky L, Krasteva M (1990) Studies on contact dermatitis in stomatological staff. Dermatol Monatschr 176: 15–18

Condé-Salazar L, Llinas MG, Guimaraens D, Romero L (1988) Occupational allergic contact dermatitis from amethocaine. Contact Dermatitis 19:69–70
Rebandel P, Rudzki E (1986) Occupational contact sensitivity in oculists. Contact Dermatitis 15:92

16. *p*-Amino-*N,N*-Diethylaniline Sulfate

1,4-Benzenediamine, *N,N*-Diethyl-para-Phenylenediamine Sulfate

CAS Registry Number [6065–27–6]

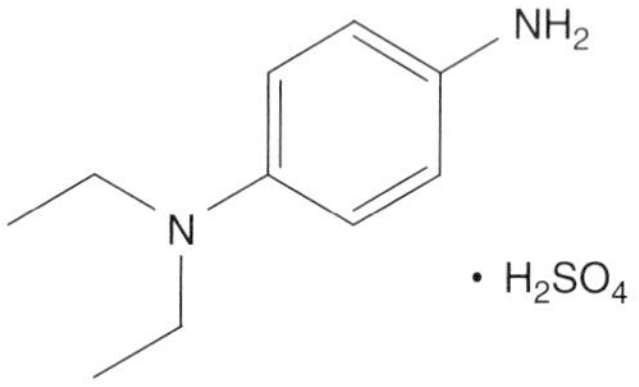

This color developer can induce sensitization in photographers.

Suggested Reading

Aguirre A, Landa N, Gonzalez M, Diaz-Perez JL (1992) Allergic contact dermatitis in a photographer. Contact Dermatitis 27:340–341

17. 4-Amino-3-Nitrophenol

3-Nitro-4-Aminophenol

CAS Registry Number [610–81–1]

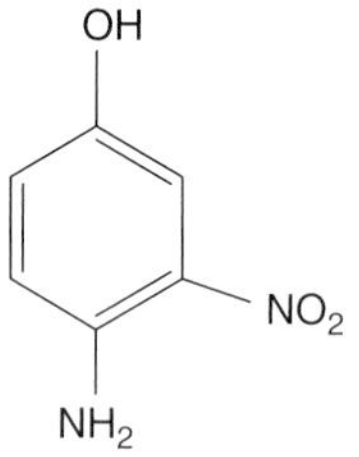

This hair dye used for semipermanent colors seems to be a rare sensitizer.

Suggested Reading

Sánchez-Pérez J, García del Río I, Alvares Ruiz S, García Diez A (2004) Allergic contact dermatitis from direct dyes for hair coloration in hairdressers' clients. Contact Dermatitis 50:261–262

18. *p*-Aminoazobenzene

Solvent Yellow 1, C.I. 11000, Solvent Blue 7

CAS Registry Number [60–09–3]

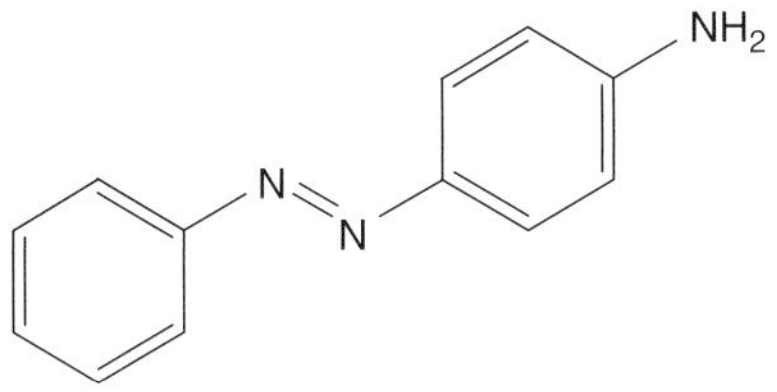

This azoic coloring can be reduced in *para*-phenylene-diamine (PPD). It can be found in some semi-permanent hair dyes and patch tests are frequently positive (about 30%) in hairdressers with hand dermatitis. Because of hydrolysis of the azo bond, the detection of sensitization to *p*-aminoazobenzene may be assumed by a PPD test.

Suggested Reading

Condé-Salazar L, Baz M, Guimaraens D, Cannavo A (1995) Contact dermatitis in hairdressers: patch test results in 379 hairdressers (1980–1993). Am J Contact Dermat 6:19–23

19. *p*-Aminodiphenylamine (Hydrochloride)

4-Aminodiphenylamine (HCl), CI 76086 (CI 75085)

CAS Registry Number [101–54–2] (CAS Registry Number [2198–59–6])

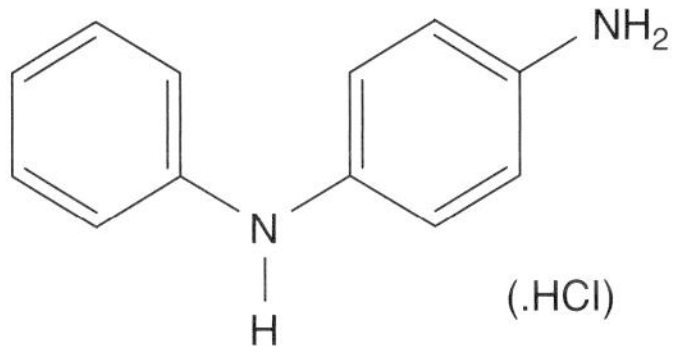

This substance was formerly used as a hair dye. Sensitization, when detected by patch testing, is relatively low in hairdressers.

Suggested Reading

Frosch PJ, Burrows D, Camarasa JG, Dooms-Goossens A, Ducombs G, Lahti A, Menné T, Rycroft RJG, Shaw S, White IR, Wilkinson JD (1993) Allergic reactions to a hairdresser's series: results from 9 European centers. Contact Dermatitis 28:180–183

20. Aminoethylethanolamine

N-(2-Hydroxyethyl)Ethylenediamine

CAS Registry Number [111–41–1]

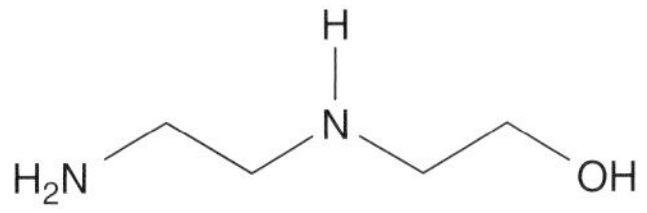

Aminoethylethanolamine is a component of colophony in soldering flux, which may cause contact and airborne contact dermatitis in workers in the electronic industry or cable jointers.

Suggested Reading

Crow KD, Harman RRM, Holden H (1968) Amine-flux sensitization dermatitis in electricity cable jointers. Br J Dermatol 80:701–710

Goh CL (1985) Occupational contact dermatitis from soldering flux among workers in the electronics industry. Contact Dermatitis 13:85–90

Goh CL, Ng SK (1987) Airborne contact dermatitis to colophony in soldering flux. Contact Dermatitis 17:89–91

21. *o*-Aminophenol

2-Aminophenol, CI 76520

CAS Registry Number [95–55–6]

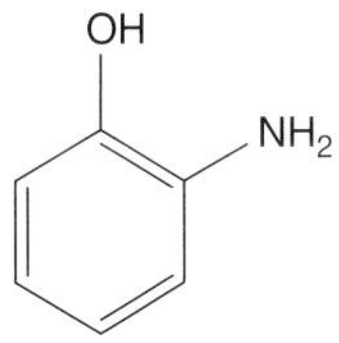

It is contained in hair dyes and can cause contact dermatitis in hairdressers and consumers.

Suggested Reading

Matsunaga K, Hosokawa K, Suzuki M, Arima Y, Hayakawa R (1988) Occupational allergic contact dermatitis in beauticians. Contact Dermatitis 18:94–96

22. *p*-Aminophenol

4-Aminophenol, Amino-4 Hydroxybenzene, Hydroxy-4 Aniline, CI 76550

CAS Registry Number [123–30–8]

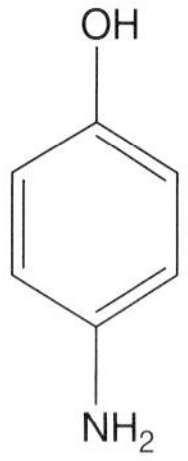

58

This hair dye is frequently implicated in contact dermatitis in hairdressers, customers, or people sensitized to *para*-phenylenediamine, by the way of "black-henna" temporary tattoos.

Suggested Reading

Guerra L, Tosti A, Bardazzi F, Pigatto P, Lisi P, Santucci B, Valsecchi R, Schena D, Angelini G, Sertoli A, Ayala F, Kokeli F (1992) Contact dermatitis in hairdressers: the Italian experience. Gruppo Italiano Ricerca Dermatiti da Contatto e Ambientali. Contact Dermatitis 26:101–107

Le Coz CJ, Lefebvre C, Keller F, Grosshans E (2000) Allergic contact dermatitis caused by skin painting (pseudotattooing) with black henna, a mixture of henna and *p*-phenylenediamine and its derivatives. Arch Dermatol 136:1515–1517

23. Aminophylline

Theophylline Ethylenediamine

CAS Registry Number [317–34–0]

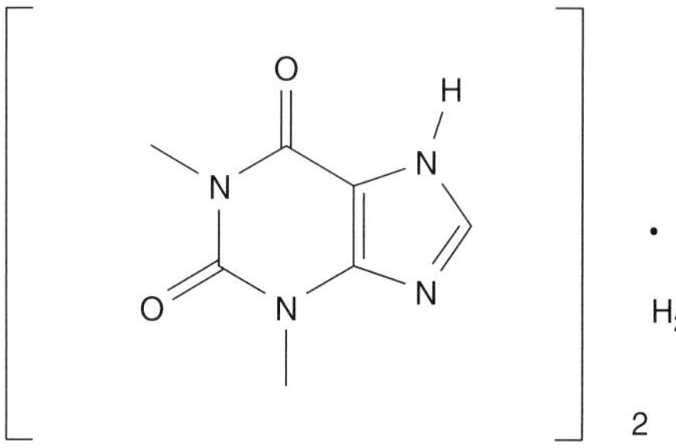

This drug is a 2:1 mixture of the alkaloid theophylline and ethylenediamine (see below). It caused contact dermatitis in industrial plants, pharmacists, and nurses. Ethylenediamine is the sensitizer and patch testing is generally positive to both ethylenediamine and aminophylline and negative to theophylline.

Suggested Reading

Corazza M, Mantovani L, Trimurti L, Virgili A (1994) Occupational contact sensitization to ethylenediamine in a nurse. Contact Dermatitis 31:328–329

Dias M, Fernandes C, Pereira F, Pacheco A (1995) Occupational dermatitis from ethylenediamine. Contact Dermatitis 33:129–130

24. *N,N*-bis-(3-Aminopropyl) Dodecylamine

N-(3-Aminopropyl)-*N*-Dodecyl-1,3-Propanediamine

CAS Registry Number [2372–82–9]

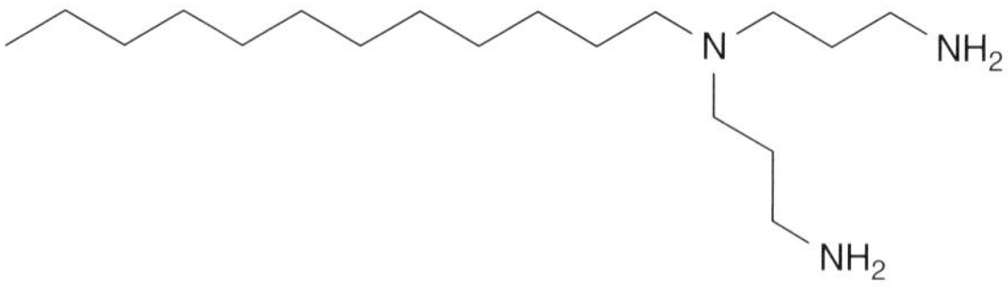

This alkylamine is contained in detergent-disinfectants solutions for medical instruments. It is also contained in association with 3-aminopropyl dodecylamine in liquid laundry disinfectants such as Aset® aqua (Johnson Wax SpA, Rydelle).

Suggested Reading

Dibo M, Brasch J (2001) Occupational allergic contact dermatitis from *N,N*-bis(3-aminopropyl)dodecylamine and dimethyldidecylammonium chloride in two hospital staff. Contact Dermatitis 45:40

25. Ammonium Persulfate

Ammonium Peroxydisulfate

CAS Registry Number [7727–54–0]

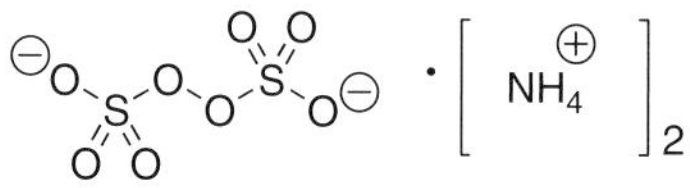

Persulfates are strong oxidizing agents widely used in the production of metals, textiles, photographs, cellophane, rubber, adhesive papers, foods, soaps, detergents, and hair bleaches. Ammonium persulfate is used as a hair bleaching agent. It may induce irritant dermatitis, (mainly) nonimmunologic contact urticaria, and allergic contact dermatitis and represents a major allergen in hairdressers. People reacting to ammonium persulfate also react to other persulfates such as potassium persulfate.

Suggested Reading

Frosch PJ, Burrows D, Camarasa JG, Dooms-Goossens A, Ducombs G, Lahti A, Menné T, Rycroft RJG, Shaw S, White IR, Wilkinson JD (1993) Allergic reactions to a hairdresser's series: results from 9 European centers. Contact Dermatitis 28:180–183

Le Coz CJ, Bezard M (1999) Allergic contact cheilitis due to effervescent dental cleanser: combined responsibilities of the allergen persulfate and prosthesis porosity. Contact Dermatitis 41:268–271

Van Joost T, Roesyanto ID (1991) Sensitization to persulphates in occupational and nonoccupational hand dermatitis. Contact Dermatitis 24:376–377

26. Ammonium Thioglycolate

Ammonium Mercaptoacetate

CAS Registry Number [5421–46–5]

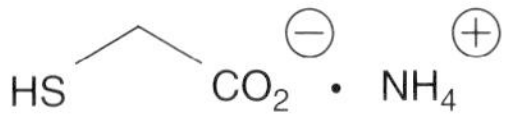

This substance is contained in "basic" permanent waves solutions and causes contact dermatitis in hairdressers.

Suggested Reading

Frosch PJ, Burrows D, Camarasa JG, Dooms-Goossens A, Ducombs G, Lahti A, Menné T, Rycroft RJG, Shaw S, White IR, Wilkinson JD (1993) Allergic reactions to a hairdresser's series: results from 9 European centers. Contact Dermatitis 28:180–183

Guerra L, Tosti A, Bardazzi F, Pigatto P, Lisi P, Santucci B, Valsecchi R, Schena D, Angelini G, Sertoli A, Ayala F, Kokeli F (1992) Contact dermatitis in hairdressers: the Italian experience. Gruppo Italiano Ricerca Dermatiti da Contatto e Ambientali. Contact Dermatitis 26:101–107

27. Amoxicillin

CAS Registry Number [26787–78–0]

Amoxicillin Trihydrate

CAS Registry Number [61336–70–7]

Amoxicillin Sodium Salt

CAS Registry Number [34642–77–8]

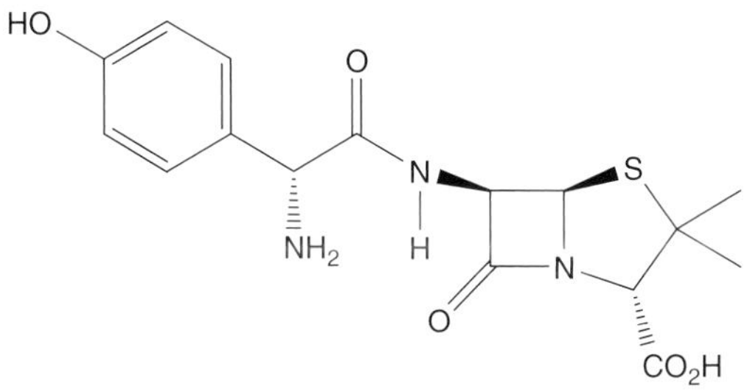

Amoxicillin is both a topical and a systemic sensitizer. Topical sensitization occurs in health care workers. Systemic drug reactions are frequent, such as urticaria, maculo-papular rashes, baboon syndrome, acute generalized exanthematous pustulosis, or even toxic epidermal necrosis. Cross-reactivity is common with ampicillin, and can occur with other penicillins.

Suggested Reading

Gamboa P, Jauregui I, Urrutia I (1995) Occupational sensitization to aminopenicillins with oral tolerance to penicillin V. Contact Dermatitis 32:48–49

Rudzki E, Rebandel P (1991) Hypersensitivity to semisynthetic penicillins but not to natural penicillin. Contact Dermatitis 25:192

28. Ampicillin

CAS Registry Number [69–53–4]

Ampicillin Trihydrate

CAS Registry Number [7177–48–2]

Ampicillin Sodium Salt

CAS Registry Number [69–52–3]

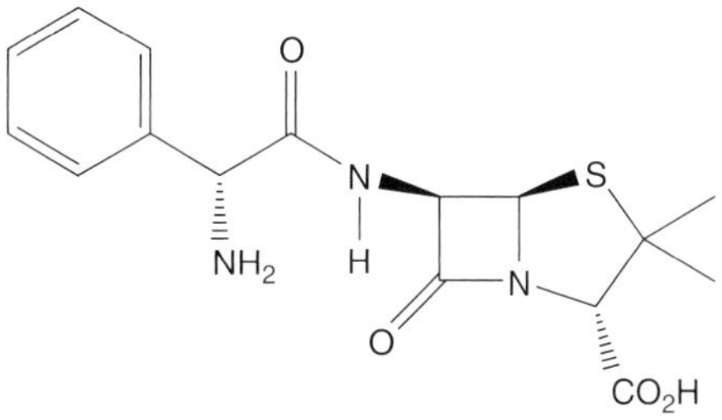

Ampicillin caused contact dermatitis in a nurse also sensitized to amoxicillin (with tolerance to oral phenoxymethylpenicillin) and in a pharmaceutical factory worker. Systemic drug reactions are common. Cross-reactivity is regular with ampicillin and can occur with other penicillins.

Suggested Reading

Gamboa P, Jauregui I, Urrutia I (1995) Occupational sensitization to aminopenicillins with oral tolerance to penicillin V. Contact Dermatitis 32:48–49

Rudzki E, Rebandel P (1991) Hypersensitivity to semisynthetic penicillins but not to natural penicillin. Contact Dermatitis 25:192

29. Amprolium (Hydrochloride)

CAS Registry Number [121–25–5] (CAS Registry Number [137–88–2])

Amprolium is an antiprotozoal agent used for the prevention of coccidiosis in poultry.

Suggested Reading

Mancuso G, Staffa M, Errani A, Berdondini RM, Fabbri P (1990) Occupational dermatitis in animal feed mill workers. Contact Dermatitis 22:37–41

30. Amyl Cinnamyl Alcohol

2-Pentyl-3-Phenylprop-2-en-1-ol, Pentyl-Cinnamic Alcohol, α-Amyl-Cinnamic Alcohol, Buxinol

CAS Registry number [101–85–9]

This scented molecule is very close to α-amyl-cinnamic aldehyde. Its presence is indicated by name in cosmetics within the EU.

Suggested Reading

Rastogi SC, Johansen JD, Menné T (1996) Natural ingredients based cosmetics. Content of selected fragrance sensitizers. Contact Dermatitis 34:423–426

31. Amylcinnamaldehyde

α-Amyl Cinnamic Aldehyde, Ammylcinnamal, 2-Benzylideneheptanal, 2-Pentylcinnamaldehyde, Jasminal

CAS Registry Number [122–40–7]

α-Amyl-cinnamic aldehyde is an oxidation product of amylcinnamic alcohol, a sensitizing fragrance, and one component of the "fragrance mix." It can also be a sensitizer in bakers. It has to be mentioned by name in cosmetics within the EU.

Suggested Reading

Nethercott JR, Holness DL (1989) Occupational dermatitis in food handlers and bakers. J Am Acad Dermatol 21:485–490

32. Anacardic Acids

Anacardic acids are mixtures of several analog molecules with alkyl chain (-R) of 13, 15, 17, or 19 carbons, and 0–3 unsaturations. They are the main cashew nut shell liquid component with cardol and can cause contact dermatitis in cashew nut workers. See also 405. Urushiol; Chap. 46.

Suggested Reading

Diogenes MJN, de Morais SM, Carvalho FF (1996) Contact dermatitis among cashew nut workers. Contact Dermatitis 35:114–115

33. Anethole

1'-Methoxy-4-(1-Propenyl)-Benzene

CAS Registry Number [104–46–1]

Anethole is the main component of anise, star anise, and fennel oils. It is used in perfumes, food and cosmetic industries (toothpastes), bleaching colors, and photography, and as an embedding material.

Suggested Reading

Garcia-Bravo B, Pérez Bernal A, Garcia-Hernandez MJ, Camacho F (1997) Occupational contact dermatitis from anethole in food handlers. Contact Dermatitis 37:38

34. Anisyl Alcohol

4-Methoxybenzyl Alcohol,
Methoxybenzenemethanol, Anise Alcohol

CAS Registry Number [105–13–5]

Blend of o-, m-, and p-Methoxybenzyl Alcohol

CAS Registry number [1331–81–3]

As a fragrance allergen, anisyl alcohol has to be mentioned by name in cosmetics within the EU.

Suggested Reading

Budavari S, O'Neil MJ, Smith A, Heckelman PE, Kinneary JF (eds) (1996) The Merck Index, 12th edn. Merck, Whitehouse Station, NJ, USA

35. Antimony Trioxide

CAS Registry Number [1309–64–4]

$$Sb_2O_3$$

This hard shiny metal is often alloyed to other elements. It is used in various industrial fields such as batteries, printing machines, bearing, textile, and ceramics. It caused positive patch test reactions in two workers in the ceramics industry.

Suggested Reading

Motolese A, Truzzi M, Giannini A, Seidenari S (1995) Contact dermatitis and contact sensitization among enamellers and decorators in the ceramics industry. Contact Dermatitis 28:59–62

36. Arsenic and Arsenic Salts (Sodium Arsenate)

CAS Registry Number [7440–38–2] and CAS Registry Number [7778–43–0]

$$As \quad AsO_4H_2Na$$

Arsenic salts are sensitizers, but most often irritants. They are used in copper or gold extraction, glass, feeds, weedkillers, insecticides, and ceramics. A recent case was reported in a crystal factory worker with positive patch tests to sodium arsenate.

Suggested Reading

Barbaud A, Mougeolle JM, Schmutz JL (1995) Contact hypersensitivity to arsenic in a crystal factory worker. Contact Dermatitis 33:272–273

37. Articaine (Hydrochloride)

Carticaine (Hydrochloride)

CAS Registry Number [23964–58–1] (CAS Registry Number [23964–57–0])

58

This local amide-type anesthetic is seldom reported as allergenic even in patients sensitized to other amide-type molecules like lidocaine, prilocaine, mepivacaine, or bupivacaine.

Suggested Reading

Duque S, Fernandez L (2004) Delayed-type hypersensitivity to amide local anesthetics. Allergol Immunopathol (Madr) 32:233–234

38. Atranol

2,6-Dihydroxy-4-Methyl-Benzaldehyde

CAS Registry number [526–37–4]

Atranol has been identified as a potent and frequent allergen, occurring from the fragrance material oak-moss absolute, which is of botanical origin.

Suggested Reading

Johansen JD, Andersen KE, Svedman C, Bruze M, Bernard G, Giménez-Arnau E, Rastogi SC, Lepoittevin JP, Menné T (2003) Chloroatranol, an extremely potent allergen hidden in perfumes: a dose response elicitation study. Contact Dermatitis 49:180–184
Rastogi SC, Bossi R, Johansen JD, Menné T, Bernard G, Giménez-Arnau E, Lepoittevin P (2004) Content of oak moss allergens atranol and chloroatranol in perfumes and similar products. Contact Dermatitis 50:367–370

39. Azaperone

4-Fluoro-4-[4-(2-Pyridyl)-1-Piperazininyl] Butyrophenone

CAS Registry Number [1649–18–9]

Azaperone is a sedative used in veterinary medicine to avoid mortality of pigs during transportation. This alternative substance to chlorpromazine is a sensitizer and a photosensitizer.

Suggested Reading

Brasch J, Hessler HJ, Christophers E (1991) Occupational (photo)allergic contact dermatitis from azaperone in a piglet dealer. Contact Dermatitis 25:258–259

40. Azathioprine

6-(1-Methyl-4-Nitroimidazol-5-ylthio)Purine

CAS Registry Number [446–86–6]

This immunosuppressive and antineoplastic drug is derived from 6-mercaptopurine. It caused allergic contact dermatitis in a mother crushing tablets for her leukemic son, and occupational dermatitis in a pharmaceutical reconditioner of old tablet packaging machines, and in a production mechanic working in packaging for a pharmaceutical company.

Suggested Reading

Burden AD, Beck MH (1992) Contact hypersensitivity to aza-thioprine. Contact Dermatitis 27:329–330

Lauerma A, Koivuluhta M, Alenius H (2001) Recalcitrant allergic contact dermatitis from azathioprine tablets. Contact Dermatitis 44:129

Soni BP, Sherertz EF (1996) Allergic contact dermatitis from azathioprine. Am J Contact Dermat 7:116–117

41. Basic Red 22

Synacril Red 3B

CAS Registry Number [12221–52–2]

This monoazoic dye was reported as allergenic in a PPD-free hair coloring mousse. See also Chap. 40.

Suggested Reading

Salim A, Orton D, Shaw S (2001) Allergic contact dermatitis from Basic Red 22 in a hair-coloring mousse. Contact Dermatitis 45:123

42. Basic Red 46

CAS Registry Number [12221–69–1]

This monoazoic textile dye seems to be an important cause of foot dermatitis, being a frequent allergen in acrylic socks. It caused contact dermatitis in two workers in the textile industry. See also Chap. 40.

Suggested Reading

Opie J, Lee A, Frowen K, Fewings J, Nixon R (2003) Foot dermatitis caused by the textile dye Basic Red 46 in acrylic blend socks. Contact Dermatitis 49:297–303

Soni BP, Sherertz EF (1996) Contact dermatitis in the textile industry: a review of 72 patients. Am J Contact Dermat 7:226–230

43. Befunolol

CAS Registry Number [39552–01–7]

Befunolol was implicated in allergic contact dermatitis due to beta-blocker agents in eye-drops. Cross-sensitivity has been described with levobunolol.

Suggested Reading

Giordano-Labadie F, Lepoittevin JP, Calix I, Bazex J (1997) Allergie de contact aux β-bloqueurs des collyres: allergie croisée ? Ann Dermatol Venereol 124:322–324

Nino M, Balato A, Ayala F, Balato N (2007) Allergic contact dermatitis due to levobunolol with cross-sensitivity to befunolol. Contact Dermatitis 56:53–54

44. Benomyl

CAS Registry Number [17804–35–2]

Benomyl is a fungicide, derived from benzimidazole. Cases of sensitization were reported in horticulturists and florists. It is however, at most, a weak sensitizer, with possible false-positive patch reactions, or with cross-reactions after previous exposure to other fungicides.

Suggested Reading

Jung HD, Honemann W, Kloth C, Lubbe D, Pambor M, Quednow C, Ratz KH, Rothe A, Tarnick M (1989) Kontaktekzem durch Pestizide in der Deutschen Demokratischen Republik. Dermatol Monats 175:203–214

58

Larsen AI, Larsen A, Jepsen JR, Jorgensen R (1990) Contact allergy to the fungicide benomyl? Contact Dermatitis 22:278–281

O'Malley M, Rodriguez P, Maibach HI (1995) Pesticide patch testing: California nursery workers and controls. Contact Dermatitis 32:61–62

45. Benzalkonium Chloride

CAS Registry Number [8001–54–5]

This quaternary ammonium cationic surfactant is a mixture of alkyl, dimethyl, and benzyl ammonium chlorides (-R). It is an irritant rather than a sensitizer, but may cause allergic contact dermatitis from creams, detergents/antiseptics, ophthalmic preparations, and in nursing, veterinary, dental, and medical personnel. Its presence was observed in plaster of Paris.

Suggested Reading

Basketter DA, Marriott M, Gilmour NJ, White IR (2004) Strong irritants masquerading as skin allergens: the case of benzalkonium chloride. Contact Dermatitis 50:213–217

Corazza M, Virgili A (1993) Airborne allergic contact dermatitis from benzalkonium chloride. Contact Dermatitis 28:195–196

Klein GF, Sepp N, Fritsch P (1991) Allergic reactions to benzalkonium chloride? Do the use test! Contact Dermatitis 25:269–270

Stanford D, Georgouras K (1996) Allergic contact dermatitis from benzalkonium chloride in plaster of Paris. Contact Dermatitis 35:371–372

46. Benzisothiazolone

1,2-Benzisothiazolin-3-one, BIT, Proxan, Proxel PL

CAS Registry Number [2634–33–5]

BIT, both an irritant and a skin sensitizer, is widely used in industry as a preservative in water-based solutions such as pastes, paints, and cutting oils. Occupational dermatitis has been reported mainly due to cutting fluids and greases, in paint manufacturers, pottery mold-makers, acrylic emulsions manufacturers, plumber,

printers and lithoprinters, paper makers, analytical laboratory, rubber factory, and employees manufacturing air fresheners. It is also a preservative in vinyl gloves.

Suggested Reading

Aalto-Korte K, Ackermann L, Henriks-Eckerman ML, Välimaa J, Reinikka-Railo H, Leppänen E, Jolanki R (2007) 1,2-benzisothiazolin-3-one in disposable polyvinyl chloride gloves for medical use. Contact Dermatitis 57:365–370

Burden AD, O'Driscoll JB, Page FC, Beck MH (1994) Contact hypersensitivity to a new isothiazolinone. Contact Dermatitis 30:179–180

Chew AL, Maibach H (1997) 1,2-Benzisothiazolin-3-one (Proxel®): irritant or allergen? A clinical study and literature review. Contact Dermatitis 36:131–136

Dias M, Lamarao P, Vale T (1992) Occupational contact allergy to 1,2-benzisothiazolin-3-one in the manufacture of air fresheners. Contact Dermatitis 27:205–206

Greig DE (1991) Another isothiazolinone source. Contact Dermatitis 25:201–202

Sanz-Gallén P, Planas J, Martinez P, Giménez-Arnau JM (1992) Allergic contact dermatitis due to 1,2-benzisothiazolin-3-one in paint manufacture. Contact Dermatitis 27:271–272

47. Benzophenones

Benzophenone (BZP) and substituted BZP numbered 1–12, trade mark Uvinul®, are photo-screen agents widely used in sunscreens and in cosmetics, such as "antiaging" creams and hair sprays and shampoos, paints and plastics. The hypolipemiant drug fenofibrate is also a substituted BZP.

Benzophenone, Unsubstituted

CAS Registry Number [119–61–9]

Unsubstituted benzophenone is largely used in chemical applications. It acts as a marker for photoallergy to ketoprofen.

Benzophenone 1

Benzoresorcinol, Uvinul 400

CAS Registry Number [131–56–6]

BZP-1 is used, for example, in paints, plastics, and nail varnishes.

Benzophenone-2

2,2,4,4-Tetrahydroxybenzophenone

CAS Registry Number [131–55–5]

BZP-2 is widely used in perfumes to prevent their degradation due to light. It can cause allergic contact dermatitis.

Benzophenone-3

Oxybenzone

CAS Registry Number [131–57–7]

BZP-3 is used as a direct sunscreen agent and in anti-aging creams. Allergic reactions have been reported. Cross-reactivity is expected in an average of one in four patients photoallergic to ketoprofen.

Benzophenone-4

Sulisobenzone

CAS Registry Number [4065–45–6]

BZP-4 is widely used in cosmetics, particularly shampoos and hair products. Cross-reactivity is rarely expected in patients photoallergic to ketoprofen.

Benzophenone-10

Mexenone

CAS Registry Number [1641–17–4]

BZP-10 is exceptionally positive in ketoprofen-photosensitive patients.

Suggested Reading

Alanko K, Jolanki R, Estlander T, Kanerva L (2001) Occupational allergic contact dermatitis from benzophenone-4 in hair-care products. Contact Dermatitis 44:188

Collins P, Ferguson J (1994) Photoallergic contact dermatitis to oxybenzone. Br J Dermatol 131:124–129

Guin JD (2000) Eyelid dermatitis from benzophenone used in nail enhancement. Contact Dermatitis 43:308–309

Jacobs MC (1998) Contact allergy to benzophenone-2 in toilet water. Contact Dermatitis 39:42

Knobler E, Almeida L, Ruzkowski AM, Held J, Harber L, DeLeo V (1989) Photoallergy to benzophenone. Arch Dermatol 125:801–804

Le Coz CJ, Bottlaender A, Scrivener JN, Santinelli F, Cribier BJ, Heid E, Grosshans EM (1998) Photocontact dermatitis from ketoprofen and tiaprofenic acid: cross-reactivity study in 12 consecutive patients. Contact Dermatitis 38:245–252

Matthieu L, Meuleman L, van Hecke E, Blondeel A, Dezfoulian B, Constandt L, Goossens A (2004) Contact and photocontact allergy to ketoprofen. The Belgian experience. Contact Dermatitis 50:238–241

Ramsay DL, Cohen HJ, Baer RL (1972) Allergic reaction to benzophenone. Simultaneous occurrence of urticarial and contact sensitivities. Arch Dermatol 105:906–908

48. Benzoyl Peroxide

CAS Registry Number [94–36–0]

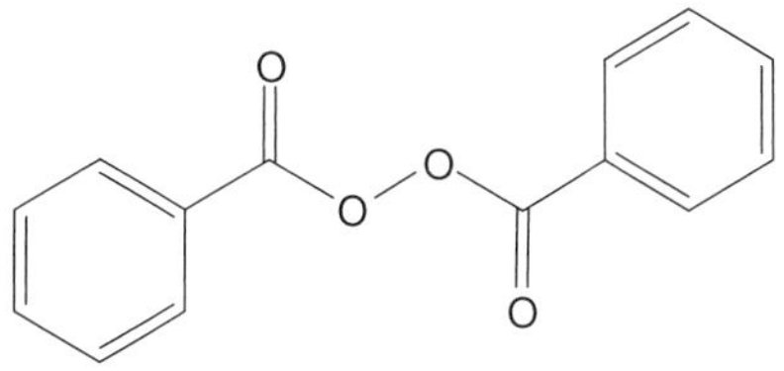

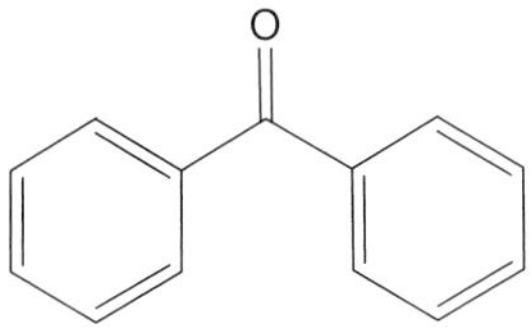

BZP

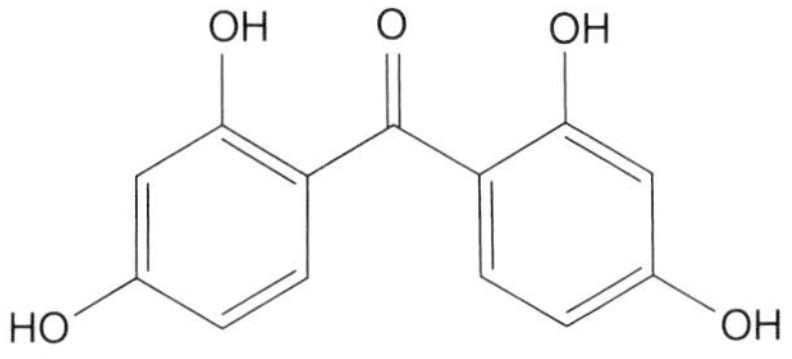

BZP-2

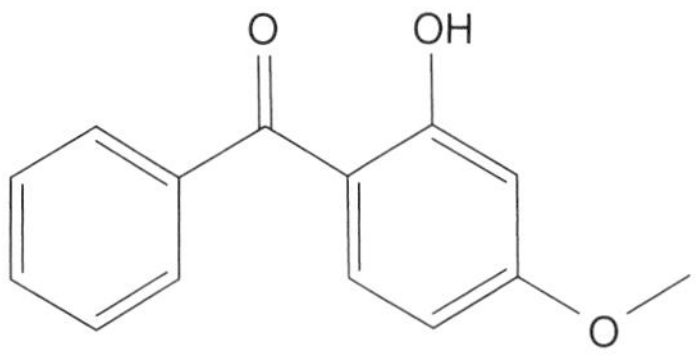

BZP-3

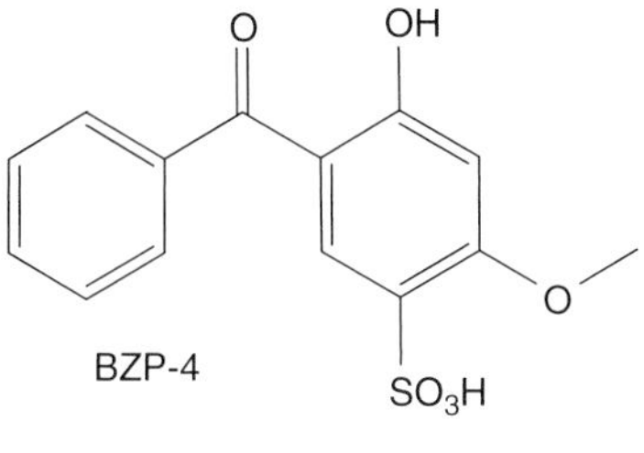

BZP-4

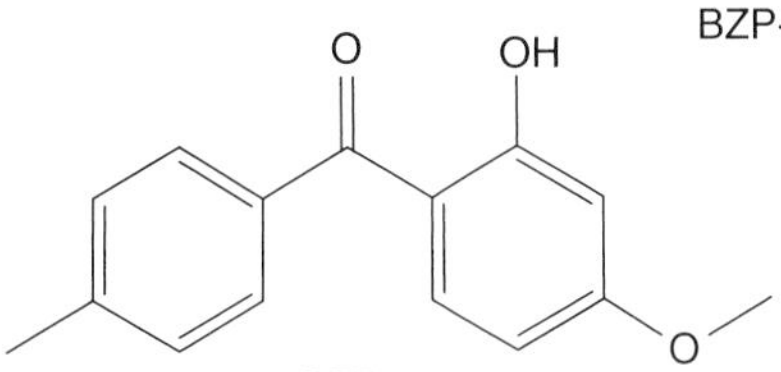

BZP-10

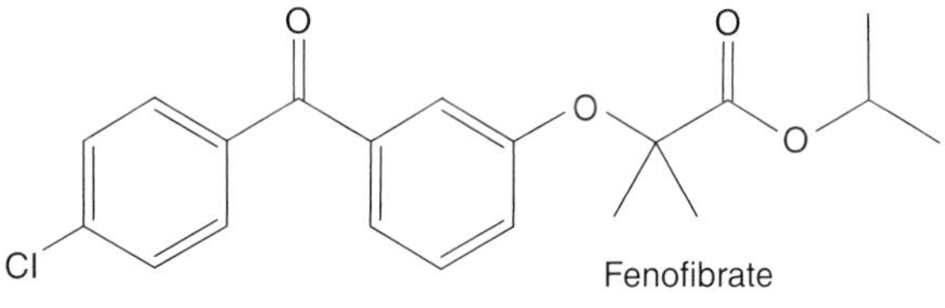

Fenofibrate

Benzoyl peroxide is an oxidizing agent widely employed in acne topical therapy. It is also used as a polymerization catalyst of dental or industrial plastics and as a decolorizing agent of flours, oils, fats, and waxes. Irritant or allergic dermatitis may affect workers in the electronics and plastics (epoxy resins and catalysts) industries, electricians, ceramic workers, dentists and dental technicians, laboratory technicians, bakers, and acne patients. As it was contained in candles, it also induced contact dermatitis in a sacristan. Patch tests may be irritant.

Suggested Reading

Balato N, Lembo G, Cuccurullo FM, Patruno C, Nappa P, Ayala F (1996) Acne and allergic contact dermatitis. Contact Dermatitis 34:68–69

Bonnekoh B, Merk H (1991) Airborne allergic contact dermatitis from benzoyl peroxyde as a bleaching agent of candle wax. Contact Dermatitis 24:367–368

Quirce S, Olaguibel JM, Garcia BE, Tabar AI (1993) Occupational airborne contact dermatitis due to benzoyl peroxide. Contact Dermatitis 29:165–166

Rustemeyer T, Frosch PJ (1996) Occupational skin diseases in dental laboratory technicians. (I). Clinical picture and causative factors. Contact Dermatitis 34:125–133

49. Benzydamine Hydrochloride

CAS Registry Number [132–69–4]

It is a nonsteroidal anti-inflammatory drug used both topically and systemically. It has been reported as a sensitizer and a photosensitizer.

Suggested Reading

Foti C, Vena GA, Angelini G (1992) Occupational contact allergy to benzydamine hydrochloride. Contact Dermatitis 27:328–329

Lasa Elgezua O, Egino Gorrotxategi P, Gardeazabal García J, Ratón Nieto JA, Díaz Pérez JL (2004) Photoallergic hand eczema due to benzydamine. Eur J Dermatol 14:69–70

50. Benzyl Alcohol

CAS Registry Number [100–51–6]

Benzyl alcohol is mainly a preservative, mostly used in topical antimycotic or corticosteroid ointments. It is also a component catalyst for epoxy resins and is contained in the color developer C-22. As a fragrance allergen, it has to be mentioned by name in cosmetics within the EU.

Suggested Reading

Lodi A, Mancini LL, Pozzi M, Chiarelli G, Crosti C (1993) Occupational airborne allergic contact dermatitis in parquet layers. Contact Dermatitis 29:281–282

Scheman AJ, Katta R (1997) Photographic allergens: an update. Contact Dermatitis 37:130

Sestini S, Mori M, Francalanci S (2004) Allergic contact dermatitis from benzyl alcohol in multiple medicaments. Contact Dermatitis 50:316–317

51. Benzyl Benzoate

Benzoic Acid Phenylmethyl Ester

CAS Registry Number [120–51–4]

Benzyl benzoate is the ester of benzyl alcohol and benzoic acid. It is contained in *Myroxylon pereirae* and Tolu balsam. It is used in acaricide preparations against *Sarcoptes scabiei* or as a pediculicide. Direct contact may cause skin irritation, but rarely allergic contact dermatitis. As a fragrance allergen, benzyl benzoate has to be mentioned by name in EU cosmetics.

Suggested Reading

Meneghini CL, Vena GA, Angelini G (1982) Contact dermatitis to scabicides. Contact Dermatitis 8:285–286

52. Benzyl Salicylate

Benzyl-*o*-Hydroxybenzoate, 2-Hydroxybenzoic Acid Phenylmethyl Ester

CAS Registry Number [118–58–1]

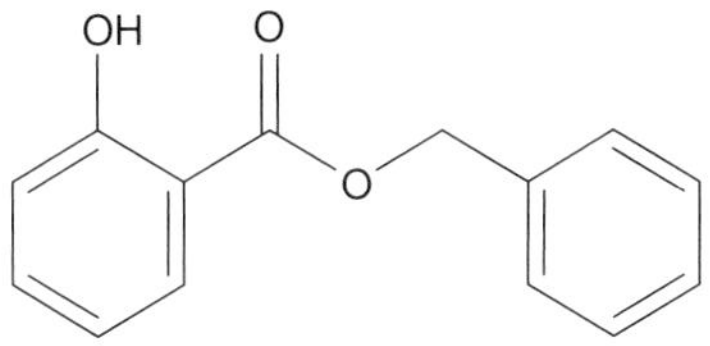

Benzyl salicylate is used as fixer in perfumery and sunscreen preparations. As a (weak) perfume sensitizer, it has to be listed by name in cosmetic preparations in the EU.

Suggested Reading

Larsen W, Nakayama H, Lindberg M, Fischer T, Elsner P, Burrows D, Jordan W, Shaw S, Wilkinson J, Marks J Jr, Sugawara M, Nethercott J (1996) Fragrance contact dermatitis: a worldwide multicenter investigation (Part I). Am J Contact Dermat 7:77–83

53. Benzylpenicillin

Penicillin G

CAS Registry Number [61–33–6]

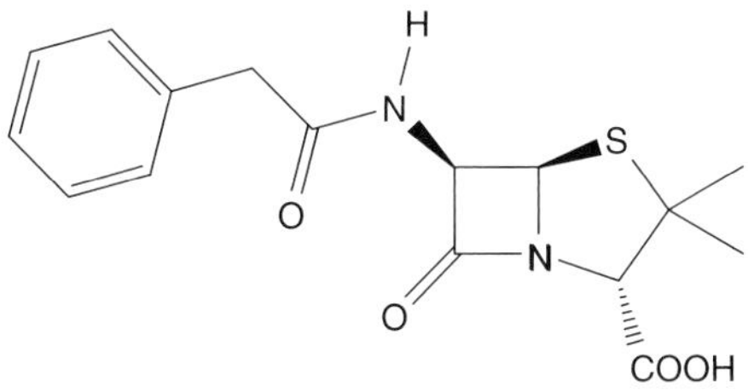

Benzyl penicillin is actually used only intravenously. It was formerly a frequent cause of contact allergy in health care workers. Facial contact dermatitis was recently reported in a nurse.

Suggested Reading

Pecegueiro M (1990) Occupational contact dermatitis from penicillin. Contact Dermatitis 23:190–191

54. BHA

Butylated Hydroxyanisole

CAS Registry Number [25013–16–5]

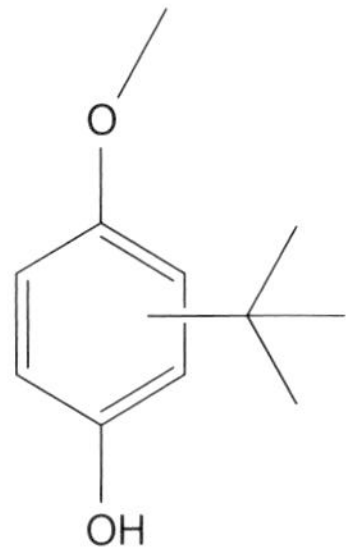

BHA is an antioxidant widely used in cosmetics and food. Contained in pastry, it can induce sensitization in caterers.

Suggested Reading

Acciai MC, Brusi C, Francalanci Giorgini S, Sertoli A (1993) Allergic contact dermatitis in caterers. Contact Dermatitis 28:48

55. BHT

Butylated Hydroxytoluene, 2,6-di-(tert-Butyl)-*p*-Cresol

CAS Registry Number [128–37–0]

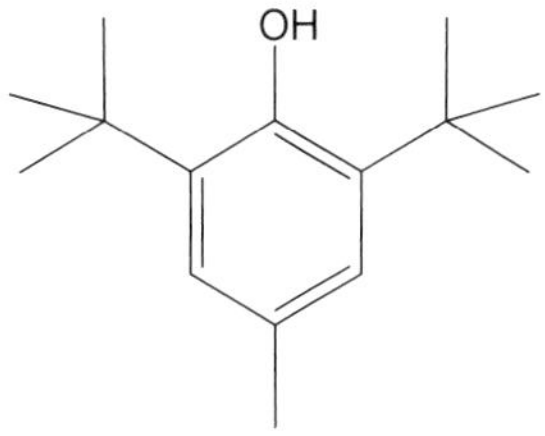

This antioxidant is contained in food, adhesive glues, industrial oils, and greases, including cutting fluids. Sensitization seems very rare.

Suggested Reading

Flyvholm MA, Menné T (1990) Sensitizing risk of butylated hydroxytoluene based on exposure and effect data. Contact Dermatitis 23:341–345

58

56. Bioban CS-1135

3,4-Dimethyloxazolidine + 3,4,4-Trimethylox-
azolidine

CAS Registry Number [81099–36–7] (CAS Registry
Number [51200–87–4] + CAS Registry Number
[75673–43–7])

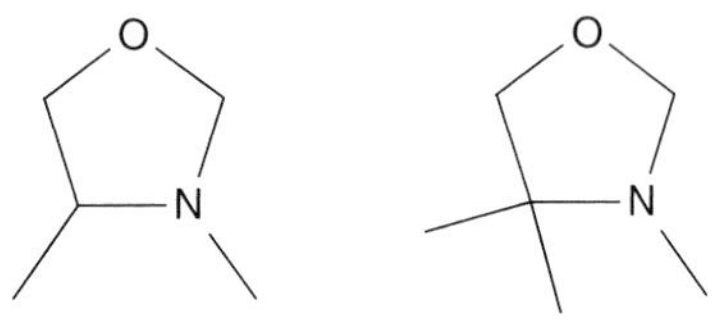

Bioban® CS-1135 is the trade name for the two compounds 3,4-dimethyloxazolidine (74.8%) and 3,4,4-trim-
ethyloxazolidine (2.5%). It is a formaldehyde releaser
used as a preservative in latex paints and emulsions and
in cooling fluids. Dimethyl oxazolidine is found in some
cosmetics. Bioban® CS-1135 can be a sensitizer per se,
in patients without formaldehyde allergy.

Suggested Reading

Brinkmeier T, Geier J, Lepoittevin JP, Frosch PJ (2002) Patch
    test reactions to Biobans in metalworkers are often weak and
    not reproducible. Contact Dermatitis 47:27–31
Kanerva L, Estlander T, Jolanki R (1994) Occupational allergic
    contact dermatitis caused by thiourea compounds. Contact
    Dermatitis 31:242–248

57. Bioban® CS-1246

Oxazolidine, 5-Ethyl-1-aza-3,7-Dioxa-Bicyclo-3,3,0
Octane

CAS Registry Number [7747–35–5], [504–76–7]

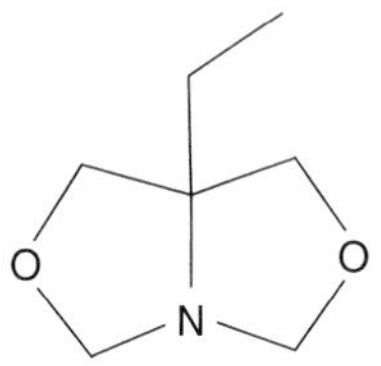

Bioban® CS-1246 is a relatively old formaldehyde
releaser, used in cutting oils. Bioban® CS-1248 is a
mixture of Bioban® CS-1246 and Bioban® P-1487.

Suggested Reading

Brinkmeier T, Geier J, Lepoittevin JP, Frosch PJ (2002) Patch
    test reactions to Biobans in metalworkers are often weak and
    not reproducible. Contact Dermatitis 47:27–31

58. Bioban® P-1487

4-(2-Nitrobutyl)Morpholine + 4,4-(2-Ethyl-2-
Nitrodimethylene)Dimorpholine

CAS Registry Number [37304–88–4] (CAS Registry
Number [2224–44–4] + CAS Registry Number
[1854–23–5]

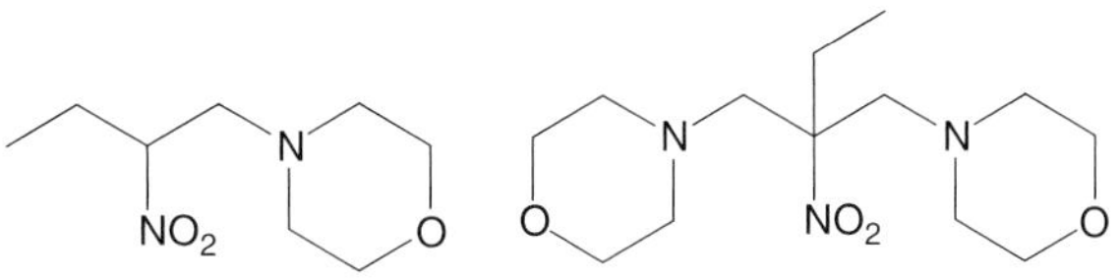

Bioban® P-1487 is a mixture of 4-(2-nitrobutyl)mor-
pholine CAS Registry Number [2224–44–4] 70%,
and 4,4-(2-ethyl-2-nitrodimethylene)dimorpholine or
4,4-(2-ethyl-2-nitro-1,3-propanediyl)-bis-morpholine
CAS Registry Number [1854–23–5] 20%. Both ingredients can be the sensitizers. It is used as a preservative
in metalworking cutting fluids. Bioban® CS-1248 is a
mixture of Bioban® CS-1246 and Bioban® P-1487.

Suggested Reading

Brinkmeier T, Geier J, Lepoittevin JP, Frosch PJ (2002) Patch
    test reactions to Biobans in metalworkers are often weak and
    not reproducible. Contact Dermatitis 47:27–31
Gruvberger B, Bruze M, Zimerson E (1996) Contact allergy to
    the active ingredients of Bioban P 1487. Contact Dermatitis
    35:141–145
Niklasson B, Björkner B, Sundberg K (1993) Contact allergy to
    a fatty acid ester component of cutting fluids. Contact
    Dermatitis 28:265–267

59. Bisphenol A

Diphenylolpropane, Isopropylidene Diphenol

CAS Registry Number [80–05–7]

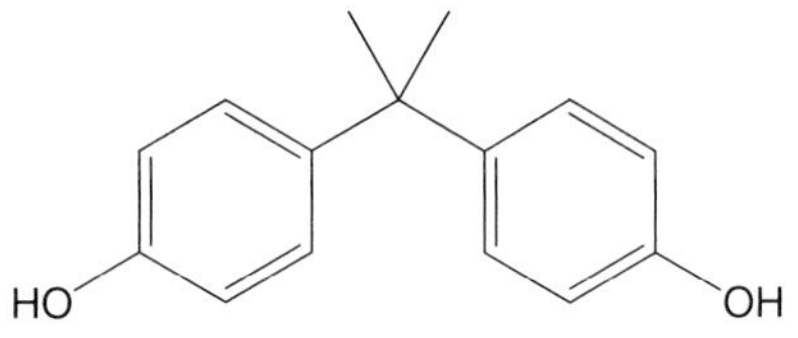

Bisphenol A is used with epichlorhydrin for the synthesis of epoxy resins bisphenol-A type, for unsaturated polyester and polycarbonate resins, and epoxy di(meth)acrylates. In epoxy resins, it leads to bisphenol-A diglycidyl ether, which is the monomer of bisphenol-A-based epoxy resins. Reports of bisphenol-A sensitization are rare and concern workers at epoxy resin plants, after contact with fiber glass, semi-synthetic waxes, footwear, and dental materials. It is also a possible sensitizer in vinyl gloves.

Suggested Reading

Jolanki R, Kanerva L, Estlander T (1995) Occupational allergic contact dermatitis caused by epoxy diacrylate in ultraviolet-light-cured paint, and bisphenol A in dental composite resin. Contact Dermatitis 33:94–99

Matthieu L, Godoi AFL, Lambert J, van Grieken R (2004) Occupational allergic contact dermatitis from bisphenol A in vinyl gloves. Contact Dermatitis 49:281–283

Van Jost T, Roesyanto ID, Satyawan I (1990) Occupational sensitization to epichlorhydrin (ECH) and bisphenol-A during the manufacture of epoxy resin. Contact Dermatitis 22:125–126

60. Bisphenol A Diglycidyl Ether (DGEBA)

BADGE

CAS Registry Number [1675–54–3]

Most epoxy resins result from polymerization of bisphenol A diglycidyl ether (BADGE). Delayed hypersensitivity is caused by the low-molecular-weight monomer BADGE (Molecular Weight 340 g/mol), the dimer having much a lower sensitization power. This allergen caused contact dermatitis in six workers in a plant producing printed circuits boards made of copper sheets and fiber glass fabric impregnated with a brominated epoxy resin. It can be contained in adhesives.

Suggested Reading

Bruze M, Almgren G (1989) Occupational dermatoses in workers exposed to epoxy-impregnated fiberglass fabric. Dermatosen 37:171–176

Bruze M, Edenholm M, Engenström K, Svensson G (1996) Occupational dermatoses in a Swedish aircraft plant. Contact Dermatitis 34:336–340

Hansson C (1994) Determination of monomers in epoxy resin hardened at elevated temperatures. Contact Dermatitis 31:333–334

61. o,p-Bisphenol F and p,p-Bisphenol F

2,4-Dihydroxy-Diphenylmethane and 4,4-Dihydroxy-Diphenylmethane

CAS Registry Number [2467–03–0] and CAS Registry Number [620–92–8]

o,p-Bisphenol F and p,p-bisphenol F are allergenic components of phenol-formaldehyde resins resol-type.

Suggested Reading

Bruze M, Fregert S, Zimerson E (1985) Contact allergy to phenol-formaldehyde resins. Contact Dermatitis 12:81–86

62. Bisphenol F Diglycidyl Ether (DGEBF)

(a) p,p-Diglycidyl Ether of Bisphenol F

CAS Registry Number [2095–03–6]

(a) o,p-Diglycidyl Ether of Bisphenol F

CAS Registry Number [57469–08–5]

(b) o,o-Diglycidyl Ether of Bisphenol F

CAS Registry Number [39817–09–9], [54208–63–8]

Epoxy resins based on Bisphenol F, also called phenolic Novolac, contain bisphenol F diglycidyl ether,

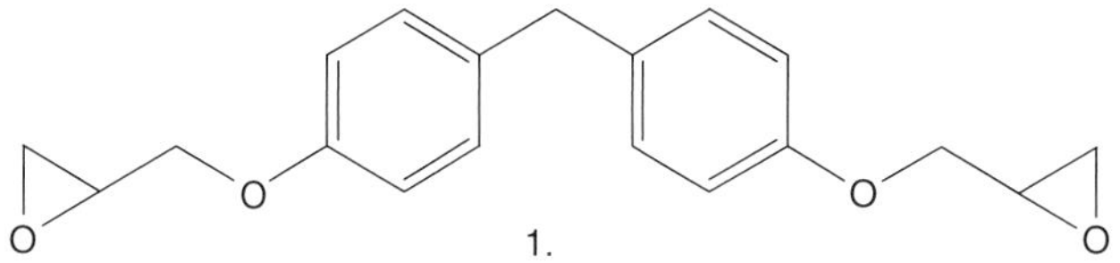

1.

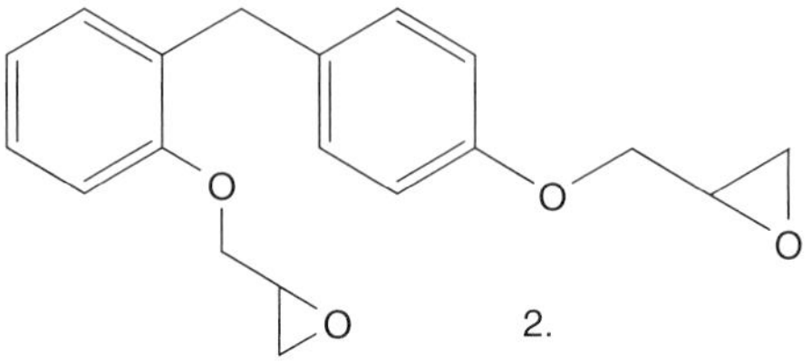

2.

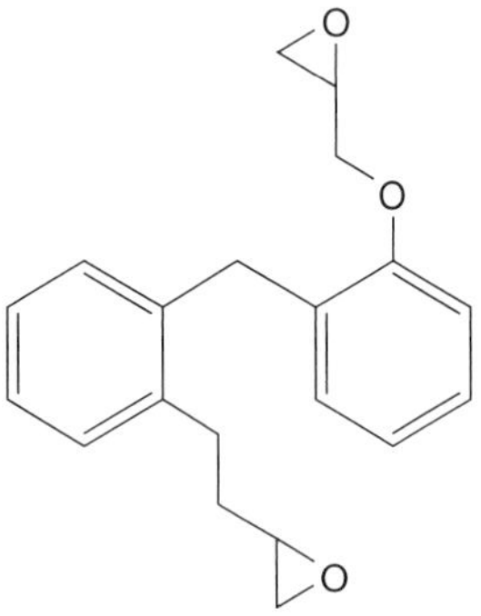

3.

which has three sensitizing isomers. DGEBF has a greater resistance than DGEBA. Contact allergy to bisphenol-F-based epoxy resins is rarer than that due to bisphenol-A-based resins and is frequently acquired with flooring materials and putty.

Suggested Reading

Bruze M, Edenholm M, Engenström K, Svensson G (1996) Occupational dermatoses in a Swedish aircraft plant. Contact Dermatitis 34:336–340

Pontén A, Bruze M (2001) Contact allergy to epoxy resin based on diglycidyl ether of Bisphenol F. Contact Dermatitis 44:98–99
Pontén A, Zimerson E, Bruze M (2004) Contact allergy to the isomers of diglycidyl ether of bisphenol F. Acta Derm Venereol (Stockh) 84:12–17

63. Brominated Epoxy Resin

As a component of nondiglycidyl ether of bisphenol A epoxy resins, brominated epoxy resin caused contact dermatitis in a cleaner of worksites in a condenser factory, where condensers were filled with a mixture made of an epoxy resin.

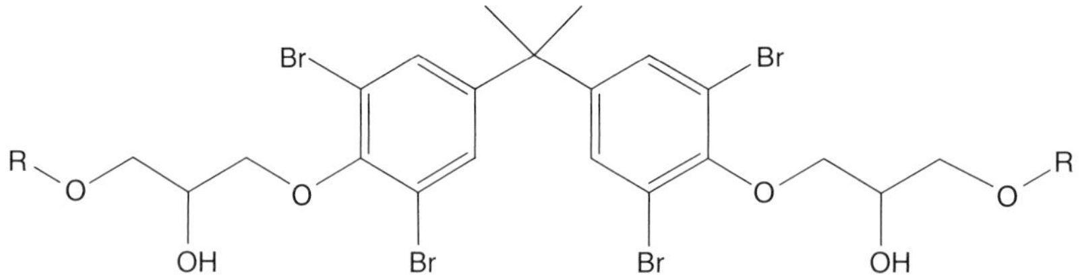

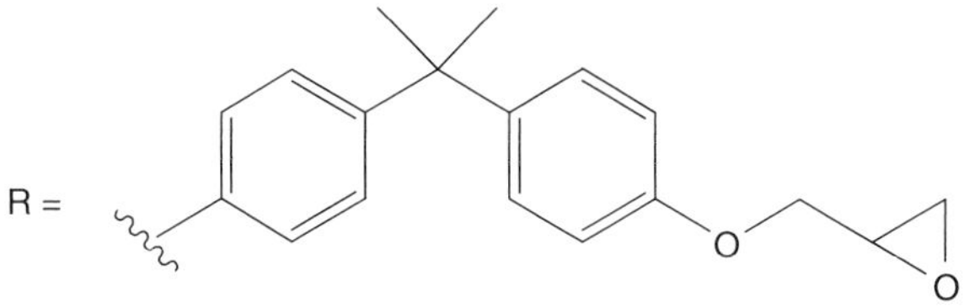

R =

Suggested Reading

Kanerva L, Jolanki R, Estlander T (1991) Allergic contact dermatitis from nondiglycidyl-ether-of-bisphenol-A epoxy resins. Contact Dermatitis 24:293–300

64. 1-Bromo-3-Chloro-5,5-Dimethylhydantoin

Di-Halo, 1-Bromo-3-Chloro-5,5-Dimethyl-2,4-Imidazolidinedione, Agribrom, Slimicide C 77P

CAS Registry Number [16079–88–2]

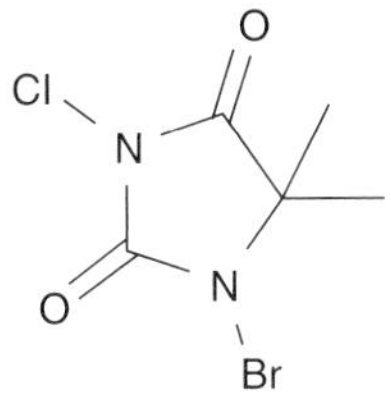

This chlorinated and brominated product is employed in agriculture as a fungicide, for wood preservation. When used to sanitize pools and spas, releasing both chlorine and bromine derivatives, it can induce irritant or allergic contact dermatitis.

Suggested Reading

Rycroft RJG, Penny PT (1983) Dermatoses associated with brominated swimming pools. Br Med J (Clin Res Ed) 287:462
Sasseville D, Moreau L (2004) Contact allergy to 1-bromo-3chloro-5, 5-dimethylhydantoin in spa water. Contact Dermatitis 50:323–324

65. Bromohydroxyacetophenone

(a) 2-Bromo-4-Hydroxyacetophenone, 1-(4-Hydroxyphenyl)-2-Bromoethanone

CAS Registry Number [2491–38–5]

(a) 2-Bromo-2-Hydroxyacetophenone, (6Cl, 7Cl, 8Cl)

CAS Registry Number [2491–36–3]

(b) 5-Bromo-2-Hydroxy-Acetophenone (6Cl, 7Cl, 8Cl), 1-(5-Bromo-2-Hydroxyphenyl)Ethanone

CAS Registry Number [1450–75–5]

Those substances are biocides used in emulsions, paints, adhesives, waxes, and polishes. They are both irritants and sensitizers. 2-Bromo-4-hydroxyacetophenone used as a slimicide provoked sensitization after an accidental spillage and recurrent allergic contact dermatitis at a workplace.

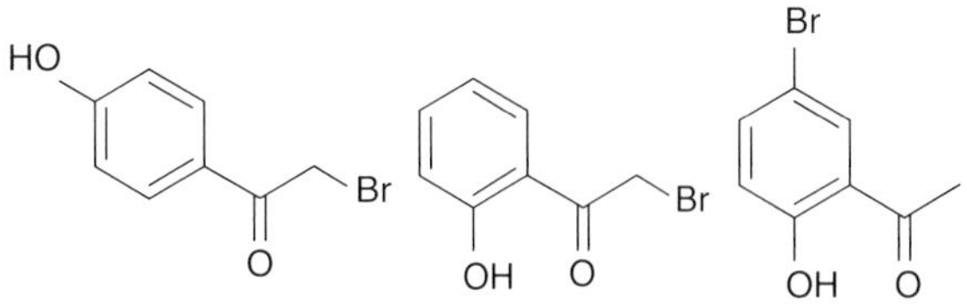

Suggested Reading

Jensen CD, Andersen KE (2003) Allergic contact dermatitis from a paper mill slimicide containing 2-bromo-4-hydroxy-acetophenone. Am J Contact Dermat 14:41–43

66. Bronopol

2-Bromo-2-Nitro-1,3-Propanediol

CAS Registry Number [52–51–7]

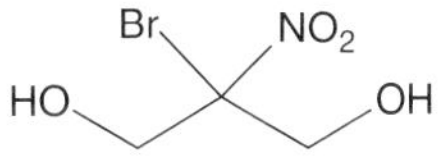

Bronopol is a preservative sometimes considered as a formaldehyde releaser. It was reported to be an allergen in cosmetics, cleaning agents, dairy workers, and a lubricant jelly used for ultrasound examination.

Suggested Reading

Grattan CEH, Harman RRM, Tan RSH (1986) Milk recorder dermatitis. Contact Dermatitis 14:217–220
Wilson CL, Powell SM (1990) An unusual cause of allergic contact dermatitis in a veterinary surgeon. Contact Dermatitis 23:42–43

67. Budesonide

Budesonide

CAS Registry number [51333–22–3]

R-Budesonide

CAS Registry Number [51372–29–3]

S-Budesonide

CAS Registry Number [51372–28–2]

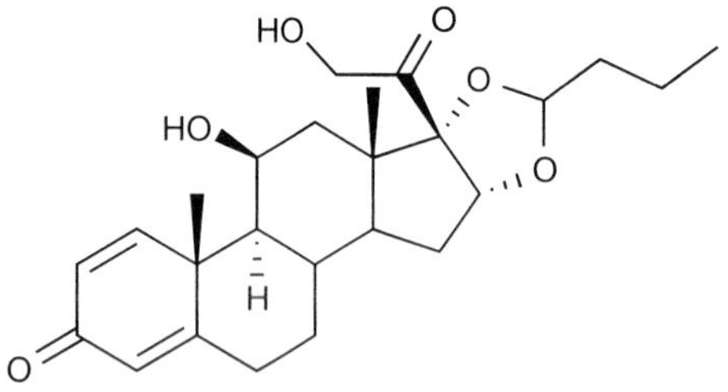

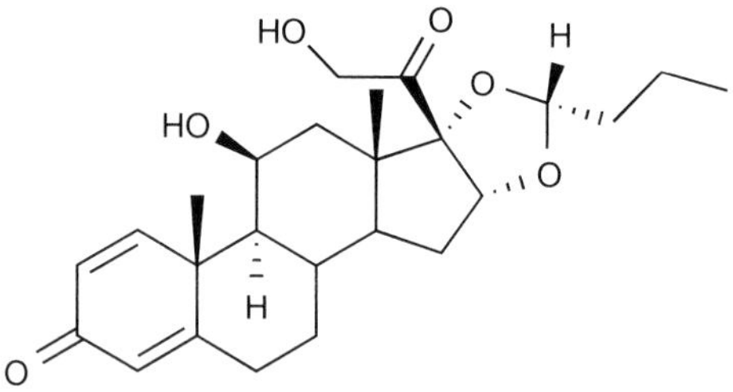

R-Budesonide

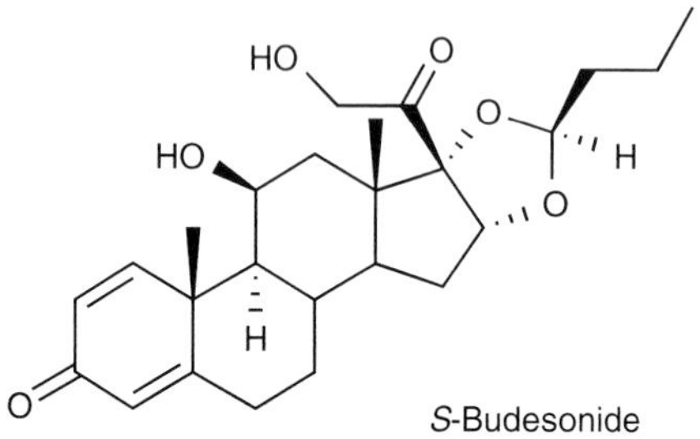

S-Budesonide

Budesonide is a corticosteroid, a blend of two diastereosiomers.

R-Budesonide is a marker of the B group of corticosteroids. Such molecules have a *cis*-diol moiety or an acetal moiety on the C_{16} and C_{17} of the D cycle. One side chain is possible on C_{21}. The B group comprises amcinonide, budesonide, desonide or prednacinolone, flunisolide, fluocinolone and its acetonide, fluocinonide, fluclorolone and its acetonide, halcinonide, and acetonide, benetonide, diacetate and hexacetonide of triamcinolone.

S-Budesonide is a marker of the D2 group of corticosteroids. Such molecules are nonmethylated in C_{16} and have an ester function in C_{17}. They comprise hydrocortisone 17-butyrate, hydrocortisone-17-valerate, hydrocortisone aceponate, methylprednisolone aceponate, and prednicarbate.

Suggested Reading

Lepoittevin JP, Drieghe J, Dooms-Goossens A (1995) Studies in patients with corticosteroid contact allergy. Understanding cross-reactivity among different steroids. Arch Dermatol 131:31–37

Le Coz CJ (2002) Fiche d'éviction en cas d'hypersensibilité aux corticoïdes. Ann Dermatol Venereol 129:346–347

Le Coz CJ (2002) Fiche d'éviction en cas d'hypersensibilité au 17 butyrate d'hydrocortisone. Ann Dermatol Venereol 129:931

Le Coz CJ (2002) Fiche d'éviction en cas d'hypersensibilité au budésonide. Ann Dermatol Venereol 129: 1409–1410

68. Bufexamac

CAS Registry Number [2438-72-4]

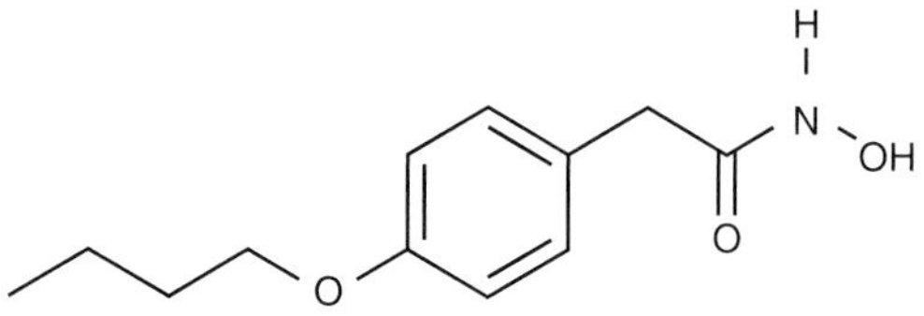

Bufexamac is an arylacetic nonsteroidal anti-inflammatory drug. It induces allergic contact dermatitis, eczematous or erythema multiforme like type, and even generalized eruptions like acute generalized exanthematous pustulosis.

Suggested Reading

Belhadjali H, Ghannouchi N, Njim L, Mohamed M, Moussa A, Bayou F, Chakroun M, Zakhama A, Zili J (2008) Acute generalized exanthematous pustulosis induced by bufexamac in an atopic girl. Contact Dermatitis 58:247–248

Kurumaji Y (1998) Photo Koebner phenomenon in erythema-multiforme-like eruption induced by contact dermatitis due to bufexamac. Dermatology 197:183–186

69. Buprenorphine

CAS registry Number [52485-79-7]

This semisynthetic opioid analgesic drug is derived from thebaine. It can be used parenterally, orally, and topically with transdermal systems (TDS). In case of localized or generalized allergic contact dermatitis due to buprenorphine in TDS, TDS containing fentanyl can be safely used.

Suggested Reading

Van der Hulst K, Parera Amer E, Jacobs C, Dewulf V, Baeck M, Pujol Vallverdú RM, Giménez-Arnau A, Tennstedt D, Goossens A (2008) Allergic contact dermatitis from transdermal buprenorphine. Contact Dermatitis 59:366–369

Pérez-Pérez L, Cabanillas M, Loureiro M, Fernández-Redondo V, Labandeira J, Toribio J (2008) Allergic contact dermatitis due to transdermal buprenorphine. Contact Dermatitis 58:310–312

70. 1,4-Butanediol Diglycidyl Ether

CAS Registry Number [2425–79–8]

This substance is a reactive diluent in epoxy resins.

Suggested Reading

Jolanki R, Estlander T, Kanerva L (1987) Contact allergy to an epoxy reactive diluent: 1,4-butanediol diglycidyl ether. Contact Dermatitis 16:87–92

Jolanki R, Kanerva L, Estlander T, Tarvainen K, Keskinen H, Henriks-Eckerman ML (1990) Occupational dermatoses from epoxy resin compounds. Contact Dermatitis 23:172–183

71. *N-tert*-Butyl-bis-(2-Benzothiazole) Sulfenamide

CAS Registry Number [3741–80–8]

This mercaptobenzothiazole-sulfenamide chemical is used as an accelerator in rubber vulcanization.

Suggested Reading

Le Coz CJ (2004) Fiche d'éviction en cas d'hypersensibilité au mercaptobenzothiazole et au mercapto mix. Ann Dermatol Venereol 131:846–848

72. Butyl Carbitol

Diethylene Glycol Monobutyl Ether

CAS Registry Number [112–34–5]

This organic solvent belongs to the carbitols group and is included in waterbased liquids such as paints, surface cleaners, polishes, and disinfectants. It is considered to be an exceptional allergen.

Suggested Reading

Berlin K, Johanson G, Lindberg M (1995) Hypersensitivity to 2-(2-butoxyethoxy)ethanol. Contact Dermatitis 32:54

Schliemann-Willers S, Bauer A, Elsner P (2000) Occupational contact dermatitis from diethylene glycol monobutyl ether in a podiatrist. Contact Dermatitis 43:225

73. *p-tert*-Butyl Catechol

CAS Registry Number [98–29–3]

58

p-tert-Butyl catechol is specially prepared by reacting the impure catechol fraction with tertiary butyl alcohol. It is used for its various properties (inhibitor of polymerization and antioxidizing agent) in the manufacture of rubber, plastics, and paints, in the preparation of petrolatum products, and as an antioxidant in oils. It may induce vitiligo.

Suggested Reading

Gawkrodger DJ, Cork MJ, Bleehen SS (1991) Occupational vitiligo and contact sensitivity to para-tertiary butyl catechol. Contact Dermatitis 25:200–201

74. *n*-Butyl Glycidyl Ether

CAS Registry Number [2426–08–6]

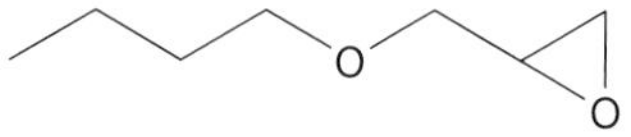

A reactive diluent used to reduce viscosity of epoxy resins Bisphenol A type.

Suggested Reading

Holness DL, Nethercott JR (1993) The performance of specialized collections of bisphenol A epoxy resin system components in the evaluation of workers in an occupational health clinic population. Contact Dermatitis 28: 216–219
Jolanki R, Kanerva L, Estlander T, Tarvainen K, Keskinen H, Henriks-Eckerman ML (1990) Occupational dermatoses from epoxy resin compounds. Contact Dermatitis 23: 172–183

75. *tert*-Butyl-Hydroquinone

2-*tert*-Butylhydroquinone, TBHQ

CAS Registry Number [1948–33–0]

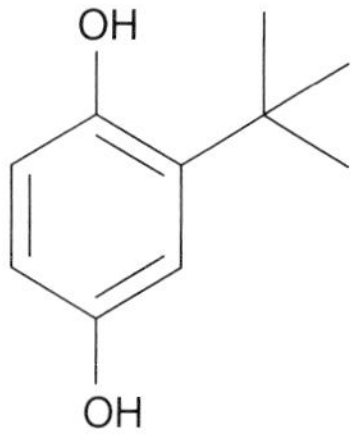

This antioxidant has seldom been reported as a sensitizer, mainly in cosmetics (lipsticks, lip-gloss, hair dyes) or in cutting oils. Simultaneous/cross-reactions have been described to butylhydroxyanisole (BHA) and less frequently to butylhydroxytoluene (BHT), but not to hydroquinone.

Suggested Reading

Aalto-Korte K (2000) Allergic contact dermatitis from tertiary-butylhydroquinone (TBHQ) in a vegetable hydraulic oil. Contact Dermatitis 43:303
Le Coz CJ, Schneider GA (1998) Contact dermatitis from tertiary-butylhydroquinone in a hair dye, with cross-sensitivity to BHA and BHT. Contact Dermatitis 39:39–40

76. *p-tert*-Butyl-alpha-Methylhydrocinnamic Aldehyde

Lilial®, 2-(4-*tert*-Butylbenzyl)Propionaldehyde, 4-(1,1-Dimethylethyl)-α-Methyl-Benzenepropanal, *p-tert*-Butyl-α-Methylhydrocinnamaldehyde, Lilestral

CAS Registry Number [80–54–6]

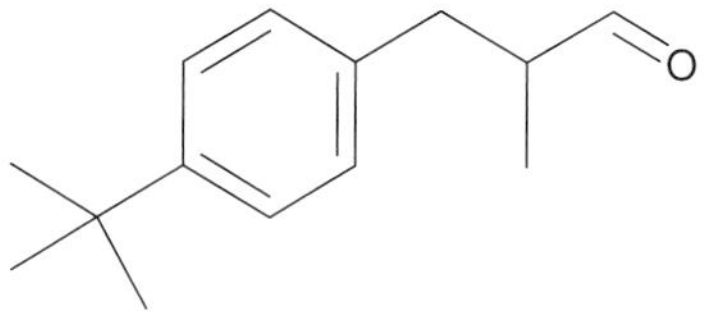

Lilial® is a synthetic compound listed as a fragrance allergen. Its presence is indicated on cosmetics within the EU.

Suggested Reading

Giménez-Arnau E, Andersen KE, Bruze M, Frosch PJ, Johansen JD, Menné T, Rastogi SC, White IR, Lepoittevin JP (2000) Identification of Lilial as a fragrance sensitizer in a perfume by bioassay-guided chemical fractionation and structure-activity relationships. Contact Dermatitis 43:351–358

77. Butylene Glycol

1,3-Butylene Glycol, 1,3-Butanediol

CAS Registry Number [107–88–0]

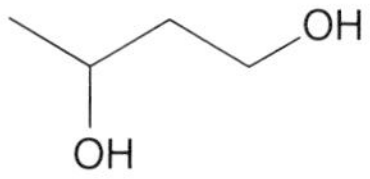

This dihydric alcohol is used for its humectant and preservative potentiator properties in cosmetics, topical medicaments and polyurethane, polyester, cellophane, and cigarettes. It has similar properties, but is less irritant than propylene glycol. Contact allergies seem to be rare.

Suggested Reading

Diegenant C, Constandt L, Goossens A (2000) Allergic contact dermatitis due to 1,3-butylene glycol. Contact Dermatitis 43:324–235
Matsunaga K, Sugai T, Katoh J, Hayakawa R, Kozuka T, Itoh J, Tsuyuki S, Hosono K (1997) Group study on contact sensitivity of 1,3-butylene glycol. Environ Dermatol 4:195–205

78. *Para-tert*-Butylphenol

CAS Registry Number [98–54–4]

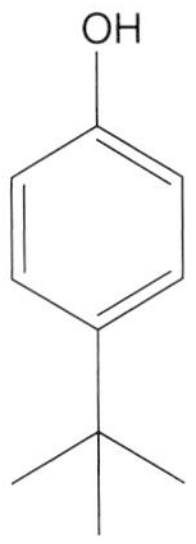

Para-tert-butylphenol is used with formaldehyde to produce the polycondensate *p-tert*-butylphenol-formaldehyde resins (PTBPFR). Major occupational sources are neoprene glues and adhesives in industry, in the shoemaking and leather industries or in car production. It is also used as a box preservative in box and furniture manufacture and in the production of casting molds, car brake linings, insulated electrical cables, adhesives, printing inks, and paper laminates. *Para-tert*-butylphenol seems to be the sensitizer.

Suggested Reading

Handley J, Todd D, Bingham A, Corbett R, Burrows D (1993) Allergic contact dermatitis from *para-tertiary*-butylphenol-formaldehyde resin (PTBP-F-R) in Northern Ireland. Contact Dermatitis 29:144–146
Mancuso G, Reggiani M, Berdondini RM (1996) Occupational dermatitis in shoemakers. Contact Dermatitis 34:17–22
Shono M, Ezoe K, Kaniwa MA, Ikarashi Y, Kohma S, Nakamura A (1991) Allergic contact dermatitis from para-tertiary-butylphenol-formaldehyde resin (PTBP-FR) in athletic tape and leather adhesive. Contact Dermatitis 24:281–288

Tarvainen K (1995) Analysis of patients with allergic patch test reactions to a plastics and glue series. Contact Dermatitis 32:346–351

79. Caffeic Acid Dimethyl Allylic Ester

3-Methyl-2-Butenyl-Caffeate

CAS Registry Number [108084–13–7]

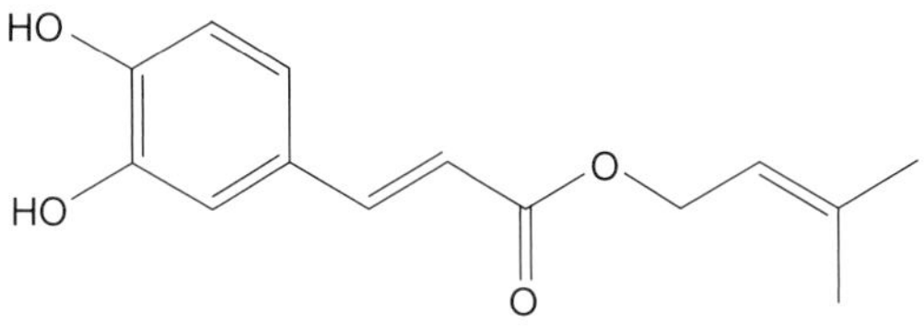

This is the major allergen of poplar bud resins and of propolis, the bee glue derived almost exclusively from poplar buds.

Suggested Reading

Lamminpää A, Estlander T, Jolanki R, Kanerva L (1996) Occupational allergic contact dermatitis caused by decorative plants. Contact Dermatitis 34:330–335
Oliwiecki S, Beck MH, Hausen BM (1992) Occupational contact dermatitis from caffeates in poplar bud resin in a tree surgeon. Contact Dermatitis 27:127–128

80. Captafol

CAS Registry Number [2425–06–1]

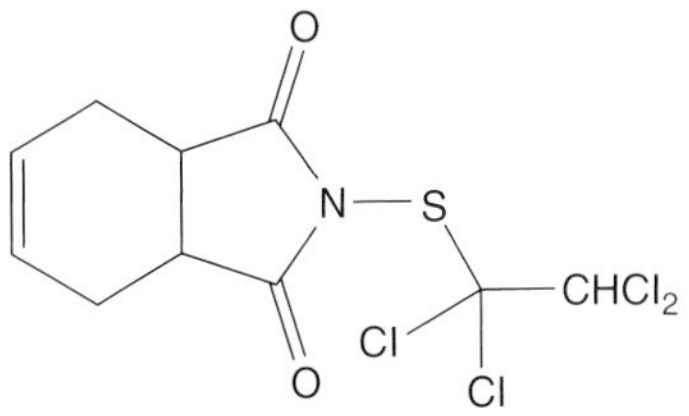

Captafol is a pesticide, belonging to thiophthalimide group. Occupational contact dermatitis was reported in an agricultural worker who had multiple sensitizations.

Suggested Reading

Peluso AM, Tardio M, Adamo F, Venturo N (1991) Multiple sensitization due to bis-dithiocarbamate and thiophthalimide pesticides. Contact Dermatitis 25:327

81. Captan

Captane, N-Trichloromethylmer-
captotetrahydrophtalimide

CAS Registry Number [133–06–2]

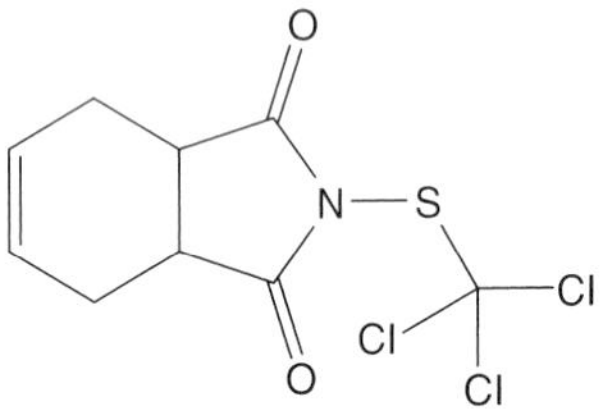

A pesticide, belonging to the thiophthalimide group, mainly affects agricultural workers. Being sensitizer and photosensitizer, it can induce contact urticaria. It is used as a fungicide and a bacteriostatic agent in cosmetics and toiletries, particularly in shampoos. Cases of contact dermatitis were reported in painters, polishers, and varnishers.

Suggested Reading

Aguirre A, Manzano D, Zabala R, Raton JA, Diaz-Perez JL (1994) Contact allergy to captan in a hairdresser. Contact Dermatitis 31:46
Moura C, Dias M, Vale T (1994) Contact dermatitis in painters, polishers and varnishers. Contact Dermatitis 31:51–53
O'Malley M, Rodriguez P, Maibach HI (1995) Pesticide patch testing: California nursery workers and controls. Contact Dermatitis 32:61–62
Peluso AM, Tardio M, Adamo F, Venturo N (1991) Multiple sensitization due to bis-dithiocarbamate and thiophthalimide pesticides. Contact Dermatitis 25:327
Vilaplana J, Romaguera C (1993) Captan, a rare contact sensitizer in hairdressing. Contact Dermatitis 29:107

82. Carbaryl

CAS Registry Number [63–25–2]

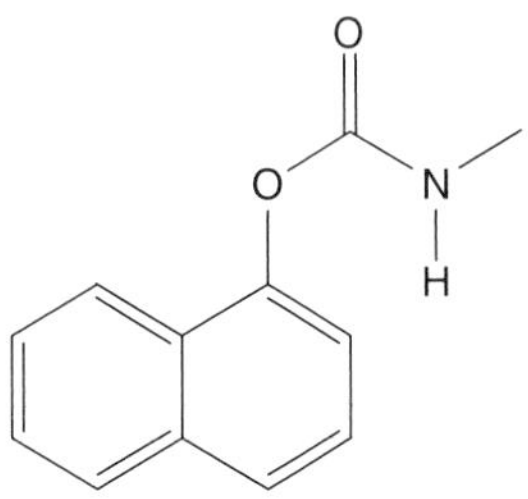

Carbaryl is a pesticide and insecticide of the carbonate group. It induced sensitization in a farmer.

Suggested Reading

Sharma VK, Kaur S (1990) Contact sensitization by pesticides in farmers. Contact Dermatitis 23:77–80

83. Carbodiimide

Cyanamide

CAS Registry Number [420–04–2]

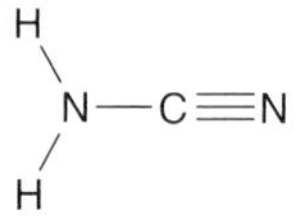

Cyanamide and its salts are used in various occasions such as in chemistry, in antirust solutions, or in a drug (Come®) for treating alcoholism (inhibition of alcohol deshydrogenase).

Suggested Reading

Goday Bujan JJ, Yanguas Bayona I, Arechavala RS (1994) Allergic contact dermatitis from cyanamide: report of 3 cases. Contact Dermatitis 31:331–332

84. Carbofuran

CAS Registry Number [1563–66–2]

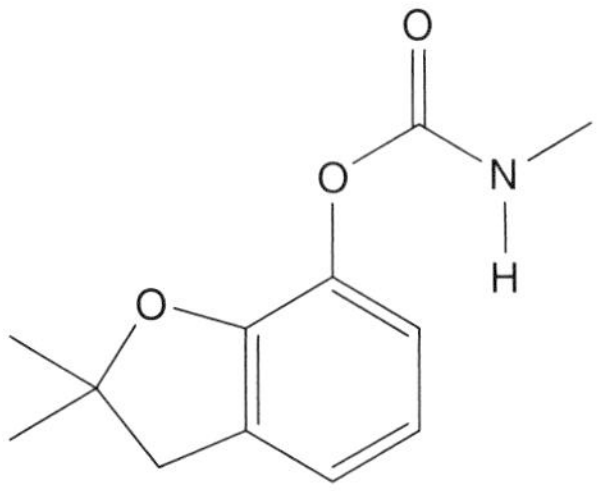

It is a pesticide with insecticide properties, of the carbamate group. It was implicated as a sensitizer in two farmers.

Suggested Reading

Sharma VK, Kaur S (1990) Contact sensitization by pesticides in farmers. Contact Dermatitis 23:77–80

85. Cardols

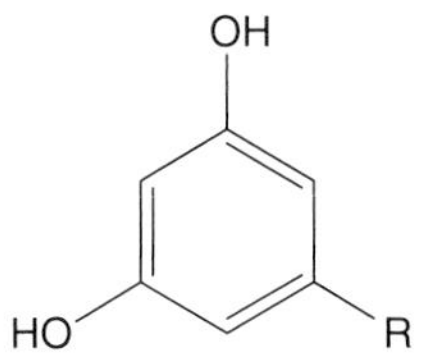

Cardols are a mixture of several analog molecules with an alkyl chain (-R) with 13, 15, 17, or 19 carbon and 0–3 unsaturations. It is one of the main cashew nut shell liquid components, along with anacardic acid. Sensitization occurs in cashew nut workers. See also Chap. 46.

Suggested Reading

Diogenes MJN, De Morais SM, Carvalho FF (1996) Contact dermatitis among cashew nut workers. Contact Dermatitis 35:114–115

86. Δ-3-Carene

CAS Registry Number [13466–78–9]

Hydroperoxides of Δ-3-carene are allergens contained in turpentine. Occupational exposure occurs in painters, varnishers, or ceramic decoration. The percentage of Δ-3-carene is higher in Indonesian than in Portuguese turpentine.

Suggested Reading

Lear JT, Heagerty AHM, Tan BB, Smith AG, English JSC (1996) Transient reemergence of oil turpentine allergy in the pottery industry. Contact Dermatitis 35:169–172

87. Carteolol

CAS Registry Number [51781–06–7]

Carteolol was implicated in allergic contact dermatitis due to beta-blockers agents in eye-drops. It seems that this molecule can be safely used in some patients with hypersensitivity to other topical beta-blockers agents.

Suggested Reading

Giordano-Labadie F, Lepoittevin JP, Calix I, Bazex J (1997) Allergie de contact aux â-bloqueurs des collyres: allergie croisée? Ann Dermatol Venereol 124:322–324
Nino M, Balato A, Ayala F, Balato N (2007) Allergic contact dermatitis due to levobunolol with cross-sensitivity to befunolol. Contact Dermatitis 56:53–54

88. CD1

N,N-Diethylparaphenylenediamine Monochlorhydrate

CAS Registry Number [2198–58–5]

A color film developer. It is an allergen and an irritant in photographers. Cross-reactivity is possible with Disperse Blue 124, Disperse Blue 106, and Disperse red 17, but not with *para*-amino compounds.

Suggested Reading

Aguirre A, Landa N, Gonzalez M, Diaz-Perez JL (1992) Allergic contact dermatitis in a photographer. Contact Dermatitis 27:340–341
Galindo PA, Garcia R, Garrido JA, Feo F, Fernandez F (1994) Allergic contact dermatitis from color developers: absence of cross-sensitivity to para-amino compounds. Contact Dermatitis 30:301
Hansson C, Ahlfors S, Bergendorff O (1997) Concomitant contact dermatitis due to textile dyes and to color film developers can be explained by the formation of the same hapten. Contact Dermatitis 37:27–31

Lidén C, Brehmer-Andersson E (1988) Occupational dermatoses from color developing agents. Clinical and histopathological observations. Acta Derm Venereol (Stockh)
68:514–522

89. CD2

4-*N*,*N*-Diethyl-2-Methyl-1,4-Phenylenediamine
(Hydrochloride)

CAS Registry Number [2051–79–8]

A color film developer. It acts as an allergen and an
irritant in photographers. Cross-reactivity is possible
with Disperse Blue 124, Disperse Blue 106, and
Disperse Red 17, but not to *para*-amino compounds.

Suggested Reading

Aguirre A, Landa N, Gonzalez M, Diaz-Perez JL (1992) Allergic
contact dermatitis in a photographer. Contact Dermatitis 27:
340–341
Galindo PA, Garcia R, Garrido JA, Feo F, Fernandez F (1994)
Allergic contact dermatitis from color developers: absence
of cross-sensitivity to para-amino compounds. Contact
Dermatitis 30:301
Hansson C, Ahlfors S, Bergendorff O (1997) Concomitant contact dermatitis due to textile dyes and to color film developers can be explained by the formation of the same hapten.
Contact Dermatitis 37:27–31
Lidén C, Brehmer-Andersson E (1988) Occupational dermatoses from color developing agents. Clinical and histopathological observations. Acta Derm Venereol (Stockh) 68:
514–522
Rustemeyer T, Frosch PJ (1995) Allergic contact dermatitis
from color film developers. Contact Dermatitis 32:59–60

90. CD3

4-(Ethyl-*N*-2-Methan-Sulfonamidoethyl)-2-Methyl-
1,4-Phenylenediamine (*1,5H$_2$SO$_4$ *H$_2$O)

CAS Registry Number [25646–71–3]

A color film developer. It caused some allergic reactions in
photographers. Cross-reactivity is possible with Disperse
Blue 124, Disperse Blue 106, and Disperse Red 17.

Suggested Reading

Aguirre A, Landa N, Gonzalez M, Diaz-Perez JL (1992) Allergic
contact dermatitis in a photographer. Contact Dermatitis
27:340–341
Galindo PA, Garcia R, Garrido JA, Feo F, Fernandez F (1994) Allergic
contact dermatitis from color developers: absence of cross-sensitivity to para-amino compounds. Contact Dermatitis 30:301
Hansson C, Ahlfors S, Bergendorff O (1997) Concomitant contact dermatitis due to textile dyes and to color film developers can be explained by the formation of the same hapten.
Contact Dermatitis 37:27–31
Lidén C, Brehmer-Andersson E (1988) Occupational dermatoses
from color developing agents. Clinical and histopathological
observations. Acta Derm Venereol (Stockh) 68:514–522
Rustemeyer T, Frosch PJ (1995) Allergic contact dermatitis
from color developers. Contact Dermatitis 32:59–60
Scheman AJ, Katta R (1997) Photographic allergens: an update.
Contact Dermatitis 37:130

91. CD4

4-(Ethyl-*N*-Hydroxyethyl)-2-Methyl-1,4-
Phenylenediamine (*H$_2$SO$_4$*H$_2$O)

CAS Registry Number [25646–77–9]

Color film developer. It is both an allergen and an irritant in
photographers. Cross-reactivity is possible with Disperse
Blue 124, Disperse Blue 106, and Disperse Red 17.

Suggested Reading

Aguirre A, Landa N, Gonzalez M, Diaz-Perez JL (1992) Allergic contact dermatitis in a photographer. Contact Dermatitis 27:340–341

Galindo PA, Garcia R, Garrido JA, Feo F, Fernandez F (1994) Allergic contact dermatitis from color developers: absence of cross-sensitivity to para-amino compounds. Contact Dermatitis 30:301

Hansson C, Ahlfors S, Bergendorff O (1997) Concomitant contact dermatitis due to textile dyes and to color film developers can be explained by the formation of the same hapten. Contact Dermatitis 37:27–31

Lidén C, Brehmer-Andersson E (1988) Occupational dermatoses from color developing agents. Clinical and histopathological observations. Acta Derm Venereol (Stockh) 68:514–522

Rustemeyer T, Frosch PJ (1995) Allergic contact dermatitis from color developers. Contact Dermatitis 32:59–60

Scheman AJ, Katta R (1997) Photographic allergens: an update. Contact Dermatitis 37:130

92. CD6

4-Amino-N-Ethyl-N-(2-Methoxyethyl)-2-Methyl Paraphenylenediamine di-p-Toluene Sulfonate

CAS Registry Number [50928–80–8]

This color film developer rarely induced contact dermatitis in photographers.

Suggested Reading

Lidén C (1989) Occupational dermatoses at a film laboratory. Contact Dermatitis 20:191–200

Lidén C, Brehmer-Andersson E (1988) Occupational dermatoses from color developing agents. Clinical and histopathological observations. Acta Derm Venereol (Stockh) 68:514–522

93. Cefaclor

CAS Registry Number [70356–03–5]

Cefaclor is a semisynthetic cephalosporin antibiotic, related to cefalexin, and a frequent inducer of serum sickness-like reactions.

Suggested Reading

Hebert AA, Sigman ES, Levy ML (1991) Serum sickness-like reactions from cefaclor in children. J Am Acad Dermatol 25:805–808

94. Cephalosporins

All cephalosporins have a 7-amino-cephalosporanic group (cephem nucleus). They differ by a C_7 and a C_3 substitution. The cause of an allergic reaction to cephalosporins can be the cephem nucleus itself, but this seems to be rare. Allergic contact dermatitis from cephalosporins is uncommon and mainly occurs in health care, pharmaceutical, and veterinary professions. Systemic drug reactions are more frequent and can involve an immuno-allergic mechanism or not. Some of them are severe and life threatening.

Cefaclor is frequently responsible for serum thickness diseases. Cefotaxime, ceftizoxime, ceftazidime, ceftriaxone and cefodizime, several third-generation cephalosporins, caused positive patch reactions in a sensitized nurse. Cefazoline, cefoxitin, ceftriaxone, and ceftazidime were responsible for contact dermatitis in a nurse. Sensitivity to cephalothin, cephamandol, and cephazolin, cephalosporins of the first and second generation, was reported in a pharmaceutical laboratory analyst. Ceftiofur sodium, a third-generation veterinary cephalosporin, caused contact dermatitis in two chicken vaccinators. No cross-sensitivity was observed to other cephalosporins. Cephalexin hypersensitivity was reported in three cases, and to cefuroxime in one case with cross-reaction to cephalotin and cephaloridine.

Suggested Reading

Condé-Salazar L, Guimaraens D, Romero LV, Gonzales MA (1986) Occupational dermatitis from cephalosporins. Contact Dermatitis 14:70–71

Filipe P, Soares Almeida RSL, Guerra Rodrigo F (1996) Occupational allergic contact dermatitis from cephalosporins. Contact Dermatitis 34:226

Foti C, Vena GA, Cucurachi MR, Angelini G (1994) Occupational contact allergy from cephalosporins. Contact Dermatitis 31:129–130

Garcia-Bravo B, Gines E, Russo F (1995) Occupational contact dermatitis from ceftiofur sodium. Contact Dermatitis 33:62–63

Romano A, Pietrantonio F, Di Fonso M, Venuti A (1992) Delayed hypersensitivity to cefuroxime. Contact Dermatitis 27:270–271

95. Cetearyl Isononanoate

Cetearyl Hexadecyl Isononanoate

CAS Registry Number [84878–33–1]

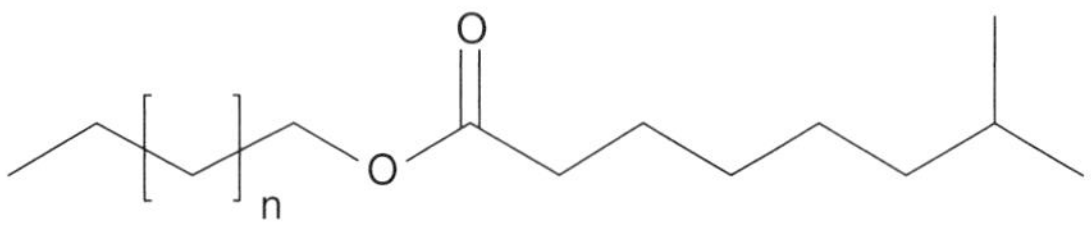

n: 14 to 16

This substance results from esterification of a saturated C_{16}–C_{18} alcohol, namely cetyl or stearyl alcohol, and a branched chain isononanoic acid. It is used as a hair conditioning agent, a skin conditioning agent, and an emollient, and is found in several moisturizing creams.

Suggested Reading

Le Coz CJ, Bressieux A (2003) Allergic contact dermatitis from cetearyl isononanoate. Contact Dermatitis 48:343

96. Chloramphenicol

CAS Registry Number [56–75–7]

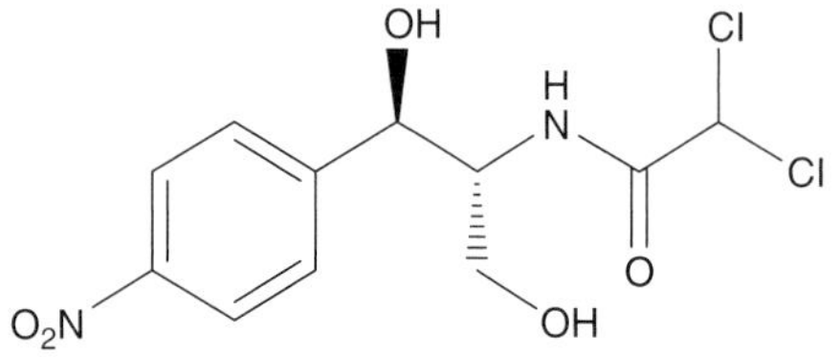

This broad spectrum phenicol group antibiotic has been implicated in allergic contact dermatitis. Cross-sensitivity to thiamphenicol is possible, but not systematic.

Suggested Reading

Le Coz CJ, Santinelli F (1998) Facial contact dermatitis from chloramphenicol with cross-sensitivity to thiamphenicol. Contact Dermatitis 38:108–109

97. Chlorhexidine (Digluconate)

CAS Registry Number [55–56–1] (CAS Registry Number [18472–51–0])

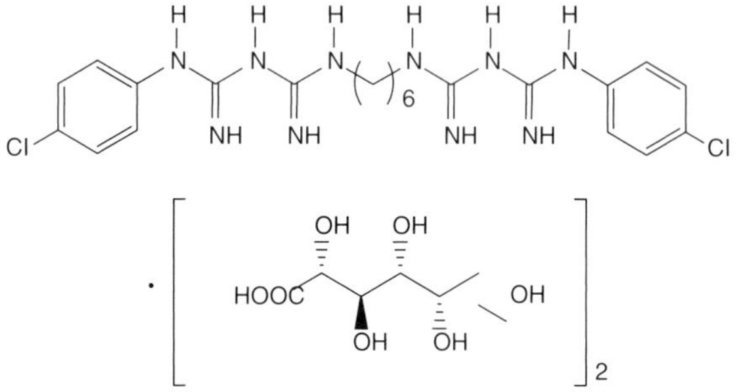

Chlorhexidine is a broad-spectrum antimicrobial agent, a synthetic biguanide antiseptic, and disinfectant, available under different forms (diacetate, dihydrochloride, and mostly digluconate). It is also used as a biocide in several topicals and cosmetics. It may cause allergic contact dermatitis, photosensitivity, or even fixed drug eruption, mainly after prolonged and repeated applications in health workers, leg ulcer, and leg eczema patients. Immediate-type reactions have been reported: contact urticaria, asthma, and anaphylactic shock.

Suggested Reading

Aalto-Korte K, Mäkinen-Kiljunen S (2006) Symptoms of immediate chlorhexidine hypersensitivity in patients with a positive prick test. Contact Dermatitis 55:173–177

Krautheim AB, Jermann THM, Bircher AJ (2004) Chlorhexidine anaphylaxis: case report and review of the literature. Contact Dermatitis 50:113–116

Rudzki E, Rebandel P, Grzywa Z (1989) Patch tests with occupational contactants in nurses, doctors and dentists. Contact Dermatitis 20:247–250

98. 5-Chloro-1-Methyl-4-Nitroimidazole

CAS Registry Number [4897–25–0]

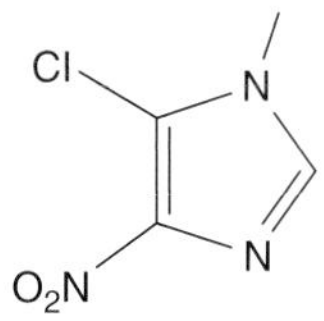

This intermediate in azathioprine synthesis is also present in the end product. It induced contact dermatitis in a man working on azathioprine synthesis. Cross-reactivity is possible with imidazoles tioconazole and econazole.

Suggested Reading

Jolanki R, Alanko K, Pfäffli P, Estlander T, Kanerva L (1997) Occupational allergic contact dermatitis from 5-chloro-1-methyl-4-nitroimidazole. Contact Dermatitis 36:53–54

99. Chloroacetamide

CAS Registry Number [79–07–2]

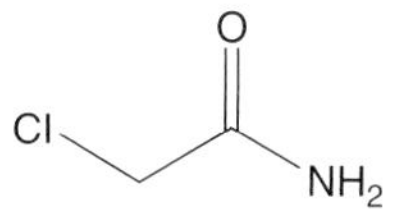

Chloroacetamide as a preservative is used in several applications as in cutting metalworking fluids, in paints or in glues. It can induce contact dermatitis in hairdressers or in shoemakers, being used as a leather preservative.

Suggested Reading

Katsarou A, Koufou B, Takou K, Kalogeromitros D, Papanayiotou G, Vareltzidis A (1995) Patch test results in hairdressers with contact dermatitis in Greece (1985–1994). Contact Dermatitis 33:347–348
Mancuso G, Reggiani M, Berdondini RM (1996) Occupational dermatitis in shoemakers. Contact Dermatitis 34: 17–22

100. Chloroacetophenone

CAS Registry Number [532–27–4]

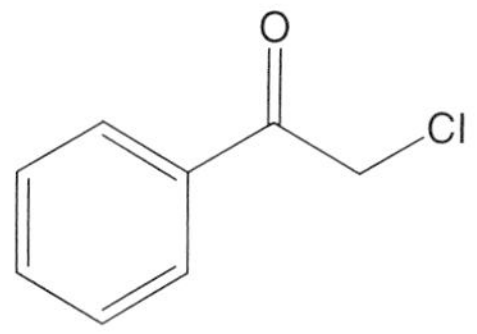

ω-Chloroacetophenone is contained in tear gases (lacrimators). This substance has important irritative potential, but can also be a sensitizer.

Suggested Reading

Brand CU, Schmidli J, Ballmer-Weber B, Hunziker T (1995) Lymphozytenstimulationstest, eine mögliche Alternative zur Sicherung einer Cloracetophenon-Sensibilisierung. Hautarzt 46:702–704

101. Chloroatranol

CAS Registry Number [57074–21–2]

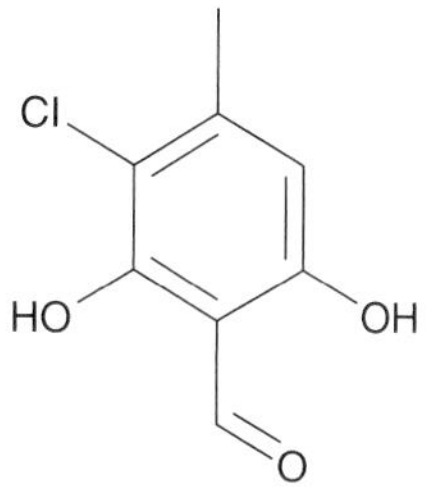

Chloroatranol has recently been identified as a constituent and major allergen in oak moss absolute, a frequent allergen in people sensitized to perfumes. This potent allergen gives reactions with concentrations down to 5 ppm in sensitized patients. It may cross-react with atranol.

Suggested Reading

Bernard G, Giménez-Arnau E, Rastogi SC et al (2003) Contact allergy to oak moss: search for sensitizing molecules using combined bioassay-guided chemical fractionation, GC-MS and structure-activity relationship analysis (part 1). Arch Dermatol Res 295:229–235
Johansen JD, Andersen KE, Svedman C, Bruze M, Bernard G, Giménez-Arnau E, Rastogi SC, Lepoittevin JP, Menné T (2003) Chloroatranol, an extremely potent allergen hidden in perfumes: a dose response elicitation study. Contact Dermatitis 49:180–184

102. Chlorocresol

4-Chloro-3-methylphenol, Parachlorometacresol, 2-Chloro-5-hydroxytoluene

CAS Registry Number [59–50–7]

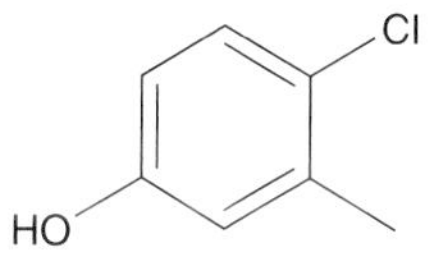

Chlorocresol is a biocide used for its disinfectant and preservative properties, in topicals or cutting fluid.

Suggested Reading

Le Coz CJ, Scrivener Y, Santinelli F, Heid E (1998) Sensibilisation de contact au cours des ulcères de jambe. Ann Dermatol Venereol 125:694–699

Walker SL, Chalmers RJ, Beck MH (2004) Contact urticaria due to *p*-chloro-*m*-cresol. Br J Dermatol 151:936–937

103. Chlorophorin

CAS Registry Number [537–41–7]

Chlorophorin is the allergen in iroko, kambala (*Chlorophora excelsa*). Occupational dermatitis can occur in woodworkers. See also Chap. 46.

Suggested Reading

Lamminpää A, Estlander T, Jolanki R, Kanerva L (1996) Occupational allergic contact dermatitis caused by decorative plants. Contact Dermatitis 34:330–335

104. Chlorothalonil

2,4,5,6–1,3-Tetrachloroisophtalonitrile, 1,3-Dicyano Tetrachlorobenzene, Daconil®

CAS Registry Number [1897–45–6]

Chlorothalonil is a fungicide widely used in the cultivation of ornamental plants and flowers, rice, and onions. In banana plantations it is used in fumigations by airplanes. It can be used as a preservative of paints and woods. It can induce contact urticaria, irritant and allergic contact dermatitis, erythema dyschromicum perstans, or folliculitis mainly in agricultural workers, wood-related professions, or in horticulturists.

Suggested Reading

Boman A, Montelius J, Rissanen RL, Lidén C (2000) Sensitizing potential of chlorothalonil in the guinea pig and the mouse. Contact Dermatitis 43:273–279

Meding B (1986) Contact dermatitis from tetrachloroisophtalonitrile in paint. Contact Dermatitis 15:187

O'Malley M, Rodriguez P, Maibach HI (1995) Pesticide patch testing: California nursery workers and controls. Contact Dermatitis 32:61–62

Penagos H, Jimenez V, Fallas V, O'Malley M, Maibach HI (1996) Chlorothalonil, a possible cause of erythema dyschromicum perstans (ashy dermatitis). Contact Dermatitis 35:214–218

105. Chlorpromazine

CAS Registry Number [50–53–3]

This phenothiazine with sedative properties is used in human medicine and induced contact dermatitis in nurses or those working in the pharmaceutical industry. It is also used in veterinary medicine to avoid mortality of pigs during transportation. It is a sensitizer and a photosensitizer.

Suggested Reading

Brasch J, Hessler HJ, Christophers E (1991) Occupational (photo)allergic contact dermatitis from azaperone in a piglet dealer. Contact Dermatitis 25:258–259

106. Cinnamal

Cinnamic Aldehyde, Cinnamaldehyde, 3-Phenyl-2-Propenal

CAS Registry Number [104–55–2]

This perfumed molecule is used as a fragrance in perfumes, a flavoring agent in soft drinks, ice creams, dentifrices, pastries, chewing-gum, etc. It can induce both contact urticaria and delayed-type reactions. It can be responsible for dermatitis in the perfume industry or in food handlers. Cinnamic aldehyde is contained in "fragrance mix." As a fragrance allergen, it has to be mentioned by name in cosmetics within the EU.

Suggested Reading

Nethercott JR, Holness DL (1989) Occupational dermatitis in food handlers and bakers. J Am Acad Dermatol 21:485–490
Seite-Bellezza D, El Sayed F, Bazex J (1994) Contact urticaria from cinnamic aldehyde and benzaldehyde in a confectioner. Contact Dermatitis 31:272–273

107. Cinnamyl Alcohol

Cinnamic Alcohol, 3-Phenyl-2-Propenol

CAS Registry Number [104–54–1]

Cinnamyl alcohol occurs (in esterified form) in storax, *Myroxylon pereirae*, cinnamon leaves, and hyacinth oil. It is obtained by the alkaline hydrolysis of storax and prepared synthetically by reducing cinnamal diacetate with iron filings and acetic acid, and from cinnamaldehyde by Meerwein–Ponndorf reduction with aluminum isopropoxide. Cinnamic alcohol is contained in the "fragrance mix." As a fragrance allergen, it has to be mentioned by name in cosmetics within the EU. Occupational cases of contact dermatitis were reported in perfume industry. Patch tests can be positive in food handlers.

Suggested Reading

Gutman SG, Somov BA (1968) Allergic reactions caused by components of perfumery preparations. Vestn Dermatol Venereol 12:62–66
Nethercott JR, Holness DL (1989) Occupational dermatitis in food handlers and bakers. J Am Acad Dermatol 21: 485–490

108. Citral

3,7-Dimethyl-2,6-Octadien-1-al, Blend of Neral and Geranial, Blend of (*Z*)-3,7-Dimethyl-2,6-Octadienal and (*E*)-3,7-Dimethyl-2,6-Octadienal

CAS Registry Number [5392–40–5] (CAS Registry Number [141–27–5] + CAS Registry Number [106–26–3])

Neral   Geranial

Citral is an aldehyde fragrance and flavoring ingredient, a blend of isomers *cis* (Neral) and *trans* (geranial). As a fragrance allergen, citral has to be mentioned by name in cosmetics within the EU.

Suggested Reading

Frosch PJ, Johansen JD, Menné T, Pirker C, Rastogi SC, Andersen KE, Bruze M, Goossens A, Lepoittevin JP, White IR (2002) Further important sensitizers in patients sensitive to fragrances. Contact Dermatitis 47:78–85

109. Citronellol

3,7-Dimethyl-6-Octen-1-ol, Cephrol

CAS Registry Numbers [106–22–9] and [26489–01–0]

L-Citronellol is a constituent of rose and geranium oils. D-Citronellol occurs in Ceylon and Java citronella oils. As a fragrance allergen, citronellol has to be mentioned by name in cosmetics within the EU.

Suggested Reading

Frosch PJ, Johansen JD, Menné T, Pirker C, Rastogi SC, Andersen KE, Bruze M, Goossens A, Lepoittevin JP, White IR (2002) Further important sensitizers in patients sensitive to fragrances. Contact Dermatitis 47:78–85

110. Clindamycin

Clindamycin

CAS Registry Number [18323–44–9]

Clindamycin Hydrochloride

CAS Registry Number [21462–39–5]

Clindamycin Phosphate

CAS Registry Number [24729–96–2]

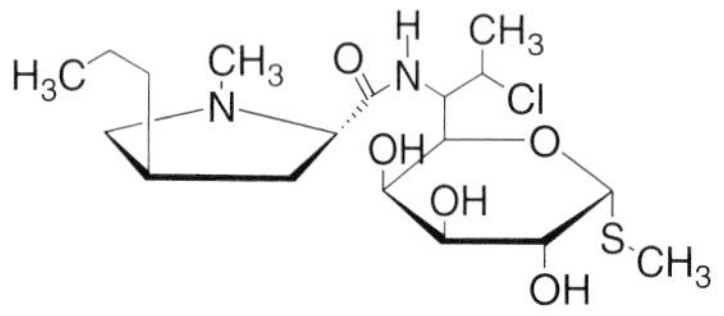

This lincosanide antibiotic is used in topical form for acne, or systemically has been responsible for exanthematous rashes and acute generalized exanthematous pustulosis.

Suggested Reading

Lammintausta K, Tokola R, Kalimo K (2002) Cutaneous adverse reactions to clindamycin: results of skin tests and oral exposure. Br J Dermatol 146:643–648
Valois M, Phillips EJ, Shear NH, Knowles SR (2003) Clindamycin-associated acute generalized exanthematous pustulosis. Contact Dermatitis 48:169

111. Clopidol

Methylchlorpindol, 3,5-Dichloro-2,6-Dimethyl-4-Pyridinol

CAS Registry Number [2971–90–6], [11116–46–4], [68821–99–8]

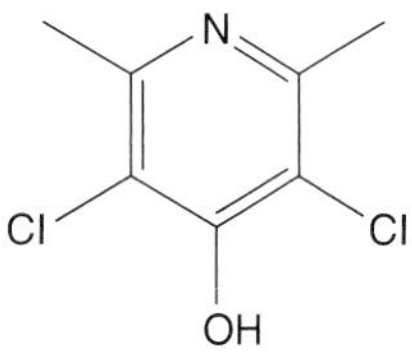

This drug is used for the prevention of coccidiosis in poultry.

Suggested Reading

Mancuso G, Staffa M, Errani A, Berdondini RM, Fabri P (1990) Occupational dermatitis in animal feed mill workers. Contact Dermatitis 22:37–41
Pang GF, Cao YZ, Fan CL, Zhang JJ, Li XM, MacNeil JD (2003) Determination of clopidol residues in chicken tissues by liquid chromatography: collaborative study. J AOAC Int 86:685–693

112. Cloxacillin

CAS Registry Number [61–72–3]

Cloxacillin Sodium Monohydrate

CAS Registry Number [7081–44–9]

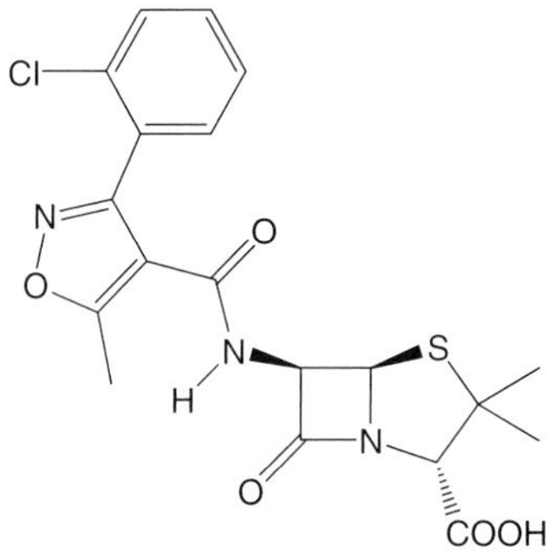

Cloxacillin is a semisynthetic penicillin close to oxacillin. It induced contact dermatitis in a pharmaceutical factory worker with positive reactions to ampicillin, but not to penicillin. In cutaneous drug reactions such as acute generalized exanthematous pustulosis due to amoxicillin, cross-reactivity is frequent to cloxacillin (personal observations).

Suggested Reading

Rudzki E, Rebandel P (1991) Hypersensitivity to semisynthetic penicillins but not to natural penicillin. Contact Dermatitis 25:192

113. Cobalt Naphthenate

Naphthenic Acids, Cobalt Salts

CAS Registry Numbers [61789–51–3], [161279–65–8]

Cobalt naphthenate is made by treating cobalt hydroxide or acetate with naphthenic acid. It is an accelerant in rubber, unsaturated polyester, and vinyl ester resins.

Suggested Reading

Shena D, Rosina P, Chieregato C, Colombari R (1995) Lymphomatoid-like contact dermatitis from cobalt naphthenate. Contact Dermatitis 33:197–198
Tarvainen K, Jolanki R, Forsman-Gronholm L, Estlander T, Pfäffli P, Juntunen J, Kanerva L (1993) Exposure, skin protection and occupational skin diseases in the glass-fiber-reinforced plastics industry. Contact Dermatitis 29: 119–127

114. Cocamidopropyl Betaine

Cocoamphodipropionate, Cocamidopropyl Dimethyl Glycine, Cocoamphocarboxypropionate, Cocoyl Amide Propylbetaine, N-(2-Aminoethyl)-N-[2-(2-carboxyethoxy)ethyl] beta-Alanine

CAS Registry Numbers [61789–40–0], [83138–08–3], [86438–79–1]

Cocamidopropyl betaine is a pseudo-amphoteric zwitterion detergent derived from long-chain alkylbetaines. It is available from many suppliers under more than 50 trade names (including Tego-betain L7 and Ampholyt JB 130). Exposure occurs via rinse-off products such as liquid soaps, shampoos, and shower gels, but also via leave-on products (for example, roll-on deodorant). Occupational sources are mainly in hairdressing. The first synthesis step consists of the reaction of coconut fatty acids with 3-dimethylaminopropylamine, giving cocamidopropyl dimethylamine. This amido amine is converted into cocamidopropyl betaine by reaction with sodium monochloroacetate. Both dimethylaminopropylamine and cocamidopropyl dimethylamine are thought to be the sensitizers.

Suggested Reading

Angelini G, Foti C, Rigano L, Vena GA (1995) 3-Dimethylaminopropylamine: a key substance in contact allergy to cocamidopropylbetaine? Contact Dermatitis 32:96–99
De Groot AC, van der Walle HB, Weyland JW (1995) Contact allergy to cocamidopropyl betaine. Contact Dermatitis 33:419–422
McFadden JP, Ross JS, White IR, Basketter DA (2001) Clinical allergy to cocamidopropyl betaine: reactivity to cocamidopropylamine and lack of reactivity to 3-dimethylaminopropylamine. Contact Dermatitis 45:72–74

115. Cocamidopropyl Dimethylamine

N-[3-(Dimethylamino)Propyl]Coco Amides, 1-(N,N-Dimethylamino)-3-(Coconut Oil Amido)-Propane, Coconut Fatty Acid, Dimethylaminopropylamide

CAS Registry Number [68140–01–2]

This amido amine may be the allergen in cocamidopropyl betaine.

Suggested Reading

McFadden JP, Ross JS, White IR, Basketter DA (2001) Clinical allergy to cocamidopropyl betaine: reactivity to cocamidopropylamine and lack of reactivity to 3-dimethylaminopropylamine. Contact Dermatitis 45:72–74

116. Coconut Diethanolamide

Cocamide DEA, Coconut Oil Fatty Acids Diethanolamide, N,N-bis(2-Hydroxyethyl)Coco Fatty Acid Diethanolamide, Cocoyl Diethanolamide

CAS Registry Number [68603–42–9]

58

Cocamide DEA, manufactured from coconut oil, is widely used in industry and at home as a surface-active agent. It is contained in hand gels, hand washing soaps, shampoos, and dish-washing liquids for its foam-producing and stabilizing properties, and in metal working fluids and polishing agents as an anticorrosion inhibitor.

Suggested Reading

Fowler JF Jr (1998) Allergy to cocamide DEA. Am J Contact Dermat 9:40–41
Kanerva L, Jolanki R, Estlander T (1993) Dentist's occupational allergic contact dermatitis caused by coconut diethanolamide, *N*-ethyl-4-toluene sulfonamide and 4-tolydietahnolamine. Acta Derm Venereol (Stockh) 73:126–129
Pinola A, Estlander T, Jolanki R, Tarvainen K, Kanerva L (1993) Occupational allergic contact dermatitis due to coconut diethanolamide (Cocamide DEA). Contact Dermatitis 29:262–265

117. Codeine (Phosphate, Hydrochloride)

Methylmorphine

CAS Registry Number [76–57–3] (CAS Registry Number [52–28–8], CAS Registry Number [1422–07–7])

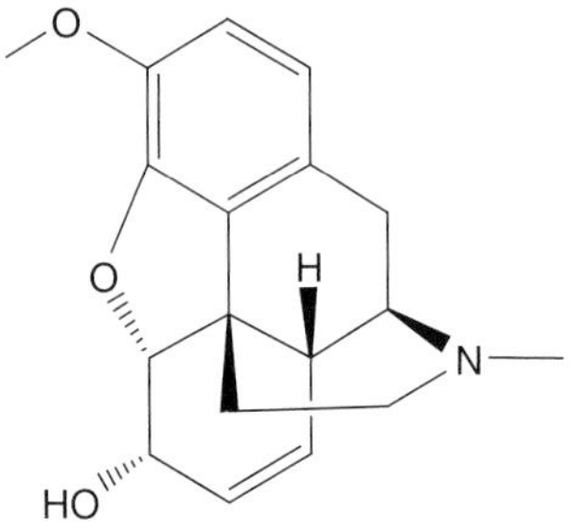

Codeine has been reported as an occupational sensitizer in workers in the production of opium alkaloids. Codeine has been responsible for fixed drug eruptions or generalized dermatitis. Cross-sensitivity is expected to morphine.

Suggested Reading

Condé-Salazar L, Guimaraens D, Gonzalez M, Fuente C (1991) Occupational allergic contact dermatitis from opium alkaloids. Contact Dermatitis 25:202–203

Estrada JL, Alvarez Puebla MJ, Ortiz de Urbina JJ, Matilla B, Rodríguez Prieto MA, Gozalo F (2001) Generalized eczema due to codeine. Contact Dermatitis 44:185
Waclawski ER, Aldridge R (1995) Occupational dermatitis from thebaine and codeine. Contact Dermatitis 33:51

118. Costunolide

CAS Registry Number [553–21–9]

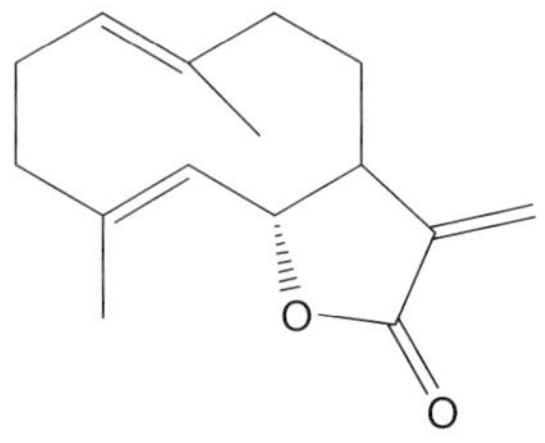

This germacranolide sesquiterpene lactone is extracted from costus oil. With alantolactone and dehydrocostunolide, it is a component of lactone mix used to elicit reactions in patients sensitive to Asteraceae–Compositae. An erythema-multiform-like occupational contact dermatitis case occurred in a chemical student after an accidental exposure to costus oil.

Suggested Reading

Ducombs G, Benezra C, Talaga P, Andersen KE, Burrows D, Camarasa JG, Dooms-Goossens A, Frosch PJ, Lachapelle JM, Menné T, Rycroft RJG, White IR, Shaw S, Wilkinson JD (1990) Patch testing with the "sesquiterpene lactone mix": a marker for contact allergy to Compositae and other sesquiterpene-lactone-containing plants. Contact Dermatitis 22:249–252
Le Coz CJ, Lepoittevin JP (2001) Occupational erythema-multiforme-like dermatitis from sensitization to costus resinoid, followed by flare-up and systemic contact dermatitis from beta-cyclocostunolide in a chemistry student. Contact Dermatitis 44:310–311

119. Coumarin

1-Benzopyran-2-one, *cis-o*-Coumarinic Acid Lactone

CAS Registry Number [91–64–5]

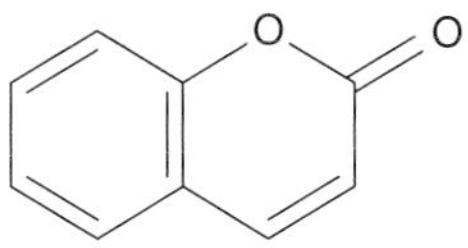

Coumarin is an aromatic lactone naturally occurring in Tonka beans and other plants. As a fragrance allergen, it has to be mentioned by name in cosmetics within the EU.

Suggested Reading

Frosch PJ, Johansen JD, Menné T, Pirker C, Rastogi SC, Andersen KE, Bruze M, Goossens A, Lepoittevin JP, White IR (2002) Further important sensitizers in patients sensitive to fragrances. Contact Dermatitis 47:78–85

120. Cresyl Glycidyl Ether

CAS Registry Number [26447–14–3]

It is a reactive diluent added in epoxy resins Bisphenol A type.

Suggested Reading

Chieregato C, Vincenzi C, Guerra L, Farina P (1994) Occupational allergic contact dermatitis due to ethylenediamine dihydrochloride and cresyl glycidyl ether in epoxy resin systems. Contact Dermatitis 30:120
Daecke C, Schaller J, Goos M (1994) Acrylates as potent allergens in occupational and domestic exposures. Contact Dermatitis 30:190–191
Holness DL, Nethercott JR (1993) The performance of specialized collections of bisphenol A epoxy resin system components in the evaluation of workers in an occupational health clinic population. Contact Dermatitis 28:216–219
Jolanki R, Kanerva L, Estlander T, Tarvainen K, Keskinen H, Henriks-Eckerman ML (1990) Occupational dermatoses from epoxy resin compounds. Contact Dermatitis 23:172–183

121. Cyclohexanone

CAS Registry Number [108–94–1]

Used as a polyvinyl chloride solvent, cyclohexanone caused contact dermatitis in a woman manufacturing PVC fluidotherapy bags. Cyclohexanone probably does not cross-react with cyclohexanone resin. A cyclohexanone-derived resin used in paints and varnishes caused contact dermatitis in painters.

Suggested Reading

Bruze M, Boman A, Bergquist-Karlson A, Björkner B, Wahlberg JE, Woog E (1988) Contact allergy to cyclohexanone resin in humans and guinea pigs. Contact Dermatitis 18:46–49
Sanmartin O, de la Cuadra J (1992) Occupational contact dermatitis from cyclohexanone as a PVC adhesive. Contact Dermatitis 27:189–190

122. 2-Cyclohexen-1-one

CAS Registry Number [930–68–7]

This strong sensitizer has been responsible for chemical burning followed by sensitization in a chemistry student.

Suggested Reading

Goossens A, Deschutter A (2003) Acute irritation followed by primary sensitization to 2-cyclohenen-1-one in a chemistry student. Contact Dermatitis 48:163–164

123. N-Cyclohexyl-2-Benzothiazylsulfenamide

CAS Registry Number [95–33–0]

A rubber accelerator chemical. The most frequent occupational categories are metal industry, homemakers, health services and laboratories, and the building industry.

Suggested Reading

Condé-Salazar L, Del-Rio E, Guimaraens D, Gonzalez Domingo A (1993) Type IV allergy to rubber additives: a 10-year study of 686 cases. J Am Acad Dermatol 29:176–180

Kiec-Swierczynska M (1995) Occupational sensitivity to rubber. Contact Dermatitis 32:171–172

Von Hintzenstern J, Heese A, Koch HU, Peters KP, Hornstein OP (1991) Frequency, spectrum and occupational relevance of type IV allergies to rubber chemicals. Contact Dermatitis 24:244–252

124. *N*-Cyclohexyl-*N*-Phenyl-*p*-Phenylenediamine

N-Phenyl-*N*-Cyclohexyl-*p*-Phenylenediamine, CPPD

CAS Registry Number [101–87–1]

CPPD is a rubber chemical used as an antioxidant. Cross-reactions are frequently observed with *N*-isopropyl-*N*-phenylparaphenylenediamine (IPPD).

Suggested Reading

Hervé-Bazin B, Gradiski D, Duprat P, Marignac B, Foussereau J, Cavelier C, Bieber P (1977) Occupational eczema from *N*-isopropyl-*N*-phenylparaphenylenediamine (IPPD) and *N*-dimethyl-1,3 butyl-*N*-phenylparaphenylenediamine (DMPPD) in tyres. Contact Dermatitis 3:1–15

Von Hintzenstern J, Heese A, Koch HU, Peters KP, Hornstein OP (1991) Frequency, spectrum and occupational relevance of type IV allergies to rubber chemicals. Contact Dermatitis 24:244–252

125. *N*-Cyclohexyl-Thiophthalimide

CAS Registry Number [17796–82–6]

N-Cyclohexyl-thiophthalimide is a rubber chemical, widely used as a vulcanization retarder. Sensitization sources are often protective gloves.

Suggested Reading

Huygens S, Barbaud A, Goossens A (2001) Frequency and relevance of positive patch tests to cyclohexylthiophthalimide, a new rubber allergen. Eur J Dermatol 11: 443–445

Kanerva L, Estlander T, Jolanki R (1996) Allergic patch test reactions caused by the rubber chemical cyclohexyl thiophthalimide. Contact Dermatitis 34:23–26

126. Cymene

Cymol, Methyl-Isopropyl-Benzol

CAS Registry Number [25155–15–1]

Terpenes, constitutive of essential oils, are hydrocarbons with the general formula $C_{10}H_{16}$. They are structurally related to cymol.

Suggested Reading

Selvaag E, Holm JO, Thune P (1995) Allergic contact dermatitis in an aroma therapist with multiple sensitizations to essential oils. Contact Dermatitis 33:354–355

127. Cymoxanil

2-Cyano-N-[(Ethylamino)Carbonyl]-2-(Methoxyimino)Acetamide

CAS Registry Number [57966–95–7]

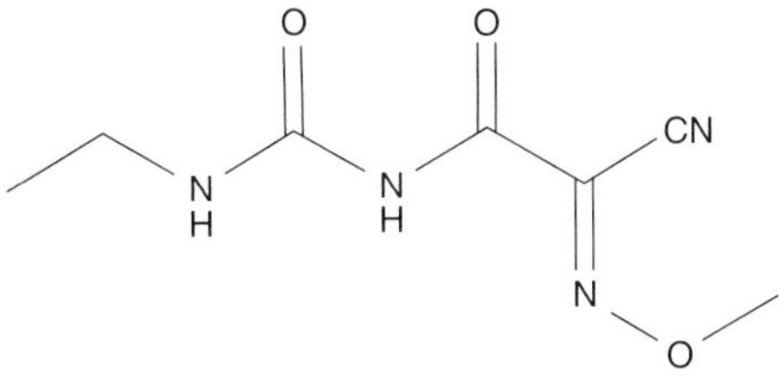

Cymoxanil, an urea derivative, is included (10%) with dithianone (25%) in Aktuan®. It is a fungicide agent, possibly sensitizing agricultural workers.

Suggested Reading

Koch P (1996) Occupational allergic contact dermatitis and airborne contact dermatitis from 5 fungicides in a vineyard worker. Cross-reactions between fungicides of the dithiocarbamate group? Contact Dermatitis 34:324–329

128. Dazomet

3,5-Dimethyltetrahydro-1,3,5(2H)Thiadiazine-2-Thione, DMTT

CAS Registry Number [533–74–4]

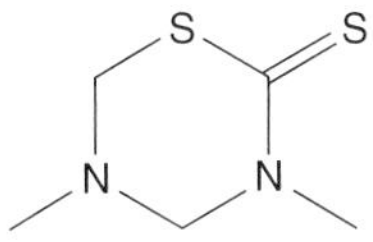

Dazomet is a biocide used to control bacterial and fungal growth in a pulp and paper system, and also in agriculture for soil disinfection. It is contained in Busan 1058, Mylone, and Fungicide 974 (Crag™). Sensitization, rarely reported, occurred in a paper mill worker.

Suggested Reading

Warin AP (1992) Allergic contact dermatitis from dazomet. Contact Dermatitis 26:135–136

129. DDT

Dichlorodiphenyltrichloroethane

CAS Registry Number [50–29–3]

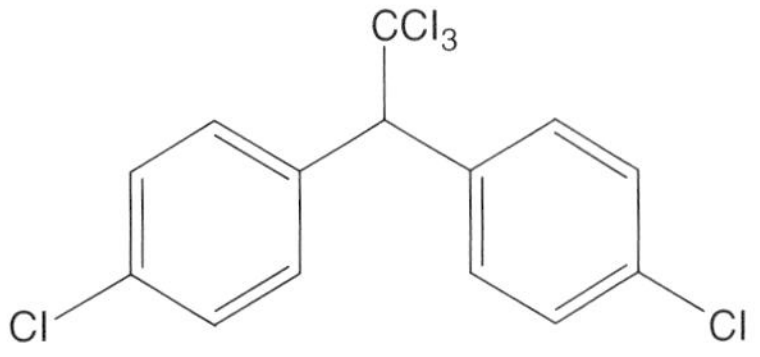

This insecticide was formerly reported as a sensitizer in farmers or agricultural workers.

Suggested Reading

Sharma VK, Kaur S (1990) Contact sensitization by pesticides in farmers. Contact Dermatitis 23:77–80

130. Decyl glucoside

CAS Registry Numbers [58846–77–8], [68515–73–1], [141464–42–8], and [54549–25–6]

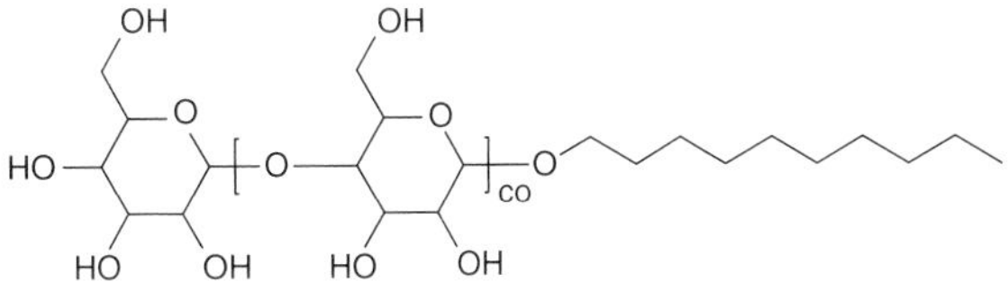

CAS : 54549-25-6   CO : 1 to 3

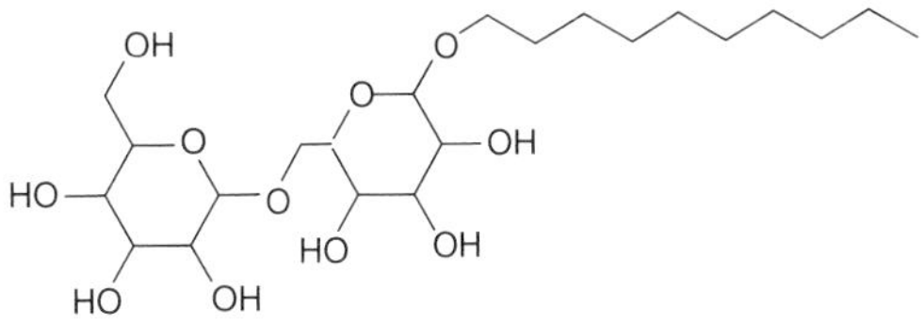

CAS : 68515-73-1

Decyl glucoside or decyl D-glucoside, also named decyl-beta-D-glucopyranoside, belongs to the alkyl glucosides family and is obtained by condensation of the fatty alcohol decyl alcohol and a D-glucose polymer. This nonionic surfactant and cleansing agent has been widely used for several years, due to its foaming power and good tolerance in rinse-off products such as shampoos, hair dyes and colors, and soaps. Decyl glucoside is also employed in leave-on products such as no-rinsing cleansing milks, lotions, and several sunscreen agents and is contained as a stabilizing surfactant of organic microparticles in sunscreen agent Tinosorb® M.

Suggested Reading

Blondeel A (2003) Contact allergy to the mild surfactant decyl-glucoside. Contact Dermatitis 49:304–305

Le Coz CJ, Meyer MT (2003) Contact allergy to decyl glucoside in antiseptic after body piercing. Contact Dermatitis 48:279–280

131. Dehydrocostuslactone

CAS Registry Number [477–43–0]

A guaianolide sesquiterpene lactone extracted from costus oil. It is one of the components of Lactone mix, with costunolide and alantolactone, used to detect Compositae-sensitive patients.

Suggested Reading

Ducombs G, Benezra C, Talaga P, Andersen KE, Burrows D, Camarasa JG, Dooms-Goossens A, Frosch PJ, Lachapelle JM, Menné T, Rycroft RJG, White IR, Shaw S, Wilkinson JD (1990) Patch testing with the "sesquiterpene lactone mix": a marker for contact allergy to Compositae and other sesquiterpene-lactone-containing plants. Contact Dermatitis 22:249–252

132. Deoxylapachol

CAS Registry Number [3568–90–9]

Deoxylapachol is the main allergen identified in teak (*Tectona grandis*). Sensitization often concerns people involved in woodwork. See also Chap. 46.

Suggested Reading

Lamminpää A, Estlander T, Jolanki R, Kanerva L (1996) Occupational allergic contact dermatitis caused by decorative plants. Contact Dermatitis 34:330–335

Meding B, Ahman M, Karlberg AT (1996) Skin symptoms and contact allergy in woodwork teachers. Contact Dermatitis 34:185–190

133. Diallyl Disulfide

CAS Registry Number [2179–57–9]

Diallyl disulfide is one of the major allergens in garlic (*Allium sativum*) and onions. Among patients patch-test-positive to garlic, all 13 who were tested had positive reactions to diallyl sulfide 5% pet. See also Chap. 46.

Suggested Reading

Bruynzeel DP (1997) Bulb dermatitis. Dermatological problems in the flower bulb industries. Contact Dermatitis 37:70–77

Lamminpää A, Estlander T, Jolanki R, Kanerva L (1996) Occupational allergic contact dermatitis caused by decorative plants. Contact Dermatitis 34:330–335

McFadden JP, White IR, Rycroft RJG (1992) Allergic contact dermatitis from garlic. Contact Dermatitis 27:333–334

134. Diaminodiphenylmethane

4,4-Diaminodiphenylmethane,
4,4-Methylenedianiline

CAS Registry Number [107–77–9]

4,4-Diaminodiphenylmethane is an aromatic diamine used as a curing agent in epoxy resins of the bisphenol A type and in the production of plastics, isocyanates, adhesives, elastomers, polyurethane (elastic and rigid foams, paints, lacquers, adhesives, binding agents, synthetics rubbers, and elastomeric fibers), and butyl rubber. 4,4-Diaminodiphenylmethane is also a byproduct in azo dyes. It is also possibly formed by hydrolysis of diphenylmethane-4,4-diisocyanate.

Suggested Reading

Bruynzeel DP, van der Wegen-Keijser MH (1993) Contact dermatitis in a cast technician. Contact Dermatitis 28:193–194

Condé-Salazar L, Gonzalez de Domingo MA, Guimaraens D (1994) Sensitization to epoxy resin systems in special flooring workers. Contact Dermatitis 31:157–160

Holness DL, Nethercott JR (1993) The performance of specialized collections of bisphenol A epoxy resin system components in the evaluation of workers in an occupational health clinic population. Contact Dermatitis 28:216–219

Jolanki R, Kanerva L, Estlander T, Tarvainen K, Keskinen H, Henriks-Eckerman ML (1990) Occupational dermatoses from epoxy resin compounds. Contact Dermatitis 23:172–183

Jolanki R, Kanerva L, Estlander T, Tarvainen K (1994) Concomitant sensitization to triglycidyl isocyanurate, diaminodiphenylmethane and 2-hydroxyethyl methacrylate from silk-screen printing coatings in the manufacture of circuit boards. Contact Dermatitis 30:12–15

Kiec-Swierczynska M (1995) Rubber chemical. Occupational sensitivity to rubber. Contact Dermatitis 32:171–172

Mancuso G, Reggiani M, Berdondini RM (1996) Occupational dermatitis in shoemakers. Contact Dermatitis 34:17–22

Tarvainen K (1995) Analysis of patients with allergic patch test reactions to a plastic and glues series. Contact Dermatitis 32:346–351

135. Diammonium Hydrogen Phosphate

CAS Registry Number [7783-28-0]

A flame retardant caused contact dermatitis in surgical personnel. It was due to excessive residual concentrations in surgical garbs.

Suggested Reading

Belsito DV (1990) Contact dermatitis from diammonium hydrogen phosphate in surgical garb. Contact Dermatitis 23:267–268

136. Diazodiethylaniline Chloride

CAS Registry Number [148-90-3]

It is a well-known allergen in diazo copy paper. This product is allergenic until exposed to light and inactivated by UV radiations.

Suggested Reading

Foussereau J, Benezra C (1970) Les eczémas allergiques professionnels. Masson, Paris

Pambor M, Poweleit H (1992) Allergic contact dermatitis due to diazo copy paper. Contact Dermatitis 26:131–132

137. Diazolidinyl Urea

Germall II

CAS Registry Number [78491-02-8]

Diazolidinyl urea, a formaldehyde releaser, is contained mainly in cosmetics and toiletries and can be found in barrier creams.

Suggested Reading

Le Coz CJ (2005) Hypersensibilité à la Diazolidinyl urée et à l'Imidazolidinyl urée. Ann Dermatol Venereol 132: 587–588

Van Hecke E, Suys E (1994) Where next to look for formaldehyde? Contact Dermatitis 31:268

138. Dibenzothiazyl Disulfide

CAS Registry Number [120-78-5]

This rubber chemical of the mercaptobenzothiazole group is used as a vulcanization accelerator. The most frequent

58

occupational categories are metal industry, homemakers, health services and laboratories, and the building industry.

Suggested Reading

Condé-Salazar L, Del-Rio E, Guimaraens D, Gonzalez Domingo A (1993) Type IV allergy to rubber additives: a 10-year study of 686 cases. J Am Acad Dermatol 29:176–180

Le Coz CJ (2004) Fiche d'éviction en cas d'hypersensibilité au mercaptobenzothiazole et au mercapto mix. Ann Dermatol Venereol 131:846–848

Von Hintzenstern J, Heese A, Koch HU, Peters KP, Hornstein OP (1991) Frequency, spectrum and occupational relevance of type IV allergies to rubber chemicals. Contact Dermatitis 24:244–252

139. Dibucaine (Hydrochloride)

Cincaine, Cinchocain(e), Percaine, Sovcaine

CAS Registry Number [85–79–0] (CAS Registry Number [61–12–1])

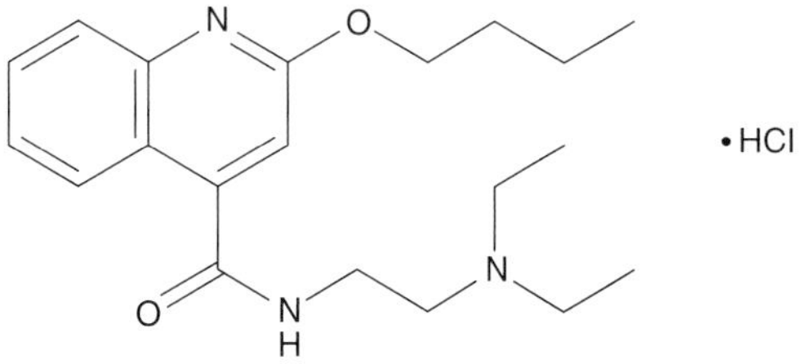

Dibucaine hydrochloride is an amide group local anesthetic that can induce allergic contact dermatitis.

Suggested Reading

Erdmann SM, Sachs B, Merk HF (2001) Systemic contact dermatitis from cinchocaine. Contact Dermatitis 44: 260–261

Nakada T, Iijima M (2000) Allergic contact dermatitis from dibucaine hydrochloride. Contact Dermatitis 42:283

140. Dibutyl Phthalate

CAS Registry Number [84–74–2]

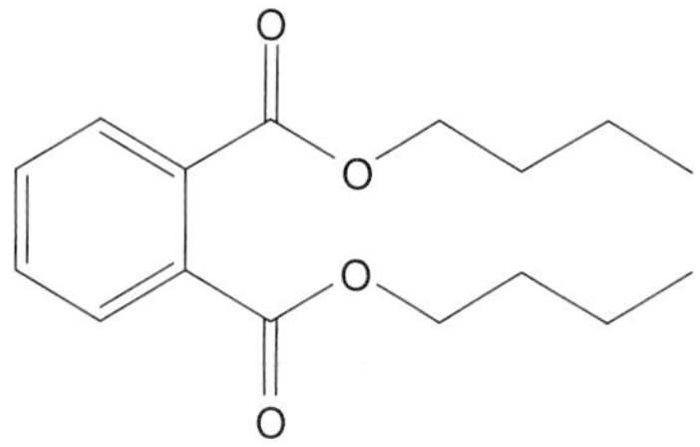

It is mainly used as a nonreactive epoxy diluent.

Suggested Reading

Capon F, Cambie MP, Clinard F, Bernardeau K, Kalis B (1996) Occupational contact dermatitis caused by computer mice. Contact Dermatitis 35:57–58

Chieregato C, Vincenzi C, Guerra L, Farina P (1994) Occupational allergic contact dermatitis due to ethylenediamine dihydrochloride and cresyl glycidyl ether in epoxy resin systems. Contact Dermatitis 30:120

141. Dibutylthiourea

1,3-Dibutyl-2-Thiourea

CAS Registry Number [109–46–6]

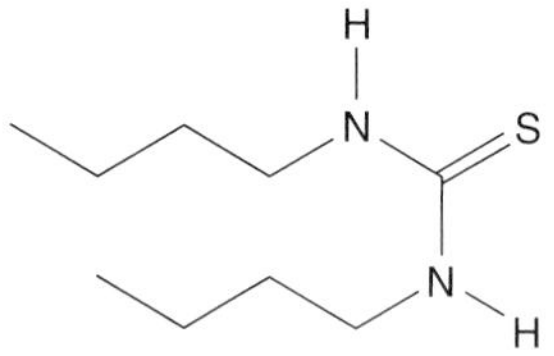

Dibutylthiourea is used in the vulcanization of rubber, in paints, and glue removers as an anticorrosive, and in phonecards as a component of the thermocoating sprayed over the optically read layer of the card. Cross-sensitivity to other thiourea derivatives is possible.

Suggested Reading

Kanerva L, Estlander T, Jolanki R (1994) Occupational allergic contact dermatitis caused by thiourea compounds. Contact Dermatitis 31:242–248

Kiec-Swierczynska M (1995) Occupational sensitivity to rubber. Contact Dermatitis 32:171–172

Schmid-Grendelmeier P, Elsner P (1995) Contact dermatitis due to occupational dibutylthiourea exposure: a case of phonecard dermatitis. Contact Dermatitis 32:308–309

142. 4,5-Dichloro-2-*n*-Octyl-4-Isothiazolin-3-one

Kathon® 930

CAS Registry Number [64359–81–5]

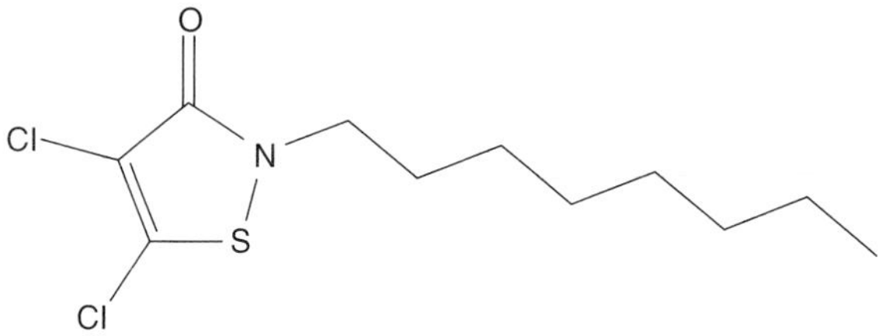

Irritant and sensitizer, Kathon® 930 caused contact dermatitis in employees of a textile finishing factory.

Suggested Reading

Kawai K, Nagakawa M, Sasaki Y, Kawai Y (1993) Occupational contact dermatitis from Kathon® 930. Contact Dermatitis 28:117–118

143. 1,3-Dichloropropene

1,3-Dichloro-1-Prop(yl)ene, 1,3-Dichloro-2-Prop(yl)ene, DD-95

CAS Registry Number [542–75–6]

This nematocide is used as a soil fumigant prior to crop cultivation. Farmers and process operators employed at pesticide plants are mainly exposed.

Suggested Reading

Bousema MT, Wiemer GR, van Joost T (1991) A classic case of sensitization to DD-95. Contact Dermatitis 24:132

144. Dichlorvos

CAS Registry Number [62–73–7]

Cases of sensitization to this organophosphorus compound with several commercial names (Benfos, Brevinyl, Chlorvinphos, DDVP, Equigard, Fly fighte, Nogos, and Unifos) were occupationally seen in chrysanthem growers, horticulturists, technicians, and in a chemist.

Suggested Reading

Cleenewerck MB, Martin P (1990) Dermite de contact au Dichlorvos. Rev Fr Allergol 30:38
Mathias CG (1983) Persistent contact dermatitis from the insecticide dichlorvos. Contact Dermatitis 9:217–218

145. *N,N*-Dicyclohexyl-2-Benzothiazole Sulfenamide

CAS Registry Number [4979–32–2]

This substance is a rubber accelerator of the mercaptobenzothiazole-sulfenamide group.

Suggested Reading

Le Coz CJ (2004) Fiche d'éviction en cas d'hypersensibilité au mercaptobenzothiazole et au mercapto mix. Ann Dermatol Venereol 131:846–848

146. Dicyclohexyl Carbodiimide

CAS Registry Number [538–75–0]

Used in peptide chemistry as a coupling reagent. It is both an irritant and a sensitizer and has caused contact dermatitis in pharmacists and chemists.

Suggested Reading

Poesen N, de Moor A, Busschots A, Dooms-Goossens A (1995) Contact allergy to dicyclohexyl carbodiimide and diisopropyl carbodiimide. Contact Dermatitis 32:368–369

147. Didecyldimethylammonium Chloride

Bardac-22

CAS Registry Number [7173–51–5]

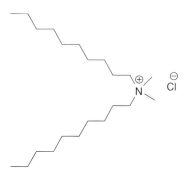

This quaternary ammonium compound is used as a detergent-disinfectant in hospitals, as an algaecide in swimming pools, as a fungicide, and against termites in wood. We observed severe contact dermatitis in a slaughterhouse worker using a liquid soap containing this product (personal observation). Immediate-type manifestations like urticaria and dyspnoea have been reported.

Suggested Reading

Dejobert Y, Martin P, Piette F, Thomas P, Bergoend H (1997) Contact dermatitis from didecyldimethylammonium chloride and bis-(aminopropyl)-laurylamine in a detergent-disinfectant used in hospital. Contact Dermatitis 37:95–96
Houtappel M, Bruijnzeel-Koomen CA, Röckmann H (2008) Immediate-type allergy by occupational exposure to didecyl dimethyl ammonium chloride. Contact Dermatitis 59:116–117

148. Diethanolamine

CAS Registry Number [111–42–2]

Diethanolamine is contained in many products, as a metalworking fluid. Traces may exist in other ethanolamine-containing fluids.

Suggested Reading

Blum A, Lischka G (1997) Allergic contact dermatitis from mono-, di- and triethanolamine. Contact Dermatitis 36:166

149. Diethyl Sebacate

Ethyl Sebacate, Diethyl Decanedioate

CAS Registry Number [110–40–7]

This emulsifier has rarely been reported as a sensitizing agent, mainly in topical treatments.

Suggested Reading

Tanaka M, Kobayashi S, Murata T, Tanikawa A, Nishikawa T (2000) Allergic contact dermatitis from diethyl sebacate in lanoconazole cream. Contact Dermatitis 43:233–234

150. Diethyleneglycol Diglycidyl Ether

Ether, bis[2-(2,3-Epoxypropoxy)Ethyl]

CAS Registry Number [4206–61–5]

Diethyleneglycol diglycidyl ether was contained in a reactive diethyleneglycol-based diluent of epoxy resins and caused contact dermatitis in three workers at a ski factory.

Suggested Reading

Jolanki R, Tarvainen K, Tatar T, Estlander T, Henriks-Eckerman ML, Mustakallio KK, Kanerva L (1996) Occupational dermatoses from exposure to epoxy resin compounds in a ski factory. Contact Dermatitis 34:390–396

151. Diethylenetriamine

CAS Registry Number [111–40–0]

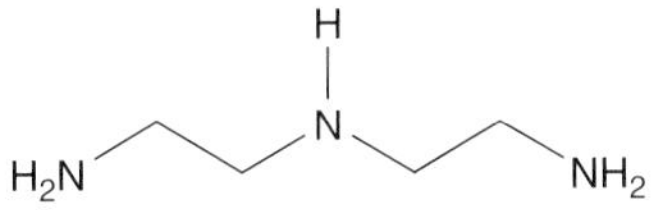

Diethylenetriamine is a hardener in epoxy resins of the Bisphenol A type. It has been reported to be a sensitizer when used in an ultrasonic bath for cleaning jewels, in synthetic lubricants, or in carbonless copy paper.

Suggested Reading

Holness DL, Nethercott JR (1993) The performance of specialized collections of bisphenol A epoxy resin system components in the evaluation of workers in an occupational health clinic population. Contact Dermatitis 28:216–219

Jolanki R, Kanerva L, Estlander T, Tarvainen K, Keskinen H, Henriks-Eckerman ML (1990) Occupational dermatoses from epoxy resin compounds. Contact Dermatitis 23:172–183

Kanerva L, Estlander T, Jolanki R (1990) Occupational allergic contact dermatitis due to diethylenetriamine (DETA) from carbonless copy paper and from an epoxy compound. Contact Dermatitis 23:272–273

152. Diethylphthalate

CAS Registry Number [84–66–2]

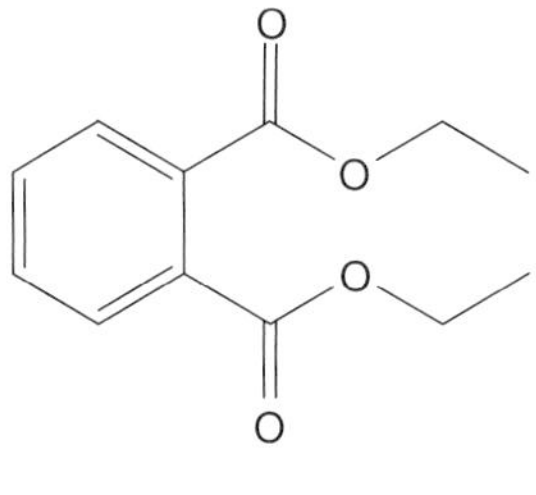

This plasticizer increases the flexibility of plastics. It is also contained in deodorant formulations, perfumes, emollients, and insect repellents. It can cross-react with dimethyl phthalate.

Suggested Reading

Capon F, Cambie MP, Clinard F, Bernardeau K, Kalis B (1996) Occupational contact dermatitis caused by computer mice. Contact Dermatitis 35:57–58

153. Diethylthiourea

Diethylthiocarbamide

CAS Registry Number [105–55–5]

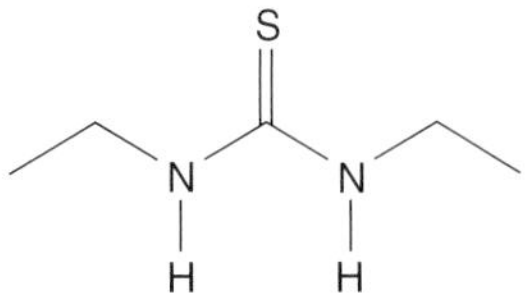

Diethylthiourea, a thiourea derivative, is used mainly as a rubber chemical, particularly in solid neoprene products.

Suggested Reading

Kanerva L, Estlander T, Jolanki R (1994) Occupational allergic contact dermatitis caused by thiourea compounds. Contact Dermatitis 31:242–248

154. Diisopropyl Carbodiimide

N,N-Methanetetraylbis-2-Propanamine

CAS Registry Number [693–13–0]

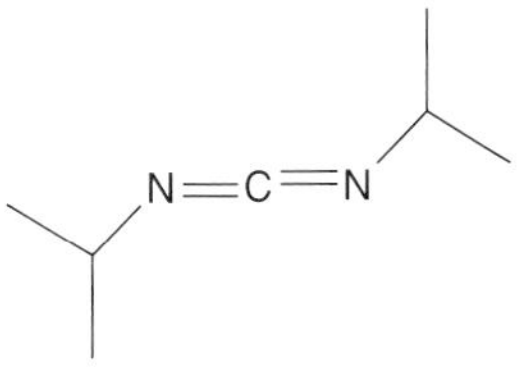

It is used in peptide chemistry as a coupling reagent. It is very toxic and causes contact dermatitis in laboratory workers.

Suggested Reading

Poesen N, de Moor A, Busschots A, Dooms-Goossens A (1995) Contact allergy to dicyclohexyl carbodiimide and diisopropyl carbodiimide. Contact Dermatitis 32:368–369

155. Diisopropylbenzothiazyl-2-Sulfenamide

CAS Registry Number [95–29–4]

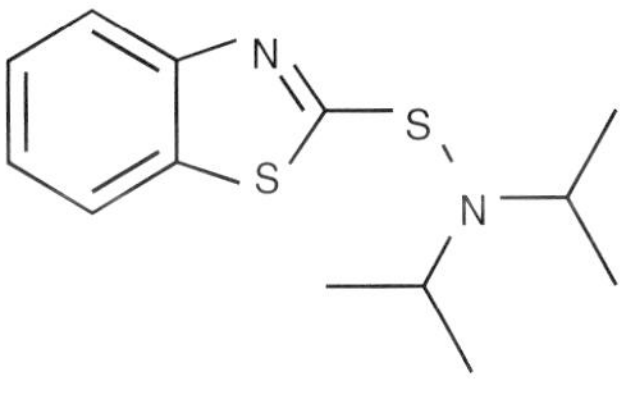

This chemical is a mercaptobenzothiazole-sulfenamide used in rubber vulcanization.

Suggested Reading

Le Coz CJ (2004) Fiche d'éviction en cas d'hypersensibilité au mercaptobenzothiazole et au mercapto mix. Ann Dermatol Venereol 131:846–848

156. 2,5-Dimercapto-1,3,4-Thiadiazole

DMTD

CAS Registry Number [1072–71–5]

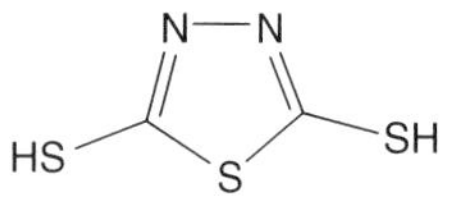

This low-molecular-weight aromatic compound is used in the production of copper corrosion inhibitors for engine oils, flame retardants, and photographic development chemicals. Seven cases of industrial allergic sensitization were reported in a manufacturing plant.

Suggested Reading

O'Driscoll JO, Beck M, Taylor S (1990) Occupational contact allergy to 2,5-dimercapto-1,3,4-thiadiazole. Contact Dermatitis 23:268–269

157. Dimethoate

CAS Registry Number [60–51–5]

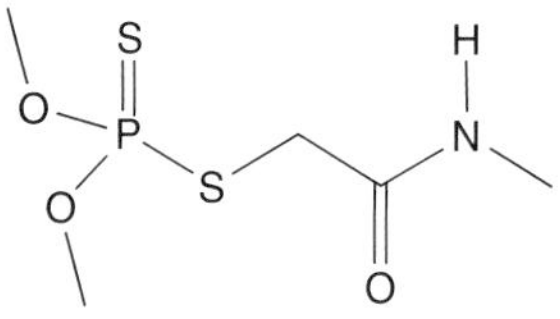

This organophosphorus compound is used as a contact and systemic insecticide and acaricide. It induced an erythema-multiform-like contact dermatitis in a warehouseman in an agricultural consortium.

Suggested Reading

Haenen C, de Moor A, Dooms-Goossens A (1996) Contact dermatitis caused by the insecticides omethoate and dimethoate. Contact Dermatitis 35:54–55

Schena D, Barba A (1992) Erythema-multiforme-like contact dermatitis from dimethoate. Contact Dermatitis 27:116–117

158. Dimethoxon

Omethoate

CAS Registry Number [1113–02–6]

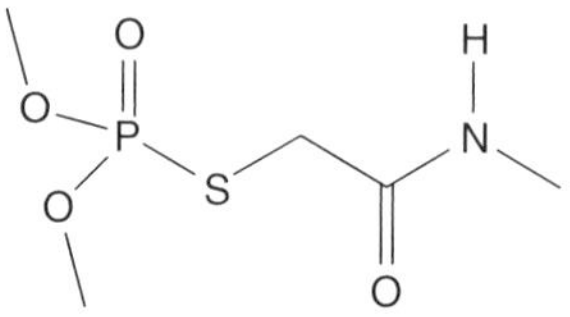

Contact dermatitis from omethoate–dimethoxon is rare.

Suggested Reading

De Moor A, Dooms-Goossens A (1996) Contact dermatitis caused by the insecticides omethoate and dimethoate. Contact Dermatitis 35:54–55

159. 2,6-Dimethoxy-1,4-Benzoquinone

CAS Registry Number [530–55–2]

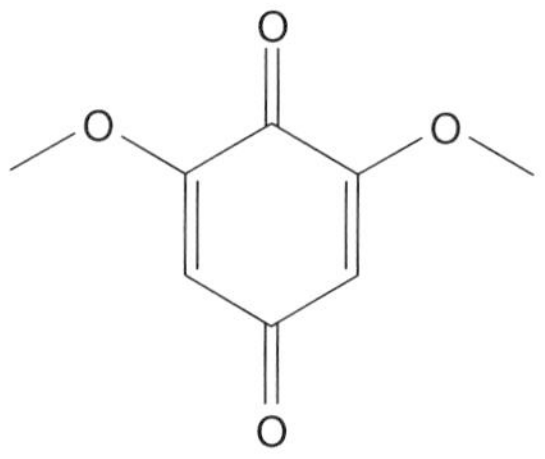

2,6-Dimethoxy-1,4-benzoquinone is an allergen in more than 50 different plants and wood species, e.g., mahogany, macore, sipo, wenge, oak, beech, elms, and poplar. With acamelin, it is one of the allergens of *Acacia melanoxylon*. Sensitization can occur in woodworkers such as carpenters, joiners, and sawyers. See also Chap. 46.

Suggested Reading

Correia O, Barros MA, Mesquita-Guimaraes J (1992) Airborne contact dermatitis from the woods *Acacia melanoxylon* and *Entandophragma cylindricum*. Contact Dermatitis 27:343–344

Lamminpää A, Estlander T, Jolanki R, Kanerva L (1996) Occupational allergic contact dermatitis caused by decorative plants. Contact Dermatitis 34:330–335

160. (*R*)-3,4-Dimethoxy-Dalbergione

CAS Registry Number [37555–64–4]

This quinone is the main allergen of *Machaerium scleroxylum* Tul. (Santos rosewood, *Pao ferro*, *Caviuna vermelha*, *Santos palissander*). Occupational sensitization mainly concerns woodworkers. See also Chap. 46.

Suggested Reading

Chieregato C, Vincenzi C, Guerra L, Rapacchiale S (1993) Occupational airborne contact dermatitis from *Machaerium scleroxylum* (Santos rosewood). Contact Dermatitis 29:164–165

Lamminpää A, Estlander T, Jolanki R, Kanerva L (1996) Occupational allergic contact dermatitis caused by decorative plants. Contact Dermatitis 34:330–335

161. (*S*)-4,4'-Dimethoxy Dalbergione

CAS Registry Number [4646–87–1]

It is an allergen of *Dalbergia nigra,* also contained in *Dalbergia latifolia* Roxb. (East Indian rosewood, palissander). Occupational dermatitis can occur in timberworkers such as carpenters, sawyers, joiners, or knifegrinders. See also Chap. 46.

Suggested Reading

Gallo R, Guarrera M, Hausen BM (1996) Airborne contact dermatitis from East Indian rosewood (*Dalbergia latifolia* Roxb.). Contact Dermatitis 35:60–61

162. 5,8-Dimethoxypsoralen

Isopimpinellin

CAS Registry Number [482–27–9]

Psoralens are natural photoactivable compounds in plants and can cause phototoxic contact dermatitis. For example, *Cachrys libanotis* L., Apiaceae-Umbelliferae family, contains 5,8-dimethoxypsoralen. See also Chap. 46.

Suggested Reading

Ena P, Cerri R, Dessi G, Manconi PM, Atzei AD (1991) Phototoxicity due to *Cachrys libanotis*. Contact Dermatitis 24:1–5

163. Dimethyl Phthalate

CAS Registry Number [131–11–3]

Phthalates are plasticizers and increase the flexibility of plastics. They are also found in deodorant formulations, perfumes, emollients, and insect repellents.

Suggested Reading

Capon F, Cambie MP, Clinard F, Bernardeau K, Kalis B (1996) Occupational contact dermatitis caused by computer mice. Contact Dermatitis 35:57–58

58

164. 4-*N*,*N*-(Dimethylamino) Benzenediazonium Chloride

p-Diazodimethylaniline zinc Chloride Double Salt

CAS Registry Number [100–04–9]

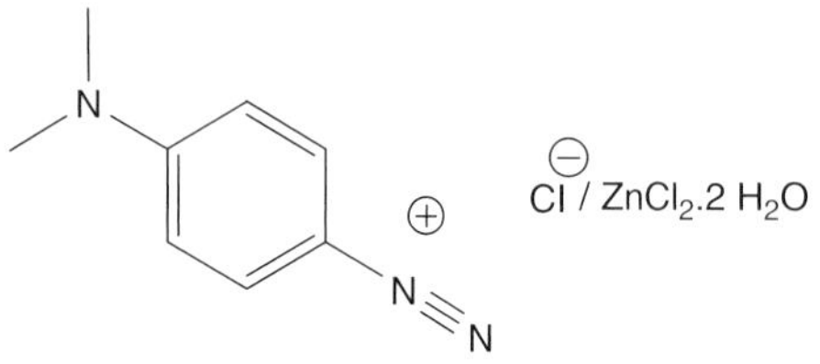

It is a diazo compound found in diazo copy paper. It is allergenic only when unexposed.

Suggested Reading

Geier J, Fuchs T (1993) Contact allergy due to 4-*N*,*N*-dimethylaminobenzene diazonium chloride and thiourea in diazo copy paper. Contact Dermatitis 28:304–305

165. 3-Dimethylaminopropylamine

CAS Registry Number [109–55–7]

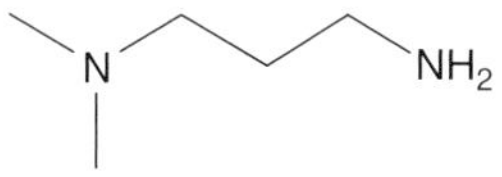

Dimethylaminopropylamine is an aliphatic amine present in amphoteric surfactants such as liquid soaps and shampoos. It is present as a residual impurity thought to be responsible for allergy from cocamidopropylbetaine. It is structurally similar to diethylaminopropylamine. It is also used as a curing agent for epoxy resins and an organic intermediate in chemical syntheses (ion exchangers, additives for flocculants, cosmetics and fuel additives, dyes and pesticides). Patch test has to be carefully interpreted, since the 1% aqueous solution has pH > 11 (personal observation).

Suggested Reading

Angelini G, Foti C, Rigano L, Vena GA (1995) 3-Dimethylaminopropylamine: a key substance in contact allergy to cocamidopropylbetaine? Contact Dermatitis 32:96–99

Kanerva L, Estlander T, Jolanki R (1996) Occupational allergic contact dermatitis from 3-dimethylaminopropylamine in shampoos. Contact Dermatitis 35:122–123
Speight EL, Beck MH, Lawrence CM (1993) Occupational allergic contact dermatitis due to 3-dimethylaminopropylamine. Contact Dermatitis 28:49–50

166. Dimethyldiphenylthiuram disulfide

CAS Registry Number [53880–86–7]

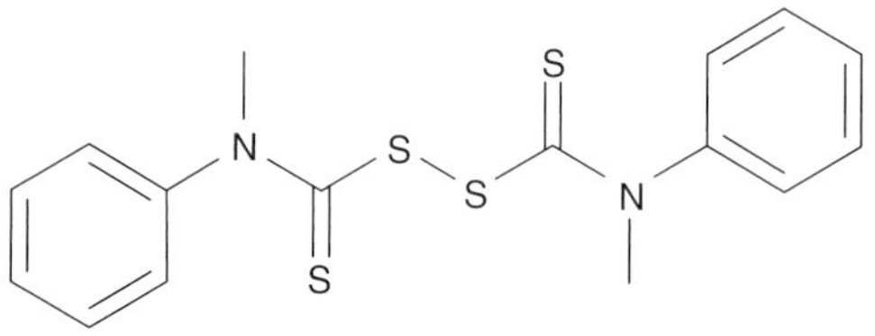

This thiuram compound is used as an accelerator for rubber vulcanization.

Suggested Reading

Le Coz CJ (2004) Fiche d'éviction en cas d'hypersensibilité au thiuram mix. Ann Dermatol Venereol 131:1012–1014

167. Dimethylformamide

CAS Registry Number [68–12–2]

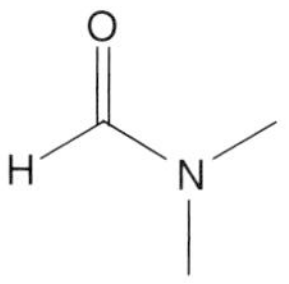

This is an organic solvent for vinyl resins and acetylene, butadiene, and acid gases. It caused contact dermatitis in a technician at an epoxy resin factory and can provoke alcohol-induced flushing in exposed subjects.

Suggested Reading

Camarasa JG (1987) Contact dermatitis from dimethylformamide. Contact Dermatitis 16:234
Cox NH, Mustchin CP (1991) Prolonged spontaneous and alcohol-induced flushing due to the solvent dimethyl formamide. Contact Dermatitis 24:69–70

168 bis. Dimethyl fumarate

CAS Registry Number [624-49-7]

Dimethylfumarate, a strong irritant, is used as an industrial wide spectrum biocide in Asia and mainly in China, for textiles, leather, seeds, food, and cosmetic ingredients. It provoked a worldwide epidemic of severe contact dermatitis, initially from Chinese sofas sold in Finland, Great Britain, and France. It also induced severe burning and contact allergy due to shoes, and to contaminated clothing as well. This chemical, presents as is (white powder) or as tablets contained in little bags disposed in/or around the materials to protect, progressively evaporates and contaminates the environment. It is forbidden in the European Union since 2008.

Suggested Reading

Rantanen T (2008) The cause of the Chinese sofa/chair dermatitis epidemic is likely to be contact allergy to dimethylfumarate, a novel potent contact sensitizer. Br J Dermatol 159:218–221

Imbert E, Chamaillard M, Kostrzewa E, Doutre MS, Milpied B, Beylot-Barry M, Le Coz CJ, Fritsch C, Chantecler ML, Vigan M (2008) Allergie au fauteuil chinois: une nouvelle dermite de contact. Ann Dermatol Venereol 135:777–779

Vigan M, Biver C, Bourrain JL, Pelletier F, Girardin P, Aubin F, Humbert P (2009) Eczéma aigu d'un pied au diméthylfumarate. Ann Dermatol Venereol 136:281–283

Foti C, Zambonin CG, Cassano N, Aresta A, Damascelli A, Ferrara F, Vena GA (2009) Occupational allergic contact dermatitis associated with dimethyl fumarate in clothing. Contact Dermatitis 61:122–124

169. 2,4-Dimethylol Phenol

CAS Registry Number [2937–60–2]

2,4-Dimethylol phenol in a compound of resins based on phenol and formaldehyde. Cross-reactivity is possible with other phenol derivative molecules.

Suggested Reading

Bruze M, Zimerson E (1997) Cross-reaction patterns in patients with contact allergy to simple methylol phenols. Contact Dermatitis 37:82–86

Bruze M, Zimerson E (1985) Contact allergy to 3-methylol phenol, 2,4-dimethylol phenol and 2,6-dimethylol phenol. Acta Derm Venereol (Stockh) 65:548–551

170. 2,6-Dimethylol Phenol

CAS Registry Number [2937–59–9]

This substance is contained in resins based on phenol and formaldehyde. Cross-reactivity is possible with other phenol derivative molecules.

Suggested Reading

Bruze M, Zimerson E (1985) Contact allergy to 3-methylol phenol, 2,4-dimethylol phenol and 2,6-dimethylol phenol. Acta Derm Venereol (Stockh) 65:548–551

Bruze M, Zimerson E (1997) Cross-reaction patterns in patients with contact allergy to simple methylol phenols. Contact Dermatitis 37:82–86

171. Dimethylthiourea

Dimethylthiocarbamide

CAS Registry Number [534–13–4]

Dimethylthiocarbamide, an antioxygen agent, is responsible for sensitization, when unexposed to light from diazo papers.

Suggested Reading

Geier J, Fuchs T (1993) Contact allergy due to 4-*N,N*-dimethylaminobenzene diazonium chloride and thiourea in diazo copy paper. Contact Dermatitis 28:304–305

Kanerva L, Estlander T, Jolanki R (1994) Occupational allergic contact dermatitis caused by thiourea compounds. Contact Dermatitis 31:242–248

172. Dinitrochlorobenzene

DNCB, 2,4-Dinitrochlorobenzene, 2,4-Dinitro-1-Chlorobenzene, 4-Chloro-1,3-Dinitrobenzene, 6-Chloro-1,3-Dinitrobenzene

CAS Registry Number [97–00–7]

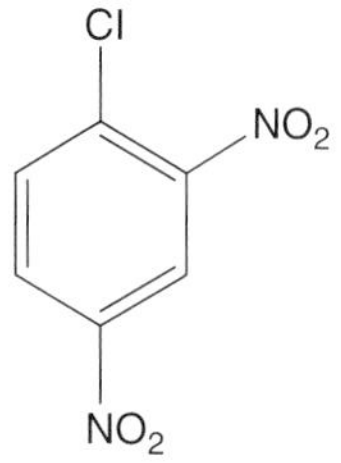

This substance is one of the strongest primary skin irritants known, and a universal contact allergen. Occupational dermatitis has been reported, but current use is decreasing or performed with completely closed systems. DNCB is sometimes used for topical treatment of alopecia areata, severe warts, and cutaneous metastasis of malignant melanoma.

Suggested Reading

Adams RM, Zimmerman MC, Bartlett JB, Preston JF (1971) 1-Chloro-2,4-dinitrobenzene as an algicide. Report of four cases of contact dermatitis. Arch Dermatol 103:191–193

173. Dinitrofluorobenzene

DNFB, FDNB, 2,4-Dinitro-1-Fluorobenzene, Sanger's Reagent

CAS Registry Number [70–34–8]

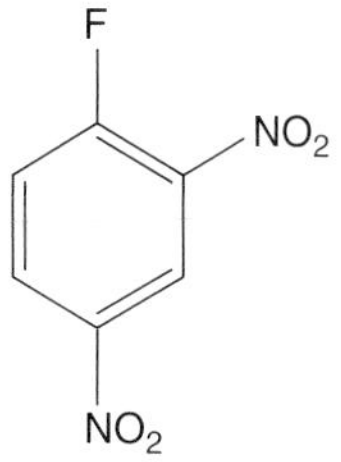

DNFB is a strong skin irritant and a universal contact allergen. It is used as an intermediate in the synthesis of pesticides and pharmaceuticals such as flurbiprofen, a chemical reagent, and as a topical sensitizer for the treatment of alopecia areata.

Suggested Reading

Perez A, Narayan S, Sansom J (2004) Occupational contact dermatitis from 2,4-dinitrofluorobenzene. Contact Dermatitis 51:314

174. 2,4-Dinitrotoluene

CAS Registry Number [121–14–12]

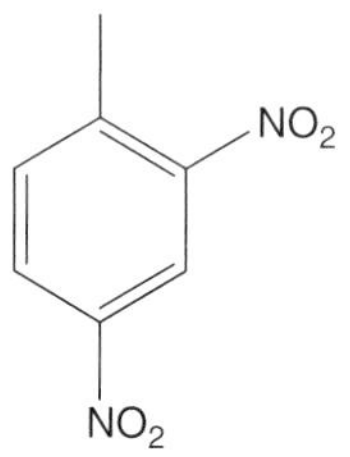

Dinitrotoluene induced sensitization in a worker for an explosives manufacturer, also sensitized to nitroglycerin.

Suggested Reading

Kanerva L, Laine R, Jolanki R, Tarvainen K, Estlander T, Helander I (1991) Occupational allergic contact dermatitis caused by nitroglycerin. Contact Dermatitis 24:356–362

175. Dipentamethylenethiuram Disulfide

CAS Registry Number [94–37–1]

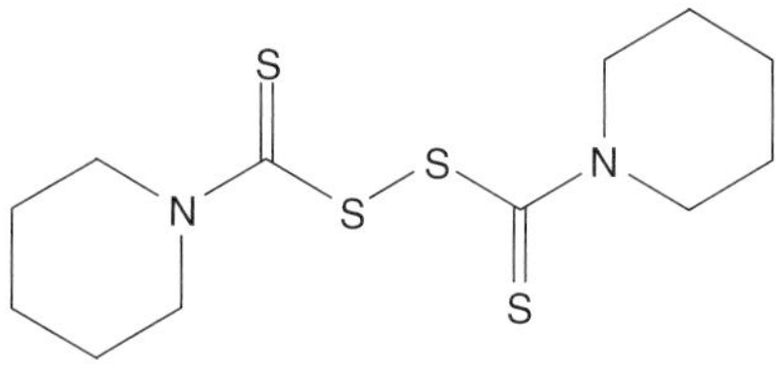

A rubber chemical contained in "thiuram mix." The most frequent occupational categories are the metal industry, homemakers, health services and laboratories, and the building industry.

Suggested Reading

Condé-Salazar L, Del-Rio E, Guimaraens D, Gonzalez Domingo A (1993) Type IV allergy to rubber additives: a 10-year study of 686 cases. J Am Acad Dermatol 29:176–180

Condé-Salazar L, Guimaraens D, Villegas C, Romero A, Gonzalez MA (1995) Occupational allergic contact dermatitis in construction workers. Contact Dermatitis 35:226–230

Kiec-Swierczynska M (1995) Occupational sensitivity to rubber. Contact Dermatitis 32:171–172

Von Hintzenstern J, Heese A, Koch HU, Peters KP, Hornstein OP (1991) Frequency, spectrum and occupational relevance of type IV allergies to rubber chemicals. Contact Dermatitis 24:244–252

176. Dipentamethylenethiuram Hexasulfide

CAS Registry Number [971–15–3]

This thiuram compound is used as an accelerator for rubber vulcanization.

Suggested Reading

Le Coz CJ (2004) Fiche d'éviction en cas d'hypersensibilité au thiuram mix. Ann Dermatol Venereol 131:1012–1014

177. Dipentamethylenethiuram Tetrasulfide

CAS Registry Number [120–54–7]

Dipentamethylenethiuram tetrasulfide is a thiuram compound used as an accelerator for rubber vulcanization.

Suggested Reading

Le Coz CJ (2004) Fiche d'éviction en cas d'hypersensibilité au thiuram mix. Ann Dermatol Venereol 131:1012–1014

178. Dipentene

CAS Registry Number [138–86–3]

Dipentene corresponds to a racemic mixture of D-limonene and L-limonene. Dipentene can be prepared from wood turpentine or by synthesis. It is used as a solvent for waxes, rosin and gums, in printing inks, perfumes, rubber compounds, paints, enamels, and lacquers. An irritant and sensitizer, dipentene caused contact dermatitis mainly in painters, polishers, and varnishers.

Suggested Reading

Martins C, Gonçalo M, Gonçalo S (1995) Allergic contact dermatitis from dipentene in wax polish. Contact Dermatitis 33:126–127

Moura C, Dias M, Vale T (1994) Contact dermatitis in painters, polishers and varnishers. Contact Dermatitis 31:51–53

179. Diphencyprone

2,3-Diphenylcyclopropenone

CAS Registry Number [886–38–4]

Diphencyprone is a potent contact allergen used in topical immunotherapy to treat some severe alopecia areata. It is responsible for occupational contact dermatitis in chemists and dermatology department staff.

Suggested Reading

Sansom JE, Molloy KC, Lovell CR (1995) Occupational sensitization to diphencyprone in a chemist. Contact Dermatitis 32:363

Temesvári E, González R, Marschalkó M, Horváth A (2004) Age dependence of diphenylcyclopropenone sensitization in patients with alopecia areata. Contact Dermatitis 50:381–382

180. Diphenhydramine (hydrochloride)

CAS Registry Number [58-73-1] (CAS Registry Number [147-24-0])

This antihistaminic drug with sedative properties is mainly sold over the counter. It can be used both topically (treatment of pruritis) and orally for its antiallergic, antiemetic, sedative, and anticough properties. Allergic or photoallergic contact dermatitis and fixed-drug eruption seem to be rare.

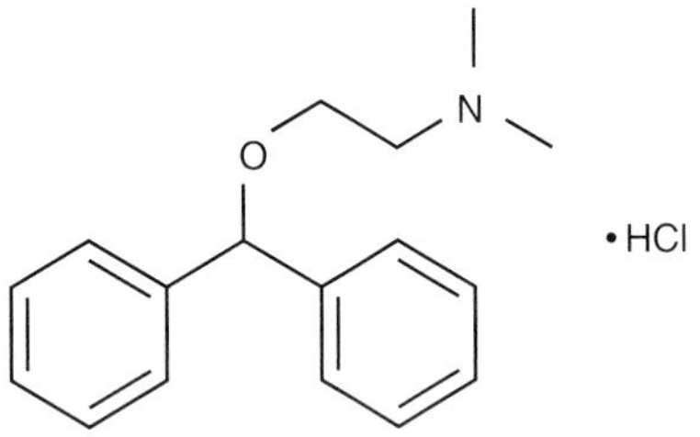

Suggested Reading

Rodríguez-Jiménez B, Domínguez-Ortega J, González-García JM, Kindelan-Recarte C (2009) Dimenhydrinate-induced fixed drug eruption in a patient who tolerated other antihistamines (2009) J Investig Allergol Clin Immunol 19:334–335

Fernández-Jorge B, Goday Buján J, Fernández-Torres R, Rodríguez-Lojo R, Fonseca E (2008) Concomitant allergic contact dermatitis from diphenhydramine and metronidazole. Contact Dermatitis 59:115–116

Yamada S, Tanaka M, Kawahara Y, Inada M, Ohata Y (1998) Photoallergic contact dermatitis due to diphenhydramine hydrochloride. Contact Dermatitis 38:282

181. N,N′-Diphenyl-4-Phenylenediamine

DPPD

CAS Registry Number [74–31–7]

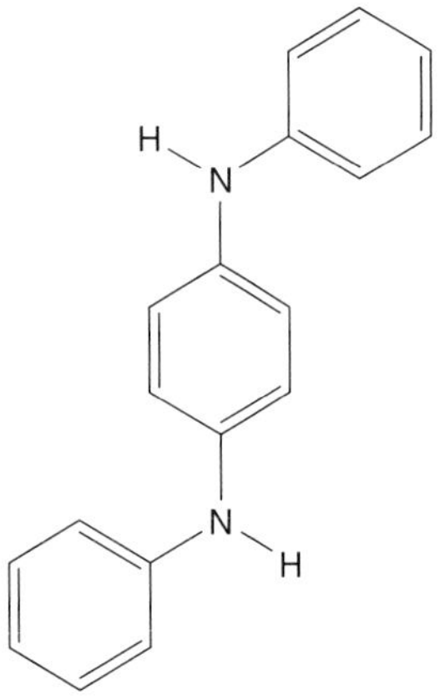

A rubber accelerant, formerly contained in "black-rubber mix." The most frequent occupational categories are in the metal industry, homemakers, health services and laboratories, and the building industry.

Suggested Reading

Condé-Salazar L, Del-Rio E, Guimaraens D, Gonzalez Domingo A (1993) Type IV allergy to rubber additives: a 10-year study of 686 cases. J Am Acad Dermatol 29: 176–180

Kiec-Swierczynska M (1995) Occupational sensitivity to rubber. Contact Dermatitis 32:171–172

Von Hintzenstern J, Heese A, Koch HU, Peters KP, Hornstein OP (1991) Frequency, spectrum and occupational relevance of type IV allergies to rubber chemicals. Contact Dermatitis 24:244–252

182. 1,3-Diphenylguanidine

CAS Registry Number [102–06–7]

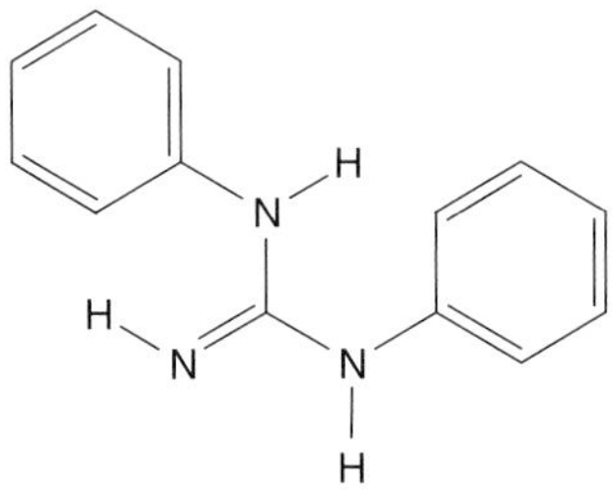

Diphenylguanidine is a rubber sensitizer that can induce immediate-type reactions and delayed-type contact allergy. It was formerly contained in "carba mix." Occupational exposure concerns finished rubber items and the rubber manufacturing industry. The most frequent occupational categories are metal industry, homemakers, health services and laboratories, and the building industry.

Suggested Reading

Bruze M, Kestrup L (1994) Occupational allergic contact dermatitis from diphenylguanidine in a gas mask. Contact Dermatitis 31:125–126

Condé-Salazar L, Del-Rio E, Guimaraens D, Gonzalez Domingo A (1993) Type IV allergy to rubber additives: a 10-year study of 686 cases. J Am Acad Dermatol 29:176–180

Kiec-Swierczynska M (1995) Occupational sensitivity to rubber. Contact Dermatitis 32:171–172

Mancuso G, Reggiani M, Berdondini RM (1996) Occupational dermatitis in shoemakers. Contact Dermatitis 34:17–22

Von Hintzenstern J, Heese A, Koch HU, Peters KP, Hornstein OP (1991) Frequency, spectrum and occupational relevance of type IV allergies to rubber chemicals. Contact Dermatitis 24:244–252

183. 4,4'-Diphenylmethane-Diisocyanate

MDI

CAS Registry Number [101–68–8]

MDI is used in the manufacture of various polyure-thane products: elastic and rigid foams, paints, lac-quers, adhesives, binding agents, synthetic rubbers, and elastomeric fibers.

Suggested Reading

Estlander T, Keskinen H, Jolanki R, Kanerva L (1992) Occu-pational dermatitis from exposure to polyurethane chemi-cals. Contact Dermatitis 27:161–165

Mancuso G, Reggiani M, Berdondini RM (1996) Occupational dermatitis in shoemakers. Contact Dermatitis 34:17–22

184. Diphenylthiourea

CAS Registry Number [102–08–9]

It is a rubber chemical used as an accelerator and sta-bilizing agent in neoprene.

Suggested Reading

Kanerva L, Estlander T, Jolanki R (1994) Occupational allergic contact dermatitis caused by thiourea compounds. Contact Dermatitis 31:242–248

Kiec-Swierczynska M (1995) Occupational sensitivity to rub-ber. Contact Dermatitis 32:171–172

185. Disperse Blue 106

This clothing dye used in synthetic fibers is one of the most potent sensitizers in clothes. Allergic contact dermatitis is relatively frequent in consumers. Occupational textile dye dermatitis was reported in a ready-to-wear shop. Constant concomitant reactions with Disperse Blue 124 are due to their chemical similarities, as with photograph developers CD1, CD2, CD3, and CD4. See also Chap. 40.

Suggested Reading

Menezes-Brandão F, Altermatt C, Pecegueiro M, Bordalo O, Foussereau J (1985) Contact dermatitis to Disperse Blue 106. Contact Dermatitis 13:80–84

Mota F, Silva E, Varela P, Azenha A, Massa A (2000) An out-break of occupational textile dye dermatitis from Disperse Blue 106. Contact Dermatitis 43:235–236

186. Disperse Blue 124

CAS Registry Number [15141–18–1]

This clothing dye used in synthetic fibers is one of the most potent sensitizers in clothes. It is a textile dye responsible for occupational contact dermatitis in the textile industry. A positive patch test reaction was observed in a painter sensitized to phthalocyanine dyes, with no occupational relevance. Constant con-comitant reactions with Disperse Blue 106, and even to photographic developers CD1–4, are due to their chemical similarities. See also Chap. 40.

Suggested Reading

Raccagni AA, Baldari U, Righini MG (1996) Airborne dermati-tis in a painter. Contact Dermatitis 35:119–120

Soni BP, Sherertz EF (1996) Contact dermatitis in the textile industry: a review of 72 patients. Am J Contact Dermat 7:226–230

187. Disperse Dyes

Disperse dyes are so called because they are partially soluble in water. These synthetic dyes have either an anthraquinone (disperse anthraquinone dyes) or an azoic structure (disperse azo dyes). They are the most commonly employed dyes, sometimes as hair dyes, but chiefly in the textile industry to color synthetic fibers such as polyester, acrylic and acetate, and sometimes nylon, particularly in stockings. They are not used for natural fibers. These molecules are the main textile sensitizers. See Chap. 40.

188. Disperse Orange 3

CI 11005

CAS Registry Number [730–40–5]

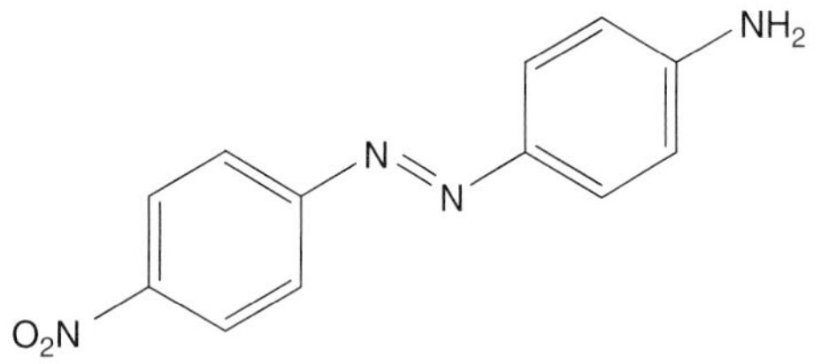

Disperse Orange 3 is an azo dye that can induce contact dermatitis in workers in the textile industry. It is positive in a great majority of PPD-positive people, because of hydrolysis in the skin into PPD. Disperse Orange 3 can also be found in some semipermanent hair dyes. See also Chap. 40.

Suggested Reading

Balato N, Lembo G, Patruno C, Ayala F (1990) Prevalence of textile dye contact sensitization. Contact Dermatitis 23:126–127
Condé-Salazar L, Baz M, Guimaraens D, Cannavo A (1995) Contact dermatitis in hairdressers: patch test results in 379 hairdressers (1980–1993). Am J Contact Dermat 6:19–23
Soni BP, Sherertz EF (1996) Contact dermatitis in the textile industry: a review of 72 patients. Am J Contact Dermat 7:226–230

189. Disperse Orange 31

CI 111135

CAS Registry Numbers [61968–38–5] (and [68391–42–4]?)

The synthetic azo dye Disperse Orange 31 was wrongly substituted by Disperse Orange 3 in patch test materials from Chemotechnique. This situation explains why a relatively low percentage of patients positive to PPD were positive to Disperse Orange 3, although a coreaction is explained to be very frequent because of skin transformation of Disperse Orange 3 into PPD. See also Chap. 40.

Suggested Reading

Goon AT, Gilmour NJ, Basketter DA, White IR, Rycroft RJ, McFadden JP (2003) High frequency of simultaneous sensitivity to Disperse Orange 3 in patients with positive patch tests to para-phenylenediamine. Contact Dermatitis 48:248–250
Le Coz CJ, Jelen G, Goossens A, Vigan M, Ducombs G, Bircher A, Giordano-Labadie F, Pons-Guiraud A, Milpied-Homsi B, Castelain M, Tennstedt D, Bourrain JL, Bernard G, GERDA (2004) Disperse (yes), Orange (yes), 3 (no): what do we test in textile dye dermatitis? Contact Dermatitis 50:126–127

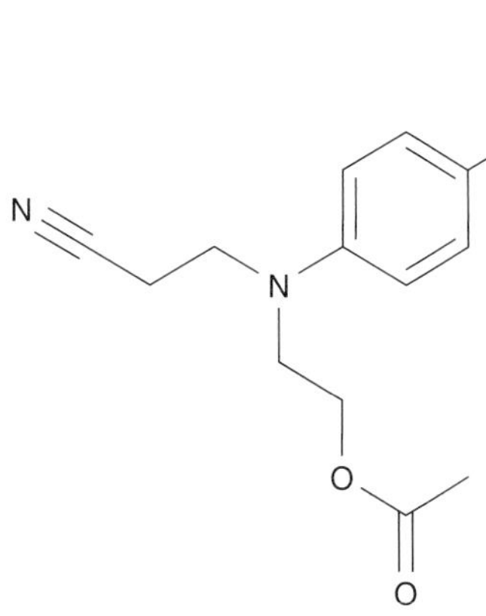

Disperse Orange 31

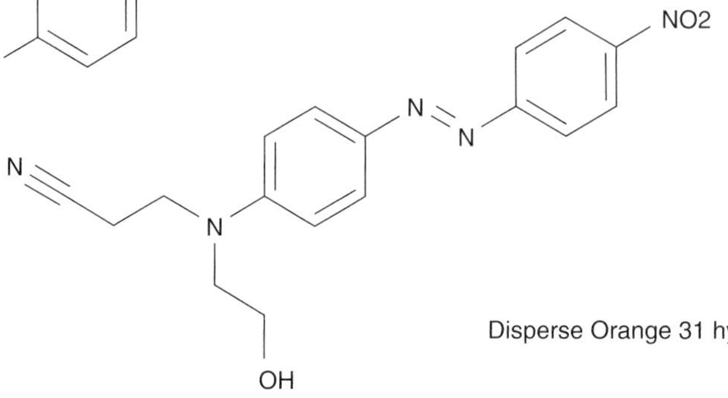

Disperse Orange 31 hydrolyzed

190. Disperse Red 11

CI 62015

CAS Registry Number [2872–48–2]

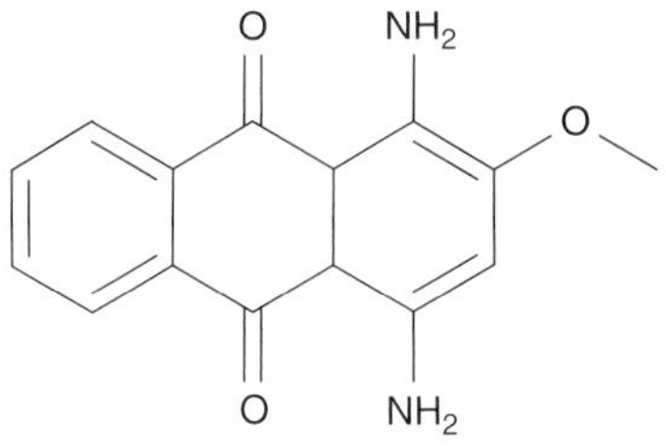

Disperse Red 11 is an example of disperse dye anthraquinone type. See also Chap. 40.

Suggested Reading

Cronin E (1980) Contact dermatitis. Churchill Livingstone, Edinburgh, pp 36–92

191. Disperse Yellow 3

CI 11855

CAS Registry Number [2832–40–8]

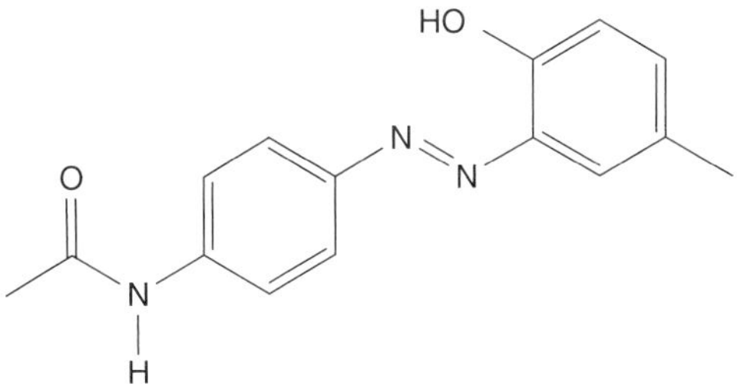

This azoic dye is responsible for textile dermatitis from stockings and occupational contact dermatitis in workers in the textile industry. It can be found in some semipermanent hair dyes. See also Chap. 40.

Suggested Reading

Condé-Salazar L, Baz M, Guimaraens D, Cannavo A (1995) Contact dermatitis in hairdressers: patch test results in 379 hairdressers (1980–1993). Am J Contact Dermat 6:19–23
Soni BP, Sherertz EF (1996) Contact dermatitis in the textile industry: a review of 72 patients. Am J Contact Dermat 7:226–230

192. Dithianone

CAS Registry Number [3347–22–6]

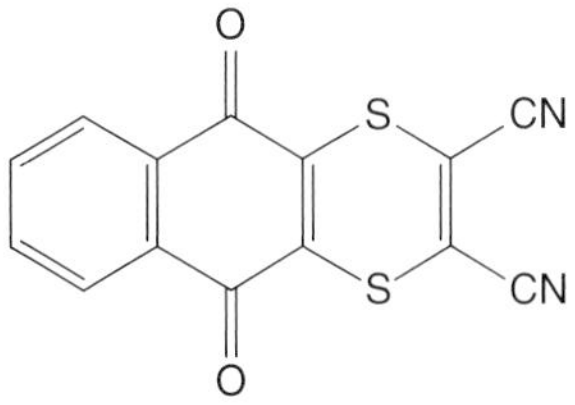

Dithianone is an anthraquinone derivative, used as a fungicide agent. With cymoxanil, it is contained in Aktuan®. Cases in agricultural workers were reported sparsely.

Suggested Reading

Koch P (1996) Occupational allergic contact dermatitis and airborne contact dermatitis from 5 fungicides in a vineyard worker. Cross-reactions between fungicides of the dithiocarbamate group? Contact Dermatitis 34:324–329

193. Dodecyl Gallate

Lauryl Gallate

CAS Registry Number [1166–52–5]

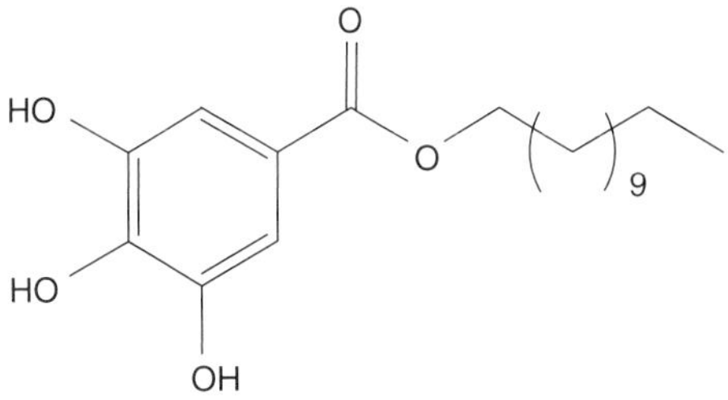

This gallic acid ester (E 310) is an antioxidant added to food and cosmetics to prevent oxidation of unsaturated fatty acids. Cases were reported in workers of the food industry, gallate being contained in margarine, and from washing powder.

Suggested Reading

De Groot AC, Gerkens F (1990) Occupational airborne contact dermatitis from octyl gallate. Contact Dermatitis 23:184–186
Mancuso G, Staffa M, Errani A, Berdondini RM, Fabri P (1990) Occupational dermatitis in animal feed mill workers. Contact Dermatitis 22:37–41

194. Doxepin

CAS Registry Number [1668–19–5]

This benzoxepin tricylcic drug has antidepressant, anticholinergic, antiitching, and antihistamine properties. After oral use, it has been developed as a topical antiitching agent. Allergic contact dermatitis is not infrequent.

Suggested Reading

Buckley DA (2000) Contact allergy to doxepin. Contact Dermatitis 43:231–232
Taylor JS, Praditsuwan P, Handel D, Kuffner G (1996) Allergic contact dermatitis from doxepin cream. One-year patch test clinic experience. Arch Dermatol 132:515–518

195. Epichlorhydrin

1-Chloro-2,3-Epoxypropane

CAS Registry Number [106–89–8]

Epoxy resin of the Bisphenol A type is synthesized from epichlorhydrin and bisphenol A. It leads to bisphenol A diglycidyl ether, which is the monomer of bisphenol-A-based epoxy resins. Sensitization to epichlorhydrin occurs mainly in workers of the epoxy resin industry. Sensitization in individuals not working at epoxy resin plants is rare. It has, however, been described to occur following exposure to a soil fumigant, due to solvent cement, and in a worker in a pharmaceutical plant, in a division of drug synthesis. Epichlorhydrin was used for the production of drugs propranolol and oxprenolol.

Suggested Reading

Holness DL, Nethercott JR (1993) The performance of specialized collections of bisphenol A epoxy resin system components in the evaluation of workers in an occupational health clinic population. Contact Dermatitis 28:216–219
Rebandel P, Rudzki E (1990) Dermatitis caused by epichlorhydrin, oxprenolol hydrochloride and propranolol hydrochloride. Contact Dermatitis 23:199
Van Jost T, Roesyanto ID, Satyawan I (1990) Occupational sensitization to epichlorhydrin (ECH) and bisphenol-A during the manufacture of epoxy resin. Contact Dermatitis 22:125–126

196. Epoxy Resins of the Bisphenol A Type

These resins are synthesized from bisphenol A and epichlorhydrin. Hardeners are added, such as amines (ethylenediamine, diethylenetriamine, triethylenetetramine, isophoronediamine, triethylenetriamine and 4,4-diaminophenylmethane) or acid anhydrides (phthalic anhydride). Reactive diluents may be added, such as allyl glycidyl ether, butanediol diglycidyl ether, n-butyl glycidyl ether, o-cresyl glycidyl ether, hexanediol diglycidyl ether, neopentyl glycol diglycidyl ether, phenyl glycidyl ether, glycidyl ester of synthetic fatty acids, and glycidyl ether of aliphatic alcohols (Epoxide-8).

Suggested Reading

Holness DL, Nethercott JR (1993) The performance of special-ized collections of bisphenol A epoxy resin system compo-nents in the evaluation of workers in an occupational health clinic population. Contact Dermatitis 28:216–219

Jolanki R, Kanerva L, Estlander T, Tarvainen K, Keskinen H, Henriks-Eckerman ML (1990) Occupational dermatoses from epoxy resin compounds. Contact Dermatitis 23:172–183

197. 2,3-Epoxypropyl Trimethyl Ammonium Chloride

EPTMAC, Glycidyl Trimethyl Ammonium Chloride, Oxiranemethanaminium, N,N,N-Trimethyl Chloride

CAS Registry Number [3033–77–0]

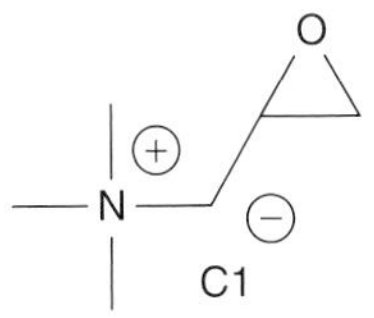

Used in the production of cationic starch for the paper industry; EPTMAC caused contact dermatitis in workers.

Suggested Reading

Estlander T, Jolanki R, Kanerva L (1997) Occupational allergic contact dermatitis from 2,3-epoxypropyl trimethyl ammo-nium chloride (EPTMAC) and Kathon R LX in a starch modification factory. Contact Dermatitis 36:191–194

198. Estradiol

17-β-Estradiol, (17β)-Estra-1,3,5(10)-Triene-3,17-diol

CAS Registry Number [50–28–2]

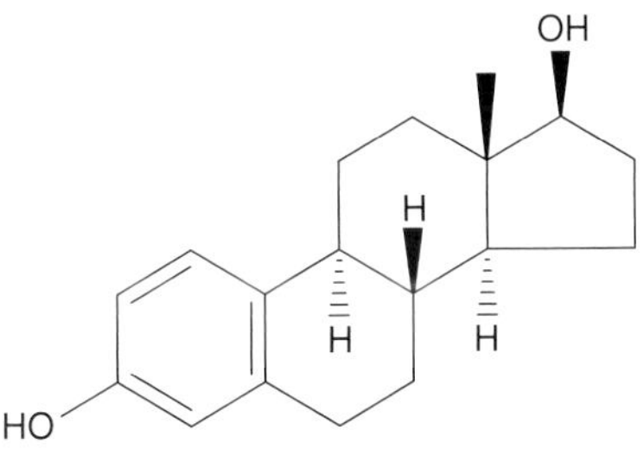

Natural estradiol, used in transdermal systems for hor-monal substitution, can induce allergic contact derma-titis, with the risk of systemic contact dermatitis after oral reintroduction.

Suggested Reading

Gonçalo M, Oliveira HS, Monteiro C, Clerins I, Figueiredo A (1999) Allergic and systemic contact dermatitis from estra-diol. Contact Dermatitis 40:58–59

199. Ethoxyquin

1,2-Dihydro 6-Ethoxy 2,2,4-Trimethylquinolein, Santoquin®, Santoflex®

CAS Registry Number [91–53–2]

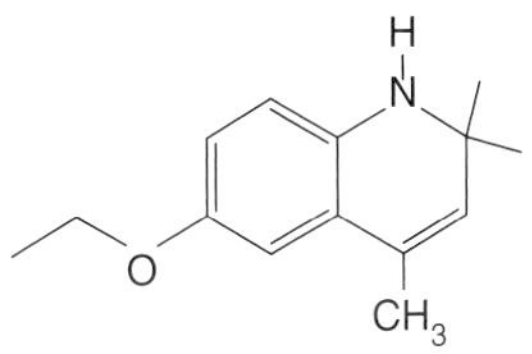

Ethoxyquin is used as an antioxidant in animal feed and caused contact dermatitis in a worker at an animal feed mill.

Suggested Reading

Mancuso G, Staffa M, Errani A, Berdondini RM, Fabri P (1990) Occupational dermatitis in animal feed mill workers. Contact Dermatitis 22:37–41

200. Ethyl Alcohol

Ethanol

CAS Registry Number [64–17–5]

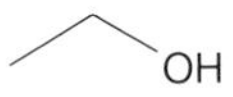

Ethanol is widely used for its solvent and antiseptic properties. It is rather an irritant and sensitization has rarely been reported.

Suggested Reading

Ophaswongse S, Maibach HI (1994) Alcohol dermatitis: allergic contact dermatitis and contact urticaria syndrome. Contact Dermatitis 30:1–6

Patruno C, Suppa F, Sarraco G, Balato N (1994) Allergic contact dermatitis due to ethyl alcohol. Contact Dermatitis 31:124

201. 4-Ethyl-Pyridine

CAS Registry Number [536–75–4]

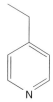

4-Ethyl-pyridine is used as a monomer in polymer chemistry.

Suggested Reading

Sasseville D, Balbul A, Kwong P, Yu K (1996) Contact sensitization to pyridine derivatives. Contact Dermatitis 35:101–102

202. Ethylbutylthiourea

CAS Registry Number [32900–06–4]

Ethylbutylthiourea is an accelerator used with other thiourea derivatives in the production of neoprene rubber. It is also contained in glues, mainly neoprene type.

Suggested Reading

Bergendorff O, Persson CML, Hansson C (2004) HPLC analysis of alkyl thioureas in an orthopedic brace and patch testing with pure ethylbutylthiourea. Contact Dermatitis 51:273–277

Kanerva L, Estlander T, Jolanki R (1994) Occupational allergic contact dermatitis caused by thiourea compounds. Contact Dermatitis 31:242–248

Roberts JL, Hanifin JM (1980) Contact allergy and cross-reactivity to substituted thiourea compounds. Contact Dermatitis 6:138–139

203. Ethylene Oxide

CAS Registry Number [75–21–8]

Ethylene oxide is a very strong irritant widely used in the chemical industry, and as a sterilizer of medical supplies, pharmaceutical products, and food. It can produce immediate (urticaria, asthma, anaphylaxis) or delayed reactions (irritant rather than allergic contact dermatitis). For example, residues in masks or dressings can produce irritant contact dermatitis. In delayed contact allergy, it seems that cross-reaction can be observed to epichlorhydrin or epoxypropane.

Suggested Reading

Birnie AJ, English JS (2006) Ethylene oxide allergy may have been confirmed by patch testing to a similar epoxy compound. Contact Dermatitis 55:126

Kerre S, Goossens A (2009) Allergic contact dermatitis to ethylene oxide. Contact Dermatitis 61:47–48

Lerman Y, Ribak J, Skulsky M, Ingber A (1995) An outbreak of irritant contact dermatitis from ethylene oxide among pharmaceutical workers. Contact Dermatitis 33:280–281

204. Ethylenediamine

CAS Registry Number [107–15–3]

Ethylenediamine is used in numerous industrial processes as a solvent for casein or albumin, as a stabilizer in rubber latex, and as a textile lubricant. It can be found in epoxy resin hardeners, cooling oils, fungicides, and waxes. Contact dermatitis from ethylenediamine is almost exclusively due to topical medicaments. Occupational contact dermatitis in epoxy resin systems is rather infrequent. Ethylenediamine can cross-react with triethylenetetramine and diethylenetriamine. Ethylenediamine was found to be responsible for sensitization in pharmacists handling aminophylline suppositories, in nurses preparing and administering injectable theophylline, and in a laboratory technician in the manufacture of aminophylline tablets.

Suggested Reading

Chieregato C, Vincenzi C, Guerra L, Farina P (1994) Occupational allergic contact dermatitis due to ethylenediamine dihydrochloride and cresyl glycidyl ether in epoxy resin systems. Contact Dermatitis 30:120

Corazza M, Mantovani L, Trimurti L, Virgili A (1994) Occupational contact sensitization to ethylenediamine in a nurse. Contact Dermatitis 31:328–329

Jolanki R, Kanerva L, Estlander T, Tarvainen K, Keskinen H, Henriks-Eckerman ML (1990) Occupational dermatoses from epoxy resin compounds. Contact Dermatitis 23:172–183

Mancuso G, Reggiani M, Berdondini RM (1996) Occupational dermatitis in shoemakers. Contact Dermatitis 34:17–22

Sasseville D, Al-Khenaizan S (1997) Occupational contact dermatitis from ethylenediamine in a wire-drawing lubricant. Contact Dermatitis 3:228–229

205. Ethylenethiourea

CAS Registry Number [96–45–7]

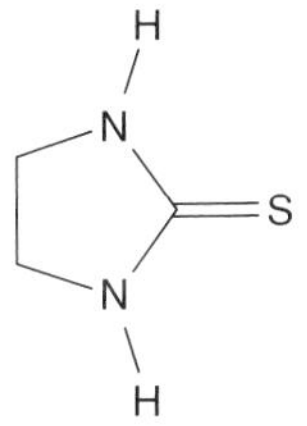

Ethylenethiourea, a thiourea derivative, is a rubber chemical. It caused contact dermatitis mainly in rubber workers.

Suggested Reading

Bruze M, Fregert S (1983) Allergic contact dermatitis from ethylenethiourea. Contact Dermatitis 9:208–212

Kanerva L, Estlander T, Jolanki R (1994) Occupational allergic contact dermatitis caused by thiourea compounds. Contact Dermatitis 31:242–248

206. Ethylhexylglycerin

Octoxyglycerin

CAS Registry Number [70445–33–9]

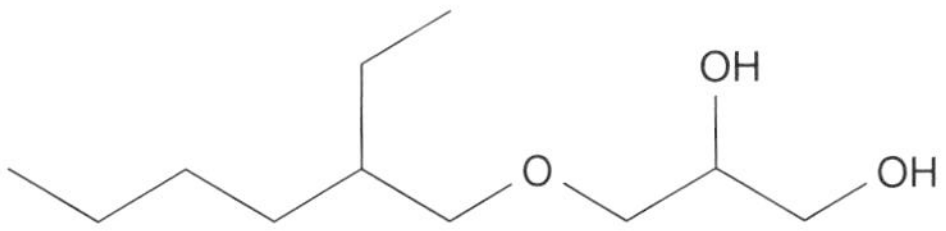

This glycerol monoalkylether is used as a skin conditioning agent, with bactericidal properties against Gram-positive bacteria.

Suggested Reading

Linsen G, Goossens A (2002) Allergic contact dermatitis from ethylhexylglycerin. Contact Dermatitis 47:169

207. Eugenol

CAS Registry Number [97–53–0]

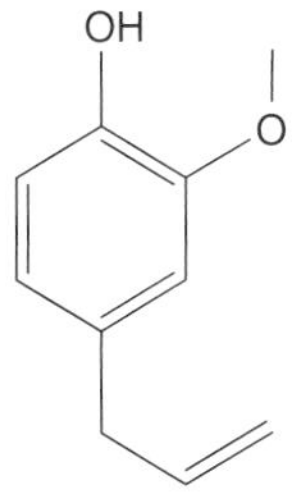

Eugenol is a fragrance allergen obtained from many natural sources. Occupational sensitization to eugenol may occur in dental profession workers. Eugenol is contained in "fragrance mix" and has to be listed by name in cosmetics within the EU.

Suggested Reading

Berova N, Stranky L, Krasteva M (1990) Studies on contact dermatitis in stomatological staff. Dermatol Monatsschr 176:15–18

Rudzki E, Rebandel P, Grzywa Z (1989) Patch tests with occupational contactants in nurses, doctors and dentists. Contact Dermatitis 20:247–250

208. Euxyl®K 400 (see 284. subentry 1,2-Dibromo-2,4-Dicyanobutane and 322. Phenoxyethanol)

Euxyl®K 400 is a mixture of 1,2-dibromo-2,4-dicyanobutane 20% and phenoxyethanol 80%, widely utilized as a preservative in cosmetics, hand creams, and toiletries, but also in water-based paints, glues, metalworking fluids, and detergents. Sensitization was reported in masseurs, in a beautician, an offset printer, and a hospital cleaner. We observed four cases of hand contact dermatitis in metalworkers, due to the so-called Euxyl® K 400 contained in barrier creams. No sensitization was observed to phenoxyethanol (personal cases).

Suggested Reading

Aalto-Korte K, Jolanki R, Estlander T, Alanko K, Kanerva L (1996) Occupational allergic contact dermatitis caused by Euxyl K 400. Contact Dermatitis 35:193–194

209. Famotidine

CAS Registry Number [76824–35–6]

Contact dermatitis in a nurse from famotidine, an H2-receptor agonist, was described. In industry, three cases were reported due to intermediates of the synthesis of 2-diamino-ethylene-amino-thiazolyl-methylenethiourea-dichloride, and 4-chloromethyl-2-guanidinothiazole-nitrochloride.

Suggested Reading

Guimaraens D, Gonzales MA, Condé-Salazar L (1994) Occupational allergic contact dermatitis from intermediate products in famotidine synthesis. Contact Dermatitis 31:259–260
Monteseirin J, Conde J (1990) Contact eczema from famotidine. Contact Dermatitis 22:290

210. Farnesol

3,7,11-Trimethyldodeca-2,6,10-Trienol (Four Isomers)

CAS Registry Numbers [4602–84–0] for the mixture, [106–28–5] for the trans/trans, [3790–71–4] for the cis/trans, [3879–60–5] for the trans/cis, and [16106–95–9] for the cis/cis

Farnesol is one of the most frequent contact allergens in perfumes. It is contained in small amounts in *Myroxylon pereirae* and poplar buds. It is a blend of four diastereosiomers *trans/cis*. As a fragrance allergen, farnesol has to be mentioned by name in cosmetics within the EU.

Suggested Reading

Frosch PJ, Johansen JD, Menné T, Pirker C, Rastogi SC, Andersen KE, Bruze M, Goossens A, Lepoittevin JP, White IR (2002) Further important sensitizers in patients sensitive to fragrances. Contact Dermatitis 47:78–85
Schnuch A, Uter W, Geier J, Lessmann H, Frosch PJ (2004) Contact allergy to farnesol in 2021 consecutively patch tested patients. Results of the IVDK. Contact Dermatitis 50:117–121

211. Fenvalerate

CAS Registry Number [51630–58–1]

Fenvalerate is an insecticide of the synthetic pyrethroid group, which induced sensitization in farmers.

Suggested Reading

Sharma VK, Kaur S (1990) Contact sensitization by pesticides in farmers. Contact Dermatitis 23:77–80

212. Fluazinam

Shirlan®, 3-Chloro-*N*-(3-Chloro-5-Trifluoromethyl-2-Pyridyl)-Trifluoro-2,6-Dinitro-*p*-Toluidine

CAS Registry Number [79622–59–6]

Fluazinam is a pesticide with a broad spectrum of antifungal activity. It caused sensitization in employees in the tulip bulb industry and in farmers. Fluazinam induced contact dermatitis in a worker in a plant where it was manufactured.

Suggested Reading

Bruynzeel DP, Tafelkruijer J, Wilks MF (1995) Contact dermatitis due to a new fungicide used in the tulip bulb industry. Contact Dermatitis 33:8–11
Van Ginkel CJW, Sabapathy NN (1995) Allergic contact dermatitis from the newly introduced fungicide fluazinam. Contact Dermatitis 32:160–162

213. Flutamide

2-Methyl-*N*-[4-Nitro-3-(Trifluoromethyl)Phenyl] Propanamide, Trifluoro-2-Methyl-4-Nitro-*m*-Propionotoluidide, 4-Nitro-3-Trifluoromethylisobutyranilide, Niftolid

CAS Registry Number [13311–84–7]

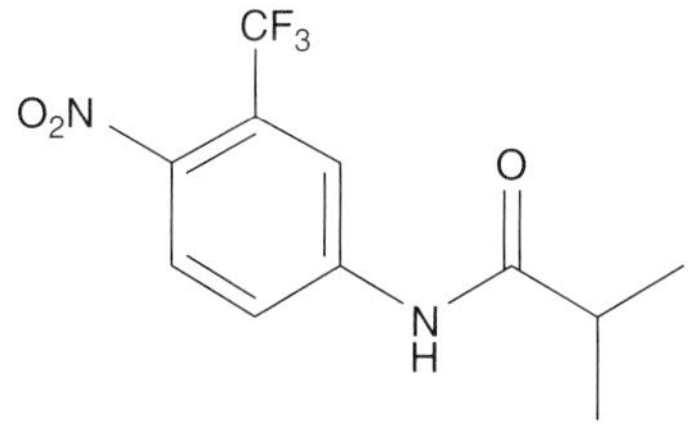

Flutamide is an antiandrogenic hormonal antineoplastic drug that can induce photosensitivity and porphyria-like eruption.

Suggested Reading

Borroni G, Brazzelli V, Baldini F, Borghini F, Gaviglio MR, Beltrami B, Nolli G (1998) Flutamide-induced pseudoporphyria. Br J Dermatol 138:711–712
Martín-Lázaro J, Goday Buján J, Parra Arrondo A, Rodríguez Lozano J, Cuerda Galindo E, Fonseca Capdevila E (2004) Is photopatch testing useful in the investigation of photosensitivity due to flutamide? Contact Dermatitis 50:325–326

214. Folpet

Folpel, Phthalane, Trichloromethylthiophthalimide

CAS Registry Number [133–07–3]

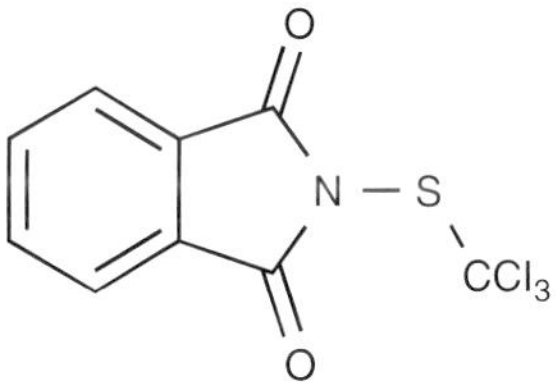

Folpet is a pesticide, fungicide agent of thiophthalimide group. Occupational exposure occurs mostly in agricultural workers or in florists. Photosensitivity has been reported.

Suggested Reading

Lisi P, Caraffini S, Assalve D (1987) Irritation and sensitization potential of pesticides. Contact Dermatitis 17:212–218
Mark KA, Brancaccio RR, Soter NA, Cohen DE (1999) Allergic contact and photoallergic contact dermatitis to plant and pesticide allergens. Arch Dermatol 135:67–70
Peluso AM, Tardio M, Adamo F, Venturo N (1991) Multiple sensitization due to bis-dithiocarbamate and thiophthalimide pesticides. Contact Dermatitis 25:327

215. Formaldehyde

Methanal, Formalin

CAS Registry Number [50–00–0]

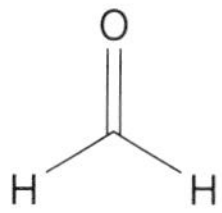

Sources and uses of formaldehyde are numerous. Exposed people are mainly health workers, cleaners, painters, metalworkers, but also photographers (color developers) and carbonless copy paper users. Formaldehyde can induce contact urticaria. Formaldehyde may be the cause of sensitization to formaldehyde releasers: benzylhemiformal, bromonitrodioxane, bromonitropropanediol (?), chloroallylhexaminium chloride or Quaternium-15, diazolidinylurea, dimethylol urea, dimethyloldimethylhydantoin or DMDM hydantoin, hexamethylenetetramine or methenamine, imidazolidinylurea, monomethyloldimethylhydantoin or MDM hydantoin, *N*-methylolchloracetamide, paraformaldehyde and trihydroxyethylhexahydrotriazine or Grotan BK.

Formaldehyde is used for the synthesis of many resins. Some of them, such as formaldehyde-urea and melamine-formaldehyde resins, can be used in textiles and secondarily release free formaldehyde (see Chap. 40).

Other resins, such as *p-tert*-butylphenol formaldehyde resin or tosylamine formaldehyde resin, do not release formaldehyde.

Suggested Reading

Flyvholm MA, Menné T (1992) Allergic contact dermatitis from formaldehyde. A case study focussing on sources of formaldehyde exposure. Contact Dermatitis 27:27–36

Murray R (1991) Health aspects of carbonless copy paper. Contact Dermatitis 24:321–333

Pabst R (1987) Exposure to formaldehyde in anatomy: an occupational health hazard? Anat Rec 219:109–112

Rudzki E, Rebandel P, Grzywa Z (1989) Patch tests with occupational contactants in nurses, doctors and dentists. Contact Dermatitis 20:247–250

Scheman AJ, Katta R (1997) Photographic allergens: an update. Contact Dermatitis 37:130

Torresani C, Periti I, Beski L (1996) Contact urticaria syndrome from formaldehyde with multiple physical urticaria. Contact Dermatitis 35:174–175

216. Frullanolide

l-(–)-Frullanolide

CAS Registry Number [27579–97–1]

d-(+)-Frullanolide

CAS Registry Number [40776–40–7]

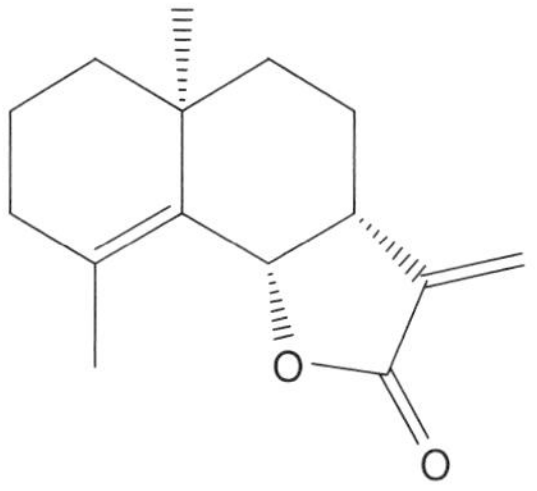

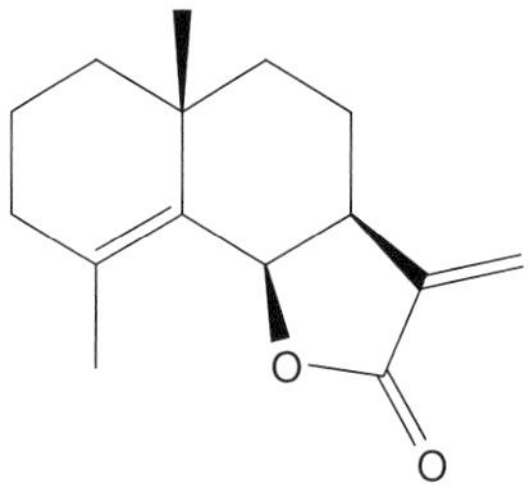

Frullanolide is a sesquiterpene lactone, contained in *Frullania tamarisci* Dum. (*l*-Frullanolide) and *Frullania dilatata* Dum. (*d*-frullanolide), a lichen that grows on lobed-leaf trees such as oak and beech. Sensitivity causes airborne and sometimes severe polymorphous erythema-like allergic contact dermatitis, mainly in foresters and in people using firewood, lumbermen, sawyers, carpenters, and merchants in rough timber.

Suggested Reading

Ducombs G, Lepoittevin JP, Berl V, Andersen KE, Brandão FM, Bruynzeel DP, Bruze M, Camarasa JG, Frosch PJ, Goossens A, Lachapelle JM, Lahti A, Le Coz CJ, Maibach HI, Menné T, Seidenari S, Shaw S, Tosti A, Wilkinson JD (2003) Routine patch testing with frullanolide mix: an European Environmental and Contact Dermatitis Research Group multicenter study. Contact Dermatitis 48:158–161

Quirino AP, Barros MA (1995) Occupational contact dermatitis from lichens and *Frullania*. Contact Dermatitis 33:68–69

Tomb RR (1992) Patch testing with frullania during a 10-year period: hazards and complications. Contact Dermatitis 26:220–223

217. Furaltadone

5-Morpholinomethyl-3 (5-Nitrofurfurilidenamine)-2-Oxazolidinone

CAS Registry Number [139–91–3]

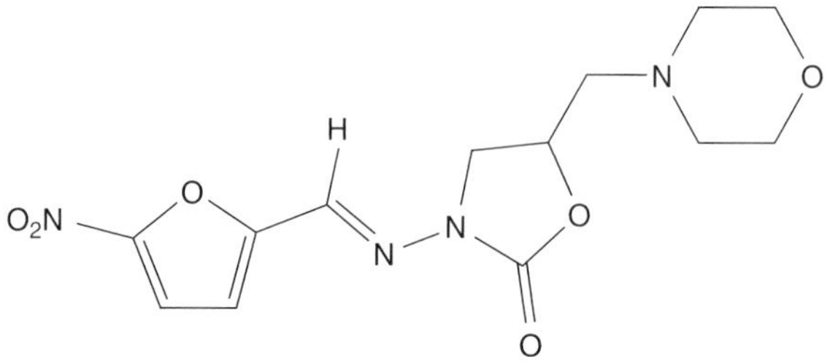

This nitrofuran derivative can be added in animal feed or in eardrops.

Suggested Reading

Sánchez-Pérez J, Córdoba S, Jesús del Río M, García-Díes A (1999) Allergic contact dermatitis from furaltadone in eardrops. Contact Dermatitis 40:222

Vilaplana J, Grimalt F, Romaguera C (1990) Contact dermatitis from furaltadone in animal feed. Contact Dermatitis 22:232–233

218. Furazolidone

3-(5-Nitrofurfurylideneamino)-2-Oxazolidinone

CAS Registry Number [67–45–8]

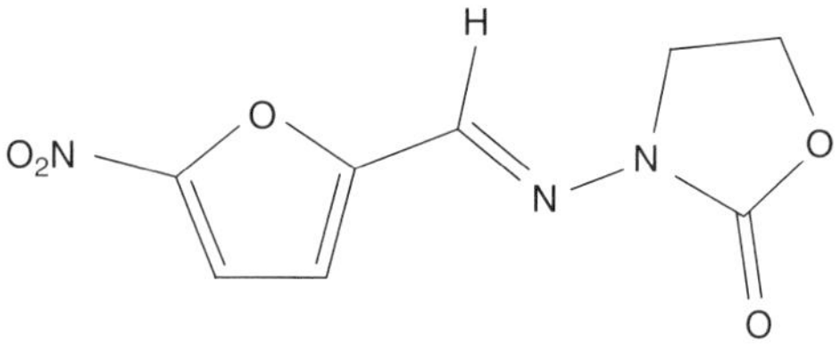

Furazolidone belongs to the group of nitrofurans. This antimicrobial (antibacterial and antiprotozoal) agent is used in veterinary medicine both topically and orally, particularly in animal feed. Reactions are reported in workers exposed to it in animal feeds. Cross-reactions with other nitrofuran derivatives are rare.

Suggested Reading

Burge S, Bransbury A (1994) Allergic contact dermatitis due to fura-zolidone in a piglet medication. Contact Dermatitis 31:199–200

De Groot AC, Conemans MH (1990) Contact allergy to furazoli-done. Contact Dermatitis 22:202–205

219. Geraniol

3,7-Dimethyl-2,6-Octadien-1-ol

CAS Registry Number [106–24–1]

cis-Geraniol: Nerol

CAS Registry Number [106–25–2]

trans-Geraniol: Citrol

CAS Registry Number [624–15–7]

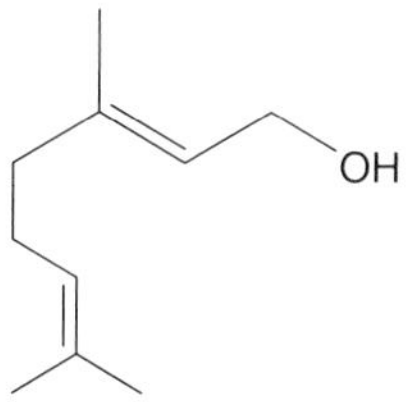

Geraniol is an olefinic terpene, constituting the chief part of rose oil and oil of palmarosa. It is also found in many other essential oils such as citronella, lemon grass, or ylang-ylang (*Cananga odorata* Hook.f. and Thoms.). It is contained in most fine fragrances and in "fragrance mix." As a fragrance allergen, geraniol has to be mentioned by name in cosmetics within the EU.

Suggested Reading

Frosch PJ, Johansen JD, Menné T, Pirker C, Rastogi SC, Andersen KE, Bruze M, Goossens A, Lepoittevin JP, White IR (2002) Further important sensitizers in patients sensitive to fragrances. Contact Dermatitis 47:78–85

Kanerva L, Estlander T, Jolanki R (1995) Occupational allergic contact dermatitis caused by ylang-ylang oil. Contact Dermatitis 33:198–199

220. Glutaraldehyde

Glutaral, Pentanedial, Glutaric Dialdehyde

CAS Registry Number [111–30–8]

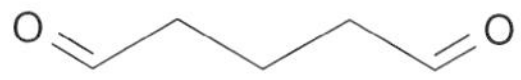

Glutaraldehyde is a well-know sensitizer in cleaners and health workers. It can also be found in X-ray developers or in cosmetics.

Suggested Reading

Cusano F, Luciano S (1993) Contact allergy to benzalkonium chloride and glutaraldehyde in a dental nurse. Contact Dermatitis 28:127

Nethercott JR, Holness DL, Page E (1988) Occupational contact dermatitis due to glutaraldehyde in health care workers. Contact Dermatitis 18:193–196

Scheman AJ, Katta R (1997) Photographic allergens: an update. Contact Dermatitis 37:130

Stingeni L, Lapomarda V, Lisi P (1995) Occupational hand dermatitis in hospital environments. Contact Dermatitis 33:172–176

Taylor JS, Praditsuwan P (1996) Latex allergy. Review of 44 cases including outcome and frequent association with allergic hand eczema. Arch Dermatol 32:265–271

221. Glyceryl Thioglycolate

Glyceryl Monothioglycolate, Glycerol Monomercaptoacetate

CAS Registry Number [30618–84–9]

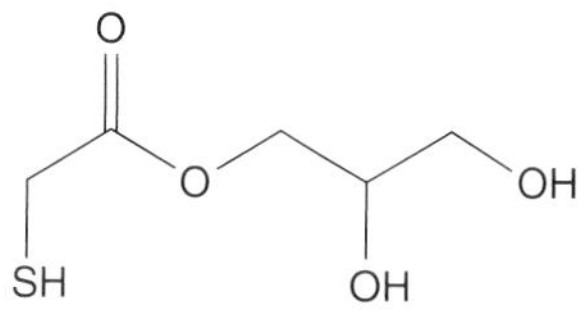

It is an acid permanent-wave ingredient, which induces contact dermatitis in hairdressers.

Suggested Reading

Frosch PJ, Burrows D, Camarasa JG, Dooms-Goossens A, Ducombs G, Lahti A, Menné T, Rycroft RJG, Shaw S, White IR, Wilkinson JD (1993) Allergic reactions to a hairdresser's series: results from 9 European centers. Contact Dermatitis 28:180–183

Guerra L, Tosti A, Bardazzi F, Pigatto P, Lisi P, Santucci B, Valsecchi R, Schena D, Angelini G, Sertoli A, Ayala F, Kokelj F (1992) Contact dermatitis in hairdressers: the Italian experience. Gruppo Italiano Ricerca Dermatiti da Contatto e Ambientali. Contact Dermatitis 26:101–107

Van der Walle HB, Brunsveld VM (1994) Dermatitis in hairdressers (I). The experience of the past 4 years. Contact Dermatitis 30:217–220

222. Glycidyl 1-Naphthyl Ether

1-Naphthyl-Glycidyl Ether

CAS Registry Number [2461–42–9]

Glycidyl ethers are used as reactive diluents for epoxy resins. Alpha-naphthyl glycidyl ether is formed by adding epichlorhydrin and NaOH to alpha-naphthol. Contact dermatitis was reported in workers of a chemical plant.

Suggested Reading

De Groot AC (1994) Occupational contact allergy to alpha-naphthyl glycidyl ether. Contact Dermatitis 30:253–254

223. 3-Glycidyloxypropyltrimethoxysilane

Gamma-Glycidoxypropyltrimethoxysilane, [(3-(Trimethoxysilyl)Propoxy)methyl]Oxirane

CAS Registry Numbers [2530–83–8], [108727–79–3], [120026–01–9], [138590–36–0] [163035–07–2], [26348–10–7], [51938–40–0], [53029–18–8], [65323–93–5], [88385–40–4]

An impurity such as allyl glycidyl ether seemed to be the sensitizing agent contained in 3-glycidyloxy-propyltrimethoxysilane.

Suggested Reading

Dooms-Goossens A, Bruze M, Buysse L, Fregert S, Gruvberger B, Stals H (1995) Contact allergy to allyl glycidyl ether present as an impurity in 3-glycidyloxypropyltrimethoxysilane, a fixing additive in silicone and polyurethane. Contact Dermatitis 33:17–19

224. Grotan BK

Hexahydro-1,3,5-Tris-(2-Hydroxyethyl)Triazine

CAS Registry Number [4719–04–4]

Grotan BK is a triazine derivative contained as a biocide in cutting fluids. It is a formaldehyde releaser. Dermatitis, delayed-type allergic conjunctivitis, and asthma were described.

Suggested Reading

Rasschaert V, Goossens A (2002) Conjunctivitis and bronchial asthma: symptoms of contact allergy to 1,3,5-tris(2-hydroxyethyl)-hexahydrotriazine (Grotan BK). Contact Dermatitis 47:116
Veronesi S, Guerra L, Valeri F, Toni F (1987) Three cases of contact dermatitis sensitive to Grotan BK. Contact Dermatitis 17:255

225 bis. HC Blue No. 7

CAS Registry Numbers [83732-72-3], [90817-34-8]

6-Methoxy-N-2-methylpyridine-2,3-diamine dihydrochloride

6-methoxy-2-methylamino-3-aminopyridine HCl

This substance, with EINECS Nr. 280-622-9, is used in two component (oxidation) hair dyes.

Suggested Reading

Søsted H, Nielsen NH, Menné T (2009) Allergic contact dermatitis to the hair dye 6-methoxy-2-methylamino-3-aminopyridine HCl (INCI HC Blue no. 7) without cross-sensitivity to PPD. Contact Dermatitis 60:236–237

Anon (2006) Commission decision of 9 February 2006 amending Decision 96/335/EC establishing an inventory and a common nomenclature of ingredients employed in cosmetic products. Official Journal of the European Union, L97/1, 5.4.2006 (2006/257/EC)

226. HC Yellow No. 7

Hair Color Yellow No. 7

CAS Registry Number [104226–21–3]

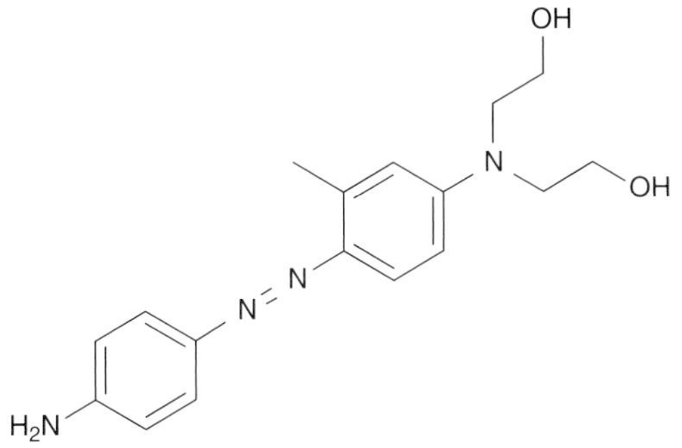

HC Yellow no. 7 is a direct azo dye used in semipermanent hair dye preparation. Since this dye leads to PPD after hydrolysis, it explains the allergic reaction in PPD-positive patients.

Suggested Reading

Sánchez-Pérez J, García del Río I, Alvares Ruiz S, García Diez A (2004) Allergic contact dermatitis from direct dyes for hair coloration in hairdressers' clients. Contact Dermatitis 50:261–262

227. Hexamethylene Diisocyanate

1,6-Hexamethylene Diisocyanate, HDI, HMDI

CAS Registry Number [822–06–0]

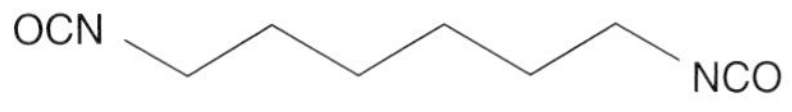

This diisocyanate compound is used in the manufacture of various polyurethane products: elastic and rigid foams, paints, lacquers, adhesives, binding agents, synthetics rubbers, and elastomer fibers.

Suggested Reading

Estlander T, Keskinen H, Jolanki R, Kanerva L (1992) Occupational dermatitis from exposure to polyurethane chemicals. Contact Dermatitis 27:161–165

228. Hexamethylenediamine

1,6-Diaminohexane

CAS Registry Number [124–09–4]

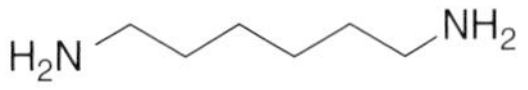

Hexamethylenediamine is used with adipic acid in the synthesis of polyamide plastics.

Suggested Reading

Michel PJ, Prost J (1954) Lésions provoquées par l'hexaméthylènediamine. Bull Soc Fr Dermatol Syphiligr 61:385

229. Hexamidine

CAS Registry Number [3811–75–4]

Hexamidine Diisethionate

CAS Registry Number [659–40–5]

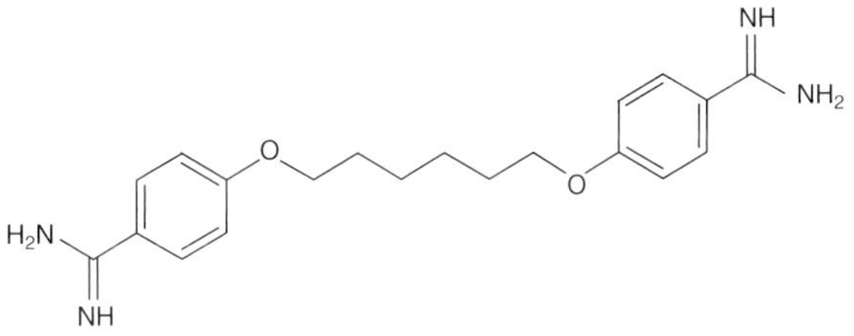

Hexamidine is an antiseptic active against Gram-positive bacteria and fungi, used as a disinfectant and a preservative in cosmetics. It induces papulo-vesicular and diffuse allergic contact dermatitis.

Suggested Reading

Dooms-Goossens A, Vandaele M, Bedert R, Marien K (1989) Hexamidine isethionate: a sensitizer in topical pharmaceutical products and cosmetics. Contact Dermatitis 21:270

Le Coz CJ, Scrivener Y, Santinelli F, Heid E (1998) Sensibilisation de contact au cours des ulcères de jambe. Ann Dermatol Venereol 125:694–699

Revuz J, Poli F, Wechsler J, Dubertret L (1984) Dermatites de contact à l'hexamidine. Ann Dermatol Venereol 111: 805–810

230. Hexanediol Diglycidyl Ether

1,6-Hexanediol Diglycidyl Ether

CAS Registry Number [16096–31–4]

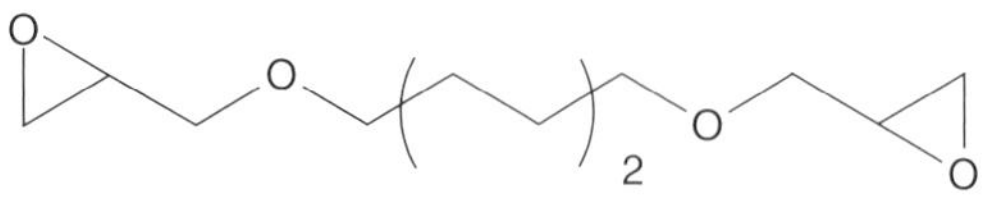

This chemical is a reactive diluent in epoxy resins.

Suggested Reading

Jolanki R, Kanerva L, Estlander T, Tarvainen K, Keskinen H, Henriks-Eckerman ML (1990) Occupational dermatoses from epoxy resin compounds. Contact Dermatitis 23:172–183

231. Hexyl Cinnamic Aldehyde

Hexyl Cinnamaldehyde, Alpha-Hexyl-Cinnamaldehyde, 2-(Phenylmethylene)Octanal, 2-Benzylideneoctanal

CAS Registry Number [101–86–0]

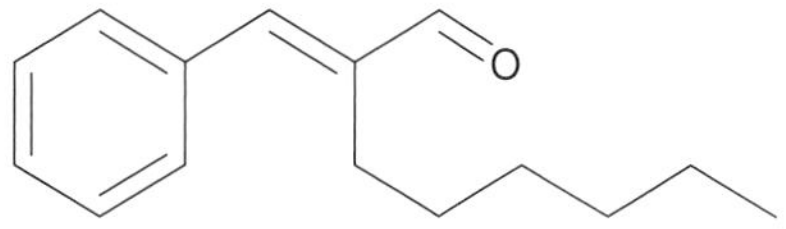

Hexyl cinnamic aldehyde is a fragrance allergen. Its presence has to be mentioned by name in cosmetics within the EU.

Suggested Reading

Frosch PJ, Johansen JD, Menné T, Pirker C, Rastogi SC, Andersen KE, Bruze M, Goossens A, Lepoittevin JP, White IR (2002) Further important sensitizers in patients sensitive to fragrances. Contact Dermatitis 47:78–85

Rastogi SC, Johansen JD, Menné T (1996) Natural ingredients based cosmetics. Content of selected fragrance sensitizers. Contact Dermatitis 34:423–426

232. Hydralazine

CAS Registry Number [86–54–4]

Hydralazine Hydrochloride

CAS Registry Number [304–20–1]

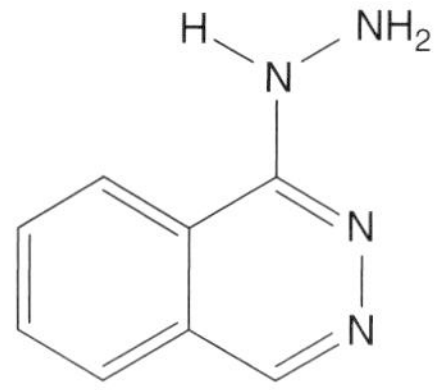

Hydralazine is a hydrazine derivative used as a antihypertensive drug. Skin rashes have been described during treatment. Exposure occurs mainly in the pharmaceutical industry. Cross-sensitivity is frequent with hydrazine, which is considered to be a potent sensitizer.

Suggested Reading

Pereira F, Dias M, Pacheco FA (1996) Occupational contact dermatitis from propranolol, hydralazine, and bendroflumethiazide. Contact Dermatitis 35:303–304

233. Hydrangenol

CAS Registry Number [480–47–7]

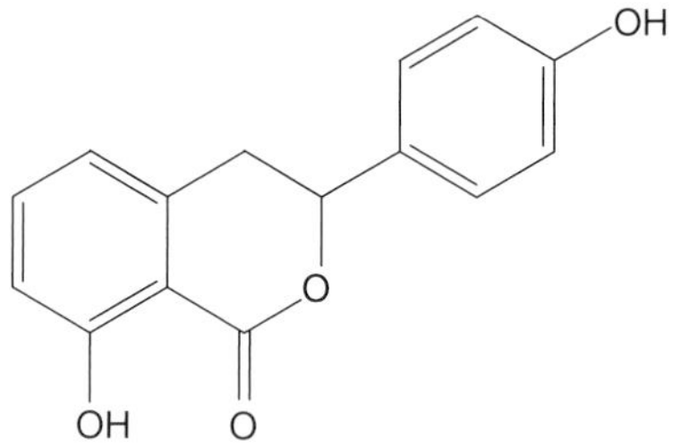

Hydrangenol is the allergen of hydrangea (*Hydrangea macrophylla* Thunb, Hydrangeaceae family). See also Chap. 46.

Suggested Reading

Avenel-Audran M, Hausen BM, Le Sellin J, Ledieu G, Verret JL (2000) Allergic contact dermatitis from hydrangea – is it so rare? Contact Dermatitis 43:189–191

Kuligowski ME, Chang A, Leemreize JHM (1992) Allergic contact hand dermatitis from hydrangea: report of a 10th case. Contact Dermatitis 26:269–270

234. Hydrazine

CAS Registry Number [302–01–2]

$$H_2N — NH_2$$

Hydrazine sulfate CAS Registry Number [10034–93–2], dihydrobromide CAS Registry Number [23268–00–0] and hydrochloride [14011–37–1] have been reported as occupational sensitizers, mainly in soldering flux.

Suggested Reading

Frost J, Hjorth N (1959) Contact dermatitis from hydrazine bromide in soldering flux. Acta Derm Venereol (Stockh) 39: 82–85

Goh CL, Ng SK (1987) Airborne contact dermatitis to colophony in soldering flux. Contact Dermatitis 17:89–91

Wheeler CE, Penn SR, Cawley EP (1965) Dermatitis from hydrazine hydrobromide solder flux. Arch Dermatol 91: 235–239

Wrangsjö K, Martensson A (1986) Hydrazine contact dermatitis from gold plating. Contact Dermatitis 15:244–245

235. Hydrocortisone

Cortisol

CAS Registry Number [50–23–7]

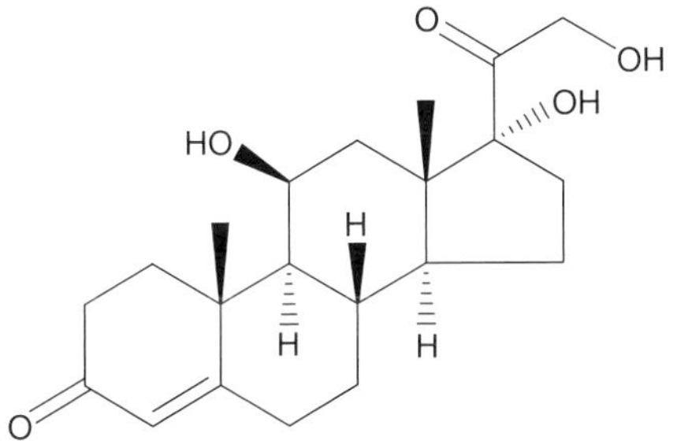

Hydrocortisone is the principal glucocorticoid hormone produced by the adrenal cortex and is used topically or systemically. It belongs to the allergenic A group. Marker of allergy is tixocortol pivalate.

Suggested Reading

Lepoittevin JP, Drieghe J, Dooms-Goossens A (1995) Studies in patients with corticosteroid contact allergy. Understanding cross-reactivity among different steroids. Arch Dermatol 131:31–37

Le Coz CJ (2002) Fiche d'éviction en cas d'hypersensibilité au pivalate de tixocortol. Ann Dermatol Venereol 129: 348–349

236. Hydrocortisone 17-Butyrate

CAS Registry Number [13609–67–1]

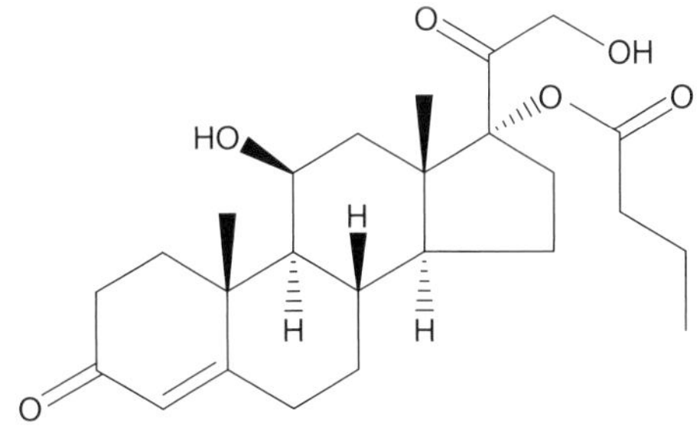

Hydrocortisone 17-butyrate is a C_{17} ester of hydrocortisone. It represents the D2 group of corticosteroids, non C_{16} methylated with a C_{17} ester: hydrocortisone 17-butyrate, hydrocortisone 17-valerate, hydrocortisone aceponate (17-propionate and 21-acetate), methylprednisolone aceponate, and prednicarbate. It is sometimes hydrolyzed in vivo into hydrocortisone, giving allergic reactions to group-A-sensitized people.

Suggested Reading

Le Coz CJ (2002) Fiche d'éviction en cas d'hypersensibilité au 17 butyrate d'hydrocortisone. Ann Dermatol Venereol 129:931

Lepoittevin JP, Drieghe J, Dooms-Goossens A (1995) Studies in patients with corticosteroid contact allergy. Understanding cross-reactivity among different steroids. Arch Dermatol 131:31–37

237. Hydrogen Peroxide

H_2O_2

CAS Registry Number [7722–84–1]

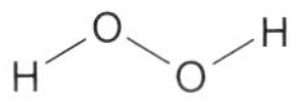

Hydrogen peroxide is an oxidizing agent used as a topical antiseptic, and as part of permanent hair-dyes and color-removing preparations, and as a neutralizing agent in permanent waving. The concentration of the hydrogen peroxyde solution is expressed in volume or percentage: Ten volumes correspond to 3%. It is an irritant.

Suggested Reading

Aguirre A, Zabala R, Sanz De Galdeano C, Landa N, Diaz-Perez JL (1994) Positive patch tests to hydrogen peroxide in 2 cases. Contact Dermatitis 30:113

58

238. Hydroquinone

1,4-Benzenediol

CAS Registry Number [123–31–9]

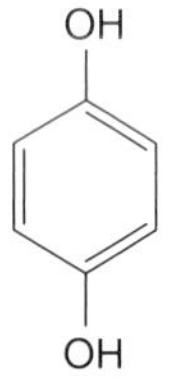

Hydroquinone is used in photography developers (black and white, X-ray, and microfilms), in plastics, in hair dyes as an antioxidant and hair colorant. Hydroquinone is found in many skin bleaching creams.

Suggested Reading

Barrientos N, Ortiz-Frutos J, Gomez E, Iglesias L (2001) Allergic contact dermatitis from a bleaching cream. Am J Contact Dermat 12:33–34

Gebhardt M, Geier J (1996) Evaluation of patch test results with denture material series. Contact Dermatitis 34:191–195

Lidén C, Brehmer-Andersson E (1988) Occupational dermatoses from color developing agents. Clinical and histopathological observations. Acta Derm Venereol (Stockh) 68:514–522

Scheman AJ, Katta R (1997) Photographic allergens: an update. Contact Dermatitis 37:130

239. (S)-4-Hydroxy 4-Methoxydalbergione

CAS Registry Number [3755–63–3]

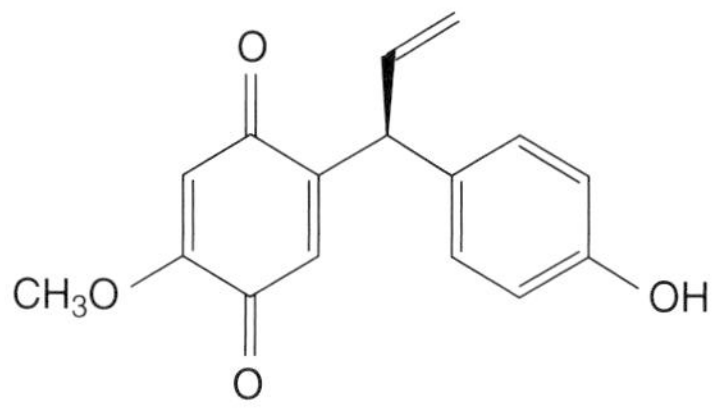

(S)-4-Hydroxy 4-methoxydalbergione is one of the allergens Brazilian rosewood or Palissander (*Dalbergia nigra* All., Papillionaceae family), cocobolo (*Dalbergia retusa* Hemsl., *Dalbergia granadilla*, and *Dalbergia hypoleuca*), or grenadil (*Dalbergia melanoxylon* Guill. and Perr.). See also Chap. 46.

Suggested Reading

Hausen BM (1981) Wood injurious to human health. A manual. De Gruyter, Berlin

240. Hydroxycitronellal

7-Hydroxycitronellal, Citronellal Hydrate, Laurine, Muguet Synthetic

CAS Registry Number [107–75–5]

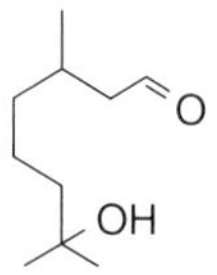

Hydroxycitronellal is a classical fragrance allergen, found in many products. It is contained in "fragrance mix." It has to be listed by name in the cosmetics of the EU.

Suggested Reading

Rastogi SC, Johansen JD, Frosch P, Menné T, Bruze M, Lepoittevin JP, Dreier B, Andersen KE, White IR (1998) Deodorants on the European market: quantitative chemical analysis of 21 fragrances. Contact Dermatitis 38: 29–35

Svedman C, Bruze M, Johansen JD, Andersen KE, Goossens A, Frosch PJ, Lepoittevin JP, Rastogi S, White IR, Menné T (2003) Deodorants: an experimental provocation study with hydroxycitronellal. Contact Dermatitis 48:217–223

241. Hydroxylamine and Hydroxylammonium Salts

Hydroxylamine

CAS Registry Number [7803–49–8]

Hydroxylammonium Chloride: Hydroxylamine Hydrochloride, Oxammonium Hydrochloride

CAS Registry Numbers [5470–11–1]

Hydroxylammonium Sulfate: Hydroxylamine Sulfate, Oxammonium Sulfate

CAS Registry Number [7803–49–8]

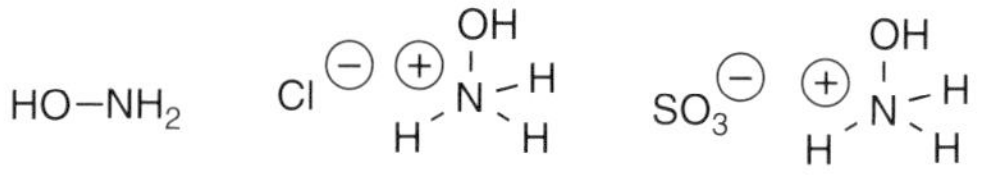

Hydroxylamine and its salts are used in various branches of industry, as reducing agents in color film developers or as reagents in laboratories.

Suggested Reading

Aguirre A, Landa N, Gonzalez M, Diaz-Perez JL (1992) Allergic contact dermatitis in a photographer. Contact Dermatitis 27:340–341

Estlander T, Jolanki T, Kanerva L (1997) Hydroxylammonium chloride as sensitizer in a water laboratory. Contact Dermatitis 36:161–162

Goh CL (1990) Allergic contact dermatitis and onycholysis from hydroxylamine sulfate in color developer. Contact Dermatitis 22:109

242. Hydroxymethylpentacy- clohexenecarboxaldehyde

Lyral®, Hydroxyisohexyl 3-Cyclohexene Carboxaldehyde, 4-(4-Hydroxy-4-Methylpentyl)-3- Cyclohexene-1-Carboxaldehyde, 4-(4-Hydroxy-4- Methylpentyl)Cyclohex-3-ene-Carbaldehyde

CAS Registry Number [31906–04–4]

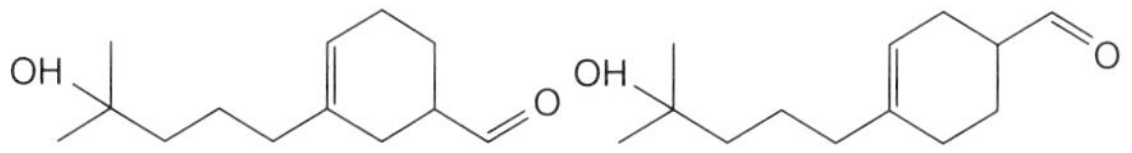

Lyral® is a synthetic blend of two isomers, and one of the most frequently encountered allergen in perfumes. It has to be listed by name in the ingredients of cosmetics in the EU, according to the seventh amendment of the cosmetic directive 76/768/EEC.

Suggested Reading

Johansen JD, Frosch PJ, Svedman C, Andersen KE, Bruze M, Pirker C, Menné T (2003) Hydroxyisohexyl 3-cyclohexene carboxaldehyde – known as Lyral: quantitative aspects and risk assessment of an important fragrance allergen. Contact Dermatitis 48:310–316

243. Hypochlorous Acid and Hypochlorites

Hypochlorous Acid

CAS Registry Number [7790–92–3]

Sodium Hypochlorite

CAS Registry Number [7681–52–9]

Sodium Hypochlorite Hydrate

CAS Registry Number [55248–17–4]

Sodium Hypochlorite Pentahydrate

CAS Registry Number [10022–70–5]

Sodium Hypochlorite Heptahydrate

CAS Registry Number [6431–03–9]

Calcium Hypochlorite

CAS Registry Number [7778–54–3]

Calcium Hypochlorite Dihydroxide

CAS Registry Number [12394–14–8]

Calcium Hypochlorite Dihydrate

CAS Registry Number [22464–76–2]

Calcium Sodium Hypochlorite

CAS Registry Number [53053–57–9]

Lithium Hypochlorite

CAS Registry Number [13840–33–0]

Potassium Hypochlorite

CAS Registry Number [7778–66–7]

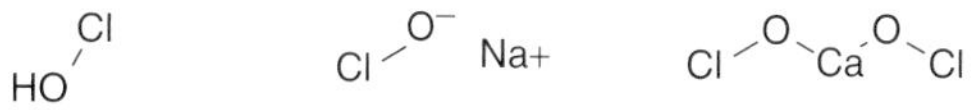

Hypochlorites are derived from hypochlorous acid. They are bleaching agents and have large-spectrum antimicrobial activity. Calcium hypochlorite is used for disinfection in swimming pools and in industrial applications and for pulp and textile bleaching. Sodium hypochlorite is used as household laundry bleach, in commercial laundering, in pulp and paper manufacture, in industrial chemical synthesis, and in the disinfection of drinking water. Lithium hypochlorite is used in swimming pools for disinfection and in household detergents. Hypochlorites have caused hand, diffuse, or periulcerous dermatitis, due to bleach settings and detergents, swimming pool water, endodontic treatment solution, or ulcer treatment.

Suggested Reading

Salphale PS, Shenoi SD (2003) Contact sensitivity to calcium hypochlorite. Contact Dermatitis 48:162
Sasseville D, Geoffrion CT, Lowry RN (1999) Allergic contact dermatitis from chlorinated swimming pool water. Contact Dermatitis 41:347–348

244. Imidazolidinyl Urea

Germall® 115, IMIDUREA®

CAS Registry Number [39236–46–9]

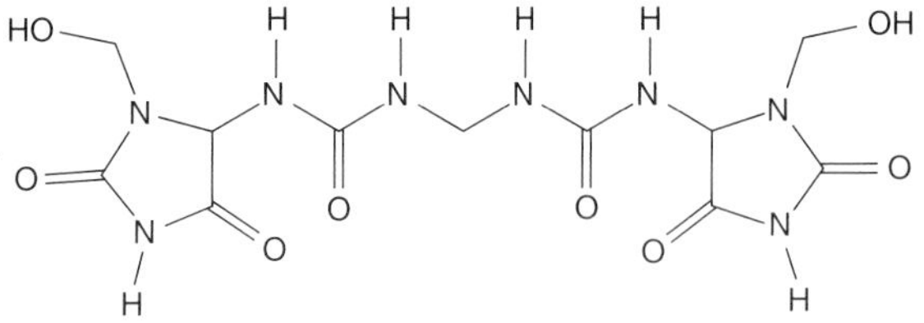

Imidazolidinyl urea, a formaldehyde releaser related to diazolidinyl urea (see above), is used as an antimicrobial agent very active against Gram-positive and Gram-negative bacteria, used as a synergist in combination with parabens. It is used as a preservative in aqueous products, mainly in cosmetics, toiletries, and liquid soaps.

Suggested Reading

Karlberg AT, Skare L, Lindberg I, Nyhammar E (1998) A method for quantification of formaldehyde in the presence of formaldehyde donors in skin-care products. Contact Dermatitis 38:20–28
Lachapelle JM, Ale SI, Freeman S, Frosch PJ, Goh CL, Hannuksela M, Hayakawa R, Maibach HI, Wahlberg JE (1997) Proposal for a revised international standard series of patch tests. Contact Dermatitis 36:121–123
Le Coz CJ (2005) Hypersensibilité à la Diazolidinyl urée et à l'Imidazolidinyl urée. Ann Dermatol Venereol 132:587–588
Van Hecke E, Suys E (1994) Where next to look for formaldehyde? Contact Dermatitis 31:268

245. Iodopropynyl Butylcarbamate

3-Iodo-2-Propynyl-Butyl Carbamate

CAS Registry Number [55406–53–6]

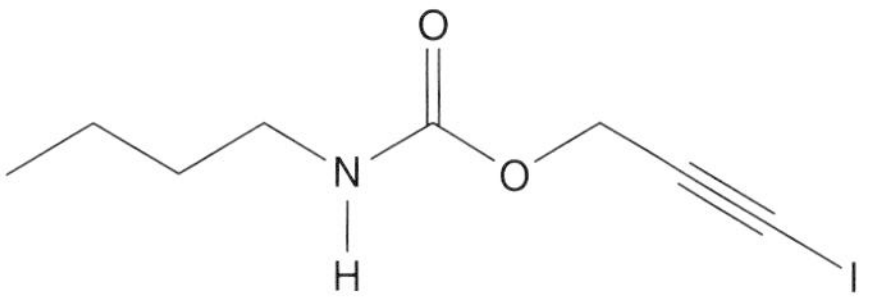

Iodopropynyl butylcarbamate (IPBC) is a broad-spectrum preservative used for years because of its wide field of application, in polymer emulsions and pigment dispersions such as water-based paints and adhesives, cements and inks, as a wood preservative, in metal-working fluids, household products, and cosmetics. Allergic contact dermatitis to IPBC was reported due to cosmetics, from sanitary wipes, and in metalworkers.

Suggested Reading

Badreshia S, Marks JG Jr (2002) Iodopropynyl butylcarbamate. Am J Contact Dermat 13:77–79

Bryld LE, Agner T, Rastogi SC, Menné T (1997) Iodopropynyl butylcarbamate: a new contact allergen. Contact Dermatitis 36:156–158
Majoie IM, van Ginkel CJW (2000) The biocide iodopropynyl butylcarbamate (IPBC) as an allergen in cutting oils. Contact Dermatitis 43:238–239

246. Isoeugenol

Isoeugenol

CAS Registry Number [97–54–1]

cis-isoeugenol

CAS Registry Number [5912–86–7]

trans-Isoeugenol

CAS Registry Number [5932–68–3]

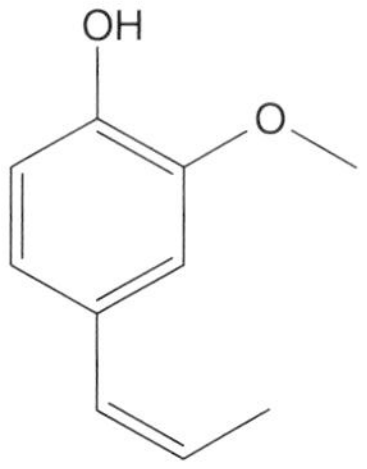

Cis-Isoeugenol

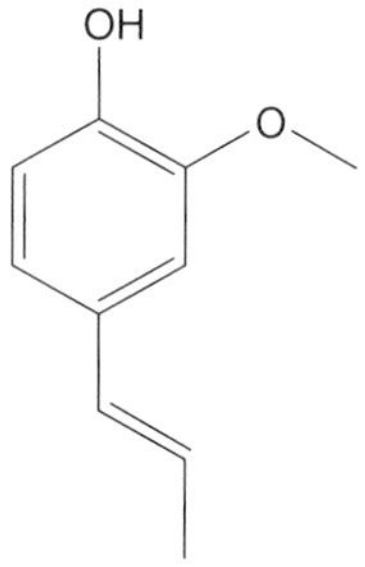

Trans-Isoeugenol

Isoeugenol is a mixture of two *cis* and *trans* isomers. It occurs in ylang-ylang and other essential oils. It is a common allergen of perfumes and cosmetics such as deodorants and is contained in fragrance mix. Its presence in cosmetics is indicated in the INGREDIENTS series. Substitution by esters such as isoeugenyl acetate (not indicated on the package) does not always resolve the allergenic problem, because of the in vivo hydrolysis of the substitute into isoeugenol.

Suggested Reading

Rastogi SC, Johansen JD, Frosch P, Menné T, Bruze M, Lepoittevin JP, Dreier B, Andersen KE, White IR (1998) Deodorants on the European market: quantitative chemical analysis of 21 fragrances. Contact Dermatitis 38:29–35
Tanaka S, Royds C, Buckley D, Basketter DA, Goossens A, Bruze M, Svedman C, Menné T, Johansen JD, White IR, McFadden JP (2004) Contact allergy to isoeugenol and its derivatives: problems with allergen substitution. Contact Dermatitis 51:288–291

58

247. Alpha-Isomethylionone

3-Buten-2-one, 3-Methyl-4-(2,6,6-Trimethyl-2-
Cyclohexen-1-yl), 3-Methyl-4-(2,6,6-Trimethyl-2-
Cyclohexen-1-yl)-3-Buten-2-one, Cetone Alpha

CAS Registry Number [127–51–5]

As a fragrance allergen, α-isomethylionone has to be
mentioned by name in cosmetics within the EU.

Suggested Reading

Frosch PJ (1998) Are major components of fragrances a problem? In: Frosch PJ, Johansen JD, White IR (eds) Fragrances.
Beneficial and adverse effects. Springer, Berlin, pp 92–99

248. Isophorone Diamine

1-Amino-3-Aminomethyl-3,3,5-
Trimethylcyclohexane, 3-Aminomethyl-3,5,5-
Trimethylcyclohexylamine

CAS Registry Number [2855–13–2]

Isophorone diamine is widely used in urethane and
epoxy coatings for light-stable, weather-resistant properties. It is used in water proofing and paving concret-
ing, and in the manufacture of diisocyanates and
polyamides as an epoxy resin hardener. It is a strong
sensitizer and can cause airborne contact dermatitis.

Suggested Reading

Guerra L, Vincenzi, Bardazzi F, Tosti A (1992) Contact sensitization to isophoronediamine. Contact Dermatitis 27:52–53
Kelterer D, Bauer A, Elsner P (2000) Spill-induced sensitization
to isophorone diamine. Contact Dermatitis 43:110
Lodi A, Mancini LL, Pozzi M, Chiarelli G, Crosti C (1993)
Occupational airborne allergic contact dermatitis in parquet
layers. Contact Dermatitis 29:281–282

249. Isopropyl Myristate

Tetradecanoic Acid 1-Methyl Ethyl Ester

CAS Registry Number [110–27–0]

Despite wide use in cosmetics, perfumes, and topical
medicaments, isopropyl myristate is a very weak sensitizer and a mild irritant.

Suggested Reading

Uter W, Schnuch A, Geier J, Lessmann H (2004) Isopropyl
myristate recommended for aimed rather than routine patch
testing. Contact Dermatitis 50:242–244

250. *N*-Isopropyl-*N*-Phenyl-4-Phenylenediamine

IPPD, *N*-Isopropyl-*N*-Phenyl-*p*-Phenylenediamine,
N-(1-Methylethyl)-*N*-Phenyl-1,4-Benzenediamine

CAS Registry Number [101–72–4]

This rubber chemical is used as an antioxidant and
antiozonant. The main occupational sources are tires.

Suggested Reading

Condé-Salazar L, Del-Rio E, Guimaraens D, Gonzalez Domingo
A (1993) Type IV allergy to rubber additives: a 10-year
study of 686 cases. J Am Acad Dermatol 29:176–180
Hervé-Bazin B, Gradiski D, Duprat P, Marignac B, Foussereau
J, Cavelier C, Bieber P (1977) Occupational eczema from
N-isopropyl-*N*-phenylparaphenylenediamine (IPPD) and
N-dimethyl-1,3 butyl-*N*-phenylparaphenylenediamine (DMPPD)
in tyres. Contact Dermatitis 3:1–15
Von Hintzenstern J, Heese A, Koch HU, Peters KP, Hornstein
OP (1991) Frequency, spectrum and occupational relevance
of type IV allergies to rubber chemicals. Contact Dermatitis
24:244–252

251. Ketoprofen

CAS Registry Number [22071–15–4]

Ketoprofen is an anti-inflammatory drug, used both topically and systemically. It is above all a photoallergen, responsible for photoallergic or photo-worsened contact dermatitis, with sun-induced, progressive, severe, and durable reactions. Recurrent photosensitivity is possible for many years. Photosensitivities are expected to thiophene-phenylketone derivatives such as tiaprofenic acid and suprofen, to ketoprofen esters such as piketoprofen, and to benzophenone derivatives (see above) such as fenofibrate and benzophenone-3. Concomitant photosensitivities – without clinical relevance – have been observed to fenticlor, tetrachlorosalicylanilide, triclosan, tribromsalan, and bithionol.

Suggested Reading

Durbize E, Vigan M, Puzenat E, Girardin P, Adessi B, Desprez P, Humbert P, Laurent R, Aubin F (2003) Spectrum of cross-photosensitization in 18 consecutive patients with contact photoallergy to ketoprofen: associated photoallergies to nonbenzophenone-containing molecules. Contact Dermatitis 48:144–149
Le Coz CJ, Bottlaender A, Scrivener JN, Santinelli F, Cribier BJ, Heid E, Grosshans EM (1998) Photocontact dermatitis from ketoprofen and tiaprofenic acid: cross-reactivity study in 12 consecutive patients. Contact Dermatitis 38:245–252
Le Coz CJ, El Aboubi S, Lefèbvre C, Heid E, Grosshans E (2000) Topical ketoprofen induces persistent and recurrent photosensitivity. Contact Dermatitis 42(suppl 2):46
Le Coz CJ, El Aboubi S, Lefèbvre C, Heid E, Grosshans E (2000) Photoallergy from topical ketoprofen: a clinical, allergological and photobiological study. Contact Dermatitis 42(suppl 2):47

252. Labetalol

CAS Registry Number [36894–69–6]

This beta-adrenergic and alpha-1 blocking agent caused contact dermatitis and a contact anaphylactoid reaction during patch testing in a nurse.

Suggested Reading

Bause GS, Kugelman LC (1990) Contact anaphylactoid response to labetalol. Contact Dermatitis 23:51

253. Lactucin

CAS Registry Number [1891–29–8]

Lactucin, as lactucopicrin, is a sesquiterpene lactone contained in lettuce (*Lactuca sativa* L.).

Suggested Reading

Paulsen E, Andersen KE, Hausen BM (1993) Compositae dermatitis in a Danish dermatology department in one year (I). Results of routine patch testing with the sesquiterpene lactone mix supplemented with aimed patch testing with extracts and sesquiterpene lactones of Compositae plants. Contact Dermatitis 29:6–10

254. Lactucopicrin

Intybin

CAS Registry Number [6466–74–6]

Lactucopicrin, as lactucin, is a sesquiterpene lactone extracted from various *Lactuca* spp. and *Cichorium intybus* L., Asteraceae–Compositae family.

Suggested Reading

Bischoff TA, Kelley CJ, Karchesy Y, Laurantos M, Nguyen-Dinh P, Arefi AG (2004) Antimalarial activity of lactucin and lactucopicrin: sesquiterpene lactones isolated from *Cichorium intybus* L. J Ethnopharmacol 95: 455–457

255. Lapachenol

CAS Registry Number [573–13–7]

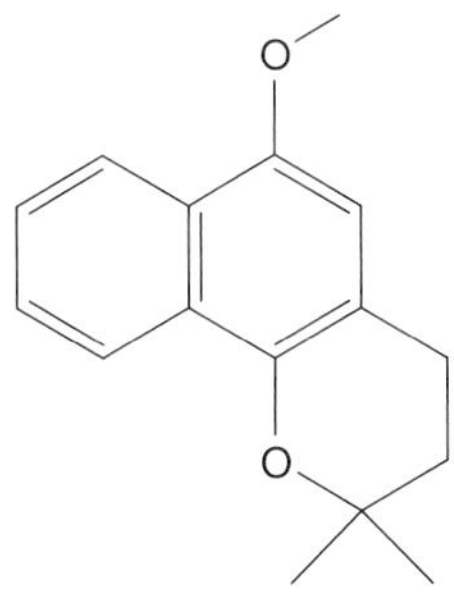

Lapachenol is contained in the heart-wood of Lapacho wood (*Tabebuia avellanedae* Lorentz, Bignoniaceae family). It is a secondary allergen, after lapachol and deoxylapachol, and likely a prohapten transformed in vivo into a quinone hapten.

Suggested Reading

Hausen BM (1981) Wood injurious to human health. A manual. De Gruyter, Berlin

256. Lapachol

2-Hydroxy-3-(3-Methyl-2-Butenyl)-1,4-Naphthoquinone, CI 75490, CI Natural Yellow 16

CAS Registry Number [84–79–7]

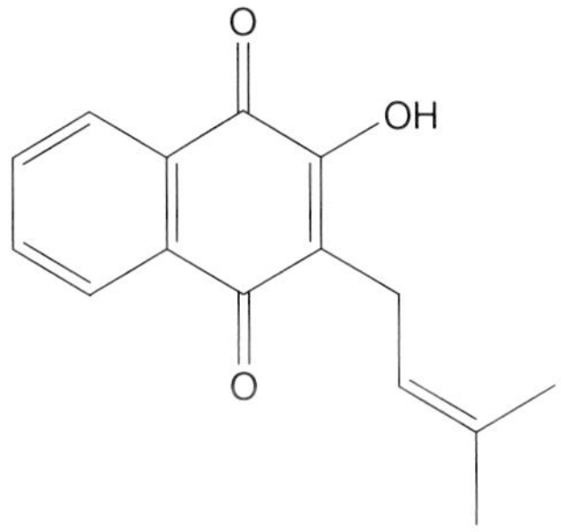

Lapachol, a benzoquinone, is a secondary allergen in teak (*Tectona grandis* L., Verbenaceae family), a wood largely used for various indoor and outdoor applications (doors, windows, etc.) because of its strong durability. It has similar reactivity to deoxylapachol. See also Chap. 46.

Suggested Reading

Estlander T, Jolanki R, Alanko K, Kanerva L (2001) Occupational allergic contact dermatitis caused by wood dusts. Contact Dermatitis 44:213–217
Lamminpää A, Estlander T, Jolanki R, Kanerva L (1996) Occupational allergic contact dermatitis caused by decorative plants. Contact Dermatitis 34:330–335

257. Lawsone

2-Hydroxy-1,4-Naphthalenedione, Henna

CAS Registry Number [83–72–7]

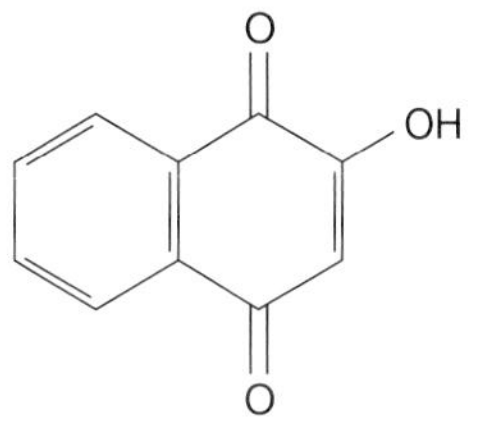

Henna, prepared by powdering the dried leaves of henna plant (*Lawsonia inermis* L.), is used for coloring and conditioning hair and nails, particularly by Muslims or Hindus. It contains Lawsone, which very rarely induces contact allergy. Most dermatitis caused by "black henna" is due to PPD and derivatives.

Suggested Reading

Le Coz CJ, Lefebvre C, Keller F, Grosshans E (2000) Allergic contact dermatitis caused by skin painting (pseudotattooing) with black henna, a mixture of henna and *p*-phenylenediamine and its derivatives. Arch Dermatol 136: 1515–1517
Pasricha JS, Gupta R, Panjwani S (1980) Contact dermatitis to henna (*Lawsonia*). Contact Dermatitis 6:288–290

258. Lidocaine

Lidocaine

CAS Registry Number [137–58–6]

Lidocaine Hydrochloride Monohydrate

CAS Registry Number [6108–05–0]

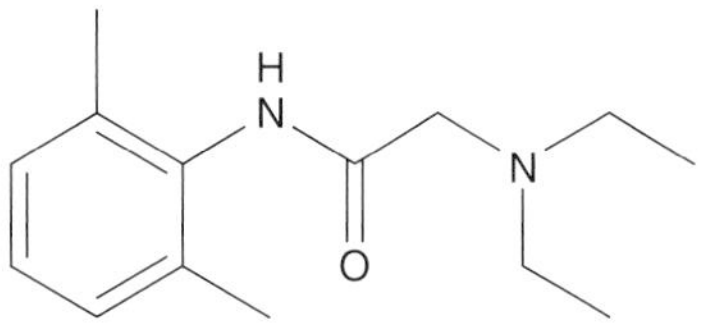

Lidocaine is an anesthetic of the amide group, like articaine or bupivacaine. Immediate-type IgE-dependent
reactions are rare, and delayed-type contact dermatitis
is exceptional. Cross-reactivity between the different
amide anesthetics is not systematic.

Suggested Reading

Duque S, Fernandez L (2004) Delayed hypersensitivity to amide
    local anesthetics. Allergol Immunopathol (Madr) 32:233–234
Waton J, Boulanger A, Trechot PH, Schmutz JL, Barbaud A (2004)
    Contact urticaria from Emla® cream. Contact Dermatitis
    51:284–287

259. Lilial®

See 76. *p-tert*-Butyl-alpha-Methylhydrocinnamic
Aldehyde.

260. Limonene

Limonene: *D*-Limonene + *l*-Limonene

CAS Registry Number [138–86–3]

D-Limonene: (+)-Limonene, *R*-Limonene,
α-Limonene, (*R*)-*p*-Mentha-1,8-Diene, Dipentene,
Carvene, Citrene

CAS Registry Number [5989–27–5]

l-Limonene: (−)-Limonene, *S*-Limonene, β-Limonene,
4-(*S*)-1-Methyl-4-(1-Methylethenyl)-Cyclohexene

CAS Registry Number [5989–54–8]

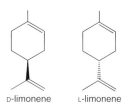

Limonene is a racemic form of D- and L-limonene.
D-Limonene is contained in *Citrus* species such as citrus, orange, mandarin, and bergamot. L-Limonene is
contained in *Pinus pinea*. The racemic form (D- and
L-limonene) is also named dipentene. D-limonene, used
as a solvent, may be found in cleansing or in degreasing agents. Its sensitizing potential increases with prolonged air contact, which induces oxidation and leads
to oxidation products. The presence of D-limonene has
to be mentioned by name in cosmetics of the EU.

Suggested Reading

Karlberg AT, Magnusson K, Nilsson U (1992) Air oxidation of
    d-limonene (the citrus solvent) creates potent allergens.
    Contact Dermatitis 26:332–340
Karlberg AT, Dooms-Goossens A (1997) Contact allergy to oxi-
    dized d-limonene among dermatitis patients. Contact
    Dermatitis 36:201–206
Meding B, Barregard L, Marcus K (1994) Hand eczema in car
    mechanics. Contact Dermatitis 30:129–134

261. Linalool

3,7-Dimethyl-1,6-octadien-3-ol, Linalyl alcohol,
2,6-Dimethyl-2,7-octadien-6-ol

CAS Registry Number [78–70–6]

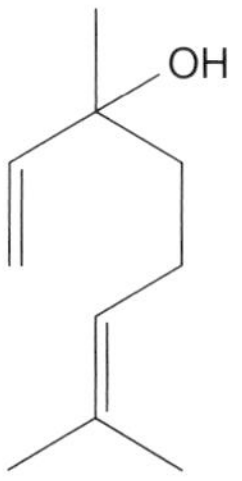

Linalool is a terpene chief constituent of linaloe oil,
also found in oils of Ceylon cinnamon, sassafras,
orange flower, bergamot, *Artemisia balchanorum*,
ylang-ylang. This frequently used scented substance is
a sensitizer by the way of primary or secondary oxidation products. As a fragrance allergen, linalool has to
be mentioned by name in cosmetics within the EU.

Suggested Reading

Kanerva L, Estlander T, Jolanki R (1995) Occupational allergic contact dermatitis caused by ylang-ylang oil. Contact Dermatitis 33:198–199

Skold M, Borje A, Harambasic E, Karlberg AT (2004) Contact allergens formed on air exposure of linalool. Identification and quantification of primary and secondary oxidation products and the effect on skin sensitization. Chem Res Toxicol 17:1697–1705

262. Linalyl acetate

CAS Registry Number [115-95-7]

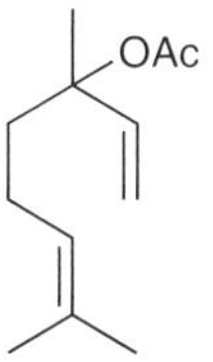

Structurally close to linalool, linalyl acetate is the main component of lavender oil and is commonly used in fragrances and toiletries, and in household cleaners and detergents as well. By autoxidation, it leads mainly to hydroperoxides, with a high sensitizing potent.

Suggested Reading

Sköld M, Hagvall L, Karlberg AT (2008) Autoxidation of linalyl acetate, the main component of lavender oil, creates potent contact allergens. Contact Dermatitis 58:9–14

263. Lincomycin (Hydrochloride Monohydrate)

Lincomycin

CAS Registry Number [154–21–2]

Lincomycin Hydrochloride Monohydrate

CAS Registry Number [7179–49–9]

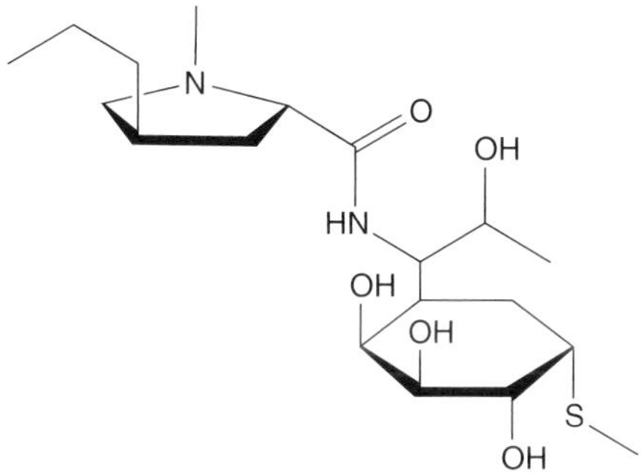

Lincomycin is an antibiotic of the lincosanide group, active against Gram-positive bacteria. Occupational exposure occurs in poultry and pig breeders.

Suggested Reading

Vilaplana J, Romaguera C, Grimalt F (1991) Contact dermatitis from lincomycin and spectinomycin in chicken vaccinators. Contact Dermatitis 24:225–226

264. Lindane

γ-1,2,3,4,5,6-Hexachlorocyclohexane

CAS Registry Number [58–89–9]

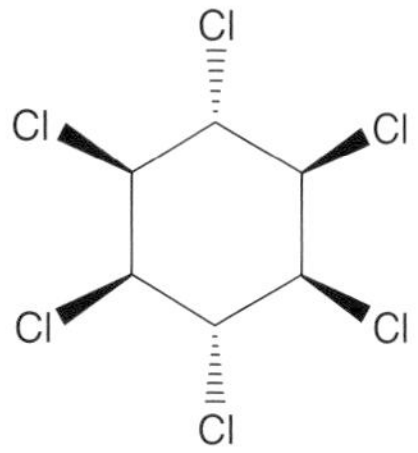

Lindane is a pesticide used for its antiinsect properties in agriculture, wood protection, in antiinsect paints, and veterinary and human medicine against many insects such as spiders, mosquitoes, ticks, scabies, lice, and demodicidosis. Its use is controlled, particularly because of neurological toxicity.

Suggested Reading

Anon (1992) Fiche toxicologique n 81. Cahiers documentaires de l'INRS

Sharma VK, Kaur S (1990) Contact sensitization by pesticides in farmers. Contact Dermatitis 23:77–80

265. Lyral®

See 242. Hydroxymethylpentacyclohexenecarboxaldehyde.

266. Malathion

Carbetox, Carbofos, Chemathion, Cimexan, Dorthion, Extermathion, Fosfotion

CAS Registry Number [121–75–5]

This organophosphorus pesticide is used as an insecticide and an acaricide, particularly against head lice. Sensitization was reported in farmers.

Suggested Reading

O'Malley M, Rodriguez P, Maibach HI (1995) Pesticide patch testing: California nursery workers and controls. Contact Dermatitis 32:61–62

Sharma VK, Kaur S (1990) Contact sensitization by pesticides in farmers. Contact Dermatitis 23:77–80

267. Mancozeb

Zinc Manganese Ethylenebisdithiocarbamate

CAS Registry Number [8018–01–7]

Mancozeb is a fungicide of the ethylene-bis-dithiocarbamate group. It is present in Rondo-M® with pyrifenox. Occupational exposure occurs mainly in agricultural workers, in vineyard workers, or in florists.

Suggested Reading

Crippa M, Misquith L, Lonati A, Pasolini G (1990) Dyshidrotic eczema and sensitization to dithiocarbamates in a florist. Contact Dermatitis 23:203–204

Iliev D, Elsner P (1997) Allergic contact from the fungicide Rondo-M® and the insecticide Alfacron®. Contact Dermatitis 36:51

Jung HD, Honemann W, Kloth C, Lubbe D, Pambor M, Quednow C, Ratz KH, Rothe A, Tarnick M (1989) Kontaktekzem durch Pestizide in der Deutschen Demokratischen Republik. Dermatol Monatsschr 175:203–214

Koch P (1996) Occupational allergic contact dermatitis and airborne contact dermatitis from 5 fungicides in a vineyard worker. Cross-reactions between fungicides of the dithiocarbamate group? Contact Dermatitis 34:324–329

268. Maneb

Ethylenebisdithiocarbamate Manganese

CAS Registry Number [12427–38–2]

Maneb is a pesticide with fungicide properties, belonging to the dithiocarbamate group. Sensitization occurs mainly in farmers and agricultural workers.

Suggested Reading

Crippa M, Misquith L, Lonati A, Pasolini G (1990) Dyshidrotic eczema and sensitization to dithiocarbamates in a florist. Contact Dermatitis 23:203–204

Jung HD, Honemann W, Kloth C, Lubbe D, Pambor M, Quednow C, Ratz KH, Rothe A, Tarnick M (1989) Kontaktekzem durch Pestizide in der Deutschen Demokratischen Republik. Dermatol Monatsschr 175:203–214

Koch P (1996) Occupational allergic contact dermatitis and airborne contact dermatitis from 5 fungicides in a vineyard worker. Cross-reactions between fungicides of the dithiocarbamate group? Contact Dermatitis 34:324–329

O'Malley M, Rodriguez P, Maibach HI (1995) Pesticide patch testing: California nursery workers and controls. Contact Dermatitis 32:61–62

Peluso AM, Tardio M, Adamo F, Venturo N (1991) Multiple sensitization due to bis-dithiocarbamate and thiophthalimide pesticides. Contact Dermatitis 25:327

Piraccini BM, Cameli N, Peluso AM, Tardio M (1991) A case of allergic contact dermatitis due to the pesticide maneb. Contact Dermatitis 24:381–382

Sharma VK, Kaur S (1990) Contact sensitization by pesticides in farmers. Contact Dermatitis 23:77–80

269. Melamine and Melamine-Formaldehyde Resins

Melamine: 2,4,6-Triaminotriazine

CAS Registry Number [108–78–1]

Melamine-formaldehyde resin (MFR) results from condensation of melamine and formaldehyde. It is an active ingredient of strong (reinforced) plasters, such as industrial or some dental plasters used for molding. It is also used as a textile finish resin. MFR acts as an allergen generally because of formaldehyde releasing (see Chap. 40).

Suggested Reading

Aalto-Korte K, Jolanki R, Estlander T (2003) Formaldehyde-negative allergic contact dermatitis from melamine-formaldehyde resin. Contact Dermatitis 49:194–196

Garcia Bracamonte B, Ortiz de Frutos FJ, Iglesias Diez L (1995) Occupational allergic contact dermatitis due to formaldehyde and textile finish resins. Contact Dermatitis 33:139–140

Lewis FM, Cork MJ, McDonagh AJG, Gawkrodger DJG (1993) Allergic contact dermatitis from resin-reinforced plaster. Contact Dermatitis 28:40–41

Rustemeyer T, Frosch PJ (1996) Occupational skin diseases in dental laboratory technicians. (I). Clinical picture and causative factors. Contact Dermatitis 34:125–133

270. Mercaptobenzothiazole

2-Mercaptobenzothiazole, MBT

CAS Registry Number [149–30–4]

MBT is a rubber chemical, accelerant of vulcanization, and contained in "mercapto-mix." The most frequent occupational categories are the metal industry, homemakers, health services and laboratories, the building industry, and shoemakers. It is also used as a corrosion inhibitor in cutting fluids or in releasing fluids in the pottery industry.

Suggested Reading

Condé-Salazar L, Del-Rio E, Guimaraens D, Gonzalez Domingo A (1993) Type IV allergy to rubber additives: a 10-year study of 686 cases. J Am Acad Dermatol 29:176–180

Mancuso G, Reggiani M, Berdondini RM (1996) Occupational dermatitis in shoemakers. Contact Dermatitis 34:17–22

Von Hintzenstern J, Heese A, Koch HU, Peters KP, Hornstein OP (1991) Frequency, spectrum and occupational relevance of type IV allergies to rubber chemicals. Contact Dermatitis 24:244–252

Wilkinson SM, Cartwright PH, English JSC (1990) Allergic contact dermatitis from mercaptobenzothiazole in a releasing fluid. Contact Dermatitis 23:370

271. Mercaptobenzothiazole Salts

Mercaptobenzothiazole, Sodium Salt

CAS Registry Numbers [2492–26–4]

Mercaptobenzothiazole, Zinc Salt

CAS Registry Number [155–04–4]

Such mercaptobenzothiazole hydrosoluble salts are used as antioxidants and biocides in cutting fluids and greases, paints, or glues.

Suggested Reading

Le Coz CJ (2004) Fiche d'éviction en cas d'hypersensibilité au mercaptobenzothiazole et au mercapto mix. Ann Dermatol Venereol 131:1012–1014

272. MESNA

Sodium 2-Mercaptoethane Sulfonate

CAS Registry Number [19767–45–4]

Mesna is used as a mucolytic agent, and as an antidote to chloro-acetyl-aldehyde and acrolein (a bladder toxic metabolite of ifosfamide or cyclophosphamide). It has been reported as a cause of occupational allergic (hand and airborne) dermatitis in nurses.

Suggested Reading

Benyoussef K, Bottlaender A, Pfister HR, Caussade P, Heid E, Grosshans E (1996) Allergic contact dermatitis from mesna. Contact Dermatitis 34:228–229

Kiec-Swierczynska M, Krecisz B (2003) Occupational airborne allergic contact dermatitis from mesna. Contact Dermatitis 48:171

58

273. Metacresol

3-Cresol, 3-Methylphenol, *m*-Cresol

CAS Registry Number [108–39–4]

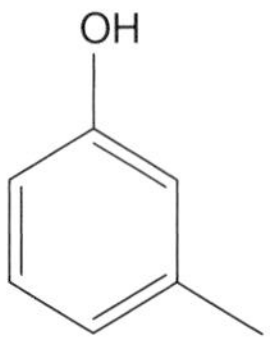

Metacresol is contained as a preservative in almost all human insulin. It has been reported as a cause of allergic reaction due to injected insulin.

Suggested Reading

Clerx V, van den Keybus C, Kochuyt A, Goossens A (2003) Drug intolerance reaction to insulin therapy caused by metacresol. Contact Dermatitis 48:162–163

274. Metanil Yellow

Acid Yellow 36, CI 13065

CAS Registry Number [587–98–4]

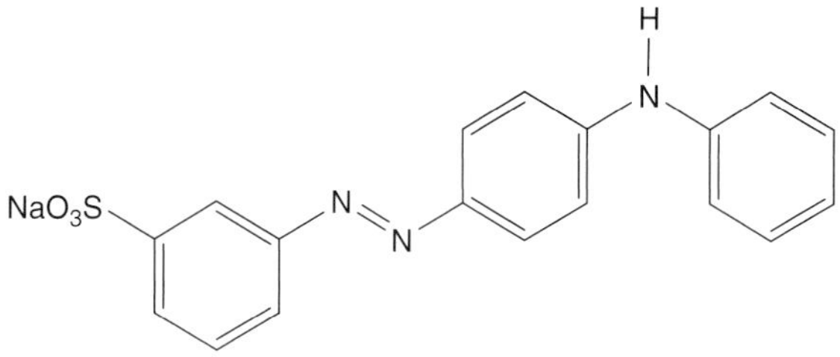

Metanil yellow is a yellow monoazoic dye. This coloring agent is used in leather and wood stains, and is also employed as a food dye in India.

Suggested Reading

Hausen BM (1994) A case of allergic contact dermatitis due to metanil yellow. Contact Dermatitis 31:117–118

275. Methenamine

Hexamethylenetetramine

CAS Registry Number [100–97–0]

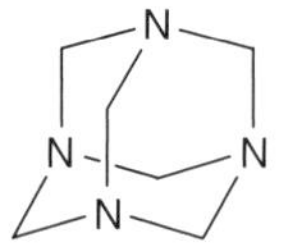

Hexamethylenetetramine is used in the foundry, tire and rubber, and phenol formaldehyde resins industries and in other applications such as a hardener in epoxy resins Bisphenol A type and as an anticorrosive agent. It is an ammonia and formaldehyde releaser sometimes used in topical medicaments and cosmetics.

Suggested Reading

Gonzalez-Perez R, Gonzalez-Hermosa R, Aseginolaza B, Luis Diaz-Ramon J, Soloeta R (2003) Allergic contact dermatitis from methenamine in an antiperspirant spray. Contact Dermatitis 49:266
Holness DL, Nethercott JR (1993) The performance of specialized collections of bisphenol A epoxy resin system components in the evaluation of workers in an occupational health clinic population. Contact Dermatitis 28:216–219

276. Methidathion

Somonil, Supracid, Suprathion, Ultracid

CAS Registry Number [950–37–8]

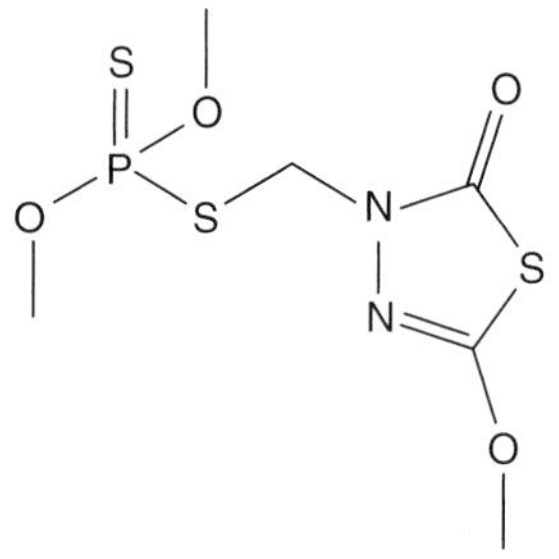

Methidation is an organophosphorus compound used as an insecticide. Cross-sensitivity was described to Dichlorvos.

Suggested Reading

Ueda A, Aoyama K, Manda F, Ueda T, Kawahara Y (1994) Delayed-type allergenicity of triforine (Saprol®). Contact Dermatitis 31:140–145

277. Methiocarb

3,5-Dimethyl-4-(Methylthio)Phenol Methylcarbamate, Mesurol

CAS Registry Number [2032–65–7]

Methiocarb is an insecticide or molluscicide with a cholinesterase inhibiting effect. A case of contact dermatitis was reported in a carnation grower.

Suggested Reading

Willems PWJM, Geursen-Reitsma AM, van Joost T (1997) Allergic contact dermatitis due to methiocarb (Mesurol). Contact Dermatitis 36:270

278. Methomyl

S-Methyl-N-(Methylcarbamoyloxy)-Thioacetimidate, Lannate

CAS Registry Number [16752–77–5]

Methomyl is a pesticide agent, a carbamate insecticide with anticholinesterase activity. This mixture of two stereoisomers is used as a foliar spray to control field crops, in stables and poultry houses, and in glasshouses on ornamentals and vegetables, or in flypapers. Cases were reported in chrysanthemum growers and in two women working in a plant nursery.

Suggested Reading

Bruynzeel DP (1991) Contact sensitivity to Lannate®. Contact Dermatitis 25:60–61

279. (R)-4-Methoxy Dalbergione

CAS Registry Numbers [4640–26–0] [28396–75–0]

(R)-4-Methoxy dalbergione is the main allergen of *Dalbergia nigra* All. (Brazilian rosewood, palissander) and *Dalbergia latifolia* Roxb. (East Indian rosewood). Occupational sensitization occurs in timber workers. See also Chap. 46.

Suggested Reading

Gallo R, Guarrera M, Hausen BM (1996) Airborne contact dermatitis from East Indian rosewood (*Dalbergia latifolia* Roxb.). Contact Dermatitis 35:60–61
Hausen BM (2000) Woods. In: Kanerva L, Elsner P, Wahlberg JE, Maibach HI (eds) Handbook of occupational dermatology. Springer, Berlin, pp 771–780

280. Methoxy PEG-17/Dodecyl Glycol Copolymer

CAS Registry Number [88507–00–0]

Methoxy PEG-17/dodecyl glycol copolymer is one of the numerous copolymers recorded in the International Nomenclature of Cosmetics Ingredients (INCI) inventory system. It belongs to the chemical class of alkoxylated alcohols. It is utilized as an emulsion stabilizer, a skin-conditioning, and a viscosity-increasing agent in cosmetics.

Suggested Reading

Le Coz CJ, Heid E (2001) Allergic contact dermatitis from methoxy PEG-17/dodecyl glycol copolymer (Elfacos® OW 100). Contact Dermatitis 44:308–309

281. Methoxypsoralens

5-Methoxypsoralen, Bergapten(e)

CAS Registry Number [484–20–8]

8-Methoxypsoralen, Methoxsalen, Meladinin, Xanthotoxin

CAS Registry Number [298–81–7]

5-MOP   8-MOP

These fur(an)ocoumarins are phototoxic compounds that cause phototoxic dermatitis. Many plants of the Apiaceae–Umbelliferae and most of the Rutaceae family contain 5-methoxypsoralen and 8-methoxypsoralen. Their spectra is in the UVA range (300–360 nm). They are used in combination with UVA to treat various skin disorders such as psoriasis. See also Chap. 46.

Suggested Reading

Ena P, Camarda I (1990) Phytophotodermatitis from *Ruta corsica*. Contact Dermatitis 22:63
Ena P, Cerri R, Dessi G, Manconi PM, Atzei AD (1991) Phototoxicity due to *Cachrys libanotis*. Contact Dermatitis 24:1–5

282. Methyl aminolevulinate

CAS Registry Number [33320-16-0]

Suggested Reading

Korshøj S, Sølvsten H, Erlandsen M, Sommerlund M (2009) Frequency of sensitization to methyl aminolaevulinate after photodynamic therapy. Contact Dermatitis 60:320–324

Jungersted JM, Dam TN, Bryld LE, Agner T (2008) Allergic reactions to Metvix (ALA-ME). Contact Dermatitis 58:184–186

283. Methyl-2,3-Epoxy-3-(4-Methoxyphenyl) Propionate

3-(-Methoxyphenyl)Glycidic Acid Methylester, Methyl 3-(p-Methoxyphenyl)Oxirane-2-Carboxylate

CAS Registry Number [42245–42–1]

Methyl 2,3 epoxy-3-(4-methoxyphenyl)propionate is an intermediate product in the synthesis of diltiazem hydrochloride. Contact dermatitis was observed in several laboratory technicians.

Suggested Reading

Rudzki E, Rebandel P (1990) Dermatitis from methyl 2,3 epoxy-3-(4-methoxyphenyl)propionate. Contact Dermatitis 23:382

284. Methyl Gallate

CAS Registry Number [99–24–1]

This ester of gallic acid is used as an antioxidant agent. A case was reported by using a reprography paper.

Suggested Reading

Degos R, Lépine J, Akhoundzadeh H (1968) Sensibilisation cutanée due à la manipulation de papier reprographie. Bull Soc Fr Dermatol 75:595–596

285. Methyl Heptine Carbonate

Methyl oct-2-ynoate, Folione

CAS Registry Number [111–12–6]

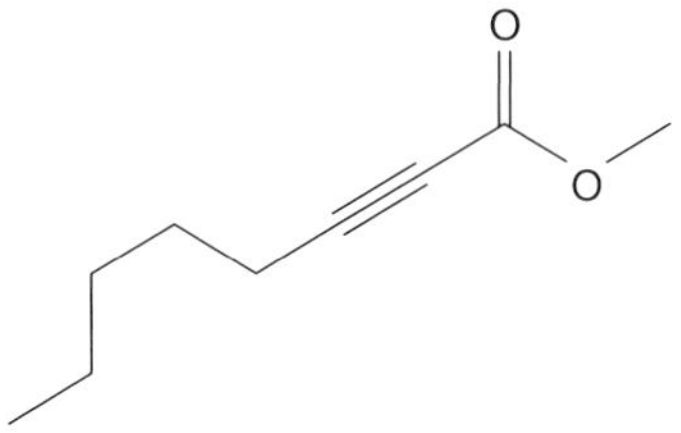

This perfumed molecule belongs to the list of 26 allergens that have to be indicated by name on the ingredients list of cosmetics in the EU.

Suggested Reading

English JS, Rycroft RJ (1988) Allergic contact dermatitis from methyl heptine and methyl octine carbonates. Contact Dermatitis 18:174–175

286. Methyl Octine Carbonate

Methyl non-2-ynoate

CAS Registry Number [111–80–8]

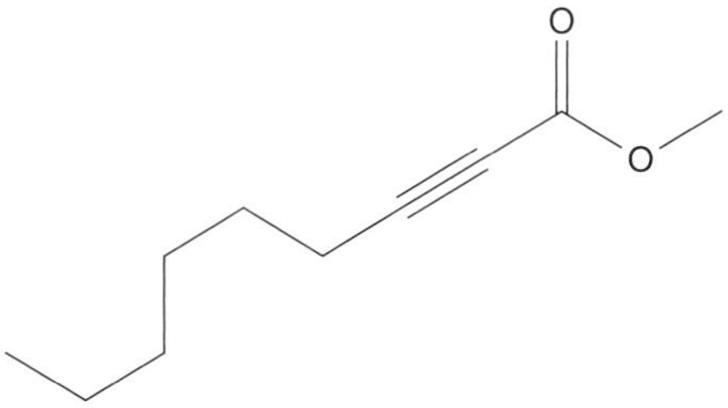

This perfumed molecule is related to methyl heptine carbonate. Cross-reactivity is frequent.

Suggested Reading

English JS, Rycroft RJ (1988) Allergic contact dermatitis from methyl heptine and methyl octine carbonates. Contact Dermatitis 18:174–175

287. Methyl Salicylate

CAS Registry Number [119–36–8]

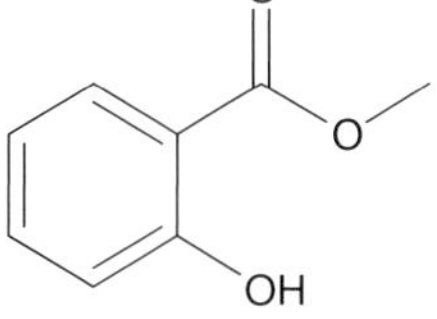

This anti-inflammatory agent is found in a wide number of ointments and can induce allergic contact dermatitis.

Suggested Reading

Hindson C (1977) Contact eczema from methyl salicylate reproduced by oral aspirin (acetyl salicylic acid). Contact Dermatitis 3:348–349
Oiso N, Fulai K, Ishii M (2004) Allergic contact dermatitis due to methyl salicylate in a compress. Contact Dermatitis 51:34–35

288. Methyl-Terpyridine

2,2:6,2,-(4-Methyl)-*ter*-Pyridine), 4-Methyl (2,2,2-Terpyridine)

CAS Registry Number for 2,2,2-Terpyridine [1148–79–4]

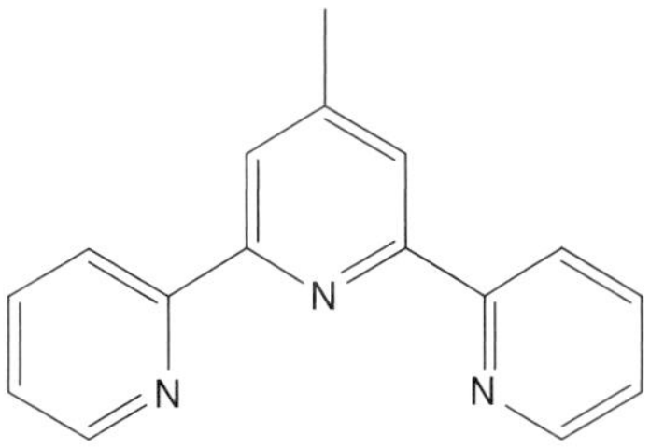

This molecule is a terpyridine with a 4-methyl substitution. A case of occupational dermatitis was reported in a chemical technician with no cross-reactivity to pyridine derivatives.

Suggested Reading

Le Coz CJ, Caussade P, Bottlaender A (1998) Occupational contact dermatitis from methyl-*ter*-pyridine in a chemistry laboratory technician. Contact Dermatitis 38:214–215

58

289. 2-Methyl-4,5-Trimethylene-4-Isothiazolin-3-one

CAS Registry Number [82633–79–2]

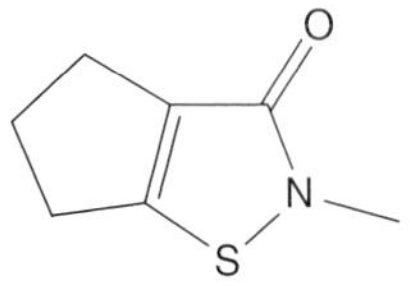

This biocide induced contact dermatitis in a laboratory technician, also sensitive to the other isothiazolinone BIT.

Suggested Reading

Burden AD, O'Driscoll JB, Page FC, Beck MH (1994) Contact hypersensitivity to a new isothiazolinone. Contact Dermatitis 30:179–180

290. Methylchloroisothiazolinone

Chloromethylisothiazolinone, 5-Chloro-2-Methyl-4-Isothiazolin-3-one, MCI

CAS Registry Number [26172–55–4]

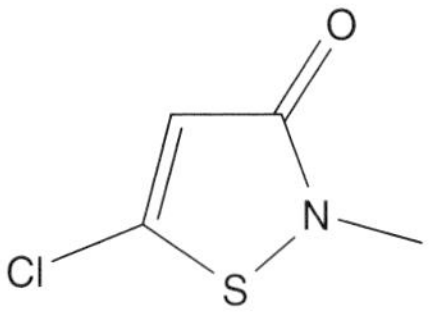

MCI is mainly associated with methylisothiazolinone for its bactericidal and fongistatic properties. It is found in Kathon® CG or derivatives. MCI is found in water-based products such as cosmetics, paints, and glues. Pure MCI is highly irritant and may cause active sensitization.

Suggested Reading

Nielsen H (1994) Occupational exposure to isothiazolinones. A study based on a product register. Contact Dermatitis 31: 18–21
Schubert H (1997) Airborne contact dermatitis due to methylchloro and methylisothiazolinone (MCI/MI). Contact Dermatitis 36:274
Tay P, Ng SK (1994) Delayed skin burns from MCI/MI biocide used in water treatment. Contact Dermatitis 30:54–55

291. Methylchloroisothiazolinone + Methylsiothiazolinone (MCI/MI)

CAS Registry Numbers [55965–84–9], [96118–96–6]

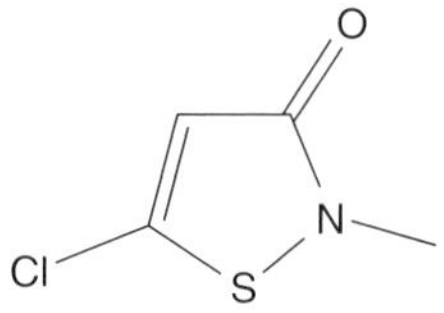

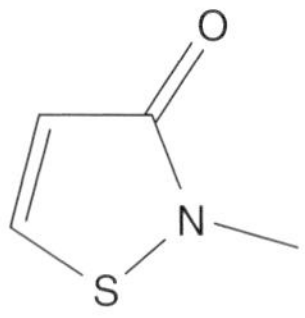

Kathon® CG (CG=cosmetic grade) is a 3:1 mixture of CMI and MI, at a 1.5% concentration. It is used for cosmetics and toiletries, metalworking fluids or paints, in which it can be added only periodically or in color film developers. Kathon® 886 MW (MW=metalworking fluids) is a mixture CMI/MI mixture at a 13.9% concentration, mainly contained in metalworking fluids. Kathon® FP 1.5 contains MCI/MI at 1.5% concentration in propylene glycol. Kathon® LX (LX=LateX) contains MCI/MI at a tenfold concentration of Kathon® CG. Kathon® WT (WT=water treatment) is a MCI/MI mixture used in the paper industry. Parmetol® K40, Parmethol® DF 12 and Parmetol® DF 35, Parmetol® A 23, Parmetol® K50, and Parmetol® DF 18 are other brand names of MCI/MI.

Suggested Reading

Björkner B, Bruze M, Dahlquist I, Fregert S, Gruvberger B, Persson K (1986) Contact allergy to the preservative Kathon® CG. Contact Dermatitis 14:85–90
Fernandez de Corres L, Navarro JA, Gastaminza G, del Pozo MD (1995) An unusual case of sensitization to methylchloro and methyl-isothiazolinone (MCI/MI). Contact Dermatitis 33:215
Pazzaglia M, Vincenzi C, Gasparri F, Tosti A (1996) Occupational hypersensitivity to isothiazolinone derivatives in a radiology technician. Contact Dermatitis 34:143–144
Scheman AJ, Katta R (1997) Photographic allergens: an update. Contact Dermatitis 37:130

292. Methyldibromoglutaronitrile

1,2-Dibromo 2,4-Dicyanobutane

CAS Registry Number [35691–65–7]

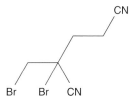

Methyldibromoglutaronitrile is a biocide widely used as a preservative agent in cosmetics, toiletries, and metalworking fluids. It is a potent allergen, banned in all cosmetics in the EU since 2007.

Suggested Reading

Aalto-Korte K, Jolanki R, Estlander T, Alanko K, Kanerva L (1996) Occupational allergic contact dermatitis caused by Euxyl K 400. Contact Dermatitis 35:193–194

Kynemund Pedersen L, Agner T, Held E, Johansen JD (2004) Methyldibromoglutaronitrile in leave-on products elicits contact allergy at low concentration. Br J Dermatol 151:817–822

Le Coz CJ (2005) Hypersensibilité au méthyldibromoglutaronitrile (Dibromodicyanobutane). Ann Dermatol Venereol 132:496–497

293. Methylhexahydrophthalic Anhydride

1,3-Isobenzofurandione, Hexahydromethyl

CAS Registry Numbers [19438–60–9] [39363–62–7], [86403–41–0], [95032–44–3]

Methylhexahydrophthalic anhydride is an epoxy hardener, irritant to skin and mucous membranes. It is included in nondiglycidyl-ether-of-bisphenol-A epoxy resins. It can induce both allergic contact dermatitis and immunologic contact urticaria. It is structurally close to methyltetrahydrophthalic anhydride, which can also cause sensitization.

Suggested Reading

Kanerva L, Jolanki R, Estlander T (1997) Allergic contact dermatitis from nondiglycidyl-ether-of-bisphenol-A epoxy resins. Contact Dermatitis 36:34–38

Tarvainen K, Jolanki R, Estlander T, Tupasela O, Pfäffli P, Kanerva L (1995) Immunologic contact urticaria due to airborne methylhexahydrophthalic and methyltetrahydrophthalic anhydrides. Contact Dermatitis 32:204–209

294. Methylisothiazolinone

2-Methyl-4-Isothiazolin-3-one, MI

CAS Registry Number [2682–20–4]

MI is generally associated with MCI, in Kathon® CG, MCI/MI, and Euxyl® K 100. This preservative is currently used in water-based products such as cosmetics, paints, and glues. Skin contact with concentrated solution can cause severe irritant dermatitis.

Suggested Reading

Schubert H (1997) Airborne contact dermatitis due to methylchloro and methylisothiazolinone (MCI/MI). Contact Dermatitis 36:274

Tay P, Ng SK (1994) Delayed skin burns from MCI/MI biocide used in water treatment. Contact Dermatitis 30:54–55

295. Methylol Phenols

2-Methylol Phenol: 2-Hydroxymethyl-Phenol

CAS Registry Number [90–01–7]

3-Methylol Phenol: 3-Hydroxymethyl-Phenol, 3-Hydroxybenzyl Alcohol

CAS Registry Number [620–24–6]

4-Methylol Phenol: 4-Hydroxymethyl-Phenol

CAS Registry Number [623–05–2]

Methylol phenols are sensitizers contained in resins based on phenol and formaldehyde of the resol type. Cross-reactivity is possible with other phenol derivative molecules.

Suggested Reading

Bruze M, Zimerson E (1997) Cross-reaction patterns in patients with contact allergy to simple methylol phenols. Contact Dermatitis 37:82–86

Bruze M, Fregert S, Zimerson E (1985) Contact allergy to phenol-formaldehyde resins. Contact Dermatitis 12:81–86

58

296. 1-Methylpyrrolidone

N-Methyl-2-Pyrrolidone, 1-Methyl-2-Pyrrolidone

CAS Registry Number [872–50–4]

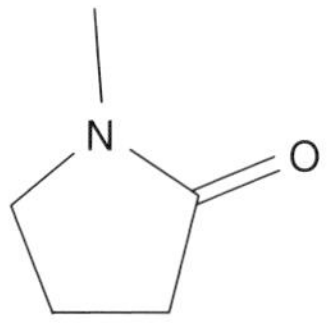

1-Methylpyrrolidone is an aprotic solvent with a wide range of applications: petrochemical processing, surface coating, dyes and pigments, industrial and domestic cleaning compounds, and agricultural and pharmaceutical formulations. It is mainly an irritant, but it can cause severe contact dermatitis due to prolonged contact.

Suggested Reading

Jungbauer FH, Coenraads PJ, Kardaun SH (2001) Toxic hygroscopic contact reaction to *N*-methyl-2-pyrrolidone. Contact Dermatitis 45:303–304
Leira H, Tiltnes A, Svendsen K, Vetlesen L (1992) Irritant cutaneous reactions to *N*-methyl-2-pyrrolidone (NMP). Contact Dermatitis 27:148–150

297. Metol (Sulfate)

4(Methylamino)Phenol

CAS Registry Number [150–75–4]

4(Methylamino)Phenol Sulfate

CAS Registry Numbers [1936–57–8] (unspecified sulfate), [51–72–9] (sulfate[1:1]), [55–55–0] (sulfate[2:1])

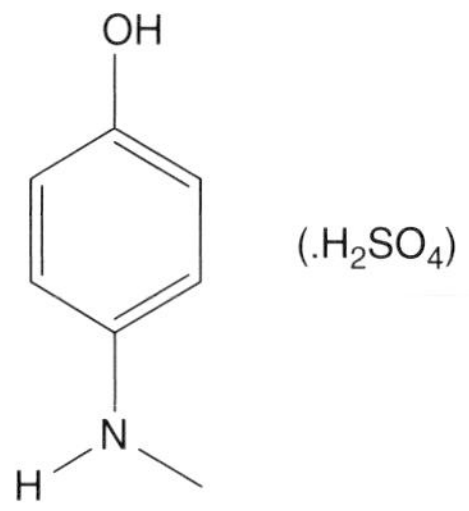

(.H$_2$SO$_4$)

Metol is contained in black and white film developers and caused contact dermatitis in photographers.

Suggested Reading

Liden C, Brehmer-Andersson E (1988) Occupational dermatoses from color developing agents. Clinical and histopathological observations. Acta Derm Venereol (Stockh) 68:514–522
Scheman AJ, Katta R (1997) Photographic allergens: an update. Contact Dermatitis 37:130

298. Metronidazole (hydrochloride)

CAS Registry Number [443-48-1] (CAS Registry Number [69198-10-3])

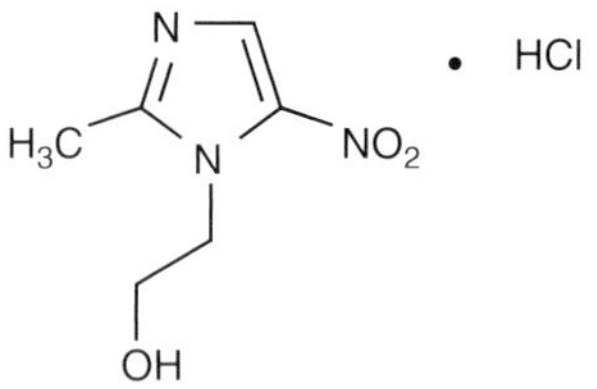

H$_3$C · HCl · NO$_2$ OH

Metronidazole is a nitro-5-imidazole compound with antiprotozoal and antibacterial properties. Topical exposure may induce allergic contact dermatitis. Sensitization is mainly observed with the treatment of rosacea and rarely occurs from handling of tablets in nurses. Systemic intake may provoke fixed drug eruption.

Suggested Reading

Madsen JT, Lorentzen HF, Paulsen E (2009) Contact sensitization to metronidazole from possible occupational exposure. Contact Dermatitis 60:117–118
Madsen JT, Thormann J, Kerre S, Andersen KE, Goossens A (2007) Allergic contact dermatitis to topical metronidazole – 3 cases. Contact Dermatitis 56:364–366
Vila JB, Bernier MA, Gutierrez JV, Gómez MT, Polo AM, Harrison JM, Miranda-Romero A, Muñoz CM (2002) Fixed drug eruption caused by metronidazole. Contact Dermatitis 46:122

299. Mevinphos

CAS Registry Number [7786–34–7]

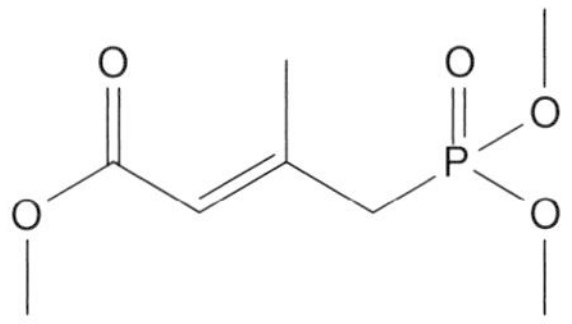

Sensitization to mevinphos (also named Duraphos, Phosdrin, and Phosfene), an organophosphate cholinesterase inhibitor that is used as an insecticide, was rarely reported.

Suggested Reading

Jung HD, Ramsauer E (1987) Akute Pesticid-Intoxication kombiniert mit epicutaner Sensibilisierung durch den organischen Phosphorsäureester Mevinphos (PD5). Aktuel Dermatol 13:82–83

300. Mezlocilin

CAS Registry Number [51481–65–3]

Mezlocillin Sodium Salt Monohydrate

CAS Registry Number [59798–30–0]

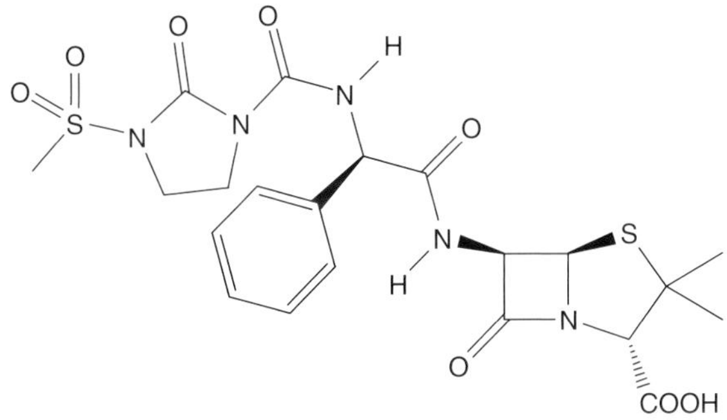

Mezlocillin is an acylaminopenicillin, which caused both immediate and delayed hypersensitivity in a nurse.

Suggested Reading

Keller K, Schwanitz HJ (1992) Combined immediate and delayed hypersensitivity to mezlocillin. Contact Dermatitis 27:348–349

301. Monoethanolamine

Ethanolamine, 2-Aminoethanol

CAS Registry Number [141–43–5]

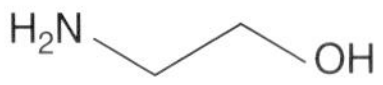

Monoethanolamine is contained in many products, such as metalworking fluids. It is mainly an irritant. Traces may exist in other ethanolamine fluids.

Suggested Reading

Bhushan M, Craven NM, Beck MH (1998) Contact allergy to 2-aminoethanol (monoethanolamine) in a soluble oil. Contact Dermatitis 39:321

Blum A, Lischka G (1997) Allergic contact dermatitis from mono-, di- and triethanolamine. Contact Dermatitis 36:166

302. Morphine (Morphine Hydrochloride, Morphine Tartrate)

CAS Registry Number [57–27–2] (CAS Registry Number [52–26–6], CAS Registry Number [302–31–8])

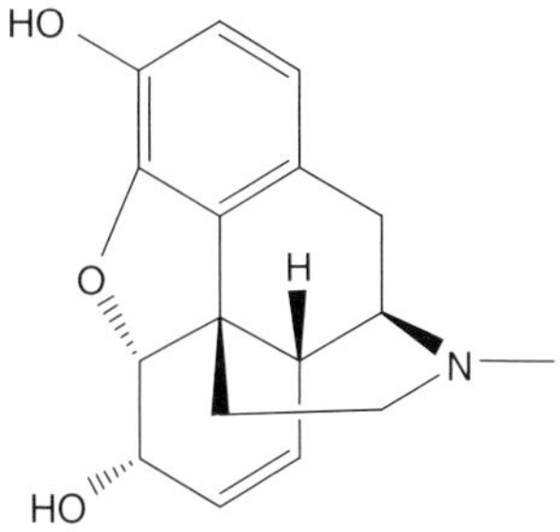

Morphine bitartrate caused contact dermatitis in a worker at a plant producing opium alkaloids. Morphine hydrochloride and morphine bitartrate showed patch-test-positive reactions in another patient with contact dermatitis working in the production of concentrated poppy straw. We observed a concomitant reaction between a morphine base and a codeine base in a patient with drug skin eruption due to codeine.

Suggested Reading

Condé-Salazar L, Guimaraens D, Gonzalez M, Fuente C (1991) Occupational allergic contact dermatitis from opium alkaloids. Contact Dermatitis 25:202–203

303. 4-Morpholinyl-2-Benzothiazyle Disulfide

2-(Morpholinodithio)Benzothiazole, Benzothiazole, 2-(4-morpholinyldithio)

CAS Registry Number [95–32–9]

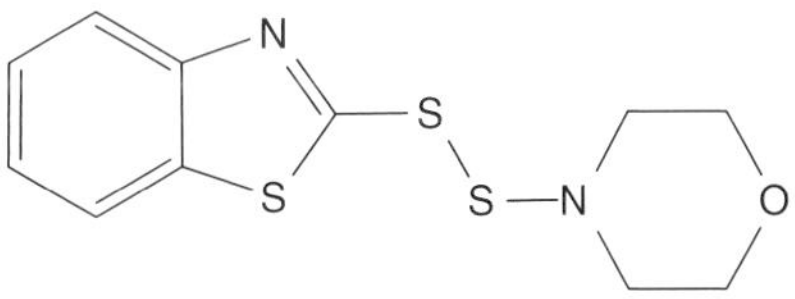

58

This chemical is a mercaptobenzothiazole-sulfenamide compound, used as moderate accelerator in rubber vulcanization.

Suggested Reading

Le Coz CJ (2004) Fiche d'éviction en cas d'hypersensibilité au mercaptobenzothiazole et au mercapto mix. Ann Dermatol Venereol 131:1012–1014

304. Morpholinyl Mercaptobenzothiazole

2-(4-Morpholinylthiobenzothiazole), 2-Morpholin Benzothiazyl Sulfenamide, Benzothiazole, 2-(4-Morpholinylthio)

CAS Registry Number [102–77–2]

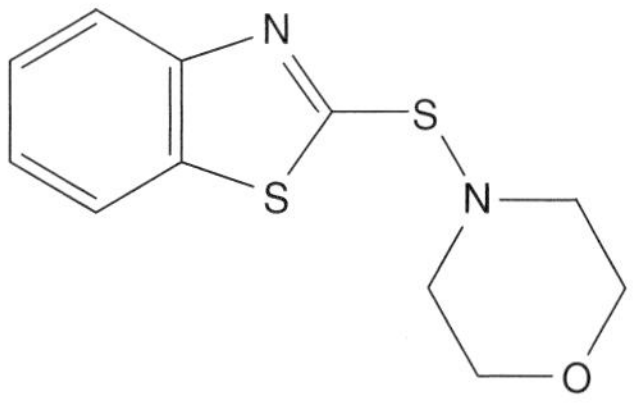

This rubber vulcanization accelerator belongs to the mercaptobenzothiazole-sulfenamide group. It is used as a chemical in the rubber industry, especially in the production of synthetic rubber articles. It is contained in "mercapto mix." As a corrosion inhibitor, it can be found in cutting fluids or in releasing fluids in the pottery industry. It induces mainly delayed-type hypersensitivity, but a case of immediate-type hypersensitivity was reported in a dental assistant.

Suggested Reading

Brehler R (1996) Contact urticaria caused by latex-free nitrile gloves. Contact Dermatitis 34:296
Condé-Salazar L, Del-Rio E, Guimaraens D, Gonzalez Domingo A (1993) Type IV allergy to rubber additives: a 10-year study of 686 cases. J Am Acad Dermatol 29:176–180
Le Coz CJ (2004) Fiche d'éviction en cas d'hypersensibilité au mercaptobenzothiazole et au mercapto mix. Ann Dermatol Venereol 131:846–848

305. Naled

CAS Registry Number [300–76–5]

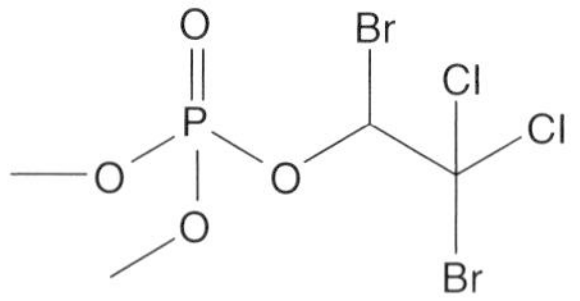

Naled is an organophosphate cholinesterase inhibitor that is used as an insecticide and acaricide. Sensitization seems to be very rare.

Suggested Reading

Edmundson WF, Davies JE (1967) Occupational dermatitis from naled. Arch Environ Health 15:89–91
Mick DL, Gartin TD, Long KR (1970) A case report: occupational exposure to the insecticide naled. J Iowa Med Soc 60:395–396

306. 1-Naphthol

Alpha-Naphthol, CI 76605, CI Oxidation Base 33

CAS Registry Number [90–15–3]

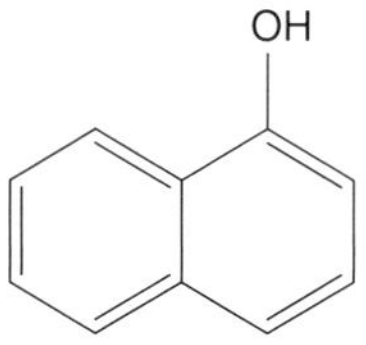

Alpha-naphthol can be used in dye manufacture and is classified as a hair dye. Combined with epichlorhydrin and NaOH to form alpha-naphthyl glycidyl ether, it caused sensitization in one of three workers in a chemical plant.

Suggested Reading

De Groot AC (1994) Occupational contact allergy to alpha-naphthyl glycidyl ether. Contact Dermatitis 30:253–254

307. Naphthol AS

CI 37505, CI Azoic Coupling Component 2

CAS Registry Number [92–77–3]

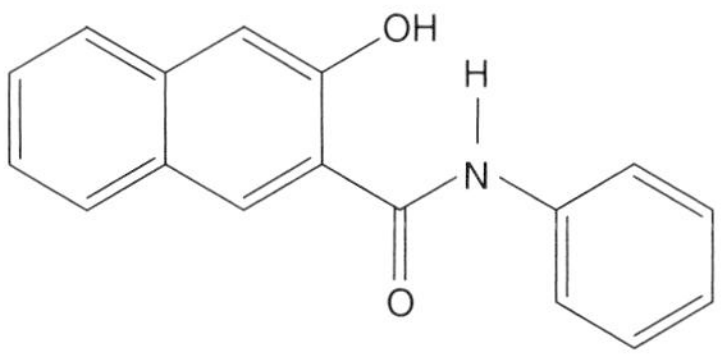

Naphthol AS is a coupling agent in cotton dyeing, inducing occupational dermatitis or contact allergy in consumers in contact with cotton-dyed clothing. It has been indirectly reported as a cause of occupational allergy due to its coupling with Diazo Component 51, or as a cross-sensitizer or sensitizer associated with Pigment Red 23 in red parts of tattoos. Pigmented contact dermatitis is usual in patients with a high phototype.

Suggested Reading

Le Coz CJ, Lepoittevin JP (2001) Clothing dermatitis from Naphthol AS. Contact Dermatitis 44:366–367
Roed-Petersen J, Batsberg W, Larsen E (1990) Contact dermatitis from Naphthol AS. Contact Dermatitis 22:161–163

308. Neomycin (Neomycin B Hydrochloride, Neomycin B Sulfate)

Framycetin, Soframycin®

CAS Registry Number [1404–04–2] (CAS Registry Number [25389–99–5], CAS Registry Number [1405–10–3])

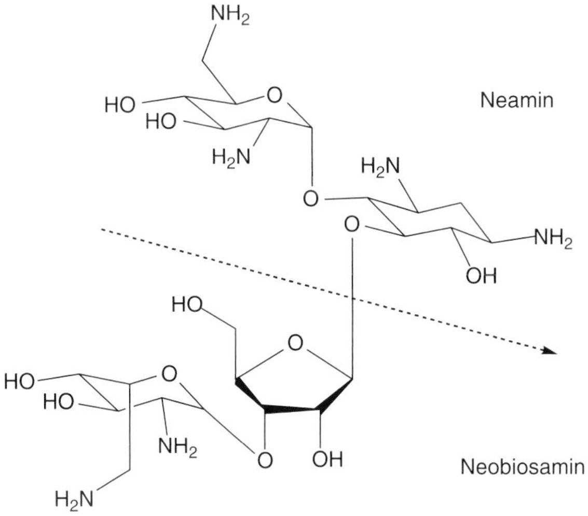

Neomycin is an antibiotic complex of the aminoglycosides group, extracted from *Streptomyces fradiae*. It is composed of neomycin A (neamin) and an isomer neobiosamin, either

neomycin B (framycetin or Soframycin®) or neomycin C. Its use has been progressively forbidden in cosmetics and as an additive for animal feed. Occupational contact dermatitis occurs in workers at animal feed mills, in veterinaries, or in health workers. Nonoccupational dermatitis mainly concerns patients with chronic dermatitis, leg ulcers, or chronic otitis. Cross-sensitivity is usual with other aminoglycosides (amikacin, arbekacin, butirosin, dibekacin, gentamicin, isepamicin, kanamycin, paromomycin, ribostamycin, sisomycin, tobramycin), is rare with netilmicin and streptomycin, but nonexistent with spectinomycin.

Suggested Reading

Le Coz CJ (2001) Fiche d'éviction en cas d'hypersensibilité à la néomycine. Ann Dermatol Venereol 128:1359–1360
Mancuso G, Staffa M, Errani A, Berdondini RM, Fabri P (1990) Occupational dermatitis in animal feed mill workers. Contact Dermatitis 22:37–41
Rebandel P, Rudzki E (1986) Occupational contact sensitivity in oculists. Contact Dermatitis 15:92

309. Nicotine

CAS Registry Number [55–11–5]

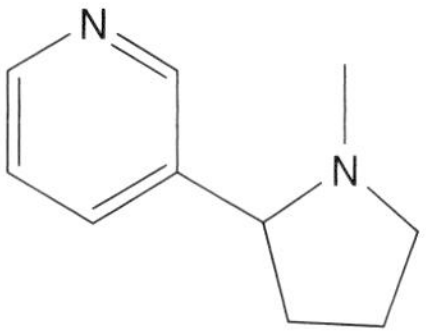

Nicotine is an alkaloid found in tobacco and is responsible for its pharmacological effects and addiction. Contact dermatitis from nicotine, considered as rare, has been more frequent since its use in transdermal systems. Irritant dermatitis is mainly encountered, as contact urticaria seems to be rare. Allergic contact dermatitis, sometimes generalized, has been reported, with positive patch testing to nicotine base (10% ethanol or petrolatum). No consequences have been reported in patients who start smoking again after skin sensitization.

Suggested Reading

Bircher AJ, Howald H, Rufli T (1991) Adverse skin reactions to nicotine in a transdermal therapeutic system. Contact Dermatitis 25:230–236
Vincenzi C, Tosti A, Cirone M, Guarrera M, Cusano F (1993) Allergic contact dermatitis from transdermal nicotine systems. Contact Dermatitis 29:104–105

58

310. 3-Nitro-4-Hydroxyethylaminophenol

4-[(2-Hydroxyethyl)Amino]-3-Nitrophenol

CAS Registry Number [65235–31–6]

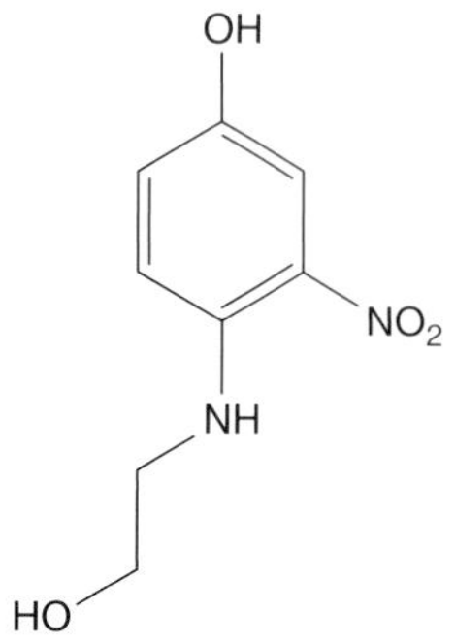

This dye belongs to the aminophenol class and is used as a hair colorant, particularly in semipermanent hair dye preparations.

Suggested Reading

Le Coz CJ, Kühne S, Engel F (2003) Hair dye allergy due to 3-nitro-*p*-hydroxyethyl-aminophenol. Contact Dermatitis 49:103

311. 2-Nitro-4-Phenylenediamine

o-Nitro-*p*-Phenylenediamine, ONPD, CI 76070

CAS Registry Number [5307–14–2]

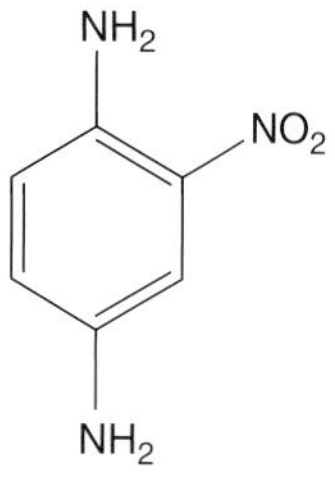

ONPD is a hair dye and a sensitizer in hairdressers and consumers who are generally sensitive to PPD too.

Suggested Reading

Frosch PJ, Burrows D, Camarasa JG, Dooms-Goossens A, Ducombs G, Lahti A, Menné T, Rycroft RJG, Shaw S, White IR, Wilkinson JD (1993) Allergic reactions to a hairdresser's series: results from 9 European centers. Contact Dermatitis 28:180–183

Guerra L, Tosti A, Bardazzi F, Pigatto P, Lisi P, Santucci B, Valsecchi R, Schena D, Angelini G, Sertoli A, Ayala F, Kokelj F (1992) Contact dermatitis in hairdressers: the Italian experience. Gruppo Italiano Ricerca Dermatiti da Contatto e Ambientali. Contact Dermatitis 26:101–107

Van der Walle HB, Brunsveld VM (1994) Dermatitis in hairdressers (I). The experience of the past 4 years. Contact Dermatitis 30:217–220

312. Nitrofurazone

Nitrofural, Nitrozone, Aldomycin

CAS Registry Numbers [59–87–0], [60051–85–6], [8027–71–2]

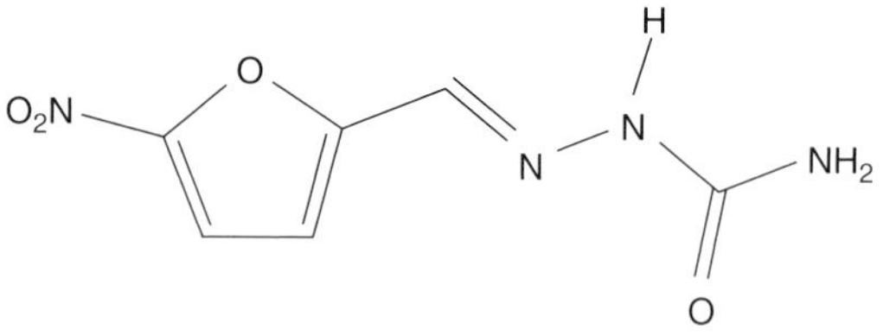

Nitrofurazone is an antibacterial agent used in animal feeds. Occupational dermatitis was reported in cattle breeders or farmers.

Suggested Reading

Condé-Salazar L, Guimaraens D, Gonzalez MA, Molina A (1995) Occupational allergic contact dermatitis from nitrofurazone. Contact Dermatitis 32:307–308

Vilaplana J, Grimalt F, Romaguera C (1990) Contact dermatitis from furaltadone in animal feed. Contact Dermatitis 22:232–233

313. Nitroglycerin

Glyceryl Trinitrate, Glycerol Trinitrate

CAS Registry Number [55–63–0]

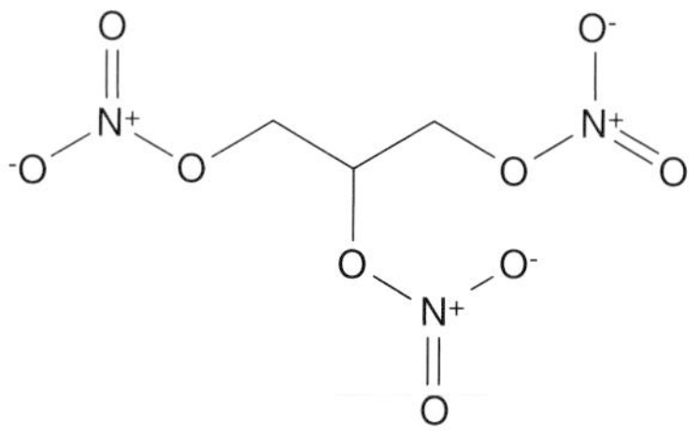

Nitroglycerin is an explosive agent contained in dynamite and an antianginal and vasodilator treatment available in systemic and topical forms. It is a well known irritant agent in dynamite manufacture. It can also cause allergic reactions in employees of explosives manufacturers and in the pharmaceutical industry. Transdermal systems are the main source of iatrogenic sensitization. Nitroglycerin can cross-react with isosorbide dinitrate.

Suggested Reading

Aquilina S, Felice H, Boffa MJ (2002) Allergic reactions to glyceryl trinitrate and isosorbide dinitrate demonstrating cross-sensitivity. Clin Exp Dermatol 27:700–702

Kanerva L, Laine R, Jolanki R, Tarvainen K, Estlander T, Helander I (1991) Occupational allergic contact dermatitis caused by nitroglycerin. Contact Dermatitis 24: 356–362

Machet L, Martin L, Toledano C, Jan V, Lorette G, Vaillant L (1999) Allergic contact dermatitis from nitroglycerin contained in 2 transdermal systems. Dermatology 198: 106–107

314. Nonoxynols

Nonylphenol Ethoxylates, PEG-(*n*) Nonyl Phenyl Ether, Polyoxyethylene (*n*) Nonyl Phenyl Ether

CAS Registry Number [26027–38–3] and more than 25 other numbers

Their general formula is $C_9H_{19}C_6H_4(OCH_2CH_2)_nOH$. Each nonoxynol is characterized by the number (*n*) of ethylene oxide units repeated in the chain; for example, nonoxynol-9, nonoxynol-14. They are present in detergents, liquid soaps, emulsifiers for creams, fabric softeners, photographic paper additives, hair dyes, lubricating oils, spermicides, and antiinfective agents. They are irritants and sensitizers. Nonoxynol-6 was reported as a sensitizing agent in an industrial hand cleanser and in a crack-indicating fluid in the metal industry. Nonoxynol-9 is the most commonly used, as a preservative in topical antiseptics or in spermicides, acting as a iodophor in PVP-iodine solutions. Nonoxynol-10 was reported as a UVB-photosensitizer. Nonoxynol-12 caused contact dermatitis in a domestic cleaner who used a polish containing it.

Suggested Reading

Dooms-Goossens A, Deveylder H, de Alam AG, Lachapelle JM, Tennstedt D, Degreef H (1989) Contact sensitivity to nonoxynols as a cause of intolerance to antiseptic preparations. J Am Acad Dermatol 21:723–727

Meding B (1985) Occupational contact dermatitis from non-ylphenolpolyglycolether. Contact Dermatitis 13:122–123

Nethercott JR, Lawrence MJ (1984) Allergic contact dermatitis due to nonylphenol ethoxylate (nonoxynol-6). Contact Dermatitis 10:235–239

Wilkinson SM, Beck MH, August PJ (1995) Allergic contact dermatitis from nonoxynol-12 in a polish. Contact Dermatitis 33:128–129

315. Octocrylene

Octocrilene

CAS Registry Number [6197–30–4]

Octocrylene is an anti-UVB filter used in cosmetics that may induce photoallergic contact dermatitis.

Suggested Reading

Carrotte-Lefebvre I, Bonnevalle A, Segard M, Delaporte E, Thomas P (2003) Contact allergy to octocrylene. Contact Dermatitis 48:46–47

316. Octyl Gallate

CAS Registry Number [1034–01–1]

Octyl gallate, a gallate ester (E 311), is an antioxidant added to food and cosmetics to prevent oxidation of unsaturated fatty acids. Cases were sparsely reported in food industry or from lipsticks. Patch tests are frequently irritant.

Suggested Reading

De Groot AC, Gerkens F (1990) Occupational airborne contact dermatitis from octyl gallate. Contact Dermatitis 23: 184–186

Giordano-Labadie F, Schwarze HP, Bazex J (2000) Allergic contact dermatitis from octyl gallate in lipstick. Contact Dermatitis 42:51

317. 2-*n*-Octyl-4-Isothiazolin-3-one

Kathon® LM, Kathon® 4200, Kathon® 893, Pancil, Skane M-8

CAS Registry Number [26530–20–1]

This isothiazolinone, contained in relatively few products compared to other isothiazolinones, is used in cleaning and polishing agents, latex paints, stains, adhesives, wood and leather preservatives, metalworking fluids (cutting oils), and plastic manufacture.

Suggested Reading

Oleaga JM, Aguirre A, Landa N, Gonzalez M, Diaz-Perez JL (1992) Allergic contact dermatitis from Kathon 893. Contact Dermatitis 27:345–346

Young HS, Ferguson JEF, Beck MH (2004) Contact dermatitis from 2-*n*-octyl-4-isothiazoline-3-one in a PhD student. Contact Dermatitis 50:47–48

318. Olaquindox

N-(2-Hydroxyethyl)-3-Methyl-2-Quinoxalinecarboxamide-1,4-Dioxide

CAS Registry Number [23696–28–8]

Olaquindox is an antibacterial agent derivative of quinoxaline, used as a growth promoter of pigs. It can be found in Bayo-N-Ox® and Proquindox® and numerous other pig feeds. It is a photosensitizer that forms reactive photoproducts on light exposure. It can induce photoallergic contact dermatitis and persistent light reactions.

Suggested Reading

Belhadjali H, Marguery MC, Journe F, Giordano-Labadie F, Lefebvre H, Bazex J (2002) Allergic and photoallergic contact dermatitis to Olaquindox in a pig breeder with prolonged photosensitivity. Photodermatol Photoimmunol Photomed 18:52–53

Kumar A, Freeman S (1996) Photoallergic contact dermatitis in a pig farmer caused by olaquindox. Contact Dermatitis 35:249–250

Schauder S, Schröder W, Geier J (1996) Olaquindox-induced airborne photoallergic contact dermatitis followed by transient or persistent light reactions in 15 pig breeders. Contact Dermatitis 35:344–354

319. Oxacillin

CAS Registry Number [66–79–5]

Oxacillin Sodium Salt Monohydrate

CAS Registry Number [7240–38–2]

Oxacillin is a semisynthetic penicillin of the group M. It is closely related to cloxacillin.

Suggested Reading

Budavari S, O'Neil MJ, Smith A, Heckelman PE, Kinneary JF (eds) (1996) The Merck Index, 12th edn. Merck, Whitehouse Station, NJ, USA

320. 7-Oxodehydroabietic Acid

CAS Registry Number [18684–55–4]

7-Oxodehydroabietic acid is an autooxidation product of dehydroabietic acid, and an allergen contained in colophony.

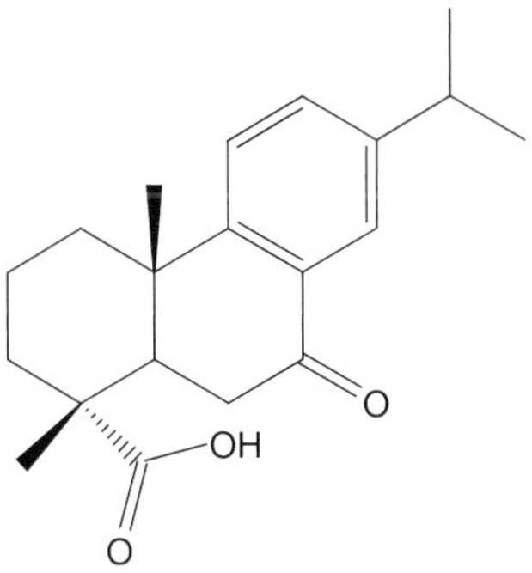

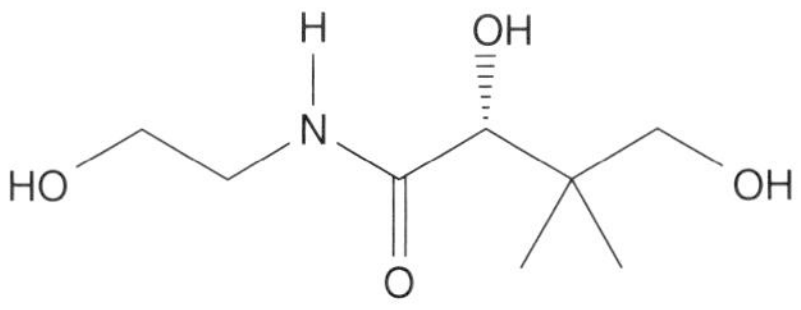

Pan(to)thenol is the alcohol corresponding to pantothenic acid, of the vitamin B5 group. It is used as a food additive, and in skin and hair products as a conditioning agent. Contact dermatitis and urticaria have been reported.

Suggested Reading

Schalock PC, Storrs FJ, Morrison L (2000) Contact urticaria from panthenol in hair conditioner. Contact Dermatitis 43:223
Stables GI, Wilkinson SM (1998) Allergic contact dermatitis due to panthenol. Contact Dermatitis 38:236–237

Suggested Reading

Bergh M, Menné T, Karlberg AT (1994) Colophony in paper-based surgical clothing. Contact Dermatitis 31: 332–333

321. Oxprenolol

CAS Registry Number [6452–71–7]

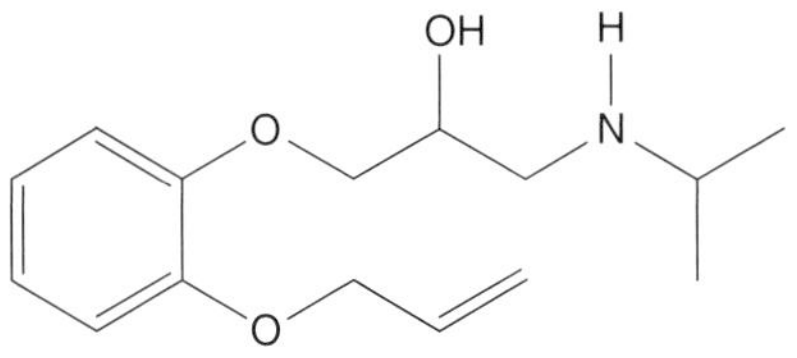

The beta-blocker oxprenolol induced contact dermatitis in a worker at a pharmaceutical plant, in a division for drug synthesis. Epichlorhydrin was also used for the production of drugs propranolol and oxprenolol.

Suggested Reading

Rebandel P, Rudzki E (1990) Dermatitis caused by epichlorhydrin, oxprenolol hydrochloride and propranolol hydrochloride. Contact Dermatitis 23:199

322. Pantothenol

2,4-Dihydroxy-*N*-(3-Hydroxypropyl)-3,3-Dimethylbutanamide, Pantothenylol, *N*-Pantoyl-3-Propanolamine, Panthenol, Pantothenyl Alcohol

CAS Registry Number [81–13–0]

323. Parabens (Parahydroxybenzoic Acid Esters)

Methylparaben, E218, E219 (Sodium Salt)

CAS Registry Number [99–76–3], E219 (Sodium Salt), CAS Registry Number [5026–62–0]

Ethylparaben, E214, E215 (Sodium Salt)

CAS Registry Number [120–47–8], E215 (Sodium Salt), CAS Registry Number [35285–68–8]

Propylparaben, E216, E217 (Sodium Salt)

CAS Registry Number [94–13–3], E217 (Sodium Salt), CAS Registry Number [35285–69–9]

Isopropylparaben

CAS Registry Number [4191–73–5]

Butylparaben

CAS Registry Number [94–26–8]

Isobutylparaben

CAS Registry Number [4247–02–3]

Phenylparaben

CAS Registry Number [17696–62–7]

Benzylparaben

CAS Registry Number [94–18–8]

Phenoxyethylparaben

CAS Registry Number [55468–88–7]

Parabens are esters formed by *p*-hydroxybenzoic acid and an alcohol. They are largely used as biocides in cosmetics and toiletries, medicaments, or food. They have synergistic power with other biocides. Parabens can induce allergic contact dermatitis, mainly in chronic dermatitis and wounded skin.

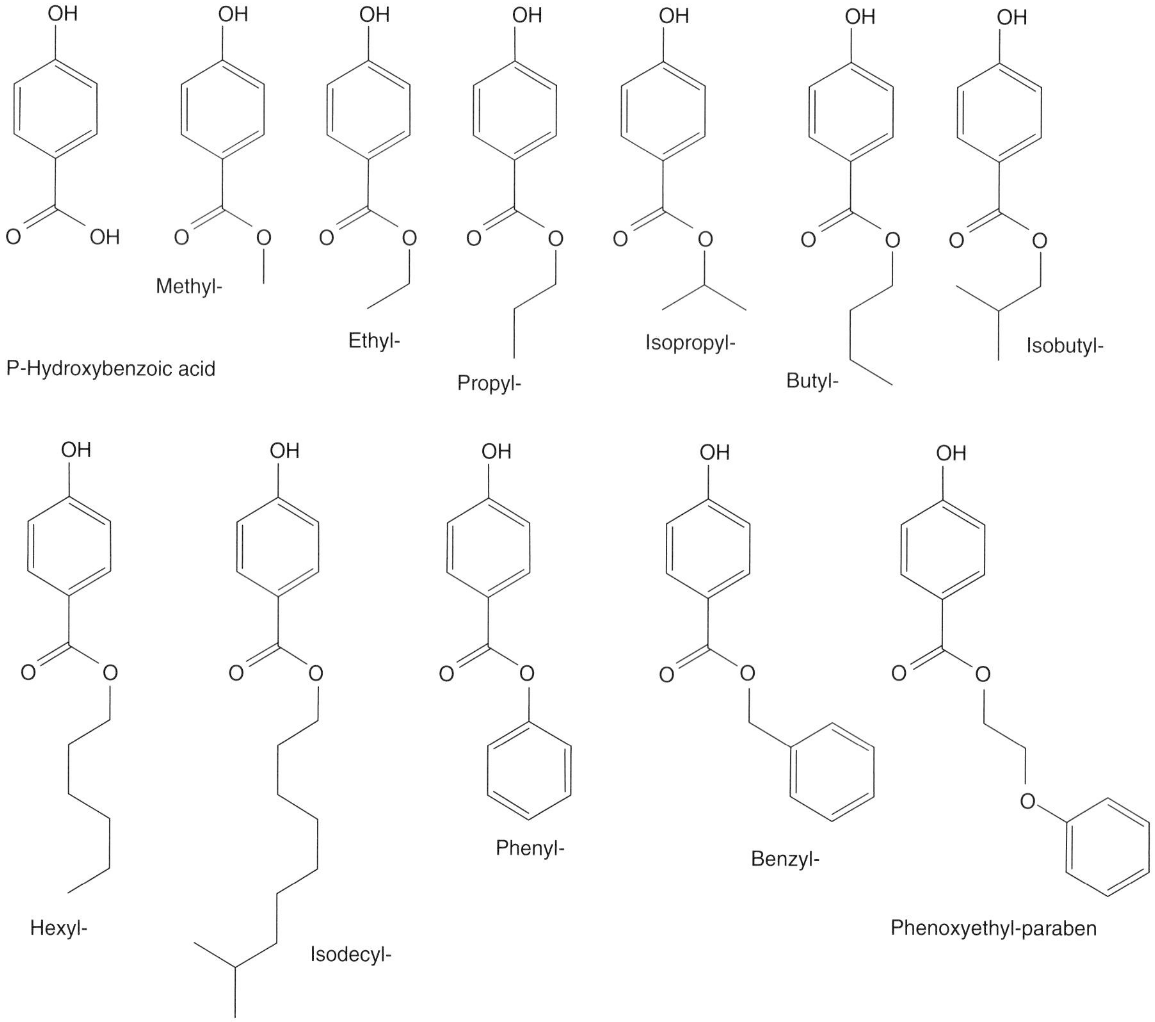

58

Methyl-

Ethyl-

Propyl-

Isopropyl-

Butyl-

Isobutyl-

P-Hydroxybenzoic acid

Hexyl-

Isodecyl-

Phenyl-

Benzyl-

Phenoxyethyl-paraben

Suggested Reading

Le Coz CJ (2004) Fiche d'éviction en cas d'hypersensibilité aux esters de l'acide *para*-hydroxybenzoïque (parahydroxybenzoates ou parabens). Ann Dermatol Venereol 131: 309–310

324. Paraphenylenediamine

PPD, *p*-Phenylenediamine, 4-Phenylenediamine

CAS Registry Number [106–50–3]

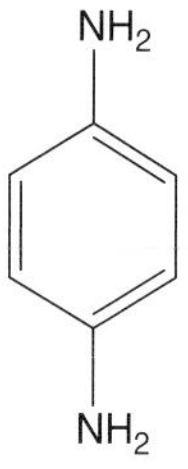

PPD is a colorless compound oxidized by hydrogen peroxide in the presence of ammonia. It is then polymerized to a color by a coupling agent. Although a well-known allergen in hair dyes, PPD can be found as a cause of contact dermatitis in chin rest stains or in milk testers. It is also a marker of group sensitivity to *para* amino compounds such as benzocaine, some azo dyes, and some previous antibacterial sulphonamides.

Suggested Reading

Bork K (1993) Allergic contact dermatitis on a violinist's neck from para-phenylenediamine in a chin rest stain. Contact Dermatitis 28:250–251

Frosch PJ, Burrows D, Camarasa JG, Dooms-Goossens A, Ducombs G, Lahti A, Menné T, Rycroft RJG, Shaw S, White IR, Wilkinson JD (1993) Allergic reactions to a hairdresser's series: results from 9 European centers. Contact Dermatitis 28:180–183

Guerra L, Tosti A, Bardazzi F, Pigatto P, Lisi P, Santucci B, Valsecchi R, Schena D, Angelini G, Sertoli A, Ayala F, Kokelj F (1992) Contact dermatitis in hairdressers: the Italian experience. Gruppo Italiano Ricerca Dermatiti da Contatto e Ambientali. Contact Dermatitis 26:101–107

Le Coz CJ, Lefebvre C, Keller F, Grosshans E (2000) Allergic contact dermatitis caused by skin painting (pseudotattooing) with black henna, a mixture of henna and *p*-phenylenediamine and its derivatives. Arch Dermatol 136:1515–1517

Rebandel P, Rudzki E (1995) Occupational allergy to *p*-phenylenediamine in milk testers. Contact Dermatitis 33:138

325. Paraquat (Dichloride, Methosulfate)

1-1-Dimethyl-4,4-Bipyridinium Salt

CAS Registry Numbers [4685–14–7], [116047–10–0] (CAS Registry Number [1910–42–5], CAS Registry Number [2074–50–2])

Paraquat is a quaternary ammonium compound with herbicide properties, as diquat. It is contained in Cekuquat® or Dipril®. It can cause contact and phototoxic contact dermatitis, acne, and leukoderma mainly in agricultural workers.

Suggested Reading

Vilaplana J, Azon A, Romaguera C, Lecha M (1993) Phototoxic contact dermatitis with toxic hepatitis due to the percutaneous absorption of paraquat. Contact Dermatitis 29:163–164

326. Parathion

Parathion-Ethyl: Parathion, Ethylparathion, Corothion, Dantion, Folidol

CAS Registry Number [56–38–2]

Paration-Methyl: Methylparathion, Matafos, Paratox, Folidol M

CAS Registry Number [298–00–0]

One case was reported of a bullous contact dermatitis due to ethylparathion. A case of sensitization to methyl-parathion was described in a female agricultural worker with multiple sensitization.

Suggested Reading

Jung HD, Holzegel K (1988) Akute Toxisch-bullöse Kontaktdermatitis durch den Phosphorsäurester Parathionethyl im Follidel-Öl. Aktuel Dermatol 14:19–31

Pevny I (1980) Pestizid-Allergie. Dermatosen 28:186–189

327. Parthenolide

CAS Registry Number [20554–84–1]

Parthenolide is a sesquiterpene lactone found Asteraceae–Compositae such as feverfew (*Tanacetum parthenium* Schultz-Bip.) or congress grass (*Parthenium hysterophorus* L.).

Suggested Reading

Hausen BM, Osmundsen PE (1983) Contact allergy to parthenolide in *Tanacetum parthenium* (L.) Schultz-Bip. (feverfew, Asteraceae) and cross-reactions to related sesquiterpene lactone containing Compositae species. Acta Derm Venereol (Stockh) 63:308–314

Lamminpää A, Estlander T, Jolanki R, Kanerva L (1996) Occupational allergic contact dermatitis caused by decorative plants. Contact Dermatitis 34:330–335

Paulsen E, Andersen KE, Hausen BM (1993) Compositae dermatitis in a Danish dermatology department in one year (I). Results of routine patch testing with the sesquiterpene lactone mix supplemented with aimed patch testing with extracts and sesquiterpene lactones of Compositae plants. Contact Dermatitis 29:6–10

328. Penicillins

CAS Registry Number [1406–05–9]

for penicillin

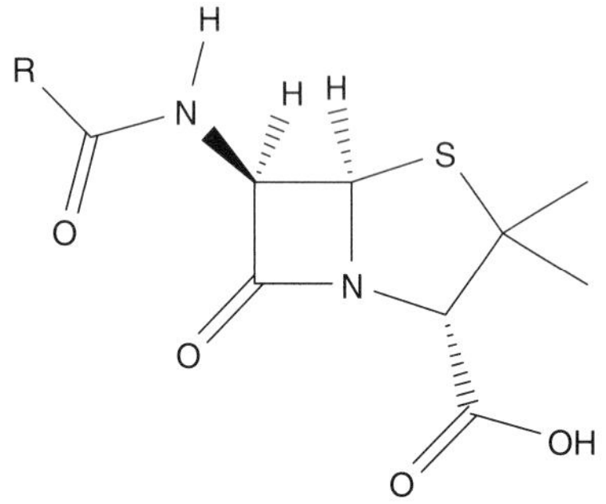

Penicillins can induce contact dermatitis, contact urticaria, and systemic and sometimes severe reactions. Occupational sensitivity to penicillins concerns health workers, workers in the pharmaceutical industry, and veterinaries, since these antibiotics are used by veterinarians and cattle breeders as medications and animal feed antibiotic. All penicillins contain the 6-aminopenicillanic acid moiety. Penicillins of G, V, A, and M groups are characterized by a specific C_7 side chain. Cross-reactivity is possible between several penicillins, but is not systematic since both immediate- and delayed-type sensitivity can implicate the 6-aminopenicillanic acid moiety, or be specific to the 7-side-chain.

Suggested Reading

Guerra L, Venturo N, Tardio M, Tosti A (1995) Airborne contact dermatitis from animal feed antibiotics. Contact Dermatitis 32:61–62

Rudzki E, Rebandel P, Grzywa Z (1989) Patch tests with occupational contactants in nurses, doctors and dentists. Contact Dermatitis 20:247–250

329. Pentachloronitrobenzene

Quintozene, PCNB, Brassicol, Terrachlor®

CAS Registry Number [82–68–8]

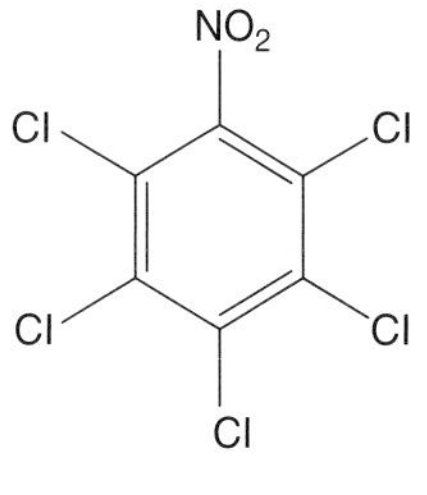

Pentachloronitrobenzene is a pesticide and a fungicide. Sensitization can occur in farmers or in chemical plants.

Suggested Reading

O'Malley M, Rodriguez P, Maibach HI (1995) Pesticide patch testing: California nursery workers and controls. Contact Dermatitis 32:61–62

Sharma VK, Kaur S (1990) Contact sensitization by pesticides in farmers. Contact Dermatitis 23:77–80

330. Pentadecylcatechol

3-Pentadecylcatechol, Hydrourushiol, Tetrahydrourushiol

CAS Registry Number [492–89–7]

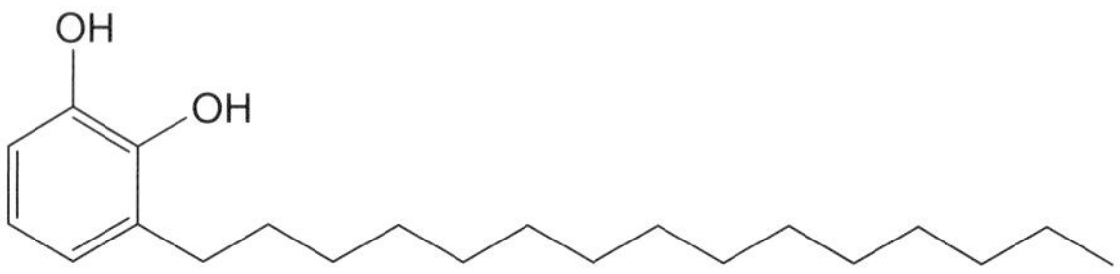

Pentadecylcatechol belongs to the urushiols and is the main allergen of the Anacardiaceae poison ivy (*Toxicodendron radicans*) and of Poison oak (*Toxicodendron diversiloba*, *Rhus diversiloba*).

Suggested Reading

Epstein WL (1994) Occupational poison ivy and oak dermatitis. Dermatol Clin 12:511–516

331. Phenoxyethanol

2-Phenoxyethanol

CAS Registry Numbers [122–99–6], [37220–49–8], [56257–90–0]

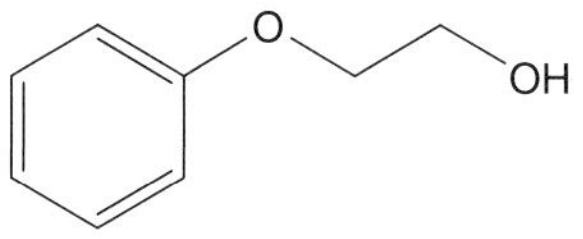

Phenoxyethanol is an aromatic ether-alcohol used mainly as a preservative, mostly with methyldibromoglutaronitrile (in Euxyl® K 400) or with parabens. Sensitization to this molecule is very rare.

Suggested Reading

Vigan M, Brechat N, Girardin P, Adessi B, Meyer JP, Vuitton D, Laurent R (1996) Un nouvel allergène: le dibromodicyanobutane. Etude sur 310 patients de janvier à décembre 1994. Ann Dermatol Venereol 123:322–324

332. Phenyl Glycidyl Ether

CAS Registry Numbers [122–60–1], [66527–93–3]

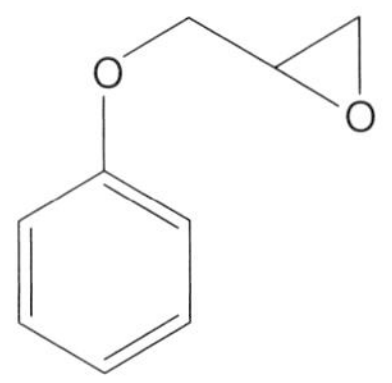

This monoglycidyl derivative is a reactive diluent in epoxy resins Bisphenol A type. It is a component of epoxy paints, epoxy glues, and epoxy resins. Sensitization has been observed in many professions, such as in construction workers, marble workers, ceramic workers, and shoemakers.

Suggested Reading

Angelini G, Rigano L, Foti C, Grandolfo M, Vena GA, Bonamonte D, Soleo L, Scorpiniti AA (1996) Occupational sensitization to epoxy resin and reactive diluents in marble workers. Contact Dermatitis 35:11–16

Condé-Salazar L, Gonzalez de Domingo MA, Guimaraens D (1994) Sensitization to epoxy resin systems in special flooring workers. Contact Dermatitis 31:157–160

Jolanki R, Kanerva L, Estlander T, Tarvainen K, Keskinen H, Henriks-Eckerman ML (1990) Occupational dermatoses from epoxy resin compounds. Contact Dermatitis 23:172–183

Mancuso G, Reggiani M, Berdondini RM (1996) Occupational dermatitis in shoemakers. Contact Dermatitis 34:17–22

Seidenari S, Danese P, di Nardo A, Manzini BM, Motolese A (1990) Contact sensitization among ceramics workers. Contact Dermatitis 22:45–49

Tarvainen K (1995) Analysis of patients with allergic patch test reactions to a plastic and glues series. Contact Dermatitis 32:346–351

333. Phenyl-Alpha-Naphthylamine

Neozone A, CI 44050

CAS Registry Number [90–30–2]

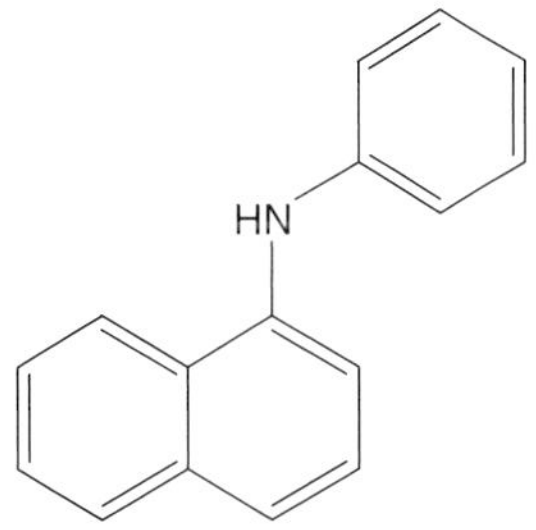

Phenyl-alpha-naphthylamine is contained in some rubbers and oils as an antioxidant of the amine group. It is closely related to phenyl-beta-naphthylamine and to di-beta-naphthyl-*p*-phenylenediamine, but without cross-reactivity.

Suggested Reading

Carmichael AJ, Foulds IS (1990) Isolated naphthylamine allergy to phenyl-alpha-naphthylamine. Contact Dermatitis 22:298–299

Svedman C, Isaksson M, Zimerson E, Bruze M (2004) Occupational contact dermatitis from a grease. Dermatitis 15:41–44

334. Phenyl-Beta-Naphthylamine

N-Phenyl-2-Naphthylamine, Neozone

CAS Registry Numbers [135–88–6], [52907–17–2], [84420–28–0]

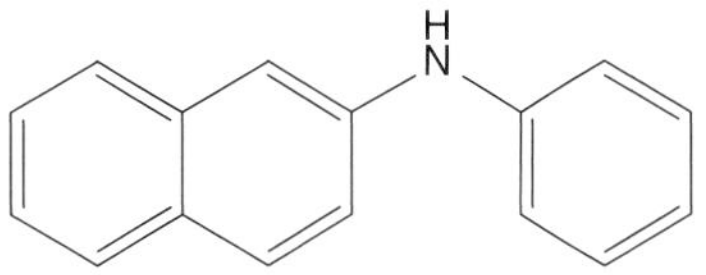

Phenyl-beta-naphthylamine is an amine compound. Sensitization was reported in patients with hypersensitivity from rubber.

Suggested Reading

Condé-Salazar L, Guimaraens D, Romero LV, Gonzalez MA (1987) Unusual allergic contact dermatitis to aromatic amines. Contact Dermatitis 17:42–44

Condé-Salazar L, Del-Rio E, Guimaraens D, Gonzalez Domingo A (1993) Type IV allergy to rubber additives: a 10-year study of 686 cases. J Am Acad Dermatol 29:176–180

Kiec-Swierczynska M (1995) Occupational sensitivity to rubber. Contact Dermatitis 32:171–172

58

335. Phenylephrine (Hydrochloride)

CAS Registry Number [59–42–7]

Phenylephrine Hydrochloride

CAS Registry Number [61–76–7]

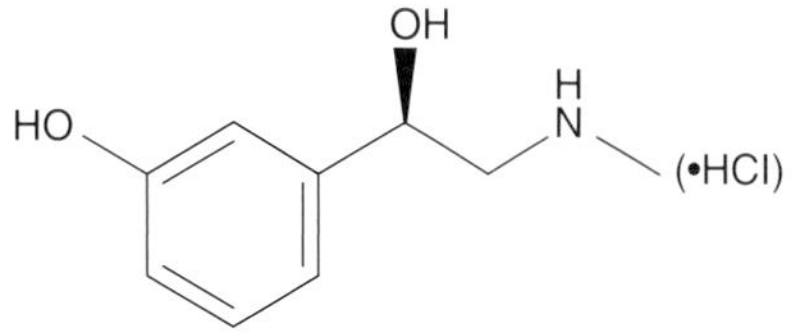

Phenylephrine hydrochloride is an alpha-adrenergic agonist, used as a mydriatic and decongestant in eyedrops.

Suggested Reading

Narayan S, Prais L, Foulds IS (2002) Allergic contact dermatitis caused by phenylephrine eyedrops. Am J Contact Dermat 13:208–209

336. Phenylethyl Caffeate

Caffeic Acid Phenethyl Ester, Capee

CAS Registry Number [104594–70–9]

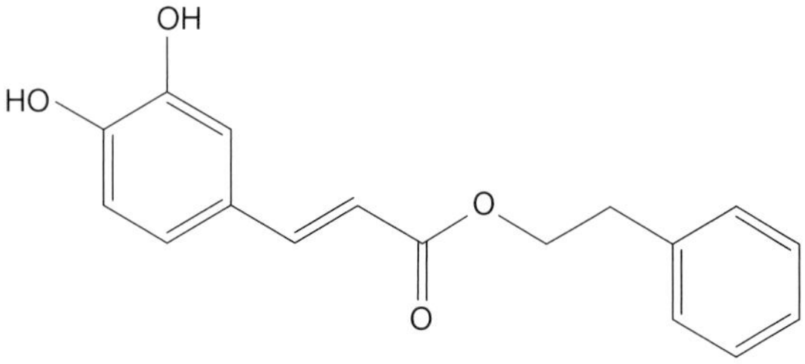

Capee is one of the allergens of propolis (bee glue). It is also contained in poplar bud secretions.

Suggested Reading

Lamminpää A, Estlander T, Jolanki R, Kanerva L (1996) Occupational allergic contact dermatitis caused by decorative plants. Contact Dermatitis 34:330–335
Oliwiecki S, Beck MH, Hausen BM (1992) Occupational contact dermatitis from caffeates in poplar bud resin in a tree surgeon. Contact Dermatitis 27:127–128

337. Phthalic Anhydride

CAS Registry Numbers [85–44–9], [39363–63–8]

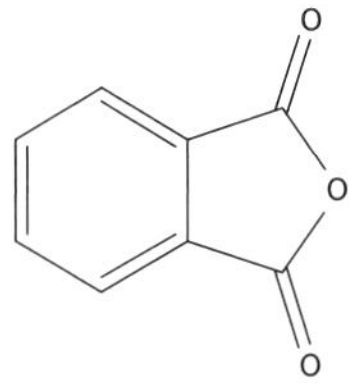

Phthalic anhydride is used in the manufacture of unsaturated polyesters and as a curing agent for epoxy resins. When used as a pigment, it can be responsible for sensitization in ceramic workers. Phthalic anhydride per se is not responsible for the sensitization to the resin used in nail varnishes phthalic anhydride/trimellitic anhydride/glycols copolymer, CAS Registry Number [85–44–9].

Suggested Reading

Seidenari S, Danese P, di Nardo A, Manzini BM, Motolese A (1990) Contact sensitization among ceramics workers. Contact Dermatitis 22:45–49
Tarvainen K, Jolanki R, Estlander T, Tupasela O, Pfäffli P, Kanerva L (1995) Immunologic contact urticaria due to airborne methylhexahydrophthalic and methyltetrahydrophthalic anhydrides. Contact Dermatitis 32:204–209

338. Picric Acid

CI 10305

CAS Registry Number [88–89–1]

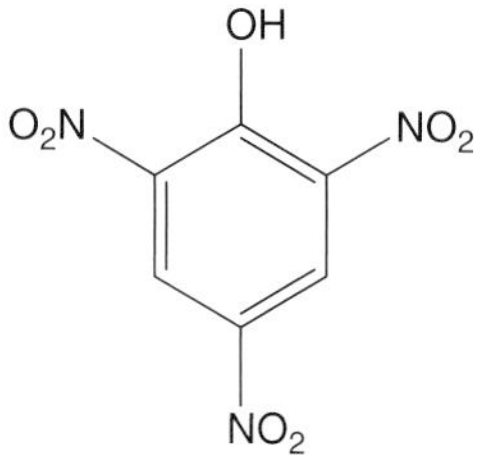

Contact dermatitis occurred primarily in the explosives industry.

Suggested Reading

Aguirre A, Sanz de Galdeano C, Oleaga JM, Eizaguirre X, Diaz Perez JL (1993) Allergic contact dermatitis from picric acid. Contact Dermatitis 28:291
Hausen BM (1994) Letter to the editor. Picric acid. Contact Dermatitis 30:59

339. Alpha-Pinene

CAS Registry Numbers [80–56–8], [2437–95–8]

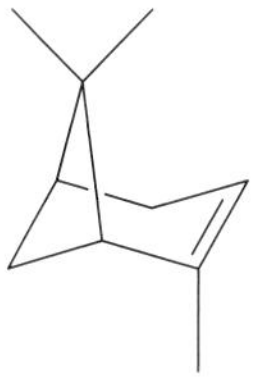

Alpha-pinene is the major constituent of turpentine (about 80%). It exists in levogyre form in European turpentine and in dextrogyre form in turpentine found in North-Americans. Sensitization occurs mainly in painters, polishers, and varnishers, and in those in the perfume and in the ceramics industry.

Suggested Reading

Lear JT, Heagerty AHM, Tan BB, Smith AG, English JSC (1996) Transient reemergence of oil turpentine allergy in the pottery industry. Contact Dermatitis 35:169–172

Moura C, Dias M, Vale T (1994) Contact dermatitis in painters, polishers and varnishers. Contact Dermatitis 31:51–53

340. Beta-Pinene

Nopinene, Terebenthene

CAS Registry Number [127–91–3]

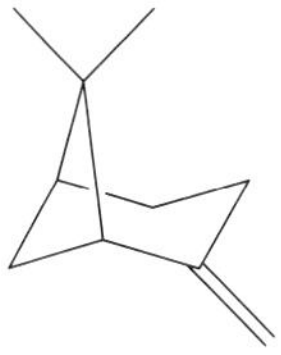

Beta-pinene is a component of turpentine. Concentrations vary with the source and seem higher in European (Portuguese) than in Asian (Indonesian) turpentine.

Suggested Reading

Lear JT, Heagerty AHM, Tan BB, Smith AG, English JSC (1996) Transient reemergence of oil turpentine allergy in the pottery industry. Contact Dermatitis 35:169–172

341. Piperazine

Diethylenediamine

CAS Registry Number [110–85–0]

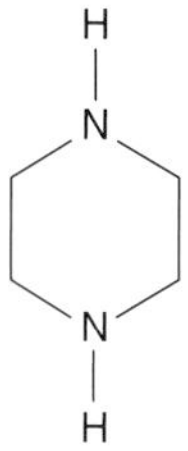

Piperazine is contained in pyrazinobutazone, an equimolar salt of piperazine and phenylbutazone. Among occupational cases, most were reported in the pharmaceutical industry or laboratory workers, in nurses, and in veterinarians.

Suggested Reading

Dorado Bris JM, Montanes Aragues M, Sols Candela M, Garcia Diez A (1992) Contact sensitivity to pyrazinobutazone (Carudol®) with positive oral provocation test. Contact Dermatitis 26:355–356

Rudzki E, Rebandel P, Grzywa Z, Pomorski Z, Jakiminska B, Zawisza E (1982) Occupational dermatitis in veterinarians. Contact Dermatitis 8:72–73

342. Piroxicam

CAS Registry Number [36332–90–4]

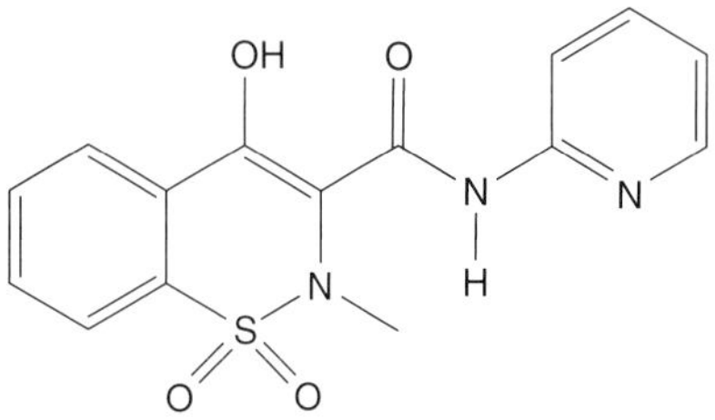

This nonsteroidal anti-inflammatory drug belongs to the oxicam class. It induces photoallergic contact dermatitis rather than contact allergy. Systemic photosensitivity is frequent, in patients previously sensitized to thiomersal. Thiosalicylic acid, the nonmercurial moiety of thiomersal, is a marker of photoallergy to piroxicam. Reactions are expected with piroxicam β-cyclodextrin, but cross-sensitivity is generally not observed to tenoxicam or meloxicam (personal observations).

Suggested Reading

Arévalo A, Blancas R, Ancona A (1995) Occupational contact dermatitis from piroxicam. Am J Contact Dermat 6:113–114
De la Cuadra J, Pujol C, Aliaga A (1989) Clinical evidence of cross-sensitivity between thiosalicylic acid, a contact allergen, and piroxicam, a photoallergen. Contact Dermatitis 21:349–351

343. Pivampicillin

CAS Registry Number [33817–20–8]

Pivampicillin Hydrochloride

CAS Registry Number [26309–95–5]

Pivampicillin is a prodrug of ampicillin. It caused sensitization in 56 workers at a penicillin factory. Pivampicillin and pivmecillinam were responsible for contact dermatitis in pharmaceutical production workers. Ampicillin, mecillinam or amdinocillin, penicillin V and penicillin G were also implicated in cross-reactions.

Suggested Reading

Moller NE, von Würden K (1992) Hypersensitivity to semisynthetic penicillins and cross-reactivity with penicillin. Contact Dermatitis 26:351–352
Moller NE, Nielsen B, von Würden K (1990) Changes in penicillin contamination and allergy in factory workers. Contact Dermatitis 22:106–107

344. Polymyxin B (sulfate)

CAS Registry Number [1404-26-8] (CAS Registry Number [1405-20-5])

Polymyxin, CAS Registry Number [1406-11-7], is a polypeptidic antibiotic complex (Polymyxin A to E) produced by *Bacillus polymyxa*. Polymyxin E is known as Colistin. Active against Gram-negative bacteria, Polymyxin B is a mixture of Polymyxin B_1 and B_2. Sensitization occurs by topical, ophthalmic, and otic preparations. Cosensitization is frequent with other topical antibiotics like neomycin or bacitracin.

Suggested Reading

Jiaravuthisan MM, DeKoven JG (2008) Contact dermatitis to polymyxin B. Contact Dermatitis 59:314–316

345. Potassium Metabisulfite

Sodium Pyrosulfite, Disodium Disulfite, E224

CAS Registry Number [16731–55–8]

Potassium metabisulfite is an antioxidant used as an antifermentative agent in breweries and wineries, as a preservative of fruits and vegetables, and to bleach straw. Reactions to both sodium and potassium metabisulfite are expected.

Suggested Reading

Budavari S, O'Neil MJ, Smith A, Heckelman PE, Kinneary JF (eds) (1996) The Merck Index, 12th edn. Merck, Whitehouse Station, NJ, USA

346. Povidone-Iodine

Polyvinylpyrrolidone-Iodine, PVP-Iodine

CAS Registry Number [25655–41–8]

Povidone-iodine is iodophor, used as a topical antiseptic. A 10% povidone-iodine solution contains 1% available iodine, but free-iodine is at 0.1% concentration. Skin exposure causes irritant rather than allergic contact dermatitis. In such a situation, however, iodine seems to be the true hapten.

Suggested Reading

Lachapelle JM (2005) Allergic contact dermatitis from povidone-iodine: a reevaluation study. Contact Dermatitis 52:9–10

Tosti A, Vincenzi C, Bardazzi F, Mariani R (1990) Allergic contact dermatitis due to povidone-iodine. Contact Dermatitis 23:197–198

347. Prilocaine (Hydrochloride)

CAS Registry Number [25655–41–8] (CAS Registry Number [1786–81–8])

Prilocaine in a local anesthetic of the amide group. It can induce allergic contact dermatitis, particularly from EMLA® cream.

Suggested Reading

Le Coz CJ, Cribier BJ, Heid E (1996) Patch testing in suspected allergic contact dermatitis due to Emla® cream in haemodialyzed patients. Contact Dermatitis 35:316–317

348. Primin

CAS Registry Number [15121–94–5]

Primin is the major allergen of *Primula obconica* Hance (Primulaceae family). Allergic contact dermatitis is mainly occupational, occurring in florists and horticulturists.

Suggested Reading

Christensen LP, Larsen E (2000) Direct emission of the allergen primin from intact *Primula obconica* plants. Contact Dermatitis 42:149–153

Lamminpää A, Estlander T, Jolanki R, Kanerva L (1996) Occupational allergic contact dermatitis caused by decorative plants. Contact Dermatitis 34:330–335

349. Pristinamycin

Pristinamycin

CAS Registry Number [270076–60–3]

Pristinamycin IA (Streptogramin B, Mikamycin IA, Ostreogrycin B, Vernamycin B$_{alpha}$)

CAS Registry Number [3131–03–1]

Pristinamycin IIA (Mikamycin A, Ostreogrycin A, Pristinamycin II$_A$, Staphylomycin M$_1$, Streptogramin A, Vernamycin A, Virginiamycin M$_1$)

CAS Registry Number [21411–53–0]

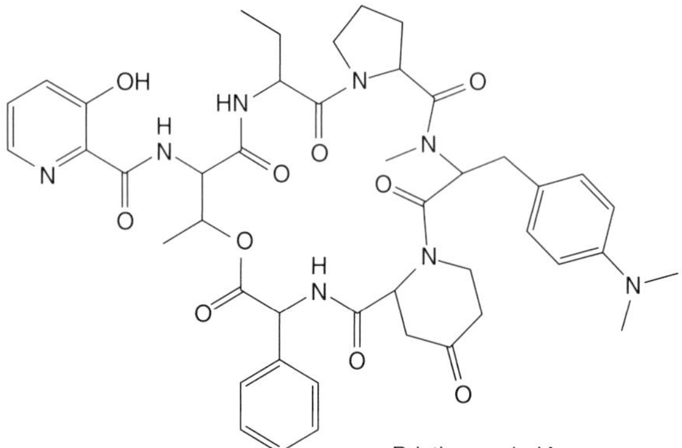

Pristinamycin IA

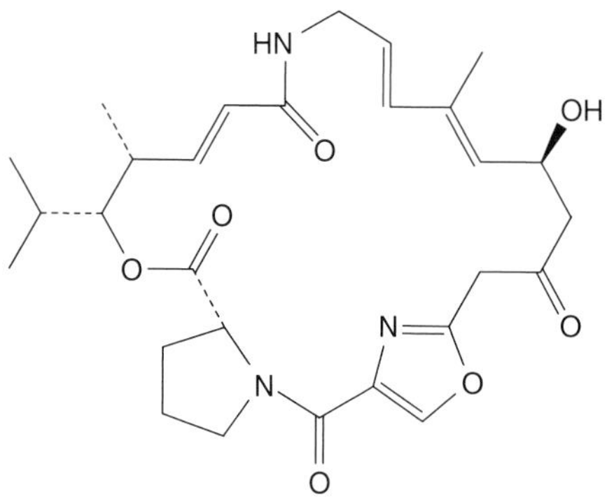

Pristinamycin IIA

Pristinamycin is a systemic antibiotic of the synergistins/streptogramins class, composed of two subunits: pristinamycin IA and pristinamycin IIA. It induces several types of drug reactions such as maculo-papular exanthema, systemic dermatitis, or acute generalized exanthematous pustulosis. Some patients have been previously skin-sensitized by virginiamycin (see below). Cross-reactivity is expected to virginiamycin CAS [11006–76–1] and to the associated dalfopristin (CAS [112362–50–2]) and quinupristin (CAS [120138–50–3]).

Suggested Reading

Barbaud A, Trechot P, Weber-Muller F, Ulrich G, Commun N, Schmutz JL (2004) Drug skin tests in cutaneous adverse drug reactions to pristinamycin: 29 cases with a study of cross-reactions between synergistins. Contact Dermatitis 50:22–26

350. Procaine (Hydrochloride)

2-Diethylaminoethyl 4-Aminobenzoate, Novocaine®

CAS Registry Number [59–46–1]

Procaine Hydrochloride

CAS Registry Number [51–05–8]

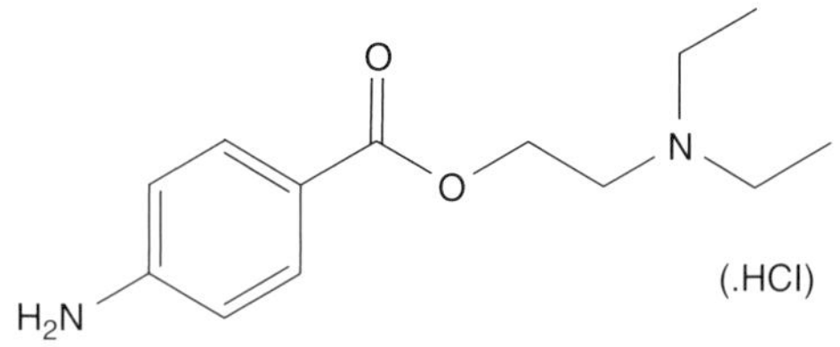

(.HCl)

Procaine is a local anesthetic with *para*-amino function. Sensitization mainly concerns the medical, dental, and veterinary professions.

Suggested Reading

Berova N, Stranky L, Krasteva M (1990) Studies on contact dermatitis in stomatological staff. Dermatol Monatschr 176:15–18
Rudzki E, Rebandel P, Grzywa Z, Pomorski Z, Jakiminska B, Zawisza E (1982) Occupational dermatitis in veterinarians. Contact Dermatitis 8:72–73

351. Propacetamol

4-Acetamidophenyl *N,N*-Diethylglycinate Hydrochloride

CAS Registry Number [66532–85–2]

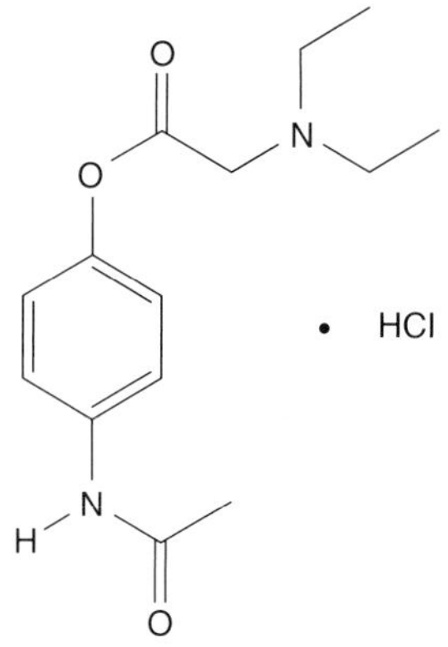

HCl

Propacetamol is a prodrug of paracetamol (acetaminophen) used for intravenous administration. It results from the combination of paracetamol and diethylglycine. It caused contact (hand and airborne) dermatitis in nurses and acute systemic dermatitis (pompholyx and nummular dermatitis, generalized eczema, urticaria-like eruption) in nurses who had became sick and received intravenous propacetamol. Allergenic properties are due to the *N,N*-diethylglycine moiety, and not to the paracetamol moiety. Propacetamol is now substituted by a solution of paracetamol in mannitol (Perfalgan®).

Suggested Reading

Barbaud A, Trechot P, Bertrand O, Schmutz JL (1995) Occupational allergy to propacetamol. Lancet 30:902
Berl V, Barbaud A, Lepoittevin JP (1998) Mechanism of allergic contact dermatitis from propacetamol: sensitization to activated *N,N*-diethylglycine. Contact Dermatitis 38:185–188
Le Coz C, Collet E, Dupouy M (1999) Conséquences d'une administration systémique de propacétamol (Pro-Dafalgan®) chez les infirmières sensibilisées au propacétamol. Ann Dermatol Venereol 126(suppl 2):32–33

352. Propargite

Omite®

CAS Registry Number [2312–35–8]

The pesticide omite principally acts as an irritant. Contact dermatitis was reported in 40 of 47 agricultural workers using Omite®.

Suggested Reading

Nishioka K, Kozuka T, Tashiro M (1970) Agricultural miticide (BPPS) dermatitis. Skin Res 12:15
O'Malley M, Rodriguez P, Maibach HI (1995) Pesticide patch testing: California nursery workers and controls. Contact Dermatitis 32:61–62

353. Propranolol

CAS Registry Number [525–66–6]

Propranolol is a beta-blocking agent that was responsible for the sensitization of workers in drug synthesis. In one case, epichlorhydrin was used for the production of drugs propranolol and oxprenolol. Cross-reactivity is expected between beta-blockers.

Suggested Reading

Pereira F, Dias M, Pacheco FA (1996) Occupational contact dermatitis from propranolol, hydralazine and bendroflumethiazide. Contact Dermatitis 35:303–304
Rebandel P, Rudzki E (1990) Dermatitis caused by epichlorhydrin, oxprenolol hydrochloride and propranolol hydrochloride. Contact Dermatitis 23:199

354. Propyl Gallate

CAS Registry Number [121–79–9]

This gallate ester (E 311) is an antioxidant frequently used in the food, cosmetic, and pharmaceutical industries to prevent the oxidation of unsaturated fatty acids into rancid-smelling compounds. It causes cosmetic dermatitis mainly from lipsticks and induced contact dermatitis in a baker, and in a female confectioner, primarily sensitized by her night cream, who fried doughnuts – the margarine probably containing gallates.

58

Suggested Reading

Bojs G, Niklasson B, Svensson A (1987) Allergic contact dermatitis to propyl gallate. Contact Dermatitis 17:294–298

Marston S (1992) Propyl gallate on liposomes. Contact Dermatitis 27:74–76

Serra-Baldrich E, Puig LL, Gimenez Arnau A, Camarasa JG (1995) Lipstick allergic contact dermatitis from gallates. Contact Dermatitis 32:359–360

355. Propylene Glycol

1,2-Propanediol

CAS Registry Number [57–55–6]

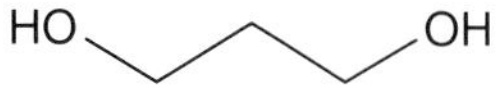

HO⌒⌒OH

Propylene glycol is used as a solvent, a vehicle for topical medicaments such as corticosteroids or aciclovir, an emulsifier and humectant in food and cosmetics, and as antifreeze in breweries, in the manufactures of resins. It was present as an occupational sensitizer in the color film developer Flexicolor®. Patch tests in aqua are sometimes irritant.

Suggested Reading

Claverie F, Giordano-Labadie F, Bazex J (1997) Eczéma de contact au propylène glycol. Ann Dermatol Venereol 124:315–317

Connoly M, Buckley DA (2004) Contact dermatitis from propylene glycol in ECG electrodes, complicated by medicament allergy. Contact Dermatitis 50:42

Scheman AJ, Katta R (1997) Photographic allergens: an update. Contact Dermatitis 37:130

356. Propylene Oxide

CAS Registry Number [75–56–9]

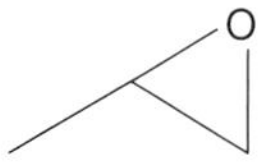

Propylene oxide is an allergic and irritant agent, used as a solvent and raw material in the chemical industry, as the starting material and intermediate for a broad spectrum of polymers. It can be used as a dehydrating agent for the preparation of slides in electron microscopy. Occupational dermatitis was also reported following the use of a skin disinfectant swab.

Suggested Reading

Steinkraus V, Hausen BM (1994) Contact allergy to propylene oxide. Contact Dermatitis 31:120

Van Ketel WG (1979) Contact dermatitis from propylene oxide. Contact Dermatitis 5:191–192

357. Pseudoephedrine

CAS Registry Number [90–82–4]

Pseudoephedrine Hydrochloride

CAS Registry Number [345–78–8]

Pseudoephedrine Sulfate

CAS Registry Number [7460–12–0]

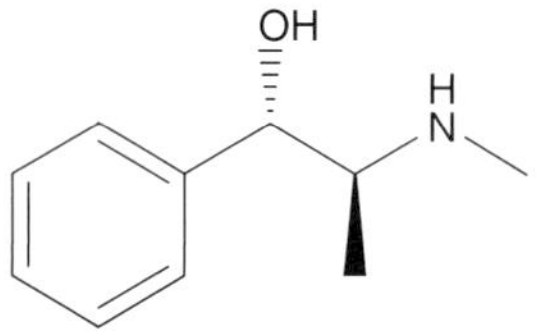

This sympathomimetic α-adrenergic agonist is found in plants of the genus *Ephedra* (Ephedraceae) and is systemically used as a nasal decongestant. It can induce drug skin reactions such as acute generalized exanthematic pustulosis or generalized eczema.

Suggested Reading

Assier-Bonnet H, Viguier M, Dubertret L, Revuz J, Roujeau JC (2002) Severe adverse drug reactions due to pseudoephedrine from over-the-counter medications. Contact Dermatitis 47:165–182

Padial MA, Alvarez-Ferreira J, Tapia B, Blanco R, Manas C, Blanca M, Bellon T (2004) Acute generalized exanthematous pustulosis associated with pseudoephedrine. Br J Dermatol 150:139–142

358. Pyrethroids

Cypermethrin(e)

CAS Registry Number [52315–07–8]

Permethrin(e)

CAS Registry Number [52645–53–1]

Deltamethrin(e)

CAS Registry Number [52918–63–5]

Bioalletrhin(e), Depalethrin(e)

CAS Registry Number [584–79–2]

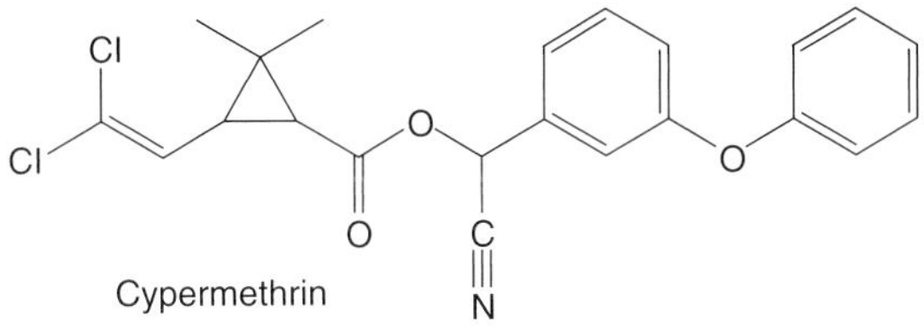

Cypermethrin

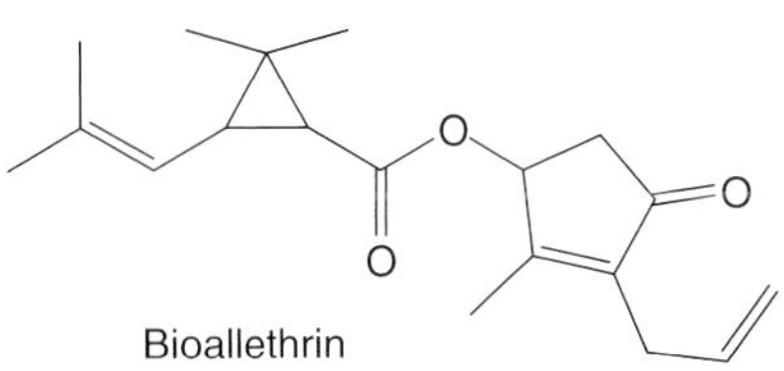

Bioallethrin

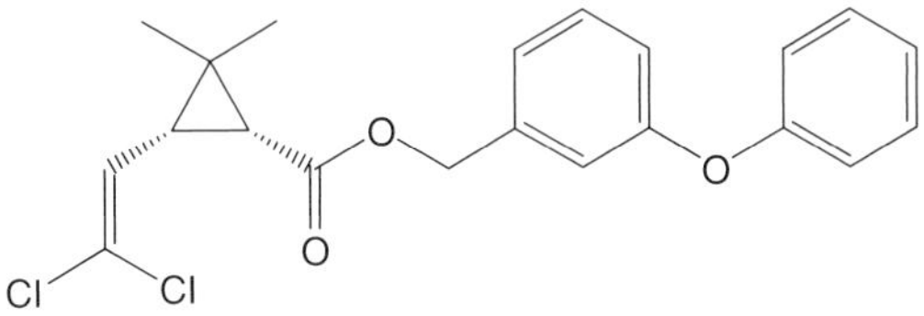

Permethrin

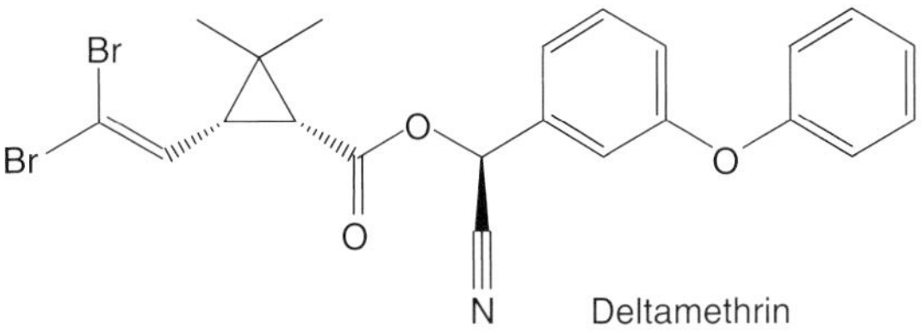

N   Deltamethrin

Pyrethroids, also called pyrethrinoids, are neurotoxic synthetic compounds used as insecticides, with irritant properties. Cypermethrin and fenvalerate have been reported as causing positive allergic patch tests, but only fenvalerate was relevant in an agricultural worker.

Suggested Reading

Flannigan SA, Tucker SB, Key MM, Ross CE, Fairchild EJ 2nd, Grimes BA, Harrist RB (1985) Primary irritant contact dermatitis from synthetic pyrethroid insecticide exposure. Arch Toxicol 56:288–294

Lisi P (1992) Sensitization risk of pyrethroid insecticides. Contact Dermatitis 26:349–350

359. Pyrethrosin

CAS Registry Number [28272–18–6]

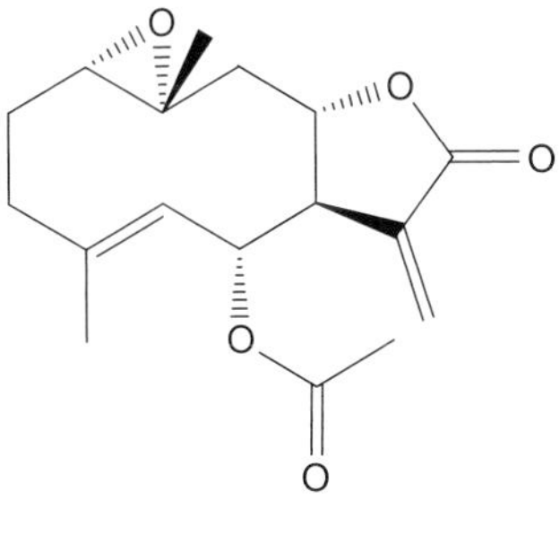

Pyrethrosin is an allergen of Asteraceae–Compositae such as *Chrysanthemum cinerariifolium* Vis.

Suggested Reading

Mitchell JC, Dupuis G, Towers GHN (1972) Allergic contact dermatitis from pyrethrum (*Chrysanthemum* spp.). The roles of pyrethrosin, a sesquiterpene lactone, and of pyrethrin II. Br J Dermatol 86:568–573

Paulsen E, Andersen KE, Hausen BM (1993) Compositae dermatitis in a Danish dermatology department in one year (I). Results of routine patch testing with the sesquiterpene lactone mix supplemented with aimed patch testing with extracts and sesquiterpene lactones of Compositae plants. Contact Dermatitis 29:6–10

360. Pyridine

CAS Registry Number [110–86–1]

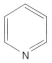

Pyridine (unsubstituted pyridine) and its derivative (substituted pyridines) are widely used in chemistry. Pyridine is a solvent used for many organic compounds and anhydrous metallic salt chemicals. Contained in Karl Fischer reagent, it induced contact dermatitis in a laboratory technician. No cross-sensitivity is observed between those different substances.

Suggested Reading

Knegt-Junk C, Geursen-Reitsma L, van Joost T (1993) Allergic contact dermatitis from pyridine in Karl Fischer reagent. Contact Dermatitis 28:252

361. Pyrithione

Pyrithione, Omadine

CAS Registry Number [1121–30–8]

Sodium Pyrithione, Sodium Omadine

CAS Registry Numbers [1121–30–8], [15922–78–8]

Zinc Pyrithione, Zinc Omadine

CAS Registry Number [13463–41–7] and more than 20 others

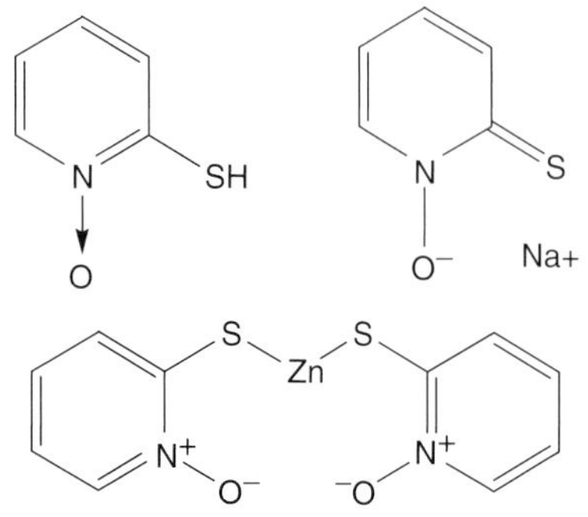

The sodium salt of *N*-hydroxy-2-pyridinethiones has germicidal activity against yeasts and fungi. Sodium omadine is a 40% aqueous solution of sodium pyrithione. It is used in the metallurgical industry as a component of water-based metalworking fluids, of aceto-polyvinyl lattices, water-based printer's ink, a lubricant for synthetic fibers, and antidandruff shampoos.

Zinc pyrithione is widely used in antidandruff shampoos and is a classic allergen. Concomitant reactions are expected to both zinc and sodium pyrithione.

Suggested Reading

Le Coz CJ (2001) Allergic contact dermatitis from sodium pyrithione in metalworking fluid. Contact Dermatitis 45:58–59
Tosti A, Piraccini B, Brasile GP (1990) Occupational contact dermatitis due to sodium pyrithione. Contact Dermatitis 22:118–119

362. Pyrogallol

1,2,3-Benzenetriol, CI 76515, Pyrogallic Acid

CAS Registry Number [87–66–1]

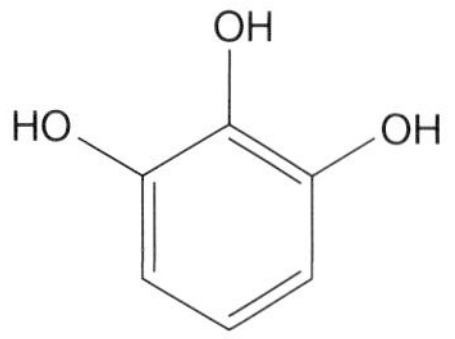

Pyrogallol belongs to the phenols group. It is an old photograph developer and a low sensitizer in hair dyes.

Suggested Reading

Frosch PJ, Burrows D, Camarasa JG, Dooms-Goossens A, Ducombs G, Lahti A, Menné T, Rycroft RJG, Shaw S, White IR, Wilkinson JD (1993) Allergic reactions to a hairdresser's series: results from 9 European centers. Contact Dermatitis 28:180–183
Guerra L, Tosti A, Bardazzi F, Pigatto P, Lisi P, Santucci B, Valsecchi R, Schena D, Angelini G, Sertoli A, Ayala F, Kokelj F (1992) Contact dermatitis in hairdressers: the Italian experience. Gruppo Italiano Ricerca Dermatiti da Contatto e Ambientali. Contact Dermatitis 26:101–107

363. PVP

Polyvinylpyrrolidone, Polyvidone, Povidone, 2-Pyrrolidinone, 1-Ethenyl-, Homopolymer

CAS Registry Number [9003–39–8]

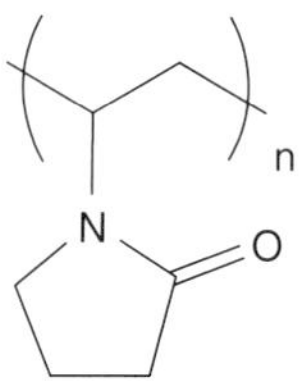

Polyvinylpyrrolidone is widely used as is in cosmetics such as hair care products and in medical products. It acts as iodophor in iodine-polyvinylpyrrolidone. PVP is an irritant and has been claimed as the allergen in some cases of dermatitis from iodine-polyvinylpyrrolidone (although iodine is more likely the hapten). It may cause type I contact urticaria or anaphylaxis.

Suggested Reading

Adachi A, Fukunaga A, Hayashi K, Kunisada M, Horikawa T (2003) Anaphylaxis to polyvinylpyrrolidone after vaginal application of povidone-iodine. Contact Dermatitis 48:133–136
Ronnau AC, Wulferink M, Gleichmann E, Unver E, Ruzicka T, Krutmann J, Grewe M (2000) Anaphylaxis to polyvinylpyrrolidone in an analgesic preparation. Br J Dermatol 143:1055–1058

364. PVP/Eicosene Copolymer

Polyvinylpyrrolidone/Eicosene Copolymer

CAS Registry Numbers [28211–18–9], [77035–98–4]

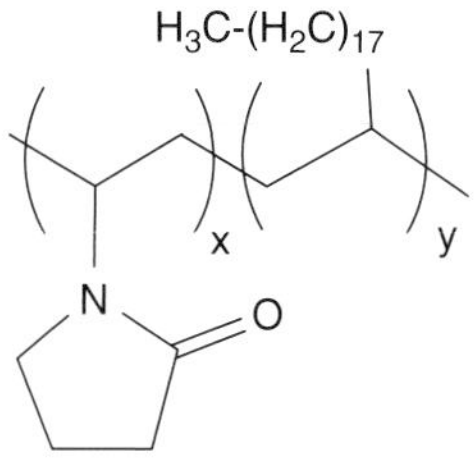

PVP/eicosene copolymer is the polymer of vinylpyr-rolidone and of 1-eicosene, and one of the 11 PVP copolymers recorded in the International Nomenclature of Cosmetics Ingredients inventory system. This substance is utilized in cosmetics, in sunscreens to enhance their water resistance, and is an inert ingredient in pesticides. Contact sensitization to a close compound VP/eicosene copolymer was also reported.

Suggested Reading

Gallo R, dal Sacco D, Ghigliotti G (2004) Allergic contact dermatitis from VP/eisosene copolymer (Ganex® V-220) in an emollient cream. Contact Dermatitis 50:261

Le Coz CJ, Lefebvre C, Ludmann F, Grosshans E (2000) Polyvinylpyrrolidone (PVP)/eicosene copolymer: an emerging cosmetic allergen. Contact Dermatitis 43:61–62

365. PVP/Hexadecene Copolymer

CAS Registry Number [32440–50–9]

PVP/hexadecene copolymer, another PVP copolymer used for identical applications as PVP/eicosene copolymer, has been rarely implicated in contact dermatitis.

Suggested Reading

De Groot AC, Bruynzeel DP, Bos JD, van der Meeren HL, van Joost T, Jagtman BA, Weyland JW (1988) The allergens in cosmetics. Arch Dermatol 124:1525–1529

Scheman A, Cummins R (1998) Contact allergy to PVP/hexadecene copolymer. Contact Dermatitis 39:201

366. Quaternium-15

N-(3-Chloroallyl)Hexaminium Chloride, Hexamethylenetetramine Chloroallyl Chloride, Dowicil 200

CAS Registry Numbers [4080–31–3], [103638–29–5], [60789–82–4]

Quaternium-15 is a quaternary ammonium compound, used as a broad-spectrum formaldehyde-releasing bactericide agent. It is contained as a preservative in cosmetics, toiletries, and aqueous products. Allergy is mainly due to formaldehyde and not to Quaternium-15 itself. Occupational case reports concerned hairdressers, a beautician, an engineer working on the maintenance of machinery in a chicken processing plant, and an employee carrying out photocopying tasks.

Suggested Reading

Finch TM, Prais L, Foulds IS (2001) Occupational allergic contact dermatitis from quaternium-15 in an electroencephalography skin preparation gel. Contact Dermatitis 44: 44–45

Marren P, de Berker D, Dawber RP, Powell S (1991) Occupational contact dermatitis due to quaternium 15 presenting as nail dystrophy. Contact Dermatitis 25:253–255

O'Reilly FM, Murphy GM (1996) Occupational contact dermatitis in a beautician. Contact Dermatitis 35:47–48

Tosti A, Piraccini BM, Bardazzi F (1990) Occupational contact dermatitis due to quaternium 15. Contact Dermatitis 23:41–42

Zina AM, Fanan E, Bundino S (2000) Allergic contact dermatitis from formaldehyde and quaternium-15 in photocopier toner. Contact Dermatitis 43:241–242

367. Quaternium-22

CAS Registry Numbers [51812–80–7], [82970–95–4]

This quaternary ammonium compound, used as a film former and conditioning agent, was reported as a co-sensitizer in eyelid dermatitis due to shellac-based mascara.

Suggested Reading

Le Coz CJ, Leclere JM, Arnoult E, Raison-Peyron N, Pons-Guiraud A, Vigan M, Members of Revidal-GERDA (2002) Allergic contact dermatitis from shellac in mascara. Contact Dermatitis 46:149–152

Scheman AJ (1998) Contact allergy to quaternium-22 and shellac in mascara. Contact Dermatitis 38:342–343

368. Ranitidine

CAS Registry Number [66357–35–5]

Ranitidine Hydrochloride

CAS Registry Number [66357–59–3]

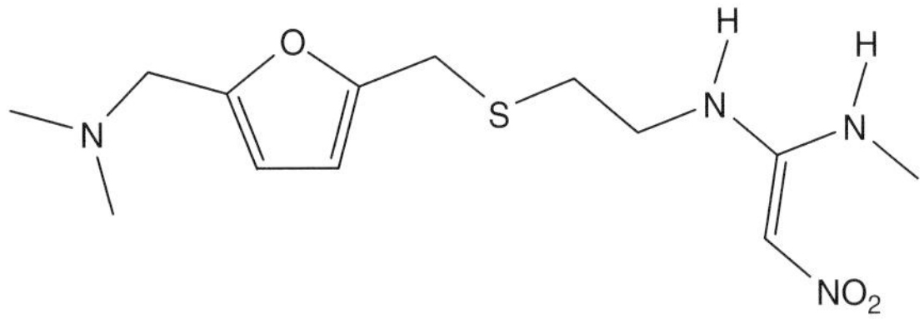

Ranitidine, an H2-receptor antagonist, can cause contact dermatitis within the pharmaceutical industry and
in health care workers, or may induce systemic drug
reactions in patients.

Suggested Reading

Martinez MB, Salvador JF, Aguilera GV, Mas IB, Ramirez JC
(2003) Acute generalized exanthematous pustulosis induced
by ranitidine hydrochloride. Contact Dermatitis 49:47
Romaguerra C, Grimalt F, Vilaplana J (1988) Epidemic of occupational contact dermatitis from ranitidine. Contact
Dermatitis 18:177–178

369. Resorcinol

1,3-Benzendiol, CI 76505

CAS Registry Number [108–46–3]

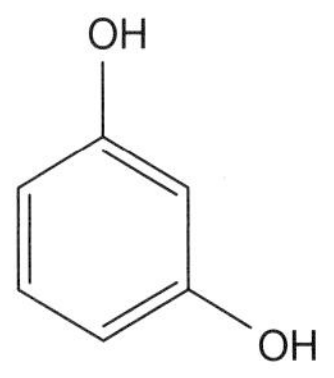

Resorcinol is used in hairdressing as a modifier (or a
coupler) of the PPD group of dyes. It is the least frequent sensitizer in hairdressers. It is also used in resins, in skin treatment mixtures, and for tanning. Severe
cases of dermatitis due to resorcinol contained in wart
preparations have been reported.

Suggested Reading

Barbaud A, Modiano P, Cocciale M, Reichert S, Schmutz JL
(1996) The topical application of resorcinol can provoke a
systemic allergic reaction. Br J Dermatol 135:1014–1015
Frosch PJ, Burrows D, Camarasa JG, Dooms-Goossens A, Ducombs
G, Lahti A, Menné T, Rycroft RJG, Shaw S, White IR, Wilkinson
JD (1993) Allergic reactions to a hairdresser's series: results
from 9 European centers. Contact Dermatitis 28:180–183
Tarvainen K (1995) Analysis of patients with allergic patch test
reactions to a plastics and glue series. Contact Dermatitis
32:346–351
Vilaplana J, Romaguera C, Grimalt F (1991) Contact dermatitis
from resorcinol in a hair dye. Contact Dermatitis 24:151–152

370. Silane

Monosilane

CAS Registry Number [7803–62–5]

$$SiH_4$$

Various silane derivatives are used as bonding agents
between glass and the resin used as a coating agent of
glass filaments. Organosilanes have been implicated as
sensitizers in workers at a glass filament manufactory.

Suggested Reading

Heino T, Haapa K, Manelius F (1996) Contact sensitization to
organosilane solution in glass filament production. Contact
Dermatitis 34:294

371. Sodium Bisulfite

Sodium Acid Sulfite, E222

CAS Registry Number [7631–90–5]

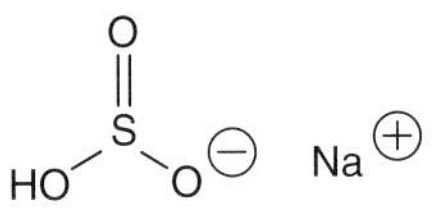

Sodium bisulfite is mainly used as an antioxidant in
pharmaceutical products, as a disinfectant or bleach,
and in the dye industry. The bisulfite of commerce
consists chiefly of metabisulfite and possesses the
same properties as the true bisulfite. So, the allergen to
be tested in products containing disulfite is the corresponding metabisulfite.

Suggested Reading

Budavari S, O'Neil MJ, Smith A, Heckelman PE, Kinneary JF (eds) (1996) The Merck Index, 12th edn. Merck, Whitehouse Station, NJ, USA

372. Sodium lauryl sulfate

SLS, Sodium Dodecyl Sulfate

CAS Registry Number [151–21–3]

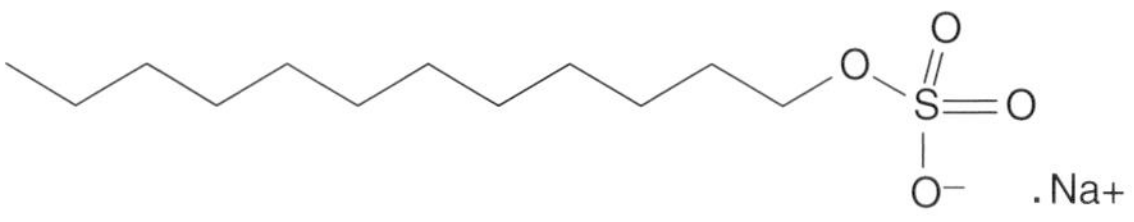

This anionic detergent is widely used in cosmetics and industry. As a skin irritant agent, SLS can be used in several dermatological applications. It is also a good indicator of excited skin during patch testing.

Suggested Reading

Geier J, Uter W, Pirker C, Frosch PJ (2003) Patch testing with the irritant sodium lauryl sulfate (SLS) is useful in interpreting weak reactions to contact allergens as allergic or irritant. Contact Dermatitis 48:99–107

373. Sodium Metabisulfite

Sodium Pyrosulfite, Disodium Disulfite, E223

CAS Registry Number [7681–57–4]

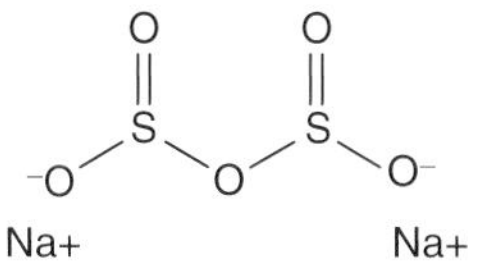

This agent is frequently used as a preservative in pharmaceutical products, in the bread-making industry as an antioxidant, and it can induce contact dermatitis. It can be used as a reducing agent in photography and caused dermatitis in a photographic technician, probably acting as an aggravating irritative factor. Sodium metabisulfite contains a certain amount of sodium sulfite and sodium sulfate.

Suggested Reading

Acciai MC, Brusi C, Francalanci Giorgini S, Sertoli A (1993) Allergic contact dermatitis in caterers. Contact Dermatitis 28:48

Jacobs MC, Rycroft RJG (1995) Contact dermatitis and asthma from sodium metabisulfite in a photographic technician. Contact Dermatitis 33:65–66
Riemersma WA, Schuttelaar ML, Coenraads PJ (2004) Type IV hypersensitivity to sodium metabisulfite in local anesthetic. Contact Dermatitis 51:148
Vena GA, Foti C, Angelini G (1994) Sulfite contact allergy. Contact Dermatitis 31:172–175

374. Sodium Methyldithiocarbamate

Metham-Na, Carbathion, Sodium-*N*-Methyldithiocarbamate

CAS Registry Number [137–42–8]

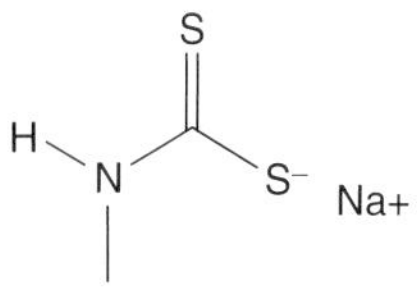

Metham-Na is a fungicide nematocide of the dithiocarbamate group. Sensitization occurs among agricultural workers.

Suggested Reading

Koch P (1996) Occupational allergic contact dermatitis and airborne contact dermatitis from 5 fungicides in a vineyard worker. Cross-reactions between fungicides of the dithiocarbamate group? Contact Dermatitis 34:324–329
Pambor M, Bloch Y (1985) Dimethoat und Dithiocarmabat als berufliche Kontaktallergene bei einer Agrotechnikerin. Dermat Monatsschr 171:401–405
Schubert H (1978) Contact dermatitis to sodium-*N*-methyldithiocarbamate. Contact Dermatitis 4:370–371
Wolf F, Jung HD (1970) Akute Kontaktdermatitiden nach Umgang mit Nematin. Z Ges Hyg 16:423–426

375. Sodium Sulfite

E225

CAS Registry Number [7757–83–7]

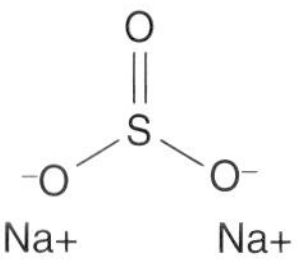

Sodium sulfite is mainly used in photographic developers, for fixing prints, bleaching textile fibers, as a

58

reducer in manufacturing dyes, as a remover of Cl in bleached textiles and paper, and as a preservative in the food industry for meat, egg yolks, and so on.

Suggested Reading

Budavari S, O'Neil MJ, Smith A, Heckelman PE, Kinneary JF (eds) (1996) The Merck Index, 12th edn. Merck, Whitehouse Station, NJ, USA
Vena GA, Foti C, Angelini G (1994) Sulfite contact allergy. Contact Dermatitis 31:172–175

376. Solvent Red 23

Sudan III, CI 26100, D and C Red No. 17

CAS Registry Number [85–86–9]

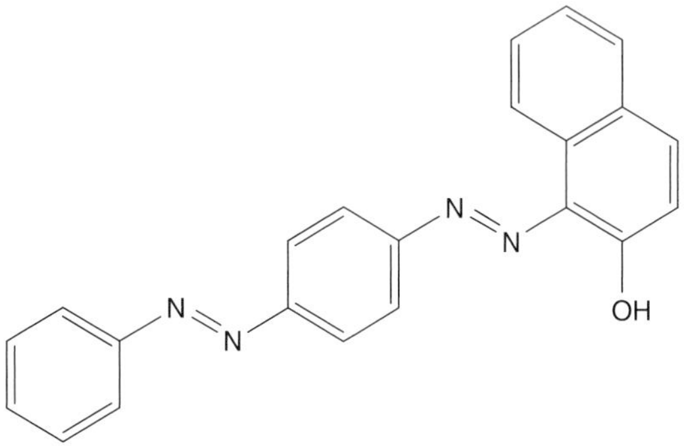

Solvent Red 23 is an oil-soluble red azo-dye used in cosmetic products in Japan. Cases were reported in hairdressers, who also reacted to PPD (the molecule is likely to be hydrolyzed into PPD) and to *p*-aminoazobenzene. One case of contact dermatitis was reported in the metal industry.

Suggested Reading

Fregert S (1967) Allergic contact dermatitis due to fumes from burning alcohol containing an azo-dye. Contact Dermat Newslett 1:11
Matsunaga K, Hayakawa R, Yoshimura K, Okada J (1990) Patch-test-positive reactions to Solvent Red 23 in hairdressers. Contact Dermatitis 23:266

377. Sorbitan Sesquioleate

Sorbitan 9-Octadecenoate (2:3), Arlacel 83, Anhydrohexitol Sesquioleate

CAS Registry Number [8007–43–0], [37318–79–9]

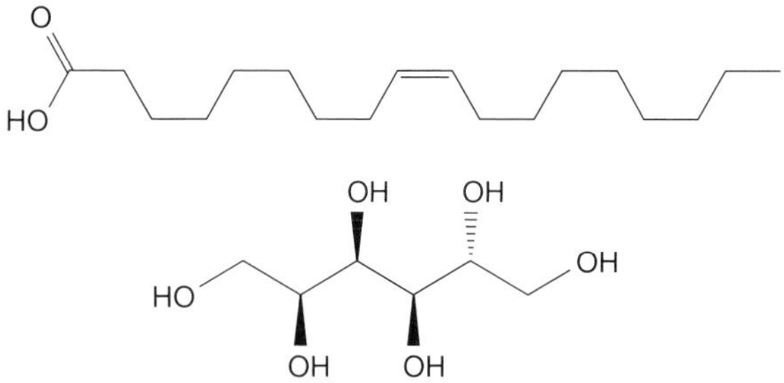

Sorbitan sesquioleate is a mixture of mono and diesters of oleic acid and extol anhydrides derived from sorbitol. It is used as a surfactant and an emulsifier in cosmetics. It acts sometimes as a contact allergen, particularly in leg ulcer patients. It is also responsible for false-positive patch test reactions to haptens, with which some allergen providers emulgated, such as parabens mix, fragrance mix, Amerchol L101, and ethylene-urea /melamine formaldehyde.

Suggested Reading

Orton DI, Shaw S (2001) Sorbitan sesquioleate as an allergen. Contact Dermatitis 44:190–191
Pasche-Koo F, Piletta PA, Hunziker N, Hauser C (1994) High sensitization rate to emulsifiers in patients with chronic leg ulcers. Contact Dermatitis 31:226–228

378. Spectinomycin

CAS Registry Number [1695–77–8]

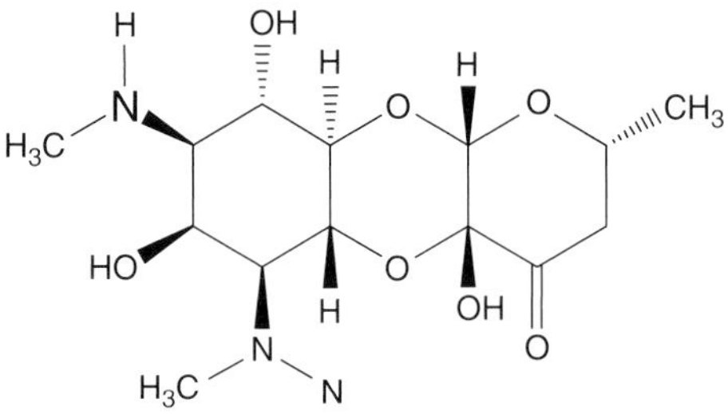

Spectinomycin is an aminocyclitol antibiotic. It is used in human medicine against *Neisseria gonorrhoeae* and in veterinary medicine, especially for poultry, pigs, and cattle. Cases of dermatitis have been reported in veterinary practice.

Suggested Reading

Dal Monte A, Laffi G, Mancini G (1994) Occupational contact dermatitis due to spectinomycin. Contact Dermatitis 31:204–205

Vilaplana J, Romaguera C, Grimalt F (1991) Contact dermatitis from lincomycin and spectinomycin in chicken vaccinators. Contact Dermatitis 24:225–226

379. Tetrabenzylthiuram Disulfide

TBzTD

CAS Registry Number [10591–85–2]

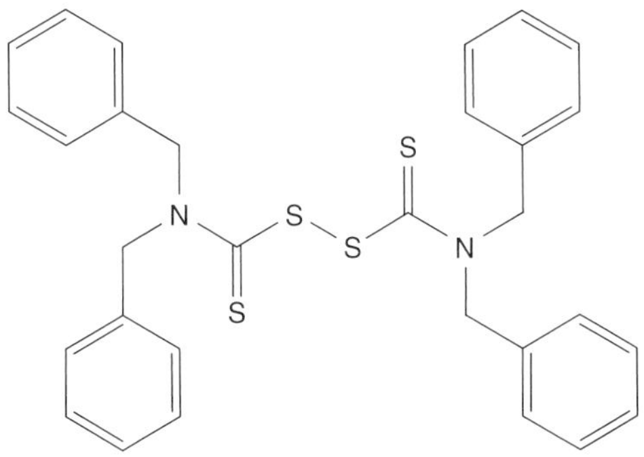

TBzTD is a rubber vulcanization accelerator.

Suggested Reading

Le Coz CJ (2004) Fiche d'éviction en cas d'hypersensibilité au thiuram mix. Ann Dermatol Venereol 131:1012–1014

380. Tetrabutylthiuram Disulfide

TBTD

CAS [1634–02–2]

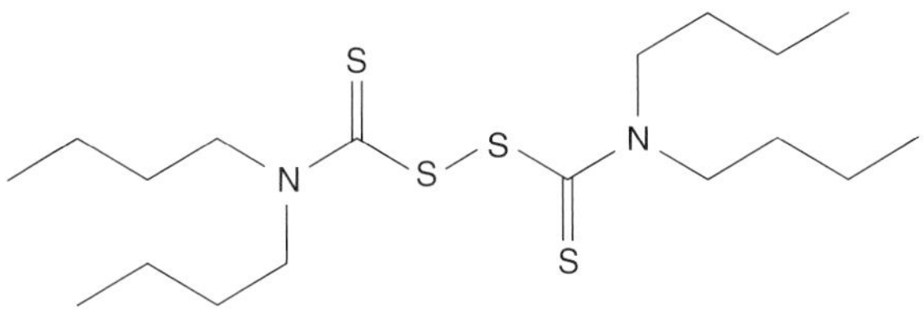

TBTD is a rubber vulcanization accelerator.

Suggested Reading

Le Coz CJ (2004) Fiche d'éviction en cas d'hypersensibilité au thiuram mix. Ann Dermatol Venereol 131:1012–1014

381. Tetrabutylthiuram Monosulfide

TBTM

CAS Registry Number [97–74–5]

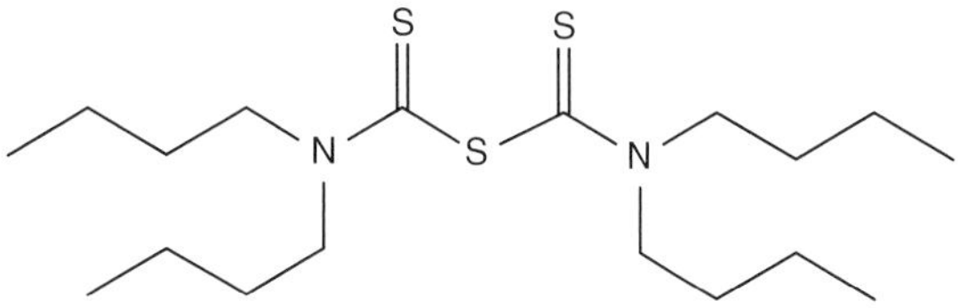

TBTM is a rubber vulcanization accelerator.

Suggested Reading

Le Coz CJ (2004) Fiche d'éviction en cas d'hypersensibilité au thiuram mix. Ann Dermatol Venereol 131:1012–1014

382. Tetrachloroacetophenone

CAS Registry Number [39751–78–5]

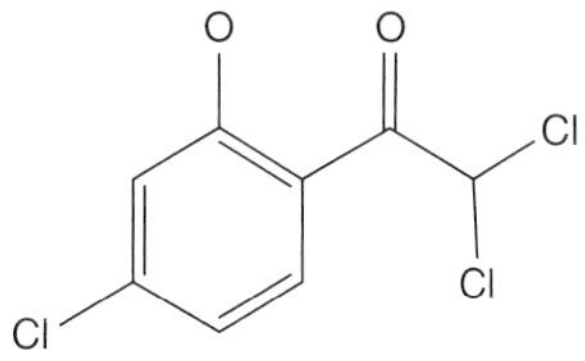

Tetrachloroacetophone was combined with triethyl phosphate to form an organophosphate insecticide. It induced contact dermatitis in a process operator in an insecticide plant.

Suggested Reading

Van Joost T, Wiemer GR (1991) Contact dermatitis from tetra-chloroacetophenone (TCAP) in an insecticide plant. Contact Dermatitis 25:66–67

383. Tetraethylthiuram Disulfide

Disulfiram, TETD, Antabuse, Esperal®

CAS Registry Number [97–77–8]

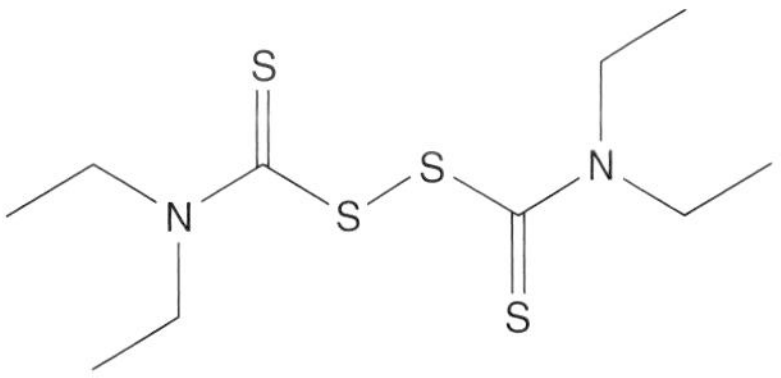

58

TETD is a rubber accelerator of the thiuram group, contained in "thiuram mix." It can cross-react with other thiurams, especially TMTD. TETD is used to aid those trying to break their dependence on alcohol. The disulfiram-alcohol reaction is not allergic but due to the accumulation of toxic levels of acetaldehyde. The implanted drug can, however, lead to local or generalized dermatitis, for example ingested disulfiram, mainly in previously rubber-sensitized patients. As an adjunctive treatment of alcoholism, it caused occupational contact dermatitis in a nurse.

Suggested Reading

Condé-Salazar L, Del-Rio E, Guimaraens D, Gonzalez Domingo A (1993) Type IV allergy to rubber additives: a 10-year study of 686 cases. J Am Acad Dermatol 29:176–180
Kiec-Swierczynska M, Krecisz B, Fabicka B (2000) Systemic contact dermatitis from implanted disulfiram. Contact Dermatitis 43(4):246–247
Le Coz CJ (2004) Fiche d'éviction en cas d'hypersensibilité au thiuram mix. Ann Dermatol Venereol 131:1012–1014
Mathelier-Fusade P, Leynadier F (1994) Occupational allergic contact reaction to disulfiram. Contact Dermatitis 31: 121–122
Webb PK, Bibbs SC (1979) Disulfiram hypersensivity and rubber contact dermatitis. JAMP 241:2061

384. Tetraethylthiuram Monosulfide

Sulfiram, TETM, Tetraethylthiodicarbonic Diamide

CAS Registry Number [95–05–6]

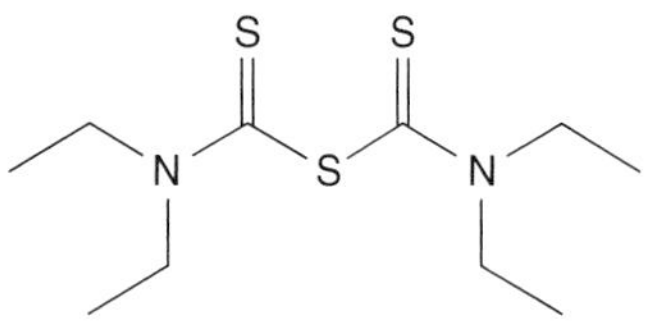

This rubber vulcanization accelerator is also used as an ectoparasiticide against *Sarcoptes scabiei*, louses, or in veterinary medicine.

Suggested Reading

Le Coz CJ (2004) Fiche d'éviction en cas d'hypersensibilité au thiuram mix. Ann Dermatol Venereol 131:1012–1014

385. Tetraisobutylthiuram Disulfide

TITD, Thioperoxydicarbonic Diamide, Tetrakis (2-Methylpropyl)

CAS Registry Number [137–26–8]

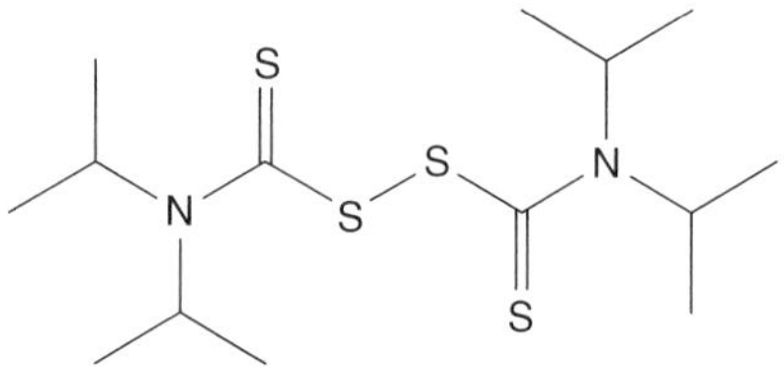

TITD is a rubber vulcanization accelerator.

Suggested Reading

Le Coz CJ (2004) Fiche d'éviction en cas d'hypersensibilité au thiuram mix. Ann Dermatol Venereol 131:1012–1014

386. Tetramethylthiuram Disulfide

Thiram, TMTD

CAS Registry Number [137–26–8]

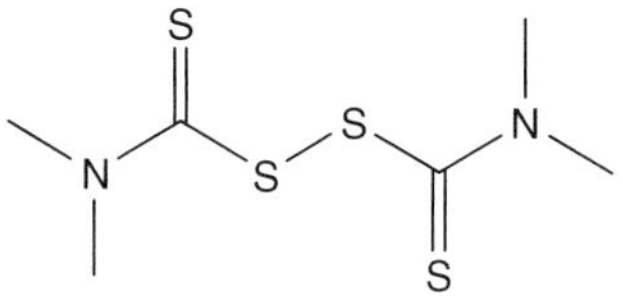

This rubber chemical, accelerator of vulcanization, represents the most commonly positive allergen contained in "thiuram mix." The most frequent occupational categories are the metal industry, homemakers, health services and laboratories, the building industry, and shoemakers. It is also widely used as a fungicide, belonging to the dithiocarbamate group of carrots, bulbs, and woods, and as an insecticide. Thiram is the agricultural name for thiuram.

Suggested Reading

Condé-Salazar L, Guimaraens D, Villegas C, Romero A, Gonzalez MA (1995) Occupational allergic contact dermatitis in construction workers. Contact Dermatitis 35:226–230
Kiec-Swierczynska M (1995) Occupational sensitivity to rubber. Contact Dermatitis 32:171–172
Le Coz CJ (2004) Fiche d'éviction en cas d'hypersensibilité au thiuram mix. Ann Dermatol Venereol 131:1012–1014

Mancuso G, Reggiani M, Berdondini RM (1996) Occupational dermatitis in shoemakers. Contact Dermatitis 34:17–22

Sharma VK, Kaur S (1990) Contact sensitization by pesticides in farmers. Contact Dermatitis 23:77–80

387. Tetramethylthiuram Monosulfide

TMTM

CAS Registry Number [97–74–5]

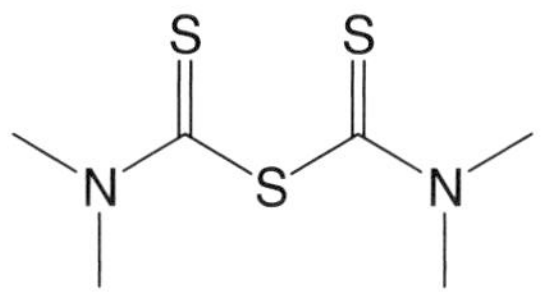

This rubber accelerator is contained in "thiuram mix." The most frequent occupational categories are the metal industry, homemakers, health services and laboratories, and the building industry.

Suggested Reading

Condé-Salazar L, Del-Rio E, Guimaraens D, Gonzalez Domingo A (1993) Type IV allergy to rubber additives: a 10-year study of 686 cases. J Am Acad Dermatol 29:176–180

Condé-Salazar L, Guimaraens D, Villegas C, Romero A, Gonzalez MA (1995) Occupational allergic contact dermatitis in construction workers. Contact Dermatitis 35:226–230

Le Coz CJ (2004) Fiche d'éviction en cas d'hypersensibilité au thiuram mix. Ann Dermatol Venereol 131:1012–1014

Von Hintzenstern J, Heese A, Koch HU, Peters KP, Hornstein OP (1991) Frequency, spectrum and occupational relevance of type IV allergies to rubber chemicals. Contact Dermatitis 24:244–252

388. Tetrazepam

CAS Registry Number [10379–14–3]

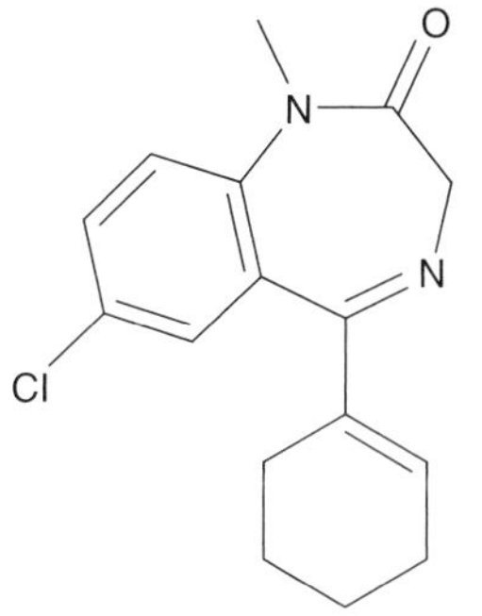

Tetrazepam is a benzodiazepine compound used systemically as a myorelaxant. It may induce skin rashes such as maculo-papular eruption, Stevens–Johnson syndrome, or photosensitivity. Occupational sensitization can be observed in pharmaceutical plants. Sensitization generally does not concern other benzodiazepines.

Suggested Reading

Barbaud A, Girault PY, Schmutz JL, Weber-Muller F, Trechot P (2009) No cross-reactions between tetrazepam and other benzodiazepines: a possible chemical explanation. Contact Dermatitis 61:53–56

Barbaud A, Trechot P, Reichert-Penetrat S, Granel F, Schmutz JL (2001) The usefulness of patch testing on the previously most severely affected site in a cutaneous adverse drug reaction to tetrazepam. Contact Dermatitis 44:259–260

Choquet-Kastylevsky G, Testud F, Chalmet P, Lecuyer-Kudela S, Descotes J (2001) Occupational contact allergy to tetrazepam. Contact Dermatitis 44:372

389. Thebaine

CAS Registry Number [115–37–7]

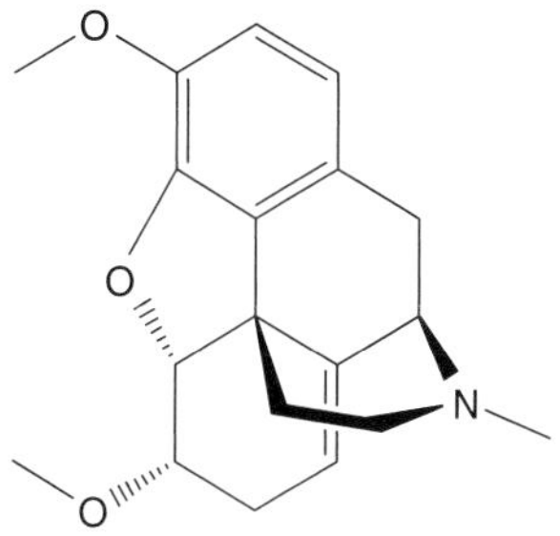

The naturally occurring opiate alkaloid thebaine is present in concentrated poppy straw, and in small concentrations in codeine alkaloid. It is used in the manufacture of other opiate pharmaceuticals, such as buprenorphine and morphine, and caused contact dermatitis in a laboratory worker at an opiates manufacturing pharmaceutical company, also sensitive to codeine.

Suggested Reading

Waclawski ER, Aldridge R (1995) Occupational dermatitis from thebaine and codeine. Contact Dermatitis 33:51

58

390. Thiabendazole

CAS Registry Number [148–79–8]

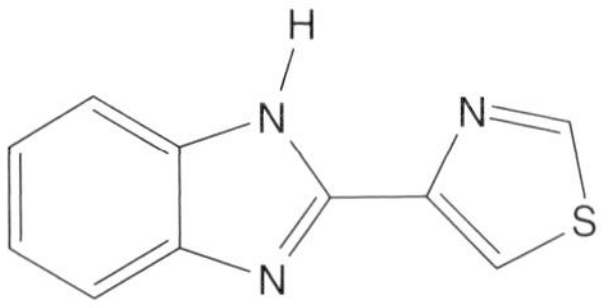

This fungicide and vermifuge agent is widely used in agriculture (for example, forcitrus fruits), and in medical and veterinary practice as an anthelmintic drug.

Suggested Reading

Izu R, Aguirre A, Goicoechea A, Gardeazabal J, Diaz Perez JL (1993) Photoaggravated allergic contact dermatitis due to topical thiabendazole. Contact Dermatitis 28:243–244

Mancuso G, Staffa M, Errani A, Berdondini RM, Fabri P (1990) Occupational dermatitis in animal feed mill workers. Contact Dermatitis 22:37–41

391. Thimerosal

Thiomersal, Thiomersalate, Merthiolate, Mercurothiolic Acid Sodium Salt

CAS Registry Number [54–64–8]

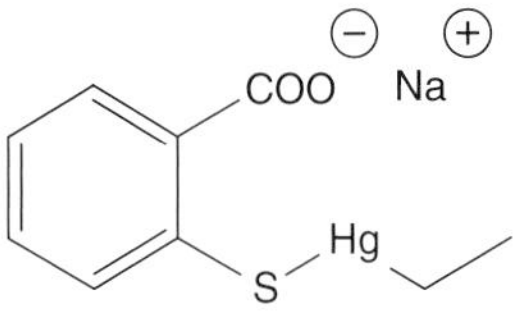

Thiomersal is an organic mercury salt prepared by reacting ethylmercuric chloride (or ethylmercuric hydroxide) with thiosalicylic acid. It is still used as a disinfectant and a preservative agent, but less commonly than previously, especially in contact lens fluids, eyedrops, and vaccines. The ethylmercuric moiety is the major allergenic determinant, sometimes associated with mercury sensitivity. Thiomersal is an indicator of photosensitivity to piroxicam, through its thiosalicylic moiety.

Suggested Reading

Arévalo A, Blancas R, Ancona A (1995) Occupational contact dermatitis from piroxicam. Am J Contact Dermat 6:113–114

De Groot AC, van Wijnen WG, van Wijnen-Vos M (1990) Occupational contact dermatitis of the eyelids, without ocular involvement, from thimerosal in contact lens fluid. Contact Dermatitis 23:195

Rudzki E, Rebandel P, Grzywa Z, Pomorski Z, Jakiminska B, Zawisza E (1982) Occupational dermatitis in veterinarians. Contact Dermatitis 8:72–73

392. Thiourea

Thiocarbamide

CAS Registry Number [62–56–6]

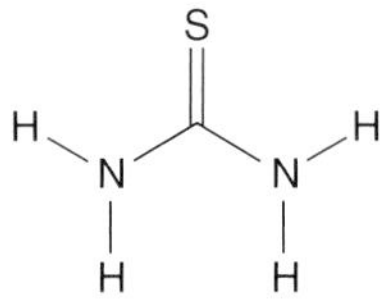

Thiourea is used as a cleaner agent for silver and copper, and as an antioxidant in diazo copy paper. It can induce (photo-) contact dermatitis.

Suggested Reading

Dooms-Goossens A, Debusschère K, Morren M, Roelandts R, Coopman S (1988) Silver polish: another source of contact dermatitis reactions to thiourea. Contact Dermatitis 19:133–135

Geier J, Fuchs T (1993) Contact allergy due to 4-*N*,*N*-dimethylaminobenzene diazonium chloride and thiourea in diazo copy paper. Contact Dermatitis 28:304–305

Kanerva L, Estlander T, Jolanki R (1994) Occupational allergic contact dermatitis caused by thiourea compounds. Contact Dermatitis 31:242–248

393. Thymoquinone

CAS Registry Number [490–91–5]

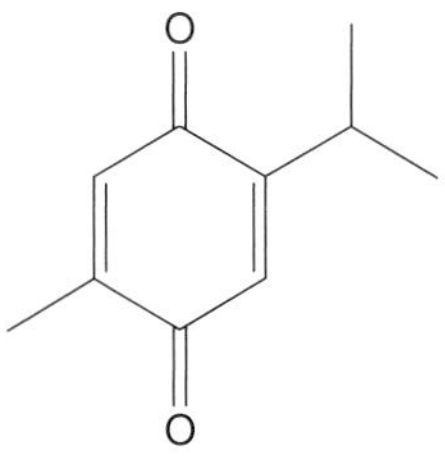

Thymoquinone is an allergen in different cedar species, Cupressaceae family, such as incense cedar (*Calocedrus decurrens* Florin) used for pencils, chests or toys, and western cedar (*Thuja plicata* Donn.) as used for hard realizations such as construction or boats. See also Chap. 46.

Suggested Reading

Hausen BM (2000) Woods. In: Kanerva L, Elsner P, Wahlberg JE, Maibach HI (eds) Handbook of occupational dermatology. Springer, Berlin, pp 771–780

Lamminpää A, Estlander T, Jolanki R, Kanerva L (1996) Occupational allergic contact dermatitis caused by decorative plants. Contact Dermatitis 34:330–335

394. Timolol

CAS Registry Number [26839–75–8]

Timolol was implicated in allergic contact dermatitis due to beta-blocker agents in eyedrops.

Suggested Reading

Giordano-Labadie F, Lepoittevin JP, Calix I, Bazex J (1997) Allergie de contact aux â-bloqueurs des collyres: allergie croisée? Ann Dermatol Venereol 124:322–324

395. Tixocortol Pivalate

Tixocortol 21-Pivalate, Tixocortol 21-Trimethylacetate

CAS Registry Number [55560–96–8]

Tixocortol 21-pivalate is a 21-ester of tixocortol, widely used in topical treatments. It can induce severe allergic contact dermatitis. This corticosteroid is a marker of the allergenic A group that includes molecules without major substitution on the D cycle (no C_{16} methylation, no C_{17} side chain). A short-chain C_{21} ester is possible. Molecules are cloprednol, cortisone, fludrocortisone, fluorometholone, hydrocortisone, methylprednisolone, methylprednisone, prednisolone, prednisone, tixocortol, and their C_{21} esters (acetate, caproate or hexanoate, phosphate, pivalate or trimethylacetate, succinate or hemisuccinate, *m*-sulfobenzoate).

Suggested Reading

Le Coz CJ (2002) Fiche d'éviction en cas d'hypersensibilité au pivalate de tixocortol. Ann Dermatol Venereol 129:348–349

Lepoittevin JP, Drieghe J, Dooms-Goossens A (1995) Studies in patients with corticosteroid contact allergy. Understanding cross-reactivity among different steroids. Arch Dermatol 131:31–37

396. Tocopherol, Tocopheryl Acetate (*Dl-*, *D-*)

Vitamin E

CAS Registry Number [1406–66–2]

Vitamin E Acetate *Dl*, Vitamin E Acetate *D*

CAS Registry Number [7695–91–2], CAS Registry Number [58–95–7]

Tocopherol and tocopheryl acetate are used mainly as antioxidants. Tocopheryl acetate, an ester of tocopherol (vitamin E), can induce allergic contact dermatitis.

Suggested Reading

De Groot AC, Berretty PJ, van Ginkel CJ, den Hengst CW, van Ulsen J, Weyland JW (1991) Allergic contact dermatitis from tocopheryl acetate in cosmetic creams. Contact Dermatitis 25:302–304

Matsumura T, Nakada T, Iijima M (2004) Widespread contact dermatitis from tocopherol acetate. Contact Dermatitis 51:211–212

397. Toluene-2,5-Diamine

p-Toluylenediamine, *p*-Toluenediamine

CAS Registry Number [95–70–5]

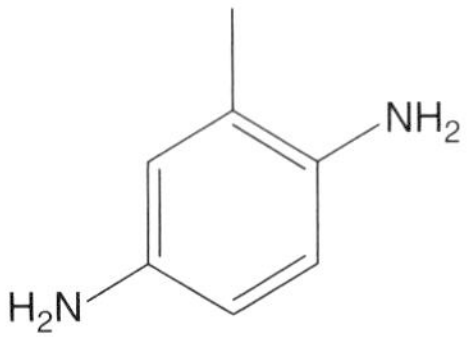

Toluene-2,5-diamine is a permanent hair dye involved in contact dermatitis in hairdressers and consumers. It does not cross-react with PPD, but cosensitization is frequent.

Suggested Reading

Frosch PJ, Burrows D, Camarasa JG, Dooms-Goossens A, Ducombs G, Lahti A, Menné T, Rycroft RJG, Shaw S, White IR, Wilkinson JD (1993) Allergic reactions to a hairdresser's series: results from 9 European centers. Contact Dermatitis 28:180–183

Guerra L, Tosti A, Bardazzi F, Pigatto P, Lisi P, Santucci B, Valsecchi R, Schena D, Angelini G, Sertoli A, Ayala F, Kokelj F (1992) Contact dermatitis in hairdressers: the Italian experience. Gruppo Italiano Ricerca Dermatiti da Contatto e Ambientali. Contact Dermatitis 26: 101–107

Le Coz CJ, Lefebvre C, Keller F, Grosshans E (2000) Allergic contact dermatitis caused by skin painting (pseudotattooing) with black henna, a mixture of henna and *p*-phenylenediamine and its derivatives. Arch Dermatol 136: 1515–1517

398. Toluene Diisocyanate

Toluene Diisocyanate (Mixture)

CAS Registry Number [26471–62–5]

Toluene 2,4-Diisocyanate

CAS Registry Number [584–84–9]

Toluene 2,6-Diisocyanate

CAS Registry Number [91–08–7]

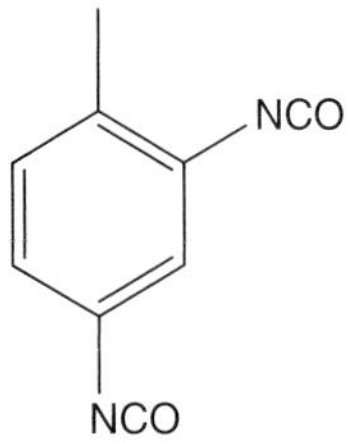

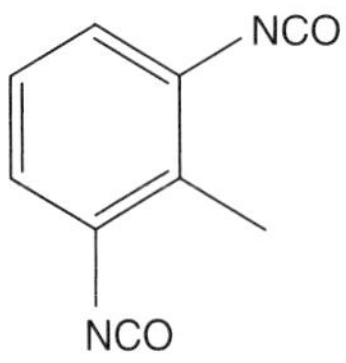

Toluene diisocyanate is a mixture of 2,4-TDI and 2,6-TDI. It is used in the manufacture of various polyurethane products: elastic and rigid foams, paints, lacquers, adhesives, binding agents, synthetics rubbers, and elastomeric fibers.

Suggested Reading

Estlander T, Keskinen H, Jolanki R, Kanerva L (1992) Occupational dermatitis from exposure to polyurethane chemicals. Contact Dermatitis 27:161–165

Le Coz CJ, El Aboubi S, Ball C (1999) Active sensitization to toluene di-isocyanate. Contact Dermatitis 41:104–105

399. Tosyl Chloride

p-Toluene Sulfonyl Chloride, *p*-Toluene Sulfochloride

CAS Registry Number [98–59–9]

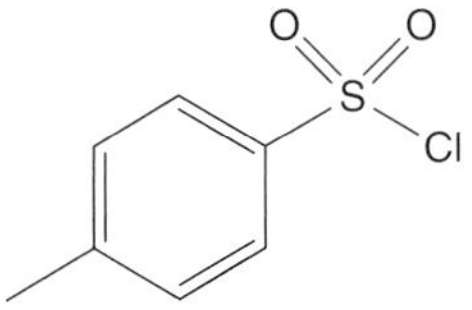

Tosyl chloride is used mainly in the preparation of chemical derivatives in the pharmaceutical, plastics, and organic chemical industries.

Suggested Reading

Watsky KL, Reynolds K, Berube D, Bayer FJ (1993) Occupational contact dermatitis from tosyl chloride in a chemist. Contact Dermatitis 29:211–212

400. Triacetin

Glyceryl Triacetate

CAS Registry Number [102–76–1]

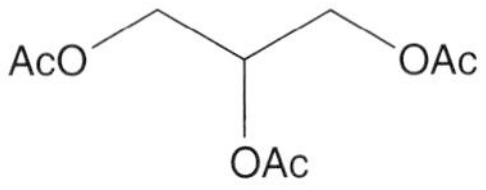

Triacetin is a component of cigarette filters, which induced a contact dermatitis in a worker at a cigarette manufactory.

Suggested Reading

Unna PJ, Schulz KH (1963) Allergisches Kontaktekzem durch Triacetin. Hautarzt 14:423–425

401. Tribenoside

CAS Registry Number [10310-32-4]

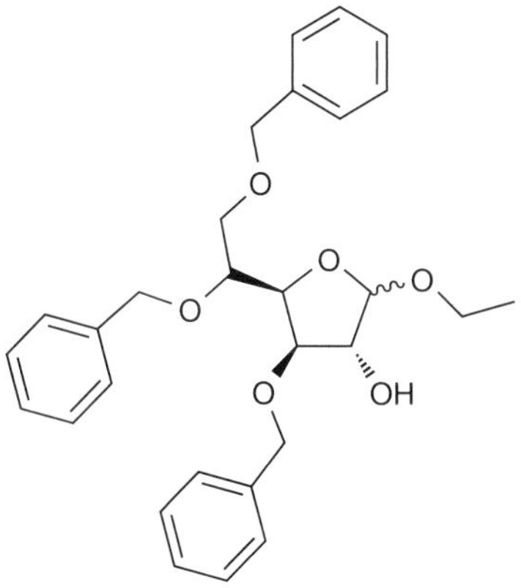

This drug is used for the treatment, both topical and oral, of hemorrhoids. It leads to benzoïc acid, that is contained in *Myroxylon pereirae* as well, and could be the sensitizer.

Suggested Reading

Inoue A, Tamagawa-Mineoka R, Katoh N, Kishimoto S (2009) Allergic contact dermatitis caused by tribenoside. Contact Dermatitis 60:349–350
Endo H, Kawada A, Yudate T, Aragane Y, Yamada H, Tezuka T (1999). Drug eruption due to tribenoside. Contact Dermatitis 41:223

402. Tributyltin Oxide

CAS Registry Number [56–35–9]

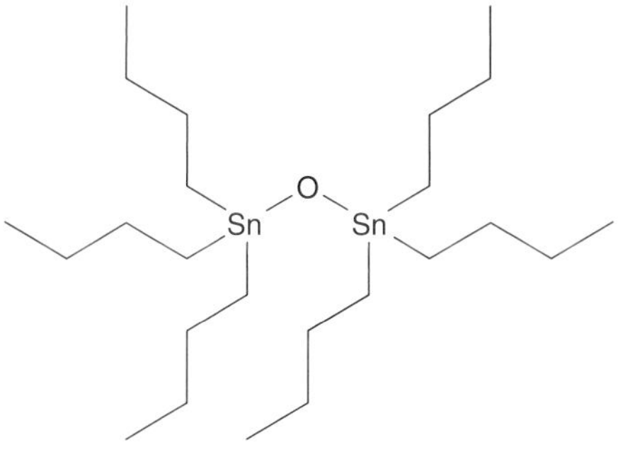

Tributyl tin oxide is used as an antifouling and biocide agent against fungi, algae, and bacteria, particularly in paints. Sometimes used in chemistry, tributyltin oxide is a strong irritant.

Suggested Reading

Goh CL (1985) Irritant dermatitis from tri-*N*-butyl tin oxide in paint. Contact Dermatitis 12:161–163
Grace CT, Ng SK, Cheong LL (1991) Recurrent irritant contact dermatitis due to tributyltin oxide on work clothes. Contact Dermatitis 25:250–251

403. Trichloroethane

1,1,1-Trichloroethane, Methylchloroform

CAS Registry Numbers [71–55–6], [25323–89–1]

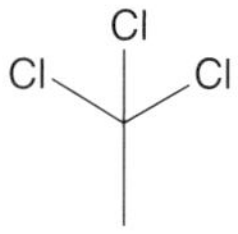

Trichloroethane is a solvent that has wide applications in industry, such as for cold type metal cleaning and in cleaning plastic molds. It is mainly an irritant, but can also provoke allergic contact dermatitis.

Suggested Reading

Mallon J, Tek Chu M, Maibach HI (2001) Occupational allergic contact dermatitis from methyl chloroform (1,1,1-trichloroethane)? Contact Dermatitis 45:107

404. Trichloroethylene

Trilene, Triclene, Trethylene

CAS Registry Number [79–01–6]

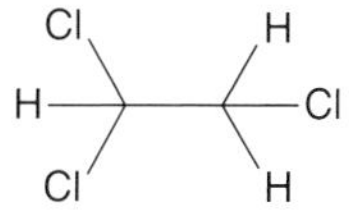

Trichloroethylene is a chlorinated hydrocarbon used as a detergent or solvent for metals, oils, resins, sulfur, and as general degreasing agent. It can cause irritant contact dermatitis, generalized exanthema, Stevens–Johnson-like syndrome, pustular or bullous eruption, scleroderma, as well as neurological and hepatic disorders.

58

Suggested Reading

Goon AT, Lee LT, Tay YK, Yosipovitch G, Ng SK, Giam YC (2001) A case of trichloroethylene hypersensitivity syndrome. Arch Dermatol 137:274–276
Puerschel WC, Odia SG, Rakoski J, Ring J (1996) Trichloroethylene and concomitant contact dermatitis in an art painter. Contact Dermatitis 34:430–431

405. Triethanolamine

Trolamine

CAS Registry Number [102–71–6]

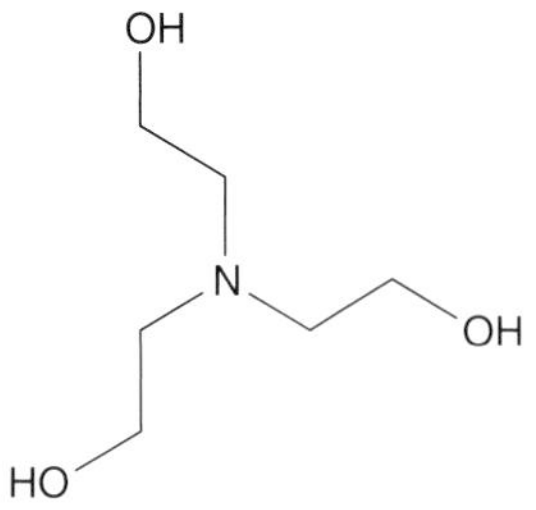

This emulsifying agent can be contained in many products such as cosmetics, topical medicines, metalworking cutting fluids, and color film developers. Traces may exist in other ethanolamines such as mono- and diethanolamine. Contact allergy seems to be rarer than previously thought.

Suggested Reading

Blum A, Lischka G (1997) Allergic contact dermatitis from mono-, di- and triethanolamine. Contact Dermatitis 36:166
Le Coz CJ, Scrivener Y, Santinelli F, Heid E (1998) Sensibilisation de contact au cours des ulcères de jambe. Ann Dermatol Venereol 125:694–699
Scheman AJ, Katta R (1997) Photographic allergens: an update. Contact Dermatitis 37:130

406. Triethylenetetramine

CAS Registry Number [112–24–3]

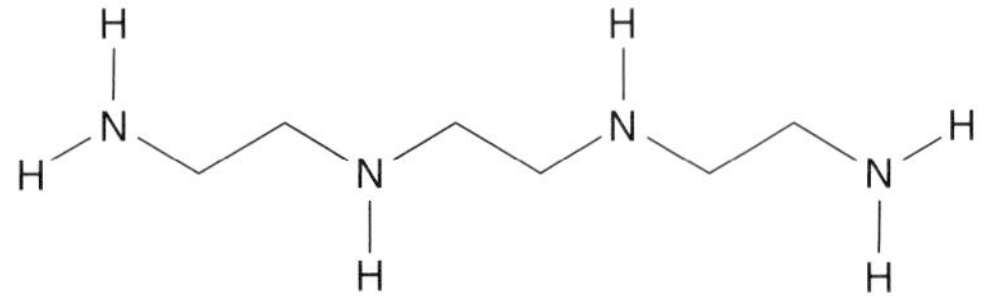

Triethylenetetramine is used as an amine hardener in epoxy resins of the bisphenol A type. Cross-sensitivity is possible with diethylenetriamine and diethylenediamine.

Suggested Reading

Jolanki R, Kanerva L, Estlander T, Tarvainen K, Keskinen H, Henriks-Eckerman ML (1990) Occupational dermatoses from epoxy resin compounds. Contact Dermatitis 23:172–183

407. Triforine

Saprol®, 1,4-bis(2,2,2-Trichloro-1-Formamidoethyl) Piperazine

CAS Registry Number [26644–46–2]

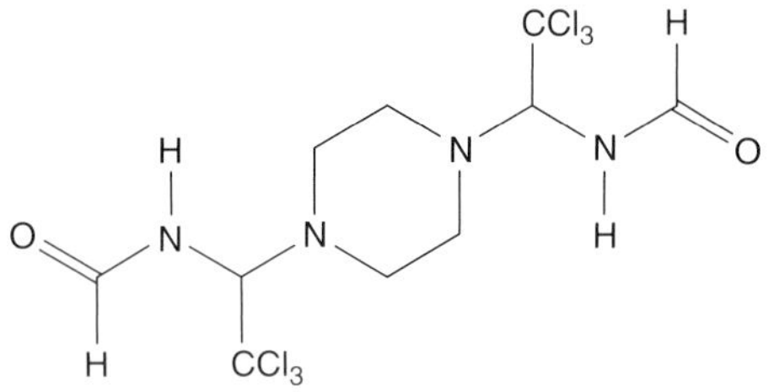

This pesticide is widely used in flower growing. Cross-reactions are expected to dichlorvos.

Suggested Reading

Ueda A, Aoyama K, Manda F, Ueda T, Kawahara Y (1994) Delayed-type allergenicity of triforine (Saprol®). Contact Dermatitis 31:140–145

408. Triglycidyl Isocyanurate

1,3,5-Triglycidyl-s-Triazinetrione

CAS Registry Number [2451–62–9]

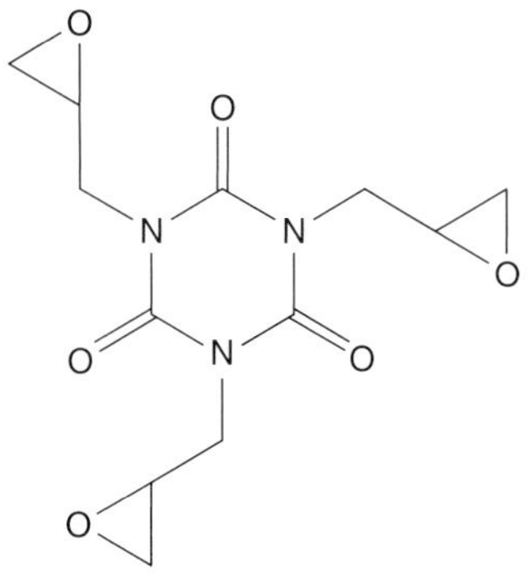

Triglycidyl isocyanurate is a triazine epoxy compound used as a resin hardener in polyester powder paints, in the plastics industry, resin molding systems, inks, and adhesives. Occupational contact dermatitis can occur

in people producing this chemical, in those producing the powder coat paint, and in sprayers. Respiratory symptoms have been observed.

Suggested Reading

Erikstam U, Bruze M, Goossens A (2001) Degradation of triglycidyl isocyanurate as a cause of false-negative patch test reaction. Contact Dermatitis 44:13–17

Foulds IS, Koh D (1992) Allergic contact dermatitis from resin hardeners during the manufacture of thermosetting coating paints. Contact Dermatitis 26:87–90

McFadden JP, Rycroft RJG (1993) Occupational contact dermatitis from triglycidyl isocyanurate in a powder paint sprayer. Contact Dermatitis 28:251

Munro CS, Lawrence CM (1992) Occupational contact dermatitis from triglycidyl isocyanurate in a powder paint factory. Contact Dermatitis 26:59

409. *N*-[3-(Trimethoxysilyl)Propyl] -*N*-(Vinylbenzyl)Ethylenediamine Monohydrochloride

1,2-Ethanediamine, *N*-[(Ethenylphenyl)Methyl]-*N*-[3-(Trimethoxysilyl)Propyl]-, Monohydrochloride

CAS Registry Number [34937–00–3]

This amine-functional methoxysilane silane compound, referenced as vinylbenzylaminoethyl aminopropyltrimethoxysilane, was implicated in the production of glass filaments.

Suggested Reading

Heino T, Haapa K, Manelius F (1996) Contact sensitization to organosilane solution in glass filament production. Contact Dermatitis 34:294

Toffoletto F, Cortona G, Feltrin G, Baj A, Goggi E, Cecchetti R (1994) Occupational contact dermatitis from amine-functional methoxysilane in continuous-glass-filament production. Contact Dermatitis 31:320–321

410. *N*-(3-Trimethoxysilylpropyl)-Ethylenediamine

Z 6020

CAS Registry Number [1760–24–3]

This amine-functional methoxysilane, referenced as aminoethyl aminopropyltrimethoxysilane, was implicated in the production of glass filaments.

Suggested Reading

Heino T, Haapa K, Manelius F (1996) Contact sensitization to organosilane solution in glass filament production. Contact Dermatitis 34:294

411. 2,4,6-Trimethylol Phenol

CAS Registry Number [2937–61–3]

Trimethylolphenol is an allergen in resins based on phenol and formaldehyde. Cross-reactivity is possible with other phenol-derivative molecules.

Suggested Reading

Bruze M, Zimerson E (1997) Cross-reaction patterns in patients with contact allergy to simple methylol phenols. Contact Dermatitis 37:82–86

Bruze M, Fregert S, Zimerson E (1985) Contact allergy to phenol-formaldehyde resins. Contact Dermatitis 12:81–86

412. Trimethylthiourea

CAS Registry Number [2489–77–2]

Trimethylthiourea is a thiourea derivative used, for example, for polychloroprene (neoprene) rubber vulcanization. Patients sensitized to ethylbutyl thiourea can also react to trimethylthiourea.

Suggested Reading

Kanerva L, Estlander T, Jolanki R (1994) Occupational allergic contact dermatitis caused by thiourea compounds. Contact Dermatitis 31:242–248

413. Tulipalin A and Tulipalin B

α-Methylene-γ-Butyrolactone and β-Hydroxy-α-Methylene-γ-Butyrolactone

CAS Registry Number [547–65–9] and CAS Registry Number [38965–80–9]

Tulipalin A   Tulipalin B

Tulipalin A is the unsubstituted α-methylene-γ-butyrolactone contained in the sap of damaged tulips (Liliaceae family) and Alstroemeria (Alstroemeriaceae family). Tulipalin B, due to hydrolysis of tuliposide B, seems to have a weak sensitizing capacity.

Suggested Reading

Bruynzeel DP (1997) Bulb dermatitis. Dermatological problems in the flower bulb industries. Contact Dermatitis 37:70–77
Gette MT, Marks JE (1990) Tulip fingers. Arch Dermatol 126:203–205

414. Tuliposide A

CAS Registry Number [19870–30–5]

Tuliposide A is a glucoside prohapten contained in tulip bulbs and in Alstroemeria (*Tulipa* spp.; *Alstroemeria* spp.; *Lilium* spp.). It is rapidly hydrolyzed to tulipalin A and represents a common occupational problem among workers in the European tulip industry. Tuliposide can be present as 1-tuliposide A, but is more frequently identified as 6-tuliposide A.

Suggested Reading

Christensen LP, Kristiansen K (1995) A simple HPLC method for the isolation and quantification of the allergens tuliposide A and tulipalin A in *Alstroemeria*. Contact Dermatitis 32:199–203
Gette MT, Marks JE (1990) Tulip fingers. Arch Dermatol 126:203–205
Lamminpää A, Estlander T, Jolanki R, Kanerva L (1996) Occupational allergic contact dermatitis caused by decorative plants. Contact Dermatitis 34:330–335

415. Tylosin

CAS Registry Number [1401–69–0]

Tylosin is a macrolid antibiotic used in veterinary medicine. Occupational exposure concerns farmers, breeders, animal feed workers, and veterinarians.

Suggested Reading

Barbera E, de la Cuadra J (1989) Occupational airborne allergic contact dermatitis from tylosin. Contact Dermatitis 20:308–309

Carafini S, Assalve D, Stingeni L, Lisi P (1994) Tylosin, an airborne contact allergen in veterinarians. Contact Dermatitis 31:327–328

Guerra L, Venturo N, Tardio M, Tosti A (1991) Airborne contact dermatitis from animal feed antibiotics. Contact Dermatitis 25:333–334

Tuomi ML, Räsänen L (1995) Contact allergy to tylosin and cobalt in a pig-farmer. Contact Dermatitis 33:285

Suggested Reading

Epstein WL (1994) Occupational poison ivy and oak dermatitis. Dermatol Clin 12:511–516

Kawai K, Nakagawa M, Kawai K, Konishi K, Liew FM, Yasuno H, Shimode Y, Shimode Y (1991) Hyposensitization to urushiol among Japanese lacquer craftsmen. Contact Dermatitis 24:146–147

Kullavanijaya P, Ophaswongse S (1997) A study of dermatitis in the lacquerware industry. Contact Dermatitis 36: 244–246

416. Urushiol

CAS Registry Number [492–89–7], [53237–59–5]

Urushiol is a generic name that indicates a mixture of several close alkylcatechols contained in the sap of the Anacardiaceae family such as *Toxicodendron radicans* Kuntze (poison ivy) or *Anacardium occidentale* L. (cashew nut tree). The R-side chain generally includes 13, 15, or 17 carbons. A urushiol with a C_{15} side chain is named pentadecylcatechol (a term sometimes employed in medical literature for poison ivy urushiol), and a urushiol with a C_{17} side chain is a heptadecylcatechol (mostly encountered in poison oak urushiol).

417. Usnic Acid (*D*-Usnic Acid, *l*-Usnic Acid)

CAS Registry Number [125–46–2] (CAS Registry Number [7562–61–0], CAS Registry Number [6159–66–6])

Usnic acid is a component of lichens, also used as a topical antibiotic. Allergic contact dermatitis from lichens occurs mainly occupationally in forestry and horticultural workers, and in lichen pickers.

58

Suggested Reading

Aalto-Korte K, Lauerma A, Alanko K (2005) Occupational allergic contact dermatitis from lichens in present-day Finland. Contact Dermatitis 52:36–38

Hahn M, Lischka G, Pfeifle J, Wirth V (1995) A case of contact dermatitis from lichens in southern Germany. Contact Dermatitis 32:55–56

418. Vinylpyridine

2-Vinylpyridine

CAS Registry Number [100–69–6]

4-Vinylpyridine

CAS Registry Number [100–43–6]

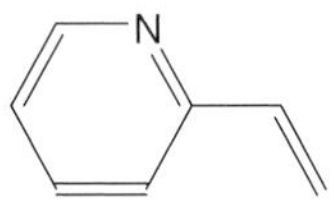

2-VP 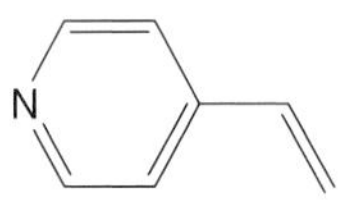   4-VP

4-Vinyl pyridine was used as a monomer in polymer chemistry and induced nonimmunological contact urticaria and allergic contact dermatitis. No cross-reactivity is observed between pyridine derivatives.

Suggested Reading

Bergendorff O, Wallengren J (1999) 4-Vinylpyridine-induced dermatitis in a laboratory worker. Contact Dermatitis 40:280–281

Foussereau J, Lantz JP, Grosshans E (1972) Allergic eczema from vinyl-4-pyridine. Contact Dermat Newslett 11:261

Sasseville D, Balbul A, Kwong P, Yu K (1996) Contact sensitization to pyridine derivatives. Contact Dermatitis 35:101–102

419. Virginiamycin

CAS Registry Number [11006–76–1]

Virginiamycin S1: Staphylomycin S

CAS Registry Number [23152–29–6]

Virginiamycin M1: Pristinamycin IIA, Mikamycin A, Ostreogrycin A, Staphylomycin M1, Streptogramin A, Vernamycin A

CAS Registry Number [21411–53–0]

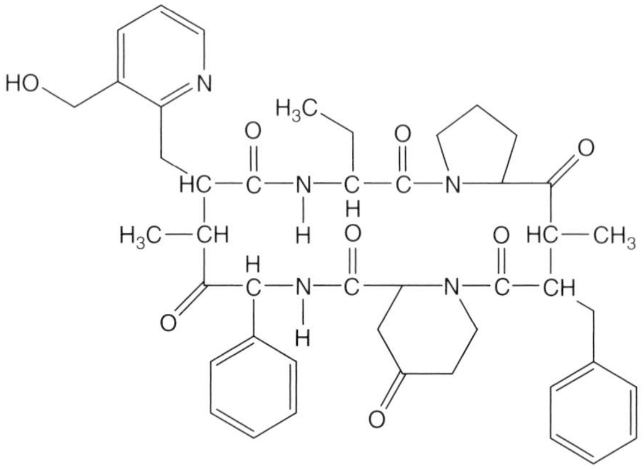

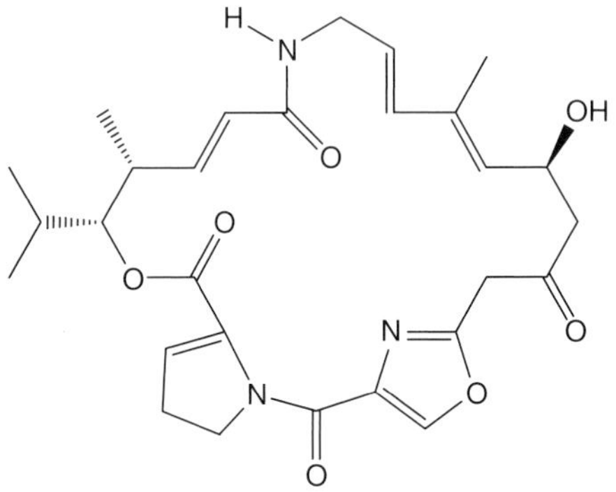

Like the other streptogramin, pristinamycin, virginiamycin is made of two subunits, virginiamycin S1 and virginiamycin M1. Dermatitis was quite common in people using the formerly available topical virginiamycin. Occupational dermatitis was observed in the pharmaceutical industry, in breeders, and in a surgeon who used topical virginiamycin on postoperative wounds (personal observation).

Suggested Reading

Rudzki E, Rebandel P (1984) Contact sensitivity to antibiotics. Contact Dermatitis 11:41–42

Tennstedt D, Dumont-Fruytier M, Lachapelle JM (1978) Occupational allergic contact dermatitis to virginiamycin, an antibiotic used as a food additive for pigs and poultry. Contact Dermatitis 4:133–134

420. Zinc bis-Dibutyldithiocarbamate

Zinc *N,N*-Dibutyldithiocarbamate

CAS Registry Number [136–23–2]

A rubber chemical, used as a vulcanization accelerator. It can also be contained in paints, glue removers, and anticorrosive. It was contained in "carba-mix."

Suggested Reading

Condé-Salazar L, Del-Rio E, Guimaraens D, Gonzalez Domingo A (1993) Type IV allergy to rubber additives: a 10-year study of 686 cases. J Am Acad Dermatol 29:176–180
Condé-Salazar L, Guimaraens D, Villegas C, Romero A, Gonzalez MA (1995) Occupational allergic contact dermatitis in construction workers. Contact Dermatitis 35:226–230
Kiec-Swierczynska M (1995) Occupational sensitivity to rubber. Contact Dermatitis 32:171–172

421. Zinc *bis*-Diethyldithiocarbamate

Zinc *N,N*-Diethyldithiocarbamate, Diethyldithiocarbamic Acid Zinc Salt

CAS Registry Number [14324–55–1]

Diethyldithiocarbamate zinc is a rubber component used as a vulcanization accelerator. Oxidation of this carbamate leads to tetraethylthiuram disulfide. It can be responsible for rubber dermatitis in health personnel. It was contained in "carba-mix."

Suggested Reading

Chipinda I, Hettick JM, Simoyi RH, Siegel PD (2008) Zinc diethyldithiocarbamate allergenicity: potential haptenation mechanisms. Contact Dermatitis 59:79–89
Condé-Salazar L, Del-Rio E, Guimaraens D, Gonzalez Domingo A (1993) Type IV allergy to rubber additives: a 10-year study of 686 cases. J Am Acad Dermatol 29:176–180
Kiec-Swierczynska M (1995) Occupational sensitivity to rubber. Contact Dermatitis 32:171–172
Vaneckova J, Ettler K (1994) Hypersensitivity to rubber surgical gloves in healthcare personnel. Contact Dermatitis 31:266–267
Von Hintzenstern J, Heese A, Koch HU, Peters KP, Hornstein OP (1991) Frequency, spectrum and occupational relevance of type IV allergies to rubber chemicals. Contact Dermatitis 24:244–252

422. Zinc bis-Dimethyldithiocarbamate

Ziram

CAS Registry Number [137–30–4]

Ziram is a rubber vulcanization accelerator of the dithiocarbamate group. Sensitization was reported in several patients. Ziram is also used as a fungicide and can cause contact dermatitis in agricultural workers.

Suggested Reading

Kiec-Swierczynska M (1995) Occupational sensitivity to rubber. Contact Dermatitis 32:171–172
Manuzzi P, Borrello P, Misciali C, Guerra L (1988) Contact dermatitis due to Ziram and Maneb. Contact Dermatitis 19:148

423. Zinc Ethylene-bis-Dithiocarbamate

Zineb, Zinc *N,N*-Ethylenebisdithiocarbamate

CAS Registry Number [12122–67–7]

Zineb is a pesticide of the dithiocarbamate group. Sensitization can occur in gardeners and florists.

Suggested Reading

Crippa M, Misquith L, Lonati A, Pasolini G (1990) Dyshidrotic eczema and sensitization to dithiocarbamates in a florist. Contact Dermatitis 23:203–204

Jung HD, Honemann W, Kloth C, Lubbe D, Pambor M, Quednow C, Ratz KH, Rothe A, Tarnick M (1989) Kontaktekzem durch Pestizide in der Deutschen Demokratischen Republik. Dermatol Monatsschr 175:203–214

O'Malley M, Rodriguez P, Maibach HI (1995) Pesticide patch testing: California nursery workers and controls. Contact Dermatitis 32:61–62

424. Zinc Propylene-bis-Dithiocarbamate

Propineb, Zinc *N,N*-Propylene-1,2-bis-Dithiocarbamate

CAS Registry Number [12071–83–9]

Propineb is a dithiocarbamate compound, which is used as a fungicide. Sensitization was reported in agricultural workers.

Suggested Reading

Jung HD, Honemann W, Kloth C, Lubbe D, Pambor M, Quednow C, Ratz KH, Rothe A, Tarnick M (1989) Kontaktekzem durch Pestizide in der Deutschen Demokratischen Republik. Dermatol Monatsschr 175:203–214

Nishioka K, Takahata H (2000) Contact allergy due to propineb. Contact Dermatitis 43:310

Index